# LIFESPAN
# NEUROREHABILITATION

## A Patient-Centered Approach
## from Examination to Intervention
## and Outcomes

# LIFESPAN NEUROREHABILITATION

## A Patient-Centered Approach from Examination to Intervention and Outcomes

**Dennis W. Fell, PT, MD**
Vice-President, APTA Academy of Neurologic Physical Therapy
Professor and Chair
Department of Physical Therapy
Pat Capps Covey College of Allied Health Professions
University of South Alabama
Mobile, Alabama

**Karen Y. Lunnen, PT, EdD**
Associate Professor and Head *(Retired)*
Department of Physical Therapy
College of Health and Human Sciences
Western Carolina University
Cullowhee, North Carolina

**Reva P. Rauk, PT, PhD, MMSc, NCS**
Director of Clinical Education and
Assistant Professor (Clinical)
University of Utah, College of Health
Department of Physical Therapy and Athletic Training
Salt Lake City, Utah

F.A. Davis Company • Philadelphia

# Compendium of Adult and Pediatric Neuromuscular Diagnoses

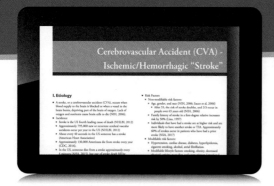

## FIND A SUMMARY OUTLINE

for each of the most common neuromuscular adult and pediatric medical diagnoses and their expected impairments and functional limitations—all in one place.

## I. Etiology

- A stroke, or a cerebrovascular accident (CVA), occurs when blood supply to the brain is blocked or when a vessel in the brain bursts, depriving part of the brain of oxygen. Lack of oxygen and nutrients cause brain cells to die (NIH, 2006).
- Incidence
  - Stroke is the US fourth leading cause of death (NHLBI, 2012)
  - Approximately 795,000 new or recurrent cerebral vascular accidents occur per year in the US (NHLBI, 2012)
  - About every 40 seconds in the US some (American Heart Association)
  - Approximately 130,000 Americans die f (CDC, 2014).
  - In the US, someone dies from a stroke a 4 minutes (AHA, 2015), but rate of stro 21.2% from 2001-2011 (AHA, 2015).
- Prevalence (NHLBI, 2008)
  - Increases markedly with age
    - Those individuals age < 44 suffer from than ischemic (NIH, 2006)
  - Higher in blacks than in whites at all ag
    - Incidence among African-Americans white Americans, whereas Hispanics, Americans incidence and mortality ra (NIH, 2006).
  - Higher in males than in females but stre severe in women, with a 1-month case f compared with 19.7% for men (Appelre
    - Men are 1.25 times more at risk than women will die from stroke (NIH, 20 southeastern US (Mozaffarian, 2015)
    - "Stroke belt and stroke buckle": 12 state death rates >10 % higher than the rest o 2006; NSA, 2006).
- Stroke Precursor: Transient ischemic attac
  - Caused by a temporary cerebral artery b symptoms to occur rapidly and last less causing no permanent injury to the brai
  - Not a stroke, but precursor to stroke an tially a more serious and debilitating str

> **Etiology** summarizes known etiologic factors, risk factors, and pathogenesis to ensure that you understand the basis of each disorder.

## II. Diagnostic Procedures

- The diagnosis of a stroke is based on history and physical examination (Ferro, 1998).
- Signs and Symptoms by location (NSA, 2006):
  - Cerebral stroke (depending on specific location of infarction)
    - Contralateral hemiplegia, hemiparesis, and hemianesthesia, aphasia, depression, post-stroke fatigue, memory deficits, severe headaches, behavioral changes (i.e., personality changes or emotional lability), balance impairment (McGeough, 2009, Stroke Association, 2012), perceptual impairment;
  - Posterior cerebral artery stroke
    - Visual field deficits (contralateral homonymous hemianopsia) if occipital lobe or optic radiations are affected, visual inattention; L hemisphere damage may result in alexia (inability to read)
    - most common impairments: motor paresis (65%), followed by visual field deficits (54%), and confusion or agitation (43%) (Ng, 2005).
  - Anterior cerebral artery stroke
    - Predominant lower extremity contralateral hemiparesis/hemiplegia, some sensory loss possible in lower extremities, incontinence, problems with bimanual tasks, apraxia
  - Middle cerebral artery stroke (most common)
    - Predominant contralateral hemiparesis and hemisensory loss of upper extremity, trunk, and face (may also affect lower extremities if deep white matter of corona radiata and posterior limb of internal capsule affected)
    - Possible dysarthria and dysphagia
    - Contralateral homonymous hemianopsia (may occur from optic radiation damage)

> **Diagnostics** guide your examination and evaluation and help you to anticipate possible underlying impairments and functional activity limitations.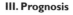

## III. Prognosis

- Stroke is nonprogressive, and is a leading cause of long term disability in the US (CDC, 2009; Smith, 2016)
- 50% of stroke survivors experience ongoing disability, and 30% require assistance for activities of daily living (Smith, 2016)
- Following a cerebral insult, the CNS can undergo reorganization or plasticity during the recovery process, with variable recovery. Prognosis depends on patient's pre-morbid condition, age, sex, lesion location, degree of damage, and rehabilitation treatment. Other long-term deficits may include:
  - Physical deficits
    - Hemiparesis on contralateral side, speech deficits, incoordination, weakness, gait deviations, pain
    - Some studies have shown that up to 85% of stroke survivors experience long-lasting hemiparesis (Yavuzer, 2008)
    - Following a stroke, women have greater disability than men (American Heart Association)
  - Muscle tone
    - Initially hypotonus due to neurogenic shock. Some remain hypotonic, most develop spastic hypertonus after weeks to months
  - Muscle performance
    - UE usually biased toward flexion with LE biased toward extension movement patterns
    - Impaired force production (eccentric and concentric), speed, and power impaired
    - Abnormal synergies may develop
  - Absence of voluntary control of the LE within the first week following the stroke and no development of normal UE synergies after 4 weeks is associated with a poor outcome at 6 months (Kwakkel, 2003)
  - Up to 2 years following the stroke there may still be some potential for improvements (Donaldson, 2009)

> **Prognosis** describes trends of progression and expected sequelae, including secondary body structure impairments and functional limitations, to help you determine appropriate short-term and long-term goals.

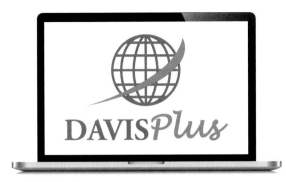

**Medical/Surgical Management** outlines the commonly used medical/ pharmaceutical interventions and surgical procedures that may be used to address primary deficits or secondary sequelae.

## IV. Medical and Surgical Management

- Most important intervention is education and prevention
  - Light physical activity such as walking is not beneficial at preventing stroke. However, moderate to vigorous physical activity can be associated with decreased incidence of stroke (Go, 2013).
- Acute stroke needs immediate medical intervention-dissolving the blood clot if ischemic stroke or stopping the [...] for hemorrhagic stroke (NIH, 2006)
  - Before administering any type of treatment fo[...] stroke, the physician must determine whether [...] an ischemic stroke or hemorrhagic stroke usin[...] imaging, and evaluating signs/symptoms. Som[...] such as sepsis, space-occupying lesions, and sei[...] mimic stroke, and should be ruled out (Golds[...]
  - Ischemic Stroke
    - Emergency room procedures
      - TPA administered directly into the cereb[...] clot, mechanical removal of clot using a [...] device to grab clot to pull it out (Mayo C[...]
    - Thrombolytic: Tissue Plasminogen Activat[...] ischemic stroke only (Stanford, 2006)
      - tPA works by dissolving the clot and rest[...] blood flow to the part of the ischemic br[...] be given emergently within 3-4.5 hours [...] symptoms.
      - Brain hemorrhage is a possible complicat[...] administration in an acute ischemic strok[...] 2014).
    - Anticoagulant: heparin and warfarin
      - Risk from long-term anticoagulant thera[...] non-cardioembolic ischemic stroke or tra[...] attack may outweigh benefit (Sandercock[...]
    - Antiplatelet: aspirin
      - "Treatment with aspirin is associated wit[...] deaths and nonfatal strokes over the ensu[...] per 1,000 persons treated." (Goldstein, 2[...]
      - Low-dose aspirin therapy (anti-platelet) t[...] recurrent ischemic stroke (Mant, 2007)
    - Surgical treatment:
      - Embolectomy and revascularization
      - Carotid endarterectomy (preventive):
        - Surgical removal of fatty plaques from[...] a potential source of emboli. Stents: i[...] the vessels containing plaques (Short term prevention) (Mayo Clinic 2013)
      - Thrombectomy is another treatment option in which the large blood clot is removed by a stent retriever. Results show that mechanical thrombectomy in acute stroke due to internal carotid artery and middle cerebral artery occlusion displays high rate of recanalization and favorable functional outcomes (Yu, 2016).

## V. Implications for Therapeutic Management

- Possible Physical Therapy Preferred Practice Patterns:
  - 5D- Impaired Motor Function and Sensor Integrity Associated with Non-Progressive Disorders of the Central Nervous System - Acquired in Adolescence or Adulthood
  - 5A: Primary prevention/risk prevention for loss of balance and falling
  - 5I- Impaired Arousal, Range of Motion, and Motor Control Associated with Coma, Near Coma, or Vegetative State.
- Role of the PT:
  - Treat symptoms of stroke including underlying impairments and their impact on functional activity, education, maintai[...] ROM, skin integrity, posture, strength; enhance motor control, self-care, ADLs. Monitor ventilation and pain. Assess for assistive device and/or splinting. (Furie 2010, Rodgers 1999)
  - Therapeutic treatment goal— functional recovery.
- General Physical Therapy Guidelines
  - Early rehabilitation intervention enhances recovery process and to prevent a quick decline (Duncan et al, 2004; Polloc[...] 2006).
    - "Initiating post-stroke rehabilitation soon after the onse[...] of an acute stroke appears to be the most important fact[...] associated with early discharge from the hospital; in addition, earlier admission is recognized as a relevant and favorable prognostic factor." (Safer, 2015)
    - Late rehabilitation using reinforced feedback (6 months post-stroke) may also be effective in improving motor performance. (Piron, 2010)
  - Multidisciplinary Team Approach to Rehabilitation
    - Speech, occupational, and psychological therapy. Stroke unit care, home health (Stroke Unit, 2006, Schouten 2008).

**Key Implications for Therapeutic Management** specifies the likely "Preferred Practice Pattern(s)" from the "Guide to Physical Therapist Practice" (APTA, 2017), the roles of the interprofessional rehabilitation team, and the rehabilitation therapy likely to be included in the plan of care, as well as contraindications/ precautions for those interventions.

## VI. Consumer and Professional Resources

- American Stroke Association
  - http://www.strokeassociation.org/STROKEORG/AboutStroke/About-Stroke_UCM_308529_SubHomePage.jsp
  - This a website dedicated to explaining a stroke, the effects, the associated risk factors, treatment options, and various other facts about strokes. Primarily used for a general understanding of the diagnosis.
  - Support group contact available
- Evidence-Based Review of Stroke Rehabilitation
  - http://www.ebrsr.com
  - A website by Heart and Stroke Foundation Canadian Partnership for Stroke Recovery to review current evidence based stroke rehabilitation techniques
- National Stroke Association
  - http://www.stroke.org/site/PageNavigator/HOME
  - A website designed to describe a stroke and to help raise awareness about the diagnosis.
  - Support group contact available
  - StrokeSmart Magazine provides tips on money, life after a stroke, and wellness.
  - Stroke Help Line to answer questions about stroke prevention, treatment, and recovery.

**Consumer and Professional Resources** lists online resources and specific agencies and associations that support individuals with the diagnosis.

# Compendium of Adult and Pediatric Neuromuscular Diagnoses

## CONTENTS
Alphabetical Listing of Common Neuromuscular Diagnoses

- Acquired Immune Deficiency Syndrome (AIDS) (A) (P)
- Amyotrophic Lateral Sclerosis (A)
- Angelman Syndrome (P)
- Arthrogryposis Multiplex Congenita (P)
- Autism Spectrum (Pervasive Developmental Disorder) (P)
- Bell's Palsy (A)
- Benign Paroxysmal Positional Vertigo (BPPV) (A)
- Brachial Plexus Injury (Obstetrical Birth Palsy) (P)
- Cerebellar Disease and Tumor (A) (P)
- Cerebral Palsy (P)
- Cerebral Tumor (A) (P)
- Cerebrovascular Accident (ischemic/ hemorrhagic) / Stroke (A) (P)
- Cerebrovascular Accident —Arteriovenous Malformation (A) (P)
- Charcot-Marie-Tooth (A)
- Complex Regional Pain Syndrome (Reflex Sympathetic Dystrophy) (A)
- Congenital Limb Deficiency (P)
- Conversion Disorder (A) (P)

- Delirium (A) (P)
- Dementia / Alzheimer's disease (A)
- Developmental Coordination Disorder (P)
- Down's Syndrome (P)
- Dystonia (A)
- Encephalitis (A) (P)
- Fetal Alcohol Syndrome (P)
- Fibromyalgia (A)
- Friedreich's Ataxia (A)
- Guillain-Barré Syndrome (A)
- High Risk Infant / Prematurity (Intraventricular Hemorrhage) (P)
- Huntington's Disease (A)
- Ischemic Encephalopathy (Near Drowning) (A) (P)
- Lyme Disease (A) (P)
- Ménière's Disease (A)
- Multiple Sclerosis (A)
- Muscular Dystrophy (P)
- Myasthenia Gravis (A)
- Myelominingocele / Spina Bifida (P)
- Myotonia (A)
- Neurofibromatosis (A) (P)
- Normal Pressure Hydrocephalus (A)

- Osteogenesis Imperfecta (P)
- Parkinson's Disease (A)
- Pediatric Infectious Diseases (P)
- Peripheral Neuropathy (A)
- Poliomyelitis / Post-polio Syndrome (A) (P)
- Prader Willi Syndrome (P)
- Progressive Bulbar Palsy (A)
- Rett's Syndrome (P)
- Reyes Syndrome (P)
- Seizure Disorder (Epilepsy) (A) (P)
- Spinal Cord Tumors (A) (P)
- Spinal Muscular Atrophy (P)
- Syringomyelia (A)
- Transverse Myelitis (A) (P)
- Traumatic Brain Injury / Diffuse Axonal Injury (A) (P)
- Traumatic Spinal Cord Injury (A) (P)
- Trigeminal Neuralgia (A)
- Vestibular Hypofunction (Unilateral) (A)

(P) Denotes primarily Disorder in Pediatrics

(A) Denotes primarily Adult-Onset Disorder

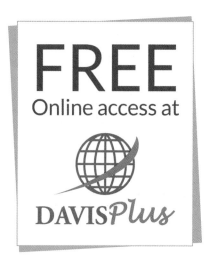

**FREE** Online access at **DAVIS**Plus

# IN CLASS, CLINICAL OR PRACTICE.

Put 57 quick-reference summaries of the most common adult and pediatric neuromuscular diagnoses at your fingertips whenever you need them.

Visit **www.DavisPlus.com** today!

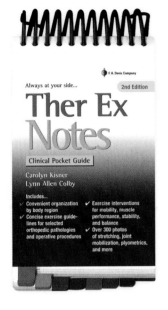
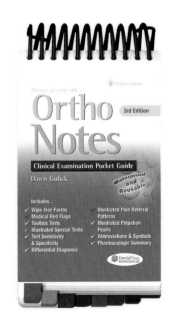

F. A. Davis Company
1915 Arch Street
Philadelphia, PA 19103
www.fadavis.com

Printed in the United States of America

Last digit indicates print number: 10 9 8 7 6 5 4 3 2

*Senior Acquisitions Editor:* Melissa A. Duffield
*Director of Content Development:* George W. Lang
*Senior Developmental Editor:* Jennifer A. Pine
*Manager of Design and Illustration:* Carolyn O'Brien
*Illustration Coordinator:* Katharine L. Margeson
*Production Manager:* Sharon Lee

As new scientific information becomes available through basic and clinical research, recommended treatments and drug therapies undergo changes. The author(s) and publisher have done everything possible to make this book accurate, up-to-date, and in accord with accepted standards at the time of publication. The author(s), editors, and publisher are not responsible for errors or omissions or for consequences from application of the book, and make no warranty, expressed or implied, in regard to the contents of the book. Any practice described in this book should be applied by the reader in accordance with professional standards of care used in regard to the unique circumstances that may apply in each situation. The reader is advised always to check product information (package inserts) for changes and new information regarding dose and contraindications before administering any drug. Caution is especially urged when using new or infrequently ordered drugs.

**Library of Congress Cataloging-in-Publication Data**

Names: Fell, Dennis W., author. | Lunnen, Karen Y., author. | Rauk, Reva P., author.
Title: Lifespan neurorehabilitation : a patient-centered approach from examination to interventions and outcomes /
  Dennis W. Fell, Karen Y.
  Lunnen, Reva P. Rauk.
Description: Philadelphia, PA : F.A. Davis Company, [2018] | Includes bibliographical references.
Identifiers: LCCN 2017040096 | ISBN 9780803646094 (hardcover)
Subjects: | MESH: Nervous System Diseases—rehabilitation | Physical Therapy Modalities | Patient-Centered Care | Child |
  Adolescent | Adult
Classification: LCC RC349.8 | NLM WL 140 | DDC 616.8/046—dc23 LC record available at https://lccn.loc.gov/2017040096

# Dedication

**From Dennis Fell:**

*Dedicated to God's everlasting, undeserved love and grace; and in gratitude to my wife, Noel, and children, Nathan (and his wife Elana) and Hannah, who have continually loved me and bring life-enjoyment and meaning to all that I do; and in memory of my father, Thomas ("Wix"), who taught me to cherish family, my mother, Norma, who taught me to love God above all else, my father-in-law, Milton ("Bud"), who taught me to respect others and to give generously, and my mother-in-law, Dorothy ("Dot"), who taught me to enjoy the joy in family!*

**From Karen Lunnen:**

*Dedicated to family and friends who supported my long-term commitment to the book and to my parents who instilled their value of lifelong learning and the importance of strong written communication. Special thanks to those who have shaped my professional and personal development, especially the children and families who were the focus of my clinical work, my colleagues in various employment settings, and students who regularly challenged and inspired me. Gratitude to Dennis for his vision and leadership and to Reva for her consistent support and positive attitude.*

**From Reva Rauk:**

*Dedicated to God, without whose grace, love, and forgiveness this text could not have been accomplished, and to the many patients I have served and will serve. Deep thanks and appreciation to my husband, Bob, and children, Kirsten, Anders, and Ane, whose persistent love supported this effort; in memory of my parents, who taught me the value of education and hard work and who always gently nudged me onward; and with gratitude to Dennis and Karen who envisioned what could be and saw potential in my contributions.*

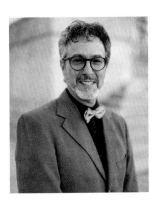

Dr. Dennis W. Fell is Professor and Chair of Physical Therapy at the University of South Alabama (USA) DPT program in Mobile, Alabama, where he has served since 1992, and loves teaching neuroscience and neuromuscular physical therapy examination and intervention. He has served APTA as a *JOPTE* Editorial Board member, Neurology Section Treasurer, Vice President of the Academy of Neurologic Physical Therapy for the Alabama Chapter, and peer reviewer for *Pediatric Physical Therapy*. He has taught in China, South Korea, South Africa, and Taiwan, and has led PT service trips to China, Belize, the Dominican Republic, and the Republic of Trinidad and Tobago. He has presented at every WCPT International Congress since 1995, and taught as a Visiting International Professor in South Korea during a 2010 to 2011 sabbatical. His numerous awards for leadership, service, and teaching include the University of South Alabama "Excellence in Teaching Award" and "50 Outstanding Faculty" from the University's 50-year history, and the 2017 APTA "Lucy Blair Service Award."

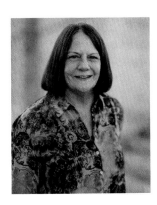

Dr. Karen Lunnen retired in 2017, drawing her 44-year professional career to a close as Head of the Department of Physical Therapy at Western Carolina University. She earned a Master of Science degree in Physical Therapy from Duke University and a Doctor of Education degree from North Carolina State University. As a young physical therapy faculty member at The University of North Carolina at Chapel Hill, with major responsibilities in maternal and child health, she was privileged to be mentored by exceptional professionals. Her clinical work primarily involved children and their families in multiple settings. Her accomplishments include awards for innovative teaching, mentorship of student research, and leadership in service-learning.

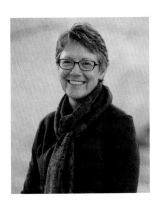

Dr. Reva P. Rauk is the Director of Clinical Education and an Assistant Professor (Clinical) in the Department of Physical Therapy and Athletic Training at the University of Utah. She received her PhD in Education from the University of Minnesota, a Master of Medical Science degree in Clinical Neuroscience Physical Therapy from Emory University, and her professional physical therapy degree from the Mayo Clinic School of Health Sciences. Dr. Rauk currently serves on the Credentialed Clinical Instructor Workgroup and is a trainer and faculty member for both APTA Credentialed Clinical Instructor Programs. Dr. Rauk served previously on the ABPTS Neurology Specialty Council, Specialty Academy of Content Experts, and as study coordinator for the 2004 Neurology Specialty Practice Analysis. Her clinical and research interests include student clinical reasoning, professionalism, interventions for cerebellar degenerative disease, and human experiences in health care.

This neurorehabilitation textbook was born from the need for a textbook that is built around the International Classification of Function (ICF) framework, which drives the way therapists make clinical decisions. This book for physical therapists and occupational therapists is **unique** in that it is organized by the constructs of body structure/function and functional activity rather than specific medical diagnoses. The book also focuses on patient management from an evidence-based perspective, with application across the lifespan because neuromuscular impairments can affect patients similarly, regardless of age.

With contributions from approximately 60 educators and professionals affiliated with the APTA Academies of Neurologic Physical Therapy, Pediatric Physical Therapy, and Geriatric Physical Therapy; occupational therapy faculty; and authors from other countries, the book represents the professional life-work of the textbook editors. Developed over a decade, this text has been a monumental task of scholarly synthesis and coordination of the conceptualizing, preparing, writing, editing, and illustrating that led to the final product; it could not have been completed without the significant contributions of many individuals. Each chapter author integrated available evidence with knowledge, understanding, energy, and enthusiasm to make this textbook an academic endeavor. The authors synthesized the most recent rehabilitation evidence for students, faculty, and clinicians to support clinical decision-making while maintaining a focus on practical clinical application, and will also be useful for those preparing for specialization.

Despite the many challenges that delayed publication, including publisher transition, disruption from a major hurricane, battles with cancer, and loving our parents through end-of-life care, the necessary revisions and updates over this period propelled the textbook to a stronger finish than could otherwise have been possible.

Two important conceptual models, (1) the APTA's Patient/Client Management Model and (2) the World Health Organization's (WHO's) ICF, are central throughout the text. The sections of the book are organized using the APTA *Patient/Client Management Model* (with sections on decision-making, examination/evaluation, intervention principles, and specific interventions/plan of care). The chapters of the examination and intervention sections are structured by *WHO ICF* constructs (with some chapters focusing on underlying impairments of body structure/body function, and other chapters focusing on functional activity limitations and participation). Because we think about and design patient care in this way—not simply providing intervention based on the medical diagnosis—we have similarly organized the book to assist in teaching students. This text organization provides a sound basis for selecting each component of patient examination and planning interventions that are based on the examination results. It also eliminates redundancy, which is inherent in chapters organized by medical diagnoses. For example, in other books, the information on balance intervention may be found primarily in the brain injury chapter, but similar balance interventions are also essential in rehabilitation for individuals with stroke, multiple sclerosis, and other neurologic diagnoses. The book is also unique in its application of neuromuscular examination and intervention techniques *across the lifespan,* from pediatrics to adulthood and geriatrics. And equally important, key content is always built upon the available *evidence.*

Section I chapters review the basis and process for making sound, patient-centered clinical decisions when managing patients with neuromuscular disorders, including the Hypothesis-oriented Algorithm for Clinicians (HOAC). Section II addresses examination/evaluation processes for specific impairments and functional activities/limitations common to neuromuscular disorders. Section III presents general therapeutic intervention concepts, principles, and approaches, as well as topics pertinent in all patients with neuromuscular disorders, such as health promotion/prevention and assistive/adaptive equipment. Each chapter of Section IV focuses on interventions for a specific impairment, presenting a variety of methods to specifically address that impairment. We can refer to these impairment-based interventions as "preparatory" interventions because they are often applied early in rehabilitation to directly improve the known impairments that underlie and contribute to functional deficits. However, these impairment-based interventions are aimed ultimately at enhancing the patient's functional skill/activity and participation. Each chapter in Section V focuses on task-specific functional interventions to directly improve a specific functional skill/activity and participation of the patient.

The writing style is intentionally reader friendly, with use of direct active voice to explain any techniques or methods (e.g., "Place your hands on...") for clear instruction, while avoiding passive voice whenever possible. In addition to the rationale for specific applications, each chapter provides specific methods and techniques with stepwise instructions that "you" can apply in clinical practice. Chapters include "Patient Application" case studies, introduced early in the chapter, that are pertinent to the content and are progressively developed throughout the chapter. Each "Patient Application" case feature is followed by "Contemplate Clinical Decisions" questions to facilitate thinking about key concepts in the case. The case study and questions serve as a reference point for considering the impairment or functional limitation in the context of the person with a disability and both current and future implications for the individual and the family.

Each chapter contains "Think About It" boxes with probing questions to guide the reader's thinking or concise "nuggets" or "pearls" to highlight essential information. The Examination and Intervention chapters include references to evidence-based "Focus on Evidence" (FOE) tables summarizing the more important studies for that topic. The FOE tables are available in the online supplemental material.

In some intervention chapters, more comprehensive case studies are included in the online supplemental material. These case studies address the more complex clinical decision-making required for patients with multiple impairments and comorbidities. Guiding questions lead the reader through a process of developing a patient-centered, evidence-based, comprehensive plan for evaluation and intervention of the

person with a neuromuscular disorder. In addition, the instructor has access to supplemental material online, including a test bank of multiple choice questions with answer key, an Instructor's Guide with answers to or discussions about the chapter case questions, answers to the "Let's Review" exercises, and suggested in-class learning activities.

The scientific literature guiding rehabilitation is immense and is growing daily. As a result, knowledge of all aspects of neurorehabilitation is beyond the capacity of any individual; so this textbook can serve as a long-term resource for clinicians. Even as this first edition debuts, the second edition is germinating in the authors' minds as new information becomes available to support clinical practice. We welcome any suggestions for improvement or corrections to the content moving forward. Here's to providing the best possible, most effective therapeutic care to restore movement, function and meaning to life!

# Contributing Editors

**Megan Danzl, PT, DPT, PhD, NCS**

Assistant Professor and Assistant Chair
Doctor of Physical Therapy Program
School of Movement and Rehabilitation Sciences
College of Health Professions
Bellarmine University
Louisville, Kentucky

**Heather Knight, PT, DPT, NCS, CBIS**

Assistant Professor
Director, Geriatric PT Residency Program
Department of Physical Therapy
Creighton University
Omaha, Nebraska

**Blair P. Saale, PT, DPT, NCS**

Assistant Professor
Department of Physical Therapy
University of South Alabama
Mobile, Alabama
Department of Physical Therapy
Pat Capps Covey College of Allied Health Professions
University of South Alabama Mobile, Alabama

**Rachel T. Wellons, PT, DPT, NCS**

Assistant Professor
Department of Physical Therapy
LSU Health Sciences Center New Orleans
New Orleans, Louisiana

# Compendium of Common Adult and Pediatric Neuromuscular Diagnoses Contributing Editors (Online at Davis*Plus*)

## Adult Diagnoses

**Dennis Fell, PT, MD**

Vice-President, APTA Academy of Neurologic Physical Therapy
Professor and Chair
Department of Physical Therapy
Pat Capps Covey College of Allied Health Professions
University of South Alabama
Mobile, Alabama

**Diane H Pitts, PT, DPT, RN BSN**

Senior Therapist, Vestibular and Physical Therapy
Beth M Rouse Rehabilitation and Wellness Center, Providence
    Hospital,
Mobile, Alabama

**Blair P. Saale, PT, DPT, NCS**

Assistant Professor
University of South Alabama
Department of Physical Therapy
Mobile, Alabama

## Pediatric Diagnoses

**Janet Tankersley, PT, DPT, PCS**

Assistant Professor
Augusta University
Department of Physical Therapy
Augusta, Georgia

**Karen Y. Lunnen, PT, EdD**

Associate Professor and Head (Retired)
Department of Physical Therapy
College of Health and Human Sciences
Western Carolina University
Cullowhee, North Carolina

# Contributors

**Amy Barnes,** MSOT, OTR/L, SWC
Occupational Therapy Clinical Specialist
Stanford Health Care
Stanford, California

**Francisco X. Barrios,** PhD
Professor and Dean
College of Liberal Arts
Southeast Missouri State University
Cape Girardeau, Missouri

**Bassam A. Bassam,** MD, FAAN
Professor of Neurology
Director of Neuromuscular and EMG Laboratory
Department of Neurology
University of South Alabama
Mobile, Alabama

**Mary T. Blackinton,** PT, EdD, GCS, CEEAA
Associate Professor, Physical Therapy Department
Nova Southeastern University-Tampa
Director, Professional DPT Program
Tampa, Florida

**Beth Cardell,** PhD, OTR/L
Associate Professor (Clinical)
Department of Occupational & Recreational Therapies
University of Utah
Salt Lake City, Utah

**Randy Carson,** PT, DPT, NCS, CCCE
University of Utah Healthcare
Rehabilitation Services
Salt Lake City, Utah

**Holly Cauthen,** PT, DPT
Physical Therapist II
Vanderbilt University Medical Center – Pi Beta Phi
    Rehabilitation Institute
Nashville, Tennessee

**Deborah Nervik Chamberlain,** PT, DPT, MHS, DHS, PCS
Associate Professor
Franklin Pierce University
Concord, New Hampshire

**Jill Champley,** PhD, CCC-SLP
Speech Language Pathologist
VA Nebraska Western Iowa
Omaha, Nebraska

**David Chapman,** PT, PhD
Associate Professor
Doctor of Physical Therapy Program
St Catherine University
Minneapolis, Minnesota

**Jennifer Braswell Christy,** PT, PhD
Associate Professor
Department of Physical Therapy
The University of Alabama at Birmingham
Birmingham, Alabama

**R. Barry Dale,** PT, PhD, OCS, SCS, ATC, CSCS
Professor, Department of Physical Therapy
University of South Alabama
Mobile, Alabama

**Megan Danzl,** PT, DPT, PhD, NCS
Assistant Professor and Assistant Chair
Doctor of Physical Therapy Program
School of Movement and Rehabilitation Sciences
College of Health Professions
Bellarmine University
Louisville, Kentucky

**Wesley Blake Denny,** PhD, MT (ASCP)
Senior Scientist
Northeast Georgia Biodiagnostics
Gainesville, Georgia

**Monica Diamond,** PT, MS, NCS, C/NDT
Board-Certified Neurologic Clinical Specialist
Ascension | Sacred Heart Rehabilitation Institute
Milwaukee, Wisconsin
Adjunct Instructor
Concordia University
Mequon, Wisconsin
Marquette University
Milwaukee, Wisconsin

**Heidi Dunfee,** PT, DScPT
Operations Manager, Mayo Clinic School of Continuous
    Professional Development
Mayo Clinic
Rochester, Minnesota

**Carina Eksteen,** PT, PhD
Professor
Sefako Makgatho Health Sciences University
University of Pretoria
Pretoria, South Africa

**Rebecca I. Estes,** PhD, OTR, CAPS

OT Program Director and Campus Director
OT Department
University of St. Augustine for Health Sciences, Austin Campus
Austin, Texas

**Andrea Fergus,** PT, PhD

Professor, Division of Physical Therapy
Shenandoah University
Winchester, Virginia

**Cheryl Ford-Smith,** PT, DPT, MS

Board-Certified Specialist in Neurological Physical Therapy
Associate Professor in Physical Therapy
Department of Physical Therapy
Virginia Commonwealth University, MCV Campus
Richmond, Virginia

**Noi Bernabe Mavredes Fraker,** PT

Director of Rehabilitation Services
Tennova Healthcare-Harton
Tullahoma, Tennessee

**Jane Mertz Garcia,** PhD, CCC-SLP

Professor
Communication Sciences and Disorders
Kansas State University
Manhattan, Kansas

**Denise Gobert,** PT, MEd, PhD, NCS, CEEAA

Associate Professor
Department of Physical Therapy
College of Health Professions
Texas State University
San Marcos, Texas

**Ruth Lyons Hansen,** PT, MS, DPT, CCS

Associate Professor
Doctor of Physical Therapy Program
School of Health and Natural Sciences
Mercy College
Dobbs Ferry, New York

**Jason Boyd Hardage,** PT, DPT, DScPT

Board-Certified Clinical Specialist in Geriatric Physical Therapy
Board-Certified Clinical Specialist in Neurologic Physical
    Therapy
Registered Yoga Teacher (RYT 200), Yoga Alliance
Associate Professor
Department of Physical Therapy
Samuel Merritt University
Oakland, California

**Cathy C. Harro,** PT, MS, NCS

Assistant Professor-Physical Therapy Department, College of
    Health Professions
Grand Valley State University
Assistant Director, Mary Free Bed Rehabilitation Hospital and
    Grand Valley State University Residency in Neurologic
    Physical Therapy
Grand Rapids, Michigan

**Jeffrey M. Hoder,** PT, DPT, NCS

Associate Professor
Doctor of Physical Therapy Division
Department of Orthopedic Surgery
Duke University School of Medicine
Durham, North Carolina

**John R. Jefferson,** PT, PhD, OCS, COMT

Chair and Associate Professor
Department of Physical Therapy
University of Arkansas for Medical Sciences
Fayetteville, Arkansas

**Lisa K. Kenyon,** PT, DPT, PhD, PCS

Associate Professor
Department of Physical Therapy
Grand Valley State University
Grand Rapids, Michigan

**Patricia Kluding,** PT, PhD

Chair and Professor, Department of Physical Therapy and
    Rehabilitation Science
University of Kansas Medical Center
Kansas City, Kansas

**Wei Liu,** PhD

Associate Professor
Research Director of Rehabilitation and Biomechanics
Edward Via College of Osteopathic Medicine, Auburn
    (VCOM)
Auburn, Alabama

**Renee G. Loftspring,** PT, EdD

Daniel Drake Center for Post-Acute Care
Cincinnati, Ohio

**Marilyn MacKay-Lyons,** BSc(PT), MSc(PT), PhD

Professor, School of Physiotherapy, Dalhousie University
Affiliated Scientist, Nova Scotia Health Authority
Halifax, Nova Scotia, Canada

**Michael J. Majsak,** PT, EdD

Associate Professor and Chair
Department of Physical Therapy
School of Health Sciences and Practice
    and Institute of Public Health
New York Medical College
Valhalla, New York

**Heather Mattingly,** PT, MS

Program Director, Physical Therapist Assistant Program
McLennan Community College
Waco, Texas

**Kathy L. Mercuris,** PT, DHS

Associate Professor
Department of Physical Therapy
Des Moines University
Des Moines, Iowa

David M. Morris, PT, PhD, FAPTA

Professor and Chair
Department of Physical Therapy
The University of Alabama at Birmingham
Birmingham, Alabama

Jonathan B. Mullins, MD

Diagnostic Radiology Specialist
Memorial Hospital
Gulfport, Mississippi

Rick Nauert, PhD, MHA, MHF, PT

Adjunct Associate Professor
College of Natural Sciences
Public Health and Health Information Technology
The University of Texas at Austin
Austin, Texas

Esther Munalula Nkandu, BSc (Hons), MSc, MA, PhD

Dean and Associate Professor of Physiotherapy
School of Health Sciences
The University of Zambia
Lusaka, Zambia

Tracy O'Connor, OTD, OTR/L

Assistant Professor/Academic Fieldwork Coordinator
Department of Occupational Therapy
University of South Alabama
Mobile, Alabama

Roberta Kuchler O'Shea, PT, DPT, PhD

Professor
Physical Therapy Program
Governors State University
University Park, Illinois

Diane H. Pitts, PT, DPT, RN BSN

Senior Therapist, Vestibular and Physical Therapy
Beth M Rouse Rehabilitation and Wellness Center, Providence
    Hospital
Mobile, Alabama

Rebecca E. Porter, PT, PhD

Interim Dean
Indiana University
School of Health and Rehabilitation Sciences
Indiana University—Purdue University
Indianapolis, Indiana

Aaron B. Rindflesch, PT, PhD, NCS

Assistant Professor
Director of Clinical Education and Assistant Program Director
Program in Physical Therapy
Mayo Clinic School of Health Sciences
Rochester, Minnesota

Blair P. Saale, PT, DPT, NCS

Assistant Professor
Department of Physical Therapy
University of South Alabama
Mobile, Alabama

Susan Diane Simpkins, PT, EdD

Associate Professor, Southwestern School of Health
    Professions
University of Texas Southwestern Medical Center
Dallas, Texas

Martha Freeman Somers, MS, DPT

Assistant Professor
Department of Physical Therapy
Duquesne University
Pittsburgh, Pennsylvania

Brad Steffler, MD

Associate Professor
Department of Radiology
University of South Alabama
Mobile, Alabama

Jeannie B. Stephenson, PT, PhD, NCS

Assistant Professor
School of Physical Therapy and Rehabilitation Sciences
USF Health Morsani College of Medicine
University of South Florida
Tampa, Florida

Mike Studer, PT, MHS, NCS, CEEAA, CWT, CSST

Northwest Rehabilitation Associates
Salem, Oregon

Marisa L. Suarez, MS, OTR/L, SWC

Occupational Therapist/Clinical Specialist
Stanford Health Care
San Jose, California

Laura K. Vogtle, PhD, OTR/L, FAOTA

Professor
Department of Occupational Therapy
School of Health Professions
The University of Alabama at Birmingham
Birmingham, Alabama

Bridgett Wallace, PT, DPT

President, 360 Balance & Hearing
Austin, Texas

Rachel T. Wellons, PT, DPT, NCS

Assistant Professor of Physical Therapy
LSU Health Sciences Center New Orleans
New Orleans, Louisiana

Laura White, PT, DScPT, GCS

Assistant Professor
Department of Physical Therapy
University of South Alabama
Mobile, Alabama

Kim Curbow Wilcox, PT, MS, PhD, NCS

Professor and Director, Residency Program in Neurologic
    Physical Therapy
University of Mississippi Medical Center, School of Health
    Related Professions
Jackson, Mississippi

**Donna A. Wooster,** PhD, OTR/L

Associate Professor in Occupational Therapy
Chair, Department of Occupational Therapy
University of South Alabama
Mobile, Alabama

**Genevieve Pinto Zipp,** PT, EdD

Professor, Department of Interprofessional Health Sciences
& Health Administration
Director, Center for Interprofessional Education in Health
Sciences
Seton Hall University
School of Health and Medical Sciences
South Orange, New Jersey

# Acknowledgments

**Sincere thanks and deep gratitude to:**

*The Chapter and Compendium Authors*, whose dedication, perseverance, and patient-centered focus brought excellence to each page.

*The Team of Contributing Editors and Blinded Reviewers* who carefully appraised and edited content, adding clinical insights and pearls to clarify the content for clinical and classroom readers.

*The Photographers and Photo Subjects*
- Mr. Jason Torres, whose photographs embody professional quality, focused composition, creative framing, and staging—the product of an exciting and fun photoshoot—and produced images that brought the message of our words to life!
- Mr. Myoungho Choi for his photographic skill in taking many patient photos, especially for the Examination chapters for Balance and Cranial Nerves, and Nathan Fell for his action shot.
- All who served as photo models, including Norma Fell; Hyopil Jeon; Deokhoon Jeon; Youngsu Kim; Elana Fell and Maddie; Kim, Bailey, and Seth Baxter; Corey Irby; Amanda Schermerhorn; Judy Smith; Del Baum; Margaret Anderson; James Nelson; Orlando Warner; Porter Hancock; Anthony Tucker; Carole Canter; William Smith; Robert Oaks; Jenny, Ryan, Ellioni, Alora, and Sadie Durrant; Jaquelyn Johnson; Rachel Porubek; Erin Longhurst; Geoff Buchanan; Danica Dummer; Katharine Kilbourne; and Randy Carson.

*The Facilities and People*
- The physical therapy clinics and laboratories at University of Utah Sugar House Rehabilitation Clinic, University of Utah Balance & Mobility Clinic, University of Utah Rehabilitation Center, University of South Alabama Physical Therapy Department, and Western Carolina University and the therapists, patients, professors, students, friends, and family members in these institutions who agreed to model for photographs and videos.
- The University of South Alabama Physical Therapy students who assisted in researching and preparing portions of the evidence-based tables and diagnosis outlines (see the complete list with the online Compendium).

*F. A. Davis Editors and Staff*
- Who enthusiastically saw the potential in this novel evidence-based textbook concept and patiently facilitated throughout the process: Margaret, for believing in us from the very beginning; Melissa, for energizing in the developmental stages; and Jennifer with her eagle eye for detail, who gently pushed, guided, and ever kept us on track toward success!

# Contents

# Clinical Decision Making for Patient-Centered Care

# Foundations for Making Clinical Decisions in Neuromuscular Rehabilitation

Dennis W. Fell, PT, MD    CHAPTER 1

## CHAPTER OUTLINE

## CHAPTER OBJECTIVES

Upon completion of this chapter, the learner should be able to:
1. Outline the clinical decisions a therapist must make.
2. Discuss the underlying principles and assumptions that are the basis for clinical decision-making.
3. Contrast models of function and disablement and describe the important terminology for each.
4. Discuss the values incorporated into all clinical decisions.

# ■ Introduction

*Mrs. Driver is fearful that she may never be able to move her right arm and leg the way she could before the stroke. She states, emotionally, "Other than an occasional cold, I had never been ill in all my 86 years until this…" As the therapists who will be directing her rehabilitation, we have multiple decisions to make. From the first moment of our encounter with Mrs. Driver, we must intentionally begin to determine the examination tests and measures that are appropriate. Mrs. Driver wants to know if she'll ever be able to walk again or cook meals for her family, the things to which she most wants to return. We must use the history and examination data along with Mrs. Driver's personal goals to make our individualized decisions about her prognosis and the intensity of intervention that will be best for her. Finally, based on the data from her examination, in the context of her prognosis, we must determine the specific intervention techniques to restore or optimize her body functions and maximize her ultimate recovery of functional activity. This book will guide the entire process!*

# ■ The Therapist's Role in Rehabilitation

There are multiple aspects of rehabilitation for individuals with neuromuscular disorders that are fascinating to consider and study. This book is designed to be a resource for the student initially gaining the knowledge and skill for neurological rehabilitation and for the practicing clinician who wants to update knowledge and skill of neurological rehabilitation. Each chapter of this book addresses specific aspects of the practical clinical decisions therapists make in daily practice for adult and pediatric patients who have neuromuscular disorders. Chapter 1 will present the principles and assumptions that are the basis for clinical decision-making, while Chapter 2 will present a framework for the process of clinical decision-making. **Physical therapists (PTs)** are the health-care experts in human movement. PTs improve a person's ability to move and function through individualized examination, evaluation, and interventions, and practice "the science of healing and the art of caring" (APTA, 2008) while also promoting general fitness and health. **Occupational therapists (OTs)** employ "the therapeutic use of occupations, including everyday life activities with individuals, groups, populations, or organizations to support participation, performance, and function in roles and situations in home, school, workplace, community, and other settings (AOTA, 2015)." This includes evaluation of factors affecting activities of daily living (ADLs) and approaches and specific interventions to promote or enhance safety and performance in ADLs, instrumental ADLs, rest and sleep, education, work, play, leisure, and social participation. As summarized in the *Guide to Physical Therapist Practice* (APTA, 2015), PTs practice as part of a health-care team but practice with autonomy; i.e., they independently decide when to examine and which tests and measures to use, individually formulate the evaluation of examination data, make decisions regarding rehabilitation prognosis and goals, develop the physical therapy intervention, and ultimately measure patient outcomes. OTs, according to the American Occupational Therapy Association, "help people live life to its fullest… by helping people relearn the skills of daily living. By focusing on the physical, psychological, and social needs of patients, OT helps people function at the highest possible level" (AOTA, 2008). OTs also make autonomous decisions within the health-care team, in consultation, and in the community. Each step in the decision-making process, as described in Chapter 2, involves practical critical decisions. Therefore, it is imperative that therapists learn to make each of these decisions, including early choices regarding examination and the judgments involved in evaluation, to the intentional and individualized design of the plan of care and intervention.

**Physical rehabilitation,** the wide array of therapeutic treatment for individuals with physical disabilities, is multidisciplinary. Its purpose is to restore the individual to optimal life and capacity for participation, including therapeutic intervention procedures and education. PTs and OTs have the unique pleasure and responsibility of providing individualized therapeutic intervention. The **intervention,** "the interactions and procedures used in managing and instructing patients/clients" (APTA, 2015), must be customized for the individual patient, family, and support system and designed and implemented by the therapist based on the therapist's own examination. The intervention is often intensive and manually delivered and must be carefully designed for the individual patient. Particularly in the context of neuromuscular disorders, patient care usually takes place in an environment that allows for significant interpersonal contact with the patient that leads to an "intense, focused connection" with patients (Jensen, 1992). The intervention schedule in this population often provides many opportunities to positively impact the patient's life in physical, psychological, and social dimensions, making a real and observed difference in the person's life. The therapist's positive impact is delivered through skilled, "evaluative, hands-on, cerebrally produced care" (Moffatt, 1993), encouraging and motivating the patient and helping the patient to focus on the strengths and positive aspects of the current situation as well as the expectation of future recovery. Sometimes the therapist must also help the patient grasp the reality of a prognosis that is less than expected and wanted. Concurrent with the joys and personal pleasures of these health-care professions, the therapist's primary responsibility is to provide optimal, effective care and rehabilitation for each patient.

As further explained later in this chapter, *optimal care* includes therapy or intervention based on individualized evaluation, is delivered with an overriding genuine concern for the patient, and is driven by functional goals. Optimal care is also patient-centered and holistic and is congruent with the best current evidence from the scientific literature. The goal or intention of delivering optimal care is achievement of optimal functional improvement in the individual, i.e., the highest level of functional skill of which a person is capable given the degree of impairment. At the outset of initiating optimal care, the therapist must collect and synthesize information in an examination, evaluate data from the examination and prioritize significant findings from the patient, and then use this information to make clinical decisions and judgments in developing the individualized intervention plan. This process is described in more detail in Chapter 2.

Guidance and principles for clinical reasoning at each step across the entire patient/client management process will be provided throughout this textbook. For specific techniques that are described, the authors will address you, the reader/learner, using active direct voice, providing clear step-by-step instructions in addition to the rationale.

# Clinical Decision-Making

**Clinical decision-making** can be defined as the process to determine appropriate examination methods and to design and customize specific intervention techniques and treatment activities for an individual patient or client. The clinical decision-making process begins when the clinical question or problem is identified. Information gathering and analysis then follow as a basis upon which the decisions or judgments are made. Clinical decision-making is also referred to as clinical reasoning or clinical problem-solving, implying a procedure, a process, and a series of cognitive steps. This process, actually a continuous, interconnected stream of thought processes, is described in detail in Chapter 2 and results in decisions toward best practice and delivery of optimal therapeutic intervention. **Best practice** could be defined as the delivery of customized and efficient care using the most helpful resources, working toward optimal recovery of function (Fell, 2004a), while doing no harm. Chapter 1 will explore the principles of clinical decision-making, while Chapter 2 will detail the process and steps of clinical decision-making, which takes place continually from first examination to the final contact with the patient. The therapist should never be cognitively disengaged during delivery of care. Rather, the therapist is constantly evaluating the situation and the patient's response and asking new questions related to how the therapeutic plan should be adjusted (Fell, 2004a). Therefore, there is always a question to be asked and an answer to be sought.

## There Is Always a Question to Answer

Every patient presents a series of clinical problems...a sequence of clinical questions that must be answered. In fact, each treatment session exposes new issues, new questions to be answered, or clinical problems to be solved. So the therapist must always be thinking. As the patient's status and abilities change, improving or declining, there are new aspects that must be addressed, and of necessity, the intervention must be delivered in a different way than before, adjusting to the patient's new level of ability (Fell, 2004a; APTA 2015). Consequently, the therapist must reconsider the patient's situation and be prepared to change the treatment plan. For example, consider George, whose rehabilitation in the early recovery after his stroke has focused mostly on transfers and sit-to-stand. As these skills improve, he begins to spend more treatment time in standing and walking activities, and these new activities reveal new issues and problems to be solved. The challenge to the clinician is to identify the continually emerging problems and be able to synthesize available information to generate a set of solutions.

## Clinical Decisions Throughout the Patient-Management Process

Clinical decision-making is necessary at the initial examination and evaluation but also with the ongoing emergence of clinical issues. It is clear that clinical decision-making is a process requiring ongoing adaptations and adjustments to the therapeutic plan. The process requires constant reevaluation of the patient and the clinical scenario, including the impact of personal factors and the environment, and a willingness to change previous plans, especially to keep pace as the patient improves.

The result of the initial decision-making process is a determination of the labels to describe the condition to be addressed. While the physician usually labels using a medical diagnosis (disease-specific label related to the cell- or tissue-level pathology), the therapist must decide on the **physical therapy diagnosis,** a label that clearly specifies the movement-related problem(s) for which the therapist will provide intervention, and must do so early in the process. *The Guide to Physical Therapist Practice 3.0* states that PTs "use labels that identify the impact of a condition on function at the level of the system (especially the movement system) and at the level of the whole person" (APTA, 2015, Chapter 2). Decisions by the clinician are required continually throughout the process of patient management and are the focus throughout this book, which is organized according to the sequence of therapist decisions.

- The general framework, principles, and process of clinical decision-making are discussed in Chapters 1 and 2 (Section I).
- Chapters 3 to 13 (Section II) will describe the tests and measures useful for patient examination for relevant body systems and functional activity, as well as the resulting evaluation and will discuss the issues of clinical decision-making based on examination data.
- Chapters 14 to 17 (Section III) discuss the clinical decisions that can relate generally to any therapy or intervention, including underlying principles of neurological rehab, general, broad approaches to intervention, health promotion and prevention, and adaptive equipment/assistive technology. The principles and specific information in these chapters apply generally to all interventions discussed in Sections IV and V of the text.
- Chapters 18 to 32 (Section IV) will explore clinical decisions to select appropriate intervention for impairments of body structure and body function.
- Chapters 33 to 37 (Section V) will present the clinical options and intervention decisions for functional limitations to optimize functional activity and participation in social roles.

While it is assumed that the reader has already been exposed to the medical aspects of neurological disorders in a pathophysiology course, the Compendium, at the end of the book, contains focused diagnosis outlines, which cover the major adult and pediatric medical diagnoses and highlight important background information on the disorders. Outlines for additional neurologic and developmental medical diagnoses, for a total of more than 50 diagnoses, are found in the online supplemental material. For each medical diagnosis, whether traumatic, vascular, degenerative, developmental, or other cause, a comprehensive summary of etiology/pathogenesis, signs/symptoms, diagnostic testing, prognosis, medical/surgical management, and the most common general objectives and options for rehabilitation in individuals with that medical diagnosis are presented and will lead the reader to appropriate sections of the textbook content.

## Toward Expert Clinical Decisions

The early career of a student or novice clinician is characterized by development and refinement of basic clinical reasoning skills. Differences between expert and novice clinicians have been carefully examined in a variety of medical professions. A **novice clinician** is an individual with little experience in their field or practice, while an **expert clinician** is experienced and possesses optimal content knowledge with the ability to reason in order to solve clinical problems identified in the patient, including reflection on their own experience (Jensen, 2000). The characteristics of the expert clinician serve as a model or target for professional development and provide implications for students and novice therapists committed to achieving more advanced clinical decision-making skill. Therapists in rehabilitation use a clinical reasoning process similar to that of physicians and formulate preliminary hypotheses early in the examination (Payton, 1985; Rothstein, 2003) about what testing to perform, the underlying causes for deficits they observe, and optimal intervention strategies and tactics. Expert clinicians draw on their years of experience (Unsworth, 2001; Hallin, 1995; Jensen, 1992), but understanding the factors described in the following might help students advance to this expert level more quickly with intentional study and practice. A number of factors characterizing the expert clinician have been identified and are summarized in Box 1-1. For example, an expert PT would take a careful history from a patient with multiple sclerosis regarding the circumstances surrounding recent falls and with just that information would develop a hypothesis about what systems need full examination (each examination result leading to more specific examination) and which functional activities should be measured as well as a hypothesis about what they will likely find (e.g., posterior falls due to lack of dorsiflexion range of motion, lack of dorsiflexion strength/control, or spastic tone in the plantar flexors). All therapists should purposefully strive to achieve these characteristics and can intentionally accelerate their own progress toward this level of practice. Expert clinicians are also known to practice reflectively (Gould, 1994). **Reflective practice** is defined generically as "those intellectual and affective activities in which individuals engage to explore their experience in order to lead to new understandings and appreciations" (Gould, 1994). Reflective practice, as demonstrated by expert clinicians, is proposed to assist in developing such practice-embedded knowledge (Cross, 1993; Clouder, 2000; Jensen, 2000).

---

**BOX 1-1 Common Characteristics of the Expert or Experienced Clinician**

- Uses a patient-centered approach to care (Resnik, 2003)
- More likely to use patient history and physical examination as part of the evaluation framework (Jensen, 1992)
- Recognizes and "intuitively grasps" cues that are important during the examination/evaluation process (Benner, 1982)
- Better at revising the plan of care according to ongoing changes (Unsworth, 2001; Mattingly, 1993)
- Listens more intently to the patient and is more responsive to the patient (Jensen, 1990)
- Better able to store and retrieve knowledge (Case, 2000)
- Exhibits a higher frequency of instances of clinical reasoning (Unsworth, 2001)
- Forms tentative hypothesis early in the examination (Elstein, 1978)
- More aware of their own mistakes (self-assessment) (Chi, 1988; Embrey, 1996) and use of reflection (Resnik, 2003)
- Performs skills with greater efficiency and proficiency (Riolo, 1996)
- Better able to predict achievement of discharge goal location (Blackman-Weinberg, 2005)
- Characterized by four identified dimensions: "(1) a dynamic, multidimensional knowledge base that is patient-centered and evolves through therapist reflection, (2) a clinical reasoning process embedded in a collaborative, problem-solving venture with the patient, (3) a central focus on movement assessment linked to patient function, and (4) consistent virtues seen in caring and commitment to patients" (Jensen, 2000).

---

## ■ Human Function and Disablement: A Unified Framework for Making Clinical Decisions

Certain functions inherent to human existence, including skills, tasks, and abilities, allow us to "take care of ourselves," to uniquely interact with the environment, and to function in distinctly human ways. Human function, as a composite, is much more complex than that of other animals, considering the complex interactions uniquely possible in physical, psychological, and social domains. Human function is dependent on the coordinated actions of multiple organ/systems. For example, balance in an upright walking task requires contributions of multiple sensory systems, many processing and regulation centers of the central nervous system (CNS) (many of which act at subconscious levels), reciprocal pathways transmitting all this information back and forth between neural structures, and multiple systems that execute the motor plans for balance reactions. As another example, driving a vehicle requires certain upper extremity and lower extremity motor skills concurrent with cognitive abilities that allow appropriate judgments and decisions for safety.

It is clear that damage to tissues, organs, or systems, particularly from disease or trauma, can result in inabilities to perform in any of these domains of function. For this text we are specifically concerned with the results of damage to the nervous and muscular systems.

*Consider Olivia, who has had a stroke and now cannot move the left side of her body. She has sensory losses on her left side and cannot see objects in her left visual field; as a result, she is currently unable to walk or do her gardening. Or consider Melvin, who sustained a traumatic brain injury resulting in poor motor control, particularly of the right side of his body, and cognitive impairment that together prevent him from driving.*

Current models describing function and the process of disablement are in contrast to the earlier "medical model" of disease, consistent with the International Classification of Disease (ICD) that has existed since 1893, with a focus on classification of "disease." This medical model as a basis for understanding disease proposed that an etiology, either an internal or external cause, leads to a particular pathology with resulting disease manifestations. By this model, within the realm of medical care, treatment resulted in cure of the disease, living with some results of the disease, or death. This model did not adequately explain the concept of managing signs and symptoms outside of the realm of cure; nor did it delineate between disease manifestation at different levels or, most importantly, the impact of those signs and symptoms on function. Therefore, this textbook is organized around a model of body functions and functional activity rather than around medical diagnoses.

Models that specifically describe the impact of neurological disorders on function and ability can provide a useful framework for making clinical decisions. The *Nagi model*, developed in 1965, includes four dimensions: pathology, impairment, functional limitation, and disability (Nagi, 1969; Nagi, 1991). The World Health Organization (WHO) developed the *International Classification of Impairment, Disabilities, and Handicaps (ICIDH) model* in the 1970s to shift focus away from disease and onto effects, especially in chronic and disabling conditions. This model includes four dimensions: disease, impairment, disability, and handicap (WHO, 1980). The *National Center for Medical Rehabilitation Research (NCMRR) model* blends these two models into one with five dimensions: pathology, impairment, functional limitation, disability, and handicap (NIH, 1993) with common terminology used in identification of disability.

In 2001, the WHO made major revisions to the ICIDH resulting in the *International Classification of Functioning, Disability, and Health* (ICF) (WHO, 2001), which changes the focus to health and functioning instead of a negative viewpoint focusing on disability. The new framework emphasizes what the patient "can" do as an initial basis on which the plan of care is built and focuses on the normal system function and abilities that the therapist intends to restore through rehabilitation. It identifies actions at three levels, defined later in this chapter: body structure and function, whole person activity, and participation of the whole person in social context (Figure 1-1). In the schematic representation of the framework, the bidirectional arrows mean that each construct can contribute to any other segment of the framework in any direction. The schematic also indicates that everything takes place in the context of environmental and personal factors. Environmental factors include the physical, social, and attitudinal environment in which people live and complete their daily activities (*WHO ICF Beginner's Guide*, 2011, p. 10). Figure 1-1 shows the major components

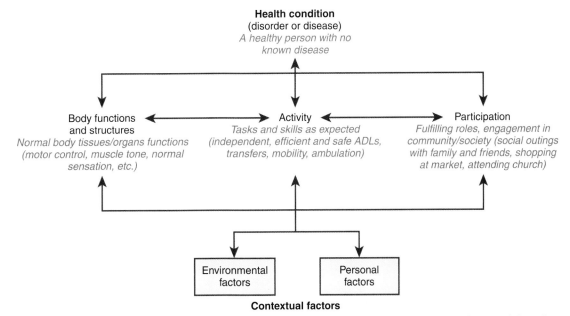

**FIGURE 1-1** International Classification of Function (ICF) Framework with examples of normal function. Adapted from World Health Organization. International Classification of Function. ICF Beginner's Guide. Available at: http://www3.who.int/icf/ Accessed October 6, 2016.

of the framework in black letters with examples of normal function shown in blue letters. Figure 1-2 provides examples, in red, of abnormal, impaired expressions for each dimension that can result from disorders or disease.

Comparisons between the different models are illustrated in Figure 1-3. The APTA, for its *Guide to Physical Therapists Practice* (2015), uses a framework that focuses on the dimensions within which PTs provide intervention: pathology, impairment, functional limitation, and disability. Over the past decade, the APTA (2008) and many other international professional health organizations have transitioned to the ICF model (Jette, 2009). Throughout this book, the terminology of both ICF and NCMRR models will be used depending on, respectively, whether the discussion is in regard to normal functioning of a system or the deficits that result from injury and disease. In summary, the text will focus on improving the impairments of body structure/body function and restoring activities and participation when functional limitations result from neurological disorders.

## Considering Frameworks of Function and Disablement

The NCMRR model of disablement focuses on the deficits that result from disease or disorders, the abnormal results that the therapist identifies on physical examination of the patient. The NCMRR model includes five dimensions of the person useful as a classification scheme for making a physical therapy diagnosis: pathology, impairment, functional limitation, disability, and societal limitation (NIH, 1993), describing, from a negative perspective, patient deficits that result from injury or disease. In contrast, the ICF framework focuses, from a positive perspective, on the positive expressions of these same constructs, i.e., the ultimate goal or the functions to be restored: body (system) functions, body activity, and societal participation. All of these new ICF concepts reflect the goal of our therapeutic intervention (identifying what systems/body segments currently do work, what those systems should be able to do, and what skill we will work to restore) as opposed to focusing on the problems and deficits we see at the beginning of rehabilitation. The integration of both models is discussed here as a framework useful to therapists.

**Pathology** is the abnormality that occurs at the cell, tissue, or organ level. Nagi (1991) defined pathology as an interruption or interference of normal body processes. The ICIDH model uses the term "disease" to describe changes at the level of the organ (WHO, 1980). The ICF uses the term **health condition** to describe "diseases, disorders, and injuries" that impact function at body function and whole person levels (WHO, 2001). Because of disruption to cell or tissue expression, pathology can often be detected by observation or diagnostic testing, including laboratory tests, direct visualization of tissue in surgery, observation of pathological specimens, and radiographs or other imaging. Examples of pathology in specific tissues include inflammation, tumors, atherosclerosis, diabetes, and pneumonia. In each case, the cell, tissue, or organ is anatomically or microscopically disturbed or not functioning properly. This dimension is not one that the therapist directly addresses very often but is most commonly addressed by the physician/physician assistant/nurse, especially through medication or surgical intervention. The therapist administering dexamethasone through

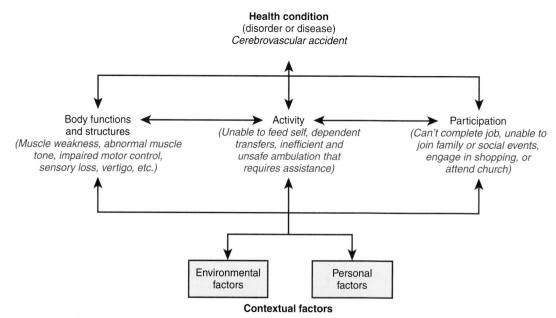

**Health condition**
(disorder or disease)
*Cerebrovascular accident*

**Body functions and structures**
*(Muscle weakness, abnormal muscle tone, impaired motor control, sensory loss, vertigo, etc.)*

**Activity**
*(Unable to feed self, dependent transfers, inefficient and unsafe ambulation that requires assistance)*

**Participation**
*(Can't complete job, unable to join family or social events, engage in shopping, or attend church)*

**Environmental factors**

**Personal factors**

**Contextual factors**

**FIGURE 1-2** ICF Framework illustrating how a disorder or disease can impact normal expression of body function, activities, and participation. These are the problems that the therapist would detect in a patient examination. Adapted from World Health Organization. International Classification of Function. ICF Beginner's Guide. Available at: http://www3.who.int/icf/ Accessed October 6, 2016.

| Process of disablement | | | | | |
|---|---|---|---|---|---|
| **NCMRR:** (composite of Nagi and ICIDH) | **Pathology** *Example: Disease or injury such as cerebrovascular accident or traumatic brain injury* | **Impairment** *Example: Sensory deficits, lack of selected/isolated movement (abnormal synergies), limited joint range of motion, spastic hypertonicity, muscle weakness, disequilibrium/ imbalance* | **Functional limitations** *Example: Slow and inefficient in bed mobility, needs assistance to transfer from wheelchair to chair, unable to reach/grasp/ manipulate with upper extremity, unable to ambulate* | **Disability** *Example: Unable to return to work or school* | **Handicap** *Example: Architectural barriers or societal attitudes that prevent the individual from participation in some societal role, activity, or location* |
| **Nagi:** | **Pathology** • Interruption of normal bodily processes or structures | **Impairment** • Loss of structure or function | **Functional limitations** • Decreased ability to perform action or activity | **Disability** • Limitation in performing socially defined activities | |
| **ICIDH:** | **Pathology** • Changes at level of organ/tissue | **Impairment** • Disruption of function at organ/ system level | | **Disability** • Decreased ability to perform common activities at person level | **Handicap** • Limitations at social level that are imposed by society or the environment |
| **ICF:** (emphasizes the positive viewpoint and aspects to restore through physical rehabilitation) | **Body structure/body function** • Body structures: "Anatomical parts of the body such as organs, limbs and their components." • Body functions: "Physiological functions of body systems (including psychological functions)." *Examples include, but are not limited to: The pancreas produces insulin normally. The brain is able to send a signal to cause an intended muscle action and maintain normal muscle tone. The brain is able to receive, process sensory information resulting in perception, awareness, and appropriate action.* | | **Activity** • "The execution of a task or action by an individual." *Example: The person is able to perform bed mobility independently, can transfer with supervision, can reach/grasp/manipulate, and can ambulate with an assistance device and hands-on assist for balance.* | **Participation** • "Involvement in a life situation." *Example: A child can participate/play with peers at the park. A child or young adult can return to the role of student. A young adult can return to the role of student. A young woman can return to the role of being a mother or volunteer at a local school/organization. An older adult can do everything necessary for their own grocery shopping or attending senior center events.* | |

**FIGURE 1-3** Comparison of disability-based models (NCMRR, Nagi, ICIDH) that focus on abnormal findings to the function-based ICF model with a focus on normal expressions of system and total body function. Overlap and contrast between ICIDH and NCMRR models of disability can be seen. The ICIDH model includes four dimensions: "disease," which correlates with *pathology;* "impairment," which is synonymous with Nagi's *impairment;* "disability," including inability to perform common activities at the person level, which is similar to Nagi's *functional limitation;* and "handicap," emphasizing societal and physical limitations, which overlaps partially with Nagi's *disability.* The NCMRR, Nagi, and ICIDH models all describe the components from a negative view with labels describing deficits that result from disease or injury, while the ICF describes the positive aspects of system function—the goals of rehabilitation.

iontophoresis or phonophoresis is providing intervention at the pathology level. But while the direct purpose is to decrease pain or inflammation (pathology), the intended outcome of this treatment is to improve the related motion limitation as a related impairment. A recent focus of medical care within the pathology dimension has been prevention and health promotion, which is certainly a role of the therapist.

As an example of health emphasis, Nagi (1991) states that, with each occurrence of pathology, the body simultaneously generates an effort to return to the normal state (Nagi, 1991).

**Impairment** is dysfunction at the organ/system level in which the function of the specific organ or system is either diminished or lost, globally or locally, depending on the extent of the pathology. The term **primary impairment** is used when the impairment results directly from a pathology, e.g., sensory loss, hypotonia, poor motor control, and impaired balance that follow a cerebrovascular accident (CVA). Impairment is one of the dimensions specifically addressed through therapeutic intervention and is defined as "alterations of physiological, psychological, or anatomical structure or function" (APTA, 2015). In this definition, "alterations" can include incomplete or complete loss and therefore can be expressed as either partial or complete loss of the organ function. The opposite, positive term from the ICF model is **body structure/body function,** which again focuses on the normal system function (i.e., that which the therapist wants to restore) instead of focusing on the deficit that results from the health condition. Force generation is one normal function of the neuromuscular system; weakness, impaired motor control, and paralysis are related examples of neuromotor impairment. Sensory reception is a normal function of the somatosensory system; hyper- or hyposensation, pain syndromes, and complete anesthesia are some related examples of sensory impairment that might be seen among populations with neuromuscular disorders. When impairments of limited range of motion and joint immobility occur, the therapist will work to restore motion and mobility as normal functions of muscles and skeletal joints. Cardiopulmonary impairments include arrhythmia, ischemia, dyspnea, and ventilatory arrest. Because of the complex structure and function of the nervous system, related impairments are numerous with tremendous variety and include incoordination (ataxia), impaired motor control, joint or segment instability, involuntary movements, abnormal muscle tone, hemiplegia, complete sensory loss, diminished or hypersensibility, abnormal pain, altered consciousness, impaired judgment and memory, perceptual abnormalities, dizziness, vertigo, and impaired balance.

**Indirect impairments** or **secondary impairments,** also termed **sequelae,** are those organ/system deficits that develop not as an immediate and direct result of the disease process but as secondary complications (Schenkman, 1989). For example, contracture/adaptive shortening of a muscle does not develop as a direct result of the damage to brain tissue in a stroke; it develops slowly over time because of impaired movement at the joint and inability to move into the end-range. Decubitus ulcerations of skin do not develop as a direct result of the damage to brain tissue in a stroke but develop slowly over time because of lack of movement and mobility and the inability to offload the skin. *Composite impairments* are impairments that are more complex and have multiple underlying, contributing impairments (Schenkman, 1989). The best example of a composite impairment is balance impairment or dysequilibrium. Balance is not in itself a total-body function or activity; rather it is a required component of many functional tasks, including sitting, standing, transfers/transitions, reaching, walking, and stair-climbing. It is a complex, composite impairment because many sensory and motor systems contribute to balance as will be seen in the discussion on examination of balance (see Chapter 9). Impairment in any of those systems, including somatosensory, visual, vestibular, or motor, for example, can result in balance impairment.

The third dimension is the ability to complete a total body task, skill, or action termed **activity** in the ICF model. From a disablement standpoint, **functional limitation** refers to inability at a total-body, whole-person, or task level. As a major dimension appropriate for therapeutic intervention, the APTA defines functional limitation as "restriction of the ability to perform a physical action, task, or activity in an efficient, typically expected, or competent manner" (APTA, 2015). Nagi (1991) explains functional limitation as a decreased or absent ability to perform an action or activity in a normal manner or range. Notice again the possibilities of complete inability (cannot complete a task even with assistance) or partial limitations (needs assistance, performs slowly or inefficiently) in this dimension. Consider any of the daily human tasks that you perform: all ADLs, self-care tasks, purposeful tasks of child's play, the actions required in your daily routine of work or school, and the highly skilled tasks of sports and the arts. An inability, or decreased ability, to perform any of these tasks or skills is a functional limitation and is perhaps the most important reason for implementing rehabilitation intervention.

Most functional tasks require contributions from multiple body systems. For example, a simplified analysis of the task of kicking a ball ultimately includes a CNS motor plan that uses the muscles of the leg to carry out movement of the skeleton at prescribed joints while dynamic balance prevents falling so the foot can make contact with the ball. In addition, cognitive components contribute to motivation and other affective components of kicking the ball, like the enjoyment of kicking the ball, and the approach and timing of the kick, while coordination is required for controlled grading on and off of opposing muscles of the leg, motor control for the accuracy and timing of the contact with the ball, and co-contraction of the trunk muscles for stability. In addition, vision and other sensory information, including joint position sense, is used to modify the plan as the movement is carried out. It is easy to see from this example that even a task as "simple" as kicking a ball is a highly complex, multisystem task.

An inability or limited ability to perform any one of the specific functional activities listed in Table 1-1 would be a functional limitation. Across the spectrum, functional limitation could include a complete inability to walk or walking that exhibits abnormal gait deviations or parameters such as having to use an assistive device, slow gait velocity, asymmetric step lengths, or inefficiency in gait. In rehabilitation, functional limitations are at least partially addressed by correcting or improving underlying impairments that are identified and hypothesized to be contributing to the functional limitation and then providing repetitions of meaningful practice of the task to improve the task. While more studies are needed in this area, there is some evidence that an increase in function results from remediation of underlying impairments, including range of motion (Wang, 2002; Singer, 2003) and balance (Bonan, 2004; Badke, 2004). Additional studies are presented in the chapters of Section II. However, we will see later that intervention for impairments only does not result in optimal functional improvement.

| **TABLE 1-1** | **Summary of Three Areas of Physical Function in Rehabilitation With Examples** | |
|---|---|---|
| **1. FUNCTIONAL MOBILITY** | **2. ACTIVITIES OF DAILY LIVING** | **3. COMMUNICATION** |
| Bed mobility (rolling, scooting in bed, supine-to-sit, scooting on edge of the mat…) | *Basic ADLs* | Expressive speech production |
| Horizontal mobility (crawling/creeping, especially in pediatric population) | Feeding | Written communication |
| Transfers (bed-to-chair, chair-to-toilet) | Dressing | Nonverbal communication: facial expression, upper extremity gestures |
| Transitions (sit-to-stand, stand-to-sit, floor-to-stand) | Hygiene (including toileting, bathing, grooming) | *[Receptive communication is not listed because it is not physical.]* |
| Ambulation | | |
| Climbing stairs/ramps | | |
| Running | *Instrumental ADLs* | |
| Wheelchair locomotion | Managing personal affairs | |
| | Cooking | |
| | Shopping | |
| | Home chores | |
| | Driving | |

An individual's involvement or engagement in society, including the ability to fulfill life roles and experience life situations, is termed **participation** in the ICF model. **Disability,** from NCMRR, is just the opposite and describes an inability to fulfill certain life roles at a social level beyond the person level. Nagi (1991) emphasizes roles within a social environment. Disability includes restriction of abilities in occupational roles, relational and family roles, and usual recreational roles. The APTA's *Guide to Physical Therapist Practice* (2015) defines disability as "the inability or restricted ability to perform actions, tasks, and activities related to required self-care, home management, work (job/school/play), community, and leisure roles in the individual's sociocultural context and physical environment." For example, a person may be unable to keep a job, fulfill her role as a mother, or complete her current role as a student. Disability is addressed in the rehabilitation process by restoring the specific skills or functional abilities necessary to complete the role or using alternate means and methods to accomplish the tasks necessary for the role if the underlying causes cannot be remediated. This may include use of compensatory devices, assistive devices, orthotics, and technology. In permanent deficits, disability may be addressed by employing aides or attendants or technology to complete the parts of the role that the individual cannot. Participation is optimal when disability and handicap are minimized.

A **handicap,** as in NCMRR and ICIDH, is a societal limitation, constraint, or barrier imposed by society or the environment, including any societal attitude, which prevents full involvement of the individual at a social level. On the positive end of the spectrum, absence of a handicap contributes to participation, as does correction of disability. Physical and architectural barriers of the environment, including curbs without wheelchair cut-outs or ramps, home bathrooms with doors too narrow for wheelchairs, restaurants and movie theaters that are not handicap accessible, and even beaches without handicap access, can create handicaps. Social and policy constraints, including occupational settings that cannot make necessary accommodations or policies of facilities or agencies that might prevent involvement of individuals with certain conditions such as incontinence or infections, can also result in a handicap. Therapists may address handicaps by advocating for changes in social policy or addressing environmental (especially architectural) barriers to allow individuals with disability greater opportunities to participate in a broad array of social experiences.

These models should not be viewed as strictly linear, though in some cases a linear relationship does exist. Pathology can lead to impairment that contributes to functional limitations, with resulting disability and associated handicap (Figure 1-4A). For example, the demyelinating plaques of multiple sclerosis (pathology of *body structure*) can result in weakness and perhaps poor motor control (impairments of *body function*). These system losses can prevent individuals from walking independently (functional limitation at an *activity* level), so they cannot maintain their usual job or completely fulfill their role as a parent (disability at a *participation* level) for a period of time. It is important to note, however, that expression in one dimension does not necessarily lead to expression in the next dimension. For example, mild lower-extremity weakness, commonly seen with aging, may occur but without causing a functional limitation to gait, but once strength decreases below a particular threshold, functional limitations, especially in ambulation, will be observed. As another example, full knee-extension range is critically important to work on standing but is not essential once standing is no longer feasible.

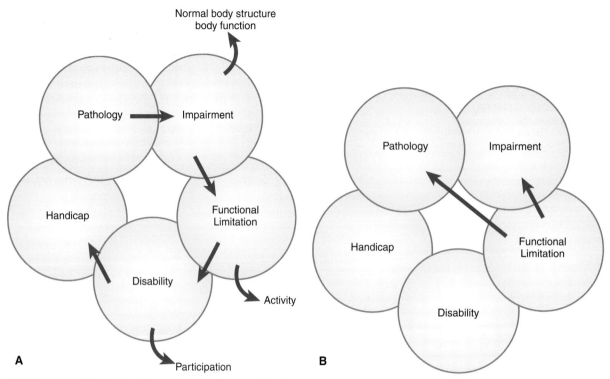

**FIGURE 1-4  A AND B:** Possible interactions between disablement components (labeled in black in the center of the figure) when normal function, as emphasized in the ICF, is disrupted.

A) Linear interactions include, for example, stroke (P), which can directly cause motor control impairment (I) on one side of the body. Impaired motor control along with other impairments contribute to an inability to ambulate (F) or use the arm for grasp and manipulation tasks (F). The composite effect of all functional limitations, including gait abnormalities, now prevents the person from being able to fulfill life roles such as attending school or doing one's work (D). This makes the person more susceptible to societal and architectural barriers such as an inability to access a public building (H) or to social stigma that limits interaction in public settings (H). However, as therapeutic intervention and treatment activities bring positive changes, the individual is more likely to move out of this cycle (as shown with the blue lines and blue labels of the ICF) with more normal expressions, as emphasized in the ICF. The person begins to exhibit improved body structure/body function of body systems and organs, increased activity and skill, and enhanced participation and engagement in life.

B) Nonlinear interactions during disablement may include components with impact that can flow in multiple directions. For example, a person with a stroke may develop habitual inactivity and insufficient ambulation following prolonged bedrest (F), which can contribute to cardiovascular deconditioning (I) and limited range of motion at particular joints (I). Prolonged bedrest with insufficient mobility can also contribute to decubitus ulcers of the integumentary system (P).

P = Pathology; I = Impairment; F = Functional Limitation; D = Disability; H = Handicap

Multiple interactions may take place across all five dimensions as illustrated in Figure 1-4B. As an example of the nonlinear relationships, consider a case of atherosclerotic CVA or stroke. The cerebral ischemia and infarction (pathology) may directly result in impaired motor control of extremities and generalized weakness of the affected side (both impairments), which may contribute to difficulty with bed mobility and dependence in ADLs (functional limitations) and inability to perform self-care (disability). So far, the process described still represents a linear relationship. On continuing the analysis, though, this inability to change position in the bed (functional limitation) can cause excessive and prolonged skin pressure at bony prominences, which can cause skin breakdown and decubitus ulceration (secondary pathology) with associated pain (secondary impairment) or decreased range of motion (secondary impairment), all of

which will likely contribute to further decreases in functional mobility (functional limitation).

Figure 1-3 will eliminate some of the confusion when comparing the models. ICIDH uses the term "disability" regarding what the *Guide to Physical Therapist Practice* (2015) and this text considers functional limitation, including daily activities of self-care, mobility, and communication. ICIDH's "disability" is basically the same component as Nagi's "functional limitation" at the person level. "Disability" as used by Nagi at the social role level is very different from "disability" as described by ICIDH as occurring at the person level. The ICIDH term "handicap" correlates with Nagi's term "disability" because of the emphasis on social roles. For the purposes of this text, the NCMRR model is used.

Impairments, functional limitations, and disability are the primary dimensions of disablement that are most commonly and specifically examined and addressed by therapists in the rehabilitation process to improve or restore body structure/body function, increase activity, and enhance participation, respectively. In some cases, the therapist may occasionally provide intervention at a pathology level. Sometimes, remediation or improvement of underlying impairments must take place before functional abilities can improve (Rothstein, 2003). However, improving an impairment is not the chief end of rehabilitation; it is only a means to the end of helping the patient increase functional ability to enable participation in life. Improving function and the ability to optimally fulfill social roles is the therapist's primary objective.

## ■ Clinical Decision-Making Is Based On...

### Knowing Patients Are People

The terms "patient" and "client" have distinctive meanings in this book. "Patient" is used, as a respectful and personal title, most often throughout this text to describe the person who comes to the therapist or other health-care professional for rehabilitation or intervention for a health- or movement-related problem. A **patient** is defined simply as "a person who is ill or who is undergoing treatment for disease" (MerckSource, 2008) or a "recipient of physical therapy examination, evaluation, diagnosis, prognosis, and intervention, and who has a disease, disorder, condition, impairment, functional limitation, or disability" (APTA, 2015). The term "patient" can connote the interpersonal, caring, and professional aspects of care delivery into the context of the professional knowledge possessed by the therapist. It is also important to note that, throughout this textbook, when referring to patient management and decision-making, the term "patient" is generally used in the broader sense to include patient and family/caregiver. The caregiver is a crucial part of the process, particularly in pediatrics, as family participation is federally mandated in the Individuals with Disabilities Education Act (IDEA) and in geriatrics, where family support becomes paramount. The recognition of therapists' knowledge and expertise is supported by the fact that the most preferred characteristics of the therapist identified by patients included "informativeness," "humaneness," and "competence/accuracy" (Wensing, 1998). Some professionals have preferred the term "client" over "patient" because the latter could imply a passive, recipient role on the part of the individual as opposed to the actively involved health-care consumer, while others have simply proposed the term "people" (Turner, 2002). The term "**client**" may be the more appropriate term when referring to a person without disease or disability who seeks care or advice from the therapist related to health promotion or wellness (APTA, 2015). The term "patient" has been preferred by a number of medical professionals (Shum, 2000; Ellard, 1994; Nair, 1998; Nair, 2000; Turner, 2002) and among one sample of home care patients (McGuire-Snieckus, 2003). As discussed in detail later in this chapter, it is essential that the therapist engage the patient and/or caregivers in the decision-making process, but the therapist is the one with the expertise, knowledge, and experience to guide rehabilitation, while considering all of the values, needs, desires, and goals of the patient.

It is essential that the therapist considers and refers to each patient as an individual person, not as a diagnosis (Jones, 1993; Woodend, 2003; Isenberg, 2001). The American Physical Therapy Association (APTA) and its journal *Physical Therapy* have long supported the use of such **people-first language** (APTA, 1991; Rothstein, 1997). All APTA members are expected to "put people first, not their disability, when communicating about a patient/client" (APTA, 1991). Guidelines for communication about individuals with disabilities have been developed (Guidelines, 2001) suggesting that therapists should not refer to their patients using the diagnostic label. For example, do not state that "Mr. Jones is a C-6 spinal cord injury." Such terminology is too frequently used in casual clinical discussions and verbal team reports. In this example, Mr. Jones is not a spinal cord injury; he is a 24 year-old male who sustained a spinal cord injury at the C-6 level. Similarly, Billy is not "a C.P."; he is a child with a diagnosis of cerebral palsy. And Mrs. Smith is not "a stroke"; she is a person who had a stroke and is now dealing with the resulting effects.

For a novice individual with little experience in dealing with persons with disability, a person-first focus is a greater challenge with patients who are profoundly or severely disabled in the physical domain. On the outside, the individual may look and move very differently, but the challenge for the therapist is to remember that, on the inside, the patient is a person. And the severity of physical disability may not correlate at all with the degree of cognitive ability. These individuals and families have many of the same issues of life as other people in addition to dealing with the stresses added by their disease or disability.

### A Focus on Function

In the rehabilitation of individuals with neuromuscular disorders, *function* of the patient is the essential and ultimate realm to be considered and should be the first consideration when defining outcomes pursued by the patient and the therapist. Think of **function** in terms of the ability of a person to perform whole-body tasks or skills that are part of the usual performance of human individuals, consistent with the individual's purpose and priorities (Wensing, 1998). Ask yourself: "What tasks or actions should the patient be able to perform upon completion of the therapeutic rehabilitation?" "What do they want to be able to do?" For an adult, some examples of function include self-care tasks, reaching, grasping, standing, sitting down on the toilet seat, sitting independently, cooking, walking, getting in and out of the car, climbing stairs, and specific skills required for jobs. The primary work and therefore function of children is simply to play. So for a child, function often initially emphasizes play skills; later, they develop self-feeding skills, tasks to explore and interact with the environment (crawling/creeping), and ultimately physical skills that support study and work. The *Guide to Physical Therapist Practice* (APTA, 2015) defines function as "those activities identified by an individual as essential to support physical, social, and psychological well-being and to create a personal sense of meaningful living."

In the earlier history of the PT profession, it seems the therapeutic emphasis, even in patients with neurological disorders, was almost exclusively on correcting specific organ/system impairments that might interfere with proper functioning, most commonly weakness and limited range of motion. Therefore, therapy often emphasized strengthening and stretching of specific muscle groups almost exclusively, with only adjunctive and cursory functional activities; the expectation was that improvement in function would result. Recently, especially since the early 1990s, the focus has shifted to more emphasis on function and functional activity while still considering underlying impairments (Rothstein, 2003). In fact, there is evidence that refutes the notion that strictly treating impairments without attention to function can improve function (Winstein, 1989; Light, 1995). While in some cases correcting weakness was shown to improve function (e.g., lower extremity strengthening, improved sit-to-stand) (Bohannon, 2007), functional training itself has been shown in some settings to provide strength gains that are comparable to direct strength training (Krebs, 2007). Additionally, a focus on functional training, at least in some situations, may improve power generation for some activities more specifically than just strength training (Puthoff, 2007). The functional focus of intervention is also supported by the evidence for specificity of learning discussed in detail in the motor-learning section of Chapter 14.

The detail regarding the process and priorities of clinical decision-making is provided in Chapter 2. The intervention chapters in Section IV will demonstrate the importance of direct intervention, particularly early in rehab, to address underlying impairments. The greatest focus on addressing impairments will occur in early phases of intervention, while an ongoing, growing, and ultimate focus on function is essential throughout rehabilitation and should be progressively emphasized throughout the continuum of therapy beginning with the initial examination.

Function in rehabilitation has been categorized in at least three domains: physical, psychological, and social; it includes the tasks and skills that allow us to physically live our lives and interact day by day. Some specific functions in the physical domain are categorized in Table 1-1 and include functional mobility activities such as crawling, transfers, ambulation, and stairs, which are a primary focus of the PT, as well as self-care tasks or ADLs, including hobbies and driving (often OT), and the physical aspects of speech production and communication. Function in the psychological domain includes mental function (attention, concentration, judgment, memory, and problem-solving as discussed in Chapter 4) and affective function (anxiety, depression, coping strategies, self-attitude, and self-esteem), which may be directly addressed by the psychologist, the PT, the speech and language pathologist, or the OT. Realize that the level of cognitive functioning has profound implications for all rehabilitation and will affect the functional mobility intervention provided by the PT and overall outcome. The social domain of function includes participation in such social activities as recreation and social interaction and fulfilling social roles, including all levels of interpersonal

relationships. It is important to note that altered function in the physical domain can both influence and be influenced by changes in psychological and social function. For example, onset of depression can precipitate a drastic decline in motivation for physical activity and mobility. If the limited movement and ambulation is not addressed, physical declines in the musculoskeletal and cardiovascular systems will result because of the patient's immobility and lack of activity.

Physical therapists are the movement and mobility specialists among rehabilitation professionals. Carr and Shepherd (1987) first used the term "movement scientists" to describe PTs, emphasizing the scientific basis of analysis and treatment of movement problems in individuals with neuromuscular disorders. The scientific knowledge base for understanding human movement and therapeutic intervention has grown immensely in recent decades as demonstrated throughout this textbook, particularly with numerous studies involving analysis of biomechanical and neuromuscular components of specific ADLs and specific functional tasks (see Chapter 10), including rolling, sit-to-stand, ambulation, and others. Details will be included throughout all chapters of Section II. As we learn more about components and principles of normal movement patterns in function, we are better able to recognize and document existing problems and then design treatment plans and incorporate components of activities that will improve function.

When a patient first arrives for the initial session of neurological rehabilitation, the clinical decision-making process immediately begins in the therapist's mind upon first visual observation of the patient. In neuromuscular rehabilitation, the combined effect of neuromuscular diseases or trauma and the usual aging process has caused a decline in the domains previously described. Suddenly, or in some cases gradually, the person is unable to do the things they were able to do earlier. In the case of pediatric developmental disabilities, the child usually does not lose function but rather may not develop those skills in the normal expected time frame. Therapists then develop a plan of care to either restore or remediate function, if possible, or teach compensation in cases where little true recovery is expected (Schenkman, 2006). Regardless of the treatment plan, the focus of clinical decision-making should always be improvement toward functional outcomes and greater independence.

## Expecting Functional Recovery—Neural Plasticity—The Brain Can Change

Our clinical decision-making is also based on an expectation that significant functional recovery is possible and that functional recovery is the result of expected positive changes in the brain. The brain can change! The functioning of the human brain and the entire nervous system is amazing! In fact, while our comprehension of the nervous system has grown significantly, complete understanding of the complex interactions and links of neuroscience to functional activity currently surpasses human capability. This section cannot be a comprehensive discussion on neural plasticity because of page constraints but rather a reminder from previous neuroscience study that neural plasticity is an essential occurrence that explains the functional recovery in the patient. You should have already learned many details of the anatomy and physiology of the CNS and its varied, highly specialized functions. Much has been discovered about CNS function in recent decades, yet there is so much that we do not understand. The CNS was once thought to be completely static and permanent, i.e., neural cells could not regenerate, reproduce, or repair themselves, or establish new connections (Chen, 2002). So after CNS injury—for example, a stroke or CVA—therapeutic efforts rarely aimed to significantly restore function. Consequently, some patients in earlier decades had to cope with the deficits that resulted from neurological injury without expectations for great recovery. Now, however, there is significant evidence indicating that the CNS can undergo positive change and reorganization, especially related to certain environmental conditions and experience, and even following CNS pathology or injury (Buonomano, 1998; Schallert, 2000; Nudo, 2003; Chen, 2002; Kleim, 2002; Kleim, 2003; Cauraugh, 2005; Carmichael, 2006; Hosp, 2011). In fact, there is evidence that some neurons do possess the capability to reproduce new cells or regenerate even in experimental, in-vitro environments (Gould, 1999; Nakatomi, 2002; Gould, 2002). This CNS reorganization can result from certain interventions (Liepert, 2000) and has been linked to recovery of function (Johnston, 2003; Rosenzweig, 2003; Ackerley, 2015). A brief review of the evidence for neural plasticity will be presented.

Plasticity implies that an object or system possesses the inherent capability for change. **Neural plasticity** can be thought of as reorganization within the CNS and includes "the tendency of synapses and neuronal circuits to change because of activity" (Cauraugh, 2005, p. 310) and the "brain's capacity to be shaped or molded by experience ... and the ability to reorganize and recover after injury" (Johnston, 2003). Built on prior exposure to the details of neural plasticity in a previous neuroscience course, the purpose of this section of the chapter is to emphasize that neural plasticity is the bridge that connects our physical interventions to the functional improvement seen in the patient after neurological injury. Neural plasticity may occur by a number of mechanisms (Hallett, 2001; Warraich, 2010; Hosp, 2011), including (1) modification of synapses, development of increased dendritic branching, and development of new synaptic connections with nearby neurons (Bear, 1987; Lee, 1995); (2) sprouting of new fibers from surviving neurons, which can synapse with distant neurons (Lee, 1995); and (3) neurotransmitter and neural receptor changes (Malenka, 2003). Some recovery may occur within the CNS following partial damage to a particular neural substrate. However, following complete destruction of a substrate of the CNS, the only possibility for plasticity is substitution by a surviving functionally related substrate (Seitz, 1997). All of these mechanisms allow for new interactions among surviving neurons with the capability for improved performance. Plasticity will be explored in (1) the intact nervous systems following practice, for example, in musicians (Elbert, 1995; Schlaug, 2001; Munte, 2002) and

in athletes (Casabona, 1990), and (2) the cortical reorganization and enhanced capability for movement that follows practice in individuals with a stroke (Ashburn, 1997; Nudo, 1998; Hallett, 2001).

## Neural Plasticity in Intact CNS

Studies have demonstrated neural plasticity in the unimpaired nervous system with changes in the functional mapping of the cortex as a result of motor experience (see Box 1-2). These changes are most often associated with increased use (practice) of a part of the body or changes that allow increased sensory feedback from the body segment. Box 1-2 summarizes examples of cortical map changes as evidence of activity-induced neural plasticity of the unimpaired and the impaired nervous systems. Interestingly, even mental practice of a task in the early stages of learning a complicated finger exercise has been reported to enhance change of neural circuits (Pascual-Leone, 1995). There is ample evidence that the intact nervous system is capable of neural reorganization. But now there is growing evidence of reorganization in the pathological nervous system.

## Neural Plasticity Following CNS Pathology

A growing body of evidence supports the potential for neural plasticity following cerebral injury such as stroke or brain injury, particularly related to the challenging practice of a motor task (Nudo, 2003). Obviously this reorganization takes place

---

**BOX 1-2  Evidence of Activity-Induced Neural Plasticity in the Unimpaired and Impaired Nervous System**

**Studies in Unimpaired Nervous System**
- Following increased use of fingers in monkeys (Jenkins, 1990)
- With skilled Braille reading in humans with the enhanced sensory feedback (Pascual-Leone, 1993)
- Following amputation, perhaps because of increased use of remaining portion of the limb (Hall, 1990)
- Following practice of a novel task (three-ball cascade juggling) (Draganski, 2004)

**Studies in Impaired Nervous System**
- CVA: Following challenging practice of a motor task (Nudo, 2003; Hosp, 2011)
- CVA: Following constraint-induced movement therapy (Liepert, 2000; Ishida, 2015)
- CVA: Following virtual reality in chronic stroke (You, 2005)
- SCI: Supralesional and sublesional reorganization of spinal cord locomotor pattern generators following body weight-supported treadmill training in spinal cord injury (Grasso, 2004)
- SCI: Neuroplasticity after spinal cord injury (review article) (Behrman, 2006)

among surviving brain tissue. It has long been suggested that cerebellar function can compensate for some cortical lesions (Evarts, 1980) and that the intact hemisphere can partially assume some of the functions of a damaged hemisphere (Glees, 1980). More recent studies have utilized positron emission tomography (PET) to demonstrate functional changes in cortical mapping with cortical motor fields extending and shifting into undamaged areas following recovery from CVA (Asanuma, 1991; Weiller, 1993), and some have suggested the essential role of rehabilitation activity to promote neuroplasticity (Dimyan, 2011; Kleim, 2008; Mang, 2013). There is also evidence of neural reorganization following spinal cord injury (Grasso, 2004; Behrman, 2006; Leech, 2016) and even related to functional recovery in chronic CVA (You, 2005).

For clinical decision-making, the key implication of the concept of neural plasticity is that, with most CNS disorders, the therapist expects some degree of CNS reorganization, especially in younger brains (Chen, 2002; Benecke, 1991; Carr, 1993). When neural plasticity is expected, the therapist works more aggressively toward significant recovery of functional skill. This will profoundly affect the overall therapeutic plan of care that the therapist designs and implements. Rather than immediately resorting to compensation as a permanent means of functional adaptation after brain pathology, the therapist will provide opportunities for meaningful practice of movement of dysfunctional parts, including educating the patient in a variety of pertinent home activities incorporating the target patterns of use to further enhance neural plasticity. The role of neural plasticity from motor learning and the principles and techniques to enhance neural plasticity are more specifically addressed in the motor-learning section of Chapter 14.

On the other hand, some neuromuscular diseases have, in fact, little or no expected long-term recovery, and the natural history includes a progressive degeneration with deterioration in symptoms and, consequently, a progressive decline in function. In such conditions, the clinical decision-making often does not include goals or intervention for dramatic improvement. Parkinson disease, Huntington disease, Alzheimer disease, and the progressive forms of multiple sclerosis are examples of progressive disorders. In these progressive disorders, is the therapist's role to help the patient cope with resulting deficits, or is it to enhance functional abilities? The potential may exist for reorganization and refinement of intact neuromotor systems that may result in some functional improvement. In these progressive disorders, early intervention after the initial diagnosis can help optimize function and should include general fitness and endurance activities and health promotion (Birleson, 2003; Kirsch, 1999; Sullivan, 2000; Shabas, 2000; Petzinger, 2010). Researchers have suggested that rehab-generated stimulation of neural plasticity should be expected (Farley, 2008; Levin, 2006; Mang, 2013). The graph in Figure 1-5 illustrates one potential positive effect of early intervention on long-term function in the context of a progressive disorder. Depending on the rate of progression for the specific disease and the extent of the pathology at the time therapy is initiated, the top (dark) line shows

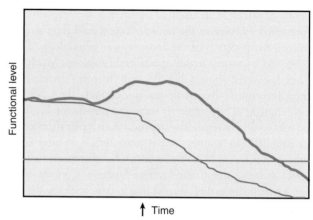

↑ Time

**FIGURE 1-5** For a patient with a progressive neuromuscular disorder, the thin line represents the expected progressive decline in physical function over time without physical rehabilitation. The dark line at the top shows the potential positive effect on function that could result from early intervention initiated at the point in time shown by the arrow. The horizontal gray line indicates some hypothetical critical level below which the person would be dependent in function. Therefore, therapeutic intervention, causing even minimal improvement, could result in delay of functional decline related to optimizing movement-related systems before the progressive declines, thereby delaying the loss of independence.

that optimizing function in the early stages of a progressive disease could sustain optimal levels of activity and participation for a longer period of time. For exacerbating conditions such as multiple sclerosis, it is also important to intervene soon after each exacerbation, especially early in the remission, to encourage and promote optimal nervous system reorganization or plasticity and functional recovery. Therefore, even in progressive neuromuscular disorders, therapy to promote neural plasticity may play a role in maximizing function in early rehabilitation that may delay the onset of significant disability.

To promote neural plasticity, it is important to enforce or encourage use of and practice with the affected/dysfunctional limbs as part of therapeutic intervention in neuromuscular disorders (Kleim, 2008; Opie, 2016; Livingston-Thomas, 2016), as will be discussed in Chapter 14, to optimize neural reorganization and functional recovery. Increasing the frequency of intentional and practiced movement, particularly skilled tasks, allows the brain to experience and practice control of the part and, as a result, enhances neural growth and new synapses as a basis for functional improvement. A younger brain, which undergoes change as a usual course of development, could be expected to have greater degrees of neural plasticity than the brain of the older individual. In fact, the capacity for reorganization within the brain is most pronounced in the postnatal period (Stiles, 2000) and decreases in older age. From a cognitive standpoint, however, it has been shown that severe traumatic brain injury (TBI) in early childhood or moderate or severe TBI in infancy increases vulnerability to significant residual cognitive impairment (Anderson, 2005).

## THINK ABOUT IT 1.1

The bottom line is that PTs and OTs do not just observe and take advantage of neural plasticity but actually create and enhance neural plasticity through the activities and physical engagement they design for the patient. In other words, we don't just watch the *train of neural plasticity* go by and jump on-board; we actually *drive the train* and can influence both speed and direction. If we challenge the patient with engaging and demanding tasks, not just performing easy tasks over and over, we are more likely to encourage more robust neural plasticity, which enhances the physical recovery. You'll get more detail later in Chapter 14, but just thinking about it, what could you as the therapist do in an intervention session to optimize the neural plasticity?

## ■ Skilled Clinical Decision-Making Incorporates These Values...

To make optimal clinical decisions, the therapist must have a mindset that incorporates functional goals from the onset of patient management, intentional preventive steps, decisions that center on the patient, a holistic approach to the person, evidence-based practice, and an emphasis on carryover to real life activity.

### Functional Goals From the Beginning

Central to the clinical decision-making process is the formulation of functional goals that are meaningful to the patient. **Functional goals** are specific behavioral objectives that describe the functional performance projected to occur by the end of your intervention or in a specified time period (Quinn, 2003, p. 34). The general approach and intensity of the therapy must be linked to the functional goals, which are an expression of the optimal, expected functional level. Functional goals are customized individually for each patient, predicting the maximal level of functional recovery based on:

1. Current functional level and presence or absence of recent improvement.
2. **Prognosis,** or the degree of recovery expected (prognosis is often dependent on such factors as a) the prior level of function; b) medical diagnosis; c) severity, extent, or stage of progression of the disorder; d) patient engagement in the rehab process; and e) presence of comorbidities).
3. Degree of neural plasticity expected (related to medical diagnosis and patient age).
4. Individual patient factors including motivation and compliance/adherence.
5. The environmental context, including resources, roles, and caregivers.

The specific components of therapeutic intervention selected by the therapist are largely determined based on the current level of functional skill and that to which the patient aspires. This applies throughout the course of rehabilitation. In other words, it is essential that the clinician *think about the end from the very beginning.* For example, even in early stages, therapy for the patient who is expected to reach independent sitting as the highest level of function will be very different from therapy for the patient who is expected to reach a functional level of independent ambulation. The thought process for goal setting is similar to that applied to many other areas of human behavior and performance, including management of time and other resources, job performance and career mapping, sports and fitness training, and dieting and weight loss. If the rehabilitation goal for a patient is set too low, the patient may be less likely to achieve the optimal level of functional recovery. Goals must be set at a high but attainable level.

## THINK ABOUT IT 1.2

It is essential that the clinician think about the end from the very beginning. So while you will be concerned about the presence of spasticity or decreased range of motion from the very beginning, your ultimate focus is on the functional skills and tasks that you want your patient to improve or gain.

Determination of functional goals at the initiation of rehabilitation is also essential in preparation for assessing **functional outcomes.** *Outcomes* are "changes in impairments, functional limitations, and disabilities and the changes in health, wellness, and fitness needs that are expected as the result of implementing the plan of care" (APTA, 2015). Functional outcomes are the actual changes observed in function that result from intervention and other factors. The term is often used to refer to projected or predicted outcomes. **Outcome measures** are the tools and methods (tests and measures) used to measure the functional outcomes. Tests and measures may be either (1) **subjective measures,** which include patient reports or therapist observations that depend on perceptions, feelings, opinions, or judgments (e.g., ratings, observations, or scales based on opinion) or (2) **objective measures,** including actual instrumental readings or counts that are more likely to be free of bias and based on facts (e.g., timed measures and distance measures). Examples of subjective measures include rating scales for balance, manual muscle testing for strength, and documenting that "gait is slow," while related objective measures include computerized center of gravity measures for balance, dynamometry for strength, and measurement of gait velocity. Objective measures, if available, are usually preferred over subjective measures because of repeatability, enhanced reliability, and providing measures that are sensitive to change. Subjective measures do contribute to the evaluative process, especially if standardized, which is preferred over purely subjective observations. The tests and measures of the initial examination as well as the functional goals provide measures of a baseline function and a projected degree of functional recovery, respectively. These measures can be compared with functional performance at any time during the rehabilitation process to document change, especially if objective measures are used. So, while functional goals help guide the intervention, they are also an important step in the process of measuring or evaluating functional outcomes as evidence of the effectiveness of the therapeutic intervention. Because the ultimate purpose of therapeutic intervention is optimizing functional outcomes, the therapist must clearly explore the link between functional goals and intervention and focus on functional outcomes from the very beginning.

## Intentional Prevention for Optimal Health

Patient goals should also include goals for optimal health promotion and wellness and introduction of prevention strategies, including issues discussed in detail in Chapter 16, such as safety related to fall risk, polypharmacy, and primary prevention of related disease such as heart disease and stroke. The therapist must focus on the person holistically, and therapy cannot focus strictly on treating existing problems. As a primary health-care provider, the therapist must always consider the long-term functional goal of maintaining optimal function through intentional prevention. The APTA's *Guide to Physical Therapist Practice* (2015) states that "Prevention services; programs that promote health, wellness, and fitness; and programs for maintenance of function are a vital part of the practice of physical therapy." In addition to treating primary problems detected in the examination, the therapist should address any potential health problems for which the patient is found to be at risk (Campbell, 1997). Chapter 32 will specifically address intervention and prevention related to cardiovascular endurance and deconditioning in the context of neuromuscular disorders. *Risk,* as explained in Chapter 16, may be related to factors intrinsic to the individual, to impairments, to disease processes, or to recent health behavior. Intentional prevention should include counseling regarding primary prevention of disease as well as prevention of expected secondary complications for the condition, as discussed in the Section IV chapters. The therapist should fulfill the role of health promoter as an advocate for healthy patient behavior and encourage behavioral change with specific suggestions. The details of planning a prevention strategy are addressed specifically in Chapter 16.

## Patient-Centered/Family-Centered Decisions

A **patient-centered focus** to the clinical decision-making process, individualized for the particular patient, has been strongly advocated for rehabilitation (Ozer, 2000; Schenkman, 2006). In fact, from beginning to end—examination/evaluation to intervention and outcomes—the whole process should be centered on the patient and the caregiver/family, specifically their priorities, needs, and values. Patient-centered care, also called *client-centered* therapy, requires an individualized therapeutic plan (Whitley, 1991) that is customized

for the individual with patient/caregiver involvement in every aspect of the intervention process, including treatment decisions (Wensing, 1998; Platt, 2001). Patient-centered care also includes placing patient/caregiver needs at the highest level, altruistically over those of health-care providers and even third-party payers (Kreitner, 1994). Ideally, the rehabilitation exclusively revolves around the patient. The patient is truly at the center of all decisions. Patient-centered care is not based on what is personally best or most convenient for the therapist or for the facility but rather what would be best for the patient.

A patient-centered approach to therapy is *individualized,* as specific examination measures and all clinical intervention decisions are customized for the individual. In neurology more than most other areas of rehabilitation, a group of patients with the same diagnosis can express widely varied clinical presentations and distribution of symptoms. For example, a CVA can manifest in a myriad of diverse clinical expressions/symptoms. Because the nervous system is so specialized, subtle differences in the location of a pathological lesion can result in widely varied symptoms and signs, including almost limitless combinations of impairments and functional limitations and infinite degrees of restriction to activity and participation. In **progressive neuromuscular disorders,** those that have a progressive worsening of impairments and progressive decline in activity as part of the expected course of the disease, a patient could exhibit any number of different impairments and functional limitations commensurate with the current stage of the disorder. For example, while cognitive deficits are common among those with Alzheimer disease, "each person is unique and requires different interventions at different times" (Francese, 1997). Consider two patients: one a retired farmer with strong family support and the other an urban-dwelling businessman who lives alone. While the two patients may have identical sensorimotor symptoms, each may have very different functional goals. Consequently, for any situations where a particular medical diagnosis lacks complete homogeneity, there can be no protocol or standardized prescription of intervention that applies to any patient with that diagnosis. Even when a treatment has been shown to be effective in a certain population through randomized, controlled trials, the treatment may fail "if a client's (patient's) characteristics do not conform to those of the (study) group" (Riddoch, 1991).

Patient-centered care starts with an individualized examination and evaluation, and strongly considers the individual's personal goals and concerns as emphasized in the Hypothesis Oriented Algorithm for Clinicians (HOAC) (Rothstein, 2003). Early in the HOAC process, as described in Chapter 2, the therapist considers the goals of the patient or family and then focuses the examination on the areas pertinent to those goals, which enforces an emphasis on meaningful, function attainment. Patient-centered examination requires the therapist to select the specific tests and measures from all examination methods available that are most appropriate to quantify the patient's areas of dysfunction (Moriearty, 1998). Goals should also be patient centered as well as functional (Randall, 2000). A focus on patient goals has been shown to specifically reduce anxiety, even without any other specific intervention (McGrath, 1999). Patient-centered care also involves the patient in treatment planning, especially by considering the personal goals and considering the patient as a partner (Lowes, 1998). Encourage patients to "take responsibility for their own health," which has been suggested to increase patient adherence, at least to medical treatment (Lowes, 1998).

## A Holistic Approach to the Person With Disability

A holistic approach to rehabilitation must include consideration of the person as a whole. The *Occupational Therapy Guidelines for Client Centered Practice* defines **holism** as "the perception of the client as a whole person... [whose] overall state of health... [is] a result of a complex interaction of factors including physical, mental, socio-cultural, and spiritual components" (CAOT, 1991). As emphasized earlier, it is essential that the therapist purposely regard each patient as a person complexly composed of these multiple dimensions. The very basis of holism is viewing the human organism as an indivisible and integrated whole (McColl, 1994). The therapist should not focus only on the patient's medical condition or isolate just the physical impairments or the specific anatomic regions involved. Rather, the therapist must also consider the inherent strengths of the individual that will be the key to initiating efforts toward long-term goals. The total combination of dimensions of human function interact together to create the unique framework from which a patient thinks, behaves, and moves and which helps us to recognize each other as individuals.

When looking at a patient as a whole, consider potential interactions of all the aspects of function, including physical function, psychological function including cognition, and social function. Though the PT will focus on physical function, particularly mobility, ADLs and psychological and social aspects must be considered to identify possible influences on physical function and interactions with the whole person. And while the OT focuses on occupations and tasks of daily living, the impact of physical function and mobility must be considered. Debility of any kind has been said to challenge two aspects of our holism: our doing and our being (Bridle, 1999). With onset of disability, there are certain things an individual cannot "do," which contributes to a disruption in "being." For example, declining self-esteem can profoundly limit motivation and physical performance. Fear, particularly the fear of falling, can severely decrease physical activity, which can then result in impaired cardiovascular endurance as a long-term sequela.

A major result of viewing patients holistically is that the therapist will be better positioned to notice the influence of affective domains on the rehabilitation process. For example, depression is commonly observed with physical disability, and the therapist will need to personally encourage such patients or refer them to other professionals as indicated.

## Evidence-Based Practice

**Evidence-based practice,** another essential principle of clinical decision-making, requires that the delivery of rehabilitation care be based on the best available scientific evidence. Jutai (2003) stated "Evidence-based practice attempts to implement the results of research trials (evidence) and to translate those results into clinical practice, with the presumed goal of improving the effectiveness of clinical care." This section discusses why evidence-based practice is important. Chapter 2 will explain the actual steps to incorporate evidence-based practice in clinical decision-making. For comparison, evidence-based practice has been contrasted with common, usual practice. Current usual practice has often been based on opinion of an authority or expert alone or based on clinical experience and anecdotes of what has worked in the past, perhaps with little scientific literature to support the decisions (Duncan, 1996). Sackett (2000) described three components to evidence-based practice: (1) the evidence, (2) practitioner expertise, and (3) patient values. Regarding the evidence, evidence-based practice requires the clinician to obtain, interpret, synthesize, and apply information from scientific studies to daily practice in the process of solving clinical problems that arise. A five-step strategy has been suggested to assure evidence-based practice in the clinical decision-making of therapeutic rehabilitation professionals (Norton, 2000):

1. Define the clinical question.
2. Find the evidence in the literature.
3. Analyze the evidence for reliability, validity, effectiveness, etc.
4. Summarize the evidence.
5. Apply the evidence in clinical practice by combining the evidence with clinical experience and patient values (Sackett, 2000).

The problem is that it is impossible for a clinician to know all the current information about every aspect of patient management in neuromuscular rehabilitation, much less the thousands of articles published every month on a topic. Therefore, in determining evidence-based practice, the emphasis is not on always *knowing* all the information but rather on knowing *where to find* the information. Fortunately, in this computer age, access to and retrieval of the scientific literature is easier than ever. With the rapidly growing knowledge base, it is impossible to keep current in every area of practice, even within a single specialty. Therefore, it is essential to know how to search the literature through a number of online databases and how to access the literature, including online journals (Fell, 2004b).

Evidence-based practice includes basing all aspects of rehabilitation (selection of examination methods, planning of intervention strategies and techniques, and assessing outcomes) on (1) evidence available from the scientific literature, in addition to (2) expert opinion and (3) patient values (Sackett, 2000). In examination and evaluation methods, evidence-based practice implies use of measures that are preferable to others because they are valid and reliable, regardless of whether they are objective measurements, norm- or criterion-referenced tools, interview-based functional assessments, or others. It is important for the therapist to understand the purpose for each type of test, as will be explained in Chapter 3. Emphasis in examination methods is shifting from subjective measures and informal observational analysis to measures that are more standardized and objective (measurable and repeatable). Not only does this apply to initial examination measures but also in selecting outcome measures that are shown to be valid and reliable.

Regarding therapeutic intervention, therapists should select treatment approaches, methods, and techniques that have been shown to be effective and are supported by scientific research whenever possible. Most often, when intervention studies examine changes related to intervention over time, the evidence is strengthened if a comparison is made to a control group that did not receive the intervention. Some studies compare two treatment techniques over time to see if one produces a significantly better result. There are several limitations of such intervention studies, including:

1. While PT intervention is delivered by human individuals, the rigors for analysis of intervention trials evolved specifically for studying drug intervention where dosage and administration can be precisely standardized.
2. Comparisons among interventions for patients in neurorehabilitation are difficult because of the lack of precise methods to categorize patients and the difficulty in designing standardized interventions that can apply meaningfully across an entire sample of patients with variable neurological deficits. When the same methods are used to compare types of therapeutic intervention, the quantity and quality of administration of hands-on care cannot be so carefully controlled as the amount of medication in a pill.
3. If the study doesn't have an appropriate control group, it is impossible to know whether the improvement observed would have occurred anyway in similar circumstances even without the intervention.
4. There are emotional, relational, and affective components to the interpersonal delivery of intervention that are difficult to control.
5. In a well-designed study, the sample is very homogeneous such that, even if the intervention is shown to be highly effective in the sample, it may be difficult to actually extrapolate the findings to patients with the same diagnosis but with a different clinical presentation or to patients with a similar or very different neurological diagnosis.

Among the different types of experimental and pseudoexperimental studies, the strength of the evidence found in results and conclusions varies for each type of study and sample size (Table 1-2). Randomized controlled trials (RCT), originally developed for medication trial research, are truly experimental studies with sufficient sample size to allow true randomization of subjects to experimental and control groups and where manipulation of independent variables occurs with the control group not receiving the intervention being investigated. Generally, RCTs are considered to have the greatest strength among primary studies. But a meta-analysis of a group of related RCTs carries even greater strength. Pseudoexperimental or quasi-experimental designs are less rigorous because either randomization or control is lacking. Therefore, the evidence presented has less strength because the results may not generalize and are susceptible to outside influences. Common examples of pseudoexperimental research are the uncontrolled intervention study and the case report. While RCT results are touted as having the greatest strength for generalizability, in applying research to the clinical setting, the therapist must always consider how closely the patient to be treated fits the characteristics of the studied sample. If the patient has different characteristics than the sample, the application of the results to this patient may not be appropriate.

| TABLE 1-2 | Summary Box of Strength of Evidence by Study Category and Type. Study Types at the Top of the Table Have Greater Strength of Evidence. | |
|---|---|---|
| *Systematic Reviews* | • Including meta-analysis of multiple RCTs | Highest evidence strength |
| *Experimental*<br>• Randomization<br>• Control<br>• Manipulation | • Randomized controlled trial | |
| *Quasi-experimental*<br>• Manipulation necessary<br>• No randomization<br>• No control | • Subjects as own controls<br>• Sample of convenience<br>• Single-case experiment<br>• Case study<br>• Clinical practice improvement | |
| *Nonexperimental*<br>• No manipulation<br>• Control not possible<br>• Randomization not possible | • Descriptive, observational research<br>• Investigation of fixed variables<br>• Examine postfacto variables<br>• Examine relationship between existing variables | Lowest evidence strength |

Because human understanding is incomplete, we are always in the process of gaining knowledge and understanding. We must remember that "evidence-based practice" is not "proof-based practice," especially in the realm of human experimentation. This is illustrated, for example, in the placebo effect. In manual intervention delivered by human hands compared with pharmaceutical intervention, it is difficult to eliminate interpersonal and attention effects of therapeutic intervention. It is well accepted that evidence from the scientific process does not prove anything but rather gives a strong indication as to the hypothesized relationship or conclusion, thus supporting the need for multiple studies in a variety of populations to support any particular intervention. To illustrate the point, if the result of "intervention A" is shown to be better than the result of an alternate "intervention B" at $p = 0.03$ ($p = 0.05$ significance level) in a specific, homogeneous sample of sufficient sample size, the $p = 0.03$ means that such a difference could be reported in 3 of 100 similar experiments (3%), even though no true difference exists (Portney, 2009, p. 419–420) or that the observed difference could have occurred by chance. So, in this case, does that mean that "intervention B" has no value and should never be used? Not necessarily, especially if the patient you are treating does not exactly fit the demographic characteristics or clinical presentation or the study sample. In some studies, a randomized, controlled trial with a large number of subjects may reveal a significant improvement in the study group, while no improvement is shown in the control group. In this case, one cannot assume that the particular treatment will be effective in every individual patient, even if they meet the strict inclusion criteria of the study group. The complexities of the human body and mind appear to make such universal conclusions problematic. Until more replication studies are completed to validate and reinforce previous studies with additional studies to broaden the application of research findings, care should be taken before completely rejecting specific examination or intervention methods. The bottom line is that, until multiple studies are completed on a topic with substantiation of previous results (or meta-analyses), results need to be interpreted and applied cautiously to areas of physical rehabilitation, especially if the study sample does not precisely match your patient.

However, it is essential that rehabilitation professions continue to move toward defining and refining the knowledge base and application of the knowledge base to daily clinical practice. If evidence does exist regarding a certain topic, therapists need to explore the implications for change in clinical practice while watching for more definitive studies and replications to confirm the necessary changes in practice. Understanding the scientific basis for each examination and intervention method will help to support our services in discussion with third-party payers, lawmakers, and others as we defend, promote, and advance our profession. Evidence-based practice also probably limits personal and employer liability because the therapist can report or testify that an intervention was delivered in a manner consistent with the best current practice, or the standard of care, as supported by the recent scientific literature and can provide references if necessary.

Evidence basis is essential in clinical decision-making, especially in examination and intervention, and needs to be applied by clinicians to each individual patient as part of a patient-centered approach. Therefore, a "Focus on Evidence" (FOE) table for each examination and intervention chapter (Sections II–V) can be found in the online resources made available to readers. The FOE table will summarize the most important published studies related to the chapter topic. Each table will include current information from studies related to the topic, including characteristics of the study sample, methods employed in the study (examination or intervention), the type of study, and results and significance of the study with implications for patient management. This summarized information can be used in developing treatment plans that are optimally effective and also for ready comparison with future studies. Box 1-3 provides evidence-based resources to assist in finding evidence-based information on specific clinical problems that arise.

## THINK ABOUT IT 1.3

Consider your expectations for patient outcomes in two scenarios:

1. If the therapist performs the "usual" intervention methods that are "popular" without regard to whether an intervention is supported by research
2. If the therapist is continually adapting their clinical reasoning and plan of care to incorporate tests/measures and interventions that are most clearly supported by the research literature

### Emphasis on Carryover to Home Activities

Finally, for all phases of rehabilitation, it is very important for the therapist to consider what the patient is doing in nontherapy hours and to encourage intentional physical movement. On weekdays, patients admitted to rehabilitation may spend less than 20% of the day involved in therapeutic movement (Esmonde, 1997), and when alone, they are inactive nearly two-thirds of their time (Ada, 1998). Even during intervention time following a stroke, functional upper extremity movements have been documented in only 51% of inpatient and outpatient sessions that addressed upper limb rehabilitation, with an average of 32 repetitions/session (Lang, 2009). Systematic reviews have concluded that people with a stroke are physically active for an average of 60% of their intervention session (Kaur, 2012) and are inactive most of the day (median 48.1%) (West, 2012). Too often, patients are inactive when not in structured therapy (Keith, 1980; Keith, 1987), and observation within the first 14 days after a stroke indicates they spend greater than 50% of time resting in bed, more than 28%

---

**BOX 1-3 Tools to Support Evidence-Based Practice**

MEDLINE database via PubMed
<www.pubmed.gov>

Cumulative Index to Nursing and Allied Health Literature database (CINAHL)
<http://www.ebscohost.com/cinahl/>
[also available to APTA members through APTA PTNow.org Article Search at http://www.ptnow.org/ArticleSearch/ Default.aspx]

Cochrane Database of Systematic Reviews
<http://www.thecochranelibrary.com/view/0/index.html>
[also available to APTA members through APTA PTNow.org Article Search at http://www.ptnow.org/ArticleSearch/ Default.aspx]

Hooked on Evidence: An APTA database that summarizes research evidence on the effectiveness of physical therapy interventions
<www.hookedonevidence.org>

Physiotherapy Evidence Database (PEDro): A database of randomized trials, systematic reviews and clinical practice guidelines in physiotherapy, including quality ratings for each study
<http://www.pedro.org.au/>

PTNow Article Search: APTA's Portal to Evidence Based Practice (APTA member-only service)
<http://ptnow.org/ArticleSearch/>

StrokEngine: An evidence-based site that focuses on stroke rehabilitation, including a section on examination/assessment and a section on intervention.
<http://strokengine.ca/>

Evidence Database to Guide Effectiveness (EDGE) documents developed by the Neurology Section (APTA) include recommendations for use of outcome measures in people with stroke (StrokEDGE), Multiple Sclerosis (MS-EDGE), Traumatic Brain Injury (TBI-EDGE), Spinal Cord Injury (SCI EDGE), Parkinson Disease (PDEDGE), and Vestibular Disorders (VEDGE).
<http://www.neuropt.org/professional-resources/neurology-section-outcome-measures-recommendations>

---

of time sitting out of bed, and only 13% of time engaged in functional activities (Bernhardt, 2004). Experienced therapists describe the task of "teaching patients" as one of their most important clinical skills (Jensen, 1992), and this should include teaching the patient specific applications of the intervention to everyday activities, especially in ways that will be easy to remember and incorporate. Effective motor learning requires appropriate and sufficient amounts of practice, and it cannot all happen during therapy time. A patient who practices therapeutic activities only during therapy time misses important opportunities for practice and improvement. It

therefore seems that, particularly in neuromuscular rehabilitation, an emphasis on nontherapy time is essential to achieve optimal outcomes and carryover to function. In each chapter of this text, watch for key features of patient education and the home exercise program that will be highlighted.

Studor (email communication, Nov. 12, 2011) has highlighted the importance of motivating patients toward compliance with the home exercise program (HEP). He delineated three recommendations for optimizing compliance/adherence and related patient attendance and for assuring patient "buy-in" from the start of therapy, even from the initial examination. He assumes that people want to get better, but they do not always believe that therapists can help them get better, so proof or evidence becomes an important factor for motivation as well as an essential part of measurement. According to Studor's recommendations, the therapist should:

1. Perform objective testing during initial examination. This will demonstrate that the therapist is serious about getting the patient better and has a specific measure that will be used (with a focus on functional ability).
2. Explain why. Describe exactly how each HEP activity relates to the tests/measures and will work toward improving the outcome measures.
3. Make eye contact as you communicate expectations to the patient: "This is what I found in your examination... By doing these (3–4) activities in your time at home, you will be helping to achieve these goals... I will be re-testing you with these measures to see that we made a difference in your life" (M. Studor, email communication, Nov. 12, 2011).

---

*It's About Time:* There are 24 hours in a day or 168 hours in a week. In the most optimal situation, you might see an individual for in-patient rehabilitation therapy 2 hours a day or 10 hours a week. More commonly in outpatient settings, the therapist may see the patient only 1 to 3 hours a week. If we assume that individuals get an average of 8 hours of sleep each night, that still leaves 112 waking hours during a week. If the patient is "in therapy" only 10 of those waking hours, that leaves 102 waking hours that are "nontherapy times." You may be providing great opportunities for motor learning during the therapy sessions, but what is the patient practicing and learning in those 102 nontherapy hours?

---

Consider the time comparisons in relation to therapy hours presented in the "It's About Time" feature. The **home exercise program,** or home activity program, is a set of prescribed exercises/activities conducted by the patient at home that is essential to optimal rehabilitation. They could be performed either alone or with the assistance of a caregiver and should be easily and naturally incorporated into the routine at home. The therapist must also provide **patient education,** giving the patient information and instruction to optimize their rehabilitation and health status through helping them understand their disease process and emphasizing the essential nature of their personal involvement in the rehabilitation process, including changes in daily behavior and home exercises/activities. In one study of patients with a stroke in six rehabilitation facilities, education was reported in only about 7% of overall sessions, and only 84% of the patients or their families received any educational intervention (Jette, 2005). Patient education will enhance the individual's rehabilitation and health status by including specifics about the disease/disorder, the rehabilitation prognosis for the patient, explanation of therapeutic procedures, and informed consent, including the purpose and expected results, precautions, and contraindications to home activity and health promotion information as discussed in Chapter 16. It is also important to assess and address the individual's **self-efficacy,** the degree to which an individual believes in personal capability to achieve change (Bandura, 2007). Self-efficacy, discussed as a general principle of neurological rehabilitation in Chapter 14, can certainly influence whether the individual will change behavior and engagement in the rehabilitation. Regarding the home program, the therapist should clearly explain options for activities and posture and positioning of the affected extremities during all usual home activities, including watching television, riding in a vehicle, sitting at the dinner table, walking to the mailbox, and other activities that are functionally meaningful to the patient and regularly incorporated in the day.

It is also important to incorporate other individuals from the home setting into the home program, including family, caregivers, and peers. For the pediatric patient, parents or other caregivers are essential partners (Cunningham, 1985), and siblings can also be very helpful. Family members and caregivers can provide some consistency and often play a role in assuring the frequency and correct performance of activities, especially when the patient has cognitive impairments. Higher motor development score improvements have been associated with more supportive and stimulating home environments (Abbott, 2000), including significant parental involvement. Family, peer, and sibling involvement can also be a motivating

factor to encourage the patient to participate in therapeutic activities at home.

Home activities should be incorporated into the established daily routine as naturally as possible (Levitt, 1990; Forster, 1990; Ross, 1993; Gordon, 2004). It may therefore be helpful, before developing specific home exercises or activities, to ask the patient/caregiver, "What are the things you currently do every day or would like to do every day?" For example, stretching as a home activity for infants is often convenient and timely during each diaper change. For the elderly female with a stroke who enjoys helping her daughter do the dishes each evening while standing and supporting at the kitchen counter, the therapist could develop therapeutic activities in standing with tasks that address the identified problems. Consider the schedule and responsibility of the family and caregivers, and match these with the frequency and duration of home activities. It is important that the home program not be overwhelming to the home setting in an already stressful and overloaded home situation.

It is also essential to incorporate motivating factors for the patient in the home program. So, you might ask, "What things are important to you? What do you like to do?" A common example in the elderly population might be the motivation of play and interaction with grandchildren or leisure and recreation activities with peers. In treating a grandparent, the primary personal goal might be to be able to sit on the floor or at least at a table and play with grandchildren or enjoy a game of cards with friends again. Or a particular person may be highly motivated to be able to squat again or sit on a stool to work in the flowerbed. When the patient is personally and intrinsically motivated to perform the activity, and if they really believe they can get better, there is a much greater likelihood that they will perform greater numbers of repetitions in nontherapy times. Activities for which the patient is self-motivated can increase patient compliance or adherence to the therapeutic plan. Incorporating motivating settings and activities in the home program also emphasizes a patient-centered approach to rehabilitation.

## Let's Review

1. What are the primary decisions and basis for the decisions that a therapist must make when:
   a. selecting appropriate examination tests/measures and outcome measures?
   b. designing a plan of care to include education, direct interventions, and home activities?
   c. making changes to the intervention plan to keep pace with advancing patient capability?

2. What are the reasons that the therapist recognizes and measures impairments and functional limitations and not just normal body structure/body function and activity?

3. State some specific ways that the therapist can foremost acknowledge the patient as a person.

4. Because functional activity and skill are the ultimate goals of intervention, why does the therapist devote energy and time, particularly in early rehab, to assess and provide intervention for underlying impairments?

**5.** Can the therapist, through physical activity/intervention, stimulate neural plasticity? If so, how can the therapist structure the intervention to optimize and drive neural plasticity?

**6.** Describe at least three things that would make a rehab session "patient centered."

**7.** Why is exercise and activity at home (or outside of therapy hours) so important?

---

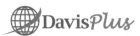 For additional resources, including Focus on Evidence tables, case study discussions, references, and glossary, please visit http://davisplus.fadavis.com

---

## CHAPTER SUMMARY

Before the therapist can successfully complete the process of making clinical decisions, the foundational basis of clinical decisions must be understood and embraced. All clinical decisions that arise daily in each patient should emphasize what is best for the patient. This includes formulation of functional goals that are priorities for the patient/family/caregiver and using examination and intervention methods with a scientific evidence-basis wherever possible. The purpose of all clinical decisions is to develop a plan that will optimize functional recovery. In the next chapter, we will discuss the process of clinical decision-making.

### PATIENT APPLICATION

*In conclusion, let's consider a case that highlights decisions to be made in a child with a developmental disability. Shane is a 6-month-old boy who was born 12 weeks premature. The physician has identified neurosensorimotor deficits in bilateral lower extremities and motor delay, and his mother is concerned that, when supported, he has great difficulty holding his head upright. He is not even attempting to sit upright, even with assistance. After deciding which examination tools and techniques to utilize, the therapist will have to decide how to interpret the resulting examination data, including prioritization, determine the impairment or function diagnoses to be addressed and the prognosis for recovery, develop the plan of care, design the specific interventions, and make decisions regarding the ongoing adjustments and progression to the intervention plan. The details of this process are described in Chapter 2 and will be explored progressively through each chapter of this book.*

# Making Clinical Decisions: A Path to Optimal Therapeutic Plan and Outcomes

Genevieve Pinto Zipp, PT, EdD ▪ Susan Diane Simpkins, PT, EdD
Dennis W. Fell, PT, MD      CHAPTER 2

**CHAPTER OBJECTIVES** ____ Upon completion of this chapter, the learner should be able to:

1. Discuss the steps associated with making clinical decisions.
2. Analyze and interpret patient data using a patient management model to make sound clinical decisions.
3. Design appropriate goals and objectives based on specific patient data.

## ◼ Introduction

As more people across the country have direct access to rehabilitation services, therapists are becoming a frequent point of entry into the health-care system for patients with neurological disorders. The responsibility of autonomous practice means that, today more than ever, physical therapists (PTs) and occupational therapists (OTs) must be prepared to make sound clinical decisions including independently determining appropriate examination, evaluation, diagnosis, plan of care (POC), specific interventions, and appropriate referral. The processes involved in **clinical decision-making** are complex and include aspects of clinical reasoning, judgment, and problem-solving. In addition to these cognitive processes, decision-making requires a therapist to possess the discipline-specific knowledge and skills needed to manage the range of problems seen in patients with neurological conditions. Of course, the patient also plays an important role in this process as discussed in Chapter 1; indeed, it is the patient's goals and values that establish the context for how a therapist gathers the information needed to develop the best plan for patient management. As

a therapist gains practical experience, the ability to recognize similarities and differences between patients' problems and diagnoses is also incorporated into the decision-making process. Thus, decision-making by therapists is a multidimensional, patient-centered process based on a therapist's ability to use both discipline-specific and practical knowledge to weigh, prioritize, and draw conclusions about a patient's functional problems. While Chapter 1 covered the principles and foundations that underlie effective clinical decisions, this chapter will explore the overall process and specific steps involved in making sound clinical decisions.

## ◼ Elements of Clinical Decision-Making

While Chapter 1 described the foundations and principles of making clinical decisions, this chapter will describe the process of making clinical decisions. How does the PT or OT make sound clinical decisions? Before this question can be answered, one must understand the elements that contribute to clinical decision-making. **Clinical reasoning** is one element of clinical decision-making that has been described by Benamy (1996) as a cognitive process that guides the ongoing acquisition, recall, sorting, and prioritizing of information regarding the clinical situation. This process enables the therapist to draw conclusions and make the judgments and decisions that lead to the POC and outcomes assessment. The resulting decisions also contribute to modification of intervention plans that occur from the time a therapist first sees a patient until the patient is discharged from services, in one episode of care. Clinical reasoning is not outwardly visible to observers. It is an ongoing process and the basis for the decision-making that takes place at every point in the patient management process. **Patient management** is the ongoing decision process that guides development and adjustment of the patient's POC.

According to Dowie and Elstein (1988), clinical decisions theory suggests that clinical judgment is a vastly complex process that requires the use of mathematic **algorithms** (a procedure or process of rules for decision-making or problem-solving) and decision models that use available data related to clinical problems rather than solely relying on clinicians' judgments. Consistently, studies have demonstrated that using algorithms, as compared to unstructured clinicians' judgments, increases reliability in diagnostic decision-making (Dowie, 1988; Dawes, 1989). Goldberg and Deb (1991) proposed that clinicians frequently use intuition, hunches, and personal clinical experiences to formulate their clinical decisions, which may lead to bias. The use of decision algorithms based on data from standardized assessments and intervention can help guard against bias in clinical judgment and provide guidance in the problem-solving process. However, the process is highly complex in populations with neurological disorders in which patients with similar medical diagnoses can present with very different clinical constellations of **symptoms,** the information reported by the patient or caregiver, and **signs,** the observations or objective measures made by the clinician. In PT and OT practice, the decisions regarding who requires intervention and the strategies used during intervention frequently revolve around the patient's diagnosis and individual degree of motor dysfunction as measured by a standardized assessment tool. While therapists have grown comfortable with the use of many standardized assessments, their validity for use in patients with neurological conditions remains uncertain in many cases. This has led practicing therapists, clinical researchers, and educators to seek out new conceptual frameworks for the construction of valid and reliable measurement tools and the processes for making clinical decisions.

## ■ Models That Guide PT Practice

The responsibility for making decisions that have a significant effect on the lives of others can be daunting, especially for students and those new to clinical practice. Fortunately, a number of frameworks and models exists to guide therapists through the clinical decision-making process. In Chapter 1, clinical decision-making was defined as a deliberate, ongoing process or set of processes that result in decisions toward the delivery of optimal patient-centered intervention. The focus in this chapter is on the steps of the clinical decision-making process.

One model used by PTs and OTs to direct patient management is the disablement model (see Fig. 1-3 in Chapter 1). The term "disablement" refers to the effects of acute and chronic disease on human functioning at the system, individual, and societal levels (Jette, 2006). The Nagi model (Fig. 1-3) (Nagi, 1969), which is currently used in the second edition of the *Guide to Physical Therapists Practice* (APTA, 2015), is an example of a disablement model used in patient management. Another example of a disablement model is one proposed by The National Center for Medical Rehabilitation Research (NCMRR) (Fig. 1-3), which classifies a patient's problems using a framework similar to the Nagi model (NIH, 1993; Nagi, 1969). Both models consider the consequences of pathology on an individual by determining the impairments, functional limitations, and disability associated with a disease or injury. The NCMRR model includes the category *societal limitations* to capture how social policy can present a barrier to one's ability to fulfill individual roles and responsibilities in light of disease or injury (NIH, 1993). Information gathered using a disablement model can serve as a basis for organizing an examination, intervention, and outcomes assessment. However, the differences in terminology used in these and other disablement models complicates communication between members of the health-care team, including the patient.

Quinn and Gordon (2003) extended the Nagi model by describing rehabilitation as the "reverse and mirror image of disablement." Here, patient management starts by determining the consequences of disease or injury on the patient's participation and role requirements. This information leads to an examination of the specific skills the patient needs for participation and the resources that support or hinder the performance of these skills. This approach to patient management is termed a "top-down approach" because clinical decision-making begins by first defining the patient's desired outcome and then determining the specific factors interfering with the patient's function.

The International Classification of Functioning Disability and Health (ICF) is the second version of a model developed by the World Health Organization (WHO) (Fig. 2-1). The model, as explained in Chapter 1, classifies the effects of health-related conditions on the domains of body structure and body function, activity, and participation in addition to how personal and environmental factors act as barriers or facilitators of function (WHO, 2001). The ICF has been adopted by more than 71 countries worldwide and will replace the Nagi model in the third edition of the *Guide to Physical Therapist Practice* (WHO, 2009; Nagi, 1969; APTA, 2009). The ICF has emerged as a universal model of health that offers standardized terminology and a construct to operationally define disability. In contrast to other models, the ICF is a *biopsychosocial model* where disability is defined by an interaction between the individual, environment, and society (Jette, 2006). For example, if a bus is not equipped with a wheelchair lift, commuting options for someone using a wheelchair for mobility are limited. The bus becomes as much a barrier to an individual's ability to participate in work or school as the

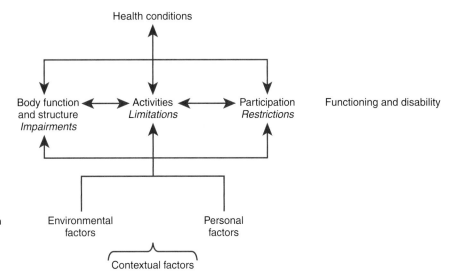

FIGURE 2-1 International classification of function, disability, and health (ICF, 2001). Adapted from World Health Organization. International Classification of Function. ICF Beginner's Guide. Available at: http://www3.who.int/icf/ Accessed March 28, 2011.

individual's mobility status. PTs and OTs are highly skilled at assessing the influence of environmental factors on a patient's functional skills. The ICF model can be used to guide the selection of tests and measures to assess each domain as well as the influence of contextual factors on function.

In addition to the decision-making models described in this chapter, other sources of information may be used to guide PT and OT practice. For example, **clinical practice guidelines** may also be used to direct the management of specific problems or diagnoses such as low back pain or fibromyalgia (Bekkering, 2005; Brosseau, 2008). Clinical practice guidelines are based on current best evidence and expert opinion and offer a systematic approach to treatment (Jewell, 2008). Although clinical practice guidelines are not available for the management of most neurological conditions, some initial guidelines have been developed for the management of acute stroke, use of constraint-induced movement therapy, and fall prevention (RCP, 2009; Brosseau, 2006; Moreland, 2003). Of course, therapists must critically evaluate the credibility of clinical practice guidelines before incorporating these recommendations into clinical practice; as the body of evidence continues to grow, it is expected that clinical practice guidelines will change over time.

To assist therapists as they engage in the clinical decision-making process, the Academy of Neurologic Physical Therapy of the American Physical Therapy Association (APTA) has led a process for reviewing available literature on outcome measures that has led to the development of recommendations for outcome measure to be used in clinical practice and in entry-level PT education (Academy of Neurologic Physical Therapy, 2015). Outcome measure recommendations are categorized by five practice settings—acute care hospital, inpatient rehabilitation, home health, skilled nursing facility, and outpatient—as well as by acuity level. To assist with entry-level PT education, measures are also characterized into three skill levels, those: (1) students should learn to administer (practical application), (2) students should be exposed to (knowledge of), and (3) not recommended for entry level. Additionally, measures are categorized as appropriate for research or not. Currently, the Academy has completed recommendations for outcome measures use in people with various diagnoses including stroke, multiple sclerosis, traumatic brain injury, spinal cord injury, Parkinson disease, and vestibular. Using available evidenced-based recommendations can assist therapists in our process toward making sound clinical decisions.

## Structured Process of Patient Management for Clinicians

Guiding the POC for a patient requires ongoing decision-making. The Hypothesis-Oriented Algorithm for Clinicians (HOAC), initially proposed by Rothstein and Echternach (1989) and revised by Rothstein (2003), is an example of a top-down decision-making model. This model is an algorithm that uses both patient-identified and nonpatient-identified problems to guide the therapist through the patient management process. The process includes developing hypotheses about the patient's problems and the underlying factors (particularly body structure and body function impairments) most likely contributing to the problems. The hypotheses then direct the therapist's examination strategy and ultimately help to determine the approach to and specific tactics of the intervention.

Schenkman (2006) proposed a clinical decision-making framework that incorporates several models that can be used to guide patient management in individuals with neurological disorders. For PTs, the *Guide to Physical Therapist Practice* (APTA, 2015), the HOAC II (Rothstein, 2003), and the ICF (WHO, 2001) collectively provide a comprehensive structure for organizing information throughout a patient's episode of care. Using a structured framework is a means to ensure that all relevant information is gathered from the patient, the patient's family, and other professionals and is used in the decision-making process. This information is the basis for formulating the questions and hypotheses used to make clinical decisions. Experienced clinicians may use cues and patterns noted from prior experiences to make clinical decisions, thereby using a forward-reasoning approach. Alternately, novice clinicians with limited prior knowledge and experience rely on a hypothetico-deductive approach (backward reasoning) when making clinical decisions. The hypothetico-deductive approach provides the novice with a directed process for gathering data, generating a hypothesis, assessing the data, and executing a goal-directed action. Decision-making frameworks assist clinicians in making decisions when managing patient problems.

Clearly, the ultimate goal when working with patients is reaching optimal functional improvement. However, the question arises, "How can we as novices or less-experienced therapists assist our patients in reaching this goal?" The first step is to utilize a decision-making framework that enables the therapist to develop an evidence-based treatment plan tailored (patient-centered) to meet the individual needs of each patient.

## Patient Management Model

The "patient management model" from the *Guide to Physical Therapist Practice* presents and describes six interrelated steps that assist therapists in making clinical decisions for optimal patient outcomes (APTA, 2015; Fig. 2-2). Other rehabilitation

professionals, including OTs, can use these steps when making clinical decisions.

### Step 1. Examination

**Examination** of the patient includes patient history, relevant systems review, and tests and measures (APTA, 2015). Reviewing medical records and conducting the patient interview provide information about the patient's past and current health status. Figure 2-3 offers a schematic outline of the types of data that may be obtained from a detailed patient history. Therapists must be sensitive to cultural differences and ethnicity that may influence patient and family/caregiver interactions when securing patient history. The *Guide to Physical Therapist Practice* provides the Documentation Template for Therapist Patient/Client Management for securing patient information (APTA, 2015). The use of brief screening tools provides a quick scan of relevant body systems (see Chapter 3) and aids in determining areas of intact function and dysfunction.

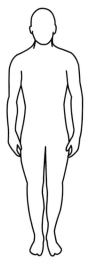

**Diagnosis**
Both the process and the end result of evaluating examination data, which the physical therapist organizes into defined clusters, syndromes, or categories to help determine the prognosis (including the plan of care) and the most appropriate intervention strategies.

**Evaluation**
A dynamic process in which the physical therapist makes clinical judgments based on data gathered during the examination. This process also may identify possible problems that require consultation with or referral to another provider.

**Prognosis (Including Plan of Care)**
Determination of the level of optimal improvement that may be attained through intervention and the amount of time required to reach that level. The plan of care specifies the interventions to be used and their timing and frequency.

**Examination**
The process of obtaining a history, performing a systems review, and selecting and administering tests and measures to gather data about the patient/client. The initial examination is a comprehensive screening and specific testing process that leads to a diagnostic classification. The examination process also may identify possible problems that require consultation with or referral to another provider.

**Intervention**
Purposeful and skilled interaction of the physical therapist with the patient/client and, if appropriate, with other individuals involved in care of the patient/client, using various physical therapy methods and techniques to produce changes in the condition that are consistent with the diagnosis and prognosis. The physical therapist conducts a reexamination to determine changes in patient/client status and to modify or redirect intervention. The decision to reexamine may be based on new clinical findings or on lack of patient/client progress. The process of reexamination also may identify the need for consultation with or referral to another provider.

**Outcomes**
Results of patient/client management, which include the impact of physical therapy interventions in the following domains: pathology/pathophysiology (disease, disorder, or condition); impairments, functional limitations, and disabilities; risk reduction/prevention; health, wellness, and fitness; societal resources; and patient/client satisfaction.

**FIGURE 2-2** The six interrelated steps from the APTA Patient Management Model (APTA, 2015) that assist therapists in making clinical decisions for optimal patient outcomes.

**General demographics**
- Age
- Sex
- Race/ethnicity
- Primary language
- Education

**Social history**
- Cultural beliefs and behaviors
- Family and caregiver resources
- Social interactions, social activities, and support system

**Employment/work (job/school/play)**
- Current and prior work (job/school/play), community, and leisure actions, tasks, or activities

**Growth and development**
- Developmental history
- Hand dominance

**Living environment**
- Devices and equipment (e.g., assistive, adaptive, orthotic, protective, supportive, prosthetic)
- Living environment and community characteristics
- Projected discharge destinations

**General health status (self-report, family report, caregiver report)**
- General health perception
- Physical function (e.g., mobility, sleep patterns, restricted bed days)
- Psychological function (e.g., memory, reasoning ability, depression, anxiety)
- Role function (e.g., community, leisure, social, work)
- Social function (e.g., social activity, social interaction, social support)

**Social/health habits (past and current)**
- General health perception
- Physical function (e.g., mobility, sleep patterns, restricted bed days)
- Psychological function (e.g., memory, reasoning ability, depression, anxiety)
- Role function (e.g., community, leisure, social, work)
- Social function (e.g., social activity, social interaction, social support)

**Family history**
- Familial health risks

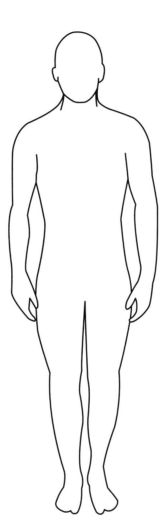

**Medical/surgical history**
- Cardiovascular
- Endocrine/metabolic
- Gastrointestinal
- Genitourinary
- Gynecological
- Integumentary
- Musculoskeletal
- Neuromuscular
- Obstetrical
- Prior hospitalizations, surgeries, and preexisting medical and other health related conditions
- Psychological
- Pulmonary

**Current condition(s)/ chief complaint(s)**
- Concerns that led the patient/client to seek the services of a physical therapist
- Concerns or needs of the patient/client who requires the services of a physical therapist
- Current therapeutic interventions
- Mechanisms of injury or disease, including date of onset and course of events
- Onset and patterns of symptoms
- Patient/client, family, significant other, and caregiver expectations and goals for the therapeutic intervention
- Previous occurrence of chief complaint(s)
- Prior therapeutic interventions

**Functional status and activity level**
- Current and prior functional status in self-care and home management, including activities of daily living (ADLs) and instrumental activities of daily living (IADLs)
- Current and prior functional status in work (job/school/play), community, and leisure actions, tasks, or activities

**Medications**
- Medications for current condition
- Medications previously taken for current condition
- Medications for other conditions

**Other clinical tests**
- Laboratory and diagnostic tests
- Review of available records (e.g., medical, education, surgical)
- Review of other clinical findings (e.g., nutrition and hydration)

**FIGURE 2-3** Schematic outline of the types of data that may be obtained from a detailed patient history (APTA, 2015).

Tests and measures provide more definitive and objective data to further assess the degree of dysfunction. The *Guide* identifies several categories that should be addressed by the tests and measures (Box 2-1 lists the categories). Details of the tests and measures appropriate in neuromuscular applications of physical therapy are described in the specific examination chapters of Section II (Chapters 4 to 13).

### Step 2. Evaluation

The **evaluation** step is a dynamic process where the therapist makes clinical judgments based on the data gathered from the examination (APTA, 2015). The evaluation is a process of synthesis that occurs within the therapist's mind. The therapist generates hypotheses based on the examination data from which measurable outcomes/goals are developed. It is also important at this stage to identify and list the patient's strengths and assets by determining what the patient can do and what abilities he or she has, not just focusing on impairments and what they cannot do. Identifying patient strengths and assets helps the therapist to identify where to start in developing the earliest aspects of the treatment plan. Building on the patient strengths and working toward more and more challenging task modifications facilitates functional goal attainment.

---

### BOX 2-1   Categories for Tests and Measures

Aerobic Capacity/Endurance
Anthropometric Characteristics
Arousal, Attention, and Cognition
Assistive and Adaptive Devices
Circulation (Arterial, Venous, Lymphatic)
Cranial and Peripheral Nerve Integrity
Environmental Home and Work (Job/School/Play) Barriers
Ergonomics and Body Mechanics
Gait, Locomotion, and Balance
Integumentary Integrity
Joint Integrity and Mobility
Motor Function (Motor Control and Motor Learning)
Muscle Performance (Including Strength, Power, and Endurance)
Neuromotor Development and Sensory Integration
Orthotic, Protective, and Supportive Devices
Pain
Posture
Prosthetic Requirements
Range of Motion (Including Muscle Length)
Reflex Integrity
Self-Care and Home Management (Including Activities of Daily Living and Instrumental Activities of Daily Living)
Sensory Integrity
Ventilation and Respiration/Gas Exchange
Work (Job/School/Play), Community and Leisure Integration or Reintegration (Including Instrumental Activities of Daily Living)

Adapted from APTA's *Guide for Physical Therapist Practice.*

---

In some circumstances, therapists must decide to delegate to other health-care providers based on the evaluation process. The concept of delegating patient care tasks to others dates back to the early nursing efforts of Florence Nightingale (LeVasseur, 1998). Delegation continues to be an important component of a therapist's knowledge base and ability to practice efficiently. As novice therapists continue to enhance their decision-making skills and gain advanced clinical experience, their ability to efficiently and effectively delegate must continue to develop. Any structured process for patient management therefore must include role delegation in the patient's POC.

### Step 3. Diagnosis

The identification of the impact of a health condition on function at the level of the system and at the level of the whole person is referred to as the physical therapy **diagnosis,** which is distinct from a medical diagnosis. The process of diagnosis uses the information obtained from the examination to guide the prognosis and POC to ultimately determine the most appropriate intervention strategy for each patient (APTA, 2015).

The *Guide to Physical Therapist Practice* presents main categories of conditions, each with Preferred Practice Patterns based on the specific cluster of deficits identified (APTA, 2015). These practice patterns help to guide the therapist when planning interventions for musculoskeletal, neuromuscular, cardiovascular/pulmonary, and integumentary conditions. The five elements of patient/client management are used to present the practice patterns that were developed by the collaborative efforts of experienced physical therapists utilizing an evidence-based approach to practice. If a practice pattern cannot be identified by the therapist via the diagnostic process, then the therapist must use critical thinking skills to develop an intervention based on the observed patient deficits. Using a hypothetico-deductive approach such as the HOAC, which is explained later, can assist the therapist in critically thinking when gathering data, generating a hypothesis, assessing the data, and executing a goal directed action (Rothstein, 2003).

### Step 4. Prognoses and POC

**Prognosis** is "a broad statement that predicts a patient's likely status or degree of change, at some time in the future" (Beattie, 2007). Prognosis is defined in the *Guide to Physical Therapist Practice* as, "the predicted optimal level of improvement in function and amount of time needed to reach that level" (APTA, 2015). For many patients, the prognosis can be determined at the onset of treatment. For other patients, the predicted level of functional improvement can only be determined incrementally throughout the rehabilitative process as new information is assessed, including the observed rate of improvement, to help guide the POC. Predicting time frames for optimal patient recovery and the extent of functional improvement is always a challenge to the therapist as it must be individualized based on the patient's characteristics and severity of disease and requires data integration and clinical reasoning. With the lack of experience, determining prognosis for a particular patient is particularly challenging for the novice therapist, but it gets easier with experience.

The therapist must begin to make judgments early in the evaluation process about which functional tasks are realistic as long-term goals (LTGs) for a specific patient. A variety of prognostic indicators can assist with clinical decision-making, specifically prediction of outcomes, and should be considered. These factors include the nature and extent of the pathology, patient age, acuity, duration of amnesia, and the rate, pattern and quality of recent recovery, among others. For example, regarding younger age, if cerebrovascular accident (CVA) occurs in a 12 year-old girl and an 82 year-old grandmother, with same relative size and location of the lesion, the 12 year-old would likely have a much greater recovery of function. As another example, traumatic brain injury that destroys a 1-cm area of precentral gyrus has much better prognosis than a traumatic brain injury that destroys a 5-cm area of the same region of precentral gyrus and underlying white matter. While prognosis for further improvement may be better if CVA or traumatic brain injury (TBI) occurred within the recent 6 months, certainly significant improvement can still occur years after cerebral damage has occurred, given stimulating therapeutic environment and activity.

Trends in recent improvement of functional activities for the individual versus a plateau of functional improvement may be among the best predictors of continued improvement. Some of the more common prognostic factors, positive and negative, are summarized in Table 2-1. It is important to note that as you gain clinical experience and expertise, with a larger sample of patients seen in your career, it is easier to determine an appropriate prognosis for any given patient. In other words, after seeing many patients over years, with careful observation and reflection, you will be better able to predict how much a particular person with a specific degree of impairment from stroke will recover.

The **plan of care (POC)** culminates in the establishment of goals and outcomes, specified planned interventions, actual intervention duration and frequency, and discharge criteria (APTA, 2015). Goals and outcomes express predicted changes in the patient's degree of activity and participation. Time frame is the key factor differentiating these two terms. **Outcomes** are the anticipated level of functioning at the end of the episode of care. **Goals** are the intermediate steps that assist the patient in meeting the final outcome, and they must be specifically measurable. Goals can be further expressed as either short-term (within 2 to 3 weeks) or long-term (often

| TABLE 2-1 | Factors That Assist in Determining Patient Prognosis in Neuromuscular Rehabilitation | |
|---|---|---|
| | **POSITIVE PROGNOSTIC FACTORS** | **NEGATIVE PROGNOSTIC FACTORS** |
| **Progressive nature of pathology** *(and degree of progression):* | Nonprogressive pathology (e.g., CVA, TBI, SCI, Guillian Barré, Polio, CP, Myelomeningocele) has a higher expectation that actual body system and activity improvement will occur. | Progressive pathology (e.g., ALS, progressive forms of MS, Parkinson disease, Huntington disease, spinal muscular atrophy, Duchenne muscular dystrophy) include expectations that the patient will continually get worse over the course of the disease and, therefore, prognosis is poor for functional recovery. |
| **Extent (size and distribution) of pathology:** | Narrow or focused area of injury (e.g., a relatively small CVA affecting cortex only or Guillain Barré that primarily affects lower extremities). | Broad extent of injury (e.g., a larger area of cortex damage in CVA: frontal lobe, parietal lobe cortex, and deep white matter and brainstem or Guillain Barré that progresses to involve lower extremity, upper extremity, neck, and face). |
| **Age-related neural plasticity:** | Younger (infants, children) is associated with greater neural plasticity (Barnes, 1985; Nieto-Sampedro, 2005). | Older (geriatric, especially older old). |
| **Number of systems impaired/comorbidities:** | Single or few systems involved (e.g., only neurological impairment). | Multisystem comorbidities. |
| **Acuity of the disorder:** | Less than 6 months since injury (esp. in CVA and TBI). | Greater than 6 months since injury. |
| **Initial level of physical functioning:** *(Korner-Bitensky, 1989; Sanchez-Blanco, 1999)* | High physical function. | Low physical function. |

*Continued*

| TABLE 2-1 Factors That Assist in Determining Patient Prognosis in Neuromuscular Rehabilitation—cont'd | | |
|---|---|---|
| | **POSITIVE PROGNOSTIC FACTORS** | **NEGATIVE PROGNOSTIC FACTORS** |
| **Glasgow Coma Scale** *after traumatic brain injury (includes eye opening, best motor response, best verbal response):* | High score. | Low score. |
| **Sensation:** | Intact sensation. | Absent sensation in addition to motor impairments. |
| **Degree of impairment:** | Mild degree of neurological symptoms/signs. | Severe degree of neurological symptoms/signs. |
| **Prior intellectual** *and behavioral characteristics:* | Higher premorbid intelligence. | Lower intelligence. |
| **Prior level of physical function:** | Very active without physical limitations before cerebral damage. | Difficulty walking or limited activity before cerebral damage. |
| **Duration of amnesia** *at time of injury:* | Short-duration. | Long-duration. |
| **Current cognitive status:** | Optimal arousal, attention and cognition (including memory and judgment). | Decreased arousal, attention, cognition. |
| **Motivation** *level:* | Individual highly motivated to improve. | Individual poorly motivated. |
| **Family/Social support:** | Strong family/social support. | Limited family/social support. |
| **Recent trends of recovery** *(rate, pattern, and quality of recent recovery):* | Recent, ongoing, continued improvement in status of body systems or functional activities. | No recent improvement in body systems or activities (i.e., plateau). |

greater than 3 weeks) to help guide therapeutic intervention and monitor the patient's progress. Both outcomes and goals should be objectively measurable and time referenced. Mager (1984) formulated the acronym ABCD (Audience, Behavior, Conditions, and Degree) to describe instructional objectives. Each goal must include the following (Randall, 2000):

A. AUDIENCE (Who?): Who will perform the specified behavior? The audience of the goal is most often the patient, "Mr. Smith will …" or "Nathan will …," but could be the patient and spouse, "Mr. Smith and his wife will …," or the spouse alone, "Mr. Smith's wife will …," or in the case of pediatric patients or dependent adults, the audience of the goal could be the parent or caregiver, "Johnny's mother will …."

B. BEHAVIOR (What?): What is the actual behavior that must be demonstrated? This component of the goal states the expected and observable action, motor behavior, or movement skill to be performed by the goal audience. It usually includes the word "will" (but the phrase "be able to" is not necessary) and must include an active verb that describes the target function (e.g., will crawl, will walk, will run, will rise-to-stand, etc.) and may include a verb with object (e.g., will step up to the curb, will reach for and grasp a can of cola). For LTGs, the behavior will focus on a functional activity or skill and not on an underlying impairment or performance of a specific exercise that itself is not functional.

C. CONDITIONS (How?): What are the conditions under which the behavior must take place or occur? These circumstances, under which the behavior will be measured, include any set-up or specific activities of the therapist, such as assistance required, equipment needed, environment features, type of surface, or antecedent/preparatory events. In the written goal, it is best to be consistent and list these conditions immediately after the verb and not after the word "will" before the verb.

D. DEGREE or CRITERIA (How well?): How will you measure success of the goal? Usually the goal ends with the criteria that will be used to determine success of the goal—that the goal has been completed—and time frame for successful completion. Examples of measurable criteria could include specific distance (of crawling, ambulation, or reaching), a specific velocity of a task (e.g., gait speed), a specific time to perform a discrete task, a count or number of successful repetitions of an action, a count of number of errors in a discrete activity, the weight with which a functional activity can be performed, a specific muscle grade or force produced (if part of a short-term, nonfunctional goal), the degrees of range of motion that can be completed (if part of a short-term, nonfunctional goal), or a specific percentage or ratio of attempts an activity is completed according to the other conditions and criteria (the percentage is understood to be 100% of attempts if no percentage is stated in the goal and the percentage should always be 100% for any LTG that involves safety issues–see example below). All of these criteria could easily be used to document the change in functional performance from initial examination to the reexamination or discharge examination. You wouldn't write a LTG that says "Mrs. Smith will ambulate without assistive device for 150 feet, without falling 80% of the time." If your expectation is that she would fall 20% of the time, then the long-term goal should be written including the use of an assistive device or assistance.

For consistency, it is wise to construct your goals with the goal components always in this order. This will help you to assure that you have included all of the necessary components in each goal and help everyone locate specific components within the written goal. A common mistake is to place a "condition" such as "independently" before the action verb. Table 2-2A provides a sample **objective** with related **long-term goals (LTGs)** and **short-term goals (STGs)** for an adult patient with neurological dysfunction, including the ICF levels that each addresses. Table 2-2B provides a sample objective with related long-term and short-term school-based goals for a pediatric patient with neurological dysfunction. When designing goals and outcomes one must ensure that the criteria for success are explicit, thus enabling the goal to

be objective and measurable. Implied goals and objectives lack the ability to measure change and monitor the effects of the POC.

## THINK ABOUT IT 2.1

- How would the prognostic factors listed in the previous section, negative or positive, influence the expectations you would express in your long-term patient goals?
- What are some potential limitations that would result if you wrote a long-term patient goal but did not include the expected degree or criteria of success?

### Step 5. Intervention

Once the goals and outcomes have been written, the next step is to design a **treatment intervention** based on the available evidence that is most likely to effectively address the patient's needs, remediate deficits, and promote participation (APTA, 2015). Thus, interventions must be patient-centered, not diagnosis driven. The diagnosis, however, may contribute to selecting the general approach for initial intervention and certainly to determining the prognosis. The effectiveness of the intervention must be continually reexamined to modify the intervention as necessary. The intervention process must address three distinct key aspects of intervention (APTA, 2015): (1) coordination, communication,

| TABLE 2-2A   Sample Outcome and Related Long-term and Short-term Goals for an Adult Patient | |
| --- | --- |
| *Outcome (to be achieved within 8 weeks)* | *ICF Level Addressed* |
| • Nathan will ambulate using a straight cane in his left hand independently on level and unlevel surfaces in the community without distance restrictions. | Activity; Participation |
| *Long-term Goal (to be achieved within 4 weeks)* | |
| • Nathan will ambulate using a quad cane in his left hand on level surfaces for 50 feet with supervision within 4 weeks. | Activity |
| • Nathan will ambulate using a quad cane in his left hand on unlevel surfaces for 50 feet with contact guard within 4 weeks. | Activity |
| *Short-term Goal (to be achieved within 2 weeks)* | |
| • Nathan will ambulate using a quad cane in his left hand on level surfaces for 20 feet with contact guard within 1 week. | Activity |
| • Nathan will ambulate using a quad cane in his left hand on unlevel surfaces for 10 feet with minimal assistance for right leg advancement as needed within 1 week. | Activity; Body structure and function |
| • Nathan will exhibit increased PROM in the right ankle to 10 degrees ankle dorsiflexion within 1 week. | Body structure and function |
| • Nathan will ambulate using a quad cane in his left hand on unlevel surfaces for 10 feet with minimal assistance for right leg advancement as needed and verbal cues to assist in recognizing relevant environmental features while walking within 2 weeks. | Activity; Body structure and function |
| • Nathan will ambulate using a quad cane in his left hand on unlevel surfaces for 10 feet with contact guard and verbal cues to assist in recognizing relevant environmental features while walking within 2 weeks. | Activity |

| TABLE 2-2B | Sample Outcome and Related Long-term and Short-term Goals for School-Based Pediatric Population* | |
|---|---|---|

| Outcome (to be achieved within I academic year) | ICF Level Addressed |
|---|---|
| • Hannah will ascend and descend a 15-step staircase, taking reciprocal steps, independently, to accompany her peers to the cafeteria each day (variable environment) while carrying a backpack weighing 8 pounds on bilateral shoulders. | Activity; Participation |

| Long-term Goal (to be achieved by completion of the second marking period, about 15 weeks) | |
|---|---|
| • Hannah will ascend and descend a 15-step staircase leading to the cafeteria, taking reciprocal steps, holding the railing, with standby assistance, during crowded transition between class periods (variable environment), while carrying a backpack weighing 4 pounds on bilateral shoulders within 12 weeks. | Activity; Participation |
| • Hannah will ascend and descend a 15-step staircase leading to the cafeteria, taking reciprocal steps, without holding the railing, with standby assistance, while classes are in session (nonvariable environment), while carrying a backpack weighing 6 pounds on bilateral shoulders within 15 weeks. ["Classes are in session" implies the stairwell is less crowded.] | Activity; Participation |

| Short-term Goals (to be achieved within 8 weeks) | ICF Level Addressed |
|---|---|
| • Hannah will ascend a single stationary step (7-inch height × 20-inch length, 10-inch depth) and descend the other side with hand-held assist while maintaining upright postural stability and motor control stability in the lower extremity within 1 week. | Activity; Body structure and function |
| • Hannah will ascend and descend three steps (7-inch height) on training stairs, holding onto the railing, with standby assistance within 4 weeks. | Activity |
| • Hannah will ascend and descend three steps (7-inch height) on training stairs, touching the railing, with standby assistance, carrying a backpack weighing 4 pounds on bilateral shoulders, within 4 weeks. | Activity |
| • Hannah will ascend and descend three steps (7-inch height) on training stairs, without holding onto the railing, with standby assistance, within 8 weeks. | Activity |
| • Hannah will ascend and descend three steps (7-inch height) on training stairs, without holding onto the railing, with standby assistance, carrying a backpack weighing 4 pounds on bilateral shoulders, within 8 weeks. | Activity |

*Working toward a variety of related goals (not stated here), including ambulation on level surfaces to unlevel/compliant/unstable surfaces, in progressively increasing distances, and in progressively distracting environments, and single-limb stance activities, will also enhance the ability to maneuver on stairs. A variety of treatment strategies might be utilized to accomplish the stated goals. As an example, Hannah might kick a moving soccer ball to promote weight shift, balance, and strength during single-limb stance as required to ascend/descend stairs.

and documentation; (2) patient/client-related instruction/ education; and (3) procedural intervention.

### (1) Coordination, Communication, and Documentation

Therapists must effectively *communicate* both verbally and nonverbally to effectively implement and promote the patient's POC, including communication with the patient, family, caregiver, physician, and other health-care professionals. *Coordinating* the efforts among all members of the health-care team is also an important role of the therapist to ensure that the POC is administered effectively and efficiently. Finally, *documenting* the actions taken and specific interventions employed, including

specific parameters, in the POC is extremely important for effective communication among the team working on the POC, to the third-party payers, and to the patient and family.

The POC can be documented in many different ways depending on the facility's needs. One frequently used documentation style is the **FITT equation** (frequency, intensity, time, and type) (Sullivan, 1995). Using the FITT documentation style, therapists can compartmentalize essential information and enhance data organization. Sullivan and Markos suggest organizing information into the following: (1) posture and activity, (2) technique used, and (3) required elements (Sullivan, 1995). Regardless of the style of documentation used, therapists must ensure that they document the goals and expected outcomes based on the patient's needs, the actual interventions used, and the required elements necessary to address the identified impairments. Given the time constraints in today's healthcare settings, it is imperative that therapists choose interventions that address more than just one goal at a time, if they are appropriate for the patient and address key points of concern first. Figure 2-4 offers essential elements needed for effective POC documentation.

### (2) Patient/Client-Related Instruction

Therapists provide instruction not only to the patient but to family members and caregivers as an essential part of the intervention. Every therapist is a teacher. Instructions may be provided one-on-one or in a group format. Instructions may be provided verbally in person, or, in the case of the home exercise program, additional instructions may be given in a written format, sometimes illustrated with figures or photographs, as a reminder of the important details of the exercise and to increase compliance/adherence. It is through these instructions that the therapist interacts with the patient to ensure that the patient or caregivers are capable of participating in the safe and efficient execution of the POC.

### (3) Procedural Intervention

**Procedural interventions,** the actual procedures and technique applied by the therapist to the patient and used to execute a POC and bring about change in the patient, encompass a wide variety of tactics to promote the participation level of the patient. The therapist must use both "evidence-based practice" and "practice-based evidence" approaches to effectively develop, manage, and evaluate the treatment strategies used in a POC. As explained in Chapter 14, it is imperative to always have the patient work at the optimal level, always intentionally progressing the intervention, for the patient to reach their maximum potential (Fell, 2004). The ability to critically assess the information available on effectiveness of numerous intervention strategies is imperative to ensuring that good decisions are being made regarding the use of intervention.

### *Step 6. Outcomes*

The final step in patient management is the ongoing process of evaluating the patient's progress, including reexamination of the patient and the POC. The POC is a fluid statement of

the patient's progress in meeting the established goals and outcomes. The POC is modified as needed to further address the patient's goals. All modifications to the POC must be documented, and the patient's response to the modifications should be noted as well to objectively measure his or her status and specific improvement or lack of improvement. The patient's progress report reflects reassessment of the POC and the patient's progress toward reaching the set goals.

Discharge planning is part of the POC and is usually initiated early in the rehabilitation process. It includes instruction of the patient, family, and caregivers in appropriate home care activities, referral options, equipment needs, and follow-up procedures if needed.

The term "discharge prognosis" noted in the discharge plan reflects the therapist's perception of the patient's ability to maintain their current functional level without continued intervention.

## THINK ABOUT IT 2.2

- How are outcomes and the initial patient examination related?

## Evidence-Based POC

When developing a POC, therapists should adhere to evidence-based medicine (EBM) or the expanded term, evidence-based practice (Sackett, 2000). Sackett and colleagues described five essential steps associated with evidence-based practice (EBP) that therapists can use when developing an evidence-based POC (Sackett, 2000). Figure 2-5 offers essential steps associated with EBP.

In Step 1, identify a clinical problem and generate a question that could be answered as part of the intervention decision-making. In Step 2, conduct a systematic review of the literature to identify sources of evidence. In Step 3, critically analyze the evidence. In Step 4, integrate the evidence with the therapist's expertise and the patient's characteristics. Finally, in Step 5, reassess the process utilized to ensure that it was efficient and effective to bring about positive change in the patient's condition. Professional organizations have begun to develop databases to house systematic reviews of evidence. The Hooked on Evidence project supported by the APTA

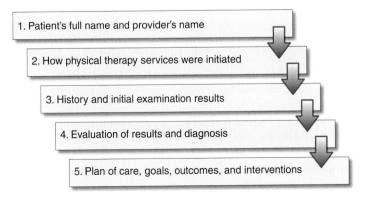

**FIGURE 2-4** An example of the essential elements needed for effective plan of care documentation.

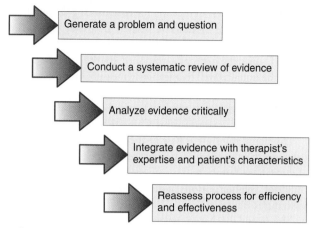

**FIGURE 2-5** Essential steps associated with evidence-based practice.

offers links to Evidence in Practice (www.ptjournal.org) to assist therapists in developing an evidence-based POC. The Canadian Stroke Network sponsors the "StrokEngine" (http://strokengine.ca) website that focuses on evidence-based stroke rehabilitation and intervention. APTA Academy of Neurologic Physical Therapy outcome measures recommendation (www.neuropt.org/professional-resources/neurology-section-outcome-measures-recommendations) offers evidence-based data on diagnostic-specific measurement tools that can be used across the ICF domains. OTseeker (www.otseeker.com) is a database that maintains evidence-based data on topics relevant to OT. PEDro (www.pedro.org.au) Physiotherapy Evidence Database offers website access to systematic reviews and evidence-based guidelines in physical therapy that can support clinical decision-making.

## Hypothesis-Oriented Algorithm for Clinicians (HOAC)

Rothstein and Echternach (1986) published the **Hypothesis-Oriented Algorithm for Clinicians (HOAC)**. The HOAC was developed for clinician use as a systematic method for decision-making as well as a guide to documentation. The HOAC was developed for use independently from any specific assessment method or treatment philosophy. This makes the HOAC useful for patients with a wide range of diseases or conditions, but particularly for neuromuscular rehabilitation where there are typically no established intervention protocols that apply to every person with a particular diagnosis. The algorithmic, hierarchical branching of the HOAC provides a format to organize a therapist's decision-making process (Rothstein, 1986). The decision-making branches associated with the algorithm were based on the scope of practice at that time. A revision to the model—HOAC II— (Rothstein, 2003) included updates to meet the needs of contemporary practice and to complement APTA's *Guide to Physical Therapists Practice* (APTA, 2015). In the revised model, HOAC II provides a means not only for using evidence in decision-making but also for documenting the nature and extent of

the evidence used (Rothstein, 2003). When designing this revision, Rothestein (2003) acknowledged the two types of patient problems that therapists face in today's health-care settings. The first includes those problems that are currently observed and require remediation, and the second includes problems that may occur in the future and therefore require the implementation of preventative strategies. Decision-making by therapists must effectively address both types of patient problems.

### Overview of the HOAC II Elements

The HOAC II outlines two ways to distinguish between the two types of patient problems—**existing problems** and **anticipated problems** (Rothstein, 2003). In Part 1 of the HOAC II, the two types of problems are pinpointed for the individual: **patient-identified problems (PIPs)** and **non–patient-identified problems (NPIPs)** (Rothstein, 2003). PIPs are usually functionally based problems, including symptoms identified by the patient and therefore of importance to them. These PIPs also provide the information a therapist uses to generate initial hypotheses about the cause and extent of the problem. Some patients may voice concerns only about current problems (existing), whereas others may express concerns about the development of future problems (anticipated).

NPIPs are problems that are not identified by the patient but rather are identified by the therapist and can be anticipated (Schenkman, 2006). It is important to note that support for anticipated, future problems, whether they are PIPs or NPIPs, must be theory or evidence based (best available evidence). Hypotheses that guide intervention to eliminate problems (PIPs or NPIPs) are testable because a change in the problem can be measured (Rothstein, 2003). By using the algorithm, the process of asking and answering questions and generating hypotheses is explicit rather than implicit, which offers the opportunity for an open dialogue and discussion among all potential parties associated with the POC (Rothstein, 2003). As one proceeds through the algorithm, the NPIPs are added to the PIPs to form a single problem list. Next in the algorithm, the therapist plans and evaluates activities designed for both existing and anticipated (preventative care) problems. Goals that are clearly articulated with expected time frames for achievement are developed as part of following the algorithm. This approach allows the therapist an opportunity to document what therapeutic activities are needed and the potential consequences if the patient does not adhere to the activities or if the intervention is not authorized by third-party payers. Part 1 of the HOAC II (Fig. 2-6 and Fig. 2-7) deals with the five elements described in the *Guide to Physical Therapy Practice* and earlier in this chapter as the "patient management model": examination, evaluation, diagnosis, prognosis, and intervention (tactics) (APTA, 2015). As noted earlier, the algorithm does not dictate the extent or breadth of information that must be obtained but rather requires the therapist to identify the processes employed in developing a POC and outcomes, providing an environment for further clinical decision-making.

Intervention, which includes ongoing reassessment of the POC, is addressed in Part 2 of the HOAC II and is illustrated

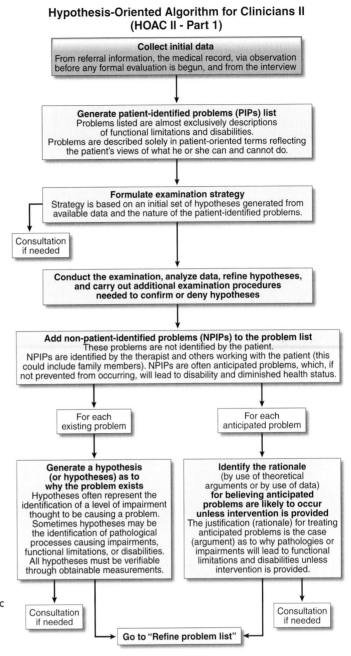

**FIGURE 2-6** Initial steps of Part 1 of the HOAC II: Schematic illustration of the initial steps (patient history, examination, evaluation) within the HOAC II, Part 1 *(Adapted from Rothstein, 2003).*

in Figure 2-8 and Figure 2-9. Part 2 of the HOAC II elaborates regarding what the *Guide* refers to as intervention, including monitoring and revision of hypotheses and goals based on the patient's response to intervention (Rothstein, 2003). In Part 2, two flow diagrams are presented to guide the reassessment of both existing and anticipated problems. Although one needs evidence-based data to report that the intervention led to goal attainment, utilizing the HOAC II provides therapists some insight into the benefit of the intervention/tactics used and appropriateness of the hypotheses set. One feature not explicitly present in the HOAC II is task analysis. **Task analysis** is the process of analyzing a specific skill to identify the abilities that underlie the performance of the skill. For example, to successfully pick up a

cup, a person must effectively perform the components of the skill, including reaching and grasping. Utilizing a systematic method of task analysis that examines performance problems from the perspective of (1) the learner's abilities, (2) the task requirements, and (3) the environmental constraints would strengthen the clinical usefulness of this algorithm to academicians, students, clinicians, and researchers.

## An Integrated Model of Patient Management

Schenkman (2006) developed an integrated framework for clinical decision-making that incorporates the *Guide to Physical Therapist Practice* (APTA, 2015), elements of the

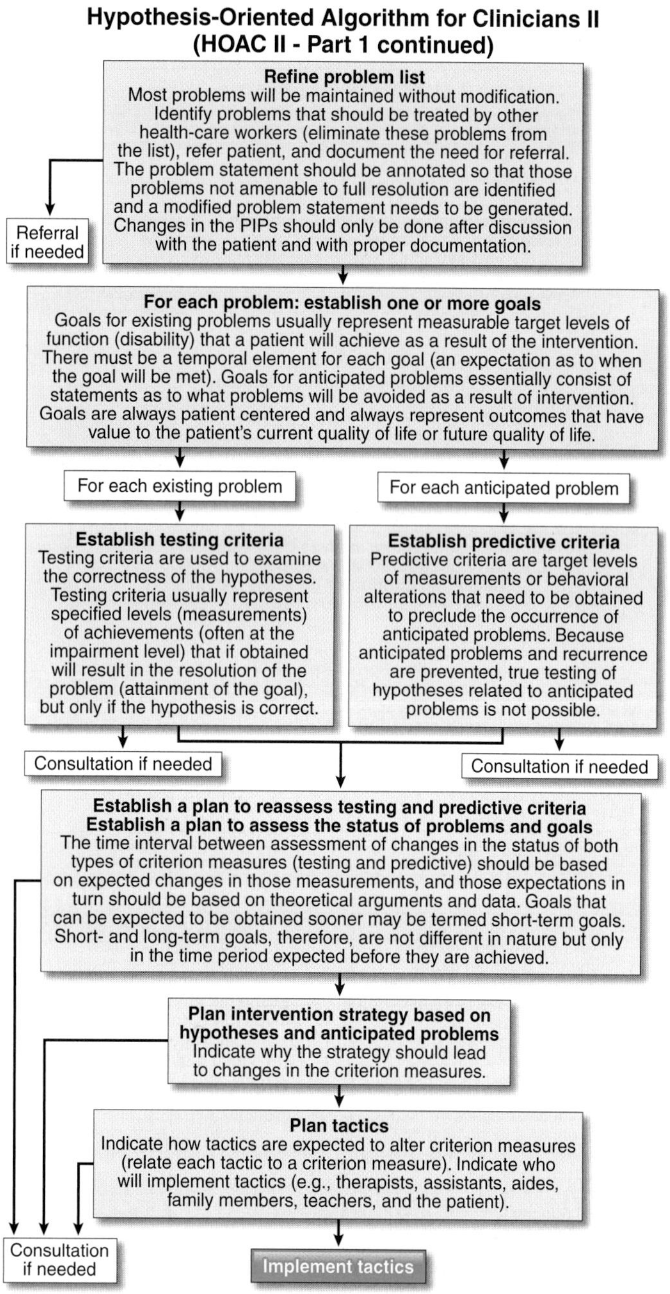

**Hypothesis-Oriented Algorithm for Clinicians II
(HOAC II - Part 1 continued)**

**Refine problem list**
Most problems will be maintained without modification. Identify problems that should be treated by other health-care workers (eliminate these problems from the list), refer patient, and document the need for referral. The problem statement should be annotated so that those problems not amenable to full resolution are identified and a modified problem statement needs to be generated. Changes in the PIPs should only be done after discussion with the patient and with proper documentation.

Referral
if needed

**For each problem: establish one or more goals**
Goals for existing problems usually represent measurable target levels of function (disability) that a patient will achieve as a result of the intervention. There must be a temporal element for each goal (an expectation as to when the goal will be met). Goals for anticipated problems essentially consist of statements as to what problems will be avoided as a result of intervention. Goals are always patient centered and always represent outcomes that have value to the patient's current quality of life or future quality of life.

For each existing problem

For each anticipated problem

**Establish testing criteria**
Testing criteria are used to examine the correctness of the hypotheses. Testing criteria usually represent specified levels (measurements) of achievements (often at the impairment level) that if obtained will result in the resolution of the problem (attainment of the goal), but only if the hypothesis is correct.

**Establish predictive criteria**
Predictive criteria are target levels of measurements or behavioral alterations that need to be obtained to preclude the occurrence of anticipated problems. Because anticipated problems and recurrence are prevented, true testing of hypotheses related to anticipated problems is not possible.

Consultation if needed

Consultation if needed

**Establish a plan to reassess testing and predictive criteria
Establish a plan to assess the status of problems and goals**
The time interval between assessment of changes in the status of both types of criterion measures (testing and predictive) should be based on expected changes in those measurements, and those expectations in turn should be based on theoretical arguments and data. Goals that can be expected to be obtained sooner may be termed short-term goals. Short- and long-term goals, therefore, are not different in nature but only in the time period expected before they are achieved.

**Plan intervention strategy based on hypotheses and anticipated problems**
Indicate why the strategy should lead to changes in the criterion measures.

**Plan tactics**
Indicate how tactics are expected to alter criterion measures (relate each tactic to a criterion measure). Indicate who will implement tactics (e.g., therapists, assistants, aides, family members, teachers, and the patient).

Consultation
if needed

Implement tactics

**FIGURE 2-7** Final steps of Part I of the HOAC II: Schematic illustration of the final steps (evaluation, treatment planning tactics, and implementation of intervention tactics) within the HOAC II, Part I (*Adapted from Rothstein, 2003*).

HOAC II, concepts (Rothstein, 2003) from enablement and disablement models, and aspects of a task-analysis framework (Fig. 2-10). This integrated model offers a comprehensive, step-by-step approach to patient management that is patient centered and focused on function. This model fits well with the perspective advanced in this text that clinical decision-making is a process of asking and answering questions and supporting or revising hypotheses regarding the clinical problems that will drive the patient's individualized POC. Further, the model includes prevention as an intervention option in keeping with the current perspective that maintaining long-term function often requires the intentional prevention of disease and disability.

This integrated framework proposed by Schenkman (2006) incorporates four key elements previously presented in other models. First, the patient/client management model from the *Guide to Physical Therapists Practice,* as discussed earlier in this chapter, is a key feature and is a backdrop from which other key elements branch (APTA, 2015). As an example, using the patient as the central point from which key elements emerge is similar to the conceptual framework used when developing a mind map. A **mind map** is a tool used by educators to help students learn to organize information and promote learning. Figure 2-11 shows an example of a mind map from a rehabilitation perspective. It was created by a student after review of a chapter written on stroke

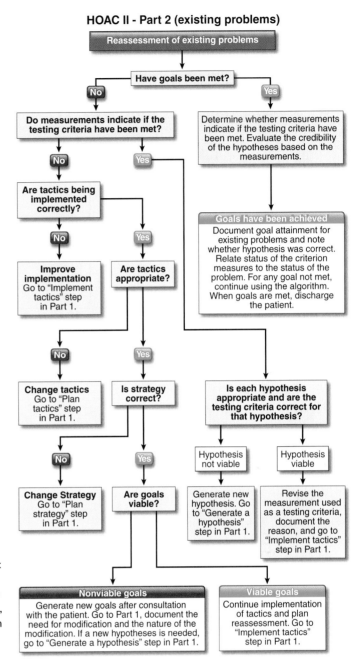

**FIGURE 2-8** Initial steps of Part 2 of the HOAC II: Schematic illustration of the reassessment steps associated with the existing problems (ongoing reassessment of the plan of care including reassessment of tactics and intervention strategies, and viability of goals, and resulting in adjustments to the plan of care) within the HOAC II, Part 2 *(Adapted from Rothstein, 2003).*

rehabilitation and focuses on the examination/evaluation and intervention for stroke. In a mind map, the placement of the central image, the patient in the Schenkman et al model, allows the therapist 360 degrees of freedom to develop the structure of the mind map to serve as the framework for making clinical decisions regarding the patient (Schenkman, 2006). Next, in constructing the mind map, main branches with key words are drawn extending from the central image. These branches represent the different categories relevant to the theme of the mind map. From these main branches, relevant subbranches are created. The use of this branch-like architecture, usually in a superoinferior direction, helps to organize and associate information

and in this case represents the decisions to be made by the therapist (Pinto Zipp, 2009).

In the Schenkman et al framework, the secondary branches stemming from "the patient" at the center (the central ring) depict the components of the patient management model from the *Guide to Physical Therapist Practice:* interview history, systems review, examination, evaluation, diagnosis and prognosis, POC interventions, and outcome (Schenkman, 2006; APTA, 2015). Imbedded within these secondary branches is the HOAC II framework that prompts generation of hypotheses at each step of the patient management model. By generating hypotheses at these points in the rehabilitation process, you have the opportunity to not

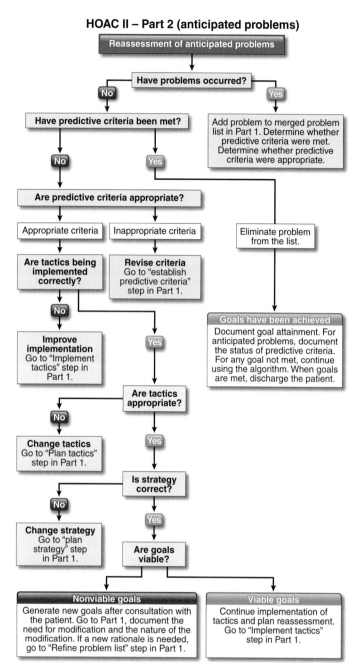

**HOAC II – Part 2 (anticipated problems)**

FIGURE 2-9 Final steps of Part 2 of the HOAC II: Schematic illustration of the reassessment steps associated with the anticipated problems (ongoing reassessment of the plan of care including reassessment of tactics and intervention strategies, and viability of goals, and resulting in adjustments to the plan of care) within the HOAC II, Part 2 *(Adapted from Rothstein, 2003).*

only develop a new clinical hypothesis but to also test the existing hypothesis.

Hypothesis testing is a crucial aspect of clinical decision-making because the outcome will either support the existing hypotheses or compel reformulation of one or more of the hypotheses. To test a hypothesis, you must first ensure that you can objectively measure the outcome needed to demonstrate a change in the patient's problem and thus support the hypothesis. The level of change required to remove a problem from a patient's problem list has been termed "testing criteria."

The tertiary branches that extend from the secondary branches in the Schenkman et al framework encompass two systematic approaches to *task analysis* and concepts from the **enablement model** and **disablement model** (as discussed in Chapter 1) (Schenkman, 2006). The data obtained from this

integrated framework for decision-making in neurological PT practice is then used to shape the patient's POC by addressing movement problems as they relate to function.

The first systematic approach to task analysis incorporated into the Schenkman model addresses the conditions under which tasks are performed (Gentile, 1972). Gentile's original model was modified to include 4 of the original 16 categories (Gentile, 1972). The four categories explore tasks that require body stability in a stationary environment, body stability in a moving environment, body transport in a stationary environment, and body transport in a moving environment. Utilizing only 4 of the 16 categories of Gentile's **Taxonomy of Tasks** (Table 2-3) limits the application of Gentile's model by eliminating tasks that require limb manipulation and the degree of variability encountered in many performance environments. Using all

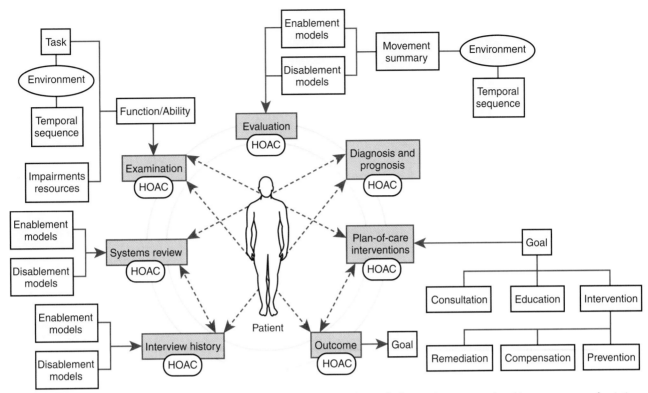

**FIGURE 2-10** Schenkman's integrated framework for clinical decision-making, which is patient-centered and integrates several existing conceptual models *(Schenkman, 2006).*

16 categories would enable a more thorough motor and functional examination and lead to a more comprehensive POC.

Although Gentile's Taxonomy of Tasks provides a thorough analysis of the task and environmental constraints on function, it does not identify *where* within the task that movement problems arise. A model offered by Hedman and colleagues outlines the temporal sequence of a task and can be used to determine where the movement control problem arises (Hedman, 1996). Figure 2-12 outlines the five stages of the Hedman et al **temporal stages model:** initial conditions, preparation, initiation, execution, and termination. During your observation and examination of the patient, identifying the *key features* in each of the stages enables an in-depth analysis of the temporal sequence of task performance for the individual patient (Hedman, 1996). Using this model enables the clinician to directly focus on the stage or stages within the sequence compromising the patient's overall function. It should be noted, however, that the Hedman et al approach to task analysis does not provide information about underlying impairments as emphasized by the HOAC framework, which is needed to further develop a specific, individualized POC (Hedman, 1996). Yet, through keen observation of movement with an understanding of both enablement and disablement models, clinicians can formulate hypotheses about the underlying impairments and select the tests and measures needed to gather the additional information required to develop an effective POC and optimize functional abilities at an activity level.

A variety of frameworks to guide clinical decision-making have been reviewed in this chapter. Each framework supports a patient-centered, decision-making process. Only the integrated framework proposed by Schenkman et al addresses the need and importance of task analysis (Schenkman, 2006). However, while it incorporates a framework for analyzing tasks, this aspect of the model is incomplete as it does not include all of the categories in Gentile's Taxonomy of Tasks (Gentile, 1972). Clearly, Schenkman and colleagues view their framework as one that is evolving and therefore could be modified to better address needs of the clinical or academic community (Schenkman, 2006). To date, the Schenkman model appears to offer one of the most comprehensive and user-friendly frameworks for clinical decision-making for both students and experienced clinicians (Schenkman, 2006). For students, it enhances understanding of the patient management process and provides a method to ensure that all aspects of patient-centered decision-making are addressed. For clinicians, it provides a process for expressing and quantifying clinical intuitions.

For the following case, the patient management model from the *Guide to Physical Therapist Practice* is used as a framework to outline the process and present the patient with information and the decision-making of the therapist (APTA, 2015). The HOAC model is used in this patient case study as a strategy to practice and develop clinical decision-making. After reading the case study information provided here, give some thought as to how you would handle this case. Then review Appendix 2-A and 2-B, which provide one example of a clinician's potential response to the case using the HOAC as a framework for clinical decision-making.

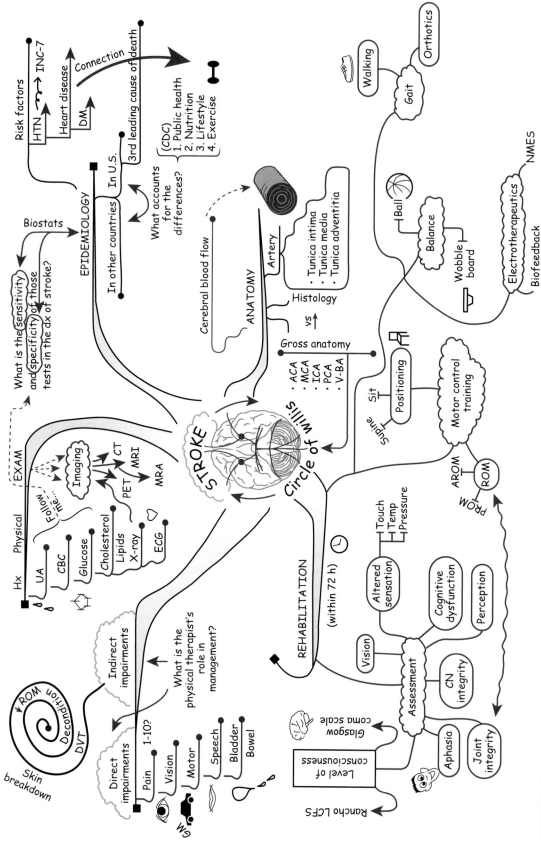

**FIGURE 2-11** An example of a mind map focusing on the assessment and treatment of stroke from a rehabilitation perspective created by a student. [Adapted from D'Antoni AV, Pinto Zipp G. Applications of the mind map learning technique in chiropractic education: A pilot study and literature review. J Chiropr Humanit 2006;13:2–11.]

**TABLE 2-3   Gentile's Taxonomy of a Task**

| | ACTION FUNCTION | | | |
| --- | --- | --- | --- | --- |
| **Body Stability Body Transport** | | | | |
| **Environmental ↓Context** | Body Stability — No Object Manipulation | Body Stability — Object Manipulation | Body Transport — No Object Manipulation | Body Transport — Object Manipulation |
| Stationary Regulatory Conditions and No Intertrial Variability | **1A** Body Stability / No Object / Stationary regulatory conditions / No intertrial variability<br>• Standing alone in a room<br>• Practicing a basketball free-throw shot without a ball | **1B** Body Stability / Object / Stationary regulatory conditions / No intertrial variability<br>• Brushing teeth standing alone at sink each day of the week<br>• Shooting basketball free-throws | **1C** Body Transport / No Object / Stationary regulatory conditions / No intertrial variability<br>• Climbing stairs<br>• Running through a basketball play several times without a ball | **1D** Body Transport / Object / Stationary regulatory conditions / No intertrial variability<br>• Climbing stairs while holding a book<br>• Running through a basketball play several times with a ball |
| Stationary Regulatory Conditions and Intertrial Variability | **2A** Body Stability / No Object / Stationary regulatory conditions / Intertrial variability<br>• Standing on different surfaces<br>• Swinging a baseball bat at different ball locations without a bat or ball | **2B** Body Stability / Object / Stationary regulatory conditions / Intertrial variability<br>• Washing dishes while standing at sink<br>• Putting golf balls from various locations on a putting green | **2C** Body Transport / No Object / Stationary regulatory conditions / Intertrial variability<br>• Walking on different surfaces<br>• Running through several basketball plays without a ball | **2D** Body Transport / Object / Stationary regulatory conditions / Intertrial variability<br>• Walking on different surfaces while carrying a grocery bag<br>• Running through several basketball plays with a ball |
| In-Motion Regulatory Conditions and No Intertrial Variability | **3A** Body Stability / No Object / Regulatory conditions in motion / No intertrial variability<br>• Walking on a treadmill at a constant speed<br>• Passing basketballs to a moving player running the same pattern several times, without a ball | **3B** Body Stability / Object / Regulatory conditions in motion / No intertrial variability<br>• Walking on a treadmill at a constant speed while reading a book<br>• Catching a series of softballs thrown at the same speed by a pitching machine | **3C** Body Transport / No Object / Regulatory conditions in motion / No intertrial variability<br>• Standing on a moving escalator at a constant speed<br>• Running through a basketball play without a ball but with moving defenders | **3D** Body Transport / Object / Regulatory conditions in motion / No intertrial variability<br>• Standing on a moving escalator while holding a cup of water<br>• Running through a basketball play with a ball and moving defenders |
| In-Motion Regulatory Conditions and Intertrial Variability | **4A** **Body Stability** / **No Object** / Regulatory conditions in motion / Intertrial variability<br>• Walking on a treadmill at different speeds<br>• Passing basketballs to a moving player running different patterns, without a ball | **4B** **Body Stability** / **Object** / Regulatory conditions in motion / Intertrial variability<br>• Walking on a treadmill at different speeds while reading a book<br>• Catching softballs thrown at various speeds by a pitching machine | **4C** **Body Transport** / **No Object** / Regulatory conditions in motion / Intertrial variability<br>• Walking in a crowded mall<br>• Practicing several soccer plays without a ball but with defenders | **4D** **Body Transport** / **Object** / Regulatory conditions in motion / Intertrial variability<br>• Walking in a crowded mall carrying a baby<br>• Practicing several soccer plays with a ball and defenders |

**Source:** From Magill RA. *Motor Learning Concepts and Applications*, 9th ed. New York, NY: McGraw-Hill; 2006:12; Carr J, Shepherd R. *Movement Science: Foundations for Physical Therapy in Rehabilitation*, 2nd ed. Austin, TX: PRO-ED; 2000:132.

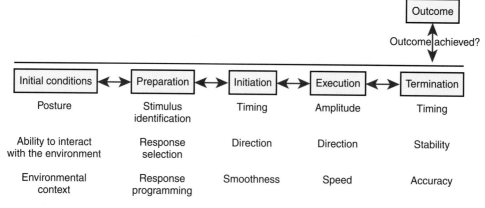

**FIGURE 2-12** Illustration of the sequence of the five stages of the Hedman et al temporal model for task analysis, including initial conditions, preparation, initiation, execution, and termination. Key features for each stage are listed *(From Hedman, Rogers, and Hanke, Neurologic professional education: Lining the foundation science of motor control with physical therapy intervention for movement dysfunction. Journal of Neurologic Physical Therapy, 1996, 20:9-13.).*

## PATIENT APPLICATION

**Case Study:** *Applying the HOAC Model*

*J.M. is a 63 year-old retired firefighter with a diagnosis of Parkinson disease (PD). Mr. M. is married and lives in a two-story home with his wife, who is a school teacher. About a month ago, Mr. M. fell in his yard while gardening. Two weeks later, he saw his neurologist to discuss concerns about his balance. The neurologist adjusted Mr. M.'s medication and recommended he see a PT regarding his mobility skills. Mr. M. was referred to a hospital-based outpatient clinic for a physical therapy examination and intervention. He was accompanied to the examination by his wife and married daughter.*

*Before seeing Mr. M., the therapist reviewed medical records forwarded from the neurologist. The therapist learned that the diagnosis of PD was made 13 months ago, shortly after he retired. Early symptoms included intermittent tremor of the right arm, bradykinesia (slowness of movement), and intermittent blurring of vision. Mr. M. takes Sinemet, 100 mg/tid. He sprained his wrist when he fell but was not otherwise injured. Mr. M. has no comorbidities and was in general good health before developing PD. Patient Interview: Mr. M. stated that his greatest concern was falling again. He described difficulty standing from a chair and climbing stairs (his bedroom is on the second floor). He also indicated that his balance was poor, especially when walking on uneven surfaces such as grass in his yard. This balance problem and an inability to squat and stand prevent him from gardening. He mentioned that he experiences periods of blurred vision. Mr. M. reported minor problems with bed mobility and difficulty sitting up from bed. He can still manage his activities of daily living (ADLs), although it now takes longer for him to groom and dress. Mr. M.'s goal is to improve his balance and walking abilities so he can resume gardening and playing with his two grandchildren.*

*Additional information was provided by Mrs. M. who indicated that, since falling about a month ago, Mr. M. spends most of his time sitting and has lost interest in socializing with friends and family. Mr. M.'s daughter is available to transport him to therapy sessions as Mr. M. does not drive and Mrs. M. works.*

## Contemplate Clinical Decisions [Related to HOAC case]

*Stop for a moment now and reflect on the information you have regarding Mr. M. from his medical record and from the responses he provided along with his wife and daughter. Now consider these questions:*

1. *Based on what you know, are there other follow-up questions you would like to ask or further information from the medical record that you would investigate?*
2. *From his statements, you have an idea of his functional activity limitations. So as you begin the neurological examination, what areas do you anticipate will be a focus, both in examination for system impairments and for functional limitations?*
3. *What hypotheses could you formulate now regarding underlying impairments that might contribute to the activity limitations? (You will be able to test those hypotheses as you move into the patient examination.)*

## PATIENT APPLICATION

**Examination**

*Participation Measures* PDQ -39 34/100: impact of PD on health and well-being (0 = perfect; 100 = worst)
ABC 60%: indicates moderate level of balance confidence (Mak, 2009)

**Activity Measures:**

| Multidirectional FRT | (in) Mr. M. | Norms older adults (Newton, 2001) |
|---|---|---|
| Forward | 6.90 | 8.89 |
| Backward | 3.35 | 4.64 |
| Right | 5.88 | 6.15 |
| Left | 5.75 | 6.61 |

*10-Meter Walk Test: 53 m/min 62% of age-normed gait velocity (Bohannon, 1997)*

***Functional Mobility Skills:*** *Slow movements increase the time it takes for Mr. M. to complete the following functional mobility tasks:*

***Sit-to-stand:*** *Mr. M. stands using the arm rests bilaterally for assistance. He tends to position his feet too far forward to initiate sit-to-stand. Mr. M. has difficulty in the extension phase due to problems extending his hips and knees.*

***Bed mobility:*** *Mr. M. can independently roll supine to prone and prone to supine. Mrs. M. reported that he has more difficulty rolling when under bedding. Mr. M. needs intermittent assistance to sit up from bed. He turns from supine to his side but can initiate movement to sit by pushing up with his arms only one out of five attempts.*

***Stair climbing:*** *Mr. M. uses a handrail to ascend and descend stairs. He has difficulty extending his hips and knees to move his body forward in the stance phase of stair ascent and particularly with raising the foot up to the next step.*

### Impairment Measures:

*Balance*
*m-CTSIB*
*Standing:*

| | |
|---|---|
| *Standing eyes open* | *30/30 sec independently* |
| *Standing eyes closed* | *30/30 sec increased postural sway* |
| *Standing on foam EO* | *12/30 seconds – assistance needed to regain balance* |
| *Standing on foam EC* | *Unable to complete* |

*Range of Motion:*
*Active*
  *Able to move all joints through available ROM*
*Passive*
  *Mild rigidity noted during passive ROM of both UEs and LEs*
  *Limitations in PROM and flexibility are as follows:*

| | |
|---|---|
| *Bilateral hip flexion* | *10–90 degrees (10-degree hip flexion contracture)* |
| *Bilateral hip extension* | *10–5 degrees* |
| *Bilateral knee extension* | *135–10 degrees (10-degree knee flexion contracture)* |
| *Hamstring flexibility* | *55 degrees* |
| *Gastrocnemius flexibility* | *0 degrees* |

*All other values are within functional limits.*
*Muscle Strength:*
  *Limitations in strength are as follows:*

| | |
|---|---|
| *Bilateral hip extensors* | *3–/5* |
| *Bilateral knee extensors* | *3+/5* |
| *Bilateral ankle dorsiflexors* | *3/5* |

*Posture*
  *Rounded shoulders and mild trunk, hip, and knee flexion*
*Pain*
  *Visual analog scale 0/5*

**Evaluation:** *Mr. M. is in Stage III on the Hoehn and Yahr Scale. Based on his responses on the PDQ-39, Mr. M. indicates he is functioning fairly well. The bradykinesia*

*with mild rigidity results in an overall slowness of all functional activity. He ambulates independently with a slow velocity. Other functional mobility skills are also accomplished slowly or with assistance. Mr. M. is at risk for falls and has a moderate level of confidence in his balance ability. His ability to organize sensory information for balance is impaired. His self-limiting of activity will hasten deconditioning. Although Mr. M. shows signs of depression, he is motivated to improve his mobility level so he can participate in leisure activities. Mr. M. has a supportive family who will provide transportation to therapy sessions and assist with his home exercise program (HEP). Secondary impairments including limitations in ROM and strength have begun to develop.*

*Mr. M. was referred to a mental health specialist for depression and an ophthalmologist to assess visual disturbances. The family was provided with information on a local PD support group. The therapist will consult with an OT about the increased time it takes for Mr. M. to complete basic ADLs.*

### Diagnosis and Functional Implications

*Physical Therapy Diagnosis: Impaired motor and sensory function associated with progressive CNS disorder (Preferred practice pattern 5E)*
**Functional Implications:**
*Participation restrictions: Unable to garden and play with grandchildren*
*Activity limitations: Mobility skills performed slowly, moderate fall risk*
*Impairments in body structure/function: Limitations in ROM and strength, decreased limits of stability, possible depression*
*Contextual factors: Patient motivated to improve mobility skills, supportive family, lives in two-story home*

## Contemplate Clinical Decisions [Related to Patient Application Examination]

1. For all of the information presented in this case thus far, can you clearly distinguish between information that is examination data collected by the therapist and evaluation reasoning that reflects the therapist's judgments and decisions about the patient?
2. If you were writing documentation of a patient's initial examination/evaluation, would you know which parts go in examination and which parts go in evaluation?
3. Use a highlighter to code/match information in the evaluation section of this case with the specific portions of the examination on which that evaluation statement was based.
4. Throughout the rest of this textbook you will be taught, with examples and illustration, how to make clinical decisions based on the examination and evaluation to determine the appropriate POC and ongoing adjustments to the POC. For now, as you read through the rest of this case, can you see how the examination/evaluation results led the therapist to the conclusions that follow (are there obvious links to you)?

**Prognosis and Plan of Care (POC):** *Outcomes and goals were developed in collaboration with Mr. M. and his family.*

### Expected Outcomes

*Mr. M. will return to preferred leisure time activities of gardening and play with grandchildren.*

### Anticipated Goals

1. *Mr. M. will transition from sitting to standing with toes under knees independently in 1 month to improve safety and efficiency.*
2. *Mr. M. will walk on grassy surfaces using a cane without loss of balance for 3 minutes in 2 months to enable return to gardening.*
3. *Mr. M. will walk on level surfaces independently for 10 meters at a velocity of 65 m/min in 3 months to improve functional ambulation skills.*
4. *Mr. M. will increase his anterior limits of stability (on multidimensional reach test) by 1.5 inches in 3 months to reduce fall risk.*

*Goals are written in measurable terms and focus on improving Mr. M.'s functional mobility skills.*

### Plan of Care

*Based on the extent of disease progression, current level of function, family support, and patient interest, Mr. M. has good potential to increase his waking velocity and improve his balance. This will enable Mr. M. to resume participation in leisure interests. POC will include:*

- *Family education on modifying home environment to increase safety. Recommendations include moving bedroom to the first floor, modifying bathrooms with grab bars and raised toilet seats, removing scatter rugs, taping wires to the floor, and limiting clutter.*

- *HEP of active and passive ROM, walking on level surfaces outdoors at least once a day with supervision, and task-specific practice of sit-to-stand from various types of chairs with supervision.*

*Evidence-based intervention to improve balance and mobility:*

- *Range of motion and flexibility exercises*
- *Functional muscle-strengthening exercises*
- *Balance activities with manipulation of sensory input, standing on various surfaces with and without vision to improve static balance control*
- *Standing while engaged in manual tasks to improve ability to divide attention between two tasks (dual task control)*
- *Standing and reaching in all directions to increase balance/limits of stability*
- *Walking over ground with pacing cues from therapist to increase walking velocity*
- *Auditory cues such as metronome to increase gait velocity*
- *Use of standard walking obstacle course to improve gait adaptations*
- *Visual cues such as tape markers on floor to increase step length*
- *Instruction in use of cane for ambulation on uneven surfaces*
- *Direct practice of sit-to-stand from various chairs with instruction on safe foot placement*

### Outcomes Assessment

*Mr. M. will be assessed on a regular basis. Reexamination will occur in 3 months unless an earlier time period is indicated. Outcomes will be measured using several of the tests administered during the initial examination: ABC, PSQ-39, 10-meter walk, multidirectional FRT, and active and passive ROM. Based on outcomes assessment, recommendations for discharge or modifying goals will be discussed with the family.*

Now review Appendix 2-A and 2-B to see a sample of a clinician's response to the case, documented within the HOAC as a framework for clinical decision-making.

# HANDS-ON PRACTICE

After reading this chapter, you should be able to:

- Define elements associated with clinical decision-making.
- Compare and contrast the models that guide physical therapy practice.
- Apply a reflective evidence-based integrated model of patient-centered management.
- Develop objectively measurable and time-referred patient-centered outcomes and goals (long-term and short-term).
- Assess the sufficiency and accuracy of links made between examination/evaluation data and POC.

## *Let's Review*

1. Why is the judgment of PTs and OTs so important?

2. As we seek to make judgments that will help us develop sound patient-centered POCs, what role does clinical reasoning play?

3. How can PTs and OTs use clinical practice guidelines?

4. Do practice guidelines negate the need for clinical reasoning in the development of a POC?

5. Given that goals and outcomes express predicted changes in a patient's degree of activity and participation, how can we use them to shape and assess the effectiveness of our treatment interventions?

6. What is the purpose of linking outcomes and goals to ICF level?

7. Using the FITT equation, document in written format a POC for a third-party payer for Mr. M., and communicate your POC verbally to Mr. M. Reflect on the difference and similarity in your written and verbal communication of the POC based on the audience.

8. How might the use of the mind map strategy aid you in integrating your thoughts as you seek to ensure an integrated model of patient management?

9. As we look at Gentile's taxonomy of motor skills, why is it helpful as we develop the POC to understand the different levels of the function of the action and the environmental context proposed?

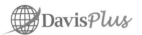 **DavisPlus**    For additional resources, including Focus on Evidence tables, case study discussions, references, and glossary, please visit http://davisplus.fadavis.com

## CHAPTER SUMMARY

With such a complex clinical reasoning structure, how do we put it all together in a meaningful way to enhance our clinical decision-making for the patient's good? Obviously, clinical decision-making is something that improves with years of practice, intentional effort, and lots of questioning and self-reflection. Ultimately, clinical decision-making will become natural and rather intuitive for the expert therapist. The specific information presented in the "Examination" chapters (3 to 13), "General Intervention" chapters (14 to 17), "Specific Impairment Intervention" chapters (18 to 32), and "Functional Intervention" chapters (33 to 37) will help the reader begin to develop these clinical decision-making skills in each area. Toward that end, Table 2-4 provides some practical tips to help guide you in honing your clinical decision-making skills associated with each element of the patient management model.

Consider a patient who incurred a stroke 3 years ago. The patient comes to your clinic seeking physical therapy services. Why is the patient seeking physical therapy services at this time? Has there been a recent change in the patient's functional abilities? What outcome does the patient expect to achieve? Will the patient's family be involved in the rehabilitation process? Answers to these and other targeted questions asked during the initial interview begin to define the PIPs and

the patient's concerns and values. The initial interview is also a time when the therapist starts to generate hypotheses about the patient's problems. Hypotheses are based not only on the information provided by the patient and data from specific tests/measures of the examination, but also on the therapist's prior clinical experience with other, similar patients and knowledge gained from a critical analysis of research. At this point in the patient management process, the hypotheses are used to determine the scope of the examination. The selection of the tests and measures that will lead to a better understanding of why the patient experiences difficulty performing specific functional activities is a key clinical decision made at the beginning of a patient's care. The functional activities tested in an examination, whether from a standardized or nonstandardized assessment tool, can be further assessed using Gentile's Taxonomy of Tasks and Hedman et al's temporal stages model (Gentile, 1972; Hedman, 1996). The data gathered during the physical examination process leads to the evaluation, a dynamic cognitive process where the clinician makes judgments about the nature and extent of the patient's problems (APTA, 2015). Throughout this dynamic process, the explicit nature of asking and answering questions fosters the development of effective decision-making. Finally, the therapist's evaluation results in development of the POC, the therapist-determined PT diagnosis, and the prognosis for the presenting disorder, all specific to the individual patient. Functional patient-centered goals and outcomes are identified and used as a frame of reference for treatment planning with the patient's current status, current abilities, and strengths used as the basis for the starting point of intervention activities. Ongoing reassessment of the patient's abilities toward achieving the set goals and outcomes is used to test hypotheses to determine the effectiveness of the POC or

the need to revise the POC. Ultimately, the goal is to optimize the patient's physical function in activities and participation in life. As we make assertions about how we understand and reason through clinical situations, we must ask ourselves if these assertions are true. Using an evidence-based, rich, integrated framework for clinical decision-making assists us as we seek to become aware of the spontaneous activities in our minds as we struggle to solve a problem or answer a question. This leads us to reflective insight as we design patient-centered evidence-based POCs.

| TABLE 2-4 | Practical Tips to Guide Each Step of the Decision-making Process |
|---|---|
| **PATIENT MANAGEMENT ELEMENTS** | **TIPS TO HELP YOU EFFECTIVELY MANAGE THE PROCESS** |
| *Examination* | • **Organization** is the key to success for the entire clinical decision-making process.<br>• Be certain you understand and explore your **patient's/goals** needs (patient-centered).<br>• Take a **top-down** approach so the examination is focused on the patient's desired outcomes.<br>• **Select tests/measures that can be used as outcome measures** during retesting at the end of the episode of care.<br>• Collect your data (implement your **examination**) **in a logical sequence** to assure a complete examination (e.g., logical sequence of anatomical regions: head, neck, shoulders, arms, forearms, hands, fingers, upper trunk, lower trunk, pelvis, thigh, leg, foot, toes, or sequence of dermatomes or myotomes).<br>• Carefully collect examination results from **right and left side for appropriate comparison.**<br>• Evidence-Based Practice: Select examination tools (tests/measures) that are optimally **valid, reliable, sensitive, and specific.** |
| *Evaluation* | • Expect certain patient problems based on patient medical diagnosis and history; **confirm or eliminate patient problems** with thoughtful evaluation of your patient-centered examination data.<br>• **Integrate clinical** observations with your quantitative findings to develop a well-rounded, holistic picture of the patient's strengthens and deficits.<br>• Evaluate the examination data in the **context of lifespan.**<br>• Evidence-based practice: Be able to **defend your conclusions** with evidence. |
| *Diagnosis* | • Use **preferred practice patterns** when available to assist in clinical decision-making. |
| *Prognosis/Plan Of Care (POC)* | • Evidence-Based Practice: Consider the evidence related to **prognostic factors** for the specific patient scenario.<br>• Develop **time-determined, measurable, and objective goals** and outcomes for an effective POC. |
| *Intervention* | • Evidence-Based Practice: Emphasize intervention methods that have a demonstrated positive influence on patient outcomes (**effectiveness/efficacy, improvement that is significantly greater than another related interventions**).<br>• **A POC must be patient-centered,** focusing on the specific patient problems.<br>• **A POC is dynamic** and may be modified as needed at any point in the patient's episode of care.<br>• The **POC must be intentionally progressed,** continually placing optimal demand on the patient's system, each time the patient's body structure/body function or functional activity level improves (Fell, 2004).<br>• **Education** of the patient/family/caregiver is essential to insure the patient and family fully understand the nature of the patient's condition.<br>• **Educate the patient/family/caregiver** so they will know why it is important to practice the therapeutic exercises and activities to enhance motivation and compliance/adherence.<br>• Remember that relationships are **influenced by many things;** therefore, during intervention and patient education, listen carefully to the questions and comments from the patient and family/caregiver. |

| TABLE 2-4 | **Practical Tips to Guide Each Step of the Decision-making Process—cont'd** |

| PATIENT MANAGEMENT ELEMENTS | TIPS TO HELP YOU EFFECTIVELY MANAGE THE PROCESS |
|---|---|
| | • The rehab process will often include an **early focus on preparatory interventions to improve or address underlying impairments** that are hypothesized to contribute to limitations to functional activity. <br> • However, the therapist **always has greatest focus on functional intervention activities** (even the impairment-based interventions must obviously contribute to functional improvement) and the therapist is always moving the patient toward optimal functional activity and participation. |
| *Outcomes* | • **Reassessment** of patient's response to intervention is an ongoing process. <br> • Choose outcomes that are **patient-centered, practical, and meaningful/clinically significant**. <br> • Documentation of outcomes provides **support for reimbursement.** <br> • Reassessment of outcome measures used at the initial examination will allow **specific comparison of the patient pre- and post-intervention** (evidence of the individual patient). <br> • Consistent use of outcome measures for specific populations will allow for **analysis of outcomes** for any specific therapist or across an entire practice or practice setting, which can contribute evidence to the professional body of knowledge. |

**HOAC II—Part I**

---

**Collect initial data**

Therapist: reviews Mr. M. 's medical records and conducts initial interview. Interview questions are based on: 1) need to clarify and expand on the information provided in medical record, 2) reason for the referral, 3) therapist's knowledge of Parkinson disease and 4) therapist's prior clinical experience

↓

**Generate Patient-Identified Problem (PIPs) List**

Therapist: develops PIP list from what patient reports during the initial interview. Mr. M.'s problems include: poor balance when walking on uneven surfaces such as grass, slow walking velocity, and inability to squat and stand which interferes with gardening, difficulty standing from a chair and climbing stairs.

↓

**Formulate Examination Strategy**

Therapist: Examination strategy based on information gathered from medical record, and patient/family interview. Therapist forms patient-identified problem list and generates hypotheses about extent and nature of the problems.

Systems Review: Musculoskeletal, neuromuscular, cardiopulmonary, integumentary systems. Purpose is to screen for problems (yellow/red flags) and need for outside referral.

Based on information from the interview and systems review the therapist selects valid and reliable Tests & Measures. The therapist selects: active and passive ROM & muscle strength, 10-meter walk, Multidirectional functional reach test (FRT), m-CTSIB. The therapist also has the patient complete the Parkinson's Disease Questionnaire (PDQ-39) and the Activities Specific Balance Confidence Scale (ABC).

↓

**Non-Patient Identified Problems (NPIPs)**

Mrs. M. and her daughter are concerned that Mr. M. may be depressed. She stated that since incurring the fall Mr. M. spends his day sitting and watching television. He was an avid reader but has complained about occasional blurring of vision.

Mr. M. may be experiencing fear of falling—self-limiting his activity. Sedentary lifestyle is a risk factor for development of secondary impairments.

↓

**Update Problem List (PIP & NPIP)**

Existing Problems
1) Slowness of movement and impaired motor control initiation of movement that affect all functional mobility skills
2) Mild rigidity L>R side
3) AROM & PROM limitations
4) Decreased limits of stability in all directions

5) Impaired sensory organization in balance blurred vision
6) Weakness-trunk & LE extensors
7) Flexed posture
8) Fear of falling
9) Apparent depression

↓

**Anticipated Problems**

Due to progressive nature of diagnosis, existing problems are expected to increase in severity.
Pt is self-limiting his mobility more than necessary due to fear of falling.
Immobility in the earlier stages of PD will hasten physical and cardiopulmonary deconditioning and compromise general health condition.

↓

---

**Left margin annotations:**

Hypotheses
1) Condition is progressing. Patient developing bradykinesia.
2) Bradykinesia and impaired motor control (movement initiation) is interfering with patient's functional mobility skills—not able to garden or play with grandchildren—*participation restriction.*
3) Increased fall risk due to balance system *impairment.*
4) *Activity limitations* in basic mobility skills—transitions and locomotion.
5) In stage III—Hoehn & Yahr Classification.

Revised Hypotheses

1) Bradykinesia, impaired motor control initiation of movement, and poor balance are contributing to activity limitations and participation.

2) Fear of falling may be contributing to sedentary lifestyle.

3) Blurred vision may be factor in balance system impairment.

4) Mr. M. may be depressed.

**Refined Problem List**

1) Bradykinesia (slowness of movement) and impaired motor initiation affecting walking skills, & functional mobility skills
2) Mild rigidity
3) Limitations in ROM and strength
4) Impaired balance—poor sensory organization
5) Decreased limits of stability
6) Low balance confidence

At risk for falls

**Refer pt to:**
- Ophthalmologist
- Mental health professional
- PD support group

**Assets/Resources**

1) Limited cognitive impairment

2) Strong family support

3) Patient wants to improve his mobility skills

4) Fairly good general health

**Expected Outcomes:**
Mr. M. will return to preferred leisure activities.

Anticipation Goals
1) Mr. M. will transition from sitting to standing with toes under knees independently in 1 month to improve safety and efficiency.
2) Mr. M. will increase his anterior limits of stability (on multidirectional reach test) by 1.5 inches in 3 months to reduce fall risk.
3) Mr. M. will walk on level surfaces independently for 10 meters at a velocity of 65 m/min in 3 months.
4) Mr. M. will walk on grassy surfaces using a cane without loss of balance for 3 minutes in 2 months.

**Establish Testing Criteria**

1) Walking velocity of 65m/min
2) Forward FR of 8.4 inches
3) ABC of 75
Activity—Walking outdoors on a daily basis
Participation—Gardening with some modifications; playing with grandchildren

**Establish Predictive Criteria**

Mr. M. will increase his daily activity level and resume participation in leisure activities to slow development of secondary impairments.

**Plan to Reassess Testing and Predictive Criteria**

Mr. M.'s level of function will be reassessed in three months unless response to intervention requires an earlier reassessment. Tests and measures used in examination will be readministered to determine if goals have been attained.

**Plan Intervention**

Mr. M.'s intervention, including education, consultation and treatment strategies, will be evidence-based, reflecting patient's values and therapist's expertise.

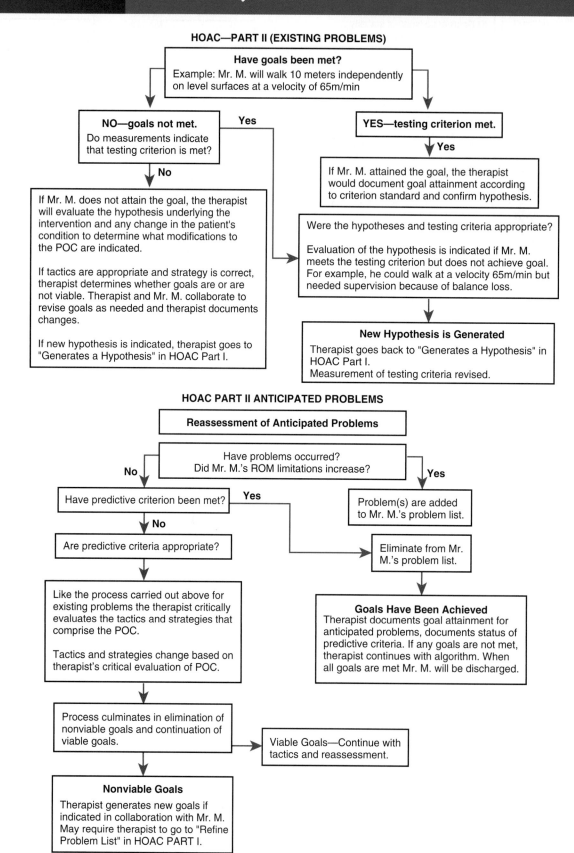

**HOAC—PART II (EXISTING PROBLEMS)**

**Have goals been met?**
Example: Mr. M. will walk 10 meters independently on level surfaces at a velocity of 65m/min

**NO—goals not met.**
Do measurements indicate that testing criterion is met?

Yes

**No**

If Mr. M. does not attain the goal, the therapist will evaluate the hypothesis underlying the intervention and any change in the patient's condition to determine what modifications to the POC are indicated.

If tactics are appropriate and strategy is correct, therapist determines whether goals are or are not viable. Therapist and Mr. M. collaborate to revise goals as needed and therapist documents changes.

If new hypothesis is indicated, therapist goes to "Generates a Hypothesis" in HOAC Part I.

**YES—testing criterion met.**

Yes

If Mr. M. attained the goal, the therapist would document goal attainment according to criterion standard and confirm hypothesis.

Were the hypotheses and testing criteria appropriate?

Evaluation of the hypothesis is indicated if Mr. M. meets the testing criterion but does not achieve goal. For example, he could walk at a velocity 65m/min but needed supervision because of balance loss.

**New Hypothesis is Generated**
Therapist goes back to "Generates a Hypothesis" in HOAC Part I.
Measurement of testing criteria revised.

**HOAC PART II ANTICIPATED PROBLEMS**

**Reassessment of Anticipated Problems**

Have problems occurred?
Did Mr. M.'s ROM limitations increase?

**No**

**Yes**

Have predictive criterion been met?

Yes

Problem(s) are added to Mr. M.'s problem list.

**No**

Are predictive criteria appropriate?

Eliminate from Mr. M.'s problem list.

Like the process carried out above for existing problems the therapist critically evaluates the tactics and strategies that comprise the POC.

Tactics and strategies change based on therapist's critical evaluation of POC.

**Goals Have Been Achieved**
Therapist documents goal attainment for anticipated problems, documents status of predictive criteria. If any goals are not met, therapist continues with algorithm. When all goals are met Mr. M. will be discharged.

Process culminates in elimination of nonviable goals and continuation of viable goals.

Viable Goals—Continue with tactics and reassessment.

**Nonviable Goals**
Therapist generates new goals if indicated in collaboration with Mr. M. May require therapist to go to "Refine Problem List" in HOAC PART I.

# Examination and Evaluation in Neuromuscular Disorders

# The Neurological Examination and Evaluation: An Overview

David Chapman, PT, PhD ▪ Rebecca E. Porter, PT, PhD

CHAPTER 3

---

## CHAPTER OUTLINE

## CHAPTER OBJECTIVES

Upon completion of this chapter, the learner should be able to:

1. Describe the purpose of the neurological examination.
2. Select the components of the examination appropriate to the individual patient.
3. State the components of a screening neurological examination.
4. Describe the process of testing the seven key areas of the screening examination.
5. Discuss the differences between a screening examination and the examination of a patient with a known or suspected neurological diagnosis.
6. Perform and document an evaluation based on screening examination data.

## ■ Introduction

When first confronted with learning the details of conducting a neurological examination, students often feel that the amount of information to be processed is overwhelming. If, however, this task is approached as a systematic investigation in which the therapist sorts out the systems that are functioning appropriately from those demonstrating potential impairments, activity limitations, and participation restrictions, the process can flow quite easily. The purpose of this chapter is to describe the objective of the neurological examination, the overall procedure and categories of the neurological examination, and the components of the neurological screening examination. The subsequent chapters in Section II will provide the details of examining the specific actions of the nervous system (including underlying impairments and resulting functional activity limitations), describe abnormal results expected in the presence of **dysfunction,** and provide the foundation needed to interpret what the specific findings mean. The first step must be to understand the purpose of the neurological examination, the overall perspective gained from a screening examination, and the role the information gathered will play in refining and focusing the remainder of the neurological examination and in developing a specific plan of care for each patient.

The neurological examination can function as a screening tool or an investigative tool (Fuller, 2008). When interacting with a patient not suspected of having neurological involvement, the screening examination provides a brief process of reviewing selected functions of the nervous system to confirm that the system is intact. In the presence of suspected or known neurological pathology, the examination process is more detailed to confirm the type and extent of the neuromotor and related impairments. Within the process of examining a single patient, the screening and investigative approaches may be intertwined. For example, during the examination of a patient with a known peripheral nerve lesion, the therapist will utilize the screening process to verify that cerebral and cranial nerve functions are intact while using more detailed processes to document the extent of the disruption of the peripheral functions. Any abnormality detected during the screening examination will lead to a more detailed examination of that subsystem as described in Chapters 4 to 13.

The neurological **examination** includes asking questions (review of the patient's medical record, history, and review of systems) and performing tests (observation of the patient, specific tests and measures of all neuromotor systems, and measures of **activity limitations** and participation restrictions). The data collected in the examination provides the basis for the **evaluation,** the cerebral process and resulting clinical judgments that are the foundation for each intervention incorporated into the patient's plan of care (APTA, 2015). Examination, evaluation, and intervention should be consistently and continually intertwined throughout an episode of care as well as during each particular treatment session (APTA, 2015). Thus, the therapist is constantly engaged in making clinical judgments about the patient's performance and function throughout an episode of care and as skilled care is provided in real time. Due to the important role this process plays in providing optimal care for patients with neurologically based **impairments, functional limitations,** and **participation restrictions,** this chapter is organized into three sections (ESCAP, 2010; APTA, 2015). The first provides an overview of the examination process and a review of the types of tests and measures to be used during the neurological examination process. Instruction on how to conduct a neurological screening examination is covered in the second section of this chapter. The final section provides the format for the neurological examination process (details presented in Chapters 4 to 13) of a patient with a known or suspected neurological diagnosis.

## ■ Purpose of the Neurological Examination

The focus of the neurological examination, either in the form of a screening process or a more in-depth examination, is to obtain information and data from the patient regarding the individual's neurological status and the impact on functional tasks and activities. The intent or purpose of the examination is to identify the patient's functional limitations and underlying impairments (APTA, 2015; Rothstein, 1986; Riddle, 2003). Both types of information must be gained efficiently and in the context of the patient's age, personal goals, lifestyle choices, occupational/educational requirements, recreational interests, and living conditions. The gathering of information can occur through observation of functional limitations, such as a patient's inability to walk up and down a flight of stairs, whereas other elements may require the use of selected tests and measures as well as disability/participation measures and functional tools (ESCAP, 2010; Rothstein, 1986; Riddle, 2003).

Once the patient's functional limitations are identified, either by observation and/or patient self-report, the therapist develops a list of suspected or possible impairments that will then be examined directly via appropriate tests and measures (Rothstein, 1986; Riddle, 2003). In the previous example, the patient's limited ability to ascend and descend a flight of stairs could be due to right-sided spastic paralysis as a result of left-sided damage in the brainstem (Goldberg, 2004). The location and extent of this type of lesion would need to be verified during the administration of selected tests and measures. For instance, you can test lesions in the medulla of the brainstem by asking the patient to push the tongue against resistance (cranial nerve XII).

The results obtained from observation and testing of selected systems will allow the therapist to identify, as efficiently as possible, the most important challenge(s) the patient faces as well as develop a thorough understanding of the patient's impairments of body systems/structures and functional limitations in tasks and activities. This collection of information will lead to the provision of optimal interventions designed to help the patient reach higher levels of functioning. It is important for the clinician to be able to distinguish between primary impairments, the symptoms and signs that are the direct result of the patient's disease or pathology, versus secondary impairments. **Secondary impairments** are abnormal changes in the structure or function of a given system that may occur as a consequence of the patient's initial pathology and related impairments and/or as a result over time of some other type of influence, such as aging or lifestyle choices (APTA, 2015). For example, a patient with cerebral palsy may demonstrate a decreased ability to extend the leg at the knee joint due to the primary impairment of spasticity (higher than average muscle tone) and decreased motor control of the knee extensors, resulting in decreased extensibility of the knee flexors over time (secondary impairment). An adult with a cerebrovascular accident (CVA) may have primary impairments of impaired motor control and impaired balance that both directly resulted from the stroke, but after several weeks of inactivity, the individual is likely to develop cardiovascular deconditioning and muscle atrophy as secondary impairments. Functional limitations, such as labored and slow ambulation with gait deviations and decreased overall mobility, can also result in secondary impairments if prolonged over an extended period,

including lower extremity weakness, cardiovascular deconditioning, and range of motion (ROM) restrictions.

Correctly identifying and categorizing the patient's impairments is required to determine appropriate interventions. Preventing secondary impairments is an important component of every treatment plan developed for patients who present with neurologically based impairments and functional limitations. Addressing secondary impairments can also enhance function; however, the gains may be limited if the interventions are not designed with a thorough understanding of the patient's underlying pathology and primary impairments. Table 3-1 presents examples of common expected primary (1°) and secondary (2°) impairments associated with CVA and spinal cord injury (SCI).

Table 3-2 presents an example of how a primary impairment, in this case the result of a CVA in the left precentral gyrus, may lead to a secondary impairment.

Figure 3-1 provides a representation of the cyclic process of the neurological examination as a component of an ongoing episode of care. Treatment is provided after the initial

| TABLE 3-1 | Common Examples of 1° and 2° Impairments Related to CVA and SCI | |
|---|---|---|
| **EXAMPLE** | **CEREBROVASCULAR ACCIDENT** | **SPINAL CORD INJURY (COMPLETE: ASIA IMPAIRMENT SCALE A)** |
| *Anticipated Primary Impairments* | • Contralateral motor control impairment (limitation in producing isolated movement)<br>• Contralateral spasticity<br>• Contralateral sensory deficits<br>• Cognitive or attention deficits | • Paralysis of muscle groups below lesion level<br>• Spasticity below lesion level<br>• Sensory deficits at and below level of lesion<br>• Bowel, bladder, and sexual function impairments |
| *Anticipated Secondary Impairments* | • Range of motion deficits from lack of full-range movement<br>• Muscle atrophy in affected muscles from decreased muscle activation<br>• Impaired cardiovascular/pulmonary endurance (deconditioning) | • Range of motion deficits from lack of full-range movement<br>• Muscle wasting from lack of muscle activation<br>• Impaired cardiovascular/pulmonary endurance (deconditioning) |
| *Functional Limitations (May Be Related to 1° or 2° Impairments)* | • Asymmetrical functional limitations in any functional skill, including upper extremity reach and manipulation tasks<br>• Gait deviations and slow gait velocity related to underlying impairments<br>• Unable to stand from sitting, or asymmetrical sit-to-stand<br>• Limited, asymmetrical ability to perform transfers, step on curbs/ramps, or walk stairs | • Requiring assistance or special equipment for upper extremity reach and manipulation tasks<br>• Requiring assistance, or requiring assistive equipment, with functional transfers and bed mobility<br>• Limited functional locomotion (including dependence on bracing and assistive equipment or mandatory use of wheelchair) |

| TABLE 3-2 | An Example of Some Specific Primary Impairments Leading to Secondary Impairments | |
|---|---|---|
| **PATHOLOGY** | **PRIMARY IMPAIRMENT** | **SECONDARY IMPAIRMENT** |
| Ischemia/infarction of left precentral gyrus → | • Spasticity of right biceps that results in reduced elbow extension<br>• Impaired motor control of elbow extensors with inability to fully extend right elbow | → • Contracture of right biceps with inability to achieve full right elbow extension, even passively |

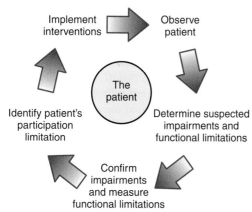

**FIGURE 3-1** Cyclic Process of the Neurological Examination. This figure illustrates the repeating, cyclical process of the neurological examination/evaluation with the patient at the center of all activity. Note that the patient has to be an integral part of the cycle at all points with an essential role in decision-making. The screening, examination, and hypothesis portions of the process must be completed before interventions can be implemented.

observation and examination during which suspected impairments are confirmed and functional limitations are identified. As the patient responds to intervention(s), the examination process continues to confirm the patient's status and provide the basis for making decisions about modifying components of the intervention(s) (Rothstein, 1986; Riddle, 2003).

## ■ Overview of the Neurological Examination

The initial neurological examination, within the framework of the overall initial examination of the patient/client, consists of four primary components: patient observation, patient/client history, review of relevant systems, and appropriate tests and measures. Patient observation should begin immediately upon meeting the patient and continue throughout the episode of care. As a result, the task of observing the patient is referenced throughout the entire discussion of the neurological examination.

### Patient Observation

Patient observation is a critical component of the initial patient encounter from the very start. The first moments of observation can provide important information that will guide the remainder of the examination and provide direction for subsequent intervention. Key elements include noting the quality and quantity of the patient's movements during the examination session, particularly movements that occur as part of a natural action, how the patient enters the examination area, how the patient spontaneously changes position, or how clothes are adjusted, rather than movements that occur based on requests from the therapist. For

example, what is the patient's sitting posture while the interview questions are answered during the examination? How did the patient move when rising from sitting to standing? Is the gait asymmetrical (i.e., did the patient spend equal or unequal amounts of time in stance and swing on the left and right legs)? Is some type of motor incoordination present (e.g., ataxia, as the patient moves into a standing posture and then begins to walk)? Are the antigravity movements of the body segments fluid and dynamic in terms of timing and power? Answers to questions like these will provide insight regarding the integrity of the neuromotor system while performing more automatic movements and will facilitate being able to fine-tune the history-taking and ROS.

### History

The information gathered during the history is the foundation upon which the neurological examination is crafted and from which patient/therapist rapport is established. Careful interview of the patient, supplemented with referral information and the results of previous diagnostic testing that might be available, can provide sufficient information to guide which subsequent sections of the examination can be addressed by a quick screening test and which areas will require more detailed examination. Do not completely rely on the referral diagnosis as sometimes the diagnosis is recorded in error (for example, a patient whose referral stated "T-6 Spinal Cord Injury" actually had a T-6 vertebral fracture without SCI). Patient-centered intervention decisions should be based on the examination results specific for the patient, including measurements of vital signs and a thorough systems review. During the interview, you may begin to gather sufficient information to generate a hypothesis for the location of the disorder and the underlying cause of the impairments with the remainder of the examination to focus on confirming or refuting elements of the hypothesis (Rothstein, 1986; Riddle, 2003).

During the history, you need to identify the patient's health risk factors, health restoration and prevention needs, current medications, and comorbidities that may affect the course of therapy (APTA, 2015). These pieces of information can be obtained from the patient, family members, significant others, caregivers, via a comprehensive review of the medical record, consultation with other health-care providers, and selected other involved persons, such as a rehabilitation counselor or a representative from a worker's compensation program (APTA, 2015).

To obtain a patient-centered history, the focus should be on the following categories of information: the patient's demographics (including race, gender, age, level of education, marital status, etc.), chief complaint/concern, history of the current condition, current and past medical history, social history, social habits, functional status, and related diagnostic tests (Boissonnault, 2010; Bickley, 2013). Be attentive to indicators of neurological dysfunction such as numbness, tingling, weakness, visual changes, alterations in speech production, cognitive changes, or dizziness when assessing the neurological status of the patient. Ask more specific questions to better understand the nature of the problem(s), the time course since the date of onset, and factors that precipitate or relieve the patient's symptoms. In some settings, a general health checklist as well as a more detailed and thorough health history questionnaire completed by the patient and/or caregiver before the initial patient interview will provide you with a basis for selecting specific areas to be covered during the neurological examination (Boissonnault, 2010). Additionally, this information may indicate potential multisystem disorders and identify constellations of symptoms that may require communication or additional follow-up with another health-care provider. Often these are symptoms the patient may not connect with the chief concern or presenting condition. By using checklists and questionnaires to obtain this information before the examination, you will save time and be able to review the information gained with the patient and/or caregiver early in the initial patient session. Obtaining this information early in the patient's examination session allows a focus on completing a thorough review of the patient's systems as well as assisting in the selection of appropriate tests and measures.

During the process of collecting information to construct the patient's history, you can assess the status of various components of the nervous system. The ability to verbally respond to questions may reflect the patient's cognitive level as well as indicate the integrity of the cranial nerves involved with speech. The ability to easily manipulate a writing instrument to complete a written questionnaire reflects integrity of the sensory and hand functions as well as related cognitive processes. The use of observations to either clear components of the nervous system or to suggest additional tests are appropriate will be incorporated in the presentation of the screening examination.

## Review of Systems

It is imperative to complete a neurological screen or a more detailed neurological examination within the framework of the Review of Systems (ROS). The ROS is an organized inquiry regarding all of the major body systems and related symptoms that should be completed during the initial patient visit (Nolan, 1996; Boissonnault, 2010). The ROS, in addition to the patient's health history, allows the therapist to identify symptoms that may be minimized by the patient and/or caregiver but are related to the patient's chief complaint (Nolan, 1996; Bickley, 2013; Swartz, 2002). During the ROS, additional knowledge about the patient's general health status is gained, which aids in the formulation of the diagnosis, prognosis, and plan of care (APTA, 2015). It may also provide guidance in the selection of appropriate interventions (APTA, 2015).

For any patient, the systems to be reviewed include the physiological and anatomic status of the patient's cardiovascular/pulmonary, integumentary, musculoskeletal, neuromuscular, gastrointestinal, genitourinary/reproductive, hematologic/lymphatic, psychological, nervous, and endocrine systems

(Swartz, 2002; APTA, 2015). The patient's ability to communicate as well as affect, cognition, language, and learning styles should also be reviewed (APTA, 2015). For instance, many patients prefer and/or need to have a written and pictorial description of their home exercise program activities after they have practiced their exercises in the clinic with the therapist. Of course, knowing the patient's primary language is essential to providing written descriptions meaningful to the patient.

In summary, the information gathered during the initial patient interview, including the ROS, provides valuable information regarding the selection of suitable tests and measures as well as insight into how to sequence the patient examination. You must choose tests and measures, including standardized tools and objective measures where possible, that will identify the location and severity of the patient's impairments, activity limitations, and participation restrictions.

## THINK ABOUT IT 3.1

- Why is it important to complete a systems review (ROS) with each patient?
- What questions will be helpful to rule out multisystem involvement?

## Tests and Measures

Multiple factors should be considered when selecting appropriate tests and measures for an individual patient. The knowledgable therapist has a wide variety of tools, tests, and measures from which to choose, such as those described in Chapters 4 to 13, and the therapist must thoughtfully and intentionally select the most appropriate measures for a particular patient. Information gained during the patient observation and history-taking are two important factors that should influence the specific tests and measures selected for a given patient (APTA, 2015; Boissonnault, 1995). In addition, consideration should be given to how each patient presents relative to the following areas (Randall, 2000):

1. What is the patient's current functional status? Is the patient ambulatory or nonambulatory? Does the person work outside the home? Does the person require assistance to complete activities of daily living (ADL)?
2. What is the patient's current cognitive status? Is the patient's cognition intact, or is the patient confused, disoriented, or exhibiting difficulty following directions?
3. What is the clinical setting in which the patient will be treated? For example, is the setting inpatient, acute rehabilitation setting, outpatient, home health, or extended care facility or school?
4. What are the patient's chief concerns? For example, why did the patient come to therapy? What does the patient most want to accomplish in terms of movements?
5. What are the patient's goals and reasonable expectations for recovery? Is this an acute, chronic, or progressive

disorder? Is there a support system in the form of family members or nonfamily caregivers?

6. What is the living situation like? Will the person return home or live in a supported environment such as an assisted living facility? Does the person live alone? Are there stairs within the home or at the entrance to the home?

The therapist, whenever possible, should also select measurement tools that yield standardized outcome data such as the Functional Independence Measure (FIM) (Cournan, 2011; Ravaud, 1999; Stineman, 1996; Linacre, 1994) that is commonly used in the inpatient rehabilitation setting, the Five- Times Sit To Stand Test (Wang, 2011; Bohannon, 2007; Mong, 2010; Paul, 2012), and the Dynamic Gait Index (Medley, 2006; Wrisley, 2010; Kadivar, 2011; Lin, 2010; Landers, 2008). Relevant outcome measures enable the clinician to set realistic treatment goals, monitor the patient's progress during the course of therapy, facilitate the therapist's ability to develop efficient and effective intervention strategies, and predict the length of treatment needed to achieve the identified goals.

Measurement tools can generally be categorized as: (1) tests/measures that are developed to provide objective information about the status of impaired body systems/structures, e.g., decreased ROM or decreased muscle strength, (2) functional tools with functional skill items, or (3) tools that include a combination of both. For example, tools such as the Functional Reach Test and Berg Balance Test are designed to measure the patient's performance of a specific ability or skill as a reflection of the person's equilibrium and balance (Blum, 2008; Muir, 2008; Conradsson, 2007; Zwick, 2000; Duncan, 1990; Weiner, 1992; Berg, 1993; Berg, 1989; Berg, 1995; Berg, 1992; Keith, 1987). The Unified Parkinson's Disease Rating Scale (UPDRS) is an example of a measurement tool that provides a mixture of impairment and functional items that yields a standardized score for the patient (Goetz, 2003). These types of measures often provide a score or set of scores used to reflect the patient's progress during therapy.

The more comprehensive the selected functional tool is the longer it will take to administer. For example, the FIM, a comprehensive multiskill instrument, takes much longer to administer than the relatively quick Functional Reach Test (Cournan, 2011; Linacre, 1994; Stineman, 1996; Ravaud, 1999; Duncan, 1990; Weiner, 1992; Berg, 1993). The time involved with giving the FIM may be justified, given the relatively rich supply of information it provides about the patient's ability to complete several important functional skills, including gait, stair-climbing, using the toilet, and completing transfers. The FIM has also been used to evaluate the effectiveness and efficiency of rehabilitation programs and compare across facilities nationwide. Ultimately, you must choose wisely in terms of the time needed to administer a given tool, and the priority should be given to tests and measures that will provide the results needed to develop optimal intervention strategies. In addition, keep in mind the information required in relation to the practice setting. An acute inpatient rehabilitation setting versus an outpatient clinic will have different challenges due to the timing of the examinations relative to the onset of patient symptoms.

In many cases, impairment-based testing, such as manual muscle testing (MMT), may be much more familiar to practicing clinicians than specific functional examination tools. Despite this familiarity, the clinicians must be vigilant when completing impairment testing to ensure that the assessment procedure(s) lead to reliable results. For example, MMT must be accomplished according to standardized MMT-testing procedures and positions, assuming the patient can create a selective isolated movement, or with the use of tools with objective measures such as dynamometry to measure force production. It is also necessary to link impairment test results to the patient's ability to complete functional skills, the most important focus of the intervention. For example, limited or decreased shoulder ROM may only be important enough to treat if it prevents a patient from completing ADL or functional skills that involve the arm. If the reduced shoulder ROM is a secondary impairment and does not negatively influence the patient's ability to complete functional activities, it may not warrant being a priority focus in therapy.

Functional assessment results coupled with the information obtained from testing specific body systems provide the foundation for the development and provision of an optimal plan of care. In completing the examination process, have systematic or specific sequences in mind (e.g., superior to inferior, involved side versus uninvolved side, or dermatomes followed by myotomes). Also note the characteristics of any deficits as well as the relative quality of the observed abnormality. This implies that it is important to carefully document observations regarding the extent of the deficits including specific distribution over the body, the quality of the movement dysfunction, and the degree of the deficit (hyper-, hypo-, or absent).

Over time and with experience, each therapist will develop a comprehensive repertoire of tests and measures. Therapists need to consider selected psychometrics of the tests and measures they choose to use with their patients, which can be understood more completely from a review of research textbooks. For example, the reliability of each test and measure used should be established at a level acceptable for use with the intended patient population. **Reliability,** in its most basic form, provides an expression of the degree to which measurements are consistent when they are repeated over time. Therapists should consider specific forms of reliability as they select tests and measures, including intrarater, interrater, test-retest, and intrasubject reliability. These forms of reliability are summarized in Table 3-3.

A statistical trait linked to reliability is validity. **Validity** is the extent to which a test or measure truly measures what it intends to measure. The types of validity include: construct, content, and criterion validity, which includes the concepts of concurrent and predictive validity. These types are described in Table 3-4 and should be considered by the therapist before selecting a given test or measure with a particular patient.

Also, it is important to consider whether or not the tests and measures chosen are subjective or objective in nature,

| Table 3-3 | Types of Reliability |
|---|---|
| **TERM** | **DEFINITION** |
| Reliability | An expression of the degree to which measurements are consistent when they are repeated |
| Intrarater Reliability | How consistently one rater assigns scores to a single set of responses on separate occasions |
| Interrater Reliability | How consistently different raters are in assigning scores to the same responses |
| Test-retest Reliability | How consistently a subject performs on the same test or measure over time |
| Intrasubject Reliability | How consistently a subject performs over time |

| TABLE 3-4 | Types of Validity |
|---|---|
| **TERM** | **DEFINITION** |
| Validity | The extent to which a test or measure truly measures what it is intended to measure and provides meaningful information |
| Construct | The validity of the abstract construct(s) that underlie tests and measures |
| Content | The extent to which a test or measure is a complete representation of the construct being measured |
| Criterion | The extent to which one test or measure is systematically related to some particular outcome (includes concurrent and predictive) |
| Concurrent | The extent to which a new test or measure is related to an established or standard test or measure |
| Predictive | The extent to which a test or measure is able to predict future function or performance |

and if they are designed to provide qualitative or quantitative examination data. Subjective tests and measures, like some sensory tests and pain-rating scales, provide the therapist with the patient's perceptions of the signs and symptoms present or the therapist's judgment about the degree of impairment. Alternatively, objective measures of functional abilities and impairments provide a quantifiable basis for the therapist to establish patient goals, to develop appropriate intervention strategies, and to provide a method for measuring patient progress. Further, *qualitative* measures enable the therapist to assess if the patient's response is absent, diminished, or excessive and describe characteristics of the performance, whereas tests and measures that are more *quantitative* in nature provide examination data that is objective and more easily linked to measuring patient progress and establishing appropriate outcomes. Consider all four traits when selecting the tests and measures to be used with each patient.

Consideration of these statistical properties will enable the therapist to select a comprehensive array of tests and measures that are holistic and provide accurate, reliable, and valid data regarding the ability of each of the patients to move and function in their world. Chapters 4 to 13 will detail the specific examination procedures and evaluation processes for each neuromotor system involved in neuromuscular disorders. These chapters will also discuss measures to assess activity limitations resulting from neurological disorders and related impairments. However, you must first decide which components

merit more detailed assessment based on the information gathered during the process of the patient interview and the screening examination described in the next section of this chapter.

## THINK ABOUT IT 3.2

- What factors should you consider when selecting appropriate tests and measures?
- What is the value to the therapist of using standardized tests and measures?
- How can subjective measures provide you with helpful information?
- How can objective measures specifically provide you with helpful information?

## ■ Neurological Screening Examination

In the absence of a known or suspected neurological lesion, it is often appropriate for the clinician to perform a neurological screening examination after the completion of the patient's history. The purpose of the screening examination is to "rule-in" or "rule-out" the need for a more in-depth neurological examination.

Although the entire screen should be completed with patients who have a nonneurological medical diagnosis, the attention to the various components will differ in patients who have had a recent medical examination versus those who have not. In a patient with a neurological diagnosis, portions of the screen can be used to confirm the integrity of the nervous system components that should be intact given the diagnosis while a more detailed examination will be conducted to evaluate those areas with known or suspected dysfunctions. For instance, a patient with a diagnosis involving recent cerebellar lesion often presents with normal strength, but the therapist may observe awkward movements characterized by intention tremors and ataxia. In this case, the therapist would want to conduct a more thorough examination of the patient's coordination following a quick screen of their strength and sensation. By knowing which systems are operational, you can identify what treatment activities might be feasible for the patient and develop treatment plans more specific to the patient's impairments and functional limitations.

The screening examination should be completed as quickly as possible. With practice, an examiner should be able to conduct the neurological screening examination in 4 minutes (Goldberg, 2004). The skillful examiner collects information from observations in addition to specific tests to determine whether a more detailed assessment is warranted. If a deficit is detected, the parameters and characteristics of the finding need to be documented. The extent and distribution of the deficit provides clues to the pathophysiological and anatomical basis of the dysfunction, which can help to explain related symptoms and constellations or groupings of findings. For example, the distribution of a sensory loss differentiates between a peripheral nerve lesion and a spinal-level dermatomal dysfunction. The quality of the abnormality must also be recorded to differentiate between a partially impaired function (hypo-), an absent response, or an excessive (hyper-) response. Because some areas of the neurological examination are subjective, such as the sensory examination, it is important to provide quantitative and qualitative descriptors.

Several key areas are the focus of the neurological screening examination (Goldberg, 2004). These include:

1. Mental status
2. Cranial nerves
3. Motor
4. Reflexes
5. Sensation
6. Coordination
7. Stance and Gait

Table 3-5 provides a summary of the process or flow of conducting a screening neurological examination.

## Mental Status

A screening examination of the patient's mental status should focus on assessing the patient's alertness, orientation, memory (especially recent memory as it deteriorates more rapidly than older memories in the presence of brain damage), and general cognitive function (Goldberg, 2004). Refer to Chapter 4 for a more detailed discussion of the cognitive examination. Use the acronym "FOGS" as a guide to this mental status segment of the neurological screening examination (Goldberg, 2004). The acronym FOGS stands for **F**amily story of memory loss, **O**rientation of the patient, **G**eneral information, and **S**pelling.

To begin, determine whether the patient is "foggy" (Goldberg, 2004) by assessing the patient's basic level of arousal and ability to attend to a task. Is the patient attentive? Is the patient lethargic or showing a tendency to "drift off" from the current situation? Is the patient in a semicoma (aroused with noxious stimuli, but not awake enough to answer questions)? Is the patient in a comatose state (not aroused with noxious stimuli)? If either of the last two conditions is present, the screening examination process is terminated, and a detailed neurological examination is in order. In most cases, this detailed information will be available in the patient's chart, so selectively examine the functions relevant to the patient's presentation.

The family story can play a critical role in uncovering the patient's current condition and in understanding how the individual presents during the initial physical therapy session. Family members or support persons can relay information about the pattern of memory loss the patient has demonstrated. You may find it helpful to ask the family if the memory loss is relatively recent or if there has been a general decline in memory over a longer period of time.

The patient's orientation to person, place, and time is a starting point in the screen of cognition. This can be done indirectly or directly, being tactful to avoid insulting or embarrassing the patient (Goldberg, 2004). If you choose to address the patient directly about this information, it should be done in the context of asking the patient to respond to routine questions as quickly as possible rather than focusing on the actual answers to each question (Goldberg, 2004).

If the patient's responses to questions during the standard history interview raise questions about the individual's recall of information, the standard procedure is to assess the patient's ability to recall general information. This can be accomplished by asking the patient to name the President and Vice-President of the United States or asking the patient to describe recent current events.

The last section of the FOGS approach is spelling. Ask the patient to spell the word "world" forward and backward. If the patient can spell "world" forward, it indicates that the patient can spell and, in the absence of organic neurological deficits, the patient should then be able to spell the same word backward (Goldberg, 2004). However, if the patient cannot spell, ask the patient to count backward from 100 by 3s, or ask the patient to repeat a seven-digit number to assess the patient's ability to perform mental manipulations of information.

During the interview process, information can be gathered regarding communication and the quality of the patient's speech (an indication of the status of cranial nerves VII, IX, X, and XII), the content of the responses (cortical level functions), and visual acuity for comprehension as the patient completes questionnaires or is asked to identify objects at a distance in the examination area. Note the

| TABLE 3-5 | Brief Neurological Screening Examination |
|---|---|

**(CONDUCTED WITH SEATED INDIVIDUAL UNTIL FINAL SECTION)**

*History-taking*
During the interview portion, the examiner will assess:
• Mental status
• Speech (content—cortical and quality—cranial nerves)
• Vision (acuity)

*Cranial Nerves*
• Check visual fields (CN II)
• Check eye movements (CN III, IV, VI), note any nystagmus
• Test touch sensation of 3 divisions of trigeminal (CN V)—defer to Sensory Testing section
• Palpate masseter/temporalis or protrude lower jaw (CN V)
• Test facial muscles: smile, pucker, then eye closure, eyebrow elevation (CN VII-upper and lower)
• Rub fingers next to ear (CN VIII)
• Ask individual to open mouth, say "Ah," then protrude tongue (CN IX, X/CN XII)

*Motor Functions*
• Check for upper extremity drift
• Test deltoids, biceps, triceps, wrist extensors, grip
• Test hip flexors, knee flexors and extensors, ankle dorsiflexion
• Test hip extensors (in coming to standing) and plantar flexors in standing (bilateral or unilateral rise of toes or hop)—defer to Stance and Gait section

*Reflexes*
• Test deep tendon reflexes (biceps, triceps, brachioradialis, knee, ankle)
• Test Babinski (if indicated)
• Test reflex development for infants and children (e.g., early tonic reflexes and equilibrium, protective and righting responses)

*Sensation*
• Test touch bilaterally on face, tip of shoulder, forearm, hand, thigh, lateral side of foot, great toe, up medial aspect of lower leg
• Test stereognosis

*Coordination*
• Test finger-to-nose and heel-to-shin tests
• Test rapidly alternating movements—upper and lower extremities

*Stance and Gait*
• Note hip/knee strength in moving from sitting to standing
• Observe normal and heel-toe (tandem) walking
• Perform the Romberg test

patient's facial expression to assess the functions of cranial nerve VII.

## Cranial Nerves

The next segment of the neurological screen is the assessment of the integrity of the cranial nerves. The depth and precision of the assessment will depend on the patient's history and other indications suggesting that the functions are intact or impaired. As previously mentioned, consider an orderly or sequential test sequence before beginning this portion of the examination. This section presents an overview of key tests that may be used to assess the integrity of the cranial nerves along with normal cranial nerve function. Table 3-6 provides a summary of this information; however, a screening

examination may not require testing of each function depending on the information gathered during the initial interview process. Note that the cranial nerves are not presented in numerical order in Table 3-6. Rather, they are "linked together" by function and ease of patient examination. Chapter 7 (Cranial Nerve Examination) and Chapter 8 (Vestibular Examination) present detailed information on the assessment of cranial nerve functions.

Dysfunction of cranial nerve I (Olfactory) may be indicated by a patient's report that the taste of food has changed because loss of the sense of smell interferes with the perception of taste (Deems, 1991). In the preponderance of individuals, assessment of olfaction is not performed. Because loss of the sense of smell is more common in older adults, in individuals with Alzheimer disease, and after a head trauma, a screening

| TABLE 3-6 | **Cranial Nerve Screen*** | |
|---|---|---|
| **CRANIAL NERVE** | **NORMAL FUNCTION** | **KEY SCREENING TEST** |
| I – Olfactory | Sense of Smell | Ask the patient to identify the odor of mild agents, e.g., scented soap, coffee, vanilla, orange, and mints with each nostril. |
| II – Optic | Visual Acuity (Central Vision) Peripheral Vision | Ask the patient to read from the Snellen Eye Chart or from the Rosenbaum Pocket Card. Ask the patient to look at your nose with one eye covered and tell you which finger(s) you are wiggling. Move your hand to screen each visual field – superior and inferior; repeat for each eye. |
| III – Oculomotor | Pupillary Reaction to Light | Observe how the patient's pupils respond to a brief light source. Observe the position of the eyelids for symmetry and an absence of drooping. |
| IV – Trochlear | Eye Position and Alignment | Ask the patient to follow a moving object with movement of the eyes – focus on both for the left and right eye. Observe the position of the patient's eyes. |
| VI – Abducens | Eye Position | Observe the position of the patient's eyes. |
| V – Trigeminal | Sensation of Face  Motor Function of Jaw (Chewing) | Lightly move your fingers simultaneously down the sides of the patient's face starting at the forehead and ending under the jaw. Palpate the masseter and temporalis muscles while the patient is asked to clench the teeth, then ask the patient to protrude the jaw forward with the mouth slightly open. |
| VII – Facial | Facial Expressions | Ask the patient to smile, pucker the lips, puff out the cheeks, close the eyes tightly, and raise the eyebrows. |
| VIII – Vestibulocochlear | Hearing Acuity | Rub your index finger and thumb together just outside of the patient's ears and ask the patient to point to the ear in which the sound is heard. |
| IX – Glossopharyngeal | Voice Quality/Vocal Cord Strength  Gag reflex | Listen to the patient's voice quality.  Elicit a gag reflex. |
| X – Vagus | Elevation of the Palate | Ask the patient to say "Ah." |
| XII – Hypoglossal | Tongue Movements | Ask the patient to stick out the tongue or push the tongue against the sides of the cheeks. |
| XI – Accessory Nerve | Shoulder Elevation | Ask the patient to shrug the shoulders against manual resistance – (beginning of motor examination). |

*NOTE: The order of the cranial nerves is listed in the order/grouping to be screened.

assessment may be appropriate in these individuals. This is particularly true for individuals who will spend periods of time alone and may need the sense of smell to alert them to signals of danger, such as the smell of smoke.

Screening of the cranial nerves associated with the functions of the eye (cranial nerves II-Optic, III-Oculomotor, IV-Trochlear, and VI-Abducens) can start while the patient information is being collected. If the patient is unable to read the forms used to collect information, visual acuity may be inadequate (CN II function), although inability to read, not the lack of visual acuity, may be the source of the problem. When looking directly at the patient's face, if the eyelids are symmetrical, and drooping is not noted (no ptosis), then

cranial nerve III function is likely intact. If the pupil sizes are unequal, additional testing of the functions of cranial nerves II and III is indicated.

Specific screening of cranial nerve II (Optic nerve) is performed by evaluating central vision and peripheral vision. Assessment of far-vision acuity can be performed formally via the Snellen chart or informally by asking the patient to state the time on a clock across the room. The Rosenbaum pocket card can be used for near-vision, although asking the patient to read the smallest type legible in printed material from a newspaper or magazine provides a quick method of gathering information. The request needs to be tailored to the patient based on whether or not the patient can read. Only one eye at a time should be tested to prevent a misinterpretation of the patient's central vision.

Peripheral vision can be checked by having the patient cover one eye while looking at your nose. It is important that the patient not move the eye. Wiggle the index finger of both your hands in the superior visual fields and ask the patient to state or point to the side that moved. This is repeated for the lower fields. Repeat with the patient covering the other eye while maintaining the gaze at your nose. For this eye, place both of the hands in the superior field, but wiggle only your right index finger. This will prevent the patient from assuming or guessing that you are wiggling both index fingers. Finally, ask the patient to identify which finger wiggled after both index fingers wiggled in the lower field.

The screening assessment of the integrity of cranial nerves III, IV, and VI can be completed by simply asking the patient to follow a moving object such as the tip of a pen, finger, or light as it moves through each of the visual field sections (right and left, upper, middle, and lower). Difficulty abducting one eye would warrant further assessment of cranial nerve VI. A brief pause at the end range in each section allows the therapist to screen for gaze-evoked nystagmus. It is also important to observe the position of the patient's eyes as the patient looks straight ahead (CNs IV/VI). (See Chapter 7 for additional information.)

Examination of the face provides a quick assessment of the functions of cranial nerves V (Trigeminal) and VII (Facial). The sensory function of cranial nerve V can be tested by lightly moving your index fingers simultaneously down the sides of the face starting at the lateral aspects of the forehead, across the cheeks, and ending under the jaws. The patient is asked to report if the touch is felt continuously in all areas and if it feels the same on both sides. Any indications of differences should be followed up with a more detailed examination (Chapter 7). For efficiency, the sensory testing of the face can be combined with the testing of sensation of the body described later in this chapter.

The motor functions of the Trigeminal nerve can be quickly screened by palpating the masseter and temporalis muscles while the patient is asked to clench the teeth. If the two sides do not feel symmetrical or the muscle mass is smaller than expected, additional tests are indicated. Ask the patient to protrude the lower jaw forward with the mouth slightly open while you look for any deviations. Alternatively ask the patient to open the mouth while you resist the movement, placing your hand under the patient's jaw. The movement should occur smoothly. Chapter 7 details additional assessments, such as the Jaw Jerk Test that can be performed if you have questions on the integrity of cranial nerve V.

The upper and lower divisions of cranial nerve VII (Facial) can be tested by asking the patient to smile, puff out the cheeks, close the eyes tightly, and raise the eyebrows. Observation should focus on whether or not there is asymmetry or weakness on one or both sides of the patient's face, which would necessitate testing the function of the specific facial muscles.

To quickly test the hearing function of the vestibulo-cochlear nerve (cranial nerve VIII), rub your thumb and index fingers together just outside of the patient's ears and ask the patient to point to the ear in which sound is heard. If there is a deficit, the determination will need to be made of whether the loss is conductive or sensorineural. Refer to Chapters 7 and 8 for additional details.

Suggestions of problems with the vestibular portions of cranial nerve VIII may be raised during the patient interview if the patient reports problems with dizziness or balance. It is important to ask questions about the patient's reports of dizziness to differentiate between indicators of vestibular dysfunction and use of the word "lightheaded" which may indicate hypoperfusion or hypoglycemia. During the motor portion of the screening examination, problems with balance during activities such as heel-toe walking or performing five quick horizontal head turns while sitting or standing could indicate the need for specific assessments of vestibular function described in Chapter 8.

Unless there are suggestions of brainstem level involvement, which would necessitate more detailed assessment of specific functions of cranial nerves IX (Glossopharyngeal), X (Vagus), and XII (Hypoglossal), a screen can be performed by listening to the patient's voice quality (CN IX), asking the patient to open the mouth and say "Ahh," followed by protruding the tongue (CN XII). Eliciting a gag reflex (CN IX) is an unpleasant procedure and is not typically included in the cranial nerve screen.

Although still a component of the cranial nerve screening sequence, testing the Accessory nerve (CN XI) becomes the first component of the screen for motor functions. The quick assessment of Accessory nerve function is performed by asking the patient to elevate (shrug) the shoulders against your manual resistance.

Specific cranial testing is challenging in infants, young children, and in older children who lack the cognitive or language ability to follow directions. In these cases, adaptations are required.

## Motor Examination

The motor examination within the screening neurological examination is relatively simple and straightforward. Visual inspection of the extremities provides background information. Noting the presence of muscle wasting, fasciculations, abnormal positioning in any of the joints, or an inability to normally move a limb against gravity provides indications for more in-depth assessment. If the patient's movements appear normal, including the ability to walk to the examination room and descend to sitting in a chair, the screening examination can progress quickly.

The quick screen for the upper extremities is conducted by having the patient, with eyes closed, hold the arms at 90 degrees of shoulder flexion with elbows extended and the palms up for approximately 15 to 30 seconds. This screening tool is formally called the Pronator Drift Test. If there is weakness in the upper extremity, the involved hand will slowly drop or pronate (palm rotating toward midline). If both arms drop, the weakness is bilateral. If one of the arms rises, cerebellar dysfunction may be present and should be investigated. Proprioceptive deficits may also contribute to difficulty maintaining the arm in a steady position.

With the patient seated, progress through conducting a gross screen of upper extremity muscle strength by performing the simultaneous bilateral tests of the deltoid (axillary nerve, C5 innervation), biceps (musculocutaneous, C5-6), triceps (radial, C7), wrist extensors (radial, C6-8), and grip (median and ulnar, C7-T1). The intent of these tests is not to establish a specific strength grade but to determine whether there are gross areas of weakness or asymmetries. Bilateral testing increases the efficiency of the testing as well as providing a basis for comparison. While conducting the strength testing, note any indications of abnormalities in tone that would require further testing.

With the patient remaining seated, continue with the motor screens of the lower extremity musculature. Typically, the strength tests for the lower extremity muscles are performed unilaterally to decrease the demands. Then the gross strength of the two sides is compared. Screening includes tests performed on the hip flexors (lumbar sacral plexus, L1-2), knee extensors (femoral nerve, L3-4), knee flexors (sciatic, L5-S1), and ankle dorsiflexors (deep peroneal, L4-5). As with the upper extremities, note any abnormal movement patterns in addition to altered muscle tone while moving the joints to position the limbs for the strength tests. Any indications of muscle wasting or fasciculations should also be noted.

The strength of the hip extensors (inferior gluteal, L5-S1) and the plantar flexors (posterior tibial, S1) is assessed as the patient moves from sitting to standing then performing a unilateral or bilateral rise on the toes. Because this assessment requires the patient to move into a standing position, it can be deferred until the final section of the screen, which addresses stance and gait.

If the patient is positioned in prone for the purpose of conducting other tests, the lower extremity counterpart to the upper extremity Pronator Drift Test is conducted by having the patient bend the knees so that bilateral lower legs are pointing vertically. If weakness is present, the weak side will show a tendency to deviate from the vertical position after about 30 seconds. The presence of pain or loss of proprioceptive sense may also contribute to the inability to maintain the vertical position.

If abnormalities are noted during the motor screening previously described, a more detailed neuromotor examination is indicated. Chapter 6 provides information on conducting a thorough neuromotor examination including considerations of ROM, muscle tone, motor control, coordination, strength, and endurance with a focus on the neuromuscular patient population.

## Reflexes

With the patient seated, the screen can progress to testing major reflexes. Note whether deep tendon reflexes are absent, diminished, or excessive and investigate any asymmetry in responses. The appropriate sequence that will provide systematic assessment of the major nerves and spinal roots is highlighted in Table 3-7. If any portion of this screen or the history suggests that an upper motor neuron lesion may be present, you may also test for ankle clonus and assess the plantar response to determine whether a positive Babinski response is present. (See Chapter 6 for additional details.)

## Sensory Examination

The screening examination for sensation is quick and starts at the forehead, lightly dragging the index and middle fingers of right and left hands simultaneously, using equal pressure bilaterally, down the right and left side of the patient's forehead, cheek, neck, upper arm, forearm, hands, lateral thighs, lateral lower legs, lateral feet, great toes, and up the medial aspects of the lower legs. Ask the patient to report any areas where the touch is not felt or where the two sides feel different during the double simultaneous stimulation. Modification to the screening may need to occur for patients with communication limitations such as difficulty with word finding or dysarthria. In this case, it may be useful to have the patient nod the head or point a finger when a sensation is identified.

Test stereognosis by placing a small object such as a coin, a key, a closed safety pin, or a paper clip into the patient's palm while the patient's eyes are closed. If the patient can easily manipulate and then identify the object, the sensory pathways and parietal lobe are intact and detailed proprioceptive examination is not necessary for the hand (Campbell, 2012).

As indicated previously, if the patient is able to maintain the extended position of the upper extremities used as a quick screen for upper extremity strength, upper extremity proprioception is probably intact. Proprioceptive deficits in the lower extremities would contribute to difficulties performing functions during the Stance or Gait tests and may be observed during other functional activities in any age patient as the person would be unable to incorporate proprioceptive information into real-time adjustments of movement.

If impairments related to proprioception, light touch, or discriminative sensation are suspected, a more detailed assessment is indicated. Details on the examination of tactile and discriminative sensation are presented in Chapter 5.

| TABLE 3-7 | Deep Tendon Reflex Testing | |
|---|---|---|
| **MUSCLE** | **NERVE TESTED** | **SPINAL ROOT** |
| Biceps | Musculocutaneous | C5–6 |
| Triceps | Radial | C7 |
| Brachioradialis | Radial | C6 |
| Finger Flexors | Median/Ulnar | C8 |
| Quadriceps | Femoral | L3–4 |
| Achilles/Ankle Jerk | Tibial | S1–2 |

## Coordination

Coordination of the upper extremities is screened by asking the patient to position the upper extremities in 90 degrees of abduction, close the eyes, and repeatedly touch the tip of the nose with the fingertip of alternating index fingers (left and right). Ask the patient to increase the speed of movement with each repetition. An alternative version of the finger-to-nose test can be performed by asking the patient to alternately touch your finger and the tip of the patient's nose. The heel to shin test provides an assessment of lower extremity coordination by asking the patient to slide the heel of one foot along the shin of the other leg, from a position in front of the knee to the front of the ankle and back to the knee. While typically described as being performed in supine, for the purposes of the screening assessment, the patient can be asked to perform the task while seated. It is important to keep in mind that, in addition to coordination, strength and flexibility will affect the ability to successfully complete the task when in the seated position. If the original attempts of the finger-to-nose or heel-to-shin test are accurate, but performance degrades with repetition, the problem may be an impairment of joint position sense or muscular endurance (Fuller, 2008).

The ability to perform rapidly alternating movements can also be used to assess coordination (diadochokinesia). A variety of tests can be used. A simple test for the upper extremities is to ask the patient to rapidly tap the thumb and index fingers against one another using both hands at the same time. Test the lower extremities by asking the patient to rapidly tap the forefoot on the floor while the heel remains on the ground/floor, testing both feet at the same time. Normally, the tapping should be rapid with an even rhythm. More detailed information on the assessment of coordination is presented in Chapter 6.

## Stance and Gait

An assessment of the patient's gait can be performed as the patient walks into the examination area and may be sufficient if the rest of the screening results are normal and there are no indications of issues from the patient interview. Assessment of the strength of the hip and knee extensors is made when the patient moves from sitting to standing. If indicated, the status of the plantar flexors can be checked by asking the patient to perform a bilateral or unilateral rise on the toes, assuming balance is adequate to safely perform the task.

If balance is thought to be a concern based on observations made when the patient was sitting, standing, or walking, the patient can be asked to tandem walk (i.e., walk heel-to-toe with careful guarding, including the use of a transfer or gait belt). Additionally, if balance deficits are suspected, the response of the patient to a posterior perturbation when standing may provide insights into the origin of the problems. The patient's response to perturbations can also allow insight into the movement strategies the patient utilizes to maintain balance. If the patient has difficulty with tandem walking, the Romberg test can be administered to gather additional information on the cause of the balance deficit. During this test, ask the patient to maintain static standing balance with feet together and eyes closed for up to 30 seconds.

Difficulty with any of the functional screening items previously described is indicative of a need for further balance assessment. Chapter 9 provides detailed information on the assessment of balance and equilibrium.

## ■ Examination/Evaluation in Patients With Known or Suspected Neurological Diagnosis

When conducting the examination of a patient with a known neurological diagnosis, you first complete a process of confirming the available information from the referral source and medical chart to ensure they are consistent with the given medical diagnosis. In addition to confirming the presence and extent of the expected impairments, also look for any signs or symptoms that would not be expected and/or would indicate a progression of the pathology, an overlay of an additional neurological disorder, or dysfunctions missed in a previous examination.

When conducting the examination of a patient with a suspected neurological diagnosis, the approach becomes that of an investigator attempting to determine whether there is a disorder present involving the nervous system and how widespread the effect is. If so, the nature of the disorder must be determined, including whether multisystem involvement is present, so the appropriate intervention plan or referral can be made.

### Based on History and ROS

As presented earlier in this chapter, the patient history is the critical element in planning the remaining components of the examination. Gathering information on the time course of the symptoms (onset, progression, and pattern of occurrence) is useful in determining that the description is consistent with the stated diagnosis or in suggesting a possible diagnosis if one has not been established. The ROS provides the opportunity to determine the nonneurological factors that will need to be considered in developing the plan of care. Individuals with neurological diagnoses, particularly if the condition is not acute, may have secondary musculoskeletal impairments due to impaired motor control and/or diminished cardiovascular endurance due to prolonged inactivity.

By the end of the information-gathering process during the history, one can typically generate a working hypothesis of where the lesion/dysfunction is located and what the source of the lesion or dysfunction is (vascular, neoplasm, infection, impingement, etc.). This will help determine the subsequent tests/measures to be implemented with the patient (Rothstein, 1986; Riddle, 2003).

### Examination

When a known or suspected neurological diagnosis is present, the therapist should be cued into the neuromuscular impairments most likely to be present so that appropriate tests are performed. Table 3-8 presents examples of common neurological impairments (adapted from Shumway-Cook, 2017). The Diagnosis Outlines in the Compendium section at the end of the book will provide a summary review regarding which neurological impairments are most expected with each major neuromuscular medical diagnosis.

The remaining chapters in Section II present the details for examination processes for each specific neuromuscular-related system and each category of functional activity, in the evaluation of neuromuscular disorders.

## Evaluation of Examination Data: Identify, Prioritize, Predict

All information collected in the patient examination is important, both for systems that are operating normally and for identified problems. As described in Chapter 2, once the specific examination data has been collected (and even as it is being collected), the therapist must: (1) *identify* the most important examination results and the interrelationships between identified impairments and activity limitations, (2) *prioritize* which functional problems should be addressed earliest, and (3) considering the patient's prognosis, *predict* the degree of improvement the patient will experience during the episode of intervention/care for each problem area. All of these will serve as the basis for determining the plan of care and the specific intervention to be implemented for the patient.

The therapist must synthesize the patient's **problem list,** that is, a list emphasizing the patient's functional limitations and participation restrictions. The problem list should be prioritized in collaboration with the patient and the patient's family/support person(s). This process will help the therapist determine which functions to address first. Through clinical reasoning and judgment, the therapist will identify and systematically link the patient's impairments to the patient's functional limitations. Details regarding the potential impact of underlying impairments on specific functions are described in the *Impact on Function* section of Section IV chapters (Chapters 18 to 32) and the *Possible Impairments* section of Section V chapters (Chapters 33 to 37), along with implications for rehabilitation interventions.

In addition to identifying the impairments, functional limitations, and participation restrictions, it is also very important to develop a list of the patient's current assets or strengths. The patient's assets, functional limitations, and impairments all need to be considered in the development of the patient's plan of care. Acknowledging the patient's assets/strengths provides a starting point from which functional intervention can begin. Strengths provide the therapist with the components needed to build treatment sessions designed to assure greater patient success early in therapy. They also help the patient and the family/support persons focus on the positive aspects of how the patient is currently able to move and function. Particularly during the examination phase of patient care the

| TABLE 3-8 | Selected Neurological Impairments and Impact on Movement | |
|---|---|---|
| | **EXAMPLES OF NEUROLOGICAL IMPAIRMENTS** | **IMPACT ON THE QUALITY OF MOVEMENTS** |
| *Muscle Tone Impairments* | • Hypertonicity: Spasticity/Rigidity (including cogwheel and lead-pipe)<br>• Hypotonicity<br>• Dystonia | • Stiff movements (usually with hypertonicity)<br>• Floppy movements (usually with hypotonicity)<br>• Choreiform movements |
| *Abnormal Reflexes* | • Hyperreflexia<br>• Hyporeflexia<br>• Areflexia<br>• Pathological reflexes | • Akinesia (usually with areflexia)<br>• Delayed motor development in children |
| *Sensory/Perceptual Impairments* | • Impaired tactile awareness or proprioceptive sense<br>• Astereognosis<br>• Contralateral homonymous hemianopsia<br>• Spatial relationship disorders | • Impaired placing and positioning (usually with loss of position sense)<br>• Impaired motor control in any task (usually with loss of movement sense)<br>• Lack of gaze stability and postural imbalance<br>• Dizziness |
| *Cognitive Impairments* | • Apraxia<br>• Memory deficits | • Difficulty initiating movement<br>• Attention deficits<br>• Arousal deficits |
| *Motor Impairments* | • Weakness<br>• Impaired coordination<br>• Poor postural control | • Bradykinesia<br>• Resting tremor<br>• Dyskinesia<br>• Impaired fractionation of movement<br>• Abnormal synergies |

spotlight can appear to only shine on what is wrong or the negative. Thus, it is very beneficial to remind the patient and ourselves of body structure(s) and body function(s) that are intact and basic activities that can be performed. This process provides the basis for providing the patient with early positive outcomes.

Chapter 14 will provide the bridge between the processes of examination/evaluation and the principles of neurological intervention.

## THINK ABOUT IT 3.3

- What body structures and functions do you anticipate to be involved in your patient with a known neurological diagnosis?
- How are you going to determine which activity limitations and participation restrictions to place at the top of your problem list?
- How will you utilize your patient's strengths in developing your prognosis and plan of care?

## ■ Pediatric General Considerations

The basic content and procedures for neurological examination and neurological screening examination as previously described are applicable to infants and children. Adaptation, including techniques to elicit responses and motivation of the child, will be required for many of the examination procedures depending on the age and capabilities of the infant or child. Knowledge of normal child development and age-appropriate activities should guide the necessary adaptation customized to the individual child. For example, the examiner cannot expect a toddler to understand or comply with specific directions for testing cranial nerve function related to eye movement, but the examiner can entice the child to look in a particular direction with a colorful toy and observe the toddler's ability to visually track the toy.

Parents or other caregivers will be important contributors to the patient's history. Parent/caregiver interaction with the infant/child should also be carefully observed and may affect how the examination is conducted and how the plan of care is developed. The parent/caregiver may be able to get the child to do something the therapist cannot. Additional population-specific information may be helpful when taking a history pertinent to an infant or child, including any difficulties during the mother's pregnancy, or during the birth or postnatal period. It is important to describe the infant's or child's behavior or state of alertness (see Chapter 4 for Brazelton states) during the examination and to interpret the influence of behavior on functional abilities. Did the toddler just awake from a nap, sleepy and withdrawn, clinging to his

mother? Is a premature infant irritable and fussy with handling? Does the infant or child have adequate self-regulatory behaviors? In other words, if the infant can self-calm, this would facilitate meaningful interaction and function for the examination. These positive behaviors would suggest valid observation of motor activity and responses. On the other hand, if mild distress easily escalates to full-blown crying, the child's typical voluntary actions and motor behavior may be difficult to observe.

When examining infants and children, it is important to determine whether functional activity is age-appropriate. It is also important to know at what age each functional activity initially develops in a child (see Chapter 13) and apply that knowledge to the evaluation of the examination observations and data. For example, an 8-month-old infant would not be expected to walk independently, but concern would arise if an 18-month-old was not yet walking. A starting point is to ask the caregiver when the infant/child attained certain developmental milestones such as sitting up, standing, and walking and/or to test the infant/child's ability to perform basic motor tasks like these. Motor milestones are building blocks for functional motor ability but must be evaluated within a broader context. It is critical to observe the variability of the child's performance and the adaptation to changing demands of the task. If delay in motor development is suspected, it is often advisable to test motor function using a standardized, norm-referenced screening or examination instrument appropriate to the age of the child and the purpose of the testing. Chapter 13 provides comprehensive information on assessing motor development.

Screening the related areas of function such as fine motor, cognitive, and language skills may best be accomplished with a standardized, norm-referenced screening instrument to assure that the child has age-appropriate abilities. Especially with infants and children, these related areas of function affect the expression of motor abilities. A child with attention deficit-hyperactivity disorder or severe cognitive impairment will not likely understand or follow instructions to walk heel-toe on a taped line despite an inherent ability to perform that motor task. Examination results must be interpreted with such influences in mind.

The educational environment creates unique challenges for the child, and adherence to the guidelines of the Individuals with Disabilities Education Act (IDEA, 2004) requires specificity in the examination process. Depending on the circumstances, it may be helpful to use an instrument specifically designed for the educational environment, such as the School Function Assessment. Interpretation of the examination results and development of an appropriate plan of care will depend on the services necessary for a child with disabilities to benefit from special education in a particular educational environment.

# HANDS-ON PRACTICE

Be sure to practice the following skills from this chapter. With further practice, you should be able to:

- Complete a patient interview, including questions pertinent to the patient's history and ROS.
- Complete a neuromuscular screening examination including:
  - Using FOGS to screen mental status.
  - Cranial nerve screen.
  - Using the Pronator Drift Test to screen upper extremity weakness.
  - Seated lower extremity strength screen, including identifying components in sitting versus standing.
- A sensory screen assessing light touch, and stereognosis.
- A systematic order for reflex assessment.
- Using toe tapping and repeated finger-to-thumb to assess coordination.
- Screening balance using perturbations, the Romberg test, or a falls assessment.
- Complete screening items previously described while integrating play activities for pediatric populations.

## Let's Review

1. What are the four main components of the neurological examination? How are they important to you as an occupational or physical therapist?

2. What information should you collect during your patient interview and why?

3. How would you determine the need for a neurological screening examination versus a more in-depth neurological examination?

4. Describe how you would screen each of the following components of the neuromuscular system: mental status; cranial nerves; motor, reflexes, and sensation coordination; and stance and gait.

5. How might your neurological examination have to be modified for patients with cognitive impairments?

6. In the presence of a known neurological diagnosis, how will you identify the appropriate components of the neurological examination on which to focus?

7. Once the neurological examination is completed, how will you compose your prioritized problem list?

8. How will the outcomes from the neurological examination help drive the plan of care?

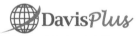 For additional resources, including Focus on Evidence tables, case study discussions, references, and glossary, please visit http://davisplus.fadavis.com

# CHAPTER SUMMARY

Like a detective in a mystery novel or criminal investigation, methodically gathering information to unravel the case and reach the final solution, the therapist moves through the process of interviewing the patient, gathering information from the history including the current condition and ROS, and then systematically evaluating the clues to determine the origin and extent of the problems.

Based on the therapist's knowledge of anatomy, functions of the nervous system, observational skills, and successful administration of the appropriate screening and detailed tests and measures, information is gathered and used to design interventions that will successfully address the individual patient's problems and customize the plan of care. The sample neurological examination form provided in Appendix 3-A illustrates one possible system that can be used to guide the screening/examination process and to collect, record, and document the examination data, as well as the resulting clinical decisions. A sample pediatric examination form with greater detail specific to the pediatric examination can be found as an appendix with Chapter 13. Refer to these appendices frequently as you read through the remainder of this book. Viewing the entire examination holistically will help put the examination and clinical decision-making in context.

## PATIENT APPLICATION

*Sal, a 38 year-old mother of three, is hospitalized with bilateral paralysis of her lower extremities, trunk, and hands/wrists along with sensory deficits in those same regions resulting from Guillain–Barré Syndrome. After 2 weeks of disease progression, she is now starting to have early, but minimal, motor recovery in her hands/wrists. She was referred for an inpatient physical therapy examination and evaluation. The specific referral reads, "P.T. eval and Rx." As you pull together your thoughts, you have already begun the process of determining how you will gather her history, review her systems, and apply selected tests and measures to verify her impairments of body systems and functional limitations of activities in order to develop an appropriate plan of care for her.*

## Contemplate Clinical Decisions

1. As the PT or OT for this patient, how will you have to adapt your examination because of the significant paralysis in this patient, including positioning the patient and what you will and won't be able to ask her to do?

2. Based on the general information provided, which categories of the physical examination will be most important to help guide the therapeutic intervention?

3. What will be the most important questions to ask to gain the patient's perspective and expectations/hopes?

# Sample Neurological PT Examination Form

Physical Therapy Department

## I. Demographic Information:

Date of Exam_____

Name_____ Age _____ Birthday_____ Race_____ Gender_____

Address_____Phone #_____ (R/L) handed

## II. History: Diagnosis:_____ Physician: _____

- Date of onset:_____
- Circumstances of occurrence:


- Previous medical history (including pregnancy and birth history for infants/children):
- Prior functional status (including achievement of motor milestones for infants/children):
- Equipment or assistive technology used or owned:
- Social situation including home, school/employment, and family support:

- Prior intervention (including involvement of various other disciplines):

- Review of systems:

- Goals of the patient or caregivers:

## III. General:

- Vital signs at rest (note position):
- Vital signs with activity:
- General observation (motor function in various positions including transitions and mobility/walking, W/C use?):

- Patient status:
- Abnormal appearance, posture, non-use:


## IV. Arousal, Alertness, Cognition (Mental Status)/Communication/Perceptual:

- Consciousness: alert, lethargic, obtunded
- Oriented (person, place, and date), confused
- Memory deficit (3 item recall)
- Communication dysfunction
- Screen for perceptual deficits
- Can summarize using some standard Mental Status questions:

| |
|---|
| 1. What is the date today?  ___/___/___ |
| 2. What day of the week is it?_____ |
| 3. What is the name of this place?_____ |
| 4. What is your telephone number? Or what is your address?_____ |
| 5. How old are you?_____ |
| 6. When were you born?_____ |
| 7. Who is the President of the US now?_____ |
| 8. Who was the President before him?_____ |
| 9. What was your Mother's maiden name?_____ |
| 10. Subtract 3 from 20 and keep subtracting 3 from each number all the way down (20, 17, 14, 11, 8, 5, 2). |
| Total number of errors_____ |
| 0—Oriented at all times (0–2 errors) |
| 1—Mild intellectual impairment (3–4 errors) |
| 2—Moderate intellectual impairment (5–7 errors) |
| 3—Severe intellectual impairment (8–10 errors) |

## V. Sensation: Note deficits as appropriate for:

A. **Tactile (superficial)** usually tested by dermatome:  Light touch, pressure, pain/temperature, and tactile localization (which can be tested with any of the above)
B. **Deep sensation** usually tested by body region: Proprioception (position sense), kinesthesia (movement sense), two-point discrimination (with a paper clip, making sure to use equal pressure on both points), and vibration (tuning fork over bony prominences & joint spaces)

C. **Perception**: stereognosis (identifying familiar objects by touch)

|          | Right | Left |
|----------|-------|------|
| Face     |       |      |
| Shoulder |       |      |
| Elbow    |       |      |
| Wrist    |       |      |
| Fingers  |       |      |
| Trunk    |       |      |
| Hip      |       |      |
| Knee     |       |      |
| Ankle    |       |      |

**VI. Motor:** note deficits as appropriate for

     1. **ROM**  2. **Muscle Tone**  3. **Motor Control (stability, movement, coordination)**  4. **Strength**

|          | Right | Left |
|----------|-------|------|
| Face     |       |      |
| Neck     |       |      |
| Shoulder |       |      |
| Elbow    |       |      |
| Wrist    |       |      |
| Fingers  |       |      |
| Trunk    |       |      |
| Hip      |       |      |
| Knee     |       |      |
| Ankle    |       |      |

*[For infants and children, examine ability to perform age-appropriate movement skills in prone, supine, sitting, standing, and walking.]*

**General comments:**

**VII. Cranial Nerves**

|              | Right | Left |
|--------------|-------|------|
| CN II        |       |      |
| CN III, IV, VI |     |      |
| CN V         |       |      |
| CN VII       |       |      |
| CN VIII      |       |      |
| CN XI        |       |      |
| CN XII       |       |      |

**VIII. Equilibrium/Balance**

• Document observations for each position (i.e., independence, upper extremity support, perturbations)

|          | Static | Dynamic |
|----------|--------|---------|
| Sitting  |        |         |
| Standing |        |         |

• Standardized balance assessment tools such as Tinetti (balance and mobility) or Berg _____
• Objective measures:     "Timed Up-and-Go" Test (3m) _____ (s)
                                       Functional reach test sitting_____    standing_____
                                       Force platform data (limits of stability, excursion of center of pressure) _____

*[For infants and children, include assessment of righting and protective responses.]*

**IX. Vestibular Examination** (patient report of symptoms in "history" above)

- Oculomotor and VOR testing

- Positional testing (after VBI clearance ___)

- Vestibular influence on balance and function

**X. Cardiovascular/Pulmonary Support**

- Endurance testing
- Breath support for phonation

**XI. Functional Skills**

- Analyze components of movement and grade level of assistance, assist devices used, and deviations noted
    - Bed mobility: roll to R, roll to L, scooting in bed, supine-to-sit, sit-to-supine, sitting balance, long sitting, lateral scooting
    - Transitions and transfers: scoot in wheelchair, sit-to-stand, stand-to-sit, transfer to bed, toilet, shower, car, floor
    - Wheelchair handling: lock brakes, manage wheelchair parts, feet on/off, pressure relief, propelling, turns, curb, door, wheelie, power drive
    - Developmental progression: prone, quadruped, crawling, kneeling, half-kneeling, standing
    - Gait: temporal and spatial descriptors, distance, assist, gait deviations at each joint
    - Stairs: temporal and spatial descriptors, height of step, number of steps, railings, and assistive devices used

| | |
|---|---|
| Bed mobility | |
| Transfers | |
| Sit-to-stand | |
| Wheelchair handling | |
| Developmental progression | |
| Gait | |
| Stairs | |

*[For infants and children, assess specific age-appropriate functional activities and developmental milestones, including unsupported sitting, creeping/crawling, pull-to-stand, cruising, etc.]*
- <u>Standardized</u> functional outcome measures such as Barthel, Fugl-Meyer, or FIM _____
- As much as possible, emphasize <u>objective</u> measures of pertinent functions (including timed tests) that can be repeated later to document functional improvement such as:

Gait velocity_____     Three-minute walk test_____     Dynamic Gait Index _____
30-Second Chair Stand Test or 5x Sit-to-Stand Test _____

**A: Write a general "Assessment" statement:**

**Rehab potential:**

Functional problem list (prioritize):      Underlying impairments (link to activity limitations):
1.                                          1.
2.                                          2.
3.                                          3.
4.                                          4.
5.                                          5.

**Patient strengths:**

**Potential barriers to progress/discharge from facility:**

Possible long-term goals (ultimate functional skills the patient is expected to achieve) and short-term goals (regarding underlying impairments or stepwise progressions toward the ultimate functional skill) for each functional problem:
LTG 1:
        STG:    1.1.
                   1.2.
LTG 2:
        STG:    2.1.
                   2.2.
LTG 3:
        STG:    3.1.
                   3.2.
LTG 4:
        STG:    4.1.
                   4.2.

P: Plan of care—frequency/duration of skilled intervention:
  Plan of care—components of direct, skilled therapeutic Intervention:
  Plan of care—education of patient and family:
  Plan of care—specific therapeutic activities/exercises to be incorporated at home:

# Screening of Attention, Cognition, Perception, and Communication

Mary T. Blackinton, PT, EdD, GCS, CEEAA
Lisa K. Kenyon, PT, DPT, PhD, PCS ▪ Dennis W. Fell, PT, MD
Mike Studer, PT, MHS, NCS, CEEAA, CWT, CSST

CHAPTER 4

## CHAPTER OUTLINE

## CHAPTER OBJECTIVES

Upon completion of this chapter, the learner should be able to:

1. Describe the rationale for screening attention, cognition, perception, and communication in all patients, including those with neurological dysfunction.
2. Compare and contrast the signs and symptoms of cognitive dysfunction across common neurological disorders.
3. Differentiate valid and reliable tests and measures that can be used to assess attention, cognition, depression, perception, and communication.
4. Describe the procedures used to administer and document cognitive tests and measures.
5. Discuss the therapeutic implications of impairments in attention, cognition, depression, perception, and communication, including the selection of motor-learning strategies, modification of patient/ client-related instruction, and referral to other health-care practitioners.
6. Given a case study, be able to (a) identify what type of screening is needed, (b) select appropriate screening tools, (c) perform the screening, (d) interpret the results, and (e) modify the plan of care based on this interpretation.
7. Describe multidisciplinary and developmental screening tools used to assess attention and cognition in pediatric populations.
8. Discuss the therapeutic implications of impaired cognition and attention in the pediatric population.

# ■ Introduction

*Mr. J* is a 68 year-old male with Parkinson disease who has been referred to outpatient physical therapy for examination and treatment after falling three times in the last month. He has been to this clinic on previous occasions. During the initial examination, it is noted that Mr. J is awake and alert but seems somewhat disheveled and distracted. For example, he opens and closes his wallet several times during the history portion of the examination as if searching for something he lost, and he is wearing his sweatshirt inside out. Mr. J knows his name and date of birth, the correct time, and that he is in the physical therapy clinic at University Hospital. He sheepishly admits however that he got lost trying to get there.

As a physical therapist or future physical therapist, what concerns do you have given this description of Mr. J? Is it normal to appear disheveled and distracted or to get lost? Should you assume if he drove to the hospital himself he has normal cognition? What tests or measures can you use to objectively determine whether Mr. J has attention, cognition, perception, or communication deficits? Would the statement "the patient was alert and oriented times 3" be accurate given this scenario? Would it be thorough? Does it give you enough information on how to best work with Mr. J?

The previous questions can help guide your clinical reasoning regarding cognition when working with patients who have neurological conditions. The *Guide to Physical Therapist Practice* (APTA, 2015) identifies "arousal, attention, and cognition" as one of 24 categories of tests and measures used by physical therapists. Testing arousal, attention, and cognition is especially important when working with patients who have neurological disorders as evidenced by the special issue of the *Journal of Neurological Physical Therapy* (JNPT, 2007) devoted to the understanding of attention and cognition in neurological physical therapy practice. As our knowledge and understanding of brain function and neuroplasticity expands, our focus on attention, cognition, perception, and communication also increases. The purpose of this chapter is to provide an overview for screening attention, cognition, perception, and communication. Specifically, we will review the (a) rationale for screening attention, cognition, perception, and communication; (b) pertinent neuroanatomy and neurophysiology; (c) indications for screening including relevant neurological conditions affecting attention, cognition, perception, and communication; (d) appropriate screening tools, tests, and standardized measures; (e) therapeutic strategies for working with patients with deficits in attention, cognition, perception, and communication; and (f) pediatric considerations in attention, cognition, perception, and communication.

# ■ Rationale for Screening Attention, Cognition, Perception, and Communication

Screening attention, cognition, perception, and communication should be part of every physical therapy examination; however, it is even more important when working with patients with neurological disorders. The rationale for screening cognition, perception, and communication is multifaceted (see Box 4-1). First and foremost, cognition impacts a host of legal and ethical issues related to patient care. In particular, understanding a patient's cognitive status helps us determine the patient's ability to participate in the plan of care, provide informed consent, follow directions, understand safety guidelines, and collaborate with the therapist in developing appropriate goals and interventions (APTA, 2015). Cognitive ability also affects a patient's discharge status, including what type of environment or setting is most appropriate and what type of assistance is needed. Understanding the patient's communication skills is also essential to effectively instruct the patient and understand the patient's needs, concerns, and goals. A patient who uses a communication board or gestures will take longer to communicate his or her needs than one who can verbalize. Likewise, your word choice should vary depending on the receptive communication skills and cognitive abilities of a patient. Selecting the mode of home exercise instruction should be based on the patient's cognitive and communication skills and the patient's preferred learning style. Because not all communication or cognitive skills are apparent during social conversation, it is important to know how to recognize and screen for deficits in an efficient yet effective manner.

A second reason to screen attention, cognition, perception, and communication relates to the therapists' role in screening for disease, including early detection and differential diagnosis of the patient's neurological condition. Cognitive changes in persons with Alzheimer disease (AD), for example, can go undetected early in the disease because cognitive loss is very subtle. Early in the disease process, individuals with AD may be able to carry on a conversation normally and perform self-care tasks, yet he or she may have difficulty performing calculations, word-finding, or interpreting the meaning of a proverb such as "a stitch in time saves nine." These subtle changes are found through the use of standardized mental status examinations, cognitive assessments, and screenings. Early detection of cognitive impairments leads to earlier

---

**BOX 4-1 Why Do We Screen Attention, Cognition, Perception, and Communication?**

- Determine patient's ability to participate in examination and plan of care.
- Determine patient's ability to provide informed consent.
- Plan effective patient instruction strategies and techniques.
- Early detection of disease, including reversible conditions such as depression.
- High incidence of attention, cognition, perception, and communication deficits in patients with neurological diagnoses.
- Plan appropriate strategies that enhance motor learning/motor control.
- Identify patients that need referral to neurologists, occupational and speech therapists.

interventions that may improve quality of life for patients and their caregivers. In addition, some conditions that cause cognitive changes are *reversible* when detected early, including normal pressure hydrocephalus (NPH), electrolyte imbalances, depression in the elderly, and drug side effects/interactions. A rapid decline in a patient's mental status may also indicate a medical emergency such as an extension of stroke, brain tumor, delirium, or the presence of an undetected subdural hematoma. It is thus important to have a baseline assessment of the patient's cognitive function and relate cognitive function to other neurological signs and symptoms.

A third reason for screening these areas in the neurological patient population relates to the high incidence of attention, cognition, perception, and communication deficits in persons with neurological conditions. For example, people with traumatic brain injury (TBI), stroke, Huntington disease (HD), Parkinson disease (PD), Down syndrome, and some cases of cerebral palsy (CP), among others, have a much higher incidence of cognitive dysfunction than the neurologically intact person. There are also subtle differences in cognitive deficits seen between various neurological conditions. The person with PD, for example, typically has difficulty tolerating distractions and making decisions, whereas the individual with HD has poor judgment and behavior changes. Also, many pediatric conditions result in cognitive and attentional deficits including Down syndrome, Angelman syndrome, untreated hydrocephalus, attention deficit hyperactivity disorder (ADHD), and some forms of CP. Children with these conditions may have associated developmental delay, perhaps because of impaired motivation accompanying decreased cognition. Understanding cognitive impairment across the lifespan helps therapists better determine the patient's prognosis and select appropriate interventions. These distinctions are described in more detail later in this chapter (Table 4-2).

Another reason for screening attention, cognition, perception, and communication is the intricate link between these functions to both motor control and motor learning. Motor control results from the interaction of the task, the individual (motor, cognition, perception), and the environment (Shumway-Cook, 2017). Screening attention, cognition, and perception helps provide a complete picture of motor control when combined with functional and other assessment. Likewise, learning/relearning a motor skill (motor learning) is affected by the complexity of the skill and the attributes of the learner, including cognition, attention, perception, and communication. Two types of motor learning processes, explicit (declarative) learning and implicit (procedural) learning, occur in different areas of the brain under different conditions. Anatomically, implicit learning is a function of the cerebellum, basal ganglia, as well as premotor and supplementary motor cortices. Implicit learning occurs *over time* with practice and repetition. Explicit learning is a function of the medial temporal lobes, sensory association cortex, and hippocampus and uses *conscious recall of information and facts* (Shumway-Cook, 2012; Vidoni, 2007). A patient with AD who cannot process verbal commands may respond better to implicit strategies emphasizing practice rather than explicit strategies involving recall of information. Therapists thus need to understand the cognitive skills of all patients to appropriately choose how to provide instruction and feedback or how to organize a practice schedule to enhance motor learning.

Lastly, screening attention, cognition, perception, and communication can provide information leading to appropriate referral to other health-care providers and services. Even subtle changes in cognition should be reported to the primary care physician and may necessitate referral for neurological testing by a neurologist or a neuropsychologist. Likewise, perceptual deficits such as apraxia can be fully examined by a battery of tests performed by an occupational therapist and communication deficits adeptly assessed by a speech-language pathologist. In outpatient and home-health settings, a physical therapist might be the first rehabilitation professional to examine the patient, so it is imperative to screen for dysfunction that may necessitate additional examination and referrals.

## ▪ Arousal, Attention, Cognition

### Introduction and Terminology

Terminology and medical jargon surrounding arousal, attention, and cognition can be very confusing, especially for the novice therapist. **Cognition** is a very broad term, defined as the act of knowing (APTA, 2015). Cognition incorporates multiple functions such as awareness, reasoning, judgment, intuition, and memory; whereas **executive functions** are the cognitive skills involving planning, manipulating information, self-monitoring (recognizing and preventing errors), problem-solving, and abstract thinking (Unsworth, 2007). Dysexecutive syndromes refer to conditions in which individuals have difficulty with planning, cognitive flexibility, initiation and self-generation, response inhibition, serial ordering, and sequencing (Hanna-Pladdy, 2007).

Historically, health-care providers often use the phrase "alert and oriented times 3" to describe a patient's cognitive status in the medical record. It implies the patient is awake and can orient him or herself in at least three ways (Kipps and Hodges, 2005): person (name, age, date of birth), place (location/building), and time (time of day/year). Based on the multiple functions making up cognition, you can see this phrase does *not* reference other important components of cognition including reasoning, judgment, planning, or thinking.

The term **alertness** describes the degree to which a patient is awake, aroused, and attentive. The related term of **awareness** refers to having knowledge of something, the ability to perceive or be aware of a fact, occurrence, or event. **Arousal** is defined as the physiological readiness for activity (APTA, 2015) and can range from being comatose (unresponsive and unable to wake up) to being fully awake. The state of arousal, ranging from fully awake to comatose, is also described as **level of consciousness** (see Table 4-1).

| TABLE 4-1 | Level of Consciousness |
|-----------|------------------------|
| Alert | Awake and attentive. |
| Lethargic | Drowsy and falls asleep easily; will have difficulty maintaining attention. Loud voice needed to keep patient engaged and awake. |
| Delirium | Often seen as a person emerges from **coma**; characterized by confusion of the circumstances. May hallucinate or act as if in dream state; conversation may not make sense. |
| Obtunded | Difficult to arouse from "sleep;" requires repeated stimulation. Often needs a loud voice plus a gentle shake to open eyes. |
| Stupor | Responds only to noxious stimuli and quickly returns to unconsciousness if stimulation stops; unable to interact when aroused. |
| Coma | Patient cannot be roused even with noxious stimuli; reflex motor responses may be seen. Using Glasgow Coma Scale, patient has score of 8 or less. |

Modified from descriptions by Blumenfeld, 2002.

**Attention** is the ability to focus one's consciousness on specific information. Attention is an important component of learning and the first step in forming memories, and is therefore essential in patient-centered, patient-engaged physical rehabilitation. Attentional mechanisms are usually controlled in the nondominant (usually right) hemisphere (Blumenfeld, 2002). Without attention, memories cannot be formed. Attention is affected by consciousness, arousal, awareness, and motivation. It can be categorized into four types (see Box 4-2): selective, divided, alternating, and sustained (McDowd, 2007; Robertson, 1999).

### BOX 4-2 Types of Attention

**Selective attention:** The ability to select important/relevant information while ignoring other sources of information. An example is the ability of a patient to follow the therapist's verbal cues while ignoring nearby conversation.

**Divided attention:** The ability to process more than one source of information or to perform more than one task at a time. An example is the ability to talk while walking or to take money out of a wallet while walking. Divided attention is also referred to as the "dual-task" paradigm because the ability to do two things at once reflects the degree of automaticity of a skill.

**Attention Switching/Alternating attention:** The ability to switch attention between two tasks or sources of information as needed for the task and environment. A common example is when a patient stops conversing to perform a difficult task then resumes talking once complete.

**Sustained attention:** The ability to pay attention over a period of time without losing interest or focus. Sustained attention is also called vigilance, and it is believed to be a function of the right hemisphere. An example of sustained attention is when a therapist asks a patient to perform 15 repetitions of an exercise and the patient must pay attention for the duration of the exercise.

**Mental status testing** is the term used to describe the portion of the neurological examination that assesses mental function. Mental status testing usually includes all of the following components (Blumenfeld, 2002; Gallo, 1988):

- Level of consciousness
- Attention
- Orientation
- Language
- Memory
- Sequencing or alternating
- Logic and abstractions
- Calculation
- Right/left discrimination
- Writing
- Neglect
- Construction of figures

Lastly, **memory** is the ability to initially acquire, store, and recall (remember) information from the past. Memory can involve remembering facts or information or can involve recalling and knowing how to perform a task. Learning and memory can be of two types. **Explicit memory**, also called **declarative memory**, is a "collection of memory systems that together are responsible for the acquisition, retention, and retrieval of information that can be consciously and intentionally recollected" (LaVoie, 2007, p. 135). Examples of explicit memory include remembering a specific fact, a specific event, or the steps required to complete a task. Implicit memory, also called **procedural** or **nondeclarative memory**, cannot be accessed by conscious recall but occurs through unconscious systems such as movement or perception (LaVoie, 2007). Examples of implicit or procedural memory include remembering your phone number or the ability to do something without thinking about it such as dialing a phone number or tying your shoes. Implicit and explicit memory are distinct forms of memory/learning and can be affected differentially under certain conditions. For example, brain injury and alcohol intoxication impair explicit memory but not implicit memory (Hashtroudi, 1984). **Reasoning,** one aspect of normal cognition, involves logical thinking to understand and formulate judgments based on all available information. Using these terms appropriately will help you identify what type of problem your patient has in the medical record as well as when you communicate with other health-care professionals.

## Cognitive Dysfunction Related to Specific Anatomical Regions

Let's begin by reviewing the anatomical areas associated with attention, cognition, perception, and communication (Fig. 4-1: Where Is It?). Because cognitive function is distributed throughout many areas of the brain, cognitive *dys*function varies greatly depending on what portions of the brain are affected.

Memory loss is usually indicative of medial temporal lobe lesions, for example, while poor judgment is characteristic of impairments in the frontal lobes. Likewise, diffuse axonal injury as part of TBI can result in diffuse cognitive dysfunction, whereas a localized infarct of the posterior portion of the left superior temporal gyrus causes Wernicke aphasia. An overview of the anatomical regions of the brain with corresponding cognitive, perceptual, and communication functions and disorders is presented in Table 4-2.

### Hemispheric Specialization of Cognition

Deficits in cognition, perception, and language are also associated with either the dominant or nondominant cerebral hemisphere. The functions of each are quite different (see Table 4-3) and can vary depending on whether an individual is right- or left-hand dominant.

The left hemisphere is dominant in 90% of the population. Impairments will thus vary in function and severity depending on the lesion/disease location and which hemisphere is dominant. This is one of many reasons why two patients with the same diagnosis such as "left middle cerebral artery infarct" may have significant differences in cognitive or communication functions.

### ■WHERE IS IT?

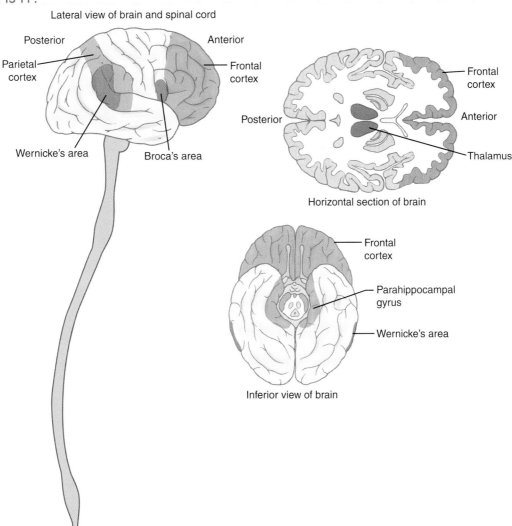

**FIGURE 4-1** The most important neuroanatomic structures related to cognition (blue), perception (green), and communication (red). The specific names of the structures are listed in Table 4-2.

| TABLE 4-2 | Cognitive, Perceptual, and Communication Function by Anatomical Region | |
|---|---|---|
| **STRUCTURE** | **COGNITIVE, PERCEPTUAL, AND COMMUNICATION FUNCTION(S)** | **DISORDERS SPECIFIC TO BRAIN REGION** |
| Frontal Cortex | Three main functions: <br> • Restraint: Includes judgment, foresight, delay of gratification, inhibiting inappropriate behavior, and self-governance <br> • Initiative: Includes curiosity, drive, creativity, mental flexibility, and personality <br> • Order: Includes planning, abstract reasoning, working memory, sequencing, and organization | Dysexecutive syndromes (Hanna-Pladdy, 2007) <br> • Acquired brain injury (ABI) <br> • Anterior or middle cerebral artery stroke <br> • Brain abscess <br> • Frontal lobe seizures <br> • Tumors <br> • Pick's disease <br> • Other diffuse damage: hydrocephalus, anoxia, toxic/metabolic disorders, Alzheimer, depression, Huntington and Parkinson disease |
| Prefrontal Cortex | Recall of long-term memories, planning & hypothesis generation <br> Supports working memory (attention), that is, ability to keep information in mind from a few seconds to several minutes before getting stored as long-term memory | • Amnesia <br> • Attention: all types. Specifically divided attention at the dorsolateral prefrontal cortex (DLPFC) |
| Broca's Area | Left hemisphere: expression of speech | • Broca's aphasia |
| Medial Temporal Lobe: Hippocampal Formation and Medial Diencephalon Anterior Temporal Lobe Superior Temporal Lobe: Primary Auditory Cortex | Primary role in declarative (explicit) memory: the conscious memory of facts, experiences, and events <br> • Merge information over minutes/years; encode/retrieve memory <br> • Loss is evident in bilateral conditions, not unilateral disorders <br> • Memory-meaning of words/knowledge <br> • Dominant hemisphere: language comprehension | • Amnesia <br> • Early Alzheimer disease <br> • Global cerebral anoxia <br> • Wernicke-Korsakoff (thiamine deficiency) <br> • Bilateral posterior cerebral artery infarcts <br><br> • Loss of semantic memory <br> • Wernicke aphasia |
| Occipital Lobe | Visual cortex | • Complete lesions posterior to optic chiasm; loss of contralateral visual field (homonymous hemianopsia). Bilateral loss leads to cortical blindness. |
| Parietal Lobe | • Spatial awareness; usually function of nondominant (right) hemisphere <br><br><br> • Motor conceptualization, planning, and execution | • Hemineglect syndromes <br> • Anosognosia; unaware of deficits <br> • Extinction: Stimulus perceived only when presented unilaterally <br> • Apraxia |
| Parietal Association Cortex | Located at junction of parietal, temporal, and occipital lobes; functions in spatial analysis; helps to localize/move visual objects in space | • Constructional difficulties; unable to draw interlocking pentagons or three-dimensional picture <br> • Contralateral hemineglect; worse in right hemisphere lesions, such that patient ignores opposite side of body and environment |
| Basal Ganglia, Cerebellum, and Thalamus | Initiation of movement, coordination of movement, timing and sequencing of movement. These processes relate to implicit or procedural learning, that is, unconscious learning of a motor task as result of repetition/practice | • Difficulty with implicit/procedural learning <br> • Deficits performing dual tasks during movement |
| Reticular Activating System | Arousal and alertness | • Difficulty staying awake and aroused; distinct from sleeping from fatigue |

Source: Blumenfeld, 2002; Hanna-Pladdy, 2007; Lundy-Eckman, 2007; Vidoni & Boyd, 2007

| TABLE 4-3 | Hemispheric Specialization in Cognitive Functions | |
| --- | --- |
| **LEFT (DOMINANT) HEMISPHERE** | **RIGHT (NONDOMINANT) HEMISPHERE** |
| Language | Visual-spatial skills |
| Skilled motor production or praxis arithmetic skills | Alignment columns/numbers in math |
| Sequencing | Emotional aspects of voice |
| Musical ability in trained musicians | Musical ability in untrained musicians |
| Attends mostly to RIGHT side of body | Attends to both sides of body |

Blumenfeld, 2002

## Cognitive Dysfunction Across Neurological Conditions

The presentation of cognitive dysfunction also varies greatly depending on the underlying disorder or condition (Table 4-4). These differences relate to the anatomical location of the disease, the speed of onset of the disorder and compensatory mechanisms, and physiological processes underlying the condition. AD, for example, has a slow, insidious onset such that early changes are subtle and often go unnoticed. In contrast, persons with severe brain injury resulting from a traumatic incident have a rapid loss of cognitive function related to diffuse axonal injury. Screening for reversible causes of cognitive dysfunction including NPH, medication side effects (see the following section), and depression in older adults can also facilitate timely medical intervention.

## Cognition and Aging

Profound cognitive loss is *not* a normal part of aging. It is important to recognize changes or abnormalities in cognitive status with older adults so further diagnostic testing can be performed. Normal age-related changes in cognition include slower information processing speed, loss of flexibility in thought, and subtle declines in executive functions that *do not* impair the ability to live independently (Hanna-Pladdy, 2007). In contrast, the term **mild cognitive impairment (MCI)** describes subtle noticeable changes in memory and can be detected by clinical tests but do not impair judgment, reasoning, or activities of daily living (Petersen, 2001). Prevalence rates for MCI range from 3% to 19% in persons over 65 and more than 50% of individuals with MCI progress to dementia within 5 years (Gauthier, 2006). It is not clear whether MCI is a precursor to dementia or a distinct clinical entity. Cognitive screening examinations are used to distinguish MCI from normal age-related changes and those associated with dementia (Guo, 2009; Hoops, 2009; Ismail, 2010). In older adults, confusion may also be the first sign of other medical conditions including (1) medication side effects from drugs such as benzodiazepines, (2) metabolic disturbances such as hyponatremia or hypoglycemia, (3) endocrine abnormality such as hypothyroidism, or (4) infectious disease including urinary tract or kidney infections (Gallo, 1988).

**Delirium** is a potentially life-threatening change in cognition affecting people of any age group but is most prevalent in older adults and in intensive care/acute settings, particularly as individuals progress into or out of a minimally conscious state. Prevalence rates reported by Fong (2009) are approximately 1% to 2% in the community but can range from 6% to 56% in hospitals. Rates of delirium for older adults in intensive care units have been reported to be as high as 70% to 87%. Delirium is an acute and transient clinical state consisting of a variety of cognitive symptoms such as confusion, inattention, altered consciousness and orientation, disorganized thought and perception, and hallucinations. The etiology of delirium is multifactorial, including neurotransmitter imbalances related to disease and/or medication, drug or alcohol withdrawal, proinflammatory cytokines, and neuronal injury (Fong, 2009). In contrast to dementia and depression, delirium has an *acute onset* and often presents with altered perception and incoherent speech (Gallo, 1988; Fong, 2009).

As stated, delirium is a potentially life-threatening condition, with mortality rates for individuals admitted to the hospital ranging from 10% to 25% (McCusker, 2002). The seriousness of delirium thus cannot be overemphasized. It underscores the need for having baseline assessments of mental status and paying careful attention to clinical findings reported by other medical practitioners in a patient's medical record. When a patient presents with a sudden change in attention, arousal, or cognition, immediate action should be taken, depending on the potential severity or risk in the situation. These steps include (1) calling 911 to activate the emergency medical system, (2) notifying the attending physician, or (3) referral for definitive neurological assessment.

Age-related changes in cognition occur slowly and can often be helped with compensatory strategies such as taking notes or using reminders. In contrast, progressive cognitive loss resulting from AD ultimately requires supervised care. Because the prevalence of AD increases with age, it is important to recognize age as a risk factor for this disorder. Consider this clinical caveat regarding cognitive function: *Never* assume cognitive decline is normal in the absence of a documented diagnosis of disease. A comparison of dementia and normal age-related changes in cognition are summarized in Box 4-3.

The incidence of AD is approximately 6% to 8% for those over 65; however, the incidence of AD doubles every 5 years after the age of 60 years. This means approximately 30% of those over 85 have AD (Bachman, 1993). Many of the

| TABLE 4-4 | Cognitive Dysfunction Related to Neurological Disorders |
|---|---|
| **DISORDER** | **TYPES OF DEFICITS IN AROUSAL, ATTENTION, OR COGNITION** |
| Acquired Brain Injury (ABI) | Rapid onset of deficits related to a defined injury to the brain. The injury can be traumatic (car accident) or nontraumatic (anoxia). Cognitive dysfunction can be diffuse or focal depending on the etiology.<br>• Disorders of executive function (see glossary)<br>• Possible changes in personality, self-awareness, self-regulation, ability to understand humor, empathize, make appropriate judgments in social behavior<br>• May have problems with declarative memory, procedural memory, or both |
| Alzheimer Disease (AD) | Initially slow, insidious onset with a subtle loss interest or withdrawal from activities and recent memory loss.<br>• As disease progresses, dysfunction includes word-finding (anomia), apraxia, and/or visual-spatial disorders<br>• Advanced stages may see behavioral changes such as wandering, paranoia, agitation, aggression, sexual disinhibition, or failure to recognize family/friends<br>• Cognitive dysfunction is usually seen in absence of other neurological functions: Motor, sensory functions and procedural memory usually spared |
| Huntington Chorea | Destruction of the striatum results in hyperkinetic movement disorder as well as emotional and cognitive disturbances.<br>• Early symptoms include clumsiness, mild chorea, and behavioral disturbances<br>• Progression: Impulsiveness, agitation, anxiety, choreiform movement, and loss of memory; in advanced cases, dementia and loss of movement occurs |
| Creutzfeldt-Jacob | Rapidly progressing dementia caused by infectious agent (prion).<br>• Symptoms include rapid progression of dementia accompanied by visual distortion, EEG changes, ataxia, and myoclonus |
| Multiple Sclerosis (MS) | The National MS Society reports that up to 50% of persons with MS may experience one or more of the following cognitive deficits:<br>• Memory loss, information processing, lack of attention—especially divided attention, difficulty planning, and loss of verbal fluency, cognitive fatigue, or visual-spatial dysfunction<br>• General intellect, long-term memory, conversation skill, and reading comprehension are likely to remain intact |
| Normal Pressure Hydrocephalus (NPH) | Slow and insidious onset; *triad* of symptoms include cognitive decline, gait disturbance, and urinary incontinence.<br>• Often confused with Alzheimer or Parkinson disease<br>• Legs are usually hyper-reflexive<br>• Symptoms can resolve after lumbar puncture or ventricle shunting |
| Parkinson Disease (PD) | Loss of dopamine in Substantia Nigra results in cardinal signs of PD (bradykinesia, rigidity, postural instability, and tremor) and cognitive changes.<br>• Deficits in planning, problem-solving, generating multiple response alternatives, tolerating distractions with a motor task (dual task)<br>• A proportion of those with PD also have AD, while others have bradyphrenia or slowness of thought<br>• Impairment of all five areas of executive function in early stage PD |
| Pick's Disease | • One form of rapidly progressing frontotemporal dementia in which deficits include inappropriate social conduct, impulsivity, disinhibition, loss of flexibility in thought, distractible, and perseveration<br>• Preserved memory and language skills early in the disease |
| Pseudo Dementia (Depression) | Reversible cause of dementia; refers to cognitive decline related to depression in older adults.<br>• Those with pseudodementia are more likely to complain of cognitive loss than those with AD; usually can pinpoint onset of difficulty and often gives up or stops trying during testing |
| Vascular Dementia | • Second-most common cause of dementia resulting from multiple infarcts or hemorrhage either cortically or subcortically<br>• Decline is described as halting or stepwise related to multiple episodes of infarct or hemorrhage |
| Wernicke-Korsakoff | Results from thiamine, niacin, or $B_{12}$ deficiency related to alcoholism or other nutritional syndromes; patients may engage in confabulation or outlandish stories to fill in missing information |

**Sources:** Blumenfeld, 2002; Gallo et al, 1988; Hanna-Pladdy, 2007; National MS Society; Kudlicka et al, 2011; www.nationalmssociety.org

---

**BOX 4-3  Alzheimer Dementia Versus Age-Related Memory Loss**

| Alzheimer Dementia | Age-Related Memory Change |
|---|---|
| Forgets entire experiences | Forgets part of an experience |
| Rarely remembers later | Often remembers later |
| Gradually unable to follow written/spoken directions | Usually able to follow written/spoken directions |
| Gradually unable to use notes as reminders | Usually able to use notes as reminders |
| Gradually unable to care for self | Usually able to care for self |

**Source:** The Alzheimer's Disease Association. Available at: http://www.alz.org/index.asp.

---

cognitive tests described in subsequent paragraphs were designed to screen for dementia.

## Principles of Screening Cognition

### Integrating Cognitive Testing in PT Examination

#### Outpatient and Home Health Settings

Screening cognition begins informally from the moment the therapist meets or observes a patient. In the outpatient and home health settings, first determine whether the patient is awake and aware of his surroundings. These early observations will determine whether further screening is required for attention and arousal. However, even individuals who are awake, socially interactive, and appropriate can have cognitive deficits, so a cognitive screening cannot be ruled out even with interactive patients. As you take the patient's medical history, ask the patient (and caregiver when appropriate) if there has been any difficulty concentrating or any changes in memory. Identify medications that might cause confusion in older adults, including antianxiety drugs such as benzodiazepines and anticholinergic or dopaminergic medications. Observe the way in which the patient answers history and demographic questions. For example, is the patient consistent in his history? Do questions have to be repeated or clarified? Does the patient have difficulty describing the problem? Does he or she avoid filling out forms or questionnaires? Does the patient use humor to deflect answering questions? Inconsistent behavior or gaps in memory are indications to further assess cognition.

#### Inpatient Settings

Therapists working in inpatient environments should begin screening cognition while scanning the patient's medical record, paying attention to medical conditions that might affect cognition, as well as descriptions of the patient's mental status in the admission, nursing, and physician notes. Pay added attention to those patients with a history of loss of consciousness, nutritional deficits, metabolic syndromes, or neurological diagnoses as the risk of cognitive impairment in those individuals is higher. The high incidence of delirium in the inpatient setting makes it important to document cognitive function so, by comparison, subsequent changes can be noted. As in the outpatient or home health setting, it is also important to review the patient's current and past medications for

potential causes of cognitive impairment. Next, compare your own impressions and observations with those recorded in the medical record. It is feasible for patients to experience a change in attention or cognition during the course of an inpatient hospital stay, thus it is imperative to compare your observations with those described by other health-care providers. Do not make assumptions about a patient's cognition and do not document anything you did not assess.

During the initial interview with the patient, begin assessing level of arousal and attention as described for the outpatient settings. Observe the patient's ability to answer questions, follow directions, and communicate his or her needs. Allow time for the weak or tired patient to respond and avoid making quick judgments because of slowed responses. Patients with PD can have bradyphrenia, meaning slowness of thought; make sure to give the patient enough response time. Many patients do not have their hearing aids in the hospital or skilled nursing facility, so also ensure the patient can hear your questions adequately. If it appears the patient has changed from previous assessments, a brief test for attention and cognition should be performed, documented, and communicated with other members of the health-care team. In older adults, the first sign of infection or dehydration is often confusion rather than the traditional signs and symptoms of infection or dehydration. Because therapists spend extended time with each patient, they are more likely to notice confusion or a change in the level of alertness.

### Precautions and Caveats While Screening Cognition

Cognitive testing can make people feel nervous, uncomfortable, or even defensive. Imagine being a patient in a hospital and being asked the following questions by five separate clinicians: "Can you tell me what day it is? What is the name of our president? What hospital are you in?" Or imagine going to an outpatient therapist after a total knee replacement and being asked to complete a cognitive examination. In both cases, the patient could become frustrated because he or she has answered the same questions before or because they don't understand how the questions relate to therapy. Furthermore, testing cognitive skills in general can cause anxiety regardless of age, intelligence, or setting. Knowing this, there are several steps you can take to ease a patient's anxiety and understanding of the screening or examination process.

First, clearly explain to the patient what you are testing in a way that does not cause alarm. For example, "Mr. Smith, I'm going to ask you some questions that will check your thinking and memory skills. Some questions might seem very easy, but others may be hard to answer. This helps me know how best to instruct you in therapy." Or, "Mrs. Smith, I would like to check your reaction time and attention skills. In this test, I would like you to tap the table like this (demonstrate) every time I say the letter 'A' aloud." At all times, maintain the dignity of the patient by using age-appropriate language, tone of voice, and maintaining eye contact.

Patients who cannot answer questions during a cognitive examination may become frustrated or upset. If this occurs, reassure the patient and document the patient's response. Individuals who do not know the right answer may act as if they are insulted or might joke about the question. When this happens, try to calmly redirect the patient to answer the question by acknowledging it might sound silly or strange. Do not continually repeat the same question over and over as it may frustrate the patient. Some cognitive tests allow you to give clues to the patient with points deducted for clues given. However, if you still do not get a response even after cluing, score that question as a zero.

### Sequencing Tests for Arousal, Attention, and Cognition

Clinically, it is impossible to accurately assess cognition when a patient is not aroused or is unable to pay attention. For example, if a patient cannot stay awake, you cannot accurately assess attention. And if the patient cannot pay attention to the examiner, it is difficult to determine cognitive skills such as short- or long-term memory (Kipps and Hodges, 2005). Therefore, it is most effective to screen this system in the following order:

1. Arousal/Alertness
2. Attention
3. Cognition and Executive Function

The tests and measures used to assess each of these areas are outlined in detail in the next section of this chapter. Tests for depression are included here because depression in older adults can manifest as cognitive decline or pseudo dementia (Abrams, 1994). Therapists should be able to competently screen this system to know when to refer for further examination and testing, especially in outpatient settings where care is not coordinated between disciplines. Never assume that another health-care provider has already screened cognition. After the examination or screen, you should document:

- Tests performed; include standardized test forms if applicable
- Patient's response and score on the examination
- Clinical interpretation/assessment of the screening including normative values or cut-off scores (in the "A" or assessment portion of the note)

- Implications for the plan of care, including referral to other specialists

## Tests and Measures for Screening Arousal, Attention, and Cognition

### Testing Arousal: Level of Consciousness

Level of consciousness (see Table 4-1) is best observed in the awake patient before and during your interaction to look for signs of drowsiness or by observing the response of the sleeping or unconscious patient to stimulation. An alert patient will stay awake during conversation even if reporting fatigue, while a **lethargic** patient might start to fall asleep even when sitting up or in midconversation.

When approaching a patient whose eyes are closed and who appears to be asleep, take the following steps:

- Approach the patient, say a *loud* "HELLO" and the patient's name to look for eye opening.
- If eyes open immediately, begin interacting with the patient to determine the ability to stay awake and interact.
- If eyes remain closed, give a gentle shake while saying a second loud "HELLO," provide more stimulation (briskly rubbing hands or arms) while talking louder if still no response. The degree of stimulation the patient needs and how long they remain awake, will determine whether the patient is rated as being **lethargic, obtunded, or in a stupor.**
- If eyes remain closed, provide a noxious stimulus (sternal rub or pinprick) and observe both the type of response such as eyes opening or flexor withdrawal and the ability to interact after the stimulus.

Document the level of consciousness as being alert, lethargic, delirious, obtunded, stupor, or coma (see Table 4-1). Include the patient's actual behavior so a clear picture of the patient's behavior is described. For example, write "Level of consciousness: Patient obtunded—needed gentle shaking to arouse and then needed frequent stimulation to keep eyes open during the physical therapy examination." Using this type of documentation ensures that everyone who reads the medical record understands the patient's behavior. If, in contrast, you are working with a patient who is awake and interactive throughout the session, you can document, "Level of consciousness: Patient alert-awake and interactive throughout session."

Impaired level of consciousness is *never* a normal neurological finding. Furthermore, a decline in level of consciousness from prior observations or compared with previous documentation should be treated as a serious clinical sign or even a potential medical emergency. Severe impairment may indicate damage to bilateral brainstem reticular formation or bilateral lesions of thalamus and cerebral hemispheres. Severe impairment can result from diffuse axonal injury in acquired brain injury, whereas mild impairment may indicate unilateral thalamic or cortical lesions. Toxic and metabolic factors can lead to diffuse changes in the brain as can diseases such as dementia or encephalitis.

## Screening Level of Consciousness in Patients with Coma

Disorders of consciousness include coma, vegetative state, and minimally conscious state. These three states can be distinguished as follows (Giacino, 2002):

- **Coma:** Complete loss of the arousal system, unable to be awakened, with reflex and postural response motor function, and no sleep/wake cycles.
- **Vegetative State:** Loss of awareness to self and environment, sleep/wake cycles, with motor function response to noxious stimuli only.
- **Minimally Conscious State:** "Partial preservation of conscious awareness" (Giacino, 2002, p. 350) including *inconsistent* localized responses to noxious stimulation or sound, verbalization, purposeful behavior such as holding objects and visual pursuit.

The level of consciousness for patients who are comatose can be further assessed using a standardized measure such as the Glasgow Coma Scale (GCS), the Expanded Glasgow Coma Scale, the Rancho Los Amigos Levels of Cognitive Function (LOCF) (Appendix 4-A), and the Coma Recovery Scale-Revised (CRS-R) (Appendix 4-B).

The *GCS* is used to monitor level of consciousness and coma in patients with brain injury, especially in the acute care or trauma setting. It is often documented by the emergency room personnel or attending physician but should be understood by physical therapists. The GCS is broken down into three components (Fischer, 2001). Scoring for each component is described in the following text with a maximum total of 15 points:

- Eye opening (4 = spontaneous opening of eyes; 3 = opening in response to speech; 2 = eye opening to pain; 1 = no eye opening response)
- Best motor response (6 = follows motor commands; 5 = localizes a motor response; 4 = withdraws specifically from a given stimulus; 3 = abnormal flexion response; 2 = abnormal extensor response; 1 = no motor response)
- Best verbal response (5 = verbal response demonstrate personal orientation to location; 4 = confused conversation is the best verbal response; 3 = inappropriate words in response to question; 2 = incomprehensible sounds; 1 = no verbal response)

Results from the GCS are used to track progress over time and to describe the severity of brain injury: ≤8: Severe Brain Injury; 9 to 12: Moderate Brain Injury; 13 to 15: Mild Brain Injury (Fischer, 2001). Factors not related to the coma can affect the patient's responses to each of the three components of the GCS. Eye opening, for example, can be affected by periorbital trauma; verbal response can be affected by aphasia, intubation, hearing loss, or sedation; motor response can be affected by spinal cord or peripheral nerve injury, medications, and pain (Fischer, 2001). The GCS is most often used in acute care and ICU environments.

The *LOCF* tool is used to describe the cognitive and emotional behaviors of a patient who is emerging from a coma or minimally conscious state. The original version of the tool described eight levels of cognitive function, while the most recent version (Hagen, 1997) describes ten levels of cognitive function (Appendix 4-A). Each level describes behaviors representing various aspects of cognitive/emotional function, including responsiveness, irritability, attention, ability to follow directions, appropriateness, verbalizations, and self-directed behaviors. To use the scale, look at the description of behaviors at each level and select the *best* description for the patient, even if not all behaviors describing a given level are present. The 10-item LOCF scale also provides a description of the amount of assistance required for each level such that levels I to III need total assistance; IV to V need maximal assistance; VI needs moderate assistance; VII needs minimal assistance for routine tasks; VIII needs stand-by assistance; and IX needs stand-by assistance on request. Level X means modified independence.

A more recent assessment scale used for patients with altered levels of consciousness is the *CRS-R*. This scale (Appendix 4-B) was developed by Giacino and colleagues in 1991 and revised in 2004. The purpose of the scale is to assist in differential diagnosis, prognosis, and treatment planning for patients in coma (Giacino, 1997; Giacino, 2004). The CRS-R can help distinguish between patients in a vegetative state and a minimally conscious state. The CRS-R consists of six subscales: auditory, visual, motor, oromotor, communication, and arousal; the subscales are structured to reflect cortical, subcortical, and brainstem responses to stimuli (Giacino, 2006). To use the CRS-R scale, clinicians should follow the *standardized instructions* for each item. The CRS-R is usually administered at regular intervals to assess changes in neurological status as patients emerge from coma.

### Testing Attention

As described in Box 4-2, there are four distinct types of attention. Although a full discussion of attention testing is outside the scope of this text, there are several simple tests that provide information regarding the patient's ability to attend. Remember, attention is tested once it has been determined the patient is awake and alert. Attention is sometimes assessed by asking the patient to spell a word backward, count backward by 7s, or say the months of the year in reverse order (Kipps and Hodges, 2005). Two tests of sustained attention, the Digit Repetition Test and the Test of Vigilance, are easy and quick to administer but assess sustained attention in different ways. It is not necessary to perform both tests on one patient. The Test for Vigilance can be used for an individual who is awake (with/without verbal communication), while the Digit Repetition Test can only be used in a person who can verbalize.

The *Digit Repetition Test* measures sustained attention by having the patient pay attention to and repeat a progressively longer series of digits, beginning with three digits and progressing to seven if the patient is capable (Strub, 2000). To perform the test, sit facing the patient and describe the purpose of the test in easy-to-understand terminology such as, "I'm going to see how well you pay attention." Then give the instructions for the test and give the patient an example (see Box 4-4). The numbers should be read as single digits and not in pairs, that is, 8-2-5-3 *not* 82, 53. The score is recorded as the highest series of digits the patient is able to repeat (three,

---

**BOX 4-4 Sample Directions for Digit Repetition Test**

"I will read you a group of numbers. After each set of numbers I read, please repeat them back to me. I will start with only three numbers in a row. Each time the list will get longer. For example, I might start with the number 276 and ask you to repeat that, then the number 3981 and I'll ask you to repeat that, until I get to seven digits in a row. Ready? Let's begin: 159 (pause for response) 2658 (pause) 47913 (pause) 628470 (pause) 9125036."

---

four, five, six, or seven). For normative comparison, adults of average intelligence are able to remember seven plus or minus two digits in a row (Strub, 2000).

The *Test of Vigilance*, also called the *a-Test*, is a test of sustained attention that asks the patient to listen and respond each time they hear the letter "A" when intermixed in a long series of random letters. The patient is instructed to tap the table with one hand each time the letter "A" is stated, and thus the patient does not need to be able to talk to take this test (see Box 4-5). The a-Test is part of the Montreal Cognitive Assessment (MoCA) presented later in this chapter. The a-Test is useful if the patient has Broca aphasia or has tubes or conditions that prevent talking. Follow the procedures previously described for telling the patient what you will do and why. Make sure the letters are read at a steady pace, and do not pause or hesitate before or after reading the letter "A."

The a-Test is scored by the number of errors, including omitting a tap or tapping when a letter other than "A" has been read (Strub, 2000). Individuals who have normal attention should be able to identify *every A in the list,* so any error is identified as inattention.

*Motor impersistence* is another sign of inattention you can observe. This is a gross test of attention that is very easy to administer for even fast screening and in any setting. However, it is a sign of inattention and not a standardized test. Ask the patient to close their eyes, stick out their tongue, or raise their arms for 30 seconds. The inability to *sustain the motor activity* can indicate inattention (Blumenfeld, 2002), although there might be other reasons affecting performance such as pain, weakness, fear, or lack of understanding. In

---

**BOX 4-5 Testing Sustained Attention Using the Test of Vigilance (a-Test)**

I will read a long list of letters from the alphabet. Every time you hear the letter "A" I want you to tap your hand on the table like this [demonstrate]. So, if you hear me say D-Z-A, then tap the table right as you hear "A" and every time after. Ready? Let's begin:

B U A I Y R A P M A N V C T A A L W X I R A Q A P Z R I M A A W T C N Q E Y A Y A L K A V X S E D R T A Z D O A U Y S A A R V X A I L C ..."

---

testing motor persistence, choose an area of the body you know is not affected by weakness, hemiparesis, or pain.

*Divided attention* can be assessed by asking the patient to do two things at once; this is also referred to as a "dual-task" condition (Hall, 2011; McCulloch, 2007; Verghese, 2002). The dual-task scenario can consist of two cognitive tasks, two motor tasks, or a combination of cognitive and motor tasks. Of particular interest to physical therapists is combining functional mobility (walking) with thinking tasks to determine the effect of divided attention on balance. The Walking While Talking Test (WWTT) times the patient while he/she walks 20 feet, turns, and returns 20 feet while performing a simple talking task (saying the alphabet aloud), then repeating the test with the more complex cognitive task (saying every other letter in the alphabet). The test was designed for older adults who are independent (although they may use an assistive device) but who do not have dementia. Verghese and colleagues found that the WWTT test could predict falls in older adults on both the simple talking test (cut score of 20 + seconds) and in the complex talking test (cut score of 33 + seconds).

More recently, Hall (2011) found that, while performance on the simple cognitive task is associated with gender, quality of life, and preferred gait speed, performance on the complex walking task is also associated with cognitive skills such as sustained attention, divided attention, and working memory. Assessing dual-task conditions during walking is thus an appropriate method to screen older patients for balance dysfunction and because of its link to cognitive function was included in this chapter. Dual-task tests can be used for patients with and without MCI, including older adults with minimal cognitive impairment (Montero-Odasso, 2009). Box 4-6 provides an example of how to apply a dual-task condition to the Timed Up and Go (TUG) test, a test of physical mobility.

Patients with brain injury typically have difficulty with attention, which may complicate an intervention session and

---

**BOX 4-6 Testing a Dual Cognitive and Motor Task Timed Up and Go-cognitive (TUG-c)**

The cognitive task in this example is the ability to subtract from 50 by 3s; the motor task is the time it takes to stand, walk 3 meters, turn around, walk back 3 meters to the chair, and sit down (back touching chair).

- Begin by measuring each skill separately:
  - Count the number of errors when subtracting by 3s from 50.
  - Measure the time it takes to complete the TUG-c, and also note overall gait characteristics such as symmetry, cadence, and rhythm.
- Next, ask the patient to count backward by 3s from 50 while performing the TUG-c.
- Calculate or describe the difference in performance between single- and dual-task conditions. For example, it might take 15 seconds to perform the TUG-c as a single task but 31.5 seconds to do so during a dual-cognitive task.

limit adherence to a home exercise program (HEP). After brain injury, deficits in attention include difficulty sustaining attention, resisting distractions, and deciding where to focus one's attention (Hart, 2008). Whyte and colleagues (2003) developed a test for attention specifically for people with brain injury called the *Moss Attention Rating Scale* (MARS) (available from the Center for Outcome Measurement in Brain Injury at http://www.tbims.org/combi/mars/index.html). The MARS is completed on a form; however, it was designed so clinicians rate the patient's behavior based on their observations over a period of time rather than from just one encounter. All 22 items on the scale should be completed to calculate a score (Hart, 2008). Each item is rated on a five-point ordinal scale, and the total score ranges from 22 to 110, with higher scores meaning better attention. The MARS can also be used to calculate three subscores: restlessness/distractibility (items 1, 10, 12, 17, and 22), initiation (items 7, 13, and 19), and sustained/consistent attention (items 6, 14, and 15).

## Testing Cognition

### Mental Status Testing

Once you have established the patient is awake, alert, and attentive, you can assess the patient's ability to think and process information cognitively. The most common mode to screen cognition in adults is also termed mental status testing. This section will compare and contrast three commonly used tests for mental status: the Mini-Mental Status Examination (MMSE), the Addenbrooke Cognitive Examination-Revised (ACE-R), and the MoCA.

First described by Folstein (1975), the *MMSE* is the most widely used tool to screen for mental status impairments (Cullen, 2007). It is no longer in the public domain, and the form can only be obtained from the current copyright owner, Psychological Assessment Resources. The MMSE was designed as a simple tool that can be used by clinicians to quickly screen for cognitive impairment. Critics of the MMSE note it is heavily weighted in the domain of orientation (person/place/time) and verbal cognition and is unable to differentiate MCI from AD (Mitchell, 2009). Analyses of the MMSE items have identified the calculation and recall items have higher sensitivity than the orientation items (Cullen, 2007). A recent meta-analysis revealed the MMSE is most accurate when confirming a diagnosis of dementia in a specialist setting (i.e., memory disorder clinic) or when ruling out dementia in nonspecialist settings (Mitchell, 2009). The MMSE lacks attention to the nondominant hemisphere and executive function.

The *ACE-R* was developed to provide a brief test sensitive to the early stages of dementia and to distinguish between the many subtypes of dementia (Mioshi, 2006). The test takes between 12 to 20 minutes to administer and score and measures 5 subscores, each representing a different domain, including attention/orientation, memory, fluency, language, and visuospatial skills. The maximum score is 100, and 88 has been identified as the standard cut-off score. When scores are ≤82, likelihood of the patient having dementia is 100:1 (Mioshi, 2006). Using a cut-off score of 88, the ACE-R has better sensitivity (72%) in detecting cognitive impairments in people

with brain injury compared with the MMSE (36%), with a cut-off score of 27 (Gaber, 2008).

The *MoCA* was also developed as a quick screening instrument for MCI and was designed to overcome some of the limitations in the MMSE by adding more items related to executive functioning (Nasreddine, 2005). The MoCA (Appendix 4-C) is available as a free download in 36 different languages from the researcher's website (http://www.mocatest.org/). The test includes items that address a broad range of cognitive function, including an alternating trail-making test, visuoconstructional skills (cube and clock drawing), naming, memory, attention including forward and backward digit span and the a-Test for vigilance, sentence repetition, verbal fluency, abstraction, delayed recall, and orientation. The MoCA takes approximately 10 minutes for experienced clinicians to administer and is available for public use by clinicians and researchers. Using a cut-off score of <26, the sensitivity for the MoCA is 90% for detecting MCI and 100% for detecting AD (Nasreddine, 2005). The MoCA also attempts to account for differences in educational levels by adding 1 point for persons who have 12 years or less of schooling. The MoCA has also been shown to be sensitive for detecting dysfunction in people with HD (Videnovic, 2010) and in people with PD (Hoops, 2009), yet the MMSE remains the most frequently used tool because of its familiarity to clinicians (Ismail, 2010).

### Staging Alzheimer Disease

If a patient already has known cognitive decline related to AD, it is not necessary to test cognition using mental status testing. There are several tools used to classify the progression of AD from a functional and cognitive viewpoint. One such tool is described in the following section, the Global Deterioration Scale (GDS). Although not a cognitive screening tool per se, the GDS is useful in characterizing the cognitive functioning of older adults with AD, to track the progression of AD, or to assist the family in making caregiving decisions. Although not typically performed by the physical therapist, it is helpful to review the stages of AD described by the GDS to appreciate the progression of the disease, communicate with other healthcare providers, and recognize the great variability in persons with AD.

The GDS is a global staging scale used to describe cognitive change over time for assessment of primary degenerative dementia based on normal aging and on AD. The six stages include (Reisberg, 1982):

- Stage 1. No Cognitive Decline
- Stage 2. Very Mild Cognitive Decline: Forgetfulness of names and where familiar objects were left.
- Stage 3. Mild Cognitive Decline: Forgetfulness of people recently introduced. Slight difficulty concentrating. Decreased work performance. Getting lost. Difficulty finding words.
- Stage 4. Moderate Cognitive Decline: Difficulty concentrating. Decreased memory of recent events. Difficulties managing finances or traveling alone to new locations. Cannot complete complex tasks efficiently or accurately. Possible denial and social withdrawal.

- Stage 5. Moderately Severe Cognitive Decline (Early Dementia): Some assistance required to survive. Memory loss more prominent, including major relevant aspects of current lives, for example, address or phone number. May not know the time or day or where they are. May have difficulty clothing themselves properly.
- Stage 6. Severe Cognitive Decline (Middle Dementia): Starts to forget names of close family and memory of most recent events. Remembers only some details of earlier life. Difficulty counting down from 10 and finishing tasks. Frequently become incontinent. Personality changes such as delusions (believing something to be true that is not), compulsions (repeating a simple behavior such as cleaning), or anxiety and agitation may occur.
- Stage 7. Very Severe Cognitive Decline (Late Dementia): Essentially no ability to speak or understand. Assistance needed with most activities (e.g., toilet, eating). Loss of psychomotor skills, for example, the ability to walk.

The GDS provides a composite picture of cognitive, functional (ADL), and emotional/psychological dimensions related to AD. Stages 1 to 4 of the GDS scale reflect normal age-related cognitive changes without dementia, while stages 5 to 7 reflect cognitive deterioration in AD termed early, middle, and late dementia (Reisberg,1982). The GDS is usually administered by mental health professionals when interviewing both the patient and a caregiver (Sclan and Kanowski, 2001). The clinician reads the descriptions of abilities and behavior in each category and selects the level that *best* describes the patient's function. For example, if your patient had memory loss of important information (address or phone number) and occasionally had difficulty dressing appropriately, you would select Level 5 on the GDS. This is very different from the patient who has difficulty remembering recent events or finding new locations: Level 4 on the GDS. Thus, the therapist or an interdisciplinary team can use these tools to grossly characterize cognitive function in the patient with a known diagnosis of dementia.

### Testing Cognition After Acquired Brain Injury

Testing cognitive skills in patients after brain injury requires a separate set of tools from those used for patients with cognitive loss and dementia. The MMSE, for example, was not intended to be used with children, young adults, or patients with acquired brain injury. The ACE-R has been tested in people with stroke, TBI, and PD (Gaber, 2008; Parsons, 2011; Rittman, 2013). The LOCF, discussed previously under the heading "Level of Consciousness," and the Cognitive Log (Cog-Log) are instruments more appropriate to patients with cognitive dysfunction after brain injury or concussion.

The *Cog-Log* (Appendix 4-E) is a tool used to monitor cognition over time after brain injury with more emphasis on memory and executive function rather than on orientation. This test was designed to be a quick screen of cognitive function that could be performed quickly during morning rounds in the inpatient environment to track change over time

(Alderson, 2003; Lee, 2004; Novack, 2004). The Cog-Log is used when its counterpart, the Orientation-Log (O-Log) yields a score of 15 or greater (Novack, 2004).

The Cog-Log has 10 items, each rated on a three-point scale and standardized instructions for the rater (see Appendix 4-E, "Administration and Scoring"). The total possible score on the Cog-Log is 30. Nonimpaired adults scored an average of 28 + 2, while a cut-off score of 25 accurately distinguished impaired versus nonimpaired 88.4% of the time (Lee, 2004; Novack, 2004). Research has confirmed usefulness of Cog-Log as a general measure of cognitive skills in patients recovering from brain injury (Novack, 2004). Following the standardized directions is important and cannot be overemphasized.

The *Galveston Orientation and Amnesia Test (GOAT)* is a screening tool used for individuals who have post-traumatic amnesia (Levin, 1979). **Post-traumatic amnesia (PTA)** is the loss of memory regarding events pre- and post-brain injury as well as a loss of ability to process information after brain injury. In fact, PTA can occur after mild injuries such as a concussion during a football game or from more serious brain injury. The GOAT was designed to monitor and track recovery of cognitive function after PTA. In addition to the focus of the GOAT on orientation to person, place, and time, it has items assessing the degree of **retrograde amnesia** (loss of memory related to events before the brain injury) and **anterograde amnesia** (loss of memory related to events after the brain trauma). Score ranges can be used to categorize patients: 76 to 100 normal, 66 to 75 borderline, and <66 impaired cognitive function (Levin, 1979; Davidoff, 1988). The GOAT was designed for use serially over several hours/days to track change over time. Scores of 78 or more on three consecutive occasions indicate the patient is out of PTA (Levin, 1979).

When performing either the Cog-Log or GOAT, pay attention to the directions on the form. The Cog-Log can be employed several times in 1 day, while the GOAT is generally performed once daily. There is no need to use both of these items for a single patient, select the test most appropriate to the patient's situation and the environment in which the test is performed.

How is the LOCF different from the Cog-Log or GOAT? The LOCF (Appendix 4-A) is a tool tracking a broad range of emotional and cognitive function as a person emerges from coma or minimally conscious state. It is not administered by asking the patient specific questions as is done with the Cog-Log or GOAT. Rather, the therapist and health-care providers make a holistic assessment of cognitive function based on cognitive and emotional behaviors displayed by the patient and observed by the therapist. The LOCF is generally used within the first year after brain injury and is less useful in higher functioning patients (McCulloch, 2013). These levels often differentiate important characteristics of individuals recovering from brain injury. For example, a patient in the Confused-Appropriate stage (Level VI-Moderate Assistance) can demonstrate goal-directed behavior with supervision, whereas a patient at Level IV (Confused-Agitated) demonstrates sometimes bizarre behavior inappropriate to the environment. These distinctions will influence the plan of care, therapeutic activities, and the environment within which the patient is treated.

Lastly, the CRS-R was designed as a test for persons with disorders of consciousness as part of differential diagnosis between three altered levels of consciousness: vegetative state, minimally conscious state, and emergence from minimally conscious state (Donnelly, 2013). The CRS-R evaluates auditory function, visual function, motor function, oral-motor/verbal function, communication, and arousal. The full instrument and directions can be accessed at http://tbims.org/combi/crs/CRS%20Syllabus.pdf.

### Quantification and Management of Agitation

Some persons with cognitive dysfunction also display agitation. Agitation is a common feature of acquired brain injury as well as late stages of Alzheimer and Pick's disease. Assessing the level of agitation can help document change in behavior over a 24-hour period or to note responses to drug or behavioral therapies and to help caregivers understand the range of behaviors occurring in one individual. The Agitated Behavior Scale (ABS) was developed to describe the degree and nature of agitation after brain injury but can also be used with other populations such as those with dementia or stroke (Bogner, 2000; Corrigan, 1995). The ABS was designed to monitor agitation over a period of time and document trends in behavior either by time of day or over the course of recovery. There are 14 behavior items on the ABS (Appendix 4-F); each of the items describes a type of agitated behavior such as "explosive and/or unpredictable anger." The total score is calculated by adding the ratings (from one "absent" to four "present to an extreme degree") on each of the 14 items. Raters are instructed to leave no blanks; but, if a blank is left, the average rating for the other 14 items should be inserted so the Total Score reflects the appropriate possible range of values. The Total Score is the best overall measure of the course of agitation (Corrigan, 1989; Corrigan and Bogner, 1994). Thus, higher scores on the ABS mean greater (worse) agitation.

Subscale scores for the ABS are calculated by adding ratings from the component items:

- Disinhibition is the sum of items 1, 2, 3, 6, 7, 8, 9, and 10.
- Aggression is the sum of items 3, 4, 5, and 14. (It is not an error that Item 3 is in both scores.)
- Lability is the sum of items 11, 12, and 13.

To allow subscale scores to be compared with each other and to the Total Score, it is recommended an average item score for each factor be calculated and multiplied by 14 (Bogner, 2000). This procedure provides subscale scores with the same range as each other and the Total Score, which is useful for graphic presentation. According to a review by Bogner, 21 or less is considered within normal limits; 22 through 28 mild agitation; 29 through 35 moderate agitation; and more than 35 is considered severe agitation.

### Therapeutic Management for Patients With Agitation

What causes agitation, and how can you minimize occurrence of agitation? Consider this metaphor: Having limited cognitive function is similar to having a limited amount of money in your wallet. If you try to purchase something and do not have enough money, you are likely to become frustrated because your needs can't be met. When cognitive function is limited, demands that surpass cognitive resources create frustration, which further taxes the limited cognitive system. Patients with cognitive dysfunction can become agitated when therapists overload the patient with too many or too difficult tasks, or even if therapists provide too much feedback. Figure 4-2 represents *preventable* causes of agitation that can emanate from a therapy session.

Many other causes of agitation exist, but the most important point is to AVOID losing rapport with your patients by making them more agitated. Patients who are still in PTA may not remember who they are but somehow might recall you have upset them recently. In addition to avoiding behaviors that can induce agitation, pay close attention to possible early warning signs of patient agitation such as avoidance of eye contact so you can modify your behavior or treatment plan accordingly (Box 4-7).

As previously mentioned, frequent feedback and task overload are common therapeutic practices and, as stimuli, can cause the patient to become agitated. Challenging patients with obvious retention tests such as "What is my name?" and asking them to self-monitor are just as likely to cause agitation. Retention testing is best completely unannounced for patients with agitation. For example, instead of saying, "Let's see if you remember how to go up the steps," instead say, "Let's go up the steps." Therapists may share the results without letting the patient realize they were secretly tested moments ago. In addition, patients who are gaining some insight to their deficits often attempt to deny the deficits, so a request for self-monitoring becomes an unwanted challenge as well.

The final two remaining items in Figure 4-2 are contrived treatments and delayed assistance. Delayed assistance refers to allowing the patient to fail to the point they perceive danger or they are being labeled inferior or ignorant. Many patients with cognitive deficits begin to develop a dependent mentality so, when faced with a problem, the therapist or nurse should recognize the dilemma and complete the task for them to prevent failure. Contrived practice refers to the use of games or simulations to improve a skill. It can cause agitation in patients who aren't aware of their deficits, so they may ask, "Why am I doing this stupid game?" In some cases, patients recognize poor performance in practice but rationalize the task was meaningless and nonsense. Therapists thus monitor

---

**BOX 4-7  Acute Warning Signs of Agitation in Patients With Brain Injury**

Restlessness
Decreased visual contact
Decreased verbal output
Increased loudness of voice
Increased distractibility
Negative, *self*-deprecating comments

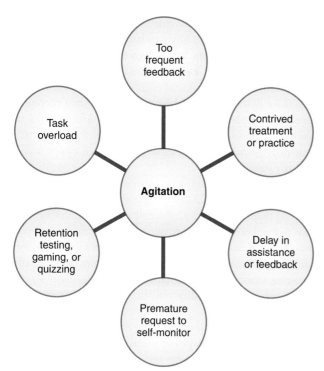

**FIGURE 4-2** Common reasons for preventable therapist-induced agitation. The therapist should observe for and avoid these factors in a treatment session.

physical and cognitive signs of intolerance when working with cognitively impaired adults.

Note that the word "self" is italicized in the list of warning signs of agitation found in Box 4-7. When patients begin to make negative comments about others, they have already crossed into the area of agitation. It is important to recognize the warning signs to prevent further progression into agitation. When a patient becomes agitated, remove the patient from the stimuli or change the stimuli promptly. Pay attention to your patient's patterns as they pertain to agitation as some patients may become agitated with direct intent to avoid therapy.

In patients with AD, agitation is believed to have four root causes: (1) pathophysiological when neural deterioration leads to disinhibition of behaviors; (2) behavioral, including people or situations (caregiver removing patient clothing for a shower) that impact the patient; (3) unmet needs such as hunger or thirst, because the patient with AD has difficulty communicating needs and thus their needs are often unmet; and (4) environmental vulnerability indicating a decreased threshold to environmental stressors such as lights or loud noises (Kovach, 2004). Therapists should keep these root causes in mind to minimize agitation. If a patient with AD becomes upset, it may be some basic need such as hunger or comfort is not being met. Therapists can assess the situation by being alert for physical signs of unmet needs such as dehydration or fatigue. Similar to the strategies suggested for people with brain injury, monitor the amount of feedback you give the patient during therapy. You can easily redirect a patient to turn left with gentle hand encouragement rather than with verbal cues. Likewise, limit background noises such as IV beeping, radio music, or construction work/hammering.

Taking the time to avoid agitated responses will greatly enhance your therapeutic environment for patients with AD.

### Screening Awareness

**Self-awareness,** the ability to recognize, perceive, and reflect on aspects of one's own personality, character, and behavior/responses, has been described as one of the most important elements of executive function in persons with brain injury because it impacts other cognitive functions such as attention, memory, and problem-solving (Studer, 2007). Impaired self-awareness can be one of the most detrimental losses a patient can sustain. It often leads to agitation, decreased motivation/participation, or unsafe behavior with regard to their "new" set of abilities. Patients with the most severe awareness deficits have no reason to attend to the therapist or remember any new information, as it does not appear to hold relevance in their lives. Awareness is often associated with right parietal and frontal lobe function. Therefore, some of the most impaired patients, those with TBI and right hemisphere stroke, have limited awareness.

The term **anosognosia** is used to describe a patient without any sense of self-awareness of their deficit; the patient with anosognosia will usually deny a problem exists. Anosognosia is considered a body scheme disorder (see proceeding section on perception), but because of its impact on attention and executive function, it will be discussed as a component of cognition at this juncture. Levels of awareness beyond anosognosia have been described by Crossen and colleagues (1989) as follows:

- *Intellectual awareness: "I can see that I have a problem."*
  - These patients recognize a new health issue but may not recognize the extent, existence, or meaning of the problem. Inability to recognize the problem can lead to agitation in patients with TBI (Studer, 2007).
  - Screen for this skill by asking the patient what difficulties he/she is having since injury/illness or ask how it has affected his life (Zoltan, 2007).
- *Emergent awareness: "A problem is occurring."*
  - A patient who has emergent awareness will recognize a shirt is inside out or that he/she has lost balance and requires the skill of self-monitoring (Studer, 2007).
  - Evaluate for this skill by noticing if the patient is able to recognize and correct a problem while it is occurring.
- *Anticipatory awareness: "I need to avoid this problem."*
  - Described as the highest level of awareness, the person with anticipatory awareness is able to remember previous attempts and problems and change behavior as a result (Studer, 2007). For example, a patient who has fallen while trying to get up off the commode will call for assistance to prevent a reoccurrence of a fall. Memory notebooks can also be used to help with future recall.
  - To evaluate this level, observe the patient in real tasks and also ask questions such as "Do you think you'll have a problem doing ___?" If the patient answers yes, ask why. Avoid cuing the patient or biasing his response (Zoltan, 2007).

## Screening for Delirium

Several tools can be used to screen or rate delirium. Because delirium occurs with much higher frequency in the acute-care and intensive-care unit (ICU) environments, many bedside tools have been developed including the Cognitive Test for Delirium (CTD), Confusion Assessment Method (CAM), Confusion Assessment Protocol (CAP), and Delirium Rating Scale-Revised-98 (DRS-R-98). The CAM is a screening tool using the presence of multiple signs of delirium (A-D following) to *identify* delirium. Of the following list of symptoms A through D, the patient must present with signs A, B, and C or signs A, B, and D to be considered delirious. Sign A is an acute confusional state that fluctuates in severity; B is inattention; C is disorganized thought or speech; and D is a change in level of consciousness such as hypoactivity or hyperactivity (Woodford and George, 2007).

In contrast, the DRS-R-98 is a scale designed to rate the *severity* of delirium. There are 13 behaviors rated on a 0 to 2 scale (higher numbers indicating worse symptoms) and 3 additional diagnosing items. The 13 characteristics rated on severity include altered sleep-wake cycle, perceptual disturbances, delusions, labile affect, language abnormalities, abnormal thought processes, motor agitation or motor retardation, orientation, attention, short- and long-term memory, and visuospatial items (Trzepacz, 2001). Therapists who work in the ICU or acute care setting may be asked to look for these characteristics during physical therapy sessions and/or participate in using the DRS-R-98.

## Screening for Depression

Depression is the most prevalent cause of pseudodementia in the elderly, and screening for depression helps distinguish between the two conditions. You should screen for depression when mild cognitive deficits are noted during the history and cognitive screen or when cognitive signs are accompanied by other signs and symptoms of depression such as irritability and sleep disturbances. Individuals with chronic health conditions such as diabetes, PD, and stroke have higher incidences of depression than other adults. Older adults who are depressed are more likely to present with signs of apathy, anhedonia (lack of pleasure and joy), and cognitive dysfunction than their younger counterparts (Krishnan, 1995). In particular, cognitive disturbances in depressed older adults include a decline in memory and executive functioning.

There are several differences between cognitive decline resulting from dementia and decline related to depression (see Table 4-4). Patients who are depressed are more likely to complain of cognitive loss than those with AD; they usually can pinpoint when the difficulty began and often give up on cognitive questions or stop trying during cognitive testing. Patients with dementia have a more insidious onset of cognitive decline and do not usually complain about forgetting.

Two tests for depression are included in this chapter, the Geriatric Depression Scale (GDS) (Appendix 4-G) and the Beck Depression Inventory-Short Form (Appendix 4-H). When screening for depression, it is important to tell the patient what you are doing and why (see Box 4-8). Allow the patient

to complete the inventory alone if he/she is able to read and use a pen or read the items and their choices to the patient if he/she needs assistance. Be careful not to intervene or interpret with the patient's response when you are reading the choices.

In both scales, higher scores indicate depression. In the *GDS*, 1 point is scored for each "depressed" response (answer in bold). Scores of 0 to 4 are considered normal, 5 to 8 indicate mild depressive symptoms, 8 to 11 indicate moderate depressive symptoms, and 12 to 15 indicate severe depressive symptoms (Krishnan, 1995). In the *Beck Depression Inventory* (short form), scores of 5 to 7 indicate mild depression, 8 to 15 indicate moderate depression, and 16 or higher indicate severe depression (Gallo, 1988). Patients with depressive symptoms should be referred to appropriate specialists in psychology, psychiatry, or social work. Therapists can remind patients that exercise is one of many treatments for depression.

## THINK ABOUT IT 4.1

Your approach to assessing arousal, attention, awareness, and cognition will vary depending on the patient, setting, and situation. A few key questions to consider regarding cognitive assessment follow. Think of a recent patient and answer these questions.

1. Does the patient's medical history, comorbidities, medications, or diagnoses potentially interfere with attention, arousal, or cognition?
2. Do your observations of the patient or interactions with the patient match the mental picture you have in your mind regarding his or her condition?
3. Do your observations of the patient or interactions with the patient match other health professionals' descriptions in the medical record or patient history?
4. Are there any unique attributes of the health-care setting that might influence this patient's cognition? For example, was the patient awakened throughout the night in an inpatient setting because of a noisy roommate or medical procedures? Could being in a new setting influence the patient's behavior or cognition? Did the patient recently lose a spouse, child, or good friend?
5. How does adapting *your* strategies influence the patient's response? For example, does the patient appear more agitated the more you talk? Do gestures work better than words? Does the patient respond better in a quiet environment?

# Therapeutic Implications for Patients With Cognitive Loss

Therapists use the information from screening arousal, attention, cognition, and depression in their clinical decision-making, including determination of the patient's diagnosis, prognosis, plan of care, and selecting interventions (APTA, 2015). These impairments may necessitate a modification in the selection of interventions, the therapy environment, or the types of motor-learning strategies used by the clinician. Findings from the screenings should be documented in the medical record and communicated with other members of the healthcare team, including the patient and caregivers. Use the "assessment" component of your note to document the clinical decisions you make based on this information. For example, you might write, "based on the patient's cognitive function, functional training will focus on skill practice with minimal verbal cues supplemented with demonstration or gestures in order to minimize patient frustration."

## Interventions for Nonalert Patients

If the patient has moderate to severe deficits in *arousal,* physical therapy interventions will emphasize prevention of secondary complications from immobility, decreasing risk of falls or injury, and instructions to caregivers on prevention and restorative techniques. The plan of care for a patient in Level I-II of the LOCF or a patient in the late stages of AD should include prevention of joint contractures, skin breakdown, or injury to self. Caregivers may need training in positioning techniques to decrease pressure on bony prominences or maximize air exchange as well as instruction on how to protect themselves from injury while caregiving. Moderate to severe deficits in arousal, attention, or cognition are most effectively addressed by a team of professionals, including nurses, respiratory therapists, occupational therapists, neurologists, speech-language pathologists, and social workers for discharge planning.

## Strategies for Patients Having Difficulty With Attention

Mild to moderate deficits in *attention* also require some modification of physical therapy interventions. When patients have impairments in attention and cognition, the treatment environment should initially have few distractions. Therapists can gradually introduce changes to the environment such as adding more people or objects in the treatment area. Therapists can also direct the patient's attention during the intervention. The "power of prediction" or error estimation is a technique used to increase a patient's attention to a task by asking him/her to predict performance (Studer, 2007). For example, you might say to the patient, "Mr. Smith, I would like you to try to stay between these two lines while you're walking." This technique focuses the patient's attention on a crucial element of the task. Clinicians can also address divided attention by beginning motor-learning sessions with single-task training and progressing to dual-task situations such as walking and talking (McCulloch, 2007; Fell, 2004). There is also some evidence that improving gait skills improves divided attention tasks such as walking and thinking (Hall and Heusel-Gillig, 2010). Retraining cognitive function, similar to retraining motor function, is enhanced with intensive practice. Patients should be allowed to make mistakes that are not dangerous to enhance the ability to problem-solve (Studer, 2007).

## Working With Patients Having Mild/Moderate Cognitive Loss

Patients with mild to moderate cognitive deficits will have more difficulty with explicit learning than with implicit learning. In this case, clinicians should emphasize procedural learning through intensive practice of the task while minimizing verbalization and feedback. Instead of staying, "I'd like you to try to have your left foot pass your right foot," the therapist could use taped lines on the floor and have the patient step over the lines, practice repeatedly, and down different hallways. Remember, talking to the patient as they perform a motor task creates a dual-task environment because the patient has to process what the therapist is saying. Feedback can be delayed until the task is completed. For example, wait until the patient has completed a transfer, then say, "Lift your bottom higher, like this."

Lastly, a *rapid* decline in a patient's arousal, attention, or cognition is NOT normal. Physical therapists should inform the primary care provider and/or the patient care team when such a change occurs. This action is potentially life-saving for some conditions and may decrease the degree of disability the patient experiences. Reexamination of arousal, attention, and cognition is thus warranted at regular intervals.

# Functional Implications of Cognitive Impairments

Patients with cognitive impairments will have difficulty performing tasks we might take for granted: balancing a checkbook, creating a grocery list, or following directions on a prescription/medication. In the rehabilitation process, the patient might have difficulty interpreting or carrying out a wordy HEP or following directions to use assistive, adaptive, or protective devices. Patients might also become frustrated or agitated if the cognitive demands exceed capacity. Chapter 31 presents a full discussion of strategies that the therapist can use in the context of cognitive dysfunction.

# THINK ABOUT IT 4.2

Think about how the following strategies will lower cognitive demand:

- Talk Less: Minimize the use of verbal cues, instructions, and feedback. Use demonstration, gestures, and physical guidance more so than talking.
- Plan Carefully: Purposefully manipulate the treatment environment based on the patient's level of function. For example, begin in a quiet room and gradually increase both the noise and/or physical movement in

the environment. Make small gradual changes rather than large sudden changes in the degree of environmental complexity.

- Repetition Matters: Emphasize intensive practice of motor tasks or skills to enhance the procedural learning process. Repeated sit-to-stand from a "circuit" of different chairs/seats is one example of intensive practice (see Chapter 36).
- Give Limited Choices: Don't bombard cognitively impaired patients with choices; use choice judiciously. For example, ask if the patient would like to stand on the red foam or the blue foam, keeping the choices simple and in line with your therapeutic goals.
- Maintain Dignity: Always maintain respect for your patient by avoiding patronizing gestures or comments. While asking a 5 year-old for a "high five" might be very appropriate and motivating, it can seem childish or demeaning to an older adult.
- Keep It Simple: HEPs and instructions should be brief and simple. Experiment with the patient to see what type of instruction is easiest to follow. Consider using a video or photographs in lieu of written directions.
- Selected Problem-solving: Give patients who are unaware of his or her own deficits (anosognosia) the opportunity to make mistakes while assuring their safety. Patients with attention and awareness deficits (such as those after a brain injury) need opportunities to recognize when there is a problem and engage in problem-solving. If the therapist continuously fixes or prevents a problem from occurring, the patient will not be able to learn or retain the information.

## PATIENT APPLICATION

**Cognition Case Study 4A: History and Reason for Referral:** *Mrs. J is a 69 year-old widowed Hispanic female who was referred to outpatient physical therapy after a transient ischemic attack (TIA) 6 weeks ago. Although she describes only mild weakness of the left arm, she reports three falls in the past month and admitted being very fearful of falling. Mrs. J was accompanied by her daughter who lives nearby and who has begun to assist the patient in her instrumental ADLs such as shopping, balancing her checkbook, and planning meals. During the history, Mrs. J communicated clearly yet often deferred to her daughter to answer medical history questions. Her past medical history (PMH) was significant for a hysterectomy at age 49, hypothyroidism, hypertension, and a TIA 1 year ago in addition to the most recent event 6 weeks ago. Her medications include Synthroid, Lopressor, Plavix, a multivitamin, and Fosamax. When the therapist asked her to describe a typical day, she just shook her head and said, "It's like everybody else's typical day." Her daughter feels that Mrs. J has had a slowly progressive decline in function, and feels she is still depressed, related to the death of her husband 2 years ago.*

## Contemplate Clinical Decisions

- *Describe what you know thus far about this patient's cognitive function. What in her history or initial interaction with the therapist raises a red flag in your mind?*
- *Given her PMH, what are the possible causes of cognitive decline?*
- *Describe what screening tools you would use with Mrs. J along with a rationale for your choice.*

*Discussion and possible answers to these questions are included in the online resources. It is important to remember the findings of these tests should not be considered in isolation of your other tests and measures. Instead, consider your results from these screens with other findings in the initial examination. For example, were there any other signs of central nervous system dysfunction such as hyperreflexia or incoordination? Did the skin turgor show any signs of dehydration? Your findings and clinical impressions should be communicated with the primary care physician and the health-care team.*

## PATIENT APPLICATION

**Cognition Case Study 4-B: History and Reason for Referral:** *LB is a 19 year-old Caucasian male who was admitted to a rehabilitation center after a TBI resulting from an all-terrain vehicle (ATV) accident 2 weeks ago. LB was in a coma for 6 days in the ICU of a regional trauma center and is now progressing out of coma. According to the medical record, he progressed in the trauma center from a GCS of 9 to 15. He has multiple facial abrasions, a left Colles fracture, and a distal fibular fracture. He was transferred to the rehabilitation center for intensive therapy. His mother states that he is often still sleepy but goes through periods of agitation and restlessness.*

## Contemplate Clinical Decisions

- *Describe what tests and measures you would select to use with LB during your initial examination to evaluate arousal, attention, and cognition and provide a rationale for your selection.*
- *How would the results of this examination affect your plan of care? For example, how would your feedback change during gait training with a patient at a Level V versus Level IX on the LOCF?*

*Discussion and possible answers to these questions can be found in the online companion material.*

## Summary on Cognition

Cognition is a very complex attribute involving arousal, attention, orientation, awareness, and executive functions such as judgment and problem-solving. Cognitive deficits, although considered impairments, greatly impact physical functional activities and skills and the ability of a person to participate in the community. Therapists play an important role in screening cognition to (a) identify problems, (b) refer patients for further testing or to other health-care providers, (c) develop treatment strategies aligned with the patient's cognitive skills, and (d) contribute to differential diagnosis of a patient's condition.

There is an implied order in cognitive testing such that, to test cognitive ability, the patient must be able to attend to the therapist and task; and for the patient to attend, then he or she must be awake/aroused. Cognitive testing should NOT be performed or documented using the phrase "alert and oriented times three" because it simply does not reflect the scope of cognitive functions such as attention, problem-solving, judgment, and awareness. While only a sample of cognitive tests have been provided in this chapter, you should be able to distinguish tests that discern emergence from a coma (GCS, LOCF, CRS-R) from those that test cognition (MMSE, ACE-R, MoCA). Furthermore, older adults who appear to have cognitive deficits should also be screened for depression.

Once cognitive deficits have been identified, your plan of care should reflect those deficits by selecting a nondistracting teaching environment, avoiding too much feedback, and engaging the patient when possible in problem-solving. Lastly, recognize the value of collaborating with other health care professionals to further assess cognitive function and/or develop intervention strategies that minimize agitation and promote functional independence.

# ■ Perception

## Introduction and Terminology

> **Roberta,** a patient with AD, thinks the black welcome mat in front of her door is a hole in the ground. When she walks with her therapist, she walks around the mat. Michael, who had a right anterior cerebral artery stroke, neglects the left side of his body and has bumped his wheelchair into the left side of the door jamb many times. Sophia is not aware that she has had a TBI and gets angry in therapy when her therapist asks her, "Do you remember my name?"

All of these individuals have perceptual deficits that can interfere with motor control, safety, and functional independence. **Perception** is the integration or use of sensory information into *meaningful information* having implications for decisions or movement (Shumway-Cook, 2017). Based on sensory input about the body, perception allows patients to understand the components and boundaries of their body and the environment as well as the relationship between the body and the environment. Screening for perceptual deficits helps therapists plan appropriate motor-relearning programs. Although occupational therapists more routinely examine and address perceptual deficits, it is important for physical therapists to assess perception because it affects motor control and safe mobility. Perceptual deficits can be broken down into four categories: (1) body image/body scheme disorders, (2) spatial relations disorders, (3) motor apraxia, and (4) agnosia. The terminology for common perceptual deficits based on these categories is summarized in Table 4-5.

## Clinical Neuroanatomy of Perception

Perception is primarily a function of the parietal association cortex (see Table 4-2), located at the intersection of the parietal, temporal, and occipital lobes. Perception is functionally distributed in other cortices as well. Contralateral neglect, for example, is associated with lesions of the right parietal or frontal cortex but also occurs in damage to the thalamus, basal ganglia, cingulate gyrus, and reticular formation. Body scheme disorders are generally related to injury to the parietal lobe but can also occur with cerebellar dysfunction (Zoltan, 2007). Perceptual dysfunction can also occur as a result of vascular infarcts. The anterior cerebral artery (ACA) supplies the medial frontal and parietal lobes as well as the basal ganglia, anterior fornix, and anterior corpus collosum. Injury to the right ACA may cause left hemineglect. The inferior portion of the middle cerebral artery (MCA) supplies the inferior-lateral temporal lobe and portions of the parietal lobe. An infarct of this portion of the right MCA can cause severe left-sided hemineglect and visual field deficits, whereas injury to the left MCA can cause right visual field deficits. The posterior cerebral artery (PCA) supplies the occipital lobe, inferior and medial temporal lobe, upper brainstem, midbrain, and thalamus. Damage to this artery can cause contralateral homonymous hemianopsia, visual agnosia, and prosopagnosia.

## Principles of Screening Perception

### Perceptual Disorders and Indications for Screening Perception

A broad range of perceptual disorders (see Table 4-5) occur in people with neurological dysfunction. Anosognosia was previously described under the heading of "awareness" in the cognition section of this chapter. It is appropriate to screen perception when there is known risk for perceptual deficits based on a patient's medical diagnosis, particularly in brain injury, AD, stroke, and any lesion such as tumor or injury to the nondominant hemisphere. Individuals with deficits in attention characteristically also have perceptual dysfunction (Zoltan, 2007).

Regardless of diagnosis, patient behaviors and performance can also prompt the need to screen perception. Screening is indicated if the individual appears to ignore one side of the body or a portion of the environment. Another perceptual "red flag" is difficulty with motor skills despite normal muscle recruitment, range of motion, and sensation. Patients who appear to be unaware of their deficits or who lack insight into the severity of their deficits are also candidates for perceptual screening. Individuals poststroke or brain injury exhibiting lateropulsion (pushing toward the more involved side) are also candidates for screening.

Perception is the integration and interpretation of multiple sensory systems: visual, auditory, and sensation. Before screening for perception, Zoltan (2007) recommends ascertaining the following information:

- Are the visual fields normal?
- Is vision accurate?
- Is hearing impaired?

| TABLE 4-5 | **Selected Perceptual Disorders** | |
|---|---|---|
| CATEGORY | DISORDERS | DEFINITION/DESCRIPTION |
| *Body Image* (Visual/mental memory of one's body, i.e., whether tall/short; slim/plump) | Autotopagnosia | Failure to recognize one's body parts and their relationship to each other. Symptoms include confusion of sides of the body, lack of differentiation between own limbs and therapist's limbs. Test with a body parts puzzle. |
| | Unilateral Spatial Neglect | Inability to integrate and use perceptions from one side. Test by asking to copy drawing, and the patient will only draw half of the image. |
| *Body Scheme* (Postural model of one's self, the body parts in relation to one another) | Anosognosia | Failure to recognize the presence/severity of the problem; may deny the problem or the part involved. Test patient's ability to identify a problem: "What problems are you having since …?" |
| | Right-Left Discrimination | Inability to discriminate between left and right. |
| | Finger Agnosia | Confusion in naming fingers. |
| *Visual Discrimination* (Process of recognizing depth, spatial relation between objects, and forms) | Figure Ground | Inability to distinguish foreground and background. Test using embedded or overlapping figures. |
| | Form Constancy | Inability to make subtle discrimination between objects of similar shape and purpose (fork and spoon). |
| | Position in Space | Inability to identify coordinates in 3-D space (up, down, near, under, over). |
| | Spatial Relationship | Difficulty with perception of two or more objects in relation to oneself or relation between the objects. "Draw a clock face and fill in the numbers." |
| | Topographical Disorientation | Difficulty understanding and remembering relation of places to one another such as the floor plan of hospital. |
| | Depth and Distance | Misjudgment causes difficulty with architecture such as stairs or filling a glass. |
| *Apraxia* (Inability to perform tasks or naturalistic actions in the absence of sensory, motor, or coordination deficits) | Constructional apraxia | Unable to reproduce a figure by drawing or copy building a block tower. |
| | Dressing apraxia | Inability to dress self even with feedback. |
| | Motor apraxia | Difficulty with complex motor tasks. |
| | Ideomotor apraxia | Can perform a task spontaneously but NOT on command. |
| | Ideation apraxia | Cannot produce movement spontaneously or on command despite absence of motor deficits. |
| *Agnosia* (Inability to recognize familiar objects) | Visual object | Unable to recognize visually, including face and colors, despite being able to recognize by sound or touch. |
| | Tactile | Includes astereognosis—when sensation is intact but objects cannot be recognized through touch. |
| | Auditory | Difficulty differentiating between similar sounds such as a vacuum cleaner versus a car motor. |

**Sources:** Zoltan, 2007; Devinsky et al., 2004; Farah & Feinberg, 1997; Sirigu et al., 1991.

- Are somatosensory and vestibular senses intact?
- Are cortical sensations (kinesthesia, stereognosis, two-point discrimination) intact?

### Rationale for Screening Perception

Deficits in perception can be dangerous. Inattention to an area of the body or the environment places the patient at risk for injury; an arm can accidentally get caught in the spokes of a wheel or bump into a physical barrier in the environment. The results of the perceptual screen can be used by the therapist to develop intervention strategies that address these safety issues

such as scanning the environment or removing obstacles from a home. Perceptual deficits will also interfere with motor control and motor learning. It is difficult to move the "nose over toes" during sit-to-stand if the patient does not understand where the toes are in relation to the rest of the body.

Lastly, understanding perceptual deficits will assist in your clinical reasoning about a patient including (a) the nature and location of the patient's neurological deficit, (b) differential diagnosis, (c) determining the patient's prognosis, and (d) developing an appropriate plan of care and discharge planning. Patients with severe perceptual deficits may require longer rehabilitation time and have ongoing restrictions in community participation. Therapists may use a restorative approach in which the goal is to promote neural plasticity as is the case with constraint-induced therapy or other forced-use paradigms. In contrast, an adaptive/compensatory approach may be employed in which the goal is to compensate for the deficit in perception by using visual or verbal cues or modification of the environment (Zoltan, 2007).

## Tests and Measures for Screening Perception

### Unilateral Spatial Neglect

**Unilateral spatial neglect (USN)** refers to inattention to the side of the body opposite of a brain lesion. It is also referred to as unilateral neglect, hemi-inattention, visual neglect, and hemispatial neglect (Menon, 2004). Before testing for USN, check the patient's visual fields and visual acuity. Begin screening for neglect by observing the patient in sitting or supine: Is the head turned or tilted primarily to the side opposite of the hemiplegia? If possible, observe a partially eaten meal. Is there asymmetry in the amount of food eaten, comparing right to left? Although there are many tests that evaluate for the presence of USN (see "Focus on Evidence," Table 4-16 ONL), three commonly used tools are presented in this chapter: Albert's Cancellation Test, the Single Letter Cancellation Test (SLCT), and the Comb and Razor Test. Another means of testing perception is to ask the patient to "Draw an Item" such as a clock or house and look for completion of both left and right portions of the object (Appendix 4-I). The Draw a Clock Test has been used as a screening tool for both cognition and spatial neglect.

*Albert's Cancellation Test* (available for download at http://www.strokengine.ca/assess/at/) is a valid and reliable screening tool for USN (Chen-Sea, 1994; Agrell, 1997; Fullerton, 1986). To take this test, the patient must be able to hold a pencil or pen. The test consists of 41 diagonal hash marks approximately 2 cm long organized in 6 lines on a white piece of paper. The orientation of the diagonal lines varies both in angle and direction of the slash. The patient is directed to make a slash through each hash mark ( / ) or ( \ ) to make an X. First, demonstrate how to make a mark through each hash mark so it looks like the letter X, then instruct the patient to do the same until all hash marks are crossed. Patients with hemineglect will *miss a portion of the hash marks such as leaving the left 1/4 of the page uncrossed.* Albert's Cancellation Test can be quantified by calculating the percentage of lines left uncrossed (Agrell, 1997). For example, if 5 of 41 lines were not crossed, then the error rate is 12%.

The *SLCT* has also been shown to be a valid and reliable test for USN (Marsh, 1993; Menon and Korner, 2004). Patients must be able to hold a pencil and recognize letters to perform the SLCT. Give the patient the piece of paper that contains 6 lines of capital letters, 52 letters in each line, including 104 of the letter H (available for download at http://www.strokengine.ca/assess_domain/assess-usn). Place the paper in midline and ask the patient to scan the letters carefully and draw a line through the letter H each time it appears. Because there are 53 on the left side of the paper and 51 on the right side, the tester can

determine whether there is a deficit and, if so, the side that is neglected. Greater than four omissions of the letter H is considered pathological (Menon, 2004).

The *Comb and Razor Test is* a functional assessment for USN (Beschin, 1997; McIntosh, 2000). Give the patient two tasks to perform for 30 seconds and record/calculate the number of times performed during each 30-second time period on the left versus the right side of the body. To perform this test, the patient must be able to use at least one upper extremity and *not* have motor apraxia. The test consists of asking the patient to (a) comb his hair for 30 seconds and (b) simulate shaving (males) for 30 seconds OR simulate applying makeup powder (females). Sit across from the patient and state, "Here is a (comb/razor/cosmetic pad). I want you to (comb your hair/pretend to shave your face/pretend to apply powder or makeup) until I tell you to stop. Do you understand the instructions? Do you have any questions? Begin when I say go." The razor is protected by a razor guard (or blade is removed), and universal precautions should be used for sanitary purposes. Then count the number of strokes on each side of the body during the 30 seconds. Quantification of this test has been described using two different formulas (Beschin, 1997; McIntosh, 2000). The method described by McIntosh (2000) is described in Box 4-9.

### Body Scheme

As described in Table 4-5, **autotopagnosia** is the failure to recognize one's body parts and their relationship to each other. The inability to recognize a body part makes it difficult for patients to distinguish between their own body and that of the external environment, and patients can even confuse their limbs with that of the therapist. For example, the patient might leave their hand on the walker thinking it is part of the walker. Therapists can screen for autotopagnosia using several different strategies (Table 4-6) but should first determine the patient does not have deficits that could mask the ability to identify body parts including aphasia, apraxia, and attentional deficits.

### Right/Left Discrimination

**Right/left discrimination** is the ability to discriminate the left and right side of the body. It incorporates several concomitant skills: spatial ability, conceptualization, and mental rotation, and it occurs developmentally around age 7 (Zoltan,

---

**BOX 4-9 Calculating Percent Bias as Described by McIntosh, 2000**

Comb and Razor Test
- Number of total strokes on LEFT side MINUS number of total strokes on RIGHT side
- Divide this number by the TOTAL strokes for both sides plus any ambiguous/unclear strokes
- Scores range between −1 to +1
  - Scores close to 0 indicates absence of neglect
  - Scores close to −1 indicates total LEFT neglect
  - Scores close +1 indicates total RIGHT neglect

| TABLE 4-6 | Screening Methods for Autotopagnosia | |
|---|---|---|
| **NAME** | **METHOD** | **INTERPRETATION** |
| Point to body parts | Ask patient to "point to" or "show me" body parts on self, therapist, doll, or body puzzle | All parts named in reasonable time frame |
| Imitate body part pointing | Tell the patient to imitate what you do. Touch 6-10 body parts on yourself. | Patient accurately imitates with same hand or mirror image |
| Draw a man test | Patient given a blank piece of paper and told to draw a man | Standardized scoring for this test exists but look for presence of all body parts |

Source: Zoltan, 2007.

2007). Tests for right/left discrimination can be performed using standardized or nonstandardized tests. As a simple non-standardized test, ask the patient to point to a body part such as "Point to your left elbow." The patient should be able to correctly point to each body part named by the therapist in a reasonable amount of time. If the patient is unable to do so in the absence of aphasia or apraxia, a referral to occupational therapy is indicated for further testing.

## Therapeutic Implications for Patients With Perceptual Deficits

Patients with perceptual deficits will have activity limitations and restrictions in their ability to participate in normal life roles, sometimes profound. Perceptual deficits may also impair safety. While each situation is unique, Zoltan (2007) recommends using both restorative and adaptive approaches. Adaptive or compensatory strategies involve modifying equipment or the environment to facilitate function. For example, a patient can wear a watch or band on the left wrist to help remember what

side is the left. Similarly, a diagram on a lap tray can show a place for each arm. Restorative intervention attempts to restore normal perceptual function through a variety of strategies, especially those that use task-intensive practice with real objects and the use of prism glasses (Table 4-7). More detailed strategies to address perceptual deficits are presented in Chapter 31.

There is some evidence that USN responds to restorative therapies. An excellent review of the evidence on USN is available at StrokEngine (http://www.strokengine.ca), a website sponsored by the Canadian Stroke Network, designed to improve translation of knowledge regarding stroke from research to clinical practice. The authors synthesized evidence from more than 60 research studies regarding the efficacy of treatments for USN (Menon-Nair, 2009). The following interventions have shown limited evidence (levels 2a or 2b) to improve USN:

- Limb activation can improve USN symptoms
- Right hemifield patches and prism glasses
- Trunk rotation
- Vibration of the head/neck

| TABLE 4-7 | Restorative and Adaptive Strategies for Perceptual Dysfunction |
|---|---|
| **RESTORATIVE** | **ADAPTIVE/COMPENSATORY** |
| Use principles of use-dependent neuroplasticity:<br>• Encourage intensive practice<br>• Decrease the intensity and frequency of feedback over time<br>• Work with real objects such as hairbrush, bottles, keyboard; include bilateral tasks<br>• Pay attention to the side and type of lesion or pathology when scheduling practice or determining interventions. For patients with visual deficits, use auditory or vibration as feedback.<br><br>Provide appropriate sensory stimulation:<br>• Graduate levels of sensory stimulation so it is not aversive or uncomfortable<br>• Incorporate functional activities that enhance sensory feedback (weightbearing)<br><br>Encourage flexible strategies:<br>• Variable practice conditions<br>• Vary the environment | Modify the environment or task as needed to address deficits:<br>• Use easy to open handles on doors/objects<br>• Apply bright-colored paint or tape to edges of stairs or change in surface<br>• Label everyday items, have cheat sheet of pictures and people's names<br>• Use reminder signs: "Did I put makeup on both eyes?"<br>• Wear a watch/band to remind right/left<br>• Provide simple instructions or diagrams on how to get from one place to another or use a global positioning device (GPS)<br>• Color-code clothing or items: button color and button hole<br>• Provide landmarks in the home/facility<br>• If visual recognition is lost, use other senses like touch to identify the item<br>• Use adapted forks/spoons to improve hand function in finger agnosia<br>• Teach patient to scan the left side of the room/environment for obstacles<br>• Stand on same side as patient, not in mirror image when giving directions |

In addition, there is limited evidence that sensory cuing (visual, auditory, verbal) *may not* improve USN and conflicting evidence (level 4) as to whether scanning techniques are effective in improving USN in patients with subacute and chronic stroke.

---

### PERCEPTION CASE STUDY

**Patient History:** DF is a 23 year-old male who underwent a right frontal/parietal lobe brain tumor resection 3 weeks ago. Before his symptoms and surgery, the patient played competitive basketball. On initial examination, he demonstrated apparent neglect on the left by bumping into doors, walls, and other people on that side. In addition, he was not aware of his deficit and became agitated, stating, "Why are you keeping me out of the game?" He is 6 feet, 6 inches, and somewhat intimidating in size/stature.

#### Contemplate Clinical Decisions

- What tests could be used to confirm unilateral neglect?
- What restorative strategies could be used with DF to increase his use and attention to the left side?
- What compensatory strategies could be used for safety purposes?

*Discussion and possible answers to these questions can be found in the online companion material.*

---

## Summary on Perception

Perception is intricately tied to motor control and should thus be screened during the initial examination of patients with neuromuscular diagnoses, before the motor control examination. Perception is dependent on intact visual, auditory, and sensory abilities, and thus screening for perceptual disorders should follow examination of the sensory systems. You should employ basic perceptual screening tests to recognize safety concerns or to appropriately refer patients for further testing and interventions.

Perceptual deficits are sometimes obvious such as the patient who routinely forgets her left arm during transfers or self-care activities. Deficits might also be subtle such as a patient who has difficulty walking up the stairs despite having the motor control to do so. Simple screening tools such as "show me your left calf" or "draw a picture of a clock" can identify deficits that might not have been identified through other testing. And, knowing that a patient has perceptual deficits will help you customize your treatment plan. Both compensatory and restorative strategies have been described so you can incorporate them into physical mobility training. As an example of an adaptive strategy, *instead* of saying "up with the good" while going up the stairs, use a brightly colored ribbon tied on the shoelace to cue the patient. A restorative strategy could include having the patient comb her hair in the mirror while counting the number of times combed on each side of the head. The clinical decision-making for perceptual deficits must incorporate safety with evidence-based strategies.

## ■ Communication

> **Rose** is a patient in an acute-care hospital who was admitted 3 days prior with the diagnosis of acute stroke with right hemiparesis. Her medical record indicated that she is having difficulty expressing herself verbally. After knocking on her door, the therapist walked into her room and stated, "Good morning. My name is Donna, and I am a physical therapist. Are you Rose?" The patient nodded her head, saying, "Well ... but ... this ... oh ..." and pointed to her mouth, clearly upset and frustrated.

### Introduction and Terminology

In the previously described scenario, both the therapist and the patient will begin their relationship having to work hard to make sure they can optimally communicate. Therapists rely on the ability to communicate with patients in all areas of patient/client management, especially when taking a history, performing an examination, implementing procedural interventions, and in patient-related instruction (APTA, 2015). Communication refers to the ability to convey and receive information through one or more of the following components of language: (1) auditory, through speech or singing; (2) nonverbal, including gestures, eye contact, body language, or sign language; and (3) writing, using words, pictures, or symbols to convey information. Impairments in communication make it difficult for the patient to comprehend instructions, receive feedback, or express their needs. Difficulty communicating can also interfere with the processes of both motor and cognitive learning. This section provides an overview of the basic communication impairments, methods of screening for communication deficits, and strategies to enhance communication in the therapeutic environment.

### Communication Disorders

#### Aphasia

**Aphasia**, also termed dysphasia, affects the ability to use, create, or understand speech because of a lesion to the dominant cerebral hemisphere. The etiology of aphasia may include cerebral contusions, hematoma, abscess, tumors, strokes, demyelinating diseases, and neurodegenerative disorders such as AD (Blumenfeld, 2002). Aphasia could be categorized in several ways, including by severity (mild to global aphasia), the nature of whether speech output is spontaneous or not (fluent versus nonfluent aphasia), the direction of communication impacted (receptive, expressive, or global), or the anatomical structures that were impacted (Wernicke's and Broca's aphasia, see Fig. 4-1, Where Is It?).

Sometimes receptive communication can be limited to one sensory type. For example, difficulty with comprehending written language is termed **alexia** whereas expressive communication limited to an inability to write is termed **agraphia**. **Fluent aphasia** describes difficulty understanding language but retaining speech production with a normal rhythm, melody, and articulation; whereas **nonfluent aphasia** describes a hesitant interruptive flow of speech with limited vocabulary (Sarno, 2007). The various types of aphasia are detailed in Table 4-8.

| TABLE 4-8 Types of Aphasia | | |
|---|---|---|
| CLASSIFICATION | TYPE | DESCRIPTION |
| *Fluent:* Lesions in posterior portion first temporal gyrus (left hemisphere*) | Wernicke Aphasia (sensory/receptive) | Loss of auditory comprehension with fluent speech and word substitutions; impaired reading and writing. |
| | Anomic Aphasia | Major word finding difficulty despite fluent speech. |
| | Pure Word Deafness | Fluent speech, but difficulty comprehending or repeating speech; retained ability to name, read, and write. In **cortical deafness**, sounds can be heard, but words cannot be interpreted (while reading and writing are preserved). |
| *Non-Fluent:* Anterior lesions, third frontal convolution (left hemisphere) | Broca Aphasia (expressive/motor) | Intact comprehension of oral and written language with difficulty producing speech, articulating, naming, and writing; limited vocabulary. |
| | Global Aphasia | Describes severe aphasia that involves loss of production and comprehension of language including writing; usually results from a large MCA infarct. |
| | Transcortical Motor Aphasia | Dysfunction in supplementary motor areas, retaining verbal and written comprehension; but characteristic difficulty repeating words or phrases. |
| *Either Fluent or Nonfluent* | Conduction Aphasia | Fluent speech with difficulty naming, repeating words while retaining written and oral comprehension. |

*Left hemisphere is the dominant hemisphere in most persons, even those who are left-handed.
Source: Sarno, 2007

## Disorders of Motor Speech: Apraxia and Dysarthria

**Verbal apraxia** is also termed aphemia and describes difficulty in producing speech in absence of a written language deficit. The etiology is usually an infarct in the dominant Broca's area, the frontal lobe "operculum." These patients have difficulty articulating speech and can sound as if they have an accent, which is also called foreign accent syndrome.

**Dysarthria**, an impairment of motor speech production, can be observed as difficulty with respiration, phonation, articulation, resonance, or prosody that occurs as a result of damage to the central or peripheral nervous system (Sarno, 2007). The major categories of dysarthria are outlined in Table 4-9 and often are associated with a range of motor-recruitment deficits seen in the trunk and extremities.

## Principles of Screening Communication

### Indications for Screening Communication

Every patient should be assessed for the ability to communicate, however, the degree of screening will vary based on the patient's medical history and/or functional presentation. Those at greatest risk for communication disorders include people poststroke, neoplasm, brain injury, basal ganglia disorders, and weakness or impaired control of the motor components of speech. During the initial history or interview, take note of whether the patient's speech is clear, spontaneous, and accurate. Low volume, poor diction, abnormal timing of speech, inappropriate word choice, abnormal spacing between words, and the absence of speech indicate that further screening is needed. In general, it is also important to know the patient's primary language, educational background, and literacy before testing. These factors affect the results of comprehension and reading tests.

| TABLE 4-9 Types of Dysarthria | |
|---|---|
| TYPE | DESCRIPTION |
| Spastic | Associated with upper motor neuron lesions, with poor articulation, monotonous pitch, poor control of exhalation, and harsh phonation. |
| Flaccid | Associated with weakness resulting from lower motor neuron lesions (Bell Palsy), muscular weakness, and hypotonicity. Symptoms include slow, hoarse, and breathy phonation; brief phrases; and poor control of exhalation. |
| Ataxic | Associated with lesions of the cerebellum, speech is irregular, may include explosive sentences and lacks precision. |
| Hypokinetic | Associated with basal ganglia lesions and people with PD; speech is slow, monotonous, hoarse, and weak. |
| Hyperkinetic | Associated with basal ganglia and people with HD, speech is variable in the ability to articulate, with long intervals between words and occasional extraneous sounds. |

Source: Sarno, 2007.

### Rationale for Screening Communication

Understanding the patient's communication abilities and/or impairments is essential for several reasons. First, therapists rely on verbal communication to instruct the patient and to provide feedback regarding the patient's performance. Communication with patients who have neuromuscular impairments is often one-sided compared with normal conversations with the clinician doing more of the talking (Marshall, 2004). The ability of the patient to listen and comprehend language will influence treatment outcomes. Second, therapy interventions often take place in noisy and distracting environments that can hamper communication in the language-impaired person. Third, impaired language and communication skills increase the time it takes to provide interventions (Marshall, 2004). Therapists must consider communication skills when determining the patient's prognosis and plan of care. Lastly, modifying communication strategies to accommodate the patient's impairments can decrease the patient's level of frustration and improve the effectiveness and efficiency of the plan of care.

## Methods to Screen Communication

Speech language pathologists (SLPs) are the experts in the examination, diagnosis, and treatment of speech and language disorders. In some settings, physical therapists and occupational therapists also contribute to physical intervention to optimize swallowing. A broad screening of communication by physical and occupational therapists helps to identify individuals who would benefit from referral to speech therapy. Attributes that can be screened are summarized in Table 4-10. Pay particular attention to (1) the quality of speech including fluency, diction, and volume, (2) the ability to comprehend the spoken and written word, and (3) the ability to write, name objects, and repeat a phrase. When speech dysfunction is identified, the therapist must modify their usual communication strategy. For example, if the patient has difficulty comprehending the

written word, use demonstration and video-taped demonstrations when developing the HEP.

## Therapeutic Implications of Communication Disorders

Patients referred to therapy for functional training, therapeutic activities, and therapeutic exercises often have speech and language deficits. In this context, how can therapists modify their communication strategies to enhance understanding?

- Whenever possible, consult with a speech language pathologist to clarify the patient's deficits and to learn strategies that maximize communication for that patient.
- Have a thorough understanding of your patient's hearing skills. Has the patient been tested by an audiologist? If hearing is diminished, can you augment with an amplification system or technology?
- Less is more: Using fewer words simplifies communication and also enhances motor learning. Make sure that you speak to adult patients as adults; simplify does not mean child-like (Marshall, 2004).
- The motor-learning literature in healthy adults discourages *frequent* extrinsic feedback because it can create a dependency on the feedback and create a loss of stability during balance tasks (Van Fliet, 2006). While further research is needed in persons with stroke, providing simultaneous feedback creates a dual-task situation in which the patient is cognitively processing commands while performing physical movement. Delaying feedback until after a task is

| TABLE 4-10 | Screening Speech/Language |
| --- | --- |
| **SPEECH ATTRIBUTE** | **METHOD OF SCREENING** |
| Spontaneous Speech | During interaction, observe spontaneous speech:<br>• Fluent speech versus halting speech?<br>• Appropriate tone and fluctuations?<br>• Correct word choice, word usage?<br>• Correct grammar, allowing for cultural and educational variations?<br>• Appropriate volume?<br>• Articulate versus slurred? |
| Comprehension | Can the patient follow simple verbal commands such as "blink your eyes"? Can the patient comprehend, for example: "If John is 28 and Christine is 23, is Christine younger than John?" |
| Reading and Writing | Reading<br>• Ask the patient to read a list of words, the title of a book, or a short paragraph.<br>• Check for comprehension after reading, such as, "What date does the juice expire?"<br>Writing<br>• Ask the patient to write a short sentence. Dictate the sentence, such as "I forgot where I put my glasses." |
| Naming | Tell me what I am pointing to:<br>• Simple objects (pen, watch, earring)<br>• Parts of objects (tip of pen, shoelace) |
| Repetition | Repeat after me:<br>• Simple and common phrase: "No ifs, ands, or buts."<br>• More difficulty: "Roberta was an expert calligrapher." |

Source: Blumenfeld, 2002.

complete decreases the need for the patient to do two things at one time such as listening while performing a skill, especially for patients who are having difficulty processing auditory information.

- Augment communication: Whenever possible, augment your verbal commands with other sensory instructions such as tactile or visual cues; allow your face to be visualized during communication as sometimes facial expressions provide cues to the patient (Marshall, 2004).

Marshall (2004) identified specific strategies for working with persons who have aphasia. The strategies include methods to (1) focus the patient's attention, (2) alter pacing or timing of the therapist's own rate of speech, and (3) modify the message content (see Table 4-11).

## PATIENT APPLICATION CASE STUDY FOR COMMUNICATION

**Three Patient Vignettes:** *Three patients were being seen poststroke in an outpatient physical therapy department. Joe was able to understand all spoken and written speech but had poor articulation. He was difficult to understand as he tended to speak quickly while exhaling. When he said, "I'll be right back," it sounded like, "I-be-rye-ba." Dora was easier to hear but could not organize her words into meaningful sentences and was easily frustrated when trying to communicate. When she wanted a drink of water, she said, "Want that/no but/can water." Jorge spoke clearly and fluently but could not interpret verbal commands. When asked to stand up, he did nothing. When given a large index card with the letters in thick marker saying, "Please stand up," he stood immediately.*

### Contemplate Clinical Decisions

- *Describe the type of communication deficits demonstrated by Joe, Dora, and Jorge. How did you come to that decision?*
- *Describe communication strategies you would use with each patient.*

*Discussion and possible answers to these questions are included in the online resources.*

The key in each of these cases is to modify how you would normally communicate to meet the individual needs of the patient. Take time to be prepared for each case; for example, have cards and a thick marker ready for Jorge, communication pictures for Dora, and a wipe-off board for Joe. Pursue communication with your patients; don't avoid it. Carefully select the best communication strategy for each situation.

## Summary on Communication

Communication is a crucial element in all aspects of patient/client management, including the therapeutic relationship. Screening communication skills is extremely important in patients with neurological conditions because of the high incidence of communication deficits related to cognitive, sensory, hearing, or motor impairments. Common communication disorders include aphasia, dysarthria, apraxia, hearing loss, and difficulty writing or interpreting the written word. There are five components to screening communication, including observation/measurement of (1) spontaneous speech, (2) comprehension of oral directions, (3) reading and writing, (4) repetition of spoken language, and (5) naming objects.

| TABLE 4-11 | Strategies for Working with Patients with Aphasia | |
| --- | --- | --- |
| **ATTENTION** | **TIMING** | **MESSAGE CONTENT** |
| Use Alerting Signals<br>"It's time to stand up now!"<br>"Let's change things a bit." | Slow Rate of Speech<br>"Walk to the door. (Pause.) Turn around. (Pause.) Come back." | Decrease Syntactic Complexity<br>Active voice: "Take large steps."<br>Phrase in the positive: "Nice-sized steps." |
| Avoid Dual Tasks<br>Don't talk during skills.<br>Save feedback until done. | Interstimulus Pauses<br>Give 30 seconds of quiet between commands to avoid overload. | Message Length<br>"Stand up." NOT "Scoot forward, lean, and push to stand up." |
| Speak Face-to-Face<br>Talk facing the patient when possible. | Give More Time<br>Wait 5 seconds between words and action. | Direct Wording<br>"Left foot first" rather than "Step with your left foot first." |
| Increase Message Saliency<br>Emphasize key words: "Take BIG steps." | | Increase Redundancy<br>*Support* your *weaker* arm.<br>Supplemental Cuing<br>Saying "nose over toes" while providing tactile or visual cuing to lean forward. |
| Clarifying Message from Patients<br>Identify topic areas. | Narrow Down Context<br>"Are you talking about eating?"<br>"Are you talking about lunch?"<br>"Are you wondering what time you go to lunch?" | |

Source: Marshall, 2004

Regardless of the communication deficit, the therapist should adapt communication strategies to meet the specific needs of the patient. When possible, work with a speech language pathologist to develop specific strategies for patients or even to integrate speech practice into your therapy session. More details are provided in Chapter 31. Evidence-basis for some of the most important communication screening and examination tools is provided in the Focus on Evidence Tables 4-13 to 4-16 ONL.

# Special Considerations in Pediatrics
## Introduction

> **Elijah** is a 6-month-old infant who was just released from the hospital following seven surgeries to correct congenital heart and intestinal defects. His therapist notes that Elijah seems irritable and unwilling to interact with the people around him. Katie is 3 years old and has Down syndrome. She often refuses to participate in therapy activities and throws herself on the floor when she does not get her way during intervention sessions. Caroline is 7 years old and has a diagnosis of developmental coordination disorder (DCD). When she arrives for outpatient therapy sessions, her therapist notices that Caroline appears lethargic and resistant to activities.

What are the unique considerations when screening attention, cognition, perception, and communication in pediatric patients? The descriptions of Elijah, Katie, and Caroline depict the wide range of cognitive and communication deficits that affect children. In addition, normal developmental changes from infancy through childhood reflect constantly changing skills in attention, cognition, perception, and communication. This section provides an overview of screening for the pediatric population, including developmental screening tools, noting behavioral state regulation in infancy, assessing alertness and attention in childhood, and therapeutic implications for working with cognitively impaired children.

Observing typically developing 5 year-olds at a community T-ball game provides many insights into the special consideration that must be given to attention, cognition, perception, and communication in pediatric patients. At the T-ball game, simple distractions such as an airplane flying overhead or a butterfly flitting through the ballfield are enough to bring play to a standstill as the children stop to watch the airplane or chase the butterfly. Difficulties remembering the principles and components of the game may be observed when a child remains standing at home plate after hitting the ball and must be reminded to run the bases. One child may start running in the wrong direction after hitting the ball and need to be redirected toward first base. Another child might lose interest in the game and start to pick dandelions growing in the ballfield. Still another might become upset but not be able to find the words to tell the coach what is wrong.

This T-ball game reminds us that all children, whether they are typically developing or have special needs, are in the process of building skills across multiple areas of cognition, perception, emotion, and communication. To maximize each child's potential, the therapist must learn to consider these areas as part of a comprehensive evaluation of motor ability and functional skills. A holistic approach to examination incorporates all aspects of function and recognizes the differences in the abilities of children at various ages and developmental stages.

## Multidisciplinary and Developmental Screening Tools

Pediatric therapy is often provided under the Individuals with Disability Education Improvement Act (IDEA) of 2004 (Public Law 108–446). This federal legislation is comprehensive in scope and stipulates that assessment, planning, and service delivery must be provided by a multidisciplinary team. Ideally practitioners from different disciplines work together under IDEA to comprehensively examine the child and develop programs to meet each child's individual needs. In this model of service delivery, screenings and specific tests related to attention, cognition, perception, and communication are typically performed by psychologists, SLPs, occupational therapists, and special education teachers. Therapists working with children should actively seek out the expertise of other team members and incorporate their suggestions into the plan of care.

In a multidisciplinary team, a comprehensive standardized assessment tool may be used to obtain a more comprehensive and holistic view of the child. For example, the *Bayley Scales of Infant and Toddler Development,* Third Edition (Bayley, 2006) includes subtests that assess skills in the following areas: (1) cognition, (2) language (both expressive and receptive), (3) motor (both gross motor and fine motor), (4) social-emotional, and (5) adaptive behavior. The physical or occupational therapist on the team might administer the motor scale and other members of the team might administer the cognitive and language portions of the test. Caregivers provide information concerning social-emotional skills and adaptive behaviors through the *Social-Emotional and Adaptive Behavior Questionnaire.* The information obtained from the components of this norm-referenced assessment provides a thorough and complete picture of a child, allowing the team to create an intervention plan that best meets the child's individual needs.

If an infant or child is referred for therapy and has not had an interdisciplinary assessment, the therapist may want to use a developmental screening tool to provide information on the child's function in the various areas of development. The *Denver II* (Frankenberg, 1992) is an example of a norm-referenced tool designed to screen children ages birth to 6 years, 6 months of age. The Denver II includes items from the following areas: (1) personal-social, (2) fine motor-adaptive, (3) gross motor, and (4) language. Five subjective items rating test behavior related to compliance, interest, fearfulness, and attention are also included in the screen. The test can typically be administered and interpreted within a 10- to 20-minute time frame and allows for the identification of developmental areas that warrant further examination or referrals to other practitioners. Using screening tools such as the Denver II helps to create a more holistic view of the child and alerts therapists to potential problems in areas such as attention, cognition, perception, and communication that may potentially affect the child's rehabilitation process.

## Behavioral State Regulation in Infancy

Although a comprehensive description of providing services in the neonatal intensive care unit (NICU) is beyond the scope of entry-level practice, many NICU graduates, at-risk infants, and infants with known developmental issues have difficulty regulating their **behavioral state** as an expression of their general cognitive function, long after discharge from the hospital. Infant behavioral state refers to the infant's level of alertness and ability to react and respond to stimuli. While the names and descriptions of behavioral states vary according to source, (Brazelton, 1995; Holditch-Davis, 1993; Als, 1986; Als, 1999) most authors include descriptors along a continuum such as quiet sleep, active sleep, sleep-wake transition, quiet alert, active alert, and crying (high stress) to illustrate the different behavioral states that may be observed in infants (see Table 4-12). Obviously, the infant's ability to receive information and to perform motor tasks incrementally decays at each end of this continuum: The baby who is sleeping doesn't sense or respond accurately, and the infant who is crying uncontrollably has decreased ability to sense and respond.

An *infant's behavioral state* is best determined by closely observing the infant. As indicated in Table 4-12, first note if the baby's eyes are open or closed, then whether eye movements are occurring under closed eyelids, the extent of extremity movements, and the infant's breathing pattern. By clustering observations in each of these areas as outlined in Table 4-12, you will be able to determine the infant's behavioral state.

An infant's behavioral state impacts his/her ability to attend to stimuli and perform motor tasks and therapists must acknowledge the influence of an infant's behavioral state on examination findings (Als, 1986; Als, 1999). An infant who is in a quiet sleep state may not respond to tactile input, but an infant who is crying may withdraw from the same stimulus or may not even recognize the stimulus. Muscle tone and movement patterns may also be affected by a baby's behavioral state, particularly with increased muscle tone and impaired movement as an infant becomes more irritable and starts to fuss or cry. Examination and intervention are provided most ideally when the baby is in a *quiet alert* state. During this state, the infant's eyes are open, minimal movements are observed, and the infant is able to appropriately attend and respond to stimuli. Unfortunately, infants who are born prematurely or who have known developmental or medical issues are often irritable and spend less time in the quiet alert, deep sleep, and active alert behavioral states.

Therapists must continually be aware of signals from the baby that may indicate onset of stress. Stressing the infant may cause the baby physiological harm and must be preempted and avoided by monitoring the infant for signs and signals of overstimulation (Als, 1999). A baby who is starting to be stressed exhibits **avoidance signals** that can typically be observed long before the baby begins to demonstrate negative physiological changes (Als, 1986; Als, 1999). Avoidance signals are natural cues the baby uses to communicate an increasing level of stress. Early avoidance signals include evading eye contact, facial grimacing, yawning, frowning, and tongue thrust. Infants who are becoming stressed may demonstrate finger splay and hold up their hand and arm similar to a "stop sign" position in an attempt to communicate to caregivers that they should stop the stressing input (see Figure 4-3).

The infant in Figure 4-3 is providing subtle cues ("stop sign") that he/she is having difficulty tolerating external stimuli. If these early signs are not noticed and the infant is furthered stressed, additional signs of stress such as hiccupping, spitting up, arching, and defecating may be observed. As the baby becomes increasingly stressed, physiological signs of overstimulation such as changes in heart and respiratory

| TABLE 4-12 | Behavioral States in Infants |
| --- | --- |
| **BEHAVIORAL STATE** | **DESCRIPTION** |
| Quiet Sleep | The infant is in a deep sleep state. The eyes are closed, and eye movements are not observed under the closed eyelids. Breathing is regular, and spontaneous movement is not observed. A relaxed facial expression is noted. |
| Active Sleep | The infant is lightly sleeping. Eyes are closed, but eye movements are noted under the closed eyelids. Breathing is somewhat irregular. Random movements and intermittent sucking may be observed. |
| Sleep-wake Transition | The infant is drowsy. The eyelids may flutter or be partially opened. Breathing is shallow and may be rapid. Variable movements are observed, and the infant may exhibit facial expressions that include grimacing or whimpering. |
| Quiet Alert | The infant is awake and alert with widely opened eyes. Minimal movement is noted, and the infant is able to focus on stimuli and process information. |
| Active Alert | The infant is very active and may be fussy but does not cry. Eyes may or may not be opened. Facial expressions indicate distress. Breathing is somewhat irregular. |
| Crying | The infant is actively crying and is in a state of high stress. Breathing is often rapid and irregular. |

**Source:** Brazelton and Nugent, 1995; Holditch-Davis, 1990; Als, 1999.

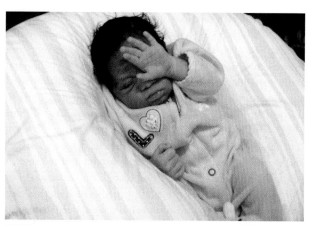

**FIGURE 4-3** An infant exhibiting the "Stop Sign Signal," an observable sign of avoidance behaviors revealing infant stress.

rate or even episodes of apnea and bradycardia may be observed. To avoid getting to the point of physiological stress, the therapist should note early signs of avoidance. If avoidance signals are noted, the therapist can help reduce the baby's sensory load by temporarily avoiding direct eye contact with the baby, limiting extraneous noise (e.g., television or talking), and avoiding coupling sensory experiences (e.g., holding the infant while rocking back and forth).

The therapist should also be aware of an infant's **approach signals** (Als, 1986; Als, 1999). Approach signals are the opposite of avoidance signals and indicate the baby is ready for interactions and optimally able to partake in examination measures and therapeutic activities. Approach signals include cooing, smiling, sustained focus, relaxed limbs, and soft pleasant facial expressions. Attending to both avoidance and approach signals allows the therapist to provide stimuli when the infant is optimally ready for the interaction.

### Screening and Regulating Levels of Alertness and Attention

In pediatric therapy, problems regulating levels of alertness or attention are not just limited to infants. The ability to focus, listen, concentrate, and perform tasks is in part dependent on one's level of alertness. The level of alertness normally varies throughout the day and ideally is specific to the demands of the particular task or activity being performed. A child may be very alert and attentive after riding a tricycle but drowsy when first waking up or getting ready to sleep. Different tasks demand varying levels of alertness and attention as well. For example, a lower level of attention is needed for watching television than for climbing up a slide ladder. The potential consequences of decreased alertness and attention are also quite different depending on the task; missing part of the storyline in a television program is not nearly as painful, and potentially dangerous, as slipping off the slide ladder.

Children who are developing typically have normal fluctuations in their level of alertness and attention. Children who have difficulty processing sensory information, however, often have difficulty matching their level of alertness or their attention to the demands of the situation and the task. A child who

is at a high level of alertness may be in constant motion, talk very rapidly, and may move quickly from activity to activity without truly attending to a specific task. A child who is at a low level of alertness may appear drowsy, resistant, or withdrawn and unable to engage. Based on the screening or examination, the therapist should describe the level of alertness and the ability to focus attention and observe whether it changes through the examination or over time.

By identifying if a child's level of alertness is too high or too low, the therapist can provide sensory inputs to help the child reach the level of alertness necessary to perform a specific task. The "How Does Your Engine Run?" program (Williams, 1996) provides a way for therapists to help increase a child's awareness of their level of alertness and to use sensory inputs to achieve the optimal level of alertness for a given activity. The program uses the analogy of an engine and helps children determine whether their engine is running too low or too high or at just the right speed. The program then teaches children to use individualized sensory strategies to achieve just the right engine speed for the particular task. A similar strategy using the same principles would be to use cartoon characters familiar to the child. For example, the therapist could directly ask if the child is feeling more like Eeyore (low level of alertness) or Tigger (high level of alertness) and then ask what would help to adjust the child toward feeling more like Winnie-the-Pooh (just the right level of alertness). Strategies like this are also helpful in explaining the concept of level of alertness to parents. Parents can easily identify with having a child who is Tigger-like, bouncing from one thing to the next, or Eeyore-like, seemingly lackluster and sluggish.

## Screening Attention With Dual-Task Activities in Children

As mentioned earlier in this chapter, dual-task conditions require divided attention (McCulloch, 2007). In typically developing children, dual-task demands such as simultaneously performing a cognitive task and a postural control or motor task have been shown to result in increased postural sway (Blanchard, 2005; Laufer, 2008; Reilly, 2008a). Blanchard (2005) studied fourth-grade students without any known motor or developmental issues and found the subjects' postural stability was negatively impacted by the demands of a concurrent cognitive task such as counting backward or reading sentences written at a second-grade level. Reilly (2008a) found that typically developing children between 4 and 6 years of age experienced interference with postural control when performing a cognitive task in both a wide-stance and a modified Romberg position. Based on these findings in children who are developing typically, it should not be surprising children with known motor problems such as CP or DCD experience difficulties with dual-task interference (Laufer, 2008; Reilly, 2008b). While tests such as the Timed Up and Go-cognitive (TUG-c) have not yet been validated for use with children, therapists should assess the impact of dual-task activities on a child's motor control and function by observing the child in various settings and under differing demands. A child with hemiplegic CP, for example, may be able to safely ascend the ladder to the slide when he and the therapist are alone on the playground, but during a busy recess period, the increased demands of attending to and interacting with other children may result in motor control issues affecting the child's safe execution of the motor task. Several authors have even suggested the dual-task conditions inherent in most functional environments may explain why improvements observed in the clinical setting do not necessarily result in improved functional performance in other environments (Blanchard, 2005; Huang, 2001).

## Therapeutic Implications for Children With Cognitive Impairments

Children with motor delays may also demonstrate problems in other areas of development. Children with motor difficulties who also have cognitive delays or cognitive deficits face inherent obstacles to learning that must be taken into account during each phase of the rehabilitation process. During the examination process, children with cognitive impairments may have difficulty following complicated directions or performing motor tasks that include a strong cognitive component. Standardized tests such as the *DeGangi-Berk Test of Sensory Integration* (Berk and DeGangi, 1983) often include motor items that may be novel to a child and that may also involve standardized directions comprised of multistep commands. For the child with cognitive deficits, these factors may impact motor performance and obscure the child's true motor function and capabilities. The presence of cognitive deficits should thus be considered when choosing a standardized test, and the results of all examination procedures should be interpreted in light of the child's functional abilities as a whole. Children with cognitive deficits have also been found to have difficulty generalizing skills and to require more practice when learning new skills (Brown, 1979). These factors must be considered when developing the plan of care and planning interventions (Parette, 1984; Horn, 1991).

Although the theories used to guide physical therapy interventions are the same regardless of whether a child has cognitive deficits or not, the learning needs of a child with cognitive impairments must be considered when applying intervention theory to practice. Several authors have suggested that the ability to address the motor needs of children with cognitive deficits can be enhanced by modifying the cognitive demands of intervention strategies (Brown, 1979; Horn, 1991).

## THINK ABOUT IT 4.3

Think about how you might incorporate the following suggestions for modifying cognitive demands in children with cognitive deficits:

- Provide opportunities for the child to be successful and praise the child's success. Frustration is often a problem for these children, and this may further hinder their learning.

- Introduce new skills slowly and one at a time. Requiring a child with cognitive deficits to learn multiple things at once may be overwhelming.
- When teaching a new skill, use strategies aimed at targeting a variety of learning avenues. Providing multimodal input through visual, kinesthetic, and auditory means will help to reinforce the new concepts being presented.
- Provide structure and consistency. Structure sessions so the child knows what to expect. Depending on the individual needs of the child, this can be accomplished by writing out a schedule of activities for the session or by simply starting each session with the same one or two activities to allow the child to transition into the session in a familiar manner.
- When appropriate, provide the child with choices. If it does not matter if the child uses the green ball or the red ball to perform a task, let the child pick which ball to use.
- On the other hand, unless you truly mean to offer a choice, make certain your instructions do not suggest that the child has a choice. Asking a child "Would you like to play this game right now?" implies that the child has a choice about playing that game. Statements such as "It is time to play this game" are more direct and do not infer that the child has a choice about participating when your treatment plan requires a particular activity.
- Providing intervention in a familiar environment may help to support the initial stages of learning. However, once a skill is learned, it should be practiced in a variety of settings under a wide range of conditions to help the child generalize skill and function.
- Provide increased opportunities to practice skills by increasing the number of repetitions performed.

In addition to these modifications, Horn (1991) further suggests coupling neuromotor and sensorimotor strategies with behavioral programming to maximize a child's rehabilitation potential. Behavioral programming involves the application of behavioral Think About principles to facilitate changes in motor behaviors (Reid, 1991). Positive reinforcements such as praise or access to a preferred activity, antecedent techniques to prompt a child's attention to a task such as tapping the stair step where you want the child to place his foot, and providing natural consequences to actions and activities are examples of how behavioral programming may be used in conjunction with traditional rehabilitation approaches. Behavioral intervention is an area where other members of the interdisciplinary team, including teachers or psychologists, may have additional experience and insights. Incorporating the suggestions of these team members will help the therapist to maximize the rehabilitation potential of each child.

## PEDIATRIC CASE STUDY

**Patient History:** BG is a 5 year-old boy who has Down syndrome. He has limited verbal communication skills and uses basic signs to help make his needs known. During therapy sessions, he frequently appears to become frustrated and refuses to participate in activities. Over the past several sessions, he has actively rejected all of his therapist's attempts to direct his activity and has thrown himself down on the floor in apparent defiance whenever the therapist even comes close to him. To his therapist, it seems that increased efforts to engage BG in therapy activities result in an increase in his out-of-control behavior. The therapist wonders if it is time to discharge BG due to his inability to cooperate with therapy activities.

## Contemplate Clinical Decisions

- What factors might be contributing to BG's apparent frustration?
- What resources does the therapist have to help find a solution to this problem?
- What strategies could be used with BG to help decrease his frustration during therapy sessions?

Discussion and possible answers to these questions are included in the online resources.

# HANDS-ON PRACTICE

- **Test arousal for the sleeping/lethargic patient**
  1. Try to rouse the patient with a loud voice.
  2. Use a gentle shake with a loud voice.
  3. Attempt a noxious stimulus such as sternal rub or pinprick.
  4. Document the results based on description using level of consciousness descriptions (Table 4-1).
- **Demonstrate performing the Digit Repetition Test AND a-Test for attention**
  1. Explain to your practice patient what you are going to do and why.
  2. Give the directions to the patient and check for understanding.
  3. Perform the Digit Repetition Test (Box 4-4) or a Test for Vigilance (Box 4-5).
  4. Score the test and interpret the results.
  5. Document the results and explain your findings to another person.
- **Perform the WWTT**
  1. Measure the time it takes for the patient to walk 20 feet, turn, and return 20 feet.
  2. Repeat this time with a simple cognitive task (patient must state aloud the letters of the alphabet).

  3. Repeat again with a complex cognitive task (patient states every other letter of the alphabet beginning with the letter B).
- **Demonstrate performing the MoCA test in its entirety**
  1. Review the test and familiarize yourself with each item, and make sure to read the scoring of each item and also how you can modify the question.
  2. Explain to your practice patient what you are going to do and why (in simple terms).
  3. Give directions to the patient for each item.
  4. Follow the directions for modifying each question (cues, prompts, etc.).
  5. Score the test and interpret the results.
  6. Document the results and explain your findings to another person.
- Practice applying restorative strategies to reduce neglect.
- Practice giving instructions to an individual with receptive aphasia. How would you modify your teaching strategies to enhance carryover?

# Let's Review

1. Describe five reasons why a therapist should screen cognition, attention, perception, and communication.

2. Compare and contrast the clinical signs and symptoms indicating a patient may have difficulty with attention, cognition, perception, or communication.

3. How can a therapist decrease a patient's anxiety about cognitive testing?

4. In what order (and why) should you screen cognition, attention, and arousal?

5. List three ways to facilitate motor learning in a patient with cognitive deficits.

6. Describe one test to screen or test each of the following:
   a. Attention
   b. Cognition
   c. Perception
   d. Communication

7. Simplify the following verbal cues using verbal and nonverbal strategies:

| Too Wordy, Cognitive, or Confusing | Simplified or Non-Verbal Strategy |
| --- | --- |
| 1. Put your "nose over toes" in order to stand up. | 1. Use tactile guidance to stand, bringing head/trunk forward. |
| 2. OK, Mrs. Jones, it's time to stand up and take a walk. | 2. _____ |
| 3. To go up the curb, put your right leg up first. | 3. _____ |
| 4. Put your hands on the walker and push it in front of you. | 4. _____ |

8. Identify developmental screening and assessment tools that may be used to provide a comprehensive view of a child's development across multiple functional domains.

9. Describe the various behavioral states of an infant. In which behavioral state should examination and intervention be provided to the baby? Why?

10. Differentiate between avoidance signals and approach signals in infants.

11. Describe five strategies that a therapist may use to modify cognitive demands during intervention sessions for children with cognitive deficits.

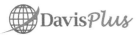 **DavisPlus**   For additional resources, including Focus on Evidence tables, case study discussions, references, and glossary, please visit http://davisplus.fadavis.com

## CHAPTER SUMMARY

Patients with neurological dysfunction frequently have difficulty with attention, cognition, perception, or communication. This chapter addressed these four areas, historically addressed by other health-care professionals. While the methods to administer the specific tests are described in this chapter, the primary evidence to support use of these tests is summarized in the Focus on Evidence (FOE) Tables (available in the online supplemental material): Table 4-13 (Mental Status Tests), Table 4-14 (Dementia-related Rating Scales), Table 4-15 (Brain Injury-related Cognitive Tests), Table 4-16 (Perceptual Tests), and Table 4-17 (Communication Screening Tests). Therapists need to be proficient in screening each of these functional areas for many reasons, including the ability to (a) make appropriate referrals to other professionals, (b) select strategies that match the patient's skills to optimize rehabilitation, (c) monitor change over time, and (d) develop a plan of care that is appropriate for the individual patient. Several key points bear repeating:

- Attention, awareness, and cognition cannot be appropriately screened using the age-old phrase "alert and oriented times three." Instead, begin by determining the patient's level of arousal, then their ability to pay attention, and

then their skills in cognition and executive function. A variety of tests and measures have been provided to screen each area.

- Deficits in attention, awareness, cognition, and executive function can be related back to specific locations in the brain, cerebral hemispheres, and specific neurological disorders. Understanding the link between neuroanatomy or pathology and function will help you know when it is appropriate to screen these areas and to what degree you should screen. For example, a patient who has known or suspected parietal lobe damage should be screened carefully for perceptual deficits.

- Perception is the interpretation of sensory information and perhaps a key "vital sign" in patients with neurological deficits. Perception screening includes checking for unilateral spatial neglect, body awareness, and awareness of one's deficits. Patients with perceptual deficits may be unable to function despite normal strength and motor recruitment, and thus identification of perceptual dysfunction and referral to occupational therapy is of prime importance.

■ Communication is critical to all aspects of rehabilitation as well as to the therapeutic relationship. Common communication deficits in patients with neurological conditions include various types of aphasia and dysarthria. Physical therapists can screen for communication dysfunction and also tailor communication strategies to meet the need of each individual patient. Strategies include focusing the patient's attention on a specific aspect of communication, modifying the rate at which communication occurs, and altering the mode of communication or message content.

Finally, the results obtained from screening attention, cognition, perception, and communication should be integrated with all other examination findings to make sound clinical decisions regarding the patient's plan of care. The findings from these screenings will be used to (a) make appropriate referrals, (b) develop communication strategies that enhance understanding, (c) determine the prognosis and plan interventions compatible with the patient's cognitive function, (d) avoid strategies that can cause agitation, and (e) modify or progress the plan of care throughout the course of treatment.

# Rancho Levels of Cognitive Functioning

| LEVEL | DESCRIPTION OF PATIENT RESPONSE/BEHAVIORS |
|---|---|
| **I. No response** | Patient appears to be in a deep sleep and is completely unresponsive to any stimuli. |
| **II. Generalized response** <br> *Total Assistance* | Patient reacts inconsistently and nonpurposefully to stimuli in a nonspecific manner. Responses are limited, often the same regardless of stimulus presented. Responses may be physiological changes, gross body movements, and/or vocalizations. |
| **III. Localized response** <br> *Total Assistance* | Patient reacts specifically but inconsistently to stimuli. Responses are directly related to the type of stimulus presented. May follow simple commands such as closing eyes or squeezing hand in an inconsistent delayed manner. |
| **IV. Confused-agitated** <br> *Maximal Assistance* | Patient is in a heightened state of activity. Behavior is bizarre and nonpurposeful relative to immediate environment. Does not discriminate among persons or objects; is unable to cooperate directly with treatment efforts. Verbalizations frequently are incoherent and/or inappropriate to the environment; confabulation may be present. Gross attention to environment is very brief; selective attention is often nonexistent. Patient lacks short-term and long-term recall. |
| **V. Confused-inappropriate** <br> *Maximal Assistance* | Patient is unable to respond to simple commands fairly consistently. With increased complexity of commands or lack of any external structure, responses are nonpurposeful, random, or fragmented. Demonstrates gross attention to the environment but is highly distractible and lacks ability to focus attention on a specific task. With structure, may be able to converse on a social automatic level for short periods of time. Verbalization is often inappropriate and confabulatory. Memory is severely impaired; often shows inappropriate use of objects; may perform previously learned tasks with structure but is unable to learn new information. |
| **VI. Confused-appropriate** <br> *Moderate Assistance* | Patient shows goal-directed behavior but is dependent on external input or direction. Follows simple directions consistently and shows carryover for relearned tasks such as self-care. Responses may be incorrect but are appropriate to the situation. Past memories show more depth and detail than recent memory. |
| **VII. Automatic-appropriate** <br> *Minimal Assist Routine ADLs* | Patient appears appropriate and oriented within the hospital and home settings; goes through daily routine automatically, but frequently robot-like. Patient shows minimal to no confusion and has shallow recall of activities. Shows carryover for new learning but at a decreased rate. With structure is able to initiate social or recreational activities; judgment remains impaired. |
| **VIII. Purposeful-appropriate** <br> *Stand-by Assist* | Patient is able to recall and integrate past and recent events and is aware of and responsive to environment. Shows carryover for new learning and needs no supervision once activities are learned. May continue to show a decreased ability relative to premorbid abilities, abstract reasoning, tolerance for stress, and judgment in emergencies or unusual circumstances. |
| **IX. Purposeful-appropriate** <br> *Stand-by on Request* | Patient shifts back and forth between tasks and completes for 2 hours, uses memory devices to assist when requested. Aware of limitations but needs stand-by assist to anticipate and correct problems before they occur. Able to think about consequences of decisions with assist, can adjust to task demands with stand-by assist, may have depression, may be easily irritated or have low frustration tolerance; able to self-monitor social appropriateness with stand-by assistance. |
| **X. Purposeful-appropriate** <br> *Modified Independence* | Able to handle multiple tasks in all environments but might need breaks; able to develop and maintain memory assistive devices; initiates and carries out all personal, leisure, household, community, and work tasks but may need more time; anticipates impact of disability and consequences of actions but may need more time to process decisions or use compensatory techniques; accurately estimates abilities; able to recognize needs of others, may have periodic depression, and irritability or low frustration level noted with fatigued, sick, or under stress. |

## JFK COMA RECOVERY SCALE–REVISED ©2oo4
### Record Form

*This form should only be used in association with the "CRS-R ADMINISTRATION AND SCORING GUIDELINES" which provide instructions for standardized administration of the scale.*

Patient:     Diagnosis:     Etiology:

Date of Onset:     Date of Admission:

| Date | | | | | | | | | | | | | | | | |
|---|---|---|---|---|---|---|---|---|---|---|---|---|---|---|---|---|
| Week | ADM | 2 | 3 | 4 | 5 | 6 | 7 | 8 | 9 | 10 | 11 | 12 | 13 | 14 | 15 | 16 |
| **Auditory function scale** | | | | | | | | | | | | | | | | |
| 4–Consistent movement to command * | | | | | | | | | | | | | | | | |
| 3–Reproducible movement to command * | | | | | | | | | | | | | | | | |
| 2–Localization to sound | | | | | | | | | | | | | | | | |
| 1–Auditory startle | | | | | | | | | | | | | | | | |
| 0–None | | | | | | | | | | | | | | | | |
| **Visual function scale** | | | | | | | | | | | | | | | | |
| 5–Object recognition* | | | | | | | | | | | | | | | | |
| 4–Object localization: reaching* | | | | | | | | | | | | | | | | |
| 3–Visual pursuit* | | | | | | | | | | | | | | | | |
| 2–Fixation* | | | | | | | | | | | | | | | | |
| 1–Visual startle | | | | | | | | | | | | | | | | |
| 0–None | | | | | | | | | | | | | | | | |
| **Motor function scale** | | | | | | | | | | | | | | | | |
| 6–Functional object use† | | | | | | | | | | | | | | | | |
| 5–Automatic motor response* | | | | | | | | | | | | | | | | |
| 4–Object manipulation* | | | | | | | | | | | | | | | | |
| 3–Localization to noxious stimulation * | | | | | | | | | | | | | | | | |
| 2–Flexion withdrawal | | | | | | | | | | | | | | | | |
| 1–Abnormal posturing | | | | | | | | | | | | | | | | |
| 0–None/flaccid | | | | | | | | | | | | | | | | |
| **Oromotor/verbal function scale** | | | | | | | | | | | | | | | | |
| 3–Intelligible verbalization* | | | | | | | | | | | | | | | | |
| 2–Vocalization/oral movement | | | | | | | | | | | | | | | | |
| 1–Oral reflexive movement | | | | | | | | | | | | | | | | |
| 0–None | | | | | | | | | | | | | | | | |
| **Communication scale** | | | | | | | | | | | | | | | | |
| 2–Functional: accurate† | | | | | | | | | | | | | | | | |
| 1–Non-functional: intentional* | | | | | | | | | | | | | | | | |
| 0–None | | | | | | | | | | | | | | | | |
| **Arousal scale** | | | | | | | | | | | | | | | | |
| 3–Attention | | | | | | | | | | | | | | | | |
| 2–Eye opening w/o stimulation | | | | | | | | | | | | | | | | |
| 1–Eye opening with stimulation | | | | | | | | | | | | | | | | |
| 0–Unarousable | | | | | | | | | | | | | | | | |
| **Total score** | | | | | | | | | | | | | | | | |

Denotes emergence from MCS†
Denotes MCS *

**Source:** *Giacino JT, Kalmar K, Whyte J. The JFK Coma Recovery Scale-Revised: Measurement characteristics and diagnostic utility. Arch Phys Med Rehabil. 2004;85(12):2020–2029.*

The Montreal Cognitive Assessment (MoCA) is available for public use; please refer to the website www.mocatest.org for test forms and instructions.

**Montreal cognitive assessment (MOCA)**
**Version 7.1 Original Version**

Name:
Education:          Date of birth:
Sex:                     DATE:

**Visuospatial/executive** — Copy cube / Draw CLOCK (Ten past eleven) (3 points) — POINTS

[ ]     [ ]     [ ]   [ ]   [ ]   ___/5
Contour  Numbers  Hands

**Naming**

[ ]     [ ]     [ ]     ___/3

| Memory | | Face | Velvet | Church | Daisy | Red | |
|---|---|---|---|---|---|---|---|
| Read list of words, subject must repeat them. Do 2 trials, even if 1st trial is successful. Do a recall after 5 minutes. | 1st trial | | | | | | No points |
| | 2nd trial | | | | | | |

**Attention**

Read list of digits (1 digit/sec.)  Subject has to repeat them in the forward order  [ ]  2 1 8 5 4
Subject has to repeat them in the backward order  [ ]  7 4 2     ___/2

Read list of letters. The subject must tap with his hand at each letter A. No points if ≥ 2 errors.
[ ]  F B A C M N A A J K L B A F A K D E A A A J A M O F A A B     ___/1

Serial 7 subtraction starting at 100     [ ] 93  [ ] 86  [ ] 79  [ ] 72  [ ] 65
4 or 5 correct subtractions: 3 pts, 2 or 3 correct: 2pts, 1 correct: 1 pt, 0 correct: 0 pt     ___/3

**Language**

Repeat: I only know that John is the one to help today. [ ]
The cat always hid under the couch when dogs were in the room. [ ]     ___/2

Fluency/name maximum number of words in one minute that begin with the letter F     [ ] ____ (N ≥ 11 words)  ___/1

**Abstraction**

Similarity between e.g. banana – orange = fruit     [ ] train – bicycle  [ ] watch – ruler     ___/2

| Delayed recall | Has to recall words WITH NO CUE | Face [ ] | Velvet [ ] | Church [ ] | Daisy [ ] | Red [ ] | Points for UNCUED recall only | ___/5 |
| Optional | Category cue | | | | | | | |
| | Multiple choice cue | | | | | | | |

**Orientation**  [ ] Date [ ] Month [ ] Year [ ] Day [ ] Place [ ] City     ___/6

© Z.Nasreddine MD          www.mocatest.org          Normal ≥ 25/30     TOTAL     ___/30
Administered by: _____                              Add 1 point if ≤ 12 yr edu

# Functional Assessment Staging (FAST) scale*

| STAGE | DESCRIPTION OF FUNCTION |
|---|---|
| 1 | No difficulties, either subjectively or objectively. |
| 2 | Complains of forgetting location of objects; subjective word finding difficulties only. |
| 3 | Decreased job functioning evident to coworkers; difficulty in traveling to new locations. |
| 4 | Decreased ability to perform complex tasks (e.g., planning dinner for guests, handling finances, marketing). |
| 5 | Requires assistance in choosing proper clothing for the season or occasion. |
| 6a | Difficulty putting clothing on properly without assistance. |
| 6b | Unable to bathe properly; may develop fear of bathing. Will usually require assistance adjusting bath water temperature. |
| 6c | Inability to handle mechanics of toileting (i.e., forgets to flush, doesn't wipe properly). |
| 6d | Urinary incontinence, occasional or more frequent. |
| 6e | Fecal incontinence, occasional or more frequent. |
| 7a | Ability to speak limited to about a half-dozen words in an average day. |
| 7b | Intelligible vocabulary limited to a single word in an average day. |
| 7c | Nonambulatory (unable to walk without assistance). |
| 7d | Unable to sit up independently. |
| 7e | Unable to smile. |
| 7f | Unable to hold head up. |

## Global Deterioration Scale (GDS) for Assessment of Primary Degenerative Dementia*

Stage 1. No Cognitive Decline

Stage 2. Very Mild Cognitive Decline
Forgetfulness of names and where familiar objects were left.

Stage 3. Mild Cognitive Decline
Forgetfulness of people recently introduced. Slight difficulty concentrating. Decreased work performance. Getting lost. Difficulty finding words.

Stage 4. Moderate Cognitive Decline
Difficulty concentrating. Decreased memory of recent events. Difficulties managing finances or traveling alone to new locations. Cannot complete complex tasks efficiently or accurately. May have denial and social withdrawal.

Stage 5. Moderately Severe Cognitive Decline (Early Dementia)
Some assistance required to survive. Memory loss more prominent including major relevant aspects of current lives, for example, address or phone number. May not know the time or day or where they are. May have difficulty clothing themselves properly.

Stage 6. Severe Cognitive Decline (Middle Dementia)
Start to forget names of close family and memory of most recent events. Remembers only some details of earlier life. Difficulty counting down from 10 and finishing tasks. Frequently becomes incontinent. Personality changes such as delusions (believing something to be true that is not), compulsions (repeating a simple behavior such as cleaning), or anxiety and agitation may occur.

Stage 7. Very Severe Cognitive Decline (Late Dementia)
Essentially no ability to speak or understand. Assistance with most activities (e.g., toilet, eating). Loss of psychomotor skills, for example, the ability to walk.

*Stages 1 to 4 describe cognitive decline without dementia. Stages 5 to 7 correspond to early, middle, and late dementia.

**Source:** *Reisberg, et al, 1982. Available at: https://images2.clinicaltools.com/?id = 5261:29351&cmestate = 3.*

# The Cognitive Log

**UAB Spain Rehabilitation Center: The Cognitive Log (Cog-Log)**   <u>Key:</u> Score 3, 2 ,1 or 0 for each item. See reverse side for scoring.

**Patient name:**                                    **Referral Reason:**

| | | | | | | | | | | | | | | | | | | | |
|---|---|---|---|---|---|---|---|---|---|---|---|---|---|---|---|---|---|---|---|
| Date | | | | | | | | | | | | | | | | | | | |
| Time | | | | | | | | | | | | | | | | | | | |
| Date | | | | | | | | | | | | | | | | | | | |
| Time | | | | | | | | | | | | | | | | | | | |
| Name of hospital | | | | | | | | | | | | | | | | | | | |
| Repeat address | | | | | | | | | | | | | | | | | | | |
| 20-1 | | | | | | | | | | | | | | | | | | | |
| Months reversed | | | | | | | | | | | | | | | | | | | |
| 30 seconds | | | | | | | | | | | | | | | | | | | |
| Fist-Edge-palm | | | | | | | | | | | | | | | | | | | |
| Go/ no-go | | | | | | | | | | | | | | | | | | | |
| Address recall | | | | | | | | | | | | | | | | | | | |

30

25

20

15

10

5

0

*Continued*

## Administration and scoring

The Cognitive Log (Cog-Log) is designed to be a quick quantitative measure of cognition for use at bedside with rehabilitation patients. It is intended for individuals who have achieved consistent accurate orientation, such as measured by the Orientation Log (O-Log). The Cog-Log can be used to document cognitive progress on a daily basis when time is short, such as when rounding on patients. All items are scored from 0 to 3 for a total possible score of 30, which can be graphed for quick reference.

**Date, Time, and Hospital Name:** These are components of orientation that may present problems for even those who otherwise are oriented. Scoring is similar to scoring on the O-Log, with 3 points given for a spontaneous correct response, 2 points for a correct response with a logical cue, 1 point for a correct response to multiple choice, and 0 points if unable to generate a correct response at all.

**Repeat Address:** The person is asked to repeat one of the following addresses based on the day of the week. The person is informed that the address is not of anyone they know, but is presented simply as a test of memory. If repeated accurately three times, 3 points is assigned. Correct repetition on two occasions is awarded 2 points and 1 point is assigned for correct performance on one occasion. Zero points are awarded for no correct repetitions. All subjects hear and repeat the address three times. After the repetition phase, advise the person that recall of the address will be expected later.

> Monday—John Brown, 42 Market Street, Chicago
> Tuesday—Tim Smith, 84 Center Ave., Cleveland
> Wednesday—Sally Jones, 23 North Blvd., Seattle
> Thursday—Bill Jackson, 16 Maple Court, Houston
> Friday—Judy Wilson, 75 Ocean Ave., Baltimore
> Saturday—Bob Taylor, 37 Main Street, Los Angeles
> Sunday—Susan Anderson, 58 River Road, Atlanta

**20-1:** The person is asked to count backwards from 20 to 1. Performance without error is assigned 3 points, one error is awarded 2 points, and two errors 1 point. More than two errors is assigned 0 points. Errors are corrected as they occur.

**Months Reversed:** The person is asked to say the months in reverse order beginning with December. The examiner can prompt the person by saying "December, November" and errors should be corrected as they occur. Prompting by the examiner to continue after stopping should be counted as an error. Performance without error is assigned 3 points, one error is awarded 2 points, two errors one point, and 3 or more errors 0 points.

**30 Second Test:** Without the benefit of a time piece the person is asked to estimate when 30 seconds has passed with the examiner stating "Beginning now." If the person attempts to see a clock or watch the examiner should make an attempt to stop the behavior, but not to an extent that generates a confrontation. If the person insists on looking at a time piece the item is scored 0. Score 3 points for an estimation from 25-35 seconds, 2 points for a response from 20-24 or 36-40 seconds, 1 point for an estimate that is from 15-19 or 41-45 seconds, and 0 points for an estimate less than 15 seconds or beyond 45 seconds.

**Fist-Edge-Palm:** The examiner demonstrates the hand positions of fist, edge, and palm two times telling the person to "Watch what I do." The person is then asked to repeat the sequence (either hand can be used) until told to stop by the examiner. Three correct repetitions is assigned 3 points, two repetitions 2 points, one repetition 1 point, and no repetitions 0 points.

**Go/No-Go:** The examiner instructs the person to "Raise your finger when I say red and then put it down. Do nothing if I say green." One practice trial is allowed. The order of presentation thereafter is: red, green, green, red, green, red. Assign 3 points for correct response on each trial, 2 points for correct response on 4 or 5 trials, and 1 point if correct on 3 or fewer trial trials, and 0 points if correct on no trial.

**Address Recall:** The person is asked to recall the address presented earlier. Give 3 points for full, accurate recall, 2 points for partial spontaneous recall, and one point if any further information is recalled after the name of the person is provided as a prompt. If the person has no recall 0 points is assigned.

*Source: Novack T. The Cognitive Log. The Center for Outcome Measurement in Brain Injury. Available at: http://www.tbims. org/combi/coglog. Accessed January 11, 2016.*

# Agitated Behavior Scale (ABS)

**Patient Period of Observation:**
**a.m.**
**Observ. Environ. From: p.m. / /**
**a.m.**
**Rater/Disc. To: p.m. / /**

At the end of the observation period, indicate whether the behavior described in each item was present and, if so, to what degree: slight, moderate or extreme. Use the following numerical values and criteria for your ratings.

**1 = absent:** The behavior is not present.

**2 = present to a slight degree:** The behavior is present but does not prevent the conduct of other contextually appropriate behavior. (The individual may redirect spontaneously, or the continuation of the agitated behavior does not disrupt appropriate behavior.)

**3 = present to a moderate degree:** The individual needs to be redirected from an agitated to an appropriate behavior but benefits from such cueing.

**4 = present to an extreme degree:** The individual is not able to engage in appropriate behavior due to the interference of the agitated behavior even when external cueing or redirection is provided.

DO NOT LEAVE BLANKS.

1. Short attention span, easy distractibility, inability to concentrate.
2. Impulsive, impatient, low tolerance for pain or frustration.
3. Uncooperative, resistant to care, demanding.
4. Violent and/or threatening violence toward people or property.
5. Explosive and/or unpredictable anger.
6. Rocking, rubbing, moaning or other self-stimulating behavior.
7. Pulling at tubes, restraints, etc.
8. Wandering from treatment areas.
9. Restlessness, pacing, excessive movement.
10. Repetitive behaviors, motor and/or verbal.
11. Rapid, loud, or excessive talking.
12. Sudden changes of mood.
13. Easily initiated or excessive crying and/or laughter.
14. Self-abusiveness, physical and/or verbal.

**\*Total Score ___**

## Scoring the ABS

According to *The Center for Outcome Measurement in Brain Injury,* "the Total Score is calculated by adding the ratings (from 1–4) on each of the fourteen items. Raters are instructed to leave no blanks; but, if a blank is left, the average rating for the other fourteen items should be inserted such that the Total Score reflects the appropriate possible range of values. The Total Score is the best overall measure of the course of agitation."

Subscale scores are calculated by adding ratings from the component items:

■ Disinhibition is the sum of items 1, 2, 3, 6, 7, 8, 9, and 10.
■ Aggression is the sum of items 3, 4, 5, and 14. (Item 3 is in both scores.)
■ Lability is the sum of items 11, 12, and 13.

**Source:** Bogner, J., 2000. The Agitated Behavior Scale. The Center for Outcome Measurement in Brain Injury. *Available at: http://www.tbims. org/combi/coglog.*

# Geriatric Depression Scale (GDS) Short Form

*(Provide the patient with a form that does not have the yes/no answers in bold.)*
For each question, choose the best answer for how you have felt over the past week:

| | | |
|---|---|---|
| **1.** | Are you basically satisfied with your life? | YES / **NO** |
| **2.** | Have you dropped many of your activities and interests? | **YES** / NO |
| **3.** | Do you feel that your life is empty? | **YES** / NO |
| **4.** | Do you often get bored? | **YES** / NO |
| **5.** | Are you in good spirits most of the time? | YES / **NO** |
| **6.** | Are you afraid that something bad is going to happen to you? | **YES** / NO |
| **7.** | Do you feel happy most of the time? | YES / **NO** |
| **8.** | Do you often feel helpless? | **YES** / NO |
| **9.** | Do you prefer to stay at home, rather than going out and doing new things? | **YES** / NO |
| **10.** | Do you feel you have more problems with memory than most? | **YES** / NO |
| **11.** | Do you think it is wonderful to be alive now? | YES / **NO** |
| **12.** | Do you feel pretty worthless the way you are now? | **YES** / NO |
| **13.** | Do you feel full of energy? | YES / **NO** |
| **14.** | Do you feel that your situation is hopeless? | **YES** / NO |
| **15.** | Do you think that most people are better off than you are? | **YES** / NO |

1 point is scored for each "depressed" response (answer in bold). Scores of 0 to 4 are considered normal. For clinical purposes, a score >5 points is suggestive of depression and should warrant a follow-up interview. Scores of >10 are almost always depression.

***Source:*** *Brink TL, Yesavage JA, Lum O, Heersema P, Adey MB, Rose TL. Screening tests for geriatric depression. Clin Gerontol. 1:37–44; 1982. (The website http://www.stanford.edu/~yesavage/GDS.html from whence this form was accessed states that, "The original scale is in the **public domain** due to it being partly the result of Federal support.")*

# The Beck Depression Inventory-Short Form

**A.** Mood
- 3 I am so sad or unhappy that I can't stand it.
- 2b I am so sad or unhappy that it is very painful.
- 2a I am blue or sad all the time and I can't snap out of it.
- 1 I feel blue or sad.
- 0 I do not feel sad.

**B.** Pessimism
- 3 I feel that the future is hopeless and that things cannot improve.
- 2b I feel that I won't ever get over my troubles.
- 2a I feel I have nothing to look forward to.
- 1 I feel discouraged about the future.
- 0 I am not particularly pessimistic or discouraged about the future.

**C.** Sense of Failure
- 3 I feel I am a complete failure as a person (parent, husband, wife).
- 2b As I look back on my life, all I can see is a lot of failures.
- 2a I feel I have accomplished very little that is worthwhile or that means anything.
- 1 I feel I have failed more than the average person.
- 0 I do not feel like a failure.

**D.** Lack of Satisfaction
- 3 I am dissatisfied with everything.
- 2 I don't get satisfaction out of anything anymore.
- 1b I don't enjoy things the way I used to.
- 1a I feel bored most of the time.
- 0 I am not particularly dissatisfied.

**E.** Guilty Feelings
- 3 I feel as though I am very bad or worthless.
- 2b I feel bad or unworthy practically all of the time now.
- 2a I feel quite guilty.
- 1 I feel bad or unworthy a good part of the time.
- 0 I don't feel particularly guilty.

**F.** Self-Hate
- 3 I hate myself.
- 2b I am disgusted with myself.
- 2a I don't like myself.
- 1 I am disappointed in myself.
- 0 I don't feel disappointed in myself.

**G.** Self-Punitive Wishes
- 3 I would kill myself if I could.
- 2c I feel my family would be better off if I were dead.

- 2b I have definite plans about committing suicide.
- 2a I feel I would be better off dead.
- 1 I have thoughts of harming myself, but I would not carry them out.
- 0 I don't have any thoughts of harming myself.

**H.** Social Withdrawal
- 3 I have lost all of my interest in other people and don't care about them at all.
- 2 I have lost most of my interest in other people and have little feeling for them.
- 1 I am less interested in other people now than I used to be.
- 0 I have not lost interest in other people.

**I.** Indecisiveness
- 3 I can't make any decisions at all any more.
- 2 I can't make any decisions any more without help.
- 1 I am less sure of myself now and try to put off making decisions.
- 0 I make decisions about as well as ever.

**J.** Body Image
- 3 I feel that I am ugly or repulsive looking.
- 2 I feel that there are permanent changes in my appearance, and they make me look unattractive.
- 1 I am worried that I am looking old or unattractive.
- 0 I don't feel I look any worse than I used to.

**K.** Work Inhibition
- 3 I can't do any work at all.
- 2 I have to push myself very hard to do anything.
- 1b I don't work as well as I used to.
- 1a It takes extra effort to get started at doing something.
- 0 I can work about as well as before.

**L.** Fatigability
- 3 I get too tired to do anything.
- 2 I get tired from doing anything.
- 1 I get tired more easily than I used to.
- 0 I don't get any more tired than usual.

**M.** Loss of Appetite
- 3 I have no appetite at all anymore.
- 2 My appetite is much worse now.
- 1 My appetite is not as good as it used to be.
- 0 My appetite is no worse than usual.

Interpretation Beck Depression Inventory-Short Form:
5 to 7: mild depression
8 to 15: moderate depression
≥16: severe depression

*Source:* Gallo JJ, Reichel W, Andersen L. Handbook of Geriatric Assessment. Gaithersurg, MD: Aspen Publishers; 1988.

# Screening for Unilateral Spatial Neglect

**Screening for unilateral spatial neglect**

### 1) Draw an item (draw a clock)

Give the patient a piece of paper with a picture of house, flower, or clock, as shown on the left and ask the patient to copy the diagrams. Patients with unilateral neglect will not incorporate components from one side of the object as shown in the three example figures on the right.

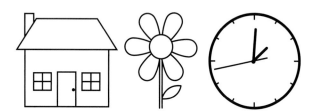 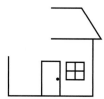 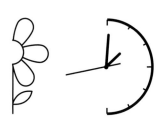

# Examination and Evaluation of Sensory Systems

Dennis W. Fell, PT, MD        CHAPTER 5

**CHAPTER OBJECTIVES**

Upon completion of this chapter, the learner should be able to:

1. Summarize the neuroanatomical regions, structures, and pathways related to sensory abilities and impairments caused by neuromuscular pathology/injury.
2. List and describe the variety of sensory modalities that can be tested.
3. Infer the impact of specific sensory deficits on functional abilities.
4. Synthesize patient factors to select the most appropriate sensory tests and measures for application to a given patient.
5. Implement each test described and document results in a patient medical record.

## ▓ Introduction

**Sensation** has been defined as "a feeling; the translation into consciousness of the effects of a stimulus exciting any of the organs of sense" (Stedman, 1982). The term sensation implies that the feeling or impression is conveyed to and processed by the central nervous system. Most sensation is processed at an awareness level and is therefore termed conscious sensation. However, some important sensory systems will be discussed (e.g., spinocerebellar "unconscious" proprioception) that are processed primarily at a subconscious or unconscious level although, with intent, one can transfer that sensory information to a conscious level. Sensation reflects information from the internal or external environment. Humans are aware of certain sensations and can purposely bring others to a level of awareness. The modalities of sensation are the specific types of sensation including pain, pressure, and joint position sense. A related term, **sensibility**, is the aspect therapists

test as part of the neurological examination and has been described as "the capability of perceiving sensible stimuli" (Stedman, 1982). Cortical sensibility processed by the cerebral cortex is the recognition of sensory information and related discrimination of sensory impression (Waylett-Rendall, 1988). In our sensory evaluation for some modalities we must determine the **threshold stimulus**, also called the limen, which is the minimal stimulus level that will produce a sensation (Jimenez, 1993). This must be determined for some of the modalities of sensation. These terms are descriptive of the stimuli we experience, the ability to feel the stimuli, or the degree to which we detect the stimuli, and they represent the content of the sensory examination.

Sensation includes all incoming information brought into the nervous system, whether processed consciously or subconsciously. In neuroscience, the term **afferent impulses** is used for sensory or incoming signals, while **efferent impulses** are those that transmit information away from the nervous system to an effector organ (muscle or gland). Sensory signals always originate from sensory receptors designed to monitor either conditions from the external environment such as pressure or temperature or internal conditions such as joint position or visceral sensation.

Examination of sensation and sensory awareness is an essential, but sometimes incomplete, portion of the neurological examination. This part of the evaluation is useful as part of the basis for clinical decision-making and to quantify sensory aspects of recovery (Cooke, 1991). Although motor integrity is a primary examination focus for rehabilitation professionals intent on improving movement, the sensory status is critical due to its profound influence on movement control. The effect of sensory impairments on motor abilities has been noted (Marsh, 1986; Dannenbaum, 1990; Bell-Krotoski, 1993; Robertson, 1994). Superficial sensation plays an obvious role in the protection of the body surface against trauma and pressure wounds (Taub, 1976; Whimster, 1976).

The important influence of sensation on movement will be explained in greater detail in the discussion of motor control theories in Chapter 14. Relative to some of the earliest reflex theories of motor control, sensory input serves as the essential basis for reflexive movements. In the more recent systems theories of motor control, sensory information is used as feedback in the control, support, and modification of movement. In addition to the effect of sensation on movement, movement can also certainly be used to alter the sensory experience of the environment. By moving the whole body or parts into certain locations, more or less sensation can be experienced.

This chapter includes discussions on sensory processing, the sensory modalities and common sensory impairments, and methods to examine the sensory system. A summary of the neuroscience basis of sensory processing is provided, but specific details are beyond the scope of this book. The examination methods described in detail in this chapter address sensory components from four categories: superficial sense, discriminative sense, proprioceptive sense, and chronic pain. These examination methods contribute to the therapist's assessment of sensory status and implications for motor function.

Evaluation of the special senses received through the cranial nerves including olfaction, vision, taste, and auditory sensation as well as tactile sensation from the face received through cranial nerve V, the Trigeminal nerve, are covered in Chapter 7. Evaluation methods for tactile and joint sensation from the head and face regions are the same as those described in this chapter but are applied to the facial skin, muscles, and joints of the head. Sensory deficits must be distinguished from perceptual deficits, which are discussed in Chapter 4. In perceptual deficits, the peripheral sensory structures may be functional, and even basic awareness of sensation may be intact; however, the person is unable to fully integrate, interpret, use, or apply meaning to specific portions of the information. Electrophysiologic testing of the sensory system, particularly nerve conduction velocity (NCV) testing is discussed in Chapter 11. The reader will find a discussion of therapeutic intervention related to the sensory deficits in Chapter 30 and a discussion of therapeutic intervention related to chronic pain in Chapter 31.

## Categories of Sensation

Sensory modalities or the types of sensory input can be generally divided into two broad categories: superficial or deep. **Superficial sensation**, also called **tactile sensation,** includes all sensations detected by receptors at the surface of the body and are usually associated with the skin or skin appendages. Some superficial sensory modalities are processed together and used to produce combined sensations. They are a subset of the discriminative general senses. The **deep sensations**, known generally as **proprioception**, may be processed consciously or subconsciously and include sensations related to position or movement of a joint or body segment or awareness of length of a specific muscle.

Superficial sensation includes pain, temperature, light touch, and pressure touch. In the examination, **pain sensibility** can be defined as the unpleasant feeling resulting from a sensory stimulus that is sharp or pinpoint, especially when the stimulus has the potential to cause tissue damage. This sensory modality, protective in nature, can also be referred to as sharp/dull discrimination. The pathological experience of *chronic pain* related to injury, inflammation, or disease is evaluated separately and is discussed later in this section. **Temperature sensibility** interprets the heat or cold state of an object or environment and also plays a protective role. **Light touch** is the sensation caused by the mildest of tactile stimulation even slight contact with separate receptor types in skin with hair and hairless or glabrous skin. In skin with hair, the stimulus usually does not even have to contact the skin surface, but the sensation can occur with only minimal application of a mechanical stimulation to a hair shaft alone (as when a mosquito lands on your arm). **Pressure touch** sensation results from mechanical stimulation due to a greater magnitude of pressures with deeper skin deformation.

Discriminative sensations include vibration, tactile localization, two-point discrimination, graphesthesia, and stereognosis. The last four of these are often considered to be perceptual processes requiring integration of numerous sensory signals and multiple sensory modalities and not purely sensory. They will, however, be included in this chapter. **Vibration** is the sensation experienced from tactile contact with an object that is shaking or oscillating at a particular frequency. **Tactile localization** is awareness of the specific skin surface site to which stimulation was applied and is characterized and documented by the distance error between the actual site of stimulus and the subject-reported site of stimulus. **Two-point discrimination** sensibility is the ability to distinguish two simultaneously applied blunt points as two discrete stimuli. The smallest interpoint distance still perceived as two points quantifies the threshold of two-point discrimination. **Graphesthesia** is the recognition of symbols traced on the patient's palm including shapes, numbers, or letters. **Stereognosis** is the ability to recognize, by tactile manipulation only, the form and characteristics of an object including size, shape, weight, consistency, and texture.

Deep sensations include joint position sense and joint movement sense and are very important components of feedback as a basis for motor control. Joint **position sense**, sometimes simply referred to with the generic term *proprioception,* is the awareness of static positions of a single joint or body segment detected without use of vision. Joint **movement sense**, often called **kinesthesia**, is awareness of the degree, velocity, and direction of movement at a single joint or body segment also internally detected through muscle and joint receptors.

In addition to alterations, deficits, or impairments of the normal sensations previously described, individuals may experience long-lasting pain that does not resolve as expected with healing. The dysfunction of prolonged or **chronic pain** is defined as the negative unfavorable sensory experience resulting from injury or pathology often related to inflammation. Chronic pain usually includes a perception of excessive and noxious sensation most often related to tissue injury. Pain, including the related noxious or negative perception of the sensation, can functionally contribute to appropriate actions to avoid continued pain or injury. Aspects of pain to be evaluated include the regional distribution and location of the pain, the intensity of the pain, aggravating and alleviating factors, and the affective dimensions of the pain. Pain may be experienced and described at the site of injury or at a site distant from the injury. **Referred pain** is the term used to describe pain that occurs at a site distant from the source of the pain. Aspects of sensory integrity and chronic pain must be appropriately evaluated in the patient with neuromuscular pathology.

## Summary Review of the Neuroscience of Sensation

Each sensory modality has specific sensory receptors (Fig. 5-1) converting the specific form of energy (mechanical, thermal, chemical, or electromagnetic) into an action potential transmitted into the central nervous system as afferent action potentials or impulses. The modalities of light touch, pressure touch, pain, vibration, and proprioception use receptors categorized as mechanoreceptors. The name mechanoreceptor refers to the receptor design that specifically responds to mechanical sources of energy as inputs. Pain impulses can be initiated by a class of receptors called nociceptors or nocioceptors, most commonly free nerve endings, but also from the effect of temperature extremes on heat and cold receptors. Temperature sensation is detected by thermal receptors. Cold and warmth receptors, located under the skin with cold receptors positioned at greater depth than warmth receptors (Morin, 1998), have concentrations varying by body region. As early as 1981, Guyton reported there are three to four times as many cold receptors as warmth receptors in most areas of the body, a figure still reported today (Jay, 2002) with greatest density in the lips (15 to 25 cold points per square centimeter) compared with fingers (3 to 5 cold points per square centimeter) and certain broad surface areas like the trunk (less than 1 cold point per square centimeter).

For each modality of sensation, Table 5-1 summarizes the major receptors utilized, the location of the receptor, the name of the related afferent pathway, the location of the afferent pathway within the spinal cord, and the location and level of crossing decussating fibers. Receptors for superficial sensations are typically located within or associated with the layers of the skin, while receptors for deep sensations, especially position and movement sense, are found within the muscle, joint surface, or capsule. Because most cerebral cortex areas control contralateral function, pathways for conscious sensation tend to decussate or cross to the opposite side as they ascend toward the cortex. It is important to know the longitudinal level at which fibers of each pathway cross (i.e., do the fibers cross in the spinal cord or in the brainstem?). Figure 5-2 highlights the major anatomic areas of the central nervous system related to sensation, and Figure 5-3 schematically represents the general path of each sensory tract listed in Table 5-1, including the longitudinal level of decussation. The geographic location of the crossing fibers within a stated horizontal section of the central nervous system are also important and are shown in Figure 5-3.

## Functional Implications

The sensory systems and the information they provide to the central nervous system are essential for optimal control and efficiency of movement. Tactile sensation provides important clues regarding the interaction of each body part with the environment, including supporting structures, perturbing objects, and external forces. For example, pressure sensation from the sole of the foot provides feedback related to center of gravity location essential for optimal balance control in standing. When leaning forward, more weight is sensed through the forefoot plantar surface. Leaning backward causes increased pressure through the heel of the foot and less through the forefoot. Joint position sense and movement sense provide feedback about muscle length and joint angles as movement occurs. Kinesthetic awareness of movement is a foundational concept in approaches such as the Feldenkrais approach to therapeutic intervention (Ruth, 1992). This proprioceptive feedback is essential for optimal motor control and the fine adjustments needed for skilled coordinated movement during tasks and activities that comprise participation.

In neuromuscular disease or trauma, damage may occur to the peripheral receptors, afferent pathways (peripheral nerve, spinal cord, brainstem, or cortical white matter), central relay nuclei (brainstem nuclei, thalamus, basal ganglia), or areas of sensory cortex (primary, secondary, or association). If dysfunction occurs in any of these structures, the person may experience partial or complete loss of sensation. Lack of pain, temperature, or pressure sensation increases the risk of injury to self and requires increased visual attention to affected areas for minimizing injury risk. Impaired joint position sense could diminish ongoing motor adjustments resulting in poorly controlled movement. Visual attention to the movement may partially compensate for such sensory loss.

**A**    **Superficial Mechanoreceptors:** detect mechanical deformation
• in the skin includes (especially for temperature, touch, and pressure):

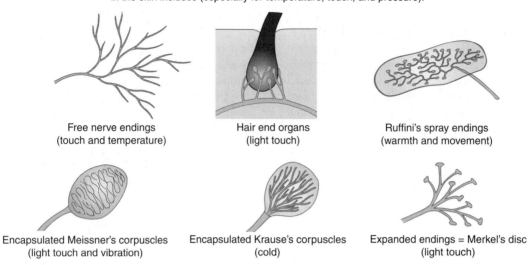

Free nerve endings
(touch and temperature)

Hair end organs
(light touch)

Ruffini's spray endings
(warmth and movement)

Encapsulated Meissner's corpuscles
(light touch and vibration)

Encapsulated Krause's corpuscles
(cold)

Expanded endings = Merkel's disc
(light touch)

**B**    **Deep Mechanoreceptors** (especially for pressure):
• in the deeper tissues include free nerve
endings, expanded nerve endings, and

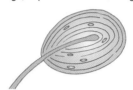

encapsulated Pacinian corpuscle
(deep pressure and vibration)

**C**

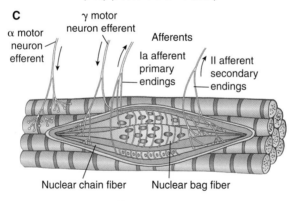

α motor neuron efferent

γ motor neuron efferent

Afferents

Ia afferent primary endings

II afferent secondary endings

Nuclear chain fiber    Nuclear bag fiber

Muscle spindles
(unconscious proprioception)

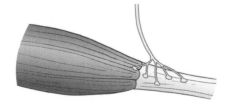

Golgi tendon organs
(unconscious proprioception)

**FIGURE 5-1** Drawing of sensory receptor types. Sensory mechanoreceptors from skin, deep tissue, and muscle. **A.** Superficial mechanoreceptors: detect mechanical deformation in the skin includes (especially for temperature, touch, and pressure): **B.** Deep mechanoreceptors (especially for pressure) in the deeper tissues include free nerve endings, expanded nerve endings, and encapsulated Pacinian corpuscles (deep pressure and vibration). **C.** Deep mechanoreceptors for proprioceptive muscle awareness.

| TABLE 5-1 | Sensory Modality Details | | |
|---|---|---|---|
| **SENSORY MODALITY** | **RECEPTORS UTILIZED** | **NAME (AND LOCATION OF SPINAL PATHWAY)** | **LEVEL AND NAME OF DECUSSATION** |
| *Pain (sharp/dull) | Free nerve endings (FNE) (also in muscle and joint capsule), thermoreceptors | Lateral spinothalamic tract (in contralateral anterolateral spinal cord) | Fibers from posterior horn cells cross within one to two levels of entry into the spinal cord through the "anterior commissure" |
| *Temperature | Free nerve endings | Lateral spinothalamic tract (in contralateral anterolateral spinal cord) | Fibers from posterior horn cells cross within one to two levels of entry into the spinal cord through the "anterior commissure" |
| *Touch | Merkel's disks*, FNE, hair follicle endings, Ruffini endings, Krause's end-bulb, and possibly Meissner's corpuscles* | Anterior spinothalamic tract (AST) (in contralateral anterolateral spinal cord) and medial lemniscal (ML) system (in ipsilateral posterior columns of spinal cord) | AST fibers from posterior horn cells cross within one to two levels of entry into the spinal cord through the "anterior commissure;" ML fibers cross from nucleus cuneatus and nucleus gracilis in low medulla as the "internal arcuate fibers" |
| *Pressure | Pacinian corpuscles, FNE (also in muscle), Ruffini endings (especially for maintained pressure), Krause's end-bulb | Medial lemniscal system: fasciculus gracilis and fasciculus cuneatus (in ipsilateral dorsal column of spinal cord); becomes the medial lemniscus (in the low medulla of the brainstem) | Fibers cross from nucleus cuneatus and nucleus gracilis in low medulla as the "internal arcuate fibers" |
| *Two-point discrimination | Merkel's disks* | (Same as pressure) | (Same as pressure) |
| *Tactile localization | Merkel's disks*, Meissner's corpuscles | (Same as pressure) | (Same as pressure) |
| *Discriminative touch (stereognosis, texture) | Meissner's corpuscles* | (Same as pressure) | (Same as pressure) |
| *Vibration | Pacinian corpuscles* Pacinian corpuscles are located subcutaneous and within deep tissues (muscle, tendon, and joint soft tissue) | (Same as pressure) | (Same as pressure) |
| *Joint Position and Movement sense (conscious) | Muscle spindles, joint receptors, golgi-type endings in ligaments, Ruffini endings in joint capsule and ligaments (for direction and velocity), free nerve ending in joint capsule (for crude awareness), Paciniform endings in joint capsule (especially for rapid joint movements) | (Same as pressure) | (Same as pressure) |
| *Tension of muscle | Golgi tendon organ (protective function for muscle) | (Same as pressure) | (Same as pressure) |

*Pacinian and Meissner corpuscles are quickly adapting receptors for moving touch. Merkel's disks, in hairy and glabrous skin, are slowly adapting to detect constant touch, low intensity, and velocity of touch.

## ■WHERE IS IT?

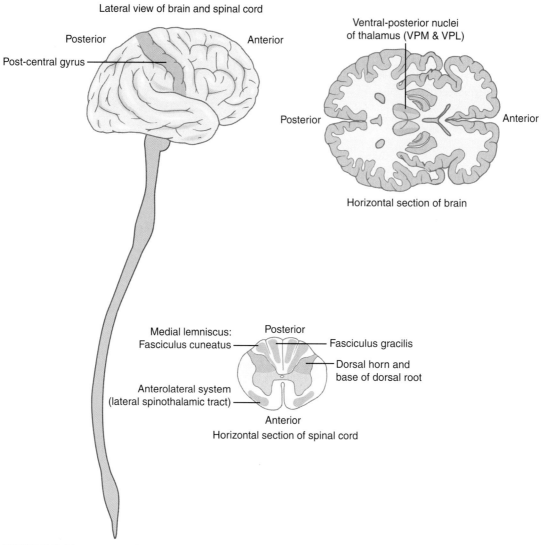

Lateral view of brain and spinal cord

Posterior          Anterior

Post-central gyrus

Ventral-posterior nuclei
of thalamus (VPM & VPL)

Posterior                    Anterior

Horizontal section of brain

Medial lemniscus:          Posterior
Fasciculus cuneatus                    Fasciculus gracilis

Dorsal horn and
base of dorsal root

Anterolateral system
(lateral spinothalamic tract)

Anterior
Horizontal section of spinal cord

**FIGURE 5-2** Major sensory locations of the central nervous system (within brain, brainstem, and spinal cord). These drawings highlight neuroanatomic sites related to sensation. In the brain, the postcentral gyrus is the primary somatosensory cortex, and ventral posteromedial (VPM) and ventral posterolateral (VPL) of the thalamus are processing and relaying nuclei for sensory information from the face and body, respectively, traveling to the cortex. In the spinal cord, the posterior funiculus carries the discriminative general senses of the medial lemniscal system, the posterior horn of the spinal cord houses most sensory nuclei, and the anterolateral system of the spinal cord carries light-touch and pain/temperature sensations.

### PATIENT APPLICATION

*Ellie is a 42 year-old white female diagnosed with multiple sclerosis (MS) 6 months ago. She has a supportive husband and two daughters who are both recently married. She has a very progressive form of MS with both motor and sensory deficits in a sporadic distribution. Here, we will focus on her sensory deficits. When she first started rehab 4 months ago, she was able to accurately report position sense and light-touch sensation throughout the upper and lower extremity, but observing her gait revealed an obvious lack of unconscious proprioception (processed by the cerebellum) in the right lower extremity, expressed with foot slap at initial contact because her body didn't have information about ankle position. Today, in addition to the loss of unconscious proprioception in the right*

*ankle, she also reports a loss of touch sensation in the right foot and calf, most of the left lower extremity, and parts of the right shoulder/arm region. Functionally, she has noticed greater difficulty with leg/foot placement. These new sensory losses are putting her at risk for extremity injury.*

### Contemplate Clinical Decisions

1. What safety concerns do you have for Ellie?
2. As the therapist, which parts of the sensory examination will you complete as a basis for treatment plan decisions and appropriate patient education?
3. Anatomically, where will you focus and be most specific with your examination?

## ■WHERE IS IT?

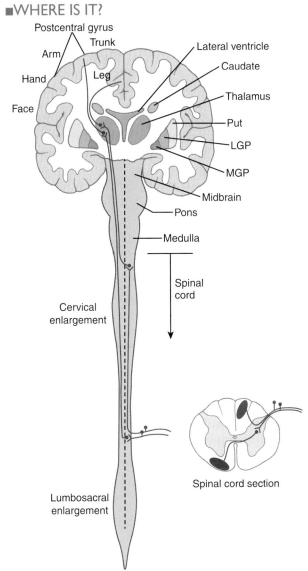

**FIGURE 5-3** Longitudinal drawing of major sensory pathways. This figure illustrates the central nervous system sensory pathways for medial lemniscus/posterior columns (carrying discriminative general senses) in blue and both lateral spinothalamic (carrying pain and temperature) and anterior spinothalamic (carrying light touch) in red. The location shown for terminus of medial lemniscus fibers on the inferior right postcentral portion of the paracentral lobule approximately represents sensation carried from the distal left lower extremity. The location shown for terminus of lateral spinothalamic fibers on the lateral surface (midportion) of the right postcentral gyrus approximately represents sensation carried from the proximal left upper extremity.

## ■ General Considerations for Sensory Examination

The general principles for sensory examination, the sequence for testing the various sensory modalities, and the parameters to investigate for each modality tested will now be discussed. This general discussion is followed by sections with specific instructions for examination of superficial sensation, discriminative

sensation, proprioceptive sensation, and chronic pain. Tests and measures may be chosen with respect to scientific evidence and the degree of support from the evidence for use of any examination method. For each test discussed in this chapter, the evidence basis available is summarized in the *Focus on Evidence* (FOE) Table 5-8 online (ONL).

## General Principles of Sensory Examination

Formal sensory examination, with the exception of electrophysiologic testing, primarily investigates the status of the consciously processed sensory modalities. For most aspects of sensory examination, you will ask the patient to respond based on his or her awareness of the sensory input given. Keep in mind, however, some essential sensory systems are not routinely processed at a conscious level and cannot be directly tested. For these systems, we can only make indirect inferences or deductions based on what we observe to be contributions those unconscious sensations make to movement. An example is the spinocerebellar system processing unconscious proprioception at the level of the cerebellum.

The sensory examination should start with screening questions such as, "Are there any areas of your skin where your feeling has changed or decreased?" In cerebrovascular pathology, with expected asymmetry, you might ask the question, "Does the skin of one side of your body feel different to you than the other side? What parts?" Obtaining this subjective information early in the evaluation has been suggested to help determine which areas are to be tested formally (Waylett-Rendall, 1988). The simple initial approach of using screening questions to guide your specific examination will quickly draw your attention to problem areas, although the whole body needs to be tested.

For each modality tested, visually demonstrate the method to the patient before you start the actual testing so the patient knows what to expect. You should explain the test you will do, show the patient what to do, and allow the patient to feel the stimulation that will be applied. Apply the stimulus first to an area where you don't expect to find impairment (for example, the "unaffected side" in a person with cerebrovascular accident or the upper extremity in a person with paraplegia) allowing the patient to watch. This simple step may help diminish anxiety in the patient (especially when you explain you are going to test "pain" sensation!) and also increase the validity of your testing as the patient knows what sensation to anticipate and what to report. At this point, as the patient watches, you should also clearly define response terms and response options with the patient: "This is sharp," "This is dull," or "We'll call this right and this left."

After demonstrating the method, vision should be eliminated during each sensory test. You can either ask the patient to close the eyes or use a blindfold if the patient is unable to keep the eyes closed. As with other aspects of examination, the patient may want to "perform well" and may, without intention, be driven to give the "right" response whether it is felt or not. In some cases, this may be a reflection of cognitive and perceptual status, including impulsivity. Elimination of vision will assure patient responses are strictly based on the sensation being tested without visual compensation. If several stimuli are presented during the course of a test and the patient has to choose a response appropriate for the stimuli presented, it is best to present the stimuli in a randomly variable sequence so the patient will not anticipate the next stimulus.

Each stimulus or test position should be maintained for several seconds and not just applied instantaneously. In fact, it is often preferable to leave the stimulus in place, if this is possible within the specific test methodology, until the patient responds, allowing sufficient time for central processing and response. Do not move too quickly from one test site to the next, especially if it is an adjacent area. This may interfere with central processing and verbal response and may have a summation effect as a previous stimulus may reinforce the current stimulus.

If the patient is unable to respond verbally, you will need to develop an alternative method for patient response such as, "Blink your eyes if 'dull,' or open your eyes wide if 'sharp.'" If cognitive deficits prevent accurate responses (also in pediatric patients), the therapist may have to infer sensibility based on the patient's nonverbal and motor response to introduced stimuli.

All parts of the sensory examination described in this chapter should be performed bilaterally for comparison of specific locations on right and left sides. This applies to superficial, deep, and discriminative senses. Bilateral testing will allow you to confirm whether or not expected differences based on diagnosis are present. However, the sequence of specific locations tested is different depending on whether you are doing superficial or deep sensation testing.

## THINK ABOUT IT 5.1

- What screening questions would you ask Ellie?
- Given Ellie's complaints of sensory loss, describe your testing process.

## Sequence of Sensory Testing

The sequence to follow for testing modalities of superficial sensation is best organized around dermatomes. A **dermatome** is a region of skin whose sensory information is received by a single spinal nerve root. Each dermatome area is named according to the spinal level of the related spinal nerve root (i.e., L2 or T10). Figure 5-4 shows a map of dermatomes suggested by Gilroy and Meyer (1979) that are typically used in sensory examination. Note the characteristic arrangement of dermatomes in the limbs. The somewhat spiral orientation is related at least in part to the rotation that the limbs undergo during normal embryological development. The dermatomes of the trunk are oriented as horizontal bands wrapping around the trunk.

Dermatomal testing is certainly not an exact science because of the variability and the overlap between adjacent dermatomes. It is important to remember the top half of one dermatome overlaps with the lower half of the dermatome above it, and the bottom half of a dermatome overlaps with the top half of the dermatome below it, as shown in Figure 5-4. Also remember that C5-T1 roots supply the brachial plexus to serve the upper extremity, and L2-S3 roots contribute to the lumbosacral plexus for the lower extremity. Therefore, T2-L1 roots are dedicated to trunk dermatomes alone. Some of the key surface landmarks associated with dermatome levels are summarized in Table 5-2 to help standardize and interpret your tactile sensory evaluation. The skin of the face and cheek mucosa is actually supplied by the Trigeminal nerve, and full assessment of this cranial nerve is discussed in Chapter 7. For sensory evaluation of the body, it will enhance consistency if you always test the dermatomes in a systematic order. For example, you could test top to bottom, for example, top and back of head for C1-2; back of neck and upper trunk for C3-4; circumferentially around each arm and forearm and across the fingertips of first, third, and fifth digits for C5-T1; paramedian along the anterior trunk for T2-L1; and circumferentially around lower extremity beginning with anterior iliac crest and including the superior surface of the foot for L2-S3. Testing anteriorly on the trunk will reveal peripheral nerve lesions there that you may miss if you test on the posterior trunk only. Careful sensory testing after a standard dermatomal sequence can help to screen for and diagnose sensory impairment in any distribution.

The testing sequence for discriminative and deep sensations is not organized around dermatomes but joints and body regions. This is primarily because of the regional differences in discrimination and the fact that joint sense testing must obviously take place joint by joint. Because these tests are performed more globally than superficial sensation tests, a chart organized by body region is ideal for documentation of these sensations. The testing sequence for discriminative and deep sensation testing as part of a comprehensive sensory evaluation therefore includes areas of the face (forehead, cheek, lips) and, for proprioception, joint regions including jaw, neck, shoulder, elbow, wrist, interphalangeal (IP) joints, spine, hip, knee, ankle, and toes.

## Parameters of Sensory Impairment to Investigate

When a sensory examination is begun, the general task is to identify, fully describe, and document all sensory impairments, especially if they interfere with activities and participation. Based on the medical diagnosis of the patient and an understanding of the related pathophysiology, the therapist will have some idea of possible sensory deficits and their expected body distribution even before starting the examination. When a sensory impairment is identified in a particular patient, the next step is to determine the parameters or characteristics of the identified sensory impairment including (1) *quantity* and (2) *quality* of the sensory impairment. The details of these two general parameters will be observed and determined through patient interview, examination techniques, and clarifying questions.

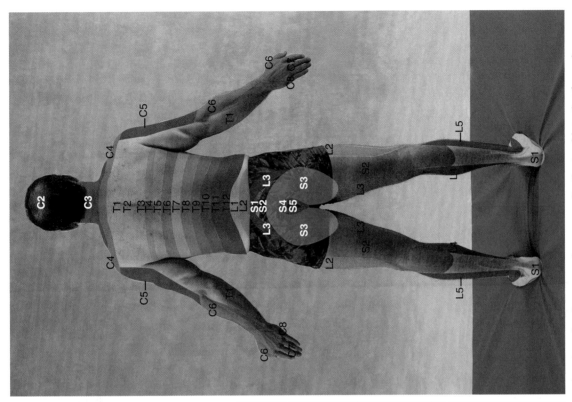

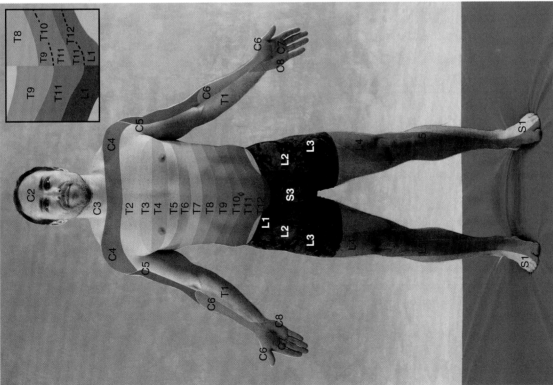

**FIGURE 5-4** Dermatome Map. A dermatome surface map showing the approximate location of each sensory dermatome distribution. Note that for each dermatome, the upper half overlaps with the next highest dermatome, and the lower half overlaps with the next lowest dermatome. The inset diagram illustrates this overlap in the lower part of the anterior trunk. Each dermatome level is present bilaterally, but for this illustration, only even-numbered dermatomes are shown on one side and odd-numbered dermatomes are shown on the other side. As shown, the top half of T10 dermatome is also innervated by the T9 root, and the bottom half of T10 dermatome is also innervated by the T11 root.

| TABLE 5-2 | Key Surface Landmarks for Sensory Testing |
|---|---|
| **DERMATOME** | **SKIN OVER THIS SURFACE STRUCTURE** |
| C2 | Posterior half of skull |
| C3 | Medial end of clavicle |
| C4 | Medial acromion and below clavicle |
| C5 | Lateral elbow (and lateral acromion) |
| C6 | 1st digit (and 2nd digit) |
| C7 | 3rd digit |
| C8 | 5th digit (and 4th digit) |
| T1 | Medial elbow |
| T2 | Anterior axilla |
| T4 | Nipple line |
| T6 or T7 | Xiphoid process |
| T10 | Umbilicus |
| T12 | Anterior iliac crest/pubic symphysis |
| L1 | Inguinal region (upper medial thigh) |
| L2 | Medial thigh–mid-distance |
| L3 | Medial knee |
| L4 | Medial malleolus |
| L5 | Base of great toe (and lateral aspect leg/plantar aspect to heel) |
| S1 | Lateral heel (base of 5th digit, fibula head, lateral malleolus, little toe) |
| S2 | Posterior knee |
| S3 | Ischial tuberosity |

*Quantity* of sensory impairment includes all characteristics related to the *extent,* size, and regional dimensions of the deficit. Assess quantity by noting the boundaries of the impairment, defining regionally where the deficit starts and where it stops. The regional distribution you determine for all sensory impairments will probably fall into one of five possible distribution patterns that each correlate anatomically with a certain hierarchical level of nervous system injury: unilateral, paraplegic/tetraplegic, dermatomal, peripheral nerve, or general peripheral neuropathy. Sensory deficits associated with cerebral or brainstem pathology (central nervous system) usually occur in a **unilateral distribution** (Fig. 5-5A) often involving both the arm and leg on the side of the body contralateral to the central nervous system pathology. Either a **paraplegic distribution** (Fig. 5-5B) (involvement of lower extremities and trunk, but arm function is unimpaired) or a **tetraplegic (quadriplegic) distribution** (lower extremities and upper extremities) of sensory loss is associated with spinal cord injury with sensory loss only in tissues innervated from below the injury level. Please note that the terms "paraplegic" and "tetraplegic" are used as adjectives to describe the distribution of sensory loss

and are not used as descriptors of the person. While paraplegia always involves some impairment of upper extremities, significant portions of the proximal limbs may also be spared if injury is to the lower cervical segments. **Dermatomal distribution** of sensory symptoms is related to nerve root lesions resulting in band-like areas of sensory loss as shown earlier in the dermatomal maps (Fig. 5-4). A peripheral nerve lesion will result in a **peripheral nerve distribution** of sensory loss characteristic of the particular cutaneous nerve distribution for the lesioned nerve (Fig. 5-5C). Peripheral nerve cutaneous distribution maps can be found in anatomy texts and atlases. A general **peripheral distribution** of sensory deficits, also described as "stocking/glove distribution," occurs generally in the distalmost parts of the limbs (feet and hands). However, this distribution does not fit a peripheral nerve distribution and anatomically such a general peripheral distribution is not a possibility with trauma to a peripheral nerve. A diagram of a classic sensory deficit distribution related to peripheral neuropathy is shown in Figure 5-5D. This type of peripheral distribution occurs most commonly with peripheral neuropathy, especially chronic diabetes and other metabolic conditions. For comparison, an L5 dermatomal distribution of sensory loss is shown in Figure 5-5E. A distribution of sensory deficits sometimes occurs that follows no pattern and is termed a **sporadic distribution**. A sporadic distribution is usually asymmetrical, perhaps affecting both sides but different regions on each side (see Fig. 5-5F). The extent or boundaries of the sensory deficit are most often related to the location of pathology in the nervous system.

*Quality* of sensory impairment includes characterization of the degree of sensory dysfunction. If sensation is unimpaired or meets some established norms for sensory function, terms like *normal* or *intact* are used in the documentation. At the opposite end of the spectrum, if sensation is completely lost and the individual has no sensibility in the affected region, the term *absent* is used. If all sensory modalities are lost, the term **anesthesia** is used. In between these two extremes are the cases where there is some degree of sensation detected in the affected region, but subjectively the patient reports a decrease in intensity compared with what is typically felt for that region or the person is less consistent in the report or performance used to demonstrate the sensory ability. In this case, the sensation is categorized as *impaired*. Several terms are used to describe abnormalities of sensory integrity. **Hypoesthesia** or **hypesthesia** is a decrease in sensibility or awareness. **Hyperesthesia** or hypersensitivity is an excessive or increased sensitivity to sensory stimuli. **Dysesthesia**, literally "difficult sensation," occurs when an ordinary stimulus results in a disagreeable sensation, and **allodynia** is an exaggerated or painful response to a stimulus that should not be painful. **Paresthesia** is an abnormal negatively perceived sensation that may include burning, pricking, tickling, tingling, or numbness without apparent cause, even in the absence of a known stimulus. Keep in mind impaired sensation from injury to a single nerve root will not result in absence of sensation in the affected dermatome, but rather hypoesthesia because of the overlap with dermatomes above and below.

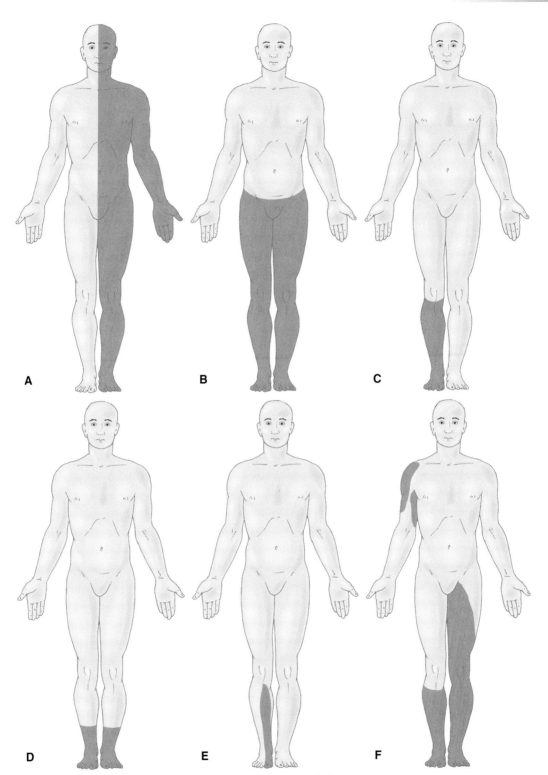

**FIGURE 5-5 A-F.** Diagrams of typical distributions for sensory deficits.
Comparison of various distributions of sensory loss: **A.** unilateral distribution (e.g., cerebrovascular accident),
**B.** paraplegic distribution (e.g., spinal cord injury), **C.** peripheral nerve distribution (e.g., lesion to any specific
nerve), **D.** general peripheral neuropathy (e.g., diabetic neuropathy), **E.** L5 dermatomal loss, and **F.** a sporadic
distribution of sensory deficits (e.g., multiple sclerosis).

## THINK ABOUT IT 5.2

- How would you describe the *quantity* and *quality* of Ellie's sensory deficits?

# Specific Sensory Examinations

The sensory evaluation is usually performed in a logical order, including tests of superficial or tactile sensibility, discriminative sensibility, and proprioceptive sensibility.

## Superficial (Tactile) Sensation

Superficial or tactile sensation includes modalities of sharp/dull (pain), temperature, light touch, and pressure touch.

### Testing Sharp/Dull Discrimination

Several methods and instruments have been described for testing pain sensibility (Cooke, 1991; Harlowe, 1985) even though it is reportedly evaluated less frequently than touch and proprioception (Van Deusen, 1997). Evaluating this *tactile ability to sense pain* differs from an evaluation of the subjective experience of chronic pain that will be discussed later in this chapter. Sharp/dull testing is used to assess integrity of the "pain" pathway (lateral spinothalamic tract).

*Equipment:* There are several instruments with both a sharp and a dull end that can be used (see Fig. 5-6):

- An opened safety pin with partially sanded point (using rounded cap for dull).
- A partially opened paperclip (using the curved end for dull).
- The pin in the handle of a commercially available neurological reflex hammer.

In each instrument, there is a pointed end for sharp input to the skin and a flat or rounded end for dull input. Care must be taken when using safety pins, gently sanding the points, as to not pierce the skin. For infection control of

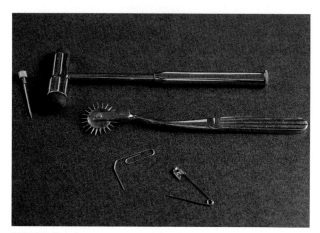

**FIGURE 5-6** Instruments used for sharp/dull testing. Several instruments useful for testing sharp/dull sensibility.

bloodborne pathogens, the safety pin or paperclip should be discarded after each patient and use of reflex hammer pins is discouraged.

*Method:* Regardless of the instrument used, deliver the inputs of sharp and dull in a variable order following a systematic dermatomal sequence as previously described. After demonstrating the sensations to be felt for the patient, the specific method and guidelines for sharp/dull testing are listed here:

1. Apply the pinpoint with enough force to indent the skin but with very slight or no blanching seen in the adjacent skin (Waylett-Rendall, 1988).
2. Hold the pinpoint in place, maintaining the stimulus for several seconds to allow time for central processing and response.
3. For each input, ask the patient to respond to the question, "Does it feel sharp or dull?"

Each time a stimulus is felt, the patient should respond "sharp," "dull," or "can't tell."

### Testing Temperature Sensation

Temperature sensation, carried by the same afferent pathway as pain sensation (lateral spinothalamic tract), is typically evaluated using test tubes of cold and hot water (Cooke, 1991; Harlowe, 1985). If your evaluation purpose is to test the integrity of the lateral spinothalamic system, there is no need to test both pain sensation and temperature sensation, and most therapists would test for sharp/dull sensation. Temperature sensation is not frequently tested as part of the neurological evaluation. Temperature sensation should be tested when preparing to apply any thermal intervention, heat or cryotherapy, especially when it is a safety issue ensuring adequate functioning of peripheral and central mechanisms of temperature sensation (e.g., incomplete spinal cord injury).

*Equipment:* There is sophisticated equipment that has been described for use in testing temperature sense (Horch, 1992; Waylett-Rendall, 1988). In the typical clinical setting, the test is accomplished with much simpler and less expensive equipment:

- Two test tubes with stoppers:
- One filled with hot water, 104°F to 113°F (40°C to 45°).
- One filled with crushed ice and water, 41°F to 50°F (5°C to 10°C).

Exceeding these temperature limits may cause a pain response that would interfere with the validity of the testing (Schmitz, 1994).

*Method:* If temperature sensation is tested as part of the neurological examination to determine distribution and severity of sensory impairment, the dermatomal sequence and general procedure for tactile sensations should be followed but with hot and cold stimuli as described:

1. First, test the temperature of the water-filled tubes on your own skin to assure safety.

**2.** Then apply hot and cold randomly following the dermatomal sequence, maintaining each contact for several seconds.

**3.** The patient is asked to verbally respond for each contact they detect with either "hot," "cold," or "can't tell."

### Testing Light-Touch Sensation

Little research has been published regarding the technique of light-touch evaluation except the Semmes-Weinstein monofilament (SWM) test discussed in the following text as a test for light touch.

*Equipment:* Several options exist clinically for light touch:

- A wisp pulled from a cotton ball is most often used.
- A thin piece of facial tissue or Kleenex.
- A camel hair brush.

*Method:* Following the general procedure and sequence for superficial sensation:

**1.** Apply the selected light-touch sensory input to the skin by very lightly and slowly stroking the surface at one small location.

**2.** Ask the patient to respond each time they feel the sensation with an affirmative response such as "O.K." or "now."

**3.** To introduce variability in testing, either alter the time interval between applications to prevent patient prediction of the next application or by asking the patient, "Do you feel anything?" at times when you are not applying a light-touch stimulation.

In skin with hair, even the fine hairs on the back of the hand and fingers, the stimulus does not have to be applied directly to the skin surface itself but lightly across the hairs only. The light-touch receptors wrapped around the base of each hair follicle are exquisitely sensitive. In glabrous or hairless skin like the palm and sole, the wisp is lightly applied to the surface of the skin.

### Testing Pressure Touch Sensation

Touch pressure sensibility is often assessed grossly using pressure through a pencil eraser or pushing deeply with a finger and asking the patient to distinguish between touch of deep and light pressures by responding to each touch with either "deep" or "light." Pressure touch has been evaluated more objectively using a system of graded weights (Sieg, 1986) but has not gained widespread clinical use. Weights of 0.5, 1, and 2 ounces were placed in a metal capsule with the blunt end placed on the skin surface to be tested. You would ask the patient to distinguish between the different weights.

A more objective method for evaluating both light touch and deep pressure uses the **SWM aesthesiometer,** which has been widely researched (Birke, 1985; Waylett-Rendall, 1988; Weinstein, 1993; Mueller, 1996; Sloan, 1998). This testing method is easy to use. It is most commonly used in populations where more specific measures of sensibility need to be monitored for change, particularly hand injuries including nerve damage, reattachments, or in peripheral neuropathies such as diabetic neuropathy.

Each aesthesiometer consists of a nylon monofilament (like fishing line) embedded near the end of a plastic rod and emerging at a right angle (see Fig. 5-7). Standardization of each filament by generating a reproducible buckling stress allows quantification of applied forces (Mueller, 1996). The color-coded number engraved on the rod, ranging from 1.65 to 6.65 (see Table 5-3), represents the logarithm to the base 10 of the force in milligrams required to bow the filament (Waylett-Rendall, 1988). The higher the assigned number, the more force is required for the filament to bend.

*Equipment:* Depending on the purpose of evaluation, there are several SWM sets commercially available:

- A full set consists of 20 filaments (ranging from 1.65 to 6.65), each with a different strength related to length and thickness of the monofilament.
- The smaller kit with five varied filaments has been reported as time-efficient and adequate for most clinical settings (Bell-Krotoski, 1993).
- The single 2.83 filament can be used alone for upper extremity screening (Bell-Krotoski, 1993; Van Deusen, 1997). This 2.83 filament has also been supported as "suitable for testing most of the body" (Bell-Krotoski, 1993).
- A single 5.07 filament, calibrated to bend at 10 grams of force, has been suggested as the best indicator of protective sensation in the feet. (Birke showed that no patient with neuropathic ulcer was able to sense the 5.07 monofilament) (Birke, 1985; Sloan, 1998; Boyko, 1999). Callous formation on the plantar surface of the foot may cause increased pressure thresholds (Bell-Krotoski, 1997).

*Method:* Have the patient seated or lying and follow the general procedures previously described (including blocking vision). One possible exception to the testing sequence is that testing may be applied from distal to proximal if the expected impairment is likely in a peripheral distribution. The method can be divided into the following steps:

**1.** Apply the filament at 90° to the skin surface with enough force to make the filament bend slightly or buckle (see Fig. 5-7) and maintain for approximately 1 second (Birke,

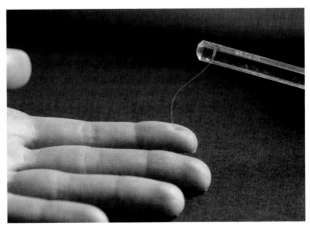

**FIGURE 5-7** Semmes-Weinstein monofilament testing. Administration of a monofilament to the second digit; note that enough pressure is being applied to cause the filament to bend.

| TABLE 5-3 | Clinical Significance of a Variety of Semmes-Weinstein Monofilaments | |
|---|---|---|
| SEMMES-WEINSTEIN FILAMENT | FORCE APPLIED WITH FILAMENT | CLINICAL SIGNIFICANCE |
| 1.65 | 4.5 mg | • The smallest filament in the complete set |
| 2.44 | | • Useful predictor of normal in females because of a lower threshold for pressure sensitivity (Bell-Krotoski, 1993) |
| 2.83 | | • Considered "within normal limits"<br>• Useful to screen for sensory abnormality anywhere in the upper extremity (Bell-Krotoski, 1993; Van Deusen, 1997)<br>• Suprathreshold for the face, subthreshold for foot callous areas (Bell-Krotoski, 1993) |
| 3.22 | 166 mg | • Threshold mapping at this level indicates an area with less than normal sensitivity (Bell-Krotoski, 1993) |
| 3.61 | 200 mg | • Pressure threshold at this level is associated with some loss of graphesthesia and texture recognition (Bell-Krotoski, 1993) |
| 3.84 | 500 mg | • Pressure threshold at this level is associated with diminished protective sensation, impaired stereognosis, and usually loss of two-point discrimination (Bell-Krotoski, 1993) |
| 4.17 | 1 gram | • Normal sensation |
| 4.31 | 4 grams | • Pressure threshold at this level is associated with absent stereognosis and protective sensation (Bell-Krotoski, 1993) |
| ≥4.56 | >4 grams | • These larger filaments simply measure degrees of deep-pressure sensation (Bell-Krotoski, 1993)<br>• One author reported, from clinical experience only, that patients who responded only to these larger filaments may have response to pinprick, but not enough protective sensation to respond to stimuli such as a hot cup fast enough to prevent injury (Bell-Krotoski, 1993) |
| 5.07 | 10 grams | • Useful to screen for sensory abnormality in the feet (Mueller, 1996; Sloan, 1998)<br>• Pressure threshold at this level is the best indicator of protective sensation in the feet (Birke, 1985). Another study concluded that 4.21 was the threshold to differentiate risk of foot ulcers (Sosenko, 1990).<br>• Useful as a predictor of foot ulceration in patients with noninsulin-dependent diabetes mellitus (compared with a neurometer, which was optimal at 2,000 Hz with high sensitivity (92.9%) and low false-positive rate (26.2%). (Olmos, 1995) |
| 6.10 | 75 grams | • Marked sensory loss if unable to feel this monofilament |
| 6.65 | 447 grams | • The largest filament in the complete set |

1985) to 1.5 seconds (Bell-Krotoski, 1997) but not at predictable intervals. A slight adaptation of the application technique shown in Table 5-4 has been suggested depending on the grade of the filament used (Waylett-Rendall, 1988).

2. Instruct the patient to say "yes" each time sensation of the application of the filament is perceived ("yes-no" method).

3. At least five trials are recommended at each site before progressing to the next location (Mueller, 1996). To avoid false-positives, stimulation with the 2.83 filament at least five times is recommended to ensure it is not felt (Bell-Krotoski, 1997).

4. Response must be correct for 80% of the trials (4/5 trials) at a site to be graded with that SWM value at that site (Mueller, 1996). A ratio of two correct responses out of three has also been suggested to be considered intact in that area (Waylett-Rendall, 1988).

5. If a patient senses less than 80% of trials at a site, proceed to test that area with the next stronger monofilament (the next higher number).

6. The threshold for a region can be determined using the psychophysical method of limits (Dannenbaum, 1993; Bell-Krotoski, 1997) by applying the filaments in several descending and ascending series, but this method is time-consuming and more applicable to research situations (Bell-Krotoski, 1997). Calculate a mean of the filament values last perceived in the descending series and the first perceived in the ascending series.

7. Compare results to normative data (see Box 5-1), especially if cerebral damage has taken place even if unilateral because of a likelihood that both hands are affected (Dannenbaum, 1993).

| TABLE 5-4 | Alternate Semmes-Weinstein Technique |
|---|---|
| **FOR FILAMENT SIZE:** | **SUGGESTED TECHNIQUE:** |
| <2.83 | bounce the filament lightly three times for a complete application |
| 3.22–4.08 | apply the filament three times with a bend |
| 4.17–6.65 | apply the filament only once with a bend |

Adapted from Waylett-Rendall J. Sensibility evaluation and rehabilitation. *Orth Clin North Am.* 1988;19(1):43–56.

---

**BOX 5-1 Expected Pressure Sensibility Ranges by Body Regions**

Hand localizes pressure between probes 2.44 to 2.83 (Waylett-Rendall, 1988)
Proximal upper extremity localizes between 4.08 to 4.17 (Waylett-Rendall, 1988)

---

## Discriminative Senses

Discriminative sensations are the group of sensations carried by the lemniscal system. These sensations require cortical processing and integrating information from more than one type of tactile sensory modality to perceive qualities of the object being explored by touch. Discriminative sensibility has been defined as the capacity for precise interpretation of sensation (Omer, 1983). For example, if you explore an object using touch only, you would use a combination of pressure touch, light touch, and position sense of the finger joints to determine the weight, size, shape, texture, and consistency of the object, then apply meaning to the perceived qualities.

### Testing Vibration Sensation

While some might not consider vibration testing to be clinically relevant in nervous system pathology (Bell-Krotoski, 1997; Dannenbaum, 1993), especially related to limited evaluation time, others have identified vibratory sense as an important screen for neuropathy (Vijay, 2001; Kastenbauer, 2004) and preferred to monofilament testing (Oyer, 2007). Testing vibration has no obvious relevance to function but may be useful to monitor sensory recovery in patients with brachial plexus injuries or high peripheral nerve lesions (Waylett-Rendall, 1988). The Automated Tactile Tester (ATT) is a reliable method for testing vibratory sensibility, both high and low frequency (Horch, 1992). Vibrometers, sometimes with fixed frequency of 120 Hz (cycles per second), are also commercially available (Waylett-Rendall, 1988). Vibration testing with a vibrometer has been reported in polyneuropathy related to repetitive stress injury of the upper extremity (Greening, 1998). Because most clinics do not have an ATT or vibrometer, a simpler screening method will be described here. Tuning forks are also used for several auditory screening methods and are described in detail in Chapter 7.

*Equipment:* A 30-Hz tuning fork has been shown to be more specific for Meissner corpuscles while 256 Hz evaluates Pacinian corpuscles (Dellon, 1981). For clinical assessment, a 128-Hz tuning fork is most often used with a moderate frequency to potentially affect both types of vibratory receptors.

*Method:* Following appropriate demonstration and general procedures for sensation evaluation, including elimination of vision, steps to evaluate vibratory sensibility include:

1. Hold the fork by the post (not the tines) (see Fig. 5-8) and strike the tines or pronged end of the tuning fork on a firm but nonsolid surface like the therapist's hypothenar eminence or heel of the palm. Allow it to quickly bounce off the striking surface to create optimal amplitude of vibration so the vibration will be stronger and last longer. Striking a solid surface like a table or chair will damage the tuning fork and the furniture.
2. Apply the post or stem of the vibrating fork to a bony prominence in the area to be tested (e.g., epicondyles, knuckles, etc.; see Fig. 5-8) following the regional sequence of testing locations described earlier. Use enough pressure to make firm contact with the underlying bone.
3. Hold the fork in place, being careful not to touch the vibrating tines because touching the tines will dampen the vibration.
4. Ask the patient, "Is it vibrating?" The patient should respond "yes," "no," or "can't tell."
5. Introduce randomization of input by occasionally and quietly touching the tines after you strike the post to stop the vibration before you apply the post to the bony prominence. They will still hear you strike the tines but will not be able to hear or see you dampen the vibration.

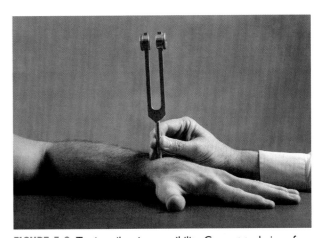

**FIGURE 5-8** Testing vibration sensibility. Correct technique for holding and placing a tuning fork at the patient's wrist. Do not contact the vibrating tines of the tuning fork because it will cause the vibration to fade rapidly.

## Testing Tactile Localization

Tactile localization or localization of touch is the ability to localize or identify the site of touch sensation on the skin. There are few references in the literature describing the method of testing (Dannenbaum, 1993; Prince, 1967; Volpe, 1979; Trombly, 1989). It may be tested simultaneously with the specific tests previously discussed, especially sharp/dull, light touch, or pressure touch since localization is actually a perceptual process that can be applied with any receptor type. Like two-point discrimination described in the next section, accuracy is probably a reflection of the density of receptors for the given region of skin. In fact, tactile localization norms appear to be related to two-point discrimination by body region (Bell-Krotoski, 1997).

*Equipment:* Equipment for tactile localization differs depending on which modality of sensation you choose to use as the test stimulus:

- A blunt probe for pressure touch (Dannenbaum, 1993)
- A paperclip, safety pin, or other pin for sharp/dull
- A cotton wisp for light touch
- And a ruler to measure the error distance

*Method:* After demonstration and vision elimination, follow these steps using a regional sequence of testing:

1. Apply the test stimulus to the skin (pressure touch with a blunt probe has been the most commonly described stimulus for tactile localization) and ask for the appropriate response for testing the primary modality as previously described ("sharp" / "dull," or "yes" / "no").
2. For each stimulus and after the patient responds, ask a second question, "Where did you feel it?" The patient may open the eyes during the response phase of the test (Trombly, 1989) because you are not testing proprioceptive ability but the ability to feel the location where the stimulus was originally applied.
3. The patient may be allowed to verbally describe the location of touch as specifically as possible, using familiar terms and including right or left.
4. For a more specific response, have the patient pinpoint the location using an open paperclip or blunt probe in the available hand. Ask the patient to touch as close to the test site as possible. Allow as many trials or touches as needed until the patient is certain the same spot has been found. If you allow the patient only one touch to the skin to localize the test site, you are probably actually testing proprioceptive joint position sense in the arm that is pointing and not tactile localization because the tactile localization is not experienced until the clip actually touches the skin. After each touch, allow the patient to adjust the position if necessary.
5. For more objective documentation, measure the error as distance in millimeters between the test site and the site indicated by the patient. Test and record this distance for each body region. Norms are not abundant for this test.

An alternative method has been described (Corkin, 1970; Weinstein, 1968) that uses a probe to apply two successive suprathreshold stimuli, then asking the patient to report whether the two stimuli were at the same place or at two different places in the palm. Usually each trial begins with a stimulus at a standard reference point followed by a second comparison stimulus applied at varying distances and different relative directions. The patient's score is the smallest distance that can be discriminated. Normative data using this method have been described for the palm of the hand where the minimal distance that can be discriminated is 3 mm (Weinstein, 1968).

## Testing Two-point Discrimination Sensation

Two-point discrimination is the ability to perceive two simultaneously applied stimuli as two discrete sensations. Light touch is the most common cutaneous stimulus for testing two-point discrimination (Nolan, 1984), while two-point vibrotactile stimulation can also be used (Tannon, 2005). Clinically, it is usually a measure of the shortest distance between two points at which two light-touch stimuli are still perceived as two distinct sensations. Among all cutaneous sensory tests, this one has been cited as "among the most practical and easily duplicated" (O'Sullivan, 1994, p.92). Concern has been raised regarding the reliability and validity with using any handheld tool to measure two-point discrimination (Bell-Krotoski, 1997). Norms from healthy adults, ages 20 to 24, have been investigated and described by Nolan. These norms are presented in Table 5-5 for face and trunk, in Table 5-6 for upper extremity, and in Table 5-7 for lower extremity. Such norms are invaluable for interpretation of two-point discrimination testing, but care must be taken when applying the values to

| TABLE 5-5 | Two-point Discrimination Limits for Face/Trunk |
|---|---|
| Over eyebrow** | 14.9 ± 4.2 mm |
| Tip of tongue* | 2 mm |
| Cheek** | 11.9 ± 3.2 mm |
| Lower lip and upper lip* | 4 mm |
| Over lateral mandible** | 10.4 ± 2.2 mm |
| Ear* | 20 mm |
| Lateral neck** | 35.2 ± 9.8 mm |
| Lateral to C7 spine** | 55.4 ± 20.0 mm |
| Lateral to nipple** | 45.7 ± 12.7 mm |
| Over inferior angle of scapula | 52.2 ± 12.6 mm |
| Side of chest* | 34 mm |
| Abdomen, lateral to umbilicus** | 36.4 ± 7.3 mm |
| Over iliac crest** | 44.9 ± 10.1 mm |
| Lateral to L3 spine** | 49.9 ± 12.7 mm |

Adapted from Weber, 1978* and Nolan, 1985**

\* Values from E.H. Weber's translation of 1834 *De Tactu*, converted to millimeters from original Paris lines. From Weber EH. *E.H. Weber: The Sense of Touch* (translated from *De Tactu* by E. H. Weber, 1834). New York, NY: Academic Press; 1978.

\*\* Mean values, among healthy 20 to 24 year-olds (n = 26–43). From Nolan MF. Quantitative measure of cutaneous sensation: Two-point discrimination for the face and trunk. *Phys Ther.* 1985;65(2):181–185.

| TABLE 5-6 | Two-point Discrimination Limits for Upper Extremity |
|---|---|
| Arm, upper lateral** | 42.4 ± 14.0 mm |
| Arm, lower lateral** | 37.8 ± 13.1 mm |
| Arm, midmedial** | 45.4 ±15.5 mm |
| Arm, midposterior** | 39.8 ± 12.3 mm |
| Forearm, midlateral** | 35.9 ± 11.6 mm |
| Forearm, midmedial** | 31.5 ± 8.9 mm |
| Forearm, midposterior** | 30.7 ± 8.2 mm |
| Over first dorsal interosseous muscle** | 21.0 ± 5.6 mm |
| Palm of hand* | 13 mm |
| Back of knuckles* | 16 mm |
| Thumb, palmar distal phalanx** | 2.6 ± 0.6 mm |
| Long finger, palmar distal phalanx** | 2.6 ± 0.7 mm |
| Little finger, palmar distal phalanx** | 2.5 ± 0.7 mm |
| Tip of 2nd finger* | 1 mm |

Adapted from Weber, 1978* and Nolan, 1982**

*Values from E.H. Weber's translation of 1834 *De Tactu*, converted to millimeters from original Paris lines. From Weber EH. *E.H. Weber: The Sense of Touch* (translated from *De Tactu* by E.H. Weber, 1834). New York, NY: Academic Press; 1978.

** Mean values, among healthy 20 to 24 year-olds (n = 43). From Nolan MF. Two-point discrimination assessment in the upper limb in young adult men and women. *Phys Ther.* 1982;62(7):965–969.

| TABLE 5-7 | Two-point Discrimination Limits for Lower Extremity |
|---|---|
| Thigh, proximal anterior** | 40.1 ± 14.7 mm |
| Thigh, distal anterior** | 23.2 ± 9.3 mm |
| Thigh, midlateral** | 42.5 ± 15.9 mm |
| Thigh, midmedial** | 38.5 ± 12.4 mm |
| Thigh, midposterior** | 42.2 ± 15.9 mm |
| Leg, proximal lateral** | 37.7 ± 13.0 mm |
| Leg, distal lateral** | 41.6 ± 13.0 mm |
| Leg, medial** | 43.6 ± 13.5 mm |
| foot top surface* | 27 mm |
| Over metatarsal interspace 1–2** | 23.9 ± 6.3 mm |
| Over metatarsal 5** | 22.2 ± 8.6 mm |
| Sole of big toe* | 13 mm |
| Tips of toes* | 9 mm |
| Great toe, tip** | 6.6 ± 1.8 mm |

Adapted from Weber, 1978* and Nolan, 1983**

*Values from E.H. Weber's translation of *De Tactu*, 1834, converted to millimeters from original Paris lines. From Weber EH. *E.H. Weber: The Sense of Touch* (translated from *De Tactu* by E. H. Weber, 1834). New York, NY: Academic Press; 1978.

** Mean values, among healthy 20 to 24 year-olds (n = 43). From Nolan MF. Limits of two-point discrimination ability in the lower limb in young adult men and women. *Phys Ther.* 1983;63(9):1424–1428.

different age groups. Because interindividual and intraindividual variation was noted, caution should be used when interpreting patients' results using these norms.

*Equipment:* This test is administered with an instrument with two points (Fig. 5-9A) that can be applied to specific areas of skin (see Fig. 5-9B) and progressively moved closer together:

- A large paperclip, opened and bent into a V-shape with two points (Nolan, 1984)
- ECG calipers with points lightly sanded to prevent skin puncture or painful stimulation (Nolan, 1984) or a geometric compass with points lightly sanded
- A ruler to measure distance between the caliper points
- The DiskCriminator includes a set of two plastic octagonal disks each containing a series of paired metal rods with interpoint intervals ranging from 1 to 25 mm apart.
- Limitations of the paperclip include burrs or rough edges on the metal points (Waylett-Rendall, 1988), which can present a problem if moving the tips across the skin.

*Method:* Methods have been described for static or moving stimuli two-point discrimination testing (Waylett-Rendall, 1988; Van Deusen, 1997). In one study, performing only the

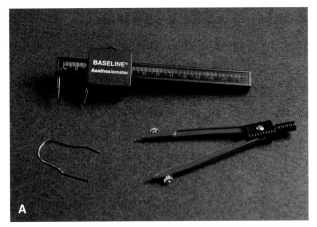

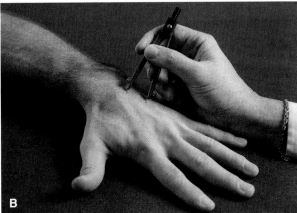

**FIGURE 5-9 A AND B.** Measuring two-point discrimination. **A.** A variety of simple tools can be used to apply two simultaneous points of tactile stimulation. **B.** Testing two-point discrimination requires simultaneous administration of two precise points of tactile stimulation, the distance between which can be measured at the closest distance that can still be discerned as two inputs.

static two-point discrimination testing was determined to be sufficient based on high correlation (r = 0.90) between scores for static and moving (Jerosch-Herold, 1993). Therefore, while following the general procedures for discriminative sensation evaluation, only the static method will be described here:

1. After visual demonstration of the test, select a distance for initial testing. A 10-mm distance is recommended to start testing of the hand (Waylett-Rendall, 1988).
2. Apply the two points parallel to the peripheral nerve trunk innervating that area. For the digits of the hand and foot, Nolan used applications perpendicular to the axis of the digit (Nolan, 1982; Nolan, 1983).
3. The two points should make contact with the skin at the same time and ensure equal pressure between the two points. Force can be monitored somewhat by observing the degree of indentation in the skin. Pressure that depresses the skin no more than 1 mm has been suggested (Nolan, 1982) or a minimum force "so as not to blanch the skin" (Waylett-Rendall, 1988).
4. Up to 20 randomly ordered one- or two-point applications should be used for each skin area with approximately two seconds allowed between each application.
5. For each application, ask the patient to respond to the question, "Do you feel one or two points?" The patient should respond with either "two" or "one."
6. If the patient is accurate at a certain interpoint distance (8 correct of 10 successive touches; Nolan, 1982; Nolan, 1983; Nolan, 1985) or five correct responses in a row (Waylett-Rendall, 1988), then narrow the distance between the two points and start the method again for the same skin area.
7. Determine and record the "smallest distance at which the patient can reliably differentiate between the application of one or two points" (i.e., 8 of 10, or 5 in a row). The placement orientation you select for the two points may depend on the expected orientation of potential impairments (i.e., peripheral nerve distribution).

### Testing Graphesthesia

Evaluation of graphesthesia is a simple but poorly studied aspect of discrimination testing. It is also difficult to quantify. No special equipment is needed.

*Method:*

1. Explain the procedure to the patient, including demonstration on the less-affected hand or other body location with intact sensation, then eliminate vision.
2. Using your fingertip or a blunt probe, trace various letters, numbers, or shapes on the person's palm.
3. Ask the patient to identify and name the symbol as they recognize it.

### Testing Stereognosis

The recognition of a familiar object involved in stereognosis is often considered to be a perceptual function and not a pure sensation, but it is often tested with the sensory evaluation and will be described here. Several methods have been described (Dellon, 1981; Pause, 1989). Recognizing an object only by touch requires the person to discern qualities of the object including size, shape, weight, consistency, and texture using both tactile sense and proprioception but not vision. The patient must have enough motor control in the hand to manipulate the object for intact stereognosis (Dannenbaum, 1993).

*Equipment:* According to the definition of stereognosis, the objects to be recognized should be items familiar to the patient and could include any of the items listed here. Clinically, it is usually sufficient to include three to five objects.

- A stopwatch to time the response.
- Objects to identify: coin (especially a quarter), house key or car key, standard wooden pencil, ballpoint writing pen, paperclip, fork or a spoon.

*Method:* After visual demonstration of the task, have the patient close the eyes as with all sensory testing. For testing stereognosis:

1. Place the objects, one at a time, in the patient's hand (each hand should be tested separately). Measure the time required to name the object correctly (Wynn Parry, 1988).
2. After the patient manipulates the object, ask them, "What is this object?" If the patient cannot state the name of the object, ask them to describe it to you.
3. If the patient is unable to respond verbally because of communication deficits, they may be able to choose the item they just felt from a group of three objects (Semmes, 1965; Weinstein, 1962), but this method does require short-term memory in the patient (Dannenbaum, 1993).
4. As related to cerebral impairment, if **anomia** or the inability to name an object is expected as a potential deficit, follow-up the tactile testing with opportunities for the patient to name the same objects based on visual exploration and input to differentiate.

Normal subjects should be able to name a familiar object within 5 seconds of contact (Wynn Parry, 1966; Klatzky, 1985). Additionally, specific tactile discrimination tests have been developed that focus on shape, texture, or size perception rather than using familiar objects (Benton, 1983; Brink, 1987; Wynn Parry, 1976; Roland, 1976; Roland, 1987).

## Proprioceptive Sensation

Proprioception is sometimes a confusing term because of its use at two different levels of meaning. Sometimes it is used in a broad sense for the category of all sensations that are considered deep, especially joint position sense and joint movement sense. Other times, the term is used to refer specifically to joint position sense. In this text, the term proprioception will be used in the general sense, and the terms "joint position sense" and "joint movement sense" will be used to refer to the specific modalities of sensory awareness of position and movement respectively of specific joints. Variability should be introduced in the testing sequence (i.e., do not use a predictable repeated pattern of positions like flexion, extension, flexion, extension, flexion, and so forth) to prevent the patient from anticipating the next test condition.

The techniques for testing position and movement sense involve passively positioning or moving the test joint (Westlake, 2006) then soliciting a response from the patient regarding the subjective sensation of the joint position or segment movement that took place. To test a joint, you will need to use one hand to stabilize the joint to be tested while your other hand grasps a joint distal to the test joint. As you passively position or move the patient's limb, you should hold and support the test joint with your fingers only on neutral surfaces (probably bony prominences). Avoid contact with skin surfaces in the plane of movement because the patient may receive tactile clues from stretch applied to these skin surfaces. For example, if you are testing elbow proprioception for flexion and extension, contact should be with medial and lateral epicondyles, avoiding contact on flexor and extensor surfaces of the arm and forearm as shown in Figure 5-10. For joint position sense, you ask the patient for a response once you have the limb positioned. For movement sense testing, you ask for the patient response during the movement.

There are at least three methods to solicit a patient response indicating the degree of proprioceptive awareness.

In the first method, which is a screening method, you move the test limb, then have the patient move the opposite limb similarly (Trombly, 1989) in a mirror position. This method only serves as a screen because, if impairment is detected using this method, you would have to do further definitive testing to determine which limb has proprioceptive impairments. It could be a problem with sensing position of the limb you moved, or it could be a problem with sensing position in the limb they are trying to move. The problem could also be a lack of motor control to reproduce the position in the test arm. The other two methods test one limb at a time.

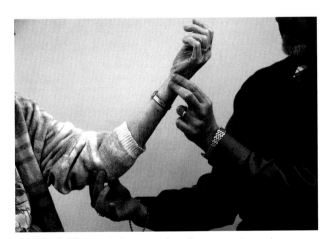

**FIGURE 5-10** Hand placement for elbow proprioception examination. When testing joint position or movement sensibility, it is important to avoid hand contact over skin surfaces where stretch or contact to the skin or active muscles may provide proprioceptive or sensory clues to the patient.

The second method uses active patient movement in the test limb to mimic the passive movement you performed earlier on the same limb.

The third method, useful especially if the patient is unable to produce a motor response because of weakness or motor deficits, requests a verbal description of the position or movement from the patient (Trombly, 1989; Dannenbaum, 1993). If you use the third method, you must establish a mutual terminology for each position, movement, or direction during the demonstration of the test procedure to the patient. This will assure you are both *speaking the same language,* especially if you use common terms familiar to the patient.

### Testing Joint Position Sense

Joint position sense has been discussed by others (Trombly, 1989; Dannenbaum, 1993). The key characteristic in testing this modality is that you position the limb and encourage patient attention to the position *while the limb is held in the position.*

*Equipment:* Often none is used, however standardization may be improved with:

- A goniometer to quantify impairment.
- A protractor has been described for use in one method.

*Method:* After explaining the test procedure to the patient, including visual demonstration and defining the response, you will request of the patient:

1. Passively position the joint to be tested very slowly, 10° per second has been suggested, (Trombly, 1989) and hold the position briefly.
2. Request a response from the patient regarding the perceived position using one of the three methods previously described. If you use the verbal response method, the terminology should be common and not medical, reflecting the static nature of this proprioceptive modality, including "up" or "down," "bent" or "straight," "in" or "out," "right" or "left," or "forward" or "back."
3. Test for at least several responses at each joint, including very subtle, small-range, random position changes. Individuals with normal proprioception should be able to detect even small changes in position (perhaps as little as several degrees of range in many joints).
4. Compare your results to normative data. Normative data is available for the IP joints of the finger, and the scores obtained can be used to classify impairment as slight, moderate, or severe (Corkin, 1970; Corkin, 1973).

A more objective method has been described and suggested for use in research but tested only for the wrist joint (Carey, 1993). This method uses a pointer device over a protractor scale to more accurately measure the patient's movement response. The score for this test is the mean absolute error or distance between the measure of test wrist position and the subject's estimate as measured with the pointer.

### Testing Joint Movement Sense

Joint movement sense utilizes the same receptors and pathways as joint position sense. The major difference is probably the requirement for additional temporal processing of the proprioceptive sensation in the central nervous system because the patient must detect *changes in position during movement*. This processing facilitates detection of the characteristics of joint movement over time including direction, speed, and magnitude.

*Equipment:* Same as joint position sense.

*Method:* Testing is similar to the method previously described for position sense but notably requires a response from the patient *while you are passively moving* the target joint.

1. Passively move the joint to be tested very slowly in a very small range.
2. Solicit a response during the movement. If using the verbal response method to test joint movement sense, the common terminology used should reflect the directional

dynamic aspects of this proprioceptive modality, including "moving up" or "moving down," "bending" or "straightening," "turning in" or "turning out."

3. Test for at least several joint movements, including slow minute-range movements and random direction changes.

## Standardized Assessment Tools for Sensory Impairment

The Fugl-Meyer Assessment was developed as an instrument to measure sensorimotor stroke recovery in individuals with stroke. It includes sensory items for light touch and position sense and has strong interrater reliability (Lin, 2004).

The American Spinal Injury Association (ASIA) has recommended a standard format for sensory testing in individuals with spinal cord injuries with substantial interrater reliability (Savic, 2007). The method includes testing light touch and pinprick (sharp/dull) at specific landmarks associated with sensory dermatomes. The ASIA sensory form is shown in Figure 5-11.

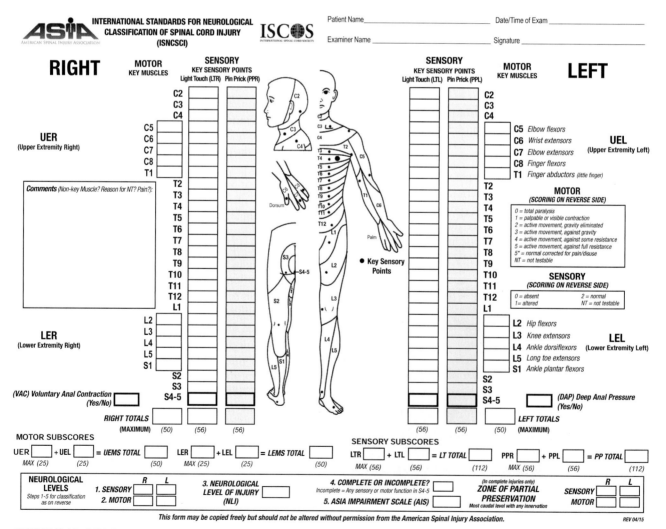

**FIGURE 5-11** ASIA Sensory Examination Form. The ASIA standardized sensory examination for patients with spinal cord injury. Reprinted from American Spinal Injury Association. Available at: http://www.asia-spinalinjury.org/elearning/isncsci_worksheet_2015_web.pdf. Accessed October 30, 2015.

## Muscle Function Grading

**0** = total paralysis

**1** = palpable or visible contraction

**2** = active movement, full range of motion (ROM) with gravity eliminated

**3** = active movement, full ROM against gravity

**4** = active movement, full ROM against gravity and moderate resistance in a muscle specific position

**5** = (normal) active movement, full ROM against gravity and full resistance in a functional muscle position expected from an otherwise unimpaired person

**5\*** = (normal) active movement, full ROM against gravity and sufficient resistance to be considered normal if identified inhibiting factors (i.e. pain, disuse) were not present

**NT** = not testable (i.e. due to immobilization, severe pain such that the patient cannot be graded, amputation of limb, or contracture of > 50% of the normal ROM)

## Sensory Grading

**0** = Absent

**1** = Altered, either decreased/impaired sensation or hypersensitivity

**2** = Normal

**NT** = Not testable

## When to Test Non-Key Muscles:

In a patient with an apparent AIS B classification, non-key muscle functions more than 3 levels below the motor level on each side should be tested to most accurately classify the injury (differentiate between AIS B and C).

| Movement | Root level |
|---|---|
| **Shoulder:** Flexion, extension, abduction, adduction, internal and external rotation **Elbow:** Supination | C5 |
| **Elbow:** Pronation **Wrist:** Flexion | C6 |
| **Finger:** Flexion at proximal joint, extension. **Thumb:** Flexion, extension and abduction in plane of thumb | C7 |
| **Finger:** Flexion at MCP joint **Thumb:** Opposition, adduction and abduction perpendicular to palm | C8 |
| **Finger:** Abduction of the index finger | T1 |
| **Hip:** Adduction | L2 |
| **Hip:** External rotation | L3 |
| **Hip:** Extension, abduction, internal rotation **Knee:** Flexion **Ankle:** Inversion and eversion **Toe:** MP and IP extension | L4 |
| **Hallux and Toe:** DIP and PIP flexion and abduction | L5 |
| **Hallux:** Adduction | S1 |

## ASIA Impairment Scale (AIS)

**A = Complete.** No sensory or motor function is preserved in the sacral segments S4-5.

**B = Sensory Incomplete.** Sensory but not motor function is preserved below the neurological level and includes the sacral segments S4-5 (light touch or pin prick at S4-5 or deep anal pressure) AND no motor function is preserved more than three levels below the motor level on either side of the body.

**C = Motor Incomplete.** Motor function is preserved at the most caudal sacral segments for voluntary anal contraction (VAC) OR the patient meets the criteria for sensory incomplete status (sensory function preserved at the most caudal sacral segments (S4-S5) by LT, PP or DAP), and has some sparing of motor function more than three levels below the ipsilateral motor level on either side of the body.
(This includes key or non-key muscle functions to determine motor incomplete status.) For AIS C – less than half of key muscle functions below the single NLI have a muscle grade ≥ 3.

**D = Motor Incomplete.** Motor incomplete status as defined above, with at least half (half or more) of key muscle functions below the single NLI having a muscle grade ≥ 3.

**E = Normal.** If sensation and motor function as tested with the ISNCSCI are graded as normal in all segments, and the patient had prior deficits, then the AIS grade is E. Someone without an initial SCI does not receive an AIS grade.

**Using ND:** To document the sensory, motor and NLI levels, the ASIA Impairment Scale grade, and/or the zone of partial preservation (ZPP) when they are unable to be determined based on the examination results.

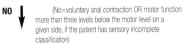

**INTERNATIONAL STANDARDS FOR NEUROLOGICAL CLASSIFICATION OF SPINAL CORD INJURY**

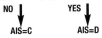

## Steps in Classification

The following order is recommended for determining the classification of individuals with SCI.

**1. Determine sensory levels for right and left sides.**
*The sensory level is the most caudal, intact dermatome for both pin prick and light touch sensation.*

**2. Determine motor levels for right and left sides.**
*Defined by the lowest key muscle function that has a grade of at least 3 (on supine testing), providing the key muscle functions represented by segments above that level are judged to be intact (graded as a 5).*
*Note: in regions where there is no myotome to test, the motor level is presumed to be the same as the sensory level, if testable motor function above that level is also normal.*

**3. Determine the neurological level of injury (NLI)**
*This refers to the most caudal segment of the cord with intact sensation and antigravity (3 or more) muscle function strength, provided that there is normal (intact) sensory and motor function rostrally respectively.*
*The NLI is the most cephalad of the sensory and motor levels determined in steps 1 and 2.*

**4. Determine whether the injury is Complete or Incomplete.**
*(i.e. absence or presence of sacral sparing)*
*If voluntary anal contraction = **No** AND all S4-5 sensory scores = **0** AND deep anal pressure = **No**, then injury is **Complete**.*
*Otherwise, injury is **Incomplete**.*

**5. Determine ASIA Impairment Scale (AIS) Grade:**

Is injury Complete? If YES, AIS=A and can record ZPP (lowest dermatome or myotome on each side with some preservation)

NO ↓

Is injury Motor Complete? If YES, AIS=B

NO ↓ (No=voluntary anal contraction OR motor function more than three levels below the motor level on a given side, if the patient has sensory incomplete classification)

Are at least half (half or more) of the key muscles below the neurological level of injury graded 3 or better?

NO ↓   YES ↓

AIS=C   AIS=D

If sensation and motor function is normal in all segments, AIS=E
*Note: AIS E is used in follow-up testing when an individual with a documented SCI has recovered normal function. If at initial testing no deficits are found, the individual is neurologically intact; the ASIA Impairment Scale does not apply.*

**FIGURE 5-11—cont'd**

---

The ATT is an automated tool used to evaluate touch-pressure, vibration, warmth, sharpness, and two-point discrimination (Horch, 1992; Jimenez, 1993). Validity, reliability, and age-related norms have been established (Horch, 1992; Jimenez, 1993). However, because it is not considered to be practical for use in many clinics yet (Van Deusen, 1997), the details of administration are not summarized here but can be found in the original references. As a standardized, reliable, and valid tool, it has potential for future clinical use.

## Chronic Pain and Perception of Pain

Chronic pain is an abnormal disturbed sensation that causes suffering or distress (APTA, 2015). It is an abnormal adverse sensation with negative affective components. In its most severe form, it is that feeling for which we do all we can to avoid and from which we urgently seek relief when it does occur. In the person with a neuromuscular disorder, pain may be related to several contributing factors: central nervous system dysfunction, trauma and increased intracranial pressure, or trauma or biomechanical causes in peripheral tissues, both peripheral nerves and musculoskeletal elements. In such cases, the therapist must measure the dimensions of the pain as the initial step in clinical decision-making.

The therapist "uses tests and measures of pain to determine the cause or a mechanism for an individual's pain and to assess the intensity, quality, and temporal and physical characteristics associated with the pain." (APTA, 2015). Because chronic pain is a subjective feeling experienced by the patient only, an observer cannot measure it externally, and evaluation occurs through methodical questioning with verbal or other responses from the patient to describe the adverse sensory experience. An excellent in-depth review of clinical assessment of pain has been written by Ross and LaStayo (1997). The essentials of evaluation of pain are discussed in the following section. The therapist will analyze and synthesize all results of these tests and measures of pain as a baseline measure for outcome comparisons and to determine the underlying causes and mechanisms of the specific pain as a first step toward developing a comprehensive individualized treatment program. A sample comprehensive pain assessment record form is included as Figure 5-12.

**Pain Assessment Record Form**

**Client's name:**                                                                                          **Date:**

**Medical diagnosis:**                                                                                  **Physical therapy diagnosis:**

**Medications:** _____        _____

_____        _____

_____        _____

**Onset of pain** (circle one): Was there an:

Accident              Injury              Trauma (violence)              Specific activity

if yes, describe:

**Characteristics of pain/symptoms:**
**Location** (Show me exactly where your pain/symptom is located):

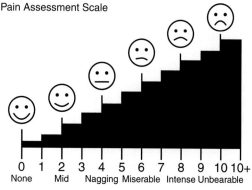

וווו Numbness
🔫 Severe pain
≋ Moderate pain
↓ Shooting pain

Do you have any pain or symptoms anywhere else?
**Description** (if yes, what does it feel like?):

**Circle any other words that describe the client's symptoms:**

| | | | |
|---|---|---|---|
| Knifelike | Dull | Aching | Other (describe): |
| Boring | Burning | Throbbing | |
| Heaviness | Discomfort | Sharp | |
| Stinging | Tingling | Stabbing | |

**Frequency** (circle one):      Constant          Intermittent (comes and goes)
If constant: Do you have this pain right now?          Yes          No
If intermittent: How often is the pain present? (circle all that apply):
Hourly      Once/daily      Twice/daily      Unpredictable      Other (please describe): _____

**Intensity:** *Numeric Rating Scale and the Faces Pain Scale*
**Instructions:** On a scale from 0 to 10 with zero meaning "No pain" and 10 for "Unbearable pain", how would you rate your pain right now?

Pain Assessment Scale

0    1    2    3    4    5    6    7    8    9    10   10+
None      Mid      Nagging  Miserable  Intense  Unbearable

**Alternately: Point to the face that best shows how much pain you are having right now.**
**Intensity:** *Visual Analog Scale*
**Instructions:** On the line below, put a mark (or point to) the place on the line between "Pain free" and "Worst possible pain" that best describes/shows how much pain you are having right now.

**Pain Free** _____ **Worst Possible Pain**

**FIGURE 5-12** Comprehensive Pain Assessment Record form. Reprinted from Goodman and Snyder. *Differential Diagnosis for Physical Therapists: Screening for Referral,* 4th ed, Philadelphia, PA: Saunders, Elsevier; 2007.

**Duration:**
How long does your pain (name the symptom) last?

| **Aggravating factors** (What makes it worse?) | **Relieving factors** (What makes it better?) |
| --- | --- |
| | |

**Pattern**
Has the pain changed since it first began?        Yes        No
If yes, please explain:

What is your pain/symptom like from morning (am) to evening (pm)?

**Circle one:**      Worse in the morning      Worse midday/afternoon      Worse at night
**Circle one:**      Gradually getting better      Gradually getting worse      Staying the same
**Circle all that apply:**
Present upon waking up           Keeps me from falling asleep           Wakes me up at night
**Therapist:** Record any details or description about night pain. See also Appendix for *Screening Questions for Night Pain* when appropriate:

**Associated symptoms** (What other symptoms have you had with this problem?)

Circle any words the client uses to describe his/her symptoms. If the client says there are no other symptoms ask about the presence of any of the following:

| | | | |
| --- | --- | --- | --- |
| Burning | Difficulty breathing | Shortness of breath | Cough |
| Skin rash (or other lesions) | Change in bowel/bladder | Difficulty swallowing | Painful swallowing |
| Dizziness | Heart palpitations | Hoarseness | Nausea/vomiting |
| Diarrhea | Constipation | Bleeding of any kind | Sweats |
| Numbness | Problems with vision | Tingling | Weakness |
| Joint pain | Weight loss/gain | Other: | |

| **Final question:** Are there any other pain or symptoms of any kind anywhere else in your body that we have not talked about yet? |
| --- |
| |

**For the therapist:**
**Follow up question can include:**
Are there any positions that make it feel better? Worse?
How does rest affect the pain/symptoms?
How does activity affect the pain/symptoms?
How has this problem affected your daily life at work or at home?
Has this problem affected your ability to care for yourself without assistance (e.g. dress, bathe, cook, drive)?
Has this problem affected your sexual function or activity?

**Therapist's evaluation:**
Can you reproduce the pain by squeezing or palpating the symptomatic area?
Does resisted motion reproduce the pain/symptoms?
Is the client taking NSAIDs? Experiencing increased symptoms after taking NSAIDs?
If taking NSAIDs, is the client at risk for peptic ulcer? Check all that apply:
☐ Age>65 years                  ☐ History of peptic ulcer disease or GI disease
☐ Smoking, alcohol use      ☐ Oral corticosteroid use
☐ Anticoagulation or use of other anticoagulants (even when used for heart patients at a lower dose, e.g., 81 to 325 mg aspirin/day)
☐ Renal complications in clients with hypertension or congestive heart failure (CHF) or who use diuretics or ACE inhibitors
☐ NSAIDs combined with selective serotonin reuptake inhibitors (SSRIs; antidepressants such as Prozac, Zoloft, Celexa, Paxil)
☐ Use of acid suppressants (e.g., $H_2$–receptor antagonists, antacids)

**Other areas to consider:**
• Sleep quality                              • Bowel/bladder habits                   • Depression or anxiety screening score
• Correlation of symptoms with peak effect of medications (dosage, time of day) • For women: correlation of symptoms with menstrual cycle
• Evaluation of joint pain (see Appendix: Screening Questions for Joint Pain)

**FIGURE 5-12—cont'd**

## Measures of Pain Intensity

Pain intensity is the dimension including the severity or magnitude of pain experienced. The information you solicit from the patient is in the form of qualitative descriptive words describing "how much" the patient hurts (Jenson, 1992). Several scales are available for evaluating pain intensity: Verbal Rating Scale (VRS), Visual Analog Scale (VAS), and Numerical Rating Scale.

The VRS (Gracely, 1978A; Gracely, 1978b) is a list of either 5 or 15 different ranked adjectives each translating as different scaled levels of pain intensity. The adjective used by the patient to describe the intensity of pain they experience is assigned a number based on the terms rank within the scale. The adjectives on the five-point scale range from none (score = 0) to very severe (score = 4). Adjectives interposed are mild, moderate, and severe. The 15-point scale is shown in Box 5-2. Because these are ordinal scales and not interval scales, the therapist must be careful to assume no magnitude of change associated with any numeric change in the scale. For example, when the number decreases from 4 to 2, the therapist can only infer that the pain intensity has decreased and not assume the same quantity of improvement as when the score decreases from 3 to 1. Problems would also be introduced if the patient has communication limitations, illiteracy, or speaks only a different language.

The VAS has also been used to quantify pain intensity. A line 10 cm long (sometimes 15 cm) is usually used with bold hash marks at each end and labels with the extremes of pain intensity (see Fig. 5-13). The patient is asked to mark the spot on the line that best represents the perceived level of pain intensity. Score the response by measuring the distance in centimeters from the end marked "no pain" to the point marked by the patient. Because measurement can be made in millimeter increments, there are potentially 101 response locations that contribute to the sensitivity of this instrument. Several authors have suggested the VAS may be more sensitive to change in chronic pain than acute pain (Carlsson, 1983; McGuire, 1984). The VAS may be particularly useful in pediatrics, especially when descriptive icons replace the labels at either end (e.g., smiling face and frowning face).

The third possibility for evaluating pain intensity is use of a Numerical Rating Scale. The patient is asked to rate the perception of pain intensity by stating or writing down a number between 0 and 10 or between 0 and 100, where 0 represents "no pain" and the highest number of the scale represents "pain as bad as it could be." Using 0 to 100 yields a 101-point scale (see Fig. 5-14) as in the VAS with great potential for sensitivity.

## Measures of Pain's Affective Dimension

The affective component of pain "involves a complex series of behaviors that an individual may employ to minimize, escape, or terminate a noxious stimulus" (Ross, 1997). The affective dimension of pain includes the patient's personal experience of the pain, the effect of the pain on behavior, and how the patient responds to it. The affective component of pain and the related concept of pain tolerance are highly variable among individuals, explaining why some people deal with severe chronic pain seemingly with ease while others with milder pain may suffer great agony.

One method for evaluating the affective dimension of pain is use of the VRS using adjectives describing the degree to which the pain is bearable or objectionable. One scale has been reported that uses a vertical listing of the 15 terms shown in Box 5-3 (Gracely, 1978).

The patient is asked to select the one word that best describes their pain experience. You then rank the response according to the order of the list. A score of 0 is assigned to the

---

**BOX 5-2 15-point Verbal Rating Scale for Pain Intensity**

| | |
|---|---|
| Extremely weak | Barely strong |
| Very weak | Slightly intense |
| Weak | Strong |
| Very mild | Intense |
| Mild | Very strong |
| Very moderate | Very intense |
| Slightly Moderate | Extremely intense |
| Moderate | |

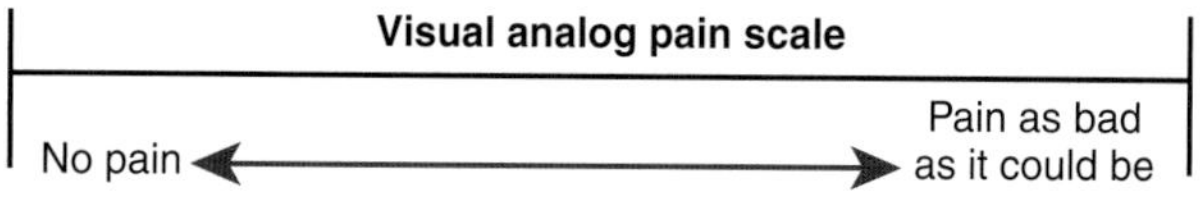

---

**Visual analog pain scale**

No pain ◄————————————► Pain as bad as it could be

FIGURE 5-13 Visual Analog Scale for Pain. A visual analog scale for the patient to rate intensity of their pain. From Van Deusen J, Foss JJ. Sensory deficits. In: Van Deusen J, Brunt D, eds. *Assessment in Occupational Therapy and Physical Therapy*. Philadelphia, PA: W.B. Saunders Co.; 1997.

---

**101 point Numeric Rating Scale (an example):**

| In the blank write the number between 0 and 100 that best describes your pain. A zero (0) would mean "no pain" and a one hundred (100) would mean "pain as bad as it could be." Please place the one best answer (number) in the blank. | _____ |
|---|---|

FIGURE 5-14 101 Numeric Rating Scale for Pain. Patients may provide a numeric rating of the intensity of their pain.

---

**BOX 5-3 Verbal Rating Scale of Adjectives Describing Pain**

| | |
|---|---|
| Bearable | Frightful |
| Distracting | Dreadful |
| Unpleasant | Horrible |
| Uncomfortable | Agonizing |
| Distressing | Unbearable |
| Oppressive | Intolerable |
| Miserable | Excruciating |
| Awful | |

first term in the list. When interpreting scores, remember such a scale is ordered, not interval, so no interpretations can be made regarding the degree of improvement.

Affective pain dimensions are commonly measured using VAS. Similar to the VAS for pain intensity, usually a 10-cm horizontal line is used to represent the possible range. For pain affect, however, the end labels of the line are "not bad at all" at the left end and "the most unpleasant feeling possible for me" at the right end (Price, 1987). As illustrated in Figure 5-15, you ask the patient to mark the line at the point along the continuum that corresponds to their experience, then measure the distance in centimeters (to one decimal place or the nearest millimeter) from the left end of the line to the point marked by the patient. This scale has been shown to be sensitive to improvements in pain affect (Price, 1987).

### Testing Pain Location and Distribution

It is also essential to explore and document the specific location and extent of the painful area. Perhaps the simplest method would be to ask the patient, "Where is your pain located?" and expect a verbal description. Response from patients may not be complete or valid if using this method.

A more valid pain location assessment can be obtained with pain drawings on a body diagram (Schwartz, 1984; Margolis, 1988). Using a human body line drawing as shown in Figure 5-16a, ask the patient to mark or shade painful areas. Additionally, after the painful areas are marked, associated abnormal sensations can be designated using visual character symbols (see Fig. 5-16b).

### Testing Pain's Temporal Characteristics and Provocations

In addition to intensity, affective, and location components, other types of information are helpful in forming a hypothesis as to the underlying cause of pain. The temporal characteristics of chronic pain and aggravating factors are essential to investigate, especially changes throughout the

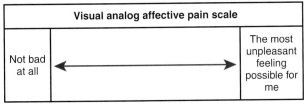

| Visual analog affective pain scale | | |
|---|---|---|
| Not bad at all | ⟷ | The most unpleasant feeling possible for me |

**FIGURE 5-15** Visual Analog Affective Pain Scale. This visual analog scale allows the patient to rate their subjective affective experience of the pain.

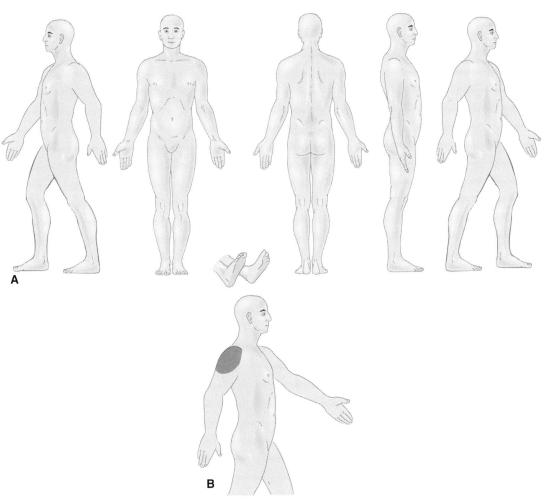

**FIGURE 5-16 A AND B.** Body diagrams for documenting pain.

24-hour cycle of a day: "Is your pain worse in the morning or at night?" It is also essential to note the relationship of pain and its intensity to certain postures or movements: "Is there a position that seems to make your pain worse?" "Is your pain worse with sitting or worse after standing or walking?" Melzack (1975) has used questions such as "What kinds of things relieve your pain?" and "What kinds of things increase your pain?"

## Documentation of Sensation Examination/Evaluation

A sample sensory section of a neurorehabilitation examination form, including superficial and discriminative sensation, is shown in Figure 5-17, highlighting a possible system for documenting superficial and deep sensory testing, including typical locations and sequences.

### Chronic Pain and Pain Perception

The McGill Pain Questionnaire is an excellent and well-researched tool that assesses all aspects of chronic pain evaluation discussed in the previous section, including location, quality, temporal characteristics and provocations, and intensity (Melzack, 1975). The questionnaire is shown in Figure 5-18. In addition to patient name and diagnostic and demographic information, the four parts of the questionnaire explore (1) pain location (using a body diagram), (2) pain quality (with a list of descriptive terms), (3) temporal changes (including relieving and provoking factors), and (4) pain intensity (with a five-point rating scale) (Melzack, 1975). The questionnaire is easy to use, but the therapist should be involved in administration. The experienced therapist should be able to administer the questionnaire in 5 minutes (Ross, 1997). The details of administering this questionnaire are beyond the scope of this text but are available from the listed references, particularly Ross.

## THINK ABOUT IT 5.3

- What pain rating scale would you suggest using for Ellie?
- What standardized assessment tools would you suggest using with Ellie?
- How would you measure pain intensity with Ellie?
- How would you measure the affective dimension of pain with Ellie?
- How would you document pain localization and distribution with Ellie?
- Once completed with your pain assessment, how would you document all the data you compiled regarding Ellie's pain?

---

**Sensory examination** (test tactile and proprioceptive sense)
A. **Tactile (superficial)** usually tested by dermatome, for one modality, usually light touch or sharp/dull. Pressure sense may also be tested and tactile localization can be tested simultaneously with any of the above.
B. **Proprioception (deep)** usually tested by body region, for one modality, usually position sense or movement sense. Other tests may include two-point discrimination (with a paper clip, making sure to use equal pressure on both points), stereognosis (identifying familiar objects by touch), vibration (tuning fork over bony prominences and joint spaces).

|  | Right | Left |
|---|---|---|
| Face |  |  |
| Shoulder |  |  |
| Elbow |  |  |
| Wrist |  |  |
| Fingers |  |  |
| Trunk |  |  |
| Hip |  |  |
| Knee |  |  |
| Ankle |  |  |

**FIGURE 5-17** Sensory sections of a sample neurorehabilitation examination form. This form is one possible configuration to document the results of the sensory examination for a patient with a neuromuscular disorder. Both tactile and proprioceptive senses should be tested.

---

### PATIENT APPLICATION

*Ellie is our patient with MS introduced earlier in this chapter. Her sensory examination confirmed areas with impaired proprioception as well as the sensory deficits she reported. Written documentation of her sensory examination could look like this:*

| Sharp/ dull testing | • Absent over entire dorsum of right foot and anterior and posterior leg up to level of tibial tuberosity<br>• Absent over entire left foot, leg, and thigh, anterior and posterior<br>• Absent in anterior right shoulder region and medial-upper humerus region |
|---|---|
| Position sense testing | • Impaired proprioception (able to sense general position but lacks accuracy) in right ankle, left ankle, left knee, and right shoulder |

*A sensory deficit map of her specific tactile sensory loss is shown in Figure 5-5D. In later chapters, you will learn how to use this information in developing a patient-centered plan for care with specific interventions that consider these sensory deficits.*

# McGill Pain Questionnaire
## Ronald Melzack

Patient's Name _____ Date _____ Time _____ am/pm

PRL:    S_____    A_____    E_____    M_____    PRI(T)_____    PPI_____
          (1-10)              (11-15)           (16)           (17-20)              (1-20)

| | | |
|---|---|---|
| 1 Flickering ____ | 11 Tiring ____ | Brief ____ |
| Quivering ____ | Exhausting ____ | Momentary ____ |
| Pulsing ____ | 12 Sickening ____ | Transient ____ |
| Throbbing ____ | Suffocating ____ | |
| Beating ____ | 13 Fearful ____ | |
| Pounding ____ | Frightful ____ | |
| 2 Jumping ____ | Terrifying ____ | |
| Flashing ____ | 14 Punishing ____ | |
| Shooting ____ | Grueling ____ | |
| 3 Pricking ____ | Cruel ____ | |
| Boring ____ | Vicious ____ | |
| Drilling ____ | Killing ____ | |
| Stabbing ____ | 15 Wretched ____ | |
| Lancinating ____ | Blinding ____ | |
| 4 Sharp ____ | 16 Annoying ____ | |
| Cutting ____ | Troublesome ____ | |
| Lacerating ____ | Miserable ____ | |
| 5 Pinching ____ | Intense ____ | |
| Pressing ____ | Unbearable ____ | |
| Gnawing ____ | 17 Spreading ____ | |
| Cramping ____ | Radiating ____ | |
| Crushing ____ | Penetrating ____ | |
| 6 Tugging ____ | Piercing ____ | |
| Pulling ____ | 18 Tight ____ | |
| Wrenching ____ | Numb ____ | |
| 7 Hot ____ | Drawing ____ | |
| Burning ____ | Squeezing ____ | |
| Scalding ____ | Tearing ____ | |
| Searing ____ | 19 Cool ____ | |
| 8 Tingling ____ | Cold ____ | |
| Itchy ____ | Freezing ____ | |
| Smarting ____ | 20 Nagging ____ | |
| Stinging ____ | Nauseating ____ | |
| 9 Dull ____ | Agonizing ____ | |
| Sore ____ | Dreadful ____ | |
| Hurting ____ | Torturing ____ | |
| Aching ____ | PPI | |
| Heavy ____ | 0 No pain ____ | |
| 10 Tender ____ | 1 Mild ____ | |
| Taut ____ | 2 Discomforting ____ | |
| Rasping ____ | 3 Distressing ____ | |
| Splitting ____ | 4 Horrible ____ | |
| | 5 Excruciating ____ | |

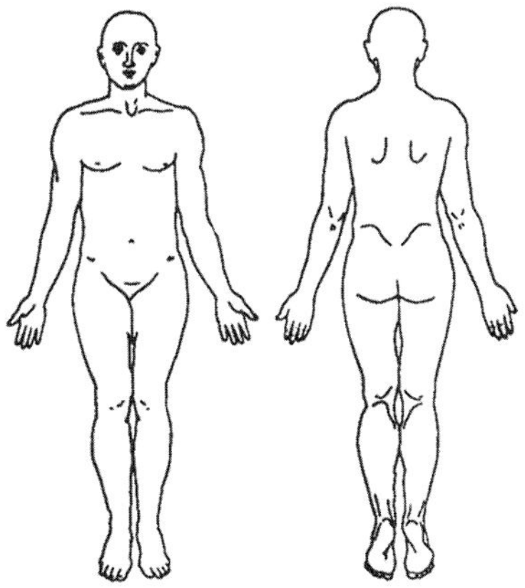

Rhythmic ____    Continuous ____
Periodic ____    Steady ____
Intermittent ____    Constant ____

E = External
I = Internal

**Comments:**

© R. Melzack, 1975

**FIGURE 5-18** McGill Pain Questionnaire. The McGill Pain Questionnaire includes four major groups of pain descriptors: sensory (S), 1 to 10; affective (A), 11 to 15; evaluative (E), 16; and miscellaneous (M), 17 to 20. The score for each item is determined by the ranked position of the selected word in each word list. For example, "flickering" would get a score of one (1) while "pounding" would get a score of six (6). The sum of rank values for all items is the pain rating index (PRI). The present pain intensity (PPI) is determined by the patient based on a scale of 0–5. © R. Melzack, 1970, 1984. Reprinted with permission from Dr. Ronald Melzack. Measure of cutaneous sensation: Two-point discrimination for the face and trunk. *Phys Ther.* 1985;65(2):181-185.

# HANDS-ON PRACTICE

Be sure to practice the following skills from this chapter. With further practice, you should be able to test:
- Sharp/dull discrimination
- Temperature sensation
- Light-touch sensation
- Deep and light pressure touch sensation using Semmes-Weinstein monofilaments
- Vibration sensation
- Tactile localization
- Two-point discrimination
- Graphesthesia
- Stereognosis
- Proprioception
- Kinesthesia

## Let's Review

1. Describe the neuroanatomical regions, structures, and pathways related to sensory abilities and impairments caused by common neuromuscular pathologies/injuries.

2. List and describe the variety of sensory modalities tested in individuals with neuromuscular pathologies/injuries.

3. Given a patient scenario, select the most appropriate sensory tests and measures.

4. Given a patient scenario, infer the impact of specific sensory deficits on functional abilities.

5. Describe what safety issues and precautions you should consider for individuals with sensory deficits and why.

6. Demonstrate the proper procedure for each sensory test described in this chapter.

7. Describe the components to include in documenting sensory test results in the medical record.

8. Given a patient scenario, appropriately document the patient's sensory test results.

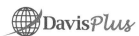 **DavisPlus**  For additional resources, including Focus on Evidence tables, case study discussions, references, and glossary, please visit http://davisplus.fadavis.com

## CHAPTER SUMMARY

### PATIENT APPLICATION

*Joe's stroke occurred 3 weeks ago. At 65 years-old, he thought he was getting ready to enjoy the freedom of retirement. Now he has to deal with a right arm and leg that will not move the way he wants them to plus complete sensory loss of the right side of his face, and he feels sharp/dull testing and tactile pressure in his right arm and leg. As part of your intervention plan, you decide he needs an ankle foot orthosis (AFO) for his right leg but realize you will have to take his sensory loss into account to minimize his risk for skin damage around the ankle*

*(intervention to be discussed in Chapter 17). His functional skill will also be severely affected by the documented lack of proprioception in the joints of his right arm and leg.*

The sensory examination is an essential part of the examination of any patient with a neuromuscular condition (Table 5-8). Synthesis of your data from this part of the examination along with the other systems and functional abilities will help to guide development of the intervention plan.

# Examination and Evaluation of Neuromotor Systems

R. Barry Dale, PT, PhD, OCS, SCS, ATC, CSCS ▪ Dennis W. Fell, PT, MD     CHAPTER **6**

## CHAPTER OUTLINE

## CHAPTER OBJECTIVES

Upon completion of this chapter, the learner should be able to:
1. Describe the normal physiology that underlies the functioning of the neuromotor system.
2. List and define the specific subcategories of muscle performance within a neuromotor examination.
3. List and define the specific subcategories of motor function within a neuromotor examination.
4. Describe the key performance-related aspects of the specific tests for each subcategory of the neuromotor examination.
5. Describe expected abnormal motor examination results in the context of specific neurological conditions.

## ▪ Introduction

Human movement is essential for the performance of functional activities and must be measured by the physical and occupational therapist across the continuum of care in any rehabilitation setting. The control of movement includes both conscious and unconscious processing utilizing a vast and complex array of neurological structures. The purposes of this chapter are to review the neuromotor concepts of human movement that underlie the motor examination in a patient with neurological pathology, focusing on motor manifestations of the nervous system, and to describe specific neuromotor examination tests/measures organized according to the *Guide to Physical Therapist Practice,* including range of motion, muscle performance, and motor function (APTA, 2015).

**Range of motion** is the ability of a joint to be moved passively or actively, and it can be restricted by abnormalities of joint capsule or ligaments as well as decreased muscle length.

**Muscle performance** includes aspects of muscle strength or force generation, power, endurance, and length or muscle extensibility (APTA, 2015). Examination of **motor function** includes tests and measures for **motor control** and motor learning. Normal functions of the neurological and musculoskeletal systems enable voluntary controlled movement. Impairments of these neuromotor functions frequently contribute to limitations in functional activity. Therefore, they must be carefully examined and are often addressed in the treatment plan.

## ▪ Neuromotor System Function: Anatomical Perspectives

### Areas of the Motor Cortex

This brief review of the motor components of the nervous system is only meant to emphasize key neurological concepts for the clinical neuromotor examination. The motor cortex, with a key role in voluntary movement, includes three portions: the primary, premotor, and supplemental areas. The *primary motor cortex,* located in the most posterior gyrus of the frontal lobe (precentral gyrus), houses a representation of the different muscle groups of the body organized regionally (Figure 6-1A: Where Is It?). The specific organization of the primary motor cortex is known as the motor homunculus and illustrates the idea that body regions over which the brain exerts more motor control, including hands and face, are represented as shown in the right half (motor cortex) of Figure 6-1B by disproportionately larger areas of cortex. Areas with less motor control are disproportionately smaller in the homunculus.  A larger representation in the homunculus shape, with a larger number of cortex cells, allows for more selective activation of motor units because there is a smaller ratio of muscle fibers to motor neurons, which results in specific discrete movements and better fine-motor control of the muscles in a region. Conversely, areas with less representation within the motor cortex, and therefore a higher ratio of muscle fibers to motor neurons, have relatively less precise motor control (Figure 6-1B). The primary motor cortex also controls absolute force and movement velocity (Evarts, 1968).

The *premotor cortex* lies adjacent and anterior to the superior portion of the primary motor cortex on the superolateral frontal lobe (see Figure 6-1A). Activity within the premotor cortex provides activation of muscles that are either directly involved or support a specific activity such as limb positioning of the humerus and forearm of the upper extremity that allows the hands to perform more discrete functions including object manipulation. The premotor cortex relies on input from other areas such as vision centers; premotor activity has been shown to increase during tasks guided by vision (Mushiake, 1991). The premotor area may either send signals to the primary motor cortex, the basal ganglia, or other extrapyramidal structures such as reticulospinal neurons and thus serves as the primary cortical influence upon these structures (Campbell, 2005). The premotor area most commonly activates the primary motor cortex indirectly by activating the basal ganglia to in turn activate the thalamus, which finally activates the primary motor cortex.

The *supplementary motor area* is the most anterior motor cortex area, lying medial and anterior to the premotor area (Figure 6-1A). Blood flow to the supplementary area does not increase during simple finger movements but does increase during mental rehearsal and actual performance of complex finger movements (Roland, 1980). This suggests that the supplementary area participates in the assembly of a motor scheme or program, particularly bilateral muscle actions. In fact, both the supplementary and premotor areas become active during planning of movement (Bear, 2007). The supplementary area also assists the premotor area in attaining trunk and extremity positions while the primary cortex area enacts more specific discrete movements during functional activities.

### Extrapyramidal System/Subcortical Motor Nuclei

The extrapyramidal system of motor control is technically all central nervous system (CNS) motor structures external to the pyramidal system, with the exception of the cerebellum, and includes pallidal, thalamopallidal, basal ganglion, and striatal levels (Campbell, 2005) (see Figure 6-1C). Extrapyramidal motor control is involuntary and considered by some to contain older phylogenic structures (Campbell, 2005). It is important to note the close functional relationships between the pyramidal and extrapyramidal systems (Campbell, 2005). Because of these complex interactions, it is inappropriate to place one system or set of structures above other structures for importance in governing the control of movement.

The basal ganglia and the dorsal thalamus are the major subcortical input areas to the premotor and supplemental motor areas. Other subcortical areas that influence motor function include the substania nigra (considered part of the

■WHERE IS IT?

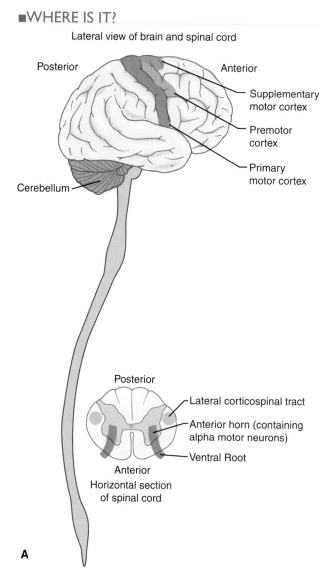

Lateral view of brain and spinal cord

**FIGURE 6-1 A.** Motor areas of the CNS showing the primary motor cortex in the precentral gyrus, premotor cortex in the superior frontal lobe just anterior to the precentral gyrus, supplementary motor cortex medial and anterior to the premotor area including part of the medial hemisphere surface, and the cerebellar cortex.

■WHERE IS IT?

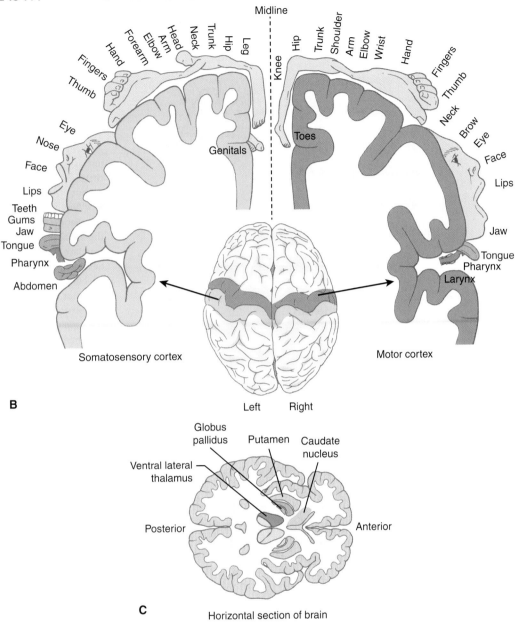

B

C   Horizontal section of brain

**FIGURE 6-1—cont'd   B.** The motor homunculus of the precentral gyrus illustrates the fact that parts of the body with the greatest motor control have a greater proportion of motor cortex controlling movement of that region. **C.** Deep CNS structures with primary motor function, which are not part of the pyramidal or corticospinal direct pathway, including parts of the basal ganglia (BG) (caudate and putamen nuclei as primary BG input and globus pallidus as primary BG output) and the ventral lateral thalamus. Damage to any of these structures will likely result in significant motor impairment.

basal ganglia), red nucleus, vestibular nuclei, and the reticular nuclei.

The basal ganglia (Figure 6-1C) contain the specific structures of the caudate, putamen, subthalamic nucleus, and the globus pallidus. Figure 6-2 illustrates an anatomical representation of the neural circuits of the basal ganglia as described by Bear (2007). At rest, the globus pallidus tonically inhibits the ventral lateral nucleus of the thalamus (Fig. 6-2A). When the motor cortex is active (Fig. 6-2B),

the caudate and putamen, together called the striatum, receive excitatory input from the cortex. The excited striatum inhibits the globus pallidus, disallowing inhibition of the ventral lateral nucleus of the thalamus (Figure 6-1C), also known as the VL (Bear, 2007). The uninhibited VL then sends excitatory information to the supplemental motor cortex, completing a complex positive feedback loop that not only assists motor function but also sends information to areas of the brain that involve memory and cognitive function

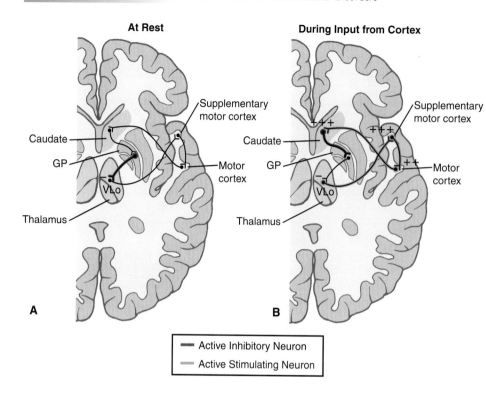

**FIGURE 6-2** The basal ganglia circuits described by Bear (2007) applied to an anatomical illustration. **A.** With the motor cortex at rest, and not stimulating the basal ganglia, the globus pallidus sends tonic inhibition to the ventral lateral thalamus to decrease motor output of the basal ganglia. **B.** When the motor cortex sends stimulation to the basal ganglia, the inhibition from the striatum (caudate or globus pallidus) decreases the globus pallidus inhibition of ventral lateral thalamus, allowing an increase in stimulation of the thalamus to the supplementary motor cortex and then primary motor cortex.

(Bear, 2007). The basal ganglia function to produce crude subconscious movements that operate in the background and refine more discrete skilled voluntary and automatic movements.

The substantia nigra is located within the cerebral peduncles of the midbrain. Intricately and reciprocally connected with the basal ganglia, the substantia nigra also functions to control subconscious movements. It is also part of the dopaminergic modulatory system and is partially responsible for the initiation of movement in response to the environment (Bear, 2007).

The red nucleus, a collection of cell bodies in the midbrain, and deep to the substantia nigra, is a subcortical area that operates similarly to the corticospinal tract. The function of the red nucleus is to provide an accessory route and modulation of motor input to the spinal cord. Direct connections exist from the primary motor cortex to the red nucleus via the corticorubral tract. The corticospinal tract also sends branching fibers to the red nucleus as it passes through the mesencephalon. The red nucleus sends signals to the spinal cord via the rubrospinal tract, which crosses to the contralateral side and runs a course parallel to the corticospinal tract down the lateral columns of the spinal cord. Connections also exist between the red nucleus and the cerebellum.

The vestibular and reticular nuclei are also subcortical areas that influence motor function. Reticular nuclei are named for their primary location in the brainstem and are divided into two major groups: pontine and medullary. Pontine nuclei are highly excitable and receive excitatory signals from the cerebellum, vestibular nuclei, and other areas of the brainstem. The vestibular and pontine reticular nuclei activate and maintain tone of antigravity musculature. The medullary reticular nuclei are antagonistic to the pontine reticular nuclei and inhibit the antigravity muscles when certain movements of antigravity limbs are desired. The medullary reticular nuclei

receive input from motor pathways, primarily the corticospinal and rubrospinal pathways.

## The Cerebellum

The cerebellum (Figure 6-1A) mainly refines movement by processing a number of unconscious senses related to muscle length and joint and body segment positions. It receives afferent information from the vestibular system, the brainstem, and spinal cord. It also sends information to the reticular formation, vestibular nuclei, and tracts, which makes it an important structure for balance and coordination (Campbell, 2005). In addition to the support of equilibrium reactions, the cerebellum contributes significantly to the regulation of muscle tone and posture (Campbell, 2005). Apart from vestibular and muscle tone regulation, the cerebellum processes unconscious proprioception by coordinating afferent signals, potentiating them by comparison of actual movement with planned movement, then passing signals on to other structures. The cerebellum is known for refining muscle activation into smooth and synchronous voluntary movements and coordination between opposing muscle groups (one shortens while the opposite lengthens). Overall, the cerebellum serves to receive, modulate, and integrate the information it receives.

## Descending Pathways

Signals arising from the motor cortex travel to the spinal cord by direct or indirect neuronal tracts. The lateral corticospinal or pyramidal tract carries signals directly from the cortex to alpha motor neurons of the spinal cord. An indirect connection occurs through bidirectional connections with the extrapyramidal motor system, including the basal ganglia, cerebellum, brainstem, and other nuclei from the brainstem.

The lateral corticospinal or pyramidal tract (see Figure 6-3) contains nerve fibers that primarily decussate to the contralateral side at the inferior medulla while some remain ipsilateral as they pass down to the spinal cord. Of all the descending nerve fibers, 80% to 90% of them decussate to the opposite side at the inferior medulla (as the pyramidal decussation) to become the lateral corticospinal tract, which descends in the posterior aspect of the lateral funiculus near the posterior horn (see Figure 6-3, Where Is It?) (Campbell, 2005). The fibers that remain ipsilateral travel in the ventral (anterior) corticospinal tract primarily arising from the supplemental motor area and affecting postural movements. Some of the largest and fastest conducting nerve fibers in the entire nervous system are found in the corticospinal tract. One corticospinal fiber innervates more than one alpha motor neuron in the spinal cord. This relationship, known as signal divergence, allows amplification of the corticospinal tract's activity (Campbell, 2005). Divergence increases the ratio of alpha motor neurons to excitatory descending pathway fibers and is particularly prevalent in large muscle groups that affect posture and perform gross movements. Divergence also occurs at the neuromuscular level concerning the ratio of alpha motor neurons to skeletal muscle fibers. An example of signal divergence is the soleus of the lower leg compared with muscles of the face or hands.

Terminal connections of the rubrospinal tract connect with the gray matter of the spinal cord along with fibers of

## ■WHERE IS IT?

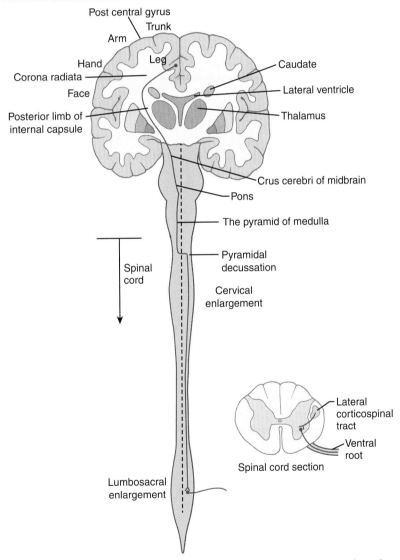

**FIGURE 6-3** Descending corticospinal tracts from primary motor cortex through corona radiata to posterior limb of internal capsule, crus cerebri of midbrain through pons to pyramids of medulla; nearly all fibers cross at pyramidal decussation (in inferior medulla) to the contralateral side, then descend on the contralateral side in lateral corticospinal tract in lateral funiculus and finally synapse on alpha motor neuron (anterior horn cell) before exiting the spinal cord through the ventral root and peripheral nerves to carry the impulse to the target muscle(s).

the corticospinal tract or directly connect with alpha motor neurons. Together, the rubrospinal and corticospinal tracts are considered the lateral motor system of the cord.

The ventromedial pathways are involved in postural control and are controlled by the brainstem. Four descending tracts comprise the ventromedial pathways: the vestibulospinal tracts, the tectospinal tract, and the medullary and pontine reticulospinal tracts. The vestibulospinal and tectospinal tracts function to keep the head postured during dynamic activities. Reticulospinal tracts, medullary and pontine, function to respectively dampen or facilitate antigravity muscle reflexes of the spinal cord depending on particular needs during motor activities.

## Muscle Activation Physiology

The motor cortex initiates voluntary skeletal muscle activation by sending efferent action potentials down the corticospinal tract (see Figure 6-3). At the appropriate spinal cord level, the action potential is carried in the corticospinal tract synapses via alpha motor neurons that carry the signal to a specific group of extrafusal skeletal muscle cells, collectively known as a motor unit. Alpha motor neurons, also known as lower-motor neurons, are analogous to wires that connect our CNS to our muscles. Thus, alpha motor neurons are an important part of the voluntary motor system. Gamma motor neurons, however, are not under conscious activation as they synapse with intrafusal fibers of skeletal muscle. Although gamma motor neurons are also efferent, their function is to match the length of the sensory intrafusal fiber to the voluntary extrafusal fiber.

The motor neuron's terminal bouton does not directly contact the muscle cell membrane (sarcolemma) as a gap (synaptic cleft) separates the two opposing membranes (motor neuron and sarcolemma). Therefore, activation passes to the sarcolemma by way of an excitatory neurotransmitter, acetylcholine, from the terminal bouton (Nielson, 2000; Sherwood, 1997).

## Clinical Manifestation of CNS Motor Pathologies

Damage to motor cortex or motor pathways in the brain or spinal cord results in both negative neurological symptoms and positive neurological symptoms. **Negative neurological signs** represent a loss or decrease of system function (i.e., you can no longer observe some normal body function that was previously present). For example, weakness, hypotonia, sensory loss, visual loss, vestibular hypofunction, or memory loss/confusion may develop. **Positive neurological signs** are body system expressions that are not normally present but increase or develop as a result of the neurological pathology (i.e., something you observe that is normally not present). For example, spasticity, rigidity, increased **deep tendon reflexes (DTRs)**, hyperesthesia (pins and needles), dystonia, tremor, or hyperactivity may develop. The resulting motor impairment of corresponding contralateral muscle groups includes varied clinical presentations ranging from **paresis**, which includes weakness or partial paralysis, or **paralysis**, a complete loss of ability to move the specified muscle group. Common pathologies affecting motor systems are summarized in Box 6-1. Contralateral motor symptoms result from

---

### BOX 6-1 Examples of Pathological Disorders Affecting Motor Areas of the Central Nervous System and Related Distribution of Motor Effects

**CVA-Anterior Cerebral Artery:** Contralateral motor symptoms primarily in lower extremity.

**CVA-Middle Cerebral Artery:** Contralateral motor symptoms primarily in face, upper extremity and trunk; lower extremity may be involved if infarction of deep subcortical white matter (corona radiata, posterior limb of internal capsule) takes place.

**CVA-Hemorrhage:** Contralateral motor symptoms depending on location of hemorrhage.

**Traumatic Brain Injury:** Variable motor symptom distribution depending on lesion location and extent; could be bilateral, but not necessarily symmetrical.

**Brain Tumors:** Contralateral motor symptoms specific to CNS area affected.

**Dementia:** Decreased movement and activity level.

**Cerebral Palsy:** Motor symptom distribution most often hemiplegia, diplegia, or quadriplegia.

---

motor cortex disorders because of decussation of motor pathways. The paralysis of cerebrovascular accident (CVA) primarily affects distal muscles and joints compared with proximal joints, which adversely influences the ability to produce movements requiring finer volitional control (Campbell, 2005). Following CVA, spasticity appears after a period of flaccidity and is more pronounced with damage of increasing severity and location (Campbell, 2005). Damage to the premotor cortex in combination with damage to the primary cortex causes severe spasticity in experimental models (Campbell, 2005). Components of pyramidal syndrome due to damage to the primary motor cortex or primary motor pathway are shown in Box 6-2 and consist of hyperreflexia, spasticity, abnormal reflexes, and impaired motor control with lack of certain isolated movements. However, experimental models suggest that spasticity associated with damage to the motor cortex may actually arise from extrapyramidal dysfunction, including imbalanced inhibition from the brainstem (Campbell, 2005).

Supplemental motor area lesions result in movement deficits during activities requiring bilateral coordinated actions of distal extremities such as the bimanual tasks (Bear, 2007).

---

### BOX 6-2 Common Contralateral Motor Manifestations of Pyramidal System Damage

- Paresis
- Impaired motor control (lack of isolated movement and impaired timing)
- Possible hypotonia (initially)
- Spastic hypertonia and hyperreflexia (typically develops later)

Lesions in the extrapyramidal areas result in signs and symptoms generally referred to as "movement disorders" (see Box 6-3) and include neurological conditions such as Parkinson and Huntington diseases. The signs of Parkinson disease include bradykinesia, disturbances in muscle tone, loss of "automatic movements," abnormal movements, and difficulty initiating movement (Campbell, 2005). Rigid hypertonicity of muscles, particularly cogwheel rigidity, and hyperkinesias in the form of resting tremors are clinical manifestations of Parkinson disease. Manifestations of Huntington disease in contrast with Parkinson disease include hyperkinesias and chorea as positive neurological signs.

Damage to the cerebellum results in numerous expressions of aberrant motor control, particularly hypotonia and ataxia (see Box 6-4). Muscle incoordination and diminished equilibrium are the principal manifestations of cerebellar dysfunction. The general term ataxia or incoordination refers to a constellation of specific motor deficits listed in Box 6-5 and described later in this chapter.

---

### BOX 6-3 Common Motor Manifestations That May Occur Following Extrapyramidal System Damage

Dystonia
Rigid hypertonicity (perhaps cogwheel)
Hyperkinesias (resting tremors)
Hypokinesias (bradykinesia)
Impaired motor control (initiation of movement)
Involuntary movements

---

### BOX 6-4 Common Motor Manifestations of Cerebellar Damage

- Muscle incoordination (ataxia; see Box 6-5)
- Hypotonia (low muscle tone)
- Asthenia (general decrease in strength or loss of energy)
- Diminished postural equilibrium
- Nystagmus (involuntary rhythmic eye movements)
- Speech disturbance (ataxic)

---

### BOX 6-5 Terms for Specific Components of Ataxia/Incoordination

- Adiadochokinesia
- Ataxia
- Dysmetria
- Dysdiadochokinesia
- Hyperkinesias
- Speech disturbances
- Hypermetria (past-pointing)

---

### THINK ABOUT IT 6.1

- If a patient has a diagnosis of Right Middle Cerebral Artery (MCA) stroke, what anatomical areas do you anticipate are affected?
- Based on these anatomical regions, what motor functions do you anticipate will be impaired?
- Based on the medical diagnosis and location of the lesion, do you anticipate the right, left, or both sides will be involved?

## Clinical Manifestation of Upper- and Lower-Motor Neuron Lesions

Neurons, cells of the nervous system, may be functionally divided into upper- and lower-motor neurons. Essentially, all neurons originating in the CNS, except those in the anterior horn of the spinal cord, are considered to be **upper-motor neurons**. **Lower-motor neurons** include the cell bodies of motor neurons in the anterior horn of the spinal cord, or motor neurons of the brainstem that contribute to cranial nerve motor functions and their axonal projections toward the periphery to innervate muscle. The term "final common pathway" is sometimes used to refer to the axons of lower-motor neurons that exit the CNS with fibers (in cranial nerves and peripheral spinal nerves) that directly stimulate motor units of muscles.

Any pathology that affects upper-motor neurons in the brain and spinal cord is categorized as an **upper-motor neuron (UMN) lesion**. Clinical manifestations of an UMN lesion include the positive neurological signs: spastic hypertonia (or spasticity) and hyperreflexia, which occur because of loss of cerebral control over voluntary and reflexive motor activity and because normal inhibitory influences from higher motor structures are discontinued. Without inhibition of intact lower-motor centers, aberrant reflexes are unregulated, causing distinctive clinical manifestations. UMN syndrome also typically includes the negative neurological signs of paralysis, impaired motor control movement, or muscle weakness. UMN lesion manifestations are detailed in Table 6-1.

Damage that occurs to the "final common pathway" is described as a **lower-motor neuron (LMN) lesion.** These disorders typically express just the opposite of UMN lesions and prevent activation of the muscles. Partial LMN lesions, with some motor units spared, cause the negative neurological signs of weakness and hypotonia. But if all motor neurons innervating a particular muscle are affected, the negative neurological sign of complete paralysis (i.e., cessation of voluntary muscle activity) will occur along with flaccidity. LMN lesion manifestations are found in Table 6-2.

## ■ Principles of Neuromotor Examination

The general sequence of a motor examination should include initial observation of the patient's posture, position, movement and intralimb coordination, a detailed history and

| TABLE 6-1 | **Common Manifestations of Upper-Motor Neuron Lesions** *(From damage to corticobulbar, corticospinal, corticorubrospinal, and corticoreticulospinal systems—cell bodies or tracts)* |
|---|---|
| Hemiplegia/Hemiparesis | • Internal capsule lesions result in lower face paralysis along with paralysis/weakness of the upper extremity and lower extremity on the contralateral side. |
| Spastic hypertonicity | • After days to weeks, spasticity (increased resistance to passive elongation that is velocity-dependent) develops accompanied by hyperactive DTRs, possibly due to loss of the normal inhibitory influence of these tracts on alpha-motoneurons.<br>• Firm resistance to passive movement, especially in UE flexors and LE extensors. The tone will often suddenly yield in the midst of the passive elongation (i.e., clasp knife). |
| Hyperreflexia | • Increased (hyperactive) DTRs, especially at wrist and sometimes at ankle. |
| Clonus | • Rhythmic oscillation of a joint, especially the ankle, is initiated by sudden, passive stretch of the spastic muscle (i.e., sudden dorsiflexion stretches the plantar flexors). Via the stretch reflex, this results in plantar flexion, which in turn stretches the dorsiflexors, beginning the cycle again. |
| Babinski sign | • Stroking the lateral plantar aspect of the foot results in hyperextension of the big toe and splaying abduction of the other toes. |

| TABLE 6-2 | **Common Manifestations of Lower-Motor Neuron Lesions** *(From damage to brainstem motor cranial nerves or anterior horn cells—cell bodies or peripheral nerve fibers)* |
|---|---|
| Paralysis/Paresis | • Loss of motor function. |
| | • Loss of coordination in muscle action. |
| | • (Decrease of motor function and decreased coordination if the LMN lesion is only partial) |
| Atrophy | • Secondary decrease in muscle mass and bulk with evident bony prominences. |
| | • Loss of automatic responses. |
| Abnormal palpation | • Soft, flabby muscle; lacks bulk. |
| Vicarious movements | • Compensatory or trick movements:<br>  • Ex: muscle substitution (long head bicep, long head tricep, clavicular pec major, supraspinatus, lat rotators can all abduct the humerus if deltoid is out).<br>  • Ex: this phenomenon may actually be helpful and useful to support compensatory actions such as tenodesis effect = flexion of the fingers passively occurs as the wrist is extended, especially in permanent losses such as individuals with quadriplegia. |
| Hyporeflexia | • Decreased or absent DTR. |
| Fasciculations | • Muscle twitches could indicate denervation injury. |

review of systems, and finally a comprehensive, patient-centered, physical examination to document the specific problems of the individual patient. See Chapter 14 for more detail.

It is also important to realize factors that may influence and affect the motor examination. Several of these factors include the patient's level of cognition and arousal, visual and sensory function, communication, the ability and willingness to cooperate, their anxiety level, the timing of the examination following injury or disease, and the influence of pharmacological agents (see Table 6-3) (Brown, 1991). The therapist should adequately document any such factors present during

the examination to enhance accurate interpretation of the present and future examination results.

## ■ Measuring Joint Range and Muscle Performance

### Joint Range of Motion

Joint range of motion and muscle flexibility directly impact the magnitude of possible movement and is covered well in other resources to which the reader has likely already been exposed (Hislop, 2007; Kendall, 2005; Norkin, 2009). It is

| TABLE 6-3 | Examples of Pharmacological Agents That May Impact Motor Function and Possible Effects |
|---|---|
| **PHARMACOLOGICAL AGENT OR CLASS** | **POSSIBLE EFFECT ON MOTOR BODY FUNCTION** |
| Antipsychotics | Extrapyramidal symptoms including tardive dyskinesia, pseudoparkinsonism, akathisia (restlessness), dystonia, and neuroleptic malignant syndrome, and sedation. |
| Baclofen | Muscle weakness. |
| Benzodiazepines | Sedation and ataxia (including Diazepam). |
| Dantrolene sodium | Generalized weakness. |
| Diruetics | Muscle weakness and/or fatigue. |
| Lithium | Sedation, lethargy, and muscle weakness. |
| Levodopa | Long-term use (3 months to 3 years) associated with dyskinesias such as ballismus, dystonia, myoclonus, tics, tremors, and choreoathetoid movements. |
| Tricyclics | Sedation, lethargy, and muscle weakness (Including Amoxapine = Ascendin: possible ataxia or tardive dyskinesia). |

Adapted from Ciccone CD. *Pharmacology in Rehabilitation.* 4th edition. Philadelphia, PA: F.A. Davis Co.; 2007.

important for the therapist to be able to distinguish between limited movements at a joint due to joint restrictions versus decreased muscle flexibility versus muscle hypertonia. Because of the profound implications for strength and motor control examination, range of motion and **flexibility (muscle flexibility)** should therefore be examined early in the motor examination of the patient with neurological dysfunction. A limitation to available motion at a joint is called a **contracture**. Details of therapeutic intervention for limitations to joint range or muscle flexibility are discussed in Chapter 23.

Joint range of motion (ROM) is the motion available at the specific joint being tested. ROM is affected directly by specific articulations of bone and the congruencies of bony surfaces. Connective tissue comprising the articular capsule also directly affects the available motion at a particular joint. Other factors that can influence joint ROM include the many structures that cross the joint such as muscles, tendons, nerves, and blood vessels. **Muscle flexibility** is a term used to describe the length and extensibility of musculotendinous structures that cross a particular joint and their influence on the ability of the joint to move. In terms of classifying joint ROM, there are three main types: active, active-assistive, and passive ROM.

Patients with neuromuscular diagnoses have impaired strength, force generation, or impaired motor control, which often prevents the person from actively moving a joint through the full available ROM. **Active ROM (AROM)** occurs when the patient uses a muscle or muscle group to independently move the joint, including antigravity movement, whereas **active-assisted ROM (AAROM)** is used when the muscle is too weak to work against gravity, and the patient receives assistance during the movement. Assistance may occur by removing the effects of gravity or by providing the patient with external assistance from another person or an object. AROM and AAROM are particularly helpful for strength assessment (see section on muscle strength) and in the individual who lacks isolated movement. AROM and AAROM are key methods for motor control movement examination (see section on motor control).

**Passive ROM (PROM)** requires no effort from the patient and is essential to assess joint mobility/range in a person who cannot actively move the limb well. The therapist provides all the movement to gauge and document the full available range. The resistance encountered at the end of the available ROM is known as an "**end feel.**" End feels are classified as soft, firm, bony, or empty (see Table 6-4).

Muscles and tendons that cross a joint will influence the ROM available at that joint. Although joint ROM and muscle flexibility are distinctly different, there is an intricate

| TABLE 6-4 | Classification of "End Feel" Associated with Passive Range of Motion |
|---|---|
| Empty | Patient prevents reaching the end of available ROM due to apprehension or pain. Also pertains to inability to assess end feel. |
| Bony | A hard stop occurs at the end of the available ROM, usually caused by bone approximation or a mechanical blockage around the articular surfaces. |
| Firm | Taut or tight feeling caused by tensile limitation of connective tissue. |
| Soft tissue approximation | Soft tissue prevents attainment of full ROM. |

relationship between the two: limitations to muscle flexibility will limit joint ROM and a range restriction inherent in a joint will eventually lead to adaptive shortening of related muscles. The kinesiological principle of passive insufficiency provides an example of how decreased muscle length affects joint ROM. Essentially, **passive insufficiency** occurs in two-joint muscles and may be described by the inability to achieve full ROM at both joints when the muscle is put on stretch (moved into the antagonistic direction). For example, the rectus femoris crosses both the hip and the knee. If a person moves the knee into flexion (the opposite of the rectus femoris action) and the hip into extension (also the opposite of its action), full flexion at the knee and full extension at the hip could not be achieved simultaneously if the muscle is short-ened. It follows then that abnormal muscle flexibility and rest-ing tone with abnormal postures will affect available joint ROM if not addressed. Increases in resting muscle tone may decrease available joint motion as muscle activation inhibits the dissociation of contractile elements and prevents full movement into the opposite end of the range. For a joint to move through its full available ROM, the antagonist of the joint motion must fully elongate. Therapeutic interventions related to ROM deficits are presented in Chapter 23.

### Basic Review of ROM Examination

Performing ROM examinations includes both active and passive movements as the reader has previously learned in detail. This section is intended only as a review with a focus on impli-cations in a population with neuromuscular disorders. Muscle flexibility can be assessed either actively or passively but differs slightly from the techniques used during ROM examination. A summary of the scientific evidence supporting use of specific measures of PROM is presented in Table 6-25 online (ONL), Focus on Evidence Table for PROM Examination.

### Arom Examination

Using basic kinesiology knowledge, have the patient perform isolated movements at each individual joint against the effects of gravity. During the active voluntary movement, you can also make observations as part of your motor control movement examination (details are described later in this chapter). Once you recognize a deficit in the available motion at a particular joint, goniometric measurements are used to quantify available joint AROM. If the patient can perform full AROM at a joint, there is no need to use PROM to test for joint integrity.

If the patient cannot complete the movement against grav-ity, you may offer assistance (AAROM) during the attempted motion by manually providing lifting force or positioning the patient in such a way that gravity assists the desired move-ment. Objects such as a dowel, pulleys, or the patient's oppo-site extremity may also provide assistance to the movement. The type of assistance (e.g., manual, dowel, etc.) provided to the AROM must be documented. If full AROM is not attain-able with assistance, a PROM assessment is warranted. Passive assessment would determine whether joint or soft tissue integrity impedes motion at the joint, but if passive mobility is full then diminished strength of associated musculature is

likely preventing full active movement. This is especially true in the case where AAROM exceeds AROM.

### PROM Examination

PROM may be tested in physiological anatomical planes, or it may be used to assess accessory joint motion. The emphasis of this section will be on physiological motion that occurs in the various anatomic planes.

To perform a general PROM assessment, place one hand proximal to or at the examined joint to optimally stabilize the joint and proximal segment. Your other hand should provide the movement force at a segment distal to the joint, making sure all your contacts are specifically over bony prominences while avoiding direct contact with muscles, especially muscles that have spasticity (see Figure 6-4). The joint should move through its entire ROM. The key component of PROM examination is determining the available amount of ROM, which is quantified with a goniometer. Details about how to perform the examination and normal findings can be found in other resources (Hislop, 2007; Norkin, 2009). As the ther-apist, you must have an awareness of the "feel" of the block or resistance at the end of the available ROM, also called the end feel, examples of which are listed in Table 6-4.

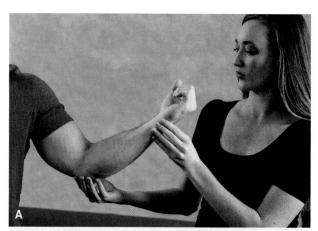
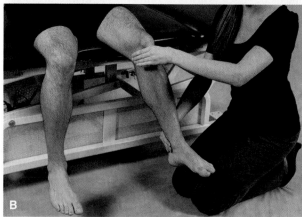

**FIGURE 6-4** Hand placements for testing ROM and muscle tone should emphasize contact with bony prominences and avoid contact with muscles, particularly those with spasticity as shown in this example of **A.** UE ROM testing for the elbow and **B.** LE ROM testing for the knee.

Finally, precautions may be necessary during the ROM examination. If spastic hypertonus is detected during passive movement, rapid movement may stimulate the stretch reflex with resulting forces that prevent moving to the full end-range. In the most extreme cases, spasticity may definitively limit ROM or could prolong the PROM examination as the therapist waits for a slow prolonged stretch to attain the true maximal joint position available. In general, when testing ROM to examine joint integrity, fast movements are unnecessary and should be avoided.

## Flexibility

A muscle elongates when the associated bone is moved in a direction opposite of the muscle action. Muscles that are flexible have greater extensibility than those that are inflexible, allowing for greater ROM at the related joints. Muscle elongation may actively occur during a terminal-range concentric muscle action by the antagonistic muscle group or passively by another external force. The soleus muscle, an ankle plantar flexor, would be stretched by active ankle dorsiflexion or forced dorsiflexion imposed by an external force such as a therapist. As a more complex example, the two-joint muscle gastrocnemius is best stretched when the knee is placed in extension while the ankle is simultaneously dorsiflexed.

Flexibility assessments may be done actively or passively, although it is usually best to perform both. For active flexibility assessments, have the patient activate the antagonist muscle group to move the joint(s) to the maximal extent possible. During passive assessments, provide external force to move the joint to the full end-range. Measure the available motion at the affected joint with a goniometer as you would for ROM assessment and compare the results to the opposite extremity. Remember that other synergistic muscles also stretch during the assessment of the targeted muscle, so it is preferable to document that a particular functional muscle group was stretched (e.g., knee flexors instead of semimembranosus). However, relatively greater emphasis may be placed on a particular muscle by moving the body segment in the opposite direction of all the particular actions of the muscle in question while placing its synergists in a shortened position, if possible. For the soleus as an example, we move the foot into dorsiflexion while placing the other primary plantar flexors, the gastrocnemius and plantaris, on slack by placing the knee in flexion. Normal flexibility data for healthy individuals is cataloged elsewhere (ACSM, 2014).

## Muscle Strength

**Muscle strength** is the ability of a muscle to generate force to cause movement and is essential for motor control. Muscle force may be produced and tested in the following modes of action: **isometric** (static) **muscle actions, isokinetic** (movement at a fixed speed, e.g., concentric or eccentric actions at 60 degrees per second) **muscle actions,** or **isotonic** (movement without a fixed speed, e.g., concentric or eccentric

actions while moving a limb with or without additional resistance) **muscle actions.** Clinical strength testing is common practice in orthopedics but is now accepted for some neurological examinations. Traditionally, some have believed strength testing to be inappropriate for some patients with UMN syndrome, because concentric muscle actions could exacerbate stretch reflexes in the antagonist, which may increase spastic tone of those muscles (Engardt, 1995). However, strength and muscle tone are distinct muscle features, and voluntary muscle actions do not necessarily result in increases in muscle tone. In fact, some argue that slow concentric actions are appropriate to assess muscle strength in patients with neurological dysfunction (Marque, 1997).

An even greater issue in the person with motor control deficits from cerebral pathology is that strength examination is not valid if the individual cannot perform an isolated movement with the target muscle. To perform traditional strength testing with the standardized protocol and position, a muscle must activate appropriately without substitution or movement compensation. Decreased force generation capability in a particular muscle or muscle group is the negative neurological sign called **weakness**. The principles and practice of therapeutic intervention for weakness in an individual with a neurological disorder are presented in Chapter 22. Certainly, strength testing is essential in patients with primary weakness related to LMN damage or hypotonia. A complete absence of the ability to generate force in a muscle is called paralysis, which occurs in complete spinal cord injury (SCI).

Isometric tests require that no joint movement occurs during the contraction. Isometric testing methods include manual muscle testing and handheld dynamometry (Andrews, 1996; Andrews, 2000; Hislop, 2007; Kendall, 2005). Isometric strength testing may be used to evaluate specific muscle/muscle groups and/or myotomes. Isometric tests for strength often occur in the midrange for two-joint muscles or at the shortened end of the available ROM for monoarticular muscles, but joint position may also depend on the specific individual's capability (Hislop, 2007; Kendall, 2005). For example, testing the quadriceps at midrange would require the knee to be placed in approximately 60 to 70 degrees of flexion (one-half of the normal 135 degrees) whereas testing at the shortened end-range would be full knee extension. Isometric tests performed with the muscle in its shortened ROM can be a problem if that particular muscle group is not able to attain its shortened position due to tightness of an antagonist muscle group or insufficient motor control. The examiner should document any lack of PROM with the accompanying muscle grade (Hislop, 2007).

In terms of a neurological assessment, myotome testing is more general than specific manual muscle testing and is particularly useful in testing in the context of SCI. A **myotome** consists of muscles or muscle groups innervated by a single spinal root that usually perform similar actions. For instance, the L3 myotome consists of the muscles that act to produce knee extension. The other major myotome levels are listed in Table 6-5. During testing, the extremity is positioned so the muscle group must work against gravity.

| TABLE 6-5 | Major Myotome Levels |
|---|---|
| **NERVE ROOT LEVEL** | **JOINT ACTIONS** |
| C5 | Elbow flexion*; shoulder abduction |
| C6 | Wrist extension* |
| C7 | Elbow extension* |
| C8 | Finger flexion*; distal phalanx of middle finger |
| T1 | Finger abduction*; little finger |
| L2 | Hip flexion* |
| L3 | Knee extension* |
| L4 | Ankle dorsiflexion* |
| L5 | Great toe extension; long toe extensors* |
| S1 | Ankle plantar flexion* |

*Designates the key muscle actions in the ASIA "Standard Neurological Classification of Spinal Cord Injury"; see Figure 5-11 (ASIA, 2011).

The additional force applied by the clinician acts in concert with gravity and against the action of the muscles being tested. Findings from the involved side are then compared with the uninvolved extremity.

**Manual muscle testing** is a method to assess muscle strength that attempts to isolate specific muscles or muscle groups by placing the patient and the tested joints in various standardized positions. Manual muscle testing results have been shown to predict short-term functional muscle recovery in patients with quadriplegia arising from a SCI (Brown, 1991). Details of manual muscle testing are described in other texts (Hislop, 2007; Kendall, 2005) but then must be applied in the context of neurological disorders. The various testing positions place the muscle in a shortened position standardized for each muscle group. Gravity's effects should be maximized in patients capable of producing large amounts of muscle force and minimized with patients who are unable to move through normal or full ROM against gravity. General principles of manual muscle testing are shown in Box 6-6.

The *Modified Research Council (MRC) grading scale* for manual strength testing, shown in Table 6-6, is the same for both specific manual muscle testing techniques and gross muscle group assessment of myotomes (Mendell, 1990). Despite being somewhat subjective, the grading scale provides good intrarater (within the same examiner) reliability (Florence, 1992; Wadsworth, 1987). The MRC manual muscle grading scale ranges from 0 to 5 with 5 considered normal, which indicates that the tested muscle group resists maximal resistance with performance and is symmetrical to the opposite extremity. The remaining grades are based upon whether the patient performs the muscle activity against gravity and how much additional force the patient is able to produce against resistance during the examination (Hislop, 2007). Some consider a functional muscle grade to be at least a 4 on the scale of 5, because one must produce more force

**BOX 6-6 Principles of Manual Muscle Testing**

- Patient must be able to assume the standard test position (adequate motor control for isolation of the muscle)
- Consider the effects of gravity
- Direct the resistance (if any) opposite the action of the muscle being tested
- Perform resistance at end of available ROM (muscle shortened)
- Build manual resistance slowly
- Allow patient to develop maximal tension
- Avoid provocation of pain
- Avoid manual contact over the tested muscle or synergistic muscle groups

than the weight of their limb during normal functional activities (Brown, 1991).

A handheld **dynamometer** (Figure 6-5) is a device that is more objective and sensitive, measuring force to detect and document muscle weakness and the improvement thereof, than the grading system associated with manual muscle testing (Crompton, 2007; Wadsworth, 1987). Test-retest and intertester reliability has been established with a handheld dynamometer (Bohannon, 1986; Bohannon, 1987), and higher test-retest values with dynamometery were observed than with manual muscle testing (Wadsworth, 1987). (See Table 6-27 online (ONL), Focus on Evidence Table for Strength Examination, for this and other evidence regarding examination of strength.) The reader can find normative data using a handheld dynamometer published by Andrews (1996) for the major extremity muscle groups in adults.

### Tests/Measures for Manual Muscle Strength

Details of muscle testing are covered well in other specific textbooks with a focus on that topic (Hislop, 2007; Kendall, 2005). Muscle strength, whether evaluated with manual muscle grades or handheld dynamometry, requires a few basic rules for proper performance. First, place the patient in a comfortable and standardized position. Testing the unaffected extremity first (if applicable), ask the patient to perform the action of the tested muscle or muscle group to first assess muscle strength related to lifting their own weight against gravity. It is important in the patient with a neurological disorder to remember that the person must be able to assume the standardized test position and perform an isolated movement without muscle substitution to obtain a valid muscle test grade. If the patient is able to move the body segment through the full available ROM, gradually apply resistance on the distal segment with one hand while stabilizing proximal segments with the other hand. Assess and document the amount of manual resistance, or use a dynamometer to document the force generated. Gradually build and release the applied resistance, being careful not to "jerk" the body segment with your force. If the person cannot perform a full isolated movement without substitution, muscle testing would not be

| TABLE 6-6 | **Modified Research Council Manual Muscle Testing Grades** | |
|---|---|---|
| **GRADE** | **VALUE** | **DEFINITION** |
| Normal | 5 | Patient has full ROM against effects of gravity. Examiner provides "maximal" resistance with no discernable difference between affected and unaffected limbs. |
| Good | 4 | Patient has full ROM against effects of gravity. Examiner provides strong resistance with slight difference noted between affected and unaffected limbs. |
| Fair | 3 | Patient has full ROM against effects of gravity, but is unable to sustain any resistance offered by examiner. |
| Poor | 2 | Gravity eliminated: patient is able to produce full AROM. |
| Trace | 1 | Gravity eliminated: patient is unable to produce full AROM, however, muscle tension is palpable to examiner. |
| Zero | 0 | Gravity eliminated: patient unable to initiate AAROM and muscle tension is not palpable. |

(Hislop, 2007; Kendall, 2005)

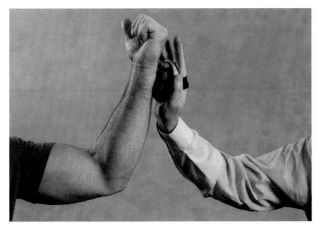

**FIGURE 6-5** Handheld dynamometer used for objective measurement of elbow extensor force.

valid, and it is more appropriate to examine for motor control movement ability as described later in the chapter.

### Assessing Paralysis and ASIA Designation

The American Spinal Injury Association (ASIA) established standards to evaluate motor function, sensation, and pain in individuals with SCI (Furlan, 2011; Priebe, 1991). The *ASIA Impairment Scale* consists of the following: "*A-Complete*" lesion occurs when no motor or sensory function is present at the lowest sacral segment (S4/5) or below the injury level; "*B-Incomplete*" occurs when sensory function is present below S4/5 without corresponding motor function; "*C-Incomplete*" happens when motor function is preserved below the neurological level but greater than one-half of the major muscle groups have a manual muscle grade less than three out of five; "*D-Incomplete*" occurs when motor function is preserved below the neurological level, and one-half of the major muscle groups have a manual muscle grade of at least three out of five; and "*E-Normal*" is when motor and sensory function are intact (El Masry, 1996; Furlan, 2011; Priebe, 1991). In addition to the ASIA Scale to assess severity of the SCI impairment, the *ASIA Standard Neurological Classification for Spinal Cord Injury* (ASIA, 2011) also include a tool to assess the specific sensory deficit and the level of motor involvement (see Figure 5-11).

Recent work substantiates the utility of the motor and sensory aspects of the ASIA scale (El Masry, 1996; Furlan, 2011).

### Tests/Measures for Isokinetic Muscle Strength

Isokinetic strength examination requires measuring force production during movement that takes place at a constant speed throughout a range of movement. Isokinetic strength assessment is performed on a piece of computerized equipment that maintains a fixed speed of movement while recording the relative amount of force produced during the movement (see Figure 6-6). Isokinetic testing, although not traditionally used to assess patients with neurological insults, has become more popular in recent years (Engardt, 1995; Marque, 1997; Pasternak-Mladzka, 2007). For isokinetic testing to be reliable, it is essential to standardize the test position, correct for gravity, and account for training effects, including learning effects that occur with patient experience with the machine (Marque, 1997). Altogether, isokinetic testing provides objectivity when assessing clinical presentations such as tonal abnormalities (see section on muscle tone) (Pasternak-Mladzka, 2007).

Isokinetic muscle strength assessment requires procedural steps that vary according to specific equipment manufacturer.

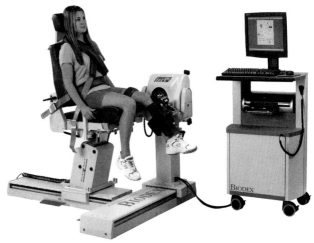

**FIGURE 6-6** Biodex® System 4 Isokinetic Dynamometer testing the knee flexors and extensors. Photograph courtesy of Biodex Medical Systems, Inc.

Nonetheless, there are general guidelines that apply regardless of the type of isokinetic equipment utilized. Calibrate the machine before testing the patient. Assist the patient to the device, if necessary, and stabilize the patient in the chair or bench with the appropriate stabilization belts or straps. Adjust the dynamometer to the patient, aligning the machine's axis of rotation with the moving joint's axis of rotation. Test the unaffected extremity first, if applicable, and then repeat for the affected extremity. Always consult manufacturer manuals for model-specific information for isokinetic testing procedures.

## Muscle Tone

**Muscle tone** is the amount of inherent neuromuscular activity present even in a resting muscle and is detected by the response, specifically the amount of resistance, to passive elongation or stretch of the muscle being tested (Masi, 2008). Muscle tone has become a controversial topic for some because it is not as easily measured as other aspects of muscle performance. Yet many research studies examine and demonstrate the ability of

medical and surgical management to alter muscle tone in patients with neurological disorders (Fehlings, 2010; Saval, 2010). Chapters 18 and 19 focus on therapeutic intervention to alter muscle tone in these populations. Damage to several neuroanatomic regions can result in abnormal expressions of muscle tone. Specifically, damage to the corticospinal (pyramidal) system in the cerebrum or the brainstem or the motor pathways of the spinal cord can result in spasticity. Damage to the extrapyramidal elements, including basal ganglia often results in rigidity or dystonia. For example, damage to the substantia nigra, either traumatic from traumatic brain injury or degenerative as in Parkinson disease, can result in rigidity. Rigidity can be differentiated from spasticity as it is not velocity dependent and is likely to be present even during PROM at slow speeds. Damage to the vestibular centers, the cerebellum, anterior horn cells, peripheral nerves, neuromuscular junction, or the muscle itself may result in decreased muscle tone.

The types of abnormal muscle tone as a continuum are shown in Table 6-7 and described in greater detail in the section later in this chapter. **Hypertoni**a **(hypertonicity)**, a

| TABLE 6-7 | Description of Variations in Muscle Tone | | | | |
|---|---|---|---|---|---|
| TONE STATE: | FLACCID | HYPOTONIA | NORMAL | SPASTIC HYPERTONIA | RIGID HYPERTONIA |
| Description of muscle resistance to passive elongation: | Complete absence of resistance to elongation | Decreased resistance to elongation | Mild and appropriate resistance to elongation | Increased resistance to elongation that increases with faster stretch (velocity-dependent), usually more predominant in muscle on one side of affected joints in stroke/TBI (or in both agonists and antagonists in affected areas following SCI), and more obvious toward the end of the range when the muscle is on maximal stretch | Increased resistance to elongation that does not increase with faster stretch (present even at slow speeds); often present in muscles on both sides of the joint and present throughout the range (though it may show a "cog-wheel" pattern) |
| Reflexes (DTRs) | Absent | Diminished (hyporeflexia) | Normal | Increased (hyperreflexia) particularly with spasticity | May be increased, but often dampened by activity of opposing muscle group |
| Common Medical Conditions | • Acute CVA<br>• Spinal shock in SCI<br>• Polio (complete)<br>• Some spinal muscular atrophy<br>• Peripheral nerve injury<br>• Guilllain Barré | • Some genetic disorders (Down syndrome, Angelman syndrome)<br>• Polio (partial)<br>• Cerebellar disorders | | • Stroke (CVA)<br>• TBI<br>• SCI<br>• Multiple sclerosis | • Parkinson disease<br>• Basal ganglia trauma or stroke |

positive neurological sign, is a muscle state with increased resistance in a muscle during passive elongation of that target muscle, whereas **hypotonia (hypotonicity)**, a negative neurological sign, is a muscle tone state in which resistance is less than normal during passive elongation of a muscle (Campbell, 2005). While this section focuses on the tests and measures for neuromotor examination including muscle tone, remember the therapist must be able to distinguish hypertonus from related joint ROM limitations/contractures such as muscle length limitations or joint capsule restrictions as described earlier in this chapter in the section on examination of "Joint Range of Motion." Therapeutic interventions related to flaccidity and hypotonia are presented in Chapter 18. Therapeutic interventions related to spastic hypertonia and rigid hypertonia are covered in Chapter 19.

Several factors can influence the clinical presentation of muscle tone, including the temperature of the muscle, the emotional and behavioral state of the patient, the speed of passive movement (faster speeds may more likely elicit activity of stretch reflexes), and cooperation of the patient. Of these factors, the patient's cooperation and relaxation are among the most important to control when performing a tonal assessment because of their effect upon the neurological examination findings. The patient must be able to voluntarily relax the limb being tested to allow optimal muscle tone testing.

Common clinical presentations associated with spastic muscle tone as part of the **upper-motor neuron syndrome** include clasp-knife resistance, scissoring gait, clonus, and the Babinski and Chaddock signs (Campbell, 2005). **Clasp-knife phenomenon** is a characteristic of spasticity, inconsistently present, in which the passive stretch results in initial resistance followed by sudden release as seen when opening a spring-loaded pocketknife. Scissoring gait is a motor control problem observed in patients with hip adductor spasticity associated with excessive abnormal synergy adduction of the leg in swing phase. **Clonus**, which is often associated with spasticity, is a rhythmic involuntary contraction and relaxation alternating between agonist and antagonist muscle groups that occurs in response to sudden passive movement of the ankle (most common), wrist, or patella (Campbell, 2005). Test for clonus by rapidly and forcefully pushing the joint up into end-range and maintaining pressure at end-range. Observe for resulting reflexive movement, counting the "beats" or oscillations of the movement. Document clonus by noting the number of "beats." If the clonus does not subside with maintained pressure at end-range, documenting "sustained clonus" may be appropriate. In spasticity, DTRs as previously described will be hyperflexive. A positive **Babinski sign** is observed by great toe extension and toe splaying (Figure 6-7) as a result of noxious stroking of the ventral aspect of the foot (starting at the base of the fifth metatarsal, sliding up the foot to the metatarsal head and then medially across to the first metatarsal head) (Campbell, 2005). The Babinski sign has a sensitivity of only 35% but specificity of 77% for predicting UMN weakness (Miller, 2005). Mass toe flexion or withdrawal of the foot and leg is considered a normal response to Babinski testing. The **Chaddock sign** is similar to the Babinski sign but

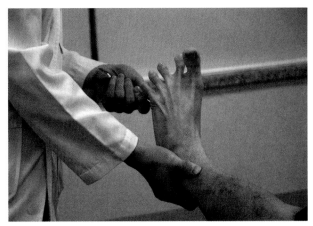

**FIGURE 6-7** Babinski sign with great toe extension and splaying of other toes in response to stroking the plantar surface of the lateral foot (along the length of the 5th metatarsal) and then along the metatarsal heads.

is great toe extension with or without splaying of toes that occurs in response to noxious stimulation of the dorsolateral aspect of the foot inferior to the malleolus (Figure 6-8) as opposed to the ventral surface (Campbell, 2005).

Tone assessment is easier and more typically tested in the extremities than the trunk, although abnormal tone is just as likely in proximal musculature following certain injuries or disease. Muscle tone examination is often difficult, and interrater reliability has been called into question because of relative subjectivity in traditional methods of tone assessment (Campbell, 2005). The traditional method for detecting abnormal muscle tone is carrying a muscle through passive elongation while the therapist "feels" or assesses how much resistance the muscle generates opposing the passive elongation. By comparing the amount of resistance to that felt when moving the limb of an individual without impairment, the therapist can determine generally whether the tone is decreased, normal, or increased. In formulating an intervention plan, the therapist will have to determine the type of abnormal tone present (i.e., flaccidity, spasticity, rigidity, etc.) and consider whether or not the

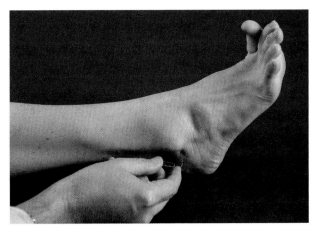

**FIGURE 6-8** Chaddock sign with toe extension, with or without splaying of the toes, in response to an inframalleolar noxious stimulus.

abnormal muscle tone is truly limiting the individual's function and activity or not. From a semantic standpoint, it is always better in conversation and documentation to specify the specific type of abnormal tone instead of making a generic and indeterminate statement such as "Billy has tone in his right biceps." An individual with a CVA may have severe spasticity that interferes with voluntary movement of the affected limbs. An individual with a complete SCI and paraplegia may have spasticity that actually contributes to lower extremity function in weight-bearing because there is no voluntary muscle control. Finally, during muscle tone testing, it is important for the therapist to compare resistance in agonist versus antagonist at each joint and compare the two sides, especially when unilateral symptoms are expected. This comparison between limbs and joints could help provide insight in the patient's baseline level of tone before the neurological event. The recent evidence regarding tests and measures of muscle tone is summarized in Table 6-28 online (ONL), the Focus on Evidence Table for Examination of Muscle Tone.

### Procedures for Measuring Muscle Tone

You will begin to formulate some hypotheses about the patient's muscle tone even when you first begin to observe their body segment posture and movement. Observe whether the muscles are bulked or atrophied and whether there appears to be any tension in the muscle at rest or during action. For example, a limb hanging limply in a gravity-dependent position may have flaccidity or severe hypotonia. A limb held in an unusual antigravity posture might, among other impairments, be related to hypertonia that you could definitively test. By definition, muscle tone is tested by passively elongating the target muscle, at both slow and fast velocities, as you gauge the amount of resistance to the elongation or stretch. When moving the limb passively, it is important to position the patient for optimal stability and to hold the patient's limb using bony prominences as much as possible to minimize contact with the potentially abnormal muscle. For example, as you test muscle tone in the elbow flexors and extensors, your proximal hand could firmly stabilize at the elbow with contact over the medial and lateral epicondyles while your distal hand uses contact over the styloid processes to provide the motion at the elbow joint. For tone testing at the wrist joint, you could contact over the styloid processes to stabilize at the wrist while contact at the lateral second metacarpal head and the medial fifth metacarpal head will allow you to control movement at the wrist joint.

In assessing muscle tone, it is important to determine muscle resistance to passive, not active, movement or elongation while the patient is relaxed (Campbell, 2005). You should also move the extremity through a full ROM and at a variety of speeds (as will be emphasized in the following section for testing spasticity). As you perform the passive elongation, use your proprioceptive awareness to determine the "feel" or resistance of the muscle throughout the movement. For spasticity, note particularly where, in the range, the resistance is first felt as this is important for grading spasticity in commonly used tests and measures. You must be keenly aware of which muscle is being

elongated during each phase of movement (the muscle being elongated is the one being tested) and feel the resistance by the muscle to assess whether the resistance to that elongation is at a normally expected level or if the resistance is decreased or increased. For example, as you move the arm into elbow extension, you are testing or feeling muscle tone (resistance) in the elbow flexor muscles as they are being elongated/stretched (see Figure 6-9). When testing muscle tone in individuals with cerebral disorders (e.g., CVA, traumatic brain injury [TBI], cerebral palsy [CP]), it is important to observe for and recognize the influence of tonic reflexes that may have reoccurred

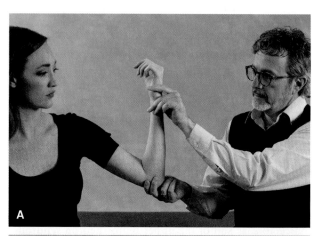

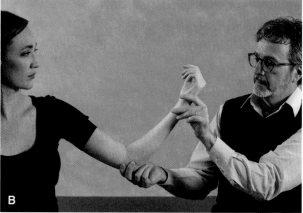

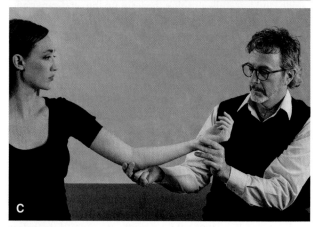

**FIGURE 6-9 A., B.,** and **C.** Testing muscle tone of the biceps by passive elongation of the biceps, moving the arm into elbow extension.

or are persistent related to the pathology. Keep the head in midline, not rotated, to avoid the influence of a recurrent asymmetrical tonic neck reflex (ATNR), which would cause increased tone in elbow extensors and knee extensors of the side toward which the neck is rotated and increased elbow flexor tone in the opposite arm. Test muscle tone in side-lying or in sitting, rather than in prone or supine, to avoid the influence of a recurrent tonic labyrinthine response, which would cause increased flexor tone while the individual is in prone and increased extensor tone while the individual is in supine.

Several tests assess general muscle tone and can be performed to confirm or corroborate the tone state detected in passive elongation testing, including clonus and DTRs (both described later in this chapter), the Arm-Dropping Test (or Drop Arm test), the Pronation Positioning Test, the Pronator Drift Test, and the Pendulum Test. The testing position for the *Arm-Dropping Test* is sitting with the arms adducted and resting comfortably (Campbell, 2005). With the patient in the sitting position, quickly elevate the patient's arms to approximately 90 degrees of shoulder flexion or abduction, then immediately drop the arms of the patient. Hypertonicity causes relative decreased rate of return to the starting position whereas hypotonicity causes an increased rate of return to the resting position compared with the uninvolved extremity. Therefore, it is advisable to assess bilateral upper extremities simultaneously. Supine is an alternate test position for patients that cannot maintain sitting during the Arm-Dropping Test; the set-up movement is passive horizontal adduction instead of abduction. The *Pronator Positioning Test* is similar to the Arm-Dropping Test in that the patient's arms are elevated to elicit abnormalities with muscle tone. However, with the Pronator Positioning Test, elevate the arms of the patient as high as possible into shoulder flexion, preferably to an overhead position. External rotation of the humerus normally accompanies overhead elevation, and supination of the forearm should accompany external rotation of the humerus when the elbow is extended (Neumann, 2009). However, patients with hypertonicity display excessive forearm pronation in the elevated humeral positions when the elbow is extended (Figure 6-10). The classic clinical presentation or positive sign for the Pronator Positioning Test is that the patient's palms face outward in the elevated humeral position with the elbows extended (Campbell, 2005).

The *Pronator Drift Test* begins with the patient's eyes closed in a standing position with the forearms in supination and the elbows, wrists, and fingers in extension. Patients with mild increased muscle tone "drift" into slight forearm pronation and elbow, wrist, and finger flexion. This test is sensitive to discern mild increases in muscle tone that may not otherwise be discernable (Campbell, 2005). Lower Extremity Pendulum Tests require the patient to sit on a plinth high enough to allow the lower extremities to dangle without touching the floor. Passively move the patient's relaxed lower extremity from a position of knee flexion into knee extension then suddenly release (Figure 6-11). Normally, the lower extremities should swing as a pendulum several times. Rigidity or spasticity causes the lower extremities

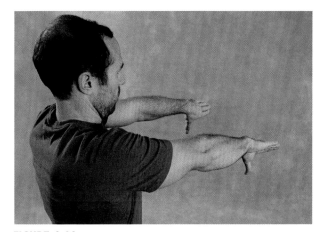

**FIGURE 6-10** Pronator-positioning test with the patient's forearm in excessive pronation while the patient tries to maintain humeral elevation and elbow extension.

to swing with diminished movement or not at all (Campbell, 2005). This test may also be performed as a general tonal assessment for hypertonicity or hypotonicity resulting in increased and decreased swing, respectively, of the lower extremity.

Another commonly used test to confirm the tone status determined by passive movement testing is DTR testing, which involves striking a muscle tendon to cause a sudden stretch/ elongation of the muscle, allowing observation for an appropriate reflexive contraction of the same muscle. As part of DTR testing, it is important to assure that the muscle being tested is either on stretch or has a partial contraction before striking the tendon. It is also essential that the patient isn't actively contracting the opposing muscle group during test. Because of the variability of tone and reflex sensitivity even among individuals without neurological impairment, it is most important to check for symmetry in the tested locations, especially in unilateral disorders. With some smaller tendons, such as the biceps brachialis, you can place your thumb over the tendon then strike your thumb (Figure 6-12A) to provide opportunities for you to feel subtle biceps contractions that might not be strong enough to elicit elbow movement. Common DTR test locations include the biceps (Figure 6-12A) and brachioradialis in the upper extremity and the patellar (quadriceps) (Figure 6-12B) and Achilles (plantar flexors) in the lower extremity (details are summarized in Table 6-8). If a person has absent or minimal response to the Patellar DTR test, the **Jendrassik maneuver** (Figure 6-13) may be used to heighten reflex reaction by increasing upper extremity tension by clasping hands and pulling them against each other (Nardone, 2008). It is not clear if this phenomenon occurs because of a heightening of the neuromotor system or if the patient occupied with the maneuver may be distracted from consciously blocking the muscle response (Nardone, 2008).

## Observations for Specific Types of Abnormal Muscle Tone

**Flaccidity** is a complete lack of muscle tone typically associated with complete or total LMN lesions when the lesion disrupts activation of the motor units of the particular muscle. LMN lesions can affect either the cell bodies located in the anterior

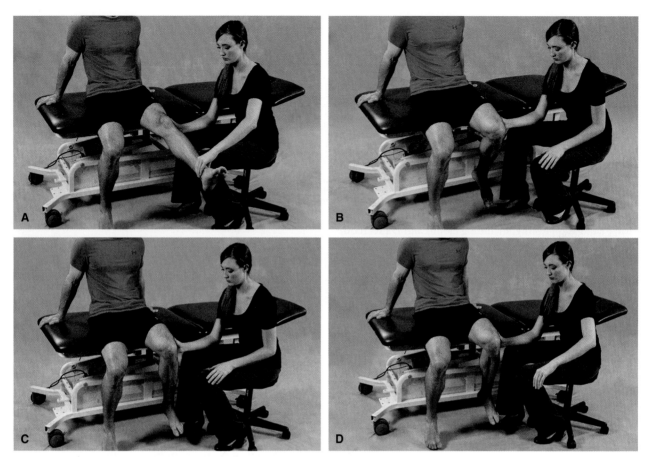

**FIGURE 6-11  A., B., C.,** and **D.** Lower Extremity Pendulum Test for muscle tone in the knee extensors. **A.** With the patient seated and extra room under the table for leg swing, the therapist releases the leg from a position of full knee extension. **B.** The leg passively swings down into knee flexion. **C.** Then the leg swings forward toward knee extension. **D.** The leg swings back into partial knee flexion and then alternates between extension and flexion movements with dampening of each cycle.

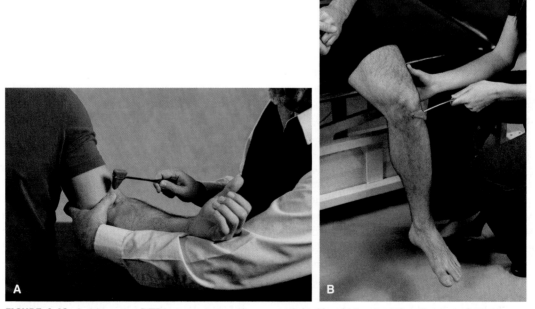

**FIGURE 6-12  A.** Measuring DTRs can sometimes be accomplished by placing your thumb over a discrete smaller tendon, then striking your thumb with the reflex hammer as illustrated in this photograph of elbow DTR testing of biceps. **B.** The patellar (quadriceps) muscle is also a common location for testing DTRs.

| TABLE 6-8 | Deep Tendon Reflex Assessment |
|---|---|
| **Biceps Tendon** (tendon lies in midline of anterior surface of arm superior to the cubital fossa) | With the patient sitting, support the patient's forearm with your forearm and position patient's elbow in less than 90-degree flexion. Palpate tendon with thumb and press thumb on tendon to add extra stretch. Then tap over your thumb and feel and observe for reaction. The reaction may vary from slight tension in tendon felt by thumb to visible movement of muscle belly or obvious elbow flexion movement. If there is difficulty in eliciting the DTR, the reaction can be heightened by increasing tension in lower extremities during test (e.g., crossing ankles with self-resistance between the lower extremities; modified lower extremity Jendrassik maneuver). |
| **Triceps Tendon** | With the patient sitting, support the humerus into abduction with internal rotation allowing the elbow to passively flex. The triceps tendon should be accessible above the tip of the olecranon; therefore, tap the tendon directly with the reflex hammer. Observe the reaction that may include no response, slight tricep muscle belly contraction, or visible elbow extension movement. |
| **Patellar Tendon** (tendon lies inferior to inferior border of the patella and superior to tibial tuberosity) | With the patient sitting with knee at 90 degrees, without foot contact to floor, palpate the tendon. Tap the tendon directly with a reflex hammer and observe for reaction that may vary from no reaction, to a slight quadriceps muscle belly contraction, to gross knee extension movement. |
| **Achilles Tendon** (tendon lies inferior to gastrocnemius/ soleus muscles and superior to calcaneous | With patient sitting, passively dorsiflex the patient's ankle slightly, palpate tendon in midline of posterior surface of the ankle, and tap it with the reflex hammer and observe for reaction. Reaction may vary from no response, to a slight contraction of the plantar flexor muscles, to gross plantar flexion movement of the ankle. |

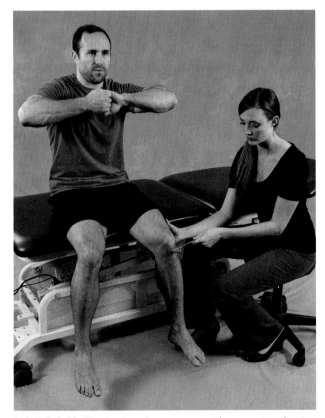

**FIGURE 6-13** The Jendrassik maneuver, with aggressive clasping of the hands with self-imposed resistance, can sometimes help to heighten a DTR that is decreased and difficult to observe.

horn of the spinal cord or peripheral motor fibers of peripheral nerves. Flaccidity may also occur temporarily early after UMN lesions of the cerebrum and brainstem such as **cerebral shock** following CVA with the flaccidity of the affected regions lasting for days to weeks (Campbell, 2005). Temporary flaccidity of affected muscle groups following traumatic SCI is called **spinal shock** and typically lasts for 24 hours, though it may last for up to 4 to 6 weeks. An absence of reflex activity, **areflexia**, is an expression of flaccidity. Flaccidity is associated with an absence of voluntary muscle activity, complete paralysis with no possibility of activation, as the affected motor neurons are unable to propagate an effective signal to the muscle or muscle group.

Hypotonia is the state in which resistance to passive elongation of the muscle is decreased below normal levels; in other words, it is easier than usual to move a joint through PROM. There is some resistance, but it is less than would be found normally. Hypotonia is most often found in a variety of genetic disorders (e.g., Down syndrome and Angelman syndrome), LMN injury in which only a portion of the motor units to a muscle are damaged (e.g., polio), neuromotor junction dysfunction (e.g., myasthenia gravis), and muscle disorders (e.g., muscular dystrophy). Hypotonia is also a common occurrence in disorders affecting the cerebellum when it is typically also accompanied by ataxia, which is discussed later in this chapter. Whereas flaccidity is associated with complete paralysis of the affected muscle group, hypotonia is most often associated with muscle weakness.

There are two common forms of hypertonicity or increased muscle tone: spastic and rigid. **Spasticity (spastic hypertonia)** associated with a UMN injury occurs as a result of damage to the pyramidal or extrapyramidal tracts. In spasticity, a key characteristic of the increased resistance to passive elongation is that the increased muscle tone is velocity dependent. Faster movements increase the resistance to stretch via an uninhibited or increased monosynaptic stretch reflex. In the milder grades of spasticity, you may not detect any increased muscle tone when moving the joint very slowly but notice an obvious increase when you move the limb more quickly. The increased excitability of the stretch reflex occurs from decreasing its threshold for activation or by diminished inhibitory control over spinal reflexes (Campbell, 2005) as damaged pyramidal tracts are unable to effectively inhibit reflexive muscle tone and normal stretch reflexes in lower-motor centers. Spasticity from cerebral lesions usually affects muscle groups on one particular side of the joint predominantly. In this case, the distribution most often includes the flexors of the upper extremities and the extensors of the lower extremities. Spasticity in an individual with SCI related to disruption of the corticospinal pathway may affect opposing muscle groups equally in the affected regions of the body. Spastic resistance decreases as tension increases in the affected muscle, such as when it is stretched at the end of its available ROM. The decrease in spastic resistance resulting from muscle elongation may be due to activity of the Golgi tendon organ (GTO), but more research is needed in this area (Nielsen, 2007). Long-term spasticity can minimize ability to move into the elongated range and can result in adaptive shortening of the spastic muscle group, which may cause permanent decreases in available ROM. The pattern of expected onset and progression of spasticity after stroke is described as one component of the Brunnstrom stages discussed later in the Motor Control Section (see Table 6-16).

Loss of joint ROM or flexibility due to spasticity differs from muscle tightness or inflexibility. The major difference is related to movement velocity. Another difference is what is felt at the beginning and end of the available ROM. During passive assessment of a spastic muscle, the clinician perceives velocity-dependent increased resistance. Resistance associated with muscle tightness or inflexibility, however, increases as the joint moves toward the end of the available range but is not velocity dependent and therefore increases even during very slow speeds of muscle elongation.

Once you have determined that there is a velocity-dependent increase in resistance to passive elongation, the **Modified Ashworth Scale (MAS)** is a scale specifically developed to rate the degree of spasticity (Bohannon, 1987; Lehmann, 1989; Mutlu, 2008; Price, 1991). Generally, the MAS grade (detail shown in Table 6-9) is determined based on the degree of resistance, what portion of the joint range exhibits the increased resistance, and how easily the resistance can be overcome. Recently, interrater reliability of Ashworth Scale and MAS has varied from moderate to good in a sample with spastic CP, and test-retest reliability ranged from poor

| TABLE 6-9 | Modified Ashworth Scale For Grading "Spasticity" |
|---|---|
| **GRADE** | **DESCRIPTION** |
| 0 | No increase in muscle tone (no spasticity). |
| 1 | Slight increase in muscle tone, manifested by a catch and release or by minimal resistance but only at the end of the ROM when the affected part(s) is moved in flexion or extension. |
| 1 + | Slight increase in muscle tone, manifested by a catch, followed by minimal resistance detected throughout the remainder (less than half) of the ROM. |
| 2 | More marked increase in muscle tone detected through most of the ROM but affected part(s) are easily moved. |
| 3 | Considerable increase in muscle tone, passive movement difficult. |
| 4 | Affected part(s) rigid in flexion and extension. |

Adapted from Bohannon RW, Smith MB. Interrater reliability of a modified Ashworth scale of muscle spasticity. *Phys Ther.* 1987;67(2): 206–207. Data from Table 1 found on p. 207.

to good (Mutlu, 2008). Limitations include lack of clear distinctions between ratings of "1" and "1 +" (Pandyan, 1999). Recommendations for more standardized methods have been presented due to reports that reliability is limited when applied to the lower extremities (Pandyan, 1999). The MAS for the adductors and the internal rotators of the hip has been found to be significantly less reliable for interrater reliability than other muscle groups (Nuyens, 1994).

The **Tardieu Scale,** originally described in 1954 (Tardieu, 1954) as a passive measure of spasticity and adapted as the Modified Tardieu Scale (Boyd, 1999) is administered by moving the client's limb passively through the available ROM and noting the precise point in range where resistance is first met or catches compared with the end of the available ROM (see Table 6-10). The Tardieu Scale has been suggested as a measure of spasticity (Ammann, 2005) with higher test-retest and interrater reliability than the MAS (Mehrholz, 2005). Specifically, you should passively stretch the muscle at three different speeds: (1) as slow as possible, (2) at the speed a limb falls under gravity, and (3) as fast as possible (greater than the speed of a limb falls under gravity) to elicit the stretch reflex. During each movement, use a goniometer to measure the point at which the muscle catch (resistance) first occurs and the end of the available range. The angle of catch of the high-velocity movement is subtracted from the angle of catch of the slowest possible movement to acquire a Tardieu spasticity angle, which indicates where the movement is influenced by the spasticity. Additionally, document the quality of the muscle reaction as the limb is moved.

| TABLE 6-10 | Modified Tardieu Scale For Grading "Spasticity" |
|---|---|
| **GRADE** | **DESCRIPTION** |
| Zero | No resistance throughout the course of the passive movement. |
| 1 | Slight resistance throughout the course of the passive movement, with no clear catch at precise angle. |
| 2 | Clear catch at precise angle, interrupting the passive movement, followed by release. |
| 3 | Fatigable clonus (<10 seconds when maintaining pressure occurring at precise angle). |
| 4 | Infatigable clonus (>10 seconds when maintaining pressure occurring at precise angle). |

From: Boyd RN, Graham HK. Objective measurement of clinical findings in the use of botulinum toxin type A for the management of children with cerebral palsy. *Eur J Neurol.* 1999;6(suppl. 4):S23–S35.

The Tardieu can be used to differentiate contractures from spasticity (Patrick, 2006), and a systematic review has concluded that the Tardieu, in some instances, may be a more accurate measure of spasticity than the Modified Ashworth Scale (Haugh, 2006).

The *Modified Tardieu Scale (MTS)* was introduced by adding standardized limb placement and alignment (e.g., supine as the starting position in the lower extremity) to the previous technique (Boyd, 2002; Boyd, 1999). The MTS is able to differentiate between neural limitations that are velocity dependent (spasticity) and passive stiffness (soft tissue limitations) while the Ashworth Scale cannot (Boyd, 2002; Damiano, 2002), and repeating measures can be used to detect change in spasticity related to medical management with botulinum toxin A in children with CP with good test-retest reliability (Boyd, 1998).

The *Triple Spasticity Scale* (TSS) (Li, 2014) was developed to consider the velocity-dependent nature of spasticity. It measures spasticity on the basis of tonic and phasic stretch reflexes, and evaluates passive resistance and dynamic muscle length. For the first item, perform a slow stretch "R2" (less than 5 degrees/sec) through full range and fast stretch "R1" (as fast as possible) of the target muscle and assess for increased resistance with the fast stretch (compared with a slow stretch) with 0 = no increased resistance, 1 = mild increase, 2 = moderate increase, 3 = severe increase, and 4 = extremely severe increase. For the second item, assess the degree of clonus: 0 = no clonus; 1 = fatigable, refers to a clonus less than 10s; and 2 = infatigable, refers to a clonus greater than 10s. And for the last item, assess dynamic muscle length (R1-R2) by noting the angle at which the increased resistance is detected for each speed and calculate the difference in the two angles, converting to this five-point scale: 0 = angle difference between R1 and R2 is 0, 1 = angle difference is <1/4 full ROM, 2 = angle difference is ≥1/4 and <1/2 full

ROM, 3 = angle difference is ≥1/2 and <3/4 full ROM, or 4 = angle difference is ≥ 3/4 full ROM. The authors suggested several scales for interpreting total scores: "mild (0 to 2), moderate (3 to 5), or severe spasticity (6 to 8) in the muscles in which clonus could not be elicited"; "mild (0 to 3), moderate (4 to 6), or severe spasticity (7 to 10) in the muscles in which clonus could be elicited" (Li, 2014). The measure has demonstrated good interrater and intrarater reliability (Li, 2014).

The *Myotonometer* (Neurogenic Technologies Inc., Missoula, MT) was developed to provide a quantitative assessment of muscle stiffness (Figure 6-14). Because muscle stiffness is thought to correlate with muscle tone, the Myotonometer has been validated as a reliable quantitative muscle tone assessment tool (see Muscle Tone Focus on Evidence Table online [ONL]) (Leonard, 2001; Leonard, 2003). It is unclear how muscle stiffness, a property inherent in the muscle itself (which presumably is not velocity dependent), correlates with abnormal muscle tone such as spasticity (which by definition is velocity dependent).

**Rigidity** or **rigid hypertonia**, a form of hypertonicity, is associated with several neurological disorders, particularly Parkinson disease. Clinical manifestations of rigidity, detected during the passive elongation testing procedure for muscle tone

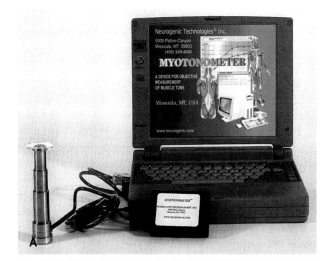

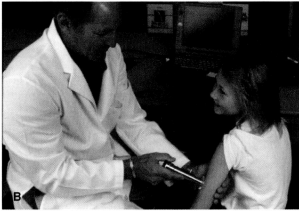

**FIGURE 6-14 A.** Myotonometer equipment. **B.** The myotonometer applied to a pediatric patient.

previously described, differ from spasticity in that muscle groups are commonly affected on both sides of the joint (opposing muscle groups, e.g., flexors and extensors, are both significantly affected), the resistance is present throughout the ROM, and it may be present even at slow speeds. In Parkinson disease, **cogwheel rigidity** is sometimes felt in which the increased muscle tone is characterized by multiple occasions of catch and release throughout the range along with rigidity and superimposed tremor. Some common types of rigidity are extrapyramidal, voluntary and involuntary, reflex, catatonic, and myotonic.

Table 6-11 contrasts the main differences between decorticate and decerebrate rigidity, actually forms of spasticity, illustrated in Figure 6-15. These postures are most often associated with very severe cerebral injury and decreased levels of consciousness, usually coma. The terms decorticate rigidity and decerebrate rigidity are misnomers, as they could be considered the most extreme forms of spasticity (see Modified Ashworth Scale, grade 4) with hypertonia predominant on one side of the joint that fixes the limb in the static posture described. On the Glasgow Coma Scale, decerebrate posturing (score 2 of the possible 5 points for the *Best Motor Response* item) is considered more severe than decorticate posturing (score 3 of the possible 5 points for the Best Motor Response item). The only lower Glasgow *Best Motor Response* score is "No Motor Response," which gets a score of 1 out of the 5 possible *Motor* points. The following special tests may be useful for rigidity assessment: the Shoulder-Shaking Test, Head-Dropping Test, and the Lower Extremity Pendulum Test (Campbell, 2005).

In clinical and research settings, rigidity is often measured using the five rigidity items of the **Unified Parkinson's Disease Rating Scale (UPDRS)** Motor Examination section (Fahn, 1987). A five-point scale score is assigned (0 to 4) with descriptors of rigidity ranging from absent to affecting five regions of the body. See Table 6-12 for a detailed UPDRS rating scale. The UPDRS motor examination section demonstrates satisfactory interrater reliability (Martinez-Martin, 1994; Richards, 1994) with high internal consistency and high correlation with Hoehn and Yahr stages (Martinez-Martin, 1994).

Perform the *Shoulder-Shaking Test* by facing the standing patient, and place your hands on the patient's shoulders.

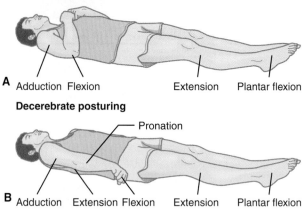

FIGURE 6-15 Characteristic posturing of **A.** decorticate and **B.** decerebrate rigidity.

| TABLE 6-12 | Qualifiers for Rating Rigidity Using the UPDRS Motor Examination |
|---|---|
| **SCORE** | **DESCRIPTION** |
| Zero | Rigidity is absent. |
| 1 | Slight rigidity or only with muscle activation. |
| 2 | Mild/moderate rigidity. |
| 3 | Marked rigidity, full ROM. |
| 4 | Severe rigidity for five regions (neck, right upper extremity, left upper extremity, right lower extremity, and left lower extremity). |

(Fahn, 1987)

Move the shoulders alternately back and forth to rotate the trunk with varying speed and force. This will result in passive swinging of the patient's arms, which may be diminished in one arm in unilateral Parkinson. Rigidity results in diminished range of movement in the affected body segments (Campbell, 2005). Starting at a speed that causes equal pendulous movements on each side, gradually and slowly reduce the force and range of the trunk movements. As the pendulous movements decrease, you may reach a point where only

| TABLE 6-11 | Decerebrate Rigidity versus Decorticate Rigidity | |
|---|---|---|
| **TYPE** | **CAUSE** | **MANIFESTATION** |
| Decerebrate Rigidity | Occurs from disruption of excitatory input to medullary reticular nuclei causing disinhibition and overactivity of pontine reticular nuclei. | Spasticity of the antigravity (extensor) muscles of the entire body: static, fixed posturing as extension of upper extremity and lower extremity (*equates to 2 points for Best Motor Response on Glasgow Coma Scale*). |
| Decorticate Rigidity | Occurs from disruption of influence from the cerebral cortex without disruption of the red nucleus or basal ganglia. | Spasticity of the flexor muscles of the upper extremity (static flexion posturing) and the extensors of the lower extremity (static extension posturing) (*equates to 3 points for Best Motor Response on Glasgow Coma Scale*). |

one arm swings. The arm with decreased swing is the one with the greater rigidity.

The *Head-Dropping Test* occurs in supine with the patient's eyes closed. There should not be a pillow between the patient's head and the plinth. Place a hand on the plinth under the patient's occiput while the other hand raises the head off the plinth. Complete the test by dropping the head into the hand under the occiput (Figure 6-16). Rigidity causes the head to lower more slowly into the awaiting

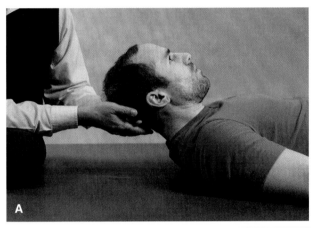

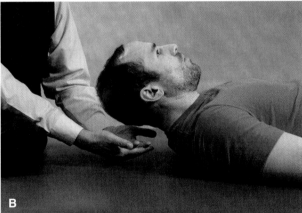

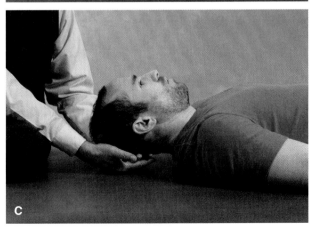

**FIGURE 6-16** Head-Dropping Test: A photo series showing **A.** the patient's head supported by the therapist's hand while the other hand waits below nearer the mat surface, **B.** sudden release of the supporting hand, and **C.** the patient's head drops gently into the therapist's lower hand.

examiner's hand whereas without rigidity the head falls more rapidly (Campbell, 2005).

## THINK ABOUT IT 6.2

- What key information are you going to be looking for during your examination to accurately identify impaired tone in your patient?
- How will you differentiate the various types of hypertonicity (spasticity, rigidity, dystonia)?
- How can you distinguish muscle stiffness or adaptive shortening of muscle from decreased movement associated with hypertonicity? What would be observed for each condition during a test like the Modified Ashworth Scale?
- How could changes in muscle tone affect your patient's functional abilities? Include some ways it could limit or assist during functional tasks in specific circumstances.
- How are you going to objectively document and track changes in tone?

## Muscle Fatigue

**Muscle fatigue,** a decline in muscle performance resulting from prolonged or sustained use of the target muscle group, may or may not in general occur during or after physical exertion. **Muscle endurance,** on the other hand, is the capacity of a muscle to sustain work and resist fatigue-related decrements of muscle performance. Fatigue associated with exertion may occur secondary to local muscle metabolism (e.g., with hydrogen ion accumulation, adenosine triphosphate depletion, and glycogen depletion). Other possible causative factors include central mechanisms or other clinical sequela affecting the individual as a whole. Overall, there are relatively few investigations concerning fatigue, and it is poorly understood compared with other physiological events (Tiesinga, 1998) especially in a population with neuromuscular disorders. For the purposes of this chapter, exertional fatigue relates to fatigue associated with physical activity whereas clinical fatigue relates to that occurring without physical exertion (Meesters, 1996; Tiesinga, 1998). The discussion will focus on local muscle fatigue primarily. However, a few standardized tests that quantify clinical as well as local muscle fatigue will be discussed.

Muscle fatigue is associated with decay of force production over time during repeated activation (Figure 6-17) such as performing a repetitive motor task. Muscles with poor endurance fatigue easily resulting in pronounced force diminution during a given activity. Muscles exposed to periods of inactivity succumb to increased fatigability due to the loss of mitochondria and aerobic enzymes in the muscle (Kasper, 1993). These changes are only part of the sequela associated with morphological changes in muscle fiber characteristics that cause them to behave more like fast-twitch muscle fibers (fast-twitch muscle fibers fatigue more readily than slow-twitch fibers).

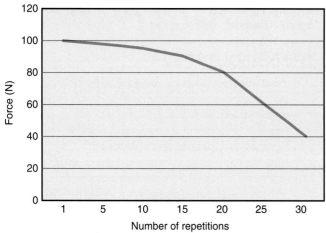

**FIGURE 6-17** Force production curve as affected by muscle fatigue during a hypothetical set of resistance exercise.

## Procedures for Measuring Muscle Fatigue

Fatigue can be assessed in a manner similar to strength assessment using isotonic or isokinetic equipment. Because the resistance is fixed with isotonic exercise, the number of repetitions that the patient can perform during an exercise set is an easily measured factor reflecting muscle endurance. The same principle applies to movements that use body weight as the resistance. Count the number of times the patient can perform the activity to quantify endurance. The number attained during the activity is recorded for future comparison. For example, a person might be able to initially perform one repetition of sit-to-stand transfer, but by the time of discharge the same person may be able to complete a series of six repetitions of sit-to-stand (Jones, 1999).

Isokinetic assessments can measure muscle fatigability using computed statistics such as total work and work fatigue. Total work is a quantification of the amount of work completed from each repetition during a set of exercise (force × distance = work). Total work portrays muscle endurance because the distance is fixed within the ROM specified during machine set up. Therefore, force production is the only variable in the equation for work because force production decreases with increased fatigue. Muscles with poor endurance will fatigue more quickly in the exercise set, which causes them to produce less force later in the set. The total work produced over the entire set would be relatively less for a muscle or muscle group with poor endurance. The work fatigue statistic can be calculated by dividing (the difference between the amount of work performed during the first and last one-thirds of the exercise set) by the amount of work performed during the first one-third of the exercise set and then multiplied by 100. This is usually calculated with isokinetic reports and provides a better indication of fatigue because it specifically captures decreases in force production that occur over the set of exercise.

An isokinetic calculation of fatigue is the determination of the specific repetition where torque diminishes by 50% (O'Sullivan, 2014). However, this method is sometimes challenging during a set of exercise because force may oscillate above and below 50% of peak torque during the bout.

Standardized tests have been developed to assess clinical fatigue and its effect upon physical functioning. The *Maastricht Interview Exhaustion (MIVE)* is a 23-item test assessing unusual fatigue and loss of energy not associated with physical exertion (Meesters, 1996). This type of fatigue is defined as "vital exhaustion," which includes irritability and feelings of demoralization (Meesters, 1996). Other valid assessments of fatigue are the *Dutch Fatigue Scale (DUFS)* and the *Dutch Exertion Fatigue Scale (DEFS)*, which assess clinical fatigue and fatigue associated with physical exertion, respectively, with particular relevance to its effect upon activities of daily living (Tiesinga, 1998). The DUFS and the DEFS include a questionnaire assessing 62 activities ranging from household activities, body care activities, and social activities. Another test, the *Fatigue Severity Scale (FSS)*, was validated in patients with multiple sclerosis (MS), systemic lupus erythematosus (SLE), and stroke (Krupp, 1989; Naess, 2005; Schepers, 2006; Tang, 2010). The FSS consists of nine questionnaire items that rank answers on a seven-point scale from one (strongly disagree) to seven (strongly agree). The Fatigue Impact Scale was also modified for use in individuals with MS (Fisk, 1994). Items of the original Fatigue Severity Scale (FSS) are described in Box 6-7 (Krupp, 1989, p. 1122).

## Muscle Activation

A specialized examination procedure to assess muscle activation requires **electromyography (EMG)** equipment. EMG instruments can be used to assess the electrical activity of a given muscle or muscle group during voluntary activation or at rest. EMG may be used as a tool to assess voluntary motor control (Wong, 2000). Drawbacks to clinical usage are the cost of EMG equipment, the expertise required to perform EMG assessments, and the time requirements for administration and data analysis. Thus, EMG assessments are not generally advocated for routine neurological examinations, but provide specific diagnostics in more complicated neuromuscular clinical cases such as neuropathies and myopathies.

Procedures for EMG assessment vary according to the type of equipment used for the analysis. A variety of equipment models measure muscle activity using a single channel that

---

**BOX 6-7  Original Items on the Fatigue Severity Scale (Krupp, 1989, p. 1122)**

1. My motivation is lower when I am fatigued.
2. Exercise brings on my fatigue.
3. I am easily fatigued.
4. Fatigue interferes with my physical functioning.
5. Fatigue causes frequent problems for me.
6. My fatigue prevents sustained physical functioning.
7. Fatigue interferes with carrying out certain responsibilities.
8. Fatigue is among my three most disabling symptoms.
9. Fatigue interferes with my work, family, or social life.

measures electrical activity at one location or multiple channels that measure electrical activity in several locations. Furthermore, EMG analysis may be performed with indwelling fine-needle electrodes or surface electrodes. The specific procedure for EMG testing is described in Chapter 12.

## ■ Measuring Motor Function

### Motor Control

Muscle strength alone does not fully define proper motor function as force gradation and the timing of activation often determine whether a muscle interacts appropriately with other muscles or muscle groups during functional activities (Shumway-Cook, 2012). **Motor control** is the process by which the brain organizes and regulates action of the muscular and skeletal systems, including movement and dynamic postural adjustments of a joint or body segment. An earlier definition provided by Shumway-Cook (2001) emphasized "the study of the nature and cause of movement, including stabilizing the body in space and moving the body in space." Therefore, motor control (1) is sometimes needed to *move* a joint or body segment with quality while other times (2) it is needed to *stabilize* a joint or body segment. This section of the chapter will discuss details for observation and measurement of both motor control for movement, which includes motor coordination in movement, and motor control for stability. Motor control takes place through volitional activation and relaxation of functional muscle groups that either move or stabilize certain joints during functional activities. Essentially, motor control is the ability of the nervous system to regulate the motor system with appropriate activation or relaxation during all normal functional activities. Motor control occurs from the collective influences of cognition or volition, cerebral motor plans (sometimes subconscious), available ROM, muscle strength, muscle tone, environmental conditions, and task characteristics that influence quality of movement including velocity, timing, and accuracy. The degree of motor control ultimately affects balance and each movement of every functional activity.

Part of the difficulty with this discussion is that there is no consensus or consistency in terminology used in publications regarding motor control. Most often, studies only label or discuss the specific control problems observed without categorizing them as movement or stability problems. The concept of motor control stability is particularly neglected in the literature. Hence, it is very important to define the terms that are used. Using the construct of the Shumway-Cook (2001) definition previous discussed, throughout this chapter and in the intervention chapters the terms *motor control for movement (MC-movement)* and *motor control for stability (MC-stability)* are used as defined in the following section. In exploring these definitions, it is important to recognize that motor control is independent and distinct from muscle tone despite frequent clinical usage of the terms as somewhat synonymous or related. It is true that deficits in motor control and muscle tone are often associated with each other, particularly in

UMN lesions. An individual who has spasticity, for example, may or may not demonstrate deficits in motor control movement. Of necessity, for any muscle group being examined, the therapist must test separately for muscle tone (a passive examination on the patient's part) and motor control (an active measure on the patient's part). Also realize that the term postural control is not synonymous with motor control. The term postural control is most often used to refer to balance or equilibrium in maintaining an upright posture as discussed in Chapter 9. It is also essential to understand that the biomechanical joint stability inherent in normal ligaments and joint capsules is also distinct from the dynamic neuromotor joint stability that results from motor control stability.

### Motor Control for Movement

**Motor control for movement (MC-movement)** can also be called **movement control** and specifically encompasses all aspects of motor control related to muscles as they create movement. The characteristics of MC-movement are summarized in the MC-movement column of Table 6-13. The therapist can observe MC-movement by looking for several specific characteristics of movement during a voluntary task, an isolated movement, or a complex multijoint movement. To test for MC-movement, ask the person to volitionally move the joint or body segment being tested and observe the quality of the movement. Perhaps most importantly, MC-movement is expressed as the person is able to perform an **isolated movement**, voluntarily activating only the intended specific muscle groups without any extraneous or unintended movement at related joints. Isolated movement has also been termed **selective motor control** (Boyd, 1999; Voorman, 2007). A controlled movement will also be *smooth,* steady, and flowing continuously without disruptions, jerks, spurts, or starts throughout the entire range of active motion as the motor units of the involved muscle fire in a precise and accurate sequence and magnitude. The smooth control includes accurate regulation of both purposeful active *initiation* of movement, from careful and timely "grading-on" of muscle units, and volitional *cessation* of a movement, from a gradual "grading-off" of the involved motor units as the joint or segment nears the end of the movement. This controlled initiation and cessation of movement allows the start and end of the motion to be gradual in timing and smooth at beginning and end. The individual will also be able to *fractionate* movement as a sign of good MC-movement. **Fractionation** is the ability of the individual, through motor control, to move the target joint through very small fragments of the available range, as small as 1 or 2 degrees, even with large gross muscle groups (by activating a small fraction of the total motor units of a muscle or group). The individual with normal MC-movement has the ability to voluntarily move the joint or segment at a *variety of velocities,* moving slowly when desired, but moving quickly when necessary. When no deficit is present, the smooth appearance of the movement, and the ability to isolate muscle action, remain intact regardless of the speed.

After cerebral injuries such as CVA and traumatic brain injury, abnormal MC-movement is often observed as the lack of

| TABLE 6-13 | Observable Characteristics of Three Aspects of Motor Control | | |
|---|---|---|---|
| | **RELATED TO MOVEMENT** | | **RELATED TO STABILITY** |
| | *MC-Movement* | *Motor Coordination* | *MC-Stability* |
| General Description of Components | **Isolated Control/Selective Motor Control:** Ability to activate and regulate *similarly acting* target muscles for *movement* at a single joint without unintended movement of other muscle groups. <br> **Timing and Sequence:** Ability to activate muscles with appropriate sequencing (coordination between muscles at multiple joints that are cooperating to complete a complex movement) and timing within the activity/task, and capability to perform movement at a variety of speeds. <br> **Initiation and Cessation:** Ability to start (initiate) and stop (cease) a particular muscle action, including grading on and grading off of muscle action. | Coordination between *opposing* muscle groups at a joint during *movement* (one grading on while the opposing group is appropriately grading off). | Cocontraction of *opposing* muscle groups when a joint or segment is *steady and unwavering* and should not move. |
| Common Abnormal Expressions | **Isolated Movement:** Abnormal movement synergies (lack of isolated movements) <br> **Timing and Sequence:** Bradykinesia <br> **Impaired initiation or cessation** | Ataxia (incoordination). | Joint instability or segment instability, particularly during closed-chain or weight-bearing actions. |

isolated voluntary movement even though the limb can often move with poor control. This inability to isolate movement at a joint is commonly called an **abnormal synergy** of movement, observed as the patient attempts to move a limb in a discrete or specific way, but instead can only move in abnormal unintended combinations of muscle groups at multiple joints. Although the person can move, the movement lacks accuracy and efficiency and therefore contributes minimally to the individual's functional ability and activity. For example, after a stroke, a person who cannot flex his right elbow in isolation may instead flex the elbow only in abnormal combination with wrist flexion, forearm supination, and shoulder adduction and internal rotation as an abnormal mass synergy. Another individual may be able to extend the elbow but only in combination with scapular elevation and shoulder abduction. The most common synergies observed during voluntary movement, illustrated in Figure 6-18 and described in Table 6-14, include flexor synergy of the upper extremity (Figure 6-18A) and extensor synergy of the lower extremity (Figure 6-18B). Less common is the upper extremity extension synergy that may occur upon voluntary shoulder elevation (Figure 6-18C). However, observation for the specific abnormal combinations of muscle activation in an individual is important.

As individuals recover from UMN lesions, particularly stroke, clinical manifestations typically emerge in stages that can be observed during examination (Brunnstrom, 1966). In 1966, Brunnstrom (1966) first described six stages of recovery following CVA and included a description of characteristic

motor control at each stage with specific observations defined separately for upper and lower extremities (see Table 6-15). Often, the patient initially exhibits flaccidity with complete absence of volitional movement (Stage 1), then progresses to weak abnormal synergies with small range movement (Stage 2), and then stronger, more obvious abnormal synergies (Stage 3). Volitional movement is first observed in Stage 4, especially in proximal muscle groups (see specifics in Table 6-22, Stage 4). In Stages 5 and 6, active movements become progressively more complex with an increased number of isolated/selective movements outside of synergy. Progressive changes in muscle tone were also described across the six stages (see Table 6-16) with progressive development and increase of spasticity in Stages 1 to 3 with a gradual diminution of spasticity from Stage 4 to 6 (Brunnstrom, 1966).

An assessment measure for determining normal voluntary motor control of the lower extremities for patients with CP is the Selective Control Assessment of the Lower Extremity (SCALE) (Fowler, 2009). The SCALE, described in the "Tests/Measures for Motor Control-Movement" section below has good content and construct validity and interrater reliability ranged from 0.88 to 0.91.

## Motor Control for Stability

**Motor control for stability (MC-stability)** can be defined as the ability of the brain to regulate muscles to precisely keep joints or body segments from moving at times when they should not move (see MC-stability column of Table 6-13).

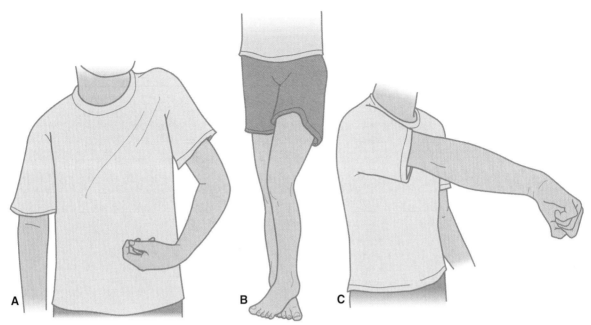

**FIGURE 6-18** Examples of the most common abnormal synergies of upper extremity and lower extremity. **A.** Upper extremity flexion synergy (left arm in this patient) commonly happens during intended flexion or antigravity movements of the upper extremity. **B.** Lower extremity extension synergy (left leg in this patient) commonly happens during intended extension of the lower extremity, for example, during the terminal portion of swing phase. **C.** Upper extremity extension synergy (right arm in this patient) that may occur during intended elevation of the arm as opposed to intended flexion of the arm.

| TABLE 6-14 | Typical Abnormal Synergies for Lower Extremity (LE) and Upper Extremity (UE) |
|---|---|
| **Typical Flexor Abnormal Synergy of UE Movement:**<br>Scapula: Elevation and retraction<br>Shoulder: Abduction and external rotation or adduction and internal rotation<br>Elbow: Flexion<br>Forearm: Supination<br>Wrist/Digits: Position varies, but usually flexion | **Typical Extensor Abnormal Synergy of LE Movement:**<br>Pelvic: Elevation and retraction<br>Hip: Adduction and extension<br>Knee: Extension<br>Ankle: Plantar flexion<br>Forefoot: Usually inversion |
| **Typical Extensor Abnormal Synergy of UE Movement:**<br>Scapula: Downward rotation and protraction<br>Shoulder: Internal rotation and adduction<br>Elbow: Extension<br>Forearm: Pronation<br>Wrist/Hand/Digits: Position varies | **Typical Flexion Abnormal Synergy of LE Movement:**<br>Pelvic: Elevation<br>Hip: Flexion<br>Knee: Flexion<br>Ankle: Dorsiflexion<br>Forefoot: Usually eversion |

This action of the brain, working through the muscles, is very different from the stability that the ligaments or skeleton provide. Motor control stabilization is often required in closed-chain activities or weight-bearing phases of tasks and most often occurs through **cocontraction** or simultaneous contraction of opposing muscle groups so the joint will not move in either direction. MC-stability, particularly examination, is a neglected concept in the evidence-based literature. Deficits of neuromotor stability following neurological conditions, such as those summarized in Table 6-16, are readily recognized and acknowledged by clinicians and in research, but there is a lack of common terminology and categorization. Most of the

research focus in motor control has been on examination and intervention of the movement aspects of motor control. It might be helpful to examine some of the most commonly observed impairments of MC-stability in specific joints. Table 6-16 provides a summary table of the most common examples of impaired MC-stability, organized by body regions, which can result from specific neurological pathologies. These problems each occur as a result of the brain's inability to cause precise activation of specific muscles, precise grading of the muscle contraction, and precise combinations of muscles as they act together. Hopefully, the examples in Table 6-16 will aid in grasping this challenging concept. In

| TABLE 6-15 | **Brunnstrom Stages of Recovery Following Stroke for the Upper and Lower Extremities** | | | |
|---|---|---|---|---|
| **BRUNNSTROM STAGE** | **TONE** | **MOTOR CONTROL** | **SPECIFIC UE ISOLATED/ SELECTIVE MOVEMENTS ON AFFECTED SIDE** | **SPECIFIC LE ISOLATED/ SELECTIVE MOVEMENTS ON AFFECTED SIDE** |
| Stage 1 • Flaccid Tone • No Movement | Flaccid; little or no resistance to passive movement | No active movement | None | None |
| Stage 2 • Increasing Spasticity • Weak Synergies | Slight spasticity | Weak synergies and weak associated reactions | None | None |
| Stage 3 • Peak of Spasticity • Basic Synergies | Spasticity, may be severe | Voluntary movement within basic synergies; demonstrates small but determinable joint movement | None | None |
| Stage 4 • Spasticity Decreasing • Earliest Isolated Motor Control | Spasticity begins to decrease | Active movement begins to occur outside of basic limb synergies | (1) Hand to sacral region (involves difficult combination of internal rotation, extension and adduction of the arm) (2) Elevation of arm to forward-horizontal position with elbow fully extended (3) Pronation/supination with elbow flexed to 90 degrees | (1) Knee flexion beyond 90° sliding foot backward on floor (2) Dorsiflexion of ankle without lifting entire foot off floor |
| Stage 5 • Spasticity Decreasing • More Isolated Motor Control | Spasticity continues to decrease | Able to perform more difficult movement combinations | (1) Shoulder abduction to 90° with elbow extended (2) Shoulder flexion past 90° with elbow extended (3) Pronation/supination with elbow extended | (1) Knee flexion with hip extension in standing (2) Ankle dorsiflexion in standing with foot in position of short step |
| Stage 6 • No Spasticity • Selective Motor Control | No spasticity with passive movement but tone may increase during faster movement velocities | Movements are generally selective, but may require performance at decreased velocities with diminished coordination | Generally selective with decreased speed and decreased coordination | (1) Hip abduction beyond pelvic elevation in standing (2) Isolated knee internal and external rotation with ankle inversion and eversion |

*Patients may progress through all stages or remain/arrest in any one stage. The extent of each manifestation and the duration of the various stages are dependent on the severity of the stroke and the age of the patient.
(Adapted from Brunnstrom, 1966)

each case, the brain is trying to regulate the musculoskeletal system to keep movement from occurring at the joint/segment for a specific purpose. The composite effect of decreased MC-stability of the hip, knee, and ankle on the affected side following a stroke will be obvious in gait as the decreased stability will result in obvious asymmetry with decreased weight-bearing on the affected side. This movement dysfunction is a result of the person being unable to trust the affected limb for weight-support. Therefore, a decreased single-support phase on the affected side and a decreased step time and step length on the unaffected side can easily be measured and documented as discussed in Chapter 10, and both directly relate, in this example, to the impaired MC-stability.

Performing a task may require MC-stability and MC-movement in different body regions depending on the context of the task. Observing John as he writes his signature provides us with an illustration of this variation. When John signs his regular signature on a piece of paper using small letters, the

| TABLE 6-16 | Common Examples of Impaired MC-Stability |
|---|---|

**Scapulothoracic Instability:**
- Following stroke, TBI, or CP (and others), scapular winging may occur because of an inability to control scapular positioning on the trunk related to decreased motor control in serratus anterior.

**Glenohumeral Instability:**
- In the UE, glenohumeral instability can result in shoulder subluxation (and subsequent pain syndromes related to the musculoskeletal consequences of prolonged subluxation), accentuated by gravity in sitting and upright positions.

**Elbow Instability:**
- Inability to stabilize the elbow in extension will severely limit UE weight-bearing through an extended arm and the ability to push with the arms.

**Wrist Instability:**
- Impaired MC-stability in the wrist/hand complex can impair grasp.

**Trunk Instability:**
- Lack of stability in intraspinal segments and abdominal muscles can result in an abnormal posture or alignment of the trunk; can also result in the trunk being an insufficient base from which the upper extremities and lower extremities can move.

**Lumbopelvic Instability:**
- Inability to stabilize the pelvis on the trunk can result in problems with maintaining stability of the pelvis (and a level position) from which lower extremity swing phase operates.

**Hip Instability:**
- If the femoral head does not stabilize against the pelvic acetabulum, the hip can go into sudden flexion or extension, or even more commonly, during weight-bearing, a Trendelenberg gait can occur during stance phase on the affected side, as the opposite side of the pelvis drops because of insufficient control from the hip abductors.

**Knee Instability:**
- Instability of the knee during the stance phase of gait can result in either genu recurvatum (sudden snapping of the knee into hyperextension during the stance phase of gait), locked knee extension in midstance as a biomechanical mechanism to provide stability in absence of control, or an unstable knee that buckles in midstance full weight-bearing.

**Ankle Instability:**
- Instability in the sagittal plane allows plantar flexion to occur during swing (any amount of plantar flexion is too much during the swing phase of gait) with foot drop or toe-drag; subtalar instability results in a medial/lateral wobble of the ankle during weight acceptance or midstance phases of gait.

shoulder and possibly also the elbow require MC-stability, whereas MC-movement is employed in the wrist and intrinsic hand muscles. However, if John signs his signature on a marker board using large letters, he must stabilize his grasp of the pen using wrist and intrinsic hand muscles for MC-stability while the shoulder and wrist muscles provide the MC-movement necessary for the skilled movement of the pen. Regardless of the size of the intended task, the outcome is similar in proportion and shape but scaled differently as appropriate for the ultimate size.

It is also essential to understand that, for any particular joint in a functional activity, there is always a dynamic interchange and interplay between the two roles of movement and stability. There are times when, for optimal function, the body needs to keep a joint or body segment from moving to accomplish a task, particularly in weight-bearing components, and there are other times when the same limb or joint needs to move with skill and precision. Depending on the task, the muscles at a particular joint may have to switch or alternate between the two forms of motor control. The gait cycle is a perfect example of body segments and specific joints that cyclically alternate between motor control stability (required in the joints of the weight-bearing stance-phase leg) and motor control movement (necessary for the precise movement of the swing phase leg). Another interesting combination can be seen in the swing phase as the trunk and pelvis must simultaneously maintain motor control stability with the motor control movement of the hip, knee, and ankle to allow the step to take place with skill and precision. The same concept applies to an upper extremity reach task as the trunk and proximal upper extremity must maintain MC-stability while the more distal joints of the arm fluidly carry out MC-movement. So in any functional activity, therapists must understand and observe which joints need to have MC-stability and which need to have MC-movement and whether some body segments require MC-stability part of the time and MC-movement part of the time throughout the activity.

### Motor Coordination

**Motor coordination** (MC-coordination) is a specific subset of MC-movement that specifically focuses on the motor control interactions and cooperation between opposing muscle groups during a movement. This control of movement requires neuromuscular coordination between agonists and antagonistic muscle groups, which requires complex regulatory interaction of the

CNS. As the agonist muscle group contracts and shortens from motor units grading-on, the opposing or antagonist group must relax by appropriately grading-off. Coordinated movements are controlled, smooth, and precise because of the cooperation between opposing muscle groups, largely mediated through action of the cerebellum. Coordination assessments may entail equilibrium and nonequilibrium examinations (Schmitz, 2014). The following paragraphs describe nonequilibrium coordination examinations, whereas equilibrium tests and measures are discussed in Chapter 9. Impairment of coordination is called **incoordination** or **ataxia** and can be observed as the following specific signs (each term is defined in Table 6-17): (1) **intention tremor,** (2) **dysmetria**, (3) **astasia**, (4) **dysdiadochokinesia**, (5) **dysynergia**, (6) **decomposition**, and (7) **overcompensation**. Note that all these specific signs occur during intended active movement and not when the limb is at rest.

Regarding motor control and motor function in general, tests and measures of motor control assess movement function by examining the collective interaction of the previously mentioned factors that affect movement. Numerous standardized tests exist to examine motor control, particularly MC-movement, and other aspects of motor function. They are discussed in the "Standardized Motor Examination Tools" section later in this chapter.

### Tests/Measures for Motor Control-Movement

To perform a motor control movement examination, one approach is to simply ask the patient to actively move the limb and carefully observe, one joint/muscle action at a time, for smoothness, initiation, cessation, fractionation, performance at a variety of speeds, and the ability to isolate movement at

the specific joint being tested. Then record your observations, including the specific abnormal muscle group combination the patient demonstrates. Because selective motor control, if limited, is most likely to be seen in the earliest parts of the range (when the muscle is on optimal stretch), Fell has conceived a method to quantify the extent of isolated MC-movement and track improvement over time: by measuring the portion of available joint range through which the individual can actively perform an isolated movement. You should stop the movement for angle measurement at the first observed sign of an abnormal synergy combination. It might also be helpful to document the position in the available range at which the isolated movement can be initiated, which will most often be at the end of range. As the individual's MC-movement improves during the period of stroke recovery and rehabilitation, the quantity of controlled isolated movements (measured as degrees of available range through which selective control is observed) will increase. It is also possible that, in the near-future, smartphone technology, through accelerometers and 2-D video capture, will be able to help document these improvements more objectively. Several standardized methods for examination of MC-movement have been described to specifically measure MC-movement. Recent evidence regarding tests and measures for motor control movement are summarized in Table 6-28 online (ONL), Focus on Evidence Table for Examination of Motor Control Movement.

### Finger Extension/Grasp Release

Grasp and release are essential components of hand function. While maintaining grasp is an example of MC-stability, release of grasp is an example of MC-movement. *Active release*

| TABLE 6-17 | Coordination Examination: Abnormal Signs of Ataxia/Incoordination |
|---|---|
| **ATAXIC SIGN** | **DEFINITION** |
| Ataxia/Incoordination | An umbrella term including all aspects of incoordination listed here. Abnormally inaccurate or uncoordinated volitional movement of skeletal muscle. |
| Intention Tremor | A specific component of ataxia: tremor occurs during voluntary (intended) movement, often in a back-and-forth direction in the plane of intended movement. |
| Dysmetria | A specific component of ataxia: the inability to judge the distance to a target during movement; results in either stopping short of the target or pass-pointing; inability to correctly position limbs relative to one another. |
| Hypermetria (pass-pointing) | A specific component of ataxia: reaching past, or overshooting, the intended target. |
| Astasia | A specific component of ataxia: an inability to maintain standing that results from incoordination during weight-bearing. |
| Dysdiadochokinesia | A specific component of ataxia: decreased ability to perform a rapidly alternating movement (e.g., forearm pronation/supination; wrist flexion/extension; ankle dorsiflexion/plantar flexion). |
| Adiadochokinesia | A specific component of ataxia: inability to perform rapidly alternating movements. |
| Dysynergia | A specific component of ataxia: the incoordination of antagonist muscle groups. |
| Decomposition | A specific component of ataxia: a movement is abnormally broken down into its component parts instead of a smooth, fluid, multijoint movement. |
| Overcompensation | A specific component of ataxia: in attempting to correct a dysmetric, ataxic error (over- or undershooting), the individual overcorrects and again passes the target. |

*of grasp* is one of the items in the Upper Extremity Motor Score section of the *Fugl-Meyer Assessment* (Fugl-Meyer, 1975) discussed later in the chapter. After stroke, individuals often have difficulty releasing an object because of limited ability to initiate isolation of finger extension movement. Finger extension/grasp release, defined as the ability to actively release a mass flexion grasp as specified by the Fugl-Meyer item, is a significant predictor of motor recovery (as measured by the Wolf Motor Function Test) (Fritz, 2005).

## The Trost Selective Motor Control Test

The *Trost Selective Motor Control examination* method (Trost, 2009) is a basic general assessment system to document isolated movement ability for a specific muscle group, generally using an absent/impaired/normal rating system. Definitions for the three grades include: 0 = "no ability to isolate movement," 1 = "partially isolated movement," and 3 = "complete isolation of movement." It does not specify a specific joint or motion and can therefore be applied at any joint/segment. A modified version of the scale with additional qualifiers, including whether the isolated movement occurs through only the early part of the range or through the entire range of movement, has been described (Voorman, 2007) with the following scale:
"0 (no selective, only synergistic movement),
1 (diminished selective movement [the first range of movement selective and later on, during the movement, no selective movement]), and
2 (full selective movement during extension of the knee and dorsiflexion of the ankle)."

In a sample of children with CP, impairment of selective motor control was found to be the most important factor in predicting a "less favorable course" of gross motor function over time (Voorman, 2007). Interrater reliability is good for the modified Trost Selective Motor Control Test (Smits, 2010).

## The Boyd and Graham Selective Motor Control Test

The *Boyd and Graham Selective Motor Control Test* (Boyd, 1999) is an attempt to define better ways to describe or quantify the extent of joint MC-movement or selective motor control. The test uses a five-point scale (0 to 4) related to active isolated MC-movement specifically of ankle dorsiflexion and how much muscle substitution occurs. Because isolated ankle dorsiflexion is accomplished by the tibialis anterior muscle, the scale assigns lower ratings if the ankle movement is accomplished primarily by involvement from extensor hallucis longus (Figure 6-19) or extensor digitorum longus while higher ratings are used when these muscle groups are not utilized. Have the person short-sit on a flat surface with hips flexed and knees comfortably extended. Ask the individual to dorsiflex to a target over the foot, one foot at a time, and observe and document overall muscle activity. A grade of 0 is assigned for "No movement when asked to dorsiflex the foot"; grade of 1 for "Limited dorsiflexion using mainly Ext Hall Longus (EHL) and/or Ext Digitorum Longus (EDL)"; grade of 2 for "Dorsiflexion using EHL, EDL, and some Tibialis Anterior (TA)"; grade

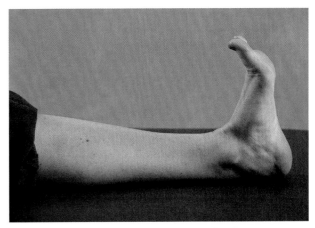

**FIGURE 6-19** An example of a deficit in isolated movement (selective control) for ankle dorsiflexion using the Boyd and Graham Selective Motor Control Test. While attempting to perform isolated ankle dorsiflexion, the extensor hallicus longus in the test leg is observed with major contribution to the active ankle dorsiflexion in this person who is unable to perform selective ankle dorsiflexion on the affected side.

of 3 for "Dorsiflexion achieved using mainly TA activity, but accompanied by hip and/or knee flexion"; and grade of 4 for "Isolated selective dorsiflexion achieved, through available range, using a balance of TA activity without hip and knee flexion" (Boyd, 1999, p. S26).

While this specific scale is for isolated control of ankle dorsiflexion, a similar scale could be developed for any specific muscle group using an understanding of muscle actions that commonly occur as abnormal synergies with the target muscle. For example, elbow flexion may be accompanied by synergistic shoulder flexion and internal rotation and wrist and finger flexion. The Boyd and Graham Selective Motor Control Test has moderate interrater reliability (Smits, 2010).

## Selective Control Assessment of the Lower Extremity (SCALE)

The *Selective Control Assessment of the Lower Extremity (SCALE)* tool was first described in 2009 as a measure of selective voluntary motor control (SVMC) of the lower extremity (LE) to take less than 15 minutes without specialized equipment (Fowler, 2009). Directions for administration, instructions for grading, and a Score Sheet are available to assess hip, knee, ankle, subtalar, and toe joints bilaterally. One representative isolated reciprocal movement that varies from the mass flexor/extensor patterns is used to assess SVMC for each joint while the patient is seated, except for hip flexion, which is tested in the side-lying position to allow for adequate hip joint excursion. Sitting and side-lying positions are intentionally implemented to allow evaluation of patients who are unable to stand, permitting observation of contralateral limb movements and to enable the patient to visualize their limb in case of proprioceptive deficits. The assessment and grading criteria are based on four factors: "(1) ability to move each joint selectively; (2) involuntary movement at other joints including the contralateral limb; (3) ability to reciprocate movement; (4) speed of movement; and (5) generation of force as demonstrated by excursion within the available range of motion" (Fowler, 2009).

First, demonstrate the joint movement passively through the desired movement sequence using a three-second verbal cadence and note the approximate PROM for comparison with the patient's active effort. Then ask the patient to perform the desired motion at approximately the same speed without moving other joints of the test extremity or the contralateral limb. If unsuccessful, feedback is provided and additional attempts are allowed.

In this protocol, four LE movement patterns are tested: knee extension and flexion, ankle dorsiflexion and plantar flexion with the knee extended, subtalar inversion and eversion, and toe flexion and extension in a reciprocating pattern to a verbal cadence (e.g., "flex, extend, flex"). Conceivably, the same system could be applied to the upper extremity. Next, grade the SVMC at each joint as "Normal" (2 points), "Impaired" (1 point), or "Unable" (0 points).

> *"A grade of 'Normal' is given when the desired movement sequence is completed within the verbal count without movement of untested ipsilateral or contralateral lower extremity joints. A grade of 'Impaired' is given when the patient isolates motion during part of the task, but demonstrates any of the following errors: movement occurs in only one direction; observed movement is less than 50% of the approximate available passive range of motion found during the passive demonstration; movement occurs at a nontested joint (including mirror movements); or the time for execution exceeds the approximate 3-second verbal cadence. A grade of 'Unable' is given when the requested movement sequence is not initiated or when it is performed using a synergistic mass flexor or extensor pattern." (Fowler, 2009)*

Fowler (2009) states that, for a patient who does not initiate the requested movement sequence, you can elicit an extensor and flexor synergy patterns using manual resistance to verify muscle force-generating capacity. Summing the points assigned to each joint results in a SCALE score for each LE limb with a maximum of 10 points per limb.

### Tests/Measures for Motor Control Stability

Among the tests and measures for motor control stability presented in the following text, the recent scientific evidence regarding this area of the neurological examination is summarized in Table 6-27 online (ONL), Focus on Evidence Table for Examination of Motor Control Stability at the end of the chapter.

### Motricity Index Pincer Grip Item

Item 1 of the Arm section of the *Motricity Index* specifically tests the patient's ability to grasp a 2.5-cm cube between the thumb and forefinger using a **pincer grip** (Collen, 1990). This action of holding the object can be used to gauge stability of the hand and fingers. The patient is scored in six increments depending on how well the individual performs the task. The Motricity Index in general has been supported as reliable with scoring that gives an objective reproducible

means of tracking a patient's progress in therapy (Collen, 1990).

### Scapula Locator System

In at least one study, scapular position was evaluated by triangulating location of the acromion, inferior angle, and root of the scapular spine using the *Scapula Locator System* (Price, 2001). Inter- and intraobserver reliability of the Scapula Locator System device was high, and the scapula was found to normally tilt downward in both healthy controls and in individuals with stroke (Price, 2001). However, about half of the 30 patients with stroke showed abnormality of glenoid fossa positioning. A portion of subjects (eight) showed stroke-affected upper extremities with increased downward tilt while six subjects had an upward-tilting glenoid fossa (Price, 2001).

### L-Shaped Jig With Calibrated Rule

An *L-shaped thermoplastic jig with an embedded 21-cm tape measure* has been described as a means of measuring impairment of MC-stability of the glenohumeral joint (Hayes, 1989). Sliding markers on the ruler portion were used to identify landmarks and to compute measurements. The acromion and a mark 20 cm above the olecranon served as landmarks. The method could be adapted using a transparent ruler to mark 20 cm above the olecranon (Figure 6-20A). Then take the initial measurement (between the two landmarks) with the subject's elbow extended and arm allowed to hang freely applying a natural gravitational distraction force at the glenohumeral joint (Figure 6-20B). Take a second measure between the two landmarks with the arm supported under the flexed elbow to reduce the subluxation (Figure 6-20C). The measure of the subluxation is documented as the difference between the two measures (Figure 6-20). Intrarater and interrater reliability for the original jig are supported by the literature (Hayes, 1989) as detailed in the MC-Movement Focus on Evidence Table online (ONL).

### Sulcus Sign for Shoulder Instability

A wide variety of clinical tests are commonly used for shoulder/glenohumeral instability. Provocation, relocation, and augmentation tests are each enhanced when **apprehension**, anxiety, and voluntary resistance result from 90-degree abduction and maximal external rotation (Tzannes, 2004). Any of these findings are considered as a positive test finding (Tzannes, 2004). It has also been concluded that the positive sulcus sign, when a depression occurs just below the acromion as the arm hangs at the side or is distracted manually away from the shoulder, is valid and reliable as a test for multidirectional shoulder instability (Tzannes, 2004).

### Inversion/Eversion Instability Observations

To explore medial/lateral stability at the ankle, a cradle device allowing the patient to support their full weight can be used to test for ankle stiffness/stability while the ankle is perturbed toward inversion or eversion. In this design, a potentiometer is used to measure lateral angular displacement at the ankle (higher amounts of displacement indicate

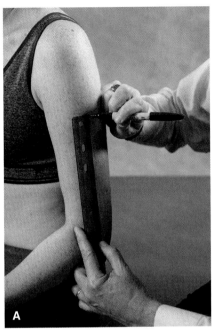 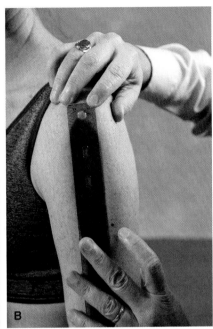 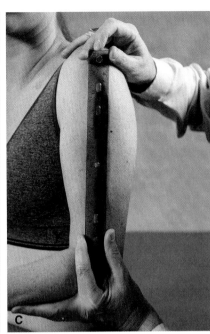

**FIGURE 6-20** Using a transparent ruler to measure glenohumeral subluxation of the shoulder using a method based on Hayes (1989). **A.** Mark a point on the skin, along the lateral humerus, 20 cm above the olecranon. **B.** With the arm hanging in a gravity-dependent position, measure the distance between two landmarks (the acromion and the point you marked). **C.** Support the arm under the flexed elbow to reduce the subluxation and remeasure the distance between the two points. The subluxation is documented as the difference between the two measures.

deficits in ankle stability) (Zinder, 2007). Without the potentiometer, you can still simply observe the lateral movements at the subtalar joint (Zinder, 2007). Video analysis of ankle position during ambulation indicates that observed ankle instability increases with faster walking speeds (Manor, 2008).

### Tests/Measures That Include Multiple Aspects of Motor Control

#### Action Research Arm Test (ARAT)

The *Action Research Arm Test (ARAT)* is a standardized assessment for upper extremity functional/motor recovery that consists of 19 items, divided into 4 subtests (grasp, grip, pinch, and gross arm movement) as shown in Table 6-18 (Hsieh, 1998). Realize that the grasp, grip, and pinch items each incorporate both MC-movement components to approach and contact the object and MC-stability components to maintain the grasp, grip, or pinch. The test is simple to administer and each item is scored on a four-point scale attending to speed, precision, and accuracy (0 = no movement possible to 3 = movement performed normally).

If the patient scores the maximum on the first item in a subtest, the most difficult item of each subtest, the patient is credited with a score of 3 on all items of the subtest. In chronic stroke, strong reproducibility, scalability, and responsiveness as well as very high interrater and test-retest reliability are reported (Lyle, 1981). The test has also been demonstrated to have very high inter- and intrarater reliability as shown in the MC-Movement Focus on Evidence Table online (ONL) and is sensitive to change (Lang, 2006). Raw

sum scores of the ARAT can be used for comparison of a patient's upper extremity functional abilities over time but cannot represent a patient's exact functioning at any one time (Koh, 2006).

#### Wolf Motor Function Test

The *Wolf Motor Function Test (WMFT)* assessment tool designed specifically for motor recovery in Constraint-Induced Movement Therapy (CIMT) trials also has a focus on upper extremity motor ability (Morris, 2001). Again, some tasks include a combination of MC-movement and MC-stability. The 15 upper extremity functional tasks (see Table 6-19) are timed while the individual performs the task as quickly as possible. The maximum time that can be recorded for each task is 120 seconds. Each task, some of which are functional, involves a dynamic combination of motor control stability in some joints while motor control-movement is predominant at other joints. In addition to timing each task, you will also assign a rating based on the five-point Functional Ability Scale of the WMFT. For the determination of normal in the scale, the uninvolved arm can be used as an available index for comparison with premorbid limb dominance taken into consideration. The reliabilities and validity of the WMFT are detailed in the MC-Movement Focus on Evidence Table online (ONL) (Morris, 2001; Wolf, 2001).

#### Chedoke Arm and Hand Activity Inventory Score Form

The *Chedoke Arm and Hand Activity Inventory Score Form (CAHAI)* (Barreca, 2005) was developed to determine upper

| TABLE 6-18 | Action Research Arm Test |
|---|---|

ACTION RESEARCH ARM TEST

Patient Name: _____

Rater Name: _____

Date: _____

Instructions

There are four subtests: Grasp, Grip, Pinch, Gross Movement. Items in each are ordered so that:

• if the subject passes the first, no more need to be administered and he scores top marks for that subtest;

• if the subject fails the first and fails the second, he scores zero, and again no more tests need to be performed in that subtest;

• otherwise he needs to complete all tasks within the subtest.

| ACTIVITY | SCORE |
|---|---|
| **Grasp** | |
| 1. Block, wood, 10-cm cube (If score = 3, total = 18 and to Grip); Pick up a 10-cm block. | _____ |
| 2. Block, wood, 2.5-cm cube (If score = 0, total = 0 and go to Grip); Pick up 2.5 cm block. | _____ |
| 3. Block, wood, 5-cm cube | _____ |
| 4. Block, wood, 7.5-cm cube | _____ |
| 5. Ball (Cricket), 7.5-cm diameter | _____ |
| 6. Stone 10 × 2.5 × 1 cm | _____ |
| Coefficient of reproducibility = 0.98 Coefficient of scalability = 0.94 | |
| **Grip** | |
| 1. Pour water from glass to glass (If score = 3, total = 12, and go to Pinch) | _____ |
| 2. Tube 2.25 cm (If score = 0, total = 0, and go to Pinch) | _____ |
| 3. Tube 1 × 16 cm | _____ |
| 4. Washer (3.5-cm diameter) over bolt | _____ |
| Coefficient of reproducibility = 0.99 Coefficient of scalability = 0.98 | |
| **Pinch** | |
| 1. Ball bearing, 6 mm, third finger and thumb (If score = 3, total = 18, and go to Grossmt) | _____ |
| 2. Marble, 1.5 cm, index finger and thumb (If score = 0, total = 0, and go to Grossmt) | _____ |
| 3. Ball bearing, second finger and thumb | _____ |
| 4. Ball bearing, first finger and thumb | _____ |
| 5. Marble, third finger and thumb | _____ |
| 6. Marble, second finger and thumb | _____ |
| Coefficient of reproducibility = 0.99 Coefficient of scalability = 0.98 | |
| **Grossmt (Gross Movement)** | |
| 1. Place hand behind head (If score = 3, total = 9, and finish) | _____ |
| 2. (If score = 0, total = 0, and finish) | _____ |
| 3. Place hand on top of head | _____ |
| 4. Hand-to-mouth | _____ |
| Coefficient of reproducibility = 0.98 Coefficient of scalability = 0.97 | |

(Adapted from Hsieh, 1998) Table taken from Appendix on p. 113.

limb function by assessing relevant upper extremity functional tasks. It consists of 13 real-life functional tasks (Table 6-20) that analyze bilateral hand activities and non-gender-specific functional tasks to determine upper limb function. The CAHAI uses a seven-point quantitative scale similar to the Functional Independence Measure (FIM). Interrater reliability, validity, and sensitivity to change in acute and chronic stroke are supported (Barreca, 2005) by the research statistics presented in the MC-Movement Focus on Evidence table online (ONL). An abbreviated nine-item version (Barreca,

2006) has been developed that shows validity and sensitivity to change. Both versions of CAHAI have a higher sensitivity to change than the Action Research Arm Test (Barreca, 2006).

## Nine-Hole Peg Test

Typically described as a test of upper extremity dexterity (MC-movement), the Nine-Hole Peg Test is a standardized test that requires the individual to place as many pegs as possible (maximum nine) into nine peg holes of a flat board

| TABLE 6-19 | Wolf Motor Function Test and Functional Ability Scale of WMFT |
|---|---|

*Wolf Motor Function Test Items*

1. Forearm to table (side): Subject attempts to place forearm on the table by abduction at shoulder.

2. Forearm to box (side): Subject attempts to place forearm on the box by abduction at shoulder.

3. Extend elbow (side): Subject attempts to reach across the table by extending the elbow (to side).

4. Extend elbow (to the side) with weight: Subject attempts to push the sandbag against outer wrist joint across the table by extending the elbow.

5. Hand to table (front): Subject attempts to place affected hand on table.

6. Hand to box (front): Subject attempts to place hand on the box.

7. Reach and retrieve (front): Subject attempts to pull 1-lb weight across the table by using elbow flexion and cupped wrist.

8. Lift can (front): Subject attempts to lift can and bring it close to lips with a cylindrical grasp.

9. Lift pencil (front): Subject attempts to pick up pencil by using a three-jaw chuck grasp.

10. Pick up paper clip (front): Subject attempts to pick up a paper clip by using a pincer grasp.

11. Stack checkers (front): Subject attempts to stack checkers onto the center checker.

12. Flip cards (front): Using the pincer grasp, patient attempts to flip each card over.

13. Turning the key in lock (front): Using pincer grasp while maintaining contact, patient turns key fully to the left and right.

14. Fold towel (front): Subject grasps towel, folds it lengthwise, then uses the tested hand to fold the towel in half again.

15. Lift basket (standing): Subject picks up basket by grasping handles and placing it on bedside table.

*Functional Ability Scale of the Modified Wolf Motor Function Test*

0 Does not attempt with the involved arm.

1 Involved arm does not participate functionally; however, an attempt is made to use the arm.

2 Arm does participate, but movement is influenced to some degree by synergy or is performed slowly and/or with effort.

3 Arm does participate; movement is close to normal but slightly slower; may lack precision, fine coordination, or fluidity.

4 Arm does participate; movement appears to be normal.

(Adapted from Morris, 2001). Data compiled from Table 1 (p. 751), Table 2 (p. 752), and Table 3 (p. 752).

(Figure 6-21) within 50 seconds. The objective measure is the number of pegs successfully placed within the 50 seconds. While the precision of peg placement reflects MC-movement, simultaneous MC-stability can also be observed in the hand intrinsic muscles (pincer grip) and the wrist and shoulder for stability. The Nine-Hole Peg Test is a valid and reliable upper extremity outcome measure to use following stroke and Charcot-Marie-Tooth (Mathiowetz, 1985; Oxford Grice, 2003). There is also evidence (details in the MC-Movement Focus on Evidence Table online [ONL]) for inter-rater reliability, test-retest reliability, and concurrent and convergent validity established against the Motricity Index (r = 0.82, n = 187) (Croarkin, 2004), very high reliability (Svensson, 2006) and sensitivity to change during recovery from stroke (Jacob-Lloyd, 2005).

### Tests/Measures for Motor Coordination

Common nonequilibrium coordination tests include the finger-to-nose test, the patient's finger-to-therapist's finger test, patient's index finger to the patient's other index finger, and the alternate heel-to-knee and heel-to-toe assessments, all described in the following text. During each requested movement, observe for smooth fluid movement with continuity throughout the movement as evidence that opposing muscle groups are cooperating, one contracting and shortening while the opposing group relaxes and elongates. A generic ordinal grading system is designed to provide standardization; however, it remains subjective based on the judgment of the examiner. The ordinal grading scale includes: 1 = the patient cannot perform the intended activity, 2 = the patient has a severe impairment, 3 = associated with moderate impairment, and 4 = minimal impairment, whereas 5 = normal.

### Motor Coordination Upper Extremity Tests

Tests of upper extremity coordination typically involve asking the patient to intentionally move the arm, particularly the finger, toward a target and observing for signs of ataxia or incoordination during the voluntary movement (DeHaven,1969). Tests of motor coordination of the upper extremity may involve either mass (large movements) or smaller (finite movement) tasks. Mass movements include the finger-to-finger test, touching their index fingers together; combining the finger-to-nose test with the finger-to-therapist's finger such that the patient alternates touching their nose with touching the therapist's

| TABLE 6-20 | Chedoke Arm and Hand Activity Inventory Score Form | | |
|---|---|---|---|
| **13 FUNCTIONAL ITEMS** | **AFFECTED LIMB (CHECK ONE):** | | **SCORE*:** |
| 1. Open jar of coffee | ☐ holds jar | ☐ holds lid | |
| 2. Call 911 | ☐ holds receiver | ☐ dials phone | |
| 3. Draw a line with a ruler | ☐ holds ruler | ☐ holds pen | |
| 4. Put toothpaste on toothbrush | ☐ holds toothpaste | ☐ holds brush | |
| 5. Cut medium consistency putty | ☐ holds knife | ☐ holds fork | |
| 6. Pour a glass of water | ☐ holds glass | ☐ holds pitcher | |
| 7. Wring out washcloth | | | |
| 8. Clean a pair of eyeglasses | ☐ holds glasses | ☐ wipes lenses | |
| 9. Zip up the zipper | ☐ holds zipper | ☐ holds zipper pull | |
| 10. Do up five buttons | | | |
| 11. Dry back with towel | ☐ reaches for towel | ☐ grasps towel end | |
| 12. Place container on table | | | |
| 13. Carry bag up the stairs | | | |
| Total Score | | | |

*Seven-point rating scale to be used for each item:
1. Total assist (weak U/L 25%)
2. Maximal assist (weak U/L 25%–49%)
3. Moderate assist (weak U/L 50%–74%)
4. Minimal assist (weak U/L 75%)
5. Supervision
6. Modified independence (device)
7. Complete independence (timely, safely)
(Adapted from Barreca, 2005). Data from Appendix 1 on p. 1620 and 1621.

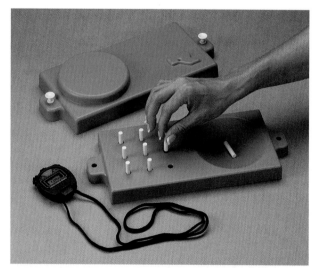

**FIGURE 6-21** Testing set-up for the Nine-Hole Peg Test. (Reprinted with permission from Patterson Medical, 28100 Torch Parkway, Suite 700, Warrenville, IL 60555-3938)

finger; pointing and pass-pointing test; and drawing geometrical shapes in the air such as figure eight or circle. Smaller finite movements include tapping the hand or fingers in a specified pattern, rapid pronation and supination, the rebound test, rapid fist development, handwriting tasks, and finger opposition movements. Remember to test both right and left sides for a built-in comparison, which is especially useful in conditions where one side of the body is affected.

Three types of tremor can be distinguished in patients with cerebellar or somatosensory ataxia, namely an intention tremor, a postural tremor, and titubation (Ropper, 2009). Intention tremor (see Table 6-17) in patients with cerebellar ataxia occurs only during intended voluntary movement (think of it as the opposing muscle groups struggling against each other in the planes of intended movement) and has a frequency of 3 to 5 Hz. The second type of tremor presenting in patients with cerebellar dysfunction is a postural tremor. Postural tremor presents when a patient is asked to adopt and maintain a posture or maintain a limb against gravity, for instance, holding an arm in 90-degree abduction. The typical frequency of postural tremor is about 3 Hz. Both the agonist and antagonist muscles contribute to the tremor. The characteristic postural tremor disappears if the limb is supported proximally. Postural tremor is only present when the patient is attempting to maintain a position. **Titubation** is a rhythmic tremor mainly of the head and/or upper trunk primarily present in the anteroposterior plane with a frequency of 3 to 4 Hz (Ropper, 2009).

The **finger-to-nose-to-finger test** assesses nonequilibrium coordination of the upper extremities and includes precision movements of the upper extremity to bring the patient's index finger into contact with either the patient's own nose, the therapist's finger, or alternating between the two (Figure 6-22). To begin the finger-to-nose test, seat the patient with their arms abducted to 90 degrees and ask the patient to flex one elbow at a time and touch the tip of their nose with their index finger. Have the patient alternate upper extremities at various speeds with and without their eyes open. Observe for dysmetria, past-pointing, intention tremor, and other components of ataxia described in Table 6-17. Recent evidence regarding tests and measures for Motor Control Coordination is summarized in Table 6-30, Focus on Evidence Table for Examination of Motor Control Coordination online (ONL).

To quantify the magnitude of inaccuracies during the finger-to-nose test, a transparent shield over the face with concentric rings centered around the patient's nose has been used (Notermans, 1994). The error is measured as the distance from the point where the patient's index finger contacts the shield to the patient's nose. The use of stopwatch measures has also been suggested to quantify the speed of finger-to-nose movement (Swaine, 1993). Another possibility is measuring the frequency of errors by counting the number of missed targets in either 10, 15, or 30 seconds (errors/second) or calculating the ratio of errors to total attempts.

The test can be expanded by asking the patient to alternate between touching the patient's own nose and the therapist's index finger as targets. This is a more complex test requiring visual input to execute the task and reach the targets appropriately, especially if the therapist moves the finger to varying locations in multiple quadrants requiring the patient to adjust the trajectory with each approach. Additionally, modify other factors such as speed, distance, and direction to challenge the patient during the examination. Another version includes the **finger-to-finger test** where the patient touches the two index fingers together (Figure 6-23). Beginning in a position with the patient's arms abducted to 90 degrees with full elbow extension, the patient is then instructed to move both upper extremities into horizontal adduction until the tips of each index finger touch in midline.

The pointing and pass-pointing test requires you to face the patient as you both place your arms in 90 degrees of shoulder flexion allowing index fingers to approximate. Next, while maintaining the position of your upper extremities in 90 degrees of shoulder flexion, have the patient move into full shoulder elevation causing the patient's index fingers to point toward the ceiling. The patient then returns their upper extremities back to the beginning position. The normal response is for the index fingers of the patient to reapproximate with

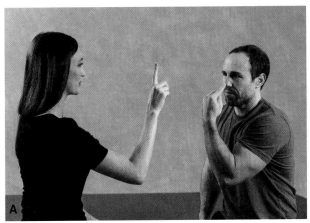

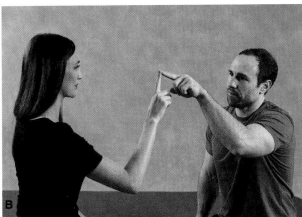

FIGURE 6-22 Coordination test for upper extremity: finger-to-nose. **A.** The patient will first touch their own nose with index finger of the hand to be tested. **B.** Then move the same finger to touch the therapist's finger, then repeat the cycle between nose and finger.

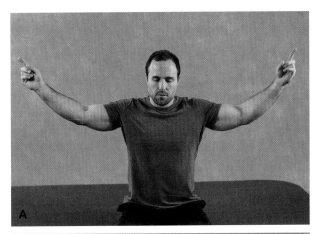

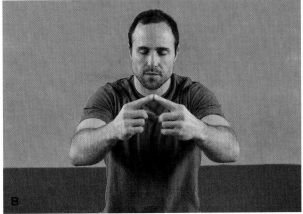

FIGURE 6-23 Coordination test for upper extremity: finger-to-finger. **A.** The patient starts with arms horizontally abducted and index fingers extended (with eyes closed). **B.** Then have the patient touch the two index fingers together in the midline.

your index fingertips, whereas an abnormal response results in "pass-pointing" in which the patient's fingers move beyond the level of your hands.

Small finite movements that require coordination between opposing muscle groups typically occur in distal joints such as the hand or forearm. Tapping the hand or fingers in a specified movement may be quantified by the use of sophisticated equipment that records the number of taps or you may employ less-sophisticated tasks such as observation of the patient during tapping of a table surface or the ipsilateral knee, which may be timed. The **rebound test** requires isometric tension in a muscle group, which is suddenly released. For example, gradually build up resistance against a muscle group such as the elbow flexors or the shoulder flexors, then abruptly release without warning. Normally, the cerebellum rapidly detects the change in velocity at the joint and the antagonistic muscle group activates to prevent excessive movement as a reflection of appropriate processing of proprioceptive information. An abnormal response is observed as the limb moves excessively in the direction of the tested muscle group's action.

Rapidly alternating movements are important to test for *dysdiadochokinesia* (see Table 6-17). Test rapid forearm pronation and supination with the patient's shoulder in adduction, the elbow in 90 degrees of flexion, and the wrist in neutral. Instruct the patient to rapidly move from full forearm pronation to full supination. Other tests for dysdiadochokinesia include repetitive patting of the hand (rapid wrist flexion/extension) on a flat surface or rapid fist development where the patient extends all fingers maximally followed by full finger flexion, forming a fist. Finally, finger opposition movements involve sequential movement of the thumb to the tip of each individual finger one at a time.

An upper extremity shape-drawing test consists of having the patient draw geometrical shapes in the air such as a "figure eight" or circle. The idea is to have the patient use large movements with the hand fixed in one position throughout the movement. Observe the quality of the movement, including the symmetry, smoothness, and speed of movement. Writing by hand on paper is similar to drawing shapes in the air, but the movement is much smaller and is supported. The therapist may draw an object or write a letter or words and have the patient trace with a performance of their own. Grade the performance by quantifying the number of errors that occur during the movement. Having the written sample documenting the errors at the time of initial evaluation will also allow for visual comparison with coordination at a later time in rehab. Accelerometer applications on smartphones can also now be used to quantify the smoothness and consistency of movement in three planes for individuals with ataxia.

## Motor Coordination Lower Extremity Tests

Lower extremity test options are similar to those described for the upper extremity, including mass movements or finite movements of multiple or single joints, respectively. Mass movements include the heel-to-shin test, touching the great toe to an examiner's finger (toe-to-finger test), picking up objects with the toes and moving them to another location,

and drawing geometrical shapes with the foot (DeHaven, 1969). Smaller finite movements include tapping tasks with the feet and toes.

The patient should assume a lying or sitting position for mass movement tests of the lower extremity coordination. Testing in standing would compromise safety and the contralateral extremity must then support the body's weight, making it an equilibrium test. Positioning in supine or supported sitting removes equilibrium requirements of the contralateral side during testing procedures and allows isolation of the lower extremity being tested. The supine position can also help minimize any confounding affects that may be due to weakness.

For the **heel-to-shin test**, ask the patient to sit or lie supine and to place the heel of the limb being tested along the anterior surface of the contralateral ankle. The patient then slides the calcaneus along the anterior surface of the contralateral tibia up toward the knee and then back down again, repeating this cycle several times (Figure 6-24). Observe the quality of the movement, such as the ability to make smooth movements or to maintain a straight path along the tibia. You might quantify errors by counting the number of times the heel moves horizontally off the tibia, the number of times the movement stops and starts (versus continuous flow of movement), and the number of times that overshooting and undershooting occurs during one cycle.

You can also ask the patient to touch their great toe to your finger in a manner similar to the upper extremity finger-to-finger test, except the great toe to finger test should occur in the supine position. As with the upper extremity, you can modify the examination by moving your target finger to change the distance, speed, or direction required to complete the task. As you move the finger in close, then away from the patient's body, relatively more flexion and extension are required for the hip and knee, respectively. It is important to test coordination at near and distant positions during a comprehensive assessment.

The patient may also use toes to pick up objects with the lower extremity and move them to another location. This test requires skills similar to the toe-to-finger test but is even more advanced because toe flexion is required to grasp an object such as a marble, crumpled towel, or small cylinder and move it to another location.

Shape drawing test for lower extremity (i.e., asking the patient to draw geometrical shapes with the lower extremity) is similar to the upper extremity test except that the patient may not be able to use the great toe to independently draw the object as in the upper extremity assessment. The patient uses the great toe as if it were a writing utensil, only the toes remain fixed such that the entire lower extremity must move to perform the task.

**Foot tapping** to test for dysdiadochokinesia occurs with rapidly alternating movements of ankle plantar flexion and dorsiflexion. While sitting, the patient begins with the knee and hip in approximately 90 degrees of flexion and the test foot flat on the floor. Ask the patient while maintaining heel contact with the floor to quickly dorsiflex and then plantarflex the ankle as the metatarsal heads (forefoot) alternately tap the floor. Tapping speeds may be increased to challenge the

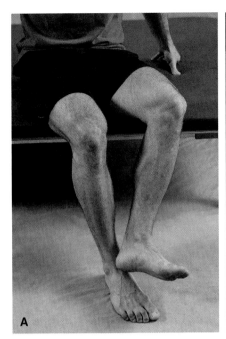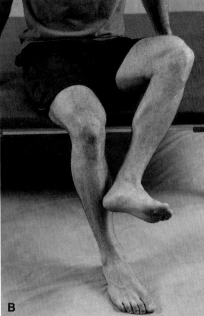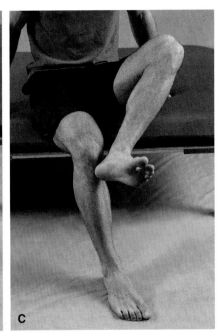

**FIGURE 6-24** Coordination test for lower extremity: heel-to-shin. **A.** The patient starts with placing the heel of the test leg anterior to the ankle of the opposite leg. **B.** Then ask the patient to slide the calcaneous of the test leg from the anterior aspect of the opposite ankle along the tibia **C.** up to the anterior aspect of the opposite knee, then repeat the movement up and down along the anterior tibia, back and forth.

patient. In ataxia, the normal response of rhythmic tapping will deteriorate to erratic arrhythmic movements with no obvious cadence. Another opportunity to observe for diadochokinesia occurs at the hip if the heel-to-shin test is performed quickly with rapidly alternating hip flexion/extension.

## Standardized Motor Examination Tools

This section discusses many clinical assessment techniques and tools that quantify and/or qualify motor function. The examination methods, particularly useful in clinical settings, are organized according to common diagnostic groups.

### Pediatric Motor Assessment Tools

The Motor Control Assessment, the Bruininks-Oseretsky Test of Motor Proficiency, the Test of Infant Motor Performance, the Peabody Developmental Gross Motor Scale, the Basic Gross Motor Assessment, the Clinical Observations of Motor and Postural Skills, and the Gross Motor Function Measure are pediatric assessment tools for diagnosis of delayed motor development (preterm and full term) and motor incoordination including that associated with CP, Down syndrome, and hydrocephalus (Han, 2010; Kolobe, 1998). These pediatric standardized assessments are summarized in Table 6-21.

The *Motor Control Assessment (MCA)* is an assessment of motor control, rather than functional ability, for children with physical disabilities (Steel, 1991). Spastic and nonspastic CP, spina bifida and other congenital abnormalities, and acquired

neurological injuries are some of the conditions suitable for assessment with the MCA. It includes 113 test items ranging from early infant reflexes to tasks requiring the coordination of a typical 5 year-old. Administration time ranges between 30 and 60 minutes depending on the capabilities and cooperation of the child. The MCA correlates well (R = 0.95 and higher) with the Physical Abilities Chart, another measure of motor ability (Steel, 1991).

The *Basic Gross Motor Assessment (BGMA)* evaluates gross motor performance of children from 5½ years of age up to approximately 12 years of age (Hughes, 1981). Nine motor tasks comprise the BGMA: (1) standing on one leg with eyes open and (2) with eyes closed, (3) stride jump, (4) tandem walking, (5) hopping on one foot, (6) skipping, (7) target throwing with bean bags, (8) yo-yo, and (9) ball handling. The following scale is used to rate each task: 3 = requires no deviations (good), 2 = one deviation (fair), 1 = two deviations (poor), and 0 = more than two deviations or if the child is unable to perform the task (Hughes, 1981).

The *Clinical Observations of Motor and Postural Skills (COMPS)* screens children with motor incoordination and is based upon clinical observation. Assessing children from 5 to 9 years of age, it consists of seven items: slow motion movements, finger-nose touching, rapid forearm rotation, postural stability or the ATNR, Schilder's arm extension (holding arms in extension while turning the patient's head with eyes closed), prone extension posture, and supine flexion posture (Wilson, 1992). The COMPS was designed to measure more than one domain of motor control including cerebellar function, postural control, and motor coordination (Wilson, 1992).

**TABLE 6-21** | **Partial List of Standardized Motor Examination Tools for Pediatric Patients**

| ASSESSMENT TOOL | POPULATION/ PURPOSE | AGE RANGE | TEST ITEM(S) | ADMINISTRATION TIME (IF REPORTED) | STATISTICS |
|---|---|---|---|---|---|
| Basic Gross Motor Assessment (BGMA) (Hughes, 1981) | Gross motor performance | 5.5 to ~12 years of age | Nine tests | | Test-retest and interrater reliabilities for the BGMA were reported to be 0.97 and 0.97, respectively. Internal consistency was 0.71 and construct validity ranged from 0.54–0.92. |
| Bruininks-Oseretsky Test of Motor Proficiency (BOTMP) (Flegel, 2002; Wilson, 1995) | Motor function based upon fine and gross motor skills | 4.5–14.5 years of age | 46 items (8 sub tests) | | |
| Clinical Observations of Motor and Postural Skills (COMPS) (Wilson, 1992) | Motor incoordination screen test | 5–9 years of age | Seven items | | Test-retest and interrater reliabilities to be 0.92 and 0.87, respectively. Internal consistency (Cronbach's alpha) was 0.75. |
| Gross Motor Function Measure (GMFM) (Kolobe, 1998) | Cerebral palsy | Infant to 3 years of age | 88 items | | |
| Gross Motor Performance Measure (GMPM) (Boyce, 1995) | Cerebral palsy | 0–12 years | 20 items | <60 minutes | Intraclass correlations ranged from 0.92–0.96 for the total score of the GMPM and 0.84–0.94 for the five attribute scores. |
| The Motor Control Assessment (MCA) (Steel, 1991) | Spastic and nonspastic cerebral palsy, spina bifida and other congenital abnormalities, and acquired neurological injuries | Early infant to 5 years | 113 test items | 30–60 minutes | Intra- and interrater reliability are 0.99 and 0.97, respectively |
| Peabody Developmental Gross Motor Scale (PDMS-GM) (Kolobe, 1998; Palisano, 1995) | Motor development | Birth to 83 months | | | |
| Test of Infant Motor Performance (TIMP) (Campbell, 1999) | Motor function | 32 weeks gestational age and 16 weeks postterm | 59 items | | Test-retest reliability was 0.89 (Cronbach's alpha) |

Another clinical motor control assessment tool in common use for children ranging from 4½ to 14½ years of age is the *Bruininks-Oseretsky Test of Motor Proficiency (BOTMP)* (Flegel, 2002; King-Tomas, 1987; Wilson, 1995). This test has 46 items overall with eight separate subtests: running speed and agility, balance, bilateral coordination, strength, upper-limb coordination, response speed, visual-motor control, and upper-limb speed and dexterity (Wilson, 1995). Although the test is useful to establish a clinical portrayal of motor function, it lacks substantial evidence to establish its reliability and its appropriateness as an evaluative tool (Wilson, 1995).

A comprehensive motor test for infants between 32 weeks gestational age and 16 weeks postterm age is the *Test of Infant Motor Performance (TIMP)* (Campbell, 1999). This test consists of 59 items divided into elicited and observed sections. Elicited items determine motor reactive responses with changes in position or to visual or auditory stimulation. Observed items rate unsolicited movement produced by the infant.

The first standardized instrument designed to measure change in gross motor function in children with CP was the *Gross Motor Function Measure (GMFM)* (Kolobe, 1998). It was validated on 136 children with CP and is weighted on motor skills that develop during the first 3 years. A total of 88 items in five different dimensions comprise the GMFM. The five dimensions are: lying and rolling; sitting; crawling and kneeling; standing; and walking, running, and jumping. The GMFM may be less appropriate for infants between 9 and 18 months of age who have behavioral problems or cannot imitate a demonstration or follow verbal commands (Kolobe, 1998). Furthermore, scores on this test are strongly influenced by the level of cooperation from the infant. Modified versions of this test (Wang & Yang, 2006) are the GMFM-66 (Han, 2010) and GMFM-66-IS (Russell, 2010).

The *Gross Motor Performance Measure (GMPM)* is similar to the GMFM except that the GMPM allows qualitative assessment of movements in children with CP (Boyce, 1995). Attributes of alignment, coordination, dissociated movement, stability, and weight shift during standing are considered with the GMPM (Boyce, 1995). The GMPM is a criterion-referenced tool based upon clinical observation. Attributes are observed and scored on a five-point scale ranging from 1 = severely abnormal to 5 = consistently normal.

The *Peabody Developmental Gross Motor Scale (PDMS-GM)* is a frequently used test of motor development in children (Kolobe, 1998; Palisano, 1995). It is standardized, normalized, and validated for children from birth up to 83 months (Kolobe, 1998; Palisano, 1995). Comparison of the PDMS-GM to the GMFM found that the PDMS-GM was similar to the GMFM in its ability to determine status changes in infants with CP or motor delay (Kolobe, 1998). Approximately 50% of the items are comparable in each test, particularly items that assess function in infants. A revised version of the PDMS-GM is the PDMS-2, which has also been shown to

have good test-retest reliability for children with CP (Wang & Liao 2006).

## Adult Motor Assessment Tools

There are numerous standardized adult motor examinations from which to choose. A few of the available adult motor examinations include the Motor sections of the Fugl-Meyer Assessment, Motricity Index, the Mayo-Portland Adaptability Inventory, the Wolf Motor Function Test, the Arm Motor Ability Test, the Physical Disability Index, the Trunk Control Test, the Canadian Neurological Scale, the Modified Motor Assessment Scale, Muscular Impairment Rating Scale, and the Mayo Test. Table 6-22 contains a summary of these standardized adult motor tests.

The *Fugl-Meyer Assessment (FMA),* specifically designed for poststroke assessment with a sensorimotor focus, includes five impairment-based subsections: joint motion, joint pain, balance, sensation, and motor function of upper extremity and lower extremity (Fugl-Meyer, 1975; Gladstone, 2002). It is useful in clinical settings to determine the patient's initial status, contribute to the intervention plan, and to document motor recovery following intervention.

The motor domain section tests for motor impairments and includes items assessing movement, coordination, and reflex action of upper extremity and lower extremity joints. The Canadian StrokEngine website (www.strokengine.ca) states that "items in the motor domain have been derived from Twitchell's 1951 description of the natural history of motor recovery following stroke and integrates Brunnstrom's stages of motor recovery." (Gladstone, 2002)

Rating each item requires direct observation of the patient's performance of the item and use of a three-point ordinal scale based on ability to complete the item (0 = cannot perform, 1 = performs partially, and 2 = performs fully). The more specific breakdown of scores is shown in Table 6-23, including the breakdown of points with a total possible scale score of 226 (100 points possible for the motor function section). Classifications for severity of motor impairment have been proposed based on the FMA Total Motor scores with a maximum 100 points (Duncan, 1994; Fugl-Meyer, 1980) and is shown in Table 6-24.

The FMA has often been used as a gold standard in studies evaluating validity of a variety of poststroke examination tools, particularly motor impairments. The sensory subsection has particularly been reported to have poor face, construct, and predictive validity and responsiveness (Lin, 2004). The very strong reliability, validity, prediction, and responsiveness to change for the FMA are summarized in Table 6-22.

The *Motricity Index (MI)* quantifies strength in patients following stroke. Muscle strength of 31 movements of the upper and lower extremities on the involved side are assessed using a six-point scale (0 to 5) ranging from 0 = "no contraction" to 5 = "movement against a resistance equal to maximum resistance overcome by the healthy side"

| TABLE 6-22 | Partial List of Standardized Motor Examination Tools for Adult Patients | | | |
|---|---|---|---|---|
| **ASSESSMENT TOOL** | **POPULATION/ PURPOSE** | **AGE RANGE** | **TEST(S)/ITEMS** | **ADMINISTRATION TIME** | **STATISTICS** |
| Arm Motor Ability Test (AMAT) (Kopp, 1997; McColloch, 1988) | Central nervous system injury; assesses ADL performance | Adult | 13 (Kopp, 1997) or 16 (McColloch, 1988) compound tasks | | Test-rest reliability was 0.99 for performance time, 0.93 for functional ability, and 0.94 for quality of movement. Intertester reliability ranged from 0.97–0.99 (Spearman correlations). |
| Canadian Neurological Scale (CNS) (Cote, 1989) | Stroke | Adult | 3 sections: mentation, and motor responses for patients with and without comprehension deficits | <5 min for most cases | Internal consistency (Cronbach's alpha) to be 0.79 while inter-rater reliability was 0.92 (Cote, 1989). Concurrent validity ranged from 0.76–0.89 (Cote, 1989). Predictive validity of the CNS using crude odd ratios for death within 6 months, additional strokes within 6 months, and independence at 6 months were 0.73, 0.70, and 1.6, respectively. |
| Fugl-Meyer Assessment (Fugl-Meyer; 1975) | Stoke; assesses five sensorimotor domains | Adult | 155 direct observation items divided into five domains: motor function (UE and LE), sensory function, balance, joint ROM, and joint pain | ~30–35 minutes for the entire FMA (Poole, 2001) ~20 minutes if just the motor scale | • Internal consistency reported as excellent, with Cronbach's alpha ranging 0.94–0.98 (Lin, 2004).<br>• Interrater reliability reported at excellent levels in multiple studies: ICC = 0.93 (Lin, 2004); ICC = 0.96 (Sanford, 1993); ICC = 0.99 for total motor score (Platz, 2005); Pearson correlations for motor domain upper extremity r = 0.96 to r = 0.97 and lower extremity r = 0.83 to r = 0.95 (Duncan, 1983); ICC for total score was 0.96 (Sanford, 1993).<br>• Test-retest reliability was also reported excellent including ICC = 0.97 for Total motor score (Platz, 2005); and Pearson correlations r = 0.98 to r = 0.99 for the total FMA score, r = 0.995 to r = 0.996 for motor domain upper extremity subscore, and r = 0.96 for motor domain lower extremity subscore (Duncan, 1983).<br>• Predictive validity evidenced by ability to predict: 1) FMA lower extremity admission subscores predicted the rehabilitation discharge Functional Independence Measure mobility r = 0.63, and locomotion scores r = 0.74 (Chae, 1995); 2) FMA admission scores predicted the rehabilitation discharge Barthel Index scores (Hsueh, 2008). |

- Construct validity is supported by excellent correlations between 1) the FMA and Barthel Index—except with FMA sensation subscale (Platz, 2005); 2) the FMA motor upper extremity subscale and Action Research Arm Test r = 0.77 at admission and r = 0.87 at discharge (Rabadi, 2006); 3) the FMA and Bobath Assessment of upper extremity r = 0.73 pre- and r = 0.85 postrehabilitation (Arsenault, 1988); 4) the FMA with Functional Independence Measure r = 0.63, FMA Motor domain upper extremity subscore to FIM self-care scores r = 0.61, and Motor domain lower extremity subscore to FIM mobility score r = 0.74 (Shelton, 2000); and 5) the FMA Motor subscale and various measures of gait (Dettmann, 1987).
- FMA is better than Motor Assessment Scale to discriminate the level of motor recovery, especially in more disabled individuals or early stage of recovery, Wilcoxon = p <0.0001 (Malouin, 1994).
- Responsive to change: responsiveness ratio was 0.41 for the FMA Motor score, but was better for the Action Research Arm test (a functional measure) (Van der Lee, 2001); STREAM and the FMA shortened versions demonstrated a moderate effect size of 0.53 and 0.51 (Hsueh, 2008).

| Test | Population | Items | Time | Reliability/Validity |
|---|---|---|---|---|
| Mayo Test (Mayo, 1991) | Traumatic Brain Injury | 165 items (51 upper extremity motor impairments, 51 lower extremity motor impairments, 51 functional mobility, and 12 equilibrium and protective extension) | | Raters were in perfect agreement on coordination and prehension scores, and all but one motor skill. Kappas ranged from 0.70–0.76 for scoring voluntary movements. However, interrater reliability was not as good for other items on the instrument, namely with scoring muscle tone, spinal reflexes, and equilibrium. |
| Mayo-Portland Adaptability Inventory (MPAI) (Bohac, 1997; Malec, 2000) | Brain injury | 22 (Malec, 2000) or 30 (Bohac, 1997) items | Actual time not reported, although 22 item version is "less lengthy"(Malec, 2000) | |

Continued

**TABLE 6-22  Partial List of Standardized Motor Examination Tools for Adult Patients—cont'd**

| ASSESSMENT TOOL | POPULATION/ PURPOSE | AGE RANGE | TEST(S)/ITEMS | ADMINISTRATION TIME | STATISTICS |
|---|---|---|---|---|---|
| Modified Motor Assessment Scale (MMAS) (Loewen, 1988) | Stroke; motor recovery | Adult | 8 items pertaining to balance, function, and upper extremity motor performance | | Intrarater reliability ranged from 0.72–0.97 (mean Kappa coefficients) whereas interrater reliability ranged from 0.73–0.96 (mean Kappa coefficients). |
| Motricity Index (MI) (Demeurisse, 1980) | Stroke | Adult | 31 movements for upper and lower extremities | | Internal consistency was 0.77 and 0.73 for the MI and handheld dynamometry, respectively. |
| Motricity Index (Modified) (MI) (Collin, 1990) | Stroke | Adult | 6 strength tests: 3 each for upper and lower extremities | <5 min. | |
| Muscular Impairment Rating Scale (MIRS) (Mathieu, 2001) | Myotonic dystrophy | Adult | 5 point ordinal scale based partly on manual muscle testing of 11 muscle groups | 10–15 minutes | Intrarater reliability was 0.84 (weighted Kappa) whereas interrater reliability was 0.77–0.79 (weighted Kappa). |
| Physical Disability Index (PDI) (Gerety, 1993) | Physical function in frail older adults without severe cognitive impairment | Adult (60–98 years of age) | 54 items include 20 ROM, 20 strength, 6 balance, and 8 mobility | Mean time of 60 min.; 36 min. for ROM and 24 min. for mobility/balance | Test-retest reliability of the overall PDI was 0.97 with the individual subscale categories ranging from 0.92–0.96. Interrater reliability was reported to be 0.92 for the overall PDI. |
| Trunk Control Test (TCT) (Collin, 1990) | Stroke | Adult | 4 mobility tests | <5 min. | Interrater reliability was 0.76. |
| Wolf Motor Function Test (WMFT) (Morris, 2001) | Stroke | Adult | 6 point functional ability scale assessing 15 functional tasks | ~30 minutes | • Interrater reliability (ICC) was 0.97 for performance time and 0.88 for functional ability. • Test-retest reliability (r) was 0.90 and 0.95 for performance time and functional ability, respectively. • Internal consistency (Cronbach's alpha) ranged from 0.86–0.92 for both measures on two different testing sessions. |

**TABLE 6-23  Breakdown of Fugl-Meyer Sections and Points**

| DOMAIN OF FUGL-MEYER | SUBSECTIONS WITHIN DOMAIN | MAXIMUM POINTS |
|---|---|---|
| Motor score | 66 pts UE and 34 pts LE | 100 points |
| Sensation score | 8 pts light touch and 16 pts position sense | 24 points |
| Balance | 6 pts for sitting and 8 pts for standing | 14 points |
| Joint ROM | | 44 points |
| Joint pain | | 44 points |

**TABLE 6-24  Classifications of Motor Severity Based on Fugl-Meyer Total Motor Score**

| FUGL-MEYER (1980) | FUGL-MEYER (1975) | DUNCAN (1994) |
|---|---|---|
| <50 = Severe | | 0–35 = Very Severe |
| 50–84 = Marked | ≤84 = Hemiplegia | 36–55 = Severe |
| 85–94 = Moderate | 85–95 = Hemiparesis | 56–79 = Moderate |
| 95–99 = Slight | 96–99 = Slight motor dyscoordination | >79 = Mild |

(Demeurisse, 1980). A modification of the MI uses six total strength assessments: three for the upper extremities (pinch, elbow flexion, and shoulder abduction) and three for the lower extremities (hip flexion, knee extension, and ankle dorsiflexion) (Collin, 1990). Scores are weighted for the quality of the individual actions, then totaled to yield a final score. For example, in a validation study, the MI was tested on the lower extremities using the following scale: A score of 33 was given for normal strength, a score of 25 for movement against resistance but weaker than the other side (corresponds with good, 4/5), 19 points for movement in the full range against gravity without resistance (corresponds with fair, 3/5), 14 points were given for movement but not against gravity or within full range (corresponds with poor, 2/5), a score of 9 points for a palpable contraction without movement (corresponds with trace, 1/5), and zero points were given for no movement or palpable contraction (corresponds with zero, 0/5) (Cameron, 2000). Approximately 100 total points were possible from all three muscle actions (33 points each possible for the actions of hip flexion, knee extension, and ankle dorsiflexion) (Cameron, 2000). The authors found high correlations (greater than 0.77) between a handheld dynamometer and the MI for the lower extremity (Cameron, 2000).

The *Mayo-Portland Adaptability Inventory (MPAI)* contains 30 items that assess areas of impairment and disability from brain injury (Bohac, 1997). The MPAI generally characterizes impairment, activity, and participation in patients with brain injuries (Malec, 2000). Mobility and use of the hands are the two primary motor control aspects assessed by the MPAI. A 22-item version of the test was compared with the 30-item MPAI using a rating scale analysis where the 22-item MPAI was found to decrease the duration of the assessment while maintaining good reliability and strong correlation with the 30-item MPAI (Malec, 2000).

The *Wolf Motor Function Test (WMFT)* was developed to determine the effects of constraint-induced movement therapy upon motor function in individuals with brain injury or stroke. Originally, the WMFT consisted of 21 simple tasks arranged according to joints involved and order of difficulty (Wolf, 1989). However, the test, as outlined in Table 6-19, has been recently modified to include 15 functional tasks using a six-point functional ability scale (Morris, 2001). Studies have documented high interrater reliability, internal consistency, and test-retest reliability (summarized in Table 6-22) for the modified WMFT.

The *Arm Motor Ability Test (AMAT)* qualitatively and quantitatively measures the ability to perform activities of daily living in patients who have CNS injury (Kopp, 1997). The AMAT is an assessment in "Constraint-Induced Movement Therapy" studies and may supplement the Wolf (Emory) Motor Function Test. The original AMAT included 16 compound activities of daily living tasks (McColloch, 1988). In a subsequent investigation, 13 tasks that assessed feeding, dressing, and grooming abilities in addition to other functional abilities were included (Kopp, 1997). The authors concluded that the AMAT has satisfactory concurrent validity, internal consistency, and sensitivity to change (Kopp, 1997).

The *Physical Disability Index (PDI)* was developed to measure multiple aspects of physical functioning in frail adults without severe cognitive impairments or neurological injury (Gerety, 1993). The PDI is purposed to differentiate levels of function among individuals and determine change in function over time within individuals (Gerety, 1993). The 54 items including ROM, strength, balance, and mobility categories (see breakdown in Table 6-22) are standardized and divided into subscale and summary PDI scores with a range of 0 to 100 for the total score. Strength was assessed with a handheld dynamometer in the supine position with gravity eliminated, balance in sitting and standing while resisting sternal nudges standardized to 1.5% of the patient's body weight, and functional mobility with bed mobility and ambulation, transfers, and turning ability. The average administration time was 60 minutes: 36 minutes for the ROM and strength subscales and 24 minutes for the mobility and balance subscales.

The *Trunk Control Test (TCT)* was derived from the Northwick Park Motor Assessment (Collin, 1990). The TCT examines four aspects of trunk movement, which allows for clinical prediction of functional recovery from stroke. The patient is asked to actively roll to the involved side from a supine position, roll to the uninvolved side, transfer to sitting from a lying position, and sit in a balanced position on the edge of the bed with the feet dangling in the air for at least 30 seconds (Collin, 1990). Scoring for the TCT uses arbitrary values: 0 = unable to perform the movement without assistance, 12 = able to perform the movement but requiring assistance from upper extremities for steadiness, and 25 points = performing the movement in a normal fashion. It generally takes less than 5 minutes to perform the TCT (Collin, 1990). When the TCT was compared with the Motricity Index and the Rivermead Motor Assessment, the tests were well correlated with each other and the TCT has sufficient predictive validity for patients recovering from stroke (Collin, 1990).

The *Canadian Neurological Scale (CNS)* is a test designed to assess mentation as well as motor function for patients recovering from a stroke (Cote, 1989). The CNS consists of three sections: mentation, motor function for patients without comprehension deficits, and motor response for patients with a comprehension deficit. Motor function for patients without comprehension deficits assesses weakness of the facial muscles and the proximal and distal arm and leg muscles using a subjective scale. Scoring for the facial muscles is 0.5 points = normal muscle responses and 0 points = weakness present (Cote, 1989). Scoring for extremities includes 1.5 points = normal, 1.0 = "mild" impairment, and 0.5 = "significant" impairment (Cote, 1989). For patients with comprehension deficits, scoring for the face is either 0.5 or zero, depending on whether symmetry is present or not, and for arm and leg symmetry, 1.5 points = equal or 0 points = unequal (Cote, 1989). The results indicated that high initial CNS scores appeared to be associated with favorable outcomes. The authors recommend the usage of the CNS because of its brevity, practicality, ability to detect differences in neurological status, its ease of use and interpretation by various medical personnel, and because it assesses factors that most affect prognostication of recovery from acute stroke (Cote, 1989).

The *Modified Motor Assessment Scale (MMAS)* assesses motor recovery of patients after a stroke based upon motor requirements to perform activities of daily living (Loewen, 1988). Eight items pertaining to balance, upper extremity motor performance, and function comprise the MMAS. These items are scored from 0 to 6 points (Loewen, 1988).

Muscle impairment in patients with myotonic dystrophy type I may be assessed with the Muscular Impairment Rating Scale (MIRS) (Mathieu, 2001). This test uses an ordinal five-point rating scale (with 1 = no muscular impairment and 5 = severe proximal weakness) based on manual muscle testing of 11 muscle groups. The test had good intra- and interrater reliability and correlated well with the Functional Status Index.

The *Mayo Test* is an instrument consisting of 165 items that evaluate neurophysical sequela following traumatic brain injury (Mayo, 1991). The instrument assesses volitional movement, muscle tone, strength, coordination, prehension, deep

tendon and spinal reflexes, and dysmetria and tremor in 51 items for each extremity, giving a total of 102 items. Another 51 items assess functional mobility, and 12 items assess equilibrium and protective reactions. The test has good reliability as shown in Table 6-22. The authors conclude that the instrument is useful for assessing items that are observable such as the assessment of muscle tone.

## THINK ABOUT IT 6.3

- How will you first suspect and notice that your patient has issues related to MC-movement, MC-stability, or MC-coordination during your examination? What specific tests/measures will be most useful for each?
- How will you prioritize motor control assessment tools to identify the ones that are most appropriate for your patient?

## ■ Documentation of Motor Examination

Regardless of the scope and duration of the motor examination and the style of the clinician, detailed neuromotor findings should be properly recorded to standardize the examination. Combined with all the other data from the neurological examination, this also facilitates future evaluations performed by different examiners and allows determination of the patient's progress and future prognosis. Documentation of the examination findings may be handwritten notes with or without specialized documentation forms, occur with voice dictation, or electronic documentation devices.

In the written documentation, it is important to assimilate and synthesize all of the neuromotor examination data with all the other impairments detected. For optimal treatment planning, it is essential to prioritize the observed impairments and formulate logical hypotheses regarding the impairments underlying or contributing to the functional limitations at an activity level for that the patient (Rothstein, 1986; Rothstein, 2003). The motor impairments are obviously such an important contributor to limitations of activity or participation, which are the ultimate focus of therapeutic intervention.

### Documentation Forms

Form documentation provides a template for the examiner and organizes information obtained from the assessment. Many standardized tests require documentation unique to the examination. An example of a documentation form, including the neuromotor aspects, is included in Chapter 3, Appendix 3-A.

# HANDS-ON PRACTICE

Be sure to practice the following hands-on skills discussed in this chapter. With practice, you should be able to perform the following:

1. Examination of range of motion
   a. Passive ROM
   b. Active ROM
   c. End feel
2. Examination of muscle flexibility
3. Examination of muscle strength by myotomes
   a. Manual muscle testing
   b. Handheld dynamometer
4. Examination of muscle spasticity
   a. Modified Ashworth Scale
   b. Tardieu Scale
   c. Triple Spasticity Scale
5. Examination of muscle rigidity
   a. the UPDRS Motor Examination
   b. Head-Dropping Test
   c. Shoulder-Shaking Test
6. Examination of deep tendon reflexes
7. Examination of pathological reflexes
   a. Clonus
   b. Babinski
8. Observational movement analysis to differentiate MC-movement and MC-stability
9. Examination of motor control movement
   a. Measure the degrees of motion through which the individual can complete selective isolated control of movement

   b. Active release of grasp
   c. Trost Selective Motor Control Examination
   d. Boyd and Graham Selective Motor Control Test
   e. Selective Control Assessment of the Lower Extremity
10. Examination of motor control stability
    a. Motricity Index Pincer Grip Item
    b. Scapular Locator System
    c. L-shaped Jig with Calibrated Rule
    d. Sulcus Sign for Shoulder Instability
    e. Inversion/Eversion Instability Observations
11. Examination of motor coordination tests for the upper extremity
    a. Finger-to-nose
    b. Finger-to-finger
    c. Rebound test
    d. Rapidly alternating movements (pronation/supination)
12. Examination of motor coordination tests for the lower extremity
    a. Heel-to-shin test
    b. Toe-to-finger
    c. Foot tapping

## Let's Review

1. Describe the normal physiology underlying the function of the neuromotor system. What happens when one or more structures does not perform its normal activities? Given a specific impaired body structure, what identifiable physical impairment might you observe in your patient?

2. List and define the specific subcategories of muscle performance within a neuromotor examination. How is muscle performance described, tested, and the findings documented?

3. What similarities and differences would you anticipate on a motor examination for a patient with a LMN injury versus an UMN injury?

4. Describe the key aspects and critical considerations of the specific tests for each subcategory of the neuromotor examination.

5. Describe expected abnormal motor examination results in the context of specific neurological conditions. What impairments are associated with the pyramidal and extrapyramidal systems? Which class of medications may mimic extrapyramidal dysfunction?

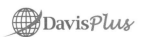 For additional resources, including Focus on Evidence tables, case study discussions, references, and glossary, please visit http://davisplus.fadavis.com

# CHAPTER SUMMARY

## PATIENT APPLICATION

Cade, a 54 year-old with a right cerebellar tumor (1 month postsurgical resection), never dreamed he'd be dealing with problems like these at this point in his life. The tumor was benign but had to be surgically removed because of the mass effect of the tumor (space-occupying lesion) that compressed local structures. He is now admitted to inpatient rehab, and you have finished your initial examination, which you did as a demonstration for your new student who has just started with you today. As you prepare the documentation, you summarize the motor impairments and their impact on Cade's functional activity for the student. While he has no ROM deficits, he does have a general hypotonicity throughout the right side with resulting proximal instability in both right limbs. He is able to perform isolated movements for all joints bilaterally without abnormal synergies, but he does exhibit intention tremor, dysmetria, and dysdiadochokinesia in the right arm and right leg. These ataxic expressions decrease his efficiency in reaching tasks with the right arm and in the right swing phase of the gait cycle. He has normal strength through the left side (4 +/5 MMT) but does have general weakness (3 + to 4-/5 MMT) for all right extremity muscle groups. His dynamic standing balance is impaired with his erratic step lengths, sometimes causing the foot to "catch" on the floor with resulting imbalance (but he has not fallen, yet). Timed Up-and-Go (TUG) test was 26 seconds. His self-selected gait speed is slow at 0.37 m/s. You have a discussion with the student about how the hypotonia, ataxia, and weakness are particularly contributing to the balance impairment and the limitations to functional reaching and gait. A treatment plan will need to be developed that addresses the underlying impairments and provides opportunities to practice repetitions with feedback to improve the functional skills.

## Contemplate Clinical Decisions

1. Can you explain why this patient with a brain tumor does not have problems with abnormal synergies (he does have selective, isolated control)?

2. How might the associated general hypotonia affect this patient's functional skills? And how would you detect it when he starts to get improvement in his muscle tone?

3. We'll discuss specific direct interventions later, but with his hypotonia/weakness/ataxia and associated gait deviations, slow ambulation, and risk for falling, will you provide intervention for underlying impairments, functional activity limitations, or both? What will be the ultimate focus?

4. How might Cade's cerebellar deficits interfere with his ability to communicate with you?

In addition to the previous examples of this chapter, Cade provides a great example of how important the neuromotor examination is to prepare optimally for developing the intervention plan. The various aspects and expressions of the neuromotor system have clear linkages to limitations in activities, tasks, and skills. Focus on Evidence Tables online (ONL) provide a summary of the recent evidence regarding examination of PROM (Table 6-25). If there are flexibility or ROM deficits, obviously the individual will not be able to control movement or perform function through the normal magnitude/range of movement. A weak muscle may be able to move a joint initially but might not be able to contract against gravity or produce enough force to contribute adequately to movement. Generalized hypotonia may contribute to proximal instability and poor antigravity posture. Hypertonia may produce elevated resting forces, accentuated by the elongation that results from antagonist contraction and therefore interfere with voluntary movement. Motor control deficits are among the most common and most problematic impairments that follow neuromuscular disorders. If the person can move and can generate force but cannot make the limb move in the precise way needed (MC-movement) or cannot stabilize the joint during a weight-bearing activity (MC-stability), the movement and force generation is of little use to them. As therapists who focus on restoring movement related to functional activities and skills, observing and measuring neuromotor deficits and their specific impact on function will assist in the paramount task of optimizing the neuromotor system to restore function.

# Examination and Evaluation of Cranial Nerves

Dennis W. Fell, PT, MD    CHAPTER 7

## CHAPTER OBJECTIVES

Upon completion of this chapter, the learner should be able to:

1. Describe the function/purpose of each cranial nerve, including motor, sensory, and autonomic function.
2. Select appropriate tests/measures for each cranial nerve.
3. Describe the effect of any specific cranial nerve deficit.
4. Correlate cranial nerve deficits to specific anatomic areas of the brainstem.

## ◼ Introduction

The term **cranial nerve (CN)** is an anatomical term for the peripheral nerves directly emerging from the brain or brainstem that provide innervation to structures around the head, face, neck, and body organs. CNs are responsible for numerous essential functional abilities, particularly sensory and motor processes for structures of the head, face, and neck as well as parasympathetic control. CN functions include the life-sustaining aspects of cardiovascular and pulmonary function, significant autonomic control, and the **special senses** of smell, vision, taste, and hearing. **Equilibrium sensibility**, the ability to sense the position and movement of the head in space, is the function of a CN. The adjective **bulbar** refers anatomically to the brainstem excluding the midbrain, especially the medulla oblongata. **Bulbar symptoms** are abnormal expressions of CN function, especially aspects of motor paralysis (bulbar paralysis) of the face, mouth, tongue, pharynx, and esophagus related to medulla pathology with impaired facial expression, speech production, and swallowing often seen with bulbar Amyotrophic Lateral Sclerosis (ALS) or progressive supranuclear palsy. Examination of CNs is often completed as a specific subset of the neurological examination because of the common aspects of head and neck functions and basic life-sustaining functions. This chapter will describe the tests and measures used to detect normal versus abnormal function of the CNs.

Examination of CN function is important as part of the evaluation of any patient with injury to the cerebrum or brainstem, whether from vascular disease, trauma, or other causes. The CN examination can reveal significant or subtle deficits often overlooked in the patient who has sustained orthopedic trauma such as a lower extremity fracture. Because of the focus on medical management of the orthopedic trauma, other health-care workers have often not previously detected such deficits. Abnormal results on a CN screen in this population, even just subtle signs, could be the first indication of brain injury related to the trauma.

# ■ Categories of Cranial Nerve Function

In general, CN function is either motor, sensory, or autonomic. With few exceptions, most CNs are "mixed" with both motor and sensory fiber components. As explained in the following sections, some motor and sensory components are designated as "special" because they carry special senses or motor innervation of structures derived from the embryonic branchial arches, particularly for motor functions related to eating and breathing.

## Motor Cranial Fiber Categories

**General somatic efferent (GSE)** describes somatic motor innervation that results in voluntary movement. GSE includes movement of the eyes through CNs III, IV, and VI, and voluntary tongue movement through CN XII.

**General visceral efferent (GVE)** is the designation used to refer to involuntary efferent input to a number of visceral structures. All these fibers emerge as preganglionic **parasympathetic** fibers, including CN III fibers to the iris constrictors of the eye, CN VII to lacrimal and salivary glands, CN IX to parotid salivary glands, and parasympathetics to thoracic and abdominal viscera and blood vessels through CN X.

**Special visceral efferent (SVE)** includes branchial motor innervation to all voluntary muscles related to eating and breathing, including voluntary muscles of the jaw and tensor tympani by CN V, facial expression and hyoid muscles by CN VII, swallowing and larynx control by CNs IX and X, and head and shoulder movement through CN XI.

## Sensory Cranial Fiber Categories

**General somatic afferent (GSA)** CN components receive general senses from the face through CN V, including proprioception from the muscles of the face and eye.

**Special somatic afferent (SSA)** refers to fibers that receive input from special sense organs. CN II carries the special sense of vision while CN VIII carries special senses related to hearing and vestibular sense.

**Special visceral afferent (SVA)** is the classification applied to special senses that process internal information. SVA includes the special sense of smell from CN I, and the special sense of taste through CNs VII, IX, and X.

**General visceral afferent (GVA)** describes the class of afferents that receive general sensory input from visceral organs including CNs VII, IX, and X.

# ■ Review of Physiology and Neuroscience of Cranial Nerve Function

CN I (Olfactory) and CN II (Optic) each exit from the cerebrum. The other 10 CNs exit from the brainstem and the most rostral part of the spinal cord. CN IV (Abducens) is the only CN to exit from the posterior brainstem. The anatomic locations of the CN nuclei and emerging nerve roots are given in Table 7-1.

Abnormal CN function can be related to disease or injury of a variety of anatomic locations. A lesion to the areas of sensory or motor cortex that process facial or CN functions (i.e., the face region of the sensory homunculus or motor homunculus) can result in abnormal CN function. Damage to cerebral or brainstem deep white matter carrying tracts related to CNs can also impair CN function. Increases in intracranial pressure from any cause can also result in CN dysfunction. The surface and deep matter of the brainstem are highly concentrated with CN nuclei and CN structures (see Figs. 7-1 A, B, and C). Damage to the brainstem is one of the most significant and common sources of CN dysfunction. Finally, CNs may be damaged at their site of exit from the cranium through the specific cranial foramen.

General central nervous system (CNS) pathology including cerebrovascular accident, traumatic brain injury, multiple sclerosis, and tumors of brain can all result in an array of varied CN symptoms if the brainstem or specific facial areas of motor or sensory cortex are affected. Pathologies related to specific CN dysfunction are discussed later in this chapter but may include visual hemianopsia and other visual field deficits, trigeminal neuralgia, Bell's palsy, hearing loss, vestibular dysfunction, and cardiac and/or respiratory deregulation.

The physiology of sensory and motor systems is covered in Chapters 5 and 6, respectively. The major aspects of physiology and neuroanatomy of several special senses will be summarized in the following text, with the exception of the vestibular system covered in Chapter 8.

## Olfaction

For **olfaction**, the special sense of smell mediated by CN I, transmission of the impulse begins at the chemical receptors, bipolar neurons with cilia extending from the dendrites. These receptors are present in the nasal mucosa of the upper nasal septum, roof of the nasal passage, and superior concha. The perception of different smells results from complex reactions of odorous substances with the receptor neuron. Once an olfactory action potential is initiated in the receptor neuron, it passes through the olfactory nerve fibers passing through the cribriform plate of the skull and synapses on mitral cells of the olfactory bulb, an extension of the telencephalon, the rostral-most portion of the brain. These fibers then pass through the olfactory tract with the signal eventually delivered by the second-order neuron to the primary olfactory cortex, the piriform cortex of the medial inferior frontal lobe for perception of smell. The mitral cell fibers also terminate in the amygdala, a deep nucleus within the uncus of the parahippocampal gyrus, which partially explains the link between olfaction and emotion and memory.

## Vision

**Vision** is a complex special sense system mediated by CN II. The receptor cells are the rods and cones located within the retinal wall. **Rods** are much more numerous than cones (20:1)

**TABLE 7-1**   **Anatomic Locations of Cranial Nerve Components**

| CRANIAL NERVE | LOCATION OF NERVE NUCLEI | NERVE LOCATION |
|---|---|---|
| Cranial nerve I<br>Olfactory | • Anterior olfactory nucleus in the olfactory stalk | Inferior frontal lobe in olfactory sulcus (forebrain) |
| Cranial nerve II<br>Optic | • Ganglion cells at retina | Optic tracts attached at lateral geniculate body; optic chiasm is superior and anterior to pituitary stalk |
| Cranial nerve III<br>Oculomotor | • Oculomotor nucleus of upper midbrain peri-aqueductal gray at the level of the superior colliculus<br>• Parasympathetic: Edinger-Westphal nucleus in midbrain | Emerges from medial cerebral peduncle (midbrain) |
| Cranial nerve IV<br>Trochlear | • Trochlear nucleus anterior to periaqueductal gray of lower midbrain (inferior colliculus level) | Emerges from posterior midbrain inferior to the inferior colliculus (the only CN to emerge from the posterior brainstem) then winds laterally around the brainstem to appear lateral to middle cerebellar peduncle |
| Cranial nerve V<br>Trigeminal | • Sensory: Tactile sense to primary sensory nucleus of CN V (discriminative sense) and spinal trigeminal nucleus (pain, temperature, and light touch)<br>• Sensory: Proprioceptive sense to mesencephalic nucleus of CN V located along the dorsolateral pontine tegmentum and midbrain lateral periaqueductal gray<br>• Motor: Motor nucleus of CN V in lateral tegmentum of rostral pons | Emerges from the lateral pons out of the middle cerebellar peduncle |
| Cranial nerve VI<br>Abducens | • Abducens nucleus in the floor of fourth ventricle at level of pons causing the surface landmark "facial colliculus" as the fibers of CN VII wrap over the surface of the CN VI nucleus | One of three nerves emerging at the pontomedullary junction; exits just superior to the pyramid of the medulla |
| Cranial nerve VII<br>Facial | • SVA: Geniculate ganglion, solitary nucleus<br>• Motor: Motor nucleus of CN VII in the pontine tegmentum | One of three nerves emerging at the pontomedullary junction; exits medial to cranial nerve VIII |
| Cranial nerve VIII<br>Vestibulocochlear | • Auditory: Ventral cochlear nucleus<br>• Dorsal cochlear nucleus<br>• Vestibular: Four vestibular nuclei and the cerebellum | One of three nerves emerging at the pontomedulllary junction; exits lateral to cranial nerve VII |
| Cranial nerve IX<br>Glossopharyngeal | • SVA: Inferior ganglion of IX, solitary nucleus | One of three nerves emerging lateral to the olive of the medulla; exits most superior of the three |
| Cranial nerve X<br>Vagus | • GVE: Dorsal motor nucleus of the vagus located in medulla just lateral to hypoglossal nucleus<br>• SVA: Inferior ganglion of X, solitary nucleus (just lateral to dorsal motor nucleus of vagus) | One of three nerves emerging lateral to the olive of the medulla; exits between the other two |
| Cranial nerve XI<br>Accessory (Spinal Accessory) | • Spinal Accessory Nucleus in C2-C5 contributes to spinal roots; nucleus ambiguous contributes to cranial root fibers, which will be recurrent laryngeal nerve | One of three nerves emerging lateral to the olive of the medulla; exits most inferior of the three and partially from upper cervical spinal cord |
| Cranial nerve XII<br>Hypoglossal | • Hypoglossal nucleus is paramedian column in medulla | Emerges from the medulla, medial to the olive and lateral to the pyramid |

and contribute very little to visual acuity. However, they exhibit high sensitivity and are therefore essential in low-light conditions. **Cones** are the color receptors and provide very high visual acuity. The weakness of cones is their low sensitivity explaining why we do not see color very well in low-light conditions. While cones are generally less common overall, the fovea centralis, a specialized area within the macula of the retina, contains only cones for optimal visual acuity in this part of the retina as the primary focal point. When light strikes

these receptors, a photochemical reaction occurs which initiates graded potentials the retinal cells use to transmit electrical signals. Bipolar retinal cells transmit to second-order ganglion cells with fibers joining to become the optic nerve.

The visual pathway is complex and multifaceted and is illustrated in Figure 7-2. The **visual field** is the "area simultaneously visible to one eye without movement" (Stedman, 2005). With the eyes looking forward, the visual field includes what you see straight ahead and the areas you can glimpse "out

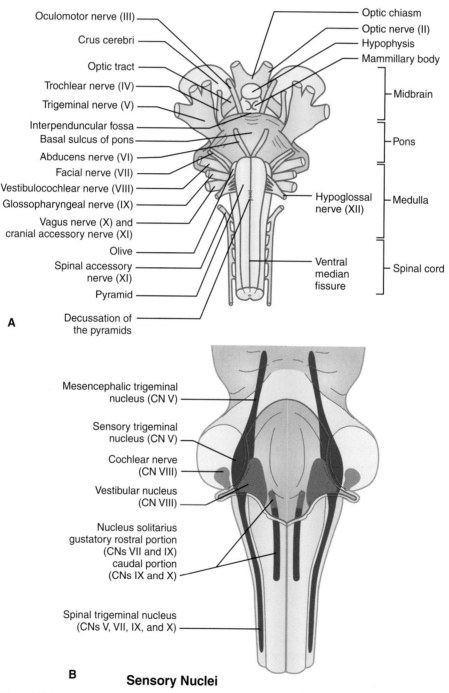

**Sensory Nuclei**

**FIGURE 7-1 A.** Diagram of the surface of the brainstem showing site where each CN emerges. **B.** Stereogram illustrating the location of the major sensory nuclei of the CNs within the brainstem.

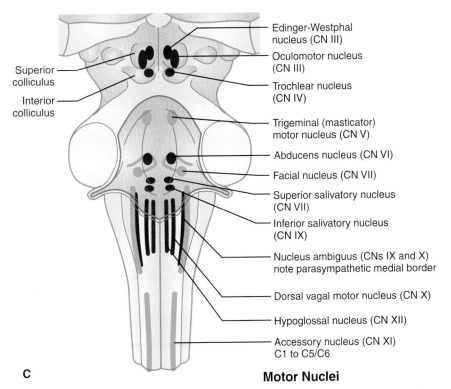

Superior colliculus

Interior colliculus

Edinger-Westphal nucleus (CN III)

Oculomotor nucleus (CN III)

Trochlear nucleus (CN IV)

Trigeminal (masticator) motor nucleus (CN V)

Abducens nucleus (CN VI)

Facial nucleus (CN VII)

Superior salivatory nucleus (CN VII)

Inferior salivatory nucleus (CN IX)

Nucleus ambiguus (CNs IX and X) note parasympathetic medial border

Dorsal vagal motor nucleus (CN X)

Hypoglossal nucleus (CN XII)

Accessory nucleus (CN XI) C1 to C5/C6

**C**

**Motor Nuclei**

**FIGURE 7-1—cont'd  C.** Stereogram illustrating the location of the major motor nuclei of the CNs within the brainstem.

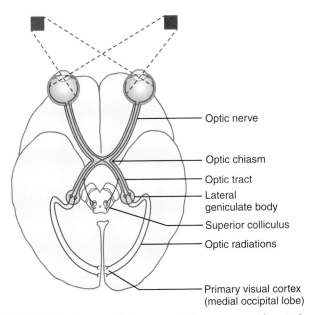

Optic nerve

Optic chiasm

Optic tract

Lateral geniculate body

Superior colliculus

Optic radiations

Primary visual cortex (medial occipital lobe)

**FIGURE 7-2** Diagram of the anatomical structures and central pathways related to vision. This diagram also illustrates the relationship of each half of the visual field to the visual pathway and where the pathways carrying lateral visual fields cross. The image of objects seen in the right visual field (red in this diagram) strike the left half of each retina and travel back through the optic nerve. At the chiasm fibers from the medial half of each retina cross to the optic track on the opposite side. This brings all the fibers of the right visual field together in the left optic tract (and left visual field in the right optic tract) to pass to the appropriate lateral geniculate body and then through the optic radiations to the primary visual cortex.

of the corner of your eye" in any direction without moving your eye. The retinal wall is actually a concave structure within the posterior surface of the eye. Because of the optics involved, the right half of each retina receives visual information from the left half of the visual field. Therefore, an object you glimpse peripherally to your left will reflect on the right half of each retina. The optic nerve running posteriorly from the eye to the optic chiasm carries signals from both halves of the retina for that eye. So damage to the optic nerve results in loss of right and left visual fields (complete blindness) from the eye in question.

Another important anatomical feature is the decussation or crossing of the optic nerve fibers that originate from the medial half of each retina through the **optic chiasm**. This decussation allows the fibers from the two eyes carrying information from the same visual field to join together for the remainder of the visual pathway. For example, an object you glimpse in your right peripheral vision, which would strike the lateral half of the left retina and the medial half of the right retina (i.e., left half of each retina), would be carried in both optic nerves. In this same example, at the optic chiasm, the fibers from the medial half of the right retina would cross through the optic chiasm (see Fig. 7-2) to join the fibers from the lateral half of the left retina. Functionally, this crossing is significant in that the visual pathway structures on each side posterior to the optic chiasm carry only information from the contralateral visual field as shown in Figure 7-2, regardless of the eye in which the signal originates.

From the optic chiasm, the **optic tract** extends posteriorly to the lateral geniculate body of the thalamus, the last relay before projection to primary cortex. Fibers from the lateral geniculate body pass through the subcortical white matter as the optic radiations that terminate in the **primary visual cortex** of the medial occipital lobe. It is important to note that, because of the optics and the pathway decussation, the right visual cortex processes all information related to the left visual field from each eye and vice versa.

## Taste

The special sense of **taste** is mediated through CNs VII, IX, and X. Taste buds are chemical receptors located on the tongue and epiglottis. Action potentials are initiated by chemical reactions of the food with the receptor cells in taste buds. CN VII carries taste impulses from the anterior two-thirds of the tongue. CN IX carries taste impulses from the posterior third of the tongue and the pharynx. CN X carries taste impulses from the epiglottis. Each nerve transmits to specific CN nuclei located in the brainstem (see Table 7-1). Ultimately, the signal from all three passes to the solitary nucleus, which sends signals that ascend ipsilaterally to the ventral posteromedial (VPM) nucleus of the thalamus as the final relay before projection to the opercular cortex, adjacent to the inferior end of the precentral and postcentral gyri. This primary taste cortex is next to but distinct from the primary somatosensory cortex for touch sensation on the tongue.

## Auditory

CN VIII carries the special sense of hearing. First, the external sensory stimulus, vibration, is transmitted into the inner ear where the receptors are located. The sound or vibration travels through the external auditory canal causing the tympanic membrane to vibrate. Vibration of the tympanic membrane conveys vibration through a series of bony ossicles in the air-filled middle ear, which each act as an amplifier of the signal as it passes from malleus to incus and finally to the stapes. The stapes then transmits the vibration through the membrane of the oval window into the fluid-filled inner ear.

The receptor cells within the cochlea of the inner ear are hair cells along the length of the membranous spiral **organ of Corti**. The organ of Corti is tonotopically organized with the basal portion of the cochlea designed to receive highest frequency/pitch and the apical portion best suited to receive lowest frequency sounds. The hair cells send their information through the bipolar spiral ganglion cells to cochlear nuclei of the upper medulla. Eventually, information passes to the inferior colliculus of the midbrain and the medial geniculate body of the thalamus before finally reaching the primary auditory cortex, the **transverse temporal gyri of Heschl,** located in the portion of the superior temporal gyrus extending into the lateral fissure.

## ■ Functional Implications

Normal operation of the CNs is important for a number of specific functions and contributes to safety and protection. The special senses of smell (CN I), vision (CN II), and taste

(CN VII, IX, and X) all have important implications related to motivation of the patient. Many patients are more motivated to move or perform certain functional tasks if their senses provide an additional basis or reason for the movement. For example, imagine the patient's motivation to walk to the other side of the room to see the grandchild. For some patients, the smell of freshly baked chocolate chip cookies and the promise of the rewarding taste may enhance their motivation to walk to the kitchen area. The sense of smell also contributes to safety, equipping the person to smell smoke from a fire. Olfaction also contributes to appetite, which may affect the quantity of food consumed and resulting energy as related to activity level. Hearing live music from a common area may entice a patient to walk to that area of the home or facility. When a person is unable to see certain parts of the visual field from one eye or both, there is decreased ability to use visual feedback and instruction. Weakness or imbalance of extraocular eye muscles (CN III, IV, and VI) can also result in disturbed vision in the form of **diplopia** or double vision. Hearing (CN VIII) is essential for the patient to receive auditory feedback and instructions regarding therapeutic exercise and therapeutic activities.

Motor production of speech is often interrupted by damage to CN structures. The basis of speech production lies in coordinated movement of the tongue (CN XII), pharynx (CN IX), lips and cheeks (CN VII), jaw (CN V), and vocal cords (CN X) with respiratory support primarily from the diaphragm supplied by the phrenic nerve (innervated by spinal levels C3, 4, and 5). In addition to the spoken message, another major part of communication results from the nonverbal cues of facial gestures and facial expression (CN VII). Neck and scapular movements can be impaired from sternocleidomastoid and upper trapezius dysfunction from CN IX damage. Protection of the face and eyes is enhanced by normal sensibility of facial skin with innervation from CN V.

### PATIENT APPLICATION

*Biova is a 48 year-old African male who sustained a traumatic brain injury (TBI) in a motor vehicle accident 2 months ago. Radiographic imaging studies confirmed that the CNS pathology was primarily confined to the right side of the brainstem, especially pons and medulla. In addition to the motor paralysis on the left side of the trunk and extremities with impaired motor control and lack of isolated movements, he has deficits of his right face/head related to several cranial nerves. Initially, the therapist must observe, measure, and document the cranial nerve deficits that we'll explore for this patient case as this chapter is developed. The intervention for Biova's specific deficits and other similar patients will be addressed within the related "Intervention" chapters of Section IV.*

## ■ Tests and Measures of Cranial Nerves

When testing the CNs, it is important to systematically organize your examination, which will enhance completeness of your testing. It is helpful to test the CNs in numerical order as described in this chapter, with some grouping, so you will not skip important components. Use the sensory and motor testing techniques as described in the two previous chapters while applying the techniques and distributions specific for the nerve being tested as described in the remainder of the chapter. For motor and sensory testing of CNs in patients with neuromuscular dysfunction, it is particularly important to test for symmetry of function in the face. Table 7-2 provides a summary of classification (motor, sensory, and special sensory) and specific functions for each CN.

## Cranial Nerve I Examination

The **olfactory nerve** consists of bipolar SVA neurons as described earlier with cell bodies and chemoreceptors in the nasal mucosa. Keep in mind there are important and significant interactions of smell with other systems including emotion,

| TABLE 7-2 | Classification and Specific Functions for Each Cranial Nerve | |
|---|---|---|
| **CRANIAL NERVE** | **CLASSIFICATION: FUNCTION** | |
| I Olfactory | Sensory (SVA) | • Special sense of smell. |
| II Optic | Sensory (SSA) | • Special sense: Visual field, visual acuity, sensory aspect of pupillary light reflex. |
| III Oculomotor | Motor (GSE) | • Extraocular movement (adduction, elevation, depression), eyelid elevation. |
| | Motor (GVE) | • Parasympathetic: Motor aspect of pupil reflex, pupil diameter. |
| | Sensory (GSA) | • Proprioception from four eye muscles. |
| IV Trochlear | Motor (GSE) | • Extraocular movement (depression of adducted eye). |
| | Sensory (GSA) | • Proprioception from superior oblique muscle. |
| V Trigeminal | Motor (SVE) | • Motor: Movement of jaw (masseter, pterygoid) and tensor tympani muscle. |
| | Sensory (GSA) | • Sensory: Facial skin sensation (three divisions), sensory aspect of corneal reflex. |
| VI Abducens | Motor (GSE) | • Extraocular movement (abduction of eye). |
| | Sensory (GSA) | • Proprioception from lateral rectus muscle. |
| VII Facial | Motor (SVE) | • Motor: Muscles of facial expression (smile, wink, pucker, close the eye), motor aspect of corneal reflex; buccinator muscle, stapedius muscle. |
| | Motor (GVE) | • Parasympathetic: Lacrimal and salivary glands. |
| | Sensory (SVA) | • Special sense: Taste from anterior two-thirds of tongue. |
| | Sensory (GVA) | • Visceral sensory. |
| VIII Vestibulocochlear | Sensory (SSA) | • Special sense: Hearing. |
| | Sensory (SSA) | • Special sense: Vestibular (sensibility regarding position of the head in space). |
| IX Glossopharyngeal | Motor (SVE) | • Motor: Stylopharyngeus muscle & motor innervation to pharynx for swallowing. |
| | Motor (GVE) | • Parasympathetic: Parotid salivary gland. |
| | Sensory (SVA) | • Special sense: Taste from posterior third of tongue. |
| | Sensory (GVA) | • Sensory: Sensation of pharynx, tonsils, and carotid; sensation from posterior third of tongue, sensation from external ear, sensory aspect of gag reflex. |
| X Vagus | Motor (SVE) | • Motor: Movement of pharynx, larynx, and soft palate, motor aspect of gag; speech (vocal quality). |
| | Motor (GVE) | • Parasympathetic GVE: To heart, vessels, lungs, and gastrointestinal systems. |
| | Sensory (GVA) | • Sensory: From respiratory, cardiovascular, and gastrointestinal systems, sensation from external auditory canal. |
| | Sensory (SVA) | • Special sense: Taste from epiglottis. |
| XI Spinal Accessory | Motor (SVE) | • C1-C5 spinal root fibers: Neck rotation (sternocleidomastoid muscle), scapular elevation and adduction (upper trapezius). |
| | | • Cranial root fibers: Form the recurrent laryngeal nerve of CN X for vocal cord control. |
| XII Hypoglossal | Motor (GSE) | • Movement of tongue contributes to articulation of spoken language and eating/swallowing. |
| | Sensory (GSA) | • Sensory: Proprioception from tongue muscle. |

*SVA = Special Visceral Afferent; SSA = Special Somatic Afferent; GVA = General Visceral Afferent; GSA = General Somatic Afferent; SVA = Special Visceral Efferent; GSE = General Somatic Efferent; GVE = General Visceral Efferent (parasympathetic).*

memory, salivation, and secretion. Regarding movement, the sense of smell can have important implications for motivation.

### CN I Special Sense: Olfactory Screening

While not typically part of the therapist's examination, olfactory testing may be helpful in identifying impairments related to feeding and swallowing. You should test the integrity of the olfactory system using items or liquids with common and recognizable smells such as coffee, orange, vanilla, or cinnamon. First, have the patient blow the nose to more clearly expose the receptors in the nasal mucosa (Barker, 1992). Avoid use of substances such as ammonia or alcohol that can irritate the mucosa. Ammonia can stimulate CN V (Trigeminal nerve) rather than the olfactory nerve and provide a false positive result. Test one open nostril at a time by presenting the substance and asking the patient, with eyes closed, to identify the recognizable smell. More specific quantitative examination of olfactory dysfunction has been described elsewhere (Doty, 1992).

### Abnormal CN I Findings

As with any sensory impairment, the loss of smell sense can be partial, retaining some ability to smell, or complete with no remaining smell sensibility. Common problems such as cigarette smoking, cocaine use, inflammation, rhinitis, or sinus problems can interfere with the ability to smell. The term **anosmia** is used to describe a complete absence of the sense of smell. Because of the location of this nerve, anosmia is often related to head injury, particularly with damage to the anterior base of the skull.

## Cranial Nerve II Examination

The **optic nerve** also consists of bipolar neurons, but fibers are classified as SSA with rod and cone receptors and their cell bodies located in the retina. While physical therapists may perform the visual screening methods described in this section, occupational therapists may perform more definitive testing and ophthalmology professionals may perform definitive acuity and visual field examinations and also test aspects such as color vision, astigmatism, and observation for retinal health.

### CN II Special Sense: Visual Acuity Screening

To screen for visual acuity, use a **Snellen chart** printed on a pocket card for portability or a Snellen wall chart as shown in Figure 7-3. Have the patient stand 20 feet from the wall chart and read the lowest line of type possible. Alternatives to the Snellen chart include charts with visual symbols that children can recognize and the use of figures such as a series of capital "E"s with the lines pointing up, down, right, or left for individuals who cannot read. Read the visual acuity measure from the chart adjacent to the lowest line the patient can read. For example, 20/40 visual acuity means the person is able to read at 20 feet what the average person can read from 40 feet.

### CN II Special Sense: Visual Field Screening

Perform screening of the visual field of each eye separately using confrontation testing. Sit in front of the patient,

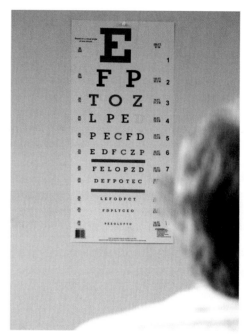

**FIGURE 7-3** Using a Snellen chart for visual acuity screening.

face-to-face to assure they do not move their eyes, and ask the patient to close one eye as the therapist closes the corresponding eye. For example, the patient closing the left eye while you close your right eye allows you to compare visual fields with the patient. The patient is asked to stare at your left eye with the open right eye and not to move the eye. In the most commonly used test, you can use a brightly colored small object or your wiggling fingers as the visual object. Start with the object placed laterally beyond the normal periphery of vision. Slowly bring the object toward midline, testing the lateral visual field of this eye, until the person reports they see the object moving (see Fig. 7-4). An alternative form of the test, to eliminate confusing the patient with the movement of the therapist's arm, involves the therapist seated in front of the patient with an assistant seated behind the patient (out of view). The assistant then moves the wiggling fingers on one side from behind the patient's ear, progressively more

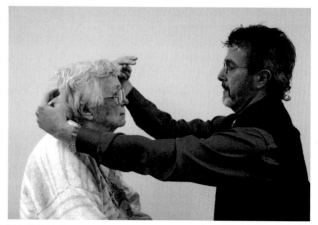

**FIGURE 7-4** Visual field testing (therapist in front of patient).

anteriorly until the patient can identify the movement. Assuming visual fields are intact in each individual, the patient and therapist should see the object at about the same time. Then, test the same eye from the opposite side of the head to test the extent of the medial visual field. Continue to test from top and from bottom of the visual field. To be more complete, you could present the confrontation object from each diagonal direction, also screening the four quadrants of the visual field (right upper, right lower, left upper, left lower). Also check for central areas of visual field loss by moving the object across the visual field while asking the patient to continue to focus on your eye and to inform you if there are any locations where they lose sight of the object. Finally, apply the examination procedure to the other eye. You will end up with a separate visual field map of the extent of intact central and peripheral vision for each eye.

### CN II Sensory Component of Pupillary Light Reflexes

A normal pupillary **light reflex** requires intact visual sense to detect light as the sensory stimulus that initiates the reflex. Test the pupillary light reflex by shining a penlight into one eye. You should see a rapid constriction of the pupil (**direct light reflex**) of the same eye followed by a prompt dilation of the same pupil when the light is eliminated. You should also see a similar response in the contralateral pupil even though the light is not shined into that eye (**consensual light reflex**) because of pathway fibers that cross in the pretectal area of the midbrain. The initial size of the pupils should be the same and the response of the two pupils to light should be equal. As with any reflex, observing the reflex requires both the sensory and motor components to be intact. The motor component of this reflex is carried out by parasympathetic fibers within the oculomotor nerve (CN III).

### Abnormal CN II and Parasympathetic CN III Findings

Abnormal visual acuity may occur related to abnormal focal lengths within the ocular structures with inability to focus clearly. Possibilities include being nearsighted (**myopia**) in which the person cannot see clearly at distances and farsighted (**hyperopia**) in which the person can see most clearly at distances but can not see things up close. Cloudy vision can result from **cataracts** in which the lens of the eyes becomes cloudy or opaque. Cataracts also allow less light from the environment to reach the retina. Any of these acuity deficits will interfere with a person's ability to see fine details with clarity, including reading written directions or observing a demonstration of an exercise or therapeutic activity.

In neurological visual field loss, the deficits often occur in half of the visual field, called *hemianopsia,* which by convention is usually named for the portion of the field of vision lost and not the portion of the retina that is dysfunctional. The most commonly encountered visual field deficit in patients with neuromuscular diagnoses is contralateral **homonomous hemianopsia** in which there is an inability to see half of the visual field in each eye (the same half from each eye) opposite

to the cerebral pathology. As an example, you could observe a right homonomous hemianopsia in a person if visual pathways or structures are affected in a left-sided stroke or brain injury.

Macular degeneration will result in a loss of central vision while vision around the peripheral field will remain intact. A patchy or sporadic distribution of visual field loss can occur from the patchy CNS demyelination of multiple sclerosis. Complete loss of vision from the entire field of one eye results from damage to the optic nerve anterior to the optic chiasm. An optic chiasm lesion, usually related to a pituitary tumor, will result in **bitemporal hemianopsia** with loss of the temporal or lateral visual field from each eye (opposite halves from each eye; i.e., right half of visual field from right eye and left half of visual field from left eye). Common visual field deficits are shown in Figure 7-5.

Considering both the sensory and motor components of the papillary light reflex, comparison of the pupillary light reflexes of each eye can help identify the location of a CNS lesion. If light shined in one eye causes a consensual reflex but no direct reflex, this indicates the afferent component of the reflex (visual sense) in the eye being tested is intact, but the effector component (parasympathetic motor fibers from CN III) is not working in the eye to which the light is directed. Disruption of the sensory component of the reflex in one eye (CN II) would result in no direct or consensual light reflex when light is shined into the affected eye, but in the same patient, light shined in the other eye would result in both direct and consensual light reflexes.

## Cranial Nerve III, IV, and VI Examination

The **oculomotor nerve** (CN III), **trochlear nerve** (CN IV), and **abducens nerve** (CN VI) will all be considered together from a testing standpoint because they each primarily contribute to GSE lower motor neuron innervation for muscles that move the eye within the orbit. The oculomotor nerve carries innervation to the levator palpebrae muscle, which elevates the eyelid to open the eye and innervates four muscles that move the eye. The oculomotor nerve also supplies parasympathetic GVE fibers to the iris to constrict pupil diameter. The trochlear nerve innervates one eye muscle and the abducens nerve innervates one eye muscle. These **extraocular muscles**, their innervation, and their actions are summarized in Table 7-3. These nerves also carry afferent proprioception (GSA) from these same muscles.

### CN III, IV, VI Motor: Testing for Extraocular Function

One of the key elements of extraocular motor function is production of **conjugate eye movements**, coordinated movement of both eyes such that the two eyes almost always move in the same direction at the same speed and to the same magnitude. The only exception in normal extraocular function is normal convergence of the eyes. Before testing for conjugate eye movements, note the relative position of the two eyes at rest. The eyes should have a parallel alignment and appear as if they are looking in the same direction. From directly in

Visual field loss

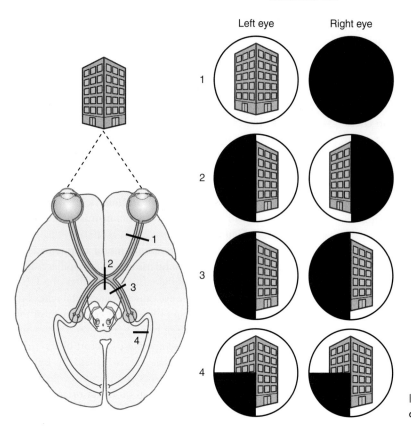

FIGURE 7-5 Diagram of common visual field deficits.

| TABLE 7-3 | **Innervation and Actions of Extraocular Eye Muscles** | |
|---|---|---|
| **EXTRAOCULAR MUSCLE** | **CN INNERVATING MUSCLE** | **ACTION OF THE MUSCLE** |
| Medial rectus | CN III | Adducts the eye |
| Superior rectus | CN III | Elevates the eye |
| Inferior rectus | CN III | Depresses the eye |
| Inferior oblique | CN III | Elevates the adducted eye; and extorts (externally rotates) the eye |
| Superior oblique | CN IV | Depresses the adducted eye and intorts (internally rotates) the eye in forward-looking position |
| Lateral rectus | CN VI | Abducts the eye |

while you observe for conjugate eye movements. Conjugate eye movement is always in the same direction, at the same speed, and in the same angular degree of movement. Conjugate eye movements will always result in parallel gaze with both eyes looking in the same direction. You can test for conjugate movement, including all three nerves at one time, by asking the patient to follow the tip of your finger with eye movement only, keeping the head straight forward with no head movement. Slowly trace an "H" pattern in front of the patient's face (see Fig. 7-6) to create conjugate eye movements

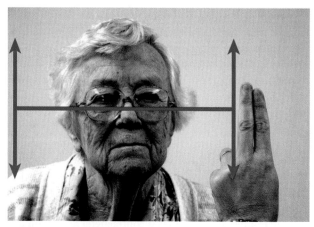

FIGURE 7-6 Photo showing the path used for oculomotor testing using an "H" pattern to test full elevation and depression at the extremes of right and left movement.

front of the patient, note the position in the pupil of light reflections from light sources in the room. Normally, the light reflections should have a similar position in each pupil.

Eye movements are tested by asking the patient to visually follow a moving test object (e.g., pen cap, finger, or eraser) following your finger. The two vertical side lines of the "H" remind you it is important that you ask for full elevation and depression of the eye while both the adducted and abducted position to look for movement deficits. Various combinations of muscles must be coordinated during these conjugate eye movements. Upward and downward movements of the eyes require that the same muscle act in each eye, but horizontal movements require unique combinations of extraocular muscles and therefore CNs. For example, moving the eyes to the right requires simultaneous and coordinated contraction of the right lateral rectus (right CN VI) and the left medial rectus (left CN III). You should also test for **convergence** by asking the patient to visually follow your fingertip with eye movement only as you progressively move your finger in the midline closer to the patient's face. This will cause the eyes to begin to angle toward each other through simultaneous contraction of the medial rectus of each eye.

Test innervation of the levator palpebrae muscle by asking the patient to open the eyes wide. Look for symmetry in eyelid elevation as an indication of equal innervation of the two sides.

### CN III Parasympathetic Motor Component of Pupillary Reflexes

Pupillary light reflex testing and implications of abnormal findings have been described earlier in this chapter. Pupil reflexes are dependent on parasympathetic motor fibers carried by CN III to cause pupil constriction. Therefore, it is important to look at pupil diameter at rest in normal lighting followed by observing pupil constriction bilaterally as an indication of CN III function as the penlight is shined into either eye. In addition, observe for the pupillary response of bilateral constriction when the patient focuses on near objects such as reading a newspaper. This normal response is described as "pupils reactive to accommodation." A normal response on a pupillary examination is often indicated in the medical record with the acronym PERRLA, which stands for "Pupils Equal Round Reactive to Light and Accommodation."

### Abnormal CN III, IV, and VI Findings

When observing resting eye positions relative to each other, you may note that the eyes are not properly aligned when the patient attempts to look straightforward. This is most often due to a specific weakness or muscle imbalance of the extraocular muscles, pulling one eye out of alignment to some degree. The unaligned eye is said to exhibit **strabismus** and can be further delineated as external or internal strabismus. External strabismus describes an affected eye that is deviated laterally while internal strabismus is directed medially. In extreme cases, a strabismus may result in blurred or double vision (diplopia). If the eyes appear to be differently aligned but the reflection of room lights are similarly placed on each cornea, then the term **pseudostrabismus** is applied.

Eye movements that are not coordinated are termed **nonconjugate** or **disconjugate** eye movements, often related to paralysis of specific extraocular muscles. The patient may be able to move the eyes conjugately in several of the planes tested, but in particular directions, movement is not possible

or weak resulting in eyes that are not aligned at the extremes of movement. For example, if a person has a CN VI palsy on the right with paralysis of the right lateral rectus, normal vision and near-normal alignment at rest may be observed. But when asked to glance toward the right, the right eye would not be able to move to the right, resulting in internal strabismus of the right eye and a horizontal diplopia with the two images side-by-side. While these signs occur with ipsilateral gaze, there would be no diplopia or abnormal alignment seen during contralateral gaze. Similarly, a CN III palsy results in horizontal diplopia when gazing to the nonaffected side as well as external strabismus because of medial rectus paralysis. If one of the muscles elevating or depressing the eye is paralyzed, a vertical diplopia would result with one of the images just above the other.

CN III damage could also result in an inability to raise the eyelid on the affected side, a condition termed **ptosis** (pronounced "toe-sis"). Ptosis most often occurs in association with a widespread motor paralysis of one side of the facial muscles related to stroke or head injury that disrupts the face portion of the primary motor cortex homunculus. Severe ptosis can result in obstruction of the upper half of the visual field in the affected eye and may require facial surgery.

Abnormal pupil size is often associated with CN III pathology. A CN III palsy would result in a dilated pupil (**mydriasis**) on the affected side and unequal pupil sizes (**anisocoria**) with the affected pupil being wider than the nonaffected side. The pupil on the affected side would not constrict during direct or consensual light reflex testing.

Incidence, etiology, and recovery of acquired eye muscle palsies have been described for a large sample (Tiffin, 1996). Among specific acquired palsy of oculomotor, trochlear, and abducens nerves, CN VI is most common (57%) followed by CN IV (21%) and CN III (17%) while mixed palsies accounted for only 5%. The same study showed 35% of cases were of unknown etiology and 32% had a vascular basis. Of all patients, 57% made a total recovery with a median time of 3 months, and 80% made at least a partial recovery.

> *Remember our patient Biova? Upon voluntary eye movement, he reports onset of diplopia, both horizontal and vertical. With specific extraoccular testing, it is determined that, for his right eye, he has impaired ability to adduct, abduct, elevate, or depress the eyeball as well as mild ptosis of the right eye.*

## THINK ABOUT IT 7.1

Given Biova's deficits on testing:

- What cranial nerves are involved?
- What muscles are involved?

## Cranial Nerve V Examination

The **Trigeminal nerve** (CN V) is a mixed motor and sensory nerve that mediates numerous functions of head and neck structures. The motor component includes SVE fibers innervating the muscles that move the jaw for chewing (**mastication**) and talking. This nerve also innervates the tensor tympani muscle that dampens vibration of the tympanic membrane to reflexively decrease the intensity of sound when loud noises occur. The three distinct sensory branches of CN V—ophthalmic, maxillary, and mandibular—each carry tactile sensation from the face, forehead, cheek/upper jaw, and lower jaw regions, respectively, and from other anterior head structures including the teeth and the cornea. In addition, CN V also carries proprioception (GSA) from the muscles of mastication.

### CN V Motor: Movement of Jaw and Jaw Jerk Reflex

Ask your patient to open and close the jaw and note the degree of active movement. Note whether both sides are moving equally. Next add mild resistance for a modified manual muscle test to jaw opening and closing to assess the relative amount of force the jaw muscles can generate for these two motions, being very careful not to let your hand slip off or allow the patient's mouth to close suddenly. To test the jaw jerk reflex, ask the patient to open the mouth slightly, then tap downward on the chin (see Fig. 7-7) watching and feeling for reflexive closure of the jaw. Jaw closure should be accomplished by symmetrical contractions of the masseter and temporalis muscles.

### CN V Sensory: Sensation of Face

Test tactile sensation of the face just as sensation in other regions of the body, usually with an open safety pin or paperclip to test sharp/dull or a cotton wisp to test light touch. With the three divisions of the nerve, you should test the face systematically, including all three divisions (see Fig. 7-8). First, test several locations on the forehead bilaterally (ophthalmic branch), then the upper jaw and cheek region (maxillary branch), and finally over the bilateral lower jaw (mandibular branch).

### CN V Sensory Component of Corneal Reflex

Before testing for the **corneal reflex**, explain the procedure to patients to minimize any anxiety they may have about something touching their eye. Prepare a wisp of several strands of

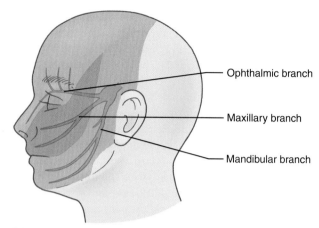

**FIGURE 7-8** Diagram showing three divisions of facial sensory innervation from the Trigeminal nerve. It is important to test sensibility in all three divisions.

cotton fibers from a clean cotton ball. With both the patient's eyes open, lightly touch the cotton fiber to the cornea of one eye. Sensory afferents from the cornea are carried through CN V. The response you should see includes rapid closure of eyelids of both eyes using orbicularis oculi muscles with motor innervation from CN VII.

### Abnormal CN V Findings

A lesion to CN V will result in anesthesia and loss of general senses of the face and anterior head on the affected side, including the ipsilateral corneal sensation. Therefore, both ipsilateral and consensual corneal reflex will be lost. A paralysis of jaw muscles will also occur with asymmetric jaw movement and jaw jerk reflex if the pathology is unilateral.

**Trigeminal neuralgia**, also called **tic douloureux**, is a pathological condition related to CN V function and characterized by brief but repeated sharp excruciating pain in the distributions of the Trigeminal nerve often accompanied by motor tics of facial muscles (through CN VII) which occur reflexively.

> *In testing facial sensation of our patient Biova with traumatic brainstem injury, he has obviously impaired, but present, tactile sensation of right face (forehead, cheek, and lower jaw).*

## THINK ABOUT IT 7.2

Take a moment to review the procedures you would use to test Biova's facial sensation.

## Cranial Nerve VII Examination

The **facial nerve**, CN VII, is primarily a motor nerve but with sensory components. The motor division of the nerve provides lower motor neuron SVE innervation for the subcutaneous muscles of facial expression and buccinator and stapedius muscles. The muscles of facial expression are extremely important for self-image and verbal communication. Parasympathetic

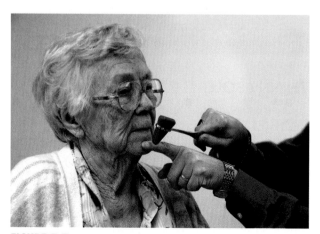

**FIGURE 7-7** Jaw jerk reflex testing.

preganglionic GVE fibers supply the lacrimal glands and the salivary glands as well as blood vessels of the head. SVA afferents of CN VII receive taste from the anterior two-thirds of the tongue.

### CN VII Motor: Facial Expression

Testing muscles of facial expression is simple but very important. Observe the patient's face with attention to symmetry and particular muscle groups with profound functional significance. Observe for wrinkles in the forehead and ask the patient to voluntarily wrinkle the forehead and compare sides. Ask the patient to close the eyes tightly, and you can provide resistance by trying to pull the eyelids open. Finally, ask the patient to close the lips tightly, to move the lips purposefully (pucker), and to "smile." Compare the angles of the mouth on each side. You can also provide resistance to the elevation at the corner of the mouth. Use Figure 7-9 to practice looking for subtle facial asymmetry (note the slight droop of the right side of the mouth and more crinkled skin of right cheek during smile).

The corneal reflex has been explained previously. Orbicularis oculi action, innervated by CN VII, closes the eye as the motor component of this reflex.

### CN VII Special Sense: Taste

The special sense of taste can be easily screened on the anterior two-thirds of the tongue with taste buds innervated by CN VII. If there is any concern about possible impaired swallowing, an appropriate referral or evaluation, perhaps by a speech-language pathologist, should be completed even though actual food items are not administered. Only minute quantities of testing material (examples in parentheses in the following section) are used and, in some cases, the tongue is only touched with a dipped cotton swab. Wear gloves for protection because of the potential exposure to blood/body fluids. The taste buds at the most anterior portions, the tip, of the tongue are most sensitive to "sweet" tastes (sugar), taste buds on the edges of the middle of the tongue are most sensitive to "salty" (salt), and taste buds located along the posterior lateral edges of the tongue are most sensitive to "sour" (vinegar) (Montmayeur, 2002). Most posteriorly are the taste buds that are most sensitive to "bitterness" (bitter strong coffee brew). You can blindfold the patient then ask to distinguish between common and recognizable tastes, naming them or at least specifying a category: sweet, salty, or sour. Do not use sugar for sweet tastes if the patient is diabetic.

### Abnormal CN VII Findings

CN VII dysfunction results in impairment of the corneal reflex. The person is unable to blink but corneal sensibility remains intact, carried by CN V. Disturbed taste sensibility may result in a decrease in appetite and nutritional health.

With **Bell's palsy** (unilateral peripheral CN VII dysfunction), paralysis of the upper and lower face on the affected side occurs (Fig. 7-10A). Bell's palsy will include loss of wrinkles in the forehead, sagging corner of the mouth with impaired smile, and increased drooling related to poor oromotor and lip function. The person will also be unable to close the eye on the affected side. However, they can open the eye and raise the eyelid on the affected side because CN III innervates the muscle that elevates the eyelid.

Facial weakness or paralysis related to cerebral hemisphere damage as opposed to peripheral nerve or nucleus damage is characterized by motor impairment primarily of the lower face, cheek, and mouth. The lower face paralysis is contralateral to the site of cortex damage. The forehead musculature will be less affected or not affected in cerebral damage due to dual innervation of the forehead musculature by motor cortex in each cerebral hemisphere. Figure 7-10B illustrates facial motor dysfunction of central etiology (cortex or deep white matter) with motor impairment primarily of the contralateral lower face. (Remember, peripheral damage of CN VII nucleus or nerve is associated with motor impairment usually of contralateral upper and lower face.)

---

#### PATIENT APPLICATION

*Biova has impaired motor control of the right facial muscles of expression because of the traumatic injury to the right medulla. Specifically, he exhibits no wrinkles in right forehead at rest and especially when he tries to raise his eyebrows; he is unable to close his right eye voluntarily; and the right side of his mouth does not rise when he smiles. The asymmetry in these voluntary facial movements is quite obvious.*

---

### Contemplate Clinical Decisions

1. *Anatomically, why do cranial nerve impairments frequently occur as one expression of TBI, as happened with Biova?*

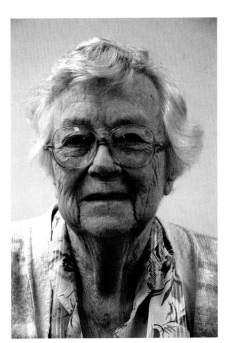

**FIGURE 7-9** Use this photograph to practice your observation skills. Can you identify the subtle asymmetries in motor function as seen in facial motor innervation, creases, and wrinkles?

2. *How could it be logical that his motor impairments are predominant on the left side of his body but the right side of his face?*

3. *In addition to the motor impairment of the right side of his face, what other cranial nerves will be important to test, and what is the functional implication of deficits of each?*

## THINK ABOUT IT 7.3

What cranial nerve(s) are involved given Biova's facial asymmetry, and is the damage likely central or peripheral?

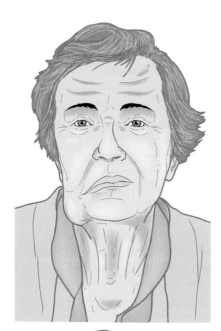

A

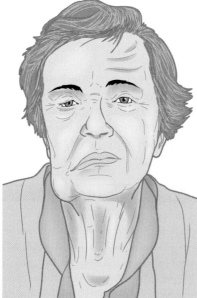

B

**FIGURE 7-10** Clinical presentation of facial motor dysfunction from: **A.** central or cortex etiology causing contralateral impairment primarily of lower face (e.g., left MCA cerebrovascular accident causing droopy right cheek and mouth) compared with **B.** peripheral etiology causing ipsilateral upper and lower face impairment (e.g., Bell's palsy with dysfunctional right CN VII causing droopy right forehead, inability to close right eye, and sagging right cheek and mouth).

## Cranial Nerve VIII Examination

The **vestibulocochlear nerve** is made up of two portions. The cochlear nerve consists of bipolar neurons transmitting auditory signals that we perceive as sound. The vestibular nerve also consists of bipolar neurons transmitting signals from the three semicircular canals, the utricle, and the saccule of the vestibular apparatus. This section of the chapter will focus on the auditory portion of this nerve as the details of the vestibular examination are covered in Chapter 8.

### CN VIII Auditory Screening

You can screen for auditory function by whispering a different number into each ear and then ask the patient to repeat the number heard, or you can rub your fingers together alternately next to each ear with equal intensity and ask, "Can you hear both equally?" In neonates and children, you can screen for auditory function by making a sudden noise (ring a bell, click a clicker, etc.) and observing the child's reaction.

Tuning forks (512-Hz or 256-Hz) can be used to test for sensorineural versus conductive deafness. For the **Weber test**, which is both sensitive and reliable (Golabek, 1979), strike the tuning fork and place the base of the vibrating fork in the middle of the patient's head just above the center of the forehead (Fig. 7-11). Ask the patient if the ringing is louder in one ear. Normally, the sound should be fairly equal in both ears. The **Rinne test** compares bone and air conduction using a tuning fork. Figure 7-12 shows (A) placing the base of a ringing tuning fork on one mastoid process and asking the patient, with eyes closed, to tell you when the sound is *no longer* heard. Then (B), immediately move the vibrating tines in front of the ear on the same side and ask the patient if the vibration is heard again. The patient should still be able to hear the sound through the air even after the bone conduction

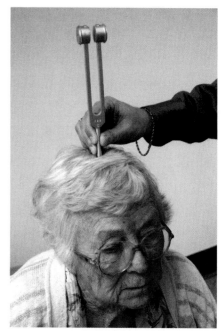

**FIGURE 7-11** Use of the tuning fork to perform Weber's test for auditory screening.

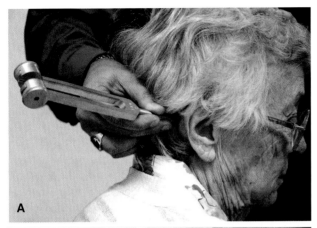

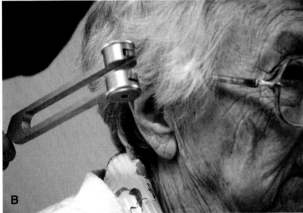

**FIGURE 7-12** The Rinne test, to screen air conduction versus bone conduction of sound. **A.** Test bone conduction by placing the post of the vibrating tuning fork on one mastoid process until the patient no longer hears the sound. **B.** Then move the tines of the vibrating fork next to the external auditory canal and the patient should be able to hear it again.

has ceased. In other words, air conduction is greater than bone conduction.

With sensorineural deficits in one ear, the Weber test will seem louder in the unimpaired ear, and for the Rinne test, air and bone conduction are both decreased but air conduction still lasts longer than bone conduction. With conduction deafness, the sound will seem louder in the affected ear because of enhanced perception by bone conduction, and on the Rinne test, bone conduction lasts longer than air conduction so the patient will not hear through air conduction after bone conduction has ceased.

### CN VIII Vestibular Examination

A detailed explanation of examination of the vestibular system is presented in Chapter 8.

## Cranial Nerve IX and X Examination

The **glossopharyngeal nerve** (CN IX) and **vagus nerve** (CN X) will be considered together because of common aspects of testing. The glossopharyngeal nerve carries sensory input from the pharynx, and taste and touch from the posterior third of the tongue, and supplies motor innervation to

the pharynx with a major role in early swallowing. The vagus nerve carries sensory information from major visceral organs plus parasympathetics to the gastrointestinal, cardiovascular, and respiratory systems. The vagus also supplies motor innervation to the soft palate, pharynx, and larynx.

### CN IX, X Motor: Pharynx/Palate Testing

While you are positioned in front of the patient with a penlight, ask the patient to vocalize a sustained "ahh…." Observe the soft palate movement for symmetry. The uvula should remain in the midline as each side of the soft palate elevates equally throughout the vocalization (Fig. 7-13). You may need to use a tongue depressor to keep the tongue down and out of the way as you observe the soft palate and uvula. You can also assess the patient's general ability to swallow through your history and review of systems. Any suspected problems with swallowing should be assessed by a speech-language pathologist. The potential impact on communication is addressed in Chapter 4.

### CN IX, X Gag Reflex Testing

Intact sensory and motor functions of the pharynx can be confirmed by testing the **gag reflex**. Sensory input from the pharynx is carried by CN IX while the motor innervation to the pharynx is carried by CN X. To test the gag reflex, touch a tongue depressor gently to the back of the pharynx. This should cause a gag and, with a penlight, allow you to observe a symmetrical contraction of the pharynx and a symmetrical contraction and rise of the soft palate with the uvula remaining midline.

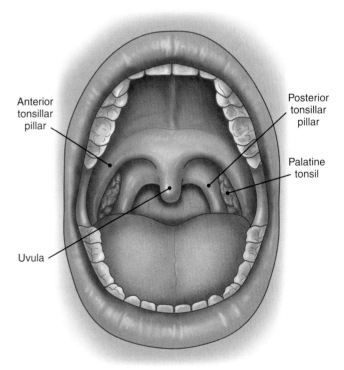

Anterior tonsillar pillar

Posterior tonsillar pillar

Palatine tonsil

Uvula

**FIGURE 7-13** Illustration of symmetrical rise of the soft palate and midline uvula, which would be seen in a normal neurological examination when the patient is asked to say "Ahh." *(From: Weaker, F. Structures of the Head and Neck. Philadelphia, PA: F.A. Davis; 2014.)*

### CN IX Special Sense: Taste

Taste through CN IX is tested just as previously described with CN VII but specifically using bitter tastes. Also, to test the taste portion of CN IX, the bitter substance must be specifically applied to the posterior third of the tongue where taste buds for "bitter" are most heavily concentrated.

### Abnormal CN X Findings

If one side of the soft palate is paralyzed from a CN X lesion, that side of the palate will rise less than the nonaffected side. You will see the uvula deviate toward the nonaffected side. Paralysis of the soft palate will also affect vocal abilities and quality. Paralysis of the pharynx will result in severe difficulty with swallowing, which is a poor prognostic sign among patients with stroke (Mann, 1999).

## Cranial Nerve XI Examination

The **Accessory nerve** is also called the **spinal accessory nerve** because it has spinal roots that emerge from C1–C5 levels of the spinal cord and ascend to join the cranial roots emerging from the medulla lateral to the olive. The cranial roots then continue with the vagus nerve and ultimately separate as the recurrent laryngeal nerve supplying the larynx. The spinal roots continue as CN XI and innervate the pair of sternocleidomastoid muscles in the neck and the upper fibers of the trapezius muscle of each scapula responsible for elevation of the scapula.

### CN XI Motor: Sternocleidomastoid

To test the integrity of the sternocleidomastoid muscles as an indication of CN XI function, ask the patient to rotate the neck fully to one side. You can also add resistance to perform a specific manual muscle test. **Dynamometry** could also be used and would particularly be helpful in comparing strength measures of one side to the other. Keep in mind, the sternocleidomastoid muscle causes lateral flexion of the neck toward the same side while rotating the neck to the opposite side.

### CN XI Motor: Upper Trapezius

The upper fibers of the trapezius elevate the scapula with adduction toward the cervical spine. You can perform a manual muscle test of the upper trapezius by asking the patient to shrug the shoulders followed by shoulder shrugging against graded resistance. Dynamometry again could be very helpful.

### Abnormal CN XI Findings

The person with an Accessory nerve lesion would exhibit the unique combination of weakness in rotating the neck to the opposite side and weakness/paralysis in elevating the scapula on the ipsilateral side.

## Cranial Nerve XII Examination

The **hypoglossal nerve** innervates the musculature of the tongue. The tongue is essential in numerous functional tasks but particularly chewing, swallowing, and speech articulation. During chewing tasks, the tongue is continually repositioning the food bolus to optimize the chewing effect on the food. Individuals have the ability to tense the tongue and move it in all directions. Some people have amazing motor control of their tongue and can perform unique actions especially after practice. To complete the act of tongue protrusion, the individual must tense the tongue musculature and then contract bilateral muscles at the base of the tongue, which draws the tongue forward as a unit.

### CN XII Motor: Tongue Movement

Test tongue movement by asking the patient to stick the tongue out, straight forward. As previously explained, this movement requires a unique and complex coordination of tongue musculature. You can also ask the patient to move the tongue from side-to-side while protruded. Visually, you can observe how tongue movement coordinates with a swallowing motion as well. You can resist tongue movement by asking the patient to push the tongue up while you push down on the tongue with a tongue blade or have the patient push out on the cheek with the tongue while you press the cheek in from the outside (Barker, 1992).

### Abnormal CN XII Findings

The person with paralysis of the tongue will have significant difficulty with speech, chewing, and swallowing. Upon specific motor testing of the tongue, the tongue will deviate toward the paralyzed side upon voluntary protrusion. This occurs because the muscles on the functional side can draw that side of the tongue forward as the tongue protrusion begins, but the affected side of the tongue does not move forward and the protruding tongue deviates toward the affected side. Remember that, because of the CNS design, paralysis of one side of the tongue might result from ipsilateral lower brainstem damage affecting the ipsilateral CN XII motor nucleus, tracts, or nerve or from damage to contralateral cerebral cortex or subcortical white matter pathways. Thus, with a unilateral medial brainstem lesion, the patient will exhibit the unique combination of contralateral limb paralysis (from corticospinal damage) and ipsilateral tongue paralysis (from CN damage).

---

**PATIENT APPLICATION**

*Thinking about our patient with TBI to the right brainstem, when Biova tries to stick out his tongue, his tongue does protrude somewhat but deviates toward the right side because the left side can translate forward but the base of the right side of the tongue cannot move forward.*

---

## ■ Documentation of Cranial Nerve Examination/Evaluation

In documenting the results of the CN examination, it is important to clearly specify and quantify, if possible, any motor or sensory deficits. At a minimum, the therapist should document when an abnormality exists and whether the abnormality is a complete absence of nerve action or just a partial impairment of the CN. It is also essential to document the effect of such impairments on functional tasks related to CN function, much of which has to do with face and neck tasks and visceral function.

Evaluation of the combinations of CN symptoms can give clues as to the location of CNS pathology. This is particularly true when comparing distribution of brainstem symptoms with general body symptoms. For example, if a patient has sensory deficits on one side of the body but on the opposite side of the face (e.g., right arm, trunk, and leg, but left face), this is a clinical scenario described as **alternating hemianesthesia**, the most likely location of pathology is a unilateral brainstem lesion, especially laterally in the brainstem. This occurs because most sensory pathways have crossed in either the spinal cord or the low medulla before they ascend through the lateral brainstem. Most sensory CN nuclei and nerve roots are also located laterally. Therefore, pathology to the lateral brainstem on the right side would affect lower motor neurons and first-order sensory neurons associated with the right side of the face while sensory pathways originating in the left side of the body would be affected.

A related situation occurs after a unilateral medial brainstem lesion because most motor CN structure lie medially and the crossed primary motor pathway, lateral corticospinal tract, also runs medially within the brainstem. Such a lesion, perhaps from basilar artery or vertebral artery infarct, would cause paralysis of the ipsilateral face and neck with a contralateral paralysis of the trunk and extremities, an **alternating hemiplegia**.

## Pediatric Examination of Cranial Nerves

Some of the methods previously described could be used in a pediatric population unable to follow specific directions or give specific verbal descriptions of deficits. In this case, the therapist will have to observe for appropriate reactions to stimuli given and observe for spontaneous voluntary muscle movement of the target muscles.

At least one specific infant assessment has been developed as a simple quantifiable examination (Haataja, 1999). This assessment includes five specific items regarding CN functions with the highest score for each item given for the following characteristics: facial appearance (smiles, closes eyes, grimaces), eye appearance (normal conjugate eye movements), auditory response (reacts to bell or rattle on both sides separately), visual response (follows a red ball for a complete arc), and sucking/swallowing (good suck and swallow).

## HANDS-ON PRACTICE

Be sure to practice the following skills from this chapter. With further practice, you should be able to:

- Test integrity of the olfactory nerve (CN I).
- Perform a visual screening examination (CN II) using a Snellen chart and adapt testing for a pediatric patient and for individuals who cannot read.
- Perform a visual field screening (CN II) with and without a second person to assist you.
- Test the pupillary light reflex (CN II).
- Test conjugate eye movements (CN III, IV, VI)–"H" pattern and convergence.
- Test innervation of the levator palpebrae muscle (CN III).
- Test sensation of the face (CN V).
- Test the jaw jerk reflex (CN V).
- Test the corneal reflex (CN V).
- Test the muscles of facial expression (CN VII).
- Perform a screening examination for taste (CN VII).
- Screen for auditory function (CN VIII).
- Perform the Weber test (CN VIII).
- Perform the Rinne test (CN VIII).
- Complete motor testing of the palate/pharynx (CN IX).
- Test the gag reflex (CN IX, X).
- Test integrity of the Accessory nerve (CN XI).
- Test tongue movement (CN XII).

## Let's Review

- For each cranial nerve, describe the purpose and function of each portion:
  - Motor
  - Sensory
  - Autonomic

- Describe the tests and measures you would choose to determine the integrity of each cranial nerve.

- Given any cranial nerve deficit, describe the effect the deficit would have on function.

- Given any cranial nerve deficit, identify the corresponding area of the brainstem affected.

- Given any cranial nerve deficit, document appropriately the results of your patient examination.

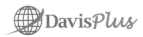 For additional resources, including Focus on Evidence tables, case study discussions, references, and glossary, please visit http://davisplus.fadavis.com

# CHAPTER SUMMARY

To summarize key aspects of the CN examination, Table 7-4 lists the major tests used for clinical examination of CN function as part of the neurological examination along with potential abnormal findings for these tests. The therapist should include CN testing for any patient with possible brainstem or cranial injury, including any traumatic injury, in addition to neurological disease of the brain or brainstem. As with all areas of neuromuscular examination, the therapist should utilize tests and measures with evidence to support their use. Table 7-5, the Focus on Evidence (FOE) Table online (ONL), summarizes some of a representative sample of research evidence for CN tools and measures, including available studies that explored reliability, validity, sensitivity, and specificity. A thorough examination of CN function will often pick up subtle signs of CNS abnormality that have been previously overlooked and may have significant implications for therapeutic intervention.

## PATIENT APPLICATION

*To explore another case with a different CNS diagnosis, consider Janie, who for all of her 33 years of life has been healthy and never hospitalized except for the labor and delivery of her boys, now 4 and 6 years old. This recent onset of symptoms expressed in the head and face region over the past 2 months has been most perplexing in its progressive development even to her physician. She was diagnosed just 2 weeks ago with multiple sclerosis, primarily with bulbar symptoms (CN symptoms related to white matter plaques of either subcortical white matter or brainstem white matter as detected on CT scan). She has recounted to you an unusual pattern of both motor and sensory loss that is bilateral but asymmetric.*

*While the motor and sensory examination for her trunk and all four extremities revealed only mild right knee weakness with knee extensor motor control stability impairment (including genu recurvatum in midstance of gait), you detect the following significant findings on the neurological examination. She has a patch of visual field deficit in the right lower quadrant of each eye. She has weakness and impaired motor control around*
*the mouth at the right corner with drooling. She has poor control of extraocular movements of the left eye with ptosis on the right and asymmetry of jaw closure with weakness on the right. The patient also reports recent onset of difficulty swallowing; in particular, swallowing now takes a longer time than usual.*

### Contemplate Clinical Decisions

*For this patient, take a moment to consider the following:*

1. *Which CN is responsible for normal function related to each of the described deficits? (visual field, facial muscles around the mouth, extraocular movements and eyelid elevation, jaw closure)*
2. *Because multiple sclerosis is a CNS demyelinating disease, the pathology is not in the cranial peripheral nerve itself, the related cortex, or the CN nuclei. So what are the possible white matter areas in which lesions could create these symptoms, including related subcortical white matter or tracks that connect the cortex to the CN nuclei or tracks from the CN before they exit the brainstem?*

| TABLE 7-4 | **Summary of Cranial Nerve Testing and Abnormal Results** | |
|---|---|---|
| **CRANIAL NERVE** | **TESTS** | **ABNORMAL TEST RESULTS** |
| I | • Sense of smell with common and recognizable odors: Coffee, vanilla, citrus, etc. | • Impaired or absent sense of smell |
| II | • Sensory component of pupillary light reflexes (direct and consensual) | • Impaired or absent pupillary light reflexes (direct and consensual) with penlight in affected eye |
| | • Visual acuity screening with Snellen chart | • Impaired visual acuity |
| | • Visual field screening by confrontation testing | • Impaired visual field (hemianopsia…) |
| III | • Eye lid elevation | • Ptosis |
| | • Extraocular eye movements (elevation, depression, adduction, and elevation of adducted eye) | • External strabismus on affected side and unable to elevate or depress the eye, unable to adduct the eye |
| | • Motor component of pupillary light reflexes | • Asymmetric pupils (anisocoria) with dilated pupil (mydriasis) on affected side; unable to constrict affected pupil to direct or consensual light reflex testing |

| TABLE 7-4 | Summary of Cranial Nerve Testing and Abnormal Results—cont'd | |
|---|---|---|
| **CRANIAL NERVE** | **TESTS** | **ABNORMAL TEST RESULTS** |
| IV | • Extraocular eye movement (depression of the adducted eye) | • Vertical diplopia when looking downward (i.e., walking down stairs) and compensatory head tilt to opposite shoulder |
| V | • Sensory testing of face (forehead, upper jaw, lower jaw) | • Impaired or absent tactile sense of face (forehead, upper jaw, lower jaw); sharp, excruciating pain associated with Trigeminal neuralgia |
| | • Sensory component of corneal reflex | • Lack of blink when touching cornea with cotton wisp |
| | • Movement of jaw | • Impaired movement (or paralysis) of jaw (lack of chewing) |
| | • Sensory and motor component of jaw jerk reflex | • Impaired or absent jaw jerk reflex |
| VI | • Extraocular eye movement (abduction of eye) | • Internal strabismus and unable to abduct eye |
| VII | • Movement of muscles of facial expression (wrinkle forehead, close eye, smile, etc.) | • Paralysis of one side of face with lack of wrinkles and folds in upper and lower face; corner of mouth sags with drooling; unable to close eye on affected side<br>• With cortex lesion, paralysis is primarily to lower half of face on the affected side. Upper face and forehead (frontalis and orbicularis oculi) are less affected because of dual innervation from the motor cortex of each hemisphere. |
| | • Motor component of corneal reflex | • Impaired corneal reflex (though corneal sensitivity is intact) |
| | • Taste to anterior two-thirds of tongue | • Loss of taste sense from anterior two-thirds of tongue |
| VIII | • Screen for hearing, including bone versus air conduction | • Loss of hearing |
| | • Vestibular function (see Chapter 8) | • Loss of awareness of position of head in space, with consequent impairment of balance |
| IX | • Swallowing and motor pharynx | • Difficulty swallowing<br>• Deviation of uvula to unaffected side |
| | • Taste to posterior third of tongue | • Loss of tactile sense and taste from posterior third of tongue |
| | • Sensory component of gag reflex | • Unilateral loss of gag reflex and carotid reflex |
| X | • Movement of palate: say "Ahh" | • Flaccid soft palate and dysphagia |
| | • Motor component of gag reflex | • Loss of gag reflex |
| | • Autonomic function | • Transient tachycardia (rapid death if bilateral) |
| XI | • Motor muscle test of sternocleidomastoid | • Inability to rotate head with chin to opposite side (sternocleidomastoid) |
| | • Motor muscle test of upper trapezius | • Inability to elevate scapula on affected side |
| | • Vocalization | • Dysphonia if cranial root or recurrent laryngeal nerve damage |
| XII | • Tongue protrusion and symmetry | • Ipsilateral paralysis of tongue, deviation to affected side with attempted protrusion |

# Examination and Evaluation of Vestibular Function

**CHAPTER 8**

Noi Bernabe Mavredes Fraker, PT ▪ Cheryl Ford-Smith, PT, DPT, MS
Bridgett Wallace, PT, DPT ▪ Dennis W. Fell, PT, MD

## CHAPTER OUTLINE

## CHAPTER OBJECTIVES

Upon completion of this chapter, the learner should be able to:

1. Describe the key aspects of anatomy and physiology of the vestibular system and the implications of specific disorders.
2. Describe the normal functions of the vestibular system.
3. Analyze clues from the medical history and clinical examination findings to differentiate between peripheral and/or central dysfunctions.
4. Select appropriate vestibular testing methods for a given patient scenario.
5. Differentiate normal from abnormal on the vestibular examination tests and measures.
6. Explain specific vestibular test results and implications for treatment decisions.

## ▮ Introduction

The vestibular system is the sensory system that plays a dominant role in postural control, eye-head coordination, and perception of our orientation in space. Dysfunction in the vestibular system may result in unsteadiness, dizziness, and/or misperceptions about movement of the body or head in space. Dizziness and balance disorders are a frequent complaint to physicians (Maarsingh, 2010; Jonsson, 2004; Tinetti, 2000; Sloane, 2001). One large epidemiological study reported an estimated 69 million Americans have experienced some form of vestibular dysfunction (Agrawal, 2009). Studies also show dizziness is the third most common complaint to physicians (Warner, 1992), and in 85% of patients reporting these symptoms, the cause is vestibular dysfunction (Guzmán, 2001). Balance impairment is one of the most important risk factors

for falls and injuries. From 1999 to 2013, more than 25,000 fall deaths occurred among people ages 65 and older resulting in the leading cause of death due to unintentional injury in the United States (CDC, 2015). Research shows declines in balance occur even in the context of typical geriatric pathological changes. Hip fractures are the most common result from a fall (Parkkari, 1999), however, the elderly rarely report falls to caregivers or family (CDC, 2003). One of the most difficult issues facing health-care providers is formulating an accurate diagnosis and effective treatment plan. Part of the challenge is that dizziness is a vague term and does not provide the examiner with any specific information about the possible pathology. Dizziness is also a common symptom secondary to a number of disease processes and is one of the most common side effects of prescription medication. Even outside the context of the effect on balance, vestibular dysfunction can result in significant fear and avoidance and even emotional distress associated with activity and participation restrictions (Yardley, 2004; Hillier, 2011) that limit an individual's engagement in society and life roles. Therefore, an efficient and effective examination is essential to identify appropriate interventions to restore activity and participation.

The purpose of this chapter is to discuss the clinical examination and evaluation of individuals with vestibular disorders. Key aspects of anatomy and physiology of the vestibular system are reviewed as well as the effect of common vestibular disorders and the most important tests and measures. By the end of this chapter, the reader should be able to analyze clues from the medical history and clinical examination to differentiate between peripheral and/or central vestibular dysfunction. First, dizziness will be categorized to provide the reader with a framework to explore the individual's symptoms and obtain clues from the initial examination to assist in formulating a working diagnosis based on the patient's subjective report.

## Getting Specific About Dizziness

**Dizziness**, a generic term referring to a sense that one is about to fall, is often the chief complaint (and referring diagnosis) in patients with vestibular dysfunction. Dizziness affects 20% to 30% of the general population (Neuhauser, 2007). Dizziness, however, is a nonspecific umbrella term that does not always have the same meaning for everyone. So, it is essential to gain a deeper more specific understanding of what the patient is experiencing and attempting to describe. The best way may be to simply ask the individual to describe the symptoms(s) without using the word dizziness. It may be helpful to ultimately categorize the symptoms into the following three categories (Karatas, 2008):

1. **Vertigo** is an illusion of movement, which always includes a subjective sensation of spinning or rotation with the individual feeling as if (1) the room is spinning, (2) the individual is spinning within the room, or (3) the individual is spinning inside his head. The individual may also describe a sudden "falling" sensation with the vertigo. Symptoms of vertigo can be associated with peripheral and/or central pathology as described in the BPPV, Vestibular Hypofunction, and Ménière's Disease outlines in the Compendium of Medical Diagnoses found after the last chapter, and later in this chapter. Asymmetric involvement of the vestibular system may lead to vertigo due to the mismatch of vestibular signals from the right and left sides.

2. **Lightheadedness** is often experienced as giddiness or feeling faint while feeling that loss of consciousness may occur and is usually a less localizing symptom. Lightheadedness is commonly associated with a nonvestibular disorder such as hypoglycemia, orthostatic hypotension, and/or anxiety.

3. **Unsteadiness** is commonly described as feeling off or almost falling usually with a fear of falling. Some individuals may relate their unsteadiness to their feet, which is suggestive of loss of sensation and/or lower extremity weakness. Some also describe a drunk-like intoxicated

feeling common in both peripheral and central vestibular disorders.

## ▮ Categories of Vestibular Testing

Testing related to the vestibular system, including the influence on balance, can be divided into three categories: **functional approach testing**, **system approach testing**, and **quantitative computerized posturography** (Nashner, 2004). Laboratory testing including rotary chair, bithermal caloric testing, or computerized dynamic visual acuity testing can also be part of the vestibular examination. The functional approach is used to identify whether or not a balance problem exists that affects function and whether it is related to vestibular dysfunction. The functional assessment tools such as the Dynamic Gait Index, Functional Gait Assessment, Berg Balance Scale, modified Clinical Test of Sensory Interaction on Balance, Fukuda Stepping Test, Balance Evaluation Systems Test, and Timed Up and Go are included in this category. These tools rate the performance of the individual during various tasks to help identify functional limitation and the capacity to do a particular task or activity in a specific context. This approach helps determine a patient's balance capacity in relation to their age. These tools are helpful in determining baseline balance and gait status and in reexamination for changes in performance after intervention. Self-assessment questionnaires help determine a client's level of participation in his or her environment and measure how the symptoms are perceived as a limitation in daily activities. The Activities-specific Balance Confidence scale (ABC) and the Dizziness Handicap Inventory (DHI) are common self-assessment questionnaires utilized with patients who have suspected vestibular impairment. Many of the functional balance assessment tools are described in detail in Chapter 9. The system approach usually refers to examination of musculoskeletal, neuromuscular, and other systems of the body related to vestibular function. This system approach is used to determine underlying body structure/body function causes of the problem and therefore can help guide intervention. Systems examination identifies the disorder subcomponents such as biomechanical factors, motor control/coordination, and sensory organization constraints. When using this approach, it is important to differentiate these primary constraints from secondary constraints (e.g., use of hip strategy due to decreased range of motion [ROM] or presence of weakness in the lower extremities). The evaluation of the systems, vestibular testing and physiological tests, fall under the system category. The quantitative posturography approach uses technology to measure forces at the surface, electromyography (EMG) patterns, and analysis of strategies for specific tasks. The rotary chair, caloric testing, computerized dynamic visual acuity (DVA) testing, and electronystagmography/videonystagmography (ENG/VNG) are also technological approaches in physiological vestibular evaluation. ENG/VNG testing can provide information on whether the dizziness and/or balance problem is caused by a peripheral (inner ear) and/or central nervous system dysfunction. While rotary chair testing assesses VOR function at slower speeds that are less associated with daily living activities, rotary chair is sensitive to detect bilateral vestibular loss. More sophisticated technology is available today through high velocity head rotation testing and can better assess higher demands of the VOR function related to quick head turns movements we perform on a daily basis. These active head rotation systems are often computerized, with recent incorporation of infrared video to more objectively measure the corrective saccades noted in the head thrust test (MacDougall, 2009). These systems can measure the smaller correct saccades (covert saccades that are not otherwise observable), and indicate vestibular disruption. Comprehensive audiometric testing is a useful diagnostic procedure helpful with the vestibular evaluation, which can often aid in determining the specific pathology and even the site of the lesion associated with dizziness. Comprehensive audiometrics should include a pure tone audiogram, tympanometry, speech, and acoustic reflex testing performed by an audiologist. Auditory Brainstem Response

(ABR) can measure how sound signals move from the external ear and along the cochlear nerve to the brainstem as well as other parts of the brain. Electrocochleography (ECoG) can measure how sound signals move from the ear along the auditory nerve and provide information about fluid fluctuations of the inner ear. Vestibular Evoked Myogenic Potential (VEMP) is used to determine whether a specific area of the inner ear (saccule) as well as the inferior vestibular nerve and the connections with the brain are functioning.

## ■ Review of Vestibular Neuroscience

You have previously learned the anatomy and physiology of the vestibular system in a neuroscience course. This section will provide a brief review of the major anatomic components associated with vestibular function. Figure 8-1 (Where Is It?) summarizes the major anatomic areas of the CNS that contribute to normal

■WHERE IS IT?

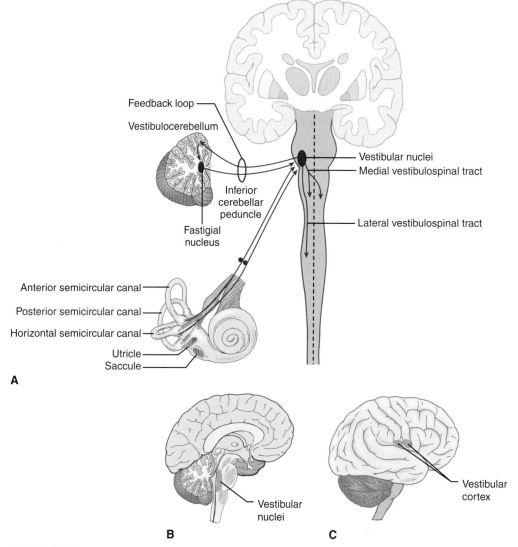

**FIGURE 8-1 A.** Peripheral vestibular apparatus (semicircular canals, utricle, saccule) connected to vestibular nuclei and then to fastigial nucleus of vestibulocerebellum, **B.** vestibular nuclei in the deep brainstem, and **C.** vestibular cortex.

vestibular function including (A) peripheral vestibular apparatus (semicircular canals, utricle, saccule) connected to vestibular nuclei, (B) vestibular nuclei in the deep brainstem, and (C) vestibular cortex. The vestibular system includes a complex dynamic interplay between the three following systems:

1. **Peripheral vestibular system** is composed of the bony labyrinth, the membranous labyrinth, and specialized sensory hair cells all within the inner ear. The inner ear has two distinct divisions: (1) the cochlea for hearing and (2) the vestibular system for sensing position and movement of the head. The bony labyrinth is a cavity located within the temporal bone on each side of the head. The membranous labyrinth is filled with endolymph and suspended in the perilymph. The endolymphatic fluid is maintained at a constant volume and contains specific concentrations of sodium, potassium, chloride, and other electrolytes although the endolymph has a higher concentration of potassium than sodium (Jacobsen, 2015). Within each labyrinth are the three semicircular canals (SCC) and otolith organs. Associated arterial blood is supplied to these peripheral structures primarily through the anterior inferior cerebellar artery. The three SCCs (anterior, posterior, and horizontal) provide the sensory neural input related to angular head acceleration, which is processed to coordinate compensatory eye and head movements via the vestibulo-ocular reflex (VOR). The two otolith organs (utricle and saccule) provide sensory neural input related to linear head acceleration. The utricle senses linear movements of the head in the horizontal plane while the saccule senses linear movements of the head in the vertical plane. Additionally, the utricle and saccule gather information to convey to spinal and leg musculature for balance strategies (ankle, hip, and stepping) via the vestibular spinal reflex (VSR) to stabilize body movement. The otoliths further convey information regarding the direction of gravity through head tilt, which is incorporated into locomotion. This function of the otolith organs is accomplished by otoconia, calcium carbonate crystals that are denser than the surrounding endolymph, which remain partially stable while the head and endolymphatic fluid moves around them. If otoconia become displaced from the utricle into the SCCs, then brief spells of vertigo are experienced related to position changes, a condition called Benign Paroxysmal Positional Vertigo (BPPV). The peripheral vestibular system sends angular and linear information to the central vestibular system via primary afferents of the vestibulocochlear nerve (CN VIII).

2. **Central vestibular system** is comprised of the vestibular nuclear complex (VNC), the group of vestibular nuclei and connections within the brainstem, spinal cord, cerebellum, reticular formation, thalamus, and cerebral vestibular cortex. The majority of the vestibular afferents end in the vestibular nuclei of the brainstem, specifically in the rostral end of the medulla and the caudal pons. The four pairs of vestibular nuclei in the brainstem include the medial, lateral, inferior, and superior vestibular nuclei associated with two important tracts: the medial vestibulospinal tract (MVST) and the lateral vestibulospinal tract (LVST). Connections between the vestibular nuclei, the reticular formation, the thalamus, and cerebral cortex contribute to arousal, conscious awareness of movement through space, and ability to distinguish between movement of the body versus the environment. The cerebellum is referred to as the adaptive processor of the vestibular system and assists in coordination, maintaining posture, and modulation of vestibular reflexes.

3. **Vestibular motor (output) system** is primarily comprised of the **vestibulo-ocular reflex (VOR)**, which produces compensatory movements to control **gaze stability** (ability to fixate on targets during head movements), and **vestibulospinal reflex (VSR)**, which contributes to postural control. The VOR is essentially a reflexive eye movement in response to head movement, which enables humans to maintain visual focus on an object in the environment during body/head motion. The primary function of the VOR is to control the eye position during head movements so as to maintain a stable visual image and therefore contribute to equilibrium. The VOR is a three-neuron arc including (1) the peripheral vestibular primary afferent to the vestibular nuclei, (2) the ipsilateral arc, and (3) contralateral oculomotor nuclei. It activates the six pairs of eye muscles for eye movements. This reflex is highly adaptive and can be modulated by changes in visual stimuli, mental set, and medications. The vestibulospinal reflex carries vestibular input to affect head and body tilt. It communicates the vestibular input, primarily from the otolith organs, to the spinal and lower limb muscles. It interacts with stretch receptor reflexes to produce appropriate muscle contractions when there is change in body position in space and/or movement of the support surface. Thus, the VSR plays a key role in postural stability by mediating use of balance strategies (e.g., ankle, hip, and stepping).

## THINK ABOUT IT 8.1

1. What physical impairments would manifest after injury to the labyrinth of one ear?
2. What are some medical diagnoses that could cause damage to the central vestibular system?
3. How would functional status be affected if the vestibulo-ocular reflex (VOR) is impaired?

## The Vestibular Vascular System

The vertebrobasilar system delivers the main arterial supply of oxygen-rich blood to the posterior aspects of the brain. The two vertebral arteries join to form the basilar artery and all together are referred to as the vertebrobasilar system. The vertebrobasilar arterial system supplies both the peripheral and central vestibular system. The posterior inferior cerebellar artery (PICA) is the largest branch of the vertebral artery, is one of the three main arteries supplying the cerebellum, and is the most important blood supply for the central vestibular system, including the vestibular nuclei of the brainstem. The PICA divides into two branches inferior to the cerebellum. The medial branch continues backward to the notch between the two hemispheres of the cerebellum. The lateral branch supplies the undersurface of the cerebellum then anastomoses with the anterior cerebellar and superior cerebellar branches of the basilar artery.

The anterior inferior cerebellar artery (AICA) arises from the basilar artery at the level of the junction between the midbrain and the pons in the brainstem. It passes backward to distribute blood to the anterior part of the inferior cerebellum, anastomosing with the posterior inferior cerebellar branch of the vertebral artery. It supplies the anterior inferior quarter of the cerebellum. The AICA also gives off the labyrinthine artery, which is the main blood supply for the peripheral vestibular system. The labyrinthine artery is a long slender branch of the AICA that accompanies the vestibulocochlear nerve through the internal acoustic meatus and is distributed to the internal ear.

## Functional Implications

Vestibular system dysfunction can have a profound impact on postural control and functional activities in daily living and participation in life. For most individuals with a vestibular disorder, movement aggravates their symptoms. Consequently, many people start to limit their activities, becoming more sedentary and adopting a rigid head position to minimize their movement-related symptoms. These individuals may also develop a fear of falling as well as anxiety and even depression. For example, in VOR dysfunction, head movement can result in visual blurriness and, in severe cases, **oscillopsia**, the false visual perception that objects are moving in space, usually as swaying back and forth or jumping. It is not uncommon for these symptoms to increase in busy visual environments such as a grocery store or when riding in a car. VSR dysfunction, on the other hand, can result in diminished postural control by decreasing the effectiveness of appropriate balance strategies (e.g., ankle, hip or stepping strategy). Difficulty walking on uneven or compliant surfaces (e.g., carpet or grass) is another common complaint among this population as well as difficulty walking in the dark, in dimly lit environments, or in wide-open spaces. In addition to limiting head movement and avoiding busy visual environments, individuals often ambulate with a wide base of support, frequently holding onto the wall or nearby objects for support. The social and even financial effects of dizziness are significantly underestimated and frequently misunderstood (Neuhauser, 2008).

### PATIENT APPLICATION

*Mrs. Park is a 67 year-old female who presents to the clinic with residual dizziness/unsteadiness since the onset of severe vertigo 5 days ago. She reports that on the day of initial onset of "spinning," she had diaphoresis that was similar to a "bad hot flash." Her symptoms resolved but in the evening she began to feel unsteady and dizzy when walking with her husband. This eventually progressed into nausea, vomiting, and vertigo. She was seen in the ER and was given a diagnosis of labyrinthitis. The severity of these symptoms gradually decreased but never completely resolved. Mrs. Park was seen by an otolaryngologist (ENT) who confirmed viral infection, and ENG revealed complete left unilateral vestibular lesion (UVL). She also had an audiogram, which revealed no significant change in hearing. After the ENT received the audiogram results, her diagnosis was changed to vestibular neuritis. She has a past medical history of allergies, diabetes mellitus Type II (DM), hypertension (HTN), high cholesterol, nodule on left thyroid, chronic anemia, and bowel obstructions. Her past surgical history includes gallbladder removal, hysterectomy, and protocolectomy.*

### Contemplate Clinical Decisions

1. *As the therapist, what is the most important subjective information you have obtained from this patient?*
2. *Based on the previously supplied information, which vestibular examination components do you think will be important to include when examining this patient?*
3. *Are there any other questions you would ask this patient at this point?*

## Principles of Examination of the Vestibular System

### General Considerations

Obviously, the purpose of the examination is to formulate a physical therapy (PT) diagnosis and, above all, a differential diagnosis to identify peripheral and/or central vestibular involvement to guide intervention. Among individuals with vertigo, it has been reported 85% have a peripheral vestibular cause and 15% have a central vestibular disorder (Paparella, 1990). In vestibular rehabilitation, an accurate diagnosis is critical to develop the most appropriate specific plan of care, which includes identifying those individuals who may not be candidates for vestibular rehabilitation and need further referral. A comprehensive initial examination, understanding of the patient's symptoms, and clinical evaluation by an experienced clinician can result in an accurate diagnosis without more extensive workup. It is generally agreed that 80% of the information needed to identify potential causes of symptoms is obtained in the patient interview (Goodman, 2007), thus establishing the basis of a working diagnosis.

Before performing the tests specific to the vestibular system, a thorough clinical examination should be done, including a screen of other body systems (e.g., cardiopulmonary, integumentary, musculoskeletal, and neuromuscular) as well as a thorough review of medical history as defined by the APTA *Guide to Physical Therapist Practice* (APTA, 2015). Providing patients/clients with a structured questionnaire has been reported to be highly predictive of the ultimate diagnosis (Zhao, 2011). Appendix 8-A presents an example of a vestibular examination intake questionnaire. Cervical range of motion should also be examined along with testing for vertebrobasilar insufficiency (VBI) before performing any vestibular tests as a number of the clinical vestibular tests involve motion of the cervical region in a variety of planes, amplitudes, and speeds.

During testing, it is important to understand that you will often intentionally provoke the symptoms the patient is trying to avoid. However, this is an essential part of the diagnostic process, which must be explained to the patient. You must also be prepared for instances of nausea and vomiting (with a trash can or garbage bag at hand). While the risk of vomiting may be minimized if the patient takes an antiemetic such as Zofran or Phenergan before your session, keep in mind that medications for dizziness and/or nausea are vestibular suppressants and will likely interfere with the reliability of your test results. It is also essential to identify what tests exacerbate the symptoms, and you should measure or grade the severity of the patient's symptoms. It is equally important to observe for the latency, timing, and duration of any symptoms that occur.

Communicating with the patient is one of the best tools to use when performing these tests. Make sure you always explain what movements you will be performing, what the examiner expects from the patient, and what the patient may experience during testing. Because your tests will most likely reproduce the very sensation/experience the individual has been earnestly trying to avoid, it is very important that you reassure the patient of the value of your tests to make a specific PT diagnosis and institute intervention. Successful treatment is built upon an accurate diagnosis, thus the examination findings will guide the selection of specific interventions (see Chapter 29) to obtain the most desirable treatment outcomes.

## Screening for Vertebrobasilar Insufficiency

As was briefly described earlier, the vertebrobasilar artery is one of the main systems supplying blood to the brain. Thrombosis, narrowing, or compression of these blood vessels can be life-threatening as it leads to hypoxia and ischemia of the brainstem, which may cause paralysis, difficulty in swallowing, respiratory arrest, or vestibular symptoms. With this in mind, it is important to note that some of the vestibular testing positions may occlude this essential arterial system. Before initiating any vestibular positional testing, particularly with cervical motion, the examiner must test for VBI. Several VBI screening methods have been described but lack validation or documented sensitivity. The United Kingdom National Health Service (2007) proposed a protocol that includes a comprehensive examination, informed consent, and a guideline for VBI testing in sitting or supine position. This VBI test includes (1) cervical rotation to the right for 10 seconds, (2) cervical rotation to the left for 10 seconds, and then (3) head and body position that provokes symptoms. During each movement, observe for and ask the patient to report abnormal responses including sweating, nausea, nystagmus, dizziness, or vertigo. The signs of VBI can be referred to as the "5 Ds and 3 Ns," which are as follows: diplopia (double vision), dizziness, dysarthria (slurred speech), drop attacks, dysphasia, nausea, numbness (unilateral), and nystagmus

(vertical nystagmus). Additional testing movements are considered optional by NHS: cervical extension, combined cervical rotation and extension, and slow simulation of any treatment positions that are anticipated (UK NHS, 2007). The guidelines also state, "It is essential that the patient is allowed 10 seconds rest between each test procedure, and that the test is suspended as soon as symptoms are provoked" (UK NHS, 2007). If VBI signs are observed, the patient should be urgently referred to the physician for medical evaluation and management.

## THINK ABOUT IT 8.2

What might the patient say to you about their symptoms that would make you suspect that they could have a symptomatic VBI test?

## Ruling Out Nonvestibular Disorders

Although vestibular dysfunction is one of the most common causes of dizziness, ruling out nonvestibular disorders should first be considered. One approach is for the examiner to initially categorize vestibular dysfunction clinically into peripheral and central vestibular disorders. As previously explained, a peripheral vestibular disorder refers to dysfunction of the labyrinth, hair cells, and/or vestibular nerve. Damage to the peripheral system may result from an inner-ear infection, a fluid problem of the inner ear, damage to the hair cells, structural problems of the inner ear, or a tumor. However, the literature strongly supports vestibular rehabilitation as effective for alleviating and, in many cases, eliminating symptoms related to peripheral vestibular disorders (Venosa, 2007). A central vestibular disorder refers to dysfunction in the brainstem (including vestibular nuclei), cerebral hemisphere areas that process vestibular function, cerebellum, or spinal cord. Damage to the CNS may be caused by a vascular event (ischemic or hemorrhage), head trauma, demyelinating diseases, and/or tumors. The literature supporting vestibular rehabilitation for central vestibular disorders is not as definitive as that for peripheral disorders. Some specific vestibular conditions are discussed in more detail in the Compendium of Neurological Diagnosis Outlines that follows Chapter 2. Regardless of location, the disorder can be further categorized into unilateral or bilateral as well as acute versus chronic and stable versus nonstable. Table 8-1 contrasts the common characteristics of vertigo as seen in peripheral versus central pathology.

The majority of individuals with dizziness will have already seen a number of health-care providers before therapy and may have frequently been misdiagnosed and misunderstood. Thus, there may be a psychological component related to their symptoms. Medications can also interfere with vestibular testing results (suppressing symptoms and nystagmus) and may actually be hindering the normal recovery process. Studies suggest less than only 50% of patients with a primary symptom of dizziness/vertigo (who have not been seen by a specialist) receive an accurate diagnosis (Squires, 1993) and greater than 70% receive a prescription of meclizine (Burke, 1995). Meclizine causes CNS depression comparable to that of an elevated blood alcohol level and frequently results in drowsiness and decreased reaction times

| TABLE 8-1 | Characteristics of Vertigo in Peripheral Versus Central Pathology | |
|---|---|---|
| | PERIPHERAL | CENTRAL |
| Onset | Sudden (and often follows an illness) | Slow, gradual (although can be sudden and without warning); sometimes associated with medications |
| Intensity | Severe | Poorly defined |
| Duration | Brief, episodic | Longer, constant |
| Nausea/ Diaphoresis | Frequent | Infrequent |
| CNS signs | Absent | Usually present |
| Tinnitus/ Hearing loss | Can be present | Absent |
| Nystagmus | Torsional/ horizontal | Vertical |
| Nystagmus | Fatigable | Nonfatigable |
| Nystagmus | Same direction even with changing head position (excluding horizontal BPPV) | Direction changing without changing direction of the head |

(Manning, 1992). Continuous use of meclizine during rehabilitation diminishes the effectiveness of vestibular rehabilitation techniques (Hain, 2003). In a more recent national survey by the Vestibular Disorders Association (VEDA), it was found that, among patients who had multiple visits to providers without an accurate diagnosis, more than 40% reported perceived limitations in daily activities and more than 52% noted having anxiety, fear, and other psychological effects (Haven, 2011).

## THINK ABOUT IT 8.3

What might be the clinical presentation of a patient with mixed central and peripheral pathology?

## Nystagmus

Another general but key principal of a vestibular examination/evaluation is the understanding of **nystagmus**. Nystagmus is an involuntary, rhythmic, rapid eye movement and is often considered the cardinal sign of vestibular dysfunction with the latency, plane, direction, and duration of nystagmus being critical factors to observe. Nystagmus is critical in differentiating peripheral versus central disorders. Nystagmus characteristically includes a fast phase movement in one direction and a slow phase in the opposite direction. The nystagmus is named based on the direction of the fast phase. For example, a patient with an acute unilateral vestibular lesion (UVL) may

present with a right-beating nystagmus, which indicates the eyes are moving quickly to the right in the horizontal plane, then slowly to the left with each cycle. The fast phase is actually a resetting mechanism that brings the eyes back to their original position while the slow phase represents the involved side of the vestibular abnormality. Therefore, a right-beating nystagmus associated with vestibular dysfunction is typically associated with a left UVL. These characteristics were originally described by Alexander in 1912 and became the basis for vestibular nystagmus known as Alexander's Law. Alexander proposed three degrees of nystagmus: (1) first-degree nystagmus is documented only on lateral gaze, and the fast phase is in the direction of gaze; (2) second-degree nystagmus is a nystagmus present in primary gaze, but the movement increases with gaze in the direction of the fast component; and, (3) third-degree nystagmus is a nystagmus present in all gaze directions. Alexander's Law does not apply to a healthy vestibular system. Nystagmus may occur in a horizontal, vertical, or rotational (also referred to as torsional) plane. A nystagmus that occurs in the same direction regardless of test positions (in reference to eye, head, or body) has a strong likelihood of being a peripheral vestibular disorder especially if the nystagmus decreases with visual fixation. The nystagmus is most intense during the acute phase and decreases over time due to natural central compensation. In other words, in the acute phases, you may be able to see the direction of the nystagmus during the clinical examination (without using more advanced technology). The central nervous system is able to suppress the nystagmus when the eyes are open and can fixate on objects, therefore methods to decrease visual fixation, as described in the following text, are helpful. Central compensation can occur within hours of the onset but, as a general rule of thumb, will subside within 1 to 2 weeks (Leigh, 2015). The nystagmus, however, may still be present or more prominent when visual fixation is prevented or suppressed. More reliable methods for observing nystagmus without fixation include Frenzel lenses, electro-oculography, or infrared video goggles.

**Frenzel lenses**, a special type of magnifying lenses within goggles, make it easier for the therapist to observe nystagmus by providing magnification of the eyes and their movement while also preventing the individual from visually fixating on specific targets in the visual field. Both of these mechanisms increase the likelihood of more accurately observing nystagmus when present. As previously noted, observing if the nystagmus is present with versus without fixation is also an important differential criteria for identifying the etiology. **Videonystagmography** (VNG) **or electronystagmography** (ENG) systems offer more advanced diagnostic information through measuring eye movement under a variety of test conditions. The ENG utilizes superficial electrodes to measure eye movements while VNG uses an infrared camera system mounted in a goggle set. VNG is more widely used today and typically considered the preferred method for vestibular diagnostics. VNG also allows for playback of video to review test findings (Pietwiewicz, 2012). Remember, nystagmus that decreases with visual fixation and/or increases when visual fixation is removed is more indicative of peripheral involvement. If the nystagmus does not decrease or abate with visual fixation, a central lesion is suspected. Two additional findings suggestive of central pathology are nystagmus that changes direction without changing the direction of the head, pure torsional and/or pure vertical nystagmus. These two findings are indicative of possible brainstem and/or cerebellar pathology.

### Functional Classes of Eye Movement

Table 8-2 summarizes the classification of eye movements that may be observed during the vestibular examination. Knowing the types of eye movements and their classifications is key in the evaluation of the vestibular patient.

| TABLE 8-2 | Functional Classification of Eye Movements |
|---|---|
| Vestibular | Eye movement that holds images steady on the retina during brief head rotations. |
| Optokinetic | Eye movement that holds images steady during sustained head rotation. |
| Smooth pursuit | Eye movement that holds the image of a small moving target on the fovea. |
| Saccades | Quick phasic, jumping, eye movements, bring images of moving objects of interest onto the fovea (or if the person is moving through space as in being a passenger of a vehicle). |
| Visual fixation | Eye movement that holds the image of a stationary object on the fovea. |

## Importance of a Thorough History to Formulate a Working Diagnosis

An accurate history is perhaps the single most important component of the vestibular examination to guide selection of tests and measures and is essential for developing the most appropriate treatment plan, especially considering that some diagnostic tests may be inconclusive. The initial history information to gather includes family history; past medical and surgical history; results of previous diagnostic tests; medications used; comprehensive list of symptoms related to dizziness and imbalance; the onset, duration, and frequency of symptoms; and description of activities that exacerbate or relieve the symptoms.

The differentiation of vestibular disorders is highly dependent on clues gained from the history, which can lead to appropriate examination tests/measures. If the individual reports dizziness, the examiner can categorize their symptoms (e.g., spinning, lightheadedness, and/or unsteadiness) then begin to ask questions about the onset, intensity, and duration. These factors can provide invaluable information, especially differentiating among peripheral vestibular disorders. Of course, it is also crucial to identify what activities may increase and/or decrease vestibular symptoms as well as additional symptoms (e.g., auditory changes, visual disturbances, etc.) associated with the individual's primary report of dizziness. As mentioned earlier, the examiner will note whether the individual's symptoms are unilateral versus bilateral, acute versus chronic, and/or stable versus fluctuating. Tables 8-3, 8-4, and 8-5 provide a summary of

| TABLE 8-3 | "Clues from the History" Related to Common Peripheral Vestibular Disorders |
|---|---|
| **PERIPHERAL VESTIBULAR DISORDER** | **COMMON SYMPTOMS** |
| Benign Paroxysmal Positional Vertigo (BPPV): Dislodged otoconia ("ear rocks") in one or more of the semicircular canals | • Short spells of vertigo that are brief in nature (could last up to several minutes)<br>• Symptoms exacerbated by movement in one particular direction, including turning head to right or to the left, lying down, rolling over, looking up, and/or bending over |
| Ménière's Disease: A progressive problem with high pressure of inner ear fluid that most often leads to vertigo spells and hearing loss | • Low frequency hearing loss<br>• Fluctuating hearing loss<br>• Fluctuating fullness/pressure in the ears<br>• Fluctuating tinnitus (noises/ringing in the ear)<br>• Spells of vertigo that are usually minutes to hours and accompanied with nausea and residual imbalance/dizziness<br>• Spells typically spontaneously recover (although may have residual symptoms between spells)<br>• Frequency may vary from years, months, days |
| Vestibular Neuritis: An inner ear infection that is typically caused by a virus | • Sudden onset that often follows another illness and/or stressful event<br>• Duration of vertigo is hours to days<br>• Nausea<br>• No hearing loss<br>• Occurs as a single event in more than 95% of individuals<br>• May have residual imbalance and dizziness with head movements |
| Vestibular Labyrinthitis | • Same as Vestibular Neuritis, but with hearing loss |

| TABLE 8-4 | "Clues from the History" Related to Less Common Peripheral Vestibular Disorders |
|---|---|
| **PERIPHERAL VESTIBULAR DISORDER** | **COMMON SYMPTOMS** |
| Acoustic Neuroma: Nerve sheath tumor found in the internal auditory canal or cerebellopontine angle, often associated with neurofibromatosis-2 | • Asymmetrical hearing loss<br>• Tinnitus<br>• Vertigo does not occur until more advanced stages |
| Ototoxicity: Bilateral peripheral pathology due to damage of the vestibular hair cells usually after receiving antibiotic treatment, particularly IV aminoglycosides | • Unsteadiness with wide-based gait pattern<br>• Vertigo is usually absent<br>• May include hearing loss<br>• Oscillopsia (objects appear to be jumping or moving) |
| Perilymphatic Fistula (PLF): An abnormal connection between the middle and inner ear through the round or oval window, allowing perilymph to leak into the middle ear space | • Dizziness/vertigo<br>• Hearing loss<br>• Oscillopsia<br>• Exacerbated by coughing, sneezing, lifting<br>• May follow head trauma, barometric pressure trauma |
| Superior Canal Dehiscence: The roof of the superior (anterior) semicircular canal is missing, resulting in hearing and balance symptoms | • Symptoms of dizziness and imbalance with loud noises and/or changes in intracranial pressure (coughing)<br>• Hennebert's sign: Eye movements induced by external auditory canal pressure in the affected ear<br>• Complaints of hearing the heartbeat in the affected ear and hearing a swishing sound with eye movements (gaze-evoked tinnitus) |

| TABLE 8-5 | "Clues from the History" Related to Nonvestibular Disorders |
|---|---|
| **NONVESTIBULAR DISORDER** | **COMMON SYMPTOMS** |
| Anxiety | • Shortness of breath<br>• Tingling sensations around the mouth and occasionally in extremities<br>• Lightheadedness |
| Mal de Debarquement Syndrome (MdDS): Etiology is uncertain (thought to be an error with internal model of sensory processing; also a migraine component is suspected) | • Primarily associated with residual "rocking" sensations after being on a boat, train, or plane<br>• Most common in women (30–40 years of age)<br>• Previous testing (including vestibular) is often normal<br>• Symptoms are typically worse with movement and improved (if not alleviated) with movement |
| Neurological Conditions | • Diplopia<br>• Symptoms are constant with difficulty describing exacerbating and alleviating factors<br>• Could have a PMH of dementia, seizures, CVA, TBI, neurodegenerative diseases, demyelinating diseases, hereditary diseases, Parkinson disease, medications, toxicity |
| Vascular Impairment (reduced blood flow to peripheral vestibular and central balance centers) | • Arrhythmias<br>• Symptoms with supine-to-sit-to-stand<br>• Cervicogenic symptoms: occur with cervical extension (and rotation)<br>• Drop attacks<br>• Headache (Migraine-Associated Vertigo) and difficulty with speech<br>• Medication |

"clues" that can be obtained from the history related to peripheral vestibular disorders.

# Specific Vestibular Examination Tests and Measures

This section includes key components of the vestibular examination/evaluation, including special vestibular tests, which should be performed as part of a comprehensive neurological examination. An example is shown in the documentation section that follows.

## Questionnaires

Determining the physical, emotional, and functional effect of any impairment is important to gain a greater understanding of the patient's perceived limitations in daily activities and to assist with intervention planning. Several self-report questionnaires provide reliable valuable background information regarding the effect of vestibular disorders. These questionnaires also provide standardized measurements that should be repeated to monitor the patient's progress throughout the rehabilitation process.

### Dizziness Handicap Inventory (DHI)

One widely used questionnaire is the Dizziness Handicap Inventory (DHI) (Table 8-6), which measures the patient's perception of their handicap (Jacobson, 1990). It could be considered a quality of life (QoL) questionnaire. The DHI consists of 25 questions answered by "yes," "sometimes," or "no," then scored using a corresponding point system of 4, 2, and 0, respectively, with total scores ranging from 0 (perceived absence of disability) to 100 (perceived maximal presence of disability). The questionnaire can be completed by the patient (before the interview/examination) or by the examiner with adequate to excellent construct validity (Jacobson, 1990; Perez, 2001; Alghwiri, 2011). However, construct validity was reported as questionable in one study (Duracinsky, 2007) because the patients had chronic pathology spanning over several years and may not have been representative of the population with dizziness. Mean DHI score ± s.d. among patients with vestibular dysfunction was 32.7 ± 21.9 (Jacobson, 1990) and 25.8±18.7 among individuals with unilateral vestibular loss (Mbongo, 2007).

### Activities-specific Balance Confidence Scale (ABC)

Another popular questionnaire is the Activities-specific Balance Confidence (ABC) scale (shown in Fig. 9-7) measuring the elderly patient's level of confidence in performing common daily activities without loss of balance and fear of falling. The ABC consists of 16 functional activities upon which the individual self-rates on a continuum scale of 0% to 100% confident with "0" representing no confidence and "100" representing complete confidence. The ABC score has been shown to be lower in elderly patients with

| TABLE 8-6 | Summary of Dizziness Handicap Inventory (Jacobson, 1990) | |
|---|---|---|
| Domain of the Dizziness Handicap Inventory | • Number of Questions<br>• Max number of points* | Areas the questions explore: |
| Functional | • 9 questions<br>• Max 36 points | Impact of the condition on function (restrict travel, difficulty getting into or out of bed, restrict social activity, difficulty reading, avoid heights, difficult to do strenuous housework or yardwork, difficult to go for a walk alone, difficult to walk around home in the dark, interfere with job/household responsibilities?) |
| Emotional | • 9 questions<br>• Max 36 points | Impact on emotions (feel frustrated, afraid to leave home without someone else, embarrassed in front of others, afraid people might think one is intoxicated, difficult to concentrate, afraid to stay home alone, feel handicapped, stress on relationships, depressed?) |
| Physical | • 7 questions<br>• Max 28 points | Specific movements that cause dizziness (looking up, supermarket aisle, strenuous activities, quick movements of head, turning in bed, walking down a sidewalk, bending over) |
| TOTAL | 100 points (minimum score is 0)<br>The higher the score, the greater the perceived handicap due to dizziness; 0 = no perceived disability | |

Total Score >18 has 94% specificity for BPPV (Whitney, 2005)
Minimal clinically important difference for DHI is 11 points. (Tamber, 2009)
Among patients with vestibular dysfunction: Mean 32.7 ± S.D. 21.9 (Jacobson, 1990)

*Each item is scored: 4 for "Yes," 2 for "Sometimes," and 0 for "No".
Jacobson GP, Newman CW. The development of the dizziness handicap inventory. *Arch Otolaryngol Head Neck Surg,* 1990;116:424-427.

decreased mobility and is highly correlated with the DHI for patients over 65 years of age (Duracinsky, 2007). Scores less than 67% indicates a risk of falling, and it can accurately classify people who fall 84% of the time (Lajoie, 2004). A minimally clinically important difference has not been determined for patients with vestibular dysfunction.

### Vestibular Disorders Activities of Daily Living (VADL)

The VADL was designed by Cohen (2000) to determine the effect of vestibular impairment on everyday activities. It includes 28 items grouped in 3 areas: functional, ambulation, and instrumental (home management and leisure activities). Each item is scored on a 10-point Likert-type scale from 1 (independent) to 10 (too difficult, no longer perform). Some researchers consider the content and wording of the items on the VADL vague and not specific to vertigo (Cohen and Kimball, 2000). Also, one must note the VADL does not discriminate patients with benign paroxysmal positional vertigo (BPPV) from patients with chronic vestibulopathy (Duracinsky, 2007).

### Vertigo Handicap Questionnaire (VHQ)

In general, the VHQ may offer the most promise as a questionnaire capable of determining the effect of vertigo on QoL indicators. It includes 22 items representing the handicapping consequences of vertigo on physical and everyday activities to the influence on social life and leisure activities (Duracinsky, 2007). Patients with episodic vertigo tend to have lower scores. The VHQ needs more research on larger samples to determine responsiveness and to confirm its psychometric properties (Duracinsky, 2007).

### Contemplate Clinical Decisions

*Which questionnaire would you use for an elderly adult with a history of falls?*

## Oculomotor Testing

Physical therapists should examine **ocular movements** because abnormalities of ocular motility can help the examiner localize disease processes. It is helpful to identify eye muscle imbalances that may impair visual function and therefore contribute to difficulties with standing and walking. Often, the eyes respond predictably to specific pathology, anatomical injury, and medications. In this section, we will discuss the primary components of oculomotor control, including smooth pursuit, saccades, and vergence as well as the importance of assessing vestibular ocular reflex function and nystagmus.

### Testing Smooth Pursuit Movement

When examining extraocular muscle function, begin by observing ocular alignment one eye at a time and then together to determine preexisting deformity or malalignment. **Smooth pursuit eye movements**, tested by having the patient keep

the head stationary while following a moving target with eye movement alone, are used to determine the integrity of cranial nerves III, IV, and VI (described in Chapter 7). Normal eye movements, when following a moving visual target occur as **conjugate eye movements** in which both eyes move exactly together with identical direction (as long as the object does not move closer to or further away from the face), amplitude, and speed. Conjugate is not the same as symmetrical because, for example, right movement of the right eye is accompanied by right movement of the left eye. Disruptions in cranial nerve function will yield ocular alignment and mobility abnormalities as explained in Chapter 7. The smooth pursuit system keeps moving targets on the fovea when the head is stationary or moving at slower speeds. The primary stimulus for voluntary pursuit eye movements is the motion of a visual target (image) across the retina. To test smooth pursuit, sit in front of the patient and ask the patient to use eye movement only (no head movement) to follow your finger as the target moving in all directions using an "H" pattern (side-to-side, then up and down at each extreme) as shown in Figure 7-6. The motion is from center to 30 degrees right and then 30 degrees left in the horizontal position, then 30 degrees up and 30 degrees down in the vertical position at each end of the horizontal movement. With a normal smooth pursuit system, you should observe eye movements that exactly match the velocity of the target and are smooth and continuous without any sudden starts, skips, or stops. Keep in mind that horizontal tracking will typically provide the most reliable results compared with vertical and diagonal movements. The onset of eye movements should occur almost as soon as the target begins to move and should easily maintain gaze on the target in all directions. Use low velocity target movements to examine this system, moving the target at around 20 degrees/second and not greater than 30 degrees in each direction. When the patient is unable to maintain visual contact with the object in motion or loses visual contact with movement in a particular direction, you should report the response as abnormal or impaired. While there is no strong supporting evidence, observing more than three saccades per smooth pursuit eye movement has been used by some to indicate a central vestibular pathology (Boot, 2012). If corrective saccades are observed, slow down the movement to rule out speed as the contributing factor. **Gain** is the ratio of eye movement to target velocity. Some patients, designated as having low gain, are slow to begin the pursuit of the moving target. Gain in relation to tracking, however, is typically associated with more advanced testing (e.g., ENG/VNG). Although abnormal smooth pursuit findings are associated with central dysfunction, tracking tends to diminish with advancing age. Thus, in the older adult, if abnormal tracking is the only central sign noted, then such a finding could be an age-related factor and is of little clinical significance.

### Smooth Pursuit and Vestibulo-Ocular Reflex (VOR) Cancellation

Information about the ability to track moving visual targets is accurately obtained by testing smooth pursuit eye movements.

However, this system has a complex interaction with the VOR during head and whole body movements. This interaction promotes precise eye movements in space to maintain visual focus. When combined eye and head movements occur in the same plane or head movement is combined with visual target movement, accurate visual tracking requires overriding the contribution of the VOR known as VOR Cancellation. Abnormalities in the pursuit system can influence VOR function in combined eye-head movements. The VOR must be suppressed during combined eye-head movement so the image can be maintained on the fovea. In most instances, a peripheral vestibular lesion will not impair smooth pursuit or VOR cancellation. A lesion in the central system, such as the cerebellum or vestibular nuclei, will lead to saccadic corrections. The VOR cancellation test is essentially a higher demand test of the smooth pursuit system. To test VOR cancellation, have the patient sit and then tilt the patient's head forward 30 degrees. Grasp the patient's head firmly with one hand on each side of the head, and ask the patient to continuously look at your nose during the testing. Shift your head to one side while moving the patient's head synchronously in the same direction your face moves, keeping your face/nose directly in front of the patient as a visual target. Observe for any saccadic eye movement or nystagmus. Any abnormality of VOR cancellation is usually associated with a central vestibular disorder. Another method is to ask the subject to clasp hands together and extend their arm with thumbs pointing upward. The head and body/arms rotate together as a single unit 30 degrees to the right and then 30 degrees to the left while the subject maintains gaze on their thumb (Fig. 8-2). Findings should be consistent with results of the smooth pursuit test with eyes smoothly and continuously following the moving thumb target. Again, observation of corrective saccades or provocation of symptoms indicates abnormal findings.

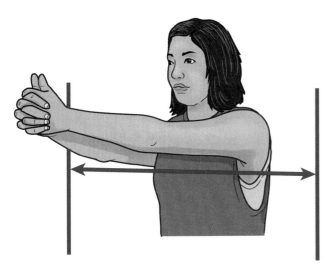

**FIGURE 8-2** A drawing to illustrate the test for VOR cancellation as the eyes attempt to follow the thumbs while the head and body/arms rotate together in an arc.

# Vestibulo-Ocular Reflex (VOR) Testing

The vestibulo-ocular system is the primary mechanism to maintain gaze stability. This system generates compensatory slow-phase eye movements in response to head movement. Therefore, this reflex keeps the visual environment stable when the head is in motion. The semicircular canals signal the acceleration and direction the head is rotating and the oculomotor system responds with equal and opposite movement of the eyes, referred to a VOR gain. The VOR gain in a normal person is 1:1, implying that the direction of head and eye movement is opposite but equal. For example, if the head turns 30 degrees to the right, then the eyes turn 30 degrees to the left to maintain stability of the stationary target image on the fovea. When hair cells of one or more canals are damaged in one ear, a static efferent firing rate imbalance is created. This static imbalance compromises gaze stability and, in the acute period within 7 days of onset, results in spontaneous nystagmus (i.e., rapid involuntary horizontal eye movements viewed by the examiner when the patient is looking straight ahead) (Thabet, 2008). Several tests examine the VOR as discussed in detail in the following sections along with possible outcomes and interpretation.

## Tests for Vestibulo-Ocular Reflex (VOR)

The VOR test is generally passive on the patient's part. Ask the patient to fixate on a stationary visual target while you gently turn the patient's head several times, first horizontally, then vertically at a rate of 60 degrees per second for 10 to 20 degrees to each side. During the head movement, carefully monitor for the provocation of vertigo and loss of gaze stability. Both these clinical signs would denote an absence of VOR and a disruption in the peripheral vestibular system. Also, you can ask the individual to perform the head movements volitionally with a stationary target held at the patient's arm length although active movement may not be as reliable as passive testing. First, perform VOR testing with slow head movements, then ask for faster velocity head movements while still maintaining gaze on the target. Individuals without vestibular pathology will be able to maintain fixation with both slow and fast head movements and should experience no symptoms of vertigo. An inability to maintain gaze on the stationary target at optimal head speeds during either passive or volitional head movement is an abnormal response.

## Head Thrust Test (HTT)

The head thrust test or head impulse test is another measure of VOR function, which is highly sensitive in diagnosing vestibular hypofunction (Schubert, 2004). The HTT is more effective when it is performed with the head pitched forward 30 degrees in neck flexion to place the semicircular canals in the plane of rotation (Schubert, 2004). Grasp the patient's head firmly with one hand on each side of the head and tilt the head forward into 30 degrees of flexion. Instruct the patient to look at a target, usually the examiner's nose. Before the test, move the patient's head gently side-to-side to make sure they are relaxed. Then progress to faster head turns at 2 Hz (2 cycles per second) but only through a small arc of motion and observe and document the patient's ability to maintain gaze on the target during head movements (Fig. 8-3). Make sure the patient is informed that the examiner will at some point move the head quickly. When you achieve a rate of 2 Hz (equivalent to 2 side-to-side cycles per second) suddenly thrust the patient's head 10 degrees to one side and observe for saccades. Repeat the test to the other side. A sudden corrective movement (saccade) back to the examiner's nose when the head stops moving to refix the gaze on the target is a positive sign of peripheral vestibular hypofunction. A positive refixation sign after left rotation indicates hypofunction of the left peripheral vestibular system while right rotation is testing the right vestibular system. Patients with vestibular hypofunction generate a corrective saccade when the head is turned toward the side of the hypofunction. An alternative method to the traditional HTT is to start with the patient's head rotated and ask them to keep their eyes on your nose. Then quickly rotate the head to midline. This technique can be particularly beneficial when the patient has neck pain and/or is guarded about rapid head movements. The clinician must keep in mind, however, if the modified technique is used then the ear being tested is the one towards the rotation. For example, if quickly moving the head from right rotation to midline then the side being tested is the left ear. If quickly moving the head from left rotation to midline then the side being tested is the right ear.

### Head Shaking Test

This test of VOR function is best performed using Frenzel goggles or infrared video goggles because visual fixation must be eliminated for test accuracy. Eye movements are observed in darkness for 10 seconds to obtain a baseline (Hain, 2007). Eyes are then closed and the neck placed in 30 degrees of flexion. Shake the head in rotation vigorously at 2 Hz left and right, around 30 to 45 degrees for 20 to 30 cycles. After 20 cycles, stop and ask the patient to open the eyes while you observe and document any nystagmus. In normal people or individuals with bilateral vestibular loss, there will be no nystagmus observed. Individuals with unilateral vestibular hypofunction or loss will exhibit nystagmus that will beat (fast component) toward the intact ear.

### Static and Dynamic Visual Acuity

Another method of determining VOR function is comparing the difference between static visual acuity (described in Chapter 7) and DVA. Most clinicians measure DVA using a Snellen eye chart as described by Bhansalie (1993) and Barber (1984). This method requires the patient to volitionally rotate their head at a consistent rate and arc or requires the clinician to move the patient's head at a consistent rate and arc of movement while the patient reads the visual chart. The Snellen chart is viewed at a distance of 6 meters, however, some clinicians utilize the Early Treatment Diabetic Retinopathy Study (ETDRS) chart viewed at 4 meters (Fig. 8-4). The standard eye chart has limitations, particularly in DVA testing because the lines with larger font have fewer letters (the top line has a single letter "E"), which affects counting the percentage of errors reading each line. The ETDRS improves this aspect by using five letters on each line with spacing commensurate with the letter size, allowing equal opportunity to make mistakes on each line.

To begin the test, have the patient wear glasses if they need them for distance correction. To measure static visual acuity, have the patient sit at the appropriate distance for the chart being utilized. Then ask the patient to read aloud the smallest line of letters that can be accurately discerned and record the

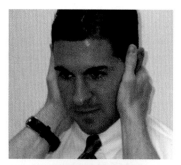
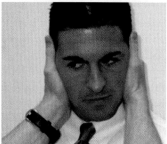

**FIGURE 8-3** Head Thrust Test. *(From Roy, S, et al. The Rehabilitation Specialist's Handbook. Philadelphia, PA: F.A. Davis; 2013.)*

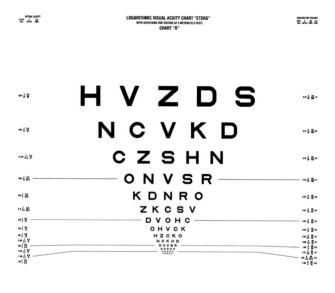
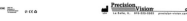

**FIGURE 8-4** ETDRS Chart. Provided courtesy of Precision-Vision.

line where this occurs to establish the patient's static visual acuity.

Next, stand behind the patient and grasp the patient's head firmly with one hand on each side of the head and tilt the head forward 30 degrees so the horizontal semicircular canals are level in the horizontal plane. Then rotate the patient's head side-to-side at a frequency of 2 Hz. Dannenbaum (2005) recommends that clients be tested in both the horizontal and vertical planes at 1.5 Hz. Speed of head movement is most accurately accomplished using a metronome. While the head is moving, ask the patient to read the eye chart aloud starting from the largest optotype (top of the chart) and progressing to the smallest optotype (bottom of the chart) that can be identified correctly. Record the smallest line the patient can read with fewer than two errors. This will be the patient's horizontal DVA. Retest the patient moving the head up and down. This will provide the vertical DVA. A difference of three lines or more between static visual acuity and DVA is often indicative of impaired VOR function usually associated with vestibular hypofunction. It is also important to ask if either direction resulted in a provocation of vestibular symptoms. Keep in mind, that vertical DVA testing is difficult, and it may be easier to have the patient actively move the head.

### Saccades System

The **saccadic system** is responsible for generating fast ballistic eye movements to scan the environment, observed as very fast changes in eye position. Stereotypical rapid eye movements are produced by the saccade system to bring a visual target back onto the fovea, allowing us to reposition our gaze to a new target in our visual field. This action may be voluntary or involuntary. The patient should be able to produce an eye movement that rapidly and accurately reaches a target and abruptly stops at the target. Shifting gaze between two stationary targets tests the patient's ability to make predictable volitional movements. To test, sit in front of the patient and hold the patient's head stationary. Position one of your fingers about 15 degrees laterally to your nose and in the same plane of the tip of your nose. (Note: The lateral aspect of each eye is a good reference point for each target.) Keep the target at least 14 inches from the patient's face. Then instruct the patient to look at your nose then quickly at your finger, repeating this sequence several times. Or you can instruct the patient to quickly shift gaze between two targets as

demonstrated in Figure 8-5. Repeat the test, including voluntary movements to the right and left sides and up and down. Observe the number of eye movements it takes for the patient's eyes to reach each target. An individual with normal saccadic movement should reach the target in less than two eye movements. Any abnormality in this test with impairment observed as slow saccadic velocity and/or saccadic dysmetria (overshooting or undershooting the target) is indicative of central pathology and has a high level of specificity for suggesting disruption in the brainstem or cerebellum (Leigh, 2006). Such findings should be referred back to the physician for more testing as central pathology warrants further consideration.

### Vergence

**Vergence**, distinct from conjugate eye movements, refers to eye movements in which the eyes move in opposite directions to allow binocular fixation of a single object (i.e., equal and opposite movements of both eyes). Vergence may be observed as **convergence**, adduction of both eyes as the visual target moves closer to the face, or **divergence**, symmetrical abduction of both eyes as the visual target moves farther from the face. To test convergence (Fig. 8-6), ask the patient to follow your finger as it slowly moves closer to and further from the patient's nose. Normally, vergence should be observed as smooth and symmetrical movements of each eye. This test is one of the less utilized clinical oculomotor tests but can provide valuable insight if the patient is also reporting difficulty reading, eye fatigue, and/or double vision. Near-point convergence (NPC) is the most commonly assessed (versus divergence). A normal NPC is noted when the eyes can symmetrically move inward less than 10 cm (4 inches) from the bridge of the nose. Abnormal NPC is noted when either the eyes move asymmetrically, you observe one eye drifting laterally, and/or the patient reports double vision with target greater than 10 cm from the bridge of their nose. NPC impairment is common following head trauma (Mucha, 2014).

## Spontaneous and Gaze-evoked Nystagmus

As stated previously, evaluation of nystagmus is of key importance in the vestibular examination because it provides insight to help identify peripheral and/or central vestibular

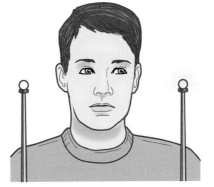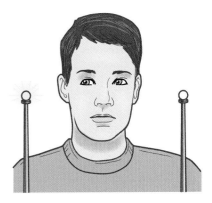

**FIGURE 8-5** Illustrates a patient quickly shifting their gaze between two targets without head movement to observe for normal saccade movement.

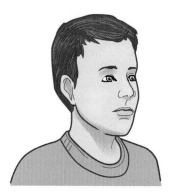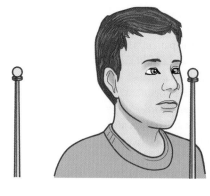

**FIGURE 8-6** Near-point convergence is tested by having the patient follow a target as it moves closer and closer to the patient's face and the eyes both adduct (normal disconjugate movement) to maintain visual focus on the object.

pathology. Examination of nystagmus begins with baseline observation of the eyes in the primary position. Primary position is defined as the eye position when the patient is looking straight ahead at the examiner's nose or a stationary target. Observe the patient for a head tilt that may compensate for lack of volitional eye movement. Also observe for an abnormal resting alignment of each eye within the orbit by comparing the relative position of the ambient room light reflection off each cornea to give some idea about resting or primary position of each eye and if each eye is "looking" in the same direction. **Visual fixation** occurs when the patient focuses on a target (e.g., your nose or a stationary target) and can interfere with vestibular testing, particularly by suppressing the degree of nystagmus that is present, which is more obvious if the nystagmus is mild. Therefore, it is important to prevent or minimize visual fixation during examination for nystagmus using Frenzel lenses or with more advanced vestibular diagnostics including ENG or VNG, discussed later in this section, which also minimize visual fixation. A key component to differentiate between central and peripheral nystagmus is observing the effects of visual fixation on the nystagmus. In central nystagmus, visual fixation typically does not decrease the intensity of nystagmus while visual fixation does typically suppress peripheral vestibular nystagmus.

Nystagmus viewed in the primary position may be called spontaneous nystagmus. **Spontaneous nystagmus** is characterized by horizontal eye movements with the slow phases directed to the side of low tonic output and quick phases away from the side of lesion, especially in the acute phase of the vertigo within the first 1 to 2 weeks. In the examination data, nystagmus is designated according to the direction of the fast phase (i.e., "right-beating spontaneous nystagmus" has the fast component beating toward the right, which often indicates a central vestibular lesion on the left, if acute). During the chronic and/or recovery phases, however, this pattern may reverse.

Several factors can help to interpret specific observations of nystagmus. If the nystagmus is greater in one eye than the other, this is more suggestive of central pathology whereas peripheral vestibular nystagmus is typically equal in intensity between each eye. Also, the intensity of the nystagmus increases when the eyes are turned in the direction of the quick phases (Alexander, 1912). Vertical nystagmus

is more suggestive of central pathology while horizontal and rotary nystagmus are more common in peripheral vestibular disorders.

**Gaze-evoked nystagmus** is the most common pathological nystagmus. This type of nystagmus is not present in primary position, but when the person looks in the affected direction, a jerk nystagmus occurs. In patients with dizziness, gaze-evoked nystagmus occurs in eccentric gaze. This jerk nystagmus follows Alexander's Law, which describes the principle that jerk nystagmus increases when the eyes move into the direction of the fast component, which is usually the active or intact side. For example, a left-beating nystagmus will become more intense when the individual looks left and less intense when the individual looks right, which is typically suggestive of a right UVL. If the nystagmus switches directions in gaze right versus gaze left, then this could be suggestive of central pathology. More advanced vestibular testing (e.g., VNG) is more sensitive in measuring gaze-evoked nystagmus, especially "end-point" nystagmus, which can be of no clinical significance.

## Positional Testing for BPPV

As in most cases, patient history is a key component in the examination and evaluation of the patient with vestibular dysfunction. The patient with **Benign Paroxysmal Positional Vertigo (BPPV)** will often complain of a spinning sensation (vertigo) resulting from specific head movements, that is brief (e.g., often less than 30 seconds) and episodic in nature. These symptoms may be associated with specific movements of lying down, rolling over, tilting head back to look up, or bending over. Episode duration can vary from several days to weeks, then can disappear and may reoccur in the future. Dizziness due to BPPV is thought to be caused by semicircular canal debris that has collected within the canals of the vestibular apparatus in the inner ear. Clinically, the debris particles are known as otoconia although they are commonly referred to as ear rocks or ear crystals, especially when explaining to patients.

### Test Vertebral Artery Sufficiency First

As stated earlier, due to the inherent risk in performing the neck motions involved in positional vestibular testing, always test first to make sure the patient has no signs of VBI, which can result in cerebrovascular accident. With the patient in sitting or supine position, passively move the patient's head in cervical extension and rotation (with slight side bending). Maintain eye contact with the patient and hold for 30 seconds while the patient counts backward from 10. Monitor for any signs of vertigo, nystagmus, or central signs (slurring of speech or motor/sensory changes on one side of the body or face) that may indicate some ischemia within the vertebrobasilar artery system. If symptoms are elicited in the position, testing should cease and the patient should be referred for immediate medical attention. As a clinician, we should always be aware of the "5 Ds" and "3 Ns" discussed earlier in the chapter.

### Dix-Hallpike Test

The most common test for confirming BPPV is the **Dix-Hallpike Test** (see Fig. 8-7). This test is used to test for anterior or posterior canal involvement. When performing the Dix-Hallpike Test, start with the patient in a long-sitting position with the back toward and close enough to the edge of the mat so that upon laying back into supine, the head and neck will be hanging off the edge. This starting location can most easily be determined before starting by using a pillow to measure the approximate distance in long-sitting from the mat surface to the top of the shoulders, then use that length of the pillow to scoot the patient that far from the edge. Before starting the maneuver, rotate the patient's head 45 degrees to one side, then quickly guide the patient from the long-sitting position to a supine position with the neck extended about 20 degrees off the edge of the mat and supported by the examiner's hands while positioning yourself to be able to see their eyes following the maneuver (see Fig. 8-8). After this sudden movement, while the patient is

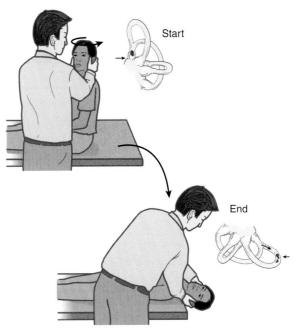

**FIGURE 8-8** This drawing illustrates the patient positioning and therapist's position during a left Dix-Hallpike maneuver, including the starting and end position.

in this position, observe for occurrence of nystagmus, which may not begin immediately after the movement and note the direction and duration (in seconds) of the nystagmus. There may be a latency of 10 to 30 seconds following the maneuver before symptoms and nystagmus begin, so don't abandon the test prematurely. If nystagmus is present, it is often accompanied by patient complaints of the room spinning, (i.e., vertigo). Make sure to instruct the patient to keep the eyes open during the test as some will have a strong tendency to close them.

Return the patient to the original position and observe for a reversal in nystagmus. A positive test for BPPV will show a burst of nystagmus in the vertical or horizontal plane that has a superimposed rotational component. Remember, it is helpful if the patient is tested with Frenzel goggles or infrared video goggles to inhibit visual fixation. Observe for these key features during the testing:

1. **Latency** (how many seconds before nystagmus begins) and **duration** (how many seconds the nystagmus lasts).
2. Nystagmus torsional component toward the involved ear.
3. Nystagmus vertical component, which is upbeating (posterior canal affected on the side being tested) or downbeating (anterior canal affected on the opposite side being tested).
4. Gradual decay in the intensity of the nystagmus and the subjective complaints of vertigo.
5. Reversal of the nystagmus when returned to sitting position.
6. Decreased intensity of the nystagmus with each repeated movement into the provoking position.

The following principles, summarized in Table 8-7, are helpful in interpreting positional testing results. With posterior canal BPPV, an upbeating nystagmus with torsional

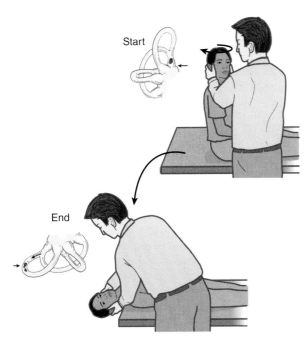

**FIGURE 8-7** This drawing illustrates the patient positioning during a right Dix-Hallpike maneuver, including the starting position (in long-sitting) and the end position with neck extension over the edge of the treatment table with 45-degree neck rotation toward the side being tested.

| CANAL (TEST) | RIGHT | LEFT |
|---|---|---|
| Posterior (Dix-Hallpike)* | Upbeat and right torsion | Upbeat and left torsion |
| Anterior (Dix-Hallpike), contralateral side* | Downbeat and right torsion | Downbeat and left torsion |
| Horizontal Cupulolithiasis (Roll Test) | Ageotropic (away from earth) | Ageotropic (away from earth) |
| Horizontal Canalithiasis (Roll Test) | Geotropic (toward earth) | Geotropic (toward earth) |

**TABLE 8-7  Nystagmus: A Summary to Help Interpret the Results of Positional Testing**

*In canalithiasis, nystagmus duration will be less than 60 seconds; in cupulolithiasis, nystagmus duration will be ≥60 seconds.

component toward the involved ear will occur. Anterior canal BPPV will have downbeating nystagmus with torsional component toward the involved ear. The duration of nystagmus helps determine whether the BPPV mechanism is **canalithiasis** (a form of BPPV in which the otoconia are freely moveable in a semicircular canal) with duration of less than 60 seconds or **cupulolithiasis**, (otoconia are adherent to the cupula) with duration of 60 seconds or greater and therefore determines the specific intervention to employ.

### Roll Test for Horizontal Canal

The **Roll Test** (Fig. 8-9) is the positional test for horizontal canal BPPV. Position the patient in supine and flex the patient's neck to 30 degrees to place the horizontal canal in the plane of movement for the following maneuver. Then rapidly turn the head (neck rotation) to one side and hold the position for up to 60 seconds while observing for any nystagmus and

symptoms. Return the head to midline for 30 seconds, then repeat the test to the other side. The nystagmus, as summarized for horizontal canal in Table 8-7, can be **geotropic**, beating toward the ground or undermost ear in the test position, which indicates canalithiasis, or **ageotropic**, beating away from the ground, which indicates cupulolithiasis. It is important to note that horizontal canal BPPV, if present, will result in a positive test when the head is turned to the right or left side. When nystagmus is geotropic, the most symptomatic side is the affected side. When nystagmus is ageotropic, the intensity is greater when the head is turned away from the involved ear (Choung, 2006). The vertigo with horizontal canal BPPV can be prolonged and is exacerbated with side-to-side head movements.

### Alternative Testing Position for Posterior

In cases where the patient cannot assume a supine position, an alternate side-lying position test may be used (Fig. 8-10). Start the patient in a sitting position with legs hanging off the side of the testing table. Turn the patient's head 45 degrees away from the testing side (e.g., if testing the right canal, turn head 45 degrees to the left). Then quickly guide the patient into a side-lying position on the testing side (e.g., down to the right to test the right canal). Observe for the same symptoms and signs (including latency and direction and duration of nystagmus) as in the Dix-Hallpike test. Figure 8-11 list decision-making steps for interpreting results of BPPV.

## Testing Balance as a Related System

Balance, or body equilibrium, is a very complex process as described in Chapter 9, and is usually disrupted by vestibular dysfunction. Balance involves tremendous interaction and cooperation between the sensory systems, motor systems, and biomechanical factors. The sensory system gives input to determine body positioning in relation to gravity and weight-bearing on the support surface. **Balance** is the

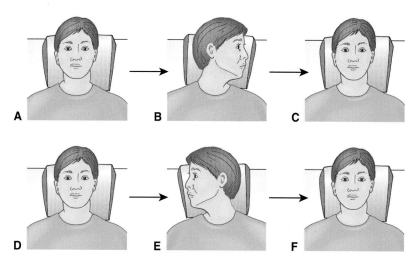

**FIGURE 8-9** This drawing illustrates the Roll Test, including the start and the end positions. A, B, and C testing to the left, and D, E, and F testing to the right.

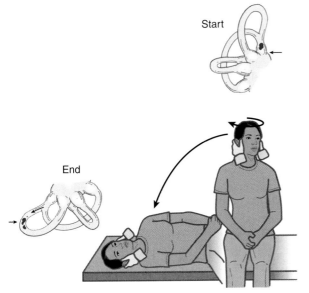

**FIGURE 8-10** The alternative Dix-Hallpike Test (side-lying) showing the procedure to test right posterior canal, by turning the head 45° to the left before lying down to the right side.

ability to control one's center of gravity over the base of support in a given environment and is required during each specific task or activity. Input from three sensory systems (vestibular, visual, and somatosensory input) is utilized to help determine body position in space in three ways. Vision detects the orientation of the eyes and head in relation to the environment, somatosensory provides input regarding orientation of body parts to each other and in relation to the base of support, and vestibular provides the gravitational, linear, and angular acceleration information regarding movement of the head. The function of the vestibular system is most importantly tested through the integration into functional output. Therefore, a variety of tests for balance/equilibrium with clinical applications and interpretation are discussed in Chapter 9.

### Modified Clinical Test for Sensory Interaction on Balance

The modified Clinical Test for Sensory Interaction in Balance (mCTSIB), explained in detail in Chapter 9, examines the capacity of the individual to adapt the use of the various senses for postural control in response to changes in the availability

**BPPV Algorithm**

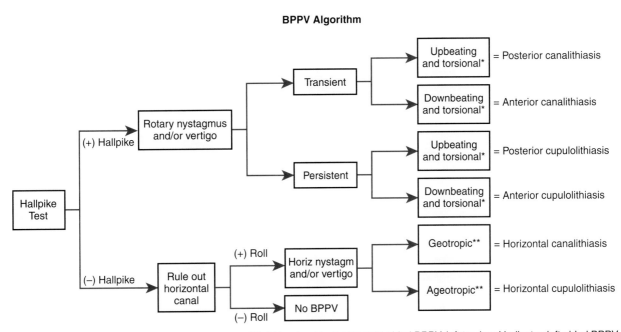

*Right torsional indicates right-sided BPPV, left torsional indicates left-sided BPPV
**For ageotrophic, the side of weakest nystagmus/symptoms is the affected side
**For geotrophic, the side of strongest nystagmus/symptoms is the affected side

| Key Definitions | Major Characteristics of BPPV: |
|---|---|
| Nystagmus—rapid rhythmic eye movement name according to the fast phase<br>Rotary nystagmus—torsional nystagmus named by movement of the superior aspect of the eye<br>Geotropic—toward the ground; most often refers to downward ear<br>Ageotropic—away from the ground; most often refers to the upward ear | Onset—latency of 2–20 seconds<br>Duration— < 30 sec = transient<br>              > 60 sec = persistent<br>Type of nystagmus—rotary or horizontal<br>Most common—transient, rotary<br>              nystagmus toward ear |

**FIGURE 8-11** This algorithm provides a decision tree for interpreting the results of positional testing for BPPV.

and accuracy of each sensory system. It is an extension of the Romberg Test and utilizes both eyes-open and eyes-closed conditions on both stable and compliant (foam) surfaces. It used to be known as the "foam and dome test" but in this modified version the visual conflict dome is no longer used. It assesses the relative influence of vestibular, somatosensory, and visual inputs on postural control. Results may determine the sensory cues on which the patient is dependent and therefore help to guide patient-centered intervention.

### Computerized Dynamic Posturography

Computerized Dynamic Posturography has gained wide acceptance as a method of measuring postural control. Nashner (1990) developed the Sensory Organization Test (SOT), which includes six sensory conditions described here (similar to CTSIB), to evaluate a person's standing balance. The SOT is administered using a computerized system with dual force plates and adjustable visual field, both of which can be stable or moving. The SOT protocol assesses the patient's ability to make effective use of visual, vestibular, and proprioceptive inputs as well as the patient's ability to suppress inaccurate sensory information. The patient is asked to stand on force plates with arms at the sides. Changes in the amount of body sway in each sensory condition are used to determine the patient's ability to organize and select the appropriate sensory information to maintain postural control (Nashner, 1990).

The SOT protocol consists of six independent sensory conditions (Table 8-8). Each condition has three 20-second trials. Condition 1 is considered a normal situation and no sensory stimuli are altered. This condition is considered the baseline measure and is used as a comparison to the remaining conditions. In Condition 2, visual stimuli are removed by instructing the patient to close the eyes or use a blindfold. In this condition, the patient must rely upon somatosensory and vestibular cues alone to remain upright. Individuals with loss of sensation in their feet will have difficulty with this condition. In Condition 3, visual stimuli are altered by a moving visual field equal to the subject's sway in the anterior/posterior planes, thus maintaining the visual field a constant distance from the patient's eyes and creating sensory conflict. Visual information in this condition is unreliable, therefore somatosensory and vestibular inputs should prevail. In Condition 4, proprioceptive stimuli are altered by rotating the standing platform with the patient's sway, thus maintaining

a constant angle at the ankle joint. Somatosensory information in this condition is not helpful so visual and vestibular cues should provide adequate information to remain upright. Patients with impaired visual acuity will have difficulty on Condition 4. In Condition 5, proprioceptive stimuli are altered and visual stimuli are absent; the patient's eyes are closed and the platform moves with the patient's sway. The only remaining accurate system in Condition 5 is the vestibular system. Patients with vestibular pathology will have difficulty with this condition. In Condition 6 of the test, proprioceptive and visual stimuli are both altered by moving the platform and visual field with the patient's sway. Both Condition 3 and 6 provided inaccurate visual stimuli thus determining whether the patient can recognize the sensory conflict and ignore this inappropriate visual-sensory information. Those patients who are unable to ignore inaccurate sensory information will have difficulty standing during these conditions. The SOT is valid and reliable for measuring standing balance across age groups (Ford-Smith, 1995).

## Physiological Testing

The purpose of physiological testing is to determine whether there is any insult to the vestibular portion of the inner ear. Dizziness not caused by the inner ear may be indicative of a disorder occurring in the brain, which can be physiological or psychological in nature. The following is a simple discussion of the physiological testing available and their main purpose.

### Electronystagmography (ENG) or Videonystagmography (VNG)

The purpose of nystagmography is to determine, by careful analysis of nystagmus, whether or not dizziness is due to inner-ear vestibular disorder. There are four main parts to the ENG. Nystagmography consists of three major components: (1) **Oculomotor testing** includes measuring nystagmus during smooth pursuit tracking, saccades, and optokinetic testing. (2) The **positional test** measures nystagmus associated with positions of the head as well as measuring eye responses to slow positional tests and fast positional tests (e.g., Dix-Hallpike); and (3) the bithermal **caloric tests** measure oculomotor responses to warm and cold water or warm and cold air circulated into the external auditory canal, one ear at a

| TABLE 8-8 | Six Conditions of the Sensory Organization Test (SOT) | |
| --- | --- | --- |
| Condition 1: Eyes open; stable floor (*baseline condition*) | Condition 2: Eyes closed; stable floor (*visual input is eliminated; patient must rely on somatosensory and vestibular cues*) | Condition 3: Eyes open; moveable visual screen; stable floor (*vision is inaccurate/unhelpful; patient must rely on somatosensory and vestibular cues*) |
| Condition 4: Eyes open; unstable, movable floor (*somatosensory information is not helpful, patients with visual acuity impairment will have difficulty*) | Condition 5: Eyes closed; unstable floor (*with visual input eliminated, and proprioception inaccurate, the vestibular input is essential*) | Condition 6: Eyes open; moveable visual screen; unstable floor (*vision and proprioception are inaccurate/unhelpful; patients who are unable to ignore inaccurate sensory information will have difficulty standing*) |

time. ENG and VNG are good diagnostic tools and are considered the gold standard for determining a disorder affecting the peripheral vestibular system of one ear, for example, **vestibular neuritis/labyrinthitis.** The positional test is useful in diagnosing BPPV while the oculomotor tests are intended to diagnose central nervous system involvement. Caloric tests measure function of the horizontal canal and are frequently found to be within normal limits even in the context of vestibular dysfunction. Limitations of caloric testing include the fact that it only measures the horizontal canal (does not include anterior or posterior canal function). Nor does it accurately capture function of the vestibular system associated with more dynamic tasks such as walking and carrying out activities of daily living. A caloric response (nystagmus and/or vertigo) is absent or diminished on the affected side when there is significant vestibular loss, which is most commonly recognized as more than 25% difference between the right and left ears. Vestibular impairment can also occur bilaterally of which rotational chair testing is considered the gold standard.

### Rotational Chair Test

Rotational chair testing is used to determine whether or not dizziness may be due to a disorder of the peripheral vestibular system or the central vestibular system. There are three parts to the test. The **rotational chair test** measures nystagmus while being turned slowly in a motorized rotating chair. Patients with an inner ear disorder become less dizzy than do normal people. The **optokinetic test** measures the nystagmus produced while the patient is viewing a moving striped optical drum. Optokinetic nystagmus is usually abolished in cases of bilateral vestibular loss. The **fixation test** measures nystagmus during visual fixation on a stationary target (a dot of light) while the patient is being rotated in the chair. Fixation

is impaired for those who have central nervous system conditions and is improved when there is bilateral vestibular loss.

### Computerized VOR Testing

Testing that involves high velocity head rotation can assess higher demands of VOR function associated with activities of daily living (ADLs) and more dynamic activities better than calorics or rotation chair. These active head rotation systems also provide additional information about canal function in the vertical plane. The tests can be performed with or without electrodes or with the use of infrared video goggles. More recently, infrared video has been incorporated, based on Halmagyi and Curthoys' (1995) work, to more objectively measure the corrective (overt) saccades noted in the head thrust test as well as identification of covert saccades, which has previously not been measurable.

## ■ Documentation of Vestibular Examination/Evaluation

Documenting the results of your examination tests is as important as performing the test itself. The documented outcome will help you determine the key problem areas and inform development of the plan of care and specific interventions to be employed. Table 8-9 provides a simple framework for documentation of your oculomotor findings for a particular patient.

In BPPV, determining which canal is affected is essential to determining which treatment options should be utilized. Binocular goggles, Frenzel glasses, or infrared nystagmography should be utilized for the testing. Table 8-10 can be used for documenting results of your positional testing.

---

| TABLE 8-9 | Oculomotor and Vestibular Testing |
|---|---|

**Spontaneous nystagmus:**
*Room light:* ☐ Absent ☐ Present-direction: _____
*Fixation blocked:* ☐ Absent ☐ Present-direction: _____

**Gaze-holding nystagmus:**
*Room light:* ☐ Absent ☐ Present-direction: _____
*Fixation blocked:* ☐ Absent ☐ Present-direction: _____

**Smooth pursuit eye movement:**
☐ Intact  ☐ Saccadic correction present
☐ Horizontal  ☐ Vertical direction

**VOR Cancellation:**
☐ Maintains visual fixation ☐ Saccadic eye movements or (☐) nystagmus

**Head Thrust:**
☐ Maintains visual fixation ☐ Refixation saccades to _____ L/ _____ R _____

**Static Visual Acuity:** _____ line
**Dynamic Visual Acuity:** _____ line
Number of line/s difference between static and dynamic visual acuity: _____ line/s

**Vergence:** ☐ Intact ☐ Abnormal

| TABLE 8-10 | Positional Testing | | | |
|---|---|---|---|---|
| POSITION | NYSTAGMUS | DIRECTION OF BEAT | DIRECTION OF TORSION | DURATION (SECONDS) |
| Head rotated 45 degrees left and extended 20 degrees | ☐ Present<br>☐ Absent | ☐ upbeat<br>☐ downbeat<br>☐ horizontal L<br>☐ horizontal R | ☐ right<br>☐ left<br>☐ no torsion | ☐ short (<60 seconds)<br>☐ long (60 seconds)<br>☐ persistent (>60 seconds) |
| Head rotated 45 degrees right and extended at 20–60 degrees | ☐ Present<br>☐ Absent | ☐ upbeat<br>☐ downbeat<br>☐ horizontal L<br>☐ horizontal R | ☐ right<br>☐ left<br>☐ no torsion | ☐ short<br>☐ long<br>☐ persistent |
| Supine with head flexed 20 degrees Roll left | ☐ Present<br>☐ Absent | ☐ Geotropic<br>☐ Ageotropic | | ☐ short<br>☐ long<br>☐ persistent |
| Supine with head flexed 20 degrees Roll right | ☐ Present<br>☐ Absent | ☐ Geotropic<br>☐ Ageotropic | | ☐ short<br>☐ long<br>☐ persistent |

## PATIENT APPLICATION

*Mrs. Park, with vestibular neuritis, was introduced earlier in this chapter. The significant portions of her physical examination include:*

*Mental Examination: Mrs. Park did not appear distressed during the examination and was attentive. She was alert and appeared to have no deficits in cognition. Her spontaneous speech was fluent with normal tone modulation. She was able to comprehend simple questions/commands.*

*Cranial Nerve Examination: Static Visual Acuity was screened at 20/20. CNs III, IV, and VI revealed equal pupils and no ptosis with normal reaction to light. (See Oculomotor for more testing.) CN VII testing revealed facial symmetry and voluntary movements of facial expression. CN VIII screening revealed symmetry in hearing between both sides and a (-) Weber's test. (See additional info in Vestibular section.) CN IX and X revealed symmetrical soft palate movement, normal cough, normal voice production, and midline uvula. CN XI and XII had no asymmetry in shoulder shrug and normal articulation, respectively.*

*Sensory Examination: Mrs. Park presents with intact sensation to vibration in right and left LE at malleolus.*

*Motor Examination: Muscle tone is normal. Gross MMT is 5/5 for UE and LE.*

*Nystagmus Examination: Mrs. Park does not exhibit spontaneous nystagmus. Head Shake Test: not performed. Dix-Hallpike/Positional Testing: (-)*

*Oculomotor Examination: Smooth pursuit and saccadic eye movements are intact in vertical, horizontal, and diagonal planes.*

*Vestibular Ocular Reflex (VOR) Examination: Head Thrust: (+) left. Dynamic Visual Acuity: 20/80 (5 line difference) with mild dizziness.*

*Coordination Examination: She does not exhibit dysmetria, dysdiadochokinesia, truncal ataxia, or overshooting.*

*Neuro Examination - Additional: Pronator Drift: negative. Tremors: not present. Reflexes: intact bilateral knee DTR is 2 +.*

*Static Balance Examination: Tandem stance (eyes open) × 15 sec with mild increased sway. Single Leg Stance (eyes open) × 5 to 7 sec. Romberg, firm × 12 sec and foam unable; Computerized Sensory Organization Test: not performed.*

*Gait: (Observation) widened base of support; normal cadence and velocity 1.2 m/s. Patient can walk on heels and toes without assistance. Dynamic Gait Index Score: 18/24.*

### Contemplate Clinical Decisions

1. What information is most significant from this examination?
2. Are there other tests you would want to perform at this point?
3. What body system/body structure impairments do you identify in this patient that will need to be addressed in the intervention?

## ■ Pediatric Applications

The vestibular system is one of the first sensory systems to develop and is believed to be at least minimally operational at 4 months gestation. Labyrinthine reflexes, mediated by the vestibulospinal system, influence tone in early infancy, and the majority of normal infants demonstrate vestibular responses to caloric and rotational stimuli (measures of VOR) by 2 months of age (Weissman, 1989). However, research has demonstrated that various components of the vestibular system and an individual's reliance on vestibular input to maintain postural control continue to mature through age 15 years and possibly longer (Hirabayashi, 1995; Rine, 1998).

One of the difficulties in assessing vestibular function in children is the absence of clearly established developmental norms across the age span. Evidence of mature vestibular function is variable in reported studies. As examples, Rine (2005) suggests that utricular-related function is mature by 4 years of age. Peterson (2005) tested 154 children (age range, 6 to 12 years) using computerized dynamic posturography to assess overall balance as well as the use of specific sensory information in maintaining stability. The study concluded that 12 year-olds achieved scores comparable to those of adults but not the younger children. All groups demonstrated mature use of somatosensory information but the younger groups did not use visual or vestibular information as effectively as adults. Children have been found to rely more heavily on visual information than vestibular information to maintain postural control (Woollacott, 1987).

Children of all ages are subject to vestibular disorders, both central and peripheral in origin. The incidence of vestibular disorders in children is low compared with adults, although it is suspected that the occurrence is underreported for various reasons, including children's inability to accurately report the abnormal sensations they are experiencing. In a 14-year study with more than 2,000 children referred for vertigo and balance disorders, Wiener-Vachner (2008) reported the most common diagnoses, in order of prevalence and as a percent of the total population, is as follows:

1. Migraine-equivalent (about 25% of total)—In children, migraine symptoms tend to be localized to frontal or periorbital region, last less than 2 hours, and may not be associated with throbbing pain typically reported by adults. About 20% of children with migraine have associated dizziness.
2. Benign paroxysmal vertigo of childhood (about 20% of total)—Typically occurs before age 4; primary symptoms include episodic attacks of vertigo lasting from seconds to minutes that result in child being unable to stand without support.
3. Cranial trauma (about 10% of total)—For various reasons, children sustain head trauma at high rates; about 10% report dizziness as one symptom.
4. Genetic malformations of the inner ear (about 10% of total).
5. Ophthalmological disorders (about 10% of total)—Reading acuity may be affected because of lack of gaze stability and oculomotor control. In a population of 523 pediatric patients with vertigo, Anoti-Tanon (2000) reported that 27 children (about 5%) presented with normal vestibular and somatic neurological examinations but with ophthalmological disorders (primarily vergence insufficiency).
6. Vestibular neuritis (about 5% of total)—Symptoms are typically the same as adult (i.e., sudden onset of vertigo and vomiting lasting for days to weeks); causative mechanism unknown but most likely viral.
7. Posterior fossa tumors (less than 1% of total).

Vestibular dysfunction has also been reported in approximately 60% of children with sensorineural hearing impairment (Horak, 1988; Rine, 2003; Wiener-Vachner, 2008), in association with central nervous system conditions (e.g., spinal cord injury or cerebral palsy), and as a complication of recurrent or chronic otitis media (Schaaf, 1985; Casselbrant, 1995). Vatovec (2003) assessed vestibular function in 110 high-risk infants (via demonstrated spontaneous symptoms and caloric testing) and reported vestibular disorders in 14.5% of the infants. The authors found a statistically significant correlation between the presence of vestibular disorders and the degree of neurological risk.

Symptoms that may indicate vestibular dysfunction in children include hearing loss or tinnitus, abnormal movement patterns, clumsiness, incoordination, falls, nystagmus, dizziness, nausea, motion intolerance, visual-spatial problems, ear pressure, or difficulty moving in the dark (VEDA, 2007). Many of these symptoms would not be readily observable and may not be reported by the child, complicating the evaluative process. Children with vestibular disorders will likely be delayed in acquisition of motor skills and equilibrium responses and will be generally uncoordinated. These motor delays and difficulties with balance will be observed in testing but perhaps more notable are the behavioral manifestations. Often, these children are hesitant to move, avoid activities that require complex motor planning/performance, become tense with challenges to balance, and "act out" rather than persist with efforts to accomplish motor tasks (e.g., falling purposely when attempting to balance on one leg). They have special difficulty with motor tasks involving alternating movements, eye-hand or eye-foot coordination (e.g., ball play), and bilateral precision. They may crave vestibular stimulation (e.g., swings, sliding boards) or avoid it. It can be challenging to distinguish the child with vestibular dysfunction from the child with sensory organization deficits (Horak, 1988).

Screening for vestibular function with appropriate referral for more in-depth testing is recommended in any of the prevalent diagnoses listed previously, especially those that are accompanied by impairments in postural control or motor delays. Because the vestibular system is an integral component of so many motor functions and the symptoms of vestibular disorders are so varied, the examination is also varied. Testing for the early tonic reflexes (e.g., asymmetrical tonic neck reflex, tonic labyrinthine reflex) in young infants or the abnormal persistence influence in older infants/children can be accomplished fairly easily and may contribute to a more comprehensive examination. To test the older child for persistent influence of the asymmetrical or symmetrical tonic neck reflex, place the child in quadruped and examine tone in the extremities as the head is moved side-to-side and up and down. To test persistent influence of the tonic labyrinthine reflex, ask the child to maintain a fully extended position while in prone ("airplane") or fully flexed position in supine.

Balance and postural control (vestibulospinal abilities) are typically assessed as part of a neurological or developmental evaluation in infants and children but the specific contribution of vestibular hypofunction is often not tested. A few of the norm-referenced standardized tests of motor function include items related to balance and vestibular function, including the Peabody Developmental Motor Scales II (Folio, 2000) and the Bruinincks-Oseretsky Test of Motor Proficiency, Second Edition (Bruinincks, 2005). Single task tests like the Functional Reach Test (FRT), which has been shown to be both a valid and reliable measure of dynamic balance in adult populations, has not been recommended for use with pediatric populations because of poor reliability (Westcott, 1997). Some researchers have recommended adjustments in the strategies used and measures taken that would improve the test's responsiveness, reliability, and applicability for children with varying levels of motor control. Volkman (2009) recommended a reaching strategy with two arms and measurement from toes-to-finger rather than finger-to-finger and found that both age and height affected the performance in the pediatric population. Bartlett (2003) recommended modifying the test to include lateral as well as forward reaching and in standing as well as sitting positions to better accommodate children with varying levels of involvement. The Berg Balance Scale (BBS) has been studied extensively with adults and found to be a useful measure of the balance required to perform everyday tasks. Children, however, lose interest in the test items, negatively impacting the results. Franjoine (2003) developed a Pediatric Balance Scale by modifying the BBS and found that the 14-item criterion-referenced measure of functional balance had excellent test-retest, interrater, and intrarater reliability when used with school-aged children with mild to moderate motor impairment. Shumway-Cook and Horak (1986) developed the Clinical Test of Sensory Interaction for Balance (CTSIB) as a means of measuring the influence of sensory information on balance and the client's adaptability in situations of intrasensory conflict. The test has been adapted for children and some normative data exist but test-retest reliability was found to be low to moderate (Westcott, 1994). These are examples of the challenges encountered when using tests of balance and vestibular function designed for use with adults in the pediatric population.

A variety of tests designed to measure vestibular function more specifically have mixed applicability with the pediatric population. Ayres (1989) developed the Southern California Post-Rotary Nystagmus Test with normative data for children ages 5 to 11 year that measures the duration and excursion of nystagmus following seated spinning on a rotary board (vestibular ocular system). Rine (2005) studied the use of the subjective visual vertical test with the pediatric population and found that it could be a reliable measure of utricular function in children as young as 4 years of age with suspected acute vestibular loss.

Many of the formal assessment measures used to diagnose vestibular dysfunction in adults have limited application in children because they are costly, may make children uncomfortable or fearful, and require a level of attention and cooperation not feasible in younger populations. Test procedures may be lengthy and complex, equipment may not be adaptable for use with children (e.g., goggles used with videonystagmography), and there may be insufficient research on sensitivity and specificity of various tests or a lack of normative data when used with children (Valente, 2011). Examples of adaptations that may make testing more "child-friendly" include using cartoon characters (e.g., on the calibrated light bar used to assess gaze-evoked nystagmus), allowing the child to sit on the parent's lap (e.g., during computerized rotary chair testing), using appealing visual stimuli (e.g., child-friendly visual surrounded in computerized dynamic posturography), decreasing the number of repetitions of a single item, or in number of items administered. Dynamic posturography testing involves two distinct tests: sensory organization test (SOT) and Motor Control Test (MCT). Normative values have been developed for the SOT for children 3 to 15 years of age (Hirabayashi, 1995; Rine, 1998) but not for the MCT. A fully functioning vestibular system is critically important for the developing infant/child, and many authors advocate for more routine screening and diagnostic testing of vestibular function in the pediatric population for early identification of problems and appropriate team-based intervention (Valente, 2011). Additional research is needed related to age-differentiated normative data and findings that assist with differential diagnosis.

## Let's Review

1. What characteristics differentiate vertigo from dizziness?

2. What are the three categories of vestibular and balance testing for patients with suspected vestibular dysfunction?

3. Considering the International Classification of Functioning, Disability, and Health (ICF) model, determine which outcome measures are best for testing participation versus activity versus body structure and function in a population with possible vestibular impairment.

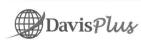 For additional resources, including Focus on Evidence tables, case study discussions, references, and glossary, please visit http://davisplus.fadavis.com

## CHAPTER SUMMARY

As shown in the previously discussed patient application, the individual vestibular examination is essential in determining what interventions should be utilized in the individualized management of the patient with dizziness and/or unsteadiness. Knowledge of the purpose and expected results for each test/measure is critical to planning the patient examination based on history and patient interview and therefore determining what intervention methods and/or other referrals are indicated. Understanding nystagmus and the various eye movements along with recognition of direction and latencies are key components to the vestibular examination, especially considering the intricate relationship between the vestibular and visual systems. Upon completion of the vestibular examination, the physical therapist should be able to identify whether a problem is of peripheral or central origin and which aspects of vestibular function and resulting activity limitations should be addressed in intervention. The Focus on Evidence (FOE) table (Table 8-11 (ONL)) provides a summary of some of the most important evidence related to tests and measures for vestibular system function. Detailed information on intervention for vestibular dysfunction is presented in Chapter 29.

# Balance and Vestibular Examination
# Intake Questionnaire

Patient Name: _____

Date: _____

MR# _____

Name and address of physician(s) you wish our report to be sent:

_____

_____

_____

**Please answer the following questions to the best of your ability. PLEASE BRING THIS QUESTIONNAIRE WITH YOU TO YOUR APPOINTMENT—DO NOT MAIL IT BACK. If you need to change or cancel your appointment please contact the clinic.**

Describe your major problem or the reason why you are seeing a physical therapist.

What do you think caused your problem?

How long have you had your problem? Give a specific date and/or event if known.

What treatment have you received for your problem?

1. **Please check the tests or evaluations that you have had in the past year.**
   - ☐ Hearing Test
   - ☐ Caloric test (water or air in the ears)
   - ☐ MRI
   - ☐ Head CAT Scan
   - ☐ Evaluation by a neurologist
   - ☐ Evaluation by an ear doctor
   - ☐ Evaluation by an eye doctor

2. **Please check the symptoms that apply to your problem.**
   - ☐ The room spins around me.
   - ☐ I feel like I am spinning.
   - ☐ I frequently feel off-balance.
   - ☐ I fall once a week.
   - ☐ I fall once a month.
   - ☐ I fall twice a month.
   - ☐ I fall 3 or more times a month.

☐ I get car sick as a passenger.
☐ I get car sick as a driver.
☐ I have my symptoms today.
☐ I have symptoms all of the time.
☐ Different head positions cause my problem to occur.

**Associated symptoms**
☐ Sweating
☐ Nausea
☐ Vomiting
☐ Queasiness
☐ Headache

**Impaired vision**
☐ Double vision
☐ Blurred vision
☐ Flashes of light
☐ Jumping of vision when walking or riding in a car

3. **To what extent is your dizziness or imbalance brought on by:**

| CHECK ONE ANSWER FOR EACH QUESTION | NONE | SOME | SEVERE |
|---|---|---|---|
| Turning over in bed | | | |
| Bending over to tie your shoes | | | |
| Looking up | | | |
| Standing up | | | |
| Rapid head movement | | | |
| Walking in a dark room | | | |
| Walking on uneven surfaces | | | |
| Loud noises | | | |
| Coughing or sneezing | | | |
| Straining | | | |
| Movement of objects in the environment | | | |
| Moving your eyes while your head is still | | | |

4. **Social History**

| PROBLEM | YES | NO |
|---|---|---|
| Have you recently traveled a long distance by train, plane, or boat? | | |
| Do or did you use alcohol? How much? | | |
| Do or did you ever smoke? | | |
| If so, how many packs/day? | | |
| Do you consume caffeinated drinks? | | |
| Do you live alone? | | |
| Do you live in a one-story home? | | |
| Do you have to negotiate steps? | | |
| Are you employed? State occupation: | | |

## 5. Past or Present Medical History

| PROBLEM | YES | NO |
| --- | --- | --- |
| High blood pressure | | |
| Diabetes | | |
| Heart Problems | | |
| HIV/AIDS infection | | |
| Arthritis | | |
| Cancer | | |
| Depression | | |

List all major illnesses, injuries, and surgeries not previously described.

_____

_____

_____

## 6. Medications

What medications are you currently taking? Please include hormones, birth control pills, special diet, etc. (Name and Amount/Day)?

1.

2.

3.

4.

5.

6.

7.

**7. Have you ever had any of the following: (If yes, please give details.)**

| PROBLEMS | YES | NO |
|---|---|---|
| Ankle sprains | | |
| Ankle fractures | | |
| Knee replacements or pain | | |
| Hip replacements or pain | | |
| Foot problems or pain | | |
| Loss of sensation in your feet | | |
| Neck problems or pain | | |
| Back problems or pain | | |
| Ear infections | | |
| Hearing loss (right ear, left ear, both ears) | | |
| Ear pain, fullness, popping, or pressure | | |
| Ringing in ears (right ear, left ear, both ears) | | |
| Head injury or concussion (with loss of consciousness) | | |
| Headaches more than 3 times per week | | |
| Migraines accompanied by vertigo | | |

**8. Review of Systems (If yes, give details.)**

| WITHIN THE LAST 6 MONTHS HAVE YOU NOTED: | YES | NO |
|---|---|---|
| Significant loss in strength | | |
| Significant loss of energy | | |
| 10 lb. or more weight change (if yes, up _____ or down _____) | | |
| Significant memory loss (amnesia) | | |
| Significant change in handwriting | | |
| Fainting or blackout spells | | |
| Pins and needles, numbness in arms or legs | | |
| Muscle or joint aches (if yes, which muscles or joints _____) | | |
| Urinary incontinence (leakage of urine) | | |
| Incoordination | | |
| Headaches (If you answered yes to headaches, please answer the following:) | | |
| Approximate age they began_____ | | |
| Number per month _____; Pain intensity (1–10 with 10 being the most severe) | | |
| Do your headaches last at least 4 hours? | | |
| Do they start on one side of the head? If yes, which side _____ | | |
| Are they throbbing or pulsatile in quality? | | |
| Are they severe enough to interfere with your schedule? | | |
| Are they aggravated by routine physical activity? | | |
| Are they associated with nausea and/or vomiting? | | |
| Are they aggravated by bright lights or loud noises? | | |

# Examination of Balance and Equilibrium

Andrea Fergus, PT, PhD ▪ Dennis W. Fell, PT, MD
Rachel T. Wellons, PT, DPT, NCS

**CHAPTER 9**

## CHAPTER OBJECTIVES

Upon completion of this chapter, the learner should be able to:

1. Distinguish between static and dynamic forms of balance with examples of each that may be identified on the problem list in patients with neurological disorders.
2. Identify safety issues that can affect the examination of balance and equilibrium.
3. Describe the critical aspects of anatomy and physiology related to motor and sensory systems that contribute to balance and equilibrium.
4. Synthesize knowledge of balance impairment with understanding of functional activity performance to determine examples of how decreased balance can contribute to functional activity limitation.
5. Analyze information from patient history in a specific patient scenario to select appropriate balance tests/measures.
6. Explain the significance and implications of specific balance test/measure results.
7. Record thorough, meaningful, and accurate documentation of balance examination results, patient problems related to balance, and goals/prognosis for recovery in a given patient scenario.

## ■ Introduction

*Mr. McMurray,* a 75 year-old man, was a fairly active golfer until 6 months ago when he was diagnosed with peripheral neuropathy related to diabetes mellitus. He now reports he has fallen three times in the past week. He and his wife report that his balance is "off" and has gradually worsened over the past couple of months. Because of his falls, now combined with significant fear of falling, Mr. McMurray even avoids many of the simple community activities he frequently enjoyed in the past, including attending the weekly Bingo game. It will be very important to determine the impact of his balance deficit on his functional activity and on his participation. Measures should be selected to optimally quantify his balance ability as a baseline and to help direct the development of the treatment plan.

**Balance** or **equilibrium**, sometimes referred to as **postural stability**, is the ability to maintain stability in an upright posture particularly keeping the body up against gravity.

Balance is an essential component of all upright tasks involving both the ability to recover from episodes of instability and the ability to anticipate and move in ways to avoid instability and falling. From the standpoint of physics, for any upright object to be stable *the center of mass must be maintained over the base of support.* The **center of mass (COM)** is the single point at which all the mass of the object can be considered to lie. The **base of support (BOS)** includes all points of body contact with the supporting surface and can be described or visualized as the area enclosed within the perimeter of all these points of contact. For example, in sitting, the BOS includes the ischial tuberosities and buttocks, probably part of the posterior thighs (depending on how far back the person is sitting on the surface), the feet, and perhaps even an upper extremity or hand. The statement relating COM to BOS implies there must be a system of sensory input to monitor the location of the COM in relation to the BOS and a system of motor output that can regulate these positional relationships. The maximum distance a person can intentionally move or displace his/her COM in each direction without losing balance is known as the **limits of stability (LOS).**

The ability to maintain balance allows an individual to maintain an upright posture during a perturbation such as getting bumped while waiting in line. In addition, anticipatory control to maintain balance would be needed in situations such as intentionally bending down to pick up an object from the floor. Dynamic balance, described in the following section, is needed to stay upright while running and kicking a soccer ball. The ability to balance can be compromised by disease, dysfunction, medications, or the processes of aging. Impaired balance can cause a significantly negative effect on a person's quality of life and should be examined thoroughly by the therapist. The level of independence in functional tasks as well as personal safety, particularly the risk for falls, are closely associated with one's balance (Shubert, 2006; Brotheton, 2005; Shumway-Cook, 1997) with fall risk clearly increasing with aging (Tinetti, 1988b).

Equilibrium or balance is a complex body function/body structure that depends on normal operation of multiple sensory and motor systems. Disequilibrium or balance impairment is considered a complex impairment because multiple body systems may be involved. Balance, in and of itself, is not an activity or functional task, but it is a required component in all specific upright functional tasks. Disequilibrium can result from impairment of any of the related systems as described later in this chapter. Limitations in balance may contribute to functional limitations in many specific tasks and activities. In adults, limitations in standing and sitting, for example, influence gait, transfers, activities of daily living (ADLs), and reaching activities. Balance also influences function in other developmental positions such as kneeling and quadruped, so deficits could affect tasks such as floor transfers and creeping in children. Limitations in balance often result in restrictions of activities due to fear of falling (Vellas, 1987; Tinetti, 1990; Tinetti, 1993; Chandler, 1996; Lachman, 1998; Murphy, 2002). The decrease in functional abilities and avoidance of activities may negatively influence a person's societal roles and result in disability or participation restrictions. The examination of balance and equilibrium is a critical component of the neurological examination across the lifespan and in multiple neuromuscular diagnoses. The patient-specific examination will help identify the degree of balance impairment, related safety concerns, underlying impairments contributing to balance deficits, limitations to functional activity that result, and fall risks each with implications for direct intervention the therapist must provide.

## ■ Categories of Balance and Equilibrium

The goals of the **postural control** systems, the systems regulating upright position of the body against gravity, are upright stability and function. A complex interaction of biomechanical components, sensory systems, motor systems, and central nervous system (CNS) integration must occur to maintain balance during both static and dynamic activities. **Static balance** is maintaining upright posture, any posture, in the absence of self-initiated movement—that is, simply maintaining a posture while not trying to move or even maintaining a posture against mild disturbance from an external source. **Dynamic balance**, whether sitting or standing, is maintaining upright posture or stability during self-initiated body or body-segment active movement. Cognition also plays an essential role in the patient's interpretation of available information and the planning of effective responses including those involved in postural control. Impairments in cognition are associated with decreased balance ability and increased fall risk (Holtzer, 2007; Kose, 2005; Blanchard, 2005). Consideration of a patient's cognition, discussed in Chapter 4, is therefore critical in the interpretation of the examination of balance and in the intervention planning that follows.

## The Process of Dynamic Equilibrium

Horak (1987) divides the postural control system into three basic functional components (biomechanical, sensory, and motor) that provide a helpful framework to keep in mind for examination and intervention decisions regarding balance. The three elements should be kept in mind also as components that can be manipulated in the intervention plan (Fig. 9-1). *Biomechanically,* it is important to consider the forces applied and the mechanical factors that contribute to body and joint/segment stability. *Sensory* components include all incoming information used to monitor the person's equilibrium status as a basis upon which to determine appropriate adjustments to maintain an upright posture. The *motor* components include

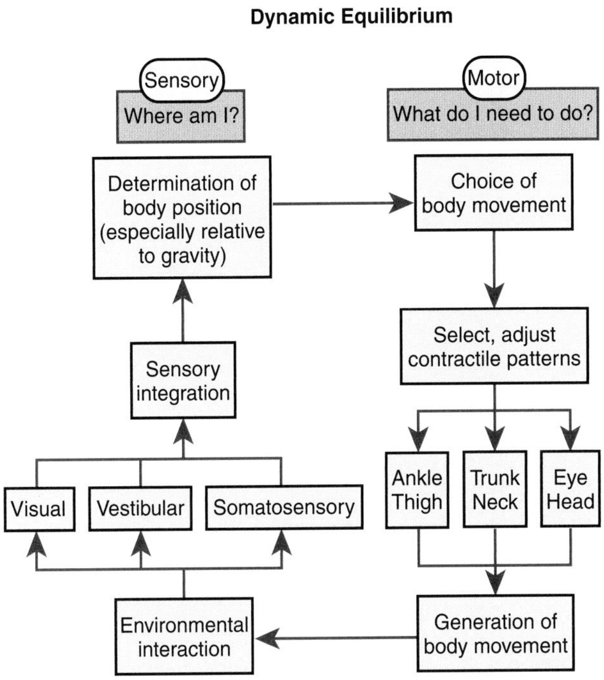

**FIGURE 9-1** Process of Dynamic Equilibrium (interaction of sensory and motor).

all parts of the neuromusculoskeletal systems that help to carry out the postural adjustments and equilibrium reactions essential to maintain balance. Obviously, *central processing* must take place in the CNS after receiving the sensory components and before implementing the motor components and for real-time adjustments and reactions during the balance reaction.

### Biomechanical Components

Force-platform studies using computerized force-platforms have contributed to the understanding of the biomechanical properties of balance, including center of pressure and LOS. The **center of pressure (COP)** or the **center of gravity** is the single location on the supporting surface where the gravitational line, passing through the COM, would strike the floor or other supporting surface as shown in Figure 9-2. When using a force platform, the COP can be displayed dynamically on a visual monitor or recorded as a string of data representing changes in the COP location. As a person's weight shifts, the COP moves in the direction of the weight shift. On the monitor, right weight-shift causes the computer cursor to move right, left weight-shift causes left cursor movement, forward shift causes upward cursor movement, and backward shift causes downward cursor movement. The LOS are the maximal distances an individual can safely lean in each direction without loss of balance (Fig. 9-3). You could envision this as the circumferential extremes within which the COP can lean with the body remaining stable. In standing, how far, without taking a step or repositioning your feet, can you incline your body forward and how far backward (Fig. 9-3A), how far to the right, and how far to the left (Fig. 9-3A)? The composite of all these movements

circumferentially would create a cone-shaped representation of a person's ability to lean in each direction, the LOS (Fig. 9-3C). Figure 9-3D illustrates the same concepts applied to a person in sitting position. Using force-platform measures of movement of COP in subjects with hemiplegic stroke, dynamic balance measures using force-platform data are supported over static balance measures as valid indicators of functional balance performance (Liston, 1996). This seems logical, since the majority of functional skills or tasks involve movement toward the extremes of the LOS to accomplish a purposeful task rather than simply maintaining a static posture safely in midline. Therefore, during balance training, we should encourage our patients to regularly move toward the edge of their LOS while in a safe guarded environment. Before this however we must observe and measure the patient's balance ability.

In standing with four inches between the feet, Nashner (1990) reported the LOS as 12 degrees in an anteroposterior direction and 16 degrees from side-to-side. Obviously, sway in a posterior direction is most limited as there is no extension of the BOS posteriorly. The greater mediolateral sway is probably related to having two separated supports (the feet) in the frontal plane and the resulting stance width. As balance abilities decline, logically the LOS decrease. It has been shown in young healthy adults that, under more challenging stance conditions (eyes closed, narrow BOS, and movement of the support surface), the COP tends to move toward the center of the BOS and spends a greater time more centrally, away from the edge of the LOS (Nichols, 1995).

### Sensory Systems

The primary sensory (afferent) systems involved in balance and equilibrium include the visual system, somatosensory system (both proprioception and superficial tactile), and the vestibular system. The CNS must integrate the information from these systems to appropriately regulate goal-directed actions and automatic postural responses to maintain balance.

The **visual** system provides information regarding the environment, in particular a reference for determining "upright" to which the individual must accurately respond to maintain balance. Visual cues regarding the orientation of the environment relative to the individual are obtained by scanning for horizontal and vertical cues such as the horizon, windows and doorframes, buildings, walls, room corners, and trees. These cues are then utilized to maintain an upright position during static tasks or dynamic movement. When standing on a ramp/incline, an individual must process information from the somatosensory system regarding the degree of the incline and integrate that information with visual input regarding what is upright against gravity, then respond to maintain balance and equilibrium. Visual processing begins very early in development, and young children learn to visually compare body position to vertical and horizontal images from the environment. Optical righting reactions, the orientation of the head in response to visual inputs, develop during childhood to allow such orientation of the head to occur. You may have experienced, as you were falling from your bicycle for example,

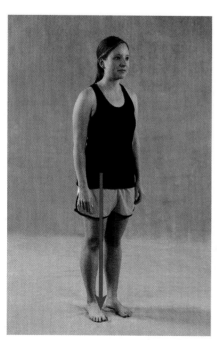

**FIGURE 9-2** An individual in standing, showing the approximate location of the Center of Pressure (COP) in relation to body position.

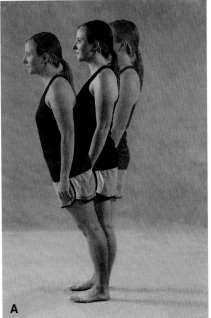

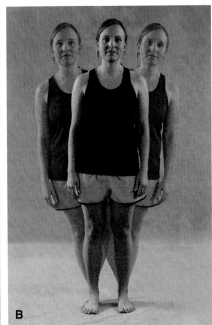

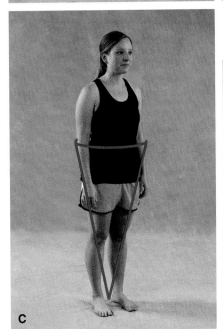

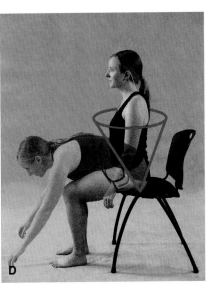

FIGURE 9-3 **A.** An individual in standing illustrating the anterior-posterior dimensions of the cone-shaped Limits of Stability (LOS) from a lateral view. **B.** An anterior view illustrating the lateral dimensions of the limits of stability. **C.** The projected cone-shaped Limits of Stability (LOS) in an adult. **D.** A possible anterior/posterior LOS for an adult in sitting position.

awareness that your personal orientation was becoming less and less upright compared with the trees, bushes, and fence posts around you. The visual system also provides information regarding obstacles to navigate and/or anticipate in the environment to maintain equilibrium. In addition to the recognition of objects within the environment, the visual system provides dynamic information regarding the movement of objects. For example, when one approaches an escalator, the visual system provides information on the height and speed of the approaching step. The individual must then anticipate the step onto the escalator with appropriate postural responses while maintaining balance. A reduction of visual cues in unstable surface conditions has been shown to increase the likelihood of balance loss 5.7-fold (Judge, 1995).

*Somatosensory* **system** information contributing to balance includes (1) cutaneous touch and pressure sensations from the body segments in contact with the supporting surface and (2) proprioceptive and kinesthetic information from muscle receptors (muscle spindles) and joint receptors (Golgi tendon organs and joint capsule receptors). The tactile information from the external environment contacting the body (e.g., differential pressure from the forefoot or heel while standing or from the ischial tuberosities, posterior thighs, and feet while sitting) provides the individual with necessary information such as the shape, orientation, and stability of the support surface or environment and whether bodyweight in standing is mostly borne at the forefoot (leaning forward) or the heel (leaning backward). Tactile receptors in the skin, especially pressure receptors along the sole of the foot in standing or the buttocks/thigh in sitting, help to self-monitor, in a general way, the location and movement of the COP. In the feet as you shift forward, you can feel most of your weight on the front of your foot, and as you shift backward most of the weight is felt at your heel. As your CNS detects extreme changes, you can use the motor system through the legs and trunk to adjust your body position accordingly.

Even more importantly for balance, proprioception, particularly subconscious position sense from muscle spindles carried by the spinocerebellar pathways, provides essential information about joint position at each body region but especially throughout the legs in standing. In standing, position sense from the ankles is most important because this joint serves as the primary pivot joint in quiet standing. For example, if excessive dorsiflexion is detected as an indication of excessive forward lean, which would be accompanied by increased pressure sense from the forefoot, the individual would use plantar flexor muscles to pull the tibia backward into plantar flexion, and the body with it, back into a more upright position. Input from the joint and muscle receptors provides the individual with information regarding joint position as well as the speed and direction of movement. This information is utilized to determine appropriate postural responses. For example, when running to kick a ball, the individual must anticipate and respond to the speed, direction, and magnitude of the lower extremity movement by activating postural responses involving the trunk and extremities.

The *vestibular* **system** apparatus consisting of the semicircular canals and the otolith organs in the inner ear provides information about the position of the head relative to gravity as well as the movement of the head in space. Even with our eyes closed, we can sense position and movement of our head primarily using vestibular input. We tend to depend on this sense most when vision and somatosensation are limited. The primary functions of this system for balance include the awareness of upright in relation to gravity, the stabilization of gaze during head movements via the **vestibulo-ocular reflex** (VOR), and the regulation of postural tone and muscle activation via the vestibulospinal pathways. During any head movement, the VOR promotes **gaze stability** by causing the eyes to move at the same speed and magnitude but in the opposite direction from the head movement. Along with the somatosensory and visual systems, the vestibular system provides essential information regarding the position of the head, communicating this information to the appropriate postural muscles to support equilibrium and to the extraocular muscles to maintain gaze. The maintenance of gaze allows the visual system to transmit accurate information to the brain even during head movement, thus further assisting the individual in maintaining equilibrium.

### Central Processing

The CNS integrates the information from all of these sensory systems as a basis for maintaining balance. The relative importance of each system varies depending on the individual, the task, and the context of the task as each piece of information

is interpreted in relation to the others. Some types of sensory information are not valid in certain circumstances. For example, the joint position at the ankle, very important sensory information while standing on a stable surface, is irrelevant if standing on an unstable surface with changing slant/incline. Perception takes place at the level of the cerebral hemispheres with the composite information serving as the basis for the motor responses that comprise the equilibrium reactions. Depending on the circumstances and environmental conditions, a person may depend on certain sensory modalities more than others as the basis for balance reactions. Under low light conditions, for instance, the somatosensory and vestibular systems would play a greater role than the visual system. The redundancy of input from the three systems allows for increased flexibility in the system across diverse environments. Individuals with a loss in one area may compensate for this loss through expanded use of another system. For example, in an individual with somatosensory loss (e.g., a person with peripheral neuropathy related to diabetes), the roles of the visual and vestibular systems would increase. The Clinical Test for Sensory Interaction in Balance (CTSIB), discussed in more detail later in this chapter, can be used to determine how well an individual utilizes each of these sensory systems to maintain balance (Shumway-Cook, 1986).

The interaction of these three sensory systems is essential in maintaining upright balance. In quiet undisturbed standing, humans depend most on the somatosensory information from the ankle and foot, primarily position sense from the ankle, but some from pressure sensation from the sole of the foot (in sitting, the brain uses position sense from the hip joint and pressure sensation from the ischial tuberosities and buttocks). When standing on an unstable or moving surface, for example standing in a rocking boat on rough seas or walking across an inflatable mattress, somatosensory input is less reliable in reflecting our relationship to upright and in fact can conflict with the other sensory systems. In fact, under such conditions, if there were a hard and fast rule that depended only on proprioception, "always maintain the ankle at zero degrees," a fall would quickly result on unstable surfaces as this rule assumes that the support surface is always horizontal. On unstable surfaces, people therefore rely more on visual cues (e.g., scanning the environment for the horizon) and vestibular information (e.g., detecting whether the head is upright or not) to help maintain equilibrium. When standing on an unstable surface with limited vision (e.g., standing in a fishing boat at night), the balance system depends primarily on vestibular input to help gauge position in relation to gravity as a prerequisite for making adjustments to maintain balance.

Declines in somatosensory (Lia, 2002), visual (Kosnik, 1988), and anatomical and physiological aspects of vestibular system (Sloane, 1989) function occur with aging (Furman, 2001). These declines affect the balance ability of elderly adults but there is no particular pattern of loss in the elderly. The elderly may be generally able to maintain balance ability when one sensory system is reduced. However, when more than one sensory modality is reduced, older adults are less able to maintain balance than younger individuals (Woolacott, 1986).

## Motor Responses

The motor plans to maintain balance are complex and vary depending on the demands and context of the task and the individual. Each individual motor plan of the balance process in standing is carried out by the neuromuscular system—specifically, motor pathways of the CNS acting upon specific muscle groups, primarily in the lower extremity, to cause the desired coordinated actions that maintain equilibrium. Upright postural stability is possible only with carefully timed complex interactions taking place between opposing muscle groups at each supporting joint and among muscles at related joints that work together to maintain balance.

Righting, protective, and equilibrium reactions are postural responses that occur in a "reflexive" or stereotypic manner to certain sensory stimuli and are developed during childhood (see Chapter 13), playing a critical role in balance. **Righting reactions** orient the head in space and the body in relation to the head and support surface and can occur in response to visual (optical righting), vestibular (labyrinthine righting), or somatosensory (body on head righting) cues. Righting reactions typically begin development at approximately 3 months of age. **Protective reactions**, including protective extension, prevent a fall after the COM moves irreparably beyond the LOS and prevent injury by one or more extremities reaching out to prop on the surface or reset/expand the BOS in the direction of the disturbance to avert a fall. Figure 9-4 illustrates protective responses in a pediatric and adult individual. In sitting, forward and sideways protective reactions typically begin between 6 and 9 months of age with backward protective reactions being the last to develop by 10 to 12 months of age. **Equilibrium (balance) reactions** are relatively sophisticated postural responses that occur in response to substantial displacement of the COM; these reactions begin to develop at the end of the first year of life. These movements generally shift the body in the direction opposite from the perturbing force to maintain balance. An equilibrium reaction typically includes trunk rotation along with extension and abduction of the extremities. As one matures to adulthood, the motor strategies involved in postural control and maintaining one's balance become much more complex and adaptable with a decline that occurs in the geriatric years.

Nashner has described and categorized the complex motor interactions of balance in standing as three levels or three balance strategies: **ankle strategy**, **hip strategy**, and **stepping strategy** (Nashner, 1976; Nashner, 1985; Horak, 1986; Nashner, 1990). The three balance strategies the therapist would observe during the examination are described in the following text from simplest (which result from mild perturbation) to most complex (which result from more severe perturbation) and illustrated in Figures 9-5A, B, and C.

1. *Ankle strategy.* If a person is quietly standing, whether conversing with a friend or visually appreciating the beauty of the great outdoors, maintaining balance would simply involve appropriate but subtle responses to the environment including the wind, the individual's perceptions, or responses to one's own movement, even something as simple as a basic arm gesture. Most often, responses to such mild perturbations occur in what Nashner calls an "ankle strategy" observed as tibial movement at the ankle joint to shift the body's COM toward the center of the BOS and enhance postural stability. This strategy in standing employs predominantly distal muscle activation of the lower extremity, using muscles at the ankle as the primary pivot joint. In sitting, the analogous response would be movement at the hip joint for anterior/posterior sway and the lower trunk muscles for lateral sway.

2. *Hip strategy.* At a more active level, if a person gets bumped, for example by someone quickly passing on the sidewalk, more forceful reactions may be required to keep from falling. This may occur when the bus or subway comes to a rapid stop while standing and facing forward. Nashner calls this a "hip strategy," which involves flexion or extension of the hip to more extremely shift the COM within the bounds of the BOS. A proximal to distal activation of muscles has been described for this strategy, and knee flexion may also be incorporated to lower the COM, which also increases stability. The analogous response in sitting could be dramatic upper-trunk movements or upper-extremity position changes to quickly reposition the COM over the BOS.

3. *Stepping strategy.* This most active balance strategy occurs following sudden and forceful disturbances that displace the COM well outside the BOS even to such a degree that the person cannot recover stability using the ankle strategy or hip strategy. In standing, this "stepping strategy," which can be considered a form of protective extension, occurs by quickly lifting and moving one foot in the same direction as the externally applied perturbation to reset a new BOS which encompasses the new COM location. If the force is applied from one side, the individual usually takes a step with the foot on the opposite side. However, if the contralateral foot is the predominant weight-bearing foot at the instant of perturbation, the step will likely be made by the ipsilateral foot moving across the midline of the body in the direction of the external force because there is insufficient time to carry out a weight-shift before the step. In response to extreme forces, as seen frequently in sports, a series of several steps may be required to regain stability.

Combinations of these strategies are utilized to maintain equilibrium (Horak, 1986) in this very flexible multicomponent system. As part of the physical examination of balance, you should note the motor strategies utilized to maintain balance. In addition to the presence of the strategies, you should document (1) whether the strategy utilized was effective and appropriate within the context of the task, (2) whether the

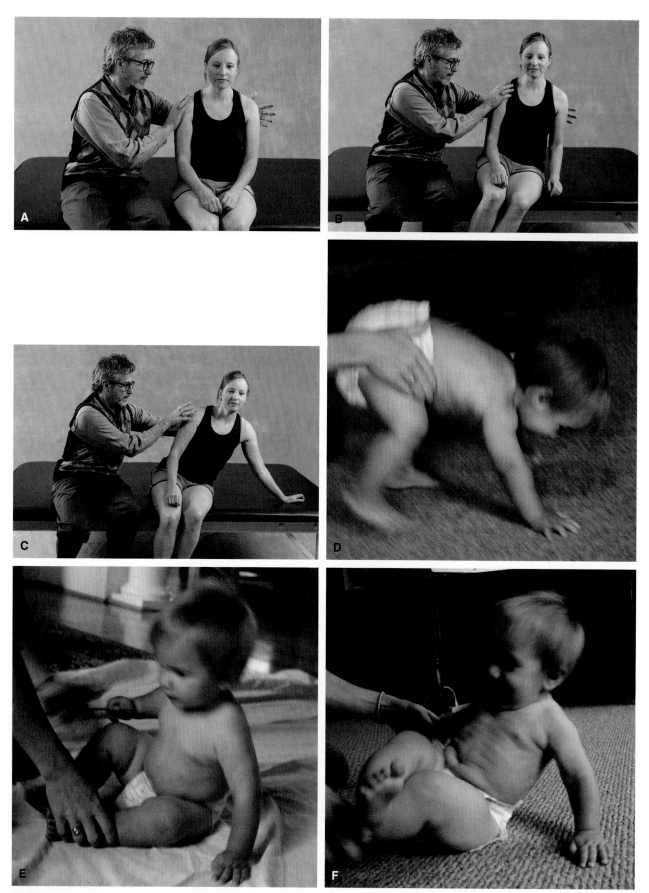

**FIGURE 9-4** Figures **A, B,** and **C.** show the sequence of protective responses in sitting in an adult. Protective extension responses in sitting for a toddler are shown for **D.** forward protective response in standing, **E.** sideways in sitting, and **F.** backward in sitting. Posterior/backward protective extension is the latest form of protective extension to develop in childhood.

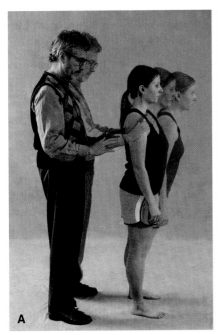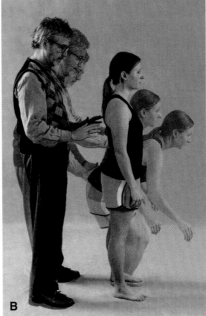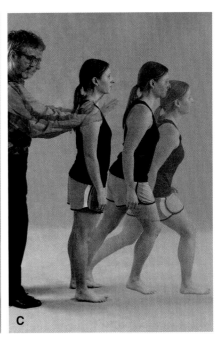

**FIGURE 9-5** These photos demonstrate typical balance strategies in standing: **A.** Ankle strategy, **B.** hip strategy, and **C.** stepping strategy.

timing of the execution of the strategy was effective to meet the demand, and (3) whether the muscles were activated in the appropriate sequence. These strategies should be tested across a variety of tasks involving both reactive and anticipatory postural control.

## Safety Concerns

During balance examination, the safety of the patient must be uppermost in the therapist's mind. Safety concerns should be inherent in any test or measure related to balance and equilibrium. As part of the initial examination, the balance test is performed because the therapist does not know the balance ability of the patient, and often before the examination, you already know the person has some known risk for falling related to the neuromuscular disorder or related system impairments such as weakness or range of motion restrictions. Also, most balance tests place the patient in a demanding or precarious position (e.g., narrow BOS, single-limb stance, etc.) that places the patient at further risk for falling. Therefore, you must carefully observe, guard (including a gait belt), and protect the patient from any risk of falling during the testing procedure. You must be prepared in any instant to fully support the patient or gently lower them to the support surface to prevent a fall if their balance reserves are overcome by the demands of the balance test.

## Physiology and Neuroscience of Balance

The group of neuroanatomical structures that intercommunicate to maintain equilibrium is complex, including the integration of several sensory systems and the motor systems previously described. The key structures in the CNS related to balance are illustrated in Figure 9-6 (Where Is It?). The somatosensory system utilizes mechanoreceptors and somatosensory motor pathways described in greater detail in Chapter 5. The visual system detects light via photoreceptors located in the retina. Visual information is transmitted via both conscious and subconscious optic pathways to the primary visual cortex to allow the brain to perceive visual images of the environment, including horizontal and vertical cues to optimize upright position. The vestibular apparatus, located in the inner ear and described in more detail in Chapter 8, consists of the bony and membranous labyrinths and the hair cells that are the vestibular sensory receptors. The bony labyrinth contains three semicircular canals that detect angular or rotary acceleration of the head in three different planes and two otolith organs that primarily monitor planar acceleration movements of the head. Vestibular inputs and outputs related to balance are described in Chapter 8. The neuroanatomical pathways and receptors of all these sensory systems relative to their roles in balance are summarized in Table 9-1.

Several motor pathways are involved in the maintenance of equilibrium, including the medial corticospinal, vestibulospinal, and tectospinal pathways. Certainly, to maintain balance there must be precise coordination, motor control, and strength of muscle activity in the limbs and axial musculature. Therefore, strength and coordination must be closely examined as potential underlying factors in impaired balance. For the purposes of the discussion here, however, the primary motor pathways considered in the maintenance of equilibrium are those pathways acting on the axial musculature. The motor system can be divided into a dorsolateral system, controlling purposeful limb movement, and a ventromedial system, controlling posture and balance. The ventromedial system includes several pathways to the lower motor neurons of axial and girdle musculature. These motor pathways are summarized in

■WHERE IS IT?

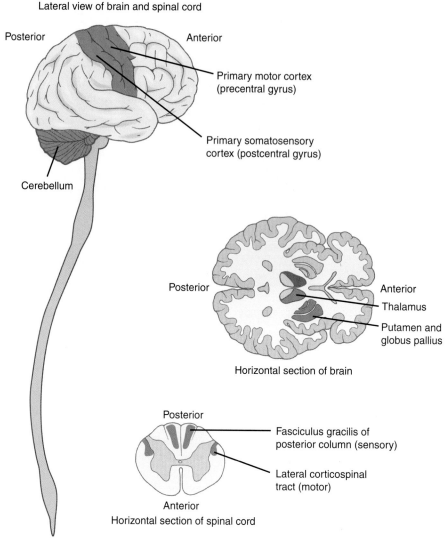

FIGURE 9-6 Major CNS locations related to balance (within brain, brainstem, spinal cord). In the brain, important areas related to balance include the primary somatosensory cortex (postcentral gyrus), primary and secondary motor cortex (precentral gyrus and posterior aspects of the superior frontal lobe), and processing centers in the cerebellum, basal ganglia, and thalamus. Lesion locations are shown on only one side of the brain but damage to either side can impair balance.

Table 9-2. Based on CNS integration of input from several sensory systems and central processing of the collective information, motor signals are sent to coordinate multiple motor pathways for implementation of the motor responses previously described to maintain balance across a variety of tasks and conditions.

## ■ Functional Implications of Balance and Equilibrium

Maintaining personal equilibrium is critical for independence and safety. Impairment of balance in either sitting or standing will decrease independence in related specific functional tasks, decrease efficiency in performance of those tasks, or prolong performance time of the task. These limitations to functional skill performance can decrease the individual's motivation to move and may result in a more sedentary lifestyle with resulting further decrements in balance.

Limitations in balance and in mobility have been identified as risk factors for falls (Hyndman, 2002; Hyndman, 2003; Lamb, 2003). The incidence of falls in community-dwelling older adults is between 11% and 30% while reported incidence in individuals who have suffered a stroke is as high as 50% (Jorgenson, 2002; Lamb, 2003; Hyndman, 2003; Graafmans, 1996). According to the Centers for Disease Control and Prevention (2016), "Injuries from falls are treated in an emergency department every 13 seconds and claim a life every 20 minutes. Every year, 1 out of 3 older adults

| TABLE 9-1 | Central Nervous System Sensory Structures and Their Roles in Maintaining Balance | | | |
|---|---|---|---|---|
| **SENSATION** | **RECEPTORS/ LOCATION** | **PATHWAYS TO CNS** | **FUNCTIONAL ROLE IN BALANCE** | **PROJECTIONS/ DECUSSATION** |
| Conscious proprioception | Muscle spindles, joint receptors, and Golgi tendon organs in muscles, tendons, and joints | Dorsal Column/Medial Lemniscus Fasciculus cuneatus and fasciculus gracilis in dorsal column of spinal cord, becomes medial lemniscal system in brainstem to parietal lobe of cerebral cortex | Conscious knowledge of position and movement of body relative to environment | Fibers cross in the low medulla through the internal arcuate fibers |
| Unconscious proprioception | Muscle spindles, joint receptors, and Golgi tendon organs in muscles, tendons, and joints | Spinocerebellar pathways to the cerebellum | Subconscious feedback regarding accuracy of movement and position | Most fibers end up in ipsilateral cerebellum (either as uncrossed fibers or tracts that cross in the spinal cord and then recross to the original side in the brainstem) |
| Visual | Photoreceptors (rods and cones) in retina of each eye | Retinotectal (Tectum) | Visual awareness of environment, including static and dynamic components Feedforward anticipation of environmental challenges Feedback responses to changes in environment and position of body relative to environment | Fibers from the medial half of each retina cross at the optic chiasm |
| | | Retinogeniculocalcarine (to visual cortex) | Conscious movement (dorsal action stream) Visual identification of objects | |
| Angular and linear acceleration | Hair cells, semicircular canals, and otolith organs of inner ear | To the neocortex via oculomotor nuclei via medial longitudinal fasciculus To the spinal cord via vestibulospinal pathways | Perception of head movement Coordination of eye movements Postural control | |
| Tactile sensation | Mechanoreceptors | Dorsal column/medial lemniscus and antero-lateral pathway (anterior spinothalamic and lateral spinothalamic tracts) to the somatosensory cortex | Provide information regarding location and movement of center of pressure | The fibers cross in low medulla (DCML) or in the spinal cord (spinothalamic) before ascending to contralateral thalamus |

falls, yet less than half tell their doctor about it." Up to 28% of individuals who have had a stroke report an injury associated with a fall (Lamb, 2003).

Relationships between mobility and balance, particularly dynamic balance, have been demonstrated in the literature (Shubert, 2006). Balance performance is a significant predictor of both gait speed and timed chair rise (Shubert, 2006). In sitting, impaired balance can decrease a person's ability to sit unsupported, cause the person to depend on external support for sitting, and impair active sitting activities such as weight-shift,

| TABLE 9-2 | Central Nervous System Motor Structures and Their Roles in Maintaining Balance | | | |
|---|---|---|---|---|
| **MOTOR** | **STRUCTURE/ LOCATION** | **PATHWAYS FROM CNS** | **FUNCTIONAL ROLE IN BALANCE** | **PROJECTIONS/ DECUSSATION** |
| Primary motor cortex | Cell bodies in precentral gyrus of cerebral cortex (head, neck, arms, and trunk cell bodies on lateral surface; lower extremity and foot cell bodies on medial surface) | Contribute to corticospinal tracts | Voluntary contralateral motor control of all skeletal muscle groups; also carries signals for all reflexive motor responses of balance and equilibrium to skeletal muscles | |
| Premotor cortex | Cell bodies in caudal portion of lateral frontal lobe cortex, just anterior to upper body portion of precentral gyrus | Interconnects to primary motor cortex | Control of axial and proximal limb musculature and initial movements to orient the body | |
| Supplementary motor cortex | Cell bodies in superomedial aspect of the caudal frontal lobe (anterior to the paracentral lobule lower extremity primary motor cortex) | Interconnects to primary motor cortex | Programming patterns and sequences of movements | |
| Lateral corticospinal tract | From cell bodies (pyramidal cells) of precentral gyrus | Fibers pass sequentially through:<br>-corona radiata<br>-internal capsule<br>-crus cerebri of cerebral peduncle<br>-through pons<br>-pyramids of medulla<br>-pyramidal decussation to cross to contralateral side<br>-then passes down through spinal cord as a tract in posterior aspect of lateral funiculus (lateral corticospinal tract)<br>-terminates on target anterior horn cells (alpha motor neurons) | Carries motor signals from primary motor cortex to skeletal muscles | Fibers cross in anterior aspects of lower medulla through pyramidal decussation |
| Final common pathway | For each spinal level, cell bodies of anterior horn of spinal cord central gray matter | Fibers pass sequentially through:<br>-ventral root<br>-spinal root<br>-spinal nerve<br>-peripheral nerve<br>-terminates at neuromuscular junction of specific target skeletal muscle | All voluntary and reflexive motor signals must pass through final common pathway to activate muscles | |

reaching, scooting in sitting, transfers, and sit-to-stand. Functional tasks in standing such as standing at a counter unsupported, standing in line, turning around to see someone, reaching for an object, walking, and stepping up ramps, curbs, or stairs, would also be negatively affected when balance is impaired.

## ■ Principles of Examination of Balance

Now, to build upon the theoretical base, certain principles and tactics always apply during administration of the balance examination. Analysis of balance is a critical component of the examination in any individual with a neuromuscular disorder, adult or pediatric, guided by a detailed history. The history should explore any falls or near-falls the patient has experienced. Then, assess whether the falls were the result of intrinsic or extrinsic factors. Factors intrinsic to the patient or **intrinsic factors** contributing to falls may include system impairments including but not limited to dysfunction of the vestibular, proprioceptive, or visual sensory systems as well as motor impairments of weakness, incoordination, poor motor control, and limited range of motion. Also ask about **extrinsic factors**, factors external to the patient that can lead to falling, for example, ice that causes slipping, an indoor throw rug that causes slipping, poor lighting in a room or hallway, a pet or toddler who can interfere with safe stance or ambulation, or a raised threshold or environmental obstacle that causes tripping. A detailed home assessment should be included as part of the patient examination so the extrinsic risk factors can be addressed to minimize future falls.

A thorough examination of balance includes an evaluation of the multiple factors contributing to the maintenance of equilibrium as described earlier in the chapter. These include sensory reception and integration, motor planning and execution, musculoskeletal integrity, cognitive abilities and allocation of attention, balance strategies, and balance-specific self-confidence. You should consider the potential influence of these factors when selecting appropriate tests and measures for balance and measure balance in all the critical positions (at least sitting and standing) and in static and dynamic tasks focusing on the functional skills that are limited by the balance deficit. As previously emphasized, carefully consider the patient's safety and potential fall risk at all times when examining balance ability.

Regardless of the tests and measures utilized, you must identify specific functional limitations that result from balance impairment including how the task is specifically affected by impaired balance, the degree to which the activity is limited, the effect of any resulting "fear of falling," and the safety risks that follow. Generally begin with an assessment of sitting balance, which has fewer risks, and proceed to standing balance. The complexity of the tasks selected in the examination of balance begins with less complex static tasks such as maintaining unsupported sitting or static standing during a conversation and progresses to more challenging dynamic tasks such as bending to put on a shoe while sitting or walking through a crowded cafeteria carrying a lunch tray.

The clinical reasoning required during the evaluation of balance is complex. The Taxonomy of Tasks by Gentile (1987) will be particularly helpful in organizing your observations of the patient and their balance ability in a variety of settings and demand levels (see Table 2-3). Tyson and Desouza (2003) analyzed the clinical reasoning of therapists in the assessment of balance and suggested there are three overarching questions that must be addressed: (1) "What can the patient do?," (2) "How do they do it?," and (3) "Why do they do it that way?" Essentially, you analyze task performance at the activity level with attention to the functional abilities and level of independence. Then, examine balance at the movement level, studying the posture and movement strategies employed to maintain equilibrium. Finally, identify the constraints and/or impairments underlying the performance and whether these are primary problems or compensations. Always incorporate objective measures when possible. Strength, motor control, range of motion, and sensation should be assessed for their potential contribution to the patient's balance impairment, related functional activity limitations, and/or the compensatory strategies utilized. Certainly, Rothstein and Echternach's clinical decision guide (2003), the Hypothesis Oriented Algorithm for Clinicians (HOAC II) described in Chapter 2, applies to the clinical decision-making regarding balance examination and development of the intervention plan and specific intervention tactics.

## ■ Tests and Measures of Balance

The clinical reasoning behind the selection of appropriate tests and measures of balance must include consideration of many factors. Tools with optimal psychometrics (e.g., sensitivity, validity, and reliability) are preferred. Although qualitative observational descriptions provide valuable information about balance strategies, objective measures should also be incorporated whenever possible. You should consider the ability of the tool to discriminate the degree of impairment and especially to detect change over time. You should also consider, when selecting tools, the purpose of the data collected. For example, one specific test may be used to screen for a fall risk while findings from another test may be used more appropriately to guide intervention. If you observe difficulty with a particular item or component of a task within the instrument, it could highlight areas on which you should focus within the plan of care. The context of the examination will also direct you in the selection of appropriate tests and measures. For example, you should consider the length of time to complete the measure relative to the other components of the patient examination, the cognitive ability of the patient to follow the instructions of the tool, and the space and equipment resources available to the therapist.

The Neurology Section of the American Physical Therapy Association (APTA) has formed various task forces to examine the psychometric properties of objective assessments and make clinical recommendations. To this date, the Neurology Section has examined the following diagnoses: stroke, multiple sclerosis, traumatic brain injury, spinal cord injury, Parkinson disease, and vestibular disorders. The task forces have identified outcome assessments for balance and other areas pertinent to the previously listed disorders. It is beyond the scope of this chapter to review all of the measures, but you are encouraged to go to www.neuropt.org for more information.

In the examination, you must consider the entire person, holistically, at multiple levels. This examination should include an analysis of the biological and psychosocial factors influencing the individual. The *International Classification of Functioning, Disability, and Health* (ICF) Model of Functioning and Disability (Chapter 1, Fig. 1-1) is useful in examining functioning and disability (WHO, 2001). Utilization of the ICF Model provides a coherent view of various dimensions of health at biological, individual, and social levels as discussed in Chapter 1.

The complete examination of balance includes measures at the body structures and function level, activity limitation level, and at the participation restriction level, and balance tests at each level are discussed in the following section. At the body structure and function level, balance-related confidence, neuromuscular impairments, and postural impairments are considered. At the activity limitation level, functional balance

measures such as the Berg Balance Scale (Berg, 1992a, b) and the Performance-Oriented Mobility Assessment (Tinetti, 1986a) could be utilized while participation level restrictions and quality of life indicators can be assessed with tools such as the 36-Item Short Form Health Survey (SF-36) developed at RAND as part of the Medical Outcomes Study (2009). The procedure for administration of each of these tests along with others is described in this chapter. Later in the chapter, Table 9-3 presents a summary of reference values/normative data and test/measurement thresholds related to fall risk for some of the most common tests of balance in adults. Table 9-4 presents a summary of reference values/normative data for some of the most common tests of balance in pediatric patients.

## Examination of Balance: Body Structure/Function and Biomechanics

### Balance-Related Confidence

Balance-related confidence is an important aspect of the examination of balance. Psychological factors such as the fear of falling are significantly associated with changes in balance and gait, decreased activity level, and increased risk for falls

| TABLE 9-3 | Reference Values for Common Tests of Balance and Equilibrium in Adults | | | |
|---|---|---|---|---|
| **TOOL** | **REFERENCE VALUES** | | | **FALL RISK** |
| Push and Release Test (Jacobs, 2006) | Group | Mean steps ± SD | Median and (Range) | |
| | Parkinson Disease (PD) | 2.10 ±1.16 | 2 (0 to 4) | • The greater the number of steps, the greater the fall risk in PD. |
| | Normal | 0.63 ± 0.74 | 0 (0 to 3) | |
| Clinical Test for Sensory Integration in Balance CTSIB (Shumway-Cook, 1986) | • Normal should maintain balance for 30 seconds on all six conditions with minimal amounts of body sway.<br>• A single fall is not considered abnormal for any condition. | | | • Two or more falls are indicative of difficulties adapting sensory information for postural control.<br>• Cut off >260 sec composite fall risk in community dwelling elderly (90% specificity, 44% sensitivity) (DiFabio,1996) |
| Romberg Test (Bohannon, 1984) | Normal: should maintain balance for 30 seconds with eyes open and eyes closed. | | | Generally, a fall or a step, when the eyes are closed, is considered a positive test indicating further testing, with a focus on proprioception, is necessary. |

| **TABLE 9-3** | **Reference Values for Common Tests of Balance and Equilibrium in Adults—cont'd** | | | |
|---|---|---|---|---|
| **TOOL** | **REFERENCE VALUES** | | | **FALL RISK** |
| Sharpened Romberg Test Right anterior tandem stance (El Kashlan,1998) | Age (years) | Eyes Open (EO) (seconds) | Eyes Closed (EC) (seconds) | |
| | 20–49 y | 29.5 ± 2.5 | 26.0 ± 8.0 | |
| | 50–59 y | 30.0 ± 0 | 21.3 ± 9.3 | |
| | 60–69 y | 29.0 ± 4.2 | 20.1 ± 10.8 | |
| | 70–79 y | 30 ± 0.2 | 16 ± 9.4 | |
| Single Leg Stance with arms crossed (Bohannon, 1984) | Age (years) | Eyes Open (EO) (seconds) | Eyes Closed (EC) (seconds) | Cut off >10 sec in subjects with PD (Jacobs, 2006) |
| | 20–29 y | 30 | 28.8 ± 2.3 | |
| | 30–39 y | 30 | 27.8 ± 5.0 | |
| | 40–49 y | 29.7 ± 1.3 | 24.2 ± 8.4 | |
| | 50–59 y | 29.4 ± 2.9 | 21.0 ± 9.5 | |
| | 60–69 y | 22.5 ± 8.6 | 10.2 ± 8.6 | |
| | 70–79 y | 14.2 ± 9.3 | 4.3 ± 3.0 | |
| Single Leg Stance Dominant and nondominant leg stance times in older adult subjects (Briggs, 1989) | Age (years) | Dominant leg stance time (seconds) | Nondominant leg stance time (seconds) | |
| | 60–64 y | 38 | 34 | |
| | 65–69 y | 24 | 24 | |
| | 70–74 y | 18 | 20 | |
| | 75–79 y | 11 | 12 | |
| | 80–86 y | 11 | 10 | |
| | All groups | 20 | 20 | |
| Timed Up and Go TUG Times for males and females in 60–69 year-old age group (Shumway-Cook, 2000) | Age (years) | TUG Time (seconds) | | Using >14 sec cut-off = 87% sensitive and 87% specific for risk for falls, >20 sec impaired functional mobility, >30 sec dependency in most ADLs |
| | 60–69 Male | 8 | | |
| | 60–69 Female | 8 | | |
| | | | | TUG >14 predicts falls in subjects with stroke (Andersson, 2006) TUG >19 predicts falls in LE limb loss (Dite, 2007) TUG >11.1 predicts falls in subjects with vestibular disorders (Whitney, 2004) • 5m TUG >30 seconds predicts falls in older women (Morris, 2007) |

*Continued*

| TABLE 9-3 | Reference Values for Common Tests of Balance and Equilibrium in Adults—cont'd |
|---|---|

| TOOL | REFERENCE VALUES | | | FALL RISK |
|---|---|---|---|---|
| **TUG** Mean times for various age groups (Wall, 2000) | Group | TUG mean ± SD (sec) | | |
| | Young controls (19–29 y) | 7.36 ± 0.945 s | | |
| | Elderly controls (>65 y) | 8.74 ± 0.851 s | | |
| | Elderly at-risk: (>65 y) with history of falls or current treatment for gait or balance disorders | 18.14 ± 4.604 s | | |
| **TUG** Times in older adults >80 years of age; risk for falls (Huang, 2006) | Group | TUG mean ± SD (sec) | 95% CI | |
| | >80 y EO, Low Risk for Falls* | 12.0 ± 3.4 | (11.2–14.1) | |
| | >80 y EO, Medium Risk for Falls* | 28.3 ± 15.4 | (22.4–34.2) | |
| | >80 y EO, High Risk for Falls* | 54.5 ± 39.1 | (40.1–69.3) | |
| **TUG Dual Task** Times in elderly without falls (Shumway-Cook, 2000) | TUG (sec) | TUG-manual (sec) | TUG-cognitive | |
| | 8.4 | 9.7 | 9.7 | |
| **Functional Reach Test FRT** (Duncan, 1990) | Age (years) | Mean Reach ± SD (inches) Males | Mean Reach Females (inches) | • Unable to reach = 28x more likely to fall |
| | 20–40 y | 16.7 ± 1.9 | 14.6 ± 2.2 | • 1–6'' = 4x more likely to fall |
| | 41–69 y | 14.9 ± 2.2 | 13.8 ± 2.2 | • 6–10'' = 2x more likely to fall |
| | 70–87 y | 13.2 ± 1.6 | 10.5 ± 3.5 | >10'' = not likely to fall |
| **FRT** Reach in inches with eyes open; subjects >80 years old; risk for falls (Huang, 2006) | Group | Mean Reach ±SD (inches) | 95% Confidence Interval (CI) | |
| | >80 y EO, Low Risk for Falls* | 9.4 ± 2.1 | (8.6–10.2) | |
| | >80 y EO, Medium Risk for Falls* | 5.2 ± 2.1 | (4.4–6.0) | |
| | >80 y EO, High Risk for Falls* | 3.2 ± 1.4 | (2.6–3.7) | |
| **Multidirectional Reach Test MDRT** Reach in inches; older adults; mean age 74 (Newton, 2001) | MDRT Direction | Mean ±SD (inch) | <Below Avg; >Above Avg | |
| | Forward | 8.9 ± 3.4 | <5.6; >12.2 | |
| | Backward | 4.6 ± 3.1 | <1.6; >7.6 | |
| | R Lateral | 6.2 ± 3.0 | <3.8; >9.4 | |
| | L Lateral | 6.6 ± 2.8 | <3.8; >9.4 | |
| **Sitting Functional Reach** measured in two directions among healthy adults (Thompson, 2007) | Age group | Forward Reach (cm) | Lateral Reach (cm) | |
| | 21–39 yo | 44.9 | 29.5 | |
| | 40–59 yo | 42.3 | 26.7 | |
| | 65–93 yo | 32.9 | 20.3 | |

| TABLE 9-3 | Reference Values for Common Tests of Balance and Equilibrium in Adults—cont'd | | |
|---|---|---|---|
| **TOOL** | **REFERENCE VALUES** | | **FALL RISK** |
| **Four Square Step Test FSST** (Dite, 2002) | • Using cut-off score of 15 seconds, 86% sensitive and 88% specific<br>• Using cut-off score of 12 seconds, 80% sensitive and 92% specific | | |

| **FSST** in individuals with balance deficits secondary to vestibular disorders (Whitney, 2007) | Group | FSST (sec) | |
|---|---|---|---|
| | All subjects | 13.6 ± 4.3 | >12 sec fall risk in subjects with vestibular disorders (Whitney, 2007) |
| | Age <65 y | 12.4 ± 4.2 | > 15 sec risk for multiple falls in community dwelling elderly (Dite, 2002)<br>> 9.68 fall risk for PD (Duncan, 2013)<br>> 15 sec or failed attempt fall risk for subjects with stroke (Blennerhassett, 2008) |
| | Age ≥65 y | 14.8 ± 4.3 | |

| **Dynamic Gait Index DGI** (Whitney, 2004a) | • Using DGI cutoff score ≤19/24 = 70% sensitive and 51% specific | | ≤19 fall risk in subjects with vestibular disorders (Whitney, 2000), community dwelling elderly (Wrisley, 2010), and subjects with PD (Dibble, 2008) |
|---|---|---|---|

| **DGI** in individuals with balance deficits secondary to vestibular disorders (Whitney, 2007) | Group | DGI Score | |
|---|---|---|---|
| | All subjects | 20.3 ± 3.5 | |
| | Age <65 y | 19.9 ± 4.1 | |
| | Age ≥65 y | 20.7 ± 2.9 | |

| **Functional Gait Assessment FGA** (Wrisley, 2004) | Age | Mean score ± SD (feet) | Range (feet) | Cut off ≤22 fall risk (85% sensitivity, 86% specificity) (Wrisley, 2010) |
|---|---|---|---|---|
| | 40–49 y | 28.9 ± 1.5 | (24–30) | Cut off ≤15 sec fall risk in subjects with PD (Leddy, 2011) |
| | 50–59 y | 28.4 ± 1.6 | (25–30) | |
| | 60–69 y | 27.1 ± 2.3 | (20–30) | |
| | 70–79 y | 24.9 ± 3.6 | (16–30) | |
| | 80–89 y | 20.8 ± 4.7 | (10–28) | |

*Continued*

| TABLE 9-3 | Reference Values for Common Tests of Balance and Equilibrium in Adults—cont'd | | |
|---|---|---|---|
| **TOOL** | **REFERENCE VALUES** | | **FALL RISK** |
| Walk While Talking Test WWT test (Verghese, 2002) | Simple – walk 40 feet and recite alphabet | | ≥20 sec fall risk |
| | Complex – walk and recite every other letter of alphabet | | ≥33 sec fall risk |
| | Velocity and cadence slowed more with focus on talking than when asked to focus on talking and walking. Verghese J, Kuslansky G, Holtzer R, Katz M, Xue X, Buschke H, Pahor M. Walking while talking: Effect of task prioritization in the elderly. *Arch Phys Med Rehabil.* 2007;88(1):50–53. | | • Individuals who slow gait velocity during a WWT test are at increased risk for falls (Verghese, 2002) |

| WWT comparing normal walk to WWT-T, asking patient to focus on talking only, and WWT-C, asking patient to focus on both talking and walking (Verghese, 2007) | Condition | Velocity (range) (cm/second) | Cadence (range) (steps/min) |
|---|---|---|---|
| | Normal walking Median | 104.7 (92.3–115.8) | 104.0 (96.4–110.4) |
| | WWT-C Median | 76.6 (58.1–94.5) | 87.9 (68.2–101.2) |
| | WWT-T Median | 72.2 (54.55–92.5) | 87.2 (67.3–100.0) |

| Berg Balance Scale BBS (Bogle, 1996) | Using cut-off score of 45 (out of maximal possible score of 56) is 53% sensitive and 96% specific. | 41–56 = low fall risk 21–40 = medium fall risk 0 –20 = high fall risk |
|---|---|---|
| BBS (Riddle, 1999) | Using cut-off score of 45 has sensitivity = 64% (correctly predicts fallers); and specificity = 90% (correctly predicts nonfallers) • Authors recommend a cut-off score of 40 for screening for fall risk. | >45 = no risk for falls (Riddle, 1999) |

| BBS by age group and assistive device use (Lusardi, 2004) | Group | Mean BBS | Confidence Intervals | |
|---|---|---|---|---|
| | 60–69 yo | 54.0 ± 1.5 | 52.4–55.6 | |
| | 70–79 yo | 52.7 ± 2.4 | 51.5–53.8 | |
| | 80–90 yo No Device | 46.3 ± 4.2 | 44.1–48.5 | |
| | 80–90 yo Device | 31.7 ± 10.0 | 28.3–35.1 | |
| | 90–101 yo No Device | 45.0 ± 4.2 | 40.9–49.1 | |
| | 90–101 yo Device | 31.8 ± 7.6 | 28.4–35.2 | |
| | | | | Cut off <29 for falls in subjects with stroke with 80% sensitivity and 78% specificity (Maeda, 2009) |

| Gait Velocity measured as relative speed (velocity / height = statures per second) (Wall, 1991) (see *also Gait Velocity in* | Group | Relative Gait Speed: The range from self-selected slow pace to self-selected fast pace (statures/sec)++ |
|---|---|---|
| | Healthy young females | 0.57–1.23 statures/sec |
| | Healthy elderly females | 0.50–1.05 statures/sec |

| TABLE 9-3 | Reference Values for Common Tests of Balance and Equilibrium in Adults—cont'd | | |
|---|---|---|---|
| **TOOL** | | **REFERENCE VALUES** | **FALL RISK** |
| *Chapter 10)*<br>*++ data in this*<br>*study was normalized*<br>*as statures per*<br>*second by dividing*<br>*the velocity (m/s)*<br>*by the person's*<br>*height (m)* | Females with Idiopathic Gait Disorder of Elderly | 0.19–0.41 statures/sec | Significantly slower than healthy groups; also very little difference between slow and fast self-selected pace |
| | Subjects with stroke (Perry, 1995) | <0.4 m/s household ambulators<br>0.4–0.8 m/s limited community ambulators<br>>0.8 m/s community ambulators | |
| **Timed Measure of Standing from a Chair**<br>(10 repetitions)<br>(Csuka, 1985) | **Age** (years) | **Mean for Women** (and upper limit) (seconds) | **Mean for Men** (and upper limit) (seconds) |
| | 60 y | 16.6 (22.6) | 16.6 (20.1) |
| | 65 y | 18.4 (23.5) | 17.6 (21.1) |
| | 70 y | 19.2 (24.3) | 18.5 (22.0) |
| | 75 y | 20.1 (25.2) | 19.5 (23.0) |
| | 80 y | 20.9 (26.1) | 20.5 (24.0) |
| | 85 y | 21.8 (27.0) | 21.5 (25.0) |
| **Five Times Sit to Stand Test**<br>Community dwelling adults<br>(Bohannon, 2007) | **Age** (years) | **Mean ± SD (sec)** | |
| | 19–49 | 6.2 ± 1.3 | Cut off >15 sec recurrent fall risk community dwelling elderly (Buatois, 2010) |
| | 50–59 | 7.1 ± 1.5 | Cut off >16 sec fall risk for PD (Duncan, 2011) |
| | 60–69 | 8.1 ± 3.1 | |
| | 70–79 | 10.0 ± 3.1 | |
| | 80–89 | 10.6 ± 3.4 | |

*Risk for falls based on Tinetti score
(Table created from multiple published sources; see references for each row) including but not limited to:
-Push and Release Test data is from Table 2, p.1409. (Jacobs JV, Horak FB, Tran VK, Nutt JG. An alternative clinical postural stability test for patients with Parkinson's disease. *J Neurol.* 2006;253:1404–1413.)
-FSST data and DGI data for vestibular patients is from Table 2, p.101. (Whitney S, Marchetti G, Morris L, Sparto P. The reliability and validity of the four square step test for people with balance deficits secondary to a vestibular disorder. *Arch Phys Med Rehabil.* 2007;88:99–104.)
-FRT data and TUG data (Huang, 2006) is from Table 1, p.5. (Huang M, Burgess R, Weber M, Greenwald NF. Performance of balance impaired elders on three balance tests under two visual conditions. *J Geriatric Phys Ther.* 2006;29(1):3–7.)
-TUG (Wall) data is from the manuscript of p.111. (Wall JC, Bell C, Campbell S, Davis J. The timed get-up-and-go test revisited: Measurement of the component tasks. *J Rehabil Res Dev.* 2000;37(1):109–114.)
-Berg Balance Scale data is from manuscript of Bogle Thorbahn, 1996.
-FGA (Wrisley) is from personal communication from Dr. Wrisley, also published.
-Gait Velocity (Wall) is from (Wall JC, Hogan DB, Turnbull GI, Fox RA. The kinematics of idiopathic gait disorder. *Scand J Rehab Med.* 1991;23:159–164.).

(Maki, 1991; Myers, 1996; Maki, 1997; Liu-Ambrose, 2006). Thirty percent of older adults report a fear of falling, and this percentage is doubled in those who have fallen (Tinetti, 1988b; Tinetti, 1994). Those who have a fear of falling tend to avoid activity, which can result in restriction in social participation (Howland, 1993) and functional decline (Cumming, 2000). Balance-related confidence can be assessed with tools such as the *Activities-specific Balance Confidence Scale* (*ABC Scale*) (Filiatrault, 2007), *Balance Efficacy Scale* (*BES*), the *Fear of Falling Avoidance Behavior*

| TABLE 9-4 | Reference Values for Common Tests of Balance and Equilibrium in Pediatric Population | | | |
|---|---|---|---|---|
| **TOOL** | | | | |
| **Pediatric Functional Reach** Mean reach in cm for various ages (Donahoe, 1994) | Age (yr) | Mean Reach (cm) | 95% Confidence Interval (cm) | Critical Reach (cm) |
| | 5–6 | 21.17 | 16.79–24.91 | 16.79 |
| | 7–8 | 24.21 | 20.56–27.96 | 20.57 |
| | 9–10 | 27.97 | 25.56–31.64 | 25.56 |
| | 11–12 | 32.79 | 29.68–36.18 | 29.68 |
| | 13–15 | 32.30 | 29.58–36.08 | 29.58 |
| **Berg Balance Scale in Pediatric Population** Spastic CP children with and without aids and control (Kembhavi, 2002) | Group | Mean BBS Score (max = 56) | SD | |
| | Spastic hemiplegia | 53.21 | 6.49 | |
| | Spastic diplegia (no aids) | 49.75 | 6.73 | |
| | Spastic diplegia (with aids) | 25.10 | 12.37 | |
| | No motor impairment | 55.86 | 0.36 | |
| **Pediatric Balance Scale** Mean score for various age groups of typically developing children (more variability in younger age groups) (Franjoine, 2010)* | Age (years and months) | Mean PBS Score (mean ± 1 SD) | Range of Scores | |
| | 2 y 0 mo to 2 y 5 mo | 26.2 ± 6.38 | (15–30) | |
| | 2 y 6 mo to 2 y 11 mo | 34.3 ± 7.72 | (23–46) | |
| | 3 y 0 mo to 3 y 5 mo | 46.0 ± 6.55 | (28–53) | |
| | 3 y 6 mo to 3 y 11 mo | 48.5 ± 5.02 | (30–54) | |
| | 4 y 0 mo to 4 y 5 mo | 49.5 ± 5.76 | (27–56) | |
| | 4 y 6 mo to 4 y 11 mo | 51.2 ± 5.07 | (31–56) | |
| | 5 y 0 mo to 5 y 5 mo | 54.0 ± 2.52 | (42–56) | |
| | 5 y 6 mo to 5 y 11 mo | 53.3 ± 3.20 | (41–56) | |
| | 6 y 0 mo to 6 y 5 mo | 53.8 ± 2.49 | (46–56) | |
| | 6 y 6 mo to 6 y 11 mo | 54.4 ± 1.89 | (47–56) | |
| | 7 y 0 mo and older | 55.2 ± 1.74 | (46–56) | |

*For the reader who wants more specific data, the Franjoine (2010) original Table 1 provides mean ± SD and ranges separately for male and female groups within each age bracket.

(This table was developed from numerous primary sources; see each citation for each row of the table) including but not limited to:

-Pediatric Functional Reach data is from Table 3, p.192. (Donahoe B, Turner D, Worrell T. The use of functional reach as a measurement of balance in boys and girls without disabilities ages 5–15 years. *Pediatr Phys Ther.* 1994;6(4):189–193.)

-Berg Balance Scale in Pediatric data is from Table 2, p.95. (Kembhavi G, Darrah J, Magill-Evans J, Loomis J. Using the Berg Balance scale to distinguish balance abilities in children with cerebral palsy. *Pediatr Phys Ther.* 2002;14(2):92–99.)

-Pediatric Balance Scale norms are from Table 1, p.354–355. (Franjoine MR, Darr N, Held SL, Kott K, Young BL. The performance of children developing typically on the Pediatric Balance Scale. *Pediatr Phys Ther.* 2010;22(4):350–359.)

*Questionnaire (FFABQ)* (Landers, 2011), and the *Falls Efficacy Scale (FES)* (Hellstrom, 2002; Belgen, 2006; Liu-Ambrose, 2006).

The *ABC Scale* (Fig. 9-7) and the *BES* (Fig. 9-8) are 16- and 18-item scales, respectively, based on patient self-report. Ask the patient to rate each item between 0% (reflecting no confidence) and 100% (reflecting complete confidence). Then, calculate the average percentage (Powell, 1995; Rose, 2003) and record the result in the patient record for current decision-making and for future comparison postintervention. There is some indication the *ABC Scale* is sensitive to change (Miller, 2003). The *ABC Scale* and *BES* were based

**The Activities-specific Balance Confidence (ABC) Scale\***

For each of the following activities, please indicate your level of self-confidence by choosing a corresponding number from the following rating scale:

0%   10   20   30   40   50   60   70   80   90   100%
no confidence                                    completely confident

"How confident are you that you will not lose your balance or become unsteady when you ...

| | |
|---|---|
| ... walk around the house? | _____% |
| ... walk up or down stairs? | _____% |
| ... bend over and pick up a slipper from the front of a closet floor? | _____% |
| ... reach for a small can off a shelf at eye level? | _____% |
| ... stand on your tiptoes and reach for something above your head? | _____% |
| ... stand on a chair and reach for something? | _____% |
| ... sweep the floor? | _____% |
| ... walk outside the house to a car parked in the driveway? | _____% |
| ... get into or out of a car? | _____% |
| ... walk across a parking lot to the mall? | _____% |
| ... walk up or down a ramp? | _____% |
| ... walk in a crowded mall where people rapidly walk past you? | _____% |
| ... are bumped into by people as you walk through the mall? | _____% |
| ... step onto or off an escalator while you are holding onto a railing? | _____% |
| ... step onto or off an escalator while holding onto parcels such that you cannot hold onto the railing? | _____% |
| ... walk outside on icy sidewalks? | _____% |

**FIGURE 9-7** The Activities-specific Balance Confidence (ABC) Scale. *(Reproduced from: Powell LE, Myers AM. The Activities-specific Balance Confidence (ABC) Scale. J Gerontol Med Sci. 1995;50(1):M28–34.)*

on Bandura's (1982) theory of **self-efficacy,** which is defined as the degree of confidence a person has in his or her ability to perform specific behaviors. Self-efficacy has been shown to predict behavior (Bandura, 1982) with low self-efficacy resulting in a decrease in the related behavior, i.e., low self-efficacy for balance would be related to a decrease in activities that require balance. The *FES* (Tinetti, 1990) is a 10-item self-administered assessment of self-efficacy in completing ADLs without falling with scores ranging from 0% ("very confident") to 100% ("not confident"). The *FFABQ* (Landers, 2011) is a 14-item self-reported assessment that quantifies an individual's avoidance of specific activities due to fear of falling. Landers (2015) reported that psychological measures (*ABC Scale* and *FFABQ*) are more predictive of fall risk than physical measures, history of falls, or presence of pathology.

## THINK ABOUT IT 9.1

What is the relationship between patients' subjective impression of their balance abilities and their actual objective performance?

### Observe Postural Control

Examine postural control through the direct observation of trunk and limb activation and ankle, hip, and stepping strategies as described earlier during a variety of tasks and in reaction to

varying degrees of perturbation, always assuring patient safety. Document the presence and quality of righting and equilibrium reactions in sitting and standing and specifically note the timing, efficiency, and appropriateness of the reactions you observe. Static and dynamic posture should be documented including asymmetries and any deviations from midline using visual observation, perhaps with a transparent posture grid, or force-platform data (next section) to reflect the symmetry of stance or sitting.

### Push and Release Test

The *Push and Release Test* (Horak, 2004) was developed to improve standardization and sensitivity of the *Pull Test,* Item #30 on the Unified Parkinson Disease Rating Scale (UPDRS), as a measure of postural stability in static stance (Horak, 2004; Jacobs, 2006). To administer the test, stand behind the patient and apply an isometric push at the upper trunk as patient leans back. Ask the patient to continue to push back into your hands until his/her hips and shoulders are just behind his/her heels but without his/her heels lifting off the ground. This extent of trunk excursion allows the COM to move outside his/her BOS. It has been demonstrated that more consistent perturbation force is applied with this Push and Release method than with the Pull Test of UPDRS (Jacobs, 2006). Then, suddenly release your hands and visually observe the number, degree, and quality of backward steps and be prepared to assist the patient to prevent falling. Then, score the patient on this five-point scale (Horak, 2004) that is reported to better

**The Balance Efficacy Scale**

Name: _____Date: _____

Listed below are a series of tasks that you may encounter in daily life. Please indicate how confident you are, today, that you can complete each of these tasks without losing your balance. Your answers are confidential. Please answer as you feel, not how you think you should feel. (Circle one number from 0 to 100%)

1. How confident are you that you can get up out of chair (using your hands) without losing your balance?
         0%   10%  20%  30%  40%  50%  60%  70%  80%  90%  100%
  not at all confident           somewhat confident        absolutely confident

2. How confident are you that you can get up out of a chair (not using your hands) without losing your balance?
         0%   10%  20%  30%  40%  50%  60%  70%  80%  90%  100%
  not at all confident           somewhat confident        absolutely confident

3. How confident are you that you can walk up a flight of 10 stairs (using the handrail) without losing your balance?
         0%   10%  20%  30%  40%  50%  60%  70%  80%  90%  100%
  not at all confident           somewhat confident        absolutely confident

4. How confident are you that you can walk up a flight of 10 stairs (not using a handrail) without losing your balance?
         0%   10%  20%  30%  40%  50%  60%  70%  80%  90%  100%
  not at all confident           somewhat confident        absolutely confident

5. How confident are you that you can get out of bed without losing your balance?
         0%   10%  20%  30%  40%  50%  60%  70%  80%  90%  100%
  not at all confident           somewhat confident        absolutely confident

6. How confident are you that you can get into or out of a shower or bathtub (with the assistance of a handrail or support wall) without losing your balance?
         0%   10%  20%  30%  40%  50%  60%  70%  80%  90%  100%
  not at all confident           somewhat confident        absolutely confident

7. How confident are you that you can get into or out of a shower or bathtub (with no assistance from a handrail or support wall) without losing your balance?
         0%   10%  20%  30%  40%  50%  60%  70%  80%  90%  100%
  not at all confident           somewhat confident        absolutely confident

8. How confident are you that you can walk down a flight of 10 stairs (using the handrail) without losing your balance?
         0%   10%  20%  30%  40%  50%  60%  70%  80%  90%  100%
  not at all confident           somewhat confident        absolutely confident

9. How confident are you that you can walk down a flight of 10 stairs (not using the handrail) without losing your balance?
         0%   10%  20%  30%  40%  50%  60%  70%  80%  90%  100%
  not at all confident           somewhat confident        absolutely confident

10. How confident are you that you can remove an object from a cupboard located at a height that is level with your shoulders without losing your balance?
         0%   10%  20%  30%  40%  50%  60%  70%  80%  90%  100%
  not at all confident           somewhat confident        absolutely confident

11. How confident are you that you can remove an object from a cupboard located above your head without losing your balance?
         0%   10%  20%  30%  40%  50%  60%  70%  80%  90%  100%
  not at all confident           somewhat confident        absolutely confident

12. How confident are you that you can walk across uneven ground (with assistance) when good lighting is available without losing your balance?
         0%   10%  20%  30%  40%  50%  60%  70%  80%  90%  100%
  not at all confident           somewhat confident        absolutely confident

**FIGURE 9-8** Balance Efficacy Scale (BES). Reproduced from: Tinetti ME, Richman D, Powell L. Falls Efficacy as a Measure of Fear of Falling. *J Gerontol.* 1990;45(6):239–243.

13. How confident are you that you can walk across uneven ground (with no assistance) when good lighting is available without losing your balance?

    0%   10%  20%  30%  40%  50%  60%  70%  80%  90%  100%
not at all confident        somewhat confident       absolutely confident

14. How confident are you that you can walk across uneven ground (with assistance) at night without losing your balance?

    0%   10%  20%  30%  40%  50%  60%  70%  80%  90%  100%
not at all confident        somewhat confident       absolutely confident

15. How confident are you that you can walk across uneven ground (with no assistance) at night without losing your balance?

    0%   10%  20%  30%  40%  50%  60%  70%  80%  90%  100%
not at all confident        somewhat confident       absolutely confident

16. How confident are you that you could stand on one leg (with support) while putting on a pair of trousers without losing your balance?

    0%   10%  20%  30%  40%  50%  60%  70%  80%  90%  100%
not at all confident        somewhat confident       absolutely confident

17. How confident are you that you could stand on one leg (with no support) while putting on a pair of trousers without losing your balance?

    0%   10%  20%  30%  40%  50%  60%  70%  80%  90%  100%
not at all confident        somewhat confident       absolutely confident

18. How confident are you that you could complete a daily task quickly without losing your balance?

    0%   10%  20%  30%  40%  50%  60%  70%  80%  90%  100%
not at all confident        somewhat confident       absolutely confident

Last, we are interested in understanding what factors affect your confidence levels. On the lines below, please provide reasons for answering the way you did on questions 1 through 18. For example, if you answered that you were "not very" confident, why do you feel that way? If you were "not very" confident about an activity because you no longer do it very often (e.g. climb stairs, walk on uneven ground), we would like to know that also.

_____
_____
_____
_____
_____
**FIGURE 9-8—cont'd**  _____

differentiate less severe balance dysfunction than the *Pull Test* (Jacobs, 2006):

**0** – recovers independently with one step of normal length and width
**1** – two to three small steps backward, but recovers independently
**2** – four or more steps backward, but recovers independently
**3** – steps but needs to be assisted to prevent a fall
**4** – falls without attempting a step or unable to stand without assistance

The response to the external force may be more consistent because the patient cannot anticipate the timing of the release. The test is reported to be valid and sensitive to change (Horak, 2004), more sensitive than the *Pull Test* to subjects with low balance confidence, and has higher interrater reliability (Jacobs, 2006). Details are shown in the Focus On Evidence table online (ONL).

## Posturography

**Posturography**, computerized balance assessment with objective data collected from a **force platform**, has become particularly popular with evidence reported in the literature (Thapa, 1994; Piirtolaa, 2006; Ruhea, 2010). The most commonly examined parameters of posturography include (1) the location of the COP as a measure of symmetry (defined earlier), (2) postural sway measures including COP movement or excursion over a given time-period and speed of COP movement, and (3) LOS measures (defined earlier) to reflect dynamic postural stability. For all posturography measures, the patient, stands (posturography measures could also be completed in sitting position) on a force platform (Fig. 9-9A). Enter age, gender, and anthropometric information regarding the patient, including weight and height into the computer to allow calculation of predicted values for the LOS.

For static balance posturography testing on the force platform, ask the patient to maintain quiet, unperturbed, upright stance while the computer measures the excursion/movement of the COP during a specified time period. The patient's goal in static balance testing, using visual feedback through the computer monitor, is to maintain the screen cursor within the central target box on the monitor, sustaining a stable symmetrical position as much as possible. If there is no deficit, the location of the COP in static testing would have very little excursion (i.e., a very short squiggly line) during the prescribed test period. An individual with balance impairment would have a more extensive back-and-forth squiggly line, like scribbling, as they attempt to maintain the central position but the COP is continually moving away from and back toward the central box. You can then compare the measured excursion of the COP to norms for subjects with similar anthropometric characteristics.

For dynamic balance posturography testing, the patient is standing on the force platform. Ask the patient to sequentially shift the COP toward the periphery of the BOS in multiple directions following the visual cues/targets provided by the computer. During this voluntary weight-shift, the patient visually observes feedback through the movement of the computer cursor on the monitor (representing the location of the COP) toward the targets at the periphery. The cursor movement is a reflection of the patient's movement (see the three forward targets, left lateral target, right lateral target, and three posterior targets shown in the monitor screenshot: top left corner of Fig. 9-9B). During the movement, the computer measures the actual length and path of active excursion of the COP (shown in the screen capture of Fig. 9-9B in the top left corner) and the velocity of the sway excursion for comparison of results to the normative data for degree of intended excursion and the accuracy in reaching each target. As an example, in addition to the monitor screenshot, the sample report in Figure 9-9B includes the computer generated data in the top right corner with results, as percentage of predicted value, that are weighted based on the target and the graphs at the bottom with graphical representation of the results with deficit measures marked in red on each graph. Another posturography measure of dynamic balance is a rhythmic weight-shift test in which the patient actively and rhythmically shifts the body weight alternately between a right lateral target and a left lateral target (monitor view in Fig. 9-9C in the top left corner) following the timing and visual cues provided by the computer at slow, moderate, and fast speeds. The test can also be repeated with alternation between forward and backward targets (Fig. 9-9C in the top right corner).

Force-platform velocity of sway excursion and mean sway in the anterior-posterior direction with eyes closed has been shown to be a valid balance measure with significant correlation to functional balance tests (Frandin, 1995). The Balance Master by NeuroCom and Biodex Balance System SD are commercial computerized dynamic posturography assessment and training systems that have been investigated and shown to have good test-retest reliability for dynamic balance measures and concurrent validity with the Berg Balance Scale and gait velocity (Liston, 1996; Hinman, 2000; Cachupe, 2001) as well as acceptable reliability and repeatability in individuals with Duchenne muscular dystrophy (Barrett, 1987).

## Examination of Sensory Systems Used in Balance

The relative contributions of the various sensory systems (somatosensory, visual, and vestibular) to maintain balance can be examined with the Clinical Test for Sensory Interaction in Balance (CTSIB). The CTSIB, developed by Shumway-Cook (1986), originally examined postural sway during quiet stance as influenced by six different test conditions (Fig. 9-10, the two conditions for visual conflict are not shown) for 30 seconds each with each condition effecting a different aspect of sensory input to balance. Position the patient for each condition with feet together, side-by-side, and with hands at the hips. Under each condition, the amount and direction of sway is documented for comparison.

Condition 1 provides full access to available visual, vestibular, and somatosensory information with eyes open while standing on a stable flat surface and provides a baseline for the other conditions. The six conditions are organized as two groups of three with Conditions 1, 2, and 3 performed on a solid floor while Conditions 4, 5, and 6 are performed standing on a 24″ × 24″ piece of medium-density Temper foam to compromise the use of proprioceptive information from the ankle (see Fig. 9-10C and 9-10D; Conditions 4 and 5). Visual conditions include "normal" for Conditions 1 and 4 (Fig. 9-10A and 9-10C) and "blindfolded" for Conditions 2 and 5 (Fig. 9-10B and 9-10D). Originally, Conditions 3 and 6 utilized a large Japanese lantern cut in half and attached by a headband as a "dome" over the face to provide visual conflict, related to the irregular diagonal lines

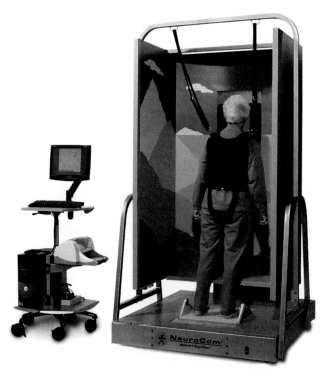

**FIGURE 9-9 A.** Patient standing on the Neurocom Balance Master SMART Equitest during dynamic posturography Limits of Stability (LOS) testing. The patient is voluntarily and actively shifting the weight toward their right side.

# Limits Of Stability

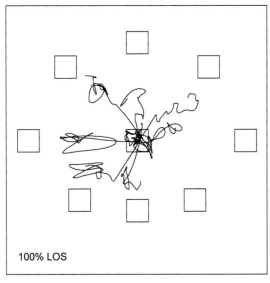

100% LOS

| Transition | RT (sec) | MVL (deg/sec) | EPE (%) | MXE (%) | DCL (%) |
|---|---|---|---|---|---|
| 1 (F) | 2.92 | 0.8 | 27 | 52 | 78 |
| 2 (RF) | 0.65 | 2.6 | 31 | 72 | 74 |
| 3 (R) | 0.25 | 1.9 | 42 | 42 | 70 |
| 4 (RB) | 1.23 | 1.8 | 29 | 29 | 0 |
| 5 (B) | 1.11 | 3.0 | 71 | 71 | 68 |
| 6 (LB) | 1.14 | 5.5 | 55 | 87 | 59 |
| 7 (L) | 1.28 | 6.2 | 70 | 71 | 89 |
| 8 (LF) | 0.51 | 3.7 | 57 | 80 | 84 |

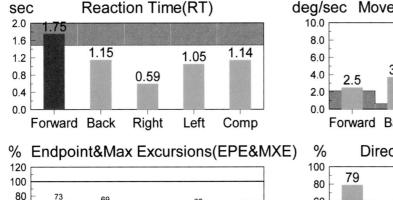

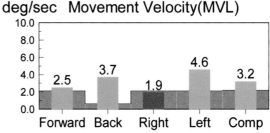

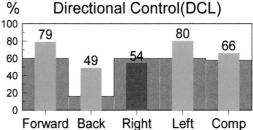

## Data Range Note:   User Data Range: 60–69

Post Test Comment:

Limited voluntary movement distance in all rightward movements (loss of 70% of safe limits).

**FIGURE 9-9—cont'd   B.** Printed sample report from Neurocom Balance Master after dynamic posturography testing with computer generated data in the top right corner and graphical representation at the bottom with abnormal results marked in red on the graph. LOS measures include Reaction Time (RT) in seconds, Movement Velocity (MVL) in deg/sec, Endpoint Excursion (EPE) as percentage of predicted, Maximum Excursion (MXE) as percentage of predicted, and Directional Control (DCL) as a percentage of predicted. In this report example, the patient exhibits significantly decreased weight-shift toward the right side compared with the left side (the patient comes much closer to the targets on the left side). Note in the data at the top that Endpoint Excursion is greatly decreased to the right compared with predicted values. *(Figures A-C used with permission from Neurocom.)*

*Continued*

# Rhythmic Weight Shift

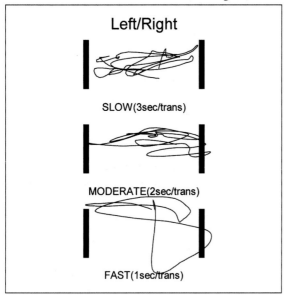

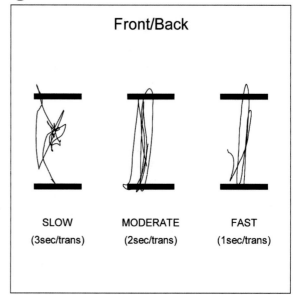

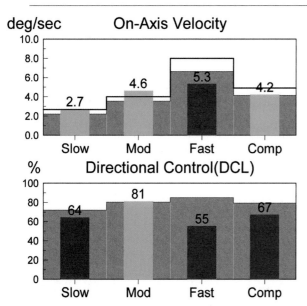

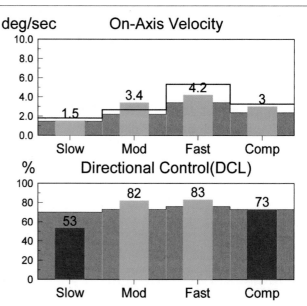

**Data Range Note:** User Data Range: 60–69

Post Test Comment:

Decreased movement control at varied functional speeds, particularly in lateral weight shift activities

**FIGURE 9-9—cont'd C.** Printed report from Neurocom Balance Master with patient data in rhythmic weight-shift (RWS) testing. This example report reflects a patient with difficulty with control of weight-shift, particularly in lateral weight-shift activity especially to the left side. *(Used with permission from Neurocom.)*

of bamboo in the interior of the Japanese lantern, which allows visual input but inaccurate, unhelpful, visual input in regard to upright position. However, because results of visual conflict dome (Conditions 3 and 6) were not significantly different from vision eliminated (Conditions 2 and 4) (Cohen, 1993) the test was modified (the modified CTSIB or mCTSIB) to include only Conditions 1, 2, 4, and 5 (Whitney, 2004b). For each condition, it is recommended additional trials be allowed if a patient is

unable to stand for 30 seconds (Horak, 1987), and an average of three trials should be calculated for each condition (Whitney, 2004b). The test can be administered with the patient barefoot or wearing shoes, as no difference is seen in the results (Whitney, 2004b).

The rationale behind the test is to systematically disadvantage the sensory systems involved. The dense foam is utilized to interfere with accurate somatosensory information from the

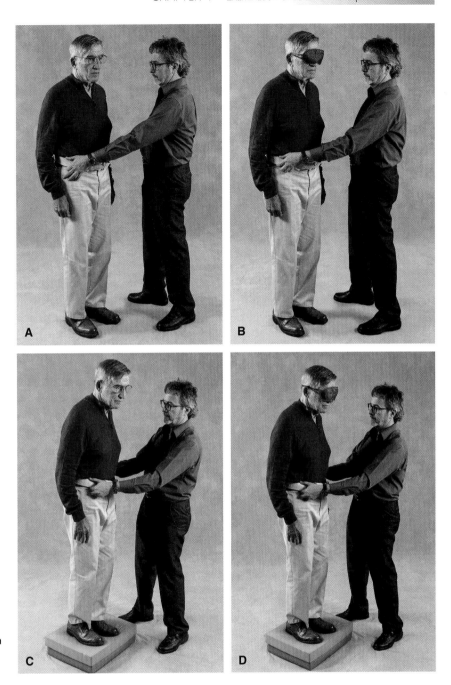

**FIGURE 9-10** The four test conditions of the Modified Clinical Test of Sensory Interaction In Balance (CTSIB): **A.** Condition #1 = firm surface, eyes open; **B.** Condition #2 = firm surface, vision eliminated; **C.** Condition #4 = foam surface, eyes open; **D.** Condition #5 = foam surface, vision eliminated.

ankle since a position of neutral ankle dorsiflexion while standing on foam does not mean the same thing as neutral ankle dorsiflexion while standing on a firm level surface. The blindfold is used to eliminate vision completely, and the visual conflict dome is placed over the head to provide irrelevant visual information. Each condition disadvantages one or more sensory systems forcing the patient to rely on the remaining system(s) to maintain balance. Record and document (1) time in balance (up to 30 seconds per condition) and (2) increased sway or loss of balance for each condition. You should also document strategies utilized and any subjective patient reports such as nausea or dizziness. An increase in instability in a particular condition or combination of conditions suggests dysfunction in the sensory system the patient is being forced to

utilize. For example, if the patient exhibits increased instability when standing on the dense foam with a blindfold, dysfunction in the vestibular system is implicated. This information can then be used to guide intervention. Specifically, you can develop a plan of care that challenges or stresses the system not adequately functioning to stimulate motor learning and recovery. Interventions developed to target the implicated system(s) including patient and family education regarding safety are discussed in Chapter 30.

Young adults without balance deficits are able to maintain balance for 30 seconds on each of the six conditions with minimal amounts of body sway (Whitney, 2004b; Shumway-Cook, 2007). Shumway-Cook (2007) has proposed a model for interpreting results of this test, categorizing patients with greater sway or loss of balance on Conditions 2, 3, 5, and 6 as "visually dependent," depending on vision for postural control. She categorizes patients with problems on Conditions 4, 5, and 6 as "surface dependent," depending primarily on somatosensory information from the feet in contact with the surface for postural control. This information has important implications for designing a customized therapeutic intervention plan.

The Sensory Organization Test (SOT) is similar to the CTSIB but used with computerized dynamic posturography to assess an individual's ability to use visual, proprioceptive, and visual cues to maintain postural stability in stance. The individual stands on dual-force plates within a three-sided surround, and anterior-posterior sway is recorded under various conditions. Conditions 1, 2, and 3 are performed on a flat stable force platform. Conditions 4, 5, and 6 are performed on a force platform that is unstable and changes its orientation. Conditions 1 and 4 are normal unrestricted vision with a fixed visual surround scene; Conditions 2 and 5 are vision eliminated with a blindfold or by having the patient close their eyes; Conditions 3 and 6 involve movement of the visual surround that corresponds to the patient's movement to provide visual feedback unrelated to true upright. For the SOT, three trials are given for each condition and the average time is recorded. This information is compared with age-related norms so your patient's performance can be appropriately analyzed. The SOT has been found to have moderately high sensitivity (85%) and specificity (77%) in identifying vestibulopathies (Cohen, 2008). Results can help guide treatment for individuals with a history of falls (Whitney, 2006).

The CTSIB has been applied to children with reliability demonstrated in a sample of 9 to 10 year-olds (Geldhof, 2006). A pediatric version of the CTSIB (P-CTSIB) has been developed with similar items but includes six feet-together and six heel-to-toe standing positions for a total of 12 different test conditions instead of six (Deitz, 1991). Among 4 and 5 year-olds, the feet-together position of the test can discriminate between children with and without balance deficits (Richardson, 1992). Adequate test-retest score agreement (Westcott, 1994) and strong interrater reliability (Crowe, 1991) have been reported. There is some indication that children with learning disabilities may have deficits in sensory organization related to balance as shown on the P-CTSIB (Deitz, 1996). The SOT has also been examined in children (Gagnon, 2006; Inder, 2005).

### Examination of Other Underlying Impairments

Any other underlying impairments that could contribute to balance impairment detected on the neurological examination must be documented in the evaluation with major implications to guide interventions that will ultimately improve balance in each functional task. For example, a plantar flexion contracture (examination techniques are covered in Chapter 6) preventing the individual from optimally bringing the body weight forward over the feet must be addressed to optimize balance. Other potential underlying impairments that must be evaluated and addressed to improve balance are lower extremity weakness, impaired coordination, impaired motor control, dystonia (Chapter 6), and cognitive deficits (Chapter 4). Use of the HOAC is highly recommended to help prioritize the examination as assessing every individual impairment may not be feasible in an appropriate clinical time frame.

## Examination at the Activity Level: Functional Balance Tests

A wide variety of functional balance tests exist to examine static and dynamic balance in individuals in the context of balance as it supports functional activity.

### Static Balance

Measures of static balance include double- and single-limb stance, the Romberg test, and Sharpened Romberg. It is critical in all tests of static balance that you clearly establish the criteria for stopping timed-measures and the position of the patient, including arm position. To perform the **Romberg test,** ask the patient to stand unaided with feet together and arms crossed on the chest with each hand touching the opposite shoulder for up to 30 seconds (see Fig. 9-11A), first with eyes open (Fig. 9-11A), then with eyes closed (Fig. 9-11B) (Romberg, 1853). Observe and record the amount of sway and the duration the patient can maintain this position without stepping or losing balance. The Romberg test can be utilized to examine sensory ataxia as a causal factor in postural imbalance (Khasnis, 2003). A positive test is indicated when the patient demonstrates increased instability or stepping in the eyes-closed position, indicating an excessive dependence on visual input. In the **Sharpened Romberg test**, the feet are placed in a tandem heel-to-toe position (see Fig. 9-11C and 9-11D) and the observation is repeated in both the eyes open (Fig. 9-11C) and eyes closed (Fig. 9-11D) conditions.

### Balance Grading Scales

Many therapists utilize an ordinal rating scale for first-round assessment of static and dynamic balance. Even though the scales are highly subjective, they can provide a general descriptor of the patient's balance ability. Although some variation exists between settings, the majority of these scales are built around a "fair" balance grade representing the individual who can maintain undisturbed balance without support but cannot tolerate any resistance or perturbation. One example of such a grading scale is presented in Table 9-5. Although such scales provide a clinical "picture" of the patient and require little time or equipment, the psychometrics of such scales have not been well established, and the descriptive terms are usually poorly defined in any given facility. Reliability and validity of a seven-level ordinal balance scale have been reported (Bohannon, 1995a) in acute rehabilitation compared with Functional Independence Measure (FIM) scores (Bohannon, 1995b). Bohannon also reported good validity with significant correlations between changes in balance and changes in three

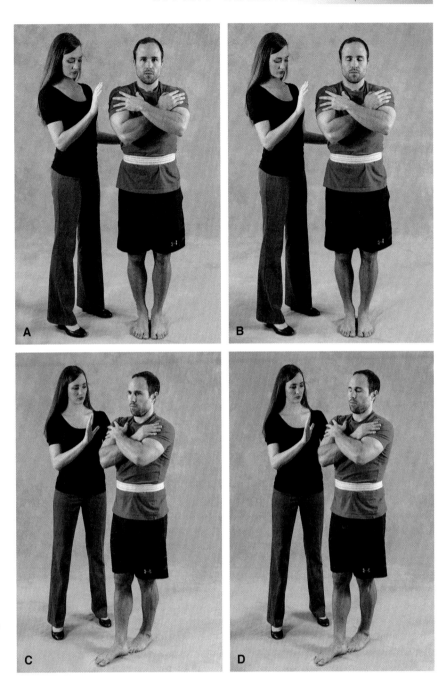

**FIGURE 9-11** Testing position for the Romberg test (**A.** with eyes open, **B.** with eyes closed); and Sharpened Romberg test (**C.** with eyes open, **D.** with eyes closed).

FIM item scores: chair-to-mat transfer, locomotion, and stair climbing.

## The Functional Reach Test and Multidirectional Reach Test

If your facility does not have a force platform, a patient's LOS can be approximated using tools such as the Functional Reach Test (FRT) (Duncan, 1990) or the Multidirectional Reach Test (MDRT) (Newton, 2001). The FRT measures the maximal distance a standing patient can reach beyond arm's length while maintaining a fixed BOS. While it could be argued whether this task in isolation is truly functional or not, obviously the ability to reach and the accompanying total body equilibrium is an important functional task. To perform the test, tape a yardstick to the wall in a horizontal position at the level of the patient's acromion (two vertical strips of Velcro attached to the wall allow for easy adjustment of the ruler height to customize position for each specific patient's height). Have the patient stand adjacent to the wall, facing parallel to the wall but not touching the wall. In preparation for the test, ask the patient to move the shoulder adjacent to the wall, flexing to 90 degrees for the start position with the elbow extended and hand either fisted (interphalangeal joint flexion) or fingers fully extended as shown in Figure 9-12A. Just make sure you use the same hand landmark, middle finger knuckle or tip of the middle phalynx, at the start and the end measurements. Make sure the patient's hand is positioned along the ruler with plenty of room such that, at the end of the reach, the fingers will still be in front of the ruler. Note the starting

| TABLE 9-5 | A Subjective Balance Scale to Rate Ability of the Patient | | | |
|---|---|---|---|---|
| RATING | SITTING STATIC BALANCE | SITTING DYNAMIC BALANCE | STANDING STATIC BALANCE | STANDING DYNAMIC BALANCE |
| 0 | Needs MAX assist to maintain sitting without support | NA | Needs MAX assist to maintain without support | Unable to move voluntarily from midline |
| Poor | Needs MOD assist to maintain without support | NA | Needs MOD assist to maintain without support | Needs MOD assist during gait |
| Poor + | Needs MIN assist to maintain without support | NA | Needs MIN assist to maintain without support | Needs MIN assist during gait |
| Fair | Maintains without assist but unable to take challenges | Cannot move trunk without losing balance | Maintains without assist but unable to take challenges | Needs contact guard during gait |
| Fair + | Sustains balance during minimal challenges from all directions | Maintains balance through minimal excursions | Sustains balance during minimal challenges from all directions | Needs close supervision during gait and able to right self with minor loss of balance |
| Good | Sustains balance during moderate challenges from all directions | Maintains balance through moderate excursions | Sustains balance during moderate challenges from all directions | Needs supervision during gait and able to right self with moderate loss of balance |
| Good + | Sustains balance during maximal challenges from all directions | Maintains balance through maximal excursions | Sustains balance during maximal challenges from all directions | Independent gait with or without assistive device |
| Normal | No deviations seen in postures held statically | No deviations seen dynamically | No deviations seen in static standing posture | No deviation seen in any standing upright dynamic activity |

position on the ruler at the end of the finger (Fig. 9-12A inset) and then have the patient reach forward as far as possible to the end position, keeping the feet in the initial position (Fig. 9-12B). The test result is the change in location from start to end, the mathematical difference between the start and end measurements. Either subtract the start measure from the end measure or subtract the end from the start; if the result is a negative number, just remove the negative sign. After a practice trial is given, measure and record three trials and calculate and document the average of the three trials with comparison to available norms (Table 9-3).

While initially developed for a geriatric population, the Functional Reach Test has been applied in pediatric samples. In this younger population, it is recommended to do one practice trial and then one test trial (Niznik, 1996). The pediatric version of the test has values significantly lower in children with lower extremity spasticity compared with children without disabilities (Niznik, 1996). The test has high intrarater reliability (Donahoe, 1994; Niznik, 1996) and acceptable interrater and test-retest reliability for children aged 5 to 15 (Donahoe, 1994). Norms are published for age groups between 5 and 15 years-old and shown in Table 9-4 (Donahoe, 1994).

In the **MDRT,** the subject should reach forward as in the FRT but also test and record the magnitude of reach in the backward direction and lateral directions, right and left (Newton, 2001). For the backward reach, the position of the patient is the same as for the FRT but the yardstick is positioned for excursion of weight-shift in the backward direction (Fig. 9-13B). The measurement is again made the same, calculating the difference between start and end positions. For the lateral reach, ask the subject to face away from the wall and hold the test arm up in an abducted position with hand in front of the beginning of the yardstick. Then, ask the subject to reach as far as possible to the side without moving the feet (see Fig. 9-13A). Then, repeat the reach using the opposite arm in the opposite direction. Results can be compared with reference values (Table 9-3). When performing this assessment, you should also record the movement strategies you observe, in addition to the difference between start and end positions.

The **Pediatric Reach Test** was developed by Bartlett and Birmingham (2003) as a modification of the multidirectional reach test. This test involves reaching in forward and lateral directions in both sitting and standing positions. Normative values for the reach tests as well as many other

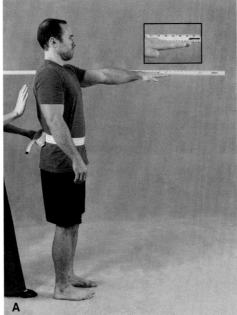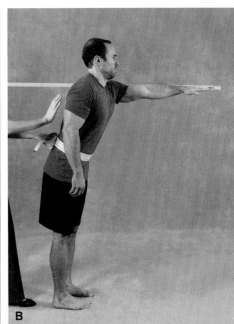

**FIGURE 9-12** The Functional Reach Test is shown with **A.** start position (inset shows close-up of hand position at ruler) and **B.** end position. The difference between the start and end position (subtract one from the other) is recorded as the test result.

balance assessment tools are presented in Table 9-3. Comparison with these normative values can help the clinician assess the severity of the patient's balance impairment and appropriate intervention.

### Berg Balance Scale

The **Berg Balance Scale (BBS)**, consisting of 14 functional tasks, is a valid functional measure of static and dynamic balance in older adults and individuals with stroke (Berg, 1992a). These tasks, listed completely in Appendix 9-A, include activities such as retrieving an object from the floor and standing with feet together. The first five items are basic balance items and the remaining nine are considered more advanced balance tasks. A score is assigned for each task on a five-point ordinal scale and the scores are then summed for a maximal possible score of 56. This scale has been extensively studied in older adult and stroke populations. Psychometric properties are very strong, including the prediction of falls in the elderly if the score is less than 45/56; however, sensitivity at this cutoff is very low at 53% (Thorbahn, 1996).

The BBS has been applied to children with cerebral palsy (Kembhavi, 2002). However, the Pediatric Balance Scale (PBS) is a version of the BBS specifically developed as a criterion-referenced, pediatric modification with 14 items assessing balance associated with everyday childhood tasks (Franjoine, 1999) and has been applied to children with cerebral palsy wearing lower extremity orthoses (Kott, 2002). It can be performed in less than 15 minutes using equipment easily obtained in schools and clinics (Franjoine, 2003). Franjoine (2003) have reported excellent test-retest, interrater, and intrarater reliability among school-age children. Performance by a sample of typically developing children ages 2 years, 4 months to 13 years, 7 months has been characterized and published (Franjoine, 2010) (Table 9-3). Neither the BBS or Timed Up and Go

(TUG) can differentiate children with mild impairments from children with normal motor function (Kembhavi, 2002). Chia-ling (2013) examined the clinimetric properties of the PBS and found moderate responsiveness to change in children with cerebral palsy and good concurrent validity with the Gross Motor Function Measure (Russell, 2002) and the Wee-FIM (Uniform Data System Medical Rehabilitation, 2011). Franjoine (2010) provides the PBS form as a downloadable appendix document at dshttp://links.lww.com/PPT/.

### Performance-Oriented Mobility Assessment

The Performance-Oriented Mobility Assessment (POMA) (Fig. 9-14), often referred to as the "Tinetti," is a measure of mobility with two subscales: (1) balance and (2) gait (Tinetti, 1986a). In a revised version, Tinetti and Ginter (1988b) eliminated step length, trunk stability, and walk stance items from the original gait subscale. To perform the test, only minimal equipment is needed: a hard armless chair, a stopwatch, and a 15-foot walkway. Consistent with the balance focus of this chapter, the balance subscale includes nine items: (1) sitting balance, (2) sit-to-stand, (3) attempts to arise, (4) immediate standing balance, (5) standing balance, (6) balance when nudged or perturbed, (7) sustained standing with eyes closed, (8) standing when turning 360 degrees, and (9) stand-to-sit (Fig. 9-14). For each balance item, typical/normal performance is awarded 1 or 2 points and 0 represents the most significant impairment for a maximum balance subscale score of 16 points (Lewis, 1993). The gait subscale (Fig. 9-14) incorporates balance components, with a focus on gait, and includes seven items: (10) initiating gait, (11) gait step length and height (foot clearance) with separate scores for right and left swing foot, (12) step symmetry, (13) step continuity while turning 360 degrees, (14) gait path, (15) trunk sway, and (16) walking stance width, each of which require balance,

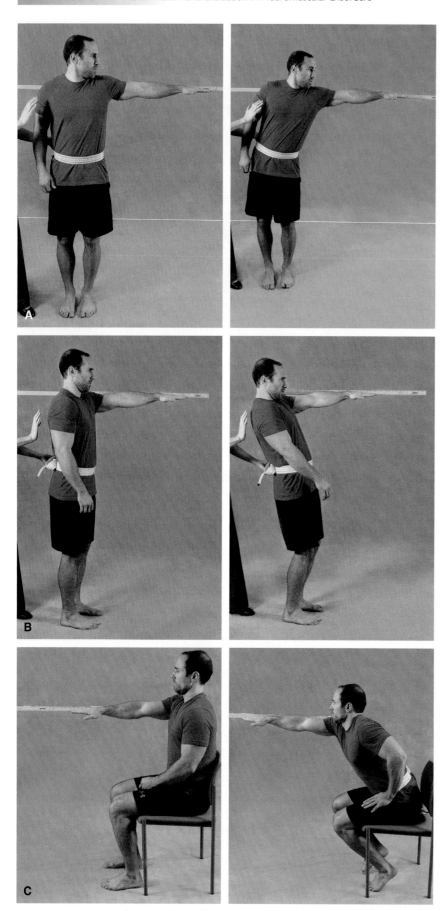

**FIGURE 9-13** Standing Multidirectional Reach Test is shown with **A.** lateral reach start and end position and **B.** backward reach start and end position. An adaptation, the Sitting Multidirectional Reach Test, is shown with **C.** forward reach start and end position and

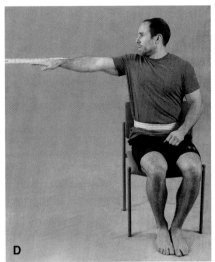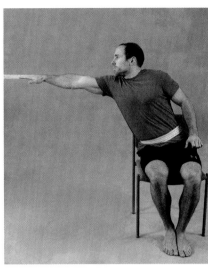

**FIGURE 9-13—cont'd  D.** lateral reach start and end position.

**Tinetti Performance Oriented Mobility Assessment (POMA)**
**Balance Tests**

Initial instructions: Subject is seated in hard, armless chair. The following maneuvers are tested.

| | | |
|---|---|---|
| 1. **Sitting balance** | Leans or slides in chair | = 0 |
| | Steady, safe | = 1 _____ |
| | | |
| 2. **Arises** | Unable without help | = 0 |
| | Able, uses arms to help | = 1 |
| | Able without using arms | = 2 _____ |
| | | |
| 3. **Attempts to arise** | Unable without help | = 0 |
| | Able, requires > 1 attempt | = 1 |
| | Able to rise, 1 attempt | = 2 _____ |
| | | |
| 4. **Immediate standing balance** (first 5 seconds) | Unsteady (swaggers, moves feet, trunk sway) | = 0 |
| | Steady but uses walker or other support | = 1 |
| | Steady without walker or other support | = 2 _____ |
| | | |
| 5. **Standing balance** | Unsteady | = 0 |
| | Steady but wide stance (medial heals > 4 inches apart) and uses cane or other support | = 1 |
| | Narrow stance without support | = 2 _____ |
| | | |
| 6. **Nudged** (subject at maximum position with feet as close together as possible, examiner pushes lightly on subject's sternum with palm of hand 3 times) | Begins to fall | = 0 |
| | Staggers, grabs, catches self | = 1 |
| | Steady | = 2 _____ |
| | | |
| 7. **Eyes closed** (at maximum position of item 6) | Unsteady | = 0 |
| | Steady | = 1 _____ |
| | | |
| 8. **Turing 360 degrees** | Discontinuous steps | = 0 |
| | Continuous steps | = 1 _____ |
| | Unsteady (grabs, staggers) | = 0 |
| | Steady | = 1 _____ |
| | | |
| 9. **Sitting down** | Unsafe (misjudged distance, falls into chair) | = 0 |
| | Uses arms or not a smooth motion | = 1 |
| | Safe, smooth motion | = 2 _____ |

**Balance Score: _____ /16**

**FIGURE 9-14** The "Tinetti" Performance-Oriented Mobility Assessment (POMA) includes a balance subscale and a gait subscale. *(Reproduced from: Faber MJ, Bosscher RJ, Van Wieringen PCW. Clinimetric properties of the Performance-Oriented Mobility Assessment. Phys Ther. 2006;86:944–954.)*

*Continued*

**Tinetti Performance Oriented Mobility Assessment (POMA)**
**Gait tests**

Initial Instructions: Subject stands with examiner, walks down hallway or across room, first at "usual" pace, then back at "rapid, but safe" pace (using usual walking aids)

10. **Initiation of gait**
(immediately after told to "go")
Any hesitancy or multiple attempts to start = 0
No hesitancy = 1 ____

11. **Step length and height**
Right swing foot
Does not pass left stance foot with step = 0
Passes left stance foot = 1 ____
Right foot does not clear floor completely with step = 0
Right foot completely clears floor = 1 ____

Left swing foot
Does not pass right stance foot with step = 0
Passes right stance foot = 1 ____
Left foot does not clear floor completely with step = 0
Left foot completely clears floor = 1 ____

12. **Step symmetry**
Right and left step length not equal (estimate) = 0
Right and left step length appear equal = 1 ____

13. **Step continuity**
Stopping or discontinuity between steps = 0
Steps appear continuous = 1 ____

14. **Path**
(estimated in relation to floor tiles, 12-inch diameter; observe excursion of 1 foot over about 10 ft. of the course)
Marked deviation = 0
Mild/moderate deviation or uses walking aid = 1
Straight without walking aid = 2 ____

15. **Trunk**
Marked sway or uses walking aid = 0
No sway but flexion of knees or back or spreads arms out while walking = 1
No sway, no flexion, no use of arms, and no use of walking aid = 2 ____

16. **Walking stance**
Heels apart = 0
Heels almost touching while walking = 1 ____

Gait Score: ____ /12
Balance Score: ____ /16
Total Score (Gait + Balance): ____ /28

**FIGURE 9-14—cont'd**

and are scored with 1 or 2 representing normal and 0 = abnormal for a total subscale score of 12 points. Greater detail for scoring is shown in Figure 9-14. The test can be completed in 5 to 10 minutes (Nakamura, 1998). The original POMA scale (Tinetti, 1986a) was developed for use in frail older adults (total maximum score of 28). The revised POMA was developed for use with community-dwelling older adults (total maximum score of 40) (Tinetti, 1988b). POMA results from the original scale have been used to rate the risk of falling: low fall risk (25 to 28); medium fall risk (19 to 24); high fall risk (less than 19) (Tinetti and Williams, 1986).

### Dynamic Gait Index and Functional Gait Assessment

The Dynamic Gait Index (DGI) was designed to examine the ability of an individual to adapt gait to changes in task demands as a predictor of falling (Shumway-Cook, 1995). Eight task

demands (see Table 10-12) are each rated on a four-point ordinal scale (0 to 3) with 0 indicating the most serious impairment and a total maximal possible score of 24. The tasks take approximately 15 minutes and include: (1) gait on level surfaces, (2) walking at different speeds, (3) walking while turning the head, (4) gait with vertical head turns, (5) gait and pivot turn, (6) stepping over and around obstacles, and (7) ascending and descending stairs. For standardization, specific instructions are provided for each item that should be read to the patient. An individual with a total score of 22 or greater is considered to be a safe ambulator, while a total DGI score of less than or equal to 19 is reported to be predictive of falls in the elderly (Whitney, 2004a). The DGI was modified to include scoring parameters for time and level of assistance (Shumway-Cook, 2013).

The Functional Gait Assessment is a 10-item gait assessment (Table 9-6) adapted from the DGI (Wrisley, 2004). It is comprised of seven of the eight DGI items and an additional

| TABLE 9-6 | **Functional Gait Assessment** |
|---|---|

Subject Code: _____ Date: _____ Rater: _____

Functional Gait Assessment

| SCORE | TASK | GRADING CRITERIA: MARK THE HIGHEST CATEGORY THAT APPLIES (I.E., THE HIGHEST CATEGORY IN WHICH THE SUBJECT MEETS ALL CRITERIA) |
|---|---|---|
| **1.**<br>FGA: _____<br>Time: _____ | **1. Gait Level Surface**<br>Walk from here to the wall at your normal speed (time for 20 ft) | (3) Normal: Walks 20 ft in less than 5.5 seconds, no assistive devices, good speed, no evidence for imbalance, normal gait pattern, deviates no more than 6 in outside of the 12-in walkway.<br>(2) Mild impairment: Walks 20 ft in less than 7 seconds but greater than 5.5 seconds, uses assistive device, slower speed, mild gait deviations, or deviates 6–10 in outside of the 12-in walkway width.<br>(1) Moderate impairment: Walks 20 ft, slow speed, abnormal gait pattern, evidence for imbalance, or deviates 10–15 in outside of the 12-in walkway. Requires more than 7 seconds to ambulate 20 ft.<br>(0) Severe impairment: Cannot walk 20 ft without assistance, severe gait deviations or imbalance, deviates greater than 15 in outside of the 12-in walkway width or reaches and touches the wall. |
| **2.**<br>FGA: _____ | **2. Change in Gait Speed**<br>Begin walking at your normal pace [5 ft]. When I tell you "go," walk as fast as you can [5 ft]. When I tell you "slow," walk as slowly as you can [5 ft]. | (3) Normal: Able to smoothly change walking speed without loss of balance or gait deviation. Shows a significant difference in walking speeds between normal, fast, and slow speeds. Deviates no more than 6 in outside of the 12-in walkway width.<br>(2) Mild impairment: Is able to change speed but demonstrates mild gait deviations, deviates 6–10 in outside of the 12-in walkway width, or no gait deviations but unable to achieve a significant change in velocity, or uses an assistive device.<br>(1) Moderate impairment: Makes only minor adjustments to walking speed, or accomplishes a change in speed with significant gait deviations, deviates 10–15 in outside the 12-in walkway width, or changes speed but loses balance, but is able to recover and continue walking.<br>(0) Severe impairment: Cannot change speeds, deviates greater than 15 in outside 12-in walkway width, or loses balance and has to reach for wall or be caught. |
| **3.**<br>FGA: _____ | **3. Gait With Horizontal Head Turns**<br>Walk from here to the next mark 20 ft away. When I tell you "look right," turn your head right and keep walking straight, when I tell you "look left," turn your head left and keep walking straight. Have subject turn head every 3 steps. | (3) Normal: Performs head turns smoothly with no change in gait. Deviates no more than 6 in outside 12-in walkway width.<br>(2) Mild impairment: Performs head turns smoothly with slight change in gait velocity (e.g., minor disruption to smooth gait path), deviates 6–10 in outside 12-in walkway width, or uses an assistive device.<br>(1) Moderate impairment: Performs head turns with moderate change in gait velocity, slows down, deviates 10–15 in outside 12-in walkway width but recovers, can continue to walk.<br>(0) Severe impairment: Performs task with severe disruption of gait, i.e., staggers 15 in outside 12-in walkway width, loses balance, stops, or reaches for wall. |
| **4.**<br>FGA: _____ | **4. Gait With Vertical Head Turns**<br>Walk from here to the next mark 20 ft away. When I tell you "look up," tip your head up and keep walking straight, when I tell you "look down," tip your head down and keep walking straight. Have subject turn head every 3 steps. | (3) Normal: Performs head turns with no change in gait. Deviates no more than 6 in outside 12-in walkway width.<br>(2) Mild impairment: Performs task with slight change in gait velocity (e.g., minor disruption to smooth gait path), deviates 6–10 in outside 12-in walkway width or uses assistive device.<br>(1) Moderate impairment: Performs task with moderate change in gait velocity, slows down, deviates 10–15 in outside 12-in walkway width but recovers, can continue to walk.<br>(0) Severe impairment: Performs task with severe disruption of gait (e.g., staggers 15 in outside 12-in walkway width, loses balance, stops, reaches for wall). |

*Continued*

| TABLE 9-6 | Functional Gait Assessment—cont'd | |
|---|---|---|
| SCORE | TASK | GRADING CRITERIA: MARK THE HIGHEST CATEGORY THAT APPLIES (I.E., THE HIGHEST CATEGORY IN WHICH THE SUBJECT MEETS ALL CRITERIA) |
| 5. FGA: _____ | 5. Gait and Pivot Turn Begin with walking at your normal pace. When I tell you, "turn and stop," turn as quickly as you can to face the opposite direction and stop. | (3) Normal: Pivot turns safely within 3 seconds and stops quickly with no loss of balance. (2) Mild impairment: Pivot turns safely in >3 seconds and stops with no loss of balance, or pivot turns safely within 3 seconds and stops with mild imbalance, requires small steps to catch balance. (1) Moderate impairment: Turns slowly, requires verbal cueing, or requires several small steps to catch balance following turn and stop. (0) Severe impairment: Cannot turn safely, requires assistance to turn and stop. |
| 6. FGA: _____ | 6. Step Over Obstacle Begin walking at your normal speed. When you come to the shoe box, step over it, not around it, and keep walking. | (3) Normal: Is able to step over 2 stacked shoe boxes taped together (9 in total height) without changing gait speed; no evidence of imbalance. (2) Mild impairment: Is able to step over one shoe box (4.5 in total height) without changing gait speed; no evidence of imbalance. (1) Moderate impairment: Is able to step over one shoe box (4.5 in total height) but must slow down and adjust steps to clear box safely. May require verbal cueing. (0) Severe impairment: Cannot perform without assistance. |
| 7. FGA: _____ # steps: _____ | 7. Gait With Narrow Base of Support Walk on the floor with arms folded across the chest, feet aligned heel to toe in tandem. The number of steps taken in a straight line are counted for a maximum of 10 steps. | (3) Normal: Is able to ambulate for 10 steps heel to toe with no staggering. (2) Mild impairment: Ambulates 7–9 steps. (1) Moderate impairment: Ambulates 4–6 steps. (0) Severe impairment: Ambulates less than 4 steps heel to toe or cannot perform without assistance. |
| 8. FGA: _____ Time: _____ | 8. Gait With Eyes Closed Walk at your normal speed from here to the next mark [20 ft] with your eyes closed. | (3) Normal: Walks 20 ft, no assistive devices, good speed, no evidence of imbalance, normal gait pattern, deviates no more than 6 in outside 12-in walkway width. Ambulates 20 ft in less than 7 seconds. (2) Mild impairment: Walks 20 ft, uses assistive device, slower speed, mild gait deviations, deviates 6–10 in outside 12-in walkway width. Ambulates 20 ft in less than 9 seconds but greater than 7 seconds. (1) Moderate impairment: Walks 20 ft, slow speed, abnormal gait pattern, evidence for imbalance, deviates 10–15 in outside 12-in walkway width. Requires more than 9 seconds to ambulate 20 ft. (0) Severe impairment: Cannot walk 20 ft without assistance, severe gait deviations or imbalance, deviates greater than 15 in outside 12-in walkway width or will not attempt task. |
| 9. FGA: _____ | 9. Ambulating Backward Walk backward until I tell you to stop. | (3) Normal: Walks 20 ft, no assistive devices, good speed, no evidence for imbalance, normal gait pattern, deviates no more than 6 in outside 12-in walkway width. (2) Mild impairment: Walks 20 ft, uses assistive device, slower speed, mild gait deviations, deviates 6–10 in outside 12-in walkway width. (1) Moderate impairment: Walks 20 ft, slow speed, abnormal gait pattern, evidence for imbalance, deviates 10–15 in outside 12-in walkway width. (0) Severe impairment: Cannot walk 20 ft without assistance, severe gait deviations or imbalance, deviates greater than 15 in outside 12-in walkway width or will not attempt task. |

| TABLE 9-6 | **Functional Gait Assessment—cont'd** | |
|---|---|---|
| SCORE | TASK | **GRADING CRITERIA: MARK THE HIGHEST CATEGORY THAT APPLIES (I.E., THE HIGHEST CATEGORY IN WHICH THE SUBJECT MEETS ALL CRITERIA)** |
| 10.<br>FGA: _____ | 10. Steps<br>Walk up these stairs as you would at home (i.e., using the rail if necessary). At the top, turn around and walk down. | (3) Normal: Alternating feet, no rail.<br>(2) Mild impairment: Alternating feet, must use rail.<br>(1) Moderate impairment: Two feet to a stair; must use rail.<br>(0) Severe impairment: Cannot do safely. |

FGA Total Score: _____

FGA modified from Wrisley DM, et al. Reliability, internal consistency, and validity of data obtained with the Functional Gait Assessment. *Phys Ther.* 2004;84: 906–918.

three items, including gait with a narrow BOS, ambulating backward, and gait with eyes closed, making it more challenging. It is potentially better able to detect subtle balance changes in individuals with vestibular dysfunction and more sensitive to change (Wrisley, 2004). Gait with eyes closed provides a condition in which the patient must rely on vestibular and somatosensory input to maintain balance and therefore examines the individual's utilization of the various sensory systems.

### The Timed Up and Go (TUG) Test

The TUG test (Podsiadlo, 1991) is a timed modification of the earlier Get Up and Go test (Mathias, 1986) and is designed as a quick screen of balance that incorporates several functional activities. The original Get Up and Go test was scored on a five-point ordinal scale from "normal" (with low risk of falls) to "severely abnormal" (high risk of falls). The TUG test was developed to improve the objectivity and psychometric properties of the test as a timed measure of the specific mobility sequence described. To perform the TUG, instruct the patient, starting from a seated position, to stand up from a chair, walk 3 meters to a mark on the floor, turn around, return to the original chair, and sit in the chair. Start timing with the stopwatch when the patient is instructed to "go" and end the timed measure when the patient returns to the seated position in the chair. Both young and older adults without deficits were able to perform the TUG in less than 10 seconds (Podsiadlo, 1991; Wall, 2000), while adults who were dependent in ADLs took more than 30 seconds (Podsiadlo, 1991). Reference values for the TUG are presented in Table 9-3. The same procedure for the TUG has been examined in children with disabilities and found to have excellent interrater reliability (Lowes, 1997). Nicolini-Panisson (2014) published normative values for the TUG test in children and adolescents and verified its use for assessment of functional mobility in individuals with Down syndrome.

Wall (2000) has developed an Expanded TUG (E-TUG) test using a 10-meter walkway (2-meter starting walkway, 6-meter central walkway to measure gait velocity, and 2-meter walkway for slow-down and turn around) instead of a 3-meter distance. Using a multimemory stopwatch to separately time each component of the TUG will help determine which specific component tasks contribute to extended time. This information can help develop a customized therapeutic plan of care with outcome measures to document improvement in the targeted portion of the task. For this purpose, the entire task was broken down into six laps for timing purposes: Lap 1, Sit-to-Stand; Lap 2, Gait Initiation (during the first two meters); Lap 3, Walk 1 (timed in central six meters); Lap 4, Turn Around (in the last two meters); Lap 5, Walk 2 (central six meters going in the opposite direction); Lap 6, Slow down, stop, turn around, and sit down (in the original two meters) (Wall, 2000). The E-TUG has demonstrated good reliability and validity (Botolfsen, 2008).

### Examination of the Allocation of Attention: Balance and Dual-task

The role of cognition in function and movement addressed in Chapter 4 and the influence of dual-task performance on balance must be considered in the examination of balance. The relationships between attention, specific cognitive function, and falls have been reported in older adults (Holtzer, 2007). Difficulties with dual-task performance are associated with a history of falls and risk of future falls in institutionalized and community-dwelling older adults. (Shumway-Cook, 1997; Shumway-Cook, 2000; Hauer, 2003; Lundin-Olsson, 1997; Lundin-Olsson, 1998). Similarly, concurrent cognitive tasks negatively influence postural sway in children (Blanchard, 2005). Younger children demonstrate more difficulty with a dual-task paradigm than older children, related at least in part to increased attentional resources associated with greater maturity (Boonyong, 2012) and a gradual shift in reliance on visual versus proprioceptive cues to maintain postural control (Peterson, 2006). Gait velocity, which is discussed in the following section, has been shown to decrease under dual task conditions (Van Iersel, 2007), which may be a strategy used to maintain balance under more difficult conditions. Clinically, there are several tools utilizing dual tasks with simultaneous motor and cognitive demands developed to examine the influence of cognition and attention on balance and risk for falls. These include the Walkie Talkie, the

TUG-manual, the TUG-cognitive, and the Walk While Talking (WWT) test.

Several procedures have been described to assess the influence of the cognitive demand of attention (during talking or communication) on ambulation and balance. The Walkie Talkie test assesses divided attention (Rose, 2010) by posing a question to the patient that requires more than a yes or no answer while walking alongside the patient and observing for the influence on walking. The test is considered positive if the patient has difficulty walking while talking. Some specific test conditions to assess the influence of divided attention during walking include (1) asking a simple question such as "What is your age?" (De Hoon, 2003), (2) reciting the alphabet or alternate letters of the alphabet (skipping the letters in between) as described in the following text (Verghese, 2002; 2007), (3) repeating random digits while walking (Sheridan, 2003), or (4) reciting names while walking (Camicioli, 1997; Bootsma-van der Wiel, 2003). The single question method was sufficient to identify the individuals who stop walking while talking and these were the same individuals who had slower walking speed and more unstable trunk control (De Hoon, 2003). Possible abnormal results for which to observe include decreased speed with the added task or, in more severe cases, loss of balance or a patient who simply stops walking to respond to the question. Hence, the original version of the test is sometimes referred to as the Stops Walking When Talking test (Lundin-Olsson, 1997; De Hoon, 2003).

The WWT test is a recent and more standardized version that can be used to examine the influence of divided attention on balance in ambulation (Verghese, 2002; Verghese, 2007; Rose, 2010; Rose, 2011). In the WWT test, you time the patient during a 40-foot walk (a 20-foot path, turning and returning). First, time the patient at a self-selected "normal" walking speed through the course, then repeat the test, asking the patient to recite the letters of the alphabet aloud (WWT-simple) or alternate letters of the alphabet (WWT-complex). Comparing the time taken to ambulate 40 feet under the three conditions, it has been shown the WWT-simple condition slows gait speed and the WWT-complex task causes even greater declines in gait velocity (Verghese, 2002; Verghese, 2007). Interestingly, asking the patient to focus on talking during the WWT test caused slower velocity and cadence than when asking the patient to focus on both talking and walking (Verghese, 2007). Older adults without dementia who slowed down during a WWT test are at increased risk of falls during the following year (Verghese, 2002). In the WWT-complex task, among a sample of older adults without disability or dementia:

- The gait velocity, during focus on walking and talking vs focus on talking only, decreased by 26.4% and 28.3%, respectively.
- The cadence, during focus on walking and talking vs focus on talking only, decreased by 17.5% and 19.2%, respectively (Verghese, 2007).

An adaptation to the TUG test, described in the previous section, includes the addition of a manual or cognitive component and is called TUG-manual or TUG-cognitive, respectively. This adaptation can be used to assess the influence of dual task attention on balance in ambulation (Lundin-Olsson, 1998). For the TUG-manual, ask the patient to perform the TUG (stand, 3-meter walk, turn 180 degrees, walk 3 meters back, sit down) while simultaneously holding a glass full of water (Fig. 9-15). For the TUG-cognitive, the patient performs the TUG while counting backward by threes from a randomly selected number between 20 and 100. In the frail elderly, a TUG-manual score increased by more than 4.5 seconds over the TUG score is associated with an increased risk for falls (Lundin-Olsson, 1998). In community-dwelling older adults, the TUG, TUG-manual, and TUG-cognitive were all able to identify individuals at risk for falling (Shumway-Cook, 2000).

### Measurement of Gait Speed

**Gait velocity** is a clinically useful outcome measure in the examination of balance and equilibrium and, in fact, slow velocity has often been used as a criterion standard (gold-standard) for validity testing associated with decreased balance (Frandin, 1995; Liston, 1996; Judge, 1995; Hill, 1996). Both self-selected gait velocity and maximal gait velocity correlate with balance in older adults, including those with stroke (Wade, 1992; Witte, 1997; Rosen, 2005). Gait velocity is useful as a screen for balance and mobility impairment in older adults especially when combined with the BBS (Harada, 1995a). It has been reported as a functional outcome measure related to standing dynamic balance used on initial assessment and reassessment (Harada, 1995b), has been shown to predict new falls as well as other adverse events in the elderly (Montero-Odasso, 2005), and is reported to be sensitive to clinically relevant change in older adults (Van Iersel, 2008). The measurement of gait velocity is so simple and quick and is such a vibrant and

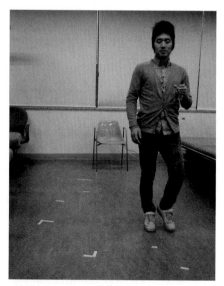

**FIGURE 9-15** TUG-manual task as individual performs two simultaneous motor tasks: The TUG while carrying a glass of water.

relevant outcome measure related to both balance and functional ambulation that it should always be incorporated as part of the neurological examination of any patient who has the ability to ambulate with or without assistance (Fritz, 2009).

Specific methods for measuring gait velocity are described in Chapter 10, but, in general, the technique of measuring temporal gait parameters involves using a stopwatch to measure the time to ambulate a given distance, often measuring the time it takes to ambulate the central 6 meters of a 10-meter walkway (Fritz, 2009). The initial and final 2 meters are not included in the calculation as these are considered acceleration and deceleration areas. Alternatively, the central 10 meters can be measured in a 20-meter straight walkway (Steffen, 2002; Perera, 2006). For each trial, gait velocity is then easily calculated as "distance divided by time," usually reported as meters/second (m/s). Ask the subject to walk first at their normal speed (self-selected pace) and then to walk at what they consider a maximal but safe speed (which will reflect their self-perceptions about their balance ability in ambulation). The bottom line is gait velocity is an objective and valid measure (see Chapter 10 for details) that is simple and quick and is related to one of the most common physical therapy intervention goals (ambulation). Gait velocity is also sensitive to change in populations with neuromuscular disorders (Goldie, 1996; Richards, 1996; Fulk, 2008). Gait velocity is broadly applicable and can be measured for any ambulatory patient in any clinical setting (acute care, inpatient rehabilitation, home health, outpatient rehabilitation, long-term care, school-settings, etc.), with or without assistive device if you can measure and mark the specified test distance on the floor. So do not neglect this important measurement. Because gait velocity is responsive to changes in equilibrium status, measuring gait velocity is an excellent way to document functional improvement as an objective functional outcome that is hard for third-party payers to refute. The result is most often reported as meters per second (m/s) and can be compared with norms as given in Chapter 10. Gait velocity values (see Gait Velocity in Table 9-3) declines with advancing age accompanied by decreased ability to vary the speed of gait while older adults with idiopathic gait disorders have an even more significant decline in gait velocity and range of gait speeds (Wall, 1991).

In addition to gait velocity, you can time other measures of specific functional upright mobility tasks as a clinical indication of balance in function including crawling, transfers, sit-to-stand, and stair negotiation as long as you have clearly defined start and end points for the measurement. Velocity of stair ascent has been described (Salem, 2000) and timed stair tests have been used as outcome measures with a variety of patient populations but standard methodology and normative values are not available across ages and diagnostic categories (Nightingale, 2014). Recommendations to improve validity include having the patient ascend and descend at least 10 steps with the instruction to do so as quickly and safely as possible using a handrail only for balance as necessary (Nightingale,

2014). The Timed Up and Down Stairs (TUDS) test has been shown to be reliable and valid in children with and cerebral palsy (Zaino, 2004). Children are asked to "quickly, but safely go up the stairs, turn around on the top step (landing) and come all the way down until both feet land on the bottom step (landing)." They may use any method they choose to ascend/descend 14 steps (wearing shoes but not orthoses) and handrails may be available.

The task of rising to stand from a starting position seated in a chair can be easily timed (Anemaet, 1999; Salem, 2000). A protocol of completing 10 repetitions of standing and sitting down as quickly as possible require less than a minute to perform (Anemaet, 1999) and can be compared with normal individuals from the age group (Csuka, 1985) (see Table 9-3). Finding two specified items on a shelf, in sitting or standing, and touching them is also part of a standardized timed assessment of ADL (Owsley, 2002).

### Use of an Obstacle Course

Balance can also be examined functionally through the use of an obstacle course. Means (1996) reported a course consisting of 12 simulated functional tasks with qualitative and quantitative individual tasks and overall scores. Taylor and Gunther (1998) developed a standardized walking obstacle course designed to quantify ambulation in an environmental context, which obviously requires balance. This course incorporates manipulation (i.e., carrying objects while walking), directional changes, negotiation past obstacles such as stepping over and around objects, changes in texture of the support surface, and response to ambulation in dimly lit conditions. Utilize such an obstacle course to gain valuable information regarding the ability of the patient to maintain balance in a functional manner under a variety of conditions.

A Standardized Walking Obstacle Course (SWOC) has also been described for the pediatric population (Kott, 2002). While the patient walks on a path (12.2 meters long × 0.9 meters wide), ask the patient to complete: (1) three directional turns, (2) stepping over an axillary crutch, (3) walking across a visually stimulating mat, (4) stepping around a trash can, (5) walking across a shag rug, and (6) moving from sit-to-stand and stand-to-sit to using an armchair and a chair without an armrest. Reliability of the method has been demonstrated (Held, 2006; Taylor, 1998). The number of steps, stumbles, and steps off the path are also recorded. The course can be repeated while carrying a lunch tray or wearing sunglasses for a dual task analysis.

### Four Square Step Test

The Four Square Step test (Dite, 2002; Whitney, 2007) is another method useful to examine dynamic standing balance in a functional setting because it requires rapid stepping sequentially forward, sideways, and backward. Four canes are placed on the floor in a "+" or cross pattern as shown in Figure 9-16A. The four squares formed by the canes are numbered one through four as shown in the figure. The subject stands in square number 1 facing square number 2. The aim is to step as quickly as possible from square 1 to the following squares in this order: 2,3,4,1,4,3,2,1, but always facing in the same direction (Fig. 9-16B). To do this, the subject steps over the canes in the following directional sequence: forward, right, backward, left, right, forward, left, and backward (see Fig. 9-16). Measure and record the time required to complete the sequence, returning to the starting square with both feet. The trial is not recorded if the subject touches a cane or does not complete the sequence. This test is quick and functional but may be very difficult for some individuals, including older adults, to complete without touching a cane. This limits its utility clinically in some settings. However, the test may also be useful in developing the plan of care through identification of specific conditions in which the patient has difficulty maintaining balance.

## THINK ABOUT IT 9.2

There are many different objective assessments which can be used to assess balance. How do you decide which assessment to use with your patient?

### Balance Evaluation Systems Test (BESTest)

Although all the balance assessments discussed previously provide clinicians with many options for evaluation and fall risk prediction, they are not able to identify the underlying postural control system which is contributing to a patient's balance dysfunction. Clinicians must be able to identify the underlying postural control system deficit to effectively treat balance dysfunction. To assist clinicians in evaluation of these

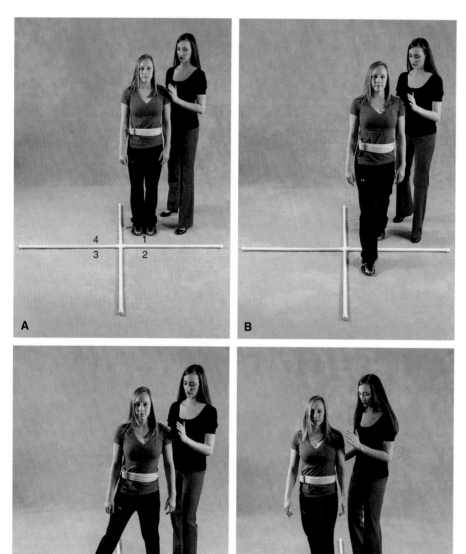

FIGURE 9-16 Four Square Step Test (FSST) **A.** showing the start position in block #1 and **B. through D.** showing the sequential steps through the first half of the test to block 2, 3, 4, respectively, and back to block #1. Then the subject would reverse direction around the squares ultimately back to the original starting square.

postural control systems, Horak (2009) and colleagues have devised the Balance Evaluation Systems Test (BESTest). The score form can be downloaded at http://ptjournal.apta.org/content/89/5/484/suppl/DC1. This test has integrated many elements of the previously discussed balance tests such as functional reach, dynamic gait, TUG and TUG-cognitive, and mCTSIB.

The test includes six subsystems of balance (Fig. 9-17):

1. Biomechanical Constraints: Functional strength, foot evaluation (BOS)
2. Stability Limits/Verticality: Excursion of the body's COM over the stationary BOS
3. Anticipatory Postural Adjustments: Movements of the body's COM before activity in preparation of a destabilizing activity
4. Postural Responses: Postural control response to a destabilizing episode
5. Sensory Orientation: Ability to integrate and use afferent information about one's body position in space
6. Stability in Gait: Balance during walking

It is important to note these balance systems work together rather than in isolation. Commonly, impairment in one subsystem will affect other subsystems. For example, if your patient has decreased lower extremity strength (biomechanical constraints), the patient will have decreased LOS as lower extremity muscles will not be strong enough to hold the weight at the edge of the BOS. The patient will also have limited anticipatory postural adjustments and postural

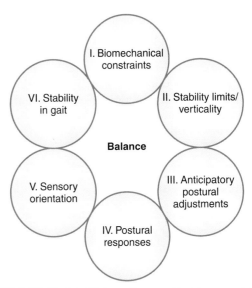

**FIGURE 9-17** Model of Balance Systems: Model summarizing systems underlying postural control corresponding to sections of the Balance Evaluation Systems Test (BESTest). Used with permission and reproduced from: Horak FB, Wrisley DM, Frank J. The balance evaluation systems test (BESTest) to differentiate balance deficits. *Phys Ther.* 2009;89:484–498.

responses as force to create these movements will be limited and the resultant movements will be decreased in amplitude. See Figure 9-18 for a table outlining the specific items of the BESTest. This test has also been shortened into two different versions: Mini-BESTest and Brief BESTest (Franchignoni, 2010; Padgett, 2012). While the shortened versions address

**Summary of Balance Evaluation Systems Test (BESTest) Items Under Each System Category**[a]

| I. Biomechanical constraints | II. Stability limits/ verticality | III. Anticipatory postural adjustments | IV. Postural responses | V. Sensory orientation | VI. Stability in gait |
|---|---|---|---|---|---|
| 1. Base of support | 6. Sitting verticality (left and right) and lateral lean (left and right) | 9. Sit to stand | 14. In-place response, forward | 19. Sensory integration for balance (modified CTSIB) Stance on firm surface, EO Stance on firm surface, EC Stance on foam, EO Stance on foam, EC | 21. Gait, level surface |
| 2. CoM alignment | 7. Functional reach forward | 10. Rise to toes | 15. In-place response, backward | | 22. Change in gait speed |
| 3. Ankle strength and ROM | 8. Functional reach lateral (left and right) | 11. Stand on one leg (left and right) | 16. Compensatory stepping correction, forward | | 23. Walk with head turns, horizontal |
| 4. Hip/trunk lateral strength | | 12. Alternate stair touching | 17. Compensatory stepping correction, backward | 20. Incline, EC | 24. Walk with pivot turns |
| 5. Sit on floor and stand up | | 13. Standing arm raise | 18. Compensatory stepping correction, lateral (left and right) | | 25. Step over obstacles |
| | | | | | 26. Timed "get up and go" test |
| | | | | | 27. Timed "get up and go" test with dual task |

[a] CoM = center of mass, ROM = range of motion, CTSIB = clinical test of sensory integration for balance, EO = eyes open, EC = eyes closed

**FIGURE 9-18** Summary of BESTest Items Under Each System Category. Used with permission and reproduced from: Horak FB, Wrisley DM, Frank J. The balance evaluation systems test (BESTest) to differentiate balance deficits. *Phys Ther.* 2009;89:484–498.

one of the main drawbacks of the test, the time it takes to complete this measure, they are not as comprehensive as the full version.

A score of 69% or less in patients with Parkinson disease differentiates fallers from nonfallers (Leddy, 2011). Also, individual items from tests such as the TUG and TUG-cognitive are built into the BESTest and can be interpreted separately for fall risk assessment.

## Examination at the Participation Restriction Level

A complete examination of balance would also include the effect of any balance deficits on one's role in society and quality of life. Although not specific to balance, these tests include ADL and Instrumental ADL (iADL) checklists or scales, Disability Rating Scale (Rappaport, 1982), Dizziness Handicap Inventory (Jacobson, 1990), and 36-item Short Form Health Survey (SF-36) (RAND Health, 1990).

## ◼ Documentation of Balance Examination/Evaluation

The documentation of the balance examination data is critical for the evaluative process and making clinical decisions about what is important to treat in the individual patient. The written documentation should clearly represent the person's balance ability. As shown in the sample examination form in Chapter 3, the balance examination should include general descriptive ratings of balance in sitting, transfers, and standing, including static and dynamic activities in each posture. More importantly, the balance examination must include reliable and valid measures, perhaps with some subjective judgments, but emphasizing objective measures when possible, particularly objective measures sensitive to change. The balance examination data in the context of the neurological and functional examination as a whole will help to determine underlying impairments needing to be addressed.

## HANDS-ON PRACTICE

The student should be able to perform the following hands-on skills for appropriate examination of a patient's balance:

- Guarding to assure patient safety for a variety of patients during static and dynamic balance activities
- Push and Release Test
- Modified Clinical Test for Sensory Integration and Balance (mCTSIB)
- Romberg test
- Single leg stance
- Timed Up and Go (TUG) , TUG-cognitive, and TUG-manual

- Functional and multidirectional reach tests (adult and pediatric)
- Four Square Step Test
- Five Times Sit-to-Stand Test and timed measure of standing from a chair
- Dynamic Gait Index
- Functional Gait Assessment
- Walking While Talking Test
- Berg Balance Scale (adult and pediatric)
- Gait velocity
- Balance Evaluating Systems Test (BESTest)

## Let's Review

For all of the questions, use the case presented at the beginning of the chapter.

Mr. McMurray, a 75 year-old man, was a fairly active golfer until 6 months ago when he was diagnosed with peripheral neuropathy related to diabetes mellitus. He now reports he has fallen three times in the past week. He and his wife report that his balance is "off" and has gradually worsened over the past couple of months. Because of his falls, now combined with significant fear of falling, Mr. McMurray even avoids many of the simple community activities he frequently enjoyed in the past, including attending a weekly Bingo game.

1. What is the BEST assessment to use to measure this patient's subjective fear of falling?
   a. Activities-specific Balance Confidence Scale
   b. Falls Efficacy Scale
   c. Gait Velocity
   d. Timed Up and Go

2. Based on the history of peripheral neuropathy related to diabetes mellitus, what impairment level test is MOST important to complete?
   a. Cognition
   b. Lower extremity muscle tone
   c. Manual muscle test of hip and knee strength
   d. Sensation assessment of the distal lower extremity

3. Which objective assessment is BEST used in this patient to assess his dynamic balance ability in the community?
   a. Berg Balance Scale
   b. Functional Gait Assessment
   c. Multidirectional Reach Test
   d. Timed Up and Go

4. Which objective assessment is MOST useful in planning interventions for this patient?
   a. Balance Evaluating Systems Test
   b. Berg Balance Scale
   c. Dynamic Gait Index
   d. Five Repetition Sit to Stand Test

5. You perform a Push and Release test and the patient takes five steps to recover. Based on the results of this test, which of the following aspects of the patient's balance do you infer is impaired?
   a. Anticipatory Postural Control
   b. Limits of Stability
   c. Reactive Postural Control
   d. Sensory Orientation

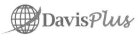 **DavisPlus**    For additional resources, including Focus on Evidence tables, case study discussions, references, and glossary, please visit http://davisplus.fadavis.com

## CHAPTER SUMMARY

Mr. Park, 85 years-old, moved to the United States after living in South Korea for 78 years and had a stroke 1 year ago. He understands English well but has difficulty finding the right English words to tell you what he is thinking and experiencing. His daughter tells you that after the stroke his right arm and leg were "completely paralyzed," but he has gradually regained some use of his right side. However, regarding his right arm and leg, she stated, "He can't make them do what he wants them to do." Today, she believes his biggest problem is that he is unsteady. Because of the way he moves, as he has tried to become more active (walking more) in the past 2 months, he has lost balance numerous times and has fallen twice but without injury. His falls usually occur when he tries to turn during walking.

General results of your examination of underlying systems pertinent to balance include impaired motor control of right leg (particularly locked knee extension in midstance biomechanically because of inability to stabilize the knee and impaired movement control of right knee extension and right ankle dorsiflexion with inadequate foot clearance during swing phase of gait) and decreased conscious proprioceptive sense at the right ankle. No cognitive deficits or abnormalities of the vestibular system were observed.

When the patient initially walked into the treatment area using his cane, you had observed, within approximately 10 meters, two occasions of the right toe catching on the floor causing him to nearly stumble but, in both instances, he recovered his balance independently. His self-selected gait velocity was 0.32 meters/sec and Berg Balance Scale was 19/56.

The TUG was 22 seconds with particular difficulty making the turns.

Based on your examination of Mr. Park, you determine he needs intervention to improve his balance/equilibrium and improve his safety (decrease fall risk).

Balance/equilibrium is essential to every form of upright functional mobility. Disequilibrium or balance impairment, especially after neurological disorders with the effect on multiple body systems, can negatively affect and limit functional skill including sitting, performing other functions in sitting, creeping (forward mobility in quadruped position), transfers, sit-to-stand, ambulation, and navigating stairs. In each skill, the balance impairment can result in decreased confidence, limited self-efficacy, slowed velocity of function, and increased risk of falling and subsequent injury. A decline in balance is a complex impairment that can be affected by numerous dimensions of body function/body structure, particularly proprioceptive, visual and vestibular sensory deficits, impaired central processing from disorders of thalamus, basal ganglia, and cerebellum, and any disruptions to the motor systems.

A discussion of the available tests for balance is presented in this chapter. While the methods for administering the tests/measures are discussed in the chapter, the Focus on Evidence Table (Table 9-7 ONL) provides a summary of some of the more important evidence supporting use of these tests. Table 9-3 provides reference values for many common balance tests and Table 9-4 provides reference values for common tests of balance in a pediatric population. From a broader perspective, there is obviously no need, nor is it feasible, to administer all these tests to any one individual. Harro (2006) has recommended how the continuum of balance examination measures may be applied across the different function levels in individuals with traumatic brain injury (TBI), listed here from lower functioning individuals to higher functioning individuals. The specific tests used will differ based on patient ability and therefore may also differ by practice setting. This recommendation may apply to individuals with other neurological conditions as well:

- Sitting and standing: BBS
- Walking: DGI/FGA
- Adaptable demands: Timed gait tasks
- Running/jumping: High Level Mobility Assessment Tool (HiMat) (Williams, 2004)
- Community mobility

Because of the wide variety of underlying contributors to balance impairment, intervention must be customized with therapeutic intervention and appropriate functional activity training. Interventions for balance impairment are presented in Chapter 30. Interventions for other related systems are presented in other chapters including cognition (Chapter 31), sensory (Chapter 27), vestibular (Chapter 29), range of motion (Chapter 23), coordination (Chapter 21), strength (Chapter 22), and motor control (Chapters 24 and 25). Functional interventions for balance related to specific functional skills are also discussed: horizontal skills and crawling/creeping (Chapter 34), sitting and sit-to-stand (Chapter 35), standing (Chapter 36), and upright mobility/ambulation/stairs (Chapter 37). The therapist must always customize the intervention for the individual patient.

# Berg Balance Scale

Berg Balance Scale
14-Item Long Form Original Version

Name: _____     Date: _____

Rater: _____

GENERAL INSTRUCTIONS: Please demonstrate each task and/or give instructions as written. When scoring, please record the lowest response category that applies for each item.

In most items, the subject is asked to maintain a given position for a specific time. Progressively more points are deducted if the time or distance requirements are not met, if the subject's performance warrants supervision, or if the subject touches an external support or receives assistance from the examiner. Subjects should understand that they must maintain their balance while attempting the tasks. The choices of which leg to stand on or how far to reach are left to the subject. Poor judgment will adversely influence the performance and the scoring.

Equipment required for testing are a stopwatch or watch with a second hand and a ruler or other indicator of 2, 5, and 10 inches (5, 12, and 25 cm). Chairs used during testing should be of reasonable height.

**1.** SITTING TO STANDING
   INSTRUCTIONS: Please stand up. Try not to use your hands for support.
   **(4) able to stand without using hands and stabilize independently**
   **(3) able to stand independently using hands**
   **(2) able to stand using hands after several tries**
   **(1) needs minimal aid to stand or to stabilize**
   **(0) needs moderate or maximal assist to stand**

**2.** STANDING UNSUPPORTED
   INSTRUCTIONS: Please stand for 2 minutes without holding.
   **(4) able to stand safely 2 minutes**
   **(3) able to stand 2 minutes with supervision**
   **(2) able to stand 30 seconds unsupported**
   **(1) needs several tries to stand 30 seconds unsupported**
   **(0) unable to stand 30 seconds unassisted. If a subject is able to stand 2 minutes unsupported, score full points for sitting unsupported. Proceed to item #4.**

**3.** SITTING WITH BACK UNSUPPORTED BUT FEET SUPPORTED ON FLOOR OR ON A STOOL
   INSTRUCTIONS: Please sit with arms folded for 2 minutes.
   **(4) able to sit safely and securely 2 minutes**
   **(3) able to sit 2 minutes under supervision**
   **(2) able to sit 30 seconds**
   **(1) able to sit 10 seconds**
   **(0) unable to sit without support 10 seconds**

**4.** STANDING TO SITTING
   INSTRUCTIONS: Please sit down.
   **(4) sits safely with minimal use of hands**
   **(3) controls descent by using hands**
   **(2) uses back of legs against chair to control descent**
   **(1) sits independently but has uncontrolled descent**
   **(0) needs assistance to sit**

**5.** TRANSFERS

INSTRUCTIONS: Arrange chairs(s) for a pivot transfer. Ask subject to transfer one way toward a seat with armrests and one way toward a seat without armrests. You may use two chairs (one with and one without armrests) or a bed and a chair.

**(4) able to transfer safely with minor use of hands**
**(3) able to transfer safely definite need of hands**
**(2) able to transfer with verbal cueing and/or supervision**
**(1) needs one person to assist**
**(0) needs two people to assist or supervise to be safe**

**6.** STANDING UNSUPPORTED WITH EYES CLOSED

INSTRUCTIONS: Please close your eyes and stand still for 10 seconds.

**(4) able to stand 10 seconds safely**
**(3) able to stand 10 seconds with supervision**
**(2) able to stand 3 seconds**
**(1) unable to keep eyes closed 3 seconds but stays steady**
**(0) needs help to keep from falling**

**7.** STANDING UNSUPPORTED WITH FEET TOGETHER

INSTRUCTIONS: Place your feet together and stand without holding.

**(4) able to place feet together independently and stand 1 minute safely**
**(3) able to place feet together independently and stand for 1 minute with supervision**
**(2) able to place feet together independently but unable to hold for 30 seconds**
**(1) needs help to attain position but able to stand 15 seconds feet together**
**(0) needs help to attain position and unable to hold for 15 seconds**

**8.** REACHING FORWARD WITH OUTSTRETCHED ARM WHILE STANDING

INSTRUCTIONS: Lift arm to 90 degrees. Stretch out your fingers and reach forward as far as you can. (Examiner places a ruler at end of fingertips when arm is at 90 degrees. Fingers should not touch the ruler while reaching forward. The recorded measure is the distance forward that the finger reaches while the subject is in the most forward lean position. When possible, ask subject to use both arms when reaching to avoid rotation of the trunk.)

**(4) can reach forward confidently >25 cm (10 inches)**
**(3) can reach forward >12 cm safely (5 inches)**
**(2) can reach forward >5 cm safely (2 inches)**
**(1) reaches forward but needs supervision**
**(0) loses balance while trying/requires external support**

**9.** PICK UP OBJECT FROM FLOOR FROM A STANDING POSITION

INSTRUCTIONS: Pick up shoe/slipper that is placed in front of your feet.

**(4) able to pick up slipper safely and easily**
**(3) able to pick up slipper but needs supervision**
**(2) unable to pick up but reaches 2 to 5cm (1 to 2 inches) from slipper and keeps balance independently**
**(1) unable to pick up and needs supervision while trying**
**(0) unable to try/needs assist to keep from losing balance or falling**

**10.** TURNING TO LOOK BEHIND OVER LEFT AND RIGHT SHOULDERS WHILE STANDING

INSTRUCTIONS: Turn to look directly behind you over toward left shoulder. Repeat to the right. Examiner may pick an object to look at directly behind the subject to encourage a better twist turn.

**(4) looks behind from both sides and weight shifts well**
**(3) looks behind one side only, other side shows less weight shift**
**(2) turns sideways only but maintains balance**
**(1) needs supervision when turning**
**(0) needs assist to keep from losing balance or falling**

**11.** TURN 360 DEGREES

INSTRUCTIONS: Turn completely around in a full circle. Pause. Then turn a full circle in the other direction.

**(4) able to turn 360 degrees safely in 4 seconds or less**

**(3) able to turn 360 degrees safely one side only in 4 seconds or less**

**(2) able to turn 360 degrees safely but slowly**

**(1) needs close supervision or verbal cueing**

**(0) needs assistance while turning**

**12.** PLACING ALTERNATE FOOT ON STEP OR STOOL WHILE STANDING UNSUPPORTED

INSTRUCTIONS: Place each foot alternately on the step/stool. Continue until each foot has touched the step/stool four times.

**(4) able to stand independently and safely and complete 8 steps in 20 seconds**

**(3) able to stand independently and complete 8 steps >20 seconds**

**(2) able to complete 4 steps without aid with supervision**

**(1) able to complete >2 steps, needs minimal assist**

**(0) needs assistance to keep from falling/unable to try**

**13.** STANDING UNSUPPORTED ONE FOOT IN FRONT

INSTRUCTIONS: (DEMONSTRATE TO SUBJECT) Place one foot directly in front of the other. If you feel that you cannot place your foot directly in front, try to step far enough ahead that the heel of your forward foot is ahead of the toes of the other foot. (To score 3 points, the length of the step should exceed the length of the other foot and the width of the stance should approximate the subject's normal stride width.)

**(4) able to place foot tandem independently and hold 30 seconds**

**(3) able to place foot ahead of other independently and hold 30 seconds**

**(2) able to take small step independently and hold 30 seconds**

**(1) needs help to step but can hold 15 seconds**

**(0) loses balance while stepping or standing**

**14.** STANDING ON ONE LEG

INSTRUCTIONS: Stand on one leg as long as you can without holding.

**(4) able to lift leg independently and hold >10 seconds**

**(3) able to lift leg independently and hold 5 to 10 seconds**

**(2) able to lift leg independently and hold = or >3 seconds**

**(1) tries to lift leg, unable to hold 3 seconds but remains standing independently**

**(0) unable to try or needs assist to prevent fall**

**(\_\_\_\_) TOTAL SCORE (Maximum = 56)**

**A person under 45 is considered to be at risk for falling.**

Adapted from: Berg K, Wood-Dauphinee S, Williams JI, Gayton D.: Measuring balance in the elderly: Preliminary development of an instrument. *Physiother Can.* 1989;41:304–311.

# Examination and Evaluation of Functional Status and Movement Patterns

Kim Curbow Wilcox, PT, MS, PhD, NCS ▪ Megan Danzl, PT, DPT, PhD, NCS
Wei Liu, PhD ▪ Dennis W. Fell, PT, MD

CHAPTER **10**

## CHAPTER OUTLINE

## CHAPTER OBJECTIVES

Upon completion of this chapter, the learner should be able to:

1. Describe the categories of function and functional measurement using key terms and definitions.
2. Explain the clinical significance of functional measures from the perspective of the patient, therapist, and facility.
3. Describe the process for selecting an appropriate functional measure.
4. Recognize the components of normal movement for rolling, come to sitting, unsupported sitting, transfers, sit-to-stand, stand-to-sit, gait and stair negotiation, wheelchair mobility, and upper extremity function.
5. Analyze movement patterns of patients with neurological deficits and determine missing movement components.
6. Discuss the characteristics of the functional measures presented.
7. Apply concepts in selecting appropriate functional measures based on specific patient problems.
8. Interpret the results of the functional examination.

## ▪ Introduction

One of the primary goals of physical and occupational therapy is to promote **functional independence**, the ability to perform daily skills or tasks without depending on help from another person. These tasks, necessary to a person's daily life, are usually referred to as **functional activities**. *Functional activities* are defined by the World Health Organization (WHO, 2002) as "the execution of a task or action by an individual." Functional activities are required for daily living and are a key component of participation in work or leisure

events. Damage to most areas of the central nervous system (CNS) will result in functional activity limitations; therefore, the "Where Is It?" feature with specific anatomical structures highlighted is not included in this chapter. To accomplish the goal of improved performance, the therapist must understand the relationship among existing pathology, impairment, functional limitation, and disability for each patient (Nagi, 1965; Nagi, 1969; Nagi, 1991) as well as interactions between the International Classification of Functioning, Disability, and Health (ICF) levels of function, body structure/body function, activity, and participation (WHO,

2002) as explained in Chapter 1. A **functional examination** includes analysis and documentation of a patient's performance of the specific activities needed in daily life such as transfers or ambulation, including aspects of balance required in executing each of those activities. Optimal tests and measures in the functional examination are required to accurately document the patient's initial functional status, document impairments that may contribute to a specific deficit in functional activity, guide development of the specific intervention plan, and document the patient's progress or lack of progress over time. Additionally, the evaluation of the data from the functional examination guides the selection of appropriate interventions to address deficit areas. Each of these aspects is facilitated through selection of appropriate functional tests and measures as explained in this chapter.

Physical and occupational therapists have long utilized observational skills to determine a person's ability to perform tasks and to identify missing movement components or abnormal movement patterns contributing to difficulty in performing a particular task. Results of this subjective observational analysis are used to determine appropriate interventions. While this method of examination is valuable, more objective methods of examination are now required to specifically document impairments and limitations to functional activity in reliable ways, as well as to document improvement attributable to intervention.

Functional measures were first published in the 1960s as illustrated by the Barthel Index, one of the earliest published measures (Mahony, 1965). The focus on reliable and valid functional measures has increased as the emphasis on documenting improvement in function and disabilities has intensified and the demand for proof of treatment effectiveness has risen. Optimally, the effectiveness of services provided is demonstrated through research studies (Kane, 1994). Standardized functional measures with acceptable psychometric properties determined through research provide one mechanism to show treatment effectiveness.

This chapter provides an introduction to standardized functional examination, including an overview of selected measures with an emphasis on performance-oriented measures. The scope of the chapter limits the number of specific measures presented. Many appropriately developed and studied measures are not presented in detail. This chapter introduces a variety of options for examination of functional tasks and movement patterns in the adult with neurological involvement as well as a brief introduction to self-assessment that may be incorporated into the examination process. Developmental and pediatric functional examination measures are discussed in Chapter 13.

## Functional Examination in Context

The qualitative and quantitative examination of a person's functional ability is an essential part of the patient examination in rehabilitation. Conduct and interpret the functional examination in the light of underlying system impairments for specific body segments, joints, muscle groups, or physiological systems during the examination of the patient. The components of the functional examination are selected based on the patient history, the patient's individual values and priorities, and the realm of the patient's abilities (not asking them to do things that are not possible). The functional measures presented in this chapter, focusing on methods to describe and document the functional ability of a patient as well as any functional deficits, may be used for examination and documentation of functional activities before, during, and after the interventions discussed in Chapters 33 to 37.

## ■ Categories of Function and Terminology

The functional tasks necessary to a person's life can be categorized in multiple ways. For this chapter, functional activities are divided into categories based on the position in which an activity is performed or the functional transitions from one position to another. The "Tests and Measures of Functional Status" section is divided according to these categories (with examples of specific functional tasks given in parentheses):

- Horizontal Mobility and Sitting (prone-to-supine, supine-to-prone, scooting in bed, crawling on belly, creeping on all fours, propped sitting, unsupported sitting, rotation and movement in sitting, reaching in sitting)
- Transitional Movements and Transfers (prone-to-sitting, supine-to-long-sit, supine-to-sitting, quadruped-to-sitting, rising-from-floor, sit-to-stand, transfer bed-to-wheelchair, transfer wheelchair-to-toilet, transfer wheelchair-to-sofa)
- Ambulation and Stair Negotiation (ambulation at various speeds, ambulation on inclines/ramps, stepping up a curb/step, stair ascent, stair descent, ladder ascent, ladder descent, running)
- Wheelchair Mobility (wheelchair propulsion, wheelchair navigation and steering, wheelchair wheelies, wheelchair ramps)
- Upper Extremity Tasks (reaching, grasp, grip, manipulation, pushing or pulling with arms)

## Functional Limitation in a Disablement Model

Functional abilities can be limited by an abnormality in any of the dimensions of the National Center for Medical Rehabilitation Research (NCMRR) disablement model as discussed in Chapter 1. According to the ICF model (WHO, 2002), the therapist will need to work toward restoring or at least improving underlying body structures/body functions and the functional abilities to which they contribute with an overarching goal of improving participation in life roles and events. A selection of possible tests and measures for examination of **functional tasks** will be presented in detail in this chapter. The presence of any impairment may negatively affect the performance of functional tasks, resulting in a functional limitation. A **functional limitation** is defined as reduced or absent ability to perform an activity with efficiency or in the typical manner (Nagi, 1965; Nagi, 1969). Limitations may be seen in the performance of **activities of daily living (ADLs)** such as walking outside, transfers, toileting, and other aspects of self care (Harris, 1986) as well as **instrumental activities of daily living (IADLs),** which include physical tasks and related cognitive abilities for tasks such as shopping, food preparation, and home management (Lawton, 1971). A functional limitation can be either a complete or partial lack of ability to perform the specific task. For example, a functional limitation of gait could be ambulation with observable gait deviations or a complete inability to walk. One functional limitation may also contribute to the development of another functional limitation. For instance, if a patient demonstrates difficulty with transfers to level or unlevel surfaces, the ability to engage in home management activities may be affected. As with impairments, a functional limitation may not be directly related to active pathology (Jette, 1994) but may occur secondarily.

A functional limitation may contribute to a **disability**, which is defined as difficulty meeting role expectations within society, including work and family responsibilities (Nagi, 1965; Nagi, 1969). It is important to realize that there is not necessarily a linear relationship in that not all impairments and functional limitations result in disability. Furthermore, patients with different active pathologies and impairments may demonstrate similar functional limitations and disabilities (Jette, 1994). A domino effect may occur, however, that influences the patient's life and possibly lifestyle. To illustrate, a person with a spinal cord injury classified as C6 ASIA A will demonstrate absent motor and sensory function below the C6 spinal level. These impairments limit unsupported sitting activities, sitting mobility, upright mobility, and hand movement among other functional limitations. Due to these functional limitations, the person would not be able to return to his previous occupation as a production line worker, resulting in a reduced income. In this example, the effects of the injury result in drastic changes in the person's life postinjury. Although physical and occupational therapists perform examination at all levels, the primary focus of this chapter is on examination of functional activity limitation.

## Functional Examination

Functional examination is the process of performing tests and measures to determine a person's ability to perform specific functional tasks (APTA, 2003). In the updated version of the *Guide to Physical Therapist Practice* (APTA, 2014), this process is referred to as an examination of "motor function" or "the ability to learn or to demonstrate the skillful and efficient assumption, maintenance, modification, and control of voluntary postures and movement patterns." The examination can include a **self-assessment** in which the patient indicates self-perception of task performance, including how performance of tasks has affected the individual's life or a **performance-based examination** in which the therapist

observes the patient performing a specific task. Tests and measures are "the means of gathering reliable and valid cellular-level to person-level information about the individual's capacity for, and performance during, movement-related functioning" (APTA, 2014). A functional measure should ideally be an objective measure and may be used as an **outcome measure,** a tool to assist in determining effectiveness of treatment or treatment approach to evaluate the overall result of care, comparing initial results to results at the time of discharge. A functional measure, which may or may not be disease-specific, often addresses one or more of the disablement levels (impairment, functional limitation, and disability) or the ICF constructs (body structure/body function, activity, participation). Depending on the specific measure used, the therapist rates the patient on either (1) actual performance or (2) the patient's capability to perform the activity. Some functional measures include items addressing cognitive and communication status since the ability to perform functional activities and to follow directions for performance of activities upon request is affected by these areas.

A performance-based examination can be accomplished through subjective measures, observational analysis, standardized measures, objective measures, or a combination of these as the patient performs the task to be measured. One of the very basic and key features to note is the level of independence or whether or not assistance is required to complete the task. An examination using **objective measures** of function is one completed using a valid instrument that allows an actual repeatable measurement of some characteristic of the task. Examples of objective measurement of functional ability include the time to complete the task, distance, velocity, number and degree of specific movement errors, and number of task completions or attempted trials (MaGill, 1993). The objective information is ideally obtained through standardized tools or methods to make them measurable and repeatable.

**Subjective measures** require some degree of judgment or estimation on the part of the therapist to characterize the task performance and may include the required level of assistance, the level of perceived exertion, qualitative movement scales, or other scales. Reliability is more questionable if tools are based simply on subjective measures. Because a subjective measure requires judgment or estimation, results are usually not as predictable or consistent as other types of measures (Portney, 1993). If subjective measures are used, reliability may be increased the more the administration and assessment of the item is standardized (see the following discussion). Subjective information included in a functional measure may include rating the degree of assistance required, a description of movement, movement quality, or other qualitative components.

An **observational analysis**, the process of observing the performance of a specific task and recording the results, can be comprised of both objective and subjective elements. Observational analysis is a valuable supplement to examination results gained from other tests and measures, such as timed measures of discrete functional tasks, range of motion, and strength, to further describe functional activities. The synthesis of data from all of these tests and measures contribute to the decision-making process for selection of the most appropriate interventions to address the deficits in functional movement. To perform observational analysis, determine the **essential components** of the particular movement or task, then observe patient performance to identify missing or abnormal movement components. Essential movement components are based on normal movement strategies and are determined through structured observation and research as described later. Gait, bed mobility, transfers, eating, grooming, and crawling/creeping are activities that are generally examined clinically using observational analysis.

A standardized functional measure rates a person's ability to perform specific purposeful activities in an efficient manner using a standardized testing protocol and standardized rating criteria. A functional examination may include objective and subjective measures as well as observational analysis. Standardized functional measurement tools, however, are published with specific instructions for administration and scoring and quoted instructions or responses to read to the patient, including reports of reliability and validity studies, making standardized measures the preferred method of examining functional activities. A standardized measure, often called a standardized assessment or a standardized tool, utilizes a set of specific **items** (measures or task variations to observe) developed for a particular activity or patient population. Such tools are frequently used as outcome measures with measures taken at initial examination and repeated just before final discharge. The protocol for administration of a standardized test, including sequence and verbal instructions, should not be altered from those specified to maximize the reliability of the test (Portney, 1993). Give preference to measures that demonstrate acceptable levels of reliability and validity. A wide range of standardized functional measures is available, and many are designed for administration by a variety of health-care professionals. In addition to variations in the areas examined and the modes of administration, diversity exists in the characteristics or **psychometric properties** of standardized measures.

Functional measures are designed to examine performance of a particular task, such as wheelchair mobility or ambulation, or can be comprehensive and examine several **domains of function**. Measures of domains of function examine several specific tasks or activities such as bed mobility, sitting balance, and transfers. Some functional measures are designed for use in certain populations, restricted by age group or medical diagnosis, while others are intended for generalized use.

Functional measures may also utilize a grading or rating system including nominal, ordinal, interval, or ratio measurement scales. A **nominal scale** classifies options in mutually exclusive categories such as male/female or ability/inability to perform a task. An **ordinal scale** uses ordered ranked categories, often assigning numerical values, but without equal spacing between the values. For example, a numerical value may be assigned according to the degree of assistance required for task performance. Because ordinal scales do not have equal

spacing between the numerical values, the difference between the values cannot be specified, which has relevance when comparing data or selecting statistical analysis. In comparison to nominal and ordinal scales, both the **interval scale** and the **ratio scale** do have equal distance between values. In addition, the ratio scale has an absolute zero point. An example of an interval scale is temperature in degrees Fahrenheit whereas height and range of motion are considered ratio scales. For these two scales, the equal distance between values allows addition or averaging of the values as in a summary or additive measure. In this type of measure, the numerical scores are added to present a "summary" of the patient's performance. Depending on the particular measure, the total score from a standardized measure may be compared with normative data to characterize the level of function or may be used for predictive purposes. For example, joint range of motion, a ratio scale, may be compared with normative data to determine whether deficits are present. Refer to Chapter 3 for a discussion on the importance of reliability and validity.

## Clinical Importance of Functional Tests and Measures

A thorough functional examination includes a variety of tests and measures, including objective measures and subjective qualitative measures as well as observational analysis. Although thorough objective and functional examinations are necessary to document progress or regression, it is also beneficial to assess the patient's perspective using a self-reported tool. One example of a commonly used self-assessment tool is the 36-Item Short Form Survey (SF-36) (www.qualitymetric.com/tabid/238/Default.aspx; a demo of the licensed SF-36v2 Health Survey is available at www.qualitymetric.com/demos/TP_Launch.aspx?SID = 100) (Ware, 1992). The SF-36, which demonstrates high reliability and validity (Stewart, 1993; McHorney, 1993; Hagan, 2003), measures self-perception on eight health attributes including physical function, social function, role function, pain, fatigue, mental health, and general perceptions of health. The 36 items are presented both positively and negatively to reduce the likelihood of falsification of answers. The results of the SF-36 may be used to document changes as the patient progresses through rehabilitation or to compare the patient to gender-, diagnostic-, or age-specific norms. The second version of the SF-36, the SF-36v2, includes both 4-week and 1-week recall versions. Norm-based scoring with linear T-score transformation results in mean = 50 and standard deviation = 10, so scores can be compared across the eight-scale profile. SF-36v2 scoring software also yields less-biased estimates of missing responses and makes it possible to estimate scores for more respondents with incomplete data (Kosinski, 2000). A shorter version of the tool, the SF-12 with only 12 items, is available. Functional measures are utilized in a variety of ways at the patient, program, and facility levels. In general, a standardized functional measure may be used to verify patient progress, to determine program effectiveness, and as a basis for reimbursement for services.

A functional measure or test is used to document patient progress or lack of progress thus determining the effectiveness of therapeutic interventions as most goals are written in functional terms. A functional measure is administered before initiation of treatment, at regular intervals during the course of treatment to document change over time, and upon discharge. Based on the results of the test, discipline-specific and interdisciplinary interventions are modified to facilitate optimal patient improvement (Fell, 2004). Depending on the specific functional measure used, the most appropriate cost-effective discharge environment and level of care can often be determined. Additionally, eligibility for federal- or state-funded programs may be determined and future outcomes predicted based on the results of standardized functional measures. In some instances, the payer may approve additional treatment sessions based on documentation of consistent objective progress toward functional independence. Furthermore, for the patient, there is an obvious link between the functional activities in a standardized measure and the activities performed in daily life that are valued by the patient. Using a functional measure to examine performance may assist the patient and family members in recognizing the relationship between the patient's needs, the examination, and the prescribed intervention. Finally, appropriate use of functional measures serves to improve communication among team members and to facilitate the continuity of care.

In addition to documenting patient progress, standardized functional measures are used to evaluate program effectiveness and the **cost/benefit ratio** as well as to document and improve program outcomes. By analyzing outcome data on specific patient groups such as diagnosis-specific groups, the strengths and weaknesses of a program can be determined and steps taken to modify the overall program as necessary. Possible modifications include reallocation of staff or resources to better meet patient needs, development of staff or additional programs, or expansion of existing programs. Favorable program outcomes are used to justify length of treatment to payers and as recruitment tools for both patients and pay sources.

At the facility level, patient and program outcomes based on standardized functional measures are used for accreditation purposes and for reimbursement. In fact, many third-party payers require functional measures because the results relate specifically to patient performance of goal activities while results of impairment measures do not necessarily indicate improvement in task performance. The value of functional examination rather than impairment examination alone is shown through studies indicating a low correlation between physical impairments and task performance and activities (Hazard, 1994; Sullivan, 2000). Examination of underlying body structure and body function, however, will be important to identify system dysfunctions contributing to the functional limitation and need to be addressed in the treatment plan.

Although there are numerous uses and benefits of functional measures, there are also some disadvantages to consider.

Specific functional measures do not always describe how a person functions in their usual daily life (Sager, 1992). Daily functioning is affected by many factors including motivation, medications, and environmental influences (Kane, 1994) and, therefore, may not be accurately reflected in any one testing. In addition, the measure may not be sensitive enough to measure change in patient status. For instance, improvement in level transfers from maximum assistance of two to maximum assistance of one may not be measurable by some functional measures. Finally, some measures may be time or cost prohibitive for a specific clinical setting.

### PATIENT APPLICATION

*Mrs. Park is an 82 year-old grandmother who experienced a right middle cerebral artery (MCA) stroke 1 month ago. Upon admission to the inpatient rehabilitation facility, you see her husband push her wheelchair into the physical therapy (PT) treatment area. As you initially observe Mrs. Park, you note that she has difficulty repositioning herself in the wheelchair and demonstrates poor trunk/head alignment as well as difficulty moving her affected extremities.*

### Contemplate Clinical Decisions

1. *In your role as therapist, you might expect her to have difficulty with which functional tasks/activities?*
2. *What components of movement do you anticipate may be affected for each of the functional activities expected?*
3. *Which parts of the functional examination will you complete as a basis for treatment plan decisions? Are there objective or timed measures you would try for these functional activities?*
4. *What underlying system impairments might be contributing to the expected functional limitations of activity and need to be examined?*

## ■ Principles of Examination of Function

### General Considerations for Functional Examination

Although functional measures examine a wide range of different activities, tasks, and skills, there are some basic aspects of functional examination to consider before and during administration of any measure. *Select a combination of self-assessment and performance-based functional measures.* For self-report tools, *distinguish between reported performance and perceived capability to perform.* Before administration, *become familiar with the measure* to facilitate scoring and ensure that all necessary equipment is readily available. Knowing or having available the specific verbal instructions and understanding equipment that may be used or the amount of assistance allowed during testing allows more accurate scoring of the test. Necessary equipment may include a stopwatch, cup, or bed as well as assistive devices. In addition, any measured distances should be clearly marked such as for ambulatory distance or wheelchair propulsion distance.

During testing, *determine the amount of assistance the patient needs* to safely perform the prescribed activities and also note the specific movement strategies and patterns the patient employs. *Determine whether the movement patterns are efficient with appropriate sequencing* and if they contribute to the person's ability to engage in activities and life roles. Recognizing and documenting specific deviations from the normal pattern (e.g., specific gait deviations) is an essential part of the therapist's clinical observation and decision-making toward designing and implementing interventions to improve the person's functional ability. *Choose functional measurement tools that would match the patient's level of function.* Note that the patient's score on a particular measure may be affected by the amount of physical or verbal assistance required to perform the functional activity. If the patient requires maximal or total assistance for a specific task, the functional measure selected may not be appropriate for that patient at that particular time. Finally, whenever possible, *incorporate objective measures* of the function that is assessed and favor measures that have reported validity, reliability, and responsiveness to change. Objective measures may include measures of time to complete a prescribed discrete task with clearly defined starting and ending points,

measures of distance for the task, amplitude of the action, and surface height among others.

## Selecting Functional Measures

Selecting a functional measure for clinical use involves investigation of several factors and can be described as a series of steps (Table 10-1). First, determine the purpose of the measure and how the data will be used. The purpose of the measure may be to track individual patient progress during rehabilitation. In the case of Mrs. Park, for example, the Trunk Control Test (Sheikh, 1980) is a suitable measure. If the purpose is to compare group outcomes in similar facilities, a national database such as that available through the Functional Independence Measure (Functional Independence Measure resource page, 2011) is appropriate. The data may be used to improve communication, facilitate program development, or develop specific interventions, depending on the needs of the facility. It is also essential, as a key step in selecting the most appropriate measure, to determine the functional activities to be examined. Some tests may examine a specific functional activity such as sitting balance while others examine several activities within one tool such as rolling over and coming to sitting. In addition to the anticipated patient population, also consider the characteristics of the facility such as availability of funding, time for training, implementation, and interpretation of the measure as well as staffing. To select the most appropriate measure, also thoroughly evaluate the psychometric properties of the selected

| TABLE 10-1 | Basic Steps in Selecting a Functional Measure |
|---|---|
| 1. Determine the purpose of the functional measure. | The purpose of the measure may include documentation of baseline function and patient progress, determination of appropriate interventions, improving communication, resource allocation, or research. |
| 2. Decide how the data will be used. | Data may be used to facilitate communication among the health-care team, pay sources, patient, and caregivers, assist in program development, and facilitate the referral process. |
| 3. Determine the specific activity to be examined. | The measure may examine a specific activity/task or multiple activities. |
| 4. Evaluate the environment. | Consider the type of health-care facility, patient population, available resources, and cost of the measure in terms of fees, training, and time to administer and interpret. |
| 5. Conduct a literature search and examine psychometric properties of the selected measure. | Determine the reliability and validity of the measure as well as scoring methods. Consider ethnic and cultural contexts and integration with the health-care environment. |
| 6. Plan and implement staff training. | Plan for initial training and follow-up training of all staff who will participate in gathering data. |
| 7. Develop a pilot test for reliability. | The purpose of the pilot test is to determine the effectiveness of the staff training and to avoid significant problems with full implementation of the measure. |
| 8. Implement the functional measure. | Following implementation, plan for continued training for staff review or new staff. |

measure. Finally, carefully prepare through staff training and pilot testing to ensure appropriate implementation of the testing and interpretation process. Considering all these factors, selecting and implementing a functional measure requires a great deal of planning and time; however, the resulting benefits are well worth the effort.

## THINK ABOUT IT 10.1

- You are scheduled to complete an examination with Mrs. Park, who is described in the "Patient Application." Think about functional measures you are familiar with and have accessible equipment to administer. Consider objective measures with good psychometric properties. Finally, think about what measures might best match the expected level of function for Mrs. Park. In addition to the Trunk Control Test suggested in the text, which self-assessment or performance-based functional measures are you considering?

## Tests and Measures of Functional Status

A section is included here for each specific functional activity to be examined. While there is tremendous variability in the way in which any functional task may be performed, the uniqueness in the way we each move, the components necessary for efficient performance of each activity are described as the components for which to watch during examination of each functional activity. Selected functional measures are presented for each functional activity. Table 10-2 lists other specific functional measures as well as diagnosis-specific measures not presented in this chapter. Table 10-3 provides a listing of reference values and cut-off scores for some of the more common functional tests and measures.

## Horizontal Mobility and Sitting

The ability to scoot in bed as well as roll from supine to side-lying and return to supine is necessary for comfortable positioning and pressure relief in bed. The ability to scoot and roll also prepares the patient to come to sitting and contributes to performance of other functional activities such as rising to standing. Movement strategies used to roll and progress to standing vary considerably among people without impairments. In fact, McCoy and VanSant (1993) found 89 different strategies for moving from supine to standing among 60 older children and adolescents; and no subjects consistently used the same strategy during 10 trials. Individuals between 20 and 60 years of age also show variability in rolling patterns (Ford-Smith, 1993; Richter, 1989).

### Essential Components of Scooting in Bed

Scooting in bed is a useful skill for proper positioning, pressure relief, in-bed self-care activities such as toileting with a bedpan

and dressing, and for preparing to transition out of bed. Scooting in bed involves lateral scooting (side-to-side), scooting toward the head of the bed, or scooting toward the foot of the bed. Individuals can scoot in bed while in a supine or hooklying position (supine, hips and knees flexed to about 60 degrees, feet flat on surface).

Bridging, which involves hip extension and lifting the pelvis from the surface, is a helpful skill in scooting. First, assess the person's ability to bridge from hooklying. The muscles of the lower trunk and hips provide stability for this action. The muscles of the lower back and hip extensors, particularly the gluteus maximus, lift the pelvis from the support surface. The hamstring muscles enable the person to maintain knee flexion and foot position on the surface. During the bridge, examine for muscle weakness (e.g., if one side of the pelvis is lower than the other during the full bridge) and controlled ascent and descent. Partial bridging can be assessed as well in which one lower extremity is in a hooklying posture and the other lower extremity is fully extended. A modification of bridging from the typical hooklying position is to assess the person's ability to bridge with both lower extremities extended. This may be the preferred method of individuals unable to assume a hooklying position or unable to bear weight through both feet during the bridge. You can also evaluate the person's ability to bridge using various positions of the lower extremities (e.g., feet wider or more narrow) and upper extremities (e.g., folded across the chest, extended at the sides). Repositioning the lower and/or upper extremities to enlarge the base of support will decrease the level of difficulty of the task.

There will be considerable variation in how one scoots laterally, or side-to-side, in bed. Typically, the action is performed segmentally. For example, to scoot to the right, one can first assume a hooklying position, bridge and place the pelvis to the right, march each foot to the right, then lift the upper trunk and head and move these to the right. The order of each segmental move may vary from person to person. The same segmental steps can be taken with bridging with both lower extremities fully extended instead of in hooklying.

Scooting toward the head of the bed is especially important to assess for individuals who use hospital beds as sliding down toward the foot of the bed can commonly occur. Scooting toward the head of the bed is achieved through a variety of methods. For example, a person can assume a hooklying position, press both heels down into the surface, and use the hip and knee extensors to push oneself up toward the head of the bed with periodic lifting of the upper trunk and head to aid the movement. Individuals may prefer to lift the head up, then segmentally and alternately move one scapula and shoulder up followed by the other side. Examples of how to incorporate the upper extremities into the movement include (1) abducting the shoulders, flexing the elbows, and pressing the palms flat on the bed to then push with; (2) abducting the shoulders, flexing the elbows, and pressing the elbows down into the surface to lift the upper trunk off the surface and up toward the head

(Text continued on page 296)

| TABLE 10-2 | Additional Functional Status Measures and Selected Diagnosis-Specific Measures That Are Not Described in the Chapter |
|---|---|
| **FUNCTIONAL MEASURE** | **DOMAINS EXAMINED** |
| ***Horizontal Mobility and Sitting*** | |
| Trunk Impairment Scale (Fujiwara, 2004) | • Perception of trunk verticality<br>• Trunk rotation muscle strength on affected side<br>• Trunk rotation muscle strength on unaffected side<br>• Righting reflex on the affected side<br>• Righting reflex on the unaffected side<br>• Stroke Impairment Assessment Set Verticality<br>• Stroke Impairment Assessment Set Abdominal Muscle Strength |
| Trunk Impairment Scale (Verheyden, 2004) | • Static sitting balance<br>• Dynamic sitting balance<br>• Coordination |
| Sit and Reach Test (Tsang, 2004) | • Forward reach in unsupported sitting |
| ***Ambulation and Stair Negotiation*** | |
| Iowa Level of Assistance Scale (Shields, 1995) | • Getting out of bed<br>• Standing from the bed<br>• Ambulating 15 feet<br>• Climbing up and down steps |
| Gait Abnormality Rating Scale (Wolfson, 1990) | • Stepping<br>• Staggering<br>• Waddling<br>• Range of Motion of Hip and Knee |
| ***Wheelchair Mobility*** | |
| Wheelchair Circuit (Kilkens, 2002) | • Figure 8<br>• Crossing a doorstep<br>• Mounting a 0.10-m platform<br>• Sprint<br>• Walking<br>• 3% slope<br>• 6% slope<br>• 5-minute wheel<br>• Transfer |
| Wheelchair mobility in patients with paraplegia (Harvey, 1998) | • Paraplegia<br>• Supine to long sitting<br>• Horizontal transfer<br>• Vertical transfer<br>• Push on level surface<br>• Push on ramp<br>• Negotiate curb |
| ***Upper Extremity*** | |
| Frenchay Arm Test (DeSouza, 1980) | • Upper extremity function |
| Functional Test for the Hemiparetic Extremity (Wilson, 1984) | • Upper extremity function |
| Wolf Motor Function Test (Wolf, 1989) | • Upper extremity function |

*Continued*

| TABLE 10-2 | Additional Functional Status Measures and Selected Diagnosis-Specific Measures That Are Not Described in the Chapter—cont'd |
|---|---|
| **FUNCTIONAL MEASURE** | **DOMAINS EXAMINED** |
| *Multidimensional Measures* | |
| Functional Mobility Profile (Platt, 1998) | • Chronic care clients<br>• Bed mobility<br>• Lie-to-sit<br>• Sitting balance<br>• Sit-to-stand<br>• Standing balance<br>• Transfers<br>• Wheelchair mobility<br>• Ambulation<br>• Stairs |
| Physical Performance and Mobility Examination (PPME) (Winograd, 1994) | • Hospitalized elderly, frail elderly<br>• Bed mobility<br>• Transfers<br>• Multiple stands from chair<br>• Standing balance<br>• Step-up<br>• Ambulation |
| Rivermead Motor Assessment (Lincoln, 1979) | • Balance<br>• Transfers<br>• Gait<br>• Lower extremity function<br>• Upper extremity function<br>• Trunk function |
| Tinetti Performance-Oriented Mobility Assessment (POMA) (Tinetti, 1986a; Tinetti, 1986b) | • Balance items:<br>  • Sitting balance<br>  • Sit-to-stand<br>  • Standing balance<br>    • Immediate<br>    • Perturbed<br>    • Standing<br>    • Eyes closed<br>    • 360-degree turn<br>  • Stand-to-sit<br>• Gait items:<br>  • Gait initiation<br>  • Gait path<br>  • Foot clearance<br>  • Step symmetry<br>  • Step continuity<br>  • Trunk sway<br>  • Base of support |
| *Diagnosis-Specific Measures* | |
| MS Impairment Scale (Ravnborgl, 1997) | • Diagnosis: Multiple Sclerosis |
| MS Functional Composite (MSFC) (Fischer, 1999) | • Diagnosis: Multiple Sclerosis<br>• Lower Extremity function: 25-foot walk test<br>• Upper Extremity function: 9-hole peg test<br>• Cognitive function: Paced auditory serial addition |

| TABLE 10-2 | **Additional Functional Status Measures and Selected Diagnosis-Specific Measures That Are Not Described in the Chapter—cont'd** |
|---|---|
| **FUNCTIONAL MEASURE** | **DOMAINS EXAMINED** |
| 12-Item MS Walking Scale (MSWS-12) (Hobart, 2003) | • Diagnosis: Multiple Sclerosis<br>• Self-report measure with higher scores indicating greater impact of MS on walking |
| Postural Assessment Scale for Stroke Patients (PASS) (Benaim, 1999) | • Diagnosis: Stroke<br>• Domains: Maintaining a Posture (sitting and standing postures), Changing Posture (bed mobility, sit to/from stand, and standing task) |
| National Institutes of Health (NIH) Stroke Scale (Wityk, 1994) | • Diagnosis: Stroke<br>• Level of consciousness including commands and questions<br>• Horizontal eye movements<br>• Visual<br>• Facial palsy<br>• Upper Extremity motor status<br>• Lower Extremity motor status<br>• Limb ataxia<br>• Sensation<br>• Language<br>• Dysarthria<br>• Extinction (Neglect) and inattention<br>• Provides specific instructions |
| SCIM: Spinal Cord Independence Measure (Catz, 1997) | • Diagnosis: Spinal Cord Injury<br>• Self-care: Feeding, bathing, dressing, grooming<br>• Respiration and Sphincter Management: Respiration, bladder sphincter management, bowel sphincter management, toilet use<br>• Mobility: To prevent pressure sores, transfers, indoors, outdoors, stairs, distances |
| Unified Parkinson's Disease Rating Scale (Fahn, 1987) | • Diagnosis: Parkinson disease<br>• Mentation, behavior, mood: intellectual impairment, thought disorder, depression, motivation<br>• Activities of daily living: Speech, salivation, swallowing, handwriting, cutting food, dressing, hygiene, bed mobility, falling, freezing, walking, tremor, sensation<br>• Motor: Speech, facial expression, resting tremor, hand tremor, rigidity, finger taps, hand movements, alternating hand movements, leg agility, come to stand, posture, gait, postural stability, brady/hypo-kinesia<br>• Complications of therapy: Dyskinesias, disability, dystonia, "off" period descriptions, nausea, sleep disturbances<br>• Modified Hoehn and Yahr stage<br>• Activities of Daily Living Scale |
| Parkinson Disease Activities of Daily Living Scale (PADLS) (Hobson, 2001) | • Diagnosis: Parkinson disease (PD)<br>• Subjective, self-report measure<br>• Description of effects of PD on daily living<br>  • Responses range from no difficulty with day-to-day activities to extreme difficulties performing daily activities |
| United Huntington Disease Rating Scale (UHDRS) (Kieburtz, 1996) | • Diagnosis: Huntington disease<br>• Components: Motor assessment, cognitive assessment, behavioral assessment, independence scale, functional assessment, total functional capacity<br>• Lower score indicates less disability |
| Amyotrophic Lateral Sclerosis Functional Rating Scale–Revised (ALSFRS-R) (Cedarbaum, 1999) | • Diagnosis: Amyotrophic Lateral Sclerosis<br>• Self-report measure; measures decline in function due to loss of muscle strength<br>• Does not test cognition |

**TABLE 10-3  Reference Values for Common Functional Tests and Measures**

| TOOL | GROUP | REFERENCE VALUES S = SECONDS | | ABNORMAL VALUES |
|---|---|---|---|---|
| Trunk Control Test (TCT) (Collin, 1990) | Individuals with stroke | Scores greater than or equal to 50 at 6 weeks poststroke have been associated with walking recovery at 18 weeks poststroke | | Scores less than 40 at 6 weeks poststroke are predictive of nonambulatory status |
| Sit-to-stand (STS) (Millington, 1992) | Typical 65–76 year-olds | Average 2.03 s | (range of 1.62–2.54 seconds) | |
| Sit-to-stand (STS) (Baer, 1995) | Typical subjects average age 61 | Average 1.67 s | (range of 1.26–2.13 seconds) | |
| Stand-to-sit (StTS) (Kralj, 1990) | Typical subjects 27–51 years | STS avg 3.33 s StTS avg 4.62 s | 2.58–5.12 s 4.01–5.38 s | |
| Stand-to-sit (StTS) (Kerr, 1997) | Typical subjects 20.1–78.3 years | STS 1.21 s StTS 1.97 s | | |
| Normal Range of Walking Speed (Oberg, 1993) | Age (yrs) | Gait Velocity mean±SD (cm/s) | 95% C.I. (cm/s) | |
| | Men (10–14) | 132.3±19.6 | 119.9–144.7 | |
| | Men (15–19) | 135.1±13.3 | 127.5–142.7 | |
| | Men (20–29) | 122.7±11.1 | 116.7–128.7 | |
| | Men (30–39) | 131.6±15.0 | 123.5–139.7 | |
| | Men (40–49) | 132.8±9.8 | 127.5–138.1 | |
| | Men (50–59) | 125.2±17.7 | 115.6–134.8 | |
| | Men (60–69) | 127.7±12.4 | 121.0–134.4 | |
| | Men (70–79) | 118.2±15.4 | 109.8–126.6 | |
| | Women (10–14) | 108.6±11.2 | 101.5–115.7 | |
| | Women (15–19) | 123.9±17.5 | 114.0–133.8 | |
| | Women (20–29) | 124.1±17.1 | 114.8–133.4 | |
| | Women (30–39) | 128.5±19.1 | 118.1–138.9 | |
| | Women (40–49) | 124.7±14.4 | 116.9–132.5 | |
| | Women (50–59) | 110.5±9.7 | 105.2–115.8 | |
| | Women (60–69) | 115.7±16.7 | 106.6–124.8 | |
| | Women (70–79) | 111.3±12.5 | 104.5–118.1 | |
| Normal Walking Speed (meta-analysis of 41 articles with 23,111 subjects) (Bohannon, 2011) | Group (age in years) | Gait Speed cm/s | Grand mean (95% CI) range cm/s | |
| | Men (20–29) | 135.8 (127.0–144.7) | 121.7–147.4 | |
| | Men (30–39) | 143.3 (131.6–155.0) | 132.0–153.8 | |
| | Men (40–49) | 143.4 (135.3–151.4) | 127.0–147.0 | |
| | Men (50–59) | 143.3 (137.9–148.8) | 112.2–149.1 | |
| | Men (60–69) | 133.9 (126.6–141.2) | 103.3–159.0 | |
| | Men (70–79) | 126.2 (121.0–132.2) | 95.7–141.8 | |
| | Men (80–99) | 96.8 (83.4–110.1) | 60.8–122.1 | |
| | Women (20–29) | 134.1 (123.9–144.3) | 108.2–149.9 | |
| | Women (30–39) | 133.7 (119.3–148.2) | 125.6–141.5 | |
| | Women (40–49) | 139.0 (133.9–141.1) | 122.0–142.0 | |

| TABLE 10-3 | Reference Values for Common Functional Tests and Measures—cont'd | | | |
|---|---|---|---|---|
| **TOOL** | **GROUP** | **REFERENCE VALUES**<br>**S = SECONDS** | | **ABNORMAL VALUES** |
| | Women (50–59) | 131.3 (122.2–140.5) | 110.0–155.5 | |
| | Women (60–69) | 124.1 (118.3–130.0) | 97.0–145.0 | |
| | Women (70–79) | 113.2 (107.2–119.2) | 83.0–150.0 | |
| | Women (80–99) | 94.3 (85.2–103.4) | 55.7–117.0 | |
| Gait Speeds (healthy versus geriatric idiopathic gait disorder) *Velocity is measured in statures/second, which equals meters/ second divided by subject height in meters (Wall, 1991) | Group | Gait Velocity*: Range of self-selected slow to fast pace | | Gait Velocity in Idiopathic Gait Disorder: Range of self-selected slow to fast pace |
| | Healthy young females (mean age 21±1.70 yrs; range 19–25) | 0.57 stat/s slow to 1.23 stat/s fast | | |
| | Healthy elderly females (mean age 75.7±5.50 yrs; range 70–85) | 0.50 stat/s slow 1.05 stat/s fast | | |
| | Females with Idiopathic Gait Disorder of Elderly (mean age 79±7.06 yrs; range 68–91) | | | 0.19 stat/s slow to 0.41 stat/s fast (note that this group has self-selected fast pace that was slower than the slow pace of the healthy elderly group) |

| Temporal and spatial parameters of gait: comparison of healthy versus stroke versus traumatic brain injury (numerical values reported as mean ± SD) (Ochi, 1999) *Male and female were reported separately by Ochi, but results were similar so only male results are presented here. | | Healthy Adult Males (Murray, 1964) | Healthy Adult Females (Murray, 1970) | Stroke (Brandstater, 1983) | Traumatic Brain Injury* (Ochi, 1999) |
|---|---|---|---|---|---|
| | Age (yrs) | 42.5 (20–65) | 20–70 | 61.4 | 31.1 ± 10.3 |
| | Gait velocity (m/s) | 1.52 | 1.30 ± 0.15 | 0.31 ± 0.21 | 0.50 ± 0.33 |
| | Stride time (s) | 1.03 ± 0.10 | 1.03 ± 0.08 | 2.3 ± 0.8 | 2.42 ± 2.00 |
| | Cadence (steps/min) | 117 | 117 | 57 | 67 ± 30 |
| | Stance time-affected limb (%) | 61% (right) | 62% | 70 | 59 ± 10 |
| | Stance time-unaffected limb (%) | 61% (left) | 62% | 83 | 72 ± 8 |
| | Step length-affected limb (cm) | 78 ± 6 (right) | 133 ± 9 (stride length) | 60 ± 25 (stride length) | 45 ± 14 |
| | Step length-unaffected limb (cm) | 78 ± 6 (left) | – | – | 36 ± 16 |
| | Step width (cm) | 8.6 ± 3.4 | 6.9 ± 2.9 | – | 9 ± 6 |

| Dynamic Gait Index (DGI) (Whitney, 2004) | | Reference Value: DGI score >22/24 = safe ambulator | | Abnormal: DGI score <19/24 is predictive of falls in the elderly |
|---|---|---|---|---|
| Stroke Rehabilitation Assessment of Movement (STREAM) (Ahmed, 2003) | To assess motor recovery in stroke | | | STREAM score <60 at 1-week poststroke correlates with a discharge location NOT home |

of the bed; or (3) gripping any rails on the bed to help pull oneself up toward the head of the bed.

### Essential Components of Rolling

Although research has documented many individual variations, rolling from supine to sidelying is generally accomplished by one of three basic methods: segmental rolling with movement initiated with the upper body, segmental rolling with movement initiated by the lower body, or the less mature nonsegmental or "log" rolling.

In segmental rolling, the upper or lower body initiates movement resulting in trunk rotation and **dissociation** (i.e., separation or independent movements of the shoulder and pelvic girdles with counterrotation of the trunk—one girdle being forward and the other girdle lagging posteriorly). A roll through left-sidelying to prone, initiated from the upper body (see Fig. 10-1), begins with cervical flexion and left rotation of the neck with simultaneous right scapular protraction, shoulder flexion, and adduction. These movements lift the right side of the upper thorax, shifting weight toward the left upper thorax, and produce initial rotation of the upper trunk on a relatively stable and lagging lower trunk (i.e., trunk dissociation). With further scapular protraction and right

upper extremity movement across midline, upper trunk rotation progresses until the right pelvis lifts off the support surface, shifting weight to the left trunk and pelvis. Finally, the right lower extremity flexes at the hip and knee to lift off the support surface and then rests on the left lower extremity (see column one of Table 10-4). Initiating a roll from the upper body, using one or both upper extremities, is considered one of the most common movement patterns to roll from supine (Richter, 1989).

A roll from supine to the left initiated by the lower body begins with flexion of the right hip and knee (see Fig. 10-2 and column two of Table 10-4). The lower extremity may then flex and adduct across midline, resulting in right pelvic protraction, trunk flexion, and trunk rotation toward the left. In an alternate method, the right foot positions on the support surface to push the pelvis forward. Either way results in right pelvic protraction and rotation to the left with trunk extension and left rotation, followed by hip flexion, knee flexion, and hip adduction to bring the leg across midline. As trunk rotation to the left progresses, the right scapula lifts off the surface while the right upper extremity horizontally adducts to cross midline. Cervical flexion and left rotation assist in completing the roll to sidelying. These methods result in lower trunk

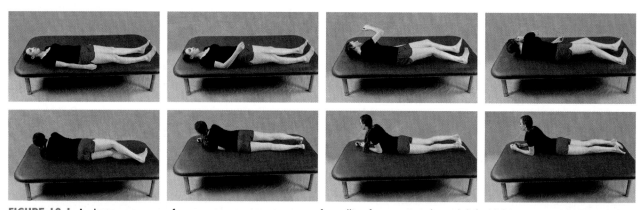

**FIGURE 10-1** A photo sequence of a common movement pattern for rolling from supine through left sidelying to prone with initiation by the upper body. *(Consistent with the work of Richter, VanSant, Newton, 1989.)*

| **TABLE 10-4** | **Essential Components: Summary of Rolling to Left Sidelying** | |
|---|---|---|
| **SEGMENTAL ROLL** | | **NONSEGMENTAL ROLL** |
| *Upper Body Initiated* | *Lower Body Initiated* | |
| 1. Cervical flexion and left rotation<br>2. Right scapular protraction with right shoulder flexion and adduction<br>3. Weightshift to left upper thorax with left rotation of upper trunk on lower trunk<br>4. Weightshift to left pelvis when right pelvis lifts and rotates left<br>5. Right hip and knee flexion with hip adduction to cross midline | 1. Right hip and knee flexion<br>2. Right LE flexion and adduction across midline OR positioned to push off surface<br>3. Lower trunk rotation to left on upper trunk<br>4. Weightshift to left as right scapula lifts off surface<br>5. Cervical flexion and left rotation | 1. No trunk rotation or dissociation (the entire trunk rolls/rotates as a single unit without any counterrotation)<br>2. Can be initiated by extremities or trunk |

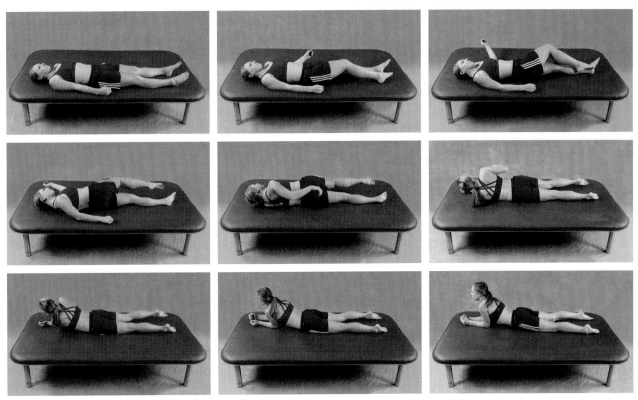

**FIGURE 10-2** A photo sequence of a common movement pattern for rolling from supine through left sidelying to prone with initiation by the lower body.

rotation on the upper trunk. From here the movement can be completed (with gravity assistance) to a prone position.

In nonsegmental rolling, also called a log-roll, the trunk moves as a unit with little rotation. A nonsegmental roll to the left may be initiated by the trunk with assistance from the extremities or exclusively by trunk action. No shoulder/pelvic girdle dissociation is evident regardless of the method of initiation (see column three of Table 10-4) so the pelvis and shoulder girdles stay in the same relative position throughout the roll. It is important to note that trunk rotation is not required to roll. Most adults without impairment, however, utilize trunk rotation initiated from the upper body or lower body when rolling supine to sidelying, whereas some nonimpaired individuals did not use trunk rotation when rolling (Richter, 1989).

### Essential Components of Coming to Sitting

Moving from horizontal to sitting is a necessary skill for an individual to achieve upright positioning and begin other transitional movements. Methods for coming to sitting from a horizontal position are as numerous and varied as methods for rolling to sidelying. As with rolling, subjects in various age groups demonstrate different methods of accomplishing the task (Ford-Smith, 1993; McCoy, 1993).

The most common method used by young adults involves moving from supine to partial sitting before moving the lower extremities off the support surface. The trunk, lower extremities, and upper extremities are involved in this functional movement; however, the trunk and extremities may not move

simultaneously or symmetrically (Ford-Smith, 1993). In addition, the supine to sitting movement shows differences with aging and level of impairment (Alexander, 1992; Alexander, 1995). The use of the upper extremities to assist trunk elevation is critical, especially in those with impairments (Alexander, 2000).

The most common method of moving from supine to sitting for 40 to 49 year-olds begins with the upper extremities positioned along the trunk with the forearms pronated and the palms in contact with the surface (see Fig. 10-3 and column one of Table 10-5) (Ford-Smith and VanSant, 1993). As the bilateral shoulders and elbows extend to push into the surface, the neck and trunk flex elevating the upper trunk off the bed, while lower extremities also flex slightly, resulting in a partial sitting position. To achieve the full sitting position, the lower extremities swing off of the supporting surface toward the floor as the trunk pivots toward the edge of the surface. The person assumes a short-sitting position on the edge of the bed or edge of the treatment table as the upper extremities assist in aligning the upper trunk over the lower trunk (see Fig. 10-3) (Ford-Smith, 1993). This method is also the most commonly used by younger and older persons; however, the upper and lower extremity sequences vary slightly (Ford-Smith, 1993).

Another method of moving to sitting is to roll to sidelying and push up with the lower arm. As with rolling, moving from sidelying to sitting and sitting to sidelying may be initiated by the upper trunk or the lower trunk. Use of the extremities to assist the trunk during this activity is critical to efficient movement (Alexander, 2000).

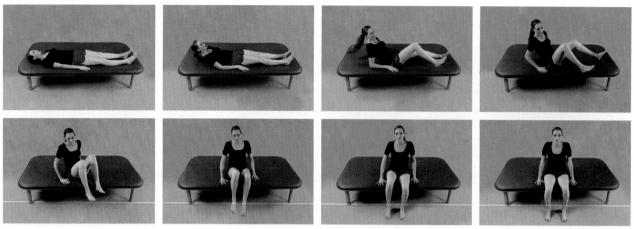

**FIGURE 10-3** A photo sequence of the most common method of moving from supine to sitting. *(Consistent with the work of Ford-Smith and VanSant, 1993.)*

| TABLE 10-5 | **Essential Components: Summary of Left Sidelying or Supine to Sitting** | |
|---|---|---|
| **SUPINE TO SITTING** | **UPPER TRUNK INITIATED** | **LOWER TRUNK INITIATED** |
| 1. Cervical flexion | 1. Cervical right lateral flexion | 1. Cervical right lateral flexion |
| 2. Trunk and lower extremity flexion | 2. Trunk flexion, left rotation, and right lateral flexion | 2. Trunk flexion to right to lift lower extremities |
| 3. Bilateral shoulders and elbows extend for partial sitting position | 3. Left shoulder abduction to push off | 3. Left shoulder abduction to push up |
| 4. Lower extremities moved from surface to floor | 4. Right shoulder adduction to push off | 4. Right shoulder adduction to push up |
| 5. Upper extremities extend to assist in aligning upper and lower trunk | 5. Bilateral elbow extension | 5. Lower extremities move off support surface |
| 6. Aligned sitting position achieved | 6. Trunk left lateral flexion to neutral as weight shifts from left to right hip | 6. Weightshift from left to right hip as feet lowered to floor |
| | 7. Upper trunk aligns over lower trunk | 7. Upper trunk aligns over lower trunk |
| | 8. Aligned sitting position achieved | 8. Aligned sitting position achieved |

One method of moving from sidelying to sitting involves upper extremity push-off from the support surface (Ford-Smith, 1993). In moving from left sidelying to sitting using the upper trunk to initiate movement, the hands are placed on the surface near the trunk and the head leads the movement with right lateral flexion of the cervical spine (Fig. 10-4). Trunk flexion, left rotation, and right lateral flexion of the trunk follow with nearly simultaneous abduction of the weight-bearing upper extremity and adduction of the opposite upper extremity to assist the trunk movement. As bilateral elbows extend, the trunk moves into left lateral flexion then neutral as weight shifts from the left hip toward the right hip. Finally, the upper trunk aligns and balances over the lower trunk as the upper extremities become nonweight-bearing (see column two of Table 10-5).

To return to left sidelying, the process is reversed. Both hands are positioned on the mat next to the left thigh as the trunk moves into flexion, left rotation, and left lateral flexion and the cervical spine laterally flexes to the right. As the upper extremities begin to bear weight and weight is shifted from the right to the left hip, the lower extremities are moved onto the mat. Using controlled flexion, the upper extremities lower the upper trunk to the mat.

Coming to sitting from left sidelying using the lower trunk to initiate the movement requires right lateral flexion of the cervical spine and trunk with simultaneous abduction of the left shoulder and adduction of the right shoulder to push up. As the upper trunk is lifted from the mat, the bilateral lower extremities move off the mat, shifting weight from the left hip toward the right hip. Sitting is achieved as the right hip and thigh contact the mat, weight is distributed equally on the bilateral hips and thighs, and the trunk assumes a neutral position (see column three of Table 10-5).

To return to left sidelying using the lower trunk method, the left hand is placed lateral to the left thigh. As weight is shifted to the left hip through lateral flexion of the trunk to the right, the bilateral lower extremities are lifted to the mat. At this point, weight-bearing occurs primarily on the left upper extremity, hip, and thigh. As the lower extremities are lifted, controlled flexion of the left upper extremity (i.e., eccentric work of the elbow extensors) lowers the trunk to the mat with assistance from the right upper extremity as necessary.

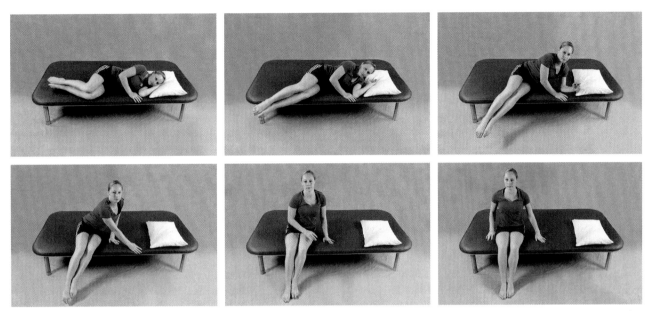

**FIGURE 10-4** A photo sequence of a common movement pattern for moving from left sidelying to sitting using upper extremity push-off initiation. The hands are used to push on the surface and the head leads the movement with right lateral flexion of the cervical spine, ending with trunk realignment over the pelvis.

Because so many variations exist, the optimal method of moving from horizontal to sitting depends on the patient. For this reason, it is necessary to determine strength and range of motion of the upper extremities, lower extremities, and trunk and existing movement patterns and preferences when retraining this task.

### Essential Components of Unsupported Sitting

**Balanced sitting** is the ability to control the center of gravity over the base of support while performing voluntary tasks in a sitting position as defined in the following text and to appropriately react to external perturbations in this position (Horak, 1987; Shumway-Cook, 2001). Balanced sitting begins with equal weight-bearing on the bilateral ischial tuberosities and posterior thighs and optionally through the feet. Positioning the patient to allow weight-bearing through the feet assists in balanced sitting by widening the base of support. However, if the goal is to challenge the patient's sitting balance as part of therapeutic intervention, the therapist may intentionally not allow the feet to be in weight-bearing thus reducing the base of support and increasing the challenge to trunk control. Slight anterior pelvic tilt and lumbar lordosis contribute to an upright trunk with the shoulders aligned over the hips. The head should be balanced on level shoulders. At least 90 degrees of hip and knee flexion is desirable while maintaining the anterior pelvic tilt to prepare the patient for transitions such as transfers or sit-to-stand. The femurs should be aligned with the hip joint without excessive adduction or abduction, and the feet should be positioned in line with the knees, approximately 2 to 4 inches apart. Finally, the bilateral upper extremities, if necessary, should rest comfortably on the thighs or bedside in preparation for functional movement.

### Standardized Functional Measures of Horizontal Mobility and Sitting

Because bed mobility is one of the most basic functional activities and is a precursor to more advanced activities, many standardized measures are available to assess patient ability. Bed mobility is considered one indication of trunk control, often predictive of future recovery in patients with stroke (Loewen, 1990; Kwakkel, 1996; Nichols, 1996; Kuys, 2009). Most relevant measures incorporate bed mobility as one or more items in a larger range of functional activities performed by the patient; however, some measures do focus primarily on bed mobility. One such measure is the Trunk Control Test, a modification of an earlier assessment (Collin, 1990; Sheikh, 1980).

The *Trunk Control Test (TCT)* uses a three-level ordinal scale to rate performance of four bed mobility activities: (1) rolling to the weak side, (2) rolling to the strong side, (3) supine to sitting, and (4) balanced sitting on the edge without foot support for at least 30 seconds. Each item is scored using the defined grading scale with 25 points maximum per item (for items 1–3: 0 = Unable to perform; requires assistance, 12 = Able to perform with nonmuscular help, 25 = Normal; for item 4: 0 = Unable to remain upright for 30 seconds, 12 = Remains upright for 30 seconds, but uses hands to steady, 25 = Remains upright for 30 seconds without support or use of hands) (Collin, 1990), then the scores are summed for an overall TCT score with maximum score of 100.

The TCT, with good construct validity, is sensitive to change in patient status (Franchignoni, 1997), has high inter-rater reliability (Collin, 1990), and is associated with walking ability in patients with stroke (Collin, 1990; Duarte, 2002). The TCT predicts recovery and hospital length of stay post-stroke, and lower admission TCT scores correlate with longer lengths of stay (Wade & Hewer, 1987; Franchignoni, 1997; Duarte, 2002). In addition, TCT scores greater than or equal to 50 at 6 weeks poststroke are associated with walking recovery at 18 weeks poststroke while TCT scores less than 40 at 6 weeks poststroke are predictive of nonambulatory status (Collin, 1990). Although the TCT is administered quickly and easily during a therapy session, it does not incorporate examination of movement quality or impairments that may contribute to movement deficits. The TCT may have a ceiling effect and therefore is recommended for use in lower functioning patients (Franchignoni, 1997). Currently, there are no ranges or norms for the TCT.

Other functional measures that include bed mobility or balanced sitting as one component of the test are summarized in Table 10-6. These include the Motor Assessment Scale (MAS) (Carr, 1985), the Physiotherapy Clinical Outcome Variables Scale (COVS) (Seaby, 1989), mobility milestones (Smith, 1999; Baer, 2003), the Mobility Scale for Patients with Acute Stroke (Simondson, 1996), Stroke Rehabilitation Assessment of Movement (STREAM) (Daley, 1997), and the Fugl-Meyer Assessment (Fugl-Meyer, 1975). These measures are discussed in the section on "multidimensional functional measures."

## Transitional Movements and Transfers

**Transitional movements**, shifting or pivoting from one position to another, are frequently assessed in the PT and occupational therapy (OT) examinations using both observations, as outlined in the following, and specific measures, including timed tasks. Transitions are also a common focus of therapeutic intervention. **Transfers**, defined as moving from one sitting surface to another closely positioned sitting surface, are typically among the first transitional movements learned after a neurological insult. Rising from a sitting position to standing, also called **sit-to-stand,** is also a common focus of the functional examination. As with rolling, the specific movement patterns used for transitional movements and transfers vary greatly among individuals without impairments. It is important to note that individuals without impairments rarely move from one surface to another without walking.

### Essential Components of Transitional Movements and Transfers

Before any transition or transfer, examine the person's ability to independently complete any preparatory actions. For example, the movement from sitting to standing is influenced by many factors including foot placement, trunk alignment, use of the arms, and seat height among others. Foot placement posterior to the knee with the knee flexed slightly more than 90 degrees is optimal for the sit-to-stand transition (Kawagoe, 2000; Shepherd, 1996). Changes in foot position of the dominant or nondominant extremity alter muscle activity and may increase demand on the extensor muscles (Brunt, 2002) and can therefore be intentionally incorporated in treatment progression. Initial trunk position also affects the sit-to-stand transition. An upright trunk with anterior pelvic tilt and slight lordosis of the lumbar spine is the most efficient position from which to initiate the sit-to-stand movement and should be maintained throughout the transition. Excess trunk flexion results in a longer extension phase (Shepherd, 1994) and longer overall movement time with delayed lift from the seating

| TABLE 10-6 | Standardized Functional Measures: Horizontal Surfaces and Sitting | | | | |
|---|---|---|---|---|
| **MEASURE** | **SUPINE TO SIDELYING** | **SIDELYING TO SITTING** | **SUPINE TO SITTING** | **BALANCED SITTING** |
| Fugl-Meyer Assessment (Fugl-Meyer, Jaasko, Leyman, Olsson, Steglind, 1975) | | | | X |
| Trunk Control Test (Collin & Wade, 1990) | X (both sides) | | X | X |
| Motor Assessment Scale (Carr, Shepherd, Nordholm, Lynne, 1985) | X | Included in supine to sitting | X | X |
| Physiotherapy Clinical Outcome Variable Scale (Seaby and Torrance, 1989) | X (both sides) | | X | X |
| Mobility Milestones (Smith and Baer, 1999) | | | | X |
| Mobility Scale for Acute Stroke (Simondson, Goldie, Brock, Nosworthy, 1996) | | | X (either side, patient selection) | X |
| STREAM (Daley, Mayo, Wood-Dauphinee, 1999) | X | | X | |

surface (Goulart, 1999). In addition to foot and trunk position, arm position and use of the arms influences sit-to-stand. If a person raises the arms using shoulder flexion near the end of the sit-to-stand movement, the center of mass moves forward (Carr, 1992). Using chair armrests for upper extremity weight-bearing to assist in coming to standing results in reduced moments at the hip and knee (Burdett, 1985; Seedhom, 1976). Seat height affects each of these factors. A lower seat height demands greater movement of the center of mass and therefore increases muscle demand and results in altered sit-to-stand strategies, including foot repositioning and trunk realignment (Hughes, 1994; Munton, 1984; Schenkman, 1996). The nature of neurological disorders can result in alterations in center of mass sway during sit-to-stand as well. For example, individuals with stroke demonstrate significantly increased mediolateral sway compared with healthy subjects (Chou, 2003).

When examining a patient's functional ability in the sit-to-stand transition, observe for the essential characteristics of the movement. The sit-to-stand transition has been studied extensively to determine typical movement sequence and force of muscle contraction (Ellis, 1984; Fleckenstein, 1988; Kralj, 1990; Millington, 1992; Stevens, 1989). There are four phases for moving from sitting to standing (see Fig. 10-5) (Schenkman, 1990). In the first phase, called *Flexion Momentum,*

forward lean of the trunk (through hip flexion of pelvis on the femur; not through trunk flexion) produces forward momentum of the upper trunk and initiates forward weight-shift from the buttocks/thighs toward the feet. The second phase, *Momentum Transfer,* begins as the buttocks lift off the support surface (the first sign of quadriceps action and the resulting knee extension) with continued momentum to assist the lift through forward tibial movement with maximal ankle dorsiflexion. During this phase, the center of mass transfers from the larger base of support (provided by the seating surface and the feet) to the smaller base of support (the feet alone). *Extension* of the hips and knees is the key aspect of the third phase as the body straightens and elongates vertically. After full hip and knee extension, the final phase of *Stabilization* occurs with completion of the rise to standing and the body achieving stability in a vertical position (Schenkman, 1990).

To interpret data from your patient, an average sit-to-stand time of 2.03 seconds (range of 1.62–2.54 seconds) in typical subjects ranging from 65 to 76 years of age is reported (Millington, 1992). An additional study of healthy subjects with an average age of 61 years showed a mean of 1.67 seconds (range of 1.26–2.13 seconds) to move from sitting to standing (Baer, 1995). The results of these studies indicate variances in sit-to-stand times among individuals without impairment.

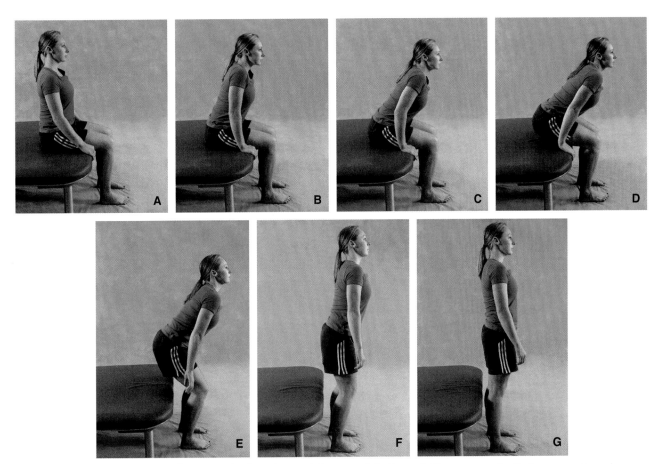

**FIGURE 10-5** A photo sequence illustrating the four phases of sit-to-stand: **A through C** represents the flexion momentum phase as the trunk inclines forward. **D** demonstrates the momentum transfer as buttocks lift-off from the surface. **E and F** illustrate the extension phase. **G** represents the stabilization phase. *(Consistent with the work of Schenkman, Berger, Riley, Mann, Hodge, 1990.)*

Individuals with stroke who can transition from sit-to-stand within 4.5 seconds have significantly better gait velocity, cadence, stride time, and single and double support (Chou, 2003). For patients who have difficulty transitioning from sit-to-stand efficiently, further examination of quadriceps strength is warranted as this variable is the most important in explaining the variance in sit-to-stand times in healthy subjects (Lord, 2002).

In **stand-to-sit**, the process is reversed as the person returns to a sitting position, primarily an eccentric activity. As the hips and knees flex, the center of mass shifts backward and must be counterbalanced by forward lean of the trunk at the hips to maintain stability throughout the transition. The body is then lowered to the support surface through controlled flexion of the lower extremities (Carr, 1987; Kralj, 1990) using eccentric contraction of the extensors until the buttocks make contact with the seating surface. The process of sitting down normally takes longer than the sit-to-stand transition. To interpret the results from your patient, Table 10-3 provides reference values for these timed measures.

Although variations exist for standing transfers, there are basically two methods: (1) a partial stand transfer or (2) a full stand-pivot transfer (see Fig. 10-6). These methods are usually initiated with leaning the trunk forward (hip flexion) as described in the previous paragraph for sit-to-stand, requiring the patient to transition to either partial or full standing. Regardless of the type of transfer, observe

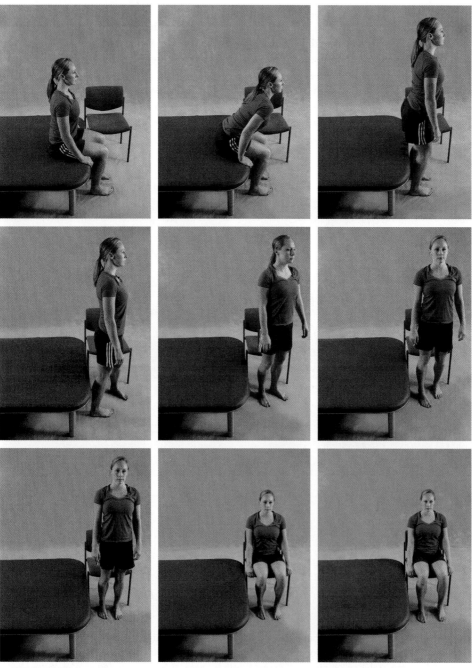

**FIGURE 10-6** A photo sequence illustrating a common movement pattern for a stand-pivot transfer.

for other necessary elements, regardless of the method of transfer, including alignment of the upper trunk over the lower trunk, balance with the center of mass maintained over the base of support (see Chapter 9), and lower extremity extensor control, concentrically in the rise to standing and eccentrically during the return to sitting. The patient must also have the ability to weight-shift from one lower extremity to the other midtransfer, maintain adequate stability of the support lower extremity to take a step with the contralateral extremity, and rotate the pelvis on the lower extremities.

Once the patient has achieved partial or full standing in the transfer, confirm that the patient can then pivot the feet or take a small step to reach the new support surface. The full stand transfer, also called a **stand-pivot transfer**, requires full hip and knee extension and therefore greater balance/equilibrium. A full stand transfer is accomplished by taking one or two small steps toward the new support surface rather than simply pivoting. During this method of transfer, the ability to laterally weight-shift and support the body weight on one lower extremity to take a step are required. In the partial stand transfer, sometimes called a **modified stand-pivot transfer or squat-pivot transfer** (see Fig. 10-7), the buttocks are lifted just enough to clear the support surface and the patient pivots on the feet, usually without taking a step, before lowering to the new support.

### Standardized Functional Measures of Transitional Movements and Transfers

The Five-Times-Sit-to-Stand Test is a standardized measure assessing a person's ability to rise from a chair and return to sitting five times as quickly as possible (Whitney, 2005). This measure focuses on the speed to complete a functional task. Instruct the person to cross arms over the chest and sit with the back against the chair. Instruct the person to stand up and sit down five times as quickly as possible and start timing when you signal the person, "Go," and stop timing when the person's buttocks touch the chair on the fifth repetition. The person should stand fully each time. There are variations in the described testing procedure. For example, some descriptions indicate that you should stop timing when the patient's back is against the backrest after the fifth repetition (Mong, 2010; Kumban, 2013). Document the procedure you use (e.g., start/stop time indicators, chair height/depth, chair type, patient arm position) to improve intra- and interrater reliability in future tests. The measure has good psychometric properties in a variety of neurological patient populations (see Table 10-24 [ONL] and the online Focus on Evidence [FOE] resources).

Although there are few functional measures that examine only the sit-to-stand movement or transfers, many incorporate these activities as one or more components of the tool. Standardized measures that include a sit-to-stand component include the MAS (Carr, 1985), the Physiotherapy Clinical Outcomes Variables Scale (COVS) (Seaby, 1989), the Mobility Scale for Acute Stroke Patients (Simondson, 1996), the STREAM (Daley, 1997; Daley, 1999) and the Functional Independence Measure (FIM) (Uniform Data System for Medical Rehabilitation) (see Table 10-24). Transfers are included in the COVS (Seaby, 1989) and FIM (Uniform Data System for Medical Rehabilitation). These measures are discussed in the section on multidimensional measures.

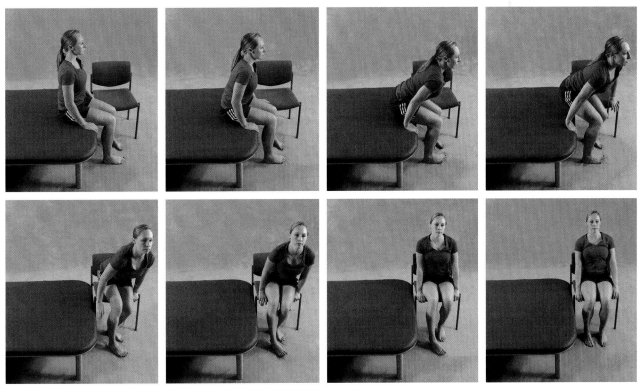

**FIGURE 10-7** A photo sequence illustrating a common movement pattern for a modified stand-pivot transfer, also known as a squat-pivot transfer.

# Ambulation and Stair Negotiation

Independently ambulatory individuals with or without an assistive device use ambulation or gait as a functional task to efficiently participate in daily activities such as homemaking, working, grocery shopping, attendance at a baseball game, and nearly every other activity of life. The ability to walk is a precursor to more advanced activities including **stair negotiation**, which is the transition from level ground ambulation to a surface at a different elevation through ascending or descending steps. Therapists who fully understand the complex interaction of joint movement and muscle demands in functional ambulation are better equipped to complete gait training with individuals with neurological disorders. The information obtained from functional measures, including ambulation, provides the foundation for therapists to understand a patient's movement strategies and therefore design effective individualized interventions.

## Essential Components of Ambulation and Stair Negotiation

Human walking is a repetitive, sequential, bipedal motion with the purpose of moving the body from one location to another. The center of mass is repetitively moving forward outside the base of support with balance carefully regained each time by resetting a new base of support (a step forward). As such, walking has been referred to as "a series of catastrophes narrowly averted" (Steindler, 1955). A single sequence of timed events of one lower extremity during walking is called the **gait cycle**. By convention, the gait cycle starts when the heel of one lower extremity contacts the ground and ends when the heel of the same limb contacts the ground the next time. The gait cycle is a basic time window for **observational gait analysis** (OGA), which serves an important role in determining specific intervention strategies to employ, in addition to objective temporal and spatial measures, which are essential for documenting change in ambulation status and response to intervention. Basically, the gait cycle has two phases: **stance phase**, when the foot is in contact with the ground, and **swing phase**, when the foot is not in contact with the ground. For example, when the left lower extremity is considered the **reference limb** or the observed limb, stance phase is the time interval when the left foot is on the ground and swing phase is the time interval when the left foot is off the ground and swinging forward in preparation for the next ground contact. Stance phase includes two **double support phases** when both feet are in contact with the ground, one at the beginning of stance and one at the end of the stance phase and one interposed **single support phase** when the opposite nonsupporting limb is swinging forward leaving the reference limb alone in contact with the ground.

A comprehensive OGA system developed by Rancho Los Amigos (RLA) National Rehabilitation Center (Rancho Los Amigos, 2001) identifies three basic functional tasks interspersed throughout the gait cycle: weight acceptance (WA), single limb support (SLS), and swing limb advancement (SLA). The gait cycle is further divided into eight specific sequential phases or critical events of gait summarized in Table 10-7. WA includes the phases of initial contact and loading response. SLS includes the phases of midstance and terminal stance. SLA, mostly consisting of swing phase, includes the phases of preswing, initial swing, midswing, and terminal swing (see Fig. 10-8). Table 10-7 describes the critical events and essential functions at each phase of gait.

As indicated earlier, the gait cycle has double support phases, which distinguishes walking from the faster form of repetitive bipedal motion called *running*. In running, there is no time period of double support such that the single support phase is followed by a period called the float phase when neither foot is on the ground. The Rancho classification of the gait cycle is also valid during stair negotiation, including the three major phases of WA, SLS, and SLA. The transition from

| TABLE 10-7 | Critical Events of the Gait Cycle (Adapted from Rancho Los Amigos, 2001) |
|---|---|
| **WEIGHT ACCEPTANCE** | |
| Initial contact | Normally in human gait, the heel of the reference foot makes initial contact. The heel rocker redirects and preserves forward progression of the body. |
| Loading response | Hip joint stability prevents unnecessary pelvic tilt. Knee flexion serves as shock absorption but is controlled to prevent excessive knee flexion. |
| **SINGLE LIMB SUPPORT** | |
| Midstance | The ankle rocker controls tibial advancement and provides support against gravity. |
| Terminal stance | The heel begins to rise and ankle plantar flexors change from eccentric to concentric contraction. |
| **SWING LIMB ADVANCEMENT** | |
| Preswing | Ankle plantar flexion is essential to produce sufficient knee flexion for foot clearance. |
| Initial swing | Knee flexion increases to approximately 60 degrees and contributes to foot clearance. |
| Midswing | The hip flexes to 25 degrees and contributes to foot clearance. |
| Terminal swing | The knee extends to neutral in preparation for weight-bearing at weight acceptance. |

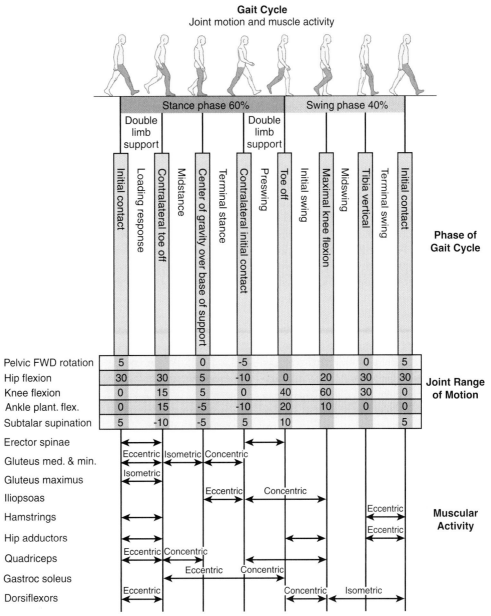

**FIGURE 10-8** Rancho Los Amigos Functional Divisions of the Gait Cycle.

walking on level surfaces to stairs or from stairs to the ground requires higher extensor moment demands on lower extremity joints in comparison to walking. For example, during WA of ascending stairs, the body must be maintained in both forward and upward directions. The hip, knee, and ankle must generate additional increased extensor moments to counterbalance gravity, which produces flexor moments. During WA of descending stairs, greater eccentric control at the hip and knee are required for a slow and controlled descent.

### Standardized Functional Measures of Ambulation and Stair Negotiation

A performance-based examination of gait can be achieved including both OGA and **instrumental gait analysis (IGA).** An IGA utilizes computer-augmented instrumentation to analyze gait and is addressed in a later section of the chapter.

OGA offers therapists a more practical clinical approach to examine a patient's gait performance because it is easier, quicker, and less expensive to use compared with IGA. Incorporate objective measures of walking such as distance, velocity, step lengths, and stride lengths in the OGA. These repeatable objective variables are commonly included as functional outcome measures. In addition, human gait may be measured by both qualitative and quantitative means.

Objective measures of gait can be classified into two general categories: kinematics and kinetics. **Kinematics** analysis is used to describe the motion of the whole body or body segments during the gait cycle but no forces are considered. **Kinetics** is the analysis of the forces or torques during movement such as the gait cycle. Most standardized functional measures focus on kinematics, which include **temporal measures** such as walking speed, walking time, step time, stride time, and

**spatial measures** such as walking distance, step length, and stride length. Other advanced measures such as angular change of individual joints, and kinetic factors such as joint forces and joint moments are reviewed in the OGA section. Counting the number of **steps per day (SPD)** describes real walking activity poststroke and could be measured with a pedometer (Roos, 2012) at the initiation of rehabilitation and upon discharge to document improvement. In a study comparing the Fitbit Ultra (Fitbit Inc., San Francisco, CA), Nike + Fuelband (Nike Inc., Beaverton, OR), StepWatch Activity Monitor (SAM) (Orthocare Innovations, Oklahoma City, OK), and the Yamax Digi-Walker SW-701 pedometer (YAMAX Health & Sports Inc., San Antonio, TX) in individuals with stroke or traumatic brain injury, the SAM was the most accurate. Given possible limitations to the clinical utility of the SAM, however, Fitbit Ultra had fair to good accuracy when measuring stepping activity in people with a stroke or traumatic brain injury who could walk at speeds of greater than or equal to 0.58 m/s, and it may be a good cost-effective and user-friendly alternative (Fulk, 2014).

Time, distance, and quality of gait are important factors to consider for functional mobility. For example, the therapist may examine how long it takes for a patient to walk a certain distance or how far the patient can walk within a specific time, thus simulating crossing the street before the traffic light changes or shopping in the grocery store. Walking speed is perhaps one of the most important functional outcomes that can be measured because both distance and time are considered and enable an efficient measurement of functional ambulation. Gait velocity declines with advancing age, particularly beyond age 80 years (Oberg, 1993; Fritz, 2009; Bohannon, 2011) and in individuals with stroke (Brandstater, 1983; Wade & Heller, 1987; Olney, 1994; Hsu, 2003), traumatic brain injury (Ochi, 1999), and multiple sclerosis (Givona, 2009). The individual without neuromusculoskeletal deficits can easily change walking speed from slow to fast to meet different task requirements with a wide variety of possible speeds. Those with neuromusculoskeletal deficits, such as stroke or cerebral palsy or idiopathic gait disorder of the elderly, usually lack this potential for variability in gait speed with "slow" speeds very similar to the individual's "fast" speed (Wall, 1991).

To measure gait velocity in a clinical setting, mark a prescribed distance on the ground (often 6 meters or 10 meters) then time the individual from the time the person walks over the start line until the person walks over the other line. Gait velocity is calculated as "distance divided by time" and is best reported in units of meters per second (m/s). In some studies, gait velocity is reported in the units of statures/second to normalize velocity to subject height (statures/second = velocity [m/s] divided by subject height [in meters]) (Wall, 1991). Measure the individual's "self-selected" pace, "slow" speed, and "fast" speed to gain valuable information about the person's ability to purposefully modify their walking speed. The range for normal walking speed is generally reported between 1.2 to 1.4 m/s (Fritz, 2009; Lerner-Frankiel, 1986). More specific ranges of human walking speed by sex and age group are shown in Table 10-3 (Oberg, 1993; Bohannon, 2011).

Three standardized measures to consider for measuring gait velocity include the 10-Meter Walk Test, Timed 25-Foot Walk test, and 4-Meter Walk Gait Speed Test. The 10-Meter Walk Test (10MWT) involves timing an individual as the person walks the set distance and subsequently calculating gait speed in m/s. Start timing when the individual crosses the 2-meter mark and stop timing when the individual crosses the 8-meter mark. These spaces enable acceleration and deceleration periods that are not included in determining speed. The Timed 25-Foot Walk test (T25FW) typically involves asking the individual to walk a total of 35 feet to enable 5 feet before and 5 feet after the timed 25-foot course. Record the number of seconds to walk 25 feet. Seconds per feet can be converted into m/s.

For both the 10MWT and T25FW tests, the person's comfortable (or preferred or self-selected) speed and fastest safe walking speed can be assessed. An assistive device is allowed for both but should be documented. Possible testing designs include: (1) a single trial walk, (2) recording the best performance of two or three trials, or (3) recording the average of two or three trials. Indicate if a practice trial was allowed for these various setups. Additional details about the 10MWT and T25FW, including patient instructions, copies of the measures, and psychometric data are available through these websites: www.rehabmeasures.org and www.neuropt.org/professional-resources/neurology-section-outcome-measures-recommendations.

The 4-Meter Walk Gait Speed Test is the recommended measure for assessing gait speed in the National Institutes of Health (NIH) Toolbox for the assessment of neurological and behavioral function (accessible at: www.nihtoolbox.org/WhatAndWhy/Motor/Locomotion/Pages/NIH-Toolbox-4-Meter-Walk-Gait-Speed-Test.aspx). Individuals walk 4 meters at a usual pace, completing one practice and two timed trials. Use the best timed trial time for scoring. In a study examining the reliability and validity of the 4-Meter Walk Test and the 10MWT in healthy older adults, both measures demonstrated excellent test-retest reliability, similar standard error of the measurement values, and similar minimal detectable change values (Peters, 2013). The lack of concurrent validity between the two tests, however, reveal shortcomings in using the two tests interchangeably. The 4-Meter Walk Test may be a valuable alternative in the home health setting when space restrictions prohibit the 10MWT.

Several temporal variables are measured based on time intervals between key events of the gait cycle. **Swing time, stance time,** and other temporal parameters are defined in Table 10-8. The specific time data from a patient should be converted to percentages of the total time of the gait cycle. Normally, when walking at a self-selected usual speed, each foot spends about 60% of the total gait cycle in the support phases (10% breaking double support, 40% single support, then 10% thrusting double support) and 40% in the swing phase. Swing phase time of one leg always coincides with single support time of the opposite leg.

During gait, the feet move or step alternatively in front of each other in the line of progression. The distance between

| TABLE 10-8 | Temporal Variables of Gait |
|---|---|
| Stance time | Time reference foot is on the ground *(seconds from initial contact to toe-off)* |
| Swing time | Time reference foot is off the ground *(seconds from toe-off to next initial contact)* |
| Double limb support time | Time both feet are on the ground that occurs twice during the gait cycle *(seconds from initial contact to contralateral toe-off; and from contralateral initial contact to toe-off)* |
| Single limb support time | Time nonreference foot is swinging forward and reference foot is on the ground *(seconds from contralateral toe-off to contralateral initial contact)* |
| Step time | Time for one foot to step forward *(seconds from initial contact of one foot to initial contact of the opposite foot)* |
| Stride time | Time for one foot to step forward and the other foot to step forward *(seconds from initial contact to initial contact of the same foot [two steps])* |

two specific points of contact of the feet (e.g., the heels) can be measured to provide information on the gait cycle. The measurements of specific distances within the gait cycle, considered **spatial variables,** which include **step length**, **stride length**, **step width,** and foot progression angle, are described in Table 10-9. The specific length data from a patient should be converted to percentages of the total length of the gait cycle (stride length). In a normal straightforward progression walking pattern, the right and left step lengths within a stride are approximately equal; for a normal walking pattern, the length of one stride is equal to the length of two steps. Clinically, this measure is important to identify gait asymmetry (e.g., in hemiplegia) and may be a useful measure to show improvement after intervention. For example, gait asymmetry in patients with stroke is characterized by a shorter step length of the nonparetic lower extremity compared with the paretic lower extremity (Wall, 1986) along with shorter step time of the nonparetic lower extremity. However, despite the presence of asymmetric step lengths, straightforward progression in gait will always be characterized by equal stride lengths on the right and left. Asymmetric stride lengths will result in a deviated or curved forward progression.

The full-body *Rancho Observational Gait Analysis* system (Rancho Los Amigos, 2001) is a comprehensive tool for examining gait. This system is basically a matrix with columns and rows (see Fig. 10-9), and the therapist uses a binary "present"

or "absent" system to document the presence of any gait deviation, the specific phase of gait during which it occurs, and the side of the occurrence. Each column represents different phases of the gait cycle. Each row indicates a different body segment or joint from the trunk to the toes and includes gait components, specifically normal joint kinematics, to be considered during gait analysis. Cells are shaded to indicate whether the specific gait deviation at a certain joint is likely to occur during the gait phase (cell is not shaded) or not (cell is shaded orange). For example, excessive knee flexion may be observed as a major gait deviation (white cell) during loading response or midstance (i.e., early- to mid-stance phase) but is not likely to occur during swing phase (orange cell). Table 10-10 summarizes commonly encountered gait deviations in a population with neurological disorders, organized by body joint.

There are few functional measures that focus only on walking, but many other functional measures incorporate walking, and sometimes stairs, as important components in the functional examination. Some standard measures that incorporate gait as one component include the FIM (Uniform Data System for Medical Rehabilitation) and the STREAM (Daley, 1997; Daley, 1999). These measures are discussed in the section on multidimensional measures. Standardized measures that focus on gait or gait components are the Dynamic Gait Index (DGI), Timed Up and Go test (TUG), the Emory Functional Ambulation Profile (E-FAP), and the 6-minute

| TABLE 10-9 | Spatial Variables of Gait |
|---|---|
| Stride length | Distance for one step and the following step of the opposite foot *(measure from initial contact of the reference foot to initial contact of the same foot)* |
| Step length | Distance that one foot steps forward *(measure from initial contact of the reference foot to initial contact of the opposite foot)* |
| Foot progression angle | Degree of inward or outward angulation of the reference foot *(compare foot angle to an imaginary line in the general forward progression during gait)* |
| Step width | Distance between the two feet—how far apart are the feet? *(measure from the midpoint of one heel to the midpoint of the opposite heel)* |

**Observational Gait Analysis Checklist**

| | Stance | | | | Swing | | |
|---|---|---|---|---|---|---|---|
| | LR | MSt | TSt | PSw | ISw | MSw | TSw |
| **Trunk** | | | | | | | |
| forward lean<br>backward lean<br>lateral lean (R/L) | | | | | | | |
| **Pelvis** | | | | | | | |
| no forward rotation (R/L)<br>no contralateral drop (R/L)<br>hiking (R/L) | | | | | | | |
| **Hip** | | | | | | | |
| inadequate extension<br>circumduction/abduction | | | | | | | |
| **Knee** | | | | | | | |
| excessive flexion<br>uncontrolled extension<br>inadequate flexion | | | | | | | |
| **Ankle/Foot** | | | | | | | |
| foot slap<br>forefoot contact<br>foot flat contact<br>late heel off<br>contralateral vaulting | | | | | | | |

**FIGURE 10-9** Rancho Los Amigos Observational Gait Analysis Checklist.

walk test (6MWT). Also, the Functional Gait Assessment (Wrisley, 2004) is described in Chapter 9.

The *DGI* is a measurement tool that includes a series of eight clinical walking tasks (Shumway-Cook, 1995). These tasks are level surface walking, walking with speed change, walking with horizontal head turns, walking with vertical head turns, walking with pivot turn, stepping over obstacles, stepping around obstacles, and walking up stairs. Each task is rated on a four-point scale with "0" indicating severe impairment, "1" representing moderate impairment, "2" signifying mild impairment, and "3" indicating normal performance (see Table 10-11). Although the four-point scale in this test is based on impairment levels, the criteria for each level for each task has to be set. The DGI is used as a functional outcome measure in people with neurological diagnoses such as chronic stroke, Parkinson disease, and multiple sclerosis (Jonsdottir, 2007; Sheau-Ling, 2011; McConvey, 2005). It shows high reliability (McConvey, 2005) and evidence of concurrent validity with other balance and

| TABLE 10-10 | **Common Gait Deviations in Individuals with Neurological Disorders, by Body Joints** |
|---|---|
| Foot and Ankle | • Toe contact with the floor during a portion of swing or entire swing (toe drag)<br>• Inadequate dorsiflexion in swing<br>• Initial contact with forefoot in early stance<br>• Medial-Lateral instability in midstance |
| Knee | • Inadequate knee flexion in swing<br>• Hyperextension of knee in stance to biomechanically compensate for weakness of the quadriceps or lack of motor control-stability of the knee muscles<br>• Excessive knee flexion during stance |
| Hip | • Hip joint rotated outward (external rotation)<br>• Hip hiking during swing phase to clear the foot<br>• Forward swing in an external arc (circumduction)<br>• Inadequate flexion of hip in early swing<br>• Inadequate extension of hip in stance<br>• Drop of the nonaffected side of the pelvis during affected side stance because of hip abductor (gluteus medius) weakness |
| Pelvis | • Pelvic retraction on the hemiplegic side |
| Trunk | • Forward flexion of trunk to compensate for weak knee extensors during stance<br>• Lateral flexion of trunk to compensate for weak hip abductors during stance |

**TABLE 10-11  Dynamic Gait Index (Shumway-Cook, 1995)**

Have this equipment available:    Box (Shoebox), Cones (2), Stairs, 20' walkway, 15'' wide

**1. Gait level surface _____**

*Instructions:* Walk at your normal speed from here to the next mark (20').

*Grading:* Mark the lowest category that applies.

(3)  Normal: Walks 20', no assistive devices, good speed, no evidence for imbalance, normal gait pattern.

(2)  Mild Impairment: Walks 20', uses assistive devices, slower speed, mild gait deviations.

(1)  Moderate Impairment: Walks 20', slow speed, abnormal gait pattern, evidence for imbalance.

(0)  Severe Impairment: Cannot walk 20' without assistance, severe gait deviations or imbalance.

**2. Change in gait speed _____**

*Instructions:* Begin walking at your normal pace (for 5'), when I tell you "go," walk as fast as you can (for 5'). When I tell you "slow," walk as slowly as you can (for 5').

*Grading:* Mark the lowest category that applies.

(3)  Normal: Able to smoothly change walking speed without loss of balance or gait deviation. Shows a significant difference in walking speeds between normal, fast, and slow speeds.

(2)  Mild Impairment: Is able to change speed but demonstrates mild gait deviations, or not gait deviations but unable to achieve a significant change in velocity, or uses an assistive device.

(1)  Moderate Impairment: Makes only minor adjustments to walking speed, or accomplishes a change in speed with significant gait deviations, or changes speed but has significant gait deviations, or changes speed but loses balance but is able to recover and continue walking.

(0)  Severe Impairment: Cannot change speeds, or loses balance and has to reach for wall or be caught.

**3. Gait with horizontal head turns _____**

*Instructions:* Begin walking at your normal pace. When I tell you to "look right," keep walking straight, but turn your head to the right. Keep looking to the right until I tell you, "look left," then keep walking straight and turn your head to the left. Keep your head to the left until I tell you "look straight," then keep walking straight, but return your head to the center.

*Grading:* Mark the lowest category that applies.

(3)  Normal: Performs head turns smoothly with no change in gait.

(2)  Mild Impairment: Performs head turns smoothly with slight change in gait velocity, i.e., minor disruption to smooth gait path or uses walking aid.

(1)  Moderate Impairment: Performs head turns with moderate change in gait velocity, slows down, staggers but recovers, can continue to walk.

(0)  Severe Impairment: Performs task with severe disruption of gait, i.e., staggers outside 15'' path, loses balance, stops, reaches for wall.

**4. Gait with vertical head turns _____**

*Instructions:* Begin walking at your normal pace. When I tell you to "look up," keep walking straight, but tip your head up. Keep looking up until I tell you, "look down," then keep walking straight and tip your head down. Keep your head down until I tell you "look straight," then keep walking straight, but return your head to the center.

*Grading:* Mark the lowest category that applies.

(3)  Normal: Performs head turns smoothly with no change in gait.

(2)  Mild Impairment: Performs head turns smoothly with slight change in gait velocity, i.e., minor disruption to smooth gait path or uses walking aid.

(1)  Moderate Impairment: Performs head turns with moderate change in gait velocity, slows down, staggers but recovers, can continue to walk.

(0)  Severe Impairment: Performs task with severe disruption of gait, i.e., staggers outside 15'' path, loses balance, stops, reaches for wall.

**5. Gait and pivot turn _____**

*Instructions:* Begin walking at your normal pace. When I tell you, "turn and stop," turn as quickly as you can to face the opposite direction and stop.

*Grading:* Mark the lowest category that applies.

(3)  Normal: Pivot turns safely within 3 seconds and stops quickly with no loss of balance.

(2)  Mild Impairment: Pivot turns safely in >3 seconds and stops with no loss of balance.

(1)  Moderate Impairment: Turns slowly, requires verbal cueing, requires several small steps to catch balance following turn and stop.

(0)  Severe Impairment: Cannot turn safely, requires assistance to turn and stop.

*Continued*

| **TABLE 10-11** | **Dynamic Gait Index (Shumway-Cook, 1995)—cont'd** |
| --- | --- |

**6. Step over obstacle** _____

_Instructions:_ Begin walking at your normal speed. When you come to the shoebox, step over it, not around it, and keep walking.

_Grading:_ Mark the lowest category that applies.

(3) Normal: Is able to step over the box without changing gait speed, no evidence of imbalance.

(2) Mild Impairment: Is able to step over box, but must slow down and adjust steps to clear box safely.

(1) Moderate Impairment: Is able to step over box but must stop, then step over. May require verbal cueing.

(0) Severe Impairment: Cannot perform without assistance.

**7. Step around obstacles** _____

_Instructions:_ Begin walking at normal speed. When you come to the first cone (about 6' away), walk around the right side of it. When you come to the second cone (6' past first cone), walk around it to the left.

_Grading:_ Mark the lowest category that applies.

(3) Normal: Is able to walk around cones safely without changing gait speed; no evidence of imbalance.

(2) Mild Impairment: Is able to step around both cones, but must slow down and adjust steps to clear cones.

(1) Moderate Impairment: Is able to clear cones but must significantly slow, speed to accomplish task, or requires verbal cueing.

(0) Severe Impairment: Unable to clear cones, walks into one or both cones, or requires physical assistance.

**8. Steps** _____

_Instructions:_ Walk up these stairs as you would at home, i.e., using the railing if necessary. At the top, turn around and walk down.

_Grading:_ Mark the lowest category that applies.

(3) Normal: Alternating feet, no rail.

(2) Mild Impairment: Alternating feet, must use rail.

(1) Moderate Impairment: Two feet to a stair, must use rail.

(0) Severe Impairment: Cannot do safely.

TOTAL SCORE: _____ / 24

Adapted from: Shumway-Cook A, Woollacott M. _Motor Control Theory and Applications,_ Baltimore, MD, 1995, Williams and Wilkins, p. 323–324.

mobility scales such as the Berg Balance Scale, the TUG Test, and the timed walk test (Jonsdottir, 2007).

The _TUG_ (Podsiadlo, 1991) includes a number of mobility tasks: coming to standing from a seated position, walking, turning, stopping, and sitting down, which are all important tasks needed for a person to be independent in daily life. For testing, the patient is asked to stand up from a standard armed chair and walk a distance of 3 meters, turn around, walk back to the chair, and sit down again. To start, the person is seated with the back against the chair and arms resting on the armrests. Using a stopwatch, timing begins when the individual starts to rise from the chair and ends when once again seated in the chair. Overall, the TUG has good interrater and intrarater reliability (Podsiadlo, 1991; Shumway-Cook, 2000; Botolfsen, 2008) with excellent intra- and interrater reliability in studies with subjects with stroke (Hafsteinsdottir, 2014). When documenting administration of this measure, note the height of the chair, direction the patient turns, use of an orthosis or assistive device, and any other conditions to enable intra- and interrater reliability (Hafsteinsdottir, 2014). The TUG also demonstrated good content and concurrent validity with scores highly correlated with scores on the Berg Balance Scale, walking speed, and the Barthel Index (Podsiadlo, 1991). The TUG is sensitive and can detect small changes in patients with stroke but may not be able to accurately predict falls in patients with stroke (Hafsteinsdottir, 2014). Wall (2000) has developed an Expanded TUG (ETUG) using a multimemory stopwatch to separately time each component of the TUG

(described in full detail in Chapter 9), which is demonstrated to be reliable and valid (Botolfsen, 2008).

The _E-FAP_ is a timed walking test (Wolf, 1999). The E-FAP (see Table 10-12) requires an individual to accomplish five common environmental tasks with challenges and allows the use of necessary orthotics and assistive devices. Five subtasks include a 5-meter walk (approximately 16 feet) on a hard-surfaced floor, a 5-meter walk (approximately 16 feet) on a carpeted floor, performance of an "up and go" task, negotiation of an obstacle course, and ascent and descent of four stairs. The total score of E-FAP is based on time to finish the task and assistance levels. The total E-FAP score demonstrated high interrater reliability and validity as correlated to the Berg Balance Scale and gait speed on the timed 10-meter walk (Wolf, 1999). A Modified E-FAP (mEFAP) was developed to incorporate the level of manual assistance the person requires for the five tasks and has excellent test-retest reliability, good convergent and predictive validity, and good responsiveness for individuals with stroke (Liaw, 2006).

The _6MWT_ was originally designed for testing exercise tolerance in patients with respiratory disease (Butland, 1982). Chapter 11 provides more information on the use of the 6MWT in cardiovascular examination. The 6MWT measures the total distance an individual can walk in 6 minutes and requires an individual to walk as fast as possible during the timed test. It has been used as a functional mobility test for other populations with high interrater reliability in patients with stroke (Flansbjer, 2005).

| TABLE 10-12 | Emory Functional Ambulation Profile |
|---|---|

### Emory Functional Ambulation Profile (E-FAP) Protocol

The E-FAP is composed of 5 subtasks: (1) Floor, (2) Carpet, (3) Up & Go, (4) Obstacles, and (5) Stairs. Each subject is given a rest period between performance of the subtasks long enough for the researcher to explain and demonstrate the next component. Each subject poststroke is instructed to use an assistive device as needed and to wear a gait belt during performance of all subtasks. The researcher designated as primary researcher demonstrates, provides instructions, and answers the subject's questions. Primary researcher and secondary researcher each record performance times for all 5 subtasks on separate data collection forms. Upon completion of the entire data collection session, each researcher calculates a total E-FAP score.

### Introduction

Primary researcher provides an explanatory overview of the 5 subtasks comprising the E-FAP. Prior to performance of each subtask, primary researcher explains and demonstrates the subtask. Subject is informed that performance of each subtask is timed and is instructed to ask clarification questions at any time.

### Floor

Setup: A 1-m strip of masking tape is placed on the hard-surfaced floor at the starting point. Five meters ahead of the starting point, a 2-cm piece of masking tape marks the endpoint. A small piece of tape is used to mark the endpoint so that subjects do not decelerate in anticipation of the finish line.

1. Primary researcher explains while demonstrating the Floor subtask: "When I say 'go,' walk at your normal, comfortable pace until I say 'stop.'"
2. Primary researcher assists subject as needed in placing toes on starting line tape.
3. Primary researcher says "go," and primary and secondary researchers simultaneously press stopwatches to begin timing.
4. Subject walks toward primary researcher, who is standing 1 m beyond the end point of the 5-m distance. Secondary researcher walks alongside the subject as the subject traverses the 5-m distance.
5. Primary and secondary researchers simultaneously press stopwatches to stop as subject's lead foot crosses the endpoint. Primary researcher tells subject to stop when he or she is beyond the endpoint.
6. Primary and secondary researchers record times on separate data collection forms.

### Carpet

Setup: A piece of short pile carpet, no less than 7 m long and 2 m wide, is taped securely to the floor. Starting point is marked with a 1-m strip of masking tape. Endpoint is marked exactly 5 m from the starting point with a 2-cm piece of masking rape. Both starting point and endpoint are at least 1 m from the edge of the carpet.

1. Primary researcher explains while demonstrating the Carpet subtask: "When I say 'go,' walk at your normal, comfortable pace until I say 'stop.'"

2. Primary researcher assists subject as needed in placing toes on starting line tape.
3. Primary researcher says "go," and primary and secondary researchers simultaneously press stopwatches to begin timing.
4. Subject walks toward primary researcher who is standing 1 m beyond the endpoint of the 5-m distance. Secondary researcher walks alongside the subject as the subject traverses the 5-m distance.
5. Primary and secondary researchers simultaneously press stopwatches to stop timing as subject's lead foot crosses the endpoint. Primary researcher tells the subject to stop when he or she is beyond the endpoint.
6. Primary and secondary researchers record times on separate data collection forms.

### Up & Go

Setup: Standard armchair with a 46-cm seat height is placed on the hard-surfaced floor. Three meters away, a 1-m strip of black tape is placed on the floor.

1. Primary researcher explains while demonstrating the Up & Go subtask: "Next, you will sit in this chair with your back against the back of the chair and your arms resting on the armrests. When I say 'go,' you will stand up from the chair, walk at your normal, comfortable pace past this line where I will be standing, turn around, walk back to the chair, and sit down, making sure your back is against the back of the chair."
2. Subject assumes sitting position in the chair. Primary researcher stands at the 3-cm point marked with masking tape. Secondary researcher stands beside the chair and prepares to walk with the subject.
3. Primary researcher says "go," and primary and secondary researchers simultaneously press stopwatches to begin timing.
4. Primary researcher monitors line to ensure both of subject's feet cross the line before turning around.
5. Primary and secondary researchers stop timing when subject is fully seated with back against the chair.
6. Primary and secondary researchers record times on separate data collection forms.

### Obstacles

Setup: A 1-m piece of masking tape is place on a hard-surfaced floor to mark the starting point. A brick is placed on the floor at the 1½-m mark and the 3-m mark. A 40-gal rubber trash can is placed at the 5-m mark.

1. Primary researcher explains while demonstrating the Obstacles subtask: "When I say 'go,' walk forward at your normal, comfortable pace and step over each brick. Then, walk around the trash can from either the left or right. Then walk back, stepping over the bricks again. Continue walking until I say 'stop.'"
2. Primary researcher assists subject as needed in placing toes on starting line.
3. Primary researcher says "go," and primary and secondary researchers simultaneously press stopwatches to begin timing.

*Continued*

**TABLE 10-12 Emory Functional Ambulation Profile—cont'd**

4. When subject begins walking, primary researcher steps back 1 m beyond the end line while secondary researcher walks with subject.
5. When subject's foot crosses the end line, primary and secondary researchers simultaneously press stopwatches to stop timing. Primary researcher tells the subject to "stop" when he or she is beyond the end line.
6. Primary and secondary researchers record times on separate data collection forms.

**Stairs**
Setup: Stairs with 4 steps, hand railings, and the following measurements are utilized: 26.04-cm stair depth, 75.57-cm stair width, 15.24-cm stair height, 76.20-cm platform depth, and 75.57-cm platform width. A 1-m piece of masking tape is placed 25 cm from the base of the first step.
1. Primary researcher explains while demonstrating the Stairs subtask: "When I say 'go,' walk up the stairs at your normal, comfortable pace to the top of the stairs, turn around, and come back down. You may use the handrails if needed. I will follow behind you for safety."
2. Primary researcher assists subject as needed in placing toes on starting line tape.

3. Primary researcher says "go," and primary and secondary researchers simultaneously press stopwatches to begin timing.
4. Primary researcher follows subject up stairs to guard.
5. Primary and secondary researchers press stopwatches to stop timing when subject's nonlead foot comes in firm contact with the floor.
6. Primary and secondary researchers record times on separate data collection forms.

**Scoring the Emory Functional Ambulation Profile**
1. Researchers multiply time recorded for each subtask by appropriate factor according to level of assistive device used during that subtask.
2. Researchers record the product in the cell corresponding to appropriate subtask and level of assistive device.
3. Researchers repeat this procedure for each column/subtask.
4. Researchers sum the 5 subtask scores to obtain the E-FAP total score.
5. All total scores also are computed without the factor for assistance device for purposes of statistical testing.

**Source:** (Wolf, Catlin, Gage, Grucharri, Robertson, Stephen, 1999)

Overall, these functional tests are useful tools for clinicians to measure an individual's mobility function. In addition to documenting functional mobility, these tests enable clinicians to predict the functional changes of an individual. For example, consider the patient with hemiparesis after a stroke. The initial severity of stroke remains the strongest predictor of stroke recovery as demonstrated in a longitudinal study in which temporal change in the Barthel Index (measurement of disability) was well approximated with stroke recovery by a logistics regression model (Kwakkel, 2003). This model indicated that the earlier a patient shows recovery, the better the outcome at 6 months with the first week of the Barthel Index measurements explaining around 50% of the variance in outcome at 6 months (Kwakkel, 2003). Another study showed that the Fugl-Meyer (measurement of function impairment) at 30 days poststroke predicted 86% of the variance in recovery of motor function at 6 months (Duncan, 1992). Other factors such as lesion location could be good predictors of motor function recovery. Cortical stroke lesions show greater probability to predict function recovery than subcortical lesions (Feys & Hetebrij, 2000). This result suggests that lesion location of stroke might involve different recovery mechanisms. These standard functional measures of DGI, TUG, and E-FAP, however, do not directly predict stroke recovery. Only the TUG shows a high correlation with the Barthel Index (Shumway-Cook, 2000), which means the TUG may have a good indirect prediction of stroke recovery.

*Instrumental Gait Analysis*

IGA is generally used in a research environment or in a facility that has access to a gait laboratory. One method for conducting IGA is to use a three-dimensional optical motion capture system that utilizes reflective markers to triangulate the 3D position of specific surface points of a human subject among multiple cameras. Marker position is used by sophisticated software to generate real-time 3D motion data such as linear and angular displacement, velocity, and acceleration of the whole body or a body part and can generate visual representation animations of the movement. Another method for conducting IGA is to use infrared technology such as the VirtuBalance system by VirtuSense Technologies (www.virtusensetech.com). This portable system uses a projector and camera system to provide a 3D markerless evaluation of gait.

The kinematic information alone does not provide sufficient analysis of abnormal gait because the kinematics such as joint angle and walking trajectory are produced by kinetics (joint moments) and muscle contraction. To address this issue, electromyography (EMG) and force plates are part of IGA to provide muscle activity and kinetic information associated with 3D motion data. This information identifies the group of muscles active at specific times during the gait cycle. Because the kinetic information, including joint moments, cannot be directly measured, a process called inverse dynamics is used to calculate the joint moment. The net joint moments that produce the observed motion are determined from equations of motion identifying the joint of interest. In this approach, the position, velocity, and accelerations derived from observed motions are put into the inverse dynamics equations. In general, the calculation procedure of this method starts from the distal body segment that includes the external force and follows the same process moving sequentially to proximal body segments.

In daily life, functional tasks such as gait involve integration of the nervous and musculoskeletal systems, and require simultaneous multijoint coordination. The CNS manages kinetic factors (muscle forces, joint moments) to produce the desired kinematics (joint angles, body segment positions). Importantly, the net moment of a muscle can accelerate all other joints and segments that it does not span (Zajac, 1989). In a multijoint system, the focus on one joint of interest by using the inverse dynamics approach could provide misleading information. This is because the inverse dynamics approach does not require the system motion equation to be in a coupled linkage. An alternative method to inverse dynamics approach is coupled dynamics.

The net moment is the net effect of the individual moments at a joint from the forces produced by muscles and other structures, including ligaments, crossing that joint. Muscles, the primary movers, are controlled by the CNS to produce the observed motion. A number of studies quantify the muscle activation patterns with the measured kinematic and kinetic data during human movement such as gait. In a coupled dynamics system, all muscles can accelerate joints that they do not span. The control strategies of a muscle during a movement are difficult to determine from only the muscle activity pattern combined with the observed motion. It is important to identify the causal relationship between muscle activity and resulting motion. The dynamic muscle-driven computer simulation based on the coupled dynamics principle proposed by Zajac and Gordon (1989) was developed to estimate the individual muscle force and how these individual muscle forces accelerate the joint. Using this method, uniarticular knee and hip extensors have been identified as muscles that generate most vertical support to the body during the beginning of stance (Neptune, 2004). Hip abductors also make a significant contribution to vertical acceleration during single limb stance (Anderson, 2003). Individual ankle plantar flexor muscles such as gastrocnemius and soleus also contribute vertical support to the body during walking (Neptune, 2001).

## Wheelchair Mobility

Some individuals who are unable to walk require use of a wheelchair for mobility in the context of lower extremity paralysis, severe coordination or motor control deficits, compromised endurance, or insufficient strength or range of motion. A wheelchair can be used for all mobility within the home and community or may be used only for community mobility, depending on a person's physical status. As individuals depend more and more on wheelchair or scooter mobility, they have decreased opportunities to practice ambulation and maintain related muscle groups thus decreasing their overall potential for regaining or maintaining ambulation. Carefully consider the individual patient's prognosis for ambulation to make decisions about wheelchair use. Base appropriate selection of a manual or power wheelchair on the person's capabilities, needs, and environment. Chapter 17 discusses examination and evaluation that leads to selecting the appropriate wheelchair, components, and dimensions. The following section focuses on the therapist's examination of a person's

functional ability in using the wheelchair for mobility and accessibility.

### Essential Components of Wheelchair Mobility

A person who uses a wheelchair must be able to manipulate wheelchair components or parts for independent wheelchair mobility. Observe the patient's ability to operate the wheelchair brakes, armrests, footrests, safety belts, and any accessories on the chair. A person with functional use of the extremities, good trunk control, and adequate balance should not have difficulty manipulating the various wheelchair parts. A person with a neurological deficit resulting in decreased strength, motor control, coordination, balance, disturbances in muscle tone, or cognitive impairment, however, frequently exhibits difficulty operating wheelchair components. A checklist can be used to document the observed abilities, including objective timed measures of specific tasks (see Table 10-13).

## THINK ABOUT IT 10.2

- Think back to Mrs. Park, who has difficulty repositioning herself in the wheelchair, demonstrates poor trunk/head alignment and difficulty moving her left upper and lower extremities. Which activities in Table 10-13 will she likely perform safely, perform with safety issues, or be unable to perform?

There are a variety of methods to propel a wheelchair, and the ability to do so independently is dependent on the person's capabilities and the type of wheelchair prescribed. Manual wheelchair propulsion can be accomplished in a variety of ways including using the bilateral upper extremities, the bilateral lower extremities, or a combination of the upper and lower extremities. A checklist or table can be used (see Table 10-14) to guide the examination of functional wheelchair skills and should include mobility through doorways and thresholds, making turns, and propulsion on outdoor surfaces, rough surfaces, ramps, and curbs. Also measure propulsion speed, an important objective and repeatable measure you can use to document patient progress. Time the patient during propulsion of the wheelchair a predetermined distance and then calculate propulsion velocity (distance/time). Heart rate and rate of perceived exertion (RPE) may also be useful components of measuring wheelchair function.

Power wheelchair mobility provides an alternative method to activate and control the chair for individuals with upper extremity dysfunction or complete paralysis. Methods include a hand-operated joystick or pad, a sip-and-puff mechanism activated by breath control, a head-operated switch using neck movements, or a device controlled with eye movements. Current and developing technology provides ever-expanding methods of power wheelchair operation. Chapter 17 describes options in power wheelchair propulsion. Determine the power wheelchair user's ability to manage the wheelchair in a variety of situations such as those included in Table 10-14.

In addition to examining the method of wheelchair mobility, consider other factors that affect a person's ability

**TABLE 10-13    Operation of Wheelchair Components**

| ACTIVITY | TIME | PERFORMS SAFELY | PERFORMS WITH SAFETY ISSUES | UNABLE TO PERFORM |
|---|---|---|---|---|
| **Balance in sitting** | | | | |
| Forward trunk lean with arm support >3 seconds | | | | |
| Forward trunk lean without arm support >3 seconds | | | | |
| Forward trunk lean to touch floor and regain upright | | | | |
| Left lateral trunk lean to unweight right hip and thigh | | | | |
| Right lateral trunk lean to unweight left hip and thigh | | | | |
| Scooting forward | | | | |
| Scooting backward | | | | |
| **Brakes** | | | | |
| Locks/unlocks right brake | | | | |
| Locks/unlocks left brake | | | | |
| **Armrests** | | | | |
| Removes right armrest | | | | |
| Replaces right armrest | | | | |
| Removes left armrest | | | | |
| Replaces left armrest | | | | |
| **Footrests** | | | | |
| Removes right foot from footpedal | | | | |
| Raises right footpedal | | | | |
| Removes right footrest | | | | |
| Replaces right footrest | | | | |
| Lowers right footpedal | | | | |
| Replaces right foot on footpedal | | | | |
| Removes left foot from footpedal | | | | |
| Raises left footpedal | | | | |
| Removes left footrest | | | | |
| Replaces left footrest | | | | |
| Lowers left footpedal | | | | |
| Replaces left foot on footpedal | | | | |
| **Safety Belts** | | | | |
| Appropriately positions safety belts | | | | |
| Fastens safety belts | | | | |
| Unfastens safety belts | | | | |
| **Accessories** | | | | |
| Specify: | | | | |
| Specify: | | | | |

| TABLE 10-14 | Wheelchair Management Checklist | | | |
|---|---|---|---|---|
| **ACTIVITY** | **PARAMETERS** | **SELECT** | | |
| **Method of propulsion** | | | | |
| Manual | Bilateral upper extremities | ☐ | | |
| | Bilateral lower extremities | ☐ | | |
| | Unilateral upper/lower extremity | ☐ | | |
| | Combination of bilateral upper and lower extremities | ☐ | | |
| Power | Specify: | | | |
| | | **PERFORMS SAFELY** | **PERFORMS WITH SAFETY ISSUES** | **UNABLE TO PERFORM** |
| Smooth level surfaces | Distance: | | | |
| | Time: | | | |
| Indoor unlevel surfaces | Distance: | | | |
| | Time: | | | |
| Outdoor unlevel surfaces | Distance: | | | |
| | Time: | | | |
| Ramp | Incline: | | | |
| | Distance: | | | |
| | Time: | | | |
| | Method to ascend: | | | |
| | Method to descend: | | | |
| Curb | Height: | | | |
| | Method to ascend: | | | |
| | Method to descend: | | | |
| Stairs: 3–5 | Height: | | | |
| | Method to ascend: | | | |
| | Method to descend: | | | |
| Doorways | Method: | | | |
| **Manual Wheelchairs: Advanced Activities** | | | | |
| Wheelies | | | | |
| Falling in WC | | | | |
| Recovering fall | | | | |
| Lateral hopping | | | | |

to operate a manual or power wheelchair. The related examination should minimally include strength, range of motion, muscle tone, endurance, vision, behavior, and cognitive functioning. Examine the person's ability to sit in a stable balanced position with equal weight distribution in the wheelchair, which requires adequate range of motion of the trunk and extremities. Adaptive seating and other accessories may be required to achieve an appropriate sitting position or supported sitting. Adequate strength and range of motion of the upper extremities to push the wheels on a manual wheelchair or to operate hand controls for a power wheelchair are required for propulsion. If the person will use a sip-and-puff mechanism or a head-operated switch, determine cervical strength and range of motion. Also determine the person's endurance level to recommend the most appropriate wheelchair and make recommendations concerning daily activities.

Other factors to consider include the person's vision, cognitive and perceptual status, and behavior. Sufficient vision enables avoidance of obstacles and negotiation of the wheelchair in a variety of environments. An examination of cognitive status includes the person's ability to follow instructions and recall procedures for operating the wheelchair and the wheelchair components safely. Determine whether the patient demonstrates any perceptual deficits including unilateral neglect or figure-ground disturbances. In terms of behavior, observe the person for any safety issues exhibited such as using the wheelchair to intentionally injure self or others, which would contraindicate independent wheelchair mobility. Chapters 4, 6, 9, 11, and 17 include information on examination of these areas.

### Standardized Functional Measures of Wheelchair Mobility

Several multidimensional measures include manual wheelchair propulsion or power wheelchair operation as a component of the assessment tool. A few measures focus only on manual wheelchair propulsion using the upper extremities. The *Wheelchair Skills Test (WST)* is a standardized measure with initial reports of reliability and validity (Kirby, 2002). Performance of wheelchair skills appears to be related to wheelchair experience with no significant difference based on medical diagnosis with a slight influence of age on performance of skills in the WST (Kirby, 2002). A pilot version of the WST included 33 wheelchair management skills ranging from manipulation of wheelchair parts to negotiation of curbs and performance of **wheelies.** The most current version of the test scores manual wheelchair users, power wheelchair users, or caregivers on up to 32 different skills using a pass/fail scale (Fig. 10-10). The WST may be used at any time during the rehabilitation process to document performance of wheelchair skills. The wheelchair management skills are not timed, and wheelchair users are allowed two attempts to complete each activity if needed. The current version of the WST, Version 4.1, including forms and additional information is available at www.wheelchairskillsprogram.ca. To date, there have been no published reports on this version.

Another reliable measure for people using a manual wheelchair is the *Wheelchair Physical Functional Performance test (WC-PFP)* (Cress, 2002). The WC-PFP was modified from the Continuous Scale for Physical Functional Performance (CS-PFP; www.coe.uga.edu/cs-pfp) (Cress, 1996) and is a performance-based measure to examine manual wheelchair use. The WC-PFP was developed using the **Easy Street environment** but has been adapted for administration in public facilities. It consists of 11 tasks classified in four domains of function. The tasks are also categorized based on level of difficulty with five basic tasks, two intermediate tasks, and four difficult tasks (Table 10-15).

Scoring of the WC-PFP is similar to the CS-PFP and includes task scores in each domain, combining four domain scores, and one total score (derived by an average of the domain scores). Each task is scored from 0 (inability to perform the task) to 100 (highest performance). The tasks are standardized by time, distance, or weight to quantify function in daily tasks. The wheelchair user is tested beginning with the most basic task and progresses to the most difficult task (Table 10-15). The WC-PFP includes specific verbal instructions to use during testing as well as specific equipment requirements such as weights, heights, and transfer belts. Additional information is available on the website at www.coe.uga.edu/cs-pfp.

No standardized functional measures that focus only on power wheelchair operation were found in an extensive literature search. The WST (Version 4.1), however, allows the use of a power wheelchair as the means of mobility as does the FIM.

Other measures that incorporate wheelchair mobility are discussed in the multidimensional measures section. These include the COVS (Seaby, 1989) and the FIM (Functional Independence Measure resources page, 2011).

## Upper Extremity Tasks

The ability to perform upper extremity tasks such as dressing, grooming, and feeding is vital to independence in daily activities. While upper extremity control cannot occur without adequate proximal stability of the trunk and scapula, sufficient movement of the hand toward the object and enough hand control to grasp, release, and manipulate are necessary to perform functional activities.

### Essential Components of Upper Extremity Tasks

Upper extremity tasks have been studied extensively due to their importance in daily living. The tasks of reaching and grasping are the most commonly studied areas as these two tasks are incorporated into most upper extremity function. Normal reaching is described in four phases (Shumway-Cook, 2001). The first phase requires visually locating the target, a process referred to as visual regard and one that requires coordination between head and eye movements (Shumway-Cook, 2001). The second phase of reaching involves proximal trunk stability with movement of the arm and hand toward the object (Shumway-Cook, 2001). The arm moves toward the object with high velocity movement. In the third phase, velocity tapers as visual feedback is used to target the object and ensure an accurate contact and grasp (Jeannerod, 1984; Marteniuk, 1987). The maximum velocity achieved during a reaching activity depends on the speed required to complete the task as well as the distance between the object and the individual (Van Vliet, 1995a). As would be expected, higher maximum velocities are achieved when the task requires greater speed of completion and when the object is further away from the individual. In the final phase, the hand manipulates the object and completes the functional task (Shumway-Cook, 2001).

The presence of pathology such as a neurological deficit affects the ability to perform reaching tasks. Individuals with stroke demonstrate greater variability in reaching patterns, shorter reach distances, and slower velocities in comparison to individuals without stroke (Kusoffsky, 2001; Tromby, 1993; Van Vliet, 1995b).

The essential components of any upper extremity task depend on four factors: (1) the goal of the task, (2) characteristics of the object, (3) location of the object, and (4) characteristics of the individual (Durward, 1999; Shumway-Cook, 2001). Goals for upper extremity tasks vary considerably. The goal may be to point to an object, touch an object with one finger

as in pushing an elevator button, grasp and move an object as in brushing teeth, or grasp and throw an object as in playing ball. The goal of the specific task determines the movement components utilized to most efficiently accomplish the goal. For example, individuals select pronation or supination depending on whether they are asked to place a small cylinder on its left or right side (Rosenbaum, 1992). Velocity required to attain the goal also affects the movement patterns selected as described in the following text.

## Wheelchair Skills Test 4.1
### Manual Wheelchair - Wheelchair User

Name: _____

Date: _____  Tester: _____

Time start: _____  Time finish: _____

**Scoring Guide** (see over for details)
✓ = pass, safe
✗ = fail, unsafe
NP = no part (only for indicated skills)
TE = testing error

**Type of Test**
❑ Objective - Capacity
❑ Questionnaire - Capacity
❑ Questionnaire - Performance

| | Individual Skills | Capacity/Performance | Safety | Comments |
|---|---|---|---|---|
| 1. | Rolls forward 10m | | | |
| 2. | Rolls forward 10m in 30s | | | |
| 3. | Rolls backward 5m | | | |
| 4. | Turns 90° while moving forward L&R | | | |
| 5. | Turns 90° while moving backward L&R | | | |
| 6. | Turns 180° in place L&R | | | |
| 7. | Maneuvers sideways L&R | | | |
| 8. | Gets through hinged door in both directions | | | |
| 9. | Reaches 1.5m high object | | | |
| 10. | Picks object from floor | | | |
| 11. | Relieves weight from buttocks | | | |
| 12. | Transfers from WC to bench and back | | | |
| 13. | Folds and unfolds wheelchair | | | |
| 14. | Rolls 100m | | | |
| 15. | Avoids moving obstacles L&R | | | |
| 16. | Ascends 5° incline | | | |
| 17. | Descends 5° incline | | | |
| 18. | Ascends 10° incline | | | |
| 19. | Descends 10° incline | | | |
| 20. | Rolls 2m across 5° side-slope L&R | | | |
| 21. | Rolls 2m on soft surface | | | |
| 22. | Gets over 15cm pot-hole | | | |
| 23. | Gets over 2cm threshold | | | |
| 24. | Ascends 5cm level change | | | |
| 25. | Descends 5cm level change | | | |
| 26. | Ascends 15cm curb | | | |
| 27. | Descends 15cm curb | | | |
| 28. | Performs 30s stationary wheelie | | | |
| 29. | Turns 180° in place in wheelie position L&R | | | |
| 30. | Gets from ground into wheelchair | | | |
| 31. | Ascends stairs | | | |
| 32. | Descends stairs | | | |
| | **Total Percentage Scores** | | | |

Additional comments: _____

**FIGURE 10-10** Wheelchair Skills Test Score Sheet (version 4.1 for manual wheelchair) *(Kirby, Swuste, Dupuis, MacLeod, Monroe, 2002; www.wheelchairskillsprogram.ca)*

*Continued*

• **Note:** The WST 4.1 Manual should be consulted for scoring details (www.wheelchairskillprogram.ca).

**Scale for Scoring Skill Capacity/Performance**

**Pass:** (on the Data Collection Form, record "P" or ✓)
• Task independently and safely accomplished. Unless otherwise specified, the skill may be performed in any manner. The focus is on the task requirements, not the method used. Aids may be used (section 2.23).
• A pass may be awarded if the subject passed a more difficult version of the same skill (e.g., if a subject successfully ascends a 15cm curb, a pass may be awarded on the 5cm level change without the subject needing to actually perform the latter).

**Fail:** (on the Data Collection Form, record "F" or ✗)
• Task incomplete.
• Unsafe performance (as defined in section 2.25).
• Likely to be unsafe in the opinion of the clinician or tester (e.g., on the basis of the subject's description of how a task will be attempted).
• Unwilling to try.
• Has failed an easier version of the same skill (e.g., if the subject cannot roll forward 10m [#5.8], he/she need not be asked to roll 100m [#5.21]).
• If a caregiver is the subject of testing, he/she may not ask the wheelchair occupant for advice or physical assistance in the performance of the skill unless specifically permitted in the caregiver section of the individual skill descriptions (section 5).
• Wheelchair part malfunction.

**Scale for Scoring Skill Safety**

**Safe:** (on the Data Collection Form, record "S" or ✓)
• None of the unsafe criteria were met.
• Although a failing capacity score will be awarded in such circumstances, a safe score can be awarded to a person who states that he/she cannot do and/or will not attempt a skill.

**Unsafe:** (on the Data Collection Form, record "US" or ✗)
• Subject requires appropriate significant spotter intervention to prevent acute injury to the subject or others (section 2.26). Performing a skill quickly is not, in and of itself, unsafe. A significant intervention is one that affects performance of the skill.
• A significant acute injury occurred. This includes sprains, strains, fractures or head injury, but does not include minor blisters, abrasions or superficial lacerations. Poor technique that may or may not lead to overuse injury at a later time should be noted in the comments section, but does not warrant awarding an unsafe score.
• During screening questions (section 3), the subject describes a method of performing a skill that the tester considers dangerous.
• If a caregiver creates more than minimal discomfort or potential harm (e.g., using excessive force with the knee against a flexible backrest of the wheelchair to help push the wheelchair through gravel).
• Specific risks and whether they warrant an unsafe score or merely a recorded comment can be found later in the section on individual skills (section 5).

**Note:** If an easier version of the skill has been failed, the skill under consideration is not objectively tested, so the tester needs to determine whether the attempt would have been safe or unsafe on the basis of interview only.

**For Both Capacity/Performance and Safety**

**No Part:** (on the Data Collection Form, record "NP")
• As for Capacity Scoring (Table 1).
**Testing Error:** (on the Data Collection Form, record "TE")
• As for Capacity Scoring (Table 1).

**Total Capacity/Performance Score** = # passed skills_____/ (32 - #NP - #TE) × 100% = _____%
**Total Safety Score** = # safe skills_____/ (32 - #NP - #TE) × 100% = _____%

**FIGURE 10-10—cont'd**

Characteristics of the object also affect selection of movement strategies for specific upper extremity tasks. Changes in the object such as size, weight, fragility, and shape result in changes in the kinematics of the tasks. In grasping an object, the hand normally opens wider than is necessary to reach around the object (Castiello, 1993) then conforms to the object size as it is grasped. The velocity of reaching for an object, as well as the force in grasping it, is less when the object is fragile, such as a light bulb, compared with something sturdy, such as a tennis ball (Marteniuk, 1987). An individual poststroke may be able to pick up and drink water from a sturdy plastic cup, but when attempting to pick up and drink water from a thin paper cup, the inability to grade the forces appropriately may cause accidental crushing of the paper cup full of water causing spillage.

The location of the object is important because different movement strategies are required to touch or pick up an object close to an individual compared with an object further away. For example, the kinematics employed to pick up and drink from a small cup placed on a table a few inches in front of a person are different from those employed to reach for a large heavy object on a high shelf.

| TABLE 10-15 | Tasks of the Wheelchair Physical Functional Performance Test | | | |
|---|---|---|---|---|
| DOMAINS | UPPER BODY STRENGTH | UPPER BODY FLEXIBILITY | ENDURANCE | BALANCE AND COORDINATION |
| **Basic Tasks** | | | | |
| Lift and transfer pan of weight (0.23 kg) for 2 meters | weight | | | time |
| Transfer and pour from a jug into a cup (1 gallon) | weight | | | time |
| Put on and remove a jacket | | time | | time |
| Put a Velcro-closed strap over a shoe | | | | time |
| Pick up four scarves from floor | | | | time |
| **Intermediate Tasks** | | | | |
| Transfer laundry (7.27 kg) from washer to dryer and from dryer to counter | time | | | |
| Place and remove a sponge from an adjustable shelf | | distance | | |
| **Difficult Tasks** | | | | |
| Carry groceries for 70 meters | weight | | | time |
| Pull open and pass through a door | time | | | time |
| Transfer to a standard chair | time | | | time |
| 6-minute wheel | | | distance | |

0.23 kg = 0.5 pounds
2 meters = 6.5 feet
7.27 kg = 16 pounds
70 meters = 230 feet or 76.5 yards
(Adapted from Cress, Kinne, Patrick, Maher, 2002; www.coe.uga.edu/cs-pfp)

Finally, the essential components of upper extremity tasks are affected by the individual's characteristics including age, experience with the specific task, starting position, and presence or absence of disability. To illustrate, a 2 year-old child, a middle-aged person without disability, and a person with a stroke demonstrate differing approaches and kinematics during reaching tasks (Konczak, 1997; Levin, 1996; Pohl, 1996).

Although the essential components of reaching vary depending on the specific environment, there are some general components to examine. Box 10-1 lists the essential components of reaching for a cup from a sitting position. In addition to the essential components of upper extremity motions described in the table, reaching from a seated or standing position may also require forward trunk flexion, lateral trunk flexion, thoracolumbar rotation, and/or lower body rotation (Cavanaugh, 1999).

## THINK ABOUT IT 10.3

- A person with a spinal cord injury at the C6 level who is unable to reach and grasp with a typical movement strategy (described in Table 10-16) may use a tenodesis grasp in which the person extends the wrist and uses the passive tension of the finger flexors to grasp an object. To observe this, place your elbow on a stable surface with your forearm vertical to the table, palm down, and fingers and thumb totally relaxed. Slowly extend your wrist and observe the action of your fingers and thumb.

### Standardized Functional Measures of Upper Extremity Tasks

The *Action Research Arm Test (ARAT)* (Lyle, 1981) is one of many standardized measures used to examine upper extremity function and control in research and clinical practice. The 19 items are designed to examine changes in upper extremity function after hemiplegia and stroke (Lyle, 1981). The items are categorized in four groups for grasp, grip, pinch, and gross movement (Table 10-16) and are scored on a 0 to 3 scale with "0" indicating no movement and "3" indicating normal movement. The grasp subtest consists of six items including picking up various-sized blocks of wood, a ball, and a stone while the grip subtest includes four items such as pouring water, picking up various-sized tubes, and placing a washer over a bolt. There are six test items in the pinch subtest, all involving picking up various objects with specific fingers and the thumb. The final subtest involves four gross movement activities ranging from hand to mouth to hand to top of head (Table 10-16). The items are tested hierarchically, testing the most difficult item within each subtest first. If the patient successfully performs the most difficult item in a category, success on the remaining items is assumed and the patient scores a "3" for each item

## BOX 10-1  Essential Components of Reaching Anteriorly in Sitting

Starting position: Sitting with hand positioned palm down on the knee

Components:

Shoulder flexion

Shoulder external rotation

Scapular protraction and upward rotation

Elbow flexion progressing to extension

Forearm supination

Wrist extension with ulnar deviation

Thumb carpometacarpal joint (CMC) abduction and opposition

Finger metacarpophalangeal joint (MCP) extension with slight interphalangeal (IP) flexion

Finger rotation toward the thumb to grasp

(Summarized from Carr and Shepherd, 1987)

| TABLE 10-16 | Subtests of the Action Research Arm Test |
|---|---|
| SUBTEST | ACTIVITY |
| Grasp | Picking up blocks of wood ranging from 10-cm cubes to 2.5-cm cubes, a ball, and a stone |
| Grip | Pouring water to various sizes of glasses and tubes; placing a washer over a bolt |
| Pinch | Picking up small round objects of various sizes, beginning with 6 mm and weights such as ball bearings and marbles |
| Gross Movement | Complete movements ranging from hand to mouth to hand to top of head |

(Lyle, 1981; Van der Lee, De Groot, Beckerman, Wagenaar, Lankhorst, Bouter, 2001)

without attempting the item. If the patient does not complete the most difficult item, then the easiest item is tested. Based on the score for the easiest item, the remaining items may or may not be tested. A score of "0" on the hardest item and the easiest item in a category results in scores of "0" for all items in that category based on the assumption that if the patient cannot perform the easiest task, the patient will not be able to perform more difficult tasks. If the patient scores "0" on the hardest item and more than "0" on the easiest task, then all items are tested. At the conclusion of the test, the scores are

summed with a maximum possible score of 57. Normative data is available for time limits on each item (Van der Lee, 2001; Wagenaar, 1990). Equipment required for testing is shown in Box 10-2.

The ARAT provides specific instructions for starting position and timing of each test item. The ARAT is reliable (Lyle, 1981; Hsieh, 1998; Van der Lee, 2001a; Wagenaar, 1990; Lin, 2009), valid (Hsieh, 1998), and sensitive to change in people with acute (De Weerdt, 1985) and chronic stroke (Hsueh, 2002; Van der Lee, 2001a; Van der Lee, 2001b). The ARAT has high concurrent validity as well as satisfactory predictive validity (Lin, 2009).

Multidimensional tools that include hand movement items or upper extremity function tests include the MAS, COVS, STREAM, FIM, and Fugl-Meyer presented in the following section.

## Multidimensional Standardized Functional Measures

Multidimensional standardized functional measures examine a wide range of functional domains using one published tool. Each measure or tool assesses several specific functional skills, and many are appropriate for use in various patient populations.

### Motor Assessment Scale (MAS)

The *MAS* is designed to examine purposeful abilities of patients with stroke and may be used at any point in the recovery process. It consists of one general muscle tone item and eight functional items: three bed mobility items, two hand-movement items, and one item each for sit-to-stand, walking, and lower extremity function (Carr, 1985). The assessment uses a seven-point scale ranging from 0 = unable to perform to 6 = optimal performance, with specific descriptors provided for each activity (see Fig. 10-11). Score the general muscle tone item (Fig. 10-11) with a different scale, using a score of four to indicate normal response and higher scores to indicate presence of hypertonus and lower scores to indicate hypotonus or flaccidity. Scores are based on task completion and time to complete the task with each task performed three times.

## BOX 10-2  Equipment for the Action Research Arm Test

1. blocks of various sizes (2.5 cm, 5 cm, 7.5 cm, and 10 cm)
2. 7.5-cm ball
3. a stone
4. tubes (2.25 cm and 1 cm)
5. washer and bolt
6. two water glasses
7. large and small marbles

*1 cm = approximately 0.5 inch
*2.5 cm = approximately 1 inch
*5 cm = approximately 2 inches
*7.5 cm = approximately 3 inches
*10 cm = approximately 4 inches
(Lyle, 1981)

The best performance of the three trials is recorded. The upper extremity tasks are also organized by increasing difficulty. In addition to specific scoring criteria, the MAS stipulates the equipment used as shown in Box 10-3.

The MAS is appropriate for use at different periods of recovery poststroke, including acute hospitalization and rehabilitation (Poole, 1988). Reliability and validity are demonstrated and details reported in the FOE table at the end of this chapter (Table 10-24). The upper limb function items may be used separately as a single composite score; this practice is shown to be reliable, valid, and responsive (Lannin, 2004). In fact, the upper extremity scores obtained at 1-week and 1-month poststroke are good predictors of upper extremity recovery (Poole, 1988) but do not relate to the functional task of upper body dressing (Williams, 2001). In patients with stroke, the MAS item of moving from

**1. Supine to Side Lying onto Intact Side**
1. Pulls himself into side lying. (Starting position must be supine lying, not knees flexed. Patient pulls himself into side lying with intact arm, moves affected leg with intact leg.)
2. Moves leg across actively and the lower half of the body follows. (Starting position as above. Arm is left behind.)
3. Arm is lifted across body with other arm. Leg is moved actively and body follows in a block. (Starting position as above.)
4. Moves arm across body actively and the rest of body follows in a block. (Starting position as above.)
5. Moves arm and leg and rolls to side but overbalances. (Starting position as above, shoulder protracts and arm flexes forward.)
6. Rolls to side in 3 seconds. (Starting position as above. Must not use hands.)

**2. Supine to Sitting over Side of Bed**
1. Side lying, lifts head sideways but cannot sit up. (Patient assisted to side lying.)
2. Side lying to sitting over side of bed. (Therapist assists patient with movement. Patient controls head position throughout.)
3. Side lying to sitting over side of bed. (Therapist gives stand-by help by assisting legs over side of bed.)
4. Side lying to sitting over side of bed. (With no stand-by help.)
5. Supine to sitting over side of bed. (With no stand-by help.)
6. Supine to sitting over side of bed within 10 seconds. (With no stand-by help.)

**3. Balanced Sitting**
1. Sits only with support. (Therapist should assist patient into sitting.)
2. Sits unsupported for 10 seconds. (Without holding on, knees and feet together, feet can be supported on floor.)
3. Sits unsupported with weight well forward and evenly distributed. (Weight should be well forward at the hips, head and thoracic spine extended, weight evenly distributed on both sides.)
4. Sits unsupported, turns head and trunk to look behind. (Feet supported and together on floor. Do not allow legs to abduct or feet to move. Have hands resting on thighs, do not allow hands to move onto plinth.)
5. Sits unsupported, reaches forward to touch floor, and returns to starting position. (Feet supported on floor. Do not allow patient to hold on. Do not allow legs and feet to move, support affected arm if necessary. Hand must touch floor at least 10 cm [4 in] in front of feet.)
6. Sits on stool unsupported, reaches sideways to touch floor, and returns to starting position. (Feet supported on floor. Do not allow patient to hold on. Do not allow legs and feet to move, support affected arm if necessary. Patient must reach sideways not forward.)

**4. Sitting to Standing**
1. Gets to standing with help from therapist. (Any method.)
2. Gets to standing with stand-by help. (Weight unevenly distributed, uses hands for support.)
3. Gets to standing. (Do not allow uneven weight distribution or help from hands.)
4. Gets to standing and stands for 5 seconds with hips and knees extended. (Do not allow uneven weight distribution.)
5. Sitting to standing to sitting with no stand-by help. (Do not allow uneven weight distribution. Full extension of hips and knees.)
6. Sitting to standing to sitting with no stand-by help three times in 10 seconds. (Do not allow uneven weight distribution.)

**5. Walking**
1. Stands on affected leg and steps forward with other leg. (Weight-bearing hip must be extended. Therapist may give stand-by help.)
2. Walks with stand-by help from one person.
3. Walks 3m (10 ft) alone or uses any aid but no stand-by help.
4. Walks 5m (16 ft) with no aid in 15 seconds.
5. Walks 10m (33 ft) with no aid, turns around, picks up a small sandbag from floor, and walks back in 25 seconds. (May use either hand.)
6. Walks up and down four steps with or without an aid but without holding onto the rail three times in 35 seconds.

**6. Upper-Arm Function**
1. Lying, protract shoulder girdle with arm in elevation. (Therapist places arm in position and supports it with elbow in extension.)
2. Lying, hold extended arm in elevation for 2 seconds. (Physical therapist should place arm in position and patient must maintain position with some external rotation. Elbow must be held within 20 degrees of full extension.)
3. Flexion and extension of elbow to take palm to forehead with arm as in 2. (Therapist may assist supination of forearm.)
4. Sitting, hold extended arm in forward flexion at 90 degrees to body for 2 seconds. (Therapist should place arm in position and patient must maintain position with some external rotation and elbow extension. Do not allow excess shoulder elevation.)
5. Sitting, patient lifts arm to above position, holds it there for 10 seconds, and then lowers it. (Patient must maintain position with some external rotation. Do not allow pronation.)
6. Standing, hand against wall. Maintain arm position while turning body toward wall. (Have arm abducted to 90 degrees with palm flat against the wall.)

**FIGURE 10-11** Motor Assessment Scale *(Carr, Shepherd, Nordholm, Lynne, 1985)*

*Continued*

**7. Hand Movements**

1. Sitting, extension of wrist. (Therapist should have patient sitting at a table with forearm resting on the table. Therapist places cylindrical object in palm of patient's hand. Patient is asked to lift object off the table by extending the wrist. Do not allow elbow flexion.)
2. Sitting, radial deviation of wrist. (Therapist should place forearm in mid pronation-supination, i.e., resting on ulnar side, thumb in line with forearm and wrist in extension, fingers around a cylindrical object. Patient is asked to lift hand off table. Do not allow elbow flexion or pronation.)
3. Sitting, elbow into side, pronation and supination. (Elbow unsupported and at a right angle. Three-quarter range is acceptable.)
4. Reach forward, pick up large ball of 14-cm (5 in) diameter with both hands and put it down. (Ball should be on table so far in front of patient that he has to extend arms fully to reach it. Shoulders must be protracted, elbows extended, wrist neutral or extended. Palms should be kept in contact with the ball.)
5. Pick up a polystyrene cup from table and put it on table across other side of body. (Do not allow alteration in shape of cup.)
6. Continuous opposition of thumb and each finger more than 14 times in 10 seconds. (Each finger in turn taps the thumb, starting with the index finger. Do not allow thumb to slide from one finger to the other, or to go backwards.)

**8. Advanced Hand Activities**

1. Picking up the top of a pen and putting it down again. (Patient stretches arm forward, picks up pen top, releases it on table close to body.)
2. Picking up one jellybean from a cup and placing it in another cup. (Teacup contains eight jellybeans. Both cups must be at arms' length. Left hand takes jellybean from cup on right and releases it in cup on left.)
3. Drawing horizontal lines to stop at a vertical line 10 times in 20 seconds. (At least five lines must touch and stop at the vertical line.)
4. Holding a pencil, making rapid consecutive dots on a sheet of paper. (Patient must do at least 2 dots a second for 5 seconds. Patient picks up a pencil and positions it without assistance. Patient must hold pen as for writing. Patient must make a dot, not a stroke.)
5. Taking a dessert spoon of liquid to the mouth. (Do not allow head to lower towards spoon. Do not allow liquid to spill.)
6. Holding a comb and combing hair at back of head.

**9. General Tonus**

1. Flaccid, limp, no resistance when body parts are handled.
2. Some resistance felt as body parts are moved.
3. Variable, sometimes flaccid, sometimes good tone, sometimes hypertonic.
4. Consistently normal response.
5. Hypertonic 50 percent of the time.
6. Hypertonic at all times.

**FIGURE 10-11—cont'd**

---

**BOX 10-3 Equipment for the Motor Assessment Scale**

1. mat or bed
2. chair
3. table
4. 10 meters of space (approximately 33 feet)
5. four stairs
6. cylinder
7. 14-cm ball (approximately 5.5 inches)
8. Styrofoam cup
9. pen with cap
10. paper
11. eight jelly beans
12. two tea cups
13. a toothbrush
14. a spoon

(Carr, Shepherd, Nordholm, Lynne, 1985)

---

supine to sitting on the side of the bed predicts walking speed upon discharge from rehabilitation (Kuys, 2009).

### Physiotherapy Clinical Outcomes Variable Scale (COVS)

The *Physiotherapy COVS* includes components of the Patient Evaluation Conference System (Harvey, 1981) with additional items recommended by therapists. The purpose of the COVS is to measure the mobility tasks of patients, and it was studied in individuals with the following: spinal cord injury (Seaby, 1989; Campbell, 2003), stroke (Seaby, 1989; Eng, 2002; Hajek, 1997), brain injury (Eng, 2002; Low Choy, 2002), adult neurological conditions (Barkley-Goddard, 2000), amputation (Seaby, 1989), multiple trauma (Seaby, 1989), general geriatric population (Przybylski, 1996; Patrick, 1996), and hip and knee replacements (Seaby, 1989). The COVS may be used for quality management, benchmarking, education, and research purposes (Institute for Rehabilitation and Development; www.irrd.ca/covs).

The most recent version of the COVS consists of 13 tasks (Fig. 10-12) measured on admission and again at discharge using a 0 to 7 scale. A score of "0" indicates that the patient is unable to perform the task or that the task was not assessed. Scores from 1 to 7 range from dependence in performing the task to normal performance with higher scores representing higher levels of function. Figure 10-12 includes specific guidelines for scoring each task. Originally six of the items were scored using a six-point scale. The COVS was modified by adding performance indicators for these tasks so each was scored on a seven-point scale (Low Choy, 2002).

The tasks of the COVS include four ambulation tasks (with and without aids, endurance, and velocity), two rolling tasks (left and right), two transfers (vertical and horizontal), two upper extremity function tasks (left and right), and one task each for supine-to-sit, sitting balance, and wheelchair

**The modified Clinical Outcome Variables Scale (COVS):  Test items and performance indicators.**

**Item 1:** Roll to right from supine lying

**Item 2:** Roll to left from supine lying

1. Dependent – two assistants required
2. One person assistance, plus device (e.g., bed rail)
3. One person assistance, no device*
4. Rolls unaided, requires assistance for comfortable position
5. Independent with device
6. Independent, no device, slow, awkward, requires effort
7. Independent, no effort, coordinated and efficient

**Item 3:** Supine lying to sitting over bed edge

1. Dependent – requires two assistants
2. One person assistance, plus device (e.g., bed rail)
3. One person assistance, no device*
4. Supervision with instructions for safety, may use device
5. Independent with device
6. Independent, no device, slow, awkward, requires effort
7. Independent, no effort, coordinated and efficient

**Item 4:** Sitting balance

1. Unable to sit unsupported
2. Able to sit unsupported (10 seconds)
3. Able to move head/trunk within base of support
4. Able to lift arm/leg within base support*
5. Able to reach outside base of support and return
6. Tolerates external displacement, slow reactions
7. Tolerates external displacement, efficient reactions

**Item 5:** Horizontal transfer

1. Dependent – requires two assistants
2. One person assistance, plus device (e.g., sliding board)
3. One person assistance, no device
4. Supervision/instructions required (may use device)
5. Independent with device (e.g., sliding board)
6. Independent, no device, slow, awkward, requires effort
7. Independent, no effort, coordinated and efficient

**Item 6:** Vertical transfer – stands up from lying on the floor (floor to chair or floor to stand on firm or soft surface)

1. Dependent – requires two assistants or hoist
2. One person assistance, plus device (e.g., chair)
3. One person assistance, no device
4. Supervision/instructions (verbal cues), may use device
5. Independent with/without device (requires effort, slow)
6. Independently stands up on a firm surface, no device (slow, awkward, requires effort)
7. Independently stands up on a soft surface (mat), no effort, coordinated and efficient

**Item 7:** Performance of ambulation

1. No functional ambulation
2. One person continuous assistance
3. One person intermittent assistance
4. Supervision required with verbal cues for safety
5. Independent, level surfaces, assistance with other surfaces and stairs
6. Independent with all surfaces, stairs require rail
7. Efficient ambulation, normal speed, stairs without rail

**Item 8:** Performance of ambulation – use of walking aids

1. Not walking
2. Parallel bars required or two continuous assist
3. Walker or hopper
4. Two aids required (eg crutches, two 4-point sticks)
5. Uses one 4-point stick or crutch
6. Uses a single stick only
7. Walks without an aid

**Item 9:** Performance of ambulation – endurance

1. Not walking
2. Walks < 10m
3. Walks < 50m
4. Walks < 100m
5. Walks < 200m*
6. Walks < 500m
7. Walks > 500m

**Item 10:** Performance of ambulation – velocity

1. Not walking/0m/s
2. Walks < 0.1m/s
3. Walks < 0.3m/s
4. Walks < 0.5m/s*
5. Walks < 0.7m/s
6. Walks < 0.9m/s
7. Walks > 0.9m/s

**Item 11:** Performance of wheelchair mobility

1. Dependent
2. Able to move chair < 10m (requires assistance)
3. Able to move chair < 30m (requires intermittent assistance)
4. Supervision only required on flat surfaces, assistance for barriers such as doors
5. Independent indoors all surfaces, manages doors
6. Independent outdoors, except grass and curbs
7. Independent outdoors, all conditions and surfaces

**Items 12 and 13:** Left and right arm function

1. Unable to actively move arm
2. Able to move arm actively, no useful movement
3. Able to use arm as a stabilizer in weight bearing
4. Able to use arm as a stabilizer in function (eg hold a jar while lid is removed with other hand)
5. Able to bring a cup to mouth
6. Functional fine movement but clumsy/ awkward (eg slides coin to table edge to pick up, then inserts coin)
7. Efficient fine motor skill (e.g., picks up a coin/inserts in money box quickly and accurately)

(The * denotes the addition of a performance indicator. Modified from Seaby and Torrance, 1989.)

**FIGURE 10-12** Modified Clinical Outcomes Variable Scale (COVS)  *(Institute for Rehabilitation and Development, Ottawa, ON, Canada; http://www.irrd.ca/covs)*

mobility. The required equipment, shown in Box 10-4, is readily available in clinical environments. For testing, verbally instruct the patient to perform a specific task, then score the first attempt. The therapist may not demonstrate the task, and the score is based on actual performance rather than what the patient is capable of doing (Seaby, 1989). At the conclusion of the test, sum the scores for all 13 tasks. The total score of the COVS ranges from 13 to 91 with higher scores

indicating better mobility and function. A training program including a videotape and a software program for data analysis are available (Institute for Rehabilitation and Development; www.irrd.ca/covs/).

The measure is reliable, and details are in the chapter FOE table (Table 10-24). The COVS demonstrates predictive capabilities in some patients, predicting mobility status at discharge, and the rehabilitation length of stay in patients with

---

**BOX 10-4 Equipment for the Physiotherapy Clinical Outcomes Variable Scale (COVS)**

1. stopwatch
2. 6-inch step or curb
3. ramp (1:12 ratio rise)
4. mat or bed
5. lightweight plastic mug
6. penny
7. can with a slot through which the penny will fit

Complete COVS Guidelines are available from Institute for Rehabilitation Research and Development, The Ottawa Hospital Rehabilitation Center, Room 1504, Smyth Rd., Ottawa, ON Canada, K1H 8M2. (Institute for Rehabilitation and Development, Ottawa, ON, Canada)

---

stroke (Eng, 2002; Salter, 2010) and brain injury (Eng, 2002). There are indications of sensitivity to change in the geriatric population (Sacks, 2010).

## Mobility Milestones

The "Mobility Milestones" measurement system was developed to provide a clinically relevant standardized outcome measure that could be quickly and easily administered to patients with stroke (Smith, 1999). The measure is based on clinical observations and research relevant to recovery after stroke and proposes a recovery profile based on the classification of stroke (anterior circulation, posterior circulation, lacunar, and intracerebral hemorrhage) (Smith, 1999).

Mobility Milestones includes specific criteria for four basic tasks: 1-minute sitting balance, 10-second standing balance, walking 10 or more steps independently, and walking 10 meters (Table 10-17) (Smith, 1999). The tasks are sequentially administered in a hierarchical order with tasks typically performed earlier in poststroke recovery examined first. Rather than a scoring system, the number of days poststroke required to achieve a specific milestone is recorded with "0" indicating the day of stroke onset. This is then compared with a proposed timescale (Table 10-18) (Smith, 1999). Although additional research is needed, initial findings are promising. The measure is reliable even when used by novice therapists (Baer, 2003). Results of reliability studies are summarized in the FOE table (Table 10-24).

## Mobility Scale for Acute Stroke

The *Mobility Scale for Acute Stroke* was designed to examine mobility in patients within the first 2 weeks poststroke when lower levels of mobility are typical (Simondson, 2003). The

| TABLE 10-17 | Mobility Milestones | | |
|---|---|---|---|
| **TESTING ACTIVITY** | **TESTING TIME/DISTANCE** | **TESTING POSITION** | **REQUIREMENTS** |
| 1-Minute Sitting Balance | Greater than 1 minute | Unsupported sitting on bed or plinth | • Feet supported on floor<br>• Hips, knees, ankles in 90-degree position<br>• Equal weight-bearing on the bilateral ischial tuberosities<br>• Trunk in midline<br>• Head in midline<br>• Hands resting on lap<br>• No associated reactions evident |
| 10-Second Standing Balance | Greater than 10 seconds | Unsupported standing balance<br>• May assist in sit-to-stand transition<br>• No assistance allowed during testing | • Equal weight-bearing on the bilateral lower extremities<br>• Aligned position of trunk and head over lower extremities<br>• No associated reactions evident |
| 10 Steps | Greater than 10 steps (5 steps right, 5 steps left) | Independent ambulation<br>• No assistance allowed during testing<br>• May provide verbal cues for normal gait parameters | • Level surface<br>• May immediately follow 10-second standing test<br>• May continue from assisted ambulation |
| 10-Meter Walk (approximately 33 feet) | • Timed Walk<br>• Measured distance of 10 meters<br>• Linear path | Independent ambulation<br>• Begins in standing position<br>• Assessor accompanies patient, walking on affected side<br>• Verbal cues should be avoided | • Self-selected, comfortable walking speed<br>• Assistive gait device may be used |

(Adapted from Smith and Baer, 1999)

| **TABLE 10-18** | **Proposed Timescales for Achieving Mobility Milestones** | | | |
|---|---|---|---|---|
| | **MOBILITY MILESTONE** | | | |
| *Stroke Classification** | *Sitting Balance* | *Standing Balance* | *10 Steps* | *10 Meters* |
| Partial Anterior Circulation Infarct | 1 day | 1 week | 2 weeks | 3 weeks |
| Lacunar Infarct | 1 day | 5 days | 2 weeks | 3 weeks |
| Posterior circulation infarct | 3 days | 1 week | 2.5 weeks | 3.5 weeks |
| Total anterior circulation infarct | 3 weeks | 8 weeks | 18 weeks | 20 weeks |
| Primary Intracerebral Hemorrhage | 2 weeks | 5 weeks | 10 weeks | 11 weeks |

*Classification of clinically identifiable subtypes of cerebral infarction: Oxfordshire Community Stroke Project (Bamford J, Sandercock P, Dennis M, Burn J, Warlow C. Classification and natural history of clinically identifiable subtypes of cerebral infarction. *Lancet.* 1991;337:1521–1526). (Adapted from Smith and Baer, 1999)

scale examines abilities in six tasks: bridging, supine-to-sit, balanced sitting, sit-to-stand, balanced standing, and 10-meter walk (about 33 feet) (Box 10-5). Rate the patient based on the level of independence and the amount of assistance required using a scoring system ranging from 1 = unable to perform to 6 = safe independent performance. Allow three trials each for bridging, supine-to-sit, and sit-to-stand, then record the best trial. Allow only one trial for the balanced sitting and ambulation items. The Mobility Scale for Acute Stroke is reliable and valid as documented in the FOE table (Table 10-24). The measure has good validity in predicting length of stay poststroke (Brock, 1997).

### Stroke Rehabilitation Assessment of Movement (STREAM)

The purpose of the *STREAM* is to assess motor recovery after stroke through examination of volitional extremity movement and mobility tasks (Daley, 1997; Daley, 1999). There are 30 items with 10 items each for volitional movement of the upper extremities, volitional movement of the lower extremities, and basic mobility (Fig. 10-13). The test was studied with patients with mild, moderate, and severe strokes (Daley, 1997; Ahmed, 2003; Mayo, 2000; Salbach, 2001).

The equipment used in the STREAM is readily available in the clinic environment and includes a mat or bed, a stool, and stairs with handrails. Precise verbal instructions are provided for each activity, and demonstrations are allowed as necessary (Fig. 10-13). In addition, you may repeat instructions if the patient does not initially understand the activity. Ask the patient to perform three trials of each item and document the score of the best performance of each using the ordinal scale. Score the upper and lower extremity items using a three-point scale ranging from 0 = unable to perform, to 2 = completes movement comparable to unaffected side. A score of "1" indicates the patient performs only a portion of the movement, and the rater must include a quality subscale. Score the mobility items using a four-point scale ranging from 0 = unable to perform, to 3 = performs independently without equipment and in a normal manner with a score of "1" indicating some movement quality and a score

### BOX 10-5 Mobility Scale for Acute Stroke

**Activities**
1. Bridging from supine, buttocks clear of bed, return to supine.
2. Sitting from supine, legs over the side of the bed, let the patient choose the side, return to supine.
3. Balanced sitting for 3 minutes maximum base of support defined as thighs in contact with the couch, flexor aspect of knees in contact with the edge of the couch, legs flexed at right angles to thighs, and feet supported on a stool/floor at right angles to the legs. The bed height may be adjusted to achieve the correct position; a footstool may be used when the patient's feet do not reach the floor.
4. Sit to vertical stand from a chair (height 43 cm) with no armrests.
5. Balance standing for 1 minute (performed from the chair), only assess standing, not sit-to-stand.
6. Gait assessed indoors on a level surface along a measured walkway of 10 m with or without a gait aid.

For activities 1, 2, and 4, the patient is asked to perform the activities three times, and the best of three attempts is recorded. For activities 3, 5, and 6, the overall assistance provided for the duration of the activity is recorded.

**Rating Scale**
1. Unable to do the activity, patient makes no contribution to the activity or is unable to complete the activity.
2. Maximum assistance of one or two people, patient makes minimal contribution to the activity.
3. Moderate assistance of one person, hands-on assistance for most of the activity. The patient is able to perform a part of the activity independently.
4. Minimal assistance, hands-on for part of the activity.
5. Supervised (verbal input, no hands on assistance, physiotherapist prepared to give assistance).
6. Unassisted and safe, no verbal input.

(From Simondson, Goldie, Greenwood, 2003)

of "2" indicating the patient was independent but required equipment to perform the activity. After the test is completed, sum the scores for a total maximum raw score of 70. Although the STREAM includes subscores for movement quality, these scores are not included in the total score (Daley, 1999).

The STREAM is a recommended measure of mobility disability in patients with stroke because of its psychometric properties (Hsueh, 2003; Chen, 2007). The STREAM is reliable and valid as detailed in the FOE table (Table 10-24). The STREAM is predictive of discharge destination and gait speed in patients with stroke (Ahmed, 2003). A STREAM score of less than 60 at 1-week poststroke correlates with a discharge environment other than the patient's home (Ahmed, 2003). There is a correlation between the STREAM and gait speed at 3 months poststroke (Ahmed, 2003). The upper extremity subscale of the STREAM has satisfactory predictive validity (Lin, 2009). A potential limitation of the STREAM is the time required to complete it. A Simplified STREAM (or S-STREAM) was developed selecting the five most validated items from each of the following: STREAM Upper Extremity, STREAM Lower Extremity, and STREAM Mobility (Hseuh, 2006). This measure contains 15 items and can be completed in 10 minutes. S-STREAM is efficient and has reliability and validity similar to the STREAM in patients with stroke (Hseuh, 2006).

### Functional Independence Measure (FIM)

The purpose of the FIM, initially developed in the 1980s, is to measure a patient's progress as well as to document severity of disability and ultimate rehabilitation outcomes (Granger, 1986; Granger & Greshman, 1993). The FIM can be used for program evaluation, research, and administrative management. The FIM is one of the most widely used measures and

---

**STroke REhabilitation Assessment of Movement (STREAM)**[a]

Assessment dates (Y/M/D)

1.
2.
3.
4.

Patient's name: _____

Date of CVA: _____  Sex:  M  F  Age: _____

Side of lesion:  L  R  Side of hemiplegia:  L  R

Comorbid conditions: _____

Type of aid(s) used: _____

Physiotherapist(s): _____

General comments: _____

_____

_____

### STREAM Scoring
### I. Voluntary Movement of the Limbs

**0 unable** to perform the test movement through any appreciable range (includes flicker or slight movement)
**1 a.** able to perform only **part** of the movement, and with **marked deviation** from normal pattern
   **b.** able to perform only **part** of the movement, but in a manner that is **comparable to the unaffected side**
   **c.** able to **complete** the movement, but only with **marked deviation** from normal pattern
**2** able to **complete** the movement in a manner that is **comparable to the unaffected side**
**X** activity not tested (specify why; **ROM**, Pain, Other **(reason)**)

### II. Basic Mobility

**0 unable** to perform the test activity through any appreciable range (ie, minimal active participation)
**1 a.** able to perform only **part** of the activity independently (requires partial assistance or stabilization to complete), with or without an aid, and with **marked deviation** from normal pattern
   **b.** able to perform only **part** of the activity independently (requires partial assistance or stabilization to complete), with or without an aid, but with a grossly **normal movement** pattern
   **c.** able to **complete** the activity independently, with or without an aid, but only with **marked deviation** from normal pattern
**2** able to **complete** the activity independently with a grossly **normal** movement pattern, but **requires an aid**
**3** able to **complete** the activity independently with a grossly **normal** movement pattern, **without an aid**
**X** activity not tested (specify why; **ROM**, Pain, Other **(reason)**)

### Amplitude of Active Movement

| Movement Quality | | None | Partial | Complete |
|---|---|---|---|---|
| | Marked Deviation | 0 | 1a | 1c |
| | Grossly Normal | 0 | 1b | 2 (3) |

**FIGURE 10-13** Stroke Rehabilitation Assessment of Movement *(Daley, Mayo, Wood-Dauphinee, 1999)*

**Score**

| 4 | 3 | 2 | 1 | |
|---|---|---|---|---|
| | | | | /2 |
| | | | | /2 |
| | | | | /2 |
| | | | | /3 |
| | | | | /3 |
| | | | | /3 |
| | | | | /2 |
| | | | | /2 |
| | | | | /2 |
| | | | | /2 |
| | | | | /2 |
| | | | | /2 |
| | | | | /2 |
| | | | | /2 |
| | | | | /2 |
| | | | | /2 |
| | | | | /2 |
| | | | | /2 |
| | | | | /2 |
| | | | | /2 |

**Supine**

1. Protracts scapula in supine
   *"Lift your shoulder blade so that your hand moves towards the ceiling"*
   Note: therapist stabilizes arm with shoulder 90° flexed and elbow extended.

2. Extends elbow in supine (starting with elbow fully flexed)
   *"Lift your hand towards the ceiling, straightening your elbow as much as you can"*
   Note: therapist stabilizes arm with shoulder 90° flexed; strong associated shoulder extension and/or abduction=marked deviation (score 1a or 1c).

3. Flexes hip and knee in supine (attains half crook lying)
   *"Bend your hip and knee so that your foot rests flat on the bed"*

4. Rolls onto side (starting from supine)
   *"Roll onto your side"*
   Note: may roll onto either side; pulling with arms to turn over=aid (score 2).

5. Raises hips off bed in crook lying (bridging)
   *"Lift your hips as high as you can"*
   Note: therapist may stabilize foot, but if knee pushes strongly into extension with bridging=marked deviation (score 1a or 1c); if requires aid (external or from therapist) to maintain knees in midline= aid (score 2).

6. Moves from lying supine to sitting (with feet on the floor)
   *"Sit up and place your feet on the floor"*
   Note: may sit up to <u>either</u> side using any functional and safe method; longer than 20 seconds=marked deviation (score la or lc); pulling up using bedrail or edge of plinth=aid (score 2).

**Sitting (feet supported; hands resting on pillow on lap for items 7–14)**

7. Shrugs shoulders (scapular elevation)
   *"Shrug your shoulders as high as you can"*
   Note: both shoulders are shrugged simultaneously.

8. Raises hand to touch top of head
   *"Raise your hand to touch the top of your head"*

9. Places hand on sacrum
   *"Reach behind your back and as far across toward the other side as you can"*

10. Raises arm overhead to fullest elevation
    *"Reach your hand as high as you can towards the ceiling"*

11. Supinates <u>and</u> pronates forearm (elbow flexed at 90°)
    *"Keeping your elbow bent and close to your side, turn your forearm over so that your palm faces up, then turn your forearm over so that your palm faces down"*
    Note: movement in one direction only=partial movement (score 1a or 1b).

12. Closes hand from fully opened position
    *"Make a fist, keeping your thumb on the outside"*
    Note: must extend wrist slightly (i.e., wrist cocked) to obtain full marks; full fist with lack of wrist extension=partial movement (score 1a or 1b ).

13. Opens hand from fully closed position
    *"Now open your hand all the way"*

14. Opposes thumb to index finger (tip to tip)
    *"Make a circle with your thumb and index finger"*

15. Flexes hip in sitting
    *"Lift your knee as high as you can"*

16. Extends knee in sitting
    *"Straighten your knee by lifting your foot up"*

17. Flexes knee in sitting
    *"Slide your foot back under you as far as you can"*
    Note: start with affected foot forward (heel in line with toes of other foot).

18. Dorsiflexes ankle in sitting
    *"Keep your heel on the ground and lift your toes off the floor as far as you can"*
    Note: affected foot is placed slightly forward (heel in line with toes of other foot).

19. Plantar flexes ankle in sitting
    *"Keep your toes on the ground and lift your heel off the floor as far as you can"*

20. Extends knee <u>and</u> dorsiflexes ankle in sitting
    *"Straighten your knee and bring your toes towards you"*
    Note: extension of knee without dorsiflexion of ankle=partial movement (score 1a or 1b).

**FIGURE 10-13—cont'd**

*Continued*

**Score**

| 4 | 3 | 2 | 1 | |
|---|---|---|---|---|
| | | | | /3 |
| | | | | /3 |
| | | | | /2 |
| | | | | /2 |
| | | | | /2 |
| | | | | /3 |
| | | | | /3 |
| | | | | /3 |
| | | | | /3 |
| | | | | /3 |

21. Rises to standing from sitting
   *"Stand up; try to take equal weight on both legs"*
   Note: pushing up with hand(s) to stand=aid (score 2); asymmetry such as trunk lean, Trendelenburg position, hip retraction, or excessive flexion or extension of the affected knee=marked deviation (score 1a or 1c)

**STANDING**

22. Maintains standing for 20 counts
   *"Stand on the spot while I count to twenty"*

**STANDING (holding onto a stable support to assist balance for items 23-25)**

23. Abducts affected hip with knee extended
   *"Keep your knee straight and your hips level, and raise your leg to the side"*

24. Flexes affected knee with hip extended
   *"Keep your hip straight, bend your knee back and bring your heel towards your bottom"*

25. Dorsiflexes affected ankle with knee extended
   *"Keep your heel on the ground and lift your toes off the floor as far as you can"*
   Note: affected foot is placed slightly forward in position of a small step (heel in line with toes of other foot).

**Standing and walking activities**

26. Places affected foot onto first step (<u>or</u> stool 18=cm high)
   *"Lift your foot and place it onto the first step (or stool) in front of you"*
   Note: returning the foot to the ground is not scored; use of handrail=aid (score 2).

27. Takes 3 steps <u>backwards</u> (one and a half gait cycles)
   *"Take three average sized steps backwards, placing one foot behind the other"*

28. Takes 3 steps sideways to <u>affected</u> side
   *"Take three average sized steps sideways towards your weak side"*

29. Walks <u>10 meters</u> indoors (on smooth, obstacle-free surface)
   *"Walk in a straight line over to ... (a specified point 10 meters away) "*
   Note: orthotic=aid (score 2); longer than 20 seconds=marked deviation (score 1c).

30. Walks <u>down</u> 3 stairs <u>alternating</u> feet
   *"Walk down three stairs; place only one foot at a time on each step if you can"*
   Note: handrail=aid (score 2); non-alternating feet=marked deviation (score 1a or 1c).

ᵃThe STREAM scoring form and criteria are presented verbatim. CVA=cerebrovascular accident, ROM=range of motion.

**FIGURE 10-13—cont'd**

is used by more than 1,400 facilities in the United States and worldwide (Functional Independence Measure resources page; www.udsmr.org). Facilities must purchase a licensing agreement to participate in FIM and the national database.

The FIM is designed for interdisciplinary use and members of the health-care team are required to attend an extensive training program before administering the FIM. The training program includes specific instructions for scoring each of the 18 items in six categories. The six categories are self-care, sphincter management, transfers, locomotion, communication, and social cognition with 13 items related to motor function and five items related to cognition (Table 10-19).

The patient's performance is scored using a seven-point ordinal scale. The scale is based primarily on level of assistance required but there are also qualifiers described in the following section. The scale, ranging from 1 = total assistance to 7 = complete independence, is used to score each item on admission, discharge, and follow-up. In addition to the level of assistance scale, some items include qualifiers such as safety in performance, speed of performance, and mobility distance completed. Specifically, the gait item in FIM is not only dependent on the level of assistance but also on walking distance.

For example, 50 feet is the minimum requirement for a score of 1 and 2, while 150 feet is the minimum requirement for score ranges from 3 to 7.

Scoring at admission, discharge, and follow-up must be completed in a designated time frame, and very specific descriptions are provided for each of the 18 items and the scoring system. Score the patient on actual performance rather than the capability to perform a particular task. When all items are completed, sum the scores. The resulting total will lie within a range of 18 to 126 with the higher scores indicating greater independence. It is possible for a patient to achieve a score of 126, however, and still demonstrate significant impairment (Williams, 2001).

In addition to the 18 mobility and social cognition items, the FIM includes demographic information and medical diagnosis as well as length of treatment and hospital charges for each patient. Although the FIM does not incorporate all possible functional activities that a patient should be able to perform, the developers believe it includes the necessary activities for independent functioning and for clinical measurement of function.

Multiple studies demonstrate reliability and validity of the FIM, and details are presented in the chapter FOE table (Table 10-24). The FIM is a good predictor of outcome

**TABLE 10-19   Functional Independence Measure (FIM)**

| | ADMISSION | DISCHARGE | FOLLOW-UP |
|---|---|---|---|
| **Self-Care** | | | |
| A. Eating | | | |
| B. Grooming | | | |
| C. Bathing | | | |
| D. Dressing-Upper Body | | | |
| E. Dressing-Lower Body | | | |
| F. Toileting | | | |
| **Sphincter Control** | | | |
| G. Bladder Management | | | |
| H. Bowel Management | | | |
| **Transfers** | | | |
| I. Bed, Chair, Wheelchair | | | |
| J. Toilet | | | |
| K. Tub, Shower | | | |
| **Locomotion** | | | |
| L. Walk/Wheelchair | | | |
| M. Stairs | | | |
| **Motor Subtotal Score** | | | |
| **Communication** | | | |
| N. Comprehension | | | |
| O. Expression | | | |
| **Social Cognition** | | | |
| P. Social Interaction | | | |
| Q. Problem Solving | | | |
| R. Memory | | | |
| **Cognitive Subtotal Score** | | | |
| **TOTAL FIM Score** | | | |

(Copyright © 1997, Uniform Data System for Medical Rehabilitation, a Division of UB Foundation Activities, Inc. Reprinted with permission.)

disability and discharge destination for patients with stroke (Ocakowski, 1993) and discriminates among patients based on age, comorbidities, and discharge location (FIM, 2005). The more difficult items of the FIM motor scale discriminate among higher functioning patients after stroke (Brock, 2002); however, the FIM is not sensitive enough to detect functional change in some patient populations (Hall, 1992; Hall, 1994), perhaps because of the wide gaps between two adjacent points on the scale for an item. For example, a patient with a brain injury may improve from requiring maximum assistance of two people to requiring maximum assistance of one person to transfer, but the FIM score will not change. And a patient with stroke walking 70 feet with a score of 2 on the "gait" item cannot increase the "gait" score further regardless of any other improvements until the walking distance surpasses 150 feet.

Actual improvement in the patient in independence or distance does not always result in an increase of the total score.

### Fugl-Meyer Assessment

The *Fugl-Meyer Assessment (FM)* was designed to examine motor function of the upper and lower extremities in patients with stroke. The FM includes impairment-based items for balance, sensation, joint motion, and joint pain (Fugl-Meyer, 1975). It was used in studies involving patients with both acute (Wood-Dauphinee, 1990) and chronic stroke (Nadeau, 1999).

The measure is comprised of 155 items in six major categories (Table 10-20). Each item is scored on an ordinal three-point scale of 0 = no function, to 2 = full function, for a total possible score of 226. Maximum possible scores within each category vary (Table 10-21). The upper and lower extremity tasks, which

*(Text continued on page 334)*

**TABLE 10-20    Fugl-Meyer Assessment**

**MOTOR FUNCTION: LOWER EXTREMITY**

| TEST | ITEM | SCORE Pre | SCORE Post | SCORING CRITERIA |
|------|------|-----|------|------------------|
| I. Reflex Activity | Achilles | | | 0-No reflex activity can be elicited<br>2-Reflex activity can be elicited |
| | Patellar | | | |
| II. A. Flexor Synergy (in supine) | Hip flexion | | | 0-Cannot be performed at all<br>1-Partial motion<br>2-Full motion |
| | Knee flexion | | | |
| | Ankle dorsiflexion | | | |
| II. B. Extensor Synergy (in sidelying) | Hip extension | | | 0-Cannot be performed at all<br>1-Partial motion<br>2-Full motion |
| | Adduction | | | |
| | Knee extension | | | |
| | Ankle plantar flexion | | | |
| III. Movement combining synergies (sitting: knees free of chair) | A. Knee flexion beyond 90° | | | 0-No active motion<br>1-From slightly extended position, knee can be flexed, but not beyond 90 degrees<br>2- Knee flexion beyond 90 degrees |
| | B. Ankle dorsiflexion | | | 0-No active flexion<br>1-Incomplete active flexion<br>2-Normal dorsiflexion |
| IV. Movement out of synergy (Standing, hip at 0 degrees) | A. Knee flexion | | | 0-Knee cannot flex without hip flexion<br>1-Knee begins flexion without hip flexion, but does not reach to 90 degrees or hip flexes during motion<br>2-Full motion as described |
| | B. Ankle dorsiflexion | | | 0-No active motion<br>1-Partial motion<br>2-Full motion |
| V. Normal Reflexes (sitting) | Knee flexors, Patellar, Achilles (This item is only tested if the patient achieves a maximum score on all previous UE items. If the person has not achieved a full score to this point, enter 0) | | | 0-At least 2 of the 3 phasic reflexes are markedly hyperactive<br>1-One reflex is markedly hyperactive or at least 2 reflexes are lively<br>2-No more than one reflex is lively and none are hyperactive |
| VI. Coordination/speed Sitting: Heel to opposite knee (5 repetitions in rapid succession) | A. Tremor | | | 0-Marked tremor<br>1-Slight tremor<br>2-No tremor |
| | B. Dysmetria | | | 0-Pronounced or unsystematic dysmetria<br>1-Slight or systematic dysmetria<br>2-No dysmetria |
| | C. Speed | | | 0-Activity is more than 6 seconds longer than unaffected side<br>1-(2–5.9) seconds longer than unaffected side<br>2-Less than 2 seconds difference |
| Lower Extremity Total | | | | Maximum = 34 |

**TABLE 10-20**  **Fugl-Meyer Assessment—cont'd**

**MOTOR FUNCTION: UPPER EXTREMITY**

| TEST | ITEM | Pre | Post | SCORING CRITERIA |
|------|------|-----|------|------------------|
| I. Reflexes | Biceps | | | 0-No reflex activity can be elicited<br>2-Reflex activity can be elicited |
| | Triceps | | | |
| II. Flexor synergy | Elevation | | | 0-Cannot be performed at all<br>1-Performed partly<br>2-Performed faultlessly |
| | Shoulder retraction | | | |
| | Abduction (at least 90°) | | | |
| | External rotation | | | |
| | Elbow flexion | | | |
| | Forearm supination | | | |
| III. Extensor synergy | Shoulder add./int. rot. | | | 0-Cannot be performed at all<br>1-Performed partly<br>2-Performed faultlessly |
| | Elbow extension | | | |
| | Forearm pronation | | | |
| IV. Movement combining synergies | Hand to lumbar spine | | | 0-No specific action performed<br>1-Hand must pass anterior superior iliac spine<br>2-Performed faultlessly |
| | Shoulder flexion to 90 degrees, elbow at 0 degrees | | | 0-Arm is immediately abducted, or elbow flexes at start of motion<br>1-Abduction or elbow flexion occurs in later phase of motion<br>2-Performed faultlessly |
| | Pronation/supination of forearm with elbow at 90 degrees and shoulder at 0 degrees | | | 0-Correct position of shoulder and elbow cannot be attained, and/or pronation or supination cannot be performed at all<br>1-Active pronation or supination can be performed even within a limited range of motion, and at the same time the shoulder and elbow are correctly positioned<br>2-Complete pronation and supination with correct positions at elbow and shoulder |
| V. Movement out of synergy | Shoulder abduction to 90 degrees, elbow at 0 degrees, and forearm pronated | | | 0-Initial elbow flexion occurs or any deviation from pronated forearm occurs<br>1-Motion can be performed partly, or, if during motion, elbow is flexed, or forearm cannot be kept in position<br>2-Performed faultlessly |
| | Shoulder flexion 90–180 degrees, elbow at 0 degrees, and forearm in midposition | | | 0-Initial flexion of elbow or shoulder abduction occurs<br>1-Elbow flexion or shoulder abduction occurs during shoulder flexion<br>2- Performed faultlessly |

*Continued*

| TABLE 10-20 | Fugl-Meyer Assessment—cont'd |
|---|---|

**MOTOR FUNCTION: UPPER EXTREMITY**

| TEST | ITEM | SCORE | | SCORING CRITERIA |
|---|---|---|---|---|
| | | Pre | Post | |
| | Pronation/supination of forearm, elbow at 0 degrees and shoulder between 30–90 degrees of flexion | | | 0-Supination and pronation cannot be performed at all, or elbow and shoulder positions cannot be attained<br>1-Elbow and shoulder properly positioned and pronation and supination performed in a limited range<br>2-Performed faultlessly |
| VI. Normal reflex activity | Biceps and/or finger flexors and triceps (This item is only tested if the patient achieves a maximum score on all previous UE items. If the person has not achieved a full score to this point, enter 0) | | | 0-At least 2 of the 3 phasic reflexes are markedly hyperactive<br>1-One reflex is markedly hyperactive, or at least 2 reflexes are lively<br>2-No more than one reflex is lively and none are hyperactive |
| VII. Wrist | Stability, elbow at 90 degrees, shoulder at 0 degrees | | | 0-Patient cannot dorsiflex wrist to required 15 degrees<br>1-Dorsiflexion is accomplished, but no resistance is taken<br>2-Position can be maintained with some (slight) resistance |
| | Flexion/extension, elbow at 90 degrees, shoulder at 0 degrees | | | 0-Volitional movement does not occur<br>1-Patient cannot actively move the wrist joint throughout the total ROM<br>2-Faultless, smooth movement |
| | Stability, elbow at 0 degrees, shoulder at 30 degrees | | | 0-Patient cannot dorsiflex wrist to required 15 degrees<br>1-Dorsiflexion is accomplished, but no resistance is taken<br>2-Position can be maintained with some (slight) resistance |
| | Flexion/extension, elbow at 0 degrees, shoulder at 30 degrees | | | 0-Volitional movement does not occur<br>1-Patient cannot actively move the wrist joint throughout the total ROM<br>2-Faultless, smooth movement |
| | Circumduction | | | 0-Cannot be performed<br>1-Jerky motion or incomplete circumduction<br>2-Complete motion with smoothness |
| VIII. Hand | Finger mass flexion | | | 0-No flexion occurs<br>1-Some flexion, but not full motion<br>2-Complete active flexion (compared with unaffected hand) |

| TABLE 10-20 | Fugl-Meyer Assessment—cont'd |
|---|---|

**MOTOR FUNCTION: UPPER EXTREMITY**

| TEST | ITEM | SCORE Pre | SCORE Post | SCORING CRITERIA |
|---|---|---|---|---|
| | Finger mass extension | | | 0-No extension occurs<br>1-Patient can release an active mass flexion grasp<br>2-Full active extension |
| | Grasp I - MCP joints extended and proximal and distal IP joints are flexed; grasp is tested against resistance. | | | 0-Required position cannot be acquired<br>1-Grasp is weak<br>2-Grasp can be maintained against relatively great resistance |
| | Grasp II - Patient is instructed to adduct thumb, with a scrap of paper interposed. | | | 0-Function cannot be performed<br>1-Scrap of paper interposed between the thumb and index finger can be kept in place, but not against a slight tug<br>2-Paper is held firmly against a tug |
| | Grasp III - Patient opposes thumb pad against the pad of index finger, with a pencil interposed. | | | 0-Function cannot be performed<br>1-Pencil interposed between the thumb and index finger can be kept in place, but not against a slight tug<br>2-Pencil is held firmly against a tug |
| | Grasp IV - The patient should grasp a can by opposing the volar surfaces of the 1st and 2nd digits. | | | 0-Function cannot be performed<br>1-A can interposed between the thumb and index finger can be kept in place, but not against a slight tug<br>2-Can is held firmly against a tug |
| | Grasp V - The patient grasps a tennis ball with a spherical grip or is instructed to place his/her fingers in a position with abduction position of the thumb and abduction flexion of the 2nd, 3rd, 4th, and 5th fingers. | | | 0-Function cannot be performed<br>1-A tennis ball can be kept in place with a spherical grasp but not against a slight tug<br>2-Tennis ball is held firmly against a tug |
| IX. Coordination/Speed Finger to nose (5 repetitions in rapid succession) | Tremor | | | 0-Marked tremor<br>1-Slight tremor<br>2-No tremor |
| | Dysmetria | | | 0-Pronounced or unsystematic dysmetria<br>1-Slight or systematic dysmetria<br>2- No dysmetria |
| | Speed | | | 0-Activity is more than 6 seconds longer than unaffected hand<br>1-(2–5.9) seconds longer than unaffected side<br>2-Less than 2 seconds difference |
| Upper Extremity Total | | | | Maximum = 66 |
| Total Motor Score (Upper + Lower Extremity) | | | | Maximum = 100 |

*Continued*

| TABLE 10-20 | Fugl-Meyer Assessment—cont'd | | | |
|---|---|---|---|---|

**SENSATION**

| TYPE OF SENSATION | AREA | SCORE | | SCORING CRITERIA |
|---|---|---|---|---|
| | | Pre | Post | |
| I. Light Touch | Upper Arm | | | 0-Anesthesia |
| | Palm of Hand | | | 1-Hyperesthesia / dysesthesia |
| | Thigh | | | 2-Normal |
| | Sole of Foot | | | |
| II. Proprioception | Shoulder | | | 0-No Sensation |
| | Elbow | | | 1–75% of answers are correct, but considerable difference in sensation relative to unaffected side |
| | Wrist | | | |
| | Thumb | | | 2- All answers are correct, little or no difference |
| | Hip | | | |
| | Knee | | | |
| | Ankle | | | |
| | Toe | | | |
| Total Sensation Score | | | | Maximum = 24 |
| Total Motor and Sensory Score | | | | Maximum = 124 |
| Comments | Pre: | | | |
| | Post: | | | |

(From Fugl-Meyer, Jaasko, Leyman, Olsson, Steglind, 1975)

| TABLE 10-21 | Maximum Score per Category for Fugl-Meyer Assessment |
|---|---|

| CATEGORY | MAXIMUM POSSIBLE SCORE |
|---|---|
| Upper extremity | 66 |
| Lower extremity | 34 |
| Sensation | 24 |
| Light touch (8) | |
| Position sense (16) | |
| Passive joint motion | 44 |
| Joint pain | 44 |
| Balance (sitting and standing) | 14 |
| Total | 226 |

(Based on Fugl-Meyer, Jaasko, Leyman, Olsson, Steglind, 1975)

include items on speed, coordination, and reflexes, are scored separately then combined for a total motor function score (Fugl-Meyer, 1975).

To administer the measure, first instruct the patient in the activities using verbal directions. Demonstration with the uninvolved extremity is allowed as necessary. Score the patient on the actual unassisted performance of the task. Assistance is allowed only to stabilize the upper extremity during testing of the wrist and hand. Examine reflexes before and at the conclusion of the motor tasks. The equipment required for the Fugl-Meyer Assessment is readily available in the clinic (Box 10-6). Allowances are made for patients who are confined to the bed. For patients tested in the bed, limit passive shoulder abduction to 90 degrees and hip extension to neutral (Fugl-Meyer, 1975).

The FM demonstrates good interrater reliability (Duncan, 1983) as well as good test-retest reliability (Beckerman, 1996; Hsueh, 2008). The FM lower extremity score at

---

**BOX 10-6 Equipment for the Fugl-Meyer Assessment**

1. sheet of paper
2. small ball (tennis ball)
3. pencil
4. small can

---

(Based on Fugl-Meyer, Jaasko, Leyman, Olsson, Steglind, 1975)

6 weeks poststroke demonstrates predictive validity in FIM mobility locomotion scores, and FM admission score is predictive of rehabilitation length of stay (Feys & Van Hees, 2000). Furthermore, the upper extremity subscale shows satisfactory predictive validity (Lin, 2009).

## Documentation of Functional Status

Examining functional status and movement patterns as described in this chapter is an essential component of the patient examination and may be used during the initial, interim, and discharge examinations. Although the measures presented are valuable in examining and documenting a person's ability to perform specific tasks, do not use these measures in isolation. Rather, the functional measures should be used in conjunction with other tests and measures, particularly objective measures where available, to determine a person's physical status and condition, develop the evaluation, and establish the diagnosis and plan of care.

Medical documentation is one means of communicating a patient's progress or lack of progress to other interested parties, including pay sources. There are numerous methods of documenting results of functional measures. Results may be presented as flow charts (Finch, 2002), as a part of a functional outcome report (Stewart, 1993; Quinn, 2003), a standardized examination form, or a "SOAP" (Subjective, Objective, Assessment, Plan) note. Regardless of the method of documentation, the results of the functional measure and the effect to the patient must be thoroughly understood by therapists, patient, physicians, nurses, and payer sources among others. Interpret the results of the functional tests/measures as part of the evaluation in addition to documenting the objective values in the examination portion of the note. For example, in the examination section, a patient may receive a score of 36 on the Trunk Control Test. In the evaluation, note that this score indicates difficulty with bed mobility activities including rolling and come to sit.

### PATIENT APPLICATION

Mrs. Park is our patient with right MCA stroke introduced earlier in this chapter. Her functional examination confirmed limitations in transfers, sit-to-stand, and ambulation. A summary of her examination, including some objective measures of her functional ability and physical impairments are in the following table. Mrs. Park's goals are to return home with limited assistance from her husband. Mr. Park reports that Mrs. Park needs to be independent in toilet transfers for a home discharge.

## Summary of Selected Examination Findings for Mrs. Park

| | |
|---|---|
| **PROM:** Full PROM throughout BUE/BLE | **Spastic hypertonicity:** left triceps (Modified Ashworth: 1+), gastroc/soleus (Modified Ashworth 1+) |
| **Motor Status:** RUE/RLE: 4/5 strength (MMT) throughout LUE: ¼ active ROM against gravity for all major muscle groups with exception of ⅛ ROM finger flexion and extension LLE: ½ to ¾ active ROM against gravity for all major muscle groups with exception of 0 active ROM for ankle dorsiflexion | **Sensation:** Impaired tactile and proprioceptive sensation throughout LUE/LLE **Perceptual:** Left unilateral inattention Decreased midline orientation |
| **Bed/Mat Mobility:** Max A roll to right I roll to left with decreased dissociation Max A come to sitting from left and right Max A repositioning in bed/mat | **Sit-to-Stand:** Max A with increased weight-bearing RLE Max A to weightshift to LLE with manual stabilization at left hip, knee, ankle Max A to weightshift all directions |
| **Short Sitting with B foot support (static)** Posture: posterior pelvic tilt with increased lumbar lordosis, increased weight-bearing right ischial tuberosity with left lateral trunk flexion, increased thoracic kyphosis, rounded shoulders, forward head with increased cervical spine extension and left lateral flexion; uses RUE to support/maintain position | **Transfers (Bed/Mat <-> Wheelchair):** Mod A SPT to right with increased Weight-bearing RLE Max A SPT to left **Standing and Ambulation:** Max A to maintain aligned standing with right-sided hemiwalker Max A ambulation x 10', level surface |

*Continued*

## Summary of Selected Examination Findings for Mrs. Park—cont'd

Mod A to correct position
Maintains ≤10 seconds with BUE support

**Gait Analysis:**

Left Stance Phase: excess ankle plantarflexion with toe first contact, knee hyperextension at midstance and terminal stance
Left Swing Phase: Excess plantarflexion with toe drag throughout, limited knee and hip flexion, hip external rotation and hip abduction

**Trunk Control Test:**
Rolling to weak side: 12
Rolling to strong side: 0
Sitting up from lying down: 0
Balance in sitting position: 12
Total: 24

**STREAM:** 24/70

## Contemplate Clinical Decisions

1. Given this specific data on this patient, what are the top priority (most important) functional limitations to address in your therapeutic plan of care? Provide justifications for your answers.

2. Which underlying impairments are hypothesized to contribute to the functional limitations that you stated are a priority and need to be addressed in the therapeutic plan of care? Explain your response.

3. Are there additional functional measures that would be appropriate to use with this patient?

4. Considering Mrs. Park's diagnosis, what are factors that may hinder her performance on the functional tests?

5. How will you integrate the examination results into the evaluation component of your documentation?

6. How will the results of the examination be used to select appropriate interventions?

7. Do you anticipate discharge to home based on Mr. and Mrs. Park's goals? Justify your response.

## ■ Organization and Documentation of Home/Work Setting Evaluation

As health-care professionals who focus on performance of functional tasks, physical and occupational therapists conduct home and work setting evaluations for individuals in rehabilitation settings in anticipation of discharge. Both home and work site evaluations may include an interview, patient examination, and an on-site or visual evaluation of the space. The purpose of the interview is to gather information on: (1) the general home or work environment such as type of flooring and presence of stairs, railings, and elevators and (2) home activities, values, and issues that are important to the patient. Obtain information on challenges the patient has experienced in the environment in the past and any problems the patient anticipates. Determine the type of physical and technical support available. Include the patient, family members, and caregivers in the home evaluation interview. Include the patient, the employer, and supervisor in a work site evaluation interview. Additional information may be needed based on information gained from the interviews. Conduct a thorough observational analysis of the physical environment with a focus on accessibility and functional use of the space. A checklist of the most commonly examined areas is shown in Table 10-22. Make recommendations for changes in the work or home environment if minimal changes are needed. If more extensive renovations are required, consultation with a local general contractor is beneficial.

| TABLE 10-22 | General Checklist for Home/Environmental Assessment |
|---|---|
| **GENERAL CHECKLIST FOR ENVIRONMENTAL ASSESSMENT** | |

| | |
|---|---|
| Method of Mobility<br>• Manual wheelchair<br>• Power wheelchair<br>• Ambulatory with assistive device<br>• Ambulatory without assistive device | Furniture arrangement to allow access:<br>• Bedroom<br>• Leisure areas<br>• Work space<br>• Meeting areas |
| Approach to Home/Work Setting<br>• Driveway<br>• Sidewalk<br>• Surface material<br>• Level/Unlevel | Height of:<br>• Bed<br>• Toilet<br>• Tub bench/chair<br>• Favorite chair<br>• Desk |

| TABLE 10-22 | **General Checklist for Home/Environmental Assessment—cont'd** |

**GENERAL CHECKLIST FOR ENVIRONMENTAL ASSESSMENT**

Entrance to Home/Work Setting
- Threshold height
- Steps
- Railing
- Ramp (width, length, rise)
- Number of accessible exits

Kitchen accessibility of:
- Refrigerator/freezer
- Dishwasher
- Stove
- Oven
- Counter
- Microwave
- Sink/faucet
- Countertop appliances

Door widths
- Entrance
- Interior
- Bathroom

Bathroom accessibility of:
- Sink/soap dispensers
- Towels
- Toilet/toilet paper
- Tub/shower
- Stalls
- Mirrors

Flooring
- Type of flooring
- Loose rugs
- Damaged
- Level/unlevel

Laundry accessibility:
- Washer
- Dryer
- Ironing board
- Detergent

Accessibility of:
- Light switches
- Lamps
- Telephone
- Thermostat
- Windows
- Closets/drawers

Elevator accessibility:
- Location
- Call buttons
- Elevator floor flush with corridor flooring
- Timing for opening/closing
- Visible/audible signals

# HANDS-ON PRACTICE

Be sure to practice the following skills from this chapter. With further practice, you should be able to:
- Observe someone move and analyze the movement pattern for the following activities:
  - Rolling (supine to/from prone; supine to/from sidelying)
  - Scooting in bed (toward the head of the bed, toward the foot of the bed, laterally)
  - Come to sitting
  - Transfers
  - Sit to/from stand
  - Stair negotiation
  - Operation of wheelchair components
  - Wheelchair mobility

- Upper extremity tasks (including reaching, grasping, releasing, manipulating)
- Complete OGA for a person with neurological disorders and identify essential components that need to be addressed in therapy
- Measure gait velocity (self-selected, slow, and fast speeds) in a clinical setting by marking a 6- or 10-meter distance and timing the person as they cross the start and end lines, then calculate gait speed in meters per second
- Administer outcome measures for functional examination (e.g., Dynamic Gait Index, Timed Up and Go, etc.)
- Conduct an environmental assessment for the home and work

## Let's Review

1. Define the following terms: functional activities, functional independence, functional examination, functional measure, and functional limitation.

2. Summarize the "General Considerations for Functional Examination" to select and administer appropriate functional measures.

3. What are the basic steps in selecting a functional measure?

4. Identify two commonly used outcome measures to assess a functional activity (e.g., horizontal skills and transfers, gait, stairs, upper extremity function). Would data from these measures be classified as nominal, ordinal, interval, or ratio?

5. For the two measures identified in number 4, describe the pros and cons of using them to examine function in a patient with a neurological diagnosis (e.g., in terms of equipment required, time to administer, if the measure matches the patient's level of function, psychometric properties of the measure).

6. Describe the essential components for scooting in bed, rolling supine to sidelying, come to sitting from supine or sidelying, unsupported sitting, transfers, sit-to-stand, stand-to-sit, stair negotiation, wheelchair mobility, and upper extremity function.

7. What are the critical events of the gait cycle as described by the Rancho Los Amigos scale?

8. Which muscles contribute to vertical support to the body during single limb stance?

9. What factors affect a person's ability to operate a manual or power wheelchair?

10. Describe the four factors that dictate the essential components of an upper extremity task.

---

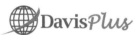 **DavisPlus**    For additional resources, including Focus on Evidence tables, case study discussions, references, and glossary, please visit http://davisplus.fadavis.com

---

# CHAPTER SUMMARY

## PATIENT APPLICATION

*Mr. Taylor is a 59 year-old male with an 8-year history of Parkinson disease. His current Hoehn and Yahr Classification of Disability is level III, indicating impaired righting reactions and difficulty with stability during turning and coming to stand (Hoehn, 1967). Administration of the Clinical Outcomes Variables Scale (COVS) results in a score of 48/91.*

## Contemplate Clinical Decisions

1. *What other physical examinations will you conduct for a thorough examination? Provide justification for your selections.*
2. *What other functional measures are appropriate for this patient in addition to those provided? Explain why you chose each measure.*
3. *What does the score on the COVS indicate? How would you use this information in your documentation?*
4. *Based on the available information, develop appropriate goals for Mr. Taylor.*
5. *What is the value of the functional measures for this patient?*

Examination of functional activity and ability is an essential foundation to determine patient status, develop the therapeutic plan of care, and monitor for significant functional improvement as the therapy is delivered. Without tests and measures of functional activity, the therapist could not develop an effective intervention plan or document improvement in functional skills. This chapter presents only a few of the many functional measures available for clinical use. Remember that Table 10-2 includes some information on other functional measures that are not presented in the chapter but may be beneficial in your clinical practice. Table 10-3 provides reference values for tests of some of the most important areas of the functional examination. Table 10-23 provides a summary of the domains addressed by the functional measures discussed. Table 10-24 provides a summary of the evidence in each category of the functional examination. It, along with, the full FOE table (Table 10-25) is located in the online resources that accompany this book and includes research results on the psychometric properties of each functional measure. FOE tables with evidence regarding outcome measures for specific medical diagnoses can be found in the online resources Table 10-26 (Outcome Measures for CVA), Table 10-27 (Outcome Measures for Multiple Sclerosis-MS),

Table 10-28 (Outcome Measures for Parkinson's Disease-PD), and Table 10-29 (Outcome Measures in Spinal Cord Injury-SCI).

New measures are continually being developed and studied for reliability and validity while more established measures are also being reviewed and studied. As such, the following resources are recommended for finding up-to-date information about outcome measures: (1) the Rehabilitation Measures Database developed by the Rehabilitation Institute of Chicago, Center for Rehabilitation Outcomes Research, and Northwestern University Feinberg School of Medicine Department of Medical Social Sciences Informatics group (www.rehabmeasures.org; accessed December 1, 2015); (2) Neurology Section Outcome Measure Recommendations for patients with stroke, multiple sclerosis, spinal cord injury, traumatic brain injury, Parkinson disease, and vestibular disorders, developed by the Neurology Section of the American Physical Therapy Association (www.neuropt.org/professional-resources/neurology-section-outcome-measures-recommendations; accessed December 1, 2015); and (3) Stroke Engine through the Heart and Stroke Foundation's Canadian Partnership for Stroke Recovery (www.strokengine.ca/find-assessment; accessed December 1, 2015).

Based on the information gathered from the body structure/function and functional activity examinations, the therapist develops a customized patient-centered treatment plan addressing underlying impairments and providing opportunities for meaningful practice with emphasis on motor learning and improving motor control for all of the functional skills that need to improve. General intervention principles and approaches are discussed in Chapters 14 to 17, and specific interventions to address underlying impairments are covered in Chapters 18 to 32. Interventions for specific functional activity limitations will be presented and illustrated in Chapters 33 to 37.

**TABLE 10-23    Summary of Domains Addressed by Functional Measures**

| MEASURE | BED MOBILITY | BALANCED SITTING | TRANSFERS | SIT-TO-STAND | GAIT | STAIRS | WC MOBILITY | UE FUNCTION | OTHER |
|---|---|---|---|---|---|---|---|---|---|
| Trunk Control Test (Collin and Wade, 1990) | X | X | | | | | | | |
| Rancho Los Amigos Observational Gait Analysis (Rancho Los Amigos, 2001) | | | | | X | | | | • Recording of gait deviations by phase |
| Dynamic Gait Index (DGI) (Shumway-Cook and Woollacott, 1995) | | | | | X | X | | | • Gait with horizontal and vertical head movement<br>• Stepping over obstacles<br>• Stepping around obstacles<br>• Change in walking speed |
| Timed Up and Go (TUG) (Shumway-Cook, Brauer, and Woollacott, 2000) | | | | X | X | | | | • Come to standing<br>• Walk 3 meters<br>• Turn<br>• Return to chair<br>• Return to sitting |

*Continued*

| TABLE 10-23 | Summary of Domains Addressed by Functional Measures—cont'd | | | | | | | | |
|---|---|---|---|---|---|---|---|---|---|
| **MEASURE** | **BED MOBILITY** | **BALANCED SITTING** | **TRANSFERS** | **SIT-TO-STAND** | **GAIT** | **STAIRS** | **WC MOBILITY** | **UE FUNCTION** | **OTHER** |
| Emory Functional Ambulation Profile (E-FAP) (Wolf, Catlin, Gage, Gurucharri, Robertson, Stephen, 1999) | | | | | X | X | | | • Allows use of necessary orthotics and assistive devices<br>• Gait on smooth and carpeted floor<br>• Obstacle course |
| Wheelchair Skills Test (Kirby, Swuste, Dupuis, MacLeod, Monroe, 2002) | | | X (into and out of WC) | | | | X | | • Part manipulation<br>• Folding<br>• Reaching<br>• Level surfaces<br>• Unlevel surfaces<br>• Wheelies |
| Wheelchair Physical Functional Performance Test (Cress, Kinne, Patrick, Maher, 2002) | | | X (WC to standard chair) | | | | X | | • Lifting<br>• Reaching up and to floor<br>• Removing Jacket<br>• Closing shoe<br>• Laundry activities<br>• Doorway negotiation<br>• Timed distance |
| Action Research Arm Test (Lyle, 1981) | | | | | | | | X | • Pinch<br>• Grasp<br>• Grip<br>• Gross movement |
| Motor Assessment Scale (Carr, Shepherd, Nordholm, Lynne, 1985) | X | X | | X | X | | | X | • General Tone<br>• Hand movement |
| Clinical Outcomes Variable Scale (Seaby and Torrance, 1989) | X | X | X Horizontal and vertical | X | X | Incorporated in gait | X | X | • Ambulation: endurance<br>• Ambulation: velocity |

| | | | | | | | | | |
|---|---|---|---|---|---|---|---|---|---|
| **TABLE 10-23** | **Summary of Domains Addressed by Functional Measures—cont'd** | | | | | | | | |
| **MEASURE** | **BED MOBILITY** | **BALANCED SITTING** | **TRANSFERS** | **SIT-TO-STAND** | **GAIT** | **STAIRS** | **WC MOBILITY** | **UE FUNCTION** | **OTHER** |
| Mobility Milestones (Smith and Baer, 1999) | | X | | | X | | | | • Standing balance<br>• Timed walk: 10 meters |
| Mobility Scale for Acute Stroke (Simondson, Goldie, Brock, Nosworthy, 1996) | X | X | | X | X | | | | • Bridging |
| STREAM (Daley, Mayo, Wood-Dauphinee, Danys, Cabot, 1997) | X | | | X | X | X | | X | • LE function<br>• Static standing balance<br>• Timed walk |
| Functional Independence Measure (FIM) (Functional Independence Measure: FIM) | In transfer category | | X | In transfer category | X | X | X | Included in other domains | • Self-care<br>• Sphincter Control<br>• Communication<br>• Social Cognition |
| Fugl-Meyer Assessment (Fugl-Meyer, Jaasko, Leyman, Olsson, Steglind, 1975) | | X | | | | | | X | • Passive ROM<br>• Active movement<br>• Pain<br>• Sensation<br>• Reflexes<br>• Speed<br>• Coordination<br>• Standing balance |

## CHAPTER 11

# Examination and Evaluation of Cardiovascular/Pulmonary Systems in Neuromuscular Disorders

Ruth Lyons Hansen, PT, MS, DPT, CCS

## CHAPTER OUTLINE

## CHAPTER OBJECTIVES

Upon completion of this chapter, the learner should be able to:

1. Gather appropriate information through history and chart review.
2. Identify risk for cardiovascular/pulmonary disease and complications in patients with neuromuscular disorders.
3. Select appropriate cardiovascular/pulmonary tests and measures for given patient characteristics.
4. Describe the test procedure for cardiovascular/pulmonary tests and measures described in the chapter.
5. Evaluate cardiovascular/pulmonary examination data to determine prioritized problems to be addressed.

## ■ Introduction

*Mrs. Norma is an 89 year-old grandmother who is 4 weeks status-post stroke. In addition to her poststroke motor and sensory deficits you note throughout her right side, it is obvious she has limited cardiovascular and pulmonary reserves. Your initial observations of the patient include shortness of breath (SOB) that occurs with any activity and feelings of faintness every time she attempts to stand up. This chapter explores some of the tests and measures of cardiovascular/pulmonary function including oxygenation, ventilation, and functional endurance.*

Physical therapists are responsible for screening and examination of four major body systems: musculoskeletal, neuromuscular, integumentary, and cardiovascular/pulmonary (APTA, 2014). The cardiovascular/pulmonary system may be negatively affected in neuromuscular disorders often as a secondary impairment related to decreased activity level. However, rehabilitation therapists often overlook examination of the cardiovascular/pulmonary system (Scherer, 2011; Village, 2011; Frese, 2002). Frese (2002) reported 38% of physical therapists did not measure heart rate (HR) and 43% did not measure blood pressure (BP) in their initial examination of new patients. Scherer (2011) reported that 65.8% of acute care patients who received gait training did not have their vital signs monitored and clients who had abnormal vital signs still received gait training, indicating results may not be used to inform clinical decision making.

Proper operation of the cardiovascular/pulmonary system is crucial to movement and functional activity because of the system's role in **oxygen ($O_2$) delivery,** extraction of $O_2$ from the blood by the body tissues, and utilization (Frownfelter, 2006). If the body is unable to effectively deliver $O_2$ to the working tissues, **aerobic capacity**, the maximum amount of $O_2$ that can be absorbed by the blood (as a measure of fitness), will be impaired. The decreased aerobic capacity will limit the patient's function and restrict progress in the rehabilitation program. Additionally, chronic diseases of the cardiovascular/pulmonary system not only affect the patient's well-being but may result in alteration of the treatment plan by the therapist. Therefore, therapists need to be proficient in selecting and performing the appropriate tests and measures to effectively examine this system. This will facilitate evaluation of how impairments of the system affect mobility, functional capacity, and health and guide development of a customized plan of care that takes into consideration the patient's cardiovascular/pulmonary status.

Cardiovascular/pulmonary system review should include, at a minimum, measuring HR, BP, **respiratory rate (RR)**, and edema. Based on this screening, a more thorough cardiovascular/pulmonary examination may be warranted (APTA, 2014). Areas that may require further examination in a population with neuromuscular disorders are respiratory pattern, breath sounds, cough effectiveness, and exercise capacity.

Patients with a primary neurological diagnosis are at high risk for developing cardiovascular/pulmonary secondary complications, particularly **deconditioning**, impaired cardiovascular endurance that results from periods of inactivity. Additionally, cardiovascular/pulmonary disease may be preexisting and/or contribute to the neurological diagnosis. Patients who have suffered an ischemic stroke have a high incidence of cardiovascular disease with 75% of all stroke survivors having some form of cardiac disease (Roth, 1993). Ischemic strokes can result from atherosclerosis of the carotid arteries, which predisposes the patient to plaques in the coronary arteries and places him/her at risk for myocardial infarction. Stroke and cardiovascular disease, both related to atherosclerosis, share common risk factors listed in Table 11-1 (Yang, 2007; American Heart Association, 2015; American Stroke Association, 2015).

Patients with long-term physical disabilities due to impairments of the neurological system, including **spinal cord injury (SCI)**, traumatic brain injury (TBI), and developmental disabilities, have a higher risk of cardiovascular disease (Yang, 2007). Patients with developmental disabilities have a higher incidence of congenital cardiovascular abnormalities. Although advances in medical science have prolonged life in these individuals, these structural cardiovascular abnormalities often become symptomatic later in life (Barnhart, 2007). Additionally, higher levels of inactivity, deconditioning, and health disparities each increase cardiovascular risk (Brown, 2005; Havercamp, 2004; McGuire, 2007).

Many neurological conditions, including **cerebrovascular accident (CVA)**, TBI, SCI, multiple sclerosis (MS), Parkinson disease (PD), Guillain-Barre syndrome (GBS), and amyotrophic lateral sclerosis (ALS), can directly affect the respiratory control centers in the brainstem and/or control of the muscles of respiration therefore impairing ventilation and gas exchange. **Ventilation** is the process by which gases are moved into and out of the lungs. In **gas exchange**, $O_2$ moves from the capillaries into the alveoli while carbon dioxide ($CO_2$) passes from the alveoli into the venous system. Careful screening and, when necessary, more thorough examination of the cardiovascular/pulmonary system is necessary to identify life-threatening complications as well as to allow the therapist to play a major role in primary disease prevention.

The purpose of this chapter is to briefly review the normal physiology of the cardiovascular/pulmonary system, present risk factors of cardiovascular/pulmonary disease for which the therapist must be alert, and describe procedures for tests and measures used to examine the cardiovascular/pulmonary system in patients with neurological impairments. Normal and abnormal cardiovascular responses to exercise and an evidence-based summary of tests and measures will be discussed.

## THINK ABOUT IT 11.1

Cardiovascular/pulmonary problems may be preexisting (e.g., heart disease causing stroke), secondary to the neuromuscular condition (e.g., deconditioning from inactivity or development of scoliosis), or will develop/worsen as part of a progressive disease process (e.g., ALS). Therapists must consider these possibilities in their assessment, intervention, and prevention planning.

## ■ Categories of Cardiovascular/Pulmonary Function

The cardiovascular/pulmonary system includes all of the operations of the heart and blood vessels, and lungs. These systems work in coordinated fashion with (1) lungs bringing necessary $O_2$ into the body and eliminating the gaseous byproducts of metabolism and (2) heart and vasculature delivering blood with essential $O_2$ and nutrients to all organs and systems in the body to support the operation of all other systems. This chapter will cover several categories of testing related to these systems.

The examination of cardiovascular and pulmonary function in individuals with neuromuscular disorders will focus on the following categories, which are presented in this chapter:

1. Vital signs, including HR, RR, BP, and temperature, may be among the simplest clinical measures to take.
2. Tests of pulmonary physiology and function include pulse oximetry, which provides an approximation of

| TABLE 11-1 | Risk Factors for Heart Disease Versus Risk Factors for Ischemic Stroke |
|---|---|
| **HEART DISEASE** | **ISCHEMIC STROKE** |
| Nonmodifiable risk factors | Nonmodifiable risk factors |
| Age >65 years old | Age >55 years old |
| Heredity (family history) | Heredity (family history) |
| Race/ethnicity–African Americans, Mexican Americans, Native Americans, Native Hawaiians | Race–African Americans |
| Male gender | Male gender |
| Personal history | Personal history of stroke or transient ischemic attack |
|  | Pregnancy and use of oral birth control (females) |
| **Modifiable Risk Factors** | **Modifiable Risk Factors** |
| Hypertension | Hypertension |
| Cigarette smoking | Cigarette smoking |
| Diabetes | Diabetes |
| High blood cholesterol | Carotid artery disease |
| Obesity | Peripheral artery disease |
| Sedentary lifestyle | Atrial fibrillation |
|  | High blood cholesterol |
| **Contributing Factors** | **Contributing Factors** |
| Stress | Cardiac abnormalities (mitral stenosis, valvular disease, structural abnormalities of patent foramen ovale, and atrial septal aneurysm) |
| Alcohol >2/day males; >1/day females | Alcohol >2/day males; >1/day females |
| Elevated inflammatory markers: homocysteine, C-reactive protein | Diet high in saturated fat, transfat, or cholesterol |
|  | Sedentary lifestyle |
|  | Obesity |

arterial blood oxygenation, and measures to assess and document dyspnea and self-perception of exertion.

3. Chest examination and auscultation will include physical examination of chest expansion and movement, and auscultation of both lung and heart sounds.

4. Various exercise testing, or stress testing, will systematically assess the physiological response of the patient to progressively increasing workloads.

## ■ Review of the Physiology and Neuroscience of the Cardiovascular/ Pulmonary System

The human body requires energy to fuel all biological processes including, and perhaps especially, movement. To meet its energy demands, the body transforms energy supplied in food sources such as carbohydrate, fat, and protein into **adenosine triphosphate (ATP)**. ATP is a compound stored as energy in cells of the body, and when the phosphate bonds

of the ATP molecule are broken, 7.3 kcal of energy are released for fuel (Berg, 2007). ATP is produced via two processes: anaerobic metabolism and aerobic metabolism. Short-term energy needs are met via **anaerobic metabolism**, the metabolic process in the body that does not require $O_2$ to generate energy. Although it may be desirable that it does not require oxygen ($O_2$), it can supply only a limited quantity of ATP. Additionally, accumulation of lactic acid, the byproduct of anaerobic metabolism, can cause an imbalance of the body's normal pH. **Metabolic acidosis**, an acidic state in which the blood pH falls below 7.4, will result from accumulated lactic acid, among other causes. For longer duration activities such as walking, running, and most functional activities, a long-term supply of energy is needed. **Aerobic metabolism** requires a continuous supply of $O_2$ but produces a steady supply of ATP to meet sustained energy needs.

Technically, the cardiovascular/pulmonary system is comprised of two systems; the cardiovascular system and the pulmonary system. The two systems work synergistically for the primary purpose of delivering $O_2$ to the tissues, where it is used for energy production. The cardiovascular system consists of the heart and blood vessels that pump and transport blood that carries $O_2$. The pulmonary system consists of the lungs, which take in air containing a relatively high concentration of $O_2$ and expel air with a higher concentration of $CO_2$, a major waste product of cellular respiration. Additionally, the lungs are dependent on optimally functioning muscles of respiration, namely the diaphragm and intercostal muscles. These muscles contract, which causes pressure changes in the lungs, driving air movement in and out of the lungs.

The continuous supply of $O_2$ needed to meet our energy demands is maintained by the cardiovascular/pulmonary system. The complex process of taking in $O_2$ from the ambient air and delivering it to the tissues where it can be used is called **oxygen transport**.

The components of $O_2$ transport include (1) diffusion of $O_2$ across the alveolar-capillary membrane where it binds to hemoglobin in red blood cells (RBC), (2) transport of $O_2$-saturated blood through peripheral circulation via the pumping function of the heart, (3) extraction of $O_2$ from the blood by the tissues ($O_2$ delivery), and (4) diffusion of $CO_2$ from the tissues into the blood. Oxygen-desaturated blood along with $CO_2$ is brought back via the venous system to the right atrium and ventricle to be pumped to the lungs where $CO_2$ is expelled and the process begins again.

## Pulmonary Ventilation

The process of bringing air into and out of the lungs is called **pulmonary ventilation** and includes inhaling and exhaling. Pulmonary ventilation is dependent on optimal functioning of the lungs, chest wall, respiratory muscles, and central respiratory control centers. Inspiration occurs when the diaphragm, the primary muscle of respiration, contracts and descends downward toward the abdomen. This action elongates the thoracic cavity, to create negative pressure within the chest, and elevates the ribs, which causes an increase in thoracic volume. This decrease in intrapulmonary pressure, below that of atmospheric pressure, causes air to passively move into the lungs. During exercise or labored breathing, the scalene and external intercostal muscles act to lift and rotate the ribs to assist in ventilation. Normal quiet expiration occurs passively due to the increase in intrathoracic pressure that occurs when the diaphragm relaxes, thoracic volume decreases, and the lungs recoil. During forced expiration, the respiratory and abdominal muscles contract to force the diaphragm back to its resting position and aid expiration by forcing air out of the lungs. If motor control of these muscles is deficient after stroke or head injury, obvious problems will develop in ventilatory capacity. In addition to their role in forced expiration, both the abdominals and the intercostal muscles play a supportive role in inspiration. The abdominal muscles act to hold the abdominal organs in place, helping to maintain the diaphragm in a normal resting position and stabilizing the central tendon, therefore aiding diaphragmatic excursion. The intercostals play a supportive role in inspiration by stabilizing the rib cage to prevent collapse during the negative pressure generated during inhalation.

### Control of Ventilation

The diaphragm is innervated by the phrenic nerve, which arises from C3-C5 spinal segments. The intercostal nerves at each level, originating from T1-T11, innervate the intercostal muscles. The abdominal muscles are innervated by thoracic spinal nerves of T7-T12. Efferent output from the cerebral cortex to the motor neurons of the respiratory muscles is transmitted via the corticospinal tract and is responsible for voluntary control of breathing. Efferent output for automatic breathing comes from the respiratory control centers of the pons and medulla in the brainstem to the motor neurons of the specified muscles via the efferent white matter pathways of the spinal cord.

Respiratory control centers, made up of distinct groups of neurons located in the pons and medulla, integrate information from central and peripheral chemoreceptors with that of the CNS to regulate breathing. The dorsal respiratory group, located on the dorsum of the medulla, is responsible for inspiration, and the ventral respiratory group plays a role in forced expiration or cough. The pneumotaxic center, located in the pons, helps to regulate the length of inspiration and breathing rate.

Central chemoreceptors are located in the medulla and are bathed by cerebrospinal fluid. These receptors are sensitive to rising levels of $CO_2$ in the cerebrospinal fluid and stimulate increase in rate and depth of breathing causing increased delivery of $O_2$ and increased release of $CO_2$. The peripheral chemoreceptors are located in the aortic and carotid bodies and are sensitive to rising levels of $CO_2$ and low levels of $O_2$ in the arterial blood. In the presence of normal arterial $CO_2$, $O_2$ levels must drop very low, below 50 mm mercury (Hg), before these receptors are stimulated. In the presence of high $CO_2$ levels, they will respond much more quickly to low levels of arterial $O_2$. Under normal conditions, the central chemoreceptors respond more quickly to rising levels of $CO_2$.

### Oxygen Uptake

Upon arrival in the tissues, $O_2$ at the cellular level diffuses across the capillary cell membrane where it is used for aerobic processes to generate ATP for energy. At the same time, $CO_2$ is released by the cell and transported back to the heart via the venous circulation. This process is called **cellular respiration**. The total amount of $O_2$ taken up by the body is referred to as $O_2$ uptake or **oxygen consumption** ($VO_2$). $VO_2$ is the product of cardiac output and the arteriovenous $O_2$ difference and is represented by the equation $VO_2 = Q \times (a-v)O_2$. In this equation, Q refers to cardiac output and is calculated by multiplying **stroke volume** (SV), which is the amount of blood ejected from the heart in one contraction, by the HR. The difference between $O_2$ content of arterial blood and venous blood is represented as $(a-v)O_2$. $VO_2$ is often used to indirectly measure energy expenditure. This is based on the assumption that $O_2$ is required for aerobic work to occur and measuring the volume of $O_2$ consumed is indirectly measuring the amount of energy expended. Resting $VO_2$ is normally 3.5 ml/kg of body weight/minute and is often referred to as one metabolic equivalent (MET). When functional activities or exercise are performed, energy demands increase, more $O_2$ is consumed, and $VO_2$ increases. The MET is often used to estimate the metabolic requirements of different types of physical activity and is an important concept to understand for exercise testing and prescription. The American College of Sports Medicine (ACSM) establishes a single MET as "equivalent to the amount of energy expended during seated rest" (Nagelkirk, 2014, p. 52) and defines "light physical activity as requiring <3 METS, moderate as 3 to ≤6 METS, and vigorous as ≥6 METS" (Thompson, 2014, p. 3). ACSM provides charts with estimates of energy consumption for various activities based on MET units (Pescatello, 2014). For example, jogging at 5 miles per hour represents 8.0 METS.

### Acute Cardiovascular Responses to Activity

The body's need for $O_2$ increases with exercise, especially in the working muscles. To meet this need, there is local vasodilation in the working muscles in an attempt to increase blood flow and $O_2$ to the muscles. To compensate for this local vasodilation, the body responds with increased sympathetic nervous system activity, which causes an increase in HR, an increase in myocardial contractility, and a generalized vasoconstriction. **Myocardial contractility** is the innate capability of the heart tissue to contract. The normal cardiovascular response to exercise, therefore, includes an increase in HR and an increase in systolic BP. Diastolic BP either remains the same or decreases slightly during exercise.

## ▌ Functional Implications of Cardiovascular/Pulmonary Function

Cardiovascular/pulmonary operations are essential to support all functional activities and participation. **Physical deconditioning** is a decline of physical fitness and strength that can result from inactivity. But, as well as resulting from inactivity, deconditioning can also contribute to progressive decrease in activity level with further development of weakness. Deconditioning is very common in physical rehabilitation. Deconditioning has been documented after onset of many neurological disorders including stroke (Ivey, 2005; Ryan, 2000; Michael, 2005; Michael, 2006), SCI (Krassioukov, 2006; Claydon, 2006), and particularly after progressive disorders such as PD (Haas, 2004). A significant component of deconditioning is related to declines in cardiopulmonary status. After a stroke, metabolic fitness levels have been documented at half of that in age-matched sedentary controls (Ivey, 2005). Even in healthy subjects, deconditioning can develop in a relatively short time; for example, after 10 days of bedrest (Convertino, 1982) or even as little as 20 hours of bedrest (Gaffney, 1985).

After neurological disorders, deconditioning is most often a secondary impairment. For example, if a stroke causes motor and sensory impairment with balance dysfunction, the activity level of the individual decreases related to decreased motor control, decreased strength, or fear of falling. Then the inactivity, particularly prolonged bedrest (Krassioukov, 2006; Convertino, 1982), can result in further declines in muscle strength, balance, and cardiovascular fitness, which contribute to deconditioning and reduced ambulation activity (Michael, 2005). Although deconditioning is usually a secondary impairment in neurology, it can occur as a primary impairment in some neurological disorders. For example, orthostatic hypotension can develop after SCI (Claydon, 2006), or ventilatory restrictions can occur after TBI.

Functionally, when cardiovascular/pulmonary deconditioning results from neurological disorders, a decline in physical function and activity will follow because of the decline in cardiovascular/pulmonary effectiveness. As an example, gait velocity after stroke correlates with $VO_2$ max (Ryan, 2000). In addition, limitations to functional activity, particularly related to weakness, decreased motor control, or fatigue (Michael, 2006), will also accentuate functional limitation. As a result of deconditioning, almost every functional skill will decline: ambulation and stair negotiation, rising to stand, transfers and transitions, sitting skills, and even horizontal skills including crawling, creeping, and rolling. Remember that functional declines can contribute to deconditioning, then deconditioning, if not addressed, will contribute to further decline in physical functional activity.

### PATIENT APPLICATION

Mr. Exline is a 68 year-old male who has suffered a left CVA with resultant right-sided hemiplegia with his UE more involved than his LE. He presents with facial droop on the right side and difficulty speaking. PMH: diabetes; Social History: lives with his wife, social drinker, quit smoking 5 years ago but smoked for 40 years.

### Contemplate Clinical Decisions

1. For what cardiovascular/pulmonary problems is Mr. Exline at risk?
2. What should the physical therapist focus on during the initial examination as it relates to the cardiovascular/pulmonary system?

## ▌ Principles of Examination of the Cardiovascular/ Pulmonary System

### Sequencing of Examination Procedures

Before examining a patient, perform a thorough chart review. In outpatient and home care settings, a medical chart is not always available, and this information must be obtained from the patient or caregiver or by phone conversations with the referring practitioner. Upon initial contact with the patient, generally observe the patient's status. Some of this observation can occur simultaneously with the patient interview. Because patients with cardiovascular/pulmonary disorders often fatigue quickly, it is important to sequence your examination in a way that minimizes change of position. Also prioritize the examination procedures should the patient fatigue and not be able to complete the session. Measure resting vital signs, conduct a baseline auscultation of heart and lung sounds, and assess body composition before any physical activity because movement and exercise can affect these results. Leave activities that can cause fatigue such as assessment of function and exercise tolerance until the end of the examination or interspersed with rest to avoid fatigue so the initial session will not have to end prematurely.

## Obtaining History

Knowing the history of the current event as well as past medical history is important for determining whether the cardiovascular/pulmonary system is impaired. In an inpatient setting, the medical record can provide most of this information. The primary diagnosis is the first thing to consider because some neurological diagnoses can cause either primary or secondary impairments to the cardiovascular/pulmonary system. TBI and CVA can cause damage to central nervous system areas of respiratory control, therefore affecting control of breathing and primary impairment of pulmonary function. Diseases such as MS, ALS, GBS, and SCI can cause paralysis or weakness of the respiratory muscles and impair the ability to ventilate. These same disease processes can cause weakness of the muscles that control expiration, cough, and swallowing, making the patient susceptible to secondary pulmonary conditions such as pneumonia or **aspiration pneumonia**, inflammation/infection of the lungs that results from particulate matter from the pharynx entering the airways, complicated by impaired airway clearance.

The medical record can alert the physical therapist to any secondary cardiovascular/pulmonary complications that might be suspected since admission. Both stroke and coronary artery disease (CAD) are related to atherosclerosis of the vascular system and share common risk factors and etiology (American Heart Association, 2015). Therefore, patients who have had a stroke are at risk for also having CAD. Table 11-1 summarizes risk factors of atherosclerosis, which contributes to both stroke and CAD. Reviewing the medical record and asking questions specifically about cardiovascular/pulmonary risk factors such as smoking history or exposure to environmental toxins and symptoms of disease are essential (see Box 11-1 and Table 11-2).

Infants and young children are at greater risk for acute respiratory failure, an impairment of gas exchange within the lungs that can become immediately life-threatening, for several reasons. They have an increased rate of respiratory tract infections because of their exposure to infectious agents (e.g., day care environment) combined with the immature immunological system. Anatomic features of the infant and young child also make them more susceptible. Even a small amount of mucus, bronchospasm, or edema can obstruct the airways because of the relatively small

---

### BOX 11-1 Signs and Symptoms of Pulmonary Disease to Assess in Screening Portion of the Examination/History

Cough
Dyspnea
Abnormal sputum
Chest pain (typically substernal or overinvolved lung)
Cyanosis
Fingernail clubbing
Altered breathing patterns

---

airway diameter. Other structural factors in the infant include decreased number of fatigue-resistant muscle fibers in diaphragm and other ventilatory muscles, greater work of breathing as a proportion of basal metabolic rate, poor cough and ability to cough on command, poor mechanical advantage for intercostal and accessory muscles of respiration because of horizontal alignment of ribs, and increased chest wall compliance (Tecklin, 2015).

## Reviewing Available Laboratory and Medical Tests

Results of certain routine laboratory and diagnostic tests found in the medical record are important when considering possible cardiovascular/pulmonary involvement, particularly arterial blood gases (ABG), hemoglobin, hematocrit, clotting factors, electrocardiogram (ECG), chest x-ray, and pulmonary function tests.

### Arterial Blood Gases

ABG provide information about the respiratory and metabolic status of the individual. The arterial sample is obtained by drawing blood directly from an artery (typically the radial artery) and is usually performed by a respiratory therapist or nurse. The partial pressure of $O_2$ ($Pa_{O_2}$) and $O_2$ saturation ($O_2$ Sat) provide an approximation of the $O_2$ content of arterial blood with information relating to how well the patient is oxygenating. Acid-base balance is determined by the pH of the blood and determines whether a patient is in a state of acidosis or alkalosis. Partial pressure of $CO_2$ ($Pa_{CO_2}$) provides information regarding the respiratory system's contribution to acid base balance, and bicarbonate ($HCO_3$) offers information relating to the kidney or metabolic contribution to acid-base balance. Analyzing the values of pH, $Pa_{CO_2}$, and $HCO_3$ within the context of the clinical presentation can help to determine the primary system contributing to the imbalance and whether the body is compensating. Tables 11-3 and 11-4 provide reference values and interpretation of arterial blood gas results.

### Medical Laboratory Values

Hematocrit represents the volume of RBC as a percentage of total blood volume. Hematocrit is important in the $O_2$-carrying capacity of the blood and the work of the heart.

| TABLE 11-2 | Signs and Symptoms of Cardiovascular Disease to Assess in Screening Portion of the Examination/History | |
|---|---|---|
| **SIGN/SYMPTOM** | **DESCRIPTION/COMMENTS** | **CAUSE/SIGNIFICANCE** |
| Chest pain/angina | • Substernal chest pressure, neck, jaw, or arm pain<br>• Discomfort above waist typically brought on by exercise, activity, or stress and relieved by rest | • Cardiac ischemia<br>• Myocardial infarction (MI)<br>• Pericarditis<br>• Endocarditis<br>• Mitral valve prolapse |
| Palpitations | Described as pounding, thumping, running, bumping, or galloping in chest, fluttering in neck | Arrhythmia/irregular rhythm<br>• Benign causes: caffeine, anxiety, mitral-valve prolapse (MVP)<br>• Lethal causes: ventricular arrhythmias, heart block, ischemia, congestive heart failure (CHF) |
| Dyspnea | • Sensation of breathlessness<br>• If cardiac in origin, felt with minimal exertion or at rest and can be accompanied by other signs of left ventricular failure (LVF): S3 heart sound, crackles that do not clear with cough<br>• Can be angina equivalent, especially in diabetics | • Fever<br>• Pain<br>• Pulmonary causes/hypoxia<br>• Cardiac: CHF/LVF; blood backs up into lung, causes pulmonary congestion, and impairs gas exchange |
| Paroxysmal nocturnal dyspnea | Shortness of breath (SOB) that wakes patient from sleep | CHF |
| Orthopnea | Inability to lie flat without SOB | CHF |
| Syncope | Fainting, loss of consciousness (LOC) | • Arrhythmia<br>• Orthostatic hypotension |
| Cough | If cardiac in origin, often accompanied by crackles that do not clear with cough or pink frothy sputum | • In CHF/LVF, fluid backs up into pulmonary vasculature<br>• Pulmonary causes |
| Edema | Often bilateral; may also have jugular vein distention and weight gain | • CHF<br>• Right ventricular failure (RVF)<br>• Peripheral vascular disease (PVD)–venous stasis |
| Cyanosis | Bluish/gray discoloration of lips and nailbeds due to inadequate $O_2$ level | • Hypoxemia/pulmonary disease<br>• Anemia |
| Claudication | Cramping or pulling sensation in the legs typically brought on by exercise, relieved with rest | PVD is primary cause, but CAD often occurs along with PVD |

| TABLE 11-3 | Reference Values: Arterial Blood Gas | |
|---|---|---|
| **LABEL** | **DEFINITION** | **NORMAL VALUE** |
| $PaO_2$ | Partial pressure of dissolved $O_2$ in blood | >80 mm Hg |
| $PaCO_2$ | Partial pressure of dissolved $CO_2$ in blood | 35 to 45 mm Hg |
| pH | Degree of acidity or alkalinity in blood | 7.35 to 7.45 |
| $HCO_3$ | Level of bicarbonate in blood | 22 to 28 mEq/liter |
| $SaO_2$ | Oxygen saturation: percent of $O_2$ that binds to the hemoglobin molecule in the arterial blood | 96% to 100% |

(Kacmarek, 2012)

| TABLE 11-4 | | Characteristics of Acid-Base Disturbances and Possible Causes | | | | |
|---|---|---|---|---|---|---|
| DISTURBANCE | pH | INITIAL CHEMICAL CHANGE | COMPENSATION | MEASURED $Paco_2$ | MEASURED $HCO_3$ | POSSIBLE CAUSES |
| Respiratory Acidosis | <7.35 | Increase in $Paco_2$ (converted to carbonic acid) | $HCO_3$ increases | >45 (a primary increase) | Normal (or compensatory increase) | COPD, upper or lower airway obstruction, neuromuscular impairment, CNS depression, hypoventilation, sleep disordered breathing, cardiac arrest, respiratory failure |
| Respiratory Alkalosis | >7.45 | Decrease in $Paco_2$ (with less carbonic acid) | $HCO_3$ decreases | <35 (a primary decrease) | Normal (or compensatory increase) | Hyperventilation, fever, pain, hypoxia, CVA, brain trauma/tumor, cerebral edema, pulmonary embolism, pneumonia, pneumothorax, pleural effusion, pregnancy, brain injury, CHF, asthma, severe anemia, hyperthyroidism |
| Metabolic acidosis | <7.35 | Decrease in $HCO_3$ | $Paco_2$ decreases | Normal (or compensatory decrease) | <22 (a primary decrease) | Diabetic ketoacidosis, lactic acidosis, poisoning (methanol, ethanol, salicylate), renal failure, diarrhea |
| Metabolic alkalosis | >7.45 | Increase in $HCO_3$ | $Paco_2$ increases | Normal (or compensatory increase) | >26 (a primary increase) | Vomiting, diarrhea, diuretic therapy, corticosteroids, Cushing disease, hypokalemia |

Modified from two sources: Kaufman DA, Interpretation of Arterial Blood Gases (ABGs), American Thoracic Society. Available at www.thoracic.org/professionals/clinical-resources/critical-care/clinical-education/abgs.php. Accessed January 2, 2016; and Carter R, Tiep B, Boatwright D. Oxygen delivery and acid-base balance. *RT for Decision Makers in Respiratory Care.* Available at www.rtmagazine.com/2010/08/oxygen-delivery-and-acid-base-balance/. Published August 6, 2010; Accessed January 2, 2016.

If the RBC count is too high, blood can become thick and viscous causing increased work demand on the heart to pump the blood and increasing myocardial $O_2$ demand. If the RBC count or hemoglobin is too low, the $O_2$-carrying capacity of the blood will be impaired and the patient may experience SOB or exhibit signs of **hypoxemia**, a low level of $O_2$ in the blood. An elevated white blood cell (WBC) count may indicate infection.

### Pulmonary Function Testing

Pulmonary function testing (PFT) is typically performed by a respiratory therapist and not a physical therapist, but a physical therapist should be able to understand and apply the results to the physical therapy plan of care. PFT results are

typically available in the medical record. PFT involves the measurement of lung volumes and capacities as well as flow rates and spirometric patterns and usually generates a graph of respiratory movements. Four lung volumes and four lung capacities are typically measured (Table 11-5). In addition to these, a flow volume loop is typically displayed as a graphical representation of gas flow over volume. In obstructive lung disease, lung inspiratory reserve volume (IRV) and functional residual capacity (FRC) are increased and flow rates are decreased (Kacmarek, 2012). In restrictive lung disease, all volumes and capacities are decreased while flow rates are usually normal (Kacmarek, 2012). Most patients with neurological impairments who do not have underlying lung disease will have restrictive impairment due to respiratory and chest wall

| TABLE 11-5 | Pulmonary Function Tests | | |
|---|---|---|---|
| **TEST** | **DESCRIPTION** | **NORMAL VALUES** | **SIGNIFICANCE OF ABNORMALITY** |
| Tidal Volume (TV) | Volume of air inspired and expired/minute | 500% smL | Can be normal or increased in obstructive disease and decreased in restrictive disease |
| Inspiratory Reserve Volume (IRV) | Volume of air that can be inspired after a normal inspiration | 3.10 L | |
| Expiratory Reserve Volume (ERV) | Amount of air that can be expired after a normal expiration | 1.20 L | • Necessary to calculate RV and FRC<br>• Normal or decreased in obstructive and normal in restrictive |
| Residual Volume (RV) | Volume of air remaining in the lungs after a maximal exhalation | 1.20 L | • Used to differentiate between obstructive and restrictive disease<br>• Increased in obstructive disease |
| Vital Capacity | Maximal amount of air that can be expired after a maximal inspiration | 4.8 L | Can be decreased in diseases that decrease distensibility of the lung and depress the respiratory centers |
| Functional Residual Capacity | Amount of air remaining in the lungs at the end of expiration | 2.40 L | Increased in obstructive disease and decreased in restrictive disease |
| Inspiratory Capacity | Maximum amount of air that can be inspired after a normal exhalation | 3.6 L | Decreased in restrictive disease (conditions affecting lung tissue as well as neuromuscular conditions that affect respiratory muscles) |
| Total Lung Capacity | Volume of air in the lung after a maximal inspiration | 6.00 L | |

Douce FH. Pulmonary function testing. In: Kackmarek RM, Stoller JK, Heuer AJ, eds. *Egan's Fundamentals of Respiratory Care,* 10th edition. Elsevier; 2013: 417–450.

muscle weakness. In addition to typical PFT, sometimes maximal inspiratory pressure (MIP) and maximal expiratory pressure (MEP) are measured, typically with a handheld bugle dynamometer. This device measures pressure generated at the mouth by the respiratory muscles and is an indirect measure of respiratory muscle strength. See Table 11-5 for a description of pulmonary function tests, normal values, and the significance of abnormal values.

# Tests and Measures of Cardiovascular/Pulmonary Systems

## General Observation/Inspection

When you first see the patient, you should observe for any medical devices used by, or attached to, the patient. These may include intravenous (IV) lines, central and arterial lines, and $O_2$ and ventilator tubes. It is important to be aware of line location to avoid accidentally dislodging the lines or injuring the patient during movement. Observe the patient for body type and posture (which influence breathing), positioning, breathing pattern, or any signs of distress. A person's body type provides an indication of his/her general health. Individuals who are overweight or obese (body mass index >25) may not be in good physical condition, are at higher risk for

developing chronic diseases, and have higher mortality rates (Centers for Disease Control and Prevention, 2016a). Individuals with excess weight also have an increased incidence of heart disease, sleep apnea, and asthma, and have double the risk for high BP. Often, patients with long standing pulmonary conditions are **cachetic**, a condition of obvious weight loss and severe wasting due to the increased energy demands needed just to breathe. A patient experiencing **dyspnea**, difficulty with breathing, may exhibit excess use of accessory breathing muscles, take on a forward flexed posture, lean on his/her arms, and have difficulty speaking in full sentences. Certain postural deformities, if severe—including **kyphosis**, abnormally increased flexion of the spine, or **scoliosis**, an abnormal lateral curvature of the spine—can change the mechanics of the respiratory muscles, making them less efficient and increasing the work of breathing. Trunk deformities can also result in compression of vital structures such as the lungs and heart, affecting $O_2$ transport. Careful observation and inspection should provide a general assessment of patient distress, the current state of health, and the ability to tolerate activity. This information will help to prioritize examination procedures.

## Vital Signs

Vital signs include HR, BP, RR, and temperature (T). Vital signs are essential examination procedures to perform and provide valuable information regarding the physiological state of an individual at rest and how the individual's system adapts to activity. Resting vital signs, vital signs immediately following exercise, and recovery vital signs, if interpreted correctly, are crucial to assess cardiovascular/pulmonary status. Physical therapists are one of the few health-care practitioners who work with patients during exercise. Despite this fact, vital sign monitoring during physical therapy is not performed frequently enough (Frese, 2002; Village, 2011). Vital signs when combined with validated exercise tests provide important objective measures of the patient's functional exercise capacity/exercise tolerance.

### Heart Rate

**Heart Rate (HR)**, the number of heartbeats per minute, is measured in beats per minute (bpm) by taking the pulse (wave of blood in the artery created by contraction of the left ventricle during a cardiac cycle) at various locations. The radial and carotid arteries are the most common sites. The radial pulse location is typically preferred over the carotid pulse because excess pressure on the carotid artery can cause vagal stimulation resulting in dizziness or loss of consciousness (LOC) due to a sudden drop in HR and BP. Palpating the pulse provides valuable information regarding the strength of heart contraction, rate and rhythm of contraction, and blood flow. To review a detailed description on how to take a pulse, the reader should refer to a text on physical examination.

Normal HR for adults ranges between 60 and 100 bpm. Table 11-6 includes reference values for HR by age group. The pulse should be regular, consistent, and strong. Slow HR below 60 bpm is termed **bradycardia** and HR above 100 bpm is termed **tachycardia**. A pulse that is irregular is indicative of an arrhythmia. The exact type and severity of the arrhythmia can only be determined with an ECG. If an irregular pulse is palpated in a patient without a previously documented arrhythmia or if other symptoms of cardiovascular disease are present, the patient should be referred for medical evaluation. A pulse that is difficult to palpate, often called "thready," or that varies between strong and weak may be indicative of poor left ventricular function or peripheral vascular disease (PVD) and is an indication for further medical evaluation.

### Respiratory Rate

**Respiratory rate (RR)**, the number of respiratory cycles per minute, is examined by counting the rate of rise and fall of the chest while the patient breathes quietly. This should be done when the patient is not aware of being watched because, if aware, the rate and pattern of breathing may change. Counting RR after taking the pulse but without removing the finger from the patient's wrist is a good way to observe without the patient's awareness. Table 11-6 includes reference values for RR by age group.

At the same time, observe and document the respiratory pattern. Patients who have suffered a stroke or TBI involving the respiratory control centers in the brainstem may exhibit pathological breathing patterns. See Table 11-7 for a description of pathological breathing patterns and possible causes. Also observe how abdominal girth changes during inspiration/expiration. Patients with SCI may utilize a paradoxical breathing pattern due to weakness or paralysis of the abdominals, intercostals, or diaphragm. In **paradoxical breathing**, the patient's upper chest collapses and the abdomen rises excessively during inspiration. Patients with hemiplegia may demonstrate asymmetrical chest motions with impaired expansion on the side of paresis/hemiplegia.

### Blood Pressure

**Blood pressure (BP)**, the pressure in arterial blood vessels, in units of millimeters (mm) of mercury (Hg), should be measured at rest, with position changes, during exercise, and in recovery along with HR to adequately assess the cardiovascular system. Arterial BP is most commonly measured with a sphygmomanometer (aneroid or Hg), BP cuff, and stethoscope. Refer to other sources for a complete description of how to perform a BP assessment. Table 11-6 includes reference values for BP by age group.

| TABLE 11-6 | Vital Signs Reference Values at Various Ages | | | | |
|---|---|---|---|---|---|
| | AGE | HEART RATE (beats/min) | SYSTOLIC BP (mm Hg) | DIASTOLIC BP (mm Hg) | RESPIRATORY RATE (breaths/min) |
| Vital signs at various ages (Kliegman, 2011) | Premature | 120–170 | 55–75 | 35–45 | 40–70 |
| | 0–3 months | 100–150 | 65–85 | 45–55 | 35–55 |
| | 3–6 months | 90–120 | 70–90 | 50–65 | 30–45 |
| | 6–12 months | 80–120 | 80–100 | 55–65 | 25–40 |
| | 1–3 years | 70–110 | 90–105 | 55–70 | 20–30 |
| | 3–6 years | 65–110 | 95–110 | 60–75 | 20–25 |
| | 6–12 years | 60–95 | 100–120 | 60–75 | 14–22 |
| | 12 years | 55–85 | 110–135 | 65–85 | 12–18 |
| | Adult | 60–90 | 110–120 | 60–70 | 14–22 |

*Continued*

**TABLE 11-6    Vital Signs Reference Values at Various Ages—cont'd**

|  | AGE | HEART RATE (beats/min) | SYSTOLIC BP (mm Hg) | DIASTOLIC BP (mm Hg) | RESPIRATORY RATE (breaths/min) |
|---|---|---|---|---|---|
| Resting heart rate (Minor, 2014) | Infant/child | 80–100 bpm |  |  |  |
|  | Adult | 60–100 bpm |  |  |  |
|  | Bradycardia | <60 bpm |  |  |  |
|  | Tachycardia | >100 bpm |  |  |  |
| Blood pressure ranges (Minor, 2014) | Normal |  | <120 | <80 |  |
|  | Prehypertension |  | 120–139 | 80–89 |  |
|  | Stage 1 hypertension |  | 140–159 | 90–99 |  |
|  | Stage 2 hypertension |  | ≥160 | ≥100 |  |

| Normal body temperature ranges for different activities (Minor, 2014) | Situation | Oral temp (°F) | Rectal temp (°F) | Oral temp (°C) | Rectal temp (°C) |
|---|---|---|---|---|---|
|  | Usual normal range | 98.6–99.5 | 96.8–99.7 | 36.0–37.5 | 36.0–37.6 |
|  | Morning/Cold weather | 95.0–96.8 | 95.9–97.0 | 35.0–36.0 | 35.3–36.1 |
|  | Hard work/Emotion | 99.7–101.0 | 99.7–101.5 | 37.6–38.3 | 37.6–38.6 |
|  | Hard exercise |  | 101.2–104.0 |  | 38.4–40.0 |

| Body temperature (U.S. National Library of Medicine, 2016) |  | Body Temp (°F) | Body Temp (°C) |  |  |
|---|---|---|---|---|---|
|  | Average normal body temperature | 98.6°F | 37°C |  |  |
|  | Elevated temp "fever" | >100.4°F | >38°C | Usually indicates infection or inflammation |  |

**TABLE 11-7    Abnormal Breathing Patterns That May Be Observed in Neuromuscular Disorders**

**ABNORMAL BREATHING PATTERNS**

| Pattern | Description | Causes |
|---|---|---|
| Apnea | Absence of breathing >15 sec | Cardiac arrest, drug overdose, alteration to respiratory control centers (in the medulla) |
| Bradypnea | Respiratory rate <12/min | Overdose of sedatives, narcotics, or alcohol, neurological disorders, metabolic disorders |
| Biot's | Irregular rate and depth of breathing with long periods of apnea | Increased intracranial pressure |
| Cheyne-Stokes respirations | Increasing rate and depth of breathing followed by period of apnea | CHF, kidney failure, elevated ICP, overdose of narcotics |
| Kussmaul respiration | Increased rate and depth of respirations | Metabolic acidosis |
| Apneustic breathing | Prolonged inspiration | CNS damage |
| Paradoxical respiration | Chest wall or abdomen moves inward with inspiration and outward on expiration | Diaphragm fatigue/paralysis, chest trauma |
| Hyperpnea | Increased depth | CHF, activity, lung infection |
| Hyperventilation | Increased rate and depth of breathing | Anxiety, pain, metabolic acidosis |

(Kacmarek, 2012)

Take care to avoid common errors in measurement that affect BP accuracy. These errors include improper cuff size, excessive pressure of the bell of the stethoscope on the artery, taking readings over clothing, and excessive inflation pressure. Proper fit of the BP cuff is essential to obtain accurate measurements (Fig. 11-1). A cuff that is too short or too narrow can lead to false high readings, and a cuff that is too large may result in false low readings (Bickley, 2013). To obtain a proper fit of the cuff, the bladder of the cuff should be approximately 40% of the width of the upper arm circumference (Bickley, 2013). Eighty percent of arm circumference should be used for the length of the bladder (Bickley, 2013), paying attention to the location markings on the cuff (Fig. 11-1). For example, if a patient's arm circumference measures 10 inches at the widest point of the upper arm, then a properly fitting BP cuff would be approximately 4 inches wide with a bladder 8 inches long.

Initially, BP should be taken at rest and ideally before ingesting caffeine products or smoking. BP should not be taken through the patient's clothing. The sleeve should be removed or rolled up. Take care to avoid allowing the sleeve to be rolled up tightly above the cuff or placing the cuff over the clothing as this can impair accuracy of the reading. Place the cuff snugly on the arm by centering the bladder (look for indicator arrow on the cuff) over the brachial artery and positioning the lower border approximately 1 inch above the antecubital fossa (Bickley, 2013). Palpate the brachial artery and position the arm resting at heart level. The patient should not independently hold the arm up because muscle contraction can cause a rise in BP. To determine how high to pump the cuff, an estimate of systolic pressure should be made by palpating the radial artery then rapidly inflating the cuff until the radial pulse disappears. This is the estimated systolic pressure. The cuff is then rapidly deflated. With the bell of the stethoscope placed over the brachial artery, taking care not to press hard enough to occlude the artery, inflate the cuff to approximately 30 mm Hg above the systolic pressure estimated in the previous step. Then slowly deflate the cuff

at a rate of 2 to 3 mm Hg per second. The point where the first two consecutive sounds are heard determines the **systolic blood pressure (SBP)**, the highest arterial pressure in the cardiac cycle. Continue to lower the pressure until there is a muffling of sound and the sound disappears. The point where the sounds disappear is the **diastolic blood pressure (DBP)**, the lowest BP in the cardiac cycle. Occasionally, particularly in the elderly, the sounds do not disappear; if this occurs, use the point of muffling of sound as the DBP (DeTurk, 2011; Irwin, 2004).

BP should initially be taken in both arms then subsequent readings taken in the arm with the higher recorded pressure. A difference of greater than 10 to 15 mm Hg between arms is abnormal and suggestive of arterial obstruction on the side with the lower BP (Bickley, 2013).

Also you should take BP related to certain position changes in the patient. Typically, when moving from sit-to-stand, SBP will momentarily drop, but the autonomic nervous system compensates by increasing HR to counteract the BP drop. **Orthostatic hypotension** is defined as a drop in SBP of >20 mm Hg that accompanies a change to more upright position or appearance of symptoms of lightheadedness or dizziness with position change (Bickley, 2013).

The *2014 Evidence-Based Guideline for the Management of High Blood Pressure in Adults,* the Eighth Report of the Joint National Committee on Prevention, Detection, Evaluation, and Treatment of High Blood Pressure (JCA-8), reports strong evidence to support treating hypertensive persons aged 60 years or older to a BP goal of less than 150/90 mm Hg and hypertensive persons 30 through 59 years of age to a diastolic goal of less than 90 mm Hg. Panel members report insufficient evidence in hypertensive persons younger than 60 years for a systolic goal or in those younger than 30 years for a diastolic goal, therefore panel members recommend a BP of less than 140/90 mm Hg for those groups based on expert opinion (James et al, 2014). An informative "2014 Hypertension Guideline Management Algorithm" is available online as part of the report at http://jamanetwork.com/journals/jama/fullarticle/1791497.

When evaluating the BP response to activity/exercise, it is important to take both resting and peak BP in the position of the exercise; for example, standing if the activity is walking. Sometimes in patients with neurological deficits, balance and fatigue make this difficult or impossible, but whenever possible this protocol should be followed to get an accurate assessment of response to exercise.

### Temperature

Body temperature is routinely measured by nursing staff in inpatient settings. In outpatient settings it is not routinely measured. If inflammatory or infectious processes are suspected or the patient exhibits other signs such as fever, chills, sweating, and/or malaise, temperature should be measured. For most adult patients, taking the temperature in the mouth or axillary region or via a tympanic thermometer is adequate and more comfortable than taking a rectal temperature. Table 11-6 includes reference values for temperature. Average oral

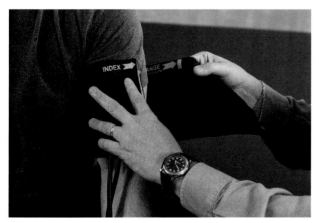

**FIGURE 11-1** Photograph showing proper fit of the BP cuff on the arm, including attention to the location markings on the cuff (indicating the range within which the "index" line should fall for an adult).

temperature is 37°C (98.6°F) but can vary throughout the day. Temperature is usually lower in the morning and highest in late afternoon. Variations in body temperature from 35.8°C (96.4°F) to 37°C (99.1°F) are not considered abnormal (Bickley, 2013). Temperatures over 100.5°F are considered elevated and the patient should be referred to the physician. Fever or pyrexia refers to an elevated body temperature and can be caused by infection, surgery, trauma, malignancy, infarctions, blood disorders, drugs, and immune disorders. Hypothermia or temperature under 35°C (95°F) is typically caused by exposure to cold but other causes can include paralysis, vasoconstriction, starvation, hypothyroidism, and hypoglycemia (Bickley, 2013).

## Other Tests

### Pulse Oximetry

**Pulse oximetry** provides an estimated measure of blood oxygenation by a noninvasive instrument that uses a light source and photodiode light detector to measure the amount of light passing through an arteriolar bed. $O_2$ saturation can be estimated with the instrument based on the light-absorbing characteristics of hemoglobin that differ depending on levels of oxygenation. Typically, pulse oximetry utilizes instrumentation with a sensor that fits comfortably over the tip of the patient's middle finger and displays an estimate of the $O_2$ saturation of hemoglobin in arterial blood and HR almost instantaneously. It is not invasive compared with direct measurement of $O_2$ saturation through ABG and can easily be performed by a physical therapist with the correct equipment. Distortion can occur for a variety of reasons (Orenstein, 1993; Yamaya, 2002), and accuracy is better with the patient at rest than during exercise, so the therapist is advised to interpret the values obtained using good clinical judgment (Lotshaw, 2011). However, as a noninvasive tool that provides a good estimation of arterial $O_2$ saturation, the pulse-oximeter is a commonly used and accepted measure with the patient at rest or while performing exercise (Escourrou, 1999; Lotshaw, 2011).

Normal values for $O_2$ saturation range from 96% to 100% (saturation of Hb) and typically should not change significantly with exercise. Patients with known chronic obstructive lung disease often have baseline $O_2$ saturations in the low 90% range. As a general rule, you should not continue exercise if $O_2$ saturation drops to 88% or below (Hillegass, 2011b). If $O_2$ saturation drops more than a few percentage points in a patient with no known lung pathology, contact the physician to discuss possible need for supplemental $O_2$. When documenting $O_2$ saturation, the therapist should document the values at rest, with change of position, and the range values during activity and recovery as appropriate. Type, intensity, and duration of activity should also be documented. If desaturation occurs, document the circumstances and specific timing within which it occurs.

### Perception of Exertion and Dyspnea

Several scales have been developed to quantify a patient's perception of exertion or dyspnea during physical activity: (1) the Borg Rating of Perceived Exertion Scale (RPE), (2) the Modified Borg Scale for Perceived Dyspnea (shortness of breath), and (3) a visual analog scale (VAS) of dyspnea (Gift, 1989; Muza, 1990). The Borg scales are widely accepted as a valid and reliable means to measure the sense of exertion and dyspnea during exercise (Meeks, 2003; Noble, 1983; Kendrick, 2000; Whaley, 1997).

The Borg RPE asks individuals to rate their perceived level of exertion on a 6- to 20-point scale ranging from 6, which means "no exertion at all," to 20, which means "maximal exertion" (extremely strenuous). The instructions are as follows: "While doing physical activity, we want you to rate your perception of exertion. This feeling should reflect how heavy and strenuous the exercise feels to you, combining all sensations and feelings of physical stress, effort, and fatigue. Do not concern yourself with any one factor such as leg pain or SOB, but try to focus on your total feeling of exertion." The RPE is available on the Centers for Disease Control and Prevention website at www.cdc.gov/physicalactivity/basics/measuring/exertion.htm. Validity for RPE is generally good, and a high correlation exists between the perceived exertion rating multiplied by 10 as an estimate of the actual HR during physical activity (Borg, 1967; Borg, 1974; Noble, 1983; Borg, 1987). For example, a perceived rating of 12 would correlate with an HR of 120. The RPE may not be valid for long-lasting exercise at constant load until exhaustion (Garcin, 1998). The RPE number multiplied by 10 may also be inaccurate in people taking heart-rate limiting drugs or those with cardiac disease. The RPE is often the preferred method to assess exercise intensity among those individuals who take medications that affect HR or pulse and is frequently used in conjunction with more formal submaximal exercise tests.

The Modified Borg Rating of Perceived Dyspnea asks individuals to rate their perceived level of SOB on a 10-point VAS ranging from "nothing at all" to "shortness of breath so severe you need to stop." Both scales have been found to correlate to minute ventilation (Muza, 1990). More lengthy scales such as the Chronic Respiratory Disease Questionnaire (Guyatt, 1987), St. George's Respiratory Questionnaire (Jones, 1991), and the Pulmonary Functional Status Dyspnea Questionnaire (Lareau, 1994; Lareau, 1998) are quality of life scales that measure the effect dyspnea has on one's functioning.

## Chest Assessment

Examine the chest for any structural abnormalities as well as abnormal breathing patterns. With a normal breathing pattern, the abdomen rises in inspiration and there is no accessory muscle use. Variations from the normal pattern can be seen in pulmonary disease and some neurological impairments and are summarized in Table 11-7.

Patients with SCI may utilize a paradoxical breathing pattern, previously described, due to weakness or paralysis of the abdominals, intercostals, or diaphragm. Patients with hemiplegia may demonstrate asymmetrical chest motions with impaired expansion on the side of paresis/plegia. These abnormalities may be observed during your inspection. Detection of subtle changes in asymmetry of breathing may require palpation of chest expansion.

Both heart sounds and breath sounds should be auscultated with a stethoscope. Prolonged bedrest (the inability to make frequent position changes), impairment of respiratory muscles, and weak cough impairing airway clearance put patients with neurological diagnoses at risk for **atelectasis**, collapse of lung alveoli that impairs gas exchange, and **pneumonia**, inflammation or infection of the lung. Diminished or absent breath sounds or the presence of inspiratory crackles may indicate the presence of these pathologies. (See Tables 11-8 and 11-9 for a summary of normal and abnormal breath sounds.)

Heart sounds should also be examined. Listen to heart sounds over four specific anterior chest locations (see Fig. 11-2). Two normal heart sounds can be heard: S1 or the first heart sound

| TABLE 11-8 | Characteristics of Normal Breath Sounds | |
|---|---|---|
| **NORMAL BREATH SOUNDS** | | |
| *Sound* | *Location* | *Description* |
| Vesicular | Periphery of lung | Low pitch; soft intensity<br>Inspiration longer and louder than expiration, continuous: no pause between inspiration and expiration |
| Bronchial | Sternum/manubrium | Loud high pitch<br>Expiration louder and longer |
| Bronchovescicular | 1st and 2nd intercostal spaces between scapulae | Moderate pitch and intensity<br>Inspiration and expiration equal in length and loudness |
| Tracheal | Over trachea | High pitch; loud intensity (like wind blowing through pipe)<br>Expiration longer than inspiration |

Source: Kallet RH. Bedside assessment of the patient. In: Kacmarek RM, Stoller JK, Heuer AJ, eds. *Egan's fundamentals of respiratory care.* 10th ed. St. Louis, MO: Elsevier; 2013: 330–355.

| TABLE 11-9 | Abnormal Adventitious Breath Sounds and Voice Sounds | |
|---|---|---|
| **ADVENTITIOUS BREATH SOUNDS** | | |
| *Type* | *Sound Quality/Description* | *Possible Pathology* |
| Fine Crackles | Fine, late inspiratory | Opening up of previously closed peripheral airways such as in atelectasis |
| Coarse Crackles | Coarse inspiratory and expiratory | Excess airway secretions moving through airways<br>Severe pneumonia; bronchitis |
| Wheeze | High pitched; usually expiratory, can be inspiratory | Rapid airflow through obstructed airways<br>Asthma, CHF |
| Stridor | High pitched; monophonic | Rapid airflow through obstructed upper airways |

Source: Kallet RH. Bedside assessment of the patient. In: Kacmarek RM, Stoller JK, Heuer AJ, eds. *Egan's fundamentals of respiratory care.* 10th ed. St. Louis, MO: Elsevier; 2013: 330–355.

| **VOICE SOUNDS** | | |
|---|---|---|
| Egophony | When patient says E, it is heard as A through stethoscope on chest | Mass, consolidation, or exudate in the lung allows greater transmission of sound than would air and sound is heard clearly. In a normal lung sound would be muffled. |
| Bronchophany | Patient says "99," and it is heard clearly through stethoscope on chest | |
| Whispered Pectoriloquy | Patient whispers, and it is heard clearly through stethoscope on chest | |

Source: Easy Auscultation: Lessons, Quizzes and Guides – Available at www.easyauscultation.com/cases?coursecaseorder=2&courseid=202. Accessed January 15, 2016.

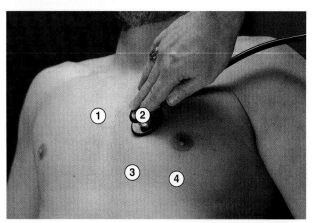

**FIGURE 11-2** Photograph showing the surface of the anterior chest and four specific locations for chest auscultation of heart sounds: 1) Aortic: in the second intercostal space, right sternal border, 2) Pulmonic: in the second intercostal space, left sternal border, 3) Tricuspid: in the fifth intercostal space, left sternal border, and 4) Mitral: in the fifth intercostal space, left mid-clavicular line.

that represents closure of the mitral valve and S2 or the second heart sound that represents closure of the aortic and pulmonic valves. Although there are several abnormal heart sounds that can occur, the two to be most concerned about are the third (S3) and the fourth (S4) heart sounds. S3 is a low frequency sound heard in early diastole, immediately after S2. It is due to poor ventricular compliance and is indicative of left ventricular failure. S4 is heard late in diastole and is the result of turbulence due to a forceful atrial contraction needed to overcome high filling pressures in the left ventricle (DeTurk, 2011). Heart sounds and breath sounds should be examined at rest, and at least initially, immediately postexercise. The detection of S3 heart sounds or crackles that do not clear with cough and were not present at rest are indicative of poor ventricular function that is exacerbated with exercise.

## Exercise Testing: Overview

Exercise testing, often referred to as stress testing, is a means of evaluating a patient's ability to tolerate increasingly progressive workloads of exercise while physiological responses (including HR and rhythm, ischemia via ECG, BP, symptoms, and RPE) are carefully monitored (Thompson, 2014). The addition of a metabolic cart provides gas analysis of expired air to calculate a measure of $VO_2$. Exercise testing can also be used to determine the presence of CAD and, if present, the prognosis (Thompson, 2014). It is also used to determine safe levels of activity post-myocardial infarction (post-MI) for functional testing to determine appropriate exercise prescription and for disability assessment (Thompson, 2014). The following section will briefly review the common types of exercise tests typically used, normal and abnormal findings, and recommendations for patients with physical disabilities due to neurological impairment.

Exercise testing can be either maximal or submaximal. In a **maximal exercise test,** the patient performs a progressive

workload and continues until the point of exhaustion or until the patient perceives an inability to continue because of symptoms such as chest discomfort, SOB, or leg fatigue or when 85% of age-appropriate maximal HR (HR max) is achieved (Thompson, 2014). Maximal testing is generally used to diagnose cardiac disease by provoking myocardial ischemia as the patient is asked to exercise at progressively higher workloads while HR, ECG, and BP are measured. The use of a metabolic cart for indirect measurement of $VO_2$, detection of the anaerobic threshold, and ventilations/minute (VE) is useful, along with $O_2$ saturation, in determining whether exercise limitations are primarily due to cardiac or pulmonary issues (Medoff, 1998). Maximal exercise testing is performed in a clinical setting with physician supervision and appropriate emergency advanced cardiac life support equipment and personnel available. The most common types of exercise equipment used in testing are the treadmill or bicycle ergometer (Noonan, 2000). Imaging techniques such as echocardiography or thallium scintigraphic scanning are often combined with maximal testing to improve sensitivity and specificity. Exercise echocardiography utilizes ultrasound imaging to observe cardiac wall motion and valve function during exercise. Wall motion abnormalities are indicative of cardiac tissue ischemia and/or infarction.

Maximal exercise testing is well established as being a valid and reliable measure of aerobic fitness (Pescatello, 2014). However, its applicability to physical therapy in the clinical environment is limited for several reasons. Maximal exercise testing is costly and requires equipment for monitoring, a high degree of technical skill to administer, and availability of emergency personnel (including a physician) and equipment (Noonan, 2000; Pescatello, 2014). Additionally, patients with pain or physical impairments are commonly unable to physically perform the maximal test (Noonan, 2000).

Another form of maximal stress testing is pharmacological stress testing. Although it is not technically an exercise test, pharmacological stress testing is frequently used for patients with significant physical disabilities that limit their ability to utilize exercise equipment or for those patients who are unable to exercise due to physical impairments or severe deconditioning. It involves injection of a drug typically used to increase HR (Pescatello, 2014). Pharmacological agents used include Dobutamine, Dipyridine, and Adenosine. Either echocardiography or thallium scintigraphic imaging is performed pretesting and posttesting (Pescatello, 2014). Pharmacological stress testing is useful in diagnosing cardiac disease in those unable to exercise but has limited value in determining functional capacity. Pharmacological testing is only carried out with physician supervision.

With **submaximal exercise testing**, the patient does not exercise to exhaustion but rather to volitional fatigue or less than 85% of age-predicted HR max. Typically, monitoring equipment is not required. $VO_2$ is not directly measured but is usually estimated by measuring some other parameter such as HR or distance walked and using those values in a regression equation to estimate $VO_2$ max. Submaximal testing is

| TABLE II-10 | Indications and Contraindications for Exercise Testing | |
|---|---|---|
| **INDICATIONS** | **ABSOLUTE CONTRAINDICATIONS** | **RELATIVE CONTRAINDICATIONS** |
| • Screening for disease<br>• Evaluation of symptoms: Chest pain/dyspnea<br>• Evaluation of treatment: Medical, surgical, exercise<br>• Determine exercise prescription<br>• Evaluate functional status/exercise tolerance/fitness | • Recent significant change in resting ECG suggesting significant ischemia<br>• Unstable angina<br>• Cardiac arrhythmias that are symptomatic or hemodynamically unstable<br>• Symptomatic severe aortic stenosis<br>• Uncontrolled symptomatic heart failure<br>• Acute pulmonary embolus or infarction<br>• Acute myocarditis/pericarditis<br>• Suspected or known dissecting aneurysm<br>• Acute systemic infection | • L main coronary artery stenosis<br>• Moderate stenotic valvular heart disease<br>• Electrolyte abnormalities<br>• Arterial hypertension >200 mm<br>• Tachy- or brady-dysrhythmias<br>• Hypertrophic cardiac myopathy<br>• Chronic infectious disease<br>• Ventricular aneurysm<br>• High degree atrioventricular block<br>• Uncontrolled metabolic disease<br>• Mental/physical impairment causing inability to exercise safely/adequately<br>• Neuromotor, musculoskeletal, or rheumatoid disorders exacerbated by exercise |

(Pescatello, 2014, p. 53)

less costly as it utilizes everyday functional activities such as walking, running, or stepping rather than equipment. Submaximal testing is the form typically done in a physical therapy environment. Instead of being used to diagnose CAD, it is primarily used for exercise prescription and/or functional testing, including preintervention and postintervention assessment (Noonan, 2000; Pescatello, 2014).

Before initiating a submaximal exercise test, you must screen the patient very carefully for cardiac risk and for contraindications to exercise testing. Table 11-10 summarizes the indications/contraindications for exercise testing. If risk factors are present, refer the patient for monitored or physician-supervised testing. Carefully select the appropriate exercise mode and protocol before initiating the test.

The different modes of submaximal exercise testing include treadmill tests, bicycle ergometer tests, and arm ergometer tests, as well as field tests such as timed walk/run tests, distance walk/run tests, shuttle tests, step tests, and sit-to-stand tests (Noonan, 2000; Pescatello, 2014). When choosing a test, consider the patient's physical capabilities or impairments including, but not limited to, balance, coordination, strength, range of motion, and use of assistive device (Noonan, 2000). Also consider the population for which the test was originally developed and the test's documented validity and reliability (see Table 11-13).

## Treadmill Protocols

Several protocols are used for exercise testing but probably the most widely used is the Bruce Treadmill Protocol (Bruce, 1969), which can be performed as a submaximal or maximal measurement. Details of the protocol are provided in Table 11-11. The Bruce Treadmill Protocol involves walking on a treadmill at a starting speed of 1.7 mph and a 10% grade with the speed and incline increasing at 3-minute intervals to a maximum of

| TABLE II-II | Standard and Modified Bruce Treadmill Protocols | | |
|---|---|---|---|
| **MODIFIED BRUCE STAGES** | **3 MINUTE STAGES** | | **STANDARD BRUCE STAGES** |
| | **MPH** | **GRADE OF INCLINE** | |
| | 5.5 | 20% | 6 |
| | 5.0 | 18% | 5 |
| | 4.2 | 16% | 4 |
| | 3.4 | 14% | 3 |
| | 2.5 | 12% | 2 |
| 3 | 1.7 | 10% | 1 |
| 2 | 1.7 | 5% | |
| 1 | 1.7 | 0% | |

5.5 mph and a 20% grade. The speeds and grade necessary to complete the Bruce Treadmill Protocol are far too rigorous for many patients to complete. The Modified Bruce Treadmill Protocol (Sheffield, 1988) starts at 1.7 mph and a 0% grade and is more appropriate for deconditioned patients and clinical populations (Noonan, 2000). The Bruce Treadmill Protocol and the Modified Bruce Treadmill Protocol have been widely used and tested (see Table 11-13). Regression equations to predict $VO_2$ have been validated and normative values have been developed (Table 11-12; Noonan, 2000; Pescatello, 2014). Although these equations provide only estimates of $VO_2$ and the validity has been questioned by some in select populations (Koutlianos, 2013; Chavda, 2013), it circumvents the necessity for more complicated and potentially dangerous protocols for actual estimation of $VO_2$.

| TABLE 11-12 | Description of Submaximal Exercise Tests | |
|---|---|---|
| **NAME OF TEST** | **DESCRIPTION/PROTOCOL** | **REGRESSION EQUATION TO ESTIMATE VO$_2$** |
| Walking Tests | | |
| 6-minute or 12-minute walk tests (ATS, 2002) | • Subjects are asked to walk at their own pace for 6 minutes (or 12 minutes). <br>• A straight 100 ft hallway with hard flat surface should be used. <br>• Subjects should be given standard instructions and standard verbal encouragement at specified points during the test. <br>• RPE, HR, and BP should be monitored. | None |
| Modified Bruce Protocol Treadmill Test (Pescatello, 2014) | • Treadmill Test <br>Stage 1: 1.7 mph @ 0% grade <br>Stage 2: 1.7 mph @ 5% grade <br>Stage 3: 1.7 mph @ 10% grade | • $VO_2 = 0.1(S) + 1.8 (S)$ (grade) $+ 3.5$ <br>S = speed |
| Single Stage Sub-maximal Treadmill Walking Test (SSTT) (Ebbeling, 1991) | • Calculate 50% and 70% age-predicted max HR. <br>• Test has three submaximal 4-minute stages: <br>Stage 1: Warm up: Walk 4 minutes at 0% grade at speed that brings person to HR between 50%–70% HR$_{max}$. <br>Stage 2: Increase grade to 5% walk for 4 minutes. Record HR in final 30 seconds of this stage. <br>Stage 3: Cool down: Decrease grade to 0% and cool down 4 minutes. | • $VO_2$ max $= 15.1 + 21.8$ (speed mph) $- 0.327$ (HR bpm) $- 0.263$ (speed × age in years) $+ 0.00504$ (HR × age) $+ 5.98$ (gender; female = 0, male = 1) <br>• HR = average steady state HR achieved in last 30 seconds of stage 2 |
| Modified Shuttle Walk Test (Singh, 1992; Campo, 2006) | • Two cones are set up 0.5 m in from each end of a 10 m course and client is asked to walk back and forth around the cones in an elliptical path. <br>• Speed is determined by audio signals played on a cassette tape so that patient is turning at each cone with each audio "beep." <br>• Start speed = 0.5 m/s and speed is increased by 0.17 m/s each minute (see detailed protocol in Table 11-13). | • $VO_2$ max $= 4.19 + 0.25$ (distance) <br>• $VO_2$ max = mL/kg <br>• Distance = meters |
| Shuttle Run Tests (SRT) for Children with Cerebral Palsy (CP) (Verschuren, 2006) | • Developed two SRT for children with CP. SRT I for children with GMFCS. <br>• Level I: Starting speed 5 km/hr speed increases 0.25 km/hr each minute and SRT II for GMFCS <br>• Level II: Starting speed 2 km/hr with speed increasing 0.25 km/hr | None |
| Arm Ergometer Protocols | | |
| Arm Cycle Ergometer Test (Werner, 2006) | • Arm ergometer may be used or modified from bicycle ergometer. <br>• Client is seated with fulcrum of handle adjusted to height of the shoulder joint. <br>• Cranking rate 60 rpm increase workload by 10 W every 2–3 minutes. | • $VO_2 = (18 \times W \times M^{-1}) + 3.5$ <br>W = workload in Watts <br>M = body mass in Kg |
| Six-Minute Arm Test (6MAT) (Hol, 2007) | • One single 6-minute stage of exercise is performed on a standard arm cycle ergometer. <br>• Initial power output is chosen to produce a steady state heart rate of 60% to 70% age-predicted max HR or 11 to 15 on Borg scale. | None |

| TABLE 11-12 | **Description of Submaximal Exercise Tests—cont'd** | |
|---|---|---|
| **NAME OF TEST** | **DESCRIPTION/PROTOCOL** | **REGRESSION EQUATION TO ESTIMATE VO$_2$** |
| | • <u>Initial Power Output Setting for Paraplegia:</u><br>Female inactive: 30 W<br>Female active/male inactive: 40 W<br>Female competitive athlete or male active: 50 W<br>Male competitive athlete: 60 W<br><u>Tetraplegia:</u><br>Power WC user or wrist ext ≤grade 4: 10 W<br>Manual WC user: 15 W<br>Manual WC user with grade 5 wrist extension<br>and active: 20 W | |
| University of Toronto<br>Arm-Crank Protocol<br>(Kofsky, 1983; Kosak,<br>2005) | • Field test using portable Vigio forearm ergometer<br>• Subjects arm pedals at cadence of: 80 rpm.<br>• Perform three 5-minute submaximal periods at<br>PO that produce 40%, 60%, 80% of age-predicted<br>max HR with 2-minute rests between workloads<br>then raise intensity at 1 minute intervals until<br>voluntary exhaustion. | Males:<br>$VO_2 = 0.18$ (W) $+ 0.40$<br>Females:<br>$VO_2 = 0.17$ (W) $+ 0.37$ |
| Wheelchair Propulsion Tests | | |
| Treadmill Exercise Test<br>for Wheelchair Athletes<br>(Knechtle, 2001) | • Wheelchair treadmill protocol with constant<br>speed and increasing inclination.<br>• Starting workload: Speed 8 km/hr and incline 1%.<br>Incline increased by 0.5% every 2 minutes. | None |
| 12-Minute Wheelchair<br>Propulsion Test<br>(12MWCT)<br>(Franklin, 1990) | • Subjects propel their wheelchair to cover the<br>most distance possible in 12 minutes. | • $VO_{2\ peak} =$ (Distance in miles −<br>0.37)/0.0337<br>• Regression equation validated with<br>Quickie II WC and 0.1-mile indoor level<br>running track.<br>• Assigned levels of aerobic fitness based<br>on distance covered. |
| Adapted Leger and<br>Boucher Test<br>(Vinet, 2002) | • Field test to predict VO$_2$ max in wheelchair<br>athletes.<br>• 400 m field marked off every 50 m with<br>a pylon.<br>• Velocity is increased when crossing a marker<br>corresponding to a sound signal.<br>• Initial velocity is 4 km/hr for 1 minute and is<br>increased every minute by 1 km/hr until<br>exhaustion. | • $VO_{2\ peak} = 0.22 Va_{max} − 0.63 \log(age) +$<br>0.05 BMI 0.25 level + 0.52<br>• Where $Va_{max}$ = velocity in last minute<br>of exercise<br>• Lesion level:<br>Paraplegia with high lesion level = 1<br>Paraplegia with low lesion level,<br>amputee, or postpolio = 0 |
| Multistage Field Test for<br>Wheelchair Users<br>(Vanderthommen, 2002) | • Indoor multistage field test where subjects wheel<br>around an octagonal course.<br>• Octagonal course has four long sides of 11 m<br>and four short sides of 2 m.<br>• Turning zones are marked by two internal cones<br>placed at the angle of the octagon and one<br>external cone located on the corner of the<br>15 m × 15 m square.<br>• Subjects wheel around the course and are paced<br>by an external auditory cue.<br>• Initial velocity is 6 km/hr. | • $VO_{2\ peak} = (18.03 + 0.78$ MFT score)<br>• Where MFT score = stage of test<br>reached.<br>• Regression equation was validated with<br>subjects utilizing their own wheelchair,<br>therefore applicable to wide variety of<br>WC types. |

*Continued*

| TABLE 11-12 | Description of Submaximal Exercise Tests—cont'd | |
| --- | --- | --- |
| **NAME OF TEST** | **DESCRIPTION/PROTOCOL** | **REGRESSION EQUATION TO ESTIMATE VO$_2$** |
| | • Velocity increases by 0.37 km/hr every minute until exhaustion.<br>• Subjects must be in the turning zone when the sound beeps.<br>• Test is terminated when subject is unable to reach the turning zone on three consecutive beeps. | |
| *All-Extremity Exercise Tests* | | |
| Power Trainer All-Extremity Submaximal Exercise Test (Loudon, 1998) | • Two 6-minute steady state exercise stages.<br>• Initial power output is determined by following: 50 W low fitness, 75 W medium fitness, 100 W high fitness.<br>• Pedaling rate self-selected between 50 to 90 rpm. Second workload increased by 25 W. | $VO_{2\,peak} = -0.01$ (age in years) $- 0.0029$ (HR 1) $- 0.0099$ (HR 2) $- 0.0029$ (PO$_1$) $+ 0.0151$ (PO$_2$) $+ 3.010$ |
| Nu-Step All-Extremity Test (Mendelsohn, 2008) | • Three constant level 4-minute stages predetermined based on responses on practice session.<br>• In the practice session, the subject completes 2 minutes of exercise at workloads ranging from 1 to 8 on Nu-Step.<br>• At the highest workload reached, subject completes 4 minutes of exercise not to exceed 75% age-predicted HR max.<br>• Workload 1 = highest workload yielding RPE of 3<br>• Workload 2 = workload midway between stage 1 and 3<br>• Workload 3 = Highest workload subject could complete in 4 minutes of exercise | • No regression equation but correlation between MET values and HR values generated by built-in software and those directly measured was moderate to high (r = .85 – .97)<br>• Test retest reliability was moderate to high (intraclass correlation coefficient = .85 – .91) |

### Single-Stage Submaximal Treadmill Test

The Single-Stage Submaximal Treadmill Test (Ebbeling, 1991) consists of three 4-minute periods. The first period is a warm-up in which the person walks at a comfortable pace to produce a HR between 50% and 70% of age-predicted HR max. During the second 4-minute period, the only one that includes exercise stimulus, the incline is increased to 5%. The final period is a cool-down. HR from the final 30 seconds of the second period is used in a regression equation to estimate $VO_2$ max (Ebbeling, 1991). Validity is established through correlations of regression equation-estimated $VO_2$ (Table 11-12) with actual $VO_2$ measured on a maximal treadmill test (Ebbeling, 1991). Other investigators have found that $VO_2$ obtained from the low 50% HR and high 70% HR were not as valid (Waddoups, 2008). The test has not been studied extensively in a variety of populations. Because it is a single-stage test, it is appropriate to test those individuals in rehabilitation who fatigue easily on more traditional treadmill tests.

Although treadmill protocols are the most popular, they are often impractical to use with patients who have neuromuscular conditions and/or physical disabilities. Additionally, most metabolic equations have been validated in the able-bodied population using no hand support but not among individuals with gait deviations who expend more energy. Validity of standardized equations to estimate $VO_2$ in the population with disabilities has not been determined (Noonan, 2000).

### Bicycle Ergometry

Exercise test protocols utilizing bicycle ergometers are also common. These may be more appropriate for people with impaired walking balance or inability to walk for prolonged periods. Disadvantages of bicycle ergometry tests include potential to cause lower extremity muscle fatigue and discomfort in some patients. Additionally, individuals need to have sufficient sitting balance to safely maintain an upright sitting posture on the bicycle seat during exercise. Because bicycle ergometry does not represent a functional activity for many people, its applicability to everyday activities may be limited.

### Timed Run/Walk Tests

Timed run/walk tests require a patient to walk or run for a set period of time and to try to cover as much distance as possible during that time frame. The 12-Minute Run Test (12MRT) was the original run test (Cooper, 1968) and a regression equation validated for healthy males (Bandyopadhyay, 2015). Normative values are published for males and females from age 13 years to 60 years or older in fitness categories ranging from "very poor" to "superior" (Cooper, 1981).

Both the 12-Minute Walk Test (12MWT) and the 6-Minute Walk Test (6MWT) evolved from Cooper's 12MRT (Solway, 2001; Steele, 1996). Walk tests such as the 6MWT and the 12MWT are more suitable to clinical rehabilitation populations because many people with physical impairments are not able to run or sustain running for 12 minutes or are unable to use a treadmill due to impairments in balance, motor control, or foot drop (Verschuren, 2006; Noonan, 2000). Walk tests incorporate a familiar functional activity that many people are able to perform. Additionally, timed walk tests allow individuals to walk at their own speed as opposed to treadmill protocols in which the treadmill enforces the pace (Enright, 2003).

Walk tests are used to measure functional status and the ability to undertake physical activity needed for daily activities (Solway, 2001) as a reflection of cardiovascular/pulmonary support of functional activities. Walk tests also provide an outcome measure for response to interventions. Various timed walk tests have been created but probably the most widely used is the 6MWT. This test has been used in populations with chronic lung disease (Noonan, 2000; Solway, 2001; Enright, 2003) and cardiac conditions (Gayda, 2004). Distance walked on the 6MWT correlates with $VO_2$ max with strength of the correlation ranging from 0.51 to 0.90 (Solway, 2001). The 6MWT has been studied in patients with chronic obstructive pulmonary disease (COPD; Turner, 2004; Bernstein, 1994), heart disease (Hamilton, 2000), stroke (Eng, 2002; Tang, 2006a; Kosak, 2005), MS (Savci, 2005; Goldman, 2008), PD (Falvo, 2009), and postpolio (Gylfadottir, 2006). Correlations between 6MWT and $VO_2$ max have been weaker in patients with neuromuscular conditions (Eng, 2002; Gylfadottir, 2006).

In patients with neuromuscular disorders, diagnosis-specific factors other than cardiorespiratory endurance, including weakness, balance, and leg length, limited the distance walked (Savci, 2005; Eng, 2002; Pang, 2005a; Tang, 2006a; Gylfadottir, 2006). When using the test in these populations, it is recommended that other measures of exertion also be measured including HR, BP, and RPE (Eng, 2002). Both the 6MWT and the 12MWT have been found to be reliable (Table 11-13). To ensure reliability, it is recommended that standard procedures and standardized patient instructions be followed as established by the American Thoracic Society (Enright, 2003; American Thoracic Society Committee on Proficiency Standards for Clinical Pulmonary Function Laboratories, 2002).

A 12-Minute Wheelchair Propulsion Test has been developed for wheelchair users with a regression equation (Table 11-12) validated using a Quickie II wheelchair (Franklin, 1990). Use of a different wheelchair may change the weight being pushed or change efficiency of propulsion thereby limiting the validity of the regression equation.

### Shuttle Tests

**Shuttle walk tests** are exercise tests in which the patient walks back and forth over a prescribed distance at a prescribed advancing pace. The 20-Meter Shuttle Run Test is a maximal exercise test (Léger, 1984) developed for physically fit adults. It involves quick changes in movement (Noonan, 2000) and is reliable and valid in a young healthy population (Liu, 1992). It has limited applicability in clinical rehabilitation populations. The Modified Shuttle Walk Test (MSWT) is an adaptation of the 20-Meter Shuttle Run Test. It was originally developed for patients with COPD to provide an incremental symptom-limited exercise test (Noonan, 2000; Singh, 1992). In the MSWT, the patient is asked to walk back and forth between two cones placed 9 m apart (0.5 m from each end of a 10 m elliptical course). Using the Modified Shuttle Walk Test parameters explained here, ask the patient to walk back and forth, around the cones, to the timing of an external audio tape that gets progressively faster, providing an incremental increase in workload (Singh, 1992). Level 1 starts with three shuttles at 0.50 m/s with each successive level increasing the number of shuttles by one and increasing the velocity by 0.17 m/s. Therefore, level 5 consists of seven shuttles at 1.18 m/s. Ultimately, level 10 is 12 shuttles at 2.03 m/s. Level 12, the most strenuous level, is 14 shuttles at 2.37 m/s (Singh, 1992). The test is stopped when the patient can no longer complete the shuttle in the time frame or the patient becomes too fatigued to go on (Singh, 1992; Lewis, 2001). Validity is supported (Table 11-13) with a high correlation to both $VO_2$ and to distance walked in 6MWT among individuals with COPD (Singh, 1994) and heart failure (Lewis, 2001). Additionally, completing 450 m on the MSWT is predictive of individuals who could achieve a $VO_2$ of over 14 mL/min/kg (Lewis, 2001).

One advantage of the MSWT is that it provides an incremental progressive increase in exercise stress. A regression equation to estimate $VO_2$ (Table 11-12) has been validated in patients with COPD (Campo, 2006). The external pacing of the audio signal can be motivating to patients and may help facilitate performance. Because the test is externally paced, it is thought to more closely resemble a maximal incremental exercise test (Campo, 2006); because of this, it is recommended that patients be carefully screened for cardiovascular disease before testing (Noonan, 2000). Some investigators have found no significant difference in peak HR on MSWT versus the 6MWT (Vagaggini, 2003; Turner, 2004). The patient's physical capabilities such as balance, ability to walk at higher speeds, and to make quick turns should also be considered before implementing the test.

Modifications of the SRT and SWT have been made to accommodate populations with physical impairments. There are two SRTs specifically for children with cerebral palsy based on severity of gross motor functional impairment as measured by Gross Motor Function Classification System (GMFCS; Verschuren, 2006). These two modifications of the

SRT are reliable and valid for measuring aerobic capacity in this population (Verschuren, 2006). The Adapted Leger and Bouchar Test (Vinet, 2002) and the Multistage Field Test for Wheelchair Users (Vanderthommen, 2002) are shuttle tests developed for individuals who utilize a wheelchair as their means of mobility.

The Endurance Shuttle Walk Test (ESWT) was developed to complement the MSWT (Revill, 1999) and to provide a constant-walking-speed measure of endurance. Other timed walking tests such as the 6MWT and 12MWT allow the patient to vary the walking speed and therefore are not true measures of **endurance** (i.e., the ability to perform a submaximal workload over a period of time; Revill, 1999). For the ESWT, ask the patient to walk the shuttle course at a pace corresponding to 75%, 85%, or 95% of the patient's maximal intensity achieved on the MSWT. Record the length of time the patient is able to continue to walk at this workload. The advantages of this test over a timed walk test are that it provides a constant walking speed, pace is regulated, and it is more standardized because patients must maintain a certain predetermined workload over time (Revill, 1999). This regulation is not possible in timed walk tests. A description of various exercise tests and regression equations is presented in Table 11-12 and a summary of current evidence-basis for exercise testing is presented in Table 11-13 after the Chapter Summary.

### Normal and Abnormal Responses

The expected normal response to exercise testing is a rise in HR and SBP with each incremental increase in workload without signs of ischemia. Signs that are suspicious for CAD include **ST segment depression** (a lowering of the ST segment below the isoelectric line) on ECG; an increase in frequency of **premature ventricular contractions (PVCs),** which are cardiac arrhythmia in which the ventricular depolarization occurs earlier than expected, or **ventricular arrhythmias,** which are abnormal heart rhythms initiated by abnormal electric activity in the ventricles; change in pulse rhythm; failure of HR to rise with increased workload; a flat SBP response or a drop in SBP; or a drop or rise in DBP of >10 mm Hg. Symptoms that are highly suspicious for CAD are occurrence of angina, SOB, fatigue, dizziness, or feeling lightheaded.

## ■ Exercise Responses and Testing in Specific Populations

These sections will summarize expected exercise responses commonly observed in patients with specific neurological conditions. Some alternate stress-test protocols for these populations will also be described.

### Stroke

Cerebral vascular accident, commonly referred to as stroke, is a condition resulting from ischemia-related infarction to the brain as a result of an embolus, thrombus, or cerebral hemorrhage. Primary impairments vary depending on the size and site of the lesion but can include paresis/paralysis, weakness,

sensory changes, aphasia, or problems with cognition or speech problems. Of these impairments, weakness and paralysis have the greatest effect on exercise testing and exercise responses (Nicola, 2009) and, if longstanding, can eventually result in deconditioning with impaired cardiovascular endurance.

As stated previously, CAD, obesity, hypertension, hyperlipidemia, and Type-2 diabetes are common comorbidities of stroke (Nicola, 2009). Seventy-five percent of patients who have experienced stroke have some form of heart disease (Roth, 1993). Loss of function and resultant deconditioning can only compound the factors and increase cardiovascular risk and negatively affect quality of life (Washburn, 2002; Nicola, 2009; Pang, 2005a). Exercise testing is strongly recommended in this population because of the high likelihood of cardiovascular comorbidities and the need to help determine interventions to optimize cardiovascular function. The physical impairments in this population make exercise testing and exercise prescription a challenge (Nicola, 2009).

Although HR can be altered by medications (e.g., beta blockers for hypertension) and presence of CAD, in general, both peak HR and peak $VO_2$ are lower in individuals with stroke versus age-matched controls (Nicola, 2009). Factors thought to contribute to the impaired aerobic capacity seen following stroke include fewer motor units available for recruitment in weak/paralyzed muscles, lower oxidative ability of weak/paralyzed muscle, and sedentary lifestyle as a result of physical impairments and comorbidities such as CAD (Nicola, 2009; Washburn, 2002). Supervised aerobic exercise programs can improve aerobic capacity in individuals with stroke (Nicola, 2009; Pang, 2005b). Before beginning an exercise program for an individual poststroke, it is recommended that a graded exercise test be performed to determine limits for safe exercise prescription. A thorough medical evaluation should be performed by the patient's physician before exercise testing (Nicola, 2009).

Modalities for exercise testing in patients with stroke can include, as described earlier, treadmill, bicycle ergometry, or upper extremity ergometry. Balance and gait abnormalities are common poststroke and make bicycle ergometry much more practical in this population than the treadmill. Bicycle ergometry is also more practical than upper extremity ergometry because of the significant upper extremity involvement after stroke. Treadmill workloads may not be consistent in the stroke population due to increased demands of ambulating with gait deviations or due to holding on to arm rails for balance. Arm cranking or upper extremity ergometry should be utilized only on patients with severe paralysis of both lower extremities because it yields significantly lower $VO_2$ than treadmill (Nicola, 2009). A ramped cycle ergometer protocol can be used for individuals with stroke starting at an initial workload of 20 watts and increasing in 10-watt increments every minute until maximal effort is achieved (Rimmer, 2000). Semirecumbent cycle ergometer can be used to test patients with acute stroke, but there is no evidence of patients achieving $VO_2$ max (Tang, 2006b).

All-extremity ergometers such as Nu-Step and Power Trainer may offer a better alternative to exercise testing in this population. Power outputs, MET levels, and HR generated by the computer software and displayed on the screen have high correlations with values directly measured via metabolic cart in frail elderly (Mendelsohn, 2008).

A modified total-body recumbent stepper exercise test has been developed for patients with stroke (Billinger, 2008). This test utilizes all four extremities at a cadence of 80 steps/minute and work intervals of 2 minutes. The starting workload is 25 watts and resistance is increased every 2 minutes by 15 watts (Billinger, 2008). Peak HR and peak $VO_2$ values correlate to those obtained from bicycle ergometry but are significantly higher (Billinger, 2008), perhaps because subjects were able to use all four extremities and therefore were utilizing more muscle mass and consuming more $O_2$. The test is supported as a valid means to measure peak HR and peak $VO_2$ in patients with stroke (Billinger, 2008). Although a regression equation to predict $VO_2$ using a total body recumbent stepper has been validated to predict $VO_2$ in the healthy adult population (Billinger, 2012), at this time a regression equation to estimate $VO_2$ in patients with stroke has not been developed.

## Spinal Cord Injury

SCI involves loss of sensory, motor, and autonomic function as the result of damage to the spinal cord. **Tetraplegia**, paralysis with involvement of all four extremities and trunk, formerly called **quadriplegia**, occurs when there is spinal cord damage between cervical segments C1-T1 and is more likely to affect respiratory function. **Paraplegia** is a result of injury at or below thoracic segment T2 and results in impairment of the trunk and legs, whereas arm function is spared (Garshick, 2005). Although there have been advances in the management of SCI, the mortality rate in this population remains high. Diseases of the cardiovascular/pulmonary system are the leading causes of death in individuals who have had SCI (Garshick, 2005; Myers, 2007). The rate of CAD and mortality due to CAD in the population with SCI is higher and occurs at an earlier age compared with that of individuals without SCI (Myers, 2007). Of particular concern, angina in this population may be silent due to autonomic denervation. Additionally the appearance of certain cardiovascular risk factors such as hyperlipidemia, truncal obesity, higher percent of body fat, elevated inflammatory markers such as C-reactive protein and diabetes occur at higher rates than in the general population (Garshick, 2005; Myers, 2007; Jacobs, 2004). The sedentary lifestyle imposed by the loss of motor function and deconditioning compounds these risks.

Patients with SCI may also have significant limitation to exercise due to loss of function of the respiratory muscles, especially above midthoracic levels. Obviously, loss of innervation to the diaphragm (C3,4,5) would require mechanical ventilation. However, even patients with intact diaphragm function can have impaired ventilation due to the lack of abdominal support. Without functioning abdominal muscles, the abdominal contents drop and no longer hold the diaphragm in a normal resting position. The diaphragm takes on a shortened resting position and diaphragmatic excursion is impaired. This leads to inefficiency of the inspiratory muscles and can cause dyspnea and limited exercise tolerance and may require external support in the form of an abdominal binder.

When injury occurs above the level of sympathetic outflow, T6, autonomic dysfunction occurs and negatively affects the cardiovascular system (Myers, 2007; Jacobs, 2004; Dela, 2003). Resting arterial BP is typically low in individuals with SCI. The normal increase in HR and contractility that occurs when changing positions from supine to sitting or standing is lost and orthostatic hypotension results (Myers, 2007). The long-term effects of low BP can significantly change heart structure and function (Myers, 2007). The combination of low BP with decreased **cardiac preload** (i.e., the stretching force the heart must overcome at the end of diastole) due to venous pooling and lack of normal responses to exercise can cause left ventricular atrophy.

SCI introduces several exercise-related complications. The first is the inability to perform large muscle aerobic activities due to lower extremity paralysis, particularly characteristic of tetraplegia. Due to loss of autonomic regulation, adaptations necessary to perform aerobic exercise are impaired. Patients with tetraplegia are unable to increase HR and contractility and exhibit venous pooling and loss of thermoregulation. This all leads to inability to increase cardiac output to support exercise and hypotension. In paraplegia, resting BP and cardiac output are normal. However, the cardiac output is characterized by lower SV and higher HR. Patients with SCI above spinal level T6 are also prone to **autonomic dysreflexia,** a life-threatening autonomic emergency, characterized by abnormal cardiovascular response including severe hypertension, headache, bradycardia, and sweating (Jacobs, 2004; Figoni, 2009).

Acute responses to exercise in SCI are characterized by blunted HR response in patients, especially in individuals with lesions above T1 who also lack a SBP response and have very low peak $VO_2$. Higher lesion levels correlate with lower peak $VO_2$ (Hjeltnes, 1986). Power output achieved is inversely related to lesion level (Jacobs, 2004; Theisen, 2012). To minimize the adverse responses of patients with SCI to exercise, the following precautions should be taken: proper trunk stabilization if needed (Figoni, 2009); "holding gloves" (Nicola, 2009); protection of the skin; emptying urinary collection devices before testing (to prevent dysreflexia); vascular support such as abdominal binders and compression stockings to minimize orthostatic response; use of a cool room; and use of an **intermittent exercise protocol**, a type of exercise test that uses periods of exercise interspersed with a short rest. Use of an abdominal binder provides abdominal muscle support and also helps improve respiratory function in patients with SCI (Huang, 1983).

Exercise testing modalities for the population with SCI include wheelchair propulsion on a specialized wheelchair treadmill or wheelchair rollers, cyclical arm-crank ergometry, and electrically stimulated exercise (Myers, 2007; Jacobs, 2004). The advantage of wheelchair testing is to allow for comparison with functional activities for a wheelchair user. However, wheelchair testing requires specialized equipment not available in most clinics and the results may be influenced by the type of wheelchair, therefore making it difficult to standardize work levels (Jacobs, 2004; Myers, 2007).

The arm-crank ergometer is frequently used for exercise testing in this population. Advantages of the arm-crank ergometer include availability of equipment in most clinical settings with ease for standardized testing and more consistent and reliable measurement of workload (Hol, 2007; Kofsky, 1983; Jacobs, 2004). The main disadvantage of arm-crank ergometry is that the movement involved does not replicate functional activity for this population, namely wheelchair propulsion (Myers, 2007).

Several wheelchair field tests have been developed with regression equations to estimate VO$_2$ and are summarized in Table 11-12. It is important to remember that validation for these regression equations was developed using a particular type of wheelchair and positioning. Any variation in wheelchair or positioning can affect the accuracy with which these equations predict VO$_2$.

## PATIENT APPLICATION

*Frank is a 42 year-old male firefighter with a diagnosis of complete T4 paraplegia (spinal cord injury) as a result of a fall from a ladder. Before his injury, he was active and in good health. He is not overweight (normal BMI) and had an annual physical examination through his fire department. He did not smoke and his medical history is negative for any preexisting medical condition. His spine has been fixated, and he has just been admitted to a rehabilitation hospital.*

### Contemplative Clinical Decisions

1. *What additional information would you like to know about this patient?*
2. *What cardiovascular/pulmonary problems is he at risk for?*
3. *What should the physical therapist focus on during the examination as it relates to the cardiovascular/pulmonary system?*

## PATIENT APPLICATION

*On examination, Frank demonstrates a weak cough. He states he "feels weak" when sitting up, and his vital sign response to position changes is as follows: resting supine HR 76, BP 118/70; change of position to sitting HR 78, BP 108/70 with complaints of feeling weak which slowly resolve.*

### Contemplative Clinical Decisions

1. *To evaluate his baseline of functional exercise tolerance, what submaximal exercise test would you choose?*
2. *What precautions should you take to avoid complications during the test and to maximize his exercise capacity?*

## Multiple Sclerosis

MS is an inflammatory demyelinating disease of the central nervous system that can cause damage in the white matter of the spinal cord, brainstem, or cerebral hemispheres. Because

of variable and unpredictable locations of the plaques, great variability exists in the presenting symptoms as well as severity from person to person. Physiological responses to acute exercise are similar to that of the general population. For most patients with MS, the HR, BP, VO$_2$, RR, and minute ventilation increase linearly with workload (Jackson, 2009). In some patients, HR and BP response to exercise may be blunted (Jackson, 2009). This blunting of HR and BP is thought to be caused by impairment in cardiovascular autonomic reflexes (Ng, 2000; Pepin, 1998) and may contribute to fatigue and poor exercise tolerance in some patients with MS (Ng, 2000; Flachenecker, 2003). VO$_2$ max differs from person to person but in general is lower in the disabled population, perhaps related to the degree of motor involvement (ACSM, 2014). Unless risk factors are present, patients with MS are able to start an exercise program without clinical exercise stress testing. Age-appropriate HR formulas, such as Karvonen's method, can be used for most patients (Swain, 2014).

## Parkinson Disease

Limited research is available regarding cardiovascular exercise responses in PD. At submaximal levels of exercise, the HR, BP, and RPE are similar to normal controls (Protas et al, 1996; Werner et al, 2006). However, for a given workload, HR responses of patients with PD are elevated, and these patients are unable to achieve the same maximal workload as normal controls, indicating diminished exercise efficiency (Protas et al, 1996). Peak workloads and VO$_2$ are diminished compared with controls (Protas et al, 1996; Reuter et al, 1999) and peak HR responses are blunted (Reuter et al, 1999; Werner et al, 2006; Protas et al, 1996). When considering exercise testing in someone with PD, apply the contraindications of exercise testing established by the ACSM (Pescatello, 2014). A thorough evaluation of gait, range of motion (ROM), flexibility, and strength should be performed to help guide the choice of modality for testing. Balance should be thoroughly examined before treadmill testing; and if balance is impaired, use of handrails on the treadmill or bicycle ergometer or arm-crank ergometer may be better choices (ACSM, 2014).

## THINK ABOUT IT 11.2

The selection of a particular exercise testing protocol will vary with the purpose of testing, safety considerations, equipment/type of exercise, underlying cardiovascular/pulmonary problems, neurological diagnosis, blunting of cardiovascular autonomic reflexes, physical ability, medications, prior activity level, and multiple other factors.

## ■ Documentation of Cardiovascular/ Pulmonary Evaluation

After collecting your data regarding the cardiovascular/pulmonary examination, it is important to carefully document the significant findings and begin to notice trends and supporting factors. All factors from the history related to cardiac and respiratory function should be carefully documented. Vital signs should not be neglected and should be carefully noted in an obvious location in the patient record. Record any available indications of hypoxia or dyspnea, and record the findings from your chest examination including auscultation of heart sounds and respiratory sounds, comparing right and left sides. Finally, carefully document the reason for selecting the specific exercise test and the results of the test so that it can be interpreted in the context of the entire set of examination data.

## HANDS-ON PRACTICE

1. Monitor vital signs: HR, BP, $O_2$ saturation, and temperature.
2. Auscultate chest and distinguish between normal and abnormal heart and lung sounds.
3. Physically examine chest expansion and movement during respiration.

4. Assess breathing patterns.
5. Administer Borg Rating of Perceived Exertion scale.
6. Conduct basic exercise testing protocols.

## Let's Review

1. For a patient with a neuromuscular diagnosis, what are some of the most important questions to ask as part of the history to initially investigate cardiovascular/pulmonary deficits?

2. Why is it essential to measure vital signs in each patient with a neuromuscular diagnosis?

3. Describe the mechanisms of aerobic metabolism, and some specific functional applications of aerobic metabolism.

4. Explain the difference between cellular respiration and pulmonary ventilation.

5. Describe the responses to exercise in blood vessels of active muscles, generalized blood vessels, heart rate, systolic BP, and diastolic BP.

6. How could you use the Borg Rating of Perceived Exertion scale? And describe how you would interpret the "Borg" rating for a particular patient.

7. List the most common forms of submaximal exercise testing used in individuals with neuromuscular disorders. And how could results of submaximal exercise testing be used for exercise prescription/progression to improve cardiovascular function?

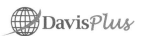 For additional resources, including Focus on Evidence tables, case study discussions, references, and glossary, please visit http://davisplus.fadavis.com

## CHAPTER SUMMARY

After disorders or dysfunction of the nervous system, the normal operation of the cardiovascular/pulmonary system can be drastically affected, as a primary impairment, from loss of appropriate nervous system signals to respiratory structures or impaired regulation of cardiac and pulmonary actions; or as a secondary impairment, with deconditioning which results from prolonged physical inactivity and impaired movement, or a musculoskeletal complication (e.g., scoliosis). Therefore, testing of cardiovascular/pulmonary operation is essential to document baseline function of the patient to determine the optimal intervention and should not be neglected in this population for either adults or children. Chapter 32 will present therapeutic intervention to address impairments of the cardiovascular/

pulmonary system. Chapters 33 to 37 will cover functional applications of intervention, which can be used as opportunities to increase endurance in specific functional skills.

Basic procedures to examine the cardiovascular/pulmonary systems in patients with neuromuscular conditions are covered in this chapter, from obtaining the patient history to observations, auscultation, and physiological measures such as pulse oximetry, and including selection of appropriate exercise testing to document patient response to physical activity. The normal response to exercise and some likely abnormal exercise responses in this population are presented. A description of submaximal exercise tests is provided in Table 11-12.

CHAPTER **12**

# Diagnostic Testing in Neurology: Lab Tests, Imaging, and Nerve/ Muscle Studies With Implications for Therapists

Dennis W. Fell, PT, MD ▪ Brad Steffler, MD
Bassam A. Bassam, MD, FAAN ▪ Wesley Blake Denny, PhD, MT (ASCP)
John R. Jefferson, PT, PhD, OCS, COMT ▪ Jonathan B. Mullins, MD

**CHAPTER OBJECTIVES**

Upon completion of this chapter, the learner should be able to:
1. Discuss the three main categories of medical diagnostic tests.
2. Discuss the main diagnostic tests within each category, including major indications and results.
3. Recognize and interpret abnormal test results on a formal test report.
4. Contrast the purposes of the different types of diagnostic imaging studies.
5. Describe the procedure and expected results for nerve conduction studies and electromyography.

## Introduction

*Celene Darby, a 46 year-old female with diabetes, is your patient in an outpatient clinic and is telling you about her hospital stay. When you ask about medical tests she had during the hospitalization for hemorrhagic stroke, she says "I can't count the number of tests I had in that hospital." Computerized tomography (CT) scans had confirmed the size and location of the cerebrovascular accident (CVA) and because of the recognized hemorrhage, verified she was not a candidate for thrombolytic intervention (tPA). She also had frequent blood tests to monitor the degree of anemia. And throughout the stay, because she was not eating or drinking well, she had numerous serum chemistries run to*

*monitor her fluid status and blood glucose. Taking this part of the patient history gives you a better understanding of some of the potential complications in this patient during her therapeutic activities.*

Physical therapists (PTs) and occupational therapists (OTs) increasingly practice in more acute settings and provide intervention to patients who are less medically stable. As explained in Chapter 2, the PT does not make a medical diagnosis in the realm of pathology, but instead the PT diagnosis consists of movement-related impairments of body structure/body function and functional limitations of activity. In any case, the therapist will be exposed to (1) printed reports of a variety of medical tests both in the patient record and (2) verbal reports by the patient. The therapist will have to make decisions regarding rehabilitation intervention and medical screening based on the available information. Therefore, it is essential for the therapist to be aware of the variety of tests, their results, and the implications of abnormal values. Medical diagnostic tests, as the name implies, most often serve the purpose of confirming or ruling out a suspected medical diagnosis. In some cases, especially with some clinical laboratory tests, medical test results can be used to (1) support or confirm a medical diagnosis, (2) determine the appropriate medical treatment (including implications for intensity of exercise), and (3) monitor the effectiveness of medical interventions.

The purpose of this chapter is to provide a brief overview for therapists and therapy students of diagnostic measures used in patients with neuromuscular disorders (both adult and pediatric). Therapists do not diagnose from these tests, but they do need to understand the terminology in each area, be able to interpret written reports, and have a working knowledge of implications of the test results for developing a plan of care for physical therapy intervention, including appropriate exercise customized for the individual patient and for explaining to the patient the prognosis for recovery of physical function. Illustrations of abnormal test results are used to support the written text.

There are three categories of diagnostic tests discussed in this chapter: clinical laboratory tests, diagnostic imaging, and electrophysiologic testing, each specifically defined later in this chapter. These tests can be used by physicians to diagnose medical disorders, the extent or localization of pathology, and to monitor results of medical intervention or progression of disease. Although PTs do not make a medical diagnosis based on any of these tests, they may initiate the referral for clinical laboratory testing, diagnostic imaging, or electrophysiological testing. PTs in the U.S. military have had referral for diagnostic imaging in their scope of practice since 1972 (Greathouse, 1994). In some countries other than the United States such as Australia and the UK (Australian Physiotherapy Association, 2006; Royal College of Nursing, 2006), PTs (called physiotherapists outside the United States) have referral for diagnostic imaging within their scope of practice. In the case of electrophysiological testing, the position of the American Physical Therapy Association (APTA) is that, after appropriate postgraduate education, PTs are prepared to perform electrophysiologic evaluations including, but not limited to, clinical electromyography (EMG), motor and sensory nerve conduction studies (NCS), and other evoked potential procedures (APTA HOD P06-96-20-04).

## Health Risk Assessment

Health risk assessment, initiated by asking the patient questions about behaviors, habits, and lifestyle issues, can help to identify risk areas. Such behaviors include smoking, alcohol abuse, drug abuse, and safety issues such as seat belt use in automobiles and helmet use on motorcycles, bicycles, and skateboards. Sometimes, clinical laboratory tests can be used to screen for health risk including cholesterol for atherosclerosis and glucose screening for diabetes.

More information on some intervention strategies to address these risk factors is presented in Chapter 16 on Health Promotion and Wellness.

## Critical Care and Physiologic Monitoring

Therapists often treat patients in the intensive care unit. The therapist in any intensive care unit must be aware of the numerous IV lines, access ports, drains, and monitor leads, and must understand how to read the basic measures displayed on the bedside monitor screen. It is essential to understand the significance, particularly of heart rate, blood pressure, respiratory rate, and central vascular pressures (pulmonary artery pressure, central venous pressure). In addition, the therapist in a neurological intensive care unit must also specifically be aware of neurological measures such as intracranial pressure monitoring (Kleinpell, 2005; Shah, 2007).

## Clinical Laboratory Tests

**Clinical laboratory tests** involve specific laboratory analysis of body fluids and tissues. Clinical laboratory test results are integral to diagnostic aspects of modern medical practice with important implications for the rehabilitation therapist. It has been estimated that 70% of all physician decisions associated with the diagnosis, treatment, and monitoring of patient pathologies are based on test results from the clinical laboratory (Forsman, 1996). By understanding laboratory test results, the rehabilitation therapist can gain valuable insight into patient health. Laboratory test results generated during the course of patient diagnosis and treatment can provide vital information about a patient's health history and current health status, which will enable more effective and safe rehabilitation of patients with neuromuscular disorders. This information is particularly important in today's clinical setting where patients are being discharged earlier after diagnosis and medical treatment or even receive a greater proportion of their medical treatment on an outpatient or home basis. The rehabilitation therapist must be aware of patient conditions that could adversely affect rehabilitation interventions and outcomes.

The clinical laboratory has traditionally been divided into four core areas: (1) chemistry, (2) hematology, (3) microbiology, and (4) immunohematology. However, advances in medical knowledge and technology have spurred the development of specialized subdivisions over time. The clinical laboratories of most large hospitals and medical centers now have additional laboratory areas dedicated to hemostasis, nonblood body fluids analysis, immunology, virology, toxicology, therapeutic drug monitoring, and flow cytometry (see Table 12-1 for a description of testing performed in these areas). The advent of molecular medicine, based on nucleic acid (DNA and RNA) technologies, has led to the introduction of yet another specialized area, molecular diagnostics. Molecular diagnostics has the potential to revolutionize medicine by allowing medical

| TABLE 12-1 | Specialized Areas of the Clinical Laboratory |
|---|---|
| **CLINICAL LABORATORY AREA** | **DESCRIPTION OF TESTING PERFORMED** |
| Chemistry | Analysis of body fluids to determine the concentration or biological activity of substances such as sugars, proteins, lipids, hormones, gases, electrolytes, and nitrogen metabolites. |
| Hematology | Analysis of whole blood for quantification of the cellular components and identification of abnormal blood cells based on cell morphology. |
| Immunohematology | Analysis of donor and recipient red blood cell antigens and antibodies, and preparation of red blood cells and other blood components (e.g., plasma, platelets, and clotting factors) for transfusion. |
| Microbiology | Analysis of tissues and body fluids for the identification of infectious pathogenic microorganisms (bacteria and fungi), and testing of cultured pathogens for antibiotic susceptibility. |
| Hemostasis | Analysis of whole blood and plasma to identify coagulopathies (blood clotting disorders) caused by abnormal platelets, clotting factor deficiencies, or autoantibodies and to assess blood clotting in patients on anticoagulant drug therapy. |
| Nonblood Body Fluids | Analysis of nonvascular organ and body cavity fluids for the identification of cellular components, infectious microorganisms, antibodies, and the quantification of certain chemistry analytes. |
| Immunology | Analysis of body fluids for the identification and quantification of antibodies, determination of viral load, and immune function testing. |
| Virology | Analysis of body fluids and tissues for the identification of infectious viruses. |
| Toxicology | Analysis of body fluids for the identification and quantification of toxins (e.g., alcohols, heavy metals, pesticides, etc.) and illegal drugs. |
| Therapeutic Drug Monitoring | Analysis of therapeutic drug concentrations in body fluids to ensure that safe and effective drug levels are achieved and maintained. |
| Flow Cytometry | Analysis of body fluids for the identification of cell population subsets using a flow cytometer, an instrument that sorts individual cells that have been labeled with fluorescent-tagged antibodies. |
| Molecular Diagnostics | Analysis of patient DNA for the identification of heritable genetic diseases, tumor characterization, assessment of multigene disease risk and therapeutic drug efficacy, and tissue-typing for organ and stem-cell transplantation. |

treatment to be tailored to an individual's genetic characteristics (Guttmacher, 2002).

Although all areas of the clinical laboratory produce test results of interest to therapists in the context of patient health history, the areas of the clinical laboratory producing results most relevant to the diagnosis and treatment of patients with neuromuscular disorders are chemistry, hematology, hemostasis, immunology, and molecular diagnostics. Each of these areas is discussed in this section of the chapter with selected test results presented in helpful tables along with implications for rehabilitation therapy activities. The **reference ranges** for tests, the array of values that represent a normal population as shown in the accompanying tables, are established independently by individual clinical laboratories through an analysis of a minimum of 100 specimens from a healthy local population, which should reflect the demographics of the population served by the facility. In addition, many test results are dependent on the type of specimen and the method used to analyze the specimen. Due to these variables, reference ranges for laboratory tests may differ somewhat from laboratory to laboratory and from the values presented in this

chapter, which are average values compiled from multiple sources.

Some tests, such as those for serum lipids, do not have reference ranges but have instead a recommended range or value established by government agencies or organizations of specialized medical professionals as associated with minimizing risk. For some, there is no agreement on what the range should be, and others provide either an upper or lower limit that is important. For example, there is still much debate about the diagnostic usefulness of measuring serum lipids. Therapists should always refer to reference ranges and values used by their facility or the laboratory that performed the analysis for the treating physician when making decisions regarding rehabilitative therapies. Many laboratory tests also have **critical values** that represent life-threatening conditions and must be reported immediately to the attending healthcare professional. Therapists in rehabilitation settings don't often encounter critical values unless therapy is conducted in an intensive care or acute care setting. As an exception, for the diabetic patient who has poorly controlled blood sugar, the therapist may see blood glucose values well outside the normal range in outpatient settings. Common units of measurement for clinical laboratory tests are shown in Table 12-2.

## Chemistry

The chemistry area of the clinical laboratory processes a large number of patient specimens that are analyzed for a wide variety of biological substances or chemical compounds. At most facilities, chemistry tests are organized into panels (e.g., general panel, cardiac panel, liver panel, renal panel, thyroid panel, etc.) according to their diagnostic potential. Table 12-3 summarizes common chemistry laboratory measures with reference ranges. Measurement of blood glucose is a routine test performed to assess a patient's glycemic status (i.e., how much glucose is accumulated in the blood), especially in diabetes. Glucose is derived from carbohydrates (sugars and starches) found in dietary foodstuffs and from body stores of glycogen, and glucose is also synthesized endogenously from the breakdown of proteins and fats. Blood glucose is normally maintained within a fairly narrow concentration range by hormones, principally insulin, glucagon, and epinephrine, under diverse conditions including after ingestion of a meal, fasting, or exercising. The most common disorder of carbohydrate metabolism is hyperglycemia (high blood glucose) caused by diabetes mellitus, which affects approximately 8% of the U.S. population (Centers for Disease Control, 2007). For diabetes, glucose levels should be measured with a glucometer, a point-of-care testing device for blood glucose, before and after exercise-based therapies, especially in the individual with brittle control of their diabetes (Peirce, 1999). This is particularly important for insulin-dependent diabetics and patients who are beginning therapy or changing established routines of physical activity (Wing, 2001).

**Enzymes** are proteins that catalyze the biochemical reactions which make life possible. Most intracellular enzymes are found in blood at low concentrations, and elevated levels of these intracellular enzymes occur when specific tissue damage has occurred. Many enzymes are specific to a cell type with different forms of the same enzyme (isoenzymes) expressed differentially from the different tissues. Measurement of serum enzymes, particularly isoenzymes, can be used to diagnose damage to those specific tissues and organs. For example, creatine kinase (CK) is an intracellular enzyme abundant in muscle tissues, especially cardiac and skeletal muscle, and normal levels of circulating CK correlate with total body muscle mass. As a result, males usually have higher values than females, and persons with sub-Saharan African ancestry tend to have higher levels than those with European or Asian ancestry.

CK isoenzymes are present at differing ratios in different tissues. CK-MM is predominant in skeletal muscle; CK-MB is most abundant in cardiac muscle; and CK-BB is most abundant in smooth muscle and the central nervous system (CNS). CK-MM is the main contributor to total CK activity and is elevated after skeletal muscle trauma, exercise, and seizures that induce extreme muscle contractions. The CK-MM fraction is significantly elevated in muscular dystrophy. The CK-MB fraction is elevated after cardiac muscle damage by conditions such as myocardial infarction (MI), trauma, congestive heart failure, and myocarditis. The timing of release after cardiac damage is very specific with serum CK-MB increasing 4 to 6 hours after

| TABLE 12-2 | Common Units of Measure for Clinical Laboratory Tests |
|---|---|
| **UNIT (ABBREVIATION)** | **DEFINITION** |
| gram (g) | Base unit of mass in the international metric system (1 gram is equivalent to 0.035273962 pounds) |
| milligram (mg) | One thousandth ($1 \times 10^{-3}$) of a gram |
| microgram (mcg) | One millionth ($1 \times 10^{-6}$) of a gram |
| nanogram (ng) | One billionth ($1 \times 10^{-9}$) of a gram |
| liter (L) | Base unit of volume in the international metric system (1 liter is equivalent to 1.056688209 quart) |
| deciliter (dL) | One tenth ($1 \times 10^{-1}$) of a liter |
| milliliter (mL) | One thousandth ($1 \times 10^{-3}$) of a liter |
| microliter ($\mu$L) | One millionth ($1 \times 10^{-6}$) of a liter |
| meter (m) | Base unit of length in the international metric system (1 meter is equivalent to 3.280839895 feet) |
| millimeter (mm) | One thousandth ($1 \times 10^{-3}$) of a meter |
| mole (mol) | A quantity representing the number of molecules in one molecular weight mass of a pure substance ($\sim 6.022 \times 10^{23}$). |
| millimole (mmol) | One thousandth ($1 \times 10^{-3}$) of a mole |
| pH | The negative logarithm of the hydrogen ion concentration ($-\log[H^+]$). |
| International Unit (IU) | The amount of enzyme required to catalyze the conversion of one micromole of substrate to product per minute under specified reaction conditions. |

**TABLE 12-3    Chemistry Reference Ranges**

| CLINICAL LABORATORY TEST | NORMAL REFERENCE RANGE | IMPLICATIONS FOR REHABILITATION |
|---|---|---|
| Glucose (fasting >8 hours) Specimen: Serum | Unit: mg/dL Neonate: 30–60 Child: 60–100 Adult: 74–100 Adult >60 yr: 82–115 | In therapy, exercise can cause a rapid drop in blood glucose resulting in hypoglycemia (low blood glucose). Hypoglycemia can also occur as a result of skipping a meal or taking too large a dose of insulin. Symptoms of hypoglycemia include headache, weakness, loss of muscle coordination, irritability, apprehension, and impaired arousal and cognition. Patients with an initial blood glucose level below 70 mg/dL should ingest carbohydrates and have their glucose rechecked after 15 to 20 minutes has passed before exercising. |
| Glycated hemoglobin (HgbA1C) Specimen: Uncoagulated whole blood Note: HgbA1C is a hemoglobin subfraction that comprises approximately 80% of the total glycated hemoglobin. | Unit: % Total Hemoglobin 4.0–6.0 | An indicator of long-term average blood glucose levels (as a measure of consistent control of diabetes). Elevated levels indicate prolonged periods of hyperglycemia (high blood glucose) associated with uncontrolled diabetes mellitus. Uncontrolled diabetic patients that experience a rapid drop in blood glucose after exercise can exhibit symptoms of hypoglycemia, even though blood glucose is still elevated. If symptoms of diabetic ketoacidosis (fruity breath odor, Kussmaul respirations, and weak, rapid pulse) are observed, give the patient a sugar-containing liquid and seek immediate medical attention. |
| Creatine Kinase (CK) Specimen: Serum Note: Total combined activity of all CK isoenzyme forms. | Unit: IU/L Male: 46–171 Female: 34–145 | CK is normally elevated after therapies that involve exercise or muscle massage. Very high levels of CK are associated with neuromuscular disorders that have a muscle-wasting component such as ALS, DMD/BMD, MG, and limb-girdle dystrophies. Electrotherapy, inflammatory myopathies, drug-induced myopathies, and metabolic disorders that cause rhabdomyolysis also increase CK. Low levels of CK can result from prolonged treatment with corticosteroids, which are often used as an anti-inflammatory agent in the treatment of inflammatory neuromuscular diseases. Low levels of CK are also associated with low muscle mass often seen in end-stage neuromuscular diseases. Total CK levels provide a reference that allows the therapist to follow the progression of patient muscle wasting as well as the effect of rehabilitative therapies. |
| CK-MB Isoenzyme Specimen: Serum | Unit: μg/L or % Total CK activity <5.0 μg/L or <3.9% | When elevated CK-MB is diagnostic for MI, patient physical activity should be curtailed and vital signs closely monitored during therapy, especially oxygenation status, heart rate, and heart rhythm. |
| Blood Urea Nitrogen (BUN) Specimen: Serum | Unit: mg/dL Neonate: 4–12 Infant/Child: 5–18 Adult: 6–20 Adult >60 yr: 8–23 | Urea is produced by the liver to eliminate nitrogen wastes generated from the catabolism of proteins and nucleic acids. More than 90% of urea is excreted via the kidneys, and elevated BUN can be an indication of impaired renal function. However, other tests that measure creatinine clearance or glomerular filtration rate are better determinants of renal function since increased BUN can also result from other conditions such as dehydration, gastrointestinal bleeding, hyperthyroidism, and increased dietary protein intake. Elevated BUN in conjunction with dehydration can cause dizziness and decreased mental function. |

| TABLE 12-3 | Chemistry Reference Ranges—cont'd | |
|---|---|---|
| **CLINICAL LABORATORY TEST** | **NORMAL REFERENCE RANGE** | **IMPLICATIONS FOR REHABILITATION** |
| Creatinine<br>Specimen: Serum<br>Note: The Jaffe test method was used to obtain reference range values. | Unit: mg/dL<br>Neonate: 0.3–1.0<br>Infant/Child: 0.2–0.7<br>Adult male: 0.9–1.3<br>Adult female: 0.6–1.1 | Creatinine is a waste product derived principally from muscle creatine, and the amount of creatinine produced is proportional to body muscle mass. Because creatinine is eliminated via the kidneys and daily creatinine production is fairly constant, the concentration of creatinine in serum is an indicator of renal function, and elevated levels of serum creatinine result when there is impaired renal function. Increased serum creatinine can also be caused by muscle-wasting associated with certain neuromuscular diseases. Low levels of creatinine are often seen in patients with low muscle mass such as the elderly and those with end-stage muscular degeneration. |
| Ferritin<br>Specimen: Serum | Unit: ng/mL<br>Neonate: 25–200<br>Infant/Child: 7–140<br>Adult male: 20–250<br>Adult female: 10–120 | Ferritin is the major iron storage protein, and serum ferritin is directly proportional to the body's total stored iron. Serum ferritin is a sensitive indicator of iron status, and decreased levels are an early indicator of iron deficiency that can lead to anemia. Decreased levels are also seen in patients with protein malnutrition. |
| Total Iron Binding Capacity (TIBC)<br>Specimen: Serum | Unit: µg/dL<br>250–450 | TIBC is a measurement of the maximum iron binding capacity of the serum iron transport protein transferrin. Serum TIBC is often increased in iron deficiency and decreased in chronic inflammatory diseases, malignancies, and hemochromatosis (iron overload). |

MI, with peak between 12 to 24 hours, and a return to normal levels 48 to 72 hours post-MI if no further damage occurs to the heart. CK-BB is elevated in CNS trauma and in neuromuscular disorders with degenerative neuropathy.

The potential results and reference ranges for other chemical tests are summarized in Table 12-3, including Hemoglobin A1C, BUN, creatinine, ferritin, and total iron binding capacity (TIBC).

## Blood Gases, Electrolytes, and Acid-Base Balance

**Blood gases** include laboratory measures of oxygen, carbon dioxide, and blood pH and related measures from the arterial blood. These are summarized in Table 12-4. Acid-base balance or homeostasis is a critical physiological process that maintains blood pH in a relatively narrow range compatible with life. The complex interplay of blood gases, electrolytes, and the organ systems involved in acid-base balance and the numerous pathologies that can alter homeostasis are beyond the scope of this text. However, some key concepts will help the therapist understand acid-base disorders and implications for therapeutic intervention. Normal metabolic processes generate acidic compounds (e.g., carbonic, sulfuric, and phosphoric acids) that are transported through the bloodstream to the lungs and kidneys, where they are eliminated. Carbonic acid

is formed when carbon dioxide ($CO_2$) dissolves in blood. Analysis of specific combinations of pH and $CO_2$ status will provide an indication of the cause of the change in acid-base status. For example, increased $CO_2$ from chronic obstructive pulmonary disease (COPD) causes an increase in carbonic acid in whole blood, which lowers blood pH. A condition of *respiratory **acidosis**,* a decrease in blood pH with excessive hydrogen ions ($H^+$) in the blood, results when $CO_2$ is retained as a consequence of impaired alveolar gas exchange or suppressed respiration. In *metabolic acidosis,* increased production or decreased renal excretion of acidic metabolites occurs, and the body attempts to compensate for low blood pH by more frequent and deeper respirations (hyperventilation) to exhale more $CO_2$. A *respiratory **alkalosis**,* an increase in blood pH from insufficient number of circulating hydrogen ions, results when the respiratory rate is increased, which eliminates $CO_2$, decreasing carbonic acid and increasing pH. In *metabolic alkalosis,* blood pH is high, and the body attempts to compensate by retaining more $CO_2$ through slower and shallower respirations (hypoventilation), increasing the concentration of hydrogen ions ($H^+$). In summary, if the pH is acidic (low) and $CO_2$ is high, then the acidosis resulted from the respiratory $CO_2$. If the pH is acidic (low) and $CO_2$ is low, the respiratory system is trying to compensate for a metabolic increase in acidity. Acid-base disorders are common, and therapists must plan treatments carefully and observe for

**TABLE 12-4** **Blood Gases and Electrolyte Reference Ranges**

| CLINICAL LABORATORY TEST | NORMAL REFERENCE RANGE | IMPLICATIONS FOR REHABILITATION |
|---|---|---|
| pH of blood<br>Specimen: Heparin-uncoagulated arterial whole blood<br>Note: pH is based on a logarithmic scale from 0–14 with 7 being neutral. | Unit: pH<br>Neonate: 7.35–7.50<br>Child/Adult: 7.35–7.45<br>Adult >60 yr: 7.31–7.42 | Values below the reference range, low pH, because of high concentration of hydrogen ions indicate a condition of acidosis. Values above the reference range, high pH, due to decreased concentration of hydrogen ions indicate a condition of alkalosis. Disturbances in acid-base homeostasis can result from either respiratory or metabolic disorders. Therapists must closely monitor patients at risk for acid-base disorders and plan treatment based on the etiology of the disorder. |
| $PCO_2$ (partial pressure of dissolved carbon dioxide in blood)<br>Specimen: Heparin-uncoagulated arterial whole blood | Unit: mm Hg<br>Neonate/Infant: 27–41<br>Adult Male: 35–48<br>Adult Female: 32–45 | Elevated $PCO_2$ occurs when there is retention of carbon dioxide due to respiratory insufficiency, hypoventilation, or compensation for metabolic alkalosis. Low $PCO_2$ values are seen when there is respiratory compensation for a metabolic acidosis or the patient is hyperventilating. |
| $PO_2$ (partial pressure of dissolved oxygen in blood)<br>Specimen: Heparin-uncoagulated arterial whole blood | Unit: mm Hg<br>Neonate: 54–95<br>Child/Adult: 83–108<br>Adult >60 yr: >80<br>Note: $PO_2$ decreases approximately 10 mm Hg with each decade of life after age 70. | $PO_2$ is dependent on cardiopulmonary function and the concentration and affinity of functional hemoglobin for oxygen. Prolonged hypoxemia ($PO_2$ <80 mm Hg) can cause dizziness, loss of coordination, impaired cognition, and life-threatening cardiac arrhythmias. Therapists should monitor patients who are at risk for developing hypoxemia with a pulse-oximeter, a noninvasive point-of-care testing device that estimates $sO_2$ from capillary blood. |
| $sO_2$ (hemoglobin oxygen saturation)<br>Specimen: Heparin-uncoagulated arterial whole blood | Unit: Percent Saturation<br>Neonate: 40–90<br>Child/Adult: 94–98 | The percentage of red blood cell hemoglobin that is saturated with oxygen. The relationship between $sO_2$ and $PO_2$ is not linear, and $PO_2$ decreases rapidly when $sO_2$ drops below 90%. Patients with anemia, COPD, pulmonary inflammation, and other conditions that impair gas exchange may require special breathing regimens or supplemental oxygen to maintain $sO_2$ above 90%, especially when exercising. |
| $HCO_3^-$ (Bicarbonate)<br>Specimen: Serum or heparinized plasma<br>Note: Determined from total carbon dioxide. | Unit: mmol/L<br>Neonate: 13–22<br>Infant/Child: 20–28<br>Adult: 22–29<br>Adult >60 yr: 23–31 | A useful indicator for determining acid-base status when used in conjunction with pH and $PCO_2$. Low levels of bicarbonate indicate a condition of metabolic acidosis such as diabetic ketoacidosis (DKA). |
| Sodium<br>Specimen: Serum | Unit: mmol/L<br>Neonate: 133–146<br>Infant: 139–146<br>Child: 138–145<br>Adult: 136–145 | Imbalances in sodium can cause changes in blood pressure and tachycardia. The therapist should closely monitor the hydration status and blood pressure of patients who have sodium imbalances. |
| Potassium<br>Specimen: Serum<br>Note: Cellular potassium concentrations are higher than serum, and specimen hemolysis will falsely elevate serum potassium. | Unit: mmol/L<br>Neonate: 3.7–5.9<br>Infant: 4.1–5.3<br>Child: 3.4–4.7<br>Adult: 3.5–5.1 | Due to potential cardiac arrhythmias, physical therapy is contraindicated in adults when potassium levels are outside the **normal reference range**. Hypokalemia is frequently seen in older adults taking diuretics and these patients should be closely observed for symptoms of hypokalemia. |
| Chloride<br>Specimen: Serum or plasma | Unit: mmol/L<br>Neonate/Infant: 98–113<br>Child/Adult: 98–107 | Chloride concentrations generally follow those of sodium, and chloride imbalances are caused by the same conditions that affect sodium. Serum chloride levels are useful in differentiating acid-base disorders. |

| TABLE 12-4 | Blood Gases and Electrolyte Reference Ranges—cont'd | |
|---|---|---|
| **CLINICAL LABORATORY TEST** | **NORMAL REFERENCE RANGE** | **IMPLICATIONS FOR REHABILITATION** |
| Calcium (Total)<br>Specimen: Serum or heparinized plasma | Unit: mg/dL<br>Adult: 8.6–10.2 | Total calcium is a measurement of both protein-bound and unbound or free calcium. Free calcium exists in its ionized form in blood. |
| Calcium (Free Ionized)<br>Specimen: Serum or heparinized plasma | Unit: mg/dL<br>Adult: 4.6–5.3 | Free ionized calcium is the biologically active form. Due to the risk of cardiac arrhythmias, cardiac arrest, and tetany, the therapist should consult the treating physician and carefully plan treatments when calcium levels are outside the reference range. Blood pressure, respiratory rate, heart rhythm, and heart rate must be closely monitored. |
| Magnesium (Total)<br>Specimen: Serum | Unit: mg/dL<br>Neonate: 1.5–2.2<br>Child: 1.7–2.2<br>Adult: 1.6–2.6 | Total magnesium is a measurement of both protein-bound and unbound or free magnesium. Free magnesium exists in its ionized form in blood. |
| Magnesium (Free Ionized)<br>Specimen: Serum | Unit: mmol/L<br>0.45–0.60 | Free ionized magnesium is the biologically active form. Due to the risk of cardiac arrhythmias, cardiac arrest, and tetany, the therapist should consult the treating physician and carefully plan treatments when magnesium levels are outside the reference range. Blood pressure, respiratory rate, heart rhythm, and heart rate must be closely monitored. |

compensatory respiratory responses when treating patients with these disorders.

Due to their volatile nature, analysis of blood gases requires proper specimen collection and handling. Samples must be analyzed immediately after collection or collected with minimal exposure to the atmosphere with arterial blood samples stored on ice until analyzed. Exposure of the specimen to the atmosphere, which has a higher concentration of oxygen and a lower concentration of carbon dioxide than blood, will falsely increase $PO_2$ and falsely decrease $PCO_2$. Placing the specimen on ice decreases cellular metabolism by the blood cells, which suppresses the production of lactic acid that can falsely lower pH. For these reasons, most facilities have blood gas analyzers at critical care points such as emergency rooms, operating rooms, and intensive care units where rapid and accurate blood gas analysis is essential. Clinical approximation of the oxygen saturation of hemoglobin can now be accomplished clinically using a noninvasive piece of equipment called a pulse-oximeter. The **pulse-oximeter** has a monitoring device that clips to the tip of the finger (with no punctures) and provides an approximation of oxygenation. It can even be used while a patient is exercising and is described in greater detail in Chapter 11.

**Electrolytes** are substances that dissociate into positively and negatively charged particles (ions) in body fluids. The positively charged electrolytes (cations) are sodium, potassium, magnesium, and calcium. The negatively charged electrolytes (anions) are chloride, bicarbonate, and phosphate. Disturbances in electrolyte homeostasis can result from excessive loss or gain of a particular electrolyte or from changes in patient hydration. Because sodium, potassium, calcium, and magnesium play such important roles in the conduction of nerve impulses and muscle contraction, alterations in the concentration of these electrolytes can have serious neural and motor consequences as summarized in Table 12-5.

## Hematology and Hemostasis

**Hematology** test results describe cellular blood composition while **hemostasis** measures provide information on clotting function of the blood. Laboratory results and clinical implications from both of these areas are summarized in Table 12-6. The complete blood count (CBC) is one of the most commonly ordered laboratory tests and is used for the detection, diagnosis, and monitoring of anemias (focus on red blood cell count), infections and leukemias (with focus on white blood cells), systemic lupus erythematosus (SLE), and arthritic disorders. The erythrocyte (red blood cell) count, hematocrit, and hemoglobin are closely related test results that give information about erythropoiesis (erythrocyte production) and red blood cell health. Abnormal blood loss including hemorrhagic CVA, anemia due to deficiencies of iron or vitamins essential to erythropoiesis, and pathologies or drug treatments that inhibit erythropoiesis or increase hemolysis (erythrocyte destruction) can be measured as decreased red blood cell count, hematocrit, or hemoglobin. When anemia is caused by vitamin $B_{12}$ deficiency, the nervous system will also be affected, resulting in symptoms of parathesia, ataxia, muscle weakness, and spasticity.

**TABLE 12-5** Causes and Common Symptoms of Abnormal Serum Electrolytes

| ELECTROLYTE ABNORMALITY | COMMON CAUSES | COMMON SYMPTOMS |
|---|---|---|
| Hypernatremia (high sodium) | Dehydration | Primarily neurological, including tremors, irritability, ataxia, confusion, convulsions, and coma |
| Hyponatremia (low sodium) | Excessive water intake, renal dysfunction, alkalosis, diarrhea, excessive sweating, certain diuretics, prolonged vomiting, and adrenal insufficiency | Nausea, muscle weakness, and mental confusion |
| Hyperkalemia (high potassium) | Renal dysfunction, acidosis, intestinal obstruction, and trauma | Mental confusion, weakness, flaccid paralysis of the extremities, cardiac arrhythmias, and cardiac arrest |
| Hypokalemia (low potassium) | Renal dysfunction, alkalosis, malnutrition, diarrhea, excessive sweating, certain diuretics, vomiting, and glucocorticoid or mineralocorticoid excess | Muscle weakness, irritability, paralysis, cardiac arrhythmias, and cardiac arrest |
| Hypercalcemia (high calcium)* | Primary hyperparathyroidism, malignancies, and thyroid hormone disorders | Decreased neuromuscular excitability including drowsiness, lethargy, irritability, confusion, muscle weakness, GI disturbances, and cardiac arrest |
| Hypocalcemia (low calcium)* | | Increased neuromuscular excitability including anxiety, hallucinations, muscle spasms, paresthesia, GI disturbances, hypotension, clotting disorders, and cardiac arrhythmias |
| Hypermagnesemia (high magnesium) | | Depression of the neuromuscular system |
| Hypomagnesemia (low magnesium) | | Increased neuromuscular excitability |

*Serum concentrations of calcium and magnesium are interrelated and tightly regulated. Calcium regulates plasma membrane permeability and excitability and thereby neuromuscular activity. Like calcium, magnesium plays a role in regulating neuromuscular excitability, and imbalances in serum magnesium have symptoms similar to those seen with calcium.

**TABLE 12-6** Hematology and Hemostasis Reference Ranges

| CLINICAL LABORATORY TEST | NORMAL REFERENCE RANGE (Reference 3) | IMPLICATIONS FOR REHABILITATION |
|---|---|---|
| Red blood cells (RBCs) Specimen: EDTA-uncoagulated whole blood | Unit: RBCs/μL<br>Neonate: $3.2–6.1 \times 10^6$<br>Infant/Child: $3.4–5.4 \times 10^6$<br>Adult male: $4.6–6.0 \times 10^6$<br>Adult female: $4.2–5.4 \times 10^6$ | Decreased RBC counts are often seen in conjunction with decreased hemoglobin and oxygen transport capacity, resulting in reduced oxygen delivery to tissues (anemia) and decreased exercise tolerance. Exercise may need to be limited, depending on the degree of anemia. Patients with increased RBC counts due to polycythemia have an increased risk of thrombosis, stroke, and MI, and treatment should be planned based on the etiology of the polycythemia. |
| White blood cells (WBCs) Specimen: EDTA-uncoagulated whole blood | Unit: WBCs/μL<br>Neonate: $5.0–37.0 \times 10^3$<br>Infant/Child: $4.5–18.0 \times 10^3$<br>Adult: $4.5–11.5 \times 10^3$ | Adults with low WBC counts are at risk for nosocomial infections, and strict adherence to Standard Precautions is mandatory. If a low WBC count is accompanied by fever, exercise is not permitted (Garritan et al, 1995). Elevated white blood cell count may indicate presence of infection. |

| TABLE 12-6 | Hematology and Hemostasis Reference Ranges—cont'd | |
|---|---|---|
| **CLINICAL LABORATORY TEST** | **NORMAL REFERENCE RANGE** (Reference 3) | **IMPLICATIONS FOR REHABILITATION** |
| Platelets<br>Specimen: EDTA-uncoagulated whole blood | Unit: platelets/μL<br>150–350 × 10³ | Due to the risk of spontaneous bleeding, exercise is not permitted in patients with platelet counts less than 20,000. Light to moderate resistive exercises are permitted when platelet counts are between 20,000 and 50,000. Patients with thrombocytosis due to polycythemia have an increased risk of thrombosis, stroke, and MI, and treatment should be planned based on the etiology of the polycythemia (Garritan et al, 1995). |
| Hemoglobin (Hgb)<br>Specimen: EDTA-uncoagulated whole blood | Unit: g/dL<br>Neonate: 12.2–21.5<br>Infant/Child: 9.6–16.4<br>Adult male: 14.0–18.0<br>Adult female: 12.0–15.0 | Exercise is not permitted in patients with Hgb concentrations less than 8 g/dL. Exercise should be restricted in patients with Hgb values between 8 and 10 g/dL (Garritan et al, 1995). |
| Hematocrit (Hct)<br>Specimen: EDTA-uncoagulated whole blood | Unit: % blood volume<br>Neonate: 38–68<br>Infant/Child: 32–51<br>Adult male: 40–54<br>Adult female: 35–49 | The percentage of total blood volume occupied by RBCs. Exercise is not permitted when the Hct is less than 25%. Exercise should be restricted in patients with Hct values between 25% and 30% (Garritan et al, 1995). |
| Erythrocyte Sedimentation Rate (ESR)<br>Specimen: EDTA-uncoagulated whole blood | Unit: mm/hour<br>Male: 0–15<br>Female: 0–20 | The ESR is used to monitor the course and treatment of many inflammatory and autoimmune disorders such as RA and SLE. The ESR usually decreases with improvement in the patient's condition. |
| Prothrombin Time (PT)<br>Specimen: Citrate-uncoagulated whole blood | Unit: seconds<br>12.6–14.6 | Increased PT values are an indication of decreased clotting ability. Due to the risk of spontaneous bleeding, therapy is contraindicated when the PT is longer than 35 seconds. |

Increases in red cell count, hematocrit, and hemoglobin can be seen with dehydration, polycythemia vera, drug-stimulated erythropoiesis, and conditions where there is reduced oxygen availability such as living at high altitude or chronic pulmonary or cardiac insufficiency. An increase in leukocyte (white blood cells) count, **leukocytosis**, can be seen with acute infection, inflammation, tissue damage, necrosis, and leukemia. In a **differential count** of a hematology report, the laboratory will report what percentage of white blood cells are lymphocytes, neutrophils, monocytes, basophils, and eosinophils, respectively. An increased neutrophil percentage on the differential count most likely implicates a bacterial source of infection. Decreased leukocyte counts are seen with chronic infections, diabetes, bone marrow deficiencies, autoimmune diseases, and immunodeficiency, including side effects of chemotherapy. Thrombocytes (platelets) initiate the clotting process, so alterations in platelet count or platelet function can impair hemostasis. A low platelet count (**thrombocytopenia**) predisposes the patient to bleeding, including hemorrhagic CVA, whereas a high platelet count (**thrombocytosis**) predisposes the patient to abnormal intravascular clotting, including thrombotic CVA. Clotting studies, including bleeding times and prothrombin times, are used to determine the patient's ability to initiate and form blood clots, identify hereditary clotting factor deficiencies, and to monitor anticoagulant drug therapy.

## Immunology

Many neuromuscular diseases have pathology caused by abnormal immune responses leading to the production of immunoglobulins (antibodies) that target and damage components of CNS neurons, peripheral nerves, muscle cells, and other organs, even host DNA itself. Immunoglobulins produced against a patient's own cellular antigens are known as **autoantibodies**. Neuromuscular myopathies associated with autoantibodies include myasthenia gravis (MG) and Lambert-Eaton myasthenic syndrome. Neuromuscular neuropathies associated with autoantibodies include amyotrophic lateral sclerosis (ALS) and multiple sclerosis (MS). In addition to autoantibodies directed toward specific cell antigens, antibodies nonspecific or directed toward unknown antigens (M-proteins) can cause polyneuropathy. Examples of these disorders include rheumatoid arthritis (RA) and SLE. Rehabilitative therapies for patients who have autoimmune neuromuscular diseases must be planned according to the type of disease, the severity of symptoms, and the rate of disease progression.

## Molecular Diagnostics

Clinical laboratory molecular diagnostics is an emerging and rapidly growing specialized laboratory area. After the discovery of the DNA molecular structure in 1953, scientists learned that DNA controls the flow of biological information from one generation to the next, and thus the field of modern genetics was born. The advent of methods used to study DNA, such as DNA sequencing in the 1970s and the polymerase chain reaction (PCR) to amplify DNA molecules in 1983, made it feasible to apply this knowledge to clinical genetic analyses. Nucleic acid technologies were first applied in the clinical laboratory in the area of microbiology where they enable more rapid identification of infectious microorganisms than traditional methods. Complete sequencing of a human genome was accomplished in 2003, opening the door to human genetic analysis. Human genetic analysis was initially confined to research laboratories and the identification of diseases caused by mutations in a single gene, but the recent development of high-throughput and low-cost DNA sequencing has enabled both clinical genetic analysis of individuals and large-scale genetic studies. Large-scale human studies have led to the identification of multiple gene combinations linked to predispositions for developing diseases that previously had unknown or complex etiologies such as diabetes and cancer. It is now widely accepted that most, if not all, human diseases have a genetic component. Many forms of muscular dystrophy are now known to be caused by inherited genetic traits, and it is highly probable that the genes or gene combinations responsible for these and many other neuromuscular diseases will be identified in the near future. Two of the most promising treatments for human genetic disease, gene therapy and stem cell therapy, will rely heavily on clinical molecular diagnostics.

In contrast to molecular diagnostics, which analyzes small segments of DNA, older genetic analysis techniques, such as karyotyping, examine gross abnormalities in DNA at the chromosome level. Chromosomal abnormalities caused by deletion, rearrangement, or duplication of normal chromosomes often cause genetic disorders with serious mental and physical disabilities as exhibited in conditions such as Down syndrome.

## Microbiology

Test results from the microbiology laboratory can provide therapists with information about the type of microorganisms causing an infection in the nervous system and other organ systems. The most common types of microbiology tests are gram stains, cultures, and antibiotic susceptibility tests. **Gram stains** enable rapid general identification of bacteria under the microscope based on color and shape of the bacterium. Gram-positive organisms stain blue and gram-negative organisms stain red. Shapes may include "cocci," which is a sphere, or "bacilli," which is a rod-shaped

bacterium. Staining also emphasizes elements of bacterial cell morphology, which also helps with identification. Definitive identification of bacteria can be accomplished by one of two techniques: (1) culture on special growth media along with biochemical testing or (2) PCR amplification of unique DNA sequences. Antibiotic susceptibility tests are performed on bacterial cultures and provide information about what type of antibiotic will be most effective in treating the infection by a specific organism. Due to the prevalence of drug-resistant bacteria (e.g. *Staphylococcus aureus, Clostridium difficile,* and *Pseudomonas aeruginosa*) in the clinical setting, therapists should always follow Standard Precautions to prevent self-inoculation and the transmission of infectious organisms to and between other patients or the general public. This is particularly important when treating patients who are immunocompromised. When treating patients, the therapist should note the presence and appearance of any pus or fluid exuding from deep wounds, surgical incisions, abscesses, or lesions and notify the treating physician.

## Nonblood Body Fluids

Test results from nonblood body fluids as outlined in Table 12-7 are often correlated with blood test results to provide additional information about patient pathologies.

## THINK ABOUT IT 12.1

Given the case at the beginning of the chapter:

- What chemistry labs would be important to track with Celene?
- What symptoms might trigger the need for further testing and referral?
- How might the results affect your therapy?

## Clinical Laboratory Testing Summary

Many resources available through the Internet can aid the rehabilitative therapist in understanding and evaluating clinical laboratory test results. One such resource is a website provided jointly by several professional clinical laboratory science and pathology organizations at www.labtestsonline.org.

**Disclaimer:** Recommendations for therapy based on abnormal laboratory test results are for reference only and should not be used in place of established protocols and guidelines at the therapist's treatment facility.

## ■ Diagnostic Imaging

Since Wilhelm Conrad Roentgen first discovered x-rays and their effects in 1895, phenomenal development has arisen out of the original field of x-ray radiography. Now radiology has grown into the broader and more complex field of **diagnostic imaging**, a term including the entire array of diagnostic imaging methods discussed in this section, some of which are computer-based, to create a view of a particular aspect of

| TABLE 12-7 | Nonblood Body Fluids Analysis | |
|---|---|---|
| **BODY FLUID** | **ANALYSES** | **IMPLICATIONS FOR REHABILITATION** |
| **Urine**<br>Specimen: Clean catch for general analysis. An In/Out catheter specimen may be necessary in females for uncontaminated culture.<br>Note: Timed collection of a urine specimen is required for direct determination of creatinine clearance and glomerular filtration rate. | Physical: Specific gravity, color, clarity, odor, and foaming<br>Chemical: pH, electrolytes, glucose, total protein, creatinine, ketones, hemoglobin/myoglobin, hormones, and drugs<br>Microscopic: Cellular components (RBCs, WBCs, epithelial cells, and bacteria), precipitates, and renal casts<br>Culture and sensitivity | Urinalysis test results are commonly used for the assessment of general health and the detection of renal and metabolic disorders. The presence of RBCs, WBCs, and bacteria are indicative of urinary tract infection and/or inflammation. Culture and sensitivity would help identify optimal antibiotic therapy. The presence of glucose (glucosuria) and ketones (ketonuria) are indicative of uncontrolled diabetes mellitus. |
| **Cerebrospinal Fluid**<br>Note: Numbness or tingling in the lower extremities, bleeding, or continued CSF leakage from the puncture site must be reported immediately to the attending health-care professional. | Physical: Color and clarity<br>Chemical: pH, electrolytes, glucose, lactic acid, total protein, immunoglobulins, and enzymes<br>Microscopic: Cellular components<br>Culture and sensitivity | Analysis of CSF is performed to diagnose CNS infections (e.g., meningitis), CNS malignancies, and inflammatory neuropathies. Symptoms of infectious meningitis can include sensory dysfunction, decreased arousal, impaired motor function, and impaired range of motion. Therapists must observe isolation procedures as required. It is essential the therapist be familiar with the acute, subacute, and chronic phases of infection associated with the type of organism causing the meningitis and may be called upon to rehabilitate resulting neurological impairments. Monitoring of patient vital signs is recommended during the acute phase. |
| **Synovial Fluid** | Physical: Color, clarity, viscosity<br>Microscopic: Cellular components, crystalline precipitates (e.g., uric acid in gout)<br>Culture and sensitivity | Analysis of synovial fluid is used to determine the cause of joint effusion and follow the progression of joint diseases. Elevated WBC counts are seen immediately after joint surgery and when there is infection and/or inflammation. Joint pain, swelling, and fever are indicators of infection and should result in referral to the physician. The therapist should apply ice and pressure to the joint to reduce pain, swelling, and excess fluid accumulation. |
| **Pleural Fluid**<br>Note: Bleeding or continued leakage of fluid from the puncture site or any onset of shortness of breath must be reported immediately to the attending healthcare professional. | Physical: Color, clarity<br>Chemical: Glucose, total protein, enzymes<br>Microscopic: Cellular components<br>Culture and sensitivity | Analysis of pleural fluid is performed to aid in the diagnosis of inflammatory and neoplastic diseases of the lung and pleura. If the patient doesn't exhibit dyspnea after collection of the pleural fluid, therapies not involving physical manipulation of the chest or thorax may be started 1 hour after the puncture site has closed. The therapist should monitor patient vital signs and assess breathing for possible pneumothorax. |
| **Peritoneal Fluid**<br>Note: Bleeding or continued leakage of fluid from the puncture site must be reported immediately to the attending health-care professional. | Physical: Color, clarity<br>Chemical: Glucose, total protein, enzymes, lipids<br>Microscopic: Cellular components<br>Culture and sensitivity | Analysis of peritoneal fluid is performed to determine the cause of peritoneal effusions. After collection of the peritoneal fluid, the therapist should monitor patient vital signs and be alert for signs of hypotension if a large volume of fluid was removed from the patient. |

internal structure of the human body. The terms medical imaging and body imaging are also sometimes used. For the purposes of therapists in neuromuscular settings, important types of imaging include plain radiographs (commonly, but inaccurately, called "x-rays"), nuclear medicine, CAT scans, ultrasound examinations, and **magnetic resonance imaging (MRI)**. Just as one would not use a hammer to turn a screw because it is not the appropriate tool, each of these types of examination should be considered a specialized tool, intended for a specific task or set of tasks. Common views and sections/slices for diagnostic images of the nervous system are summarized in Table 12-8. The specific types of diagnostic imaging useful in neurology along with some specific abnormalities that each might detect are summarized in Table 12-9 and discussed in the next section.

## Types of Imaging Examinations

Conventional plain **radiographs**, up until recently, were performed by exposing a body part to medical quality, diagnostic level radiation and recording the image on a film. The subject is exposed to a source of x-radiation with the subject as close as possible to the film or image receptor that detects the image. Because more dense tissues—bone, for example—attenuate the radiation and prevent it from reaching the film, bone and other metallic densities appear white. Tissues with progressively less attenuation (i.e., soft tissue, fat, and air being the least) show as darker areas on radiographs with air-filled spaces being black. Generally, there is no further processing of the image data. The advent of the digital computer and its ability to store large amounts of information and access the information rapidly has changed how conventional radiographic images are stored and displayed. Computerized storage and display of images is rapidly replacing film as the method of choice for recording and displaying conventional plain radiographs.

Properly speaking, "**x-rays**" are the form of radiation energy arising from the x-ray tube, not the image that results. The "film" or image receptor is the device upon which the latent image is detected, recorded, and displayed. The radiograph is the picture or image that develops on the film. This distinction is important because shorthand terminology used in a hospital setting is sometimes confusing with "x-rays" often used in a colloquial sense for "radiographs." Although not precise, "x-ray" is incorrectly but commonly used.

Since the 1990s, the ability to record images on an electronic detector has become commonplace. The image is then transferred from the detector onto a storage device such as a hard disk drive. Nowadays, a computer with a network connection to the image storage and a computer display quite often is all that is needed to view images. This type of arrangement is known as PACS, which is an acronym for Picture Archival and Communications System. In addition to the storage and display of conventional radiographs, PACS is also used to store images obtained by computed tomography (CT), MRI, nuclear medicine, ultrasound, and other specialized imaging techniques.

Conventional plain film radiography has little use in the evaluation of neurological disease and trauma, other than for detection of fractures, for example, of the spine and skull. CT and MRI have largely superseded the use of plain film radiographs in evaluation of the central nervous system, brain, and spinal cord.

**Computed tomography (CT),** also called CAT scan, is obtained by using a source of x-radiation that is rotated

| TABLE 12-8 | **Summary of Common Nervous System Diagnostic Imaging Views and Sections** |
|---|---|
| **NAME OF IMAGING VIEW** | **DESCRIPTION** |
| Plain Radiographs: | |
| Anterior/Posterior (AP) | A composite view that reflects all tissue between the source and the plate. The x-rays or other energy form pass through the body in sagittal plane, from posterior to anterior to strike the film on the other side. |
| Lateral | A composite view that reflects all tissue between the source and the plate. The x-rays pass from one side through the body to strike the film on the other side. |
| CAT, MRI, PET: | |
| Coronal sections | A planar view or **image** of the part being studied as if a slice had been made in the frontal plane, dividing the part into front and back pieces. The view is as if you are standing in front of the person, top is top, bottom is bottom, left is left, right is right. |
| Horizontal sections | A planar view or image of the part being studied as if a slice had been made in the transverse (horizontal) plane, cutting through it horizontally in top and bottom pieces. The view is as if the patient is supine and you are "viewing from the feet" so anterior is at the top of the image, posterior is at the bottom of the image, the patient's right side is at your left hand and the patient's left side is at your right hand. |
| Sagittal/parasagittal sections | A planar view or image of the part being studied as if a slice had been made in the sagittal plane, cutting it into right and left pieces. |

**TABLE 12-9** **Types of Diagnostic Imaging and Applications in Neurology**

| EXAMINATION TYPE | ENERGY TYPE | IMAGE RECEPTOR | BEST FOR IMAGING | APPLICATIONS IN NEUROLOGY |
|---|---|---|---|---|
| Plain radiograph (original modality) | x-ray tube radiation | Plain film or flat panel | Bones and joints, chest, abdomen, sinuses | Injury and fractures, pneumonia, sinusitis, abdominal pain |
| Ultrasound | High frequency sound waves above the range of human ear | Computer screen; images stored in a file | Mainly liquid imaging (blood, cyst fluid) | Antenatal and neonatal brain hemorrhage, prenatal congenital anomaly imaging |
| Computed Tomography | x-ray tube radiation | Computer screen; images stored in a file | Physical density of matter in the body; much more sensitive than plain radiographs | In brain, bony abnormalities in spine and skull, follow-up of MRI-diagnosed abnormalities, implanted prostheses. Also used when MRI cannot be used (e.g., presence of aneurysm clips, pacemaker, etc.) |
| MRI | Radiofrequency energy and a magnetic field | Computer screen; images stored in a file | Characteristics of protons in atomic nuclei and the milieu in which they are contained such as water, fat, blood, etc. | Brain tumors, small infarctions, unusual brain infections, tiny metastases, small /tiny areas of brain scarring or focal loss of brain tissue |
| PET and PET/CT | Positron emission with or without concurrent CT | Computer screen; images stored in file | Reflects metabolic rate of tissue (at present) | Detect metastatic and primary cancer; detect areas of increased or decreased metabolism seen in dementia |

around the patient for at least a 360-degree rotation and, like radiographs, also presents a visual image of relative tissue densities in the target tissue. The image receptor, located approximately 180 degrees opposite the x-ray source, is called a detector and rotates opposite the source of x-radiation around the patient. The detector measures the intensity of the received radiation and, using a complex set of algorithms running on a specialized computer, reconstructs an image of a section or "slice" of the part being studied then displays the resulting image. The information displayed, which is encoded as shades of gray on the image, reflects the varying physical densities of the subject. The source of the varying densities reflects interaction of the x-radiation with the electrons in the atoms of the patient. Because the image is computer-generated and the shades of gray arbitrarily assigned, it is possible to vary how the shades of gray are used to display the various densities in the patient. Because of this exquisite control and adjustment, visualization and analysis of very subtle differences is possible with CT (see Fig.12-1), including density of soft tissues and bone that cannot be appreciated on a conventional radiograph. In general, dense "hyperattenuated" tissue, including bone and other metallic densities, appear white and low-density tissues like fat and air both appear as dark areas. Structures with the density of water, such as muscle tissue, appear gray. Acute CNS bleeding appears as bright areas on CT

whereas water and cerebrospinal fluid (CSF) show up as dark black. One way to tell a brain CT scan from an MRI image is that the CT scan image (see Fig. 12-1 for CT and Fig. 12-2 for MRI) will have the cortex immediately adjacent to the inner surface of the "bright" skull bone without any apparent space between them.

For magnetic resonance imaging (MRI), the source of energy is radiofrequency, the same energy form used to transmit sound to your automobile radio, instead of x-radiation. MRI, therefore, eliminates the risk associated with exposure to ionizing radiation. Rather, this type of imaging is obtained by analysis of signals arising from within the patient. The patient is placed in a strong magnetic field created by a series of superconducting electromagnets. This magnetic field causes many of the protons of atomic nuclei within the patient to align themselves with the magnetic field. A source of radiofrequency energy is then applied and the alignment of the protons is changed in a predictable manner, changing the axis of proton rotation by 90°. When the radiofrequency energy is turned off, the protons, under the influence of the magnetic field, return to their position of alignment with the field. In so doing, they give off radiofrequency energy that can be detected by a metal coil, which serves as a type of "antenna." The radiofrequency energy produces signals in the metal coil, which are then analyzed by a computer to build up a "slice"

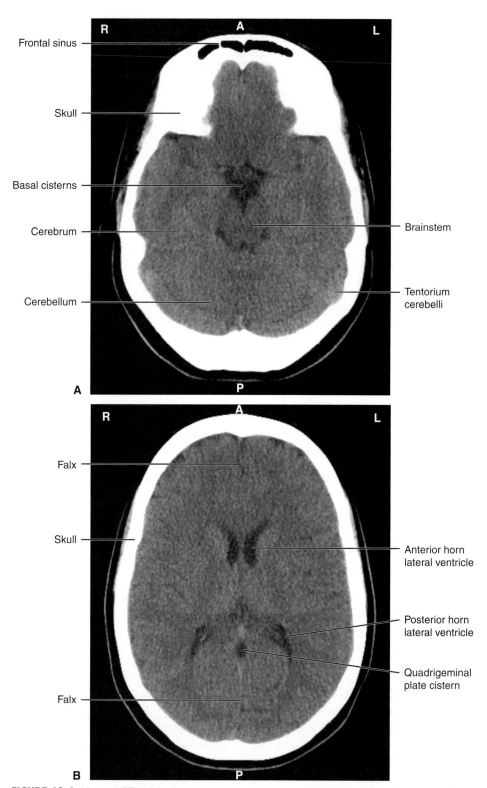

**FIGURE 12-1** Normal CTs of the brain without intravenous contrast. The patient is viewed as if he is supine on the CT table and viewed from the feet. Thus, the patient's right is to the viewer's left, and the patient's left is on the viewer's right. **A.** Axial/horizontal plane image at level of cerebellum and cerebrum. **B.** Axial image more superiorly located at level of lateral ventricles and mainly cerebrum. (A = Anterior, P = Posterior, I = Inferior, S = Superior, R = Right, L = Left)

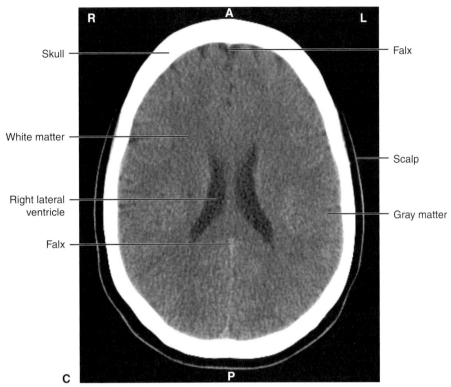

**FIGURE 12-1—cont'd  C.** Axial image at level of centrum semiovale. Observe the detail in the images. This type of detail and clarity is available everyday for evaluation of central nervous system structures. (A = Anterior, P = Posterior, I = Inferior, S = Superior, R = Right, L = Left)

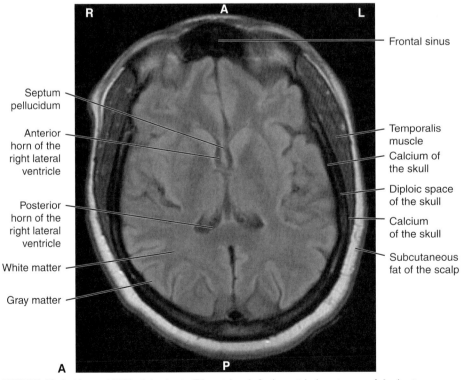

**FIGURE 12-2**  Normal MRI of the brain, T1 weighted. **A.** An axial plane image of the brain.

*Continued*

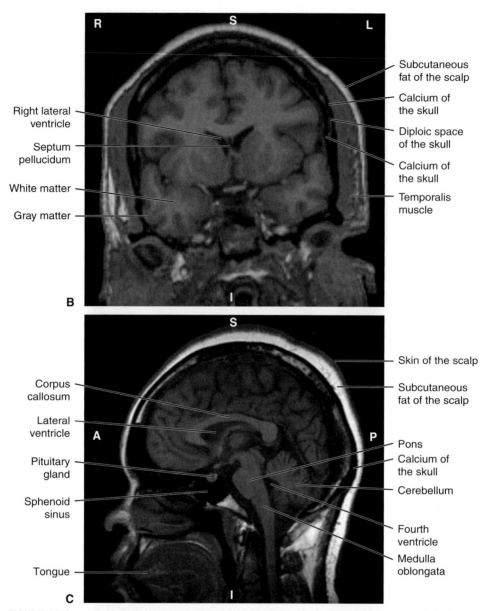

**FIGURE 12-2—cont'd B.** A coronal plane image of the brain. **C.** A sagittal plane image of the brain. Notice the exquisite detail provided by MRI. Because MRI uses electromagnetic radiation, there is no signal to be detected from ionic crystals. The calcium and bone forms an ionic crystal, and therefore yields no signal. The higher the signal level, the brighter the object. On T-1 weighted images like these, fat appears very bright. A very large percentage of the human brain is made up of fatty acids. Thus the brain is visible, and the subcutaneous fat is very bright. (A = Anterior, P = Posterior, I = Inferior, S = Superior, R = Right, L = Left)

image of the patient. The advantage of MRI is the parameters of the examination can be varied so structures not visible on CT are visible on MRI. The disadvantage is the MRI is extremely sensitive to motion, which limits its usage for imaging of moving body parts, heart, lungs, etc., and because of specialized setup, it is often not available after hours. MRI is very useful in examining soft tissues and can reveal the subtle changes, which are invisible to conventional x-radiation. Because of this sensitivity, MRI is very useful in the examination of the soft tissues of the neurological and skeletal/muscular system with great detail as well as soft tissues involved with

the joints. You can recognize an MRI of the brain by the band of dark space between the inner skull and the cortex surface in an MRI (Fig. 12-2) compared with CT (Fig. 12-1). There are a number of different types of MRI techniques, summarized in Table 12-10, often named by a variety of acronyms that are often vendor specific.

**Diagnostic ultrasound** examinations use sound frequencies as the energy source and capture the reflected sound to generate an image of the soft tissue being examined. Diagnostic ultrasound is used less frequently in neuromuscular imaging except in the fetal ultrasound examination during pregnancy

| TABLE 12-10 | **Common Types of MRI** |
|---|---|

**T1**

(Fat is bright*); Provides the best visual definition of the anatomy. If using gadolinium "Gad" contrast with T1, pathology will be bright, but you need a precontrast T1 to detect the difference.

**T2**

(Water is bright); Pathology is usually brighter on T2 compared with T1 because it has higher water content than surrounding normal tissue. CSF is also bright.

Use of both T1 and T2 sequences can distinguish blood from other pathology, and provide an estimate of the acuity of the bleed.

**FLAIR**

While similar to T2, the signal from CSF is suppressed, so a bright spot is a specific pathology and not just bright CSF, as would be seen on T2.

**STIR**

Similar to T2 fat-saturated sequence, the fat becomes dark but by a different mechanism. Useful for study of bones: because the bone marrow (mostly fat) becomes dark, pathology of bone will usually be bright in obvious contrast.

*"Bright" means tissue appears "hyperintense" compared with gray matter.

and cranial ultrasound of the **neonate** or young child. Cranial ultrasound is very useful to detect structural and developmental problems in brain and other CNS structures. Ultrasound is incapable of penetrating bone. Therefore, its utility in evaluation of the brain is limited to children whose anterior or posterior fontanelles have not yet closed.

Of all the imaging methods discussed so far—conventional radiographs, ultrasound, CT, and MRI—all of them depend on the transmission of some sort of signal through the body where the signal originates somewhere outside of the human body. These imaging methods are used mainly for imaging anatomic detail instead of physiological processes.

**Nuclear medicine** techniques, including **positron emission tomography (PET),** image radioactive substances within the body. Nuclear imaging is unique in that it allows visualization of physiological processes over time rather than just focusing on anatomic detail. In nuclear medicine, images are obtained by recording photons emitted by nuclear disintegration within a substance. Usually, the substance undergoing nuclear decay is chemically bound to a molecule or other moiety that the body uses in some specific way after it has been administered to the patient. For example, in the case of thyroid imaging, radioactive iodine is administered to the patient, which is taken up by the thyroid gland. This uptake of radioactive iodine can then be used to monitor the functional state of the thyroid gland as well as forming an image of the tissue comprising the gland. For example, normally functioning thyroid tissue takes up iodine whereas

most cancers of the thyroid gland do not take up iodine. Most cancers of the thyroid gland can thus be identified by the lack of function of the local area of cancerous tissue within the gland.

## Conventional Radiographs

Conventional radiographs, the original and most basic mode of using x-rays, serve best to provide images of bony structure. A variety of alternate terms are used for the pictures obtained: films, x-rays, pictures, or radiographic images. Because of their inherently high contrast with the soft tissues of the human body, radiographs have great value in providing images of the bones and their intervening joints. Conventional radiographs of the bones are used to determine their developmental structure, alignment (which can be altered as a secondary impairment after any neurological disorder or injury) and bony integrity, the nature and size of the intervening joints spaces, and a few associated soft tissue findings.

However, radiographs, as two-dimensional representations of a three-dimensional object, can be somewhat deceptive. Therefore, it is necessary to obtain at least two radiographs of a structure to "build up" a truer picture of the 3-D structure undergoing examination. Usually these images will be obtained at 90 degrees to each other. The observer of the radiographs then goes through a mental process of constructing the three-dimensional relationships of the imaged objects when viewing two perpendicular radiographs. When only one view or one plane is considered, it is easy to get a false idea of the true state in the patient. For instance, a single view of a fractured bone may show both fragments to be in good alignment on that particular view. However, when one looks at the 90-degree view, it can become apparent the bone segments are, in fact, grossly out of alignment. Be careful to always consider a single radiograph as a potential "liar" in this context. In neurology, plain radiographs may contribute to detecting fractures of the skull and the vertebrae as the bony cases of the brain and spinal cord.

## Diagnostic Ultrasound: Cranial and Fetal Applications

Diagnostic **fetal ultrasound** performed during pregnancy can evaluate the health of the developing and growing baby in utero and visually present the structural integrity of the child's spine and brain as well as the extremities. From a movement/developmental standpoint, current ultrasound equipment, including 4-D ultrasound, even allows detailed real-time viewing of fetal movements in the womb 2 weeks earlier than 2-D ultrasound (Kurjak, 2002). Fetal movements can be observed as early as 8 weeks gestation (the sixth week of pregnancy) for trunk movement and 9 weeks gestation (the seventh week of pregnancy) for individual limb movement (Shawker, 1980) and may be valuable to predict neonatal development (Birnholz, 1980). Neurological and developmental abnormalities that can be detected on fetal ultrasound include spina bifida (myelomeningocele), anencephaly, and some signs of

Down syndrome, to give the family and health-care team time to be optimally prepared for the transition.

To view brain structures, diagnostic **cranial ultrasound** can be performed in neonates and children as long as the anterior fontanelle is still open. The anterior fontanelle may remain open up to 4 to 24 months of age. Cranial ultrasound is particularly helpful to detect structural abnormalities of the hemispheres, cerebellum, and brainstem in the neonate. Cranial ultrasound can detect **periventricular leukomalacia (PVL)**, necrosis, and scar formation with cysts in white matter adjacent to the lateral ventricles in premature infants, the degree of which is predictive of MRI changes in cerebral palsy (de Vries, 1993). PVL is a very strong predictor of disabling cerebral palsy in low birth-weight infants (Pinto-Martin, 1995). Cranial ultrasound is also very useful to document blockage of CSF flow and the resulting hydrocephalus and the degree of **intraventricular hemorrhage (IVH)**. IVH is quantified with grades I to IV, particularly in premature neonates, as a predictor of motor function (Patra, 2006; O'Shea, 2008).

## Computerized Tomography

The imaging of soft tissue structures, including brain and spinal cord, has improved greatly with development of CT and MRI. One early name for CT, when it was first used clinically in the early to mid-1970s, was digital axial tomography (DAT), which gives us a clue as to the method of obtaining images used in CT today. For a patient lying supine or prone on a table, a complete rotation of the tube and its detectors, with the patient at the center of rotation, obtains, in the form of digital measurements, the densities of a volume of a defined thickness. This data represents the measurements of the physical density of a "slice," as it were, of a patient.

The "slice" data is obtained perpendicular to the long axis of the body in the axial plane. This data is then used to build up a picture of a "slice" of the patient. The "slices" are oriented in much the same way as a slice of bread is related to the loaf of bread itself, that is, at a right angle to a line drawn through the long axis of the loaf of bread. Slice thickness can vary from less than 1 mm to 10 mm or more. The slices are obtained by using a digital computer to calculate the physical density of a volume element, or voxel, which is a specific small volume of tissue contained in the particular "slice." Then the computer calculates the precise location of the voxel in the slice. The picture of the slice is then made up of a large number of picture elements, pixels, of varying shades of gray projected on the monitor. Each pixel represents a voxel, and the particular shade of white, gray, or black assigned to the pixel represents the physical density of the voxel. The process of turning raw scanned data into an image or slice is called **reconstruction**. Although the same basic method is used today, the raw data used to calculate the density values and develop the final image is obtained much more quickly and reconstruction is much faster because of advances in the modern digital computer and the reconstruction software. In clinical practice today, the CT examination is obtained with ease. In the early 1970s, a CT scan of the brain might take as long as 20 minutes to obtain. In 2011, the same scan can be performed in about 2 to 5 seconds.

The primary advantages of CT, when compared with MRI, are that CT takes less time, is less expensive, and is more readily available. The speed of the CT examination means greater accuracy in patients who cannot be completely still or who cannot remain in a fixed position for very long. In a modern multidetector CT scanner, slices can be obtained in 30 seconds or less for a CT of the chest or abdomen and in 10 seconds or less for a brain CT. Another advantage of CT compared with MRI is shielding from radiofrequency energy and magnetic effects is not required. This allows patients who are on life support or who require other devices, which are electrically operated, including endocardial lead pacemakers or external monitors or pumps, to be readily examined in a safe manner by CT. MRI has other advantages and limitations that will be discussed in the MRI section.

### Neurological Evaluation With CT

CT examination of the brain is the primary imaging tool used in acute stroke and in acute brain trauma (Koenig, 1998). The CT readily detects fresh blood from intracerebral hemorrhage (Kalafut, 2000) and is very sensitive and specific for extracerebral blood collections, including subarachnoid blood (shown after head trauma in Fig. 12-3 and postsurgical brain decompression in Fig. 12-4) and subdural blood (Fig. 12-5) (Marshall, 1991). With the CT examination, the health-care team can identify the location and extent of the brain lesion and begin to formulate a treatment plan and develop the prognosis almost from the time of the patient's admission to the hospital. The CT examination is also accurate in differentiating old lesions from new lesions. In general, old lesions from injury to the brain heal as areas of encephalomalacia. On the CT examination, these areas appear darker than the surrounding normal brain.

**Encephalomalacia**, an area of softening of the brain (resulting from liquefactive necrosis) secondary to infarction or injury, will often be surrounded by an area of loss of brain matter and increase in the size of normal fluid containing spaces of the brain. The density of an area of encephalomalacia is about the same as the density in the center of a dilated ventricle filled with normal CSF. Blood from a fresh hemorrhage, on the other hand, is very bright, almost white as shown in Figure 12-5, and is often associated with edema or brain swelling, which causes the brain to enlarge and encroach upon the normal fluid containing space, sometimes even obliterating those spaces. The edema itself is usually an area of brain of lower density than the surrounding normal brain.

Stroke is an injury to the brain resulting from loss of blood flow to a specific area of the brain. The lack of blood flow deprives the affected area of the brain of oxygen and the area of cell death is called an infarction. In acute stroke, the area of infarction does not appear as a bright area on the CT of the brain. Immediately after the onset of symptoms,

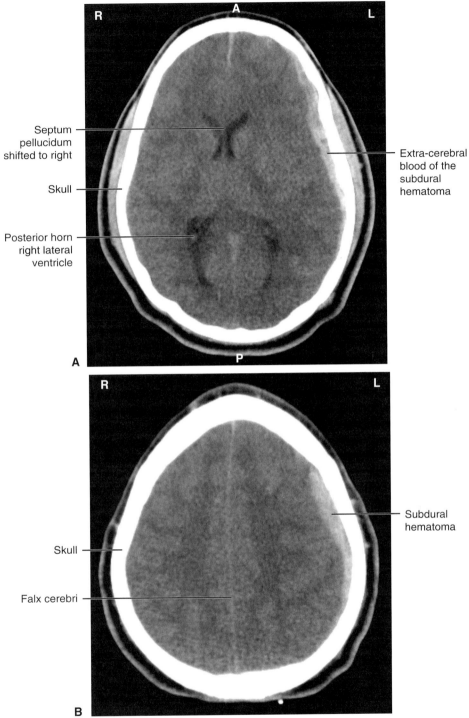

**FIGURE 12-3** Three CT images of the brain from a patient who had acute head trauma: **A.** axial plane, **B.** axial plane superior to image A, and **C.** coronal plane. These images show a subdural hematoma over the convexity of the left hemisphere of the brain. The grayish white area in each image is acute blood between the intensely white inner table of the skull and the left cerebral hemisphere, which is more gray-colored. Notice the slight deviation of the midline structures to the right caused by the space-occupying blood. Also notice the absence of the normal areas of low attenuation over the convexities of the brain, which normally represent CSF areas between sulci because of the large amount of pressure the subdural hematoma space exerts on the brain. Because the skull is solid bone, there is no way for the hematoma to expand away from the brain and it therefore compresses the brain matter.

*Continued*

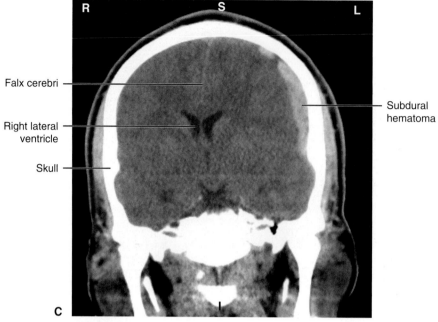

Falx cerebri

Right lateral ventricle

Skull

Subdural hematoma

C

**FIGURE 12-3—cont'd**

the injured area of the brain usually appears normal on CT (von Kummer, 2001). After a period of time, which is somewhat variable but is usually not more than 48 hours, the area of infarction begins to decrease in density, an area of hypoattenuation, on the CT examination as it becomes edematous in response to the brain injury (von Kummer, 2001). Serial CT examinations play a key role in determining the size and extent of the infarction. Knowing the location of the affected areas may be helpful in determining a specific focus of the

neuromuscular examination and specific components of the therapeutic intervention and can also provide information regarding the prognosis.

New and old stroke, intracerebral and extracerebral hemorrhage, and areas of old brain injury can be evaluated with brain CT examinations performed without intravenous contrast material. The injection of intravenous contrast material will sometimes help in the evaluation of acute stroke but has been partially supplanted by MRI examinations.

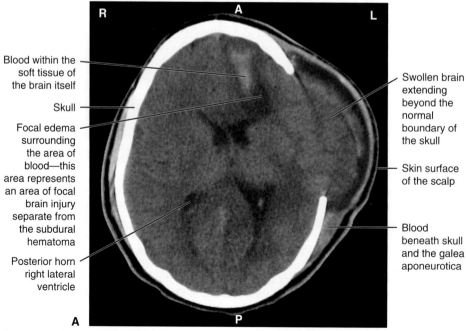

Blood within the soft tissue of the brain itself

Skull

Focal edema surrounding the area of blood—this area represents an area of focal brain injury separate from the subdural hematoma

Posterior horn right lateral ventricle

Swollen brain extending beyond the normal boundary of the skull

Skin surface of the scalp

Blood beneath skull and the galea aponeurotica

A

**FIGURE 12-4** CT images of the brain, postsurgical, for the same patient with head trauma shown in Figure 12-3. **A.** Axial plane image.

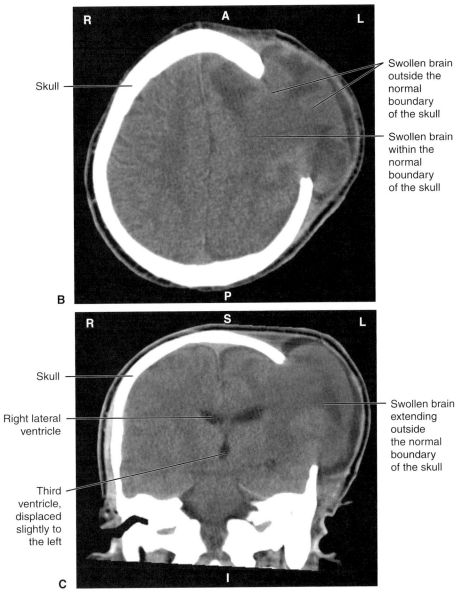

**FIGURE 12-4—cont'd B.** An axial plane image at a more superior level. **C.** Coronal plane image. A portion of the left side of the skull has been surgically removed. Note the expansion of the brain matter outside the normal boundaries of the skull and the bulging of the galea aponeurotica and the skin of the scalp superficial to it. The large area of low attenuation on the left, within what would be the normal bounds of the skull, represents edema of the brain. Compare this area with the right hemisphere to see the difference. The edema of the brain occurs as a result of the severe trauma of the left hemisphere. Imagine what damage would occur to the brain without allowing the brain to expand past the normal boundaries of the skull.

In the diagnosis and evaluation of brain tumors, both primary and metastatic, it is usually necessary to perform a CT of the brain without intravenous contrast followed by a CT examination of the brain with the injection of intravenous contrast material. The CT scans in Figure 12-6 provide examples of a brain tumor revealed by comparing brain CT with and without contrast. Different types of brain tumors will have patterns of enhancement after the injection of intravenous contrast material that sometimes make it possible to identify the type of tumor and surrounding area of brain edema. In recent years, MRI examination has become the major tool for diagnosing brain tumors (Schellinger, 1999). However, in some cases, CT is an excellent tool for follow-up of treatment of brain tumors once a definitive diagnosis by MRI has been obtained.

In some cases, CT is also an excellent tool for the detailed examination of bony structures and can supply more detail than routine radiographs. In addition, CT of the bone can

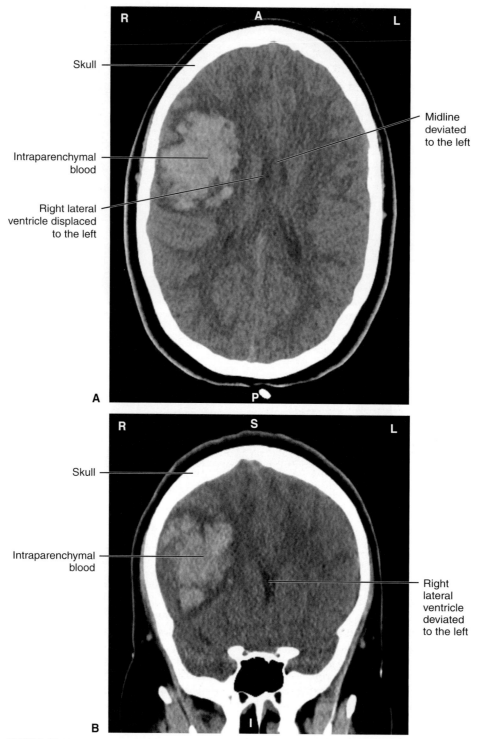

**FIGURE 12-5** CT showing intracerebral hemorrhage within the substance of the brain. **A.** Axial plane. **B.** Coronal plane.

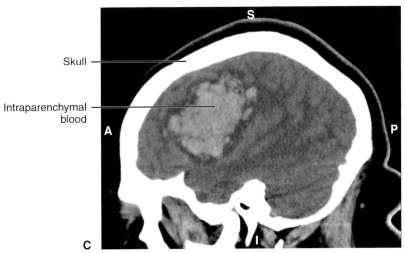

**FIGURE 12-5—cont'd  C.** Sagittal plane. The blood appears white and is surrounded by an area of low attenuation representing edema. Note the displacement of midline structures and ventricles to the left caused by the mass effect of the intracerebral hematoma.

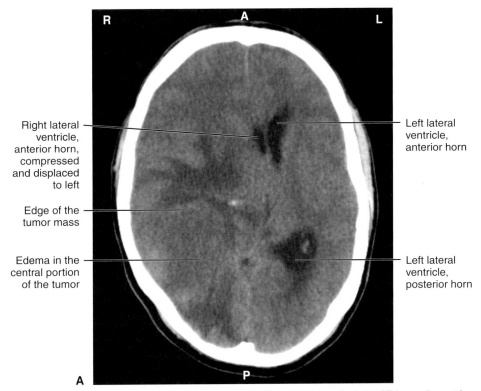

**FIGURE 12-6**  CT of the brain with a tumor in the right hemisphere. **A.** Axial CT brain slice with no intravenous contrast material given. Note the midline shift to the left so that the right lateral ventricle is to the left of the midline of the skull. Note also the compression of the right lateral ventricle compared with the left lateral ventricle, no sulci visible, and the low attenuation of the edema. The lack of visible sulci, the decrease in size of the right lateral ventricle, and the right to left shift of the midline brain structures is indicative of the large mass effect of the tumor, which is located in the right parietal occipital lobes. The edema is secondary to the tumor mass effect and extends into the temporal and frontal lobes.

*Continued*

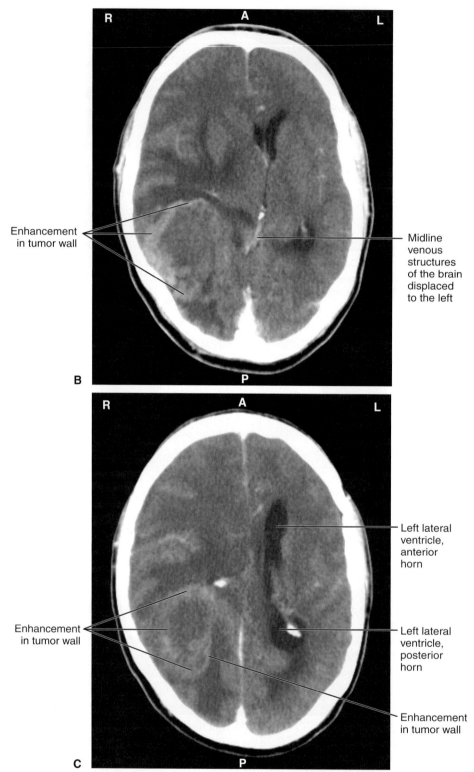

Enhancement in tumor wall

Midline venous structures of the brain displaced to the left

**B**

Left lateral ventricle, anterior horn

Enhancement in tumor wall

Left lateral ventricle, posterior horn

Enhancement in tumor wall

**C**

**FIGURE 12-6—cont'd B.** Same axial CT of the brain as seen in Figure 12-5A after administration of intravenous contrast material. Note the midline vascular structures that opacify with contrast material. Also note the opacification of a portion of the tumor outer wall. **C.** More superior axial CT slice of the brain closer to the vertex of the skull than in Figures 12-5A and 12-5B. Note how the wall of the tumor opacifies. Again note the extreme mass effect with no sulci visible because of compression of normal brain substance by the tumor.

be performed in a high-definition manner so reconstruction of the images in three planes can be performed, allowing the surgeon to better plan surgeries and to better choose which patients will benefit from surgery and which will not (e.g., Fig. 12-4).

## Magnetic Resonance Imaging

After the first MRI images were published in 1973 and the first MRI examination of a human being in 1977, MRI examinations were rapidly developed by 1987 into a very useful clinical tool. Although MRI examinations are currently a common clinical tool, MRI uses and the variety of examination types are still being researched and expanded. By comparison, conventional radiography has been used as a clinical tool for more than 110 years, and CT has been used as a clinical tool for more than 40 years.

MRI examinations are performed by placing the patient in a strong magnetic field, which causes a large percentage of the protons of atoms, usually in the nuclei of water, to align their axis of spin in the direction of the magnetic field. Radiofrequency energy is then applied to the patient to induce the protons in the atoms to change their axis of spin. When the radiofrequency energy is turned off, the protons then realign their spin axes with the applied magnetic field. In the process of realignment of the spin axes of the protons, radiofrequency energy is given off. This radiofrequency is then received by the scanner and is analyzed to determine intensity and location. The methods used for this analysis are beyond the scope of this book, but it is important to note that the nature of the MRI examination relies on energy emitted by the patient and not by energy transmitted through the patient, as is the case with conventional x-radiography and CT examinations.

Like CT, MRI units use the digital computer to analyze the energy emitted by the patient to provide the location and intensity information so a slice of the patient, representing a plane through the patient, can be reconstructed and displayed. The complexity of the analysis is an order of magnitude greater than required for CT examinations.

Because of the complexity of MRI methodology, MRI units must be shielded from external magnetic fields and external radiofrequency energy fields because the MRI unit produces its own magnetic and radiofrequency energy fields. Because of the sensitivity of the MRI units to externally produced magnetic and radiofrequency energy fields, the MRI examination is technically more limited in its application to critically ill patients who, of necessity, require multiple external electrical devices and to patients who have internally placed metallic, electromechanical, electrically operated, or radiofrequency devices such as pacemakers and defibrillators. Figure 12-7 is an MRI of the head with intravenous contrast material that demonstrates a brain tumor.

The utility of MRI, in evaluation of the neurological system (see Figs. 12-2, 12-7, 12-8) and the soft tissues of the musculoskeletal system, is unsurpassed by any other imaging

modality. By using special techniques to vary the timing of the externally applied radiofrequency energy, often called pulse sequences, and by varying the time at which the radiofrequency given off by the patient is received, it is possible to differentiate one type of soft tissue from another. This differentiation in the types of soft tissues yields the superb resolution and detail characteristic of MRI images.

MRI excels in evaluation of the brain because of its sensitivity and specificity along with the exquisite detail of the tissue it provides. The use of intravenous paramagnetic contrast material markedly increases both sensitivity and specificity of the examination of the brain in certain situations, primarily in the case of brain tumors, both primary and metastatic (Carr, 1984; Schellinger, 1999). In Figure 12-7, a brain tumor is demonstrated after the intravenous injection of paramagnetic contrast material. Diffusion-weighted MRI has been shown to be superior to both conventional MRI and CT in identifying acute brain infarction within 12 hours of onset (Mullins, 2002). MRI can be accurate for detecting acute hemorrhagic infarction with focal symptoms and is more accurate than CT for detection of chronic hemorrhage (see Fig. 12-8; Kidwell, 2004). MRI is effective in detection and identification of the MS plaques in the white matter of the central nervous system, brain, and spinal cord (Achten, 2008). Other classes of abnormalities, such as infectious diseases, may have characteristic patterns on MRI scans of the brain as well.

MRI is also an excellent method for evaluating spinal cord and its surrounding vertebral and soft tissues. MRI has revolutionized the ease with which small epidural fluid collections, such as small epidural abscesses, can be detected and characterized. MRI is also superb in the evaluation of spinal canal masses, both internal and external to the cord. Other spinal cord abnormalities such as syrinx, congenital spinal cord abnormalities, and soft tissue masses adjacent to the spine are also detected relatively easily and diagnosed by MRI.

Of course MRI is useful in orthopedic injuries because many diagnoses that used to require invasive surgical or arthroscopic procedures can now be made through noninvasive MRI studies. MRI is still in its infancy, or maybe adolescence, and new methods of imaging using the basic principles of MRI are still being developed. In addition, the theoretical basis for MRI has continued to develop and is better understood so examination parameters can be more precisely manipulated to obtain information previously not detectable. In other words, potential new and exciting examinations with and applications for MRI remain to be developed, including physiological/functional examinations, of which diffusion-weighted imaging is the first, analysis of the brain metabolic functions, distribution of different elements and/or compounds within the brain, and even analysis of endogenously generated current flow in the brain.

Other than diffusion-weighted imaging, functional MRI (fMRI) is a method of analyzing the relative rates of metabolism in the brain. The relative flow of oxygenated and deoxygenated blood can be identified with MRI techniques (Ogawa, 1990;

Kwong, 1992; Bandettini, 1992). This is called blood-oxygen-level dependence or BOLD imaging. The potential for this type of functional imaging includes prognosis for return of neurological function in therapy. This type of imaging is very complex and, at present, involves the disciplines of physics, psychology, statistics, and electrophysiology as well as the more common discipline of neuroanatomy. Other even more exotic and exciting techniques, such as arterial spin labeling (ASL),

which has the potential to determine the perfusion territory of an individual artery, diffusion tensor imaging (DTI), and magnetic resonance spectroscopic imaging (MRS) are also in development.

### MRI Limitations

The high degree of specificity and sensitivity of MRI is not obtained without cost, however. MRI units are more expensive

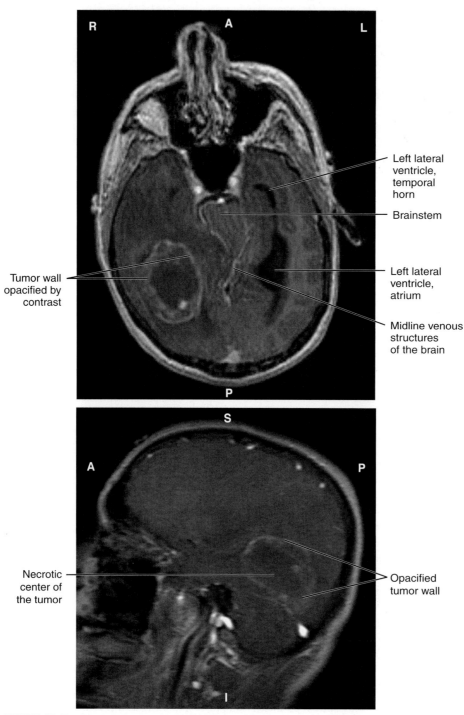

**FIGURE 12-7** MRI of the brain with intravenous contrast material for the same patient as in Figure 12-5 with right hemisphere tumor. Notice a great amount of detail, the mass effect of the tumor including the shift of the midline brain structures from the right to the left.

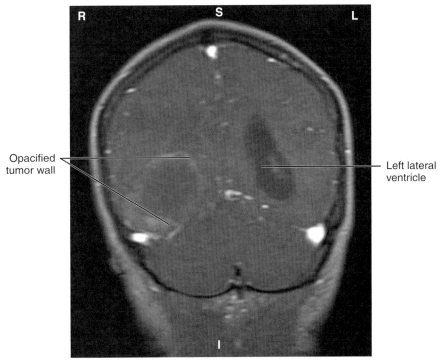

Opacified tumor wall

Left lateral ventricle

**FIGURE 12-7—cont'd**

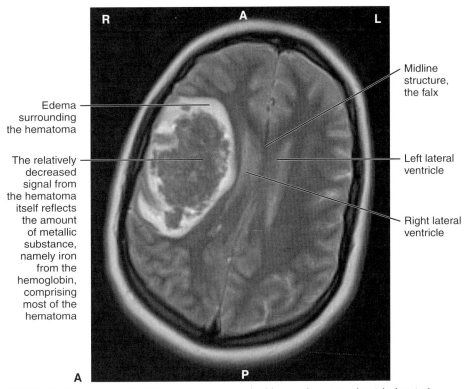

Edema surrounding the hematoma

The relatively decreased signal from the hematoma itself reflects the amount of metallic substance, namely iron from the hemoglobin, comprising most of the hematoma

Midline structure, the falx

Left lateral ventricle

Right lateral ventricle

**A**

**FIGURE 12-8  A. B.** and **C.** MRI revealing intracerebral hemorrhage into the right hemisphere. Notice the mass effect with midline shift of the structures to the left. All three of these axial images are obtained with different parameters with respect to the radio frequency pulse sequence. All these images are of the same patient at approximately the same level of the brain.

*Continued*

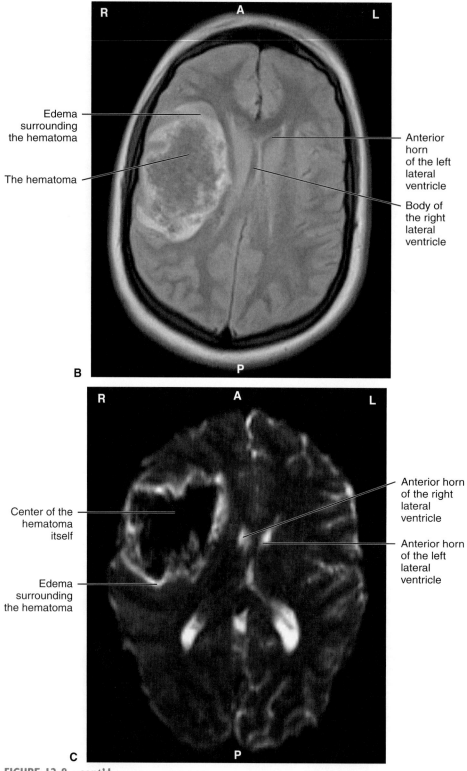

Edema surrounding the hematoma

The hematoma

Anterior horn of the left lateral ventricle

Body of the right lateral ventricle

B

Center of the hematoma itself

Edema surrounding the hematoma

Anterior horn of the right lateral ventricle

Anterior horn of the left lateral ventricle

C

**FIGURE 12-8—cont'd**

and more complex than CT units. MRI units are more confining than CT units, and claustrophobia is a significant clinical problem. Although methods are available to ameliorate claustrophobia, there are some patients who can only obtain an MRI examination while under general anesthesia. General anesthesia carries its own set of risks in addition to the risks of MRI alone.

Because of the great strength of the magnetic field used in MRI, objects made of ferrous metals can be tremendously accelerated by the magnetic field and become dangerous projectiles, much like a bullet or a thrown knife. Previously acquired ferrous metal particles in the eye, in the presence of the MRI magnetic field, can cause the otherwise stable particle to move, resulting in severe injury to the eye. The presence of metal fragments in the eye or in the orbit adjacent to the eye is not uncommon in patients who are or have been metal workers.

In the past, manufacturers have developed aneurysm clips, which are claimed to be nonmagnetic. Although the complete discussion of this clinical problem is beyond the scope of this book, there are conditions outside the control of the device manufacturer that can make an otherwise magnetically safe device become an unsafe one. One notable example would be the repeated heating and cooling of aneurysm clips. Aneurysm clips may be frequently heated and cooled by sterilization many times before being used. This is because each aneurysm presents the neurosurgeon with a unique situation in which only one or two clip shapes are usable. Clips with shapes that are rarely used may be heated and cooled many times in an autoclave before their usage. The heating of metal to a low temperature and then cooling, a process also called "annealing," is a well-recognized process in the manufacture of metals. Annealing alters the microscopic structure of a metal, which can affect its magnetic properties. In this fashion, a formerly nonmagnetic aneurysm clip, completely insensitive to strong magnetic fields, can be converted to one that can be more or less affected by strong magnetic fields. Because of the push to increase the strength of magnetic fields and because of the high variation in how aneurysm clips are stored and prepared for surgery, it is opined there is no such thing as a magnetically safe metallic aneurysm clip until complete control of clip manufacturing, storage, and handling, both in the factory and in the hospital, is rigidly standardized and enforced.

The existence of an internal pacemaker and/or defibrillator is, at this time, an absolute contraindication to an MRI examination. At present, there is at least one U.S. manufacturer that has developed a pacemaker experimentally safe in magnetic fields of a defined strength, but studies have not been published yet. Research in this area is ongoing. Likewise, devices such as deep brain stimulators, diaphragmatic pacemakers, insulin pumps, vagus nerve stimulators, cochlear implants, and many other such devices are contraindications to MRI. It is expected that research in the area of MRI-safe pacemakers can be applied, at least in part, to the safety of these other devices as well. However, in the United States in 2011, all such devices are contraindications to an MRI examination. Because of these safety considerations, MRI is not yet applicable to all patients. With further developments in technology, however, it is expected MRI will potentially be useful for any and all patients.

## Positron Emission Tomography

PET is a method of imaging utilizing the emission of photons or energy packets from within the patient. Nuclei bombarded with protons, deuterons, or helium nuclei contain excess protons and thus a positive charge. These atoms are unstable and undergo decay by positron emission. Positron emission is the process of emitting a positively charged particle from an atom. A positron is similar in mass to an electron except it has a positive charge. Scientifically, a positron is a form of antimatter and is the antimatter counterpart of the electron. Electrons have negative charge.

When a positron is emitted from an atom, it travels for a short distance, less than 2 mm, then an annihilation event occurs when the positron collides with an electron. In diagnostic PET scanning, the annihilation event results in the production of two photons that travel in exactly opposite directions (i.e., 180 degrees apart). These photons, like the photons emitted from radionuclides used in nuclear imaging, are then imaged in a special detector. Two detectors that are 180 degrees apart are used to detect the photons. To ensure the two emitted photons are from the same event, detection of a photon in one detector must be followed in quick succession by the detection of the opposite photon in the other detector. Compared with CT or MRI examination, the distance positrons travel before the photons are produced results in poor spatial resolution of the PET images.

The great utility in PET scanning of the brain is it provides an estimation of brain function by viewing metabolism of the different portions of the brain. The scans of the brain are obtained by replacing one of the oxygen atoms of a glucose molecule with fluorine-18, a cyclotron-produced positron emitter. This new molecule of glucose, containing one fluorine-18 atom, is called fluorodeoxyglucose or FDG. Because glucose is the main fuel molecule for the brain, FDG, which is handled by the brain in the same way that glucose is handled, allows imaging of the brain function by determining the levels of metabolism in different parts of the brain.

PET scanning, like nuclear medicine imaging, has dual properties of being an emission type of scan and has the ability to image function, in this case metabolism, rather than anatomic detail.

PET scanning of the brain can be very useful in the following clinical settings:

1. Separating malignant from benign tumors
2. Finding the focus of origin of an epileptic seizure
3. Separating Parkinson disease from other types of tremor

4. Evaluating the effectiveness of chemotherapy on brain tumors by separating scar tissue from areas of active metabolism
5. Evaluating certain types of movement disorders, dementia, and possible degenerative brain diseases
6. Guiding surgery by determining location of critical functional areas such as speech and movement

PET scanning of the brain is still in an early stage development with more expected from this modality in the future. Almost all positron emitters must be produced by cyclotron. Because fluorine-18 must be produced in a cyclotron, and because its half-life is 109.77 minutes, about 10 minutes short of 2 hours, PET scanning is limited in location to larger population centers that can support capital and labor costs required for cyclotron-produced radionuclides. Obviously, when there are more users in a certain geographical area, economies of scale allow the cost of cyclotron-produced radionuclides to decrease to the point that PET scanning is not prohibitively expensive provided travel times from the cyclotron source are not excessive. Many other positron-emitting radionuclides are possible but the short half-lives of most of these nuclides make them impractical for routine clinical use. At present, the main clinical use of PET scanning is in the detection, treatment, and staging of cancers and, to a lesser degree, in the evaluation of dementia.

## THINK ABOUT IT 12.2

- Conventional radiographs are best used for what purpose?
- How are 3-D relationships considered when using conventional radiographs?
- Diagnostic ultrasound is used for what purpose(s) in neurological conditions?
- CT scans are best used for what purpose(s)?
- Compare/contrast the advantages and disadvantages of CT versus MRI imaging.
- What is the quick and easy way to tell the difference between a CT versus MRI when you first glance at the image?
- PET scans are used for what purpose(s)?

## ◼ Electrophysiologic Testing

An **electrophysiologic test** is one that directly or indirectly measures physiological activity of the nervous system, peripheral nerves, or motor units/muscles (Katirji, 1998). Clinical electrophysiologic evaluation, also called electrodiagnostic testing or electroneuromyography (ENMG), plays a key role in the evaluation of many neuromuscular disorders, especially those affecting the peripheral nervous system. ENMG studies can help evaluate the status of the anterior horn cells, dorsal root ganglions (DRGs), nerve roots, brachial plexus, lumbosacral plexus, peripheral nerves, neuromuscular junctions (NMJs), and muscles. As with most diagnostic tests, ENMG

is an extension of, rather than a substitute for, the clinical examination and can provide information to confirm certain suspected diagnoses. The more detailed the clinical examination, the more specific the electromyographer can be in choosing which nerves and muscles to test. A patient with unilateral numbness and tingling on the radial side of their hand and no comorbidities would require a different ENMG evaluation than a patient with proximal muscle weakness or bilateral numbness and a history of diabetes. There are dozens of nerves and hundreds of muscles that can be tested. Because the ENMG examination is time-consuming and, in the case of needle EMG, uncomfortable for the patient, the electromyographer needs to record from as many nerves and muscles as necessary, but as few as possible, to confirm or rule out the probable diagnosis.

ENMG examination of nerve and muscle helps determine the location, magnitude, distribution, and duration of neuromuscular comprise. The two main components of ENMG studies are NCS, which assess the function of the motor and sensory nerves, and needle EMG, which assesses the electrical activity in the muscle. The NCS are usually performed first because the NCS findings aid in the planning and interpretation of the needle EMG examination. The more focused the EMG examination, the fewer needle sticks the patient receives. A primary aim of ENMG studies is to localize the lesion. Is the patient's unilateral numbness due to carpal tunnel syndrome or a cervical radiculopathy? Is the patient's bilateral numbness due to a polyneuropathy, bilateral carpal tunnel syndrome, or a myelopathy? When weakness is present, the disorder can usually be localized to the motor axon, NMJ, or muscle. Disorders of the CNS may also be indirectly implicated by ruling out peripheral nervous system dysfunction.

In the case of neuropathic disorders, ENMG studies can further delineate the diagnosis. The nerve fiber type can be identified as sensory, motor, or both. Because predominantly sensory or motor neuropathies are less common than combined sensorimotor neuropathies, the differential diagnosis can be narrowed after ENMG testing. The type of neural pathology can usually be identified as primarily **axon degeneration** or **demyelination** as discussed in detail in the following section. The acuteness of the demyelination and/or axonal loss can also be determined. There is a normal pattern of progression of both NCS and EMG findings following nerve damage. Comparing the temporal course of the patient's symptoms with the ENMG findings can alter the diagnostic impression. A patient may report a recent onset of symptoms while the ENMG findings strongly suggest a more long-standing pathology, of which the patient was unaware. On the other hand, the interpretation of the ENMG findings may change depending on the known time course. An ENMG finding found 1 week after acute trauma might indicate a different pathology than the same ENMG finding found several weeks following trauma. Only in combination with the clinical examination can the appropriate ENMG procedures be chosen and the appropriate interpretation of the ENMG findings be made.

# Nerve Conduction Studies

**Nerve conduction studies (NCS)** assess peripheral motor and sensory function by recording the **evoked response** resulting from peripheral nerve stimulation (Bertorini, 2002). NCS are divided primarily into sensory and motor conduction studies (MCS) in addition to late responses and specialized tests. Percutaneous (surface) electrical stimulation and recording is employed in all NCS. A motor response is recorded from a muscle innervated by the stimulated motor nerve, or a sensory potential is recorded from a cutaneous nerve. Both motor and sensory NCS provide very useful information to identify, localize, and differentiate various peripheral nerve disorders. For example, motor conduction abnormalities can be seen with peripheral nerve lesions but also with disorders of the anterior horn cell, NMJ, or muscle. In contrast, sensory or sensorimotor (mixed) conduction abnormalities always imply a disorder of the peripheral nerve, distal to the DRG, as sensory changes do not occur with either myopathies or disorders of the NMJ. NCS help answer the following:

- Are the peripheral nerves compromised?
- Is the compromise sensory, motor, or mixed?
- Where is the compromise located—nerve root, plexus, proximal limb, or distal limb?
- How many nerves are involved and how many limbs (local lesion versus polyneuropathy)?
- What is the magnitude of involvement—partial or complete?
- Is there evidence of recovery or further ongoing degeneration?
- Is the pathology one of axonal degeneration, demyelination, or conduction block?

## Motor Nerve Conduction Studies

**Motor conduction studies (MCS)** are performed by stimulating distal and proximal sites along the course of the peripheral nerve (see Fig. 12-9) while recording the evoked motor response with surface electrodes from a muscle innervated by

the stimulated nerve. This allows for calculation of the **motor conduction velocity (MCV)** across different segments of the limb. The recorded response during MCS, which is termed a **compound muscle action potential (CMAP)**, represents a summation of all the individual muscle fiber action potentials within the receptive field of the recording electrode. The CMAP is recorded using an active electrode (also known as G1) placed over the belly of the muscle and a reference electrode (also known as G2) placed over the tendon of that muscle. The designations G1 and G2 are terms dating back to the days when CMAP waveforms were viewed on oscilloscope grids (hence the G). Both the size and location of the active and reference electrode are essential determinants of the CMAP characteristics. Most modern EMG machines automatically measure the CMAP parameters of latency, amplitude, duration, and area (see Fig. 12-10 and Table 12-11).

The **CMAP latency** refers to the time (in msec) from the stimulus onset to the initial deflection of the CMAP. This time period is the summation of the time it takes for three separate processes to occur: (1) the conduction time along the nerve, (2) the time it takes to cross the NMJ, and (3) the time it takes for depolarization of the target muscle fibers. When the latency is obtained by stimulating the nerve at the most distal site, it is termed **distal latency (DL)**. The distance from the most distal stimulation site to the recording electrode on the muscle belly is standardized, so the motor distal latency (MDL) can be compared with normative values. The **CMAP amplitude** reflects the number of muscle fibers that have depolarized and is usually calculated (in mV) from the baseline to the peak of the waveform. **CMAP duration** is calculated from the initial deflection from baseline to the next baseline crossing. It reflects the synchrony of muscle fibers firing at

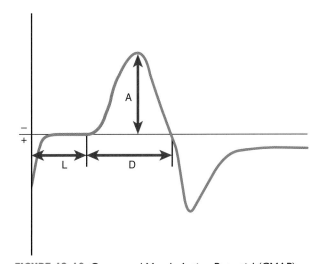

**FIGURE 12-10** Compound Muscle Action Potential (CMAP) Parameters. L = the latency (in msec) measured from the stimulus to the initial deflection from the baseline. A = amplitude (in mV) measured from the baseline to the peak of the negative spike. D = duration (in msec) measured from the initial negative deflection from baseline to when the signal crosses baseline again. Note that by convention negative is up, while positive is down.

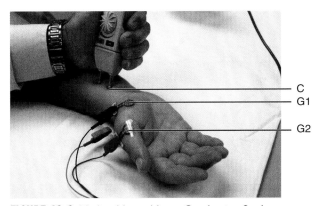

**FIGURE 12-9** Median Motor Nerve Conduction Study. The active electrode (G1) is on the belly of abductor pollicis brevis, and the reference electrode (G2) is on the tendon. The stimulator is on the median nerve with the cathode (C) located 8 cm proximal to the active electrode.

| TABLE 12-11 | Compound Muscle Action Potential (CMAP) Components |
|---|---|
| CMAP latency | • Refers to a lapsed time (in msec) from the stimulus onset to the initial deflection of the CMAP waveform from baseline.<br>• Reflects the summation of (a) conduction time along the nerve, (b) time to cross the neuromuscular junction, and (c) time for depolarization of the muscle fibers. |
| MDL | • **Motor distal latency (MDL)** is the latency obtained by stimulating the motor nerve at the most distal site.<br>• Because the distance from the most distal stimulation site to the recording electrode on the muscle belly is standardized, the MDL can be compared with normative values. |
| CMAP amplitude | • Usually calculated (in mV) from the take-off from baseline to the peak.<br>• Reflects the number of muscle fibers that have depolarized. |
| CMAP duration | • Calculated (in msec) from the initial deflection from baseline to the next baseline crossing.<br>• It reflects the synchrony of muscle fibers firing at the same time. |
| CMAP area | • The area under the waveform (in mV/msec) with correlation with the product of amplitude and duration.<br>• Useful in certain situations, particularly when conduction block or pathological temporal dispersion is suspected. |

*msec = milliseconds; mV = millivolts

the same time. **CMAP area** is the area under the waveform (in mV/msec). It is a useful measure in certain situations, particularly when conduction block or pathological temporal dispersion is suspected. MCV is obtained by stimulating the nerve at distal and proximal points, thus obtaining distal and proximal latencies, then measuring the distance between the proximal and distal stimulation points (in mm). MCV and CMAP latency both reflect the speed of the fastest conducting motor fibers only. By contrast, the other slower motor nerve fibers contribute to the CMAP amplitude and area. MCV is calculated as follows (see Fig. 12-11):

$$MCV \ (m/s) = \frac{\text{distance between stimulation sites (mm)}}{\text{proximal latency (msec)} - \text{distal latency (msec)}}$$

### Sensory Nerve Conduction Studies

To perform **sensory conduction studies (SCS),** stimulate a cutaneous sensory nerve such as the sural nerve or a mixed nerve such as the median or ulnar nerve (see Fig. 12-12A-B). Recording surface electrodes are placed along the course of the nerve to record a **sensory nerve action potential (SNAP).** Unlike MCS, which measures conduction along the nerve, NMJ, and muscle fiber, SCS only assess the nerve. Sensory nerve conduction velocity (SCV) can therefore be calculated using only one stimulation site, as there is no need to subtract the NMJ and muscle fiber depolarization times by using two stimulation sites. As with MCV, the SCV reflects the speed of the fastest conducting fibers and is calculated as follows:

$$SCV \ (m/s) = \frac{\text{distance between cathode and recording electrode (mm)}}{\text{latency (msec)}}$$

The SNAP components are described in Table 12-12. The **SNAP onset latency** reflects the time (in msec) between

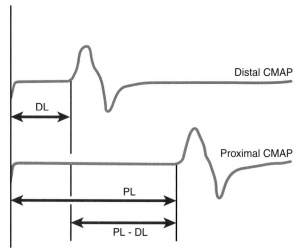

**FIGURE 12-11** Calculation of Motor Conduction Velocity. DL = distal latency (in msec), the time from the stimulus to the onset of the distal CMAP. PL = proximal latency (in msec), the time from the stimulus to the onset of the proximal CMAP. Subtracting DL from PL gives the time it takes to travel between the two stimulation sites. Dividing the distance (in mm) by the travel time (PL – DL in msec) give the motor conductions velocity (in msec).

stimulation of the nerve and the take-off of the SNAP from the baseline. Sometimes the sensory latency is measured to the peak of the SNAP, which is often more precisely defined than the take-off of the potential, in which case it is called the **SNAP peak latency** (see Fig. 12-13). Although the peak latency is easier to measure than the onset latency, as the waveform peak is often easier to locate than the onset of deflection from baseline, it cannot give an accurate measure of conduction velocity (CV). The **SNAP amplitude,** measured from

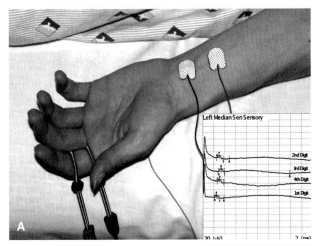

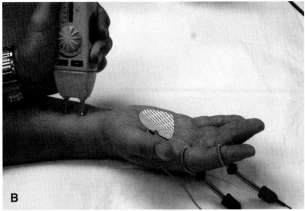

**FIGURE 12-12** Sensory Nerve Conduction Velocity Study. In **(A)**, the sensory nerves to digit 2 are stimulated with ring electrodes on the index finger while the recording electrodes are proximal to the wrist on the median nerve. The ground electrode is placed between the stimulating and recording electrodes. This is an orthodromic (distal to proximal) stimulation of the median nerve across the carpal tunnel. In **(B)**, the median nerve is stimulated and the SNAP is recorded by the ring electrodes. This is antidromic sensory stimulation.

| TABLE 12-12 | **Sensory Nerve Action Potential (SNAP) Components** |
|---|---|
| SNAP latency | • SNAP onset latency reflects the lapsed time (in msec) between stimulation of the nerve and the take-off of the SNAP from the baseline.<br>• At times, the SNAP peak latency is measured to the peak of the SNAP, which is often more precisely defined than the take-off of the potential. |
| SNAP amplitude | • Measured in µV, reflects the number of axons that conduct between the stimulation and recording sites. |

*msec = milliseconds; µV = microvolts

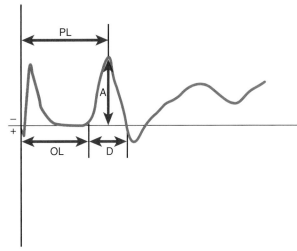

**FIGURE 12-13** Sensory Nerve Action Potential (SNAP) Parameters. Latency is recorded two ways. OL = onset latency (in msec) measured from the stimulus to the initial deflection from the baseline. PL = peak latency (in msec) measured from the stimulus to the peak of the negative spike. A = amplitude (in uV) measured from the baseline to the peak of the negative spike. D = duration (in msec) measured from the initial negative deflection from baseline to when the signal crosses baseline again. Note that by convention negative is up, while positive is down.

baseline to peak (in µV), reflects the number of axons that conduct between the stimulation and recording sites. As seen in Figure 12-13, the SNAP amplitudes are measured in µV, while CMAP amplitudes are measured in mV, a difference of a thousandfold. SNAP durations (typically 1 to 2 msec) are also shorter than CMAP durations (typically 5 to 6 msec). A normal CMAP amplitude stimulating the median nerve at the wrist would be over 4 mV compared with a normal SNAP amplitude of the median nerve of 20 uV. Low SNAP amplitudes always indicate a peripheral nerve disorder, as the SNAP is unaffected by myopathic disease or NMJ disorders.

When a nerve is stimulated, the depolarization travels in both directions. Hence SCS can be performed stimulating proximally and recording distally or vice versa. Because sensory nerves (afferents) send their information to the CNS moving from distal to proximal, stimulating distally while recording proximally is called **orthodromic** stimulation, while stimulating proximally while recording distally is called **antidromic** stimulation. Latencies should be equal in antidromic and orthodromic sensory conduction studies, as the distance between stimulation and recording is the same. However, antidromic SNAPs are larger in amplitude and therefore easier to visualize because the sensory nerves are usually closer to the skin the more distally they travel (see Fig. 12-14). The larger antidromic SNAP amplitude is particularly helpful when recording very small potentials, as occurs in many pathological conditions. The disadvantage of antidromic sensory studies, when studying mixed nerves (e.g., ulnar), is the SNAP is closely followed by a volume conducted CMAP. This could

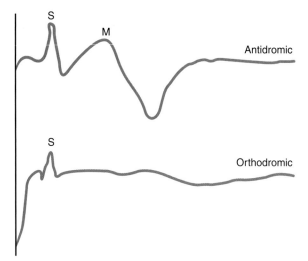

**FIGURE 12-14** Antidromic versus Orthodromic Sensory Nerve Study. Sensory nerve action potentials (SNAPs) from the median nerve. The top trace shows the waveform with antidromic stimulation. Note the higher amplitude (S), but a closely following motor response (M). The bottom orthodromic SNAP is smaller but does not create a motor response. The latencies and conduction velocities are the same with both studies, if the same stimulation sites are used.

create problems in interpreting the signal if the SNAP and CMAP latencies are similar or if the SNAP is absent and the CMAP is mistaken as a SNAP response.

There are also **mixed nerve conduction studies (MCS)** that are routinely used for entrapment syndromes (e.g., for carpal tunnel, cubital tunnel, tarsal tunnel), which stimulate both sensory and motor axons and produce a mixed nerve action potential (MNAP). Mixed studies are similar to orthodromic sensory studies in that the recording electrode is placed proximally over the nerve. The distal stimulating electrode, however, is not placed over cutaneous nerve endings; rather, it is placed over the muscle supplied by the target nerve. Hence, MCS record the Ia afferents supplying the muscle spindles, which are the largest, most myelinated, and hence the fastest conducting fibers. These are often the first fibers affected by demyelinating lesions occurring in entrapment neuropathies.

### Interpretation of Nerve Conduction Studies

In addition to determining the location of peripheral nervous system lesions, a primary diagnostic value of NCS is to determine whether the neuropathic lesion is one of axonal loss or demyelination. The differentiation is possible because the two pathologies have different effects on NCS parameters. Axonal loss (without demyelination) results in reduced amplitude but generally preserves DL and CV. Even if the fastest nerve fibers are lost, the remaining slower but still myelinated fibers will have CV values of at least 75% of normal and DL values prolonged to less than 130% of normal. The only exception to this is within a few days after an acute peripheral nerve lesion during which time NCS distal to the lesion would be normal because Wallerian degeneration has not had time to occur. In

general then, axonal loss results in decreased amplitude but not marked slowing. Demyelination, by contrast, results in marked slowing of CV (below 75% of normal) and prolonging of DL (above 130% of normal). If the demyelination is severe, no impulses will travel along the nerve resulting in a **conduction block.** Figure 12-15 illustrates the difference between axonal loss and demyelination with common clinical examples summarized in Table 12-13.

While the effect of axonal loss on conduction is consistently minimal, the effect of demyelination on amplitude is quite variable. SNAP amplitudes are generally affected more than CMAP amplitudes as the sensory fibers are less synchronous to start, and demyelination further exaggerates both the temporal dispersion and phase cancellation inherent in the SNAP response. A drop in CMAP amplitude from demyelination indicates conduction block. The conduction block can be partial or complete, localized or widespread. In the case of localized conduction block, as in entrapment syndromes, the effect on CMAP waveforms will depend on whether the lesion is proximal or distal to the stimulation

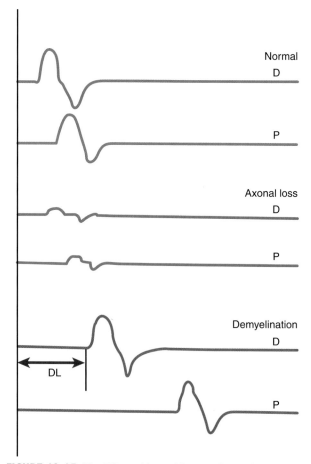

**FIGURE 12-15** The Effect of Axonal Loss vs Demyelination on CMAP parameters. With pure axonal loss (middle trace), there is decreased amplitude at both the distal (D) and proximal (P) stimulation sites. With pure demyelination without conduction block (bottom trace), there is no change in amplitude but a marked increase in distal latency (DL) and a marked slowing of conduction velocity.

| TABLE 12-13 | Hallmark Signs of Axonal and Demyelinating Neuropathies |
|---|---|
| **HALLMARK SIGNS IN NCS** | **COMMON CLINICAL EXAMPLES** |
| Axonal neuropathy:<br>• Hallmark sign is the diminution of the amplitude of the CMAP and the SNAP in the presence of normal or near-normal maximal nerve conduction velocity (NCV).<br>• In cases of severe axonal degeneration, CMAP and SNAP are unexcitable. | • Most metabolic, toxic, nutritional, and cryptogenic peripheral neuropathies with axonal degeneration |
| Demyelinating neuropathy:<br>• Hallmark sign is marked slowing in the NCVs (<75%), prolonged distal latency (>130%), possible conduction block, and abnormal temporal dispersion of the CMAP or the SNAP. | • Usually inherited such as Charcot-Marie Disease or immune-mediated such as Guillain-Barré syndrome |

site. As seen in Figure 12-16A, a conduction block proximal to all stimulation sites will have no effect on the CMAP waveform, whereas a conduction block distal to all stimulation sites (Fig. 12-16B) will result in slowing of CV and lowering of CMAP amplitude at all stimulation sites proximal to the lesion. The changes in CMAP amplitude will be similar to what is observed with axonal loss. With conduction block, however, the demyelination will also cause changes to CV and DL. When the conduction block occurs between stimulation sites (Fig. 12-16C), the CMAP from stimulation below the lesion will not be affected, while the CMAP from stimulation above the lesion will be.

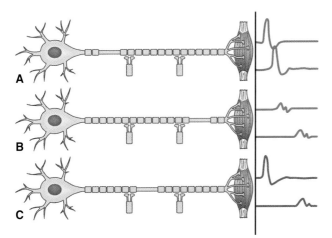

**FIGURE 12-16** Demyelination Causing Conduction Block (CB). **A.** If the CB is proximal to the stimulation sites, both the distal and proximal CMAPs will be normal, and distal latency (DL) and conduction velocity (CV) will be normal. **B.** If the CB is distal to both sites, DL will be increased and CMAP amplitudes will be decreased with temporal dispersion at both sites, but the CV between sites will be normal. **C.** If the CB is between stimulation sites, the DL and distal CMAP will be normal, while the proximal CMAP will show decreased amplitude and temporal dispersion, and CV between the two sites will be slowed. (Modified with permission from Preston, 2005, Fig. 3-19.)

In the case of demyelinating polyneuropathies, the presence of conduction block in nonentrapment sites is strongly suggestive of an acquired polyneuropathy (such as Guillain-Barré) because inherited polyneuropathies (such as Charcot-Marie-Tooth) usually show uniform slowing of CV without the presence of conduction block. The degree to which a decrease in CMAP amplitude is indicative of a conduction block is somewhat controversial with a criterion of >50% CMAP amplitude reduction currently suggested to indicate definite conduction block. Recent studies suggest changes in timing (e.g., CV, DL) are more predictive than changes in amplitude in differentiating axonal versus demyelinating pathologies (Tankski, 2007). Further complicating interpretation of conduction block is the occurrence of combined axonal loss with demyelination as frequently occurs in entrapment neuropathies. The distinction in pathologies is important for the prognosis: conduction block from demyelination is usually reversible in entrapment neuropathies while significant axonal loss suggests a longer and less complete recovery.

Because the DRG lies outside the spinal cord in the intervertebral foramen, nerve root lesions typically affect MCV but not SCV. Patients with nerve root signs and symptoms will commonly have decreased sensation but normal SCV. This suggests the lesion is proximal to the DRG. Sensory studies will always be normal in myopathic disorders and disorders of the NMJ unless there is an accompanying neuropathic lesion. Distal CMAPs will also be normal in many myopathic disorders as they primarily affect proximal muscles. In the case of NMJ disorders, it depends on whether the NMJ disorder is presynaptic or postsynaptic. In postsynaptic disorders, such as myasthenia gravis, CMAPs will usually be normal. In presynaptic disorders, such as Lambert-Eaton myasthenic syndrome, CMAP amplitudes will usually be reduced, although CV and DL will be normal. When a NMJ disorder is suspected, repetitive nerve stimulation (RNS) studies are performed as discussed in the following section.

### Late Responses

Two late responses are commonly used in daily practice in the electrophysiology laboratory, the H-reflex and F-wave response. The tibial **H-reflex**, named for Hoffman who first described it in 1918, is the electrophysiological counterpart of the ankle reflex, measuring the latency over the monosynaptic reflex arc including the afferent sensory fibers and efferent motor fibers of the S1 nerve root. If the Achilles tendon reflex is present clinically, the H-reflex should also be present. If the Achilles tendon reflex is absent, the H-reflex may still be present, but prolonged. It is obtained by stimulating the tibial nerve with submaximal stimulus at the popliteal fossa while recording over the gastrocnemius or soleus muscle. Usually, the H-reflex is obtained bilaterally for comparison purposes, particularly in suspected lumbosacral radiculopathies or peripheral polyneuropathy. H-reflexes of other peripheral nerves are not attempted due to poor reproducibility in healthy adults. The H-reflex will first appear at very low stimulus intensities with a latency of 25 to 35 msec. As the stimulation intensity is increased, the H-reflex amplitude will increase while its latency decreases. With further increase of the stimulus intensity, a motor response (CMAP) will also appear. With further increases in intensity, the motor response will grow in size while the H-reflex decreases (see Fig. 12-17).

The **F-wave** is another late response, which is evoked by supramaximal stimulation during the motor NCS. When a motor nerve is stimulated, the depolarization is propagated in both directions. The orthodromic volley travels down the nerve and across the NMJ to give the CMAP response. The antidromic volley travels up the motor nerve and excites a small percentage of motor neurons to fire again, producing a much smaller CMAP about 30 msec after the main motor response. This smaller CMAP is called the F-wave, so-named because it was first found in the foot. Because the F-wave travels the motor neurons only without a synapse, it is not a reflex. Because it represents the entire pathway to and from the anterior horn cell, the F-wave response is useful in evaluation of proximal neuropathies such as plexopathy, polyradiculopathy, or nerve root lesion. It is particularly useful in picking up polyneuropathies that begin with nerve root demyelination. While other parts of the NCS examination may be normal, increased F-wave latencies can identify early stages of disorders such as Guillain-Barré. F-waves are not useful in conditions with marked reduction of CMAP amplitude. Because they only represent 1% to 5% of motor fibers, they will probably not be seen if the CMAP is significantly reduced.

The F-wave response is easily obtained by stimulating the distal portions of commonly tested nerves such as the median, ulnar, peroneal, and posterior tibial nerves using supramaximal stimulus intensity. The most commonly employed F-wave measure is the **minimal F-wave latency**, which represents the time to fire the largest and fastest motor neurons (see Fig. 12-18). Because the subset of motor units that fire with each F-wave response differs, the minimal F-wave latency among 8 to 10 recorded potentials is measured. F-wave latency is highly dependent on the distance from stimulation site to the spinal cord. Comparison with normal values therefore requires measurement of the subject's limb length or height, which is then put into a formula to determine normal F-wave latency values for that nerve.

### Repetitive Motor Nerve Stimulation

**Repetitive motor nerve stimulation (RMNS)** is performed by stimulating a peripheral motor nerve, such as the ulnar or the axillary nerve, with a successive train of stimuli and recording the CMAP responses with an active surface electrode over the belly of the target muscle. The CMAP amplitude of each response is measured, reflecting the number of muscle fibers activated by each nerve stimulus, and is a marker of neuromuscular transmission efficiency. Current EMG machines have the capability to automatically measure and store the amplitude, area, and duration of repeated CMAPs and allow immediate analysis. In healthy NMJs, the CMAPs remain stable in amplitude and area in response to repetitive stimulation at variable stimulation rates. The low stimulation rate is typically set at about 2 to 3 Hz. The high stimulation rate can also be set (at 20 to 30 Hz) or can be obtained by having the patient perform a brief (10 sec) bout of maximum voluntary contraction (MVC), which will create a motor unit firing frequency of 30 to 50 Hz. If the patient is capable of performing a MVC, it avoids using an uncomfortable 30 to 50 Hz stimulation rate. A train of 5 to 10 pulses is used for low frequency RMNS, and a stimulus

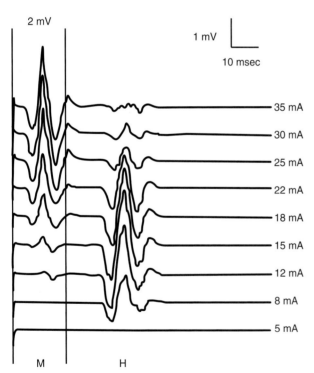

2 mV

1 mV

10 msec

35 mA
30 mA
25 mA
22 mA
18 mA
15 mA
12 mA
8 mA
5 mA

M          H

**FIGURE 12-17** The H-Reflex. Note the stimulation intensities (in mA) increasing from the bottom up. At low intensities, the H-reflex is present without a motor response (M). As intensity increases, the motor response increases, but the H-reflex starts to decrease due to collision between the H-reflex and the antidromic motor potentials. This illustrates why the H-reflex uses sub-maximal stimulation. (Reproduced with permission from Preston, 2005, Fig. 4-11.)

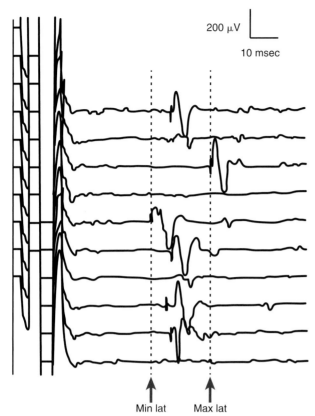

200 µV

10 msec

Min lat    Max lat

**FIGURE 12-18** The F-Wave Response. The F wave responses from ten consecutive supramaximal stimulations are shown. The much larger motor responses are on the left side. The minimal latency (Min lat) is the time to the shortest of the ten responses, reflecting the fastest conducting fibers; Max lat = the time to the slowest conducting fibers. Note that the F-wave response is absent in two of ten traces. F-wave persistence is therefore 80% in this series. (Reproduced with permission from Preston, 2005, Fig. 4-4.)

| TABLE 12-14 | Factors That Affect Nerve Conduction Test Results |
|---|---|
| Skin *temperature* | • This is the most important factor.<br>• NCV increases linearly with the temperature from 1.1–2.4 m/sec for each 1°C (Tesfaye, 1992) within the physiological temperature range.<br>• So, it is essential to measure skin temperature and adjust the NCV to the standard temperature (31°C in the lower and 32°C in the upper limbs). |
| Patient *age* | • The full-term newborn NCVs are approximately 50% of the normal adult values, reaching adult values around 4 years of age.<br>• In adults, the NCVs decline after age 60 years (a correction of 1–2 meter per second is allowed).<br>• Amplitude also decreases with age.<br>• Maybe no response with some nerves in elderly. |
| Patient *height* | • Conduction velocity varies inversely with height.<br>• Height is particularly important in measuring late responses, such as F-wave parameters, which use height to calculate normal latency values. |

of 5 to 10 seconds is given for high frequency RMNS (in patients who cannot perform 5 to 10 seconds of MVC). Decrement or excessive facilitation of the CMAPs amplitude and area occurs in various NMJ disorders. RMNS is a very useful diagnostic test in evaluation of NMJ disorders. Typically, a decrement in CMAP amplitude is seen in postsynaptic NMJ disorders, such as myasthenia gravis, whereas facilitation or increment is seen in presynaptic NMJ disorders, such as Lambert-Eaton myasthenic syndrome or botulism. Although a decremental response to RMNS is usually a sign of a NMJ disorder, other disorders can create a decrement with RMNS. For example, when testing denervated muscles that have undergone subsequent reinnervation, there may be newly formed and unstable NMJs, which also may result in a CMAP decrement during RMNS. Thus, RMNS findings must be compared with the clinical examination and findings from NCS and needle EMG.

### Factors Affecting Nerve Conduction Tests

Several factors can affect nerve conduction test results and are summarized in Table 12-14, including skin temperature, patient age, and patient anthropometrics. NCV increases linearly with the temperature from 1.1 to 2.4 m/sec for each 1°C (Tesfaye, 1992) within the physiological temperature range. Thus, it is essential to monitor and maintain a skin temperature of 31°C in the lower extremity and 32°C in the upper extremity. Alternately, NCV values obtained at a lower temperature can be mathematically converted to the standard temperature values. Age also influences conduction velocities, especially in the very young and very old. Full-term newborn CVs are approximately 50% of the normal adult values. As myelination increases, CV values reach adult values around 4 years of age. Conduction values begin to decline by 30 to 40 years of age, but CV is still at about 90% by age 60 (Kimura, 2001). What is more significant in the elderly is not a drop in CV but rather a drop in amplitude of the nerve response, which is best explained by a reduction in the number of axons. Beyond age 70, a significant percentage of the population will have absence of at least one nerve response. The sural sensory response is most vulnerable to aging, being absent in 23% of normal subjects between age 70 and 79 years and 40% of normal subjects over 80 years. By contrast, ulnar motor responses are rarely absent in normal subjects at any age (Rivner, 2001).

## Electromyography Examination

The term **electromyography (EMG)** refers to methods of studying the electrical activity of muscles. Such methods are an invaluable aid to neurological diagnosis of certain disorders. There are two main types of EMG performed in rehabilitation: surface EMG and needle EMG. **Surface EMG** measures electrical activity of muscle(s) via electrodes applied to the skin. Surface electrodes do not offer the advantage of pinpointing specific locations that indwelling electrodes provide. However, surface EMG is well suited to determine electrical activity of a functional group of muscles during a particular action. Surface EMG is commonly used in rehabilitation as a form of biofeedback to help the patient and therapist know when a muscle is contracting. Surface EMG is not commonly used for electrodiagnostic testing unless there are contraindications for needle EMG.

**Needle electromyography** examination, using a needle electrode instead of surface electrodes, tests the integrity of the muscle, NMJ, and motor neurons. A needle electrode is inserted in a selected muscle followed by multiple sampling at rest and during different degrees of voluntary contraction in each muscle of interest. The clinical examination and data from the preceding NCS determine the optimal selection of specific muscle groups for EMG testing. Because this is an invasive and uncomfortable procedure, the number of needle sticks should be kept to the minimum required to confirm or rule out the differential diagnosis.

The EMG examination helps answer the following:

- Is the muscle normally innervated, partially innervated, or denervated?
- Does evidence for reinnervation exist?
- Are EMG findings consistent with upper motor neuron, lower motor neuron, or myopathic disease?
- Is the pattern of EMG abnormalities in muscles examined consistent with a nerve root, plexus, anterior horn, or peripheral nerve lesion?
- Where along the path of the peripheral nerve is the lesion located?
- Does the problem involve muscles in the extremities (anterior rami), paraspinal muscles (posterior rami), or head/neck muscles (cranial nerve)?

Needle EMG examination is performed in three steps: (1) assessment of *insertional activity* caused by needle movement within the muscle addressed, (2) searching for *spontaneous activity* recorded with the needle stationary in a relaxed muscle, which constitutes one of the most important findings, and (3) analysis of the *motor unit potential* (MUP) parameters and recruitment during progressive voluntary muscle contraction. During these steps of the EMG examination, the electromyographer is not only looking at the resulting waveforms but listening as well. Normal and abnormal electrical activity each produce characteristic sounds

on the EMG speakers that are sometimes more meaningful to the examiner than the waveforms themselves.

In EMG tracings, downward deflections are considered positive by convention, whereas upward deflections are considered negative. **Insertional activity** is a brief burst of action potentials that follows the insertion of the needle electrode into muscle. The presence of insertional activity helps confirm the needle is in muscle. Normal insertional activity should last no longer than 200 to 300 msec (see top graph in Fig. 12-19). Increased insertional activity lasting longer than 300 msec indicates irritability of the muscle membrane. It is usually associated with denervation, myotonic disorders, and some myogenic disorders such as myositis. Decreased insertional activity indicates a reduced number of healthy muscle fibers, which occurs when muscle has been replaced by fat and connective tissue. After you insert the needle into several quadrants of the muscle, assess insertional activity from several muscle fibers by holding the needle still to record any spontaneous activity at rest. Normal muscle fibers have no spontaneous activity except at the end-plate region (bottom graph in Fig. 12-19). The normal response at rest is electrical silence

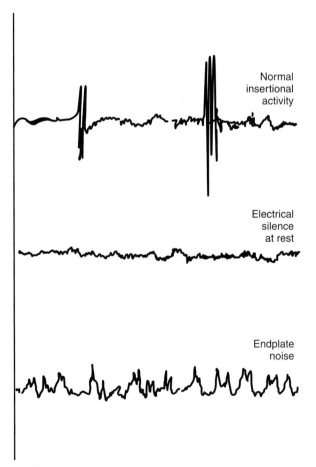

Normal insertional activity

Electrical silence at rest

Endplate noise

**FIGURE 12-19** Insertional Activity. The top trace shows normal insertional activity, brief (<300 msec) bursts of activity in response to needle movement. The middle trace shows no activity when the needle is held still, which is normal. The bottom trace shows endplate noise with the needle held still, indicating the needle is near a motor endplate.

(second graph in Fig. 12-19). If the needle is inserted at the endplate region, however, the result is **endplate noise**, irregularly firing monophasic negative potentials, 10 to 50 µV in amplitude, firing at 20 to 40 Hz, that have a characteristic sound like a seashell held to the ear. A needle inserted near a terminal nerve twig creates an **endplate spike,** an irregularly firing biphasic waveform, firing at up to 50 Hz but very irregularly with a sputtering sound like bacon in a frying pan. Both endplate noise and endplate spikes occur from needle insertion near the NMJ in healthy muscle.

Outside of the endplate zone, normal muscle is electrically silent at rest. Abnormal spontaneous activity of muscle fibers includes fibrillations, positive sharp waves, myotonic discharges, and complex repetitive discharges. A **fibrillation potential (Fib)** is the electrical activity associated with the spontaneous contraction of a single muscle fiber due to instability of the muscle fiber membrane. The duration of a fibrillation potential is very short with an amplitude from 20 to several hundred µV. Its rhythm is regular, and it makes a crisp clicking sound. A **positive sharp wave (PSW)** is a biphasic positive-negative potential recorded from a single muscle fiber at rest. It is of longer duration and higher amplitude than a fibrillation potential and makes a thud or plop sound like rain on a roof. Fibrillations and positive sharp waves often occur together and are believed to represent the same event, namely spontaneous depolarization of an unstable muscle membrane (see Fig. 12-20). They are the most common abnormal spontaneous potentials and usually suggest a lower motor neuron disorder causing denervation, although they are present in myogenic disorders as well. They are conventionally graded on a scale from 0 to + 4, wherein, for a grade of + 4, the "rain on the roof" sound would be a "downpour."

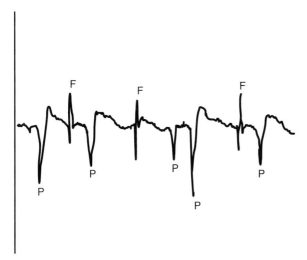

**FIGURE 12-20** Fibrillations and Positive Sharp Waves (PSWs). Both fibrillations (F) and positive sharp waves (P) represent spontaneous depolarization of muscle fibers. Fibrillations are triphasic with an initial small positive deflection, while PSWs have a larger initial positive phase followed by a smaller but longer negative phase. Both have a regular firing pattern, which distinguishes them from voluntary motor units, which lack a regular firing pattern.

A **myotonic discharge** is the spontaneous discharge of a muscle fiber (similar to a fibrillation or positive sharp wave) that waxes and wanes in both amplitude and frequency with a sound like a revving engine of a motorcycle or chainsaw. Myotonic discharges are characteristically seen in myotonic disorders, occasionally in other myopathies, and rarely in denervation. **Complex repetitive discharges (CRDs)** are bursts of repetitively discharging muscle fibers that start and stop abruptly. They originate from several muscle fibers discharging repetitively, with one muscle fiber acting like a pacemaker, spreading the depolarization from muscle membrane to membrane. Therefore, they can only occur when denervated fibers lie next to one another. Because muscle fibers from many motor units intermix, CRDs do not usually occur in acute denervation because the denervated fibers are usually spread out in the muscle. Rather they occur in cases of chronic denervation where sprouting and reinnervation has occurred, resulting in neighboring muscle fibers innervated by the same motor neuron. This can occur also in myopathies associated with denervation such as polymyositis. CRDs have a very distinct waveform, being identical in morphology from one discharge to the next, and have a distinct sound like a machine gun.

Fibrillations, positive sharp waves, myotonic discharges, and complex repetitive discharges are all abnormal muscle fiber potentials. Abnormal MUPs also occur, including fasciculations, myokymic discharges, cramps, and neuromyotonic discharges. A **fasciculation potential** is the spontaneous (i.e., involuntary) discharge of a motor unit. Fasciculations resemble normal MUPs, but they fire at a slower rate. During voluntary muscle contraction, MUPs begin to fire at 4 to 5 Hz, but fasciculations occur at less than 2 Hz. Fasciculations occur with numerous disorders affecting lower motor neurons including diseases of the anterior horn cells, motor neuron disease, and entrapment neuropathies. They also occur in normal muscle and therefore are not significant by themselves. They have the sound of corn popping. Fasciculations are brief muscle twitches that rarely produce movement except in very small muscles such as those controlling the eyelids.

Grouped spontaneous repetitive discharges of the same motor unit are called **myokymic discharges.** They occur in bursts, representing groups of involuntary fasciculations. Clinically, myokymia is involuntary quivering of the skin from underlying muscle contraction. Myokymic discharges are the EMG representation of this repetitive involuntary motor unit firing. The firing rate between bursts is quite slow, producing a marching sound on EMG speakers. Myokymic discharges are often seen in facial muscles with several disorders including multiple sclerosis, pontine tumors, and Guillain-Barré, and they are a characteristic finding of radiation-induced nerve damage. Myokymic discharges differ from tremor, which also occurs in bursts of MUPs. The bursts in myokymic discharges are the same motor unit firing repetitively within each burst, while the bursts in tremor are composed of many different motor units.

Sustained involuntary muscle contraction is called a **muscle cramp**. Electrically, cramps present as repetitive discharges of normal looking MUPs at a high frequency (20 to 150 Hz). They resemble the waveforms observed with MVCs but are occurring involuntarily. Cramps may be benign, as in postexercise cramps or nocturnal calf cramps, or may be associated with a wide range of neuropathic and metabolic conditions. They usually occur in only a few shortened muscles. They sound like normal MUPs firing at a very high rate. They commonly wax and wane for several minutes then spontaneously stop.

A more widespread continuous muscle activity called **neuromyotonia** is characterized by repetitive firing of a single motor unit at high frequency (150 to 350 Hz) that wanes before it stops. It has a characteristic pinging sound. The associated clinical signs include widespread muscle stiffness, involuntary muscle contractions that occur even during sleep, and a delay of relaxation after voluntary muscle contraction—a cluster of symptoms referred to as Isaac syndrome, pseudomyotonia, neurotonia, and continuous muscle fiber activity. The discharges are generated by peripheral motor axons and therefore should not be confused with "stiff-man syndrome," which is a separate condition of central origin.

After assessment of insertional activity and spontaneous activity at rest, the EMG examination moves on to evaluating motor unit action potentials (MUAPs) during graded voluntary contraction. Although the muscle fibers supplied by each motor nerve are not adjacent, the spread of muscle fibers from each motor unit is still over a small area of the muscle, averaging from 5 to 10 mm in cross-sectional diameter. Therefore, many different motor units need to be analyzed in a large muscle, using two to three different insertion sites and several different angles and depths of penetration at each site. Characteristic features of a normal MUAP, including amplitude, duration, and morphology, vary considerably depending on the muscle being studied and the age of the patient. In general, distal muscles have MUAPs of longer duration and MUAP amplitude increases with age. Even within each healthy muscle there is a wide range of motor unit morphology with the amplitude of MUAPs following a normal distribution (i.e., bell-shaped curve). To interpret results, for each muscle examined, the mean MUAP values for about 20 different motor units are compared with muscle-and age-specific normative data during EMG analysis. MUAPs should produce a sharp crisp sound. A dull sound indicates the MUAP is distant and it should not be analyzed.

The typical MUAP will have 2 to 3 phases, defined as the number of baseline crosses from the start of the waveform. A MUAP with more than 4 to 5 phases is considered abnormal, although polyphasia can be seen in up to 5% to 10% of MUAPs in most normal muscles and in up to 25% of MUAPs in the deltoid. **Polyphasia** is a measure of synchrony of the muscle fibers firing within a motor unit. Some asynchrony is expected within the same motor unit because of the slight variation in depolarization time required to travel the length of the different terminal axons to different muscle fibers. Excessive polyphasia, usually considered to be more than 10% (except for the deltoid), can be caused by a number of neuropathic and

myopathic pathologies, as discussed in the following section. On the EMG speaker, polyphasic MUAPs produce a high frequency clicking sound. Within one phase of the MUAP, there can be several serrations (also called turns), which are changes in direction of the potential that do not cross midline. Serrations give the normally triangular negative waveform a saw-toothed appearance. They have the same significance as polyphasia—namely they reflect less synchronous firing of the muscle fibers within the motor unit (see Fig. 12-21).

With voluntary muscle contraction against minimal resistance, the smallest motor neurons with the lowest thresholds fire first. These are generally connected to slow twitch (type I) muscle fibers and produce MUAPs with amplitudes ranging from 300 to 1,000 μV. As resistance to muscle contraction increases, progressively larger motor units fire. The largest motor neurons with the highest thresholds only fire when significant resistance to muscle contraction is given. These are generally connected to fast-twitch (type II) muscle fibers producing MUAPs with an amplitude of 1,000 to 5,000 μV.

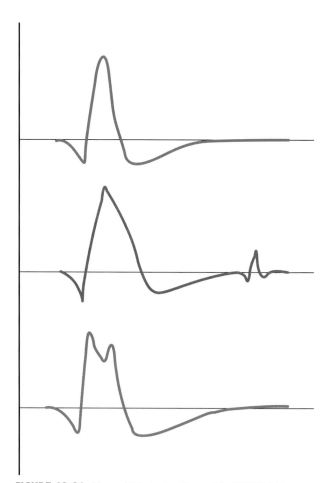

**FIGURE 12-21** Motor Unit Action Potentials (MUAPs). The top tracing shows a normal triphasic motor unit with an initial positive phase followed by a larger negative phase. The middle unit shows a satellite potential trailing the main MUAP, indicating early reinnervation. As the newly formed motor sprout matures and myelinates, it fires closer to the main potential, becoming a serration (or turn) within the main MUAP.

MUAP amplitude only represents the few fibers closest to the needle and varies widely among normal subjects. Therefore it does not accurately reflect motor unit size. By contrast MUAP duration better reflects the number of muscle fibers within a motor unit, with longer duration indicating more fibers being fired by that motor neuron. On the EMG speaker, duration correlates with pitch, with long-duration MUAPs sounding dull and thud-like while short-duration MUAPs sound more crisp and static-like. MUAP amplitude correlates with volume rather than pitch.

The normal EMG recruitment pattern exhibits a characteristic increase in MUAP amplitudes with increasing muscle contraction and also a predictable pattern of frequency of motor unit firing. With minimal contractions, a single motor unit typically begins firing at about 5 Hz. Any MUP that fires lower than 4 Hz is not under voluntary control. As muscle force output increases, the first motor unit will increase its frequency of firing to about 10 Hz and by then a second motor unit will fire. By 15 Hz, a third motor unit will fire and so forth, giving a frequency-to-motor unit ratio of about 5:1 (i.e., one motor unit firing for every 5 Hz). This continues until the muscle reaches its maximum firing frequency (around 30 to 50 Hz), which will depend on the percentage of slow-twitch versus fast-twitch fibers. With strong muscle contractions, this overlapping of motor unit firing creates an interference pattern in which no single motor unit can be distinguished. For this reason, analysis of individual motor units can only be accomplished at low levels of muscle contraction.

With a normal interference pattern, during maximal voluntary contraction (MVC), individual MUAPs cannot be identified. Incomplete interference patterns differ with neuropathic versus myopathic conditions and with upper versus lower motor neuron lesions. As seen in Figure 12-22, in myopathic lesions, the number of motor units firing is normal, but the interference pattern consists of low-amplitude, short-duration MUAPs. In neuropathic lesions, there is usually a reduced number of motor units firing at normal amplitudes, giving a picket fence appearance to the EMG trace. The space between the pickets (i.e., the firing rate) helps determine whether the neuropathy is localized to the upper or lower motor neuron. With an upper motor neuron lesion, the problem is one of motor unit activation. The MVC interference pattern may reveal only one or two motor units firing at 5 to 10 Hz, demonstrating decreased activation but a normal (5:1) recruitment pattern. The decreased activation may be from a CNS lesion (e.g., multiple sclerosis, CVA, or simply from decreased motivation secondary to pain or apprehension. With a lower motor neuron lesion, the problem is one of motor unit recruitment. The MVC interference pattern will reveal a normal firing frequency (30 to 50 Hz) but only one or two motor units firing, demonstrating decreased recruitment of motor units (15:1 to 50:1) but normal activation. This loss of MUAPs usually indicates either axonal loss or conduction block, although it could occur in end-stage myopathy when there is a marked loss of muscle fibers. Figure 12-22 illustrates the interference pattern with upper- versus lower-motor neuron disorder. Decreased activation and decreased recruitment can occur together with disorders that affect both upper and lower motor neurons such as ALS.

A more common pattern occurring with myopathies is that of early recruitment. As muscle fibers are lost, the motor unit generates less force. Subsequently, more motor units must fire to produce even small levels of force. Early recruitment can only be discerned by the electromyographer by comparing

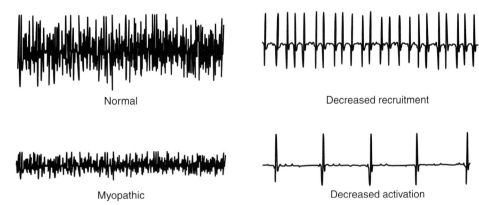

Normal

Decreased recruitment

Myopathic

Decreased activation

**FIGURE 12-22** Normal and Abnormal Interference Patterns. The upper left trace shows a normal interference pattern during maximal voluntary contraction. The bottom left shows myopathic recruitment, with normal neural drive but smaller amplitude, short duration MUAPs. The traces on the right show the "picket fence" appearance with neuropathic conditions. The top right trace shows one motor unit firing at 30 Hz, a case of decreased recruitment (30:1 ratio) but normal activation (i.e., firing rate). This suggests a lower motor neuron lesion, as in axonal loss or a conduction block. The bottom right trace shows a single MUAP firing at only 5 Hz during MVC, demonstrating a normal recruitment ratio (5:1) but decreased activation. This shows an upper motor neuron issue—either a CNS lesion or simply pain and inhibition. (Modified with permission from Preston, 2005, Figs. 15-13 and 15-14.)

the low level of muscle force being generated by the patient's muscle to the (excessive) number of MUAPs firing.

### Interpretation of EMG Studies

Although no individual EMG finding is typically diagnostic of any particular disorder, the combination of MUAP morphology and firing patterns usually can discriminate between neuropathic, myopathic, or NMJ pathology. In addition, it is usually possible to determine whether the disorder is acute or chronic and, in the case of neuropathies, whether the lesion is upper motor neuron or lower motor neuron and whether it is due to axonal loss or demyelination. With acute axonal loss, before Wallerian degeneration takes place, the MUAP is normal. The only EMG abnormality will be decreased recruitment from the loss of some of the motor axons. As denervation takes place, abnormal spontaneous potentials will appear, beginning with Fibs and PSWs. The time it takes for these denervation potentials to develop depends on the distance from the lesion to the motor endplate. Abnormal MUPs will appear much sooner with distal lesions than with proximal lesions. Fibrillation potentials may appear in the muscles of the hand within a few days of a laceration at the wrist, while they will not appear for several weeks following a lesion to the brachial plexus.

In chronic stages of axonal loss, reinnervation occurs, with subsequent changes in MUAP morphology. With gradual or partial denervation, reinnervation occurs primarily through axonal sprouting. The surviving motor units then acquire additional muscle fibers, resulting in polyphasic MUAPs of higher amplitude and longer duration. Along with reduced recruitment, these are hallmark signs of a chronic neuropathic disorder with axonal loss. In contrast, with neuropathic disorders involving demyelination only, the MUAPs will be normal. Although CV is slowed, the signals will still reach the muscle fibers and still create the same MUAP recruitment patterns. If, however, the demyelination is severe enough to create conduction block, then the number of firing motor units will be decreased, creating a decreased recruitment pattern. The findings of decreased recruitment with normal-looking MUAPs are therefore indicative of either acute axonal loss without reinnervation or demyelination causing a partial conduction block. Although the EMG findings are the same with these pathologies, the NCS will differ as demyelination will cause **conduction slowing**, decreased nerve CV, along with the EMG findings. This is an example of how the combination of NCS and EMG findings narrows the differential diagnosis more than either set of findings by themselves. In clinical practice, the electrodiagnosis is actually more difficult than this as pure demyelinating lesions are uncommon. More commonly, with entrapment neuropathies such as carpal tunnel syndrome, some axonal loss accompanies the demyelination.

Table 12-15 summarizes the NCS and EMG findings in various neuropathic disorders. Note the findings with axonal loss assume incomplete denervation (i.e., there are surviving motor units from which axonal sprouting can occur). In the case of complete denervation, as in a laceration that transects

the nerve, reinnervation can only occur through axonal regrowth. For this regrowth to occur, the anterior horn cells must be intact to create the regrowth, and an epineural sheath must be intact throughout to guide the path of regrowth. The axon will regenerate at a very slow rate (about 1 mm per day), taking months or years to reach the target muscle, depending on the location of the lesion. In this case of complete denervation, the acute findings (before Wallerian degeneration occurs) will be the same as in partial axonal loss. The chronic findings however (several weeks post onset of symptoms) will differ. Several weeks after partial denervation there will be decreased recruitment of larger polyphasic motor units, while several weeks following complete denervation there will be no recruitment with voluntary contraction until regeneration takes place.

In strictly myopathic lesions (Table 12-16), there are decreased numbers of functioning muscle fibers, but the motor drive (from anterior horn cell to NMJ) is intact. The resulting EMG pattern will show normal activation but decreased amplitudes and less synchronous firing (i.e., polyphasia). Because there are fewer functioning muscle fibers, early recruitment will also occur as more motor units fire sooner to generate the desired level of force. As the myopathy becomes more chronic, it is common to get some accompanying denervation and reinnervation. Abnormal MUAPs will then become evident, appearing similar to findings with chronic neuropathic disorders. However, with the myopathic disorder, recruitment will be either normal or early. Also, with myopathic disorders, NCS will be essentially normal, with the exception of motor NCS to the proximal muscles. Motor NCS to the distal muscles will usually be normal and sensory NCS should always be normal.

Sensory NCS will also be normal in NMJ disorders, which often present with a clinical picture similar to myopathies and with EMG patterns similar to myopathies. In presynaptic disorders (e.g., Lambert-Eaton myasthenic syndrome), baseline CMAP amplitudes are usually decreased while in postsynaptic disorders (e.g., myasthenia gravis), they are usually normal. The addition of RNS helps clarify the diagnosis. In presynaptic disorders, RMNS shows a decrement in CMAP amplitudes with low frequency stimulation but an increment with either high frequency stimulation or after 10 seconds of MVC exercise. With postsynaptic disorders, RMNS reveals a decrement with low frequency stimulation and little change with high frequency stimulation but a further decrement 2 to 3 minutes after brief MVC exercise. As with all electrodiagnostic testing, these findings should only supplement, not replace, the clinical examination. The findings of NCS and EMG for myopathic and NMJ disorders are summarized in Table 12-16.

In summary, needle EMG findings often permit the underlying lesion to be localized to the neural, muscular, or NMJ component of the motor units in question. In conjunction with NCS, needle EMG provides localization of nerve root versus plexus lesion, site of nerve injury and axonal regeneration, identification of specific myopathies such as myotonic disorders, and increased muscle activity. Thus, needle EMG

**TABLE 12-15 NCS and EMG Findings in Neuropathic Disorders**

| | NCS | | | EMG | | | |
|---|---|---|---|---|---|---|---|
| | Motor Studies | Sensory Studies | RMNS and LRs | Insertional Activity | Spontaneous Activity | MUAP Parameters | Interference Pattern |
| Axonal Loss Acute (3d-3wk)* | A: CV: ≥75% DL: ≤130% | A: CV: ≥75% DL: ≤130% | — | — | — | — | Recruitment |
| Axonal Loss Subacute (3wk-3 mo)* | A: CV: ≥75% DL: ≤130% | A: CV: ≥75% DL: ≤130% | — | Increased | Fibrillations PSWs | — | Recruitment |
| Axonal Loss Chronic (>3 mos)* | A: CV: ≥75% DL: ≤130% | A: CV: ≥75% DL: ≤130% | — | — | Fibrillations PSWs | Polyphasic Amplitude Duration | Recruitment |
| Axonal Loss Long Term (>12 mos)* | A: / — CV: / — DL: / — | A: / — CV: / — DL: / — | — | — | — | Polyphasic Amplitude Duration | Recruitment |
| Demyelination Proximal to Stimulation | A: — CV: —** DL: — | A: — CV: — DL: — | LR | — | — | — | — |
| Demyelination Distal to Stimulation | A: — CV: — DL: | A: CV: DL: | LR | — | — | — | — |
| Demyelination + Block Proximal to Stimulation | A: — CV: —** DL: — | A: — CV: — DL: — | LR | — | — | — | Recruitment |
| Demyelination + Block Distal to Stimulation | A: CV: — DL: | A: CV: DL: | LR | — | — | — | Recruitment |

*The time frames that define acute, subacute, etc., will vary depending on the distance from the lesion to the recorded muscle. Acute indicates that Wallerian degeneration has occurred but denervation potentials have not yet appeared. Subacute indicates that denervation potentials have appeared (at 2 to 6 wks) but reinnervation has not occurred. Chronic indicates that reinnervation has occurred. Long term demonstrates the end result of axonal loss with successful reinnervation and hence the loss of denervation potentials and return to close to normal CMAP parameters.

**Motor CV with demyelination will only be slowed when measured across the site of the lesion.

NCS = nerve conduction studies; EMG = electromyography; LR = late responses; RMNS = repetitive motor nerve stimulation; MUAP = motor unit action potential; Block = conduction block; A = amplitude; CV = conduction velocity; DL = distal latency; — = normal; = increased; = marked increase; = decreased; = marked decrease.

examination provides essential information of diagnostic significance in the management of patients with peripheral nerve or muscle disorders.

## Clinical Applications and Usefulness of Electrophysiologic Testing

Motor and sensory NCS and needle EMG examination are very useful diagnostic tests in the assessment of peripheral nerve, NMJ, or muscle disorders. Many neuromuscular experts consider these tests as an extension of the neurological examination. NCS has high sensitivity for diagnosis of

peripheral polyneuropathy, often at a preclinical stage (Kimura, 2001). NCS can distinguish axonal from demyelinating neuropathies, whereas clinical observations or neurological examination alone cannot make such a distinction. NCS is an essential diagnostic test to confirm and localize common entrapment neuropathies, such as carpal tunnel syndrome, and in conjunction with needle EMG examination has an indispensable role in assessment of peripheral nerve injuries.

Needle EMG examination is very helpful in differentiating neurogenic from myopathic disorders and in the diagnosis of certain muscle and nerve diseases such as ALS or myotonic

**TABLE 12-16   NCS and EMG Findings in Myopathic and Neuromuscular Junction Disorders**

| | NCS | | | EMG | | | |
|---|---|---|---|---|---|---|---|
| | Motor Studies | Sensory Studies | RMNS and LRs | Insertional Activity | Spontaneous Activity | MUAP Parameters | Interference Pattern |
| Myopathy | A: — CV: — DL: — | A: — CV: — DL: — | — | — | — | Amplitude Polyphasic | Amplitude + Early Recruitment |
| Myopathy with Denervation | A: — CV: — DL: — | A: — CV: — DL: — | — | Increased | Fibrillations PSWs CRDs | — | Amplitude + Early Recruitment |
| Myotonia | A: —/ CV: — DL: — | A: — CV: — DL: — | RMNS may show Decrement | Myotonic discharges* | Myotonic discharges* | Amplitude |
| Polymyositis | A: — CV: — DL: — | A: — CV: — DL: — | | Increased | Fibrillations PSWs | — | Amplitude |
| Presynaptic NMJ Disorder | A: —/ CV: — DL: — | A: — CV: — DL: — | RMNS Decreased postexercise | — | — / or Fibrillations PSWs | — / or Amplitude Polyphasic | Amplitude — / Early Recruitment |
| Postsynaptic NMJ Disorder | A: — CV: — DL: — | A: — CV: — DL: — | RMNS Increased Postexercise | — | — / or Fibrillations PSWs | — / or Amplitude Polyphasic | Amplitude — / Early Recruitment |
| Upper Motor Neuron Lesion | A: — CV: — DL: — | A: — CV: — DL: — | — | — | — | — | Activation |
| Lower Motor Neuron Lesion | A: CV: ≥75% DL: ≤130% | A: CV: ≥75% DL: ≤130% | — | Increased | Fibrillations PSWs | Polyphasic Amplitude Duration | Recruitment |

*Although myotonic discharges are considered a spontaneous activity, in myotonia they tend to occur in response to needle movement or voluntary muscle contraction and not predominantly at rest.

NCS = nerve conduction studies; EMG = electromyography; LR = late responses; RMNS = repetitive motor nerve stimulation; MUAP = motor unit action potential; NMJ = neuromuscular junction; A = amplitude; CV = conduction velocity; DL = distal latency; — = normal; = increased; = marked increase; = decreased; = marked decrease.

dystrophies. Needle EMG examination provides valuable prognostic and localizing information in assessment of cervical or lumbosacral radiculopathy and plexopathy. Both nerve conduction study and needle EMG examination have their limitations in certain neuromuscular disorders, such as mild pure small fiber sensory neuropathy, compressive cervical or lumbar radiculopathy where the symptoms are limited to pain or sensory disturbances, and in mild myopathies. Complications are rarely encountered in NCS, and likewise, needle EMG examination complications are rare but do include subcutaneous hematoma, infection, and local short-lived pain.

The sensitivity and specificity values of ENMG studies vary with the body region being examined as specific techniques work better in some areas than others. In general,

sensitivities are not as high as specificities. For example, in carpal tunnel syndrome, sensitivities of the ENMG examination range from 49% to 84% (AAEM, 1993; Jablecki, 1993; Kimura, 2001) while specificities are usually 95% or higher (Kuntzer, 1994; Lew, 2005). Electrophysiologic testing is based on a thorough clinical examination. The stronger the clinical findings, the higher the incidence of abnormal ENMG findings. In one study examining cervical radiculopathy, abnormal findings were found in 90% of subjects with three clinical signs, 59% of subjects with two clinical signs, and only 10% of subjects with one clinical sign (Miller, 1999). This underscores the importance of not only combining different aspects of the ENMG examination but also considering the combination of ENMG and clinical findings.

## THINK ABOUT IT 12.3

- What happens to CV with axonal loss compared with demyelination?
- How do CMAPs differ with presynaptic disorders compared with postsynaptic disorders?
- Describe the H-reflex, what it represents, and how it is used as a diagnostic test.
- Describe the F-wave, what it represents, and how it is used as a diagnostic test.
- How do NCV values change from birth through aging?
- How do CVs vary considering a patient's height?
- The EMG can help answer what clinical questions?

- Describe the characteristic sounds heard during EMG testing and why the sounds can assist with diagnosis.
- Describe the normal EMG response at rest.
- Presence of fibrillation potentials is indicative of what?
- What would a fibrillation potential look and sound like on EMG testing?
- CRDs occur with what type of denervation?
- Presence of fasciculation potentials is indicative of what neurological disorder?
- What best reflects the number of muscle fibers within a motor unit?
- What test result would be indicative of partial denervation with reinnervation?

## Let's Review

1. What are the three main categories of medical diagnostic tests?

2. Describe the main diagnostic tests within each category, including the major indications and results.

3. Describe the purposes of the various diagnostic imaging techniques.

4. Describe the advantages and disadvantages of various diagnostic imaging.

5. Describe various electrodiagnostic testing to help evaluate the status of the anterior horn cell, nerve roots, peripheral nerves, NMJ, and muscles.

6. Describe the procedure for NCS and EMG.

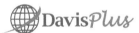 For additional resources, including Focus on Evidence tables, case study discussions, references, and glossary, please visit http://davisplus.fadavis.com

## CHAPTER SUMMARY

Therapists in rehabilitation settings must be aware of the patient holistically, including awareness of comorbid conditions in each patient and risk for any medical conditions that may develop. Although therapists don't typically order or perform clinical laboratory tests or diagnostic imaging (except in U.S. military PT practice), it is important therapists understand the reports from such tests as well as electrophysiologic nerve and muscle tests, which are commonly performed by PTs. Understanding diagnostic tests performed on a patient, including clinical laboratory tests, diagnostic imaging, and electrophysiological testing with interpretation of the reports of those tests as explained in this chapter, can help the therapist understand implications for diagnosis and appropriate referral. Understanding diagnostic testing results also informs articulation of expected patient prognosis and the individualized therapy plan of care. If a medical diagnosis must be made or if appropriate care and interventions for a suspected condition is outside the scope of practice of the therapist, the therapist should refer the patient to the appropriate medical professional.

# Development of Neuromotor Skills: Lifespan Approach

**CHAPTER 13**

Karen Y. Lunnen, PT, EdD

## CHAPTER OUTLINE

## CHAPTER OBJECTIVES

Upon completion of this chapter, the learner should be able to:

1. Describe the theoretical foundations that explain the complexity of neuromotor development and aging.
2. Apply the theoretical foundations of a lifespan perspective to examination of neuromotor development.
3. Apply knowledge of changes in various body systems with aging and their possible effects on functional activities such as ambulation.
4. Explain the concept of variability as related to neuromotor development.
5. Describe strategies for optimizing a child's performance of neuromotor or functional tasks in a testing situation.
6. Provide the rationale for selecting a specific standardized test of neuromotor development.

**Neuromotor development** is the process of change in motor behavior related to the age of the individual. Knowledge of neuromotor development is fundamental to understanding the development of functional movement and employing effective strategies for the evaluation and treatment of patients with neurological conditions across the lifespan. It is impossible to consider motor development in isolation; it must be considered within a broader context. Whole textbooks have been written on the development of functional movement or motor development across the lifespan (Cech, 2012; Gabbard 2016; Haywood, 2014; Payne, 2012). What follows is intended to create a basic framework for understanding a complex and evolving body of knowledge as it applies to the developing human from conception to death. Lifespan is categorized by periods: prenatal (conception to birth), infancy (birth to 1 year), childhood (1 to 10 years), adolescence (11 to 19 years), adulthood (20 to 59 years), and late adulthood (60 years to death). At the risk of oversimplifying, we tend to think of development in terms of maturation during the early part of the lifespan and of decline during the latter part.

Neuromotor assessment must capture the dynamic nature of the process, and measurement tools that contribute meaningfully to the overall evaluation of the patient and the long-term goals of therapeutic intervention must be utilized. Examination of other musculoskeletal and neuromuscular aspects of functional movement and the movement system covered in other chapters obviously provides an important foundation for understanding neuromotor development. Knowledge about the status of an individual's cognition and perception is also important.

The purpose of this chapter is to provide overviews of neuromotor development, the theoretical constructs that describe its complexity across the lifespan, and the principles of neuromotor examination and an introduction to selected tools for the assessment of motor development in the pediatric population. With age, the contributions of various intrinsic and extrinsic variables and their interplay with experience, culture, gender, and environment all influence motor development. The resulting complexity makes it more difficult to establish norms for motor development with increasing age. Functional measures, which rely on the interplay of multiple systems, are more meaningful and more commonly used in the assessment of older adults. Functional assessment measures are covered in depth in Chapter 10.

# Overview of Developmental and Aging Theories

Theories are formulated to explain, predict, and understand phenomena and, in many cases, to challenge and extend existing knowledge within the limits of critical bounding assumptions (Swanson, 2013). Theories attempting to explain the maturation of human capabilities from conception to adulthood, including motor development, are often categorized as developmental theories. Theories of aging attempt to explain the normal decline that is observed at the molecular, cellular, tissue, and system levels. The theoretical constructs for understanding human development typically vary with their emphasis on biological imperatives of the individual versus the environment or with the emphasis on one body system versus others. Chapter 14 provides a detailed description of various theoretical models that describe motor development. A brief summary is provided here.

Many developmental assessment tools grew out of the **neuro-maturational theory**. First proposed by Gesell in the 1930s, the theory emphasizes the predictable and orderly appearance of infant/child behavior as the nervous system matures (Gesell, 1934, 1940). According to this theory, the environment supports but does not fundamentally alter the sequence of motor development. The concept of motor milestones occurring at predictable times in development and representing markers of "normal" motor development grew out of this theoretical construct. Gesell (1940; 1934) formulated the law of developmental directions to describe the general progression of development within the human body from cephalo to caudal, proximal to distal, and radial to ulnar directions as the nervous system matures. Although Gesell described the overall process as orderly and predictable, he believed development was not a completely linear process but was more dynamic, with alternating periods of advancement and regression of skills (Gesell, 1939).

Cognitive theorists such as Piaget (1952) and Skinner (1972) recognized the importance of the maturation of cognitive-neural structures in shaping motor development but focused more on the environment. Skinner emphasized the importance of contingent learning and believed that both motor and cognitive development are shaped by the consequences of an individual's interaction with the environment. Piaget believed that cognitive functions of all types derived from knowledge gained through action. Practitioners continue to use aspects of these theoretical frameworks to understand the complex interplay between cognitive and motor domains and to shape behavior through the reinforcement of desirable behavior.

**Dynamic systems theory** as described by Thelen and colleagues (1987, 1989, 1991) seems to more accurately capture the complexity of the maturation process and is the most widely accepted theory. According to this theory, development is the result of a dynamic interplay between mechanical, neurological, cognitive, and perceptual factors within the individual and variable aspects of the environment and the task (Campbell, 2006). The theory places equal importance on the internal components of the individual and the external context of the task. Progression is influenced by motivation, experience, and practice as well as the genetically unique characteristics of the individual. Thelen perceived development not as a linear process progressing in a continuous, steady rate but rather as a cyclic process in which a critical change in one area can cause the whole system to shift, resulting in a new motor behavior. This phase shift or transition period is characterized by increased variability and is considered an ideal time for intervention because it represents a readiness for the individual to change.

## THINK ABOUT IT 13.1

Motor development is a complex process probably best described by the dynamic systems theory. Describe a motor task and how various aspects of the individual (including multiple body systems), the environment, and specific aspects of the task itself might be adapted to influence the level of successful performance.

Theories of aging attempt to address the decline seen in biological structures (from cellular to system levels) and functional performance as an individual progresses in years. **Aging** can be described in simplistic terms as the process of getting older or change as the result of the passage of time (O'Toole, 1997); however, the definition gains complexity depending on the theoretical framework applied. For example, an accepted definition by evolutionary biologists is "an age-dependent or age-progressive decline in intrinsic physiological function, leading to an increase in age-specific mortality rate (i.e., a decrease in survival rate) and a decrease in age-specific reproductive rate" (Flatt, 2012, p. 148). **Senescence**, the process of deterioration with age, is a synonym for aging.

Literally hundreds of theories have been postulated to explain the mechanisms involved in the aging process, but no one theory is widely accepted, and the complexity of the process most likely encompasses multiple theories. The process varies in how it affects different individuals and different organs within the same individual. A variety of factors influence the aging process over a lifetime, including heredity, culture, diet, environment, exercise, past illnesses, and stress (Martin, 2016). Individuals do not reach some arbitrary point in time when deterioration begins, despite the popularized concept of being "over the hill." Decline is seen in some organ systems as early as the 30s and much later in others.

Most aging theories can be conceptualized in two broad categories: (1) developmental-genetic or fundamentalist and (2) nongenetic or environmental (Lewis, 2007b; Scalise-Smith, 2013). The fundamentalist category is based on age-related changes at the tissue level of the individual including limits to cell division for specific cell types, which was first introduced by the scientists Hayflick and Moorehead (1961); evolutionary models, including the stress theory; neuroendocrine and hormonal changes caused by gradually elevated sensitivity thresholds of the hypothalamus that disrupt self-regulatory homeostasis (Dilman, 1971); the deleterious role of free radicals (i.e., reactive oxygen species) at the cellular level, both mitochondrial and nuclear (Sergiev, 2015); the accumulation of nondegradable byproducts of metabolism (Gladyshev, 2013); the cause and consequences of chronic low-grade systemic inflammation associated with aging (Woods, 2012); and the beneficial effects of caloric restriction (Kirk, 2001). Included in the environmental theories are various versions of damage to genetic material, which is accelerated with aging and influenced by various exposures (e.g., radiation); conditions (e.g., lack of sleep); imbalances (e.g., too much growth hormone and too little insulin); and mechanics at the genetic level (e.g., abnormal telomeres). Additional research is needed to capture the complex and dynamic process of aging separate from pathological processes and to understand what is normative for an age range of individuals with similar lifestyles and genetic factors.

Chronological age is the actual age in days/months/years of an individual. Biological or physiological age is affected by a variety of intrinsic and extrinsic variables and may be close to the chronological age or may differ greatly. For example, a professional athlete may have a much lower biological age than his or her chronological age, and an individual with a chronic health condition may have a much greater biological age than chronological age. A wide variety of dynamic processes, including experience, culture, gender, environment, and lifestyle influence the aging process. Some antecedents of aging are universal and species specific. Some outcomes are more likely than others, some can be made more likely, and some are not possible.

## Review of Physiology and Neuroscience of Neuromotor Development Across the Lifespan

The acquisition and performance of movement is dependent on the growth and development of multiple body systems and their efficient interplay. The Physical Stress Theory developed by Mueller and Maluf (2002) states that "changes in the relative level of physical stress cause a predictable adaptive response in all biological tissue" (p. 385). Changes in one or more body systems as part of the aging process can have a deleterious effect on the response to stress and can disturb the body's internal homeostasis, resulting in impaired motor performance among other things. In the examination of motor development from conception to death, we find that various body systems mature and deteriorate at varying rates. A brief summary of these processes over time, with an emphasis on the systems that most influence functional movement, follows.

**Nervous system:** Neural maturation does not dictate the process of neuromotor development as proposed by the early theorists, but it is certainly a critical aspect. By the eighth week of fetal development, the organs are formed through a beautifully orchestrated process of cell proliferation, growth, migration, and differentiation (Lundy-Ekman, 2013). The nervous system develops from ectoderm, the outer layer of the embryo. Development of the nervous system begins late in the third week of embryogenesis with formation of the neural plate, a thickened portion of ectoderm (Sadler, 2014; Young, 2015). The edges of the neural plate fold up, forming a neural tube, with closure of the cranial end by the 24th day of gestation and the caudal end 2 days later. Neurons in the dorsal region of the neural tube process sensory information, and those in the ventral region innervate skeletal muscle (Lundy-Ekman, 2013). The brain forms from the rostral end of the neural tube beginning at about the 28th day of gestation with three enlargements (i.e., hindbrain, midbrain, and forebrain).

The nerve cells must determine their primary function (e.g., motor or sensory) and establish a connection with the muscle or sensory tissue they will innervate. It is believed that this process is not genetically predetermined for the cell but is determined by where it migrates (Lundy-Ekman, 2013). A growth cone on the forward end of the neuron cell body actively samples the environment for molecular signals from extracellular guidance cells (either attractant or repellant) until it finds its target cell (Lundy-Ekman, 2013; Waxman, 2013). Receptor sites develop on the postsynaptic membrane of the target cell, and a functional connection forms through repeated release of neurotransmitters. In the process of brain development, it is believed that as many as two-thirds of the brain's neurons die, unable to establish an optimal connection with their target cells. Modifications can occur in the developing brain when an appropriate stimulus is applied or withheld during a critical period (Waxman, 2013). By the end of the first 3 months the brain is just more than half of adult brain volume (Holland, 2014).

Although evidence supports neurogenesis as a lifelong process, the majority of neurons (billions of them) are present in our brains by the time we are born. During the first few months of life, there is considerable dendritic branching and remodeling of other connections in response to the infant's experiences. The number of synapses is believed to peak at about 6 to 12 months of age; with further selectivity/specificity, the number gradually decreases, reaching adult levels at 5 to 10 years. Myelination of the long axons is necessary for full functionality; this begins in the fourth fetal month and is generally complete by the third year of life (Lundy-Ekman, 2013). Peripheral nervous system and cranial nerves are essentially complete at birth, but myelination of the brain continues into adulthood. The process of myelination of the corticospinal tract, one of the most important descending tracts, begins about

2 months before birth and is nearly complete by 12 months of age (Lundy-Ekman, 2013).

As the individual ages, alterations of the nervous system that have an effect on neuromotor performance and function take place at the gross anatomic, cellular, and molecular levels. Two specific aspects of nervous system function diminish over time: reaction time (a measure of nervous system efficiency during movement) and cognition (which enables interaction with the environment). A number of factors contribute to this decline.

The total weight and volume of the brain decreases with normal aging (15% decrease by 80 years of age), particularly the frontal and temporal aspects (Cohen, 1999; Young, 2015). The cortex thins, the number of glial cells increases, and the ventricles enlarge (Fox, 1999). Loss of conduction velocity in sensory and motor nerves within both the central and peripheral nervous systems, loss of myelin, damage to the DNA, accumulation of free radicals, and decreased levels of neurotransmitters have all been reported (Cohen, 1999; Gorgon, 2014). Shrinkage of white matter as a result of axonal death or degeneration of myelin may also contribute to the decreasing volume. Disuse may contribute to the loss of axonal collaterals. Myelin degeneration may be responsible for the decreases in conduction rates and potential amplitude and increases in latency periods. The production, release, and metabolism of the neurotransmitters acetylcholine, dopamine, and norepinephrine also decrease. Research suggests that after the age of 30 years, nerve conduction velocity in the peripheral nerves decreases at the rate of 1 m per second every decade (Cech, 2012). Cerebral perfusion may decrease by as much as 20% by the age of 70 years. A general decline is seen in all five senses in the neurosensory system (i.e., touch, smell, taste, vision, and hearing) as well as in proprioception/kinesthesia. Each of these sensory systems is complex and is affected by age-related changes at the cellular, molecular, and system levels.

**Cognitive system: Cognition** is a term referring to the mental processes involved in the ability to think, learn, and remember (Barnes, 2010; Scalise-Smith, 2013). It is the basis for how we reason, judge, concentrate, plan, and organize (National Institute on Aging, 2016). Critical questions remain in our understanding of cognitive aging, but experts agree that decline is not the result of loss of many, many cells but instead of minimal, selective cell loss. In addition, it is not a passive process but one in which the brain is continuously adapting at molecular, cellular, network, and behavioral levels (Barnes, 2010).

A variety of genetic risk factors as well as multidimensional lifestyle factors appear to affect the process. Exercise, especially aerobic exercise, appears to have a positive effect on cognition by reducing brain atrophy and increasing brain transfusion. Stress, genetic factors that influence the vascular state (e.g., blood pressure), metabolic syndrome factors, and inflammatory factors negatively influence cognition (Barnes, 2010).

**Musculoskeletal system:** The structural aspects of the musculoskeletal system develop early in the prenatal period, with skeletal muscle tissue and limb buds appearing during the fifth week of embryonic development and limb movements observed as early as the eighth week (Sadler, 2014). Miraculously, by the end of the third month of gestation, the fetus is capable of kicking his legs, turning his feet, bending his wrists, turning his head, opening his mouth, and swallowing; and by the end of the fourth month of gestation, the fetus may suck his thumb.

Muscle and bone continue to develop into adulthood. Differences in muscle type are seen throughout the lifespan with type I (slow-twitch) fibers predominating in infancy, consistent with the demands for postural control (Scalise-Smith, 2013). Maturity produces more type II fibers and a corresponding increase in the variability of movement patterns. Through adolescence, males display a greater increase in fiber size than girls of the same age. Girls have a steady increase in the number of muscle fibers from about the ages of 3.5 to 10 years. Boys reportedly have periods of rapid increase from birth until 2 years of age and from 10 to 16 years. Although slowed, muscle fiber development continues well into middle adulthood.

Increasing age is associated with various factors that reduce muscle protein mass and function, termed **sarcopenia** (Rolland, 2008). These factors include decreased muscle mass; infiltration of muscle by fat and nonconductive tissues; slowing of muscle contractile properties; decline in available motor neurons; motor unit remodeling; decreased fiber size; and decline in total number of fibers, fast-twitch fibers in particular (Frontera, 2014; Marcus, 2012; Scalise-Smith, 2013). Physical activity level is an important variable, and strengthening exercises can partially reverse age-related changes in muscle. However, on average, muscle mass decreases up to 40% between the ages of 50 and 80 years, with a corresponding decrease in muscle force production of approximately 30% between the ages of 60 and 90 years (Scalise-Smith, 2013).

Muscle weakness contributes to decreased physical activity, weight gain, and increased risk of falls. Muscle represents the protein reserve of the body, and decreased muscle mass diminishes the protein synthesis needed to combat disease and injury that often accompany aging (Marcus, 2012). Changes in hormone levels (including insulin, growth hormone, testosterone, and estrogen) are also thought to negatively affect muscle protein mass. The complex interplay of factors related to sarcopenia makes it the major cause of disability and frailty in older adults.

The skeletal system starts as a cartilaginous model, with the gradual appearance of ossification centers starting during the prenatal period. Primary ossification centers form at the midportion of the long bones, whereas secondary ossification centers form at the end of the bone shaft (epiphyseal plate). Almost all growth in bone length is complete by age 18 years in boys and slightly earlier in girls (Scalise-Smith, 2013). Even after bones have reached their full length, appositional growth continues throughout life.

The density of bone varies with the ratio of bone growth to bone resorption and is affected by nutrient intake, physical activity, weight-bearing, hormones, and medications. During childhood and adolescence, bone growth exceeds bone resorption; bone density increases, remains stable through middle adulthood, and then reverses, with bone resorption occurring faster than bone growth and a resultant decrease in bone density. Women begin to lose bone mass during the third decade, with a typical yearly decrease of 0.5% to 2% that doubles to about 2% per year after menopause (Brown, 2012). Bone fractures less easily in children because their bones are more flexible, porous, and strong (owing to a thick periosteum); in addition, fractures heal more quickly because of faster and stronger callus formation.

Flexibility is the result of joint mobility and the extensibility of soft tissues that cross the joint. In general, flexibility is limited at birth secondary to intrauterine positioning, referred to as *physiological flexion*. The absence of physiological flexion in preterm infants affects the course of motor development, requiring alterations in positioning and handling to support balanced development of flexor and extensor strength. Flexibility increases through adolescence and then gradually decreases through adulthood. Age-related changes at the cellular level include decreased proliferation of fibroblasts, the basic connective tissue cells and reduced responsiveness to circulating growth hormones and altered response to cyclic loading, which compromises repair (Christiansen, 2012). Collagenous tissues (including tendons, ligaments, and fasciae) gradually lose water from the cellular matrix and undergo an increase in the number of crosslink fibers and loss of elastic properties, resulting overall in decreased strength and range of motion and increased stiffness (Scalise-Smith, 2013).

Body composition also changes with age. From about the age of 30 years onward, there is a gradual loss of lean tissue and an increase of fat, with fat accumulation particularly in the midportion of the body. Research suggests that the increase in fat mass may escalate inflammation, increasing susceptibility to other problems including metabolic syndrome, heart disease, diabetes, and cancer (Brinkley, 2012; Brown, 2012). It is important to remember that flexibility, strength, and bone density are modifiable throughout the lifespan.

**Cardiopulmonary system:** Cardiac structures form between the third and eighth weeks of fetal development, and all aspects of the cardiopulmonary system make the transition to the extrauterine environment and are fully functional soon after birth. The heart doubles in size in the first year and quadruples in size by age 5 years. With increased size comes a corresponding increase in stroke volume, a decrease in heart rate, an increase in blood pressure, and an overall increase in aerobic capacity. The maximum heart rate capacity decreases from about 200 beats per minute (bpm) through young adulthood to about 170 bpm at age 65 years. The functional capacities of the cardiopulmonary system decrease with decreasing physical activity and structural changes characteristic of later adulthood. Structurally, decreased capacity is the result of decreased elasticity of the tissues (including blood vessels and ventricles), decreased efficiency of the structures, and decreased ability to increase workload.

An overall decrease in exercise tolerance is evident in the progressive decline in $VO_2$ maximum, starting at age 20 to 30 years and falling by approximately 10% per decade (Strait, 2012). Overall, individuals may demonstrate a blunted heart rate response to exercise and may take longer to recover from exercise (Voss, 2012). One age-related change in older individuals is the tendency to generate more blood lactate because work is performed less efficiently. The resulting acidosis triggers an earlier fatigue and increased rating of perceived exertion with exercise (Cohen, 2014). It is important to recognize the normal variation with age when monitoring vital signs and to be cognizant of the effects of medications prescribed to manage heart disease. See Chapter 11 for more specific information.

Crude pulmonary structures form early in the embryonic period (weeks 0 to 6); with further growth and differentiation, by the 24th week of gestation the bronchial tree is complete from the glottis to the terminal bronchioles, the diaphragm is beginning to form, and gas exchange is possible (Tecklin, 2015). A critical point in the development of independent ventilation in the infant is the presence of surfactant, which reduces surface tension within the alveolus, allowing inflation of the alveolus with less work. Surfactant is present at about 26 weeks of gestation and appears at a mature level at about 34 weeks. The first 18- to 24-month period is characterized by continued growth in the number of alveolar sacs, increasing the surface area available for gas exchange (Tecklin, 2015).

With aging, a number of mechanical factors result in increased work of breathing: decreased chest wall compliance and lung elastic recoil, progressive weakness of intercostal muscles, increased calcification of the ribs, and changes in spinal curvature (Lewis, 2007a). Slowly progressive alterations at the cellular and tissue levels with age result in decreased efficiency of ventilation, diffusion, and pulmonary circulation (Lewis, 2007a).

## ■ Overview of Key Concepts in Neuromotor Development

An understanding of the theoretical constructs underlying neuromotor development and the therapist's knowledge and abilities related to the movement system are the underpinnings of neuromotor assessment. In this section, we provide an overview of motor milestones, reflex development, general trends in the progression of motor skills, the implications of variability, the importance of variable practice, and the concept of critical periods in development.

The concept of motor milestones is a product of early theorists such as Gesell (1940), with analysis of motor skills becoming a hallmark of pediatric assessment in the 20th century. A child's attainment of motor skills or milestones can be ascertained from history and/or observation and are helpful in establishing a reference point or an initial screen. Motor milestones also form the basis for the variety of standardized measurement tools that are described later in the chapter. Table 13-1 references the mean age and range of ages for the development of key neuromotor skills or milestones based on

| TABLE 13-1 | Motor Milestones (the mean age and range, in months, for the development of key neuromotor skills useful as a broad screen) | | |
|---|---|---|---|
| **MOTOR MILESTONE** | **WHO 50th PERCENTILE (MONTHS)** | **WHO RANGE (MONTHS)** | **PDMS-2 (MONTHS)** |
| Propping on forearms | | | 4 |
| Rolling back to stomach | | | 7 |
| Sitting without support | 5.9 | (5.8–6) | 6 |
| Standing with assistance | 7.4 | (7.3–7.5) | |
| Moving forward on stomach (crawling) | | | 8 |
| Moving forward on hands and knees (creeping) | 8.3 | (8.2–8.4) | |
| Walking with assistance | 9 | (8.9–9.1) | |
| Standing alone | 10.8 | (10.7–11) | |
| Grasping (pincer) | | | 11 |
| Walking alone | 12 | (11.9–12.1) | |
| Jumping up | | | 23–24 |
| Running (30 feet in 6 seconds or less) | | | 29–30 |
| Walking upstairs without support, one foot per step | | | 35–36 |
| Walking down stairs without support, one foot per step | | | 43–44 |
| Hopping five hops on one foot, then three to five hops on other foot | | | 47–48 |
| Skipping eight steps | | | 57–58 |

Peabody Developmental Motor Scales, 2nd edition (PDMS-2; Folio, 2000); World Health Organization, Motor Development Study (2006).

data from a study by the World Health Organization (WHO) published in 2006 and also the Peabody Developmental Motor Scales, 2nd edition (PDMS-2) published in 2000 (Folio). The WHO study sampled 816 healthy children aged 4 to 24 months living in Ghana, India, Norway, Oman, and the United States and determined the age (in months) at which 50% of the sample attained six key motor milestones. The PDMS-2 reference value is based on the age at which 50% of children in a normative sample (2,003 persons residing in 46 states) mastered the selected motor skills.

Although a single reference point is helpful, it is important to remember that even in typically developing infants or children, motor skills emerge over a broad range, and not all children follow the typical sequence. For example, in the WHO (2006) study, 90% of children achieved five of the six milestones following a common sequence; 4.3% did not achieve movement forward on hands and knees. Figure 13-1 summarizes the sequence of motor skills in the first year with the mean age at which the skill occurs (based on WHO and PDMS-2 data) in parentheses.

Earlier theoretical frameworks such as the neuro-maturational theory emphasized reflexes as basic building blocks of motor behavior. Unlike voluntary motor action, **reflexes** by

definition are automatic responses to a stimulus, and the resulting movement or change in muscle tone tends to be poorly differentiated and to occur in total patterns. Various states in the individual and constraints in the environment may alter the response to a stimulus, leading some experts to question the accuracy of the automatic response terminology (Scalise-Smith, 2013). For example, the stepping response seen in a newborn typically disappears as the infant grows in size, but it may still be present in the same infant when he or she is suspended in water (i.e., decreasing relative body weight). Opinions differ about the normal time for reflexes to be present and their significance (Shumway-Cook, 2016). Over time, greater importance has been placed on self-initiated functional movement. However, a general assessment of reflexes provides a framework for understanding the influence of persistent tonic reflexes and/or delay in acquiring protective and equilibrium responses that are important for postural control. Reflexes may be absent when expected and present when they should have been integrated, exaggerated, or obligatory.

Some of the early **tonic reflexes** (mediated by the spinal cord and lower brainstem) create alterations in muscle tone in various parts of the body in response to head or body

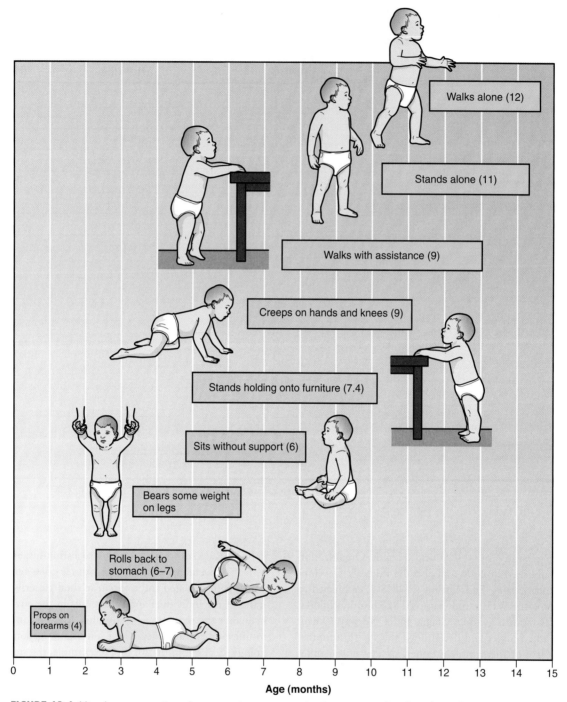

FIGURE 13-1 Visual representation of an approximate motor development timeline for a typically developing infant; mean age of motor skill attainment in parentheses based on data in Table 13-1.

position. These reflexes are normally present in the newborn but are typically suppressed or integrated by about 6 months of age and are never obligatory. These reflexes may persist with certain neurological disorders, can recur in adults after neurological injury, and may be exaggerated to the extent that they interfere with normal function.

Extensive reflex testing is not indicated, but a quick check of some basic reflexes and observation of their influence on motor performance is important so any negative influence can be minimized with handling and positioning strategies. Reflexes may contribute to neuromotor development in ways that are sometimes poorly understood, or they may interfere with function or functional development when they are exaggerated or are not integrated by an anticipated time. Table 13-2 summarizes many of the common reflexes (Ratcliffe, 1998).

With age a number of automatic reactions develop, providing a postural reflex mechanism that allows the infant/child

| TABLE 13-2 | Common Reflexes | | | |
|---|---|---|---|---|
| **REFLEX** | | **STIMULUS** | **RESPONSE** | **ONSET-INTEGRATION** |
| Asymmetrical tonic neck reflex | | Turn head (passively or actively) while positioned in supine<br>For older children:<br>Position child on hands and knees, actively have child turn head to one side | Increased extensor tone in extremities on the "face" side; increased flexor tone in extremities on the "skull" side; spine curved with convexity toward the face side<br>For older children: Arm on skull side will collapse into flexion | Birth to 6 months |
| Symmetrical tonic neck reflex | | Position child in prone: passive or active neck extension | With neck extension, increased, extensor tone is observed in the upper extremities and increased flexor tone in the lower extremities; and with neck flexion, the reverse is noted, with flexor tone in upper extremities and extensor tone in lower extremities | 6–8 months |
| Tonic labyrinthine | Tonic labyrinthine reflex<br> | Stimulus is the position of the labyrinthine in the inner ear (reflected in head position)<br>For older children:<br>Position prone and ask child to fully extend ("airplane") or position supine and ask child to curl up like a ball, flexing head onto chest | In prone position, body and extremities tend to be dominated by extensor tone; in prone position, by flexor tone<br>For older children: Persistent influence will result in difficulty sustaining fully flexed position in supine or fully extended position in prone | Birth to 6 months |

*Continued*

| TABLE 13-2 | Common Reflexes—cont'd | | | |
|------------|------------------------|---|---|---|
| **REFLEX** | | **STIMULUS** | **RESPONSE** | **ONSET-INTEGRATION** |
| Galant | | Suspend infant in prone and stroke the skin along one side of the spine from shoulder to hip | Lateral flexion of trunk to side of the stimulus | 30 weeks' gestation to 2 months |
| Moro (and startle) reflex | | Hold baby in semireclined or supine position and suddenly drop the head into extension (just a few inches) Startle reflex: similar to Moro but the stimulus is a loud, sudden noise | Response is abduction of arms with fingers open, quickly followed by adduction of the arms across the trunk in adduction Startle reflex: same as Moro | 28 weeks' gestation to 5 months |
| Palmar grasp | | Apply mild pressure to palm of hand on ulnar side | Fingers curl around stimulus | Birth to 4 months |
| Plantar grasp | | Apply mild pressure to base of toes on sole of foot | Toes curl around stimulus | 8 weeks' gestation to 9 months |

| TABLE 13-2 | Common Reflexes—cont'd | | | |
|---|---|---|---|---|
| **REFLEX** | | **STIMULUS** | **RESPONSE** | **ONSET-INTEGRATION** |
| Placing | | Stroke dorsum of hand (or foot) on ledge of a surface (e.g., table) | Lifts the hand (or the foot) and places it on the surface | Birth to 2 months |
| Positive support | | Hold infant in vertical suspension and touch balls of feet to support surface | Stiffening of legs and trunk into extension | 35 weeks' gestation to 2 months |
| Primary walking or stepping | | Hold infant in vertical suspension, touch feet to support surface, and lean infant slightly forward | Reciprocal flexion/extension of legs or stepping (poorly graded) | 38 weeks' gestation to 2 months |
| Rooting | | Stroke face starting at the corner of the mouth and moving outward | Head turns toward stimulus, and mouth opens; may be stronger in breastfed infants | 28 weeks' gestation to 3 months |

to maintain his/her balance in a variety of positions and circumstances.

- **Righting responses** – infant tries to maintain vertical orientation of the head in relation to the body or to gravity, involving two mechanisms: visual initially and then vestibular (labyrinthine)
- **Equilibrium reaction** – adjustment for changes in the body's orientation in space—initially in prone (onset 4 to 6 months), then supine (onset 8 months), sitting (onset 8 months), quadruped (onset 9 to 10 months), kneeling (onset 10 months), and upright (onset 10 to 12 months) stance
- **Protective responses** – arms and/or legs abduct or reach out to prevent fall or injury in response to a shift in the center of gravity (sometimes referred to as the *parachute reaction*), then to either side in sitting (onset 6 to 8 months) and backward (onset 9 to 11 months)

Individuals utilize different strategies depending on the extent of the perturbation to their center of mass (Fig. 13-2). Mild perturbation can usually be counterbalanced with righting reactions; moderate perturbation can usually be counterbalanced with a combination of righting and equilibrium reactions; and strong perturbation may result in loss of balance and protective responses to prevent injury. Note that the onset of these protective responses typically lags behind the respective motor milestones. For example, an infant is typically sitting independently by 6 months of age but does not develop backward protective responses until 9 to 11 months of age, resulting in the tendency to fall backward.

Motor milestones are like a snapshot, whereas motor performance is much more dynamic and complex. An assessment of an infant involves observation of motor abilities in a variety of positions, including supine, prone, sitting, horizontal suspension, standing, and walking. This is typically done first by observing spontaneous movement and then, as appropriate, facilitating postural control, adapting the demands of the task, or creating supports within the environment to determine strategies that positively affect an infant's motor abilities.

Postural control is an underlying function that is an essential component of early motor development and may be a rate-limiting factor (Shumway-Cook, 2016). For example, without external support to assist with maintaining head position, an infant may appear helpless. The same infant, given external support to maintain the head in midline, may demonstrate considerably more alerting behavior and motor control (e.g., visual regard for the examiner and intentional reach and grasp).

Marsala (1998) encouraged research on the movement patterns employed by infants/children using a component analysis as a framework for understanding the process of movement change and variability over time in the individual or among individuals. As an example, the authors analyzed the movement patterns utilized by toddlers to rise from a supine position to erect stance in three components: upper extremities, axial, and lower extremities.

A standardized developmental assessment may ask whether a child can sit independently for 30 seconds. Various qualitative aspects of children's abilities in a seated position, including the motor patterns used in component parts, may be even more important. What is their posture? Are they symmetrical? Do they have a preferred type of seating (e.g., cross-legged, side sitting, W-sitting, or long sitting)? How adaptive are they in a seated position? Do they sit stiffly? Can they move easily through a variety of sitting postures while visually regarding and reaching for objects in the vicinity? What level of support is required for them to actively engage with the people and objects in their environment while sitting? Can they sit on a variety of surfaces (e.g., the floor or a small stool)?

The text that follows and accompanying figures summarize key aspects of motor development organized by categories consistent with the first four of five dimensions used in the Gross Motor Function Measure (GMFM; Russell, 2013): (1) lying and rolling, (2) sitting, (3) crawling and kneeling, and (4) standing. The mean age when motor skills are typically attained is based primarily on normative values from the *Learning Accomplishment Profile Diagnostic Edition*, 3rd edition (Hardin, 2005) and the PDMS-2 (Folio, 2000).

1. Lying and rolling
   a. Lying (prone, supine, and sidelying)

When placed in prone, a full-term newborn is challenged when attempting to lift his/her head because of the relatively

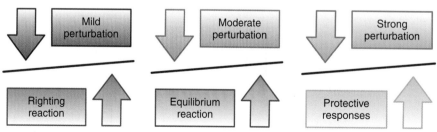

**FIGURE 13-2** Strategies utilized in response to mild, moderate, or strong perturbation of center of mass. Mild perturbation can usually be counterbalanced with righting reactions, moderate perturbation can usually be counterbalanced with righting and equilibrium reactions, and strong perturbation may result in loss of balance and protective responses to prevent injury.

large head size (about one-quarter of total body weight), physiological flexion in the hips that tends to shift weight forward onto the upper trunk and head, and possible influence of the tonic labyrinthine reflex; however, he or she is able to raise the head enough to clear the face and turn it from side to side. Gradually the hips are positioned in more extension and abduction, providing a more stable base and allowing the center of gravity to shift in a caudal direction. By 3 months, an infant can generally lift his/her head about 45 degrees but with the elbows posterior to the shoulders so there is relatively little assistance from the arms. By 4 months, the infant can prop on elbows positioned in front of the shoulders with extension into the lumbar region, can lift his or her head to 90 degrees, can turn his or her head to follow an object, and can reach forward with one arm. By 6 months, the infant can bear weight on extended arms, with good extension into the lumbar spine and emerging ability to shift weight and free one upper extremity for play with objects.

In horizontal prone suspension (sometimes referred to as *Landau* reflex or reaction, the newborn hangs limply; with increased head/neck and upper trunk extension; however, he or she is able to maintain a neutral position. The 4 month-old is able to keep his or her neck and trunk extended with the head upright to 45 degrees; and the 6 month-old is able to sustain extension in the neck and upper thoracic spine down through the hips (see Figs. 13-3 through 13-6).

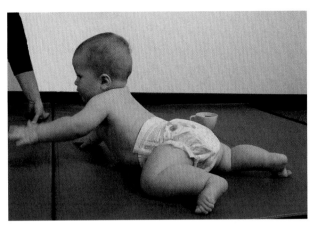

FIGURE 13-5 LYING: Prone at 6 months: able to bear weight on extended arms and shift weight to reach for toy.

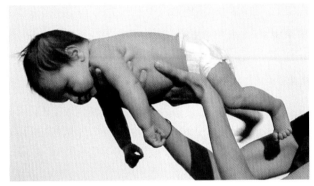

FIGURE 13-6 LYING: Prone at 1 month; Landau reaction; able to maintain head in neutral position, very little extension at hips.

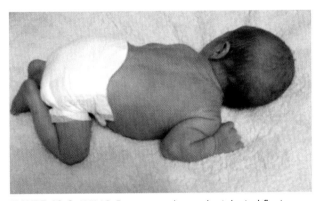

FIGURE 13-3 LYING: Prone - newborn; physiological flexion

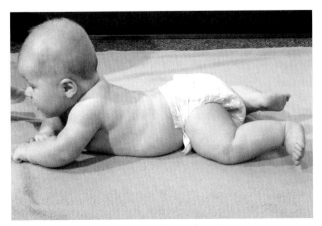

FIGURE 13-4 LYING: Prone at 4 months; able to prop on forearms and maintain head at almost 90 degrees.

In supine, the newborn has random, jerky, antigravity movements of the upper and lower extremities. Midline head control is challenging for a newborn in supine because of the lack of balanced control of flexor and extensor muscles; however, it is usually established for brief periods by 2 months of age, and the infant can track an object horizontally through a short range. With improved control, dissociation on a stable trunk, and diminishing influence of the asymmetrical tonic neck reflex, the 6 month-old infant can symmetrically lift and sustain the extremities against gravity, has good antigravity head control, and plays with his/her feet and brings the feet to the mouth. After about 6 months of age, the infant typically spends relatively little time in supine, preferring the greater function afforded by other positions (see Figs. 13-7 through 13-10).

**b.** Sidelying/rolling

By 2 months of age, an infant begins to balance activity in trunk flexor and extensor muscles and lift his or her head and upper trunk during a facilitated roll, showing lateral head righting. By 4 months, the infant uses upper arm and dissociated lower extremities to assist in facilitated roll and actively rolls to sidelying, with rotation of the head occurring as the

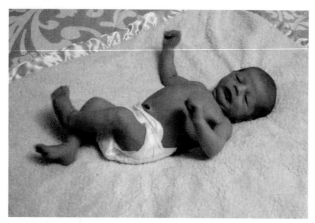

**FIGURE 13-7** LYING: Supine - Newborn: random movement of extremities; physiological flexion.

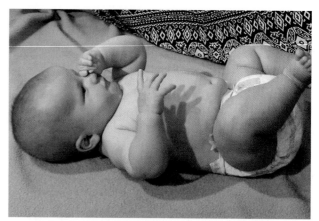

**FIGURE 13-9** LYING: Supine - 4 months: able to raise legs against gravity; plays with feet; arms and head in midline.

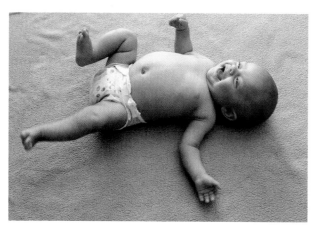

**FIGURE 13-8** LYING: Supine - 3 months: active movement of extremities; still influenced by asymmetrical tonic neck reflex.

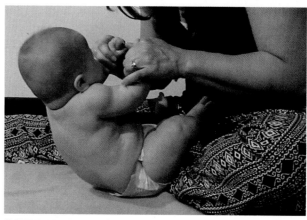

**FIGURE 13-10** LYING: Supine - 4 months: actively participates with pull to sit with at least partial activation of abdominals and hip flexors; good midline chin tuck and scapular adduction.

result of visual tracking. By 5 months, the infant actively rolls to sidelying with lateral head righting and lower extremity dissociation and may attempt rolling to prone. By 6 or 7 months, the infant rolls independently and easily from supine through sidelying into prone in either direction and shows active head righting and upper extremity pushing against the surface to raise the body while reaching with the other hand (see Figs. 13-11 through 13-14).

**2.** Sitting

When pulled to sit, the newborn may show slight activation of neck flexors but otherwise complete head lag. By 2 months, the infant demonstrates head lag until about 15 degrees from upright, uses shoulder elevation and elbow flexion to assist, and uses neck muscles to sustain midline head control when upright, with good extension through the cervical and upper thoracic spine. At 4 months, the infant maintains his/her head in midline without head

lag and with good chin tuck, lifts legs and activates trunk muscles to assist in maneuver, and pulls forward with both arms and abdominals to assist further in pull-to-sit. At 6 months, the infant responds quickly and assists in the maneuver by actively flexing his or her neck and lifting the head, uses activity in the upper extremities and abdominals to assist, and shows good symmetry in the head, neck, and upper extremities.

In supported sitting, the newborn has a posteriorly rotated pelvis and rounded back. At 1 month with trunk support, the head bobs. By 3 months with support at the hips, the infant is able to briefly hold the trunk off the legs about 30 degrees, has some upper trunk extension reinforced with scapular adduction, maintains relatively stable head position, and may elevate his or her shoulders to provide stability. By 5 months, the infant can briefly maintain head and trunk control when placed in a sitting position, propping forward on the arms. By 6 months, the infant

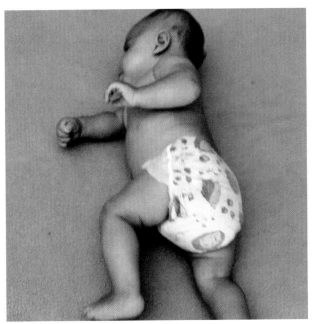

**FIGURE 13-11** LYING: Sidelying (facilitated) at 3 months: difficult to maintain position.

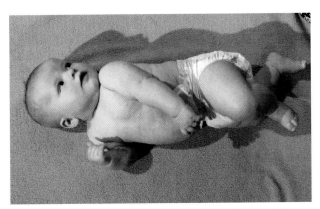

**FIGURE 13-12** LYING: Sidelying at 4 months: able to roll from supine to sidelying.

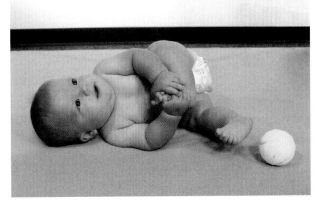

**FIGURE 13-13** LYING: Sidelying at 6 months: able to easily maintain sidelying position and play with feet.

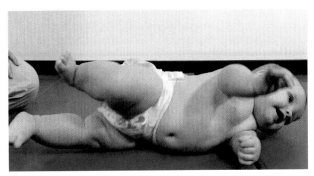

**FIGURE 13-14** LYING: Sidelying/Rolling at 6 months: able to roll from supine to prone.

can usually sit unsupported and maintain balance while reaching for and manipulating a toy. By 8 months, the infant demonstrates better trunk control, requiring less positional stability from the lower extremities and allowing considerable mobility, and as a result, moves in and out of sitting-to-quadruped, rotates through the trunk to reach for and play with toys, and varies the sitting positions used (e.g., ring sit to long sit to side sit). Protective (and equilibrium) responses to the rear typically develop at 9 to 11 months, so the infant remains vulnerable to displacement in a posterior direction (see Figs. 13-15 through 13-18).

**3.** Crawling and kneeling

Some confusion exists in the literature about the terms "creep" and "crawl." Most authors use the term "crawl" to mean gaining mobility in prone with the tummy in contact with the support surface and use the term "creep" to mean gaining mobility on hands and knees or quadruped. That terminology is used in this chapter unless specified differently. Some authors, including the authors of the GMFM (Russell, 2013), reverse the meaning of these terms.

The 7 month-old infant enjoys playing in the prone position, pivots easily in either direction, rolls actively, gains mobility with reciprocal belly crawling, can typically maintain an immature quadruped position, and may rock back and forth in quadruped. By 9 months, the infant assumes a mature quadruped position and gains mobility with reciprocal arm and leg movements as his or her preferred method of locomotion.

In a progression to standing, a child can usually move from quadruped to kneeling to half-kneeling by about 10 months of age and can maintain high kneeling (buttocks lifted off heels) while rotating the head to follow an object at about 13 months. An infant can usually gain mobility on his/her tummy by 8 months and on hands and knees, using a cross-lateral pattern (opposite arms and legs moving together), by 9 months; can creep up two steps at 14 months;

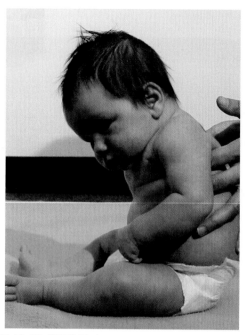

**FIGURE 13-15** SITTING (supported) at 1 month: rounded back, flexed head; unable to maintain in midline.

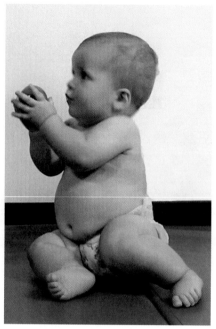

**FIGURE 13-17** SITTING (side) at 6 months: able to transition easily between variety of sitting positions with good head and trunk control.

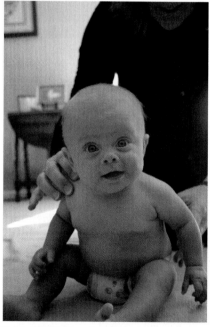

**FIGURE 13-16** SITTING at 3 months; insecure in sitting position but able to maintain erect head; only occasionally bringing arms forward for support.

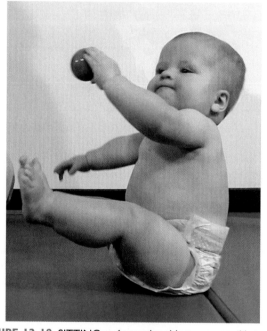

**FIGURE 13-18** SITTING at 6 months: able to use equilibrium reactions to catch self from loss of balance in posterior direction.

and can creep backward down three steps by 15 to 16 months (see Figs. 13-19 through 13-22).

4. Standing

A neonate bears partial weight on his/her legs with a narrow base of support and supinated feet and, when leaned forward, takes reflexive steps (known as *automatic stepping*). By 2 months, automatic stepping has usually disappeared, and the infant may resist weight-bearing, a phase known as *astasia-abasia*. A 5 month-old takes partial weight in supported standing with hips just behind the shoulders; has active extension into lower thoracic and lumbar spine but not

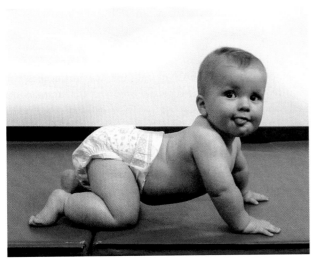

**FIGURE 13-19** CRAWLING and KNEELING at 8 months: able to attain and maintain quadruped position.

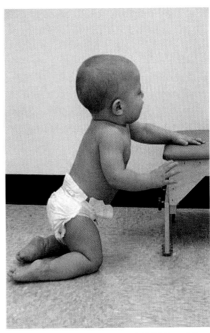

**FIGURE 13-21** CRAWLING and KNEELING at 10 months: kneeling in preparation for pulling to stand.

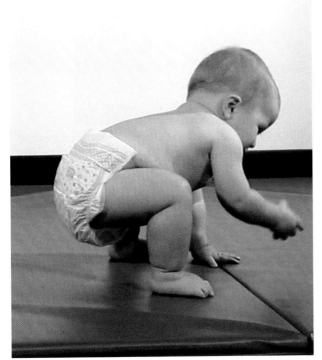

**FIGURE 13-20** CRAWLING and KNEELING: Squatting at 8 months: able to squat and play; partial support on one hand for balance.

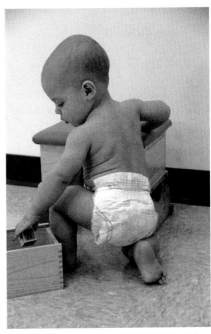

**FIGURE 13-22** CRAWLING and KNEELING at 10 months: half-kneeling for play: position allows needed flexibility to take toys from bench to floor and back.

full hip extension; has hips in moderate flexion, abduction, and external rotation with knees slightly flexed and feet pronated; can sustain standing posture; and requires minimal support at the lower trunk to aid in balance.

A 6 month-old infant exhibits immediate sustained weight-bearing on extended lower extremities; turns the head freely to look around; keeps the hips slightly flexed and somewhat behind the shoulders; and uses upper extremities to assist in

stabilizing the trunk. A 7 month-old can stand and walk with hands held and begins pulling to stand using primarily the upper extremities at 7 to 8 months. By 10 months, he or she can pull to stand at furniture; relies less on the upper extremities, transitioning from quadruped to tall kneel to half-kneel to achieve the upright position; and can lower to sitting with control. The 10 month-old enjoys playing with his newly acquired motor skills, repeatedly pulling up to furniture, sitting down, cruising, and squatting with seemingly tireless energy (see Figs. 13-23 through 13-26).

**5.** Walking/running/jumping

Cruising at furniture (starting at about 10 months of age) helps to build strength and stability at the hips and feet. Typically, the infant stands independently at 11 months and takes his or her first independent steps at 12 months. Early

attempts at walking are characterized by a high guard position of the upper extremities with scapular adduction, slightly flexed hips and knees, and a wide base of support.

Key body movement and object movement skills that develop after 12 months of age and the mean ages (in months) when they are typically observed are summarized in Table 13-3.

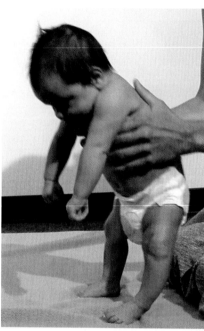

**FIGURE 13-23** STANDING at 1 month: able to bear partial weight on abducted legs and supinated feet.

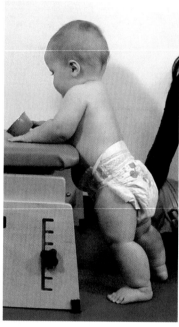

**FIGURE 13-25** STANDING at 6 months: leaning into support with chest and arms with legs abducted and feet turned out to broaden base of support.

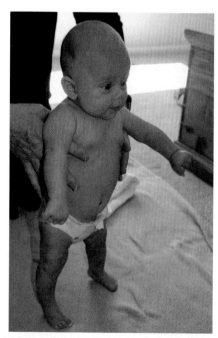

**FIGURE 13-24** STANDING at 3 months: able to support majority of weight in supported standing; recruiting variety of strategies.

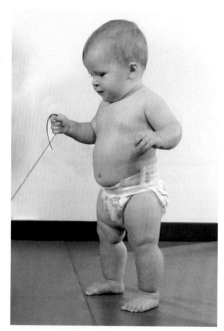

**FIGURE 13-26** STANDING at 11 months: standing independently with some scapular adduction and midguard position of arms; able to play with pull toy.

| TABLE 13-3 | Mean Age for Achievement of Higher-Level Motor Skills | |
|---|---|---|
| **AGE (IN MONTHS)** | **BODY MOVEMENT** | **PDMS-2** |
| 14 | Creeps up three steps | |
| 15 | Stoops to pick up toy from floor without falling | |
| 15–16 | Creeps down three steps (backward) | * |
| 15–16 | Walks up four steps with support from wall or rail | * |
| 17–18 | Walks down four steps with support from examiner's finger only | * |
| 18 | Seats self in small chair | |
| 19–20 | Runs forward 10 feet | * |
| 21 | Walks up and down stairs with hand held | |
| 24 | Jumps in place | |
| 25–26 | Walks backward 10 feet | * |
| 30 | Walks up and down stairs without assistance | |
| 30 | Walks on tiptoes five steps (hands on hips) | * |
| 31–32 | Jumps forward 24 inches using two-footed takeoff and landing | * |
| 36 | Balances on one foot for 5 seconds | |
| 36 | Walks on a line for 10 feet | |
| 42 | Squats in play | |
| 42 | Walks upstairs alternating feet without holding on | |
| 42 | Walks forward heel to toe | |
| 43–44 | Hops 6 feet forward on one foot or both feet | |
| 48 | Gets up from floor without using hands | |
| 51–52 | Gallops 10 feet with weight transferred smoothly and evenly; arms move freely in opposition to legs | * |
| 61–62 | Skips 10 feet maintaining balance and rhythm, using opposing arm and leg movements | * |
| 66 | Broad jumps 2 feet with running start | |
| 72 | Hops forward 10 feet on each foot separately | |
| | *Object Movement* | |
| 15 | Throws large ball forward with both hands | |
| 18 | Pushes small chair 6 feet | |
| 18 | Holds large ball while walking | |
| 21 | Kicks large ball from standing position | |
| 30 | Walks up to and kicks large ball | |
| 36 | Catches large ball with arms against body while standing | |
| 42 | Catches beanbag with arms against body while standing | |
| 42 | Kicks large rolling ball | |
| 48 | Hits large rolling ball with bat | |
| 48 | Throws small ball overhand with little body motion | |
| 54 | Catches beanbag with hands | |
| 72 | Hits large ball with bat when ball is thrown underhand | |
| 72 | Catches small ball (thrown underhand) with one hand | |

Higher level motor skills: mean ages (in months) based primarily on Learning Accomplishment Profile Diagnostic Edition and *Peabody Developmental Motor Scales, 2nd edition (PDMS-2).

The dynamic process of transitioning from one position or one motor activity to another is critical to functional movement. Transitional movements are variable in the typically developing infant (Marsala, 1998). For example, when first learning to come to a standing position, children typically rely heavily on pulling into the position with their arms and leaning into the support and/or using their arms for stability once in the standing position, limiting their ability for meaningful play. As their skill develops, they quickly transition from kneeling to half-kneeling into standing, relying minimally on their arms, and stand and play actively without the constraints that trunk/arm support imposes. Figures 13-27 to 13-30 illustrate key motor transitions in typically developing infants.

As mentioned earlier, a typically developing fetus is capable of active movement as early as 8 weeks' gestation. A newborn infant is not a passive, reflexive being but is capable of complex behaviors that involve an interplay between cognitive, motor, and perceptual systems. One of the biggest differences in the preterm and term infant is the amount of physiological flexion as a result of time spent in a flexed posture in the womb.

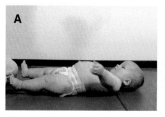 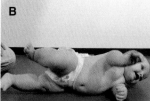 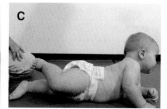 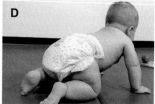

**FIGURE 13-27A-D** Rolling from supine to prone to quadruped (8 month-old).

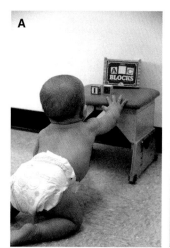 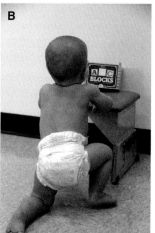 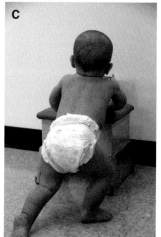 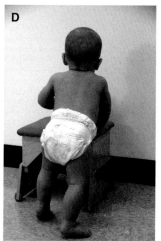

**FIGURE 13-28A-D** Quadruped to half-kneeling to standing at bench (10 month-old).

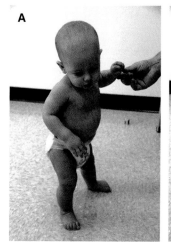 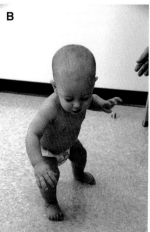 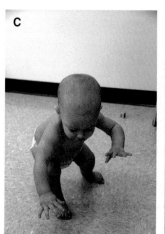 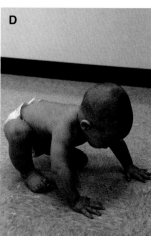

**FIGURE 13-29A-D** Lowering from standing to quadruped (10 month-old).

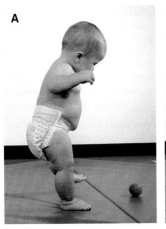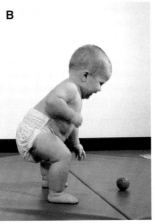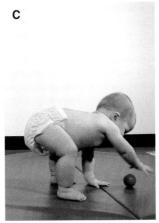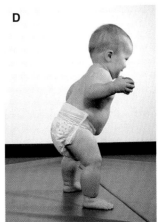

**FIGURE 13-30A-D** Lowering from standing to floor (11 month-old).

A series of videos posted on the Pathways website is a valuable resource to guide recognition of early motor delays (https://pathways.org/watch/4-month-old-baby-typical-and-atypical-development/). The videos compare the neuromotor behavior of two infants, one developing typically and one atypically, at 2, 4, and 6 months of age.

Most basic motor skills can be performed in a typically developing 5 year-old child, but the quality of performance improves with age and practice. Figures 13-31 to 13-35 illustrate sisters (aged 5 and 11 years) performing the same motor tasks: walking heel to toe on a line, kicking a ball, standing on one leg, jumping, and stepping up. Both children can perform the tasks. The quality of the older sister's performance is better. Note less extraneous, more efficient movements and better balance in the older sister. In general, the older sister demonstrates less extraneous, more efficient movements and better balance. Both would likely have earned a successful score for these items on a standardized assessment, but the scores might not reflect the quality and complexity of their performance. This emphasizes the role of the therapist in interpreting the scores and documenting the qualitative aspects of the assessment.

Our understanding of motor development and our expectations for particular motor behaviors must incorporate the concept of **variability**. In some situations, the goal is to

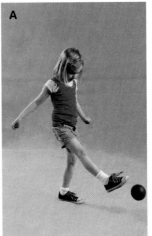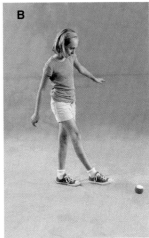

**FIGURE 13-32(A AND B)** Kicking ball.

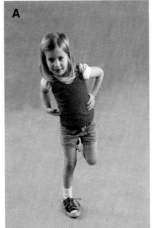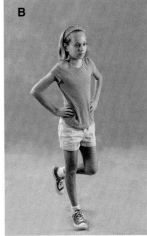

**FIGURE 13-33(A AND B)** One leg stance.

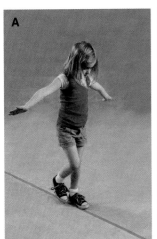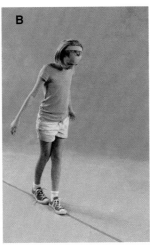

**FIGURE 13-31(A AND B)** Walking heel to toe on line.

minimize variability, resulting in more consistent outcomes. As an example, a competitive downhill skier strives to perfect various aspects of the motor abilities required to move quickly and efficiently down the slope, optimize his or her motor performance, and then practice the skills repeatedly to minimize

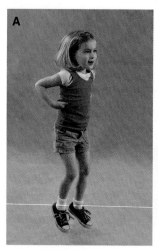
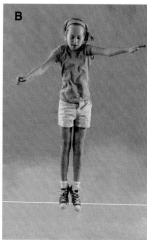

**FIGURE 13-34(A AND B)** Jumping.

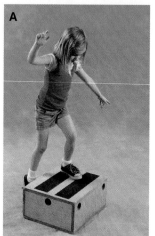
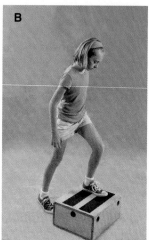

**FIGURE 13-35(A AND B)** Stepping up.

variability. Often only fractions of a second differentiate multiple trials in an individual athlete or among top athletes.

More typically, variability is a critical element allowing an individual to adapt movement strategies in response to the demands of a task or the contextual aspects of the environment (Hadders-Algra, 2010; Fetters, 2010; Shumway-Cook, 2016; Vereijken, 2010). Figures 13-36 and 13-37 illustrate variability in a 10 month-old boy's play while sitting and while standing at a bench. As an example, a child may be able to stand independently on a hard, flat surface but is challenged to stand on an inclined surface. Personality, motivation, and circumstance can all influence how children respond to the challenge, perhaps avoiding the challenge and raising their hands to be picked up or, despite repeated falls, attempting to make appropriate adjustments in their stance in multiple trials to accommodate the altered environment until it becomes part of their repertoire. As another example, agricultural workers use variability in their movement strategies to partially relieve physical stress in demanding, repetitive tasks that span long periods.

Edelman (1987) developed his theory of neuronal group selection on the premise that a newborn infant has tremendous neural diversity in the number and type of cells and their connectivity. Perceptual and motor experiences result in selection and formation of neuronal groups that are best adapted for various tasks. Hadders-Algra (2000) hypothesized that the reduced variation seen in children with developmental motor disorders was caused by a limited number of neuronal groups or impaired selection. Studies of preterm infants have suggested that diffuse damage to cerebral white matter may be the cause of decreased variability in movement strategies and increased stereotypic behavior (Hadders-Algra, 2008; Hadders-Algra, 2010; Vereijken, 2010). Assessing variability in the movement patterns of infants and children therefore gains importance as a basis for interventions that promote a more adaptive and diverse set of options to solve motor tasks.

## THINK ABOUT IT 13.2

Variability is a critical element of motor development allowing adaptability to the demands of a task and contextual aspects of the environment; it also contributes to greater success in many functional tasks (e.g., activity while sitting using a variety of positions). What are some general strategies to promote variability and adaptability in therapy sessions?

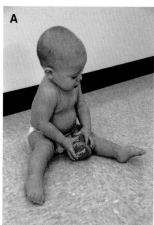
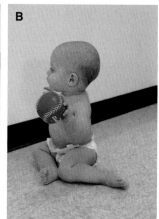
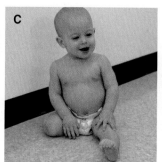
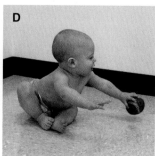

**FIGURE 13-36A-D** Variability in sitting positions for play (10 month-old).

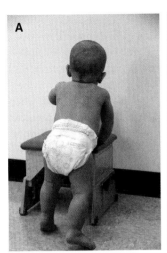 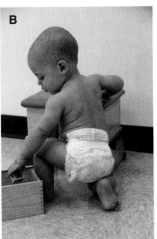 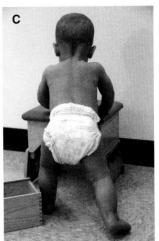 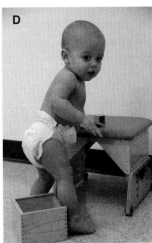

**FIGURE 13-37A-D** Variability in play while standing at bench (10 month-old).

Practice under variable conditions results in a continuous cycle of perception, feedback, and refinement of motor skills that allows infants to adapt to variations in the task and environment. For example, Adolph (2011), a developmental psychologist, and colleagues conducted a series of experiments that exposed infants who had recently acquired the ability to creep on slopes of varying degrees and discovered that with considerable practice infants became very precise about the risk posed, adapting their strategies for navigating the slope accordingly. When the perceived risk was too great, they would turn around and make the descent backward or simply move off to the side of the sloped equipment. Through these experiments, the authors also discovered that the infants did not generalize what they had learned about the risk posed in creeping down a slope to new types of motor behavior (e.g., walking). When confronted with the slope after learning to walk, they were at first totally unaware of the potential risk posed by the same slope they had previously mastered while creeping. Walking presented a whole new set of challenges.

What factors combine to stimulate an infant/child to challenge the status quo in the repertoire of motor behaviors and to progress to higher levels? This seems to happen spontaneously as infants gain motor control and discover more effective strategies. One of the more challenging transitions is from creeping to walking as a primary form of locomotion. When infants first begin to walk, the need for postural control, balance, and coordination of their limbs is very different from the demands of creeping. They have shaky steps and insecure balance and fall frequently. They may revert to creeping periodically, but in the end, they practice a lot, fall a lot, and are eventually successful. Adolph (2014) postulated that the benefits of upright locomotion outweigh the costs: Infants can cover more space more quickly, experience richer visual input, access and play more with distant objects, and interact in qualitatively new ways with their caregivers. Appreciating the benefits of upright stance requires curiosity, motivation, and cognitive ability.

The process of learning and refining motor skills occurs as the result of an immense amount of variable practice and continual interplay between sensory and motor systems. Observation of the natural, spontaneous locomotor activity of typically developing infants 12 to 19 months of age revealed that they averaged 2,368 steps and 17 falls per hour (Adolph, 2012). Children with atypical motor development need even more practice to acquire skilled motor performance. Assessment must address necessary adaptations and supports that allow opportunities for comparable levels of variable practice.

As part of his neuro-maturational theory, Gesell (1939) proposed the concept of reciprocal interweaving, viewing development as a spiral process with alternating periods of relative equilibrium and disequilibrium characterized by stable and unstable behaviors. He believed that the developmental process requires a temporary loss of equilibrium followed by reintegration at a higher level of organization (Crain, 1980). Thelen (1991 further developed this concept in dynamic systems theory. She did not conceptualize development as a linear process; movement did not develop in a continuous manner, at a steady state. Thelen realized that, consistent with the name *dynamic systems*, a small critical shift in one subsystem could cause the whole system to shift, often resulting in a new motor behavior (Smith, 1993). Often these system shifts occurred when there was too much variability in a particular movement pattern, creating instability. The resulting phase shift resulted in a new stable pattern or **attractor state**, a preferred movement pattern or posture used to perform a common activity. Thelen (1987) described these as critical periods of relative instability that represented an optimal time for therapeutic intervention. Although we tend to apply these concepts in infant/child development, critical periods exist across the lifespan. Examples in adults include shifts in hormone levels (e.g., menopause) or weight gain during pregnancy, which affects the musculoskeletal system.

## PATIENT APPLICATION: SELECTION OF APPROPRIATE PEDIATRIC ASSESSMENT TOOLS

*Angie is a 4 year-old girl with spastic diplegia (cerebral palsy) who has recently moved to your area from another state. A pediatrician has referred Angie to your interdisciplinary pediatric team at the mother's request. Angie was born at 32 weeks' gestation and spent 4 weeks in the neonatal intensive care unit (NICU) because of complications of her prematurity. The mother reports her pregnancy with Angie was uncomplicated until the early onset of labor. Angie has an older brother (5 years old) and a younger sister (2 years old). Both parents have a high school education and are employed outside the home. They seem to be loving, concerned parents who have good basic knowledge of Angie's problems, but they are stressed with the demands of supporting three children and seem very overwhelmed.*

*Angie was assessed with a variety of measures in the NICU, and a neuromotor assessment was repeated each time she returned to the Special Infant Care Clinic. She also received a battery of tests by the early intervention team who followed up with her. Her medical records include summaries of these assessments. As your team considers an assessment strategy, priorities include determining Angie's eligibility for early intervention services, a baseline measure of motor skill, and guided communication with her parents to ensure that their goals and concerns are addressed.*

*The process for developing an assessment strategy that is focused on these priorities is addressed in the next sections.*

### Contemplate Clinical Decisions

1. *What will you want to know specifically about Angie's NICU stay?*
2. *Which aspects of her history could have implications for her current motor development and prognosis for rehabilitation?*
3. *How can you ensure that the parents' goals are addressed?*

## ■ Principles of Examination of Neuromotor Development

Examination of neuromotor development is an important component of a comprehensive evaluation, especially for infants and children. Many options exist, and it is critical to clarify the purpose of the examination. Examination of neuromotor development may help to (1) document suspected delays, (2) determine eligibility for services, (3) contribute to a diagnosis and/or prognosis or determination of risk, (4) establish a baseline to measure the rate and trend of change over time, (5) justify intervention, (6) determine an intervention plan, or (7) establish the efficacy of an intervention or program (evidence-based therapy).

The Individuals with Disabilities Education Act (IDEA) states that the purpose of evaluation (under Part C) is "to determine developmental status of an infant/toddler, to identify atypical development, to make a diagnosis, and to determine eligibility for early intervention services" (IDEA, 2004). Eligibility is typically determined when delays are documented in one or more of five areas: physical, cognitive, communication, social or emotional, or adaptive. IDEA (2004) mandates that assessment be culturally appropriate and be conducted in the child's natural environment. Safeguards are in place to ensure the following: testing and evaluation materials and procedures are not racially or culturally discriminatory (including administration in a child's native language); a variety of assessment tools and strategies are used to gather relevant functional, developmental, and academic information, including information provided by parents; no single measure or assessment is the sole criterion for determining an appropriate educational program for a child; and technically sound instruments are used to assess the relative contribution of cognitive and behavioral factors, in addition to physical and developmental factors.

Examination of other systems helps to clarify why an infant, child, or adult is or is not performing at an age-appropriate level in the acquisition of motor skills. These include muscle and postural tone; strength; range of motion; reflexive responses; motor control; coordination; balance; postural control; alignment; weight-bearing; variability and adaptability of movement strategies; and biomechanical and kinesiological components of movement.

Consideration of various types of assessment is recommended to best capture the neuromotor development of children. Top-down assessments are recommended, especially for children with severe/profound delays, to focus on desired outcomes (of the child or caregivers) and current level of function related to the desired outcome(s) as a framework for identifying intervention strategies. This is in contrast to bottom-up assessments, which are typically impairment or deficit driven. **Ecological assessment** shifts the focus from artificial surroundings/situations to the child's typical environment and promotes involvement of the child and family in creating opportunities for self-initiation, choice, and problem-solving.

With some children, an accurate assessment of motor abilities requires a meaningful, perhaps playful, connection. Understanding the child's cognitive abilities helps to involve the child in tasks that are age-appropriate, motivating, and interesting. The examiner must be able to adapt the interaction to facilitate optimal performance. This may not be appropriate during administration of a standardized assessment, but outside the test parameters, the examiner should apply the principles of dynamic systems theory to probe the reasons a child might not be successful in performing a particular motor task. What are the constraints in the individual, the task, and the environment, and how might each be modified to promote success?

Each published test of neuromotor development has a unique purpose and particular strengths and limitations. Some are focused on motor development or on a particular aspect of motor development (e.g., gross motor or fine motor skills); some assess development across many areas (e.g., motor, cognitive, language, and self-help); some are focused on function, perhaps within a particular environment (e.g., the school environment); some are intended to be administered quickly as a screening test; and some are intended to help categorize or classify the level of severity.

Most tests are **standardized** to increase the likelihood that they are administered in the same way to everyone, every time they are used. The extent of standardization varies. Some tests provide comprehensive manuals with descriptions of each item, the criteria for scoring, and carefully scripted dialogues for introducing the item to the individual being tested. Some tests come with a kit containing all or most of the necessary manipulatives or test items. The Bayley Scales of Infant and Toddler Development III (Bayley, 2006) is an extremely standardized assessment instrument considered by many to be the "gold standard" for reliability and research purposes.

A test may be **norm referenced**, meaning it was given to a large representative sample of individuals, allowing a particular child's score to be compared with the average scores of the sample of children. Or the test may be **criterion referenced**, meaning the scores are interpreted on the basis of absolute criteria (e.g., the number of items performed correctly) rather than on relative criteria (e.g., how the rest of the standardized sample performed). Typically, individual items on a test are scored according to specified criteria, and the sum of these scores establishes a raw score. The raw score can be converted to (1) a **standard score** (deviation from the mean score of the normative sample), (2) a **percentile score** (number of individuals of the same age who would be expected to score lower than the individual tested), (3) an **age-equivalent score** (mean chronological age represented by a certain test score), or (4) a **developmental quotient** (an individual's age-equivalent score on a test divided by the individual's chronological age multiplied by 100). Care is needed to translate the meaning of these scores for parents who are unfamiliar with the test and to do so with sensitivity. An age-equivalent score often carries more meaning, but it can be a devastating objective reminder of the extent of a child's delays/problems.

## THINK ABOUT IT 13.3

If one purpose of testing is to determine eligibility to receive services under the IDEA, would it typically be better to select a norm-referenced test or a criterion-referenced test? Would your answer be the same if your primary purpose was to establish a baseline of motor performance that would serve as a measure of change over time and a measure of the effectiveness of an intervention?

Researchers who design tests strive for enough **sensitivity** so that the test identifies problems if there are any, as well as enough **selectivity** so that problems are not falsely identified when there are none. Tests should also be reliable. Scores should be consistent over time for one examiner (**intrarater reliability**) and consistent between examiners (**interrater reliability**). The validity of a test is also an important consideration. Does the test adhere to accepted theoretical constructs (**construct validity**)? Is the test a complete representation of the concept of interest (**content validity**)? Do the results of a particular test coincide with the results of an accepted measurement standard (**concurrent validity**)?

Meaningful involvement of various professionals in comprehensive assessment is required by the IDEA and is best practice regardless of the age of the individual being assessed or the environment. Models of team function range from contributions by multiple disciplines while in relative isolation from one another (multidisciplinary) to continual interchange and sharing across disciplines (transdisciplinary) and joint evaluation possibly using an instrument designed for that model (Ogletree, 2001). An example of a test designed for administration by a transdisciplinary team is the Transdisciplinary Play-Based Assessment, 2nd edition (Linder, 2008). Play-based assessments can be a reliable and valid option (O'Grady, 2015). The therapist must be aware of assessments that have been conducted or are planned by other members of the team, to select assessment instruments and procedures that complement those of other disciplines, and to integrate the findings across disciplines so the results are meaningful to the child and/or caregivers and form a solid foundation for intervention without duplication.

Conducting an assessment with an infant or child can be challenging, especially when using highly standardized instruments. It is important to provide an overview for the parents/caregivers about the purpose of the testing, what to expect, and how the outcomes of the testing will be used. Involve the child as much as possible depending on age and cognitive ability. If the test is highly standardized, parents need to understand that the examiner cannot deviate from the prescribed item administration and that there will be items the child is not expected to perform but that must be administered to reach a ceiling. Ensure parents that you will ask for their feedback on how well the child's performance on the test represented his/her true abilities and any skills the child might have been able to perform under different circumstances.

The examiner must determine the level of parent/caregiver involvement that will be allowed. Often this is difficult to determine, especially when the examiner is not familiar with the child and/or the family dynamic. The purpose of testing and the assessment instruments selected will affect the decision. For example, if the assessment is highly standardized and normative scores are required to determine eligibility for services, having the parents present during the testing may interfere with standardization. Regardless of caution, parents understandably want their child to be successful and may offer encouragement or otherwise negate the prescribed guidelines for item administration. On the other hand, parental presence can calm an anxious or shy child or motivate a child who is disinterested.

The testing environment should be safe with minimal distractions. Toys and test items should be cleaned before use and hidden from view until needed. Structured space should be utilized when possible. For example, fine motor items are best presented with the child seated at an appropriately sized desk (or table and chair) or held in a parent's lap with a play surface provided. Gross motor items that require focus are best administered in a relatively confined area. For example, a child will likely focus better on a one-leg stance in the corner of a testing room than in an open hallway, especially a crowded hallway. A very shy child may need to be engaged with an interesting toy that is not part of the formal assessment. For example, windup toys are often good icebreakers and can be easily concealed once the testing has begun. Generally, it is preferable to start testing with items that require focus and attention to detail, such as stringing beads, and progress to more active gross motor skills, such as running, jumping, or kicking.

The examiner is responsible for establishing rapport and developing a cooperative relationship with the child that optimizes his or her motivation to perform the desired task(s). Play is the work of children, and most neuromotor tasks can be framed as play with creativity and flexibility on the part of the therapist. Some basic guidelines include getting down to the child's eye level; speaking directly to the child when appropriate; using an accepting, nonthreatening tone of voice; having a relaxed, positive manner; reinforcing the child's effort and attention without specifically praising a certain response; and providing needed reassurance and encouragement. Use good judgment with a child who is crying. You cannot hope to get a child's best performance in this circumstance. On the other hand, you cannot always just give in. A child's behavior can be frustrating, but it is essential to remain calm and in control.

Children do not wait well and require attention to remain engaged and safe. Be familiar with the test instrument to be used so that the interaction is not constantly interrupted by referencing the test manual. Be organized and keep things moving. Know the test items, have any necessary equipment ready, and when finished with one item, replace it immediately with another. Try to remove distracting toys/equipment from view before starting the test situation and get test items you have finished with out of the way. Bursts of item administration followed by brief scoring and description may promote a more fluid test administration than scoring each item as it is administered. It is ideal to have another person available to assist, allowing the examiner to focus on interaction with the child.

When a child refuses to do an item or loses focus and does not seem to be attending, it can be difficult to know whether to persist with repeated attempts or how to comment on the refusal when documenting the test results. Children often refuse to attempt skills they know will be difficult. It requires clinical judgment and experience to know whether the child lacks the neuromotor ability or the behavior is interfering

with his/her performance. The examiner must remain flexible and creative to transition with the child's natural curiosity and interests and return to items as the testing guidelines and circumstances allow.

## ■ Tests and Measures of Neuromotor Development

A myriad of tests have been developed to assess neuromotor development. You must be knowledgeable about available tests, critically examine the test's construct and demonstrated reliability and validity, and determine the test's strengths and limitations. Consider the part physical therapy assessment will play in the team's assessment. Consider specifics about the individual: age, setting, diagnosis, presenting strengths and concerns, purpose, and constraints within the environment. If possible, testing should be conducted in a natural environment (e.g., the home or school). Standardized assessment is done at a single point and often is not repeated for many months. Therapists must be aware of the variability in infant motor performance and recognize the potential limitations of relying too heavily on standardized assessment. Another factor, particularly for infants, is their state or their behavioral organization at the time of testing (Als, 1986). Brazelton (1973), a neonatologist, described seven states of alertness in newborns: deep sleep, active (light) sleep, drowsy, awake, alert, alert but fussy, and crying. Each of these states is further described in Table 13-4. At a minimum, therapists should ask the parents or others familiar with the infant's/child's motor behavior if the performance on the test is a fair representation of his or her abilities and should document the response.

Accurate calculation of a child's age is critical and is a first step in any standardized assessment. Using numeric representation, indicate the year/month/day of the examination and below it the year/month/day of the child's birth date. Subtract, borrowing if necessary, 12 months for each year and 30 days for each month. The age is typically reported in months and days. Although rounding of days may occur in a summary report, the days should be used in the calculation (and recorded) because the manipulation of raw scores for various tests may be done using months and days. For children born prematurely, adjustments in age determination are typically done up until a chronological age of 2 years, although experts disagree about how long to continue correction. For example, some clinics adjust up until age 3 years, consistent with the transition from Part C to Part B of the IDEA. Many assessment tools specify a process or formula, and these guidelines should be adhered to. In general, an infant born before 37 weeks' gestation is considered preterm or premature (WHO, 2016), and an adjusted age, accounting for prematurity, is determined by subtracting the number of weeks premature from 40 weeks (normal gestation). Table 13-5 illustrates the age calculation (according to method specified by Bayley Scales of Infant and Toddler Development, 3rd edition) for a child who was born

| TABLE 13-4 | Six Behavioral States Described by Brazelton (1973) to Categorize the Level of Alertness in Infants |
|---|---|
| STATE | BEHAVIOR |
| Sleep state: Deep sleep | Regular breathing; eyes closed (no movement); no spontaneous activity except startles or jerky movements at quite regular intervals |
| Sleep state: Light sleep | Moves while sleeping; startles at noises; eyes are firmly closed, but there may be slow rotating movements of the eyes; bodily twitches and irregular or shallow breathing may be apparent; facial movements include frowns, grimaces, smiles, twitches, mouth movements and sucking; it is thought that brain growth and differentiation may occur during active sleep |
| Awake state: Drowsy or semidozing | Eyes may be open or closed but look glazed in appearance; may doze; arms and legs may move smoothly; breathing is regular but faster and shallower than in sleep; babies in this state may be stimulated to a more alert, responsive state |
| Awake state: Alert | Body and face are relatively quiet and inactive with bright shining eyes; sights and sounds produce predictable responses; state can be very rewarding for parents because it is the state in which the baby is most amenable to play |
| Awake state: Eyes open, but fussy | This is a transitional state to crying; available to external stimuli and may be soothed or brought to an alert state by attractive stimuli; if stimuli are too much, may break down to fussiness; movements are jerky and disorganized and may by themselves produce startles |
| Awake state: Crying | Cries, perhaps screams; sets off automatic responses of concern, responsibility, and guilt in parents; the most effective mode for attracting a caregiver; different types of cries communicate hunger, pain, boredom, discomfort, and tiredness |

Adapted from Brazelton TB. *Clinics in Developmental Medicine: No. 50: Neonatal Behavioral Assessment Scale.* Philadelphia, PA: JB Lippincott; 1973.
Brazelton TB, Cramer BG. *The Earliest Relationship; Parents, Infants, and the Drama of Early Attachment.* Boston, MA: Perseus Books Group; 1991:64–65.

| TABLE 13-5 | Age Calculation Using the Bayley Scales of Infant and Toddler Development, 3rd Edition: Child Born at 32 Weeks' Gestation | | |
|---|---|---|---|
| | YEAR | MONTH | DAYS |
| Date of testing | 2016 | 04 | 14 |
| Date of birth | 2014 | 07 | 16 |
| Calculations | 2016 – 1 year = | "Borrow" 1 year (12 months): 3 months + 12 months = | "Borrow" 1 month (30 days): 14 days + 30 days = |
| Date of testing (recalculated values) | 2015 | 15 months | 44 days |
| Date of birth | 2014 | 7 months | 16 days |
| Chronological age | 1 year | 8 months | 28 days |
| Adjust for prematurity (8 months minus 2 months) | 1 year | 6 months | 28 days |
| Convert years to months | | 18 months | 28 days |

*Adjusted Age for Purpose of Testing With Bayley: 18 months 28 days*

at 34 weeks' gestation, with a birth date of July 16, 2014 and a testing date of April 14, 2016.

A description of some of the most commonly used tests of neuromotor development follows. More complete listings are available from multiple sources, including the American Physical Therapy Association's (APTA's) Academy of Pediatrics. Additional evidence related to pediatric neuromotor assessment

instruments is presented in the Focus on Evidence (FOE) table for this chapter (Table13-6 (ONL)).

Assessment of infants/children should incorporate the basic elements of a physical therapy evaluation as described in the *Guide to Physical Therapist Practice 3.0* (APTA, 2014). Another aspect of assessment is the use of standardized tools.

# Specific Pediatric Assessment Tools (standardized tests)

## Screening Tests

Consistent with the *Guide to Physical Therapist Practice (Guide)*, "physical therapists conduct screenings to determine the need for (1) primary, secondary, or tertiary prevention services; (2) further examination, intervention, or consultation by a physical therapist; or (3) referral to another practitioner. Candidates for screening generally are not patients/clients currently receiving physical therapy services. Screening is based on a problem-focused systematic collection and analysis of data" (APTA, 2014, Introduction). Accomplishment of motor milestones within anticipated age ranges can be one aspect of screening. Several screening tests are described in the next sections. Other tests, including the Bruininks-Oseretsky Test of Motor Proficiency and the Test of Infant Motor Performance, utilize a subset of items from the complete test as a screening tool.

### Denver Developmental Screening Test II
(Frankenburg, 1992)

*Purpose:* To detect potential developmental problems in young children and monitor children who are at risk for developmental problems.

*Administration:* The test is individually administered using materials supplied in a compact kit. Standardized administration procedures are described in the manual, with key criteria and procedures on the back of the test form. The total score is based on the number of items passed or failed in relation to the age of the child. The score is categorized as "normal," "suspect," or "delayed." Five subjective items related to the child's "test behavior" are completed after administration of the test.

*Psychometric properties:*
- Norm referenced; standardization on a nonclinical sample of 2,096 children in Colorado
- Excellent interrater reliability (0.99% agreement)

*Availability:* The test is no longer available for purchase, but it is included here because it is still widely used. The test manuals and forms may be downloaded free from the following website: www.denverii.com.

| AGE RANGE | AREAS TESTED | ESTIMATED TIME | STRENGTHS | LIMITATIONS |
|---|---|---|---|---|
| 1 week to 6 years 6 months | Four areas: <br> • Gross motor <br> • Fine motor <br> • Personal-social <br> • Language | 15 minutes | • Training tapes available <br> • Comes with kit of items <br> • User-friendly scoring form provides easy-to-interpret profile of child's performance | Consistent with its purpose, limited test items in any area, especially for children at upper end of age range |

**6. The Milani-Comparetti Motor Development Screening Test, 3rd edition** (Stuberg, 1992 revised from Tremblath, 1977).

*Purpose:* Systematic examination of integration of early reflexes and emergence of volitional movement against gravity.

*Administration:* Individual observation of motor performance; manual includes drawings to facilitate scoring.

*Psychometrics:* Norm referenced; interrater and test-retest reliability good for children (n = 60) without suspected motor delays (Stuberg, 1989); reliability not determined for other populations.

*Available from:* Media Resource Center, Meyer Children's Rehabilitation Institute, University of Nebraska Medical Center, 444 S. 44th St., Omaha, NE 68131.

| AGE RANGE | AREAS TESTED | ESTIMATED TIME | STRENGTHS | LIMITATIONS |
|---|---|---|---|---|
| Birth to 2 years | 27 items <br> Spontaneous motor behaviors (locomotion, sitting, standing) <br> Evoked responses: equilibrium reactions, protective extension reactions, righting reactions, primitive reflexes | 20 minutes | One of few norm-referenced screening tests focused on motor skills | Emphasis on reflex development <br> Limited research on reliability with populations suspected of having motor delays |

## Developmental Tests

The need for more comprehensive information requires a test designed for that purpose (i.e., generally with more items).

### Alberta Infant Motor Scale (Piper, 1994)

*Purpose:* "First to discriminate those infants who exhibited immature and atypical infant motor development at the time of the assessment from those who exhibited 'normal' performance and second to evaluate small increments in performance that occur as a result of either maturation or intervention" (Piper, 1994, p. 29).

*Administration:* Observation of spontaneous movement in four positions.

*Psychometrics:*

- Norm referenced; cross-sectional sample of 2,200 infants in Alberta, Canada
- Interrater reliability (Pearson $r$ = 0.95 to 0)
- Test-retest reliability (Pearson $r$ = 0.86 to 0.99)
- Concurrent validity with PDMS (Pearson $r$ = 0.90 to 0.99 for typically developing children and 0.84 to 0.98 for abnormal and at-risk children)

*Available from:* Elsevier, Customer Service Department, 3251 Riverport Lane, Maryland Heights, MO 63043; Books CustomerService-usa@elsevier.com; 800-5452522 (phone) or 800-535-9935 (fax).

| AGE RANGE | AREAS TESTED | ESTIMATED TIME | STRENGTHS | LIMITATIONS |
|---|---|---|---|---|
| Birth to 18 months | 58 gross motor items in four positions: prone, supine, sitting, and standing<br>Each item observed for weight-bearing, posture, and antigravity movement | 20–30 minutes | • Minimal handling<br>• Caregiver can facilitate<br>• Minimal equipment needed<br>• Manual provides diagrams and photographs of each item | • Standardized on Canadian children<br>• Limited age range<br>• Dichotomous scoring (observed or not observed)<br>• Cannot be used with older children who have disabilities |

### Bayley Scales of Infant and Toddler Development, 3rd edition; Motor Scale (Bayley, 2006)

*Purpose:* The Motor Scale is just one scale used to "to identify children with developmental delays of motor functioning and provide information for intervention planning" (Bayley, 2006, p. 1). The first edition (1969) focused on motor milestones. The third edition has a Behavior Observation Inventory and Developmental Risk Indicators that contribute a qualitative component in relation to gross motor items. The Developmental Risk Indicators include brief descriptions of disorders such as atypical social behaviors, attention difficulties, vision difficulties, and motor and movement difficulties (e.g., muscle tone, posture, and coordination).

*Administration:*

- Detailed scoring guidelines are provided. Child either performs item (score of 1) or does not (score of 0). Rules for establishing basal and ceiling points are clearly described.
- Four types of norm-referenced scores are provided: (1) scaled scores, (2) composite scores, (3) percentile ranks, and (4) growth scores, as well as developmental age equivalents and confidence intervals.

- Use of the Bayley-III Motor Scale is not appropriate for obtaining a norm-referenced score for a severely physically or sensory impaired child, although the test may provide valuable qualitative information about a child's strengths and weaknesses (Bayley, 2006).

*Psychometrics:*

- Standardization sample included 1,700 children divided into 17 age groups
- One hundred children in each age group; representative sample according to selected demographic variables
- Reliability coefficient for fine motor subtest averaged 0.94 and for gross motor subtest averaged 0.98
- Overall, high degree of internal consistency in items
- Equally reliable for assessing individuals with different levels of adaptive functioning or individuals with different clinical diagnoses (Bayley, 2006)

*Available from:* Pearson, 19500 Bulverde Road, San Antonio, TX 78259-3701; 800-627-7271 (phone); http://www.pearsonclinical.com

| AGE RANGE | AREAS TESTED | ESTIMATED TIME | STRENGTHS | LIMITATIONS |
|---|---|---|---|---|
| 1–42 months | Fine Motor Subtest<br>• Prehension<br>• Perceptual motor integration<br>• Motor planning<br>• Motor speed<br><br>Gross Motor Subtest<br>• Static positioning (e.g., sitting, standing)<br>• Dynamic movement, including locomotion and coordination<br>• Balance<br>• Motor planning | 15 minutes for 12 months and younger; 20 minutes for 13 months and older | • Standardized guidelines<br>• Complete test kit<br>• User-friendly scoring form<br>• Strong validity and reliability | • Pass/Fail scoring system; therefore no credit for emerging skills<br>• Limited assessment of quality of movement<br>• No subscores available<br>• Cognitive items rely on fine motor performance<br>• Only moderate reliability for motor scale |

## Bruininks-Oseretsky Test of Motor Proficiency 2
(Bruininks, 2005)

*Purpose:*

- "To provide a reliable and efficient measure of fine and gross motor control skills and identify . . . deficits in individuals with mild to moderate motor control problems" for appropriate educational and therapeutic placement (Bruininks, 2005, p. 1)
- Screening test also available (subset of items from complete test); also norm referenced

*Psychometrics:*

- Norm referenced

- Three clinical samples for standardization study: developmental coordination disorder, high-functioning autism/Asperger disorder, and mild to moderate cognitive impairment
- Extensive reporting of reliability and validity—generally very good

*Available from:* Pearson, 19500 Bulverde Road, San Antonio, TX 78259-3701; 800-627-7271 (phone); http://www.pearsonclinical.com

| AGE RANGE | AREAS TESTED | ESTIMATED TIME | STRENGTHS | LIMITATIONS |
|---|---|---|---|---|
| 4–21 years | Complete test has four Motor Composites:<br>• Fine motor (FM) control<br>• Manual coordination<br>• Body coordination<br>• Strength and agility<br>Eight subtests:<br>• FM precision<br>• FM integration<br>• Manual dexterity<br>• Upper-limb coordination<br>• Bilateral coordination<br>• Balance<br>• Running speed and agility<br>• Strength<br>Screening test (short form)<br>• Subset of 14 items producing an overall motor proficiency score | 40–60 minutes for complete form<br>15–20 minutes for short form (screening form) | • Test kit available with almost all items<br>• Spans the range of school ages (provision of services under IDEA)<br>• Generally enjoyable items for examinees | • Requires considerable space and setup<br>• Not appropriate for children with cognitive impairment unless mild<br>• Not appropriate for children with major motor impairment |

## Gross Motor Function Measure, 2nd Edition.
(Russell, 2013)

*Purpose:* Designed and validated for use by pediatric therapists as an evaluative measure for assessing change in gross motor function of children with cerebral palsy over time; also evidence that it is valid for children and adolescents with traumatic brain injury (Linder-Lucht, 2007), Down syndrome (Russell, 1998), and osteogenesis imperfecta (Ruck-Gibis, 2001).

*Administration:* Starting position and detailed instructions are provided for each of 88 items across five domains: (1) lying and rolling, (2) sitting, (3) crawling and kneeling, (4) standing, and (5) walking, running, and jumping. A four-point scale allows the examiner to score items to reflect emerging skills. The second edition includes software for calculating outcomes on the 66-item version (based on interval rather than ordinal scales) and two abbreviated

methods of estimating GMFM-66 scores. Test allows scoring with a variety of assistive devices and comparison of total and goal scores with and without use of assistive devices. Raw scores are converted to percentages, resulting in an average percentage score for each dimension and a total score. A goal score can be calculated on the basis of domains likely to change as a result of intervention, increasing the sensitivity of the test to change.

*Psychometrics:*
- Criterion-based observational measure
- Considerable research done to establish reliability and validity with generally excellent results

*Available from:* Wiley, Inc., U.S. Distribution Center, 1 Wiley Drive, Somerset, NJ 08875-1272; 800-225-5945 (phone); 732-302-2300 (fax); E-mail: custserv@wiley.com; website: http://www.wiley.com

| AGE RANGE | AREAS TESTED | ESTIMATED TIME | STRENGTHS | LIMITATIONS |
|---|---|---|---|---|
| Appropriate for children whose motor skills are at or below those of a 5 year-old child without disability | Gross motor function in five dimensions:<br>1. Lying and rolling<br>2. Sitting<br>3. Crawling and kneeling<br>4. Standing<br>5. Walking, running, and jumping | 45–60 minutes | • Comprehensive assessment of gross motor ability<br>• Clear administration and scoring guidelines<br>• Only test designed and validated for children with cerebral palsy (CP)<br>• Goal scores allow increased sensitivity to change<br>• New scoring of 66 of original 88 items changed scoring from ordinal to interval measure, improving ability to quantify changes; can be entered into statistical program that comes with manual | Lengthy and not particularly interesting for children |

## Gross Motor Performance Measure (Boyce, 1991)

*Purpose:* To evaluate change in gross motor performance (i.e., quality of movement) in children with cerebral palsy; may be used in conjunction with the GMFM.

*Administration:* An observational measure with 20 items that assesses five attributes of gross motor performance: (1) alignment, (2) coordination, (3) dissociated movement, (4) stability, and (5) weight shift. Guidelines are provided for administration and scoring on a five-point scale; average percentage scores are calculated for attributes and total.

*Psychometrics:*
- Criterion-referenced measure
- Validated on a sample of children with cerebral palsy aged 5 months to 12 years
- Interrater (ICC = 0.93, n = 26)
- Intrarater (ICC = 0.92, n = 28)
- Test-retest reliability (ICC = 0.96, n = 28)

*Available from:* Dr. William Boyce, Director, Social Program Evaluation Group, McArthur Hall, Queen's University, Kingston, ON, Canada, K7L 3N6

| AGE RANGE | AREAS TESTED | ESTIMATED TIME | STRENGTHS | LIMITATIONS |
|---|---|---|---|---|
| 5 months to 12 years | Gross motor performance (quality of movement) in five areas:<br>1. Alignment<br>2. Coordination<br>3. Dissociated movement<br>4. Stability<br>5. Weight shift | 45–60 minutes | • Reliable assessment of movement quality<br>• Clear administration and scoring guidelines<br>• Broad age range<br>• Complements Gross Motor Function Measure | Lengthy and not particularly interesting for children |

## Movement Assessment Battery for Children, 2nd edition (Henderson, 2007)

*Purpose:* To identify children who are significantly behind their peers in motor development, assist in planning an intervention program in either a school or clinical setting, and measure change as a result of intervention.

*Administration:*

- Observational measure includes three sections: manual dexterity, aiming and catching a ball, and static/dynamic balance.

- Each section contains items for each of three age bands (3 to 6, 7 to 10, and 11 to 16 years).

*Psychometrics:* Complete test yields total standard scores and percentiles; checklist (screening test) yields percentile cut scores.

*Available from:* Pearson, 19500 Bulverde Road, San Antonio, TX 78259-3701; 800-627-7271 (phone); http://www.pearsonclinical.com

| AGE RANGE | AREAS TESTED | ESTIMATED TIME | STRENGTHS | LIMITATIONS |
|---|---|---|---|---|
| Test:<br>3 years to 16 years 11 months<br>Checklist:<br>5–12 years | 1. Manual dexterity<br>2. Aiming and catching a ball<br>3. Static and dynamic balance | Test: 20–40 minutes<br>Checklist: 10 minutes | Includes:<br>• Test and checklist<br>• Intervention manual<br>• Kit of manipulatives<br>Generally accepted as good test for children with developmental coordination disorder (Slater, 2010) | No items for handwriting<br>Assesses mild motor impairment |

## Movement Assessment of Infants (Chandler, 1980)

*Purpose:* "Provides a detailed and systematic appraisal of motor behaviors that occur during the first year of life. The test evaluates muscle tone, primitive reflexes, automatic reactions, and volitional movement" (Chandler, 1980, p. 3).

*Administration:*

- Each of the four areas has a unique scoring system:
  - Muscle tone: 1 (hypotonic), 2 (greater than hypotonic), 3 (normal), 4 (greater than normal), 5 (hypertonic), 6 (fluctuating)
  - Primitive reflexes: 1 (integrated), 2 (incomplete), 3 (complete), 4 (dominant)
  - Automatic reactions: 1 (complete), 2 (incomplete), 3 (partial), 4 (no response)
  - Volitional movement: 1 (complete), 2 (incomplete), 3 (partial), 4 (no response)
- Asymmetries are noted on the scoring form if the score for that item is at least one point different from right to left side or upper and lower portions of body

- Test is not norm-referenced, but a profile was developed for expected performance of 4 month-old infants
- Deviations from what is expected for any item generate an at-risk point
- Based on a study of 27 infants, 0 to 7 high-risk points (normal movement at 12 months); 13 to 26 high-risk points (diagnosed with cerebral palsy by 12 months)

*Psychometrics:*

- Not norm referenced
- Predictive validity of 4-month and 8-month profile for identifying infants with neuromotor dysfunction (Harris, 1984b; Swanson, 1992)

*Available from:* Infant Movement Research, PO Box 4631, Rolling Bay, WA 98061

| AGE RANGE | AREAS TESTED | ESTIMATED TIME | STRENGTHS | LIMITATIONS |
|---|---|---|---|---|
| 0–12 months | Muscle tone<br>Primitive reflexes<br>Automatic reactions<br>Volitional movement | 30–40 minutes | Predictive ability for high-risk infants assessed at 4 months of age | Manual lists the following limitations:<br>Should not be used to predict long-term motor development<br>Does not identify causes of a movement deficit and is not intended to provide a diagnosis |

## Peabody Developmental Motor Scales, 2nd Edition, and Motor Activities Program
(Folio, 2000)

*Purpose:* To assess motor development (gross and fine motor) as a basis for planning intervention. A Motor Activities Program is included with units that specifically address the skills assessed in each subtest. Each unit includes instructional objectives, reasons for teaching the skill or skills, examples of related skills as they occur in the natural environment, elements to focus on in addressing the skill or skills, and suggestions for five instructional strategies.

*Administration:* The test is designed as an observational measure with specific guidelines for the administration and scoring of each item. Scoring is based on a three-point scale: the child performs the item according to the criteria specified for mastery (scored as a 2), the child's performance shows a clear resemblance to the item mastery criteria but does not fully meet the criteria (scored

as a 1), or the child cannot or will not attempt the item or the attempt does not show that the skill is emerging (scored as a 0).

*Psychometrics:*
- First edition standardized on sample of 2,003 children in 46 states; second edition standardized on sample of 617 children from 20 states
- Reliability: test-retest and interrater reliability reported to have coefficients in the 90s for the gross and fine motor composites and for the total score
- Test yields five types of scores: (1) raw scores, (2) age equivalents, (3) percentiles, (4) standard scores, and (5) quotients for gross motor and fine motor composites

*Available from:* Pearson, 19500 Bulverde Road, San Antonio, TX 78259-3701; 800-627-7271 (phone); http://www.pearsonclinical.com

| AGE RANGE | AREAS TESTED | ESTIMATED TIME | STRENGTHS | LIMITATIONS |
|---|---|---|---|---|
| Birth through 5 years | Six subtests:<br>1. Reflexes (eight items); tested only in infants to 11 months of age<br>2. Stationary (30 items)<br>3. Locomotion (89 items)<br>4. Object manipulation (24 items)<br>5. Grasping (26 items)<br>6. Visual motor integration (72 items) | 45–60 minutes | • Many items in each subtest providing comprehensive assessment<br>• Gross and fine motor composites<br>• Scoring (0, 1, 2) allows credit for emerging skills<br>• Motor Activities Program | Test kit does not contain all required items, resulting in some loss of standardization<br>Lengthy to administer<br>Considerable training required for reliability<br>Lacks sensitivity in identifying children with mild dysfunction (Van Waelvelde, 2007) |

## Test of Gross Motor Development, 2nd edition
(Ulrich, 2000)

*Purpose:* To identify children who are significantly behind their peers in gross motor performance, to plan programs to improve skills in those children showing delays, and to assess changes as a function of increased age, experience, instruction, or intervention (Ulrich, 2000).

*Administration:* Test includes two subtests: locomotion and object control with six skills in each. The child has to perform each item twice; correct performance receives a score of 1; incorrect receives a score of 0. Standard and age-equivalent

scores for locomotion and object performance can be obtained.

*Psychometrics:* Normative information is stratified by age (in 6-month increments) relative to geography, sex, race, and residence. Reliability coefficients for the gross motor composite average 0.91; standard error of measurement is 1 at every age interval for both subtests; and content and construct validity have been investigated with good results.

*Available from:* Pro-Ed, Inc., 8700 Shoal Creek Blvd, Austin, TX, 78757-6897; 800-897-3202 (phone); http://www.proedinc.com

| AGE RANGE | AREAS TESTED | ESTIMATED TIME | STRENGTHS | LIMITATIONS |
|---|---|---|---|---|
| 3 years to 10 years 11 months | Locomotion:<br>• Running<br>• Galloping<br>• Hopping<br>• Leaping<br>• Horizontal jumping<br>• Sliding<br>Object control:<br>• Two-handed striking of a stationary ball<br>• Stationary dribbling<br>• Catching<br>• Kicking<br>• Overhand throwing<br>• Underhand rolling | 15–20 minutes | Reliable measure of gross motor performance with some qualitative assessment | No test kit; items typical of those used in physical education (lacks standardization) |

### Test of Infant Motor Performance (Campbell, 2005)

*Purpose:* Designed to examine the postural and selective control of movement needed by infants younger than 5 months for functional activity in the early months of life. A subset of items from the Test of Infant Motor Performance (TIMP) was found to be a valid screening instrument compared with concurrent performance on the TIMP (Campbell, 2008). Research continues on the ability of the TIMP to discriminate different developmental outcome groups (Barbosa, 2007).

*Psychometrics:* Validity and reliability of the TIMP have been studied and found to be strong along with the test's ability to predict motor outcome at preschool age and scores on the Alberta Infant Motor Scale. Key research is summarized in the evidence-based table at the end of the chapter.

*Available from:* Infant Motor Performance Scales, LLC, 1301 W. Madison St. #526, Chicago, IL 60607-1953; http://thetimp.com/page/mwmu/Products.html

| AGE RANGE | AREAS TESTED | ESTIMATED TIME | STRENGTHS | LIMITATIONS |
|---|---|---|---|---|
| 32 weeks postconception to 4 months corrected age | Tests infant's ability to sustain postures in a variety of spatial orientations, regain postural stability after perturbations, and make transitions between postures for orienting to interesting events and people, changing positions, and self-comforting | Average of 33 minutes to administer and score | Excellent test-retest and rater reliability; predicts 12-month motor performance with 92% sensitivity and 76% specificity and preschool motor performance with 72% sensitivity and 91% specificity; reflects demands for movement placed on infants by caregivers in daily life interactions | Limited age range |

### *Functional (Adaptive Behavior) Tests*

The assessment of neuromotor skills is complemented by an assessment of the translation of those skills to a functional context. The definition of function provided by the WHO is tied to the concept of disability. By definition, disability outcome measures appraise "any restriction or lack of ability to perform an everyday activity in a manner or within the range considered normal for the person of the same age, culture and education" (WHO, 2001). Outcome measures may be single measures (e.g., the time to complete a specific task such

as walking from the classroom to the cafeteria) or may involve the use of more comprehensive functional tools. A few of the more commonly used tools are described next.

### Canadian Occupational Performance Measure, 5th edition (Law, 2014)

*Purpose:* Designed to measure changes in self-perception of occupational performance (function) over time among patients with a variety of disabilities and across the lifespan. It produces a quantitative score calculated through a process of identifying and prioritizing meaningful functional goals with the patient or caregiver(s). Occupational performance is divided into three categories: (1) self-care, (2) productivity (work, household management, and play/school), and (3) leisure.

*Administration:* In an interview format, the patient and/or caregiver(s) are asked to think about activities that occur in a typical day, to rate the importance of the activities, to select five problems that seem to be most important, and to rate current performance and satisfaction (each on a 10-point scale).

*Psychometrics:*
- Interconsistency reliability: Pearson $r$ = 0.41 to 0.56 for performance, 0.71 for satisfaction

- Test-retest reliability: interrater correlation coefficient = 0.63 for performance score, 0.84 for satisfaction
- Responsiveness: significant change scores ($p < 0.0001$) between first assessment and reassessment with a variety of clients

*Available from:* Canadian Association of Occupational Therapists; 800-434-2268 (toll-free phone; Canada and continental United States); http://www.thecopm.ca/buy/

| AGE RANGE | AREAS TESTED | NORM OR CRITERION REFERENCED | ESTIMATED TIME | STRENGTHS | LIMITATIONS |
|---|---|---|---|---|---|
| All ages | Self-care<br>• Personal care<br>• Functional mobility<br>• Community management<br>Productivity<br>• Paid or unpaid work<br>• Household management<br>• School and play<br>Leisure<br>• Quiet recreation<br>• Active recreation<br>• Socialization | Not applicable | 30–40 minutes | Easy to administer<br>Guides caregivers or clients to participate meaningfully<br>Facilitates client-centered approach<br>Can be used on all age groups and all disabilities<br>No equipment required<br>Works well with Hypothesis-Oriented Algorithm for Clinicians (Rothstein & Ecternach, 2003); self-instructional video and workbook available | Difficult to use with clients or caregivers who have cognitive impairments |

### School Function Assessment (Coster, 1998)

*Purpose:* "To measure a student's performance of functional tasks that support his or her participation in the academic and social aspects of an elementary school program (grades K-6)" and thereby facilitate collaborative program planning for students with a variety of disabling conditions (Coster, 1998, p. 1).

*Administration:* This interview-based questionnaire can be completed by one or more school professionals who know the student well and have observed his or her typical performance of school-related tasks and activities being assessed.

*Psychometrics:*
- Summary score form provides raw scores, criterion scores, and standard scores with a criterion cut-off score for

Grades K to 3 and 4 to 6, as well as a graphic functional profile
- Internal consistency using coefficient alpha range = 0.92 to 0.98
- Test-retest reliability range = 0.82 to 0.98
- Content and construct validity examined during development of instrument on the basis of specific hypotheses (or propositions) derived from the theoretical constructs of functional performance

*Available from:* Pearson Assessments, 19500 Bulverde Road, Suite 210, San Antonio, TX 78259; 800-211-8378 (phone); http://www.pearsonclinical.com

| AGE RANGE | AREAS TESTED | ESTIMATED TIME | STRENGTHS | LIMITATIONS |
|---|---|---|---|---|
| Students in elementary school (grades K–6) | 1. Participation (in six major school activity settings) 2. Task supports (adult assistance or adaptations required to participate effectively in physical tasks and cognitive/ behavioral tasks) 3. Activity performance (21 scales providing detailed examination of activities addressed globally in the first Participation category | 1.5 to 2 hours (initial assessment by new respondents) | • Supports concept of appropriate education by helping to address barriers to participation • Supports top-down problem-solving approach • Focuses multidisciplinary team on functional tasks within school environment Facilitates incorporation of assessment results into Individual Education Plan (IEP) because items are written in measurable, behavioral terms • Summary profile form includes graph and cut-off scores (Grades K–3 and 4–6) • Manual includes helpful case studies | • Not norm-referenced • Limited examination of validity for various populations |

## Pediatric Evaluation of Disability Inventory
(Haley, 1992)

*Purpose:* Measures a child's capability and performance of functional activities in three content domains: (1) self-care, (2) mobility, and (3) social function. Separate scales within each domain measure discrete functional skills (197 items) as well as caregiver assistance and modifications (for 20 complex functional activities).

*Administration:* Interview-based assessment conducted with caregivers familiar with the child and his or her daily function.

*Psychometrics:*
- Standardized on normative sample (412 children without disabilities in New England region); can calculate normative standard scores and scaled performance scores
- Internal consistency reliability coefficients range from 0.95 to 0.99

- Interclass correlation coefficient – agreement high (ICC = 0.96 to 0.99) on all scales except Modifications for Social Function (ICC = 0.79)
- Content validity with panel of experts
- Construct validity – major assumption that change in functional behaviors is age related (strong developmental trend)
- Concurrent validity between Battelle Developmental Inventory Screening Test (range, 0.38 to 0.92 for all domains and 0.64 to 0.92 in comparisons across similar content domains) and Functional Independence Measure for Children (WeeFIM) (range, 0.54 to 0.97 and 0.80 to 0.97 across similar content domains)
- [Authors published a "lessons learned" summary that reviews the inventory's strengths and limitations; plans for revision (Haley, 2010)]

*Available from:* Pearson, 19500 Bulverde Road, San Antonio, TX 78259-3701; 800.627.7271 (phone); http://www.pearsonclinical.com

| AGE RANGE | AREAS TESTED | ESTIMATED TIME | STRENGTHS | LIMITATIONS |
|---|---|---|---|---|
| 6 months to 7 years (or older child functioning at or below the level anticipated for a 7 year-old without disabilities) | Self-care, mobility, and social function | 45–60 minutes | Comprehensive assessment of function that takes into account the amount of supervision required and/or use of assistive technology | Lengthy |

## Functional Independence Measure for Children: WeeFIM II (Uniform Data System for Medical Rehabilitation, 2009)

*Purpose:* The WeeFIM is an adaptation of the Functional Independence Measure for adults (Hamilton, 1987), designed to measure the need for assistance and the severity of disability

in children between 6 months and 7 years of age, a "measure of disability not impairment" (p. 37). The instrument has demonstrated the ability to document change in functional abilities over a 1-year period in children with chronic disabilities (Ottenbacher, 2000).

*Administration:*

- WeeFIM scoring is based on a seven-level ordinal scale representing various levels of independence according to the amount of assistance required from a helper or a device; the maximum level of independence is scored as a 7.
- Module scoring (0 to 3) is based on a three-level scale: usually, sometimes, rarely; information is obtained from the family (brief questionnaire).

*Psychometrics:* Norm referenced; extensive research on reliability and validity is included in the manual.

*Available from:* Uniform Data System for Medical Rehabilitation, Sales and Client Services, 270 Northpointe Parkway, Suite 300, Amherst, NY 14228-1897; 716 817-7800 (phone); http://www.udsmr.org

| AGE RANGE | AREAS TESTED | STRENGTHS | LIMITATIONS |
|---|---|---|---|
| 6 months to 7 years (or older child functioning at or below the level anticipated for a 7 year-old without disabilities) | WeeFIM tests three areas: 1. Self-care 2. Mobility 3. Cognition 0–3 Module tests three areas: 1. Motor (16 items) 2. Cognitive (13 items) 3. Behavioral (seven items) | • Applicable across inpatient, outpatient, and community-based settings • Can evaluate outcomes for individual patients, groups of patients, and pediatric rehabilitation programs • Subscription to WeeFIM system offers numerous benefits including access to online software | • By definition, a minimal data set; not intended to provide a comprehensive functional assessment • General functional tasks (not particular setting), which is both a strength and a limitation |

### Gross Motor Function Classification System for Cerebral Palsy – Expanded and Revised

(Palisano, 2007)

*Purpose:* To establish a mechanism for classifying children with cerebral palsy according to their functional abilities, including the need for assistive technology (handheld assistive devices for gait) or wheeled mobility. The quality of movement is not emphasized. Children are unlikely to change classification levels after 2 years of age, regardless of intervention.

*Administration:* Descriptors at each age band are based on self-initiated movement with particular emphasis on sitting (trunk control), walking, and wheeled mobility. There are five classification levels within each of five age bands: (1) before second birthday, (2) between second and fourth birthdays, (3) between fourth and sixth birthdays, (4) between sixth and 12th birthdays, and (5) between 12th and 18th birthdays.

*Availability:* CanChild Center for Childhood Disability Research, Institute for Applied Health Sciences, McMaster University, Hamilton, ON, Canada; can be downloaded from the website without cost, made possible by a grant from the United Cerebral Palsy Research and Education Foundation in the United States: https://canchild.ca/en/resources/42-gross-motor-function-classification-system-expanded-revised-gmfcs-e-r

### ■ Aging and Complexity of Alterations in Motor Behavior

As discussed earlier in the chapter, we can appreciate aging as a complex process involving both extrinsic and intrinsic factors. Life experiences, varying influences on multisystem aging

processes, and other health conditions all affect the meaning of "normal." As individuals age, normative comparisons become less and less meaningful. As a consequence, measures of motor abilities for older adults tend to be functional or designed specifically for certain conditions (e.g., stroke or Parkinson disease), and they tend to measure a limited set of skills. These measurement tools are covered in depth in other chapters related to specific underlying impairments or specific functional activity limitations.

Knowledge of anticipated age-related changes in various body systems and how these affect function should inform all aspects of an assessment of older adults. Ambulation is one example. At a sensory level, changes in visual and auditory acuity and decreased somatosensory and proprioceptive feedback may alter important feedback about environmental demands, positioning, or movement (Ries, 2012). Increased joint stiffness, decreased strength and joint range of motion, slowed reaction times, and motor control deficits may also have a negative effect. When the therapist is aware of how the various factors associated with aging affect functional mobility for specific demands (tasks) within a given environment, targeted interventions may be possible to adapt or compensate, resulting in successful outcomes.

Bohannon (2008) reported self-selected gait speed norms of community-dwelling older adults by sex and decade, which provide a useful comparison. Various other tests may contribute to the assessment: Timed Up-and-Go, Six-Minute Walk, Modified Gait Abnormality Rating Scale, Performance-Oriented Mobility Assessment, or Dynamic Gait Index.

Clinical practice guidelines and clinical guidance statements summarize best practices for a specific condition or for an area of clinical practice on the basis of the systematic review and evaluation of available scientific literature and expert opinion. These are invaluable resources that include specific recommendations for assessment. As an example, the clinical guidance statement by the Academy of Geriatric Physical Therapy (AGPT) related to the management of falls in community-dwelling older adults recommends various aspects of a comprehensive physical therapy evaluation (Avin, 2015). A task force of the AGPT, GeriEDGE, examined the "most informative, clinometrically sound, clinically feasible, and interpretable tests/measures physical therapists can use for fall risk screening and risk assessment for falls among community dwelling older adults" (Wingood, 2016). After a comprehensive review of the existing research, they recommended the following outcome measures: Berg Balance Scale, Timed Up -and-Go, Single Leg Stance (dominant leg), Five Time Sit-to-Stand, and Self-Selected Gait Speed. These and other functional assessment measures are covered in depth in Chapter 10.

## Documentation of Neuromotor Development Evaluation

Documentation of a pediatric neuromotor assessment may have to adhere to specific guidelines depending on the purpose of the assessment or funding source. For example, when testing is part of a "multidisciplinary" assessment for the IDEA, a specified format that is compatible with Individual Education Program (IEP) or Infant Family Service Plan (IFSP) guidelines may be dictated by the state or local education agency. Typically, a neuromotor assessment is part of a comprehensive physical therapy evaluation, and documentation is consistent with the *Guide* (APTA, 2014). When standardized assessment(s) are part of the evaluation process, documentation should include the following information:

- Any limitations of the test itself or the testing environment
- A summary of test conditions and infant/child behavior
- Specific findings (scores) with appropriate interpretation
- A description of qualitative aspects of neuromotor performance

Many tests have a scoring form on which the examiner records the raw score for each item as well as a portion of the score sheet or a separate sheet where the examiner can enter standard or scaled scores, age equivalents, or other summative data appropriate to the test. These separate forms should be referenced in the narrative summary and included with the evaluation.

Documentation of age-related changes in an older patient follows general guidelines for a physical therapy evaluation and a summary of any functional examination measures that were administered. In the evaluation summary, the therapist's clinical judgment is required to differentiate what are anticipated changes in neuromotor performance as a result of the "normal" aging process and what might be attributed to an abnormal condition influencing motor abilities.

## PATIENT APPLICATION: SELECTION OF APPROPRIATE PEDIATRIC ASSESSMENT TOOLS

*Angie's physical therapy evaluation (from the earlier case example) might be documented as follows.*

*Angie is a 4 year-old girl who is the product of an uncomplicated pregnancy until onset of preterm labor (32 weeks' gestation) and precipitous vaginal delivery. Angie remained in the neonatal intensive care nursery for 4 weeks for management of complications of prematurity, including an intraventricular bleed. Her family has recently moved to Jackson County. Angie has been followed by an early intervention team and has received physical therapy as a related service since early infancy.*

*Angie was seen for physical therapy evaluation at her home with both of her parents present. Her siblings were at their grandmother's house. It was midmorning, and Angie was cooperative with the examination and seemed to enjoy the interaction. The Canadian Occupational Performance Measure was used to help structure the initial interaction with the parents and to ensure that any subsequent intervention focused on goals that were meaningful for them. In that*

*process, the parents identified and prioritized goals for Angie and their family that focused on her ability to participate meaningfully in family life (see the separate form for details.) One of the first goals they identified was related to Angie's functional motor abilities: Angie will be able to navigate independently with her walker in the house so her wheelchair can be "parked" when the family gets home and she can play on the floor with her siblings and sit at the table in a regular chair at mealtimes. This goal structured the physical therapy evaluation that followed. Angie's eligibility to receive services under the IDEA was established by prior testing, so a norm-referenced assessment was unnecessary. A criterion-referenced assessment, the Gross Motor Function Measure (GMFM), was selected because it is more specific to her age and condition and would provide a measure of change over time in goal-selected areas. The GMFM was administered to establish a baseline of Angie's motor function (details are on the attached scoring form and are summarized in the following section.)*

*Per the GMFM: Angie's performance in five domains with and without the use of her posterior rolling walker (reported as average percentages):*

| DIMENSION | PERFORMANCE WITHOUT WALKER | | PERFORMANCE WITH WALKER | | GOAL AREA |
|---|---|---|---|---|---|
| | *Raw Score* | *Raw Score/Total Possible Score* × 100 | *Raw Score* | *Raw Score/Total Possible* | |
| A   Lying and rolling | 46 | (46/51) × 100 = 90% | [same] | [same] | No |
| B   Sitting | 44 | (44/60) × 100 = 73% | [same] | [same] | No |
| C   Crawling and kneeling | 23 | (23/42) × 100 = 55% | [same] | [same] | No |
| D   Standing | 22 | (22/39) × 100 = 56% | [same] | [same] | Yes |
| E   Walking, running, and jumping | 4 | (4/72) × 100 = 6% | 16 | (16/72) × 100 = 22% | Yes |
| *Total Score* | %A + %B + %C + %D + %E/5 = 56% | | %A + %B + %C + %D + %E/5 = 59% | | |
| *Goal Total Score* | (%D + %E)/2 = 31% | | (%D + %E)/2 = 39% | | |

Angie is able to ambulate for short distances with a rolling posture control (posterior) walker. She has increased extensor tone that creates a gait pattern characterized by hip adduction and internal rotation and a tendency to come up on her toes. Her gait pattern results in significant energy demands and an awkward appearance, but she can safely navigate most obstacles and surfaces. In 3 minutes, Angie was able to walk 25 feet. She is able to stand without support for 30 seconds, but she feels insecure. She cannot maintain single leg stance for more than 5 seconds on either leg.

Consistent with the family's goals and Angie's optimal level of function in both home and school settings, physical therapy intervention will emphasize safe energy-efficient ambulation. Assessment with Dimensions D and E (goal areas) of the GMFM will be repeated in 3 months as a measure of change in motor function during that time.

## Contemplate Clinical Decisions

1. Could you utilize the results of the Canadian Occupational Performance Measure as an outcomes measure? What do the results contribute to the assessment?
2. What was the rationale for selecting Dimensions D and E as goal areas on the Gross Motor Function Measure?
3. The Gross Motor Function Measure is time-consuming to administer. What other relatively quick outcome measures might you use on a regular basis?

# Let's Review

Consider the tests that were described in the chapter, and in each of the following case examples, select an assessment/screening instrument that you think is appropriate; provide a brief rationale for your choice.

1. Joe is an almost 33 month-old boy who was born at 26 weeks' gestation after a complicated pregnancy. He has spastic diplegia and has been followed since birth by a transdisciplinary early intervention team that provides services in his home. He will transition to preschool services under the IDEA and requires an assessment to determine his eligibility and as a basis for program planning.

2. Lori is an 11 year-old girl with athetoid cerebral palsy who attends a regular middle school. She is referred to you (at an outpatient clinic) to improve selected functional abilities in the home and

school settings, including short-distance ambulation. You will want to communicate with the public school physical therapist about your findings.

3. Sam is a 4 year-old (48 months) referred to you at an outpatient clinic for strengthening and gait instruction after surgical repair/casting for multiple fractures sustained in an automobile accident. You have some concerns about his expressive communication skills.

4. Ashley is a 12 year-old who has severe/profound disabilities and very limited motor abilities. She is referred to you as a school physical therapist because school employees have to lift her from her wheelchair to the changing table and are experiencing back pain. They wonder about her potential to accept at least some weight on her legs in a standing pivot transfer.

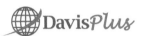 For additional resources, including Focus on Evidence tables, case study discussions, references, and glossary, please visit http://davisplus.fadavis.com

## CHAPTER SUMMARY

Neuromotor development is a complex process, and for any individual at any time, it reflects the compilation of influences from genetic makeup, the development and function of multiple systems, life experiences, personal attributes such as motivation and intelligence, and the nature of the task itself. Neuromotor development is the foundation of functional movement. The assessment of body systems and related impairments (as covered in other chapters) contributes to an understanding of neuromotor development, and neuromotor development with all of its complexities is reflected in the functional performance of individuals across the lifespan. Examination of neuromotor development with carefully selected instruments can provide an objective comparison with normative data to determine eligibility for services, contribute to a diagnosis, inform the development of an intervention plan, or provide a baseline assessment to measure change over time. Numerous tests can be used as important components of a comprehensive physical therapy evaluation. Additional evidence on interventions is presented in the Focus on Evidence (FOE) table for this chapter (Table13-6 (ONL)). Additional evidence related to pediatric neuromotor assessment instruments is presented in the Focus on Evidence (FOE) table for this chapter (Table13-6 (ONL)).

# General Therapeutic Intervention in Neuromuscular Disorders

# Concepts and Principles of Neurological Rehabilitation

Michael J. Majsak, PT, EdD

CHAPTER **14**

## CHAPTER OBJECTIVES

Upon completion of this chapter, the learner should be able to:

1. Discuss the importance of using processes of deductive and inductive reasoning in designing, implementing, testing, and validating sound strategies of neurological rehabilitation.
2. Value an integrated approach to neurological rehabilitation based on contemporary science in areas of motor control and motor learning.
3. Design intervention strategies that promote the functional competence of patients.
4. Design intervention strategies that optimally engage patients by respecting their attributes and constraints, the complexity of the tasks to be learned, and the opportunities for practice that exist.

# Introduction

The main objective of neurological rehabilitation is to help patients optimize their **functional competence**; that is, the ability to perform daily activities in a variety of environments, under different conditions, with a minimal expenditure of physical and cognitive resources. Neurological pathology alters the human condition, causing impairments of body structures and functions that limit the ability of patients to explore solutions to the functional activities they are trying to perform. During the rehabilitation process, patients learn to identify the attributes and constraints of their movement system, plan valid movement strategies and movement patterns for accomplishing tasks, and analyze and refine their motor outcomes. Through practice, they create functional coordination modes of motor output that can be refined, diversified, retained, and transferred to meet the spatial and temporal **regulatory features** of the tasks and environments they encounter. However, physical ability alone is not enough. To be functionally competent, patients must be motivated and confident in their abilities, and willing to meet the challenges they encounter when performing functional tasks. Creating and implementing comprehensive and effective therapeutic intervention strategies that empower patients with neurological pathology to optimize their functional competence can be complex and elusive processes.

The purpose of this chapter is to provide an overview of important concepts and principles of neurological rehabilitation that help patients optimize their functional competence. This involves therapists integrating the concepts of movement and function, creating meaningful interfaces for learning, progressing therapeutic interventions in a valid manner, and promoting the active role of patients in their recovery. Four major principles provide the underlying structure of this evidence-based approach to neurological rehabilitation. Hypothetical patient scenarios throughout the chapter illustrate how the concepts and principles presented apply to clinical practice. An emphasis is the importance of therapists personalizing their intervention strategies to promote patient engagement and learning. The content of this chapter complements the discussion of plasticity and the basis for making clinical decisions in Chapter 1, approaches in neurological rehabilitation in Chapter 15, prevention of secondary impairments in Chapter 16, and the indications and applications of assistive technology in Chapter 17. The principles of motor behavior and **motor learning** discussed in this chapter will apply to all interventions discussed in the chapters of Section IV of this text and to interventions designed to improve functional abilities as discussed in the chapters of Section V.

# Patient Cases

## PATIENT APPLICATION

**Case One:** *Ms. Cecilia V. Armstrong (CVA) is a 65 year-old woman you are working with in a rehabilitation hospital. Cecilia was diagnosed with a left ischemic cerebrovascular accident*

*1 month ago after an embolic infarct of the middle cerebral artery. She presents with right upper and lower limb hemiparesis and decreased tactile and proprioceptive sensation. Hyperreflexia (3+) is noted in the right elbow and wrist flexors and a mild degree of spasticity in the pronators and long finger flexors of the upper limb and the plantar flexors of the lower limb. She is able to lift her right upper limb forward and overhead 60% of normal range of motion with excessive movements in scapular elevation, internal rotation of the shoulder, flexion of the elbow, flexion and pronation of the wrist, and flexion of the hand. She shows isolated movements of her fingers and thumb with the ability to open her hand 50% of normal range of motion. Full trunk and pelvic control is present, but Cecilia shows excessive lumbar lordosis in standing, a slight hip retraction, and recurvatum of the knee, particularly during weight-bearing over her lower limb. A lack of responsiveness is noted for the intrinsic muscles of the right foot. She rolls in bed independently, occasionally pulling with her left upper limb when rolling to her right. Static sitting balance is good, but she has difficulty controlling her balance when reaching forward or to her right. Sit-to-stand requires minimal to moderate assistance with Cecilia primarily using her left lower limb. She often leans to her left and pushes off her left upper limb when attempting to stand. She does not appear to use her right upper or lower limbs to their full capacity. She requires minimal assistance to walk and is currently using a four-point cane on her left side. She walks very slowly, takes one step at a time, and shows an excessive lean to the left. Her left step length is short, and she steps only up to her left foot when advancing her right foot. She appears to have limited cardiovascular endurance because she often asks for rests. She is quickly frustrated by her functional limitations. Cecilia is a retired teacher who lives with her husband, also a retired teacher, in their ranch house. She is a gardening enthusiast and is looking forward to getting back to tending her flowers in the small greenhouse she has attached to her house. She is concerned about her ability to ambulate in the narrow space between the flower shelves and perform the tasks necessary to take care of her flowers.*

**Case Two:** *Mr. Peter Dugan (PD) is a 58 year-old gentleman you are seeing in your private practice. He was diagnosed with Parkinson disease 8 years ago. Peter reports that for the first 5 years he saw his neurologist once a year but was not experiencing any limitations. Three years ago, he began to notice his right leg occasionally dragging, particularly when walking in a hurry, when walking and talking to someone, or "trying to do two things at once." He began taking Amantadine and is now taking Sinemet, which he says is helpful. He has recently been experiencing trips and falls when walking at home and in the community, particularly when starting, stopping, or changing direction. He states he is having difficulty getting in and out of bed and standing up from his bed without falling backward. He also finds that he "gets stuck" when trying to stand up from the bathroom commode. He is beginning to have difficulty playing tennis at his club, particularly when trying to serve the ball or backpedaling to get to a hit ball. He reports that he feels a little* *stiff when walking, but that he is walking at his usual speed. He does not understand why his wife is constantly telling him to hurry up when they are walking someplace. She is also telling him to speak up when they are talking, and he feels he almost needs to yell to be heard. His goals are to be able to stand up and walk without falling, get in and out of bed more easily, and keep playing tennis.*

**Case Three:**  *Mr. Tito B. Inez (TBI) is a 28 year-old construction worker who fell from a building at a work site 6 months ago. He landed on his head and was initially unresponsive after his fall. He was brought by ambulance to the emergency room where neuroimaging showed anterior frontal lobe contusions and bilateral intracerebral hemorrhages of the supraorbital regions of the frontal lobe and the anterior temporal lobes. He was admitted to the intensive care unit (ICU). As Tito's condition improved, he was transferred from the ICU to the acute care unit and is now an inpatient on the traumatic brain injury (TBI) rehabilitation unit. The physician reports Tito is medically stable with no injuries other than his TBI. The neuropsychologist reports Tito has a deficit in his working memory as evidenced by his inability to process more than two-step commands and a short-term memory capacity limited to three items for no longer than 1 minute. He has limited problem-solving skills and is unable to fully analyze his errors and plan alternate strategies. He is described as being on Level VI of the Rancho Levels of Cognitive Functioning: Confused, Appropriate Moderate Assistance. Tito has intact tactile and proprioceptive sensation and no visual impairments. He shows no definitive signs of vestibular or visual involvement. His strength is within normal limits (WNL) for all four limbs, but he has moderately impaired coordination of his limbs and shows a slight ataxia when walking. When standing up from a sitting position, Tito does not prepare his foot position, scoot, or lean forward far enough. Instead, he pushes off both hands forcefully, propelling himself into standing. He walks independently but staggers a bit. He doesn't seem to listen when he is cued to "slow down." Tito runs into people when he is walking in the hospital hallway and has difficulty walking up stairs. Before his injury, Tito lived at home with his wife and their two children. He enjoys using his hands and carrying out home improvement projects. He wants to be able to walk well while carrying tools and construction materials and to return to work.*

## Contemplate Clinical Decisions

1. *How do the impairments of each patient pose challenges to their ability to become functionally competent?*

2. *What should therapists consider in hypothesizing the causes of the movement behaviors and functional limitations of each patient?*

3. *How should therapists set up and modify their intervention strategies for each patient to optimize patient engagement, information processing, and practice, and to promote patient self-efficacy and the potential for functional competence?*

## ■ Searching for Order in the Chaos of Neurological Rehabilitation

In the *New York Times* bestseller, *Chaos: Creating a New Science,* James Gleick (1987) reviews numerous examples of how even simple physical systems lack predictability; that small changes in conditions can have enormous effects. Gleick states, "Yet order arises spontaneously in those systems—chaos and order together" (p. 8). Neurological rehabilitation is inherently chaotic due to the variability of human motor behavior, the effect of specific types of neurological pathology, the numerous body structures and functions affected, and the innumerable tasks patients need to perform to participate in the worlds in which they live. Therapists face a daunting task of having to consider various theories of motor behavior and learning, evaluate the clinical relevance of empirical studies, integrate valid external experimental evidence with clinical experiences and patient preferences, and manage a health system that allows limited time for rehabilitation services. The purpose of this chapter is to provide therapists with insight to some patterns of order that exist within the chaos of neurological rehabilitation. Four overriding principles serve as a guide:

*Principle #1: Effective Neurological Rehabilitation Involves a Continuous Cycle of Deductive and Inductive Reasoning.* Therapists carry out processes of **deductive reasoning** when they use theories or models to guide their intervention strategies and **inductive reasoning** when they pick up, analyze, and use patient-related data to support or reformulate their theories and models. Effective neurological rehabilitation involves an ongoing cycle between these complimentary processes, unadulterated by personal bias.

*Principle #2: The Goal of Neurological Rehabilitation Is Functional Competence.* The ultimate goal of neurological rehabilitation is the ability of patients to perform activities of daily living confidently in a variety of environments, under different conditions, with a minimal expenditure of physical and cognitive resources. Although efficient activation of the motor system and a large repertoire of movement abilities are essential, these are merely the tools for accomplishing functional tasks. Patients are motivated and engage in activities that are meaningful and important to their lives. Goals of improving body structure and function often precede, but seldom supersede, the goal of functional competence.

*Principle #3: Functional Competence Is Promoted by Basing Rehabilitation Strategies on Embedded Models of Motor Behavior and Neurological Rehabilitation.* Patients cannot execute functional tasks without stabilizing and moving their body, and they cannot stabilize or move their body without activating their motor system. Thus, body structure and function and functional activity are levels of human motor behavior that are inseparable. Working with patients on these areas in isolation need not occur and is actually artificial and inefficient. Optimal rehabilitation occurs when therapists create well-designed functional tasks that require the use of desired movements in a meaningful context. Carefully conceived and manipulated motor tasks can be used to activate motor control processes at specific levels of the patient's motor system.

*Principle #4: Functional Competence Requires Motor Learning and Self-Efficacy.* Functional competence occurs when patients are confidently able to carry out motor tasks within the limits of their own abilities to meet the demands of tasks and environments. Within the domains of motor learning, this involves developing an internal model of one's motor system, creating motor plans for task performance, analyzing performance and results, revising motor plans, practicing, organizing a general coordination mode for motor tasks, and refining and diversifying motor performance. Patients must have the motivation and self-efficacy to take on the challenges of functional task performance. **Self-efficacy** is the belief that a personal challenge can be overcome and an intended behavior or activity can be performed successfully (Bandura, 1994). Therapists use rehabilitation strategies and goals that promote the retention and transfer of functional skills, not merely the initial performance of those skills. An important key to learning is to optimize patient engagement by manipulating the conditions for patient experiences and practice and building the confidence of patients in their abilities.

## Principle #1: Effective Neurological Rehabilitation Involves a Continuous Cycle of Deductive and Inductive Reasoning

A challenge for physical therapists is the ongoing need to integrate rich and diverse information in the movement sciences with clinical expertise to generate a sound model of practice (Dal Bello-Haas, 2002; Gordon and Quinn, 2001; Majsak, 1996) (see Figure 14-1). The historic role of therapists to "fix a damaged motor system" by promoting changes

in body structure and function has long since expanded to include the roles of therapists as facilitators, enablers, and educators of patients in movement, function, and participation. In addition to strengthening weak muscles, mobilizing joints, stretching tight tissues, and addressing other impairments of body structures and functions, therapists now make additional types of clinical decisions. "Should early rehabilitation prioritize the performance of specific movement patterns over the execution of functional tasks performed with compensatory movement patterns?" "What proportion of time should be spent working on impairments of body structures and functions versus the activity limitations of a patient?" "How should I use new technologies within my clinical intervention approaches?" "What is meaningful intervention for patients?" Strategies for progressing the rehabilitation of patients must be considered and the parameters on which to base these progressions (Fell, 2004; Winstein, 2014). The clinical decisions therapists make reflect how they integrate theories and models of practice with their clinical expertise, patient preferences, and clinical observation as they attempt to optimize the functional competence of patients.

## The Challenge in Carrying Out Effective Cycles of Deductive and Inductive Reasoning: Objectivity

Therapists employ deductive reasoning when they utilize theories and intervention models to guide their treatment strategies and inductive reasoning when they observe and collect clinical evidence to support, modify, or refute theories or models of practice. Neurological rehabilitation requires a continuous cycle of these two processes. Confounding factors include the way a theory or model is tested in the clinic, the type of information collected during clinical observations, and the interpretation of those observations. As illustrated in Figure 14-2 A through D, our personal biases and perceptions affect how we interpret what we observe, both in our daily world and in the clinic.

Therapists must be aware of their assumptions and biases when testing models of practice. Selecting specific patients for the testing of treatment ideas, carrying out both the delivery and outcome assessment of an intervention, deciding how to analyze the data collected, and making subjective decisions on how to test theories and models of practice all run the risk of compromising objectivity for the sake of convenience. To the extent possible, processes of deductive and inductive reasoning and clinical decision-making should be objective and free from personal bias.

## The Evolution of Concepts of Motor Behavior and Neurological Rehabilitation

A thorough understanding of human motor behavior is quite elusive. Multiple levels of motor control exist, including reflex activity at the level of the spinal cord, postural and equilibrium reactions mediated by brainstem and subcortical regions, well-learned fluid movement patterns regulated by subcortical

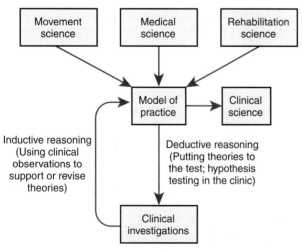

**FIGURE 14-1** The factors that contribute to the clinical science of physical therapy. Adapted from Gordon J and Quinn L, "A Model for Task-Oriented Intervention in Neurological Rehabilitation: Promoting Transfer and Functional Carry-Over." Presented at the American Physical Therapy Association Combined Sections Meeting, San Antonio, TX, February, 2001.

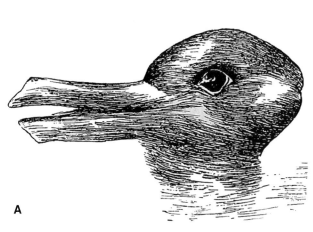
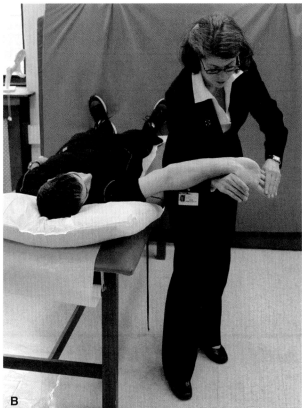
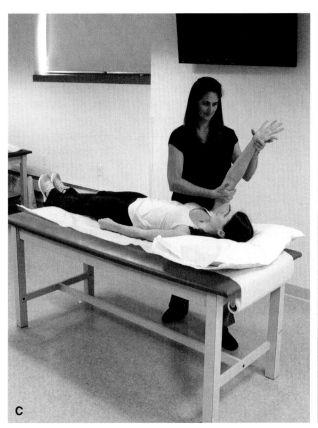
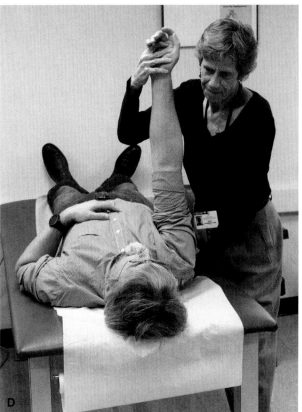

**FIGURE 14-2** What we see in the physical world and what we observe and do in the clinic is open to different interpretations. **A.** Two different interpretations exist for the duck-rabbit illusion. Is it a duck facing left or a rabbit facing right? (Source: Jastrow J. The mind's eye. *Popular Science Monthly.* 1889;54:299–312). **B through D.** Three different interpretations of the effects of using upper limb extension and abduction following stroke. **B.** Promoting a reflex-inhibiting pattern for reducing spasticity (Bobath, 1970). **C.** Creating an effective diagonal movement pattern for strengthening PNF. **D.** Promoting the learning of a functional reaching movement.

structures, and discrete voluntary movements controlled largely by cortical regions of the cerebrum. Human motor behavior emerges from the continuous interaction and differential weighting of these levels of control.

Our understanding of normal and pathological motor behavior has evolved and will continue to evolve with advances in science, clinical observations, and revolutionary theories of motor behavior. A review of the history of neurological rehabilitation illustrates how the motor behavior theories prevalent at the time and the way those theories are translated into clinical practice heavily influence principles of clinical intervention. Table 14-1 lists a number of these approaches with their theoretical foundations (refer to Chapter 15 for more details on these approaches).

The **muscle reeducation** approaches focused on the use of strengthening exercises and conditioning activities to promote the performance of functional activities with the least energy cost to the patient (Gordon, 2000; Horak, 1991). This often involved increasing the strength and control of areas of the body believed to be spared by a pathology, rather than trying to restore lost functions. Specific exercises were the therapeutic medium with little consideration of actual tasks and environments. Decreased force production was believed to be the patient's major impediment, and it was assumed an increase in strength would directly translate into improved function.

The **neurofacilitation** approaches (Bobath, 1970; Johnstone, 1978; Sawner and LaVigne, 1992; Voss, 1985) advocated that a potential for recovery existed for individuals affected by

| TABLE 14-1 | A Summary of the Theoretical Basis and Major Features and Limitations of Past Approaches of Neurological Rehabilitation | | | |
|---|---|---|---|---|
| **APPROACH** | **MAJOR PROPONENTS** | **THEORETICAL BASIS** | **MAJOR FEATURES** | **MAJOR LIMITATIONS** |
| Muscle reeducation | Jacobson; DeLorme; Goldthwait and Kendall; Kenny | Muscle physiology; Importance of patient knowledge and motivation; Conscious activation and relaxation of muscles | Use of verbal cues to motivate conscious contraction and relaxation activities; Progressive resistance exercise; Emphasis on strength and endurance; Isolated muscle strengthening exercises | Assumption that increased strength and endurance directly results in improved function; Therapist-driven approach; Little consideration for adaptation for patients with CNS lesions |
| Neurofacilitation | Rood; Knott and Voss; Bobath; Brunnstrom; Johnstone | Reflex and hierarchical models of motor control; Importance of "normal" postural reflexes and motor tone | Use of sensory stimuli and manual facilitation/ inhibition techniques to alter motor tone and promote "normal" movement patterns; "Shunting" and "normalizing" of motor tone before practicing voluntary control; Use of head and trunk "key points of control" to establish postural control; Treating proximal body points before limbs; Practicing functional tasks in "normal movement patterns"/ avoidance of compensatory movements; De-emphasis of strengthening outside of a functional context | Therapist-driven approach treating impairments before functional limitations; Emphasis on attaining specific movement patterns for functional performance; Emphasis on movement acquisition with little evidence of carryover to retention and transfer; Minimal emphasis on patient problem-solving, error correction, and planning |

| TABLE 14-1 | A Summary of the Theoretical Basis and Major Features and Limitations of Past Approaches of Neurological Rehabilitation—cont'd | | | |
|---|---|---|---|---|
| **APPROACH** | **MAJOR PROPONENTS** | **THEORETICAL BASIS** | **MAJOR FEATURES** | **MAJOR LIMITATIONS** |
| Motor Learning | Schmidt; Winstein; Gentile; Carr and Shepherd; Lee; Magill | Movement sciences; Cognitive psychology | Emphasis on patient-driven approach to motor planning, error-detection, and problem-solving; Emphasis on importance of task and environment; Use of task and environment set-up, information delivery, and structured practice for motor learning; Compensatory movements viewed as a component of learning; De-emphasis on verbal instruction and manual facilitation/inhibition of movements; Emphasis on motor skill retention and transfer | Motor learning theory based largely on studies of healthy subjects performing experimental tasks; Based largely on principles of explicit motor learning; Little offered for patients with severe motor impairments or profound functional limitations; De-emphasis of potentially effective nonfunctional treatment techniques that help to ameliorate motor impairments (strengthening, joint mobilization) |

a neurological pathology. An early assumption was that patients should relearn functional activities through practice and repetition of the normal movement patterns used by healthy individuals. Manual guidance and sensorimotor stimulation were used to elicit and strengthen motor responses, and specific movement progressions were utilized to promote the restoration of skilled motor behavior. A major assumption of these approaches was that **spasticity** and abnormal synergistic movements reflected a loss of inhibition of normal postural and spinal reflex mechanisms and that manual facilitation should be used to inhibit or shunt these "spastic patterns" into normal movements. Allowing erroneous or compensatory movements was believed to interfere with the restoration of skilled motor control (Gordon, 2000; Horak, 1991).

The perspective of task-oriented **motor learning approaches** was that the motor behavior of patients with neurological pathology reflected their best attempts to carry out functional tasks with a limited motor capacity. A major tenet was patients needed to learn to regain their motor function as independently as possible through structured exploration of motor tasks, self-assessment, **information processing**, self-correction, and practice (Carr and Shepherd, 1982; Lister, 1991). The priority of the motor learning approach was for patients to perform functional motor tasks using general and adaptable movement patterns rather than a set of kinematically specific movements.

Each of these approaches was based on a theoretical foundation that reflected the clinical issues of that time. Muscle reeducation was grounded in principles of anatomy, kinesiology,

and exercise science developed for patients with poliomyelitis or traumatic injuries acquired in World War I. Neurofacilitation approaches based on reflex, feedback, and hierarchical models of control emerged as therapists began to attempt to restore the motor control of patients with stroke, cerebral palsy, and other types of brain injury. Task-oriented motor learning approaches arose from clinical observations that the neurofacilitation of movements had limited carryover to functional tasks, and from increasing demands for evidence of the functional effectiveness of physical therapy. The motor learning approaches were based on evolving theories in biomechanics, neuroscience, cognitive and behavioral psychology, cybernetics, and human ecology. Within each of these approaches, therapists continued to create and test intervention strategies based on clinical observations and the prevalent theories at that time that supported their observations.

In several cases, intervention strategies we now believe to be sound evolved from clinical observations and expertise that preceded empirical evidence validating those observations (Bobath, 1970; Sawner and LaVigne, 1992; Johnstone, 1978). For example, Brunnstrom (Sawner and LaVigne, 1992) proposed a stereotypical staging of recovery from stroke and developed intervention approaches after years of documented clinical observation and immersion into neurophysiologic literature. Brunnstrom's stages now serve as an important foundation for the Fugl-Meyer assessment of motor recovery after stroke (Gladstone, 2002). Well before electromyographic (EMG) studies that confirmed preparatory shifts in postural activity precede voluntary limb movements (Lee, 1980; Nashner and McCollum, 1985), Berta Bobath (1970) advocated the importance of working on proximal "key points of control" of the head and trunk to better enable the limb movements of patients. Margaret Johnstone (1978) advocated the use of air splints to support and promote early use of hemiparetic limbs long before animal studies showed that forced use of a hemiparetic limb promoted **neuroplasticity** (Jenkins, 1990). Throughout the history of neurological rehabilitation, the inductive reasoning associated with clinical expertise, systematic observation and recording of patient behavior, and objective analysis of that behavior have been used to formulate rehabilitation theory. In turn, deductive reasoning processes have been used to challenge and update clinical practice. A number of clinical assumptions and motor behavior theories that continue to be relevant have been reformulated with what we know from advances in the science and practice of neurological rehabilitation.

## Advances in the Science and Clinical Practice of Neurological Rehabilitation

Major factors having a dramatic effect on the principles of neurological rehabilitation include the availability of new technology for studying motor behavior, recent advances in the basic sciences, and an expansion in the theories of motor behavior used to guide clinical practice.

### Technology

Technological advances such as the ability to record cortical motor-evoked potentials, record brain activity through functional magnetic resonance imaging, and the use of transcranial magnetic stimulation in clinical investigations has provided a means of gathering new evidence on the effects of intervention strategies (Green, 2003; Harris-Love, 2012). Virtual reality (Laver, 2012; Proffitt and Lange, 2015) and the use of interactive robotics for haptic retraining (Johnson, 2006; Lo, 2010; Mehrholz, 2007; Mehrholz, 2012) are becoming more commonplace and opening new frontiers and questions on how environments might be created to promote opportunities for rehabilitation and learning. For example, Fluet (2012) reported a hand intervention program utilizing a virtual reality environment and robot exoskeleton. However, new technology provides us only tools. It remains critically important that therapists use new technology within a sound theoretical framework. This can be seen in the work of Levac (2015), Levin (2015), and Lohse (2013), who describe how virtual reality training environments can be designed that incorporate fundamental principles of motor control and motor learning.

### Neuroplasticity

Historically, neurological pathology was commonly believed to result in a loss of central nervous system (CNS) neurons that could not be regenerated. Recovery of function was believed to be the result of compensation by spared regions of the CNS or unmasking of redundant CNS circuits rather than

actual recovery of neurological function. Specific regions of the cerebral cortex were believed to be inherently dedicated to specific functions and regions of the body with localization of function relatively fixed.

For quite some time we have been aware that mechanisms of recovery include recovery from neural shock as local vascular and metabolic events resolve, recovery of synaptic effectiveness as compression of neurons and edema-related conduction blocks subside, and changes at the neuronal level (Levere, 1988). Recruitment of silent synapses occur, and redundant axons and synapses present within the CNS are activated when the primary control pathways are damaged. It is now widely acknowledged that the human nervous system is a dynamic system with sensorimotor areas of the cerebral cortex shifting in size and function relative to the sensory experience and motor activities of individuals (Nudo, 2003). For example, Elbert (1995) reported that the finger and hand regions of the motor cortex are larger in individuals who play musical instruments for many years than in healthy individuals who do not play instruments, and the finger representations in blind individuals who learn Braille exceed those with intact vision (Pascual-Leone and Torres, 1993). Similarly, the shifting of cortical sensorimotor maps occurs in animals and humans after neurological pathology (Liepert, 2000; Nudo, 1997; Schallert and Jones, 1993).

Merzenich (1984) were among the first individuals to report the flexibility of cortical sensorimotor maps. Plautz (1995) extended this work by showing that cortical maps of animals are altered by motor skill acquisition, not by repetitive movement alone. In a series of studies, Kleim and colleagues (Adkins, 2006; Kleim and Jones, 2010; Kleim, 2007) have shown skill training in animals leads to synaptogenesis and reorganization of the motor map of the cortex, endurance training leads to angiogenesis but does not alter the cortical motor map, and strength training alters spinal motor neuron excitability and spinal cord organization, but does not affect cortical regions. Thus, it is the context of training that is critical for neuroplastic changes, not repetitive movement alone. A useful summary of principles of neuroplasticity (Kleim and Jones, 2010) is shown in Table 14-2.

The finding that high frequencies of behavioral training promote neuroplasticity in animals with neurological lesions was the impetus for two forms of clinical intervention that have been formally tested: locomotor training with body weight-support on a treadmill (Fisher and Sullivan, 2001; Mehrholz, 2007) (see Chapters 33 and 37) and constraint-induced therapy (CIT) for promoting upper limb recovery (Taub, 1980; Wolf, 2006). The seminal research in using a treadmill to drive gait recovery was animal research that showed cats with experimentally induced spinal transactions recovered the ability to step on a treadmill after training with trunk support and assistance with paw placement (Barbeau and Rossignol, 1987; de Leon, 1998). These findings were initially translated to the treatment strategies of individuals with traumatic spinal cord injury (Behrman and Harkema, 2000; Finch, 1991), and now are being applied to gait training

| TABLE 14-2 | Principles of Experience-Dependent Plasticity |
|---|---|
| **PRINCIPLE** | **DESCRIPTION** |
| 1. Use It or Lose It | Failure to drive specific brain function can lead to functional degradation. |
| 2. Use It and Improve It | Training that drives a specific brain function can lead to an enhancement of that function. |
| 3. Specificity | The nature of the training experience dictates the nature of the plasticity. |
| 4. Repetition Matters | Induction of plasticity requires sufficient repetition. |
| 5. Intensity Matters | Induction of plasticity requires sufficient training intensity. |
| 6. Time Matters | Different forms of plasticity occur at different times during training. |
| 7. Salience Matters | The training experience must be sufficiently salient to induce plasticity. |
| 8. Age Matters | Training-induced plasticity occurs more readily in younger brains. |
| 9. Transference | Plasticity in response to one training experience can enhance the acquisition of similar behaviors. |
| 10. Interference | Plasticity in response to one experience can interfere with the acquisition of other behaviors. |

Source: Reproduction of Table 1, Page S227 in Kleim JA, Jones TA. Principles of experience-dependent neural plasticity: implications for rehabilitation after brain damage. *J Speech Lang Hear Res.* 2008;51:S225–S239.

for patients with a variety of neurological pathologies, including stroke, TBI, multiple sclerosis, and Parkinson disease (Miyai, 2000; Pohl, 2002; Ruiz, 2013; Sullivan, 2002). The methodology for this training is to provide patients with sufficient body support and assistance so they can carry out high intensities of repetitive stepping on a treadmill with appropriate afferent input associated with walking. The goal is experience-dependent changes in neuroplasticity at spinal and supraspinal levels (Barbeau, 2003; Barbeau and Fung, 2001; Dobkin, 1999). Preliminary functional magnetic resonance imaging (fMRI) and transcranial magnetic stimulation data suggest treadmill-based gait training may promote neural recovery for patients with Parkinson disease (Fisher, 2008) or stroke (Fisher and Sullivan, 2001). However, the hypothesis that spinal levels of control could be enhanced through high-intensity repetitive stepping is being questioned by early advocates (Dobkin and Duncan, 2012). The Locomotor Experience Applied Post-Stroke (LEAPS) clinical trial in treadmill-based gait training for individuals with stroke (Nadeau, 2013) reported the gait outcomes of individuals with stroke who carried out an intense treadmill-based gait program were not notably different from individuals who carried out an equally intense home exercise program of strength and balance exercises.

CIT, initially referred to as "forced use," was first advocated by Taub (1980) who showed heavy bouts of practice led to functional recovery of deafferented limbs of monkeys that were not used spontaneously. Taub hypothesized that the animals had developed a **"learned nonuse"** of the deafferented limbs secondary to compensation from the intact opposite side limbs. CIT involves restricting the use of the less involved limb of a patient with stroke to emphasize use of the hemiparetic limb. Wolf (2006) showed that patients with stroke participating in CIT for 14 days had meaningful improvements in arm function that lasted for at least 1 year. Actual changes in cortical organization after CIT are reported (Levy, 2001; Liepert, 2000). However, numerous questions exist regarding the optimal dosage of CIT, the retention of the

effects attained, and the mechanisms underlying the functional improvements observed (Sirtori, 2009; Wolf, 2007). Cramer (2009) reported patients with stroke who began an intensive CIT program within 10 days of their stroke had less upper limb recovery at 90 days than patients engaged in more moderate levels of CIT or in only standard therapy. More recently, evidence has been reported that a well-structured, intensive, home program after a CIT program is far more effective in attaining optimal functional outcomes than the formal CIT training itself (Taub, 2013). Thus, the optimal timing and intensity of CIT remains unknown, and the salient element of a CIT program appears to be promoting the skilled use of an impaired limb, not restraining the contralateral limb. The findings that bilateral upper limb training leads to neuroplastic changes (Bleyenheuft, 2015) and leads to motor recovery similar to CIT (Gordon, 2007; Stoykov and Corcos, 2009) validates this proposition.

It appears that not all individuals have the same capacity for neuroplasticity. Recent advances in genomics research have revealed that the genetic profile of individuals with stroke, Parkinson disease, and other neurological pathologies affect their therapy outcomes (Goldberg, 2015). Neuroplasticity involves a series of complex cell signaling processes, with brain-derived neurotropic factor (BDNF) and Apolipoprotein E (APOE) playing import roles. Polymorphisms (genetic variants) in BDNF and APOE compromise the capacity for neuroplasticity and recovery for patients with stroke and TBI (Kleim, 2006; Pearson-Fuhrhop, 2009). Evidence exists that intense exercise (McHughen, 2011) and aerobic exercise (Mang, 2013) may help patients overcome lowered cortical responsiveness. Thus, therapeutic programs intended to promote neuroplasticity will be most effective with personalized parameters of intensity, frequency, and duration for the patients participating in those programs.

### Spasticity and Motor Production Problems Associated With Stroke

The trilogy of hypertonia, hyperreflexia, and clonus, collectively referred to as **spasticity**, previously was believed to be one of the major motor problems limiting the motor behavior of patients with stroke. Spasticity was thought to be a phenomenon that was relatively easy to explain; a release of spinal circuits from supraspinal levels of control, resulting in hyperactivity of the fusimotor system and a velocity-dependent excessive resistance to passive stretch. Limitations in isolated control of joint movements were attributed to heightened stretch reflex activity of antagonist muscles and less so to weakness of agonists.

Spasticity is still considered a result of a pathological increase in stretch reflex gain and a decrease in threshold of activation (Thilman, 1991) but is now viewed as a symptom of the initial neurological injury and a consequence of recovery. Processes of recovery that contribute to spasticity include synaptic hyper-effectiveness (increased release of acetylcholine in presynaptic fibers), denervation supersensitivity (the appearance of additional receptors in the postsynaptic membrane that increase the response to neurotransmitters), regenerative sprouting of axons that have been damaged, collateral sprouting from intact neurons adjacent damaged axons, and reorganization of spinal interneurons such as flexor reflex afferents (Levere, 1988). Craik (1991) has nicely illustrated the potential neural circuitry that can contribute to spasticity (see Figure 14-3).

Patients show altered patterns of muscle control in spastic muscles, including the inability to quickly generate and halt agonist motor activity, inadequate activation of agonist muscles, and abnormal coactivation of agonists and antagonists (Knuttson and Martenson, 1980; Sahrmann and Norton, 1977). Recent studies suggest weakness is a separate and greater limitation to movement function than spasticity (Patten, 2004). For example, Bohannon and Andrews (1990) showed that only a low correlation existed between knee extensor spasticity, muscle torque, and gait speed for

patients with stroke, and Gowland (1992) reported a low correlation between spasticity and upper limb voluntary movements.

In addition to spasticity, a number of sensorimotor factors contribute to the force production and limb coordination impairments of patients with stroke (Ada, 2006; Brown and Kautz, 1999; Kokotilo, 2009; Patten, 2004; Scheets, 2007; Schindler-Ivens, 2004; Vidoni and Boyd, 2009; Wagner, 2006). Secondary effects of neurological pathology include **stiffness**, defined as resistance to stretch due to changes in the viscoelastic and structural properties of muscles, tendons, ligaments, and joint structures. Dietz and colleagues (Dietz and Berger, 1983; Dietz and Berger, 1984) showed adults with spastic hemiplegia developed high levels of muscle tension in the gastrocnemius during passive stretch but with low EMG activity. Muscle biopsies have shown increased muscle atrophy in spastic muscles, a predominance of Type I fibers, and structural changes that contribute to muscle stiffness (Dietz and Berger, 1984). Bourbonnais and Vanden Noven (1989) provide an excellent review of changes reported in the motor neurons, nerves, and muscles of patients with stroke. Common findings include changes in the properties of agonist motor units, decreased firing rates, changes in peripheral nerve conduction, and a presence of slow-twitch, fatigable muscle fibers. Impaired force output of patients is attributed to shifts in patterns of cortical motor activity dependent on the time since stroke, extent of brain damage, and severity of stroke (Kokotilo, 2009). Sensory loss also compromises force output (Vidoni and Boyd, 2009; Wagner, 2006; Zackowski, 2004).

Although therapists previously were concerned that strengthening exercises would increase the spasticity of patients with stroke, resistance training has been shown to lead to greater muscular force output without exacerbating hypertonia (Ada, 2006; Brown and Kautz, 1998; Giuliani, 1992; Patten, 2004; Sharp and Brouwer, 1997; Teixeira-Salmela, 2001). Patients with multiple sclerosis have been shown to improve their strength and functional capacity after resistance training of moderate intensity (Cakt, 2010; Dalgas, 2008).

An important consideration in therapeutic exercise is the way strengthening activities are structured. Studies on the neural adaptation to exercise show that the effectiveness of training depends on how closely the exercises being performed replicate the muscle dynamics of the task to be learned (Gabriel, 2006; Sale, 1988). Ketelaar (2001) and Winstein (2004) showed functional task training had a greater effect than exercise alone on the restoration of functional skills for patients with neurological pathology. There may be patient cases, such as children with severe cerebral palsy or patients with severe posturing after brainstem injures, when extreme levels of spasticity might be a major factor restricting limb function. However, in many cases a therapist's time may be better spent addressing muscle stiffness, impaired agonist motor control, and weakness through functional stretching activities than addressing issues of spasticity and hypertonicity in isolation from functional contexts.

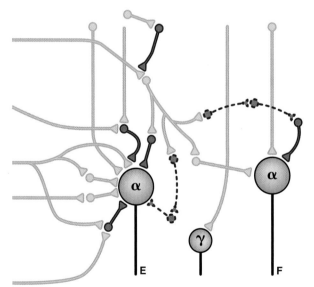

**FIGURE 14-3** An illustration of the neural mechanisms associated with spasticity. (Reprinted with permission from Craik, 1991.) Abnormalities of motor behavior. In: Lister MJ, ed. *Contemporary Management of Motor Control Problems: Proceedings of the II Step Conference.* Fredricksburg, VA: Bookcrafters; 1991, pp. 155–164 (APTA).

## Contemporary Applications of Motor Behavior Theory to Clinical Practice

In *The Structure of Scientific Revolutions,* Kuhn wrote, "Successive transition from one paradigm to another via revolution is the usual developmental pattern of mature science" (Kuhn, 1970, p. 12). Several "paradigm shifts," or changes in basic assumptions, have occurred throughout the history of neurological rehabilitation. A radical transition from the muscle reeducation to the neurofacilitation approach occurred when clinicians began to consider the possibility of "normalizing" (Bobath, 1970) or "capturing" (Sawner and LaVigne, 1992) abnormal motor tone and spastic movement patterns after stroke and restoring movement behavior in hemiparetic limbs. Another revolutionary paradigm shift occurred when clinicians became more aware of motor learning theory and began to advocate that patients be encouraged to perform functional tasks, even before high degrees of selective motor control were established. Also proposed was that patients be allowed to make and self-correct movement errors and problem-solve solutions to functional tasks rather than being facilitated or guided by therapists through specific movement patterns in an error free manner (Carr and Shepherd, 1982; Lister, 1991).

The most recent shift in neurological rehabilitation has been the transition to a more integrative system view in which the sensory and motor interactions between the performer and the environment are respected and motor control is viewed as the result of distributed control of body structures and functions across all levels of the movement system. In some task conditions, motor control may be organized in a "top-down" manner in which cognitively generated motor plans play a large role in determining the resulting motor behavior. In other contexts, the control may be "bottom-up," largely influenced by peripheral stimuli and sensory feedback. For example, when individuals are walking at a comfortable pace and talking to another person, or focusing their attention elsewhere, the control of gait may be regulated by midbrain and spinal levels of control. When the same individuals walk on ice or another type of challenging environment, cortical control and input from peripheral sensory receptors may play a larger part. The nature of an intended activity determines how body structures and functions are organized and regulated.

The reflex and hierarchical models that served as the foundation for the neurofacilitation approaches have been reconsidered in light of what we now know of human motor control. Reflexes remain an important component of the human motor system but are no longer considered to be the primary building blocks (Sherrington, 1906) or the fundamental basis for voluntary movements. Instead, complex functional assemblages of neurons that allow motor behavior to be organized at subcortical levels are described as structural units (Latash, 2002), self-organizing maps (Krishnan, 2006), or anatomical nodes (Dobkin, 2004a). Central pattern generators are a contemporary concept of reflex-like activity that can be accessed by higher centers or sensory input (Dobkin, 2004a). Similarly, traditional hierarchical models that held cortical "higher levels" controlled subcortical and spinal cord "lower levels" of motor output have been reformulated (Bernstein, 1967; Dobkin, 2004a). Although cortical areas continue to be a major organizing level of intended motor actions, the role of cortical regions is less prescriptive in specifying the details of motor output.

A number of concepts from motor behavior theory provide the foundation for our current practice of neurological rehabilitation, including **perception-action theory, biomechanics, dynamic pattern theory,** and **dynamic systems theory.** Our discussion here will be restricted to major concepts from these theories that have direct relevance to neurological rehabilitation.

### Perception-Action Theory

Perception-action theory (Gibson, 1966; Gibson, 1977; Gibson, 1988; Lee, 1989; Reed, 1984; Warren, 1984) emphasizes the motor behavior of individuals is intimately tied to an inseparable performer-environment interface, that we perceive and interact with the physical world in relation to our own morphology, scaling the external world in relationship to personal attributes such as eye height, leg length, hand size, and shoulder width. The fit between an individual and the physical world identifies certain **affordances** or possibilities for action, as well as certain constraints. Within this framework, a sitting surface is low for a patient or a step is high, based on the relationship between the height of those surfaces and the leg length of the patient. That which is low or high for an adult is not the same for a child. The perception of the individual within the environment determines the behavior that emerges. In a perception-action framework, learning involves becoming a better perceiver of the affordances and constraints that exist and the possibilities for action. Newell (1991) emphasizes the importance of exploring the **perceptual-motor workspace** for effective motor learning. Empirical evidence has been offered that the behaviors used to perform actions as diverse as picking up objects (Newell, 1989), climbing stairs (Warren, 1984), and catching moving objects (Lee, 1989; von Hofsten, 1979) are influenced by perception-action processes. These findings suggest the importance of engaging patients in valid functional tasks with actual objects so they can learn to scale the spatial dimensions of tasks to their own morphology and optimize their functional competence.

### Biomechanics

Nikoli Bernstein, a Russian movement science pioneer, observed that movement performance arises from an infinite variety of possible combinations, or degrees of freedom, of joints, muscles, and nerves. The "motor problem" as recognized by Bernstein is how we coordinate our redundant degrees of freedom to engage in the external world during the performance of specific tasks (Bernstein, 1967). Bernstein suggested we never perform a motor task exactly the same way but are guided by a movement **topology**; an internal representation of an intended action reflecting the external field forces of gravity and surface/object contact and the intrinsic mechanical characteristics of our multi-segmented musculoskeletal system. Certain aspects of our actions happen "for free," that is, due to the external and mechanical forces affecting our body in motion. For example, when walking at a normal velocity, plantar flexion of the ankle at heel strike occurs for free from the contact force of the heel hitting the floor. Similarly, knee extension during terminal swing typically occurs without activation of knee extensors because of the interaction torque generated by the femur acting on the knee and tibia. Therefore, solving the "motor problem" of gait control is not merely contracting muscles to move the body through space. It is activating muscles effectively to offset and optimize the external forces that arise during a task performance; activating dorsiflexors before heel contact to control the plantar flexion caused by ground reaction forces at loading response; and contracting hamstrings muscles at terminal swing to decelerate the forward movement of the tibia on the femur caused by the mechanical forces generated from the femur. Important clinical concepts derived from Bernstein's work include: motor activities can be performed with a variety of movement options (Ford-Smith and VanSant, 1993; Newell, 1989); optimal degrees of movement variability exist within our movements (Latash, 2002; Stergiou, 2006); and our planning and performance of actions are intimately tied to the context of the environment.

## Dynamic Pattern Theory

Dynamic pattern theory evolved from Bernstein's work and the desire to identify how the numerous neuromuscular degrees of freedom of human motor control might be organized in a coordinated fashion (Haken, 1983; Jeka, 1989; von Holst, 1973). The main proposition is that coordinated movement patterns are the primary elements of human motor behavior rather than isolated movements (Kelso, 1987). Dynamic pattern theory emphasizes that "phase shifts" occur from one preferred coordination pattern or **attractor state** to another as the conditions of the task or environment change. Attractor states are self-organized optimal coordination patterns reflecting task and environmental influences and the nature of the neuromuscular system (Fonseca, 2001; Jeng, 1996; Scholz and Schöner, 1999). Variables that cause a phase shift from one attractor state to another are termed **control parameters**, and **order parameters** are variables used to express the coordination pattern. Certain attractor states may be very strong and stable and difficult to avoid, whereas others may be transient states of coordination more open to perturbation.

Figure 14-4 shows how concepts of attractor states and control parameters can be applied to adult ambulation. A "ball in a basin" analogy shows the attraction of the movement system toward a behavior (width of a basin), the stability of that behavior (depth and slope of a basin), and areas of transition from one behavior to another when a single optimal behavior may not exist (overlap of basins). For ambulation, the control parameter is the velocity of the body moving over the support surface; the order parameter is the type of mobility pattern used. At a slow velocity, the first pattern of mobility is single steps. Although initially an optimal behavior, the attraction of single stepping exists for a small range of velocity and is not very stable. Slow walking quickly competes with stepping as an attractor state as velocity increases. Walking is a strong and stable attractor state for body mobility. The large width of the basin indicates walking is an optimal behavior over a wide range of increasing velocities. However, a loss of walking pattern stability occurs as velocity increases, as indicated by a change in the slope of the basin. At a moderate velocity skipping is possible, although as pictured in Figure 14-4, skipping emerges only for a narrow range of velocities and is not a very stable behavior. Running is an optimal behavior as velocity continues to increase. Note the overlap of the mobility basins pictured. This demonstrates that at certain velocities no one attractor state (mobility pattern) may be optimal, and inconsistent or erratic behaviors may occur as the system struggles to find stability. In dynamic pattern theory, increases in motor variability are viewed as a natural occurrence during a phase transition, not necessarily movement error. Scholz has illustrated how dynamic pattern theory can be applied to the crawling patterns of children with cerebral palsy (Scholz, 1990) and adult lifting behavior (Scholz, 1995). The emerging patterns and the stability of those patterns are dependent on the task and environmental conditions driving that pattern.

## Dynamic Systems

Thelan and colleagues (Heriza, 1991; Thelan, 1986; Thelan and Ulrich, 1991) adapted a number of concepts from dynamic pattern theory to develop a "dynamic systems" approach for understanding human motor behavior. First,

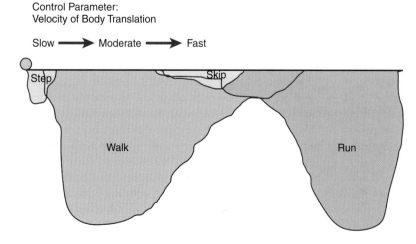

**FIGURE 14-4** Concepts of dynamic pattern theory applied to adult ambulation.

they suggested the term **collective variable** was preferable over order parameter to emphasize that the preferred coordination patterns we observe reflect the interaction of numerous underlying subsystems. Second, they suggested each contributing subsystem, including environmental influences, may act as a separate control parameter for an observed motor behavior at a given time. Third, the motor behavior of patients was considered to be a self-organizing and emergent process reflecting the effect of many influences that might change on their own course or through interactions with other subsystems. Fourth, it was suggested certain subsystems might act as **"rate limiting variables;"** that is, although changes may be occurring in one or more contributing subsystems, a change in the overall behavior of a system may not occur until one or more particularly influential subsystems reached a critical point (see Figure 14-5).

The framework put forth by Thelan and colleagues offers a particularly useful conceptual framework for considering the behavior of patients with neurological pathology. The influences of the environment and the numerous body structures and functions contributing to the behavior of patients can be defined as subsystems. Perceptual processes, biomechanical influences, cognitive processing, force production capacity, sensory processing, and emotional state can all be considered as contributing layers of the emerging motor behavior. For example, consider that patients with Parkinson disease are commonly reported to show a lack of reciprocal arm swing during gait. Although upper limb motor rigidity is often offered as the cause, the shorter step lengths and lower gait

velocities of these patients can also lead to lack of reciprocal arm swing, and a fear of falling can result in patients freezing their upper limbs in a protective mechanism. Thus, arm swing in this case can be viewed as a collective variable influenced by the patient's motor tone, biomechanics, and emotionality. The dynamic systems framework helps therapists remember the importance of evaluating the multiple subsystems that may contribute to an altered motor behavior before planning a therapeutic intervention plan. It is not helpful to simply state "everything matters" or that "every patient is different." The key is to understand how contributing body structures and functions interact and cluster as they contribute to the motor behavior of patients and to identify rate-limiting factors that preclude the ability of patients to shift from limited to more functional motor behaviors.

## The Attractor States of Patients With Neurological Pathology: The Clustering of Impairments in Body Structure and Function

The presence of neurological pathology adds additional chaos to the complexity of human motor behavior. Patients with neurological disorders often have impairments of multiple body structures and functions (see the examination measures described in Chapters 3 through 13). These impairments frequently result in altered movements that can lead to limitations in activity and participation (see examination measures described in Chapters 10 and 13). Patients with neurological pathology experience both "positive" and "negative" symptoms (Walshe, 1961). **Positive symptoms** are motor control abnormalities arising as a result of the pathology. These include abnormal movements such as ataxia, dystonia, or rigidity for patients with extrapyramidal involvement and spasticity for patients with damage to the pyramidal motor system. **Negative symptoms** are the losses or declines of body functions after neurological injury such as muscle weakness, decreased endurance, loss of sensation, visual field cuts, and loss of balance control.

Historically, therapists debated which symptoms caused the greatest limitation to recovery and created intervention strategies to address specific symptoms such as spasticity or weakness (Gordon, 2000; Horak, 1991). However, the motor problems and activity limitations of patients are not merely the result of the direct effects of a pathological condition. Patients frequently experience secondary effects from immobility such as muscle stiffness (Dietz and Berger, 1983; Thilman, 1991), deconditioning (Ivey, 2005), and learned disuse (Taub, 1999; Sterr, 2006). Many of the activity limitations patients experience arise from a combination of the direct and secondary effects of their pathological conditions (Schenkman and Butler, 1989). For example, during the swing phase of gait, patients with hemiplegia often display retraction of the trunk and pelvis, excessive external rotation of the hip, and decreased hip and knee flexion. This gait pattern may result from excessive extensor muscle tone in the trunk and lower limb muscles (a positive symptom), weakness and decreased motor control of the trunk and lower limb (negative symptom), or be a compensatory

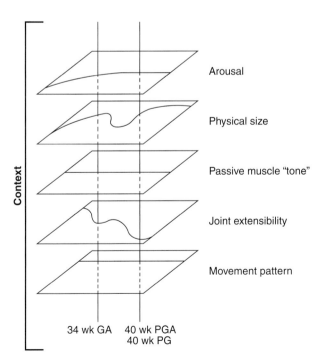

**FIGURE 14-5** A representation of Thelan's concept of dynamic systems applied to infant kicking behavior. (Reprinted with permission from Heriza, 1991.) Motor behavior: Traditional and contemporary theories. In: Lister MJ, ed. *Contemporary Management of Motor Control Problems: Proceedings of the II Step Conference.* Fredricksburg, VA: Bookcrafters; 1991, pp. 99–126 (APTA).

strategy the patient uses for dealing with both. A dynamic systems perspective helps us to consider the many factors contributing to the movement behaviors of patients and not assume that the pathological behaviors of patients are caused by one factor alone. The motor behavior of patients after neurological injury is often their best attempt to use their body structures and functions to carry out functional activities, a self-organization of body structures and functions that includes impairments, spared resources, and compensation strategies.

Patients with neurological pathology often develop attractor states self-organized around their pathology. Common pathological attractor states for patients with stroke include excessive lower limb extension and external rotation of the hip; excessive upper limb flexion at the elbow, wrist, and hand; and internal rotation and adduction of the shoulder. Patients often lack the ability to move effectively out of these attractor states. Pathological motor attractor states are common to patients with similar types of neurological pathology. For example, stereotypical spastic synergy patterns are reported in patients with stroke, and patients with Parkinson disease eventually acquire a flexed posture in standing and a shuffling gait. Therapists have recently begun to identify clusters of impairments of body structure and function that provide a means of stratifying the motor abilities and functional competence of children (Crenna, 1992) and adults with neurological pathology (Patel, 2000; Scheets, 2007).

Helping patients move from inflexible and potentially detrimental attractor states into flexible motor behaviors begins with a thorough examination and evaluation of the attractor states themselves and hypothesizing the subsystems contributing to the pathological attractor state. Therapists can then use therapeutic techniques to minimize impairments of body structures and functions and help patients shift out of detrimental attractor states. However, in doing so, therapists also need to manipulate the context of tasks and environments, optimize the information processing of patients, and promote effective practice to help patients acquire functional and flexible coordination modes of motor behavior.

## ■ Principle #2: The Goal of Neurological Rehabilitation Is Functional Competence

### Promoting Flexible Coordination Modes

How can therapists help patients achieve functional competence? That is, how can they help patients consistently and efficiently succeed in performing motor tasks under diverse conditions? It is well known that individuals carrying out functional tasks do not use the same movement strategies or movement patterns consistently (Aruntyunyan, 1968; Ford-Smith and VanSant, 1993). **Movement strategies** are the plans used to carry out a task, and **movement patterns** are the actual kinematics employed to perform the task. Ford-Smith and VanSant (1993) showed healthy subjects moving from supine to sitting on the edge of a bed used different types of

movement strategies such as pulling on the bed with one or two hands, pushing off the bed with the hands, and pushing off the bed with a lower limb. Similarly, the movement patterns used with respect to limb position and movement amplitude differed from one trial to another and one subject to another. Thus, motor behavior emerges from the interaction between the performer and the environment (Newell, 1989). When working with patients on reestablishing diverse movement patterns, effective therapists work within a task context to ensure the movements generated are indeed valid.

Functional competence involves patients performing and modifying movement strategies and patterns with efficiency. To do so, patients benefit from learning a general form of actions that can be adapted to specific tasks and environments. This form can be described in a number of ways such as a movement topology (Bernstein, 1967), an attractor state (Thelan and Ulrich, 1991), or a "schema" (Schmidt, 1975). In this chapter, the term "**coordination mode**" will be used, which is consistent with terminology used by Newell, McDonald, and Kugler (1991).

To understand the relevance of coordination modes, consider this example. The general coordination mode for moving from sitting to standing is to bring the center of mass (the trunk) over the base of support (position of the feet) and to maintain that body relationship while the lower limbs are extended. Patients with neurological pathology often fall backward when initially attempting to move from sitting to standing without upper limb support because a fear of falling if they move forward results in them keeping their weight back. Patients need to learn how they can combine different variations of scooting, foot placement, and leaning to bring their center of mass safely over their feet to succeed in moving from sitting to standing in the various environments they will encounter. Ultimately, it is the coordination mode of bringing the center of mass over the base of support that matters, not a specific foot position, strategy, or movement pattern. Certain movement strategies and patterns available to patients should be discouraged if they are dangerous or if they will lead to detrimental changes over time (e.g., equinovarus of the foot or knee recurvatum during the loading response phase of ambulation). However, movement variability should be encouraged. Functional competence requires patients be able to generate a variety of movements within flexible coordination modes when carrying out activities, not just perform a specific set of movement patterns.

## ■ Principle #3: Functional Competence Is Promoted by Basing Rehabilitation Strategies on Embedded Models of Motor Behavior and Neurological Rehabilitation: Apples Not Oranges

In the vast majority of real-world situations, the goal of motor behavior is to accomplish a functional activity. Perhaps the only time individuals carry out tasks with specific movements in mind is in certain forms of sports competition (ice skating and gymnastics), in the performing arts, and in particular social situations (walking down a fashion runway or dancing). It is indisputable that integrity of body structures and functions and the movements of patients are important. Patients cannot participate in their social contexts or carry out functional activities without activating their body structures and functions and moving. In turn, activating body structures and functions and moving is dependent on the neurophysiology of the human condition. The models of enablement and disablement that have been designed to illustrate the relationship between these levels of motor behavior have sometimes led therapists to the misconception that these levels exist in stages or in parallel, like the segments of an orange. Instead, these levels should be viewed as being embedded in one another, like the continuum of the core, pulp, and skin of an apple. Figure 14-6 A through C illustrates how the organization of motor behavior and models of rehabilitation can be illustrated within an embedded framework.

For patients to perform motor tasks successfully, they must use the affordances available and meet the **spatial** and **temporal constraints** of the task and environment. Optimal rehabilitation occurs when therapists create and use well-designed functional tasks requiring the use of desired movements in a meaningful context. Practicing limb and trunk movements in isolation may not lead to the spontaneous use of that pattern within functional tasks. For example, when therapists emphasize a particular movement pattern for gait when working with a patient, it is not unusual to find the patient "forgetting to use" that pattern as they walk out of the gym after the session. Why does this happen?

First, healthy individuals do not usually monitor the kinematics of their movements; they monitor whether or not their intended actions are successfully completed. The monitoring of movement patterns during actions impairs the automaticity, fluidity, and movement speed of actions because the self-monitoring of movements increases the information processing demands of the task. Second, the relationship between movements and actions is not one-to-one. Patients often have a variety of movement patterns they can use to accomplish an action. If a therapist imposes a specific movement pattern upon a patient for a functional activity, the patient must remember the pattern they have been given and not use alternate movement patterns that might also complete the task. If therapists truly believe the teaching of specific movement patterns is critical for functional recovery, which movements should be used? As pointed out by Bernstein (1967), with small variations in a task or environment, a completely new set of movement patterns may be appropriate.

The more movement patterns available to patients, the more strategies patients can develop and explore for a given action. If certain movement patterns appear to be dysfunctional, it certainly would make sense to try to establish viable movement patterns. Therapists can effectively work with patients on regaining movement patterns by having the patient

practice meaningful tasks created by the therapist that intrinsically require the performance of the targeted movement pattern, that is, by "**embedding**" the desired movement pattern in the task being performed. Embedding movements into tasks means structuring environments, selecting objects to manipulate, and creating task conditions in which certain desired movements will be more likely to occur. Consider the following example. Supination is a movement pattern often impaired in the upper limb of patients with a cerebral vascular accident (CVA). To reestablish supination, therapists might design a number of movement exercises while stretching and strengthening the limb musculature to improve that movement. In addition, therapists can embed supination into actions by having patients work on tasks such as turning over pages in a book or picking up and carrying a dinner tray. Therapists are sometimes concerned patients will not attain the same degree of improvement of movement in functional task training as they would in movement exercise. This is not necessarily true. Van der Weel (1991) investigated the ability of children with cerebral palsy to actively increase pronation and supination of the forearm through functional task performance. The children showed a greater active range of motion in supination and pronation when they used their limb in a drum-beating task than when attempting to maximize their pronation and supination by active exercise alone. It was not necessary for the children to prepare the limb for the task; improvement occurred during task practice. An interesting and important consideration is whether functional training alone is optimal for establishing functional competence or whether a combination of some degree of task preparation at an impairment level, followed by functionally based practice, is more effective. Schenkman (2001) reported that individuals with Parkinson disease attempting to increase functional trunk rotation benefited from trunk exercises carried out before task training.

Carefully conceived and manipulated motor tasks can be used to activate motor control processes at specific levels of the patient's motor system. For example, dual tasks shift the control of balance and gait from cortical to subcortical regions (Guerts and Mulder, 1994; Morris, 1996; Fritz, 2015). Changing the conditions for gait training from a stable walking surface to a treadmill may shift the control of gait from higher levels of motor control to spinal levels (Dobkin, 1999). Auditory cues, visual cues, and music result in increased movement speed and fluidity for patients with Parkinson disease by activating motor pathways less dependent on basal ganglia function (Ashoori, 2015; Earhart, 2010; Majsak, 1998).

Functional tasks give meaning to movement, and patient-centered task-oriented exercises lead to greater outcomes in motor control (Song, 2015) and balance (Choi and Kang, 2015) than repetitive movement training. Functional mobility is not merely the goal for therapy; it is a robust therapeutic medium for intervention. Deciding whether to emphasize functional activities, movements, or to address impairments of body structures and function is unnecessary; all can be done simultaneously.

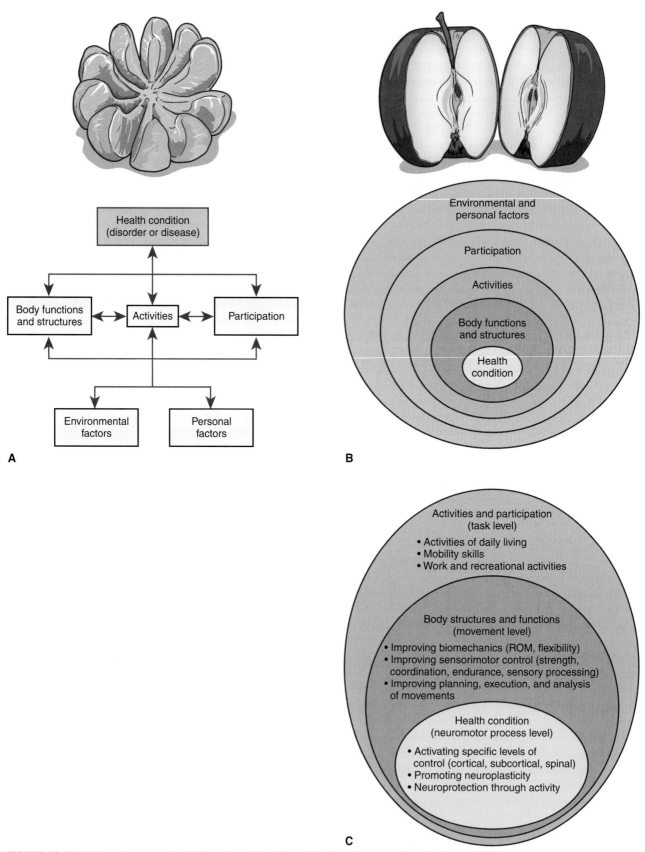

**FIGURE 14-6** Traditional versus embedded models of the ICF model of enablement and levels of motor behavior and neurological rehabilitation. **A.** An illustration of the traditional ICF model of enablement. (Source for figure A. The International Classification of Function, Disability and Health [ICF]. Reprinted from International Classification of Functioning, Disability and Health: ICF. Geneva, Switzerland: World Health Organization; 2001 with permission of the World Health Organization.) **B.** It is advantageous to conceive of the ICF model of enablement as an embedded model (b.), and levels of motor behavior and neurological rehabilitation **C.** as a set of embedded relationships.

## ■ Principle #4: Functional Competence Requires Motor Learning and Self-Efficacy

### Promoting the Capacity for Motor Learning and Functional Competence: Aerobic Exercise, Motivation, and Self-Efficacy

#### Aerobic Exercise

Aerobic exercise offers patients a wealth of benefits, including a greater capacity for motor learning and neuroplasticity (Mang, 2013), improved executive function (Tabak, 2013), and improved cardiovascular health and physical performance (Billinger, 2012). Recent advances in the study of neuroplasticity show aerobic exercise as low as 30 minutes of exercise at 60% of maximum heart rate increases production of brain-derived neurotrophic factor (BDNF), an important facilitator of motor learning and neuroplasticity (Knaepen, 2010). Aerobic exercise appears to be a strategy for "priming" patients for motor learning, particularly if task activities immediately follow aerobic exercise (Mang, 2013). Individuals with Parkinson disease and cognitive impairments reportedly show an increase in cognitive processing, quality of life, and gait function after an 8-week stationary bicycle aerobic exercise program (Tabak, 2013). An appreciation of the importance of promoting mobility and exercise for patients outside of clinic-based rehabilitation is reflected by recent publications reporting the use of shoe-based sensors (Fulk, 2012), accelerometers (Mattlage, 2015), and global positioning system technology (Evans, 2012) to monitor and encourage home and community mobility and exercise. Community wellness programs are being more strongly advocated (Rose, 2013) and innovative home exercise programs are being designed to include the use of technology for distance-based rehabilitation (Ellis, 2013b).

#### Motivation and Self-Efficacy

Patients have the greatest potential of attaining functional competence if they are motivated, confident in their abilities, and willing to meet the challenges they encounter when performing functional tasks. One of the most commonly reported barriers to exercise and mobility for patients at home and in the community is low self-efficacy (Ellis, 2013a; Robinson, 2011; Schmid, 2012). Schmid (2012) showed balance efficacy was a greater predictor of activity and participation for patients with stroke than gait speed or walking capacity. Low self-efficacy is associated with not only a higher fear of falling, but also perceptions of higher effort requirements for the performance of activities of daily living and gait (Julius, 2012). Self-efficacy is reported to be a major factor in predicting the activity levels of patients with Parkinson disease (Ellis, 2011; Ellis, 2013b), stroke (Danksl, 2016; Korpershoek, 2011; Robinson, 2011), and multiple sclerosis (Kalron, 2014; Kayes, 2011). Thus, helping patients to attain high levels of self-efficacy is an important element of effective neurological rehabilitation.

Bandura (1977; 1994) was instrumental in the development of **social cognitive theory** (SCT), which describes four elements of self-efficacy: successful performance, vicarious experience, social persuasion, and emotional arousal. This theory suggests that patients need to have early and perhaps easy task successes to build confidence and a sense of achievement, but that they also need to succeed in performing challenging tasks within their capacity in order to develop frustration tolerance and self-efficacy. Resilient self-efficacy develops when patients learn to overcome challenges through persistent effort. Social persuasion, often provided as verbal praise from a therapist, is a powerful influence for motivating patients, confirming their successes, and building their confidence. Patients benefit when they experience the psychological and affective arousal associated with their successes and mastery of tasks.

Therapists often promote patient self-efficacy by offering patients praise after successful task performance. However, building patient motivation and self-efficacy should begin even prior to the initiation of therapeutic activities. Wulf and Lewthwaite (2016) recently proposed a novel theory of motor learning, called the OPTIMAL theory of motor learning, that emphasizes explicitly the importance of priming the social-cognitive and affective motivational state of individuals prior to learning. The OPTIMAL model integrates with motor performance and practice, fundamental concepts of SCT (Bandura, 1977) and **self-determination theory** (SDT) such as patient intrinsic and extrinsic motivation, autonomy, and identification with goal content (Deci and Ryan, 1985; Teixeira, 2012). Wulf and Lewthwaite cite extensive and compelling research evidence that learning is enhanced when the motivation of patients is primed through opportunities for autonomy (patient-determined goals and plans), enhanced expectations (assuring patients of a successful learning experience), and a focus on the task goal, rather than on their movements. Patient-centered, task-oriented training is reported to lead to higher levels of self-efficacy for patients with stroke than exercise alone (Choi and Kang, 2015).

## Motor Learning: What Is Being Learned?

The causes for an improvement in the motor behavior of a patient can have multiple hypotheses. A dynamic pattern theory perspective might be that a change occurred in the mechanical properties of the patient's body; perception-action that the patient learned how to better perceive the salient aspects of the performer-environment interface and realized a different set of affordances; a Bernstein perspective could be that the patient found new ways to control or utilize his degrees of freedom or establish a new topology. A dynamic systems perspective is that a patient might be experiencing all of these and self-organizing a new emergent behavior.

Gelfand (1971) suggested the organization of human motor behavior was based on *the principle of least interaction,* meaning that to control the numerous degrees of freedom inherent to our systems, internal mechanisms are developed to compress or simplify the degrees of freedom needing to be controlled. Sensorimotor movement synergies were offered as one functional mechanism and organized pools of motor neurons as another (Easton, 1972; Gelfand, 1971). It is feasible our patients are learning how to change their motor behavior to acquire a system of least interaction. They are learning the mechanics of their new self-organized system, how to utilize mechanisms of control at various levels of their system, and how to use a variety of strategies and movements to carry out their desired activities with the least cost to their system.

## The Main Principle of Motor Learning: Optimize Patient Engagement

Schmidt (1988, p. 346) has defined motor learning as *"a set of processes associated with practice or experience leading to relatively permanent changes in the capability for responding."* This definition still rings true. Motor learning involves a set of internal processes, including perception of self, planning, motor execution, experiencing, information processing, and refinement of motor execution. Motor learning is not merely the **acquisition** of a new behavior; it is the **retention** and **transfer** of that behavior (Schmidt, 1988).

The motor behavior of patients is a marker for learning, but it is changes in the internal processes and in the capability of responding that defines motor learning. Therapists can manipulate the regulatory features of tasks, the delivery of information, and the structure of practice conditions to optimize the motor learning processes of patients. The main principle of motor learning is to optimize patient engagement in learning processes. This means helping patients to understand that they have the capacity to change their behaviors, motivating patients to engage in the challenges inherent to learning motor tasks, helping patients to understand how their altered movement system works, involving patients in ecologically valid experiences, and promoting the optimal capacity of patients for information processing and meaningful practice so they can acquire, retain, and generalize their motor behaviors for functional competence.

## ■ A Model for Applying Motor Control and Motor Learning Theory to Neurological Rehabilitation

### General Perspectives

Effective neurological rehabilitation results when therapists use sound theoretical frameworks for organizing their intervention programs. A wide variety of factors influence the motor control and motor learning of patients, including the biomechanical, neuromuscular, and psychological constraints of patients; the functional tasks patients are trying to master; the environments in which practice takes place; and the amount and type of practice carried out. The wide variety of movement strategies and patterns patients can use to perform tasks should be appreciated and patients should engage in the types of information processing they will need to accomplish on their own. Options in the structuring of practice should be kept in mind, and that it is the coordination mode or general form of motor outcome that is

desirable rather than a specific movement pattern. Figure 14-7 presents a model of motor learning that is applicable to the rehabilitation of patients with neurological pathology. The model integrates motor control and motor learning theory from a wide variety of sources, with an underlying framework derived from the seminal contributions of Newell (1985), Gentile (1987), Magill (1992), Schmidt (1991), and Winstein (1991). Three major components of motor learning are identified: (1) Perception of Self and the Environment, (2) Creating a Plan, and (3) Task Performance, Information Processing, and Practicing.

## Perception of Self and the Environment

### Intrinsic Constraints

To begin the process of attaining functional competence, patients learn the nature of their newly self-organized system and how their motor behavior reflects the interaction between their own **intrinsic constraints**, the **external constraints** of the tasks they perform, and the environments in which those tasks take place. The intrinsic constraints of individuals are defined by their inherent biomechanical, psychological, and neuromuscular attributes (see Figure 14-8). Normal and pathological motor behaviors self-organize and emerge from the interaction of all of these.

Consider that the ability to reach while standing is affected by joint mobility and muscle length at the ankles and upper limbs, perceptual-motor and cognitive processing of information, and integration of visual, vestibular, and somatosensory information. Frank and Earl (1990) suggested three types of

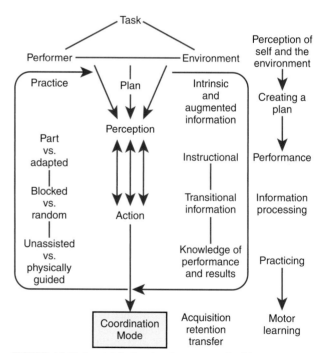

**FIGURE 14-7** A model of motor learning applicable to patients with neurological pathology. The three main stages are: (1) perception of self and the environment, (2) creating a plan, and (3) task performance, information processing, and practicing.

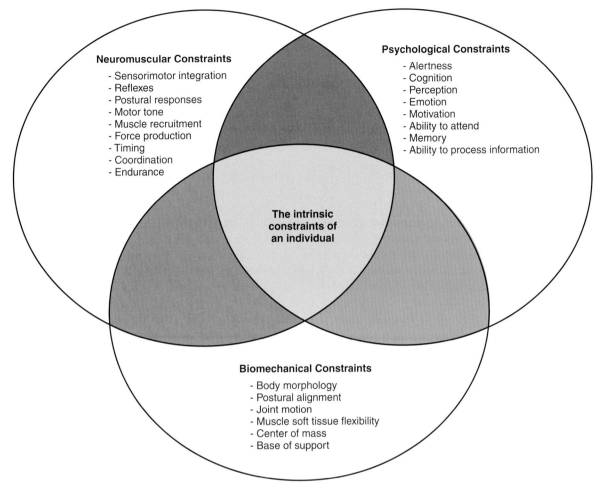

**Neuromuscular Constraints**

- Sensorimotor integration
- Reflexes
- Postural responses
- Motor tone
- Muscle recruitment
- Force production
- Timing
- Coordination
- Endurance

**Psychological Constraints**

- Alertness
- Cognition
- Perception
- Emotion
- Motivation
- Ability to attend
- Memory
- Ability to process information

**The intrinsic constraints of an individual**

**Biomechanical Constraints**

- Body morphology
- Postural alignment
- Joint motion
- Muscle soft tissue flexibility
- Center of mass
- Base of support

**FIGURE 14-8** The intrinsic constraints of individuals and patients. The attributes and limitations of both individuals and patients emerge as the sum of the interactions of biomechanical, neuromuscular, and psychological constraints.

postural strategies are used to maintain upright stance during a task (see Figure 14-9). Cognitive resources are used to preplan **postural preparations** that set a stable posture. Subcortical areas (basal ganglia, cerebellum) generate feedforward **postural accompaniments** in anticipation of and during reaching. Feedback from visual, vestibular, and somatosensory receptors trigger **postural reactions** in response to self-generated or unexpected body and limb movements. Changes in a patient's intrinsic constraints affect their balance control. A patient with hemiplegia secondary to stroke may not be able to reach very far forward because of stiffness of the plantar flexors restricting the forward motion of the tibia; a patient with traumatic brain injury and cognitive impairment may not plan and establish a stable base of support; a patient with Parkinson disease may not be able to generate a postural accompaniment in anticipation of reaching; and a patient with a peripheral neuropathy may not have functional postural reactions.

Pathological limitations in the biomechanical, psychological, and neuromuscular constraints of patients interact and cluster as their systems reorganize and their behaviors emerge (Scheets, 2007). Certain impairments or impairment combinations may be the greatest predictors for a behavior or the rate-limiting factor precluding a change to a new behavior (Patel, 2000). For

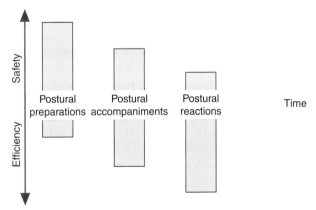

**FIGURE 14-9** Three postural strategies for maintaining standing balance during a voluntary limb movement. (Reprinted with permission from Frank JS, Earl M. Coordination of posture and movement. *Phys Ther.* 1990;70:855–863.)

example, the attractor state of hyperextension of the knee during the mid-stance phase of gait for a person with stroke may be a consequence of sensory loss, weakness, decreased flexibility of ankle plantar flexors, poor control of pelvis, a patient intention to stiffen the knee to prevent buckling, or any number of combinations of these. The relative weight of each of these influences would need to be considered in determining the cause of the knee hyperextension.

### Learning Resources: Explicit and Implicit Learning

Patients have two major types of internal resources to support motor learning: cognitive resources and perceptual-motor resources. Schmidt (1975) suggested motor learning involves the establishment of a recall schema (cognitive trace) of a motor task as well as a recognition schema (perceptual trace). Each of these involves a different type of information processing and a different mode of memory representation. **Explicit learning** occurs when cognitive skills and **episodic memories** are used to consciously plan task strategies, analyze outcomes, and problem-solve new task solutions. Anatomical correlates for explicit learning pathways have been suggested to include the temporal lobe, hippocampus, amygdala, and diencephalon structures (Squire, 1987). **Implicit learning** occurs when extended practice of motor tasks leads to an organization of motor behavior and **procedural memories** that may not be open to conscious thought. This includes the coordination of the mechanical forces of our system, the use of movement synergies, and the access of perceptual-motor linkages with our world. For example, although gait and reaching are acquired in infancy, learning how to smooth the movements used in those actions occurs over multiple years without conscious attention to the movements themselves. Learning at an implicit level requires high levels of intensity and frequency of practice. The anatomical structures associated with implicit learning include the prefrontal area, association cortices, and most importantly the basal ganglia and cerebellum (Squire, 1987).

Healthy individuals typically utilize both explicit and implicit learning processes during their stages of motor learning. Fitts and Posner (1967) suggested a three-stage model of learning involving an early **cognitive stage** (high attention, little movement automaticity), an intermediate **associative stage** (less attention, more movement automaticity), and a later **autonomous stage** (little attention, high movement automaticity). This should not be interpreted as meaning implicit learning resources are not used or important in early learning. Individuals use both explicit and implicit resources from the very first stage of learning. Explicit learning resources play a larger role when a motor task is complex or has a large cognitive component such as manipulating objects. Learning a relatively fluid motor task, such as standing up, may utilize implicit learning resources earlier in the learning process. Patients may be at different stages of learning and utilize explicit and implicit resources differently depending on the tasks they are carrying out. For example, learning to ride a bicycle might first involve a great deal of planning and problem-solving, but individuals do not master bicycle riding because they finally understand the task. Mastery occurs when the motor coordination and control of balancing on the bicycle is integrated implicitly at a level not consciously expressed. Cognitive control of motor output can actually get in the way when an individual is trying to learn a complex motor task. Green and Flowers (1991) showed healthy individuals attempting to

perform a multistep manual tracking task had greater tracking errors when they were informed of the complex pathways of the moving target than when they tracked the target without knowing the pathways. Overdependence on explicit information has also been shown to interfere with the implicit learning of motor tasks for patients with stroke (Boyd and Winstein, 2006; Orrell, 2006) and Parkinson disease (Boyd and Winstein, 2003). Orrell (2006) showed patients with stroke attempting to learn a dynamic standing balance task on a movable surface achieved greater balance control when they practiced with the surface first fixed and then allowed to move in only small increments rather than through trial and error practice of a fully moving surface. The key appears to be to not overload patients with too much explicit information. Clinically, therapists may experience this when they give a patient too many gait parameters to think about during a gait activity, and the patient shows deterioration in the ambulation pattern rather than improvement.

Interestingly, patients with pronounced cognitive impairments and deficits in explicit learning retain the ability to use their implicit learning resources to learn motor tasks (Baddeley and Wilson, 1994; Cushman and Caplan, 1987; Sullivan, 1998; Todd and Barrow, 2008). Sullivan (1998) reported a patient with stroke who had no declarative memory of practicing a tracking task actually showed improved performance over 2 days of training. Cushman and Caplan (1987) showed a similar dissociation between explicit and implicit learning for patients with stroke and cognitive impairment. Therefore, the motor learning capacity of patients cannot necessarily be predicted from their cognitive status. Patients with an inability to express their motor plan or carry out problem-solving processes may still retain the capacity to learn and perform motor tasks through extensive repetition and practice. Patients with profound cognitive impairments may benefit more greatly from high intensities of errorless learning (therapists leading patients through correct performance on every trial) than from trial-and-error learning (Baddeley and Wilson, 1994; Orrell, 2006). However, some evidence has suggested errorless learning results in fragile motor behaviors that are easily disrupted and not always adaptable to changes in task context (Baddeley and Wilson, 1994).

Therapists can promote explicit learning processes by engaging patients in planning, problem-solving, strategizing, and self-evaluating motor performance. Implicit learning can be promoted by practicing tasks at high rates of repetition within the context in which they will be performed. The integration of explicit and implicit resources leads to functional competence.

### The Extrinsic Constraints of Tasks and Environments

The motor behavior of patients is not merely a reflection of their own intrinsic attributes. The external constraints of tasks and environments must also be satisfied. External constraints are the spatial and temporal regulatory features of tasks and environments to which the performance of patients must conform. The spatial constraints of tasks and environments include the workspace that surrounds patients (i.e., the size of the support surface and the space available to carry out mobility tasks) and the size, shape, and location of the objects with which patients interact. Temporal constraints are the time limits existing when patients carry out tasks that involve moving objects or environments. Motor behavior emerges as patients generate the motor output possible within their own intrinsic constraints to meet the external constraints of tasks and environments. For patients to succeed, a great deal of information processing must take place.

Gentile (1987) developed a useful taxonomy of tasks to provide a way of categorizing, from an information-processing perspective, the different types of tasks individuals perform in natural environments. The matrix in Figure 14-10 shows environments can be categorized as either stationary or in motion and as either nonchanging or variable from one task performance to another. Motor control demands placed on an individual during task performance are categorized as body stability versus body mobility and manipulation versus no manipulation. When individuals perform acts of body mobility (e.g., walking), they must constantly take into account the features of their oncoming environment and timing issues related to motion in the environment and their own mobility. This requires a different type of information processing than when carrying out a task in a fixed posture in a stationary environment. Manipulation of objects creates additional information-processing demands as individuals need to allocate attention and motor output to what they are manipulating while simultaneously controlling their posture or gait.

The taxonomy was developed to categorize tasks by their information-processing demands. This type of task categorization can be used to describe various levels of **task complexity**. Low processing demands occur in simple tasks, whereas tasks requiring high processing demands are more complex tasks. The taxonomy does not describe a hierarchy of tasks or how tasks should be progressed for patient rehabilitation. For example, it might be assumed a simple task of standing still in a stationary environment would be less challenging for a patient than a more complex task, such as ambulating in a moving environment. However, this would not be true if the stationary task was to stand on one foot on a narrow balance beam, and the ambulation task was to walk in a quiet hospital hallway at night with only a few people slowly walking by. In this case, the dimension of the spatial constraint in the balance task is much more challenging than the spatial and temporal constraints of the ambulation task. On the other hand, if the standing surface was changed to the floor and the ambulation task took place in a crowded hospital hallway at the close of the work day, the ambulation task would now be much more challenging.

Which task categories are more difficult to perform? Task difficulty must be considered on two levels. In describing an optimal challenge point for learning, Guadagnoli and Lee (2004) astutely distinguish **nominal task difficulty**, or the characteristics of the task, from **functional task difficulty**, which is how challenging a task is in relation to the skill level of the performer and the learning conditions. In Gentile's taxonomy, task categories can be compared as being more simple or complex, but not necessarily as easier or more difficult. The nominal difficulty of a task

| Environment and task | Body stability | | Body transport | |
|---|---|---|---|---|
| | **No manipulation** | **Manipulation** | **No manipulation** | **Manipulation** |
| **Stationary** <br><br> **No intertrial variability** | Closed <br><br> Body stability | Closed <br><br> Body stability <br><br> Manipulation | Closed <br><br> Body transport | Closed <br><br> Body transport <br><br> Manipulation |
| **Stationary** <br><br> **Intertrial variability** | Variable motionless <br><br> Body stability | Variable motionless <br><br> Body stability <br><br> Manipulation | Variable motionless <br><br> Body transport | Variable motionless <br><br> Body transport <br><br> Manipulation |
| **Motion** <br><br> **No intertrial variability** | Consistent motion <br><br> Body stability | Consistent motion <br><br> Body stability <br><br> Manipulation | Consistent motion <br><br> Body transport | Consistent motion <br><br> Body transport <br><br> Manipulation |
| **Motion** <br><br> **Intertrial variability** | Open <br><br> Body stability | Open <br><br> Body stability <br><br> Manipulation | Open <br><br> Body transport | Open <br><br> Body transport <br><br> Manipulation |

**FIGURE 14-10** The taxonomy of tasks as defined by Gentile. (Carr J, Shepherd, R. *Movement Science: Foundations for Physical Therapy in Rehabilitation,* 2nd edition. Austin, TX: PRO-ED; 2000, p. 132. Copyright 2000 by PRO-ED, Inc. Reprinted with permission.)

category is defined by the spatial and temporal constraints that occur *within* each task type. If we return to the previous examples of standing on a balance beam versus the floor, it is the spatial constraint of the standing surface that makes the task more difficult, not the task category. Similarly, the need to adhere to tighter spatial and temporal constraints in a crowded environment makes that task more difficult to perform than walking in the midst of only a few people. Thus, tasks can be made more difficult without changes in task complexity. However, in considering functional task difficulty the intrinsic constraints of patients must be considered. A patient with cerebellar ataxia and difficulty maintaining a stationary posture would likely find a task involving body mobility to be far less difficult than a task of body stability, such as standing still on a single lower extremity, even if the support surface was large. A patient with multiple sclerosis and peripheral weakness who plays tennis regularly might find the complexity of playing tennis far less functionally difficult than the simple task of threading a needle. Functional task difficulty is a reflection of the interaction of the intrinsic constraints of the performer with the extrinsic constraints of tasks and environments.

In some cases, the spatial and temporal demands of tasks have a unique effect on the motor performance of patients. Morris (1996) showed how the manipulation of visual spatial cues and auditory timing cues can be used to dramatically change the gait kinematics of individuals with Parkinson disease. Majsak (1998) showed patients with Parkinson disease displayed bradykinesia when attempting to quickly reach for a stationary object but not when reaching to grasp a rapidly moving object. Similarly, Lee (1989) reported patients with stroke reached to a moving object more quickly, more directly, and with greater bilateral synchronicity than when the object was stationary. How might these findings be applied to neurological rehabilitation? If a therapist is working with a patient with the goal of increasing upper limb fluidity or reaching speed, a novice therapist might assume it would be best to start with reaching for a stationary object first and then "progress" to a moving object. In reality, it may be more prudent for the therapist to have the patient interact with moving objects first, then perhaps attempt to retain this reaching speed and fluidity while reaching for a more slowly moving or stationary object. Therapists should be careful not to create artificial task progressions.

One type of task should not be perceived as a prerequisite for another. For example, learning to ambulate in an unchanging environment with no object manipulation does not prepare a patient for learning to ambulate in a variable environment while using the upper limbs to carry an object. The key for therapists is to challenge the motor skills of patients by exposing them to many different types of tasks while manipulating the spatial and temporal constraints of those tasks. Task progressions should occur within, rather than across, different types of tasks.

## Creating a Motor Plan

The second component of motor learning is creating a plan for action. The planning of actions does not emerge from cognition alone. The movements of patients will be strongly tied to the intrinsic mechanics of their systems, access to mechanisms of movement organization not open to cognitive awareness, and perceptions of the affordances that exist in the environment. Patients benefit from practicing the creating of action plans because they must be able to create, execute, evaluate, revise, refine, and diversify their motor behavior to achieve functional competence. After stroke, important motor, attentional, and motor planning processes may be disrupted (Peters, 2015). Problem-solving and error correction are important components of the learning processes (Gentile, 1987; Hogan and Yanowitz, 1978; Fitts and Posner, 1967). Therapists can help patients explore the mechanical properties of their systems, perceptions for how tasks can be carried out, and the different movement strategies and patterns that might be employed.

Providing patients with motor solutions may be an effective method for promoting the rapid performance of a task but removes patient planning from the learning process. Although patients with pronounced cognitive or perceptual processing impairments may need the therapist to create a plan for action, therapists should ask patients what they are trying to do, share their observations of what they see, and point out factors affecting the patients' task success before giving patients specific directions of how to perform a task (see Table 14-3).

## Task Performance, Information Processing, and Practicing

The third component of motor learning is task performance, information processing, and practicing. These processes are presented together because they are largely inseparable. Before task performance patients must: (1) understand and believe they have the capacity to change their functional behaviors and be motivated to do so, (2) understand and appreciate their intrinsic constraints, (3) detect relevant information regarding the regulatory features of environments and tasks, (4) create or use previously learned movement strategies to accomplish tasks, and (5) select the appropriate movement patterns that will provide a means of carrying out their strategies. Upon completion of task performance, the process continues as patients must: (6) analyze the results of their actions, (7) assess how well they executed their motor plan, (8) create or choose appropriate corrections or alternate strategies and movements if their task performance was not successful, and (9) reassess the outcome of their next attempt. When the task is successfully performed, patients must (10) refine and diversify their movement strategies and patterns to increase their efficiency, accuracy, and consistency of task success.

### Promoting Patient Information Processing

It can be assumed patients carry out some degree of information processing as they attempt to learn motor tasks. For some patients, this may be only generating a plan for their movements. Other patients have the capacity to carry out effective performance analysis, modification of their plan, and movement refinement or diversification. The information-processing capabilities of patients are difficult to fully appreciate because we are limited by using the indirect markers of what patients tell us and the motor behaviors we see. It is

| TABLE 14-3 | Probing With Patients to Promote Learning | | | |
|---|---|---|---|---|
| **PROCESS OF LEARNING BEING PROBED** | **PATHOLOGY** | **FUNCTIONAL ACTIVITY; DIFFICULTY** | **TYPE OF PROBE** | **EXAMPLES OF PROBES** |
| Perception of Self and Environment | CVA with right hemiplegia | Reaching to pick up a plastic water cup; crushing the cup | Question | How does your hand feel when you squeeze too tight? How can you tell you are squeezing too tight without looking at your hand? |
| | | | Observation/ Suggestion | I notice your whole hand closes tightly when you squeeze too hard. What would happen if you tried using your thumb and first two fingers? |
| | Parkinson disease | Turning during ambulation; freezing | Question | What do you think happens when you get stuck? Do you feel your weight shifting over your feet? Does it happen in open spaces? |
| | | | Observation/ Suggestion | I notice your steps become very small and you stop weight shifting well when you get stuck. Can you keep a rhythmical gait going when you turn? |
| Motor Planning | Cerebellar ataxia | Moving sit-to-stand; excessive extension thrust to stand | Question | What can you do to stand up more slowly? Why do you think you thrust up? Do you feel your weight over your feet before you straighten your legs? |
| | | | Observation/ Suggestion | I notice this surface is a bit low. Maybe if you scooted forward and leaned forward more it would help. Maybe counting to 4 as you stand would help. |
| | CVA with left hemiplegia | Rolling to the less-involved side in bed; neglecting left side | Question | How did that feel? Was that pretty easy? What might you do with your left side to make it easier? How can you include your left arm and leg in rolling? |
| | | | Observation/ Suggestion | I notice your left arm and leg were left behind. How could you change that? What if you clasp your hands together and bend both knees up before rolling? |
| Performance, Information Processing, and Practice | TBI with memory deficits | Transfer from wheelchair to low couch; falling into the couch | Question | What happened that time? Could you tell that was happening when you were moving? What do you want to practice to do that better? How can I help you? |
| | | | Observation/ Suggestion | I noticed your feet were directly under you as you stood up. That makes it tough to get to the couch. You also reached back for the couch. What if you put your feet next to the couch and put your hands on your knees when you sit down? |
| | CVA with right hemiplegia | Ambulation; instability and excessively slow velocity | Question | How did that feel? Do you think that is the best speed for you to walk? Why? Is that going to work for you at home? What do you need to do to speed up a little? |
| | | | Observation/ Suggestion | I notice that you are walking so slowly you're not getting any swing in your right leg. It's sometimes harder walking slowly than a little faster... think of riding a bicycle. Maybe you can try taking bigger steps and leaning forward a bit. |

critical therapists carry out thorough cognitive and perceptual examinations to identify the processing capabilities of patients (see Chapter 4).

Patients should be involved to their full potential in planning their strategies and movement patterns, in assessing their movement performance, and in making adjustments in their task execution. For patients with limited information-processing capabilities, therapists may have to assist a great deal by instructing, cuing, and providing frequent feedback. However, for patients with the capacity to process information and internally regulate their actions, therapists must be judicious in how, when, and how much supplementary information they give to patients.

## Augmented Information

Providing patients supplementary or "**augmented information**" (AI) on task performance and task success is one way therapists promote learning. Therapists deliver AI to patients through verbal, visual, or manual cues. Information provided in relation to the way the patient performed the task is termed **knowledge of performance** (KP). Most often in therapy sessions, this is information regarding movement performance, which promotes an internal focus of patient attention. Knowledge of task success, which fosters an external focus of patient attention, is termed **knowledge of results** (KR). A review of the research related to the learning of simple and complex tasks by Wulf and Shea (2002) provides evidence that KR has stronger effects than KP on the motor behavior of learners. Similarly, for healthy adults as well as for patients with neurological pathology, focusing attention on external task-performance outcomes has been shown to be more beneficial for motor learning than concentrating on one's movements or performance in carrying out the task (Choi and Kang, 2015; Fasoli, 2002; Song, 2015; Wulf and Lewthwaite, 2016). This may not be fully appreciated by therapists; Johnson (2013) reported the feedback they observed therapists giving to patients with stroke during a series of gait rehabilitation sessions was 67% internally focused, 22% externally focused, and 11% mixed.

Newell (1985) has suggested another important type of AI they label **transitional information**. Unlike KR and KP, which are used to inform an individual on motor outcomes, transitional information is used to encourage a learner to search for an alternative task solution. For example, suppose a therapist notices a patient with lower limb weakness is attempting to stand from a low mat in the clinic by pushing off the mat with the calves to assist in standing. If the therapist believes the patient should lean forward more to get the trunk over the feet, the therapist might show the patient how to do so and then give the patient KP on the movements. An alternative is for the therapist to give the patient transitional information, telling the patient to stand up but not touch the mat with the legs. The patient might take longer to do so but would hypothetically learn that, to not push off the mat, the patient needs to lean forward more and get the weight over the feet. In the first case, the patient followed the therapist's KP. In the latter case, the patient followed the therapist's transitional information and found the same solution by

exploring different strategies and finding the coordination mode for standing up alone. Some patients will need direction and KP to shift their behaviors. Other patients may need only information that helps them explore and find different movement strategies and patterns. For purposes of simplicity, KR, KP, and transitional information will be categorized as AI for the remainder of this chapter.

The rate of learning may be accelerated when AI is provided that enhances the intrinsic information processing of the performer. Patients with impairments in information processing (e.g., decreased sensory perception, cognitive impairment) may benefit from AI, particularly if the task is complex. However, patients can become overly reliant on AI and not attend to their own intrinsic processing. This may result in improved performance in the presence of AI, but poor performance when AI is absent. This phenomenon has been offered as evidence for the *guidance hypothesis* (Salmoni, 1984). For retention and transfer of learned motor skills, it is important therapists avoid providing patients excessive feedback. The three variables therapists can manipulate in providing AI are **bandwidth**, **timing**, and **frequency**.

## The Bandwidth of AI Delivery

**Bandwidth** refers to the degree of error or deviation from a performance criterion allowed before AI is provided to patients (Magill, 1992). For example, a therapist might be working with a patient with stroke on the goal of walking over objects by flexing the hip and knee of the hemiparetic limb rather than hiking the hip and abducting the lower limb. The bandwidth decision in this case would be how much hip hiking and lower limb abduction the therapist would allow before giving the patient AI regarding "erroneous" hip hiking movements. Tight bandwidth conditions naturally result in a higher frequency of AI delivery. To allow patients to use their own information processing, wide bandwidths can be set early in practice for complex tasks or for patients with limited motor abilities. The bandwidth can then be tightened in later practice when patient performance improves. Rehabilitation approaches that use high frequencies of feedback and manual guidance to promote well-controlled movements and minimize movement errors may achieve rapid acquisition of movements but suppress patient information processing and internalization of the intended motor behavior.

## The Timing of AI Delivery

Therapists can provide AI before task performance, during a task, or after task performance (see Figure 14-11). Therapists give AI before a task when they instruct patients in how to complete a task. Another way for patients to receive AI before their performance is to observe another individual attempt the task.

Providing AI during task performance is referred to as **concurrent AI**, and **terminal AI** is information delivered after a performance. In simple motor tasks, concurrent AI is highly effective in promoting the initial acquisition of behaviors, but performance sharply declines in retention and transfer when AI is not available (Patrick and Mutlusoy, 1982; Vander

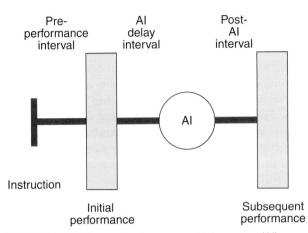

**FIGURE 14-11**  The timing of augmented information (AI) delivery.

These studies suggest the effectiveness of concurrent AI may be related to the degree to which patients are able to use AI in conjunction with their own intrinsic information processing resources. Highly complex tasks may exceed the capacity of patients to solve the task independently. Additionally, if patients are able to simultaneously process AI and their own intrinsic information, AI may be complimentary for learning. However, when intrinsic information is low or a patient has difficulty processing intrinsic information, concurrent AI may compete with a learner's intrinsic information, leading to poor retention and transfer (Buekers and Magill, 1995).

The timing of terminal AI can be manipulated to enhance the information processing of patients. If AI is given after every performance trial, patients may become reliant on AI instead of their own intrinsic sources of information. Instead, terminal AI can be given after a block of trials has been completed. This schedule of AI delivery is called **summary AI**. As a clinical example, if a patient is learning to ambulate with a longer step length, the therapist can choose to provide AI after each step for a series of steps (continuous terminal AI) or have the patient complete a block of steps before providing the AI for each step (summary AI). A number of studies have shown that, although the initial task performance is more successful with continuous AI, retention and transfer are better with summary AI (Lavery, 1962; Schmidt, 1989). Summary AI provides learners time to self-analyze their task performance before receiving AI.

When using a schedule of summary AI, considering the number of task performances a patient should carry out before receiving summary AI is important. Schmidt (1990) showed for complex tasks, summary AI may be optimal when provided after a small number of performance trials. Providing summary AI for a large number of trials is better for the learning of simple tasks. As in other methods of manipulating information delivery to patients, the goal of therapists is to

Linden, 1993). A number of studies have reported benefits of patients receiving concurrent EMG biofeedback during the acquisition of movements (Leiper, 1981; Sandweiss and Wolf, 1985; Wolf, 1983), but little evidence exists that these effects are retained or generalized. In contrast, the delivery of terminal AI does not typically result in as rapid a change in the acquisition of motor skills, but performance in the retention and transfer of those skills exceeds that of the behavior after concurrent AI (Figure 14-12). One study particularly relevant to clinical practice showed this effect for the learning of a partial weight-bearing activity (Winstein, 1996).

On the other hand, the delivery of concurrent AI has been shown to be effective for acquisition and transfer of learning in more complex motor tasks (Swinnen, 1997) and in functional tasks such as learning slalom ski movements (Wulf, 1998a) and landing skills for aircraft pilots (Lintem, 1990).

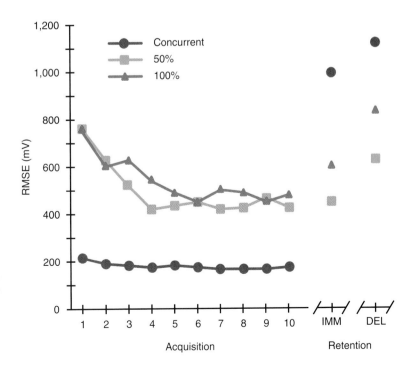

**FIGURE 14-12**  The learning effects of concurrent AI and terminal AI. (Reprinted with permission from Vander Linden DW, Cauraugh JH, Greene TA. The effect of frequency of kinetic feedback on learning an isometric force production task in nondisabled subjects. *Phys Ther.* 1993;73:79–87.)

optimize the information processing of patients, not to replace or exceed it. For a patient with a severely impaired ability to process information, for a task that is complex, and when limited practice is available, the therapist may provide concurrent AI or terminal AI in a summary fashion after only a few practice trials. On the other hand, if a patient is capable of processing information, the task being performed is not overly complex, and the patient has an opportunity for extended practice, the therapist may provide terminal AI after a greater number of trials.

Because tasks will challenge the information-processing abilities of patients to varying degrees, the summary AI therapists provide might differ from one task to another even for the same patients. For a patient learning a basic sit-to-stand task, the therapist might provide summary feedback after four or five trials. In contrast, when the same patient is learning a more complex manipulation task, the therapist might provide AI after two or three trials. The information-processing abilities of patients, the complexity of the task to be learned, and the opportunities for practice all influence the optimal schedule of AI delivery that will enhance and complement the intrinsic information processing of patients.

Therapists may be able to promote retention of task performance better if patients are asked to self-analyze their performance and are given time to intrinsically process their performance before being given terminal AI (Hogan and Yanowitz, 1978; Swinnen, 1990). Promoting self-assessment may be particularly important for patients with processing impairments who need cuing to remember to use their own intrinsic information rather than depend on the AI provided by therapists.

Considering the time between the delivery of terminal AI and when the next performance attempt is initiated is important. This is the time when patients should be comparing their own intrinsic information with the AI they received and developing a plan for the next task attempt. Although no clear guidelines have been reported on how long this delay might be, it should be long enough for patients to analyze their performance and process their own internal feedback before receiving AI.

### The Frequency of AI Delivery

Another factor to consider in providing an optimal level of AI is the frequency of delivery. Ho and Shea (1978) and Winstein and Schmidt (1990) have shown immediate and continuous AI may lead to a rapid improvement in the motor skills of healthy adults but with poor retention of these improvements. This evidence further supports the guidance hypothesis that patients become dependent on AI presented at a high frequency. With less frequent AI, patients are forced to depend on their own intrinsic information for task success. "**Fading**" refers to the process of slowly decreasing the percentage of trials in which AI is given. Fading of AI has been shown to lead to better retention of motor skill than providing continuous AI (Winstein and Schmidt, 1990).

The optimal frequency of AI for patients is difficult for therapists to predict. Given the complex interaction between the learning capacity and constraints of patients, the

nature of the tasks to be learned, and the amount of practice available, a range of frequencies may be effective. Interestingly, studies by Chiviacowsky and Wulf (2002) and Janelle (1995) showed AI is more effective for healthy individuals learning motor tasks when given upon request from the learner rather than on a predetermined schedule. Wulf (2005) extended this work by showing the AI frequency request for one individual is not necessarily the optimal frequency for another patient. AI frequency is likely best when therapists and patients are both involved in determining the timing and frequency of delivery.

## THINK ABOUT IT 14.1

- Describe how you would organize your delivery of augmented information to promote the information processing of Cecelia, Peter, and Tito as they worked on a specific task goal.
- All three patients are trying to learn to move from sitting to standing effectively. How and why would you provide AI differently to each patient even when the same task is being learned?
- How would you modify your AI bandwidth, timing, and frequency for the same individual learning different tasks?
- How would you structure the task and environment to promote valid information processing?

### Creating New Coordination Modes: Practice

Practice is inextricably linked to information processing. Patients are constantly making motor plans, executing actions, assessing their performance, and refining their motor output through the use of implicit and explicit resources. This is a cyclical process that repeats time and again until an effective coordination mode is achieved. Newell (1991) referred to the integration of these as the perceptual-motor workspace. Practice should promote explicit learning through the activation of cognitive processes necessary for identifying intrinsic and extrinsic constraints, creating a motor plan, and processing information for the conscious correction and refinement of motor output. Practice should also be structured to promote implicit learning. This requires sufficient frequency, intensity, and specificity of physical practice.

### Promoting Explicit Learning Through Practice

#### Observational Learning and Mental Imagery

One way to promote explicit learning processes is to engage patients in cognitive activities before or in addition to physical practice. Rehabilitation strategies such as promoting **observational learning** through the watching of videotaped performances (McCullagh, 1989) and having patients mentally imagine or rehearse their performance (Schmidt and Wrisberg, 2008) has been shown to promote learning. Interestingly, novice learners tend to learn tasks more quickly if they watch another person who is learning the task rather than an individual performing the task flawlessly. Observational learning is further enhanced if the learner also hears the AI being given to the learning model. More important than seeing the task solution is observing how other individuals modify their motor behavior to attain a desired motor outcome. To promote observational learning, patients can watch themselves or other patients like themselves perform a desired activity. McCullagh (1989) have provided evidence that for observational learning to be effective, the learner must be able to attend to the task being performed, create an internal representation of what they observed for their own performance, and have a physical ability to execute the task. This may not be possible for all patients. Opportunities for observational learning typically include having patients come to a treatment area early or stay after their own practice session to watch other patients working on similar task goals, working with patients in group sessions, and videotaping practice sessions so patients can watch, evaluate, and mentally practice their performance outside of physical practice sessions. One method integrating observational learning with performance is dyad training (McNevin, 2000; Shea, 1999). Dyad training involves two individuals learning the same task together, sharing the learning processes, and in some cases sharing the task performance. In addition to the benefit of observing another person learn the intended task, working with another promotes a sense of responsibility, motivation, and engagement for the learner.

To promote **mental imagery**, patients can be encouraged to imagine their performance from either an internal perspective or an external perspective. An internal perspective is to imagine the sensory experiences they would encounter performing an activity. For example, a patient mentally imaging sit-to-stand from an internal perspective might visualize the floor coming up as the patient leans forward, the pressure increase under the feet while leaning forward in preparation for standing, the floor receding and walls of the gym coming up as the patient begins to stand, and the feeling of the legs extending as a standing position is achieved. Using an external perspective, patients would imagine how it would look while watching themselves stand. Each perspective has its benefits, but in both cases, the more the imagery can replicate the look and feel of the actual performance, the more effective the imagery will be (Schmidt and Wrisberg, 2008). Using mental imagery as an adjunct to physical practice has been shown to enhance the effects of CIT (Page, 2009a), the learning of functional activities (Jackson, 2001; Liu, 2004), and the generalization of learned activities (Liu, 2009). Functional imaging studies show the brain activation patterns for mentally imaging and performing activities overlap (Gerardin, 2000) and that mental practice can actually lead to alterations in the cortical map of patients with stroke (Page, 2009b). Braun (2008) suggest the following progression in a mental practice intervention framework: (1) assess mental capacity, (2) establish the nature of mental practice, (3) teach imagery technique, (4) embed and monitor, and (5) develop self-generated treatments. The stages of embedding, monitoring, and developing self-generated treatments are repeated as the intervention framework is refined and elaborated to incorporate new activities (see Figure 14-13).

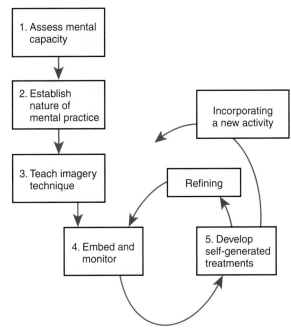

**FIGURE 14-13** Overview of steps taken in mental practice intervention framework. From Braun S, Kleynen M, Schack T, Beurskens A, Wade D. Using mental practice in stroke rehabilitation: a framework. *Clin Rehabil.* 2008;22:579–591, with permission.

### Part-Practice

In some cases, explicit learning resources can be promoted if an intended task is broken into smaller parts. This allows patients to focus their attention on specific task components and to plan and organize their movements. **Part-practice** is beneficial for tasks involving a sequence of linked components such as grooming, dressing, or preparing to transfer from a wheelchair to another surface. However, tasks involving fluid or continuous movement such as the sit-to-stand transition, reaching to grasp, or ambulating may not derive the same benefits from part-practice (Schmidt and Young, 1987).

Effective learning will occur if the task parts being practiced are naturally occurring subdivisions of the task (Lee, 1988; Schmidt and Young, 1987; Newell, 1989). For example, Winstein (1989) tested whether patients with stroke who practiced weight-shifting on a force platform showed increased weight-shifting in both standing and locomotion. Improvements were found in standing weight-shifting but not during locomotion. This is not surprising if one considers the side-by-side foot position and lateral weight-shifting subjects performed when training on the force platform were not the same foot position or weight-shift vector used during gait. Moreover, the stance and swing phases of gait are not independent from one another; each phase influences the other. Because locomotion is a continuous task not broken easily into separate components, part-practice of gait may not be a preferable strategy.

### Adaptive Practice

**Adaptive practice** involves modifying the external constraints of a task so successful performance of a modified version of the task can take place. This may include modified positions, the use of assistive devices, manual assistance, or changing the spatial or temporal demands of tasks. The difficulty level of the task is often adjusted upward during practice so an optimal level of difficulty is maintained (Kelly, 1969; Fell, 2004). The objective of adaptive practice is for patients to learn a task goal through **shaping**, that is, **successive approximation** of a desired task from more modified to less modified versions until the task itself is ultimately performed. This training technique is commonly used in CIT; patients with a hemiplegic upper limb progress in their training from working with smaller to larger objects and from slower to faster movement tasks (Mark and Taub, 2004; Sterr, 2006; Wolf, 2006).

Small modifications of a task may change the nature of the task. For example, having patients learn to ambulate independently by progressing first from parallel bars to assistive devices then to ambulation without a device may not be a valid progression. The parallel bars afford not only support but also leaning and pulling. A walker or cane will not afford pulling but will allow support and side leaning. Walking in parallel bars and with assistive devices are not naturally occurring conditions if the ultimate goal is ambulation in an open environment without a device. Assistive devices provide safety, security, and may be necessary to improve the endurance and confidence of patients. However, they afford patients a different set of practice conditions and involve a different type of information processing than walking without upper limb support. Nardone and Shieppati (1998) showed the lower limb postural responses individuals displayed when perturbed in standing were greatly reduced when upper limb support was allowed. Providing assistive devices to patients when not absolutely necessary may prevent or delay the learning of postural control necessary for walking without the device.

Excessive adaptations of motor tasks may disrupt the body movements that occur naturally in response to the forces of gravity, body inertia, and interlimb dynamics. Patients must learn to coordinate multiple-joint movements and do so in relation to the "external field forces" of gravity and contact with objects and support surfaces in the external world. Changes in biomechanics occur as the spatial and temporal conditions of tasks are modified. For example, slow walking decreases the magnitude of forces associated with gait. Walking from slow to faster gait velocities might be warranted for patients having difficulty controlling mechanical forces or perhaps fearful of falling. However, mastering the forces of slow walking will not prepare patients for the forces they will encounter when walking quickly. The timing relationships between muscle groups, contraction types, and the magnitude of forces will change with changes in gait velocity (Zernicke, 1991). Thus, the magnitude of the adaptations therapists make and the consequences of those adaptations should be considered.

### Structuring the Practice of Task Variations

The tasks patients learn and the environments in which they will take place will always possess some degree of variability. It is therefore important patients practice a number of variations of any given task. The practice of task variations can be scheduled in isolated practice blocks, in a structured order, or in a random fashion. In **blocked practice**, all of the trials of a particular task variation are completed before practice of another variation begins. In **random practice**, trials of each task variation are intermingled. Structured orders can take many forms. In **serial practice**, task variations are practiced in a set order. Lee and Magill (1983) showed the effects of serial practice are generally similar to those of random practice in simple experimental tasks.

A number of studies have shown healthy adults learning simple experimental motor tasks acquire a motor skill more quickly with blocked practice but retain and transfer a motor skill more effectively with random practice (Lee and Magill, 1985; Lee and Weeks, 1987; Lee, 1992; Magill and Hall, 1990). This paradox is referred to as the "**contextual interference effect**" (Shea and Morgan, 1979) (see Figure 14-14). Two

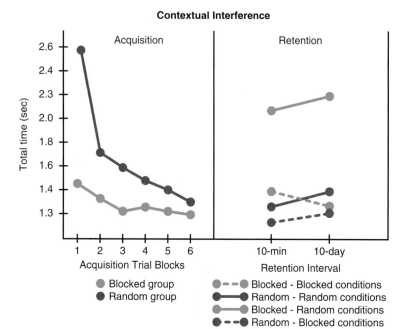

**Contextual Interference**

Blocked group
Random group
Blocked - Blocked conditions
Random - Random conditions
Blocked - Random conditions
Random - Blocked conditions

**FIGURE 14-14** The contextual interference effect as first reported by Shea and Morgan (1979). (Reprinted with permission from Shea JB, Morgan RL. Contextual interference effects on the acquisition, retention, and transfer of a motor skill. *J Exp Psychol-Learn Mem Cogn.* 1979;5:179–187.)

hypotheses have been offered for the contextual interference. The **reconstruction hypothesis** postulates random practice is beneficial to learning because learners must reconstruct their task solution on every trial, leading to greater engagement in their learning (Lee and Magill, 1985). In contrast, the **elaboration hypothesis** indicates random practice promotes the comparing and contrasting of task variations, leading to a more elaborate representation and fuller awareness of each task variation (Shea and Zimney, 1983). Both hypotheses propose blocked practice results in reproduction of a motor skill without the depth of information processing required for learning. Recent neurophysiological evidence suggests the elaboration hypothesis is a more likely explanation for the learning effects seen under random practice conditions (Lin, 2008).

Therefore, having patients practice task variations that share a common dimension or the same topology may be more effective for learning than having a patient randomly practice different types of tasks (see Figure 14-15). However, random practice is not always a more effective practice schedule for patients than blocked practice. Optimal practice schedules, like optimal patterns of delivery of AI, are determined by the constraints of the patient, the nature and complexity of the task to be learned, and the amount of practice available.

As the information-processing constraints of individuals change, the optimal practice schedule for engaging patients will also change. Del Rey (1982b) showed female college athletes experienced in sports requiring high levels of eye-hand coordination learned a manual timing task more effectively

**Finding the "10's"**

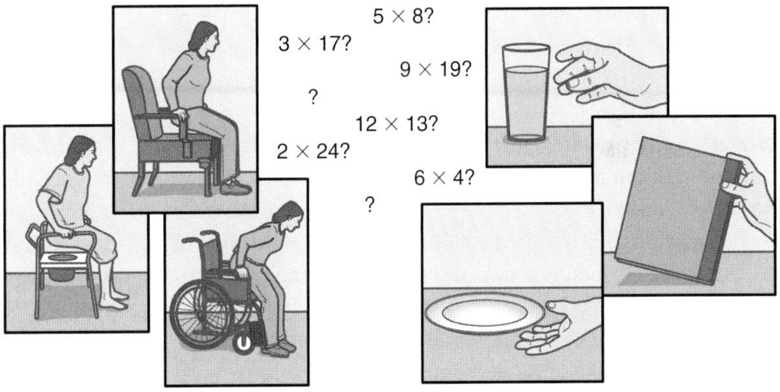

Finding the "10s"

In an elegant article titled, "What us Repeated in Repetition? Effects of Practice Conditions on Motor Skill Acquisition" Lee et al. (1991) offered the following mathematical analogy from Jacoby (1978) as an illustration of the different information processing that occurs during blocked versus random practice. If you were asked to find the sum of two large numbers, you would initially go through the process of addition. If you were asked immediately to add the same numbers you could retrieve the answer quickly, without going through the addition process. However, if a delay occurred before the question was asked again, the process of problem-solving would once again be required. This analogy has been used to suggest random practice is more conducive for engaging learners in problem-solving than blocked practice. Let's extend this mathematical analogy:

If you were given different pairs of random numbers to multiply, they would obviously require more time and processing than if you were asked to solve the same multiplication problem again and again. Let's use one of the numbers repeatedly: 8 x 12? 8 x 32? 8 x 128? Still difficult to compute. But what if the number being repeated was 10? 10 x 12? 10 x 32? 10 x 128? Although the multiplication process is still required on every attempt, the answer is attained much more quickly. Why is that? The process is the same as multiplying by 8s. The 10s are easier because a unifying pattern or rule exists for solving the problem. Learning the 'rule of 10s' provides a means of linking all random variations of multiplying by 10.

Our patients need to be able to solve motor problems in reach and grasp, standing up, and walking that they will experience in random conditions. How can their solutions be made easier? By helping them find the 10s…

Bringing the center of mass over the base of support is the "10" for sit-to-stand. Coordinating movements of the shoulder and elbow is the "10" for reaching. Promoting elaboration of functional activities within a patient's capacity is important if patients are to learn the topologies, the coordination modes…the "10s" for becoming functionally competent in a class of functional activities.

**FIGURE 14-15** Finding the "10s."

with random practice than blocked practice. However, student nonathletes learned the same task more effectively with blocked practice. A similar disparity in the benefits of random practice was shown for active versus sedentary elderly women (Del Rey, 1982a). Pinto Zipp and Gentile (2010) showed blocked practice is more effective than random practice for young children learning a novel throwing task, and Duff and Gordon (2003) reported children with cerebral palsy acquire grasp control of objects more effectively with blocked practice with no detriment to retention.

The determination of an optimal practice structure of task variations requires creativity on the part of therapists. In some cases, a hybrid practice structure may be considered. Pigott and Shapiro (1984) showed the optimal practice schedule for children learning to accurately throw bean bags of different weights to a target was a combination of blocked and random practice. In their study, the children who showed the best performance practiced their throws in a random fashion but threw the same bean bag weight twice (blocked) before randomly practicing a different weight. Patients with neurological pathology will have a wide range of information-processing abilities. Some patients will have the capacity to engage their explicit learning resources more effectively through random practice than blocked practice. Others may need to practice a motor task a few times before appreciating task variations or may learn more effectively through a blocked or combined practice structure if their explicit learning resources are limited.

A large number of practice trials may be necessary for patients to benefit from practicing task variations and to learn the coordination modes of tasks such as moving sit-to-stand, reaching for objects, and ambulation. How many trials are necessary? This will depend on the resources of the patient and the complexity of the coordination mode the patient is attempting to learn. Part of the contextual interference effect is that practice under random practice conditions requires more practice repetitions than blocked practice to reach the same level of initial performance. In fact, if learners are not provided sufficient numbers of trials, greater acquisition, retention, and transfer of motor performance occur with blocked than random practice (Shea, 1990).

An important consideration in practicing multiple task variations is the process of **consolidation,** which is the transition of initial, short-lived, fragile forms of motor memories to a long-lasting stable form (Bailey and Kandel, 1995; Brashers-Krug, 1996). When patients are learning a motor task, they are creating an internal model linking the intended task outcome to the movements and muscle forces necessary to carry out the task (Shadmehr and Mussa-Ivaldi, 1994). Newly developing internal models need to be consolidated to be retained. Studies by Shadmehr and colleagues (Shadmehr and Brasher-Krug, 1997; Shadmehr and Holcomb, 1999) showed healthy individuals learning to generate upper limb movements under two perturbing force conditions could do so if an interval of 5 hours separated the practice of the different conditions. Beginning practice of the second force condition earlier resulted in a disruption of learning. If the task variations a patient is performing

share the same coordination mode, learning should occur without interference. However, if task variations vary too greatly, they may interfere with one another, disrupting the consolidation of long-term motor memories.

The last consideration in planning the practice of task variations is the complexity of the task itself. Wulf and Shea (2002) have comprehensively described how task complexity affects the learning of motor tasks. Tasks with high demands in attention, memory, or motor coordination may make a random practice schedule erratic, and preclude a process of elaboration. Randomly presenting task variations to a patient can be a powerful path for learning as long as the task variations and task are not overly complicated. The optimal practice schedule is one that engages but does not overwhelm the patient.

### Promoting Implicit Learning Through Practice

As previously stated, implicit learning refers to a perceptual-motor organization of motor behavior occurring at a level that cannot be verbally expressed. For example, a patient who learns how to coordinate the movement components of a sit-to-stand activity or to walk rhythmically is often unable to state what they did to attain their success. Explicit learning resources often play a larger role in early learning, in complex tasks, and tasks that require a sequence of separate actions or a high degree of movement accuracy. Implicit learning resources play a larger role in the control of well-learned movements and tasks involving a fluid or coordinated movement pattern. This typically occurs only after large amounts of practice.

### Intensity of Practice

No definitive guidelines exist for how much practice is necessary to attain changes in motor behavior. However, patients typically do not carry out high levels of practice in traditional rehabilitation settings (DeWeerdt, 2000; Lang, 2007; Lang, 2009; Tinson, 1989). In fact, the low number of task-specific repetitions and practice patients typically receive may not be adequate to promote neuroplasticity (Lang, 2009). Patients with certain types of neurological pathologies certainly cannot tolerate high practice intensities. For example, individuals with stroke may have cardiovascular impairments (Ivey, 2005) and patients with multiple sclerosis or postpolio syndrome have specific pathological conditions that render the neuromuscular system susceptible to injury with excessive exercise. However, patients with the capacity to engage in aggressive physical therapy should be encouraged to do so. Evidence supports a direct relationship between the amount of practice patients have and the recovery that occurs (Byl, 2008; Fisher and Sullivan, 2001; Kwakkel, 2004; Lang, 2015; Lohse, 2014; Sterr, 2002; Sunderland, 1992). For example, Sterr (2002) reported 6-hour periods of constraint-induced movement therapy improved upper limb motor function in chronic hemiparesis more effectively than 3-hour periods.

The issue at hand is not just the total number of hours a patient has available to practice through the day but the intensity of therapy patients receive within the time they have available. Brown and Kautz (1998) showed patients with stroke participating in a bicycle-peddling program developed a greater force output in their hemiparetic lower limb when the workloads they generated while pedaling were increased. Dean (2000) provides an example of the importance of practice intensity. These investigators evaluated the immediate and 2-month retention effects of a 4-week locomotor circuit-training program for patients with chronic stroke. The program focused on strengthening exercises for the hemiparetic lower limb and functional tasks for only 1 hour a day, 3 days a week. However, within that time patients were strongly challenged with sit-to-stand activities, stepping exercises, treadmill walking, and walking over slopes, obstacles, and stairs. Patients showed immediate and retained improvement in walking speed and endurance, force production during sit-to-stand, and a greater frequency of step-ups per unit time. Highly challenging balance programs reduce the fall rate in patients with Parkinson disease (Sparrow, 2016) and improve locomotor performance for individuals with chronic stroke (Holleran, 2015).

This is not to say therapists can push patients without concern. Recent evidence shows some patients participating in high intensity rehabilitation programs may experience overtraining effects (Dromerick, 2009; Sullivan, 2007). Findings from the study of neuroplasticity in animals show early aggressive exercise for animals with unilateral brain injury may be detrimental to recovery (Kozlowski, 1996; Schallert, 1997). Moreover, high intensities of engaged practice may not necessarily lead to meaningful changes in all patients. Grattan (2016) reported only small changes in upper limb use for individuals with stroke and unilateral spatial neglect. Lang (2016) carried out an elegant study on the dose-response effects of task-specific upper limb rehabilitation for individuals at least 6 months poststroke. Despite an individualized, progressive program involving as high as 3,200–9,600 movement repetitions a day, 4 days/week for 8 weeks, individuals showed small treatment effects and no evidence of dose-response effects.

Further study is necessary to identify the levels of practice intensity optimal for patients at different times in their recovery or disease progression. Patients report five factors influencing their participation in intensive intervention programs (Merlo, 2013): (1) a manageable amount of fatigue, (2) a difficult but attainable task and intensity level, (3) sufficiently long training program to attain results, (4) enjoyment, and (5) a manageable level of muscle soreness.

### Massed and Distributed Practice

In addition to the intensity of practice, the way practice is distributed with rest is important (Schmidt and Wrisberg, 2008). **Massed practice** is repetition of a motor task with minimal rest between trials or between practice sessions. **Distributed practice** is repetition of a task with trials, blocks of trials, or practice sessions spaced over time. Massed practice often leads to rapid acquisition of a motor performance but with limited effects on the retention and transfer of that skill (Lee and Genovese, 1988). In general, tasks requiring continuous information processing or motor production, such as gait, appear to be better learned under distributed practice. Tasks that are more discrete, are conceptually simple, and of short duration can be practiced under massed conditions. The

major finding is that practicing beyond an individual's information processing or motor production capacity is ineffectual for learning. Providing patients periods of mental and physical rest may optimize their engagement. Interestingly, many of the new technologies being used in clinics such as virtual reality, robot-assisted upper limb therapy, constraint-induced therapy, and body weight-supported gait training on a treadmill employ massed practice schedules. The dosage effects of these interventions are now being explored, and the conditions in which massed or distributed practice may be optimal.

### Specificity of Practice

Another important consideration in structuring effective practice is **specificity of practice.** The traditional concept of specificity of practice was that learning best occurred when the motor characteristics of a specific task could be practiced (Henry, 1968). The major hypothesis was repeated physical performance of a task led to the formation of an internal template used as a guide for subsequent performances. The rapid acquisition of a desired motor output was believed to be an indication that learning was taking place. A more contemporary view is the acquisition of motor skills is beneficial to the retention and transfer of those skills only if those skills are acquired by the patient without excessive external cuing or guidance (Magill, 1992; Winstein and Schmidt, 1990).

The practice of motor tasks never really results in reproduction of the same motor output (Bernstein, 1967). What is learned is a topology or coordination mode of movement that can be diversified and adapted rather than an exact set of movement details. In fact, it has been suggested that skilled motor behavior is characterized by the control of movement variability, not by its elimination (Latash, 2002; Stergiou, 2006). How then is specificity of practice relevant today if the optimal motor behavior of patients involves movement variability? The answer is that specificity of practice must be redefined as practice within specific classes of actions sharing certain unifying characteristics. These characteristics may be described as the biomechanical demands of tasks, the information-processing requirements, and the nature of the task and environment.

### Biomechanical Specificity

The biomechanical nature of tasks includes internal forces patients generate and external forces to which patients must respond. Internal forces include motion-dependent torques, such as body inertia and the angular velocity of body segments around joints, and the forces patients generate through their muscle activity. External forces include gravity, contact forces with the environment, and the mass of objects. The types of forces patients must be able to generate and control during ambulation cannot be reproduced when patients are simply standing. Similarly, the interactional torques occurring during multijoint movements cannot be experienced by patients practicing single-joint movements. Lacquantiti and Soechting (1982) showed when healthy subjects reach for a stationary object, shoulder and elbow movements are tightly coupled, whereas forearm and wrist movements are independently regulated. The shoulder and elbow work in unison to transport the hand through space, whereas the forearm and wrist independently orient the hand for objects and prepare the hand for grasp. Therapists must consider the functional coupling of joints if they are to work on the movements of patients in a functionally meaningful way. Therefore, therapists might have patients practice single-joint movements of the wrist and hand separate from elbow and shoulder movements without jeopardizing upper limb coordination, but working on elbow control in the absence of shoulder movements may not be optimal. Similar concepts are applicable to lower limb function.

Neural adaptation has been shown to occur in early resistance training of healthy individuals (Sale, 1988). Changes in motor unit activity include increased recruitment, increased rate of force development, greater synchronization, and changes in reflex activity. These changes are dependent on the training methods employed. Training activities involving ballistic movements and rapid force development, such as jumping, lead to increased rates of force development but do not have as great an effect on maximal force development. In contrast, heavy resistance training leads to greater levels of maximal force development, but with little effect on the rate of force development. Therapists must consider the types of muscle activity associated with the specific types of tasks the patient will be performing. Training rapid force development may be necessary for tasks such as ascending or descending stairs or reaching quickly. Other tasks such as sit-to-stand or lifting heavy objects require training with slower but greater force output.

### Specificity of Information Processing

A second way of characterizing task specificity is the information-processing requirements of the task (Gentile, 1987) (see Figure 14-10). In single motor tasks, such as walking in an unchanging stationary environment, attention can be fully committed to one functional goal. In contrast, dual motor tasks require individuals to divide their attention between two or more task goals such as walking while carrying an object. Dual task training has recently become more popular as a therapeutic strategy for helping patients acquire the motor skills necessary for complex and compound tasks (Dorfman, 2014; Fritz, 2015; Plummer and Osborne, 2015). Some tasks require the body to be in motion, whereas others require balance in a stationary position. When individuals are walking in a moving environment, they must attend to their own motor production while they respond to the changing temporal and spatial features of the environment. Certainly, patients cannot practice all of the tasks and specific task conditions they will encounter on a daily basis. However, patients can and should practice different categories of tasks that require different types of information processing. Functional competence is the ability to carry out a diversity of tasks effectively, not high performance of a limited number of tasks.

### Specificity of Tasks and Environmental Conditions

Task specificity can also be categorized by the nature of the environment. The spatial and temporal constraints of tasks and environments have a strong effect on the motor behavior of patients. An example of this is children and adults consistently generate classes of preferred grasp patterns for objects that can be predicted by the size of the object in relation to the size of their own hand (Newell, 1989). When the goal of a practice session is for a patient to strengthen particular types of grasp patterns, it is advantageous for a therapist to have the patient manipulate objects of specific sizes or shapes to promote the grasp patterns desired. The influence of temporal constraints has been shown for individuals with Parkinson disease who have abnormally slow maximal speeds of reaching to a stationary object but not when an object is moving or available for only a limited time (Majsak, 1998; Majsak, 2008). To fully appreciate the motor capacity of patients, therapists must evaluate their motor behavior across a wide range of tasks. Practicing tasks of one class may not benefit tasks of a different class.

### Practice With Manual Guidance

A final consideration in practice is the effect of manual guidance and assistance. It is not uncommon for therapists to physically cue, guide, or assist patients with neurological pathology attempting to perform a task. In some cases, patients need physical assistance to carry out the task. In other cases, therapists may be trying to help the patient experience a specific type of movement that cannot be self-generated. Physically moving patients who cannot move their limbs and using manual guidance to show patients potential motor outcomes (delineating task solutions and goals) are uncontested therapeutic activities. More controversial is the concept of whether physical assistance enhances the ability of patients to learn to generate their own motor outcomes. First, providing physical assistance to patients changes the biomechanics of a task. Second, manual cuing is often a form of concurrent feedback that may diminish the patient's ability to analyze the intrinsic information. Third, how does a therapist determine which movement strategies or patterns should be facilitated? Patients who overly rely on the manual guidance of therapists may become dependent on the external input and not learn how to generate their own movement strategies and patterns. When manual assistance is used, patients should be given opportunities to process their own intrinsic feedback and compare the movement strategies and patterns that occur with those they planned. Opportunities for intrinsic error detection and refinement of motor output are important components of learning.

A number of studies have shown physical guidance may promote early movement performance at the expense of retention and transfer (Gordon, 1968; Hagman, 1983; Winstein, 1994). Therapists often find patients perform well within a therapy session but have a difficult time carrying-over or transferring facilitated motor skills to other contexts. Techniques leading to better retention and transfer may very well be those that result in slower and less dramatic initial change. It may be that therapists are inclined to work with patients in a way that optimizes initial performance and acquisition of movements but impairs learning.

On the other hand, a broad generalization of the effects of physical assistance on patient performance and learning cannot be made (Wulf and Shea, 2002). Physical assistance may be highly desirable for patients with limited information processing and motor abilities who are learning complex tasks. Healthy individuals show benefits in both the acquisition and retention and transfer of physically challenging tasks when provided physical assistance (Wulf and Shea, 2002; Wulf, 1998b). For example, Wulf (1998b) reported individuals learning to perform slalom skiing movements on a ski-simulator using ski poles (see Figure 14-16) generated greater movement amplitudes and more efficient patterns of force production than individuals practicing without ski poles. Moreover, when all individuals were tested without poles, those who practiced with poles showed a more efficient pattern of force production than individuals practicing without poles.

Winstein (1994) showed that individuals who practiced upper extremity point-to-point movements with a high frequency of physical guidance performed well in acquisition but had poor performance retention. However, individuals provided intermittent physical guidance performed better in both acquisition and retention than individuals who received verbal feedback at the same frequency. Manual guidance may enhance the intrinsic information processing and motor learning of individuals if the frequency of delivery does not promote dependency on the physical assistance provided. Wulf and Toole (1999) found subjects learning a complex motor task performed better when allowed to self-determine the frequency of receiving physical assistance than when receiving a comparable but externally determined frequency of physical assistance. The effects of manual cues on patient recovery have not been well tested in clinical situations. It is likely in certain task conditions that intermittent manual cuing is beneficial or even essential, while in others it may have no effect or be detrimental.

## THINK ABOUT IT 14.2

Consider the ambulation task needs and goals for Cecelia, Peter, and Tito.

- What should you consider in deciding how and when to use manual cues to promote learning?
- What would contribute to your decision whether to use a massed or distributed practice schedule to promote their learning?
- If you chose to work on complimentary tasks, how would you determine tasks of similar or different specificity?
- How would you structure the task and environment to promote skills in their ambulation goals?

## ■ Optimizing Patient Engagement and Achieving Functional Competence

It is important for therapists to appreciate that the main principle of motor learning is to optimize patient engagement in learning processes. These learning processes include perception

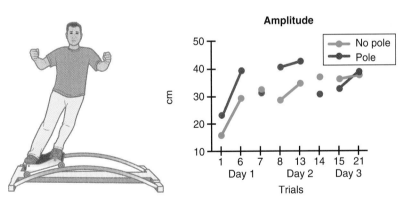

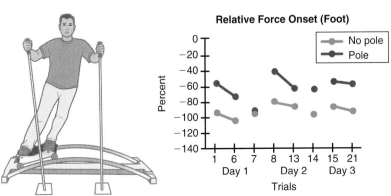

**FIGURE 14-16** Wulf et al (1998) tested ability of healthy subjects to acquire, retain, and transfer the learning of slalom-type movements on a ski-simulator. On the ski-simulator, elastic bands create a resting position of a rolling platform at the apex of a set of curved bars. By shifting weight side-to-side, the individual can move the rolling platform along the bars. The goal is to make rhythmical full-range slalom-type side-to-side movements as rapidly as possible. This task is very complex because it requires standing balance, well-timed weight-shifting, and endurance.

of self and the environment, creating a plan, generating a performance, information processing, practicing, and developing coordination modes of motor behavior that will assure functional competence. How can patient engagement be optimized? The first step is to make sure patients are motivated through a sense of autonomy and self-efficacy in their ability to achieve competent performance of meaningful and often challenging functional tasks. Optimal engagement becomes more complicated when therapists consider how they should manipulate the learning experiences of patients to promote motor learning processes. Previously held "mechanistic" principles of motor learning, such as that intermittent AI is more beneficial for learning than concurrent AI, random practice is preferable over blocked practice, and manual assistance should be avoided have been shown to not be valid across all types of patients and tasks. It is now clear that motor learning is a patient and task specific process that depends not merely on the learning experiences therapists design, but on what patients take away from those experiences. That is, the degree to which those experiences actually result in patients engaging in the intended processes of motor learning.

An "optimal challenge point" theory of learning has been suggested by Guadagnoli and Lee (2004) that emphasizes the interaction between the demands of tasks, the resources of patients, and the learning environment. Onla-or and Winstein (2008) and Pollack (2014) have described how this framework can be used favorably to evaluate and plan appropriate challenge levels of intervention. However, in addition to the dimensions of tasks and patient resources, previous research has shown that it is also important to consider a third dimension; the amount of practice available to learners. I propose a model of optimal patient engagement that suggests how therapists can manipulate learning experiences, delivery of information, and structure of practice in relation to the interaction of three major factors: 1) the intrinsic processing capacity of patients, 2) the complexity of tasks being learned, and 3) the amount of practice available. These three factors demarcate an "engagement workspace" for patients (see Figure 14-17). A useful metaphor for this model is that a golfer putting a ball cannot succeed in holing the putt without considering simultaneously the distance to the hole, the pitch of the green, and the side tilt of the green. Similarly, therapists need to consider concurrently the patient, the task, and the amount of practice a patient can carry out when determining how to create opportunities for optimal patient engagement. Just as a golf course has many types of greens, the conditions that emerge from the interaction of tasks, patients, and amount of practice available create a variety of "learning landscapes." Effectively manipulating the amount and type of guidance to provide patients is a skill therapists need to acquire to promote optimal patient engagement and learning. The amount of guidance provided may be high in some conditions, low in others, and will be relatively variable in many. Patients with limited experience or intrinsic resources who are learning relatively complicated tasks with limited practice may need a great deal of structure and guidance. In this case physical assistance, blocked practice and high frequencies of AI may be best. In contrast, patients with previous learning experience or greater processing capacity who are learning relatively simple tasks with plenty of practice available might do better with lower guidance, such as intermittent or patient-requested AI, minimal physical guidance, and a random or loose practice structure. Interaction effects will occur between these three dimensions. Given the resources of some

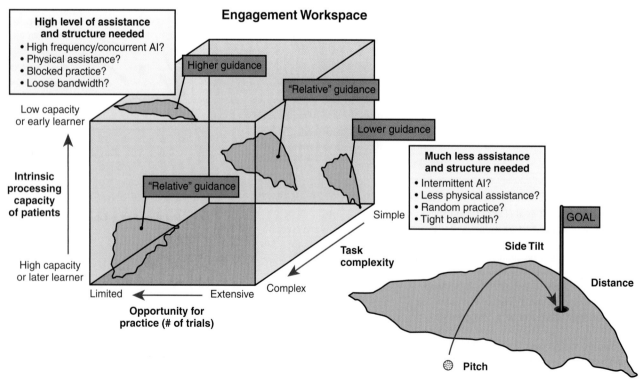

**FIGURE 14-17** The three-dimensional optimal engagement workspace.

patients, the degree of task complexity may be a greater limiting factor for learning than amount of practice, but for other patients limited practice ability may be a greater factor. Some patients with very limited resources may not be able to achieve task success in even simple tasks with large amounts of practice. As patients progress through phases of learning, the structure and assistance therapists provide to promote optimal patient engagement will change. Motor performance changes after stroke are often person-specific (DeJong, 2012). The concept of a three-dimensional engagement workspace helps therapists to remember to design effective tasks, promote the optimal information-processing abilities of patients, and structure optimal practice conditions keeping in mind that it is the motor learning processes we are promoting, not a specific structured approach for getting there.

To achieve functional competence, engaging patients in learning experiences is not enough. It is also critical that therapists consider how to promote changes in behaviors that patients will transfer into their own social communities. As cited earlier in this chapter, a major factor is helping patients achieve self-efficacy for the functional and challenging activities they will encounter on a daily basis. In addition, therapists should help patients develop home- and community-based exercise programs and use available technology to support not only patient exercise at home, but also their participation in life events. Strategies for supporting sustained exercise and participation are similar to those advocated earlier in this chapter for priming patients for learning. That is, promoting motivation and self-efficacy through concepts of SCT and SDT (Bandura, 1977, 1994; Deci and Ryan, 1985; Teixeira, 2012).

For example, Motl and Dlugonski (2011) created an internet-based 12-week program to increase the daily walking activity of individuals with multiple sclerosis. Website content was organized into 4 modules that included text and video incorporating the SCT principles of self-efficacy, goal-setting, barriers, and outcome expectations. Participants received web-based video coaching to promote program adherence, and were encouraged to wear a pedometer and record their daily steps. A 7-day accelerometer sampling was taken prior to and following the internet intervention. The program resulted in increases in physical activity, evidenced by increased self-reported activity scores on the Godin Leisure-Time Exercise Questionnaire (Godin and Shephard, 1985), higher pedometer step counts over the 12 weeks, and higher accelerometer activity shown following the termination of the program.

Another example of promoting sustained exercise and physical activity is the ENGAGE-HD program for individuals with Huntington disease (HD) proposed by Busse (2014) and further elucidated by Quinn (2016). The three main elements of the program are a physical activity coach, an exercise DVD, and a physical activity workbook. The program is intended to promote the SDT concepts of patient autonomy, motivation, enhanced expectations of goal attainment, and self-efficacy. Participants receive six home visits and intermittent phone calls by coaches over 14 weeks to develop an individualized lifestyle plan for enhancing their physical activity. The activity workbooks and exercise DVD are used to facilitate education, enablement, modeling, and goal setting. Preliminary data has been reported that program participants show greater levels of physical activity and are more mobile in their home communities than individuals not involved in the program. Therapists, coaches, patient peers and family members all play an important role in helping patients to be motivated, to develop self-efficacy, and to become functionally competent.

## ■ Designing Intervention Progressions

Therapists design the initial plan of rehabilitation by understanding the pathology, impairments, and functional limitations of patients and the ways tasks and environments, information delivery, and practice can be used to optimize patient engagement. Considerations include the interactions that occur between the intrinsic biomechanical, psychological, and neuromuscular constraints of patients and the extrinsic spatial and temporal constraints of tasks and environments, how the internal information processing of patients can be enhanced, and the optimal strategies for practice. As patients show greater degrees of functional competence in response to therapeutic intervention, therapists must continuously challenge patients to bring them to even higher levels of performance (Fell, 2004).

A number of therapeutic progressions have been suggested throughout the history of neurological physical therapy. These progressions have largely reflected the theoretical basis for the treatment philosophy advocated by specific rehabilitation approaches. Brunnstrom proposed patients be progressed "from spastic to voluntary motor stages of recovery" (Sawner and LaVigne, 1992). Advocates of the Proprioceptive Neuromuscular Facilitation (PNF) approach progressed patients through "functional movement patterns against maximal resistance" (Voss, 1985), and those following the methodology of Bobath moved patients through a "normal neurodevelopmental sequence" involving proximal to distal control (Bobath, 1970). As therapists better appreciate that the motor behavior of patients involves a self-organization of multiple levels of control, therapeutic progressions are based on multiple parameters.

Fell (2004) has suggested an excellent model of therapeutic progression in which the parameters of progression can be grouped in three categories: (1) those related to motor learning, (2) those related to characteristics of the movement or task, and (3) other considerations such as equipment used and the level of physical assistance provided. The parameters of progression related to motor learning and practice include variability in practice, part-practice, task attention, external feedback, and environmental progression. Parameters related to motor production include movement amplitude, velocity, amount of work, and endurance. Other parameters include judicious use and steady weaning from equipment and physical assistance.

Dangerous pitfalls can occur if the concept of creating progressions is overextended. For example, therapists might believe single-joint movements should be mastered by patients before they are progressed to multijoint movements. However, if one considers the biomechanics involved in these movement classes, it is readily apparent that single- and multijoint movements are quite different. It would be far more prudent to simplify or increase the difficulty of a multijoint task by varying the amplitude or velocity of the required multijoint movements than to disregard sound biomechanics properties by working instead on single-joint movements. Practice of one type of movement class prepares patients for another.

Another example of a false progression is that therapists sometimes progress patients who are first beginning gait training, from "pregait activities," to stepping activities, and then slow to fast walking. Although this might seem reasonable, one would not learn to ride a bicycle by first sitting stationary on the bicycle, then rolling very slowly, and finally peddling the bicycle only after stationary and slow speed balance activities had been mastered. The control of gait requires patients to experience and learn to use body inertia, interlimb forces, and ground reaction forces as part of the solution.

Therapists need to be cautious applying theoretical frameworks to practice such as Gentile's taxonomy of tasks. Gentile makes the point that different task types are not necessarily easier or more difficult; they are merely different. The taxonomy of tasks does not include the attributes and constraints of patients, and it is the interaction between the intrinsic constraints of patients and the spatial and temporal features of tasks and environments that determine the ease or difficulty of tasks. In and of itself, the taxonomy of tasks is not a template of how to progress patients through different tasks. Sound progressions should involve manipulations of the spatial or temporal features of a task within the same category, not across different task categories.

In a global sense, therapists create sound therapeutic progressions by manipulating the spatial and temporal constraints of tasks and environments and changing practice conditions to challenge the intrinsic constraints of patients, their information-processing capacity, and the efficiency and diversity of their movements. Table 14-4 provides a representative list of the parameters therapists can use to progress therapeutic interventions and an example of how progressions can be implemented in three different functional activities. Perhaps the two most important concepts to consider when designing progressions are the nature of the parameters being progressed and how multiple parameter progressions can be interwoven.

## THINK ABOUT IT 14.3

Develop sound treatment progressions for the following task goals:

- Cecilia's task goals of learning to use both upper limbs again for reaching, grasping, and using a variety of flower pots and garden tools
- Cecilia's goal of being able to walk and carry out gardening tasks in challenging environments
- Peter's goal of getting in and out of bed more easily
- Peter's goal of walking without falling
- Tito's goal of walking and carrying objects
  Include strategies for promoting motor planning, information processing, and practice.

| TABLE 14-4 | Treatment Progressions for Specific Task Parameters | | |
|---|---|---|---|
| **SOME FUNCTIONAL ACTIVITIES (AND PARAMETERS TO PROGRESS)** | **EARLY STAGE** | **LATER STAGE** | **CLINICAL EXAMPLE** |
| Multijoint limb control in reaching and catching (Biomechanics, force dynamics, control of multiple degrees of freedom) | Movement exercises graded in amplitude and speed that promote control of shoulder and elbow movements as a functional unit, wrist and hand movements might be practiced in isolation; Limited variability of practice with small changes in spatial/temporal task conditions | Movement exercises graded in amplitude, speed, and load (object characteristics) involving the shoulder, elbow, and wrist/hand as a functional unit; Demanding spatial and temporal task constraints | **Early** Shoulder and elbow: Wiping a table, drawing on a chalkboard, washing the face with a washcloth Wrist and hand: Picking up coins from a table, picking up a cup **Later** Shoulder, elbow and wrist/hand: Reaching to grasp a pencil, passing a cup with fluid to another person, catching and throwing a ball |

| TABLE 14-4 | Treatment Progressions for Specific Task Parameters—cont'd | | |
|---|---|---|---|
| **SOME FUNCTIONAL ACTIVITIES (AND PARAMETERS TO PROGRESS)** | **EARLY STAGE** | **LATER STAGE** | **CLINICAL EXAMPLE** |
| Sit-to-stand (Biomechanics, force dynamics, dual-task information processing) | Sit-to-stand from a stable surface at a height that does not demand large degrees of force; Limited variability of practice with small changes in spatial (sitting surface, foot surface) or temporal (stand to catch a moving object) constraints; Sit-to-stand while holding stable objects | Sit-to-stand from lower sitting surfaces and less stable sitting and standing surfaces; Demanding spatial and temporal task constraints; Sit-to-stand while holding less stable objects | **Early** Sit-to-stand from a wheelchair or a high/low mat; Use of a cane or standard walker for support **Later** Sit-to-stand from a couch or recliner chair and a carpeted surface; Use of a rolling walker for support; Holding a cup of water while moving sit-to-stand |
| Gait (Biomechanics, force dynamics, dual-task information processing) | Ambulation with spatial but no temporal constraints; Ambulation with relatively generous temporal task constraints; Ambulation with small changes in spatial (walking area) or temporal (moving environment, people) constraints; Ambulation with and without an assistive device | Ambulation with demanding spatial and temporal task constraints; Ambulation with high degrees of task variability; Ambulation with greater force demands; Ambulation while manipulating/carrying objects | **Early** Ambulation in an open area; Ambulation with a few other people walking toward the patient at a slow speed; Ambulation around small objects/over small surface changes; Ambulation with an assistive device **Late** Ambulation in a cluttered area; Ambulation in a crowded hallway; Ambulating up/down large stairs and in/out of an elevator; Pushing objects/carrying objects while ambulating |

## Let's Review

1. Describe how you use the process of deductive and inductive reasoning in designing, implementing, testing, and validating sound strategies of neurological rehabilitation. Why is this important?

2. Describe what it means to you to use an integrated approach to neurological rehabilitation based on contemporary science in the areas of motor control and motor learning.

3. What is functional competence?

4. How does acquiring flexible coordination modes or "rules" for classes of actions promote functional competence?

5. How can therapists promote functional competence?

6. Describe how therapeutic exercise, task-based practice, and the environment influence your choice of intervention strategies.

7. What does motor learning involve?

8. Describe several ways therapists can "engage" patients in the process of learning.

9. Describe what is meant by "specificity of practice."

10. Provide examples of intervention strategies that optimally engage patients by taking into account their attributes, constraints, complexity of learned tasks, and opportunity for practice.

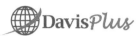 **DavisPlus**    For additional resources, including Focus on Evidence tables, case study discussions, references, and glossary, please visit http://davisplus.fadavis.com

## CHAPTER SUMMARY

This chapter provides an overview of what therapists can consider when attempting to create the most effective therapeutic conditions for neurological rehabilitation. The conceptual framework presented for applying concepts and principles of motor control and motor learning to neurological rehabilitation is supported by contemporary literature in these areas and through clinical examples that validate the utility of this framework. The integration of movement and functional training is discussed, along with specificity of practice and principles for progressing therapeutic intervention. A summary of the principles and major points for neuromuscular rehabilitation is included in Table 14-5.

Numerous major points are stressed. First, the pathological motor behavior of patients is a very complex interaction of the intrinsic resources and constraints of patients and the external regulatory features of tasks and environments. Second, the optimal therapeutic conditions for patients to attain functional competence exist when therapists understand and utilize the influence of tasks and environments within their interventions, promote the information-processing capacity of patients, and engage patients in sound practice conditions. Third, therapists promote effective neurological rehabilitation when they address the impairments and functional limitations of patients simultaneously. Therapists accomplish this by creating a therapeutic plan, including functional tasks into which desirable movements are embedded. Last, patient self-efficacy is a major determinant for functional competence.

The main objective of neurological rehabilitation is for patients to optimize their functional competence. Therapists

| TABLE 14-5 | A Summary of the Major Principles of Neurological Rehabilitation |
|---|---|
| **PRINCIPLE** | **MAJOR POINTS** |
| Neurological Rehabilitation Involves a Continues Cycle of Deductive and Inductive Reasoning | • A sound theoretical foundation and models of practice underlie effective neurological rehabilitation.<br>• Therapists test hypotheses in the clinic to confirm, revise, or reject the validity of theories and models.<br>• Objectivity and a systematic approach of analysis is important when testing hypotheses in the clinic.<br>• The motor behavior of patients reflects a self-organized interaction of multiple body structures and functions; it is important to look for clusters of impairments and rate-limiting variables to decide how to intervene most effectively. |
| The Goal of Neurological Rehabilitation Is Functional Competence | • Functional competence is the ability to perform daily activities in a variety of environments, under different conditions, with a minimal cost of physical and cognitive demands.<br>• Acquiring flexible coordination modes or "rules" for classes of actions is our patients' greatest avenue for achieving functional competence. |
| Functional Competence Is Promoted by Embedded Models of Motor Behavior and Neurological Rehabilitation | • The organization of human motor behavior and the areas of neurological rehabilitation are embedded; the health condition of patients contributes to the status of their body structures and functions. In turn, these directly affect activity, which is a necessary component of participation. All levels are engaged simultaneously, not sequentially or in parallel. |

| TABLE 14-5 | A Summary of the Major Principles of Neurological Rehabilitation—cont'd |
|---|---|
| **PRINCIPLE** | **MAJOR POINTS** |
| | • The cellular processes, movements, and actions of patients are similarly embedded.<br>• By manipulating tasks and environments skillfully, therapists can simultaneously influence the actions, movements, and cellular processes of patients. |
| Neurological Rehabilitation Involves Motor Learning | • The main principle of motor learning is to optimize patient engagement in the processes associated with learning.<br>• Motor learning involves: (1) Perception of self and the environment, (2) Making a plan, and (3) Performance, information processing, and practice.<br>• Therapists should consider the intrinsic processing capacity of patients, the complexity of the task being learned, and the opportunity for practice in determining how to create the optimal level of engagement for patients.<br>• Manipulating the delivery of augmented information and structuring the conditions for practice provide therapists multiple means for engaging patients.<br>• Specificity of practice means specificity within classes of actions, not the details of tasks.<br>• The goal of motor learning is not necessarily the rapid acquisition of task performance but the retention and transfer of motor skills. |

promote optimal function by helping patients to acquire, retain, and diversify their motor behaviors so motor tasks can be skillfully performed in a variety of environments and task conditions. Creating the most effective conditions for optimizing the functional competence of patients with neurological pathology is a daunting task. Therapists can do this by helping patients believe they have the capacity to change their behaviors, promoting patient autonomy and self-efficacy, and providing patients opportunities for identifying their constraints, motor planning, information processing, and practicing. Therapeutic exercise and task-based practice must be blended in a meaningful way through valid intervention progressions. Therapeutic programs must educate, motivate, and empower patients so they will be willing to use their full motor capacity and take on the challenges they will face as they participate in their home and community activities. An understanding and application of these factors reflects a sound application of the sciences related to neurological rehabilitation and will provide patients the greatest opportunity for attaining functional competence.

# General Approaches to Neurological Rehabilitation

CHAPTER **15**

Kathy L. Mercuris, PT, DHS ▪ Jeannie B. Stephenson, PT, PhD, NCS

**CHAPTER OBJECTIVES**

Upon completion of this chapter, the learner should be able to:
1. Discuss the evolution of neurorehabilitation models.
2. Compare and contrast the underlying principles of the neurorehabilitation models.
3. Define key terminology associated with the various neurorehabilitation models.
4. Design a therapy intervention session for a patient with neurological dysfunction, integrating the varied neurorehabilitation concepts.
5. Discuss the current evidence to support the efficacy of therapeutic interventions used in neurological rehabilitation.
6. Identify areas requiring further research on the efficacy of therapeutic interventions used in neurological rehabilitation.

## ■ Introduction

The emphasis of rehabilitation must focus on improving function to allow for a return to participation in activities of daily living (ADL), work, and leisure. In determining which of the various intervention options is best for a given patient, the therapist must work closely with the patient, family, and caregivers to identify their goals and needs. This, along with the examination results, will aid in narrowing the focus of treatment and the selection of specific exercises and activities. Some intervention approaches are more applicable to certain patient diagnoses. For example, **neurodevelopmental treatment (NDT)** was initially developed as an approach for children with cerebral palsy (CP) and was later extrapolated to adults with hemiplegia. Other approaches, such as **proprioceptive neuromuscular facilitation (PNF),** can be used with a diverse patient population with varied diagnoses. Most therapists choose to combine treatment approaches for an eclectic mix designed to meet the goals of each patient.

Therapists attempt to incorporate current research evidence into their decision-making process to determine interventions that optimize patient outcomes. The level of evidence and how it is determined varies greatly for each of the rehabilitation approaches discussed in this chapter. For example, constraint-induced movement therapy (CIMT) and locomotor training (LT) with unweighting systems use protocols that are being driven directly by experimental results. This differs from PNF and NDT approaches, which were developed from therapist observations of patients during treatment sessions, followed by research testing to verify the effectiveness of the approach. Confounding factors of the research include the quality of the study methodology, differing patient characteristics and exclusionary criteria, and the use of varied outcome measurement tools. These disparities challenge the therapist when attempting to compare treatment approaches and identify the best intervention approach for a given patient. Thus, after a critical analysis of the evidence, the patient's success is, in part, dependent on the art of therapy.

This chapter will serve as an introduction and provide a description of the treatment approaches that may be used in the care of patients with neurological dysfunction. Past and present applications and examples of integrating the models in the clinic setting will be described. Examples of clinical application for each model will be discussed. A case study at the end of the chapter will highlight the integration of the approaches for patient intervention. Discussion as to the efficacy, advantages, and disadvantages of the underlying theory of these approaches can be found in Chapter 14.

## ■ Neurofacilitation Approaches

**Neurofacilitation approaches** were developed in the 1940s and 1950s on the basis of the reflex and hierarchical models of motor control, and these approaches are still used by clinicians today. As the name neurofacilitation implies, most of these approaches were developed for individuals with abnormal sensorimotor function or muscle tone and were used to either inhibit abnormal movement or facilitate more normal motions. This section will discuss the influence of theorists Rood, Ayres, Brunnstrom, Bobath, Kabat, Knott, and Voss on patient care and rehabilitation.

### Concepts of Margaret Rood

#### Background/Overview

Margaret Rood was a physical therapist and occupational therapist who developed an approach to examination and treatment of individuals with neuromuscular dysfunction in the 1940s. She was strongly influenced by Sister Kenny's system of neuromuscular reeducation used extensively with individuals with polio at that time. A comprehensive review of the Rood approach can be found in the Northwestern University Special Therapeutic Exercise Project (NUSTEP) proceedings (Stockmeyer, 1967). According to Stockmeyer, this approach had two primary components: motor development sequences and **sensory stimulation techniques**. There was a strong emphasis on sensory function, a key component of examination and treatment in the Rood approach. Although this approach is no longer applied clinically in its entirety, it is important to understand Rood's lasting contributions to neurorehabilitation. Many concepts developed by Rood have been adapted and integrated into other approaches. For example, terminology used clinically and in the literature such as **mobility** and **stability** was first described by Rood in the context of neurorehabilitation. Sensory stimulation techniques still used with neurological populations, such as **quick tapping, quick stretch, or approximation**, were originally described by Rood and will be discussed later.

#### Principles and Concepts

The Rood approach is based on the concept that all neuromuscular function is related to one of two biological purposes: mobility or stability (Stockmeyer, 1967). Complex motor activities are thought to be variations of the interplay of these two components. Rood believed that muscles involved in mobility functions have different structural and kinesiological characteristics than those involved in stability (Stockmeyer, 1967). She distinguished the terms light work from heavy work. **Light work** refers to movement and involves reciprocal innervation of antagonist muscles. Reciprocal innervation means that during contraction of the agonist muscle there is simultaneous relaxation of its antagonist muscle. Light work or **phasic muscles** are located in superficial lateral body areas or distal body segments and they function more in voluntary movement. **Heavy work** involves cocontraction of muscles that are normally antagonists and that provide stability to a joint or body segment. Heavy work or **tonic muscles** are deep one-joint muscles that lie in medial and proximal body regions and should be stimulated early in treatment to provide stability. Some muscles are involved in both light and heavy work (Farber, 1982; Montgomery, 2003). The terms light and heavy work have contributed to our understanding of how phasic and tonic muscles have different muscular characteristics and different functions.

In the Rood approach, coordinated movement is thought to be achieved during overlapping stages of sensorimotor developmental sequences. These sequences are the foundation for identifying the patient's functional level, the requirements of coordinated movement, and the order in which intervention should progress. Sequential reeducation of the patient with neurological involvement through the stages of normal development sequences was considered critical to normal motor development and to maximum patient recovery.

Rood identified two motor developmental sequences: the skeletal function sequence and the vital function sequence. Skeletal functions included motor activities of the head, neck, trunk, and extremities whereas the vital function sequence was comprised of respiration, feeding, and speech (Montgomery, 2003). The steps of the skeletal function sequence were divided into ontogenetic motor patterns which included: withdrawal flexion in supine, rolling over, pivot prone, cocontraction of the neck, on-elbows, all-fours, standing, and walking. Four levels of motor control were thought to develop as the patient progressed through the skeletal function sequence (see Table 15-1 and Fig. 15-1). The two primary levels of control are mobility and stability. **Mobility (Level I)** is free active motion that translates a body part through space, whereas **Stability (Level II)** fixes a body part to allow for weight-bearing. By combining mobility and stability, two other levels develop that were thought to be needed for coordinated movement. The first is **Controlled Mobility (Level III)** or mobility superimposed on stability in a weight-bearing position in which the proximal part moves on a fixed distal part (e.g., weight-shifting). The second, more advanced, combined function is called **Skill (Level IV)** or mobility superimposed on stability in a nonweight-bearing position with the free distal part moving. These four levels of control were thought to develop in this

| TABLE 15-1 | Rood's Sequence of Motor Development |
| --- | --- |
| **FOUR LEVELS OF MOTOR CONTROL** | **DEFINITION ACCORDING TO ROOD** |
| Level I: Mobility | Free, flexible motion that translates the body or body part in space and includes qualities of range and speed. |
| Level II: Stability | Cocontraction of agonists and antagonists that fixes parts of the body to allow for weight-bearing and later allow for dynamic holding in Levels III and IV. |
| Level III: Controlled Mobility | The distal body parts are fixed on the support surface and the proximal segment moves over a fixed distal segment (weight-shifting). |
| Level IV: Skill | The distal part of the extremity is free from the support surface and coordinated movement of this segment is superimposed on proximal stability. |

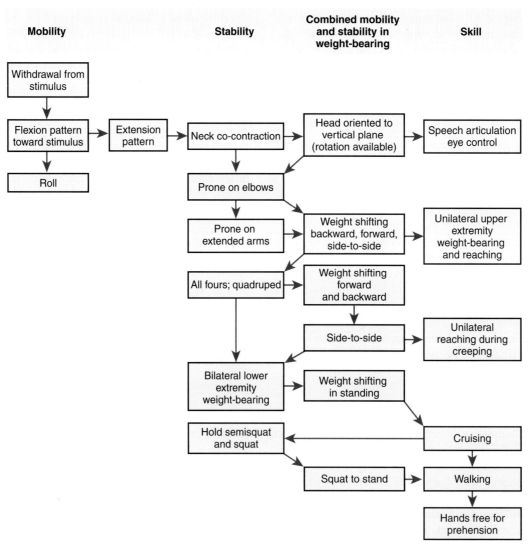

**FIGURE 15-1** Diagram of Rood's Sequence of Motor Development. This figure highlights the motor development sequence including mobility, stability, mobility superimposed on stability, and skill as described by Rood. Reproduced with permission from Case-Smith J, ed. *Occupational Therapy for Children*, 4th edition. St. Louis, MO: Mosby, 2001. Figure 14-2, p.337.

order within the skeletal function sequence and were the basis of examination in the Rood approach.

The Rood approach to intervention involved identification of lacking developmental function, developmental sequences needed to advance function, and sensory stimuli needed to facilitate appropriate responses at each level of the sequence. The goal of treatment was to restore whichever component of the sequence was missing in the order in which it normally would be acquired. Rood emphasized certain motor milestones in her developmental sequence (e.g., prone-on-elbows, rolling over) to the exclusion of other important milestones such as sitting and cruising. Other therapists have updated and added to Rood's developmental sequences (Farber, 1982).

### Clinical Applications

Rood considered the interaction of three primary systems (somatic, autonomic, and psychological) and their effect on the patient's sensorimotor function. Sensation and its relation to motor function were considered important in the analysis

of movement dysfunction and in intervention (Montgomery, 2003). Rood considered motor functions to be inseparable from sensory functions, a factor that led to a shift in treatment focus for the neurologically involved patient from a strong motor emphasis to a sensorimotor emphasis (Stockmeyer, 1967). Rood advocated the use of sensory stimulation techniques to either facilitate or inhibit patient responses. She based the use of these techniques on the reflex model of motor control previously discussed in Chapter 14. The application of each of the sensory stimulation techniques is described in Table 15-2.

Rood used techniques such as **quick (fast) brushing** or tapping of the skin over a muscle to facilitate phasic muscle responses and improve mobility (Rood, 1962). Tapping involves the therapist making brisk taps with fingertips over the muscle belly, which causes phasic contraction of this muscle. For example, tapping can be used over the triceps muscle to facilitate elbow extension and upper extremity (UE) weight-bearing in sitting as a child with CP actively attempts to extend the elbow. Muscle belly tapping activates

| **TABLE 15-2** | **Sensory Stimulation Techniques: Definitions of Sensory Stimulation Techniques Described by Rood** |
|---|---|
| **SENSORY STIMULATION–FACILITATION TECHNIQUES** | **APPLICATION OF TECHNIQUE** |
| Light Touch | Application of quick light strokes to the skin over a muscle using either fingers, cotton, or a brush facilitates contraction of the underlying muscle. |
| Tapping | Involves brisk taps with fingertips over the tendon or muscle belly of the involved muscle to facilitate phasic contraction of this muscle. |
| Quick Stretch | A quick over elongation of a muscle (often applied at its lengthened range) facilitates contraction of the muscle. |
| Quick Ice | Quick stroking with ice on the skin over the muscle belly facilitates contraction of the underlying muscle. |
| Traction | Manually applied distraction force to a joint or limb segment causes muscle relaxation and promotes movement. |
| Approximation | Compression of a joint or body segment stimulates cocontraction of muscles around the body segment and promotes stability. |
| Resistance | Manual application of force away from the axis of motion at the joints as the patient is asked to move or to stabilize. |
| **SENSORY STIMULATION–INHIBITORY TECHNIQUES** | |
| Prolonged Stretch | Application of slow passive lengthening of a muscle inhibits its contraction. |
| Deep Pressure | Manual pressure across the longitudinal axis of the muscle tendon causes relaxation of the muscle. |
| Neutral Warmth | Wrapping of body or limb in blanket, towel, or air splint for purpose of general relaxation. |
| Slow Stroking | Slow stroking with the hand along midline of the back, near the posterior rami, for 3 to 5 minutes leads to calming of patient. |
| Prolonged Cold | Application of an ice pack or ice massage over a muscle leads to its relaxation and reduction of pain. |

muscle spindles, which excite Ia afferents causing firing of alpha motoneurons and contraction of the agonist, the triceps. There is simultaneous inhibition of the antagonist, the biceps, through firing of inhibitory interneurons. Techniques such as approximation or joint compression are used to facilitate stability, tonic muscle responses, and cocontraction of muscles around a joint or body part (Stockmeyer, 1967). In the previous example, the therapist could apply approximation to the child's arm to facilitate cocontraction of muscles around the elbow and encourage UE weight-bearing. Approximation applied at the pelvis down through the thigh could be used to facilitate cocontraction of muscles around the hip joint and promote lower extremity (LE) weight-bearing in the standing position. Compression of joint surfaces facilitates static Type I joint receptors, which facilitate postural extensors and stabilizers and enhance joint awareness (Stockmeyer, 1967).

Inhibition of abnormal reflex activity and hypertonicity is accomplished through techniques such as deep pressure, prolonged stretch, or neutral warmth (see Table 15-2). For example, a therapist working with a patient in prone who has hamstring spasticity might apply pressure across the longitudinal axis of the muscle tendon to relax the muscle and allow for active or passive knee extension. The deep pressure activates Pacinian corpuscles causing inhibition of muscle tone. These inhibitory effects can be enhanced by combining with other inhibitory techniques, such as the use of deep pressure to a muscle while simultaneously providing a slow prolonged stretch to the same muscle. The therapeutic goal is to withdraw sensory stimuli and encourage the patient to control their own postures and movements. Sensory stimulation techniques are still used by therapists today but only as an adjunct to therapeutic exercise and functional training.

A therapist using the Rood approach with a child with CP could progress the child through the four levels of motor control in one motor developmental sequence position. Using function in **quadruped** (all-fours) as an example, the child is first guided to attain the all-fours position (Mobility Level I). The therapist could use sensory stimulation techniques such as tapping or quick stretch to the muscles responsible for this task to facilitate mobility into the position. Approximation can be applied down through the shoulder girdles and pelvic girdles toward the distal extremities to facilitate stability once the child has attained all-fours. This is followed by resistance to isometric contraction of the shoulder girdle and trunk muscles in the all-fours position to facilitate maintained contraction of the proximal extensors of the neck, trunk, and limb girdles (Stability Level II). The child can then be encouraged to rock back-and-forth or side-to-side in all-fours in preparation for creeping (Controlled Mobility Level III). The therapist uses handling techniques to facilitate the child's weight shift onto one UE to allow for skilled movement of the opposite UE moving forward as the child begins to creep (Skill Level IV). This is one example of a clinical application of the Rood approach.

## Concepts of Sensory Integration

### Background/Overview

**Sensory integration** is a neurobehavioral theory based on the work of Jean Ayres. Dr. Ayres was an occupational therapist and psychologist. Given her educational background, she was interested in how motor development was linked to learning and realized the importance of basing interventions on sound research evidence. She published her first material on sensory integration and learning disabilities in 1972. Ongoing research continues to expand our understanding of sensory processing and influences chosen intervention techniques.

Sensory integration is defined as "the neurological process that organizes sensation from one's own body and from the environment and makes it possible to use the body effectively within the environment" (Ayres, 1972). The individual must interpret the sensory input and organize the information to adapt motor behaviors to interact with the environment. Effective movement and environmental interaction will not only allow for survival but also for learning to occur. Ayres focused on understanding sensory processing, developing examination methods, and categorizing observed dysfunction to determine effective intervention strategies.

During development, individuals use sensory input from the tactile, vestibular, and proprioception systems. The processing and integration of this information combined with vision and hearing allows for the development of balance and postural control, utilization of both sides of the body, and eye-hand coordination. This, in turn, promotes motor planning and aids in one's self-image and body scheme. If one is not able to process and use sensory information, one is unable to motor plan and focus on learning tasks.

### Principles and Concepts

Sensory integration theory bridges the hierarchical and systems models of motor control (Short-Degraff, 1988). Ayres felt there was a hierarchy with sensory integration developing and being controlled in lower or subcortical centers followed by the development of perception, reasoning, and learning in higher cortical centers. She also advocated that processing of sensory information and interaction with the environment followed a developmental sequence. However, she was also aware of the entire holistic aspect of sensory integration and the interaction between all of the body systems. An intrinsic drive motivates one to interact, practice, and adapt to the environment for learning to occur. Multiple sensory cues enhance the learning. The plasticity of the central nervous system allows learning to occur across the lifespan (Bundy, 2002).

### Clinical Applications

Ayres thought a sensory integration deficit was a "stand-alone" problem. If a child had other neurological deficits, the sensory processing problems were considered part of the original diagnosis. This premise has been altered over time, and today a child may have a diagnosis of both sensory processing disorder and another neurological disorder such as CP or Down syndrome (DS).

Various examination tools provide objective information for sensory processing. Originally Ayres developed the *Sensory Integration and Praxis Test* (SIPT; Ayres, 1972). Although this is still used today, other tests and measures such as the *Sensory Profile* (Dunn, 1999) and *DeGange-Berk Test of Sensory Integration* have been developed (DeGange, 1988). These tests require less training for the clinician to administer and provide immediate results or scoring. Other measurement tools incorporate sensory integration components but may be more focused on motor skills or functional assessment. Motor function tests include the *Alberta Infant Motor Scale* (AIMS), *Peabody Developmental Motor Scales II,* and *Bruininks-Oseretsky Test of Motor Proficiency* (BOT 2), and the functional assessments include the *Pediatric Evaluation of Disability Inventory* (PEDI) and the *School Function Assessment* (SFA). Sensory integration is considered the basis for all learning and functional tasks that occur throughout the day in all environments. Therefore, interventions for sensory processing dysfunction require a team approach with parents, teachers, and health-care professionals. Respect for the patient and an understanding of the patient's needs are critical to enhance motivation and involvement in the therapy process. Detailed examples of interventions for individuals with **sensory integration dysfunction** can be found in Chapter 27 on Sensory Impairments.

## Concepts of Signe Brunnstrom

### Background/Overview

Signe Brunnstrom observed and defined abnormal synergistic patterns and stages in the motor recovery process after a stroke. These defined patterns and progressions were incorporated into treatment techniques (Brunnstrom, 1966) and the development of the Fugl-Meyer Assessment (Fugl-Meyer, 1980). The Fugl-Meyer Assessment is frequently used in clinical research projects. A complete description of Brunnstrom's work can be found in the text, *Brunnstrom's Movement Therapy in Hemiplegia: A Neurophysiological Approach* (Sawner, 1992).

## Principles and Concepts

**Synergies** are the actions observed when coupled muscles contract in sequence to allow efficient normal movement. However, after a central nervous system lesion, this normal coupling results in stereotypical movement patterns that do not allow for the varied movement combinations necessary for function. Brunnstrom identified these as abnormal patterns and defined a flexion and extension synergy pattern for both the UE and LE. Observation of volitional movement into an abnormal synergistic pattern is necessary to document the presence of a limb synergy.

The UE and LE abnormal synergies are described in Table 15-3 (Davies, 1985; Sawner, 1992). Dependent on the strength of the **abnormal synergy**, the UE is often observed in a resting position with the strongest components of the two patterns combined. This results in a position of shoulder internal rotation, adduction, elbow flexion, and often wrist/finger flexion. Over a prolonged period of time, pronation will be noted.

The LE extension synergy is the most prevalent pattern in individuals with hemiplegia. Therefore, most individuals will stand and ambulate with a predominance of hip adduction, knee extension, and ankle plantarflexion/inversion. A 'scissoring' gait pattern is displayed in individuals with bilateral LE extension synergy. Hip flexion in the swing phase of gait may be initiated by using the flexion synergy.

| TABLE 15-3 | Abnormal Synergy Patterns Described by Brunnstrom | |
|---|---|---|
| **SYNERGY PATTERN** | **UPPER EXTREMITY** | **LOWER EXTREMITY** |
| Flexion Synergy | Scapula: retraction and elevation<br>Shoulder: Abduction and external rotation<br>Elbow: flexion*<br>Forearm: supination<br>Wrist: flexion<br>Fingers/Thumb: flexion and adduction | Pelvis: elevation and retraction<br>Hip: flexion*, abduction, external rotation<br>Knee: flexion<br>Ankle: dorsiflexion and inversion<br>Toe: dorsiflexion |
| Extension Synergy | Scapula: Protraction and depression<br>Shoulder: Adduction*, internal rotation<br>Elbow: extension<br>Forearm: pronation*<br>Wrist: flexion or extension<br>Fingers/Thumb: flexion and adduction | Hip: extension, adduction*, internal rotation<br>Knee: extension*<br>Ankle: plantar flexion* and inversion<br>Toes: plantar flexion |

Note: For upper extremity, flexion synergy is most often observed, while for lower extremity, extension synergy is most often observed.
*Indicates the strongest positions
Adapted from: O'Sullivan, 2014, p. 671; Davies PM. *Steps to Follow-A Guide to the Treatment of Adult Hemiplegia.* Berlin Heidelberg, Germany: Springer-Verlag; 1985, 25–27.

Often, individuals with hemiplegia will move into the synergistic patterns involuntarily when another part of the body is performing a strong or forceful movement. These involuntary motions are termed **associated reactions** (Sawner, 1992). A frequently observed example is the increase in shoulder adduction and elbow flexion during ambulation or other stressful tasks. Associated reactions can also be facilitated through **overflow** such as resistance to hip abduction on the intact side facilitating hip abduction of the involved extremity. The reader is referred to Brunnstrom's text for a detailed description of additional associated reactions (Sawner, 1992).

Brunnstrom and other approaches based on the hierarchical theory of motor control incorporated the use of developmental reflexes (primitive and tonic reflexes, righting reactions). Brunnstrom notes the position of the head and/or body will often affect the synergistic responses. Body positions may be used to either inhibit an unwanted motor response or facilitate a desired response. For example, the patient may have increased difficulty initiating the LE flexion synergy while supine if the **tonic labyrinthine reflex** (TLR) is active. In supine, the TLR increases muscle tone of the extensor muscles of the body, thus preventing the LE flexion. However, turning (rotating) the head toward the side may elicit the **asymmetric tonic neck reflex** (ATNR). In this example of turning toward the non-hemiplegic side, the ATNR will increase the extension tone on the non-hemiplegic side and increase flexor tone in the hemiplegic limb, enhancing the ability to flex the hemiplegic LE.

Typically, control of movement will progress from gross to fine movement and from proximal to distal control. Brunnstrom observed six **stages of motor recovery** following stroke described in Box 15-1 (Brunnstrom, 1966). The degree

of recovery depends on several factors, including the severity of the lesion and sensory involvement. Progress or recovery may stop at any point in the described continuum.

### Clinical Applications

Brunnstrom believed an individual must move through each stage of recovery and gain active movement in both the flexion and extension synergies before a combination of movements out of the synergies could be performed (Perry, 1967). Examples of a movement combination or **isolated movement** are elbow extension with shoulder flexion during reaching or with knee extension during gait. Brunnstrom's treatment approach is rarely used alone in the clinic setting today, as some clinicians are concerned the patient will be unable to advance to isolated motions once an abnormal synergy has developed. Brunnstrom recommended an emphasis on strengthening the weaker synergy pattern to encourage a balance between the two patterns. For example, because the UE flexion synergy is typically stronger than extension, the therapist may focus on increasing the motions in the UE extension synergy by facilitating movements during a meaningful functional task. In a sitting position, the patient may rest the hemiplegic UE on a raised table. The patient is asked to dust the tabletop by extending the elbow. This is a combined motion with the shoulder maintained in 90 degrees of flexion and the elbow actively extending. The activity can be progressed by asking the patient to grasp a drinking glass in this position or decreasing the amount of shoulder support to increase shoulder flexion activation. Functional practice incorporating multiple strategies can enhance learning and carryover to daily tasks.

The previously described task of performing isolated elbow extension can be further facilitated with the use of overflow and developmental reflexes in varied body positions. By positioning the patient in supine with the shoulder flexed at 90 degrees, the TLR supports extension and may better activate the elbow extensors. Additionally, as the patient is requested to rotate the head and look toward the involved extremity, the ATNR can further enhance elbow extension. Tapping and quick icing, as described by Rood, may be used over the triceps for greater facilitation. An associated reaction for elbow extension can be elicited by asking the patient to flex the trunk and reach toward the floor while in a short sitting posture. Resisting elbow extension on the intact extremity to facilitate extension on the involved side is a technique that uses the overflow principle. A functional goal for reaching could be added to any of these tasks. Brunnstrom provides numerous examples of activities that can be used to encourage the recovery of movement (Sawner, 1992). Pandian (2012) found that individuals post-CVA had significant improvements in wrist and hand movements following Brunnstrom's treatment protocol.

## Neurodevelopmental Treatment (NDT)

### Background/Overview

Berta Bobath, PT, and her husband, Karl Bobath, MD, developed a treatment approach for children with CP that was

---

**BOX 15-1 Stages of Motor Recovery After Stroke as defined by Brunnstrom**

Stage 1: Extremities are flaccid. This typically occurs immediately after the lesion and typically persists for a few hours to a few days.

Stage 2: Minimal volitional motions are possible and associated reactions are seen in synergistic patterns. Spasticity begins to develop.

Stage 3: Voluntary control of the synergies is possible through partial range. Spasticity will peak during this stage.

Stage 4: Limited motions combining the synergistic movements are possible. Spasticity begins to decline.

Stage 5: More advanced movement combinations are possible as spasticity continues to diminish.

Stage 6: Isolated movements are possible with near normal coordination. Spasticity has declined and may only be evident with increased speed of movement.

Sawner K, LaVigne J. *Brunnstrom's Movement Therapy in Hemiplegia: A Neurophysiological Approach.* Philadelphia, PA: J.B. Lippincott; 1992: 41–42.

later applied to adults with hemiplegia. It was first described in the scientific literature in 1948 and was later termed NDT. The Bobaths anticipated changes in their approach would be necessary as advances in science occurred. Therefore, it was the intent that their approach would be a "living" concept undergoing change and improvement over time. As motor control theories evolved and more functional activities were encouraged, NDT adapted interventions with an increased emphasis on the task and environmental contexts. Therapists in the clinic, in academic classrooms, or in continuing education courses often pass the techniques orally. The intervention is not standardized, and the therapist adapts activities based on evaluation of the patient's performance and needs. The North American Neurodevelopmental Treatment Association (NDTA) based in the United States establishes changes in NDT theory and resultant techniques and provides a training regime to certify instructors to teach continuing education courses in the approach. In this way, the underlying philosophy is updated to remain current and intervention skills are performed consistently among NDT-trained therapists. NDTA offers 3-week training courses focusing on adult hemiplegia and 8-week courses focusing on babies/children.

Therapists around the world have used NDT extensively for more than 50 years. However, there had been little written information on theory changes, and there was growing confusion among clinicians as they attempted to rectify new information in the movement sciences with the NDT hierarchical approach. There were also changes in health-care delivery with decreased length of hospitalization after a stroke. This required a need for earlier ambulation training for discharge and a greater need for NDT to be provided for patients living in home settings. The Bobaths had expressed concerns about secondary complications of decreased joint mobility and weakness due to the overuse of orthotics, but again with the need for early ambulation, NDT-trained therapists are balancing the need for recovery with functional compensations (Howle, 2002). The ongoing changes in theory, application, and the health-care environment resulted in the NDTA's collaborative effort with a task force and theory committee to publish *Neurodevelopmental Treatment Approach: Theoretical Foundations and Principles of Clinical Practice* (Howle, 2002). A new text has updated Howle's original work (Bierman, 2016). These texts clarify the changes and reflect the current philosophy of NDT.

## Principles and Assumptions of NDT

The Bobath approach is based on the hierarchical theory of motor control. The principles of goal-focused intervention and the need for function are evident in the individualized approach determined by the patient's strengths and needs. Similar to other hierarchical approaches, the Bobaths recognized the need to consider patients in their entirety and examine their function from a cognitive, emotional, and social perspective. An analysis of posture and its effect on function

is a key component in the physical examination. The therapist must observe the patient to identify the constraints and underlying causes of the movement dysfunction then determine the patient needs, which will drive the choice of treatment strategies. NDT-trained therapists advocate the need for hands-on intervention to guide the patient toward normal posture and movement patterns. Therapeutic handling or **key points of control** are graded and withdrawn as the patient progresses. This hands-on approach allows the therapist to feel changing responses to the postures and movements and offer cues to facilitate optimal motions and inhibit movements that will not lead to functional movements (Howle, 2002). The therapist is continually assessing and evaluating the patient's response and adapting the intervention as needed. Practice is a common theme emphasized in all hierarchical models, but the Bobaths thought limitations are enhanced if abnormal movement patterns are practiced, thus the need for manual guidance for correct motions. Input using all sensory systems is another critical component for the development or relearning of motor tasks. In some health-care facilities all providers are trained in the NDT approach, so intervention is integrated throughout the day in all aspects of patient care to promote more practice and generalization across tasks and settings.

The Bobaths deviated from some of the principles of the hierarchical model. The Bobaths, unlike Brunnstrom, did not encourage facilitation of the abnormal synergistic patterns as a part of the recovery process but rather advocated abnormal tone should be inhibited and the patient should experience normal movement to regain function. The Bobaths used balance and equilibrium reactions as automatic movements to activate muscles, but they did not advocate the use of other developmental reflexes to facilitate movement. Although the Bobaths utilized developmental positions, they did not follow the strict sequencing of postures based on the normal developmental progression as originally described in the PNF approach. Assumptions developed by the Bobaths are found in Box 15-2 (Howle, 2002).

The review process in 2002 integrated the Bobaths' original assumptions with the current understanding of movement sciences. These revised assumptions recognize movement is a product of multiple internal systems of the individual, the task, and the environment—a reflection of the systems model of motor control. Spasticity and abnormal movement patterns need to be addressed as well as weakness and impaired postural control. Motions are best learned if they are organized around a functional outcome, which is established in collaboration with the patient and caregivers. Retention of movement patterns requires practice and experience in problem-solving. Patient education, regarding possible changes in function across the lifespan, should be considered when designing plans of care.

## Clinical Applications

NDT intervention will typically begin by addressing postural alignment. This core stability and alignment is critical for the functional use of the extremities. An example of the application

## BOX 15-2 NDT Principles

1. Impaired patterns of postural control and movement coordination are primary problems. Sensorimotor impairments will affect activity and ultimately the level of participation.

2. Motor development changes across the lifespan and recognition of general normal patterns, biomechanics of motion, deviations, and maladaptive motions provides a framework for examination, evaluation, and intervention.

3. Movements are observed and practiced in the context of task and environment. Quality of the movement and variations in practice will lead to improved efficiency.

4. Sensory feedback results from movement and is necessary to perfect motions. Currently, NDT also recognizes the effect of feed-forward controls. The therapist arranges the environment and task and prepares the patient in the best alignment or posture to link the posture and successful motion.

5. Patients must be actively involved and participate in the intervention session. The therapist will provide manual cues to facilitate or inhibit postural alignment and movement.

6. Ongoing evaluation of the patient's performance and reaction to specific tasks is critical during the intervention to allow the therapist to adapt the activities for success.

7. The goal of NDT intervention is to optimize function for the individual's return to participation in life roles. There are periods of transition in development and recovery during which individuals are more receptive to changing motor patterns.

Source: Howle, JM. *Neurodevelopmental Treatment Approach: Theoretical Foundations and Principles of Clinical Practice.* Laguna Beach, CA: Neurodevelopmental Treatment Association; 2002:3–8.

of NDT techniques for a patient to achieve midline short sitting with a neutral pelvis includes an initial request for active movement into the position. If the patient has difficulty with the posture, the therapist will facilitate the movement through a sequence of repeated demonstrations, readjustment of the patient's alignment, alteration of the environment or task, and finally tactile cues. The therapist needs to understand normal biomechanical alignment to offer the tactile cues in the appropriate location and direction. The key point of control may begin near the body part that needs to move for better postural alignment and be progressed distally as the patient gains control. Pressure of the manual contacts will be light or deep depending on the patient's need for facilitation and gradually be withdrawn as the patient gains independence. If facilitation does not result in corrected movements or postures, the therapist needs to reanalyze the problem. Soft tissue mobilization may be required to gain "passive" mobility for the activity. Once the patient has achieved midline erect sitting, he/she needs to maintain the position with isometric control, followed by slow relaxation into trunk flexion with

posterior pelvic tilt, and then a concentric contraction to return to an erect posture. Once the patient has control of moving into and out of the position, the task will be progressed by requesting an increase in speed, increase in weight shift, or altering the task and/or the environment (Al-Oboudi, 1999).

Continuing education courses have been developed that integrate joint mobilization, **therapeutic ball** exercises, or sensory integration techniques with NDT. Sensory cues such as tapping, brushing, and approximation as discussed in the Rood section can be used to facilitate muscle activation. Righting and equilibrium reactions are helpful in supporting weight-shifting postures and may be progressed through the use of a therapeutic ball. NDT concepts regarding midline orientation, trunk control for postural stability, and weight-shifting for transfers and functional tasks can be incorporated and used with a variety of patient populations as normal biomechanics underlie all of these postures and functional movements. Carr and Shepherd (2003) and Ryerson (1997) have written textbooks further demonstrating this integration of NDT activities as it relates to kinesiology and biomechanics.

Subjects with CVA, receiving individualized NDT interventions from NDT-trained therapists, show improvements in diminished tone (Kerem, 2001; Wang, 2005; Hesse, 1995), and improved ADLs (Langhammer, 2000; Wang, 2005; Lennon, 2006). NDT interventions do not appear to prevent shoulder subluxation (Fil, 2011), decrease shoulder pain (Hafsteinsdottir, 2007), or improve most gait parameters, including velocity (Eich, 2004; Hesse, 1995; Lennon, 2006). A systematic review by Kollen (2009) did not find NDT to be superior to other techniques, but there were many methodological shortcomings in the studies.

Children with spastic cerebral palsy appear to consistently improve with NDT intervention. It appears that more frequent treatments and younger children reap greater benefits of NDT (Tsorlakis, 2004; Arndt, 2008). Improvements have been measured through the Gross Motor Function Measure and the Pediatric Evaluation of Disability Inventory (Arndt, 2008; Knox, 2002).

## Proprioceptive Neuromuscular Facilitation (PNF)

### Background/Overview

PNF is an approach to therapeutic exercise originated in the 1940s and 1950s by Herman Kabat, MD; Margaret Knott, PT; and Dorothy Voss, PT. PNF includes movement patterns, basic procedures, specific techniques, and developmental or functional activities that, when used in combination, form a total approach to patient care. Dr. Kabat believed techniques based on current neurophysiologic principles and motor control theories could be applied to the treatment of patients with paralysis (Kabat, 1952). He recruited Maggie Knott, an army-trained physical therapist, to work with him in the development of this new approach to neurological rehabilitation at the Kabat-Kaiser Institute in Washington, DC. They later established a rehabilitation center and PNF training program at the Kaiser Foundation Rehabilitation Center (KFRC) in Vallejo, CA. It was not until after the basic procedures such as manual contacts and quick stretch and the PNF-specific techniques such as **rhythmic initiation (RI)** and **rhythmic stabilization (RS)** were already delineated that Kabat and Knott proposed the PNF movement patterns, a hallmark of this approach. Dorothy Voss joined them at KFRC and collaborated with Maggie Knott to propose motor developmental sequence activities, which could be applied in the rehabilitation of children and adults with neurological involvement. Knott and Voss wrote the first and second edition *Proprioceptive Neuromuscular Facilitation* textbook together (Knott, 1968). Beginning in the 1950s to the present time, 3- and 6-month training programs in PNF have been taught to therapists from all over the world at the KFRC in Vallejo, which has allowed global dissemination of this approach. Knott and Voss also traveled extensively throughout the United States and overseas to teach short courses in this concept, and their work has been carried on by therapists who trained under them (Adler, 2000; Saliba, 1990; Sullivan, 1982; Voss, 1985). These therapists have contributed to the continued growth and evolution of this approach, but this has resulted in some differences in PNF terminology. For example, some therapists may call a technique "repeated contractions" whereas others may call the same technique "**repeated quick stretch**."

The PNF approach is used extensively by therapists with patients who have musculoskeletal and/or neuromuscular dysfunction. The concepts of PNF are used in both examination and intervention and are often integrated with other approaches based on the needs of the patient. For example, rehabilitation of the patient with stroke might combine components of PNF, NDT, and task-oriented training. Comprehensive rehabilitation of a patient with shoulder dysfunction might combine soft tissue mobilization, joint mobilization, PNF for neuromuscular reeducation, and additional therapeutic exercise.

The main philosophy of the PNF approach is that all human beings, including those with disabilities, have untapped potential (Kabat, 1952). The therapist identifies the neuromuscular and musculoskeletal problems of the whole patient and guides them to attain the highest activity and participation level possible (Knott, 1968). In keeping with this overall philosophy, the therapist focuses on and capitalizes on the patient's strengths and not on the observed deficits. This is the basis on which neuromuscular reeducation and functional improvement successfully occur within this approach (Saliba, 1990). Each new movement and functional task learned by the patient is reinforced through repetition and by participation in an appropriately intensive rehabilitation program (Saliba, 1990; Kawahira, 2004).

### *Principles and Concepts*

#### PNF Basic Procedures

The PNF basic procedures are incorporated into all aspects of the approach and are used by the therapist to guide the patient to attain better kinesthetic awareness and more efficient neuromuscular control. For example, the therapist utilizes proper manual contacts and body position for effective application of the PNF movement patterns. The procedures are used to increase patient mobility or stability, guide the patient's movement, facilitate more efficient and coordinated movement through normal timing, and increase range of motion (ROM), strength, and endurance. PNF also allows therapists to incorporate important motor learning principles into intervention through the appropriate use of practice, repetition, visual guidance, and verbal commands.

Certain procedures including manual contacts, body position, appropriate resistance, verbal commands, and vision are incorporated into nearly all PNF interventions, whereas other procedures are employed based on the specific needs of the patient and goals of the task. For example, traction is used to facilitate limb movement, whereas approximation is typically used to facilitate stability of a body segment. As with any facilitation technique, the therapist should withdraw hands-on procedures as the patient begins to move and perform functional tasks more efficiently. The ultimate goal is for the patient to move and problem-solve in varying environments without the benefit of manual contact or verbal cues by the therapist.

Basic PNF procedures are described in Box 15-3.

#### PNF Movement Patterns

The PNF movement patterns are multijoint, diagonal, and rotational movements of the extremities, neck, and trunk. Multiple muscle groups are active during execution of these movement patterns. The PNF movement patterns, described by Kabat (1952) and Knott, were thought to be more characteristic of movements used in daily functional tasks, work, and sport activities than the straight plane exercises advocated in the Kenny Muscle Reeducation Method. Kabat advocated the use of these diagonal movement patterns with patients with neuromuscular or musculoskeletal dysfunction rather than exercising individual muscles in straight plane motions.

There are two diagonals of motion for the UE and two diagonals for the LE. Each diagonal is made up of two movement patterns, one flexion and one extension pattern, which are antagonistic to each other (Adler, 2000; Voss, 1985; Figs. 15-2 and 15-3). At the proximal joint, each extremity pattern has a component of flexion or extension, abduction or adduction, and rotation. The PNF extremity patterns are named for the motions occurring at the proximal joint, either the shoulder or hip. For example, UE flexion/abduction/external rotation (ER) describes the end position of the shoulder after execution of this pattern. Voss added to the nomenclature by calling the diagonals D1 or D2, so PNF UE flexion/abduction/ER pattern is also called PNF UE D2 flexion (Box 15-4). The elbow and knee joints are called intermediate pivots, meaning they can remain straight, flex, or extend during execution of the movement pattern. This allows for a great variety of possible ways to execute each pattern according to the functional needs of the patient and the task goal. Box 15-4 lists the PNF UE and LE movement patterns by their names with associated verbal commands. Figures 15-2 and 15-3 depict all components of

**BOX 15-3 PNF Basic Procedures**

| PNF Basic Procedures | Description of PNF Basic Procedures |
|---|---|
| 1. Manual Contacts | Manual contacts involve placement of the therapist's hands on the patient's body in a carefully determined manner and location. In PNF, the therapist's use of a lumbrical grip to resist and control movement facilitates the appropriate motor response while giving the patient a feeling of security without pain. A lumbrical grip means that the therapist's hand is contoured to the patient's body part with fingers together. The therapist's hand placement on the patient applies pressure in a direction opposite to the patient's motion, which affects the strength of the motor response, and the direction of patient movement. |
| 2. Body Position and Body Mechanics | Good body mechanics and body position allow the therapist to guide the direction of the patient's movement, which is essential for effective application of manual contacts and other basic procedures. The therapist's body position should be in line with the desired motion and facing the diagonal plane or direction of the motion. |
| 3. Quick Stretch | The stretch reflex is elicited by elongating a muscle or synergistic group of muscles to their lengthened range, then quickly overlengthening the muscle to facilitate muscle contraction. Eliciting a quick stretch activates the muscle spindles, which causes contraction of the agonist muscle. The quick stretch is synchronized with a verbal command and is followed immediately by appropriate resistance. |
| 4. Appropriate Resistance | The therapist's manual resistance is equal to or matches the amount of effort exerted by the patient to allow for smooth, coordinated muscle contractions and movement. The amount of resistance applied by the therapist varies through the range of motion of the particular movement pattern, and should be graded to the specific needs of the patient and specific to the type of muscle contraction desired (i.e., concentric, eccentric, or isometric). |
| 5. Verbal Command | Verbal command includes use of the therapist's words and appropriate tone and volume of voice to direct patient movement or stability. Verbal commands should be clear, simple, concise, timed to the physical demand placed on the patient, and specific to the type of muscle contraction desired; for example, push, pull, let go slowly, or hold. |
| 6. Visual Stimuli | Appropriate use of vision assists the patient to learn new activities, identify direction of their motion, identify location of their body in space, and direct motion of the extremities across midline. Vision can be used to compensate for sensory loss and increase patient awareness of involved body parts. Use of vision also encourages the patient to integrate head, neck, and trunk motions while performing functional tasks. |
| 7. Traction | Traction is the manual elongation of a body segment, which facilitates a muscular response and promotes movement. The direction of traction is away from the axis of motion of a joint. For example, traction of the upper extremity is applied by the therapist in a direction away from the shoulder joint toward the hand as the patient elevates their arm. |
| 8. Approximation | Approximation is compression of a joint or body segment, which is used to increase muscular cocontraction and promote stability (Adler, 2000). Approximation is often used to facilitate stability in weight-bearing postures and positions such as in sitting, standing, or all-fours. |
| 9. Timing | Normal timing is the efficient sequencing of muscular recruitment patterns between mobilizer and stabilizer muscles, which results in coordinated movement and function. |

each PNF movement pattern. Figures 15-4 to 15-11 show the beginning and end range position for each extremity pattern as well as hand placements and body mechanics for their implementation.

Each diagonal pattern includes either shoulder girdle or pelvic girdle motion as its most proximal component. These movements are referred to as PNF scapula and pelvic patterns. The PNF scapula and pelvic patterns are a key aspect of this approach and critical in examination and treatment of individuals with both musculoskeletal and neuromuscular dysfunction. For example, when treating a patient with

stroke in the early phases of rehabilitation, the therapist can strengthen the proximal shoulder girdle and improve proximal control and stability using scapula patterns before functional return of distal arm motion occurs. These patterns can be used with patients who have proximal muscle weakness or who lack proximal control and they can be performed in a variety of functional positions. For example, manual contacts and resistance applied at the scapula and pelvis in sitting combined with approximation can be used to improve trunk stability, alignment, and postural control. Figures 15-12 to 15-19 depict the beginning and end range

**PNF UE Movement Patterns**

| UE D1 Flexion | |
| --- | --- |
| Shoulder girdle | Anterior elevation |
| Shoulder | Flexion Adduction External rotation |
| *Elbow | Flexion |
| Forearm | Supination |
| Wrist | Flexion and radial deviation |
| Finger | Radial flexion |
| Thumb | Adduction |

| UE D2 Flexion | |
| --- | --- |
| Shoulder girdle | Posterior elevation |
| Shoulder | Flexion Abduction External rotation |
| *Elbow | Extension |
| Forearm | Supination |
| Wrist | Extension and radial deviation |
| Finger | Radial extension |
| Thumb | Extension |

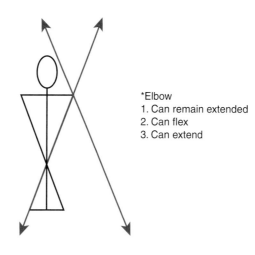

*Elbow
1. Can remain extended
2. Can flex
3. Can extend

| UE D2 Extension | |
| --- | --- |
| Shoulder girdle | Anterior depression |
| Shoulder | Extension Adduction Internal rotation |
| *Elbow | Extension |
| Forearm | Pronation |
| Wrist | Flexion and ulnar deviation |
| Finger | Ulnar flexion |
| Thumb | Opposition |

| UE D1 Extension | |
| --- | --- |
| Shoulder girdle | Posterior depression |
| Shoulder | Extension Abduction Internal rotation |
| *Elbow | Extension |
| Forearm | Pronation |
| Wrist | Extension and ulnar deviation |
| Finger | Ulnar extension |
| Thumb | Abduction |

Movement Pattern diagrams developed by Jeannie Stephenson, PT, PhD, NCS. Adapted from diagrams originally developed by Sue Adler, PT and by Greg Johnson, PT, CFMT and Vicki Saliba Johnson, PT, CFMT of the Institute of Physical Art.

**FIGURE 15-2** PNF Upper Extremity Patterns.

## PNF LE Movement Patterns

| LE D1 Flexion | |
| --- | --- |
| Pelvic girdle | Anterior elevation |
| Hip | Flexion<br>Adduction<br>External rotation |
| *Knee | Flexion |
| Ankle | Dorsiflexion<br>Inversion |
| Toe | Extension |

| LE D2 Flexion | |
| --- | --- |
| Pelvic girdle | Posterior elevation |
| Hip | Flexion<br>Abduction<br>Internal rotation |
| *Knee | Flexion |
| Ankle | Dorsiflexion<br>Eversion |
| Toe | Extension |

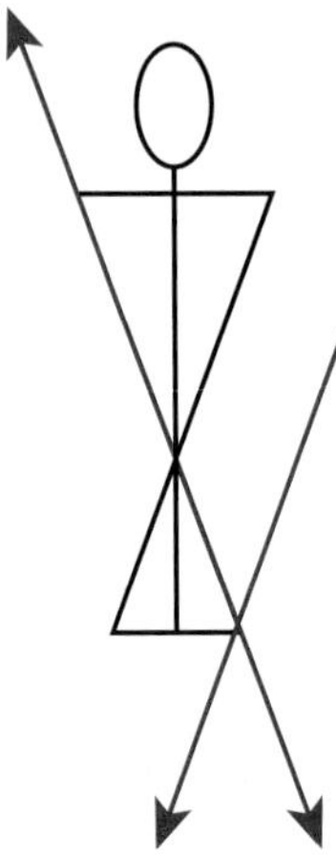

*Knee
1. Can remain extended
2. Can flex
3. Can extend

| LE D2 Extension | |
| --- | --- |
| Pelvic girdle | Anterior depression |
| Hip | Extension<br>Adduction<br>External rotation |
| *Knee | Extension |
| Ankle | Plantar flexion<br>Inversion |
| Toe | Flexion |

| LE D1 Extension | |
| --- | --- |
| Pelvic girdle | Posterior depression |
| Hip | Extension<br>Abduction<br>Internal rotation |
| *Knee | Extension |
| Ankle | Plantar flexion<br>Eversion |
| Toe | Flexion |

Movement Pattern diagrams developed by Jeannie Stephenson, PT, PhD, NCS. Adapted from diagrams originally developed by Sue Adler, PT and by Greg Johnson, PT, CFMT and Vicki Saliba Johnson, PT, CFMT of the Institute of Physical Art.

**FIGURE 15-3** PNF Lower Extremity Patterns.

positions and manual contacts for each scapula and pelvic pattern.

PNF movement patterns can be performed either unilaterally or bilaterally. A therapist can combine use of extremity patterns for the arms or legs into bilateral symmetrical, bilateral asymmetrical, or bilateral reciprocal patterns. Bilateral asymmetrical extremity patterns are used to incorporate motion of the head, neck, and trunk with those of the extremities. For example, the chopping pattern in sitting involves the lead arm moving into UE D1 extension (UE ext/abd/IR) with assist from the other arm, while the neck and trunk move into flexion with rotation. This activity is used to facilitate trunk flexion and rotation in patients with trunk flexor weakness or with patients who have difficulty reaching toward the floor, for example, to tie their shoes. The lifting pattern involves the lead arm moving

## BOX 15-4  PNF Extremity Movement Patterns

(Once the pattern has been explained and practiced, it is best to use simple single-word commands such as "push" or "pull" as appropriate.)

### PNF UE Movement Patterns—listed by name and verbal command

1. UE Flexion/Adduction/ER = UE D1 Flexion
   - Verbal command (VC) = "squeeze and pull up and in"
2. UE Extension/Abduction/IR = UE D1 Extension
   - VC = "open your hand and push down and out"
3. UE Flexion/Abduction/ER = UE D2 Flexion
   - VC = "open your hand and lift up and out"
4. UE Extension/Adduction/IR = UE D2 Extension
   - VC = "squeeze and pull down and across"

### PNF LE Movement Patterns—listed by name and verbal command

1. LE Flexion/Adduction/ER = LE D1 Flexion
   - VC = "toes up and pull your leg up and in"
2. LE Extension/Abduction/IR = LE D1 Extension
   - VC = "point your toes down and push your leg down and out"
3. LE Flexion/Abduction/IR = LE D2 Flexion
   - VC = "toes up and lift your leg up and out"
4. LE Extension/Adduction/ER = LE D2 Extension
   - VC = "point your toes and push your leg down and in"

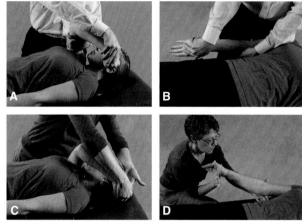

FIGURE 15-5 **A.** Beginning and **B.** end position for PNF Upper Extremity D1 Extension Pattern (UE Extension, Abduction, Internal Rotation) with the therapist standing at the patient's side and pivoting throughout the movement. Note that the end position should include a distal manual contact in which the therapist uses counter pressure of the thumb and fifth digit to create rotational torque turning the hand toward supination, while the patient pushes into pronation to complete the motion. The therapist could also stand in the diagonal at hip level with the arm as shown for the **C.** start (note that the therapist's left hand is not in contact with the patient's hand at the start of this extension pattern, but is prepared to move into contact on the lateral extensor surface after the movement is initiated) and **D.** end of the pattern with the arm moving directly toward the therapist.

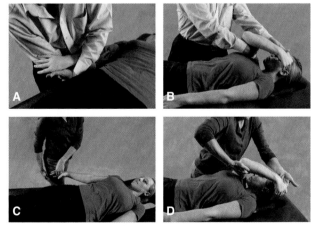

FIGURE 15-4 **A.** Beginning and **B.** end position for PNF Upper Extremity D1 Flexion Pattern (UE Flexion, Adduction, External Rotation) with the therapist standing at the patient's side and pivoting throughout the movement. The therapist could also stand in the diagonal at hip level with the arm as shown for the **C.** start (should begin the pattern in full wrist extension) and **D.** end of the pattern with the arm moving directly away from the therapist. A firmer grip on the hand will give the therapist better control throughout the pattern.

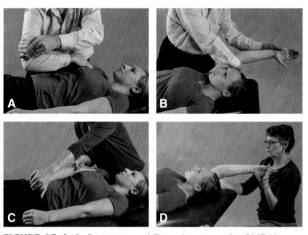

FIGURE 15-6 **A.** Beginning and **B.** end position for PNF Upper Extremity D2 Flexion Pattern (UE Flexion, Abduction, External Rotation) with the therapist standing at the patient's side and pivoting throughout the movement. Note that the proximal contact is wrapped around on the arm's lateral surface to resist abduction and extension. The therapist could also stand in the diagonal, above the patient's head, with the arm as shown for the **C.** start and **D.** end of the pattern with the arm moving directly toward the therapist. Note that for better control with the distal manual contact at end-range in 15-6D, the therapist could add a rotational resistance at the wrist/hand to turn the forearm toward pronation as the patient pushes into supination.

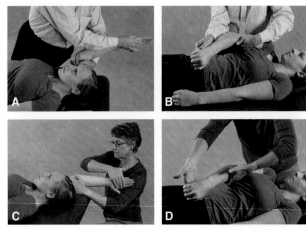

**FIGURE 15-7  A.** Beginning and **B.** end position for PNF Upper Extremity D2 Extension Pattern (UE Extension, Adduction, Internal Rotation) with the therapist standing at the patient's side and pivoting throughout the movement. Note that the distal manual contact is applying resistance with the therapist's second and third digits to push into wrist extension and counterpressure of the two digits against the thumb for supination, as the patient pushes into wrist and finger flexion, and forearm pronation. The therapist could also stand in the diagonal, above the patient's head, with the arm as shown for the **C.** start and **D.** end of the pattern with the arm moving directly away from the therapist. Note that in 15-7 C&D, a stronger distal manual contact will give the therapist greater control and increased resistance.

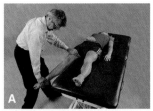
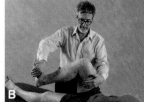

**FIGURE 15-8  A.** Beginning and **B.** end position for PNF Lower Extremity D1 Flexion Pattern (LE Flexion, Adduction, External Rotation).

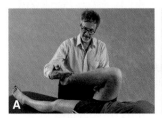
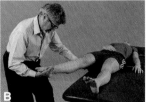

**FIGURE 15-9  A.** Beginning and **B.** end position for PNF Lower Extremity D1 Extension Pattern (LE Extension, Abduction, Internal Rotation). Note that as the leg completes the pattern in 15-9B and moves into full extension, the therapist will need to squat further to stay below the movement and in the diagonal, with use of leg muscles to power the resistance pushing toward the ceiling with proximal contact.

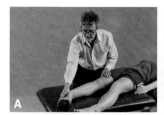
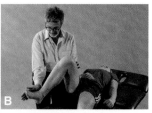

**FIGURE 15-10  A.** Beginning and **B.** end position for PNF Lower Extremity D2 Flexion Pattern (LE Flexion, Abduction, Internal Rotation).

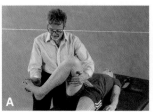
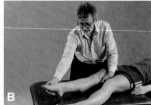

**FIGURE 15-11  A.** Beginning and **B.** end position for PNF Lower Extremity D2 Extension Pattern (LE Extension, Adduction, External Rotation). Note that the therapist should avoid contact with the medial aspect of the inferior foot. Upward resistance on the lateral inferior foot will provide a dorsiflexion, eversion force to stimulate activation of patient's plantar flexors and invertors.

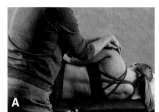
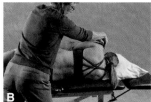

**FIGURE 15-12  A.** Beginning and **B.** end position for PNF Scapula Anterior Elevation Pattern.

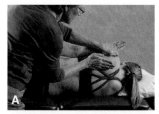
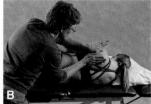

**FIGURE 15-13  A.** Beginning and **B.** end position for PNF Scapula Posterior Depression Pattern.

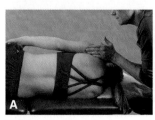
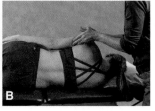

**FIGURE 15-14  A.** Beginning and **B.** end position for PNF Scapula Anterior Depression Pattern.

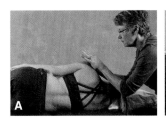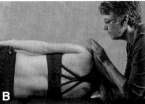

FIGURE 15-15  **A.** Beginning and **B.** end position for PNF Scapula Posterior Elevation Pattern.

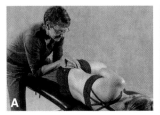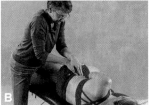

FIGURE 15-16  **A.** Beginning and **B.** end position for PNF Pelvic Anterior Elevation Pattern.

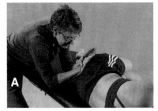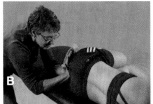

FIGURE 15-17  **A.** Beginning and **B.** end position for PNF Pelvic Posterior Depression Pattern. While difficult to see here, note that in the end position, the manual contacts include the heels of bilateral hands overlapped, directly on the ischial tuberosity.

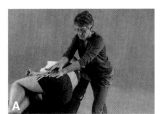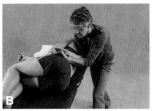

FIGURE 15-18  **A.** Beginning and **B.** end position for PNF Pelvic Posterior Elevation Pattern.

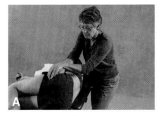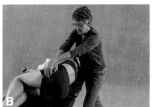

FIGURE 15-19  **A.** Beginning and **B.** end position for PNF Pelvic Anterior Depression Pattern. Note that for this pattern, the manual contacts are near the ischial tuberosity to pull up and back.

into UE D2 flexion (UE flex/abd/ER) with assist from the opposite arm, while the neck and trunk move into extension with rotation (Fig. 15-20). This activity could be used to encourage more upright sitting in patients with trunk extensor muscle weakness or rounded trunk posture, such as individuals with PD. PNF scapula and pelvic patterns can also be combined with extremity patterns for greater emphasis on the proximal component of the pattern. For example, Figure 15-21 shows the PNF pelvic posterior depression pattern combined with resistance to the LE D1 extension pattern.

## PNF Specific Techniques

PNF specific techniques are used, along with the movement patterns, to examine and treat neuromuscular control problems including difficulty initiating movement or controlling the speed, direction, or timing of movement. Depending on which technique is selected, they are used to increase muscle strength and endurance, increase ROM, and improve the ability to perform different types of muscle contractions. Ultimately, improvement in these areas allows the patient to adjust to different functional demands. Using a PNF approach, the therapist conducts a thorough history and objective examination,

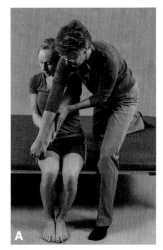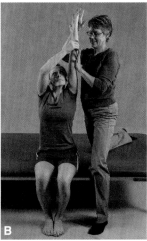

FIGURE 15-20  **A.** Beginning and **B.** end position for PNF Upper Extremity Lifting Pattern in Sitting (Example of a bilateral asymmetrical UE pattern).

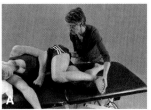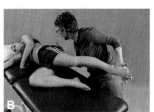

FIGURE 15-21  **A.** Beginning and **B.** end position for PNF Pelvic Posterior Depression Combined with LE D1 Extension Pattern (LE Extension, Abduction, Internal Rotation).

including assessment of functional tasks, and a plan of care is established. An important principle of PNF is that examination is an ongoing process throughout the episode of care. The therapist is continually reassessing the patient and adapting the procedures, techniques, movement patterns, and functional tasks according to the changing needs of the patient. The PNF specific techniques are described as follows:

1. **Rhythmic Initiation (RI)**—RI is a facilitating technique used to treat patients who have difficulty initiating or controlling the speed, direction, and/or quality of movement. This technique can also be used to teach the patient a new movement. Application of RI involves the therapist passively moving the patient's body part through the available ROM until complete muscular relaxation is felt. The therapist then asks the patient to gradually take over active control of the movement until the patient is able to move through the entire movement pattern against appropriate resistance. Verbal commands can be used to establish speed and rhythm of the movement. RI may be applied unidirectionally or bidirectionally (i.e., using one or both movement patterns within the same diagonal).

2. **Combination of Isotonics (COI), also called Agonist Reversals (AR)**—This facilitating technique was developed and described by Saliba, Johnson, and Wardlaw (1990). COI is used to assess and treat the patient's ability to perform and alternate between different types of muscle contractions with a focus on eccentrics. COI is used to increase joint ROM, improve strength, and improve coordination of movement. To apply this technique, the therapist resists a concentric contraction of the agonist muscle group followed by a stabilizing contraction of the same muscle group. The therapist then resists an eccentric lengthening contraction as the patient slowly moves back toward the start position.

3. **Repeated Contractions (RC)** also called **Repeated Quick Stretch (RQS)** —These facilitating techniques involve repetitive use of the stretch reflex to initiate a muscular contraction or to reinforce and strengthen an existing muscle contraction. These techniques are used to increase active ROM of the agonist, to achieve relaxation of the antagonist, and to improve strength and endurance of the agonist. There are two types of RQS techniques. Quick stretch can be applied at the initiation of the movement with the muscle in a lengthened range, followed by the therapist's manual resistance to the patient's active movement. The part is then passively returned to the elongated position and the process is repeated again to reinforce initiation of movement. Repeated quick stretch can also be applied at any point in the available ROM to strengthen a weak muscle

group and promote movement further into the diagonal pattern.

4. **Reversal of Antagonist Techniques (ROA)**—The purpose of this category of techniques is to promote coordinated control between antagonistic muscle groups and to promote smooth reversal of direction of movement. The ROA techniques (isotonic reversals, alternating isometrics, and stabilizing reversals) are based on Sherrington's principle of successive induction. In successive induction, maximum contraction of the antagonist muscle reciprocally inhibits the agonist. When the antagonist relaxes, this inhibition ceases and facilitation of the agonist occurs.

5. **Slow Reversals (SR) also called Isotonic Reversals (IR)**—This technique is designed to facilitate alternating, concentric contractions of antagonistic muscle groups within the same diagonal pattern. It is used to develop normal reversal of movement or to facilitate the agonist following contraction of its antagonist muscle. Slow reversal involves the therapist applying appropriate resistance to a concentric contraction of the agonist muscle group. The therapist then smoothly shifts manual contacts and resistance to the antagonist muscles within the same diagonal with no relaxation. Finally, the therapist shifts back to the agonist pattern to see if the patient can perform with increased active ROM or strength. There are variations of the SR technique including working in smaller to larger increments of the ROM or varying the speed of movement. The therapist may also include an isometric "holding" contraction at end range prior to the reversal of direction of movement; referred to as **Slow Reversal Hold**.

6. **Alternating Isometrics (AI)**—This technique is used to improve isometric strength of postural muscles of the trunk or proximal stabilizing muscles of the limbs. The therapist applies manual resistance in one plane on one side of the body followed by a smooth shift in resistance to the opposite side of the body or body segment. Resistance is smoothly alternated from one body surface to the opposite surface while the patient is asked to "hold" their position with no relaxation. Alternating isometrics can be applied to one or more limbs or to the trunk, often in weight-bearing positions.

7. **Rhythmic Stabilization (RS), also called Stabilizing Reversals**—This technique is used to improve patient's postural control, balance, and stability in various functional, weight-bearing positions such as sitting or standing. The therapist begins the technique by gradually increasing resistance with both hands which are placed on opposite body surfaces, using verbal commands such as "hold" or "don't let me move you." One hand then slowly releases and moves to another body surface while the therapist always maintains contact and resistance with at least one hand.

The hands are alternated gradually from one body surface to the other, with no relaxation allowed, but with a strong focus on resisting rotation.

8. **Contract Relax (CR)**—The purpose of this inhibitory technique is to achieve relaxation of muscles antagonistic to the active muscle group to increase ROM into the agonist movement pattern. For example, active contraction of the triceps results in simultaneous inhibition and elongation of shortened biceps. In this case, the antagonist is the range-limiting muscle, while the agonist refers to the muscle opposite the range-limiting muscle (Sharman, 2006). To apply this technique, the therapist moves the part passively to the point of ROM limitation in the agonist pattern. A maximum isotonic contraction of the antagonist is performed by the patient against therapist resistance. All components of the pattern are resisted but only a few degrees of motion are allowed to occur, particularly in rotation. The patient is then asked to completely relax followed by active movement into the newly acquired range of agonist motion. The CR technique is repeated until the maximum gain in ROM (tolerable to the patient) is attained.

9. **Hold Relax (HR)**—This inhibitory technique is also used to achieve relaxation and increase ROM, but of the muscles active in the agonist pattern itself, particularly when there is pain or when the patient may be able to overpower the therapist with CR. In the example of shortened biceps, HR includes an active isometric contraction of the bicep, followed by relaxation and elongation during the relaxation phase. The therapist moves the limb passively to the point of limitation of the shortened muscle, then asks the patient to perform an isometric contraction of the shortened muscle at this point of limitation. The therapist slowly increases resistance to the isometric muscle contraction, not allowing motion to occur, then asks the patient to relax completely, and finally moves the limb passively further into the newly acquired ROM of the agonist pattern until a new point of limitation is felt. As in CR, HR is repeated a few times until the maximum gain in ROM (tolerable to the patient) is attained. Resisted motion into the newly acquired agonist pattern can be used to further reinforce ROM gains attained with HR and CR. This variation on the relaxation techniques is referred to as Agonist Contraction and results in additional passive stretch to the range-limiting muscle (Sharman, 2006).

CR and HR techniques are thought to work through the neurophysiologic principles of reciprocal inhibition and autogenic inhibition in which muscle contraction by the patient can be either into the range limitation or in the opposite direction. **Autogenic inhibition** is inhibition of the agonist alpha motor neurons because of stimulation of

Golgi tendon organs (Spernoga, 2001). This decreases agonist muscle activity and allows the muscle to relax so it can be stretched, thus increasing passive and active ROM. **Reciprocal inhibition**, on the other hand, is decreased activity of the antagonist when its agonist is active, which also allows more active ROM into the agonist pattern. Recently, it has been proposed that lengthening of the range-limiting muscle and lasting improvement in ROM following PNF HR and CR techniques may be due to more complex central and peripheral neurophysiological mechanisms and effects on the musculotendinous unit (Sharman, 2006).

Research evidence exists to support the use of certain PNF movement patterns and specific techniques (Kofotolis, 2006; Kofotolis, 2008; Marek, 2005; Markos, 1979; Moore, 1991; Spernoga, 2001; Sullivan, 1980). Much of this research has focused on musculoskeletal applications of PNF and not on neuromuscular applications. For example, contract-relax and hold-relax techniques and their efficacy to increase joint ROM and flexibility in populations with musculoskeletal dysfunction has been studied extensively and substantiated (Davis, 2005; Ferber, 2002; Moore, 1991; Osternig, 1990; Spernoga, 2001; Winters, 2004; Worrell, 1994). Research evidence to support the use of PNF patterns and techniques with neuromuscular populations is more limited (Armutla, 2001; Dickstein, 1986; Duncan, 1998; Kawahira, 2004; Kim, 2011; Kraft, 1992; Nakamura, 1986; Trueblood, 1989; Wang, 1994). Wang (1994) found that gait speed and cadence improved in subjects with acute stroke after 12 sessions of resisted PNF pelvic patterns along with RI, slow reversal and agonist reversal techniques. Trueblood (1989) compared gait parameters of 20 individuals with acute stroke before and after resisted pelvic patterns. She found statistically significant improvements in stance stability and limb advancement of the involved lower extremity following treatment, but no change in gait velocity.

### Developmental and Functional Aspects of the PNF Approach

Knott and Voss described a developmental sequence of tasks that could be used clinically with patients. They described the therapeutic use of developmental sequence activities that were selected and adapted from the work of both Gesell (1947) and McGraw (1945). The PNF developmental sequence includes rolling; the prone progression as in pivoting, crawling, creeping and plantigrade walking; rising to kneeling and knee-walking; rising to stand and bipedal walking; ascending and descending stairs; running; jumping; hopping; and skipping. Progression of treatment activities was in accordance with progression through the stages of normal motor developmental sequences when working with a child (Knott, 1968). This is no longer done in lock-step fashion, but rather follows the principle of reciprocal interweaving which states that development proceeds not as a linear process, but in a continuous spiral (Heriza,

1991). For example, it is not necessary for a child to perfect rolling before working on sitting skills but rather development of the two milestones may be occurring at the same time. The goal of PNF developmental activities with a child is independence in age-appropriate sensorimotor developmental milestones and functional skills.

Adults are not expected to recapitulate the motor developmental sequence in rehabilitation but rather to practice tasks of functional importance to them in their daily lives. The focus with adults includes tasks such as rolling, sitting, sit to/from stand, walking, running, and negotiating stairs. PNF intervention involves both **part task** and **whole task training**. In other words, it is felt that working with patients on components of rolling on the mat may carry over to the whole task of rolling. Likewise, gait is sometimes broken down into component parts, such as weight-shifting onto one leg in standing and stepping forward and back with the opposite leg. This allows the patient to work on weight shift, weight acceptance, and weight-bearing on the involved leg without having to coordinate the whole gait task. The whole task of walking is then practiced within the same treatment session. There is some limited research evidence for the use of part task training and its transfer to a continuous task such as walking (Kawahira, 2004; Stephenson, 2014; Trueblood, 2003; Wang, 1994). This is in contrast to research evidence showing that only practice of the entire task of walking (whole task training) has functional carryover to gait (Langhammer, 2000; Richards, 1993; Salbach, 2004).

In the developmental aspect of the PNF approach, therapists alter patient position utilizing manual contacts and movement patterns of body parts. Balance and stability are developed in the new position before movement again leads to progression to another activity. The therapist guides the patient's assumption of a position, facilitates stability in the new position, works on weight shift in the position, and finally guides skilled mobility. For example, when treating a child with CP, the therapist guides the child's attainment of the quadruped position first. The therapist promotes stability in the all-fours position, often utilizing approximation and RS to the trunk, then resists weight shifts in quadruped as the child rocks side-to-side and forward and back. Finally, the therapist guides and resists the child's progression to creeping in the all-fours position.

### Clinical Applications

The previous example described the progression from attainment of quadruped to creeping for a child with CP. Another example of the clinical application of PNF involves a patient with acute stroke who has a functional goal of moving from lying on the bed to standing. Assumption of the position may begin with the patient in sidelying on the edge of the bed. The therapist assists or resists pelvic posterior depression pattern on the involved side as the patient lowers both legs over the edge of the bed and sits up. Once in sitting, the therapist assesses and facilitates neutral alignment of the patient's head

and trunk in sitting as well as symmetrical weight-bearing, utilizing manual contacts at the pelvis and shoulder girdles. Once neutral trunk alignment is attained, approximation and the RS technique are applied to build stability around the trunk in the sitting position. The therapist then resists the patient's forward and lateral weight shifts with manual contacts at the pelvis or shoulder girdles. The patient's lateral weight shifts to one side unweight the opposite side, allowing forward scoots of the pelvis toward the edge of the bed. The patient is then taught to flex the trunk forward at the hips to get weight forward off the sacrum onto the thighs and feet in preparation for coming to standing. The therapist can apply guidance, assistance, or resistance with manual contacts at the pelvis or shoulder girdles as the patient comes to standing. The patient is guided to keep weight progressing forward over both feet and to stand up with symmetrical LE weight-bearing. This clinical example demonstrates the combined use of PNF basic procedures, movement patterns, specific techniques, and progression of a functional task (sit-to-stand) within one therapy session with a neurological client.

## ■ Task-Oriented Approaches to Intervention

Task-oriented approaches have a common element of utilizing functional activities as a primary component of the intervention session. These activities have been utilized by therapists for a number of years as patients perform ADL, maneuver through a door with crutches, practice sit-to-stand from various surfaces, or children participate in therapeutic play activities. As the Dynamic Systems Theory became prominent in the 1980s, there was an increased focus on the individual, task, and the environment as components of the intervention. The task-oriented approach requires the patient to actively participate in defining task goals, problem-solve as needed to manipulate the environment or task for goal completion, and perform these activities in the most typical environment or surroundings where they function on a daily basis. **Task-oriented interventions** can range from repetition of component parts of functional tasks to completion of obstacle courses requiring problem-solving skills. New treatment regimes such as LT on a treadmill and **constraint-induced movement therapy (CIMT)** have been developed, and the literature refers to them as task-oriented interventions (Sterr, 2002). The similarities between supported ambulation on a treadmill versus functional ambulation outside on grass can be debated, but a progression toward completion of a functional task in the typical environment is the ultimate goal. In summary, due to the range of parameters for task-oriented activities, a critical analysis of the definitions for task-oriented interventions should be a component in any appraisal of literature to insure a clear understanding of the research. The following section will describe several approaches utilizing a task-oriented approach for functional training.

# Concepts of Motor Relearning Programme

## Background/Overview

Janet Carr and Roberta Shepherd, both physical therapists, did extensive reading of the literature from all fields of science related to movement and developed a theoretical approach for assessment and intervention called **Motor Relearning Programme** (MRP; Carr, 1987). Their early work was focused on individuals after a stroke, but later publications acknowledge its use with any individual with movement disorders. Carr and Shepherd state the primary role of physiotherapy is the "...training of motor control based on an understanding of the kinematics and kinetics of normal movement, motor control processes, and motor learning" (Carr, 1987, p. 4). The intervention techniques are eclectic, drawing from NDT with the use of weight-bearing positions and pregait activities to facilitate ambulation. Facilitation techniques of tapping, ice, and vibration described by Rood are incorporated to enhance motor relearning. Inclusion of righting and equilibrium reactions for balance may be accomplished with balance equipment such as balance discs or therapeutic ball. Carr and Shepherd describe the use of biofeedback, splinting, and unweighted ambulation in their approach. To apply the framework of the MRP into the clinic setting, Carr and Shepherd also developed a motor assessment scale for individuals with stroke (Carr, 1987).

## Principles and Assumptions of Motor Relearning Programme

The MRP is based on current research concepts of motor control and motor learning. Some of the underlying assumptions are similar to the principles of the hierarchical theory. Individuals need to understand the goal and practice the task to limit unnecessary muscle activity. Current assumptions that sensory input modulates movement, and that anticipatory feedback and postural control are critical for extremity movement have been incorporated into the approach. MRP also places a strong emphasis on practice within varied environments and the kinematics of motion. The therapist must consider the effect of the adaptations of muscle and joint alignment based on the task, environmental context, the beginning body position, the previous motor task, and gravity. MRP places a high value on the therapist's ability to critically analyze the motion and problem-solve to determine the best intervention parameters for successful goal completion. The patient must actively participate through a cognitive understanding of the goal and the ability to follow instructions and learn through practice.

Carr and Shephard's MRP is considered to be a task-oriented approach and has been called movement-science based (MSB) activities by some (van Vliet, 2005). A literature review comparing NDT to MRP approaches suggests similarities such as the need for early intervention and discouragement of compensatory movements of the nonhemiplegic extremities. Differences between the two techniques include normalization of tone and manual facilitation purported by Bobath versus the use of task-specific exercises for function and a greater use of cognitive strategies in the task-oriented intervention (Lettinga, 1999). Analyzed observed behaviors of therapists using NDT and MSB approaches revealed those using the NDT approach engaged in more social conversation, used therapeutic equipment to a larger extent, and practiced ambulation skills more than the MSB therapists. The therapists using MSB provided more detailed feedback, used everyday objects in the session, evaluated specific components of movement, and had a greater emphasis on sit-to-stand tasks (van Vliet, 2005).

## Clinical Applications

Awareness of normal kinematics of movement and the ability to observe and analyze the patterns used by patients in functional tasks is the first component of applying MRP to a patient population. The reader is referred to both Carr and Shepherd's textbooks (1987 and 2003) and *Functional Movement Reeducation* by Ryerson and Levit (1997) for a review of kinesiology and typical movement patterns of patients after a stroke. A progression of the application of MRP is evident in the newer text by Carr and Shepherd (2003) and displays the need for vigilance and constant integration of current research with interventions. Box 15-5 identifies components of MRP intervention.

Balance training will be used as an example of clinical application of MRP. Focus needs to be placed on the ability to control the body mass during voluntary actions in sitting, stance, and ambulation. The individual needs to respond quickly to both anticipated and unanticipated perturbations. A complete analysis of the underlying impairments may include vision, strength, flexibility, and sensation along with observation in stance during reaching and weight-shifting. An understanding of the causes of the dysfunction and compensatory patterns will provide insight as to what impairments need to be addressed and the amount of assistance needed. If the patient is unable to maintain support over an extended LE while standing, the therapist may utilize a knee splint or a trunk harness support system. This will allow practice without the patient's fear of falling and allow for increased sensation and strengthening of the LE. The therapist is providing ongoing verbal, visual, and manual guidance during the intervention techniques. Balance seems to be task specific and

---

**BOX 15-5 Components of the MRP Approach to Intervention**

Step 1: Observation and analysis of the task

Step 2: Practice of the missing components with feedback

Step 3: Practice of the task with feedback and ongoing reevaluation

Step 4: Transference of training in varied environments to enhance consistency

Adapted from: Carr JH, Shepherd RB. *A Motor Relearning Programme for Stroke*, 2nd edition. Rockville, MD: Aspen Publishers; 1987, pg 31.

practice is required under a variety of environmental conditions. Function will be incorporated by asking the patient to turn to look at an opening door or to look up at the ceiling or walls to locate a target. Foot position can be narrowed in standing during reaching activities in all planes as a way to progress the activity. Single leg stance is initiated by taking a step to reach an object or stepping up onto stools of varied heights, once again in all planes. As better balance is achieved, the patient is asked to ambulate in a variety of directions, pick objects up from the floor, and finally combine movements such as stepping onto a stool while reaching for an object in an overhead cupboard. A further progression is the addition of practice in an open or changing environment such as catching a ball while standing on a foam surface or carrying a cup of water through an obstacle course (Shumway-Cook, 2007).

## Constraint-Induced Movement Therapy

### Background/Overview

The concept for CIMT was introduced in 1980 by Taub and addresses the **learned nonuse** of an involved UE after a central nervous system lesion. Learned nonuse is observed in a clinic setting as the patient is unsuccessful in completing tasks with the hemiplegic extremity and learns to compensate with the noninvolved extremity. Therefore, they are learning not to use the hemiplegic UE to independently complete functional tasks. Taub's early work found that monkeys were able to regain use of a de-afferented limb after restraint of the uninvolved extremity for several days, which forced use of the involved extremity for functional activities (Taub, 1980). He transferred this design to human subjects with stroke in developing a constraint-induced protocol (Taub, 2003). Interest and use of this intervention has increased as research has continued to support its efficacy. Recent advances in the ability to measure neural plasticity after cerebrovascular accident (CVA) has provided more credence to the effectiveness of this approach as changes in the organization of the motor cortex are evident and correlate with improved patient function (Boake, 2007; Dong, 2007; Szaflarski, 2006).

The **forced use** of the hemiparetic UE is accomplished by restraining the unaffected UE with the use of a mitt, glove, hand splint, or arm sling for a specified period of time each day. The most typical protocol suggests restraint for 90% of the time the patient is awake (Taub, 2006; Taub, 2007), including therapy for 6 hours per day (with a 1-hour rest period) for 10 to 14 consecutive workdays during a 2-week period for practice in using the affected UE. The patient is asked to use the involved UE to perform repetitive gross motor and fine motor tasks, which are progressed as the patient improves. They also perform behavior **shaping activities,** described as multiple-trial practice of meaningful functional tasks such as brushing hair, drinking from a cup, picking up coins and placing them in a cup, or unlocking a door. These activities begin in achievable forms (e.g., movement through smaller range, movement of fewer joints, less work, fewer repetitions) but then gradually progress so they look more and

more like the target functional task. The therapist provides physical assistance and frequent verbal cuing and encouragement while the patient practices (Taub, 2006; Taub, 2007). The final component of CIMT is transferring the functional exercises practiced during therapy into the home or work environment. To monitor exercise and use of the constraint outside of the therapy setting, the patient may be requested to maintain a log of restraint time and activities performed with the affected UE (Bonifer, 2003; Rijntjes, 2005; Shaw, 2005; Wittenberg, 2003). Perhaps most important is the use of a behavioral contract, developed by the therapist in collaboration with the patient, which the patient/caregiver must sign to indicate their full agreement with the study protocol and the prescribed limited use of the less-affected extremity. Patient buy-in is extremely important to the consistent massed practice of using the affected extremity.

Research has indicated compliance is a concern due to the patient's level of frustration, time commitment, poor endurance, and the need for family support (Page, 2002). Therapists have commented on their hesitation to implement this approach in therapy given the lack of patients who exhibit the necessary active movement described in the protocol, the lack of staffing to offer feedback and support for 6 to 7 hours of patient practice, and concerns regarding reimbursement (Page, 2002; Page, 2008). Due to these concerns, modified CIMT (mCIMT) protocols have been suggested. One example of a mCIMT protocol is 30-minute sessions, 3 days/week of structured functional practice with a therapist while restraining the affected UE for 5 hours, 5 days/week, over 10 weeks (Page, 2002; Page, 2008). While both CIMT and mCIMT are "forced use" of the involved extremity, the literature has described an alternative protocol as forced use. Forced use calls for the restraint of the uninvolved UE and performance of various exercises and tasks with the hemiplegic UE without the intensive one-to-one training in therapy (Bonnier, 2006; Hammer, 2009; Ploughman, 2004; Willis, 2002).

### Principles and Clinical Applications

Overall, the research has indicated positive improvements, and no significant adverse effects, with the use of CIMT and mCIMT (Peurala, 2012; Stevenson, 2012; McIntyre, 2012; Shi, 2011). Additional research is needed to determine which patients would most benefit from constraint, the specific treatment protocols, and the relationship of clinical improvements to function. The side of hemiplegia, time since onset of the CVA, hand dominance, sensory deficit, previous therapy, age, sex, and ambulatory status do not affect the outcomes (Fritz, 2006; Rijntjes, 2005). This has led to the conclusion that no one should be eliminated from a trial of CIMT as it appears to be effective for a large group of individuals with CVA (Fritz, 2006). Because these demographics and factors do not affect the success of CIMT or mCIMT, does the severity of movement in the involved UE affect the outcome?

Most studies use one of two similar inclusionary criteria regarding UE function. Originally, Taub required all of the subjects to display active motion of 10 degrees in the metacarpal phalangeal joints (MCP) and the intercarpal phalangeal joints (ICP) and 20 degrees of wrist extension. Recently, other researchers have used CIMT on patients with more severely involved UEs. One study used a protocol requiring active motion of 10 degrees of wrist extension, 10 degrees of thumb abduction, and 10 degrees extension of any two other digits (Shaw, 2005). Approximately 75% of patients with CVA are expected to fall into this group. A limited number of studies have reported improvements with the most severely involved patients. The inclusion criteria were limited to the ability to lift and release a wash cloth with any available hand motion. (Bonifer, 2005a; Rijntjes, 2005). Shaping activities with the restraint are critical for the more involved individuals while subjects with better UE movement at the beginning of a study trial may benefit from restraint alone. Another study found the ability to extend the fingers and release was the only variable related to the Wolf Motor Function Test (WMFT) scores (Fritz, 2005). Wrist extension was not related to change after CIMT and, therefore, may not be a necessary inclusion criteria for patients to participate in CIMT (Fritz, 2005).

The time since the onset of the stroke does not appear to have an effect on improvement with CIMT or mCIMT, yet the question lingers as to what is the best time to initiate treatment. Early research on rats resulted in a worsening of the lesion when they were treated with CIMT shortly after the cortical lesion (Risedal, 1999). Recently Dromerick (2009) reported individuals with a mean of 9.65 days after a CVA who underwent CIMT with 3 hours/day of shaping and the use of a mitt for 90% of waking hours had significantly less motor recovery in the involved hand than those receiving a shortened application of CIMT with 2 hours/day of shaping exercises and a mitt for 6 hours/day. The specific protocol and time spent in the constraint may be a factor in people with acute stroke. A few studies agree that both CIMT and traditional therapy result in significant improvement in the acute CVA when treatment is started within 2 weeks of the stroke (Boake, 2007; Dromerick, 2009). Most of the CIMT research has been done with people 12 months or longer after the CVA (Schaechter, 2002; Shaw, 2005; Szaflarski, 2006; Tarkka, 2005; Taub, 2006; Wittenberg, 2003), and further study is needed to determine the optimal time to initiate CIMT to avoid possible harm in human subjects and optimize outcomes.

Although improvements in WMFT, **Motor Activity Log (MAL)**, Fugl-Meyer, and Stroke Impact Scale scores are significant for most of the studies, there has been minimal indication that these improvements translate to function. The MAL asks patients and caregivers to independently rate how well the patient uses the affected UE for 30 ADLs during the past week. Subjects typically report improvement in use of the UE after intervention with CIMT or mCIMT, but upon further questioning it appears the improvement may only occur with bimanual tasks (Bonifer, 2005b). A kinematic study of reaching indicates an increase in movement time, velocity, and increase consistency in trajectory, and an increase in WMFT and MAL scores indicates improved function.

However, no changes in existing trunk and elbow compensatory patterns and an increase in compensatory shoulder abduction occurred (Massie, 2009). Additional research is needed to determine the effect of CIMT on the quality of movement, carryover, and retention with functional tasks in the work and home environment.

Children with asymmetrical use of the UEs due to stroke or CP may have a "developmental disregard" for the involved extremity because they have not established typical movement patterns. Researchers have adapted the parameters used with adults to a child-friendly version of CIMT. Most of the pediatric studies use the same inclusionary criteria outlined for adult populations consisting of active wrist extension of at least 20 degrees and MCP extension of 10 degrees from full flexion, a level of cognitive understanding, and willingness to participate. In addition, children need to show a 50% difference in UE use, which may be measured by the Jebsen-Taylor Test of Hand Function (Charles, 2006; Gordon, 2006). The higher functioning UE is typically restrained for 21 days during which time the child participates in shaping activities for 6 hours/day with a therapist. The shaping activities for children have been adapted to include play and age-appropriate activities (Taub, 2004). Other researchers added a repetition of a focal or isolated component of a task before attempting the more complex movements in the shaping activities (Gordon, 2006). Evidence shows children undergoing CIMT make significant improvements in the efficiency and usage of the more involved extremity during daily activities, which persist through a 6-month follow-up (Charles, 2006; Gordon, 2006; Taub, 2004; Willis, 2002). In part, the better retention is due to parental compliance with a home program (Taub, 2007). Researchers have also found improvement in the involved UE with less time spent in the restraint and the intensive therapy sessions with shaping activities. Significant improvement has been found with 15, rather than 21, days of CIMT (Taub, 2007); use of a mitt on the less-involved hand during daily play for 2 hours over 2 months (Eliasson, 2005); and a below elbow cast for 1 month with regular therapy sessions for 30 to 60 minutes 1 to 2 times per week (Willis, 2002).

Pediatric study protocols have different inclusionary age criteria and contradicting results as to the effect of age on the success of the intervention (Eliasson, 2005; Gordon, 2006; Willis, 2002). Likewise the level of hand severity as a predictor of outcomes is controversial (Charles, 2006; Eliasson, 2005). An additional consideration in treating children is the lack of clear evidence and knowledge of periods of critical development (Charles, 2006). Therefore, more research is needed to determine the optimal age and length of constraint for children. Study limitations include small sample size, participant withdrawal due to time constraints, a child's tolerance of the restraints, an unclear diagnosis, or time of onset of the asymmetrical UE use. There is also a difference in the time spent in intervention sessions between control and experimental groups with the CIMT groups in longer therapy sessions. Some studies attempted to address this concern through a crossover design. The results were contradictory as some crossover groups had similar improvements as the original experimental group (Deluca, 2006; Willis, 2002) and others have shown no improvement in the crossover group (Charles, 2006). The conclusions of a systematic review and meta-analysis of randomized controlled trials (a total of 29 publications) were that "CIMT overall is an effective intervention to improve arm function in children with cerebral palsy" (Chen et al, 2014, p. 950). A pilot study by Zipp and Winning (2012) supports improvement in gait, balance, and functional locomotor mobility after CIMT, and the authors encourage inclusion of outcome measures for these broader motor functions.

## THINK ABOUT IT 15.1

- CIMT was developed to counteract learned nonuse that impairs task completion with the involved extremities and compensation with the noninvolved extremity. Describe some specific techniques you could use from this approach to improve symmetry in sit-to-stand.
- Because CIMT can be effective as early as 2 weeks after a stroke, describe some ways that CIMT could be implemented in the acute care/hospital setting.
- How could you apply the concept of "shaping" to a specific limitation while performing a functional task, for example, insufficient ankle dorsiflexion on the affected side during swing phase of gait?

The definition for CIMT includes repetitive extensive exercise of the involved extremity. Using this definition, LT on a treadmill could be considered CIMT for the LE due to the repetitive nature of the task.

## Locomotor Training

### Overview

**Locomotor training (LT)** is an intervention used by physical therapists to retrain people to walk after neurological injury (Behrman, 2005). LT is thought to lead to experience-dependent neural plasticity, which is the central nervous system's ability to adapt/learn from intensive task-specific repetition and practice (Kleim, 2008). This rehabilitation strategy may enhance the recovery of postural control, balance, standing, walking, and quality of life after neurologic injury or disease (Harkema, 2012). There are several types of LT. One type involves the patient walking on a motorized treadmill either with or without **body weight support (BWS)**. The BWS is provided by an overhead harness and suspension system, which supports a percentage of the person's body weight. LT on a treadmill may incorporate manual facilitation, provided by physical therapists, at the pelvis and LEs to simulate normal sensory input and kinematics of gait. Therapist-assisted LT is limited by the heavy physical requirements on the therapist. Robotic devices have also been developed to provide mechanical assistance to the LEs for stepping on the treadmill. Another type of LT encompasses overground walking training with or

without BWS. The BWS utilized during overground walking can be provided by unweighting devices on wheels or by track systems in the ceiling. The track system supports and unweights the individual, allowing them to walk on uneven surfaces and elevations in order to simulate activities necessary for participation in the community. If possible, the patient should practice overground walking after treadmill training during each therapy session.

### Background

Restoration of walking ability and improvement in gait parameters such as velocity, stride length, cadence, or symmetry are important therapeutic goals for patients with neuromuscular involvement. Gait training with this population may include part-task and/or whole-task training. **Part-task training** involves retraining components of gait, such as weight-shifting or stepping, before progressing to ongoing walking. This progression may occur within the same therapy session or across sessions. In contrast, **whole-task training** stresses practicing gait in its entirety without working on the component parts (Shumway-Cook, 2007). In this approach, patients repeatedly practice ongoing walking with or without physical assistance or assistive devices. LT on a treadmill is an example of a whole-task approach to gait training. It is task specific and involves massed practice as it allows for "multiple repetitions of complete gait cycles facilitated by the treadmill's constant rate of movement" (Trueblood, 2001). This intervention allows for intensity of walking practice, which is thought to be critical to activity-dependent neural plasticity (Behrman, 2006). LT on a treadmill with BWS enhances postural control and facilitates a more symmetrical, coordinated gait pattern with less patient effort. These responses would occur before the patient has the opportunity to develop gait deviations or learned non-use of a more involved leg, which are commonly seen when a compensatory approach is used early in rehabilitation (McCain, 2007).

The rationale underlying the use of LT on a treadmill with humans is based on extensive earlier animal studies. Research studies of adult spinalized cats demonstrated they could step independently with their hind limbs on a treadmill, but only after several weeks of "training" (Barbeau, 1987). The training involved suspension of the cat in a sling over a moving treadmill and manual assistance of their hind limbs to provide appropriate sensory input. Despite significant motor deficits, the spinalized adult cats were able to recover locomotor function of the hind limbs while walking on a treadmill (Barbeau, 1987). If the training was stopped, however, the adult cats regressed to shorter steps, inability to support their weight, and poor hind limb foot placement, indicating the importance of ongoing training. The results of these animal studies provided evidence for the existence of central pattern generators (CPGs) located in the spinal cord. These neural networks are thought to produce reciprocal lower extremity locomotor patterns in the absence of supraspinal input. Spinal CPGs are influenced by sensory and proprioceptive input coming into the system from the periphery and it is this sensory input which influences the motor output (Field-Fote, 2000). Spinal CPGs are thought to generate the basic motor patterns for walking, while supraspinal centers can activate and modulate the spinal CPGs based on functional and environmental demands (Field-Fote, 2000).

### Clinical Applications

The animal research prompted questions about the presence of spinal CPGs in humans and has led to extensive LT studies involving humans with spinal cord injury (SCI) and with stroke. Studies of LT on a treadmill have shown that rhythmic, locomotor-like electromyographic (EMG) patterns and lower extremity walking movements can be elicited in humans with cervical or thoracic spinal cord lesions even without supraspinal control (Harkema, 2001). People with incomplete SCI were able to generate independent steps on a treadmill and EMG muscle activity seen in normal locomotion after 5 to 20 weeks of LT (Behrman, 2000). The training included BWS and manual assistance to the legs while the person stepped on a moving treadmill. Some subjects with SCI also developed the ability to walk overground and demonstrated improved overground walking speed and lower extremity kinematics (Behrman, 2000). In animal and human studies, the unweighting system and treadmill provide the necessary equipment for repetitive, intensive practice of walking, but it is the manual facilitation of the pelvis and LEs and resultant sensory input that appears critical to regaining more normal locomotor patterns (Behrman, 2000).

LT on a treadmill with BWS has been shown to improve balance, gait velocity, distance walked, aerobic capacity, and level of functional independence in individuals with incomplete SCI (Behrman, 2000; Behrman, 2005; Field-Fote, 2011; Harkema, 2012). Additionally, the combined use of LT with BWS on a treadmill and LE electrical stimulation (ES) for patients with incomplete SCI has been shown to increase overground walking speed, distance, and LE muscle strength (Field-Fote, 2001; Field-Fote, 2011). In contrast, a multisite randomized controlled trial (SCILT Trial) of 145 individuals with acute incomplete SCI demonstrated no statistically significant differences in walking speed or Functional Independence Measure (FIM) scores at the end of 3 months of training, comparing subjects who received 12 weeks of treadmill training with BWS to those who received overground walking training (Dobkin, 2007). Few subjects with ASIA B SCI, but most subjects with ASIA C and D (American Spinal Injury Association Impairment levels described in Chapter 6) achieved functional walking ability after 12 weeks of either LT on a treadmill or overground walking. Field-Fote (2011) compared four different LT approaches with individuals with incomplete SCI (treadmill training with manual assistance, treadmill training with ES, overground walking training with ES, or treadmill training with robotic assistance) and reported significantly improved walking speeds for all groups except the robotic-assisted group. Interestingly, walking distance improved most in the overground walking training group. Therapist-assisted LT on a treadmill is shown to be as beneficial as robotic-assisted LT in improving gait velocity post-SCI, yet the physical demands on the therapists

were much less with robotic-assisted LT (Hornby, 2005a, 2005b).

LT on a treadmill has also been studied extensively as an intervention to improve walking post-stroke. Research has demonstrated that individuals with stroke who undergo LT on a treadmill with BWS show improved balance, increased stride length, cadence, gait speed, and distance walked (Hesse, 1994a, 1994b; Sullivan, 2002; Trueblood, 2001; Visintin, 1998); as well as increased hip and knee extension and stance time on the involved leg (Ada, 2003; Ada, 2013; Kuys, 2011; Pohl, 2007; Sullivan, 2002; Visintin, 1998). Systematic reviews exploring the efficacy of treadmill training with or without BWS for ambulatory individuals post-stroke demonstrate increased walking speed and distance walked compared to no intervention; these improvements were maintained over time, but not greater than effects of overground walking training (Mehrholz, 2014; Polese, 2013). Overground walking speeds exhibit the greatest improvement when people with stroke are trained on the treadmill at fast (0.98 m/s) compared to slow (0.22 m/s) or varied treadmill speeds (Sullivan, 2002). In addition, training at speeds comparable to normal walking velocity was most effective in improving self-selected walking velocity (Sullivan, 2002). LT on a treadmill has also been shown to be more effective for increasing gait speed and improving ADLs in individuals post-stroke than conventional therapies, cycling, or strengthening exercises (Pohl, 2007; Sullivan, 2007). The multisite, randomized, controlled "Locomotor Experiences Applied Post-Stroke" (LEAPS) trial of 408 people with stroke revealed no significant differences in walking ability between subjects who began LT on a treadmill early (2 mo.) or late (6 mo.) after stroke onset or those who received a progressive home program of strengthening exercises and balance activities (Duncan, 2011). Research results on robotic-assisted LT for stroke have not shown its benefit over other types of LT. One study indicated greater improvements in gait velocity and single limb stance time on the impaired leg in people post-stroke with therapist-assisted compared with robotic-assisted LT on a treadmill (Hornby, 2008). Additionally, subjects with stroke who received conventional overground gait training demonstrated greater improvement in walking speed and distance compared with those who were trained with robotic-assisted LT (Hidler, 2009). A split belt treadmill, in which two separate treadmill belts can be made to move at different speeds, has been used to test the ability of people with stroke to adapt and improve gait pattern symmetry (Reisman, 2009). The improved gait pattern symmetry observed following split belt treadmill training also transfers to overground walking (Reisman, 2009; Reisman, 2013).

LT on a treadmill has been used as an intervention to improve walking in other neurological populations including Parkinson disease (PD), multiple sclerosis (MS), traumatic brain injury (TBI), and ataxia; however, the evidence for LT with these populations is more limited. People with PD have demonstrated increased stride length, cadence, gait velocity, and improved balance with fewer falls after LT on a treadmill with BWS, and most improvements were retained at follow-up

(Miyai, 2000; Miyai, 2002; Toole, 2005; Nadeau, 2014). Individuals with MS showed greater improvement in gait velocity, endurance, and Kurtske Scale (EDSS) scores following 4 weeks of conventional walking therapy than those who received robotic-assisted gait training on a treadmill, while both groups improved in Berg Balance Scale (BBS) scores (Schwartz, 2012).

Promising results with adults with neurological involvement has led to LT research in pediatric populations. Neonates demonstrate a stepping reflex when held upright and inclined forward with their feet in contact with a firm surface. This reflex is usually integrated and not observed by 4 to 6 weeks after birth. Thelen (1991) demonstrated that typically developing infants were able to produce an alternating stepping pattern when held upright over a small motorized treadmill and this alternating stepping pattern persisted throughout the first year of life, if practiced. Preliminary research on infant kicking and stepping behaviors reinforced the idea of neuronal connections for locomotion and formed the theoretical basis for the application of LT on a treadmill with pediatric neurological populations (Thelen, 1991; Ulrich, 2001). A pivotal study by Ulrich (2001) demonstrated that infants with Down Syndrome (DS) who participated in daily stepping on a small, motorized treadmill at home with their parent's assistance were able to walk several months before infants with DS who did not receive treadmill walking. This study has influenced the fields of infant motor development and pediatric physical therapy, because it was the first adequately powered, randomized, controlled trial to show that the onset of walking could be accelerated several months by daily practice stepping on a treadmill. Further research demonstrated that children with DS who engage in high intensity LT on a treadmill (6 to 9 minutes/day, 5 days/week, at belt speeds of 0.18 to 0.22 meters/second, with ankle weights) achieved earlier onset of walking than children with DS who received lower intensity LT (8 minutes/day, 5 days/week, belt speed of 0.15 meters/second) (Damiano, 2009; Ulrich, 2008). Additionally, locomotor training has been studied in ambulatory and non-ambulatory children with cerebral palsy (CP). Young children with CP display increased walking speed and distance after LT on a treadmill with BWS (Dodd, 2007; Mattern-Baxter, 2009). However, another study comparing LT on a treadmill with BWS and overground walking training for school-age children with CP resulted in no significant differences in self-selected gait velocity, and the overground group showed a tendency toward increased walking distances (Willoughby, 2010).

Prior to implementing LT with a patient, therapists should consider the following questions:

1. Is this patient appropriate for LT on a treadmill or do they have medical problems that would make this contraindicated?
2. If appropriate, how soon in the course of rehabilitation should the patient begin LT? On the other hand, at what point will LT no longer benefit the person with chronic disability?

3. Which is the most appropriate type of LT to use with the patient and with what type of equipment, remembering that the equipment is just a tool to implement the intervention?
4. What parameters of LT are most appropriate for this patient such as frequency, duration, speed of the treadmill, holding the handrail, amount of BWS, and the need for manual assistance?
5. How soon can the patient begin overground walking training, a critical component of LT?

Specific guidelines for the implementation of LT are not fully delineated, but therapists can use the available published evidence and principles of application to guide their clinical decision-making (Behrman, 2000; Behrman, 2005b; Behrman, 2006; Chen, 2006). Behrman and Harkema (2000) have outlined LT principles for people with spinal cord injury based on providing sensory cues to approximate normal walking, including:

1. Generate stepping velocities on the treadmill which approximate normal walking velocities.
2. Avoid or minimize weight-bearing on the arms and facilitate reciprocal arm swing.
3. Maintain an upright extended head and trunk posture during walking.
4. Provide normal loading on the LEs in early stance phase of gait.
5. Synchronize hip extension at end stance phase and subsequent unloading of this leg as it moves into swing phase with the loading of the contralateral leg.
6. Approximate hip, knee, and ankle kinematics seen in normal walking.

The treadmill in LT affords continuous facilitation of ongoing walking and should have several features including removable handrails, speed adjustability from 0.1 to 6.0 mph at 0.1 increments, and seating for therapists to provide manual facilitation. The therapist can adjust the speed of the treadmill and should make every effort to simulate normal walking speeds as early in gait training as possible. Maximal loading of the legs during the stance phase of gait with minimal or no weight-bearing through the arms is recommended during LT, though use of handrails may be needed in certain cases. The arms should be free to allow for reciprocal arm swing, trunk rotation, and to encourage a more upright, extended head and trunk posture. If the patient is weight-bearing on the bars of the treadmill or on a gait-assistive device, they are more likely to have a forward flexed trunk posture and flexed hips. However, individuals with hemiparesis may show improved gait kinematics if allowed to hold the handrail with the less-involved arm, so therapists should consider each individual when making these decisions (Chen, 2006). LT on a treadmill reinforces appropriate timing relationships between the two legs and ensures that each hip extends during terminal stance phase of gait. Full hip extension in terminal stance phase is critical as it acts as a catalyst to facilitate hip flexion in the next swing phase of the same leg as the opposite leg moves into stance phase (Behrman, 2000). A key component of LT is that, to the extent possible, hip, knee, and ankle kinematics should approximate normal walking.

The unweighting system used in LT prevents collapse of the patient, decreases muscle force requirements and postural/balance demands on the patient, decreases lifting required by the therapist, and allows the therapist to control the amount of LE weight-bearing. This allows the patient with muscle weakness and balance deficits to practice walking, including multiple repetitions of the gait cycle, even when overground walking is not yet feasible. Visintin (1998) reported that individuals who were only 2 weeks post-stroke could benefit from LT on a treadmill with BWS without adverse effects or worsening of their condition. These patients actually walked sooner than those who did not receive early LT. The amount of body weight support provided varies based on the individual needs of the patient but should be decreased as LT progresses; for example, decreasing from 30% to 20% to 10%. It is important not to exceed 30% to 40% BWS, to avoid detracting from normal recruitment and action of the LE musculature (Richards, 2004).

Another important element of LT is the manual facilitation often provided by therapists to promote upright posture, weight shifts, and coordinated LE movements seen in normal walking. This manual guidance is important to minimize gait deviations that may develop as the patient, with significant trunk and LE muscle weakness, begins to walk. The progression of LT with a patient may begin at slow treadmill speeds with maximum BWS and constant manual assistance, gradually progressing to normal walking speeds with no BWS and no manual guidance. If the patient is able, an intensive program of LT is recommended beginning with 30-minute sessions and increasing to 60-minute sessions (with rests as needed) 3 to 5 days per week for 6-12 weeks to promote optimal motor learning (Moore, 2010). Vital signs should be monitored and the patient's medical history and aerobic capacity taken into consideration when determining the intensity of the LT program (Macko, 1997). The ultimate goal of LT on a treadmill is carryover of an improved gait pattern to overground walking, with or without an assistive device, for return to participation in the home and in the community.

In summary, research has shown the benefits of LT for both adult and pediatric neurological populations. This is a task-oriented approach to gait training, allowing for large amounts of practice of the whole task of walking afforded by the constant movement of the treadmill belt. This intervention is based on extensive animal research. Studies have demonstrated improvements in balance, gait speed and distance walked, symmetry, endurance, functional independence, and lower limb kinematics after LT on a treadmill

in neurologic populations. However, large randomized, controlled trials of LT for individuals with SCI and stroke have not shown a distinct advantage of either LT on a treadmill, overground walking training, or home-based therapy (Dobkin, 2007; Duncan, 2011). Additional research is needed to continue to establish the efficacy of this intervention and to further delineate principles of clinical application across neurologic populations.

# Complementary Movement Approaches
## Overview of Complementary Approaches

Consideration should be given to alternative or **complementary movement approaches** due to the eclectic choice of interventions used by therapists in the treatment of patients with neurological dysfunction. Peer-reviewed evidence of the efficacy of most of these interventions is limited, but they are frequently used in the clinic setting with positive anecdotal reports.

Activities on a **therapeutic** or **Swiss ball** may be combined with other approaches such as NDT or PNF. Activities on the ball may be performed slowly and rhythmically to calm the patient and inhibit abnormal tone, whereas fast bouncing movements can act through the vestibular system to excite and increase tone and alertness. Activities can be progressed through developmental sequence positions with a focus on core stability and the addition of extremity motion for fun and function. A full aerobic routine can be developed to increase endurance, incorporating learning and memory strategies to learn the sequence. Motivation on the ball can be enhanced through games requiring kicking or throwing. Treatment goals may include improved flexibility, strength, coordination, balance, and endurance.

The ball is typically fully inflated to provide a firm surface and a smaller point of contact with the floor to make the task more challenging. If the patient needs additional support, the ball can be partially deflated. Different shaped "balls" such as the peanut-shaped ball or hemi-ball with one flat surface may also decrease the balance challenge so the task is easier for the patient. The correct ball size and the patient's alignment on the ball allow for the most effective treatment and muscle activation. The ball should be sized with the patient in short sitting to allow for neutral dorsiflexion and 90 degrees of hip and knee flexion. The patient should roll forward to sit on the anterior edge of the ball to maximize LE weight-bearing, and activate muscles and balance strategies. If the focus of the intervention is to improve trunk control and/or equilibrium reactions, the patient may be placed on a large ball so the feet do not touch the floor. This position is frequently used with children. The therapist can be very creative and use a number of positions and activities on or with the ball to reach treatment goals.

The **Feldenkrais Method®** of somatic education was developed by Moshe Feldenkrais and can be administered in one of two ways. A Guild Certified Feldenkrais Practitioner may lead one-on-one sessions with guided touch and cues known as *Functional Integration* lessons. Lessons can also be provided in group settings with verbal directions/cues and are referred to as *Awareness Through Movement®* classes. The *Feldenkrais Guild®* of North America provides information about workshops and certification courses in North America and other resources, including sales of audiotapes of *Awareness Through Movement®* lessons.

The intent of the lessons is to help individuals become more aware of how they move and provide opportunities to alter habitual movement patterns, therefore allowing a greater ease of movement, decreased pain, and greater efficiency of movement with improved endurance. Classes are beneficial for all individuals and may be offered in community settings as well as within a medical model. The exercises are performed slowly within the individual's comfort level with a focus on learning new movement patterns. The person must have good cognition and the ability to follow verbal directions in order to participate in *Awareness Through Movement®* classes. The lessons focus on various areas of the body or functional activities with a progression in the level of complexity or difficulty. Typically, individuals will report feeling lighter, more symmetrical, better balanced, and with improved posture after *Feldenkrais* lessons. Over time, they may notice enhanced problem-solving and more movement alternatives.

An example of a Feldenkrais' lesson which is used frequently is known as the pelvic or scapular "clock." The patient is asked to visualize sitting on a clock. The anterior/forward position is 12:00; 3:00 is to the right; 6:00 is in the posterior/back position; and 9:00 is to the left. The patient is asked to move or tip their pelvis to 12:00 for an anterior tilt; 3:00 or 9:00 for a lateral tilt; and 6:00 or a posterior tilt. The patient may follow the numbers in sequence around the clock or they may be cued to opposite numbers of the clock, depending on the treatment goals. The concept of the clock may be performed in supine, sidelying, seated, or in stance. The same concept is commonly used for scapular movements as well. Balance may be improved in people poststroke as measured by the Berg Balance Scale and Dynamic Gait Index (Batson, 2005), and decreased stress and anxiety were noted in patients with multiple sclerosis (Johnson, 1999). As with all of the complementary approaches, further research is warranted.

**Tai chi** and **yoga** are used with patients in clinic settings, community-based exercise groups, and home exercise programs. Group classes allow for social reintegration, which is often a valuable component in the recovery process. Although tai chi and yoga each have varied forms with different objectives, they both include flexibility and strengthening with a balance component. Some of the movements/postures may need adaptation to allow an individual with neurological deficits to participate. Multiple studies on the well elderly support the benefits of yoga and tai chi for improving cardiopulmonary function and LE strength, and reducing falls (Taylor, 2012; Taylor-Piliae, 2007; Verhagen, 2004).

However, there has been little research with individuals with neurological dysfunction (Lynton, 2007).

One area of study involves 'psychological' components of mood, stress, and sleep. Studies are mixed regarding the impact of yoga on fatigue in individuals with multiple sclerosis. A few studies indicate overall less fatigue following yoga classes (Oken, 2004; Garrett, 2013). However Velikonja (2010) found no changes in fatigue, mood, executive function, or spasticity following 10 weeks of hatha yoga. It does seem tai chi qigong may improve mood and self-esteem (Blake, 2009) and decrease the use of medication (Yost, 2013) following TBI. It can also improve the quality of sleep in individuals completing rehabilitation for Guillain-Barre syndrome (Sendhilkumar, 2013). However, yoga does not appear to result in significant changes in depression or anxiety post-CVA (Chan, 2012). None of these studies included physical performance measures.

Minimal evidence indicates balance may improve in individuals with chronic CVA following 16 sessions of yoga (Bastille, 2004). In a study by Au-Yeung (2009), a short form of tai chi was effective in improving postural control in individuals with chronic stroke. However another study did not improve balance when comparing tai chi to a more traditional balance retraining program in people with stroke (Hart, 2004). A case report of three individuals with severe head injury indicated improvements in balance and gait after 2 to 4 years of tai chi chuan, but frequency of sessions and physical outcome measures were not reported (Shapira, 2001). Balance and postural stability in individuals with PD improves with tai chi as measured on computerized force plates (Li, 2012) and clinical measures such as Berg Balance Scale, TUG, tandem stance (Hackney, 2008), and functional reach (Li, 2012). Positive changes in gait velocity, stride length, and backward walking were also noted in people with PD after tai chi classes (Hackney, 2008; Li, 2012). More research is needed to determine whether the same positive effects of tai chi and yoga found in the well elderly population can be replicated in individuals after neurological injury.

Yoga has become a popular intervention for children and adolescents in educational, medical, and community settings and is used to address a variety of physical, psychosocial, and behavioral problems. Much of the research has been done with typically developing children and studies lack consistency in the type of yoga used, the intensity of the intervention, and outcome measures employed (Galantino, 2008). Therefore evidence is weak, but trends seem to support improvements in motor planning, performance of motor skills, ability to concentrate and focus, spatial and verbal memory, stress management, and socialization (Galantino, 2008).

## Aquatic Therapy

### Background/Overview

Water has been a source of healing throughout history. The full historical account and review of aquatic physics is beyond the scope of this text but the reader is referred to the text by Ruoti, Morris, and Cole (1997) or Cole and Becker (2004) for detailed information. As knowledge and different applications of therapeutic exercise have evolved, aquatic therapy has become a specialized area of rehabilitation used for patients with varying diagnoses (Kelly, 2005; Resende, 2008; Ballaz, 2011). Aquatic exercise can enhance cardiovascular fitness and endurance; improve vital capacity, strength, flexibility, and balance; normalize abnormal tone; aid in relaxation; and decrease pain (Hall, 2008). Due to the buoyancy of water, it may be one of the earliest and most supportive interventions in rehabilitation for individuals too weak to stand and initiate gait against gravitational constraints. Some patients may feel more secure in the water as the fear of falling is partially alleviated. Patients of all ages typically find water exercise enjoyable, and it may improve communication skills and socialization. Many community programs are available for water exercise, making this an appropriate leisure activity in which patients may continue to participate even after discharge from rehabilitation services.

### Clinical Approaches and Application

Currently there are three primary philosophies of aquatic therapy. The **Bad Ragaz Ring Method (BRRM)** was developed in Switzerland and has undergone several "revisions," including incorporation of PNF patterns and techniques into the philosophy. Because stabilization is difficult without the effects of gravity, the therapist must provide stability through manual contacts. The manual contacts can still be used for facilitation, but the primary force for resistance is provided by movement through the water. Proximal control, use of irradiation to weak muscles, and alternating movement patterns are all PNF principles applied in BRRM (Ruoti, 1997).

The **Halliwick Method** was founded by James McMillan. McMillan did minimal writing about his approach and most of the techniques have been promoted through continuing education coursework and secondary sources. McMillan developed his intervention based on his knowledge of competitive swimming, observations of people with disability in the water, and his engineering background. The two primary focuses of this approach are teaching individuals about their balance in the water and how to swim. To meet these objectives, he identified four principles for instruction (Ruoti, 1997; Gross, 2010). The individual must understand the forces of gravity and upward thrust of the water. When combined, these two forces result in rotation. The second principle is balance restoration which in part utilizes primitive reflexes to move the body around the midline axis. The third principle of inhibition is the ability to stabilize and control unwanted motions. Lastly, the individual achieves facilitation resulting in independent controlled movement or swimming. In the Halliwick

Method, flotation devices are typically not used, independent head control is recognized as critical for development of other skills, and breath control is an important component (Gross, 2010). A small randomized controlled trial of patients with subacute stroke demonstrated significant improvements in balance and functional gait compared with controls (Tripp, 2014).

**Watsu** or water shiatsu is based on the principles of zen shiatsu, which advocates a balance of energy flow through the meridians, applied in an aquatic environment. The one-to-one intervention is a form of meditation and was developed as a type of massage or wellness technique. Stretching is one of the primary benefits as the therapist stabilizes one body part and the drag through the water offers a stretch to the other body segment. Breathing patterns are an important element of this approach. The technique uses a sequence of movements defined as "flow," which can be adapted to individual patient needs by an experienced practitioner (Ruoti, 1997).

Aquatic therapy has been employed with children who have a wide range of diagnoses including CP, muscular dystrophy, spinal muscle atrophy, myelomeningocele, DS, juvenile idiopathic arthritis, and autism with the purpose of improving a variety of motor, social, and behavioral parameters. Research has shown positive outcomes for balance, strength, functional mobility, endurance, pulmonary function, and social participation (Blohm, 2011; Getz, 2006; Karklina, 2013; McManus, 2007). Findings suggest improved outcomes and carryover when aquatic therapy is paired with land-based therapy.

Appropriateness of aquatic therapy should be critically evaluated for patients who express fear of water or have vestibular symptoms. Acute conditions of the spine may require some level of adaptation to prevent further stress during movement in the water. Water temperature is an important factor to consider based upon the patient diagnosis. Precautions or contraindications are the same as for other hydrotherapy modalities and include fever, open wounds, infectious disease, uncontrolled seizures, incontinence of bowel or bladder, tracheotomy, or severe hypertension/hypotension.

## THINK ABOUT IT 15.2

- Describe specific components during activities on a therapeutic ball that could help to inhibit spastic hypertonus.
- Explain the mechanisms by which aquatic therapy can enhance cardiovascular endurance, strength, flexibility, and balance.
- Explain the reason for each precaution for aquatic therapy: fever, open wounds, infectious disease, uncontrolled seizures, incontinence, tracheotomy, or severe hypertension or hypotension.

# HANDS-ON PRACTICE

Skills students should be able to perform:

## ▌ Rood

- Incorporate Rood's levels of motor control (mobility, stability, controlled mobility, and skill) into interventions with neurological clients.
- Facilitation Techniques (Rood)
  - Light touch
  - Quick brushing or tapping
  - Quick stretch
  - Quick ice
  - Traction
  - Approximation or joint compression
  - Resistance
- Inhibitory Techniques (Rood)
  - Prolonged stretch
  - Deep pressure
  - Neutral warmth
  - Slow stroking
  - Prolonged cold

## ▌ Sensory Integration

- Describe the sensory inputs (tactile, vestibular, proprioceptive) necessary for a given functional task (e.g., donning a t-shirt).

## ▌ Brunnstrom

- Demonstrate both the upper extremity (UE) and lower extremity (LE) flexion and extension synergy patterns.
- Assess components of Brunnstrom synergy patterns in clients with hemiparesis.
- Provide examples of isolated movements used in daily tasks.
- Describe how developmental reflexes may be used to inhibit and facilitate recovery of movement in those with hemiparesis.

## ▌ Neurodevelopmental Treatment (NDT)

- Describe the application of NDT to a functional task (e.g., sitting, transition to stance, stance, and gait).
  - Request active movement to the posture.
  - Demonstrate.
  - Readjust the patient position or alter the environment/task.
  - Use key points of control for tactile cues to facilitate normal movement and minimize abnormal movement.
  - Use soft mobilization techniques to allow movement into the desired posture.
  - Cue patient to move into and out of posture.
  - Progress with weight shifts, increase speed, task.

## ▌ Proprioceptive Neuromuscular Facilitation (PNF)

- Select and effectively perform each of the following PNF specific techniques as appropriate for specific patient problems such as limited ROM, muscle weakness or inability to initiate movement.
  - Rhythmic initiation
  - Combination of isotonics
  - Slow reversals
  - Rhythmic stabilization
  - Repeated contractions
  - Contract relax
  - Hold relax
- Demonstrate each PNF diagonal pattern and describe how they may be applied during functional training.
  - UE D1/D2 patterns in both flexion and extension
  - LE D1/D2 patterns in both flexion and extension
  - Scapular patterns of anterior elevation/posterior depression and anterior depression/posterior elevation
  - Pelvic patterns of anterior elevation/posterior depression and anterior depression/posterior elevation
- Combine use of the PNF basic procedures, specific techniques, and movement patterns to examine and treat clients with movement disorders.
- For any functional task, such as walking, describe how PNF patterns and techniques could be used to improve task performance.

## ▌ Task/Motor Relearning Program

- Given a typical physical therapy clinic, set up an obstacle course that requires the patient to problem-solve for task completion.
- Describe ways to modify the clinic environment to allow for enhanced transference of balance and ambulation.
- Describe the component parts of a reaching task.

## ▌ Constraint-Induced Movement Therapy (CIMT)

- Design activities to constrain the more affected side.
- Describe adult parameters/recommendations for CIMT intervention sessions according to the evidence.
- Techniques of shaping

## ▌ Locomotor Therapy (LT)

- Outline principles to follow during LT.
- Outline progression of LT with specific neurological populations according to the literature.

## ▌ Complementary (e.g., therapy ball, yoga, or tai chi)

- Demonstrate how to integrate complementary or alternative therapies into treatment sessions for clients with movement disorders.

## *Let's Review*

1. Describe developmental sequence of function as it relates to the Rood approach.

2. List available Rood facilitation techniques for stimulation of muscle activity and provide examples of how these techniques were incorporated/applied in other approaches.

3. Explain the concepts outlined by Ayres that illustrate the connection between sensory information and motor learning.

4. Describe the typical stages of motor recovery post-stroke as outlined by Brunnstrom.

5. Describe flexor and extensor synergy patterns seen clinically in patients with hemiplegia.

6. What is the central focus and principles of the NDT approach?

7. Working with a patient recovering from stroke you notice decreased hip extension and knee extension during terminal stance of gait. How could you incorporate the variety of PNF diagonal patterns and techniques to develop a treatment intervention?

8. A child presents to your clinic with left hemiplegia and has difficulty transitioning from high kneeling to standing. Develop an intervention using the NDT movement patterns and techniques outlined in the chapter to progress the patient from high kneeling to walking.

9. A patient 3 weeks after an acute right CVA presents with mild left LE weakness and has difficulty ascending stairs. Describe a treatment plan consisting of several part-task interventions.

10. Why is a behavioral contract important when treating patients using CIMT?

11. When working with adults, what inclusion criteria are recommended for positive outcomes from CIMT?

12. Which variables can be adjusted when prescribing LT for a patient.

13. Describe an intervention using a therapeutic ball to work on trunk control and tone reduction in a patient with spastic cerebral palsy.

14. What are the indications and contraindications when considering a patient for aquatic therapy?

15. Compare and contrast the principles of each neurorehabilitation approach.

---

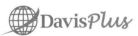 **DavisPlus**    For additional resources, including Focus on Evidence tables, case study discussions, references, and glossary, please visit http://davisplus.fadavis.com

---

## CHAPTER SUMMARY

Table 15-4 serves as an example of how the different neurorehabilitation approaches may be integrated and overlap to meet a variety of patient goals in one example. Betty has rigidity but no abnormal synergy patterns or hemiparesis. Therefore, Brunnstrom and NDT are not used as extensively with this patient.

This chapter provides an introduction to the various intervention approaches used for patients with neurological disorders. Numerous techniques have various levels of support demonstrated in published evidence, whereas others need further study. The use of these approaches, combinations of the various techniques, and the continuing search for effective interventions allows the therapist to be creative and apply the art of physical therapy in designing a treatment program with patients and families as illustrated in the previous patient scenario. Additional evidence on interventions is presented in the Focus on Evidence (FOE) tables for this chapter (available online): Table 15-5, Constraint-Induced

Movement Therapy evidence; Table 15-6, Locomotor Training evidence; Table 15-7, Neurodevelopmental Treatment evidence; Table 15-8, Proprioceptive Neuromuscular Facilitation evidence; Table 15-9, Task-Oriented Approaches evidence; and Table 15-10, Complimentary Exercise Approaches evidence.

## PATIENT APPLICATION

### Parkinson Disease

*Betty Wilson is a 66 year-old Caucasian female diagnosed with PD 5 years ago when she developed tremors in her right hand and rigidity in her left UE and LE. She is classified as Stage III on the Hoehn-Yahr Classification of Disability (Hoehn and Yahr, 1967). She has a history of hypertension, arthritis in her hands and feet, and mild clinical depression. Four weeks ago, her symptoms seemed to worsen, and she had four falls in the home. She is being seen in an outpatient clinic setting for fall prevention. Medications include Sinemet, Zoloft, hydrochlorothiazide, and a pain medication. She is 5'5" and weighs 160 pounds.*

*Social History: Betty is married and lives with her husband of 40 years. She lives in a one-level ranch home with three steps into the house. She reports she was independent with transfers, bed mobility, ambulation with a straight cane, and climbing stairs at home until 2 weeks ago. She was able to complete the laundry but has a cleaning lady twice a month. Her spouse does most of the cooking. She spends her day watching TV, reading the newspaper, and riding a stationary bike for about 20 minutes. Before the progression of PD, she enjoyed gardening, golf, and sewing. Patient reports that during the past 4 weeks her balance has worsened and she is not walking as well. She reports difficulty descending stairs and going through doorways in her home. Episodes of freezing seem to occur more frequently and may last 10 to 20 seconds. She is having increased difficulty rolling over in bed, and standing up from her bed or from chairs.*

*Subjective: Patient states her goals are to ambulate in her home safely without falling and "breaking a hip." She wants to maintain her independence in bed mobility and transfers and continue to live at home with her spouse.*

*Observation: Hearing and vision appear to be intact. Patient is alert and oriented x 3. Patient has masked facial expression. Speech is clear but she has low volume.*

*Posture: Standing posture is with trunk flexion, mild thoracic kyphosis, cervical flexion, and slight bilateral knee flexion. Patient reports a fear of falling when ambulating without UE support. Berg Balance score is 42/56, which indicates a fall risk.*

*Motor: She exhibits moderate to severe resting tremor, right greater than left hand. Bradykinesia is evident with impaired*

*righting and equilibrium reactions. Mild rigidity is noted in all four extremities and the trunk (L>R). Strength appears to be in the 4/5 range throughout.*

*Bed Mobility/Transfers: Patient requires minimal assistance with rolling to both sides in bed. She requires moderate assistance for right LE positioning and trunk flexion to move from supine to sit on the edge of the bed. She requires minimal assistance from sit to supine with right LE positioning. Periods of akinesia lasting 20 to 30 seconds were noted throughout mobility tasks. She requires minimal assist for sit-to-stand from chair and toilet. Betty requires minimal assistance for standing pivot transfers to/from the walker to bed, chair, and commode.*

*Ambulation: Betty ambulates 60 feet x 2 with a standard walker and minimal assistance of one person (assist for balance and verbal directions). Gait pattern: narrow base of support, small steps, limited foot clearance, and a flexed trunk.*

### Goals: Within 4 Weeks, the Patient Will Be Able to:

1. Roll from supine to sidelying in bed, to the left and the right, independently.
2. Move from supine to/from short sit on edge of bed independently.
3. Independently assume stance from bed, chair, and raised toilet seat to walker in 50% of trials.
4. Ambulate independently on carpet and tile in the home setting with a front-wheeled walker within 6 weeks.
5. Ascend and descend three steps using a step-to pattern and one railing with supervision in 6 weeks.

*Table 15-4 shows suggested interventions for each of Betty's goals. The intervention session can incorporate a variety of activities and an eclectic approach to reach her goals. Throughout the session, the therapist must be mindful of motor learning principles and consider the environment, specifics of the requested task, and the patient. Betty should actively participate in determining the goals and outcomes of the treatment and gradually be able to provide her own feedback of how she performed the task and how it might be improved. The therapist needs to be cognizant of the cues offered to Betty. Visual, auditory, and verbal cues can be powerful and fading feedback for Betty's independence is necessary. The use of demonstration for Betty and asking her to perform mental practice before a task may be helpful.*

**TABLE 15-4    Patient Scenario: Integrated Interventions**

**GOAL 1:** Betty will be able to roll from supine to sidelying to the left and right independently in bed within 4 weeks.

| FLEXIBILITY | STRENGTH | ACCURACY | SPEED | ADAPTABILITY | ENDURANCE |
|---|---|---|---|---|---|
| PROM (**mobility**): necessary for trunk rotation and LE mobility. **Rood/PNF:** rhythmic initiation and/or rhythmic rotation may inhibit trunk rigidity and increase ROM. **PNF:** lower trunk rotation with isotonic reversals. | **PNF:** Slow reversal to resist roll with manual contacts on the trunk or on UEs as a chop or lift pattern is used to roll. **PNF:** LE D1 flexion and extension pattern with slow reversal while rolling. **PNF:** Sitting—upper trunk rotation with slow reversal. | Practice activities to both right and left. **Rood:** controlled mobility with trunk counterrotation in sidelying. | Practice time from verbal cue to the time patient able to complete the roll. | Break down component **parts** of rolling and gradually build to practice the **whole task.** Alter LE starting position (supine, hooklying, ankles crossed). Add functional component to reach for bedside table or lamp. *Feldenkrais* lesson for rolling. | Repetition. Rolling on soft mattress will be more difficult than firm mat table. Incorporate breathing pattern with rolling task. |

**GOAL 2:** Betty will move from supine to/from short sitting on the edge of the bed independently in 4 weeks.

| FLEXIBILITY/STRENGTH | ACCURACY | SPEED | ADAPTABILITY | ENDURANCE |
|---|---|---|---|---|
| Requires combined **flexibility and strength.** If assuming sit from sidelying, complete rolling activities associated with Goal 1 above. Repetition to move from sidelying to sit with decrease PT support. If coming to sit from supine, increase in abdominal strength is needed. **PNF:** pelvic patterns and lower trunk rotation with resistance. Sitting with upper trunk rotation (may add chop or lift) with resistance. **Rood/PNF:** stability in sitting with rhythmic stabilization and focus on trunk extension. | Repetition | Practice | If allowed to initially pull or push with UE, stop UE use. Alter environment for soft and firm surfaces. Functional **task** to come to sit for drink of water or prepare for ambulation. | Repetition of abdominal strengthening and task performance. |

**GOAL 3:** Betty will independently assume stance from bed, chair, raised toilet seat to a walker 50% of trials in 4 weeks.

| FLEXIBILITY | STRENGTH | ACCURACY | SPEED | ADAPTABILITY | ENDURANCE |
|---|---|---|---|---|---|
| Necessary ankle dorsiflexion for feet to be placed back and flat on floor (may require **joint mobilization and soft tissue work**). **PNF:** resistance to upper trunk as it moves forward over lower trunk with hip flexion, LE weight-bearing. | Appropriate LE strength to push to stance. May do open chain strengthening or closed chain. **Closed chain:** bridges, sitting mini squats from bed surface, wall slides. | **NDT:** maintain trunk and pelvic alignment with hip flexion in preparation for stance. **Controlled mobility Partially stand** (mini-squat) from surface with weight shift right and sit, stand, weight shift to left and sit, etc. | Practice speed of weight shift. Use timed up and go as intervention. **Task:** Play catch in stance, gradually increasing speed. | Sitting on **therapeutic ball** with rolling, reaching, etc. **Task:** Practice standing from different surfaces, heights, and on different flooring. Alter foot position as assuming stance. Come from sit to reach for object (may require one step once in stance). Practice pulling up slacks, load | Increase time functional tasks performed. |

*Continued*

| TABLE 15-4 | Patient Scenario: Integrated Interventions—cont'd | | | | |
|---|---|---|---|---|---|
| FLEXIBILITY | STRENGTH | ACCURACY | SPEED | ADAPTABILITY | ENDURANCE |
| NDT: practice sitting in midline and maintain a neutral. pelvis with hip flexion. | | Standing: Modified Plantigrade (MP): in stride with weight shifts and resistance as tolerated, progress to stepping forward and back in MP. In stance, wt shift in all planes, add UE reciprocal movements. | | dishwasher, hang laundry, standing and donning jacket. | |

**GOAL 4:** Ambulate on carpet and tile in the home setting independently with a front-wheeled walker within 6 weeks. Multifactorial issues to address for balance in gait: ROM, strength, rigidity/abnormal tone, proprioception, vision, vestibular function. Previous exercises have incorporated weight shifts and equilibrium reactions for balance.

| FLEXIBILITY | STRENGTH | ACCURACY | SPEED | ADAPTABILITY | ENDURANCE |
|---|---|---|---|---|---|
| *Feldenkrais* for awareness of movement and improved posture. PNF: for trunk rotation needed for equilibrium reactions—sidelying trunk counterrotation, sitting upper trunk rotation, ½ kneeling with chop or lift, rotation in stance. Dissociation and isolated patterns are inherent components of the ½ kneel position. | Trunk and LE strengthening with ankle weights, Theraband, PNF LE D1 and D2 patterns. Perform in closed chain, MP, or stance. Start stepping up and down one step. | Task: Lift one LE to step to target, to different ht step, in different directions, over obstacles. Use visual cues on floor. Controlled mobility. | Task: Increase speed of stepping or ambulation. Use metronome or music as cues. Task: Kick a ball back and forth or against a wall. Task of LT on treadmill. | Sitting on therapeutic ball with activities requiring reciprocal extremity movement, trunk rotation. Balance equipment: stand on balance disks, tilt board, foam, etc., while performing reaching, PNF patterns, or functional activities. Change speed or direction of gait with VC. LT: (treadmill with or without body weight support) with changing inclines/speeds/use of UE support. Add dual task requirements or obstacle courses. Vary environment— grass, tile, carpet, lighting, curbs. | Tai chi, yoga, aquatic classes. Stationary bike (strengthening and reciprocal movement). Consider best option for gait assistive device when considering community ambulation. Skill level: Ambulation |

**GOAL 5:** Betty will ascend and descend 3 steps using a step-to pattern and one railing with supervision within 6 weeks.

| FLEXIBILITY | STRENGTH | ACCURACY | SPEED | ADAPTABILITY | ENDURANCE |
|---|---|---|---|---|---|
| Available LE ROM for task. Soft tissue and/or joint mobilization. | PNF: Half-kneel slow reversal. Combination of isotonics | Task: Step tapping or step ups on varied ht steps with | Task: Advance from step to pattern to step over step. | Task: Practice varied step patterns, with or without railings, vary height of steps, | Task: Increase number of steps. |

| TABLE 15-4 | **Patient Scenario: Integrated Interventions—cont'd** | | | | |
|---|---|---|---|---|---|
| **FLEXIBILITY** | **STRENGTH** | **ACCURACY** | **SPEED** | **ADAPTABILITY** | **ENDURANCE** |
| **PNF:** Slow reversal in tall kneel, ½ kneel, modified plantigrade to move within available range. | (eccentric strengthening) in LE diagonals or ½ kneel. **PNF:** SRH in bridging or tall kneel. **PNF:** sitting LE diagonal patterns in bilateral reciprocal motion. **PNF:** modified plantigrade with resisted LE diagonal patterns. **Closed chain** activities focusing on hip and knee extensors. | and without UE support. Reciprocal LE steps. This is a skill level activity. **NDT:** tapping different surfaces in different locations while maintaining stance. **Task:** Work on coordination with altered patterns such as up one step and down 2 steps. **Task:** Ambulation with visual cues for steps. | **Task:** Increase speed of stair climbing. **Reflex:** Practice stepping response with perturbations or large wt shifts. | ascend and descend laterally. Practice stepping on/off foam or balance disc. Practice stepping over objects on floor. **Dual task:** add cognitive, verbal, or additional physical task while performing stairs. | Carry weighted objects while performing stairs—grocery bag, laundry basket. **Tai chi, aquatic:** Increase time spent in class or progress level of difficulty. **Skill level:** ascend/descend stairs. |

# Health Promotion and Wellness in Neurology

Jason Boyd Hardage, PT, DPT, DScPT
Rick Nauert, PhD, MHA, MHF, PT ▪ Dennis W. Fell, PT, MD
Marisa L. Suarez, MS, OTR/L, SWC ▪ David M. Morris, PT, PhD, FAPTA
Esther Munalula Nkandu, BSc (Hons), MSc, MA, PhD

CHAPTER **16**

## CHAPTER OBJECTIVES

Upon completion of this chapter, the learner should be able to:

1. Define, describe, compare, and contrast terms related to health promotion.
2. Define, describe, compare, and contrast major models of health and disablement.
3. State examples of and describe health behavior theories/models.
4. Discuss issues related to adherence.
5. Identify and describe professional mandates for therapists to address health promotion.
6. Describe and discuss the role of the therapist in health promotion.
7. Describe and apply components of health promotion in neurorehabilitation.

## �\ Introduction

**Health promotion** includes all factors, information, and activities that improve the health status of an individual or population. Health promotion comprises a large body of knowledge representing many academic and clinical disciplines including education, public health, and psychology. This body of knowledge is being integrated into the health professions—including occupational therapy and physical therapy—and members of the health professions in turn are contributing to the body of knowledge as it applies to each profession's work. O'Donnell (2009) defined health promotion as "the art and science of helping people discover the synergies between their core passions and optimal health, enhancing their motivation to strive for optimal health, and supporting them in changing their lifestyle to move toward a state of optimal health." Although different disciplines have different foci and corresponding areas of expertise, health promotion is ultimately transdisciplinary as it involves researchers, academicians, and clinicians who share the common goal of improving the health of individuals and communities.

The integration of health promotion into the health professions has intersected with evidence-based practice as another major trend in health care with an explosion of evidence supporting not only the health benefits of physical activity, including exercise but also mind/body considerations, including mindfulness-based stress reduction, sleep hygiene, and cognitive-behavioral therapy. The intersection of health promotion and evidence-based practice is becoming increasingly apparent as the nation grapples with the prevalence of expensive health conditions that have the potential to strain the overall health delivery system—such as diabetes mellitus and overweight/obesity—affected by lifestyle choices.

Certainly there are many promising opportunities for rehabilitation therapists to develop and participate in niche or specialty programs in health promotion for their patients/clients. However health promotion for patients/clients does not merely comprise niche or specialty programs but rather should be inherent to clinical practice and represents best practice. Health promotion for patients/clients reflects the assertion of the *Guide to Physical Therapist Practice* (American Physical Therapy Association [APTA] *Guide*, 2015) that physical therapists are providers of primary care defined by the Institute of Medicine as "the provision of integrated accessible health care services by clinicians who are accountable for addressing a large majority of personal health care needs, developing a sustained partnership with patients, and practicing within the context of family and community." It also fits the broad perspective of the vision statement for the physical therapy profession: "Transforming society by optimizing movement to improve the human experience" (APTA, 2013).

Likewise, the American Occupational Therapy Association (AOTA) emphasizes that occupational therapists are involved in health promotion (AOTA, 2008; College of Occupational Therapists [COT], 2008; Reitz, 2013) and the prevention of disability (AOTA, 2008). Per the *Guide to Occupational Therapy Practice* (Moyers and Dale, 2007), occupational therapists encourage healthy engagement in meaningful occupations and activities to discourage the "unhealthy effects of inactivity and inappropriate activity" (p. 16). Occupational therapists promote balance of leisure, work, and rest with patients/clients, thereby contributing to health promotion. Occupational therapists also teach skills in goal-setting, pacing, and energy conservation that can be crucial in promoting the health of people with disabilities (for example, people with chronic pain; see Chapter 28). Furthermore, occupational therapists often incorporate mindfulness techniques to promote awareness of existing habits, roles, and routines to make effective lifestyle changes to reflect wellness.

The role of occupational therapy in health promotion and prevention has been further defined by AOTA's position statement *Occupational Therapy in the Promotion of Health and Well-Being* (AOTA, 2013, p. S50), identifying three critical roles:

1. To promote healthy lifestyles
2. To emphasize occupation as an essential element of health promotion strategies
3. To provide interventions not only with individuals but also with populations

Occupational therapy's domain and process within the profession's practice framework incorporates various aspects of wellness. Health management and maintenance is considered an instrumental activity of daily living (IADL); health promotion and prevention are identified as occupational therapy intervention approaches; and prevention, health and wellness, quality of life, well-being, and occupational justice are listed as potential outcomes of occupational therapy services (AOTA, 2014).

The purpose of this chapter is to provide an overview of health promotion in general as a foundation for exploring health promotion in neurology. In addition to providing information about the current state of health promotion, the chapter will also show you how to incorporate health promotion into your clinical practice in neurology. Increasingly a proactive stance is needed in the health-care system overall, including the area of rehabilitation, and occupational and physical therapists are positioned to significantly contribute to this effort. Although both disciplines can address multiple areas of health promotion and wellness to the fullest potential of their respective practice acts, occupational therapists often have a particular focus on integration of mental health considerations across all domains of daily life (reflecting the concept of *occupation* as comprising any meaningful activities in which the individual chooses to engage), while physical therapists often focus on physical fitness at all levels of ability. Ultimately health promotion recognizes the intrinsic value of health for the betterment of the individual and society.

## PATIENT APPLICATION

### Introducing Dot

*Dorothy ("Dot") is a 38 year-old female diagnosed 2 years ago with relapsing/remitting multiple sclerosis (MS). Although she has had near-complete recovery after each previous exacerbation, a week ago she had another relapse and now is referred for outpatient therapy and is already showing signs of motor and sensory recovery. Dot is very concerned about her movement and whether she'll gain full recovery. She states, "I'll do anything to get full improvement again," but she is very worried the recovery might not happen this time. During your general review of systems questions, you find out she has a history of hypertension (and recently has not been taking her medications because they make her "feel bad") and that she smokes two packs of cigarettes a day. In addition to the sporadic distribution of motor and sensory deficits, you calculate her body mass index (BMI) is 33.2 (30 and higher is categorized as "obese"). After your initial examination, you formulate the plan of care and obviously start to work toward remediation of her primary impairments and optimization of the functional activities found to be limited. Consider these questions about Dot. More information about this case will be presented as the chapter is developed with additional questions to guide your clinical decision-making.*

### *Contemplate Clinical Decisions*

1. *Do you think that Dot really understands the potential health risks of her tobacco habit?*
2. *Should you ask Dot if she has ever tried to quit smoking? If so, how might you phrase the question?*
3. *Do you think this patient sees any connection between her statement, "I'll do anything to get full improvement again" and her health risk from smoking?*

# ■ Foundations of Health Promotion

## Terms and Definitions

The numerous terms and definitions related to health promotion can be confusing, and there is not always consensus among sources. However it is important to be aware of key terms and definitions from various sources and learn how they compare and contrast to understand the critical concepts of health promotion.

Green and Kreuter (1991) defined **health education** as "any combination of learning experiences designed to facilitate voluntary actions conducive to health" and health promotion as "the combination of educational and environmental supports for actions and conditions of living conducive to health." Thus health promotion encompasses health education but also includes additional supportive components. O'Donnell (1989) further clarified, "Lifestyle change can be facilitated through a combination of efforts to enhance awareness, change behavior, and create environments that support good health practices. Of the three, supportive environments will probably have the greatest impact in producing lasting changes." Health promotion includes the element of the environment in which the person is making health decisions and engaging in health behavior and thus has a broader focus than health education.

Gochman (1982, p. 169; 1997) defined **health behavior** as "those personal attributes such as beliefs, expectations, motives, values, perceptions, and other cognitive elements; personality characteristics including affective and emotional states and traits; and overt behavior patterns, actions, and habits that relate to health maintenance, to health restoration, and to health improvement." Clearly health behavior is a complex construct! We can assess health behavior through observation or by asking questions, and its complexity makes it difficult to change.

Kasl and Cobb (1966a, p. 246; 1966b, p. 531) defined health behavior as "any activity undertaken by a person believing himself to be healthy, for the purpose of preventing disease or detecting [disease] in an asymptomatic stage." A related term is **illness behavior**, defined by the same authors as "any activity, undertaken by a person who feels ill, to define the state of his health and to discover a suitable remedy. The principal activities here are complaining and seeking consultation from relatives, friends, and from those trained in matters of health." These authors go on to make a connection between illness and psychosocial function by defining **sick-role behavior** as "the activity undertaken by those who consider themselves ill, for the purpose of getting well. It includes receiving treatment from appropriate therapists, generally involves a whole range of dependent behaviors, and leads to some degree of neglect of one's usual duties."

The definitions of health behavior, illness behavior, and sick-role behavior illustrate the integral role of psychology in health promotion. **Health psychology** is a subdiscipline within psychology with roots in both social psychology and clinical psychology defined by Taylor (2009, p.3) as "an exciting and relatively new field devoted to understanding psychological influences on how people stay healthy, why they become ill, and how they respond when they do get ill. Health psychologists study such issues and promote interventions to help people stay well or get over illness." So, it is important to realize the literature on health education and health promotion is found in a wide variety of different sources depending on the background of the researchers.

Another important term commonly used is **wellness**, defined by Dunn (1961) as "an integrated method of functioning which is oriented toward maximizing the potential of which the individual is capable." As indicated by the date of this source, wellness as a construct has existed for decades. Even this first definition emphasized the individual reaching his or her full potential rather than simply avoiding disease to maintain his or her usual state of health. Though no consensus definition of wellness exists, Bezner (2007) and other authors have outlined general characteristics of wellness as a multidimensional construct going beyond the physical domain to also include psychological, social, emotional, spiritual, and intellectual dimensions. Figure 16-1 provides a graphic representation of the dynamic interactions between the components to expand the therapist's perspective beyond just the physical problems influencing health. According to Bezner (2007), the framework's orientation is **salutogenic**, meaning it seeks ways to affirmatively maximize health rather than remediate disease (i.e., a **pathogenic** orientation) or simply maintain the normal state (i.e., a **normogenic** orientation). Wellness reflects a systems view of people and their environments while considering interrelationships among people, groups, and the environments in which they operate.

Bezner (2007) has compared and contrasted the concepts of illness, prevention, and wellness (Table 16-1) to illustrate

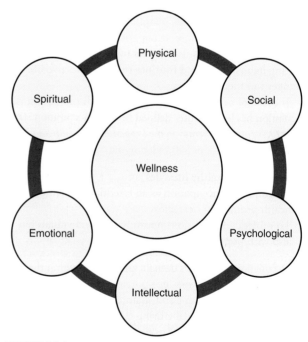

**FIGURE 16-1** A wellness model including physical domain as well as interactions of social, psychological, intellectual, emotional, and spiritual dimensions of wellness.

**TABLE 16-1** **The Wellness Matrix**

| | ILLNESS | PREVENTION | WELLNESS |
|---|---|---|---|
| View of human systems | Independent | Interactive | Integrative |
| Program orientation | Pathogenic | Normogenic | Salutogenic |
| Dependent variables | Clinical | Behavioral | Perceptual |
| Client status | Patient | Person at risk | Whole person |
| Intervention focus | Symptoms | Risk factors | Dispositions |
| Intervention method | Prescription | Lifestyle modification | Values clarification |
| The general intervention approach from a patient perspective | Fix the problems! | Avoid the future bad! | Pursue the potential good! |

Modified from Bezner, 2007, with permission.

general differences in focus. Illness, consistent with the traditional medical model, focuses on remediating disease while prevention focuses on maintaining the normal state. By contrast, wellness seeks to actively improve upon the normal state.

In addition to Bezner's model, there are other models of wellness. For example, the *Eight Dimensions of Wellness* (Swarbrick, 2006) includes dimensions of financial wellness (satisfaction with current and future financial situations) and occupational wellness (personal satisfaction and enrichment derived from one's work) as well as the six dimensions in Bezner's model.

APTA (APTA, *Physical Fitness*) has offered these definitions of the terms **physical fitness**, wellness, and **health**:

**Physical Fitness**: A dynamic physical state—comprising cardiovascular/pulmonary endurance; muscle strength, power, endurance, and flexibility; relaxation; and body composition—that allows optimal and efficient performance of daily and leisure activities.

**Wellness**: A multidimensional state of being, describing the existence of positive health in an individual as exemplified by quality of life and a sense of well-being.

**Health**: A state of being associated with freedom from disease, injury, and illness that also includes a positive component (wellness) that is associated with a quality of life and positive well-being.

These definitions of wellness and health are quite similar, which could cause confusion. However an understanding of some basic terms and definitions will decrease the likelihood of confusion from differences in terminology. For this chapter, the terms *health promotion* and occasionally *health education/health promotion* will be used. Note the definition of health promotion offered by O'Donnell (1989) incorporates multiple dimensions reflecting the concept of wellness as delineated by Bezner (2007).

A vital concept in health promotion is different levels of prevention. Consider these definitions from the *Guide* (APTA, 2015):

**Primary prevention**: Prevention of disease in a susceptible or potentially susceptible population through

specific measures such as general health promotion efforts.

**Secondary prevention**: Efforts to decrease duration of illness, severity of disease, and sequelae through early diagnosis and prompt intervention.

**Tertiary prevention**: Efforts to decrease the degree of disability and promote rehabilitation and restoration of function in patients with chronic and irreversible diseases.

To illustrate the levels of prevention, consider the management of cancer. Primary prevention entails decreasing modifiable risk factors such as tobacco use, poor diet and nutrition, alcohol use, and risky sexual and reproductive behavior (Goodman, *Oncology*, 2003). Secondary prevention encompasses early detection (e.g., mammography for breast cancer, colonoscopy for colon cancer, PSA for prostate cancer) and prompt treatment, whereas tertiary prevention entails limiting complications in established disease. The U.S. health-care system is largely geared toward secondary and tertiary prevention because most health-care services are aimed at remediating disease.

Physical therapy practice, particularly in geriatrics, is often at the level of tertiary prevention as the goal is to improve function and limit complications of acute or chronic disease or dysfunction, often in the presence of multiple comorbid conditions. For example, the physical therapy management of a patient with stroke would constitute tertiary prevention, while intervention in a patient with pneumonia would constitute secondary prevention. Screening activities can constitute primary or secondary prevention depending on the goal. Screening for risk factors (e.g., a family history of breast cancer) would constitute primary prevention, while screening for early disease (e.g., mammography) would constitute secondary prevention.

Occupational therapists can address all levels of prevention within any given population. For example, regarding risk of potential stroke, an occupational therapist might be involved with primary prevention when providing education to a group of people demonstrating risk factors for possible stroke, such as discussing healthier habits and structure to include meal planning and physical exercise. To carry out secondary prevention, occupational therapists might screen for depression in persons who have had a stroke as well as provide training regarding skills for stress management and adaptive coping strategies. Tertiary prevention might include providing rehabilitation of independent living skills or compensatory strategies in a person recovering from a stroke.

## Models of Health, Disablement, and Aging

Several important models provide some historical context for understanding the current state of the health promotion movement. The biomedical model and the biopsychosocial model represent two major theories of health and illness. In the **biomedical model**—the traditional model—illness is explained on the basis of biological factors and the focus is on disease rather than health. In philosophical terms, this model is based on reductionism and mind-body dualism reducing illness to a purely biological phenomenon studied and understood at the molecular level (Engel, 1977). By contrast the **biopsychosocial model** considers the interactions among biological, psychological, and social factors that give rise to health and illness. Thus, it is based on systems theory (Engel, 1977, 1980; Schwartz, 1982).

The Nagi (1965) model of disablement; the World Health Organization's (WHO's) International Classification of Impairments, Disabilities, and Handicaps (ICIDH); and the National Institutes of Health (NIH) National Center for Medical Rehabilitation Research (NCMRR) model (NIH, 1992) are summarized with examples in Chapter 1. For the purposes of this chapter, it is important to understand impairments may be *primary* (directly attributable to the pathology) or *secondary* (attributable to subsequent changes) (Jette, 1994). In neurology, pediatrics, and geriatrics, often the focus is on preventing or minimizing secondary impairments, which would constitute tertiary prevention.

In 2001, the WHO introduced a new substantially updated model: the International Classification of Functioning, Disability, and Health (ICF) as described in Chapter 1. The ICF model is now in wide use internationally. Because wellness reflects a systems view of persons and their environments and considers interrelationships among people, groups, and the environments in which they operate, wellness concepts are consistent with both the biopsychosocial model and the ICF. These models are mutually compatible and support the notion that health promotion is becoming integral to clinical practice.

Finally another model with face validity to clinicians is Spirduso's (1995) continuum of physical function among older adults. In this model, the individual older adult is characterized along a continuum ranging from physically elite to disabled, recognizing heterogeneity in aging. The model also illustrates geriatric disability is not the result of aging alone. Because physical function—like wellness—exists as a continuum, individuals can be found anywhere along that continuum, which is the basis of therapists' clinical practice and health promotion efforts and points to the importance of an individualized patient-centered examination and intervention.

## Professional Mandates for Therapists to Address Health Promotion

Health promotion has gained increasing focus in occupational and physical therapy and in health care. In addition to general guidelines, primarily from government sources, professional mandates for therapists to address health promotion have clarified the role of the occupational and physical therapist in health promotion. The U.S. national health objectives first outlined in the 1979 Surgeon General's report, *Healthy People: The Surgeon General's Report on Health Promotion and Disease Prevention* (U.S. Public Health Service, 1979), and *Healthy People 2000: National Health Promotion and Disease Prevention Objectives* (U.S. Public Health Service, 1991), led to the undeniably influential *Healthy People 2010: Understanding and Improving Health* (USDHHS, 2000) and its successor, *Healthy People 2020* (USDHHS, 2010). This consensus document produced by the federal government defines the nation's overall public health agenda. It has four overarching goals:

- Attain high-quality longer lives free of preventable disease, disability, injury, and premature death
- Achieve health equity, eliminate disparities, and improve the health of all groups
- Create social and physical environments that promote good health for all
- Promote quality of life, healthy development, and healthy behaviors across all life stages

These four overarching goals are supported by 12 topic areas (see Table 16-2) containing 26 Leading Health Indicators. Occupational and physical therapists can address these topic areas within clinical practice as evidence continues to support health promotion within the professions. For example, when developing an occupational profile of a patient/client,

| TABLE 16-2 | 12 Topic Areas of *Healthy People 2020* | |
|---|---|
| Access to Health Services | Nutrition, Physical Activity, and Obesity |
| Clinical Preventive Services | Oral Health |
| Environmental Quality | Reproductive and Sexual Health |
| Injury and Violence | Social Determinants |
| Maternal, Infant, and Child Health | Substance Abuse |
| Mental Health | Tobacco |

(US Department of Health and Human Services, 2010)

an occupational therapist might take note of a history of mental health or a tendency to abuse substances as means to cope with stressors. The therapist could then address these topic areas when encouraging development of daily structure and new habits, roles, and routines to promote health and wellness. Upon examination of a patient/client, a physical therapist could address physical activity, obesity, and some aspects of nutrition with education on risk factors in addition to establishment of an exercise program and referral to a nearby fitness facility and a registered dietitian. There is room for overlap between occupational and physical therapy to address the 12 topic areas, indicating the benefits of interdisciplinary care to maximize effectiveness of education to patients/clients.

Within the profession of physical therapy, several major documents address health promotion, including *A Normative Model of Physical Therapist Professional Education: Version 2004* (APTA, 2004). The *Guide* (APTA, 2015) states, "Physical therapists are involved in prevention; in promoting health, wellness, and fitness; and in performing screening activities." In the *Evaluative Criteria for Accreditation of Education Programs for the Preparation of Physical Therapists,* the Commission on Accreditation in Physical Therapy Education (CAPTE, 2016) addresses health promotion in a variety of domains as summarized in Table 16-3 along with the specific CAPTE objectives related to health promotion. Goal Eight of the APTA *Education Strategic Plan (2006–2020)* specifies "health promotion and wellness" and "healthy aging" as areas for added emphasis. Patient/client-related instruction to include "Health, wellness, and fitness programs" is specified as one of the *Minimum Required Skills of Physical Therapist Graduates at Entry-level* BOD P11-05-20-49 (APTA), which also lists "Promotion of Health, Wellness, and Prevention" as a distinct skill category with specific objectives listed in Table 16-4. Health promotion is addressed in Principle 8B of the APTA *Code of Ethics for the Physical Therapist* (APTA, *Code of Ethics*).

Also, several APTA House of Delegate positions emphasize the essential nature of health promotion in physical therapy practice (e.g., HOD P06-93-25-50, HOD P06-04-22-18, HOD P06-06-08-04). In 2008, the APTA House of Delegates passed RC 2-08, a new position on promoting physical activity including exercise that will amend APTA Position: *Promoting Physical Activity* HOD P06-03-29-28. The new position is titled *Physical Therapists and Physical Therapist Assistants as Promoters and Advocates for Physical Activity/Exercise.*

Occupational therapists also have a clear role in health promotion. The AOTA *Guide to Occupational Therapy Practice* (Moyers, 2007) clarifies that occupational therapists participate in disability prevention and health promotion both for individuals and for the larger population. The published *Scope of Practice* for occupational therapists (Brayman, 2004) includes, among other specific areas of practice, "(h)ealth promotion and wellness to enable or enhance performance in everyday life activities." Scaffa (2008) summarized three occupational therapy roles crucial in health promotion and disability prevention—"to promote healthy lifestyles; to

| TABLE 16-3 | Accreditation Criteria From the Commission on Accreditation in Physical Therapy Related to Health Promotion |
|---|---|
| 7D5 | Practice in a manner consistent with the APTA Core Values. |
| 7D16 | Determine when patients/clients need further examination or consultation by a physical therapist or referral to another health care professional. |
| 7D34 | Provide physical therapy services that address primary, secondary and tertiary prevention, health promotion, and wellness to individuals, groups, and communities. |

(CAPTE, 2016)

| TABLE 16-4 | Specific Objectives From the Skill Category "Promotion of Health, Wellness, and Prevention" in APTA Minimum Required Skills of Physical Therapist Graduates at Entry-level |
|---|---|

**Skill Category: Promotion of Health, Wellness, and Prevention**
1. Identify patient/client health risks during the history and physical via the systems review.
2. Take the vital signs of every patient/client during each visit.
3. Collaborate with the patient/client to develop and implement a plan to address health risks.
4. Determine readiness for behavioral change.
5. Identify available resources in the community to assist in the achievement of the plan.
6. Identify secondary and tertiary effects of disability.
7. Demonstrate healthy behaviors.
8. Promote health/wellness in the community.

(APTA, BOD P11-05-20-49)

emphasize occupation as an essential element of health promotion strategies; and to provide interventions"—and listed the occupational therapist's contribution to health promotion within the health-care delivery system (see Table 16-5).

## The Role of the Therapist in Health Promotion

Considering these documents collectively, it is imperative therapists focus not just on recovery from illness but also on promotion of prevention and wellness (Table 16-1). In keeping with the definition of health promotion, the role of the therapist encompasses both health education and environmental supports including advocacy. Health promotion by therapists should include not only patient/client management and screening but also community education and advocacy for policy and social change as well as research to contribute to the emerging body of knowledge.

### Two Approaches: The Wellness Model and Common Health Problems

There are multiple approaches in considering the therapist's role in health promotion. One approach is to use a wellness

| TABLE 16-5 | Contributions of the Occupational Therapist in Health Promotion |
|---|---|

**OCCUPATIONAL THERAPY PRACTITIONERS CAN**

- Evaluate occupational capabilities, values, and performance;
- Provide education regarding occupational role performance and balance;
- Reduce risk factors and symptoms through engagement in occupation;
- Provide skill development training in the context of everyday occupations;
- Provide self-management training to prevent illness and manage health;
- Modify environments for healthy and safe occupational performance;
- Consult and collaborate with health care professionals, organizations, communities, and policymakers regarding the occupational perspective of health promotion and disease or disability prevention;
- Promote the development and maintenance of mental functioning abilities through engagement in productive and meaningful activities and relationships (adapted from DHHS, 1999, p. 4); and
- Provide training in adaptation to change and in coping with adversity to promote mental health (adapted from DHHS, 1999, p. 4).

(Scaffa, 2008)

model such as Bezner's (2007), shown in Table 16-1, the therapist's perspective beyond just physical problems influencing health. Another approach is to use common health problems to organize the therapist's planning efforts. For example, Rea and colleagues (2004) addressed the physical therapist's role in health promotion using four focus areas of *Healthy People 2010* that they considered to be foundational: focus area 6 ("disability and secondary conditions" by looking at psychological well-being), focus area 19 ("nutrition and overweight"), focus area 22 ("physical fitness and activity"), and focus area 27 ("tobacco use"). They found physical therapists in three states were addressing all four areas with physical fitness and activity not surprisingly addressed most frequently but to varying degrees according to their self-efficacy in providing such education and in lower-than-desirable percentages. These statistics suggest additional education in health promotion topics is needed.

The authors suggest the role of the physical therapist in health promotion can be delineated in the following way: the physical therapist is (1) the expert on physical activity for persons with movement dysfunction and (2) a consultant on other health issues such as psychological well-being, nutrition and weight loss, and smoking cessation. This role includes referring to and collaborating with health-care providers and others to enhance the physical therapy patient/client management and recognizing circumstances necessitating a request for consultation and initiation of such consultation when in the best interest of the patient/client. As one example therapists should enhance their ability to identify mental health issues and assure patients receive the help they need. For physical therapists this role would likely be limited to recognition and referral, whereas occupational therapists often play a more integral role in provision of mental health services (Burson, 2010). In AOTA's knowledge and skills paper, *Specialized Knowledge and Skills in Mental Health Promotion, Prevention, and Intervention in Occupational Therapy Practice* (AOTA, 2010, p. 2), the goals of occupational therapy are described as "twofold: (1) to promote mental health and well-being in all persons with and without disabilities and (2) to restore, maintain, and improve function and quality of life for people at risk for or affected by mental illness."

The study by Rea and colleagues (2004) highlights a crucial aspect of the role of the physical therapist in health promotion: incorporating *health education* into routine clinical practice to include multiple areas that may often go unaddressed in contemporary practice (e.g., smoking cessation). As we will see in this chapter, there are also many other ways in which therapists can address health promotion. Examples include helping people with disabilities *transition to lifelong community-based fitness programs* (an approach strongly advocated by Rimmer, a leading researcher in the area of health promotion for people with disabilities) and *acting as consultants in chronic care*. This latter role of consulting in chronic care (i.e., for people with disabilities as they manage their care over time) fits well with the APTA position recommending annual visits to a physical therapist for everyone

(*Annual Visit With A Physical Therapist* HOD P05-07-19-20) as well as the active follow-up component of the Chronic Care Model promoted by Improving Chronic Illness Care (www.improvingchroniccare.org).

In addition, therapists now have access to condition-specific guidelines and recommendations for physical activity, an emerging critically important resource. For example, in 2004 the American Heart Association (AHA) published physical activity and exercise recommendations for people with stroke (Gordon, 2004). This document not only synthesizes evidence supporting the health benefits of physical activity in this patient population but also provides guidelines for preexercise evaluation and exercise programming. It was then updated in 2014 (Billinger, 2014). Such documents serve a dual purpose of informing health policy (at the level of public health) while also providing clinicians with evidence-based practice guidelines (at the level of patient care) consistent with the definition of health promotion. (It is interesting to note from the years of publication in this example that these types of documents comprise a fairly recent development representative of the rapid evolution of the literature in the health professions.)

### Terminology: Patients and Clients

What's in a name? The *Guide* (APTA, 2015) differentiates between **patients** and **clients** of physical therapy in this way:

> *Patients* are individuals who are the recipients of physical therapy examination, evaluation, diagnosis, prognosis, and intervention who have a disease, disorder, condition, impairment, functional limitation, or disability.
>
> *Clients* are individuals who engage the services of a physical therapist who can benefit from the physical therapist's consultation, interventions, professional advice, prevention services, or services promoting health, wellness, and fitness. Clients also are businesses, school systems, and others to whom physical therapists provide services.

This distinction emphasizes the opportunities for physical therapists to perform valuable services in such areas as consultation and personal fitness, even for individuals without diseases or disorders, outside of the traditional arena of the patient-provider relationship in health care.

The AOTA recently revised the *Occupational Therapy Practice Framework* (AOTA, 2014) to define "clients" as *persons, groups,* and *populations.* Per the AOTA's position statement on *Occupational Therapy in the Promotion of Health and Well-Being* (AOTA, 2013, p. S49), "occupational therapy practitioners can develop and implement occupation-based population health approaches to enhance occupational performance and participation, quality of life, and occupational justice." In this case, the inclusion of groups and populations shows how the way the labels are

defined can open new venues in which therapists can apply their knowledge and skills. For example, an occupational therapist might serve as an ergonomics consultant for a large corporation or teach a life-skills class to a prison population before reentry into society.

## THINK ABOUT IT 16.1

Some people believe the term "patient" is somewhat authoritarian, creating a relationship based on inequality, while the term "client" is more empowering. Others believe the term "client" is too closely associated with the service industry and is therefore not optimal in the context of health care. The APTA endorsed both terms (APTA Guide, 2015). What do you think? Do certain circumstances apply more to one term?

### Regulatory Issues

#### State Practice Acts

While health promotion is a crucial element of each profession as defined by major documents of the national associations, the practice of occupational therapists, certified occupational therapy assistants, physical therapists, and physical therapist assistants, like most of the other health professions, is governed at the state level as each state or jurisdiction has its own practice act defining the scope of practice. Both the *Model Practice Act for Physical Therapy: A Tool for Public Protection and Legislative Change* (FSBPT, 2006) of the Federation of State Boards of Physical Therapy and the *Definition of Occupational Therapy Practice for the Model Practice Act* (AOTA, 2004) specifically address health promotion. However some states have not adopted model-practice-act language. The APTA document *Wellness—Fitness—Health Promotion: Specific Language in State PT Practice Acts* (APTA, *Wellness-Fitness*) asserts health promotion is considered within the scope of practice but notes the language in each state practice act must be considered. The document summarizes language in state practice acts; however this is a rapidly changing area requiring the most up-to-date verification with the appropriate licensing authority.

#### Liability

Introductory information on risk management was given in the APTA document *Emerging PT Practice: Number 11: Senior Wellness* (APTA, *Emerging-Senior Wellness*). One key point is that wellness services may not be covered by the physical therapist's professional liability insurance; therefore it is vital for the therapist to be familiar with the coverage provided by his or her policy.

#### Reimbursement

Unfortunately many services related to health promotion are not reimbursable across professions within our healthcare system despite the obvious cost savings of maintaining a healthy population. This problem is a key target of healthcare reform efforts. Indeed a major push of the Patient

Protection and Affordable Care Act of 2010 was to integrate public health and clinical health in an attempt to move beyond the traditional model of episodic disease-oriented care to an emphasis on the achievement of quality markers and long-term health outcomes. To accomplish this aim, the health-care delivery system would be organized around accountable-care organizations reimbursed based on their performance in a patient-centered model. Thus this model has the potential to incorporate health promotion efforts into payment methodology.

The arena of reimbursement for services related to health promotion is an opportunity for therapists to engage in advocacy efforts both at the grassroots level and through their professional associations aimed at increasing reimbursement for and resisting legislative cuts to public health services. Such efforts recognize not only the intrinsic value of health but also the potential for future cost savings to the health-care system through reduction of expenditures related to care for such devastating and expensive conditions as diabetes. This potential is particularly true for large-scale efforts at the population level, which is the domain of public health, and applies even in the context of individuals with neurological health conditions.

In summary a shift in the nation's health-care system toward health promotion may well be underway, and therapists have the opportunity to help influence this process. In the meantime, consumers are often willing to pay for health promotion services out of pocket with opportunities for cash-based services and the development of niche markets. A further opportunity for therapists is the incorporation of health promotion efforts into traditional episodes of care. For instance patient/client education can be incorporated into treatment sessions in the form of discussions about health topics relevant to the individual patient/client. Such discussions can occur during routine treatment activities thus taking no extra time or additional charges.

### Non-Traditional Jobs in Health Promotion for Therapists

In addition to clinical roles in which they primarily provide patient/client services and may perform clinical-based research, therapists may also serve in regulatory and other roles within the federal government, corporations (e.g., corporate wellness programs), and academia. Although therapists often serve in academic departments of occupational and physical therapy, they may also serve in other departments and centers, including departments of health education and multidisciplinary research centers.

## Models of Practice

### Screening

According to the *Guide* (APTA, 2015):

> *Physical therapists conduct preliminary screenings to determine the need for (1) primary, secondary, or tertiary prevention services; (2) further examination, intervention, or consultation*

*by a physical therapist; or (3) referral to another practitioner. Candidates for screening generally are not patients/clients currently receiving physical therapy services. Screening is based on a problem-focused systematic collection and analysis of data.*

Some examples of the prevention screening activities in which therapists may engage are summarized in Table 16-6.

### Rimmer's Model of Health Promotion for People with Disabilities

Rimmer (1999) proposed a model of health promotion for people with disabilities in which it is not only important to consider in terms of charting the historical development of health promotion in physical therapy but also includes important practical recommendations still highly relevant to both occupational and physical therapists today in the context of disability. Rimmer advanced the idea that health promotion is for everyone—including people with disabilities—and asserted the aims of health promotion for people with disabilities are (1) to reduce secondary conditions (e.g., obesity, hypertension [HTN], pressure sores), (2) to maintain functional independence, (3) to provide an opportunity for leisure and enjoyment, and (4) to enhance overall quality of life by reducing environmental barriers to good health.

As an example of how the health-care system could better address the health needs of people with disabilities, Rimmer proposed a model for community-based health promotion in which the fitness center is the ultimate setting (Figure 16-2). In this model, a continuum of services ranges from physical therapy to fitness and takes place in corresponding settings for rehabilitation (which takes place in inpatient settings), clinically supervised health promotion (which takes places in outpatient settings), and community-based health promotion (which takes place in accessible fitness centers). The model, providing a construct for the therapist to consider throughout

| TABLE 16-6 | Examples of Preventive Screening in Which a Therapist Might Engage |
|---|---|

- Identification of lifestyle factors (e.g., amount of exercise, stress, weight) that may lead to increased risk for serious health problems
- Identification of children or adults who may need an examination for idiopathic scoliosis
- Identification of children with undiagnosed developmental delay
- Identification of elderly individuals in a community center or nursing home who are at high risk for falls
- Identification of risk factors for neuromusculoskeletal injuries in the workplace
- Preperformance testing of individuals who are active in sports

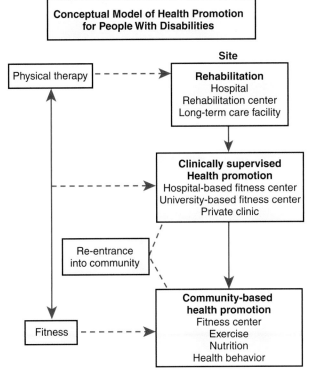

**Conceptual Model of Health Promotion for People With Disabilities**

FIGURE 16-2 **Rimmer's Model of Health Promotion for People with Disabilities.** Rimmer's model for community-based health promotion. Note the fitness center as the ultimate setting for patients with neurological dysfunction. *(Reprinted from Rimmer JH. Health promotion for people with disabilities: The emerging paradigm shift from disability prevention to prevention of secondary conditions. Phys Ther. 1999;79:495–502, with permission of the American Physical Therapy Association.)*

the rehab process, involves a partnership between rehabilitation professionals who provide clinical services and fitness professionals/fitness instructors who provide community-based services.

Although the model is noteworthy as an early effort in the arena of health promotion by physical therapists, it is problematic in that the terms "fitness professionals" and "fitness instructors" are not well-defined, though exercise physiologists and therapeutic recreation specialists are mentioned. Also the model does not allow for the possibility that physical therapists may follow an individual throughout the entire continuum of care—as indeed is possible in some outpatient clinics that offer postdischarge gym memberships. Rimmer's model invites important questions.

## THINK ABOUT IT 16.2

Should physical therapists partner with "fitness professionals" or offer aftercare/maintenance/physical fitness, wellness, and health services themselves? Who are "fitness professionals"? Certainly there are undergraduate and graduate degrees in exercise science/exercise physiology as well as numerous certifications available

through reputable bodies such as the American Sports Medicine Association; however, personal trainers are not regulated by law, leaving the consumer unprotected. Do physical therapists fit the label of "fitness professionals"?

The APTA addressed this issue in *Emerging PT Practice: Number 11: Senior Wellness* (APTA, *Senior Wellness*, p. 1):

Physical therapists have the expertise to prescribe individualized, safe, and effective exercise programs for older clients who may have a number of complicating health factors, such as osteoporosis, arthritis, joint replacement, diabetes, hypertension, and deconditioning. Physical therapists can make appropriate modifications that are not typically within the expertise of a fitness trainer. Physical therapists can also make appropriate referrals when they detect a serious medical condition.

### A Health Promotion Model for Therapists

Consider a theoretical model of health promotion by therapists (Figure 16-3). The model illustrates therapists have the opportunity to engage in health promotion activities including, but not limited to, patient/client management. Within patient/client management, therapists can improve their incorporation of health promotion by considering opportunities to address other levels of prevention (i.e., primary and secondary), other dimensions of wellness, and health issues not directly related to the presenting problem/chief complaint but nevertheless are either within the therapist's scope of practice or worthy of an appropriate referral. Note the diagram and recall from the Wellness Matrix (Bezner, 2007) (Table 16-1) that promotion of wellness (health and fitness) is distinct from prevention; the focus of wellness is on affirmative health, actually optimizing and maximizing health, rather than mere prevention of disease.

As we saw earlier, while much of therapist clinical practice probably occurs at the level of tertiary prevention (limiting the degree of disability and promoting rehabilitation and restoration of function in patients with chronic and irreversible diseases), it could also be at the level of secondary prevention (decreasing duration of illness, severity of disease, and number of sequelae through early diagnosis and prompt intervention). An example of secondary prevention in clinical practice would be prescribing exercise in an acute care setting for an older adult with a general medical condition to combat the undesirable **deconditioning** associated with both the illness and the inactivity of hospitalization. An example of primary prevention (preventing a target condition in a susceptible or potentially susceptible population) would be encouraging smoking cessation in a patient who smokes but does not have lung cancer. Another example of primary prevention would be efforts toward preventing the onset of diabetes in someone with known **risk factors**.

Consider an example of addressing other levels of prevention for the presenting problem for a patient. The therapist could educate the patient with stroke and his or her caregivers about the patient's risk factors for recurrent stroke (primary

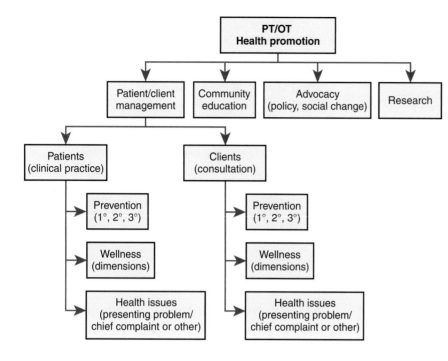

**FIGURE 16-3 A Model of Health Promotion for Occupational and Physical Therapists.** The model illustrates that PTs have the opportunity to engage in health promotion activities including patient/client management, community education, advocacy, and research. Within patient/client management, PTs can improve their incorporation of health promotion by considering opportunities to address other levels of prevention, other dimensions of wellness, and health issues that may not be directly related to the presenting problem/chief complaint.

prevention) and appropriate actions to take in the presence of signs and symptoms of recurrent stroke (secondary prevention). An example of addressing other health issues for a patient would be educating the patient with stroke and his or her caregivers about the importance of keeping an updated medication list. It is worth noting that, because many therapists develop ongoing relationships with their patients/clients, reflecting the practitioner's role in primary care, individuals may move back and forth between the categories of patient and client.

Addressing other health issues is analogous in part to the anticipated problems of the Hypothesis-Oriented Algorithm for Clinicians (HOAC II) described by Rothstein, Echternach, and Riddle (2003). The HOAC II differentiates between existing problems that require remediation and potential problems requiring prevention. Problems of either type may be identified by the patient or by another person (e.g., a caregiver or the therapist). A strength of this model is it explicitly identifies prevention as a goal. However there are also several limitations to the framework. First it does not clearly differentiate between prevention of secondary complications (a concept therapists understand well and incorporate into clinical practice but which is arguably a component of tertiary prevention) and prevention at higher levels (at which therapists may not typically operate to their full potential). Also the delineated problems —whether by the patient or by another and whether existing or potential— are focused on the presenting problem/chief complaint; thus the model does not explicitly provide a mechanism for the therapist to address health issues not related to the nature of the chief complaint. For example, the therapist who encourages smoking cessation in a patient with low back pain of musculoskeletal origin is addressing health issues not directly related to the presenting problem/chief complaint.

## Opportunities and Resources for Therapists in Health Promotion

Therapists can participate in innumerable health promotion opportunities, including the specific examples from the *Guide* (APTA, 2015) presented in Box 16-1 and examples presented by the APTA and the Academy of Geriatric Physical Therapy in their online downloadable resources summarized in Table 16-7.

## Adherence and Health Behavior Theories/Models

A major obstacle to the achievement of better health is poor adherence to healthy behavior and actions. **Adherence** is the degree to which a person's decisions, actions, and behaviors follow an established plan after participating in an episode of health education. The established plan of prescriptive intervention or healthy actions is sometimes mutually established by the health-care professional and the patient/client but, to be effective, must always be embraced by the individual. Taking medications as prescribed or participating in a customized home exercise program (HEP) are two examples of adherence. **Compliance** is a related term that may imply an authoritarian approach with the plan being established by the health-care provider rather than through a patient-centered collaboration in decision-making.

Research on HEPs for community-dwelling older adults illustrates the importance of adherence. In addition to demonstrating health benefits of an HEP, research has also found long-term adherence to be suboptimal at ~42% to 44% (Campbell, 1997; Campbell, 1999; Robertson, 2001). Suboptimal adherence is a problem because the benefits of exercise

## BOX 16-1   Examples of Health Promotion Activities, Based on *Guide to Physical Therapist Practice*

Examples of prevention activities and health, wellness, and fitness promotion activities in which therapists engage include:

- Workplace redesign, back schools, strengthening, stretching, endurance exercise programs, and postural training to prevent and manage low back pain
- Ergonomic redesign; strengthening, stretching, and endurance exercise programs; postural training to prevent job-related disabilities including trauma and repetitive stress injuries
- Exercise programs including weight-bearing and weight training to increase bone mass and bone density (especially in older adults with osteopenia and osteoporosis)
- Exercise programs, gait training, and balance and coordination activities to reduce the risk of falls—and the risk of fractures from falls—in older adults
- Exercise programs and instruction in ADL (self-care, communication, and mobility skills required for independence in daily living) and instrumental activities of daily living (IADL; activities that are important components of maintaining independent living, such as shopping and cooking) to decrease utilization of health-care services and enhance function in individuals with cardiovascular/pulmonary disorders
- Exercise programs, cardiovascular conditioning, postural training, and instruction in ADL and IADL to prevent disability and dysfunction in women who are pregnant
- Broad-based consumer education and advocacy programs to prevent problems (e.g., prevent head injury by promoting the use of helmets, prevent pulmonary disease by encouraging smoking cessation)
- Exercise programs to prevent or reduce the development of sequelae in individuals with lifelong conditions
- Develop programs for healthy lifestyle for individuals to decrease the risk of noncommunicable disease and disability

(APTA, 2015)

## TABLE 16-7   Online Resources for the Therapist Developing a Health Promotion Focus

| WEBSITE | WEB ADDRESS | RESOURCES AVAILABLE |
| --- | --- | --- |
| AOTA: Practice: Health and Wellness | www.aota.org | • Tips for Living: Brief tip sheets to help people cope with a variety of health conditions and explain how occupational therapy can help. |
| AOTA: Practice: Health and Wellness | www.aota.org | • Health and Wellness Evidence: Evidence-based practice information and the latest research to guide your practice. |
| AOTA: Practice: Health and Wellness | www.aota.org | • AOTA Official Documents: Informative documents on the role and scope of occupational therapy services. Included are *Occupational Therapy in the Promotion of Health and Well-Being; Specialized Knowledge and Skills in Mental Health Promotion, Prevention, and Intervention in Occupational Therapy Practice;* and *Occupational Therapy's Perspective on the Use of Environments and Contexts to Facilitate Health, Well-Being, and Participation in Occupations.* |
| AOTA: Practice: Health and Wellness | www.aota.org | • Fact Sheets on the Role of OT: Designed for OT practitioners and other professionals to explain the role and scope of occupational therapy. Included is *Occupational Therapy's Role in Health Promotion.* |
| AOTA: Practice: Health and Wellness | www.aota.org | • Other Resources: Suggested apps for health and wellness. |
| APTA: Practice and Patient Care: Prevention and Wellness | www.apta.org | • A section on prevention, wellness, and disease management that includes, among many other resources, resources on providing an adult fitness examination and on malpractice/professional liability in the provision of fitness services. |
| APTA: Practice and Patient Care: Physical Fitness for Special Populations | www.apta.org | • "Physical Fitness for Special Populations" features many useful links, including links to printable pocket guides for therapist use. |

*Continued*

| TABLE 16-7 | Online Resources for the Therapist Developing a Health Promotion Focus—cont'd | |
|---|---|---|
| **WEBSITE** | **WEB ADDRESS** | **RESOURCES AVAILABLE** |
| APTA Academy of Geriatric Physical Therapy: Member Resources | www.geriatricspt.org | • The document "Exercise Recommendations for Older Adults" can be downloaded.<br>• Contains patient education brochures—including such topics as fall prevention, osteoporosis, and walking—and practice resources including consumer-oriented PowerPoint presentations titled "From Frail to Fun," "So You Want to Begin Exercising," "Staying Vertical: Balance and Falls Reduction," "Osteoporosis: What You Should Know," and "Physical Activity: A Key to Wellness and Successful Aging." The Section on Geriatrics also features a special interest group on health promotion and wellness. |

depend on continued participation (Campbell, 1999). Thus efforts to maximize adherence to HEP, especially when the patient may not see the benefit, have the potential to improve patient/client outcomes, freeing the health-care system for more appropriate utilization (Hardage, 2007). Interventions and strategies to maximize adherence represent another opportunity for therapists to participate in health education/health promotion.

**Social Cognitive Theory (SCT)** is a major health behavior theory (Bandura, 1977; Bandura, 1986; Bandura, 1995; Bandura, 1997a; Bandura, 1997b) used to predict exercise adherence in older adults (Grembowski, 1993; Jette, 1998; Resnick, 2000; Resnick and Jenkins, 2000; Resnick and Spellbring, 2000; Resnick, 2001; Resnick et al, 2001; Schuster, 1995). Fundamental constructs of SCT include self-efficacy expectations, outcome expectations, and outcome expectancies. These constructs provide a language for understanding health behavior. **Self-efficacy expectations** are the belief one can successfully perform a target behavior. They are

behavior-specific and usually involve confidence in overcoming potential barriers. **Outcome expectations** are the belief that performing the target behavior will lead to the desired outcome, and **outcome expectancies** are the importance the individual places on the expected outcome of the target behavior. These constructs, as defined, are illustrated with therapy-related examples in Table 16-8.

Research into exercise nonadherence has investigated some clinical conditions, but relatively little has been done regarding individuals at risk of falls, which is particularly a problem after neurological health conditions because of their primary impairments of motor, somatosensory, vestibular, and visual systems. Research varies according to two dimensions: (1) use of specific strategies to facilitate adherence versus patient characteristics associated with adherence and nonadherence and (2) use of a theoretical framework such as SCT. Specific strategies used include examining the number of exercises comprising the HEP (Henry, 1999), the use of graphic feedback (Duncan, 2002), and the use of ongoing telephone contact

| TABLE 16-8 | Neurological-Related Examples of the Social Cognitive Theory (SCT) Constructs | |
|---|---|---|
| | **SMOKING CESSATION EXAMPLE** | **WEIGHT-LOSS (EXERCISE/DIET) EXAMPLE** |
| Self-efficacy expectations: | A person must believe that he or she can stop smoking to effectively implement a smoking cessation plan. | A person must believe that he or she can institute personal lifestyle changes that include an intentional increase in exercise and decrease in dietary caloric intake. |
| Outcome expectations: | A person must believe that smoking cessation methods, including nicotine replacement therapy, addressing the physical addiction, and behavioral strategies addressing the psychological component, do help people quit smoking. | A person must believe that increasing calorie use (through exercise) and decreasing calorie intake (through diet) do result in weight loss. |
| Outcome expectancies: | A person must believe that smoking cessation will enhance engagement in an active lifestyle and will make diseases like lung cancer and chronic obstructive pulmonary disease much less likely, and that these outcomes are important for them and their family. | A person must believe that weight loss will enhance quality and enjoyment of life and decrease the onset of multiple diseases including cardiovascular disease, diabetes, and musculoskeletal disorders. |

for encouragement and advice (Campbell, 1997; Campbell, 1999; Robertson, 2001).

Campbell and colleagues (2001) found factors associated with adherence in a sample of patients with osteoarthritis of the knee included perception of exercise effectiveness, willingness and ability to make time to perform the exercises, perceived severity of symptoms, and attitudes toward arthritis and comorbidity. Sluijs and colleagues (1993) found adherence to exercise during physical therapy was negatively affected by perceived barriers, and Biddle (1994) demonstrated adherence to exercise in university employees was influenced by self-efficacy. Jette and colleagues (1998) found positive attitudes and sense of control toward exercise, lower levels of confusion and depressive moods, and the development of fewer new medical problems were related to better adherence to home-based resistance training in community-dwelling older adults. Allison and Keller (1997) proposed a lack of support from significant others is a primary predictor of nonadherence.

Two health behavior theories/models used to examine exercise adherence in cardiac rehabilitation (Blanchard, 2003; Hellman, 1997) include the Transtheoretical Model or Stages of Change (Prochaska, 1979) and the **Theory of Planned Behavior** (Ajzen, 1991; Ajzen and Driver, 1991; Ajzen, 1985). These theories/models offer excellent examples of how therapists can use a theoretical model to promote adherence.

### Transtheoretical Model (Stages of Change)

The **Transtheoretical Model** (Prochaska, 1979), also called **Stages of Change,** is commonly used and involves six stages in the adoption of health behaviors.

- **Precontemplation**: the person has no intention to take action within the next 6 months.

- **Contemplation**: the person does intend to take action within the next 6 months.
- **Preparation**: the person intends to take action within the next 30 days.
- **Action**: the person has changed his or her overt behavior for less than 6 months.
- **Maintenance**: the person has changed his or her overt behavior for more than 6 months.
- **Termination**: the person no longer succumbs to temptation and has total self-efficacy.

Using this model can be helpful for understanding why a person might be nonadherent. The person who articulates thoughts in the precontemplation stage has no intention to take action within the next 6 months. Therefore efforts would be directed at moving the person to the contemplation stage, using education and motivation, for example, emphasizing to the person the benefits of exercise rather than prescribing exercise at that time.

### Theory of Planned Behavior

Another health promotion theory/model is the Theory of Planned Behavior (Ajzen, 1991; Ajzen and Driver, 1991; Ajzen, 1985). In this model (see Figure 16-4), behavior is determined by an individual's **behavioral intention**, which in turn is determined by the ***attitude toward the behavior, subjective norm,*** and ***perceived behavioral control.*** Each of these three theory constructs, in turn, is made up of two components, all of which offer opportunities for the therapist to intervene to promote adherence.

*Attitude toward the behavior* is influenced by ***behavioral belief*** (the belief that performing a given behavior is associated with certain attributes or outcomes) and ***evaluation of***

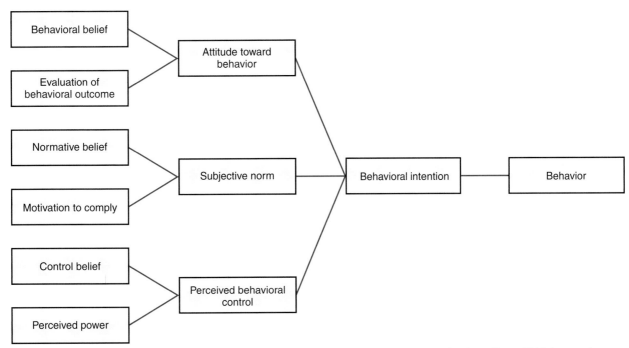

**FIGURE 16-4  Illustration of the potential interactions of the Theory of Planned Behavior.** *(Ajzen, 1991; Ajzen and Driver, 1991; Ajzen and Madden, 1986)*

*behavioral outcome* (the value attached to those attributes or outcomes). *Subjective norm* is influenced by *normative belief* (the belief about whether each of the individual's referents approves or disapproves of the behavior) and *motivation to comply* (the motivation to behave according to each referent's wishes). (A *referent* is a significant other—someone of importance to the individual.) *Perceived behavioral control* is influenced by *control belief* (the perceived likelihood of occurrence of each facilitating or constraining condition) and *perceived power* (the perceived effect of each condition in making performance of the target behavior difficult or easy).

Therefore strategies to facilitate adherence include educating the patient/client about the benefits of the activity (thus influencing behavioral belief), educating the patient's/client's referents about the benefits of exercise (thus influencing normative belief), promoting the perception of the therapist as a referent (again influencing normative belief), and maximizing facilitating conditions (thus influencing control belief). For example, promoting the use of the therapist as a referent can be as simple as communicating to the patient/client the importance to the therapist personally that the patient/client exercises. Facilitating conditions must be explored with each patient/client individually. For instance, if transportation is a barrier, then a HEP could be very important.

Using a health behavior theory/model such as the Stages of Change or the Theory of Planned Behavior can help the therapist plan patient/client education by giving direction as to what messages are important to give and to whom. Although the therapist may already routinely use elements of such an approach, using a health behavior theory/model gives the therapist a language and conceptual framework with which to approach adherence in a systematic way for maximum effect. In fact, the therapist may even choose to discuss the theory/model itself with the patient/client as a way to provide insight into his or her own behavior.

### Barriers to Adherence

Barriers to adherence in health care include poor health status and health disparities described here.

### Poor Health Status

Adherence in health care, like health behavior in general, is a complex topic and major area of research. For example, poor health status is, not surprisingly, a correlate of physical inactivity in older adults. Specific predictors include poor self-appraisal of overall health and the presence of chronic conditions, depressive symptoms, injuries, mobility limitations, pain, and fear of pain. Thus there is evidence that exercise adherence in older adults who are in poor health is influenced by different factors than in those who are well (Dominick, 2006). This is an important consideration because many of these same factors can be present in the individual with a neurological condition, and indeed many people with neurological conditions (e.g., stroke) are older adults.

Although poor health status impedes exercise adherence, it is easy to speculate older adults and those with neurological conditions who are participating in physical rehabilitation

may also actually have unique facilitating conditions. For instance, when exercise is prescribed as part of their health care, they may be biased to believe it may benefit them. They may also feel obligated to adhere. Finally they may have good self-efficacy for performing the exercise program because it was individually prescribed, customized to their level of function, and taught to them (Hardage, 2007). The therapist can capitalize on such factors by emphasizing and reinforcing them.

Zinn (2006) presents three factors making adherence in rehabilitation unique that therapists should keep in mind: (1) the presence of both an acute phase and a chronic phase, both of which have distinct characteristics; (2) the presence of high rates of physical impairments, cognitive impairments, or both; and (3) societal attitudes and particularly the social stigma attached to handicap. She cites the complexity of risk factors for nonadherence, including demographic characteristics, personality factors, the presence of mood disorders, the presence of frailty (a condition in which the individual is operating at his maximum capacity in performing IADLs and may require assistance), and level of social support. Additional research is needed to delineate factors uniquely important to exercise adherence in adults with disabilities both during and after physical rehabilitation (Hardage, 2007).

### Health Disparities

Health disparities research is a major focus within the field of public health. **Health disparities** are differences in health indicators and quality of life between specific groups of people. There are many categories of health indicators (Venes, 2009, p. 1016) including environmental (e.g., air quality advisories, pesticide levels in foods), general (e.g., birth rate, life expectancy), maternal-child (e.g., infant mortality rate, infant birth weight), prevention and screening (e.g., vaccination rates, tobacco counseling), and treatment (access to care, availability of primary care providers). Information on health disparities in general is available from the Centers for Disease Control (CDC, *Health Disparities*) at www.cdc.gov/minorityhealth/CHDIReport.html.

The CDC maintains statistics on health disparities among people with disabilities (CDC, *Injury Prevention*). For example, 40% of adults with disabilities report fair or poor health compared with only 10% of adults without disabilities. Also adults with disabilities are more likely than those without disabilities to smoke, be obese, and physically inactive (CDC, *Health Disparities*). Tips for clinicians and people with disabilities in addressing health-care access and health, wellness, and fitness are available at http://www.cdc.gov/ncbddd/disabilityandhealth/pa.html (CDC, *Increasing Physical Activity*).

Therapists, whose role has traditionally been to engage in clinical care (i.e., at the level of the individual), typically do not receive much education in health issues at the population level, which again is the province of public health. However the public-health perspective is important for clinicians to consider in the context of adherence. The effect of poverty, for example, can be a major barrier to adherence to health behaviors especially for women and children. This effect is particularly relevant with respect to diet where economics and marketing can be major challenges to meeting even the most basic health guidelines. For example, the dietary guidelines of the U.S. Department of Agriculture (USDA) and USDHHS (USDA, 2010) may be difficult to meet for a family of four living at or near the poverty level. (The guidelines, including the Executive Summary and Key Recommendations, are available at www.fns.usda.gov/dietary-guidelines-americans-2010.)

Therapists must be aware of such issues as lack of health access and the degree of vulnerability due to socioeconomic factors for some groups. This public-health perspective can help therapists promote adherence to health behaviors for their patients/clients by considering the context in which those health behaviors must take place, the barriers the individual may face, and what resources are available to help the individual overcome those barriers. It also helps members and leaders of the occupational and physical therapy professions decide how to set their policy, advocacy, and research agendas.

## PATIENT APPLICATION

### Dot, Step 2

*Over the weeks you are delivering the therapy plan of care, you get to know Dot much better. Upon questioning her about her health behavior, you learn she did try to quit smoking once about a year ago, but this effort only lasted 2 days. She says she doesn't know if she could even try to quit now with everything going on. She has never tried to go on a diet but states she is embarrassed about her weight and realizes she eats too much at each meal and snacks too much between meals.*

### Contemplate Clinical Decisions

1. How could you explore Dot's stage of change regarding smoking cessation?
2. How could you explore Dot's stage of change for nutritional changes (limiting calories and fat intake) and increasing physical exercise?
3. If Dot is still in the precontemplation stage for smoking cessation, what might you say to help her see the value and personal benefit of giving up smoking?

## ■ Health Promotion in Neurology

Having discussed health promotion as a general concept, the chapter will now focus on health promotion for people with disabilities and specifically for those with disabilities due to neurological disorders (e.g., stroke, traumatic brain injury, spinal cord injury, balance and vestibular disorders, cerebral palsy). People with disabilities are often not included in primary prevention programs to minimize risk for chronic conditions such as diabetes, cancer, heart disease, stroke (Patrick, 1994) because the focus is on fixing the problems resulting from the primary disorder. However there is growing recognition physical activity is essential for everyone, including people with disabilities.

In 2008, the USDHHS released the inaugural *Physical Activity Guidelines for Americans,* a major document for both policymakers and health professionals including key guidelines for adults with disabilities and key messages for people with chronic medical conditions (Chapter 7, available at www.health.gov/paguidelines/guidelines/default.aspx). These key guidelines with specific evidence-based recommendations for both aerobic and muscle-strengthening activities are the same as the key guidelines for adults. The document provides further clarification that individuals with disabilities who are unable to meet the specific recommendations should participate in physical activity to the best of their ability and avoid inactivity. This document reinforces the concept that all people, including people with disabilities, need ongoing physical activity for lifelong fitness.

It is worth noting too that the areas of neurology and geriatrics often overlap. This overlap can occur in at least two ways: (1) the aging of people with neurological conditions of congenital origin or acquired in infancy, childhood, adolescence, or young adulthood and (2) the occurrence of neurological conditions in older adults.

## Public Health in Individuals With Neurological Disorders

The WHO (2006) cites multiple public health challenges in the arena of neurology: (1) a "vast gap in the knowledge concerning the public health aspects of neurological disorders" (p. vii), (2) a serious underestimation of the burden of neurological disorders "by traditional epidemiological and health statistical methods that take into account only mortality rates but not disability rates" (p. 1), and (3) inadequate resources for patients with neurological disorders in most parts of the world—including the United States. For example, people with neurological disorders in the United States have problems accessing community-based fitness centers (Rimmer, 2005). Clearly there is much to be done to address the public health challenges of neurological disorders. The WHO (2006, p. 177) states "unless immediate action is taken globally, the neurological burden is expected to become an even more serious and unmanageable threat to public health."

Millions of Americans are currently affected by neurological disabilities, and the effect may rise significantly as the population ages and medical advances decrease mortality but consequently increase morbidity. Worldwide current estimates of neurological disorders and sequelae approach 1 billion lives. These numbers compel authorities to urge a call to action to mitigate an emerging public health crisis of neurological burden (WHO, 2006). Improved delivery of health promotion recommendations to people with disabilities due to neurological impairments may improve their health and quality of life.

According to the Global Burden of Disease Study (WHO, 1996), traditional epidemiological reports have underestimated the prevalence of neurological disorders because mortality statistics, rather than rates of disability, were the unit of measure. A 2004 update of the study (WHO, 2004) discovered that although mental and neurological disorders account for about 1% of deaths, they account for nearly 11% of the disease burden. The WHO suggests disease burden is a method to address "the gap between current health status and an ideal situation where everyone lives into old age free of disease and disability" (WHO, 2004, p. 3). The disparity arises from premature mortality, disability, and certain risk factors contributing to illness (WHO, 2004). An analysis in *Neurological Disorders: Public Health Challenges* (WHO, 2006) found neurological disorders cause a much higher burden than digestive diseases, respiratory diseases, and malignant neoplasms.

The emerging epidemic of neurological disability stems from the heterogeneous origins of the disorders and the fact they affect all age groups. Etiological factors include, for example, neurodevelopmental issues among neonates, degenerative disorders of the mature nervous system during midlife, and cerebrovascular accidents among older adults. Additionally, neurological disability can arise from demyelinating conditions such as MS; tumors such as glioblastomas, meningiomas, and neurofibromas; traumatic injury of brain, spinal cord, and nerves; metabolic conditions; genetics; autoimmune disorders; infections; and neuropathies.

For many individuals, life is completely different after a neurological event. Most neurological disorders are chronic and often include a progressive or incessant course (e.g., amyotrophic lateral sclerosis, Parkinson disease) with increasing functional limitations as the individual ages. For other conditions, the neurological event may become stable (e.g., spinal cord injury, stroke) although residual disability remains throughout the lifespan.

Misconceptions accompanying the perception of people with disabilities are detailed in *Healthy People 2010* (USDHHS, 2000). False beliefs include statements such as "people with disability automatically have poor health," "public health should only focus on preventing disabling conditions," and "the environment plays no role in the disabling process" (USDHHS, 2000). According to *Healthy People 2010,* "these misconceptions have led to an under emphasis of health promotion and disease prevention activities targeting people with disabilities and an increase in the occurrence of secondary conditions (medical, social, emotional, family, or community problems that a person with a primary disabling condition likely experiences)." The language of "Disability and Health" in *Healthy People 2020* (USDHHS, 2010) aims to dispel these misconceptions and highlight health disparities for people with disabilities.

In the report *The Future of Disability in America* (Institute of Medicine, 2007), an Institute of Medicine committee calls for strengthening the education of health professionals on the secondary conditions associated with disability. A specific area of concern is the transition of neurologically impaired patients/clients from childhood to adulthood. The committee calls for health professionals "to increase awareness of the secondary conditions and premature aging associated with many chronic health conditions and disabilities" (Institute of Medicine, 2007, p. 11)—that is, to educate patients/clients on healthy aging as they live with disability.

People with neurological disability are among the underserved in the area of health promotion. As mentioned previously, *Healthy People 2010* (USDHHS, 2000) and *Healthy People 2020* (USDHHS, 2010) point out having a long-term condition increases the need for health promotion, yet paradoxically individuals with disabilities receive less attention and care toward minimizing future health conditions than other groups. For people with neurological disability, performance of health-enhancing activities is critical to prevent future health problems and reduce the risk of additional disabling conditions (Rimmer, 1999). Furthermore adoption of a healthy lifestyle has far-reaching psychosocial benefits for the individual, including stress reduction and mitigation of depression.

Classically secondary and tertiary intervention has been the focus of occupational and physical therapy for individuals with neurological disorders. Therapeutic intervention has focused on improving function and limiting acute complications of the condition and, as a result, minimizes the initial disability. However upon discharge from formal rehabilitation services, subsequent care is often episodic. Counseling on health promotion activities and behaviors preventing or delaying secondary conditions is often limited if addressed at all.

Professional responsibilities for the therapist include educating all patient/clients on prevention and wellness in addition to clinical care. Therapists have an important opportunity to begin health education/health promotion efforts as they plan discharge from tertiary care. Unfortunately they have been slow to change from a clinical focus to a path of health education/health promotion (Martin and Fell, 1999). Therapists must accept the challenge of educating all patients/clients, but especially those with long-term disability, regarding a health-promoting lifestyle and the importance of making good decisions about their health. Therapists are uniquely qualified to provide health education and health behavior training, monitor and modify existing programs, and act as a lifelong consultant to the individual with a disability. This leadership role advances the emerging role of health-care providers as facilitators of care and changes the focus and responsibility of health maintenance from provider-centered care to self-care.

## Disease Management

Integral to the disease management paradigm is a transfer of health-care responsibility from the provider to the individual. Medical management of underserved individuals who suffer from a chronic illness has traditionally been hospital-based and episodic. A self-management strategy, applied to a population with chronic illness, has the potential to redirect the focus of care from episodic provider-centered intervention to individual-centered or consumer-centered acceptance of health responsibility. Unlike many medical interventions, the goal is not to eliminate or eradicate the illness, which is a chronic condition, but rather to learn effective self-management techniques to improve health and ensure appropriate utilization of community-based health-care resources.

Health-care reform is needed to expand disease management initiatives and place an emphasis on prevention of illness. Given the chronic nature of neurological impairment and the realization individuals are at high risk for subsequent or secondary medical conditions, therapists should guide the patient/client with neurological disability toward a path of wellness and healthy aging.

Therapists can adopt a prophylactic approach similar to the role adopted in the past two decades by the dental profession. People with neurological disability could be encouraged to attend regularly scheduled checkups of physical function at least annually with intervention customized to address issues identified in the annual screening. The screening appointment could involve a multidisciplinary team approach including the occupational and physical therapist along with an array of other clinicians including dietitians, nutritionists, orthotists, social workers, psychologists, pharmacists, acupuncturists, speech therapists, nurses and advanced-practice nurses, and physicians.

By taking this proactive role, therapists can improve the coordination of care, help patients/clients learn to manage their illnesses and resultant risk of secondary conditions, and ensure active follow-up for optimal outcomes. These actions are consistent with the well-respected Chronic Care Model (Improving Chronic Illness Care, available at www.improvingchroniccare.org/index.php?p=The_Chronic_Care_Model&s=2) as they address deficiencies in our current method to provide health services.

Adoption of a healthy lifestyle is a life-long challenge. The endeavor is particularly appropriate for people with neurological disability because people with some conditions are at heightened risk for secondary conditions (Rimmer, 1999). For example, individuals with cerebral palsy or spina bifida displayed risk for associated osteoporosis, osteoarthritis, weight gain, muscular weakness, decreased balance and flexibility, depression, and a host of other conditions, which can be addressed and often mitigated by appropriate health education/health promotion efforts (Marge, 1994).

Scheduled health promotion interventions would enhance an individual's self-care and self-management skills for coping with the disability. The sessions could be used to reinforce, update, or modify lifestyle behavioral adjustments as well as provide an opportunity to screen for early manifestations of secondary illness. Ongoing care is important as half of all causes of mortality in the United States are linked to lifestyle choices including smoking, diet, alcohol use, sedentary lifestyle, and accidents (McGinnis, 1993; Mokdad, 2000; Mokdad, 2004).

Promoting healthful activities to prevent subsequent health problems is an intuitive measure that has been championed for decades. As our nation and the world have witnessed a demographic transition from a society facing infectious disease to one facing chronic conditions, the benefits of health-enacting measures have gained prominence, particularly promoting health among people with disabilities (CDC, *Promoting the Health*). Many health-care disciplines include health education/health promotion interventions as a critical component of their scope of practice. Unfortunately the compartmentalization of our health-care system has resulted in discipline-specific silos of information on a variety of health measures. The isolation of disciplines is profound in areas such as health promotion. Substantial research has been accomplished in disciplines ranging from nursing and occupational and physical therapy to health education and behavioral therapy and needs to be integrated throughout the health-care system.

## Health Promotion/Integration for People With Disabilities

In 2008, Rimmer identified barriers to community-based fitness and recreation for people with stroke, reporting the five most common barriers in rank order, and that therapists can address, were (1) cost of the program, (2) lack of awareness of a fitness center in the area, (3) no means of transportation to a fitness center, (4) no knowledge of how to exercise, and (5) no knowledge of where to exercise. Simply being aware of these common barriers for people with stroke can be of tremendous help to therapists in planning for the transition in care that Rimmer (1999) envisioned from an episode of rehabilitation to ongoing participation in regular physical activity in a community-based setting. Another contribution by Rimmer et al (2004) is the development of an instrument, Accessibility Instruments Measuring Fitness and Recreation Environments (AIMFREE). Fitness facilities, as revealed by AIMFREE, tend to have low to moderate levels of accessibility constituting a major barrier to participation in community-based fitness programs for people with disabilities.

Riley and Rimmer (2008) proposed a framework for improving the accessibility of fitness and recreation facilities for people with disabilities. The framework contains three steps for the accessibility consultant—accessibility assessment, accessibility review, and accessibility transition plans—toward the objectives of (1) dispelling misperceptions about why people with disabilities do not use fitness and recreation facilities; (2) promoting collaborative relationships among consumers with disabilities, facility owners, and facility staff; (3) developing effective realistic solutions for the elimination of barriers tailored to the specific facility; (4) addressing the specific needs of consumers with disabilities who would like to use the facility and participate in its programs; (5) identifying the cost of eliminating barriers to accessibility; and (6) providing a mechanism for monitoring ongoing compliance and program evaluation. Though the proposal does not specifically name therapists as the consultant or interventionist in this framework, therapists are certainly well qualified to fulfill this role.

Although it would seem Rimmer's (1999) vision of a continuum of rehabilitation culminating in community-based fitness for people with disabilities remains largely unfulfilled at present, therapists can be part of Rimmer's vision in multiple ways. First, they can advocate for rehabilitation facilities to be made available to patients for continuing community-based fitness after discharge from an episode of rehabilitative care. Doing so may have multiple advantages such as (1) offering former patients the opportunity to continue to use facilities and equipment with which they are already familiar and (2) offering former patients the opportunity to be active in a setting that, being rehabilitation-oriented, is inherently more conducive to the needs of people with disabilities. Some clinics already use this model as a way to enhance the value of their services to the consumer and create an additional revenue stream. The owners of private clinics can opt to pursue this type of service directly (making sure to consider such compliance issues as their state practice acts and stipulations of their liability insurance carriers), and therapists who work for hospital-based facilities can propose this idea to their managers.

Second, therapists can work in community-based fitness centers (e.g., as a private contractor renting space), which may yield the same types of benefits to the consumer. Third, therapists can help patients identify appropriate community-based fitness and recreation facilities especially before discharge from physical therapy clinical services. Fourth, therapists can act as consultants to community-based fitness centers using Rimmer's framework for improving accessibility. Finally, therapists can be advocates for social change in a larger sense, which may involve participation in many types of activities from the local level to the federal level. As rehabilitation professionals, therapists are ideally suited to not only recognize the importance of lifelong physical fitness but also incorporate their knowledge of pathology-specific lifespan issues into the exercise prescription. Fundamentally, therapists must answer Rimmer's 2008 charge to identify and alleviate barriers to participation. By doing so the therapist may at times have to

function as a case manager or consult with a social worker, if available, as part of the patient's/client's health-care team. Rimmer's contributions in the area of health promotion for people with disabilities are tremendously important and provide an excellent starting point for therapists desiring to be part of this critically needed paradigm shift.

## A Growing Recognition of Health Promotion Needs in Neurology

In addition to research reports on specific aspects of fitness for the general population, pathology-specific recommendations have now been published regarding populations with neurological disorders. Some make specific fitness recommendations where enough evidence exists, whereas others make general recommendations and provide a research blueprint of topics that require further investigation. Table 16-9 summarizes published recommendations for health promotion regarding the following neurology-related specific issues and medical diagnoses: risk of falls, stroke, spinal cord injury, and cerebral palsy.

## A Systems Approach to Health Promotion in Neurology Across the Lifespan

To promote the health of people with disabilities in clinical practice (Figure 16-3), it is essential to practice in a manner consistent with the principles and procedures introduced in

**TABLE 16-9  Health Promotion Recommendations Published for Neurology-Related Specific Issues and Medical Diagnoses**

| ISSUES RAISED | RECOMMENDATIONS MADE | OTHER COMMENTS |
|---|---|---|
| **Risk of falls** (Quality Standards Subcommittee of the American Academy of Neurology. *Neurology*, 2008) | | |
| • An evidence-based review of the risk of falls in patients who are seen in neurology practices.<br>• Found that there is an established increased risk of falls in patients with stroke, dementia, and gait and balance disorders and patients who use assistive devices to ambulate and a probable increased risk of falls in patients with Parkinson disease, peripheral neuropathy, lower extremity weakness or sensory loss, and substantial vision loss.<br>• Acknowledged general risk factors for falls, including advanced age, age-associated frailty, arthritis, impairments in activities of daily living, depression, and the use of psychoactive medications including sedatives, antidepressants, and neuroleptics.<br>• A history of falls in the past year was cited as a strong predictor of future falls. | • Patients with identified risk factors should be asked about falls during the past year.<br>• Recommended assessments: The Get-Up-and-Go Test or Timed Up-and-Go Test, an assessment of the ability to stand unassisted from a sitting position, and the Tinetti Mobility Scale as screening measures as well as consideration of additional measures including the Dynamic Gait Index, timed gait, the Functional Reach Test, and the Berg Balance Scale. | The report referenced existing evidence-based guidelines for intervention: the *Guideline for the Prevention of Falls in Older Persons* of the American Geriatrics Society, British Geriatrics Society, and American Academy of Orthopedic Surgeons Panel on Falls Prevention; the Cochrane review *Interventions for Preventing Falls in Elderly People*; and a 2001 report in the *Annals of Internal Medicine*. |

| TABLE 16-9 | Health Promotion Recommendations Published for Neurology-Related Specific Issues and Medical Diagnoses—cont'd | |
| --- | --- | --- |
| **ISSUES RAISED** | **RECOMMENDATIONS MADE** | **OTHER COMMENTS** |
| **Stroke** (American Heart Association, 2004) | | |
| • Published physical activity and exercise recommendations for people with stroke, synthesized evidence supporting the health benefits of physical activity in this patient population, and provided guidelines for preexercise evaluation and exercise programming. | • A preexercise evaluation should consist of a complete medical history and physical examination and usually include graded exercise testing with ECG monitoring.<br>• Exercise testing should include selecting (e.g., arm, leg, or arm-leg cycle ergometry) and adapting (e.g., the use of handrails) the testing mode according to the needs of the individual.<br>• Exercise programming recommendations are listed by mode of exercise (aerobic, strength, flexibility, and neuromuscular); major goals; and intensity, frequency, and duration.<br>• Incorporate treadmill walking, the use of an individually tailored approach, and modifications for those who are unable to perform a graded exercise test in the form of reduced intensity with correspondingly increased frequency, duration, or both. | • Such specific evidence-based guidelines from a major organization such as the American Heart Association are an important resource for the therapist, and it is critical that we are familiar with them and use them.<br>• Another valuable evidence-based resource is the Physical Fitness for Special Populations pocket guide "Physical Fitness for Survivors of Stroke Based on Best Available Evidence," available under the "Practice" tab of the APTA website. |
| **Spinal cord injury** (Two studies:"Exercise as a Health-promoting Activity Following Spinal Cord Injury" and "Evidence-based Exercise Prescription for Individuals with Spinal Cord Injury" in *Journal of Neurological Physical Therapy,* 2005) | | |
| • Focused on the importance of exercise in people with spinal cord injury (SCI).<br>• The first report describes the benefits and barriers of participation in physical activity by people with SCI as well as the risks of exercise, including fracture, musculoskeletal overuse/injury, thermal dysregulation, autonomic dysreflexia, skin burn, and pressor decompensation during and after exercise. | • The second report provides recommendations for preexercise examination and exercise prescription in this population. | |
| **Cerebral palsy** (Section on Pediatrics Research Summit, 2007) | | |
| • The evidence base, while compelling, was incomplete, highlighting the need for additional research before definitive recommendations regarding mode, frequency, intensity, and duration can be made. | • Promotion of physical fitness for children with cerebral palsy, emphasizing both muscle strength and cardiorespiratory fitness. | |

this chapter, including the five elements of patient/client management described in Chapter 2 (Figure 2-2): examination, evaluation, diagnosis, prognosis, and intervention, which all lead ultimately to patient outcomes. Examination plays an important role in initiating the health promotion process and encompasses the history, systems review, and tests and measures; recall the systems review includes a minimum data set of patient/client responses to questions for each category (i.e., information to be gathered for all patients/clients regardless of the reason for the referral) and thus provides a basis for a systems approach to health and wellness in individuals with disability due to neurological conditions.

Body systems and issues not specifically covered in the systems review should be included as needed. For example, abuse and neglect may need to be explored and the patient's/client's temperature measured as part of the general health assessment. Optimal practice may require a level of examination higher than that required by the therapist's workplace (e.g., specific tests and measures may be required rather than simply the history and systems review).

Also, recall that although tertiary prevention is the usual level of clinical intervention in rehabilitation, it is possible for therapists to incorporate other levels of prevention into their clinical practice as well. For example, the therapist may consider performing routine screening (1) for *specific conditions/diseases/disorders* common in adults with disability of neurological origin such as depression and osteoporosis (which would constitute screening at the level of secondary prevention for early detection)

or (2) for *risk factors* for specific problems that may occur in this patient/client population such as depression, osteoporosis, and stroke (which would constitute screening at the level of primary prevention to alter risk factors and prevent disease or injury).

Primary and secondary prevention for patients can include not only screening and making appropriate referrals but also interventions including education and prescription of appropriate exercise programs. Education can include topics such as how to more effectively utilize health-care services through, for example, providing an accurate and up-to-date medication list to health-care providers; the pathophysiology of health conditions such as stroke; and specific lifestyle modifications, including the beneficial effects of exercise.

Table 16-10 provides a matrix combining the concepts of a systems approach to health promotion in neurology and the levels of prevention (APTA, 2015).

## Tips and Guidelines for Health in Neurology Across the Lifespan

Although there are a multitude of health issues of concern in neurology, both pediatric and geriatric, this section of the chapter provides a framework for considering possible interventions for the most commonly encountered health and wellness issues and serves as a starting point for discussion and illustration. Recall the multiple dimensions of wellness. Even when focusing on the physical dimension, there are many aspects including not only physical activity but also

| TABLE 16-10 | A Matrix of a Systems Approach to Health Promotion With Systems Review Items and Prevention Activities, Including Primary Prevention (1°) and Secondary Prevention (2°), in Which the Therapist May Be Involved | |
|---|---|---|
| | **SYSTEMS REVIEW ITEMS** | **PREVENTION ACTIVITIES FOR THE THERAPIST** |
| *Cardiovascular/pulmonary system* | Heart rate, respiratory rate, blood pressure, and edema. | 1° prevention: Screening for risk factors for stroke, 1° prevention and 2° prevention: Providing education on stroke. |
| *Integumentary system* | Pliability (texture), presence of scar formation, skin color, and skin integrity. | 2° prevention: Screening for skin cancer, 1° prevention and 2° prevention: Providing education on skin cancer. |
| *Musculoskeletal system* | Gross symmetry, gross range of motion, gross strength, height, and weight. | 2° prevention: Screening for osteoporosis, 1° prevention and 2° prevention: Providing education on osteoporosis. |
| *Neuromuscular system* | Gross coordinated movement, (such as balance, gait, locomotion, transfers, transitions) motor function (motor control and motor learning). | 2° prevention: Screening for peripheral neuropathy, 1° prevention and 2° prevention: Providing education on peripheral neuropathy. |
| *Communication ability, affect, cognition, language, and learning style* | Ability to make needs known, consciousness, orientation, emotional/behavioral responses, and learning preferences such as learning barriers and educational needs. | 2° prevention: Screening for abuse and neglect, depression, fear of falling, mental status, and visual changes, 1° prevention and 2° prevention: Providing education on abuse and neglect, depression, fear of falling, mental status, and visual changes. |

diet and nutrition, sleep, and general safety (e.g., the use of seat belts, the proper use of playground equipment and need for supervision of its use, the use of bicycle helmets). All of these aspects are potentially important for the therapist to address either directly or by referral.

Examples of common health issues of concern in neurology are discussed in the following section, including balance and fall prevention, safety and injury prevention, avoidance of risky personal behavior, polypharmacy issues and degree of medication adherence, infection, depression, osteoporosis, skin cancer, and recurrence of stroke. For other health promotion issues not covered in this chapter, the reader can often find government-endorsed fact sheets and guidelines through Healthfinder.gov, the online clearinghouse from the U.S. Department of Health and Human Services at www.healthfinder.gov.

Some health issues are identified during the systems review or other components of the examination. For example, HTN would be detected during the medical/surgical history component of the history and the blood pressure measurement of the cardiovascular/pulmonary systems review, and balance and falls would be initially assessed during the history and the neuromuscular systems review. Some of the other issues, however, may not typically be detected at all in the systems review or other components of the examination. For example, although the *Guide* (APTA, 2015) lists medications (e.g., medications for current condition, medications previously taken for current condition, medications for other conditions) as part of the history, it does not specifically address such medication-related issues as polypharmacy and degree of medication adherence. On the other hand, the *Occupational Therapy Practice Framework* includes "medication routines" under the IADL of "health management and maintenance" (AOTA, 2014, p. S19) demonstrating the role of occupational therapy in assessing performance patterns specific to medication management.

Also the measurement of the patient's/client's body temperature (as an indicator of possible infection) is not a component of the systems review. Affect is a component of the communication ability, cognition, language, and learning style category of systems review, but screening for depression is not specifically articulated. The patient/client may be unaware he or she has osteoporosis or skin cancer or that he or she has risk factors for osteoporosis, skin cancer, or stroke. Thus in addition to the systems review, other schemes for screening (e.g., *Minimum Required Skills of Physical Therapist Graduates at Entry-level;* APTA) and approaches to screening (e.g., the screening forms available in *Differential Diagnosis for Physical Therapists: Screening for Referral* by Goodman and Snyder (2007) may be helpful.

Regarding the following issues involving health habits, from a lifespan perspective it is important to understand many health habits, including nutritional aspects and physical activity level, are at least in part established early in life (AHA, *Top 10 Tips*). Cardiovascular disease can have its origins in childhood (Newman, 1986; Berenson, 1998; Mahoney, 1996; McGill, 2001). Logically, promotion of healthy behaviors in

childhood that carries over into early adulthood may have optimal long-term benefits. Therefore, it is essential to provide family education on every available occasion regarding nutrition, body weight, and physical activity as early and frequently as feasible. Several online resources with ideas to promote healthy behavior and wellness decisions in children are provided in Table 16-11.

Slikker and Gaylor (1995) described a two-part process: **risk assessment**, "an empirically based process used to determine the probability that adverse or abnormal effects are associated with exposure to a chemical, physical or biological agent" (p. 198) followed by **risk management**, "the process that applies information obtained through the risk assessment process to determine whether the assessed risk should be reduced and, if so, to what extent" (p.198). Martin and Fell (1999) provide examples in key areas with an emphasis on patient education to enhance health and wellness. A checklist of specific age-appropriate health promotion issues, including those discussed in this chapter, could be developed and used as part of the initial examination to quickly screen for health promotion and wellness problems. Six very important steps for implementing a health promotion focus in your therapy practice can be applied to each of the following issues and systems, including:

1. ask the patient/client or family about their current behaviors,
2. determine what pros and cons the patient/client believes are associated with current behavior and behavior change,
3. determine into what *stage of change* the patient/client falls for changing a behavior or maintaining that behavior,
4. determine the patient's/client's self-efficacy regarding a specific behavior,
5. set the treatment plan, goals, and objectives based on the patient's/client's *stage of change,* and
6. determine the best ways to help the patient/client meet goals and change behavior, again based on his or her *stage of change.*

Let's examine some specific recommendations and guidelines for the more common areas.

### Fall Prevention

Research consistently demonstrates falls are a problem for older adults, with an incidence of approximately one third (Blake, 1988; Campbell, 1989; Tinetti, 1988) and adverse events including death and injury (Berg, 1990; Sattin, 1992). Hardage (2007) found among older adults who had participated in an episode of home health physical therapy, 80% reported a history of falls with 58% reporting a history of noninjurious falls and 50% reporting a history of injurious falls. The scientific literature demonstrates the multiple interventions in which therapists can participate that are effective in decreasing the risk of falls in older adults, including exercise (American Geriatric Society, 2001; Carter, 2001; Gillespie, 2003; Howe, 2007; Hunter, 2004), home hazard assessment and modification (Gillespie, 2003), and multidisciplinary assessment and intervention (Gillespie,

| TABLE 16-11 | Health Promotion Resources on the Internet for Pediatrics and Adults | | |
|---|---|---|---|
| | | **PEDS** | **ADULT** |
| **http://www.healthfinder.gov/**<br>• U.S. government gateway/clearing house for consumer health and human services information, including publications, websites, clearinghouses. An alphabetical list or search options to discover topics including "nutrition," "physical activity," "safety," and "smoking." Also a special section "HHS for Kids" (http://www.hhs.gov/kids/). | | ✓ | ✓ |
| **http://kidshealth.org/**<br>• Nemours Foundation (dedicated to health care of children) site, includes specific category "Kids site" with info on "Staying Healthy," including: "being good to your body," sports safety, smoking, nutrition, weight, exercise. Also "Parent's site" and "Teen's site." | | ✓ | |
| **http://www.heart.org/HEARTORG/GettingHealthy/PhysicalActivity/Physical-Activity_UCM_001080_SubHomePage.jsp**<br>• American Heart Association Physical Activity site "Get Moving" includes motivation, "Tips for getting started," "AHA Guidelines," "Resources" for kids and adults, and the online "My Life Check Assessment" regarding "Life's Simple 7" (1) Get Active, (2) Control Cholesterol, (3) Eat Better, (4) Manage Blood Pressure, (5) Lose Weight, (6) Reduce Blood Sugar, (7) Stop Smoking. | | ✓ | ✓ |
| **http://www.heart.org/HEARTORG/GettingHealthy/HealthierKids/Healthier-Kids_UCM_304156_SubHomePage.jsp**<br>• American Heart Association "Healthier Kids," including "How to Make a Healthy Home," "Activities for Kids," "Understanding Childhood Obesity."<br>• "How to Make a Healthy Home" (AHA, *Top 10 Tips*). | | ✓ | |
| **http://www.choosemyplate.gov/**<br>• The site assists with online personalized eating plans and interactive tools food choices based on the U.S. Department of Agriculture "Dietary Guidelines for Americans." | | ✓ | ✓ |
| **http://www.cdc.gov/tobacco/basic_information/youth/index.htm**<br>• CDC "Youth Tobacco Prevention" site regarding smoking prevention, including fact sheets and the information sheet "You(th) and Tobacco." | | ✓ | ✓ |
| **http://www.cdc.gov/cancer/skin/**<br>• CDC "Skin Cancer" page emphasizes cancer prevention for young people, including appropriate skin cover and protection guidelines, sun safety, and the "Choose Your Cover" campaign (http://www.cdc.gov/cancer/dcpc/publications/skin.htm). | | ✓ | ✓ |
| **http://www.cdc.gov/bam/**<br>• CDC "BAM! Body And Mind" page focused on younger group with sections on diseases, food and nutrition, physical activity, your safety, your life, and your body. | | ✓ | |

2003; Tinetti, 1994). A Cochrane review, *Interventions for Preventing Falls in Elderly People* (Gillespie, 2003), found evidence supporting a professionally prescribed HEP consisting of muscle strengthening and balance training as did a series of randomized controlled trials (RCTs) (Campbell, 1997; Campbell, 1999; Robertson, 2001). These studies demonstrated an HEP as the sole intervention reducing the risk of falls by about one third in community-dwelling older adults 80 years of age and older. This HEP consisted of exercises for lower extremity strengthening and balance training with simple equipment or no equipment.

Another category of exercise receiving attention in the literature for older adults is **functional training**. Functional training differs from strength training in that it does not target muscle groups but rather focuses on muscle use in the task to be performed and uses task practice for training specificity and neuromotor control of the task (Carroll, 2001). This type of exercise appears under many names in the literature, including functional exercises (de Bruin, 2007), functional-task exercise (de Vreede, 2005), task-specific exercise (Manini, 2007), and goal-directed training (Mastos, 2007).

Emerging evidence (de Bruin, 2007; de Vreede, 2005; Manini, 2007; Mastos, 2007; Weerdesteyn, 2006) supports the efficacy of functional training. Because it uses activities of daily living and other routine mobility tasks (e.g., negotiation of obstacles), functional training targets multiple dimensions of fall prevention including avoidance, endurance, strength, balance, and cognitive skills (Manini, 2007; Weerdesteyn, 2006). Mastos (2007) noted that, because functional training involves activities often directly related to patient goals, it helps improve motivation and encourages cognitive improvement in these tasks. Manini (2007) suggested a combination of functional and resistance training may yield the best results in improving function and reducing the risk of falls in older adults.

**Fall prevention** (or **fall risk reduction**) as an intervention strategy includes patient/client education, physical intervention, and environmental adaptation to minimize the likelihood of loss of balance with resulting uncontrolled descent to the ground or other support surface. Impairment-based preparatory intervention and functional skill intervention to incorporate balance activities are central in therapist interventions. Impairment-based interventions include addressing sensory deficits (Chapter 27), range of motion deficits (Chapter 23), motor control impairment (Chapters 24 and 25), strength deficits (Chapter 22), vestibular impairment (Chapter 29), and balance deficits (Chapter 30). In addition to addressing particular underlying impairments, the therapist can use specific guidelines developed to guide the health-care provider in analysis and interventions related holistically to the patient/client and the environment. Several Web-based resources regarding fall prevention are listed in Box 16-2. Box 16-3 contains health information to prevent falls you can share with patients/clients.

### Safe Protective Behavior for Injury Prevention

It is essential therapists promote safe and protective behavior in all activities with an aim to prevent injury. For example, *Healthy People 2020* (USDHHS, 2010) identified objectives related to use of *seatbelts* (Objective 15), *child restraint /car seats* (Objective 16), and *bicycle helmets* (Objective 21 to 22). The CDC website for kids' health, "BAM! Body and Mind," has a section called "*Your Safety*" (www.cdc.gov/bam/safety/index.html) that includes kid-friendly information and specific guidelines in

---

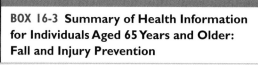

**BOX 16-3  Summary of Health Information for Individuals Aged 65 Years and Older: Fall and Injury Prevention**

**Exercise**

Regular aerobic exercise; include stretching and strengthening; walking

**Calcium and Vitamin D**

Women should take calcium (1,500 mg) and Vitamin D (750 U) daily

**Medications**

People older than 65 years should not take Valium, Dalmane, Elavil, or Tylenol PM or more than five prescription medications; consult your physician

**Footwear**

The best shoes are walking shoes with flat soles such as sneakers

**Home Hazards**

Use night-lights; have handrails or safety strips in shower/tub and on all steps; secure throw rugs; remove objects that are difficult to see

**Vision**

See an optometrist if you have trouble reading magazine print or if you have not had your eyes checked in the last 2 years

**Alcohol**

Be careful not to have more than one or two drinks a day, as drinking is associated with depression and injuries
*Summarized from Baraff, 1997 (see more detail in article).*

---

**BOX 16-2  Health Promotion Resources for Fall Prevention on the Internet**

http://www.cdc.gov/HomeandRecreationalSafety/Falls/adultfalls.html
- Fact sheet "Falls Among Older Adults" from the Centers for Disease Control and Prevention National Center for Injury Prevention and Control (NCIPC), includes a specific section titled "How can older adults prevent falls?" with references.

https://www.cdc.gov/homeandrecreationalsafety/pdf/falls/fallpreventionguide-2015-a.pdf
- The CDC document "Preventing Falls: How to Develop Community-based Fall Prevention Programs for Older Adults" provides community organizations with examples and resources regarding "Education, Exercise programs, Medication management, Vision checking and improvement, Home hazard assessment and modification."

https://www.cdc.gov/homeandrecreationalsafety/pdf/falls/fallpreventionguide-2015-a.pdf
- "Preventing Falls: What Works, A CDC Compendium of Effective Community-based Interventions from Around the World" describes 14 interventions which are grouped as either (1) exercise-based, (2) home modification, or (3) multifaceted.

---

these categories: "Gear Up," "Hard Facts about Helmets," "H2O Smartz," "Keeping Your Cool," "The Bully Roundup," "Play It Safe," "Safety Smartz," "Sun Proof," "Tick Tactics," and "Tsunami" (CDC, *Your Safety*). Another issue to be addressed in a pediatric population is safety on *playground equipment*.

In each situation, the therapist should follow the six general steps for health promotion previously described and assist and encourage the patient/client through the process of selecting and maintaining healthy behaviors. The authority and education of the health professional can have an important effect on patient/client beliefs. For example, just as emergency room physicians screen for bicycle helmet use (Cushman, 1991), therapists should also inquire about helmet use and encourage all family members to use helmets when riding.

### Avoiding Risky Personal Behavior

*Healthy People 2020* (USDHHS, 2010) included objectives to help people eliminate or avoid risky personal behavior resulting in injury or disease. Many resources for intervention, including guidelines, can be found at the CDC online clearinghouse at www.healthfinder.gov. Several of the main areas are addressed here.

### Tobacco Use

One specific *Healthy People* objective (TU-1) was a reduction of the proportion of American adults who use tobacco (any tobacco product) because of its clearly damaging effects. Other objectives, specifically regarding pediatrics, children, and teens, included reducing tobacco use among adolescents (TU-2) and reducing the initiation of tobacco use among children, adolescents, and young adults. Regarding intervention, *Healthy People 2020* objectives include (TU-9) increasing tobacco screening in health care settings and (TU-10) increasing tobacco cessation counseling in health-care settings. Given the obvious health risks of smoking, therapists should always point out the benefits of smoking cessation and specifically encourage each patient/client to stop smoking. Expressing your health-promotion opinion and reinforcing comments from many others—with the credibility your professional status brings—may cause the patient/client to reach the critical level for finally giving serious consideration to the reality of the risk and the potential effect on health and life expectancy. It might be motivating for the patient to hear that "half of all people who have ever smoked have quit" (Fiore, 1996) and although many people attempt "several times before they quit for good . . . they do succeed" (Fiore, 2008).

What can the therapist do? An online guide for clinicians (Agency for Healthcare Research and Quality, 2008) encourages all health-care professionals to perform these simple actions:

1. "Ask about tobacco use at every visit." The authors encourage a systematic collection of the data, including a response to "Tobacco use: Current, Former, Never (circle one)," recording the response as part of the patient's/client's vital signs.
2. "Advise all tobacco users (in clear, strong, and personalized language) to quit." For example, "Quitting tobacco is the most important thing you can do to protect your health." Health-care professionals carry great clout and growing influence with patients.
3. "Assess readiness to quit" including the stage of health behavior change. Each request for smoking cessation may bring the patient/client to higher realizations, moving toward the next stage of behavior change. If the patient/client is not willing to quit at this time, then provide motivation, review reasons to quit, and build confidence about quitting.
4. If the patient/client is willing to quit, "Assist tobacco user with a quit plan" including resources, assistance and referral (e.g., to a physician for medical management of the quit plan including the possible prescription of pharmacological aids), and specific tips as shown in Box 16-4. Additional Internet resources you can share with patients/clients to assist in their quit plans and strategies to "stay quit" are listed in Box 16-5.

### Distracted Driving

Because of the potential affect on driving safety, therapists should also screen for and verbally encourage safe driving behavior in all age groups. The American Automobile Association (AAA *Traffic Safety*, 2007) reports "nearly 80% of collisions involve some form of driver inattention." Numerous authors have emphasized the specific factors related to distracting the attention of the driver, particularly cell phone use

---

> ### BOX 16-4  Specific Tips to Assist Tobacco Users with a Quit Plan (AHRQ, 2008)
>
> Assist the smoker to:
> - Set a quit date, ideally within 2 weeks.
> - Remove tobacco products from their environment.
> - Get support from family, friends, and coworkers.
> - Review past quit attempts—what helped, what led to relapse.
> - Anticipate challenges, particularly during the critical first few weeks, including nicotine withdrawal.
> - Identify reasons for quitting and benefits of quitting.
>
> Give advice on successful quitting:
> - Total abstinence is essential—not even a single puff.
> - Drinking alcohol is strongly associated with relapse.
> - Allowing others to smoke in the household hinders successful quitting.
>
> Encourage use of medication:
> - Recommend use of over-the-counter nicotine patch, gum, or lozenge; or give prescription for varenicline, bupropion SR, nicotine inhaler, or nasal spray, unless contraindicated.
>
> Provide resources:
> - Recommend toll free 1-800-QUIT NOW (784–8669), the national access number to state-based quitline services.
>
> Refer to websites for free materials:
> - Agency for Healthcare Research and Quality: www.ahrq.gov/path/tobacco.htm
> - U.S. Department of Health and Human Services: www.smokefree.gov

---

and texting while driving (Hosking, 2007; McEvoy, 2006; Lee, 2007). A CDC publication, "Teen Driving: Fact Sheet" (CDC, *Teen Driving*), clearly states the risk is greatest for young teen drivers, particularly in the early years of driver eligibility. In fact, motor vehicle crashes are the leading cause of death among teens (CDC, *Teen Driving*). More specifically, a 2007 AAA survey reported that among 16 to 17 year-old drivers, 61% admit to risky driving habits, including 46% who text message while driving (AAA, *Teen Driving*).

The CDC fact sheet summarizes risk factors identified from CDC data and other research as being clearly associated with driving injury and death: being a young driver—teens ages 16 to 19 (CDC, *Teen Drivers*); being male; speeding and driving too close to the car ahead, which is accentuated when young male passengers are in the car (Simons-Morton, 2005); drinking alcohol as a vehicle driver; riding as a passenger with a driver who was drinking alcohol; poor seat belt use; late afternoon and night driving; and weekend driving. Accentuating the problem with decreased attention to the driving task is the fact that teens are also more likely than older drivers to underestimate dangerous situations or to be unable to recognize hazardous situations (Jonah, 1987).

All of these factors combined indicate that drivers, particularly teens, are placing themselves, their passengers, and other drivers at risk, especially with simultaneous tasks that distract attention. Many of these factors can obviously be addressed

## BOX 16-5  Smoking Cessation Resources for Patients Available on the Internet

http://www.smokefree.gov/

http://betobaccofree.hhs.gov/

http://www.ahrq.gov/professionals/clinicians-providers/
guidelines-recommendations/tobacco/index.html

- AHRQ guidelines includes a section of resources "For
  Tobacco Users"

http://www.ahrq.gov/health-care-information/topics/topic-
tobacco-use.html

- "You Can Quit Smoking"

http://www.ahrq.gov/professionals/clinicians-providers/
guidelines-recommendations/tobacco/clinicians/tearsheets/
helpsmokers.html

- AHRQ "Help for Smokers and Other Tobacco Users: Quit
  Smoking," a booklet that can be read online or downloadable
  as a PDF provides excellent reasons for quitting (including
  savings of $150 a month for 1 pack a day to $450 a month
  for 3 packs a day!) and practical tips for quitting.

http://www.cdc.gov/tobacco/quit_smoking/how_to_quit/
quit_tips/

- Smokers "Quit Tips" from the Centers for Disease Control

http://www.heart.org/HEARTORG/GettingHealthy/
QuitSmoking/Quit-Smoking_UCM_001085_
SubHomePage.jsp

- American Heart Association "Quit Smoking" section includes
  links for Quitting Smoking, Dealing with Urges, Your Non-
  Smoking Life, and Quitting Resources (including a calculator
  for the financial cost of smoking, and tips for family and
  friends, along with numerous online and call resources).

## BOX 16-6  Top Ten Water Safety Tips (CDC, *H2O Smartz*)

- **DO learn to swim**. If you like to have a good time doing
  water activities, being a strong swimmer is a must.
- **DO take a friend along**. Even though you may be a good
  swimmer, you never know when you may need help. Having
  friends around is safer and just more fun!
- **DO know your limits**. Watch out for the "too's"—too tired,
  too cold, too far from safety, too much sun, too much hard
  activity.
- **DO swim in supervised (watched) areas only**, and follow all
  signs and warnings.
- **DO wear a life jacket** when boating, jet skiing, water skiing,
  rafting, or fishing.
- **DO stay alert to currents** while white-water rafting. They
  can change quickly! If you get caught in a strong current, don't
  fight it. Swim parallel to the shore until you have passed
  through it. Near piers, jetties (lines of big rocks), small dams,
  and docks, the current gets unpredictable and could knock
  you around. If you find it hard to move around, head to
  shore. Learn to recognize and watch for dangerous waves
  and signs of rip currents—water that is a weird color, really
  choppy, foamy, or filled with pieces of stuff.
- **DO keep an eye on the weather**. If you spot bad weather
  (dark clouds, lightning), pack up and take the fun inside.
- **DON'T mess around in the water**. Pushing or dunking your
  friends can get easily out of hand.
- **DON'T dive into shallow water**. If you don't know how
  deep the water is, don't dive.
- **DON'T float where you can't swim**. Keep checking to see if
  the water is too deep, or if you are too far away from the
  shore or the poolside.
  (Reproduced from CDC "H2O Smarts" webpage, available
  at: www.cdc.gov/bam/safety/h2o.html)

through education regarding the consequences of not follow-ing safe behaviors, including giving full attention to the driv-ing task (e.g., not texting while driving), not driving while impaired from alcohol or drugs, using seatbelts consistently, and driving with particular care at the high-risk times noted.

### Risky Swimming/Diving

Potential injuries related to water activities include death due to drowning, anoxic brain injury due to near-drowning, and spinal cord injury due to diving accidents. Statistics show most drownings, including those of children, occur in home pools (CDC, *Unintentional Drowning*). Therapists can educate individuals regarding strategies to prevent these injuries. Tips from the CDC for water safety are shown in Box 16-6. In addition, children should always be supervised around a pool, and a pool perimeter should always be secured so children cannot enter unsupervised.

Spinal cord injuries related to diving occur when individ-uals dive into water that is too shallow or has unseen sub-merged objects, striking the head and causing compression fractures to the cervical spine. Therefore it is essential to check the water depth and underwater topography carefully before diving (Mayo Clinic, 2015) to make sure the water is not too

shallow. Generally a depth of less than 9 feet is not safe for diving (Reeves Foundation, 2010). A video, *Sudden Impact,* at www.parachutecanada.org/thinkfirstcanada, (Think First, *Sudden* Impact) has been developed in Canada to help prevent spinal cord injury caused by careless shallow water diving among teenagers in the high risk group, 15 to 24 years-old (Bhide, 2000). This public-information video is available online to share with patients/clients on YouTube at www.youtube.com/watch?v = 05ROGDsJvqQ. Swimmers and divers should also keep in mind that flowing water, like a river, could cause underwater objects such as logs to flow into deep water and pose a diving risk even in an area where others have been diving repeatedly into the same spot.

### Sun Exposure and Tanning Beds

As a lifespan cancer prevention objective, *Healthy People 2020* (USDHHS, 2010) focused on (C-20) increasing the proportion of persons who participate in behaviors that reduce their expo-sure to harmful ultraviolet (UV) irradiation and avoid sunburn.

Therapists should encourage these changes especially for those who live in regions with high sun exposure. A key strategy for limiting sun exposure is to avoid outdoor activities during peak sun hours. For example, when visiting the beach enjoy the outdoors with sun in the morning and late afternoon, but stay indoors or in the shade from 10:00 a.m. to 4:00 p.m. The CDC website *BAM! Body and Mind "Sun Proof"* (CDC, *Sun Proof*) provides other specific tips to share with patients/clients for when they go out in the sun: (1) cover up; (2) rub it on; (3) apply, reapply, and then do it again; (4) slip on sunglasses; and (5) hang in the shade. *Cover up* indicates wearing sufficient clothes to cover the skin. *Rub it on* points to the importance of using sunscreen with a sun protection factor (SPF) of 15 or higher for optimal UV protection. *Apply, reapply, and then do it again!* means even waterproof and sweatproof sunscreen should be reapplied every 2 hours. *Slip on sunglasses* refers to the importance of protecting the eyes from UV rays. *Hang in the shade* signifies looking for opportunities to avoid the sun (e.g., by going indoors, by resting in the shade). The website healthfinder.gov also has tips on sun safety at www.healthfinder.gov/HealthTopics/Category/parenting/safety/steps-to-prevent-skin-cancer.

### Nutritional Health to Avoid Overweight/Obesity

Obesity is now considered a global epidemic among adults and children (Poirier, 2006). After a decade of extreme growth in the proportion of Americans who are obese, the 2008 figures show approximately one-third of U.S. adults are obese, though the recent rate of increase may be slowing (Flegal, 2010). Data from the CDC show that, compared with whites, blacks had a 48.1% higher prevalence of obesity, and Hispanics had a 42.5% higher obesity prevalence with generally higher prevalence in the South and Midwest compared with other areas of the country (CDC, *Adult Obesity Facts*). From 2008 data (Ogden, 2010), the prevalence of obesity, defined as a high BMI, ranges from approximately 10% for infants and toddlers to approximately 18% for adolescents and teenagers with rates relatively stable over the recent 10 years. Obesity has known negative effects on other body systems, overloads and overworks the musculoskeletal system, and limits physical activity. So, it is clearly an issue therapists should address with their patients/clients.

The *Healthy People 2020* (USDHHS, 2010) nutrition and weight status objectives for adults and children include goals (NWS-8) to increase the proportion of adults who are at a healthy weight; (NWS-9–10) to reduce the proportion of adults, children, and adolescents who are considered obese; (NWS-5) to increase the proportion of primary care physicians who regularly measure BMI for their patients; (NWS-6) to increase the proportion of physician office visits that include counseling or education related to nutrition and weight; and (NWS-13–14) increase the variety and contribution of fruits and vegetables to the diets of the population aged 2 years and older. Again therapists can play an important role in reaching these goals through intervention and referral and particularly patient/client education.

Physical activity and exercise are essential components of a weight-control or weight-loss program and can easily be developed and supervised by the therapist. The specific physical interventions and exercise guidelines are, however, beyond the scope of this textbook and can be found in other exercise and physical activity resources. Although the therapist's role in nutrition is limited (e.g., the occupational therapist can assess the IADL of meal preparation and clean-up as well as the habits and routines related to meal times and nutritional management) (AOTA, 2014), guidelines from government agencies and professional associations abound. The importance of these interventions in children is undeniable (Olson, 1989; Arbeit, 1992). Many are available on the Internet as public information and can be shared with the patient/client.

Eating a healthy diet is a critical part of what the AHA (*Life's Simple 7*) calls "Life's Simple 7." These seven health and behavioral factors for ideal cardiovascular health are objectives therapists can certainly share with their patients/clients:

1. don't smoke;
2. maintain a healthy weight;
3. engage in regular physical activity;
4. eat a healthy diet;
5. manage blood pressure;
6. take charge of cholesterol; and
7. keep blood sugar, or glucose, at healthy levels.

Simple guidelines for improving nutrition in the general public, which the therapist can share, include *The American Heart Association's Diet and Lifestyle Recommendations* shown in Box 16-7. In addition, it is helpful to trim visible fat from meat before cooking it, choose skim or 1% fat milk (and nonfat or low-fat yogurt and cheeses), limit the intake of organ meats, and use cooking methods with little or no fat (e.g., broiling, baking). Box 16-8 summarizes other Internet resources providing information for optimal nutritional health; many can be shared with patients/clients.

Another superior source of consumer and health-professional information regarding healthy food consumption is the *Dietary Guide for Americans 2010* from the USDA (USDA, 2010). As well as in-depth explanations, it provides several very useful resources reproduced here. Figure 16-5 provides a comparison of the USDA Food Guide and the Dietary Approaches to Stop Hypertension (DASH) eating plan for each food category with equivalent amounts for an ideal diet. Figure 16-6 shows estimated

---

### BOX 16-7 Diet Recommendations From the American Heart Association

To get the nutrients you need, eat a dietary pattern that emphasizes:

- fruits, vegetables,
- whole grains,
- low-fat dairy products,
- poultry, fish, and nuts,
- while limiting red meat and sugary foods and beverages.

Source: www.heart.org/HEARTORG/GettingHealthy/NutritionCenter/HealthyEating/The American-Heart-Associations-Diet-and-Lifestyle-Recommendations_UCM_305855_Article.jsp.

## BOX 16-8  Nutritional Health Resources for Patients Available on the Internet

http://www.healthfinder.gov/HealthTopics/Category/health-conditions-and-diseases/diabetes/eat-healthy
- "Eat Healthy" includes basic information and action steps.

http://www.cdc.gov/bam/nutrition/index.html
CDC "BAM! Body and Mind" website for **children** has a section called "Food and Nutrition" that includes
- *Cool Treats* with quick, easy, healthy treats.
- *Dining Decisions* to help make healthy food choices.

http://www.cnpp.usda.gov/DietaryGuidelines
- "Dietary Guidelines for Americans 2010" from the Office of Disease Prevention and Health Promotion USDHHS can be downloaded as a single PDF file of the entire Dietary Guidelines that summarize what we should eat, how to optimally prepare our food, and how to keep it safe and wholesome. A consumer brochure can also be downloaded here.

http://www.health.gov/dietaryguidelines/dga2005/toolkit/DASH/default.htm
- National Heart, Lung, and Blood Institute (NHLBI) produced the DASH "Dietary Approaches to Stop Hypertension" eating plan that, in addition to reduced sodium intake, is "low in saturated fat, cholesterol, and total fat and that emphasizes fruits, vegetables, and fat-free or low-fat milk and milk products. This eating plan also includes whole grain products, fish, poultry, and nuts. It is reduced in lean red meat, sweets, added sugars, and sugar-containing beverages compared with the typical American diet. It is rich in potassium, magnesium, and calcium, as well as protein and fiber."

http://www.health.gov/dietaryguidelines/dga2005/toolkit/default.htm
- USDHHS webpage "Toolkit for Health Professionals" includes numerous dietary guidelines, resources, specific eating plans (DASH, My Plate), reproducible worksheets and tip sheets, consumer brochures and fact sheets, and older adult brochures and fact sheets, specifically assembled as a resource for health professionals.

http://www.cdc.gov/nutrition/everyone/fruitsvegetables/index.html
- CDC National Fruit and Vegetable program is a public-private partnership to increase the consumption of fruits and vegetables for improved public health. The website provides a calculator that, based on your age, sex, and physical activity level, calculates the number of servings of fruits and vegetables, respectively, that you need to consume each day. For example, a 40 year-old male with less than 30 minutes of physical activity per day should consume about two cups of fruit and three cups of vegetables every day.

http://www.heart.org/HEARTORG/GettingHealthy/GettingHealthy_UCM_001078_SubHomePage.jsp
American Heart Association Nutrition Center, also includes these links:
1. *"Heart Smart Shopping"* link includes:
   - Grocery Shopping
   - Reading Food Labels
   - Heart-Check Mark
   - Grocery List Builder (online tool)
2. *"Healthy Cooking"* link includes:
   - Healthier Preparation Methods
   - Smart Substitutions
   - Healthy Snacking
   - Summer Barbecue Tips
3. *"Recipes"* link includes numerous heart-healthy recipes categorized by Snacks/Appetizers, Soups/Salads/Side Dishes, Main Dishes, Desserts/Sweets.
4. *"Dining Out"* link includes:
   - Choosing a Restaurant
   - Deciphering the Menu
   - Eating Fast Food
   - Talking with your Server
   - Ordering your Meal
   - Tips by Cuisine

http://www.niddk.nih.gov/health-information/health-communication-programs/win/win-health-topics/Pages/default.aspx
- National Institute of Diabetes and Digestive and Kidney Diseases (NIDDK) provides an online list of webpage links and downloads for publications and resources related to nutrition, physical activity, and weight control listed by subject. Publications are categorized by those for the public, for health care professionals, promotional flyers, and en Español.

## TABLE 1. Sample USDA Food Guide and the DASH Eating Plan at the 2,000-Calorie Level[a]

Amounts of various food groups that are recommended each day or each week in the USDA Food Guide and in the DASH Eating Plan (amounts are daily unless otherwise specified) at the 2,000-calorie level. Also identified are equivalent amounts for different food choices in each group. To follow either eating pattern, food choices over time should provide these amounts of food from each group on average.

| Food groups and subgroups | USDA food guide amount[b] | DASH eating plan amount | Equivalent amounts |
|---|---|---|---|
| Fruit group | 2 cups (4 servings) | 2 to 2.5 cups (4 to 5 servings) | ½ cup equivalent is:<br>• ½ cup fresh, frozen, or canned fruit<br>• 1 med fruit<br>• ¼ cup dried fruit<br>• USDA: ½ cup fruit juice<br>• DASH: ¾ cup fruit juice |
| Vegetable group<br>• Dark green vegetables<br>• Orange vegetables<br>• Legumes (dry beans)<br>• Starchy vegetables<br>• Other vegetables | 2.5 cups (5 servings)<br>3 cups/week<br>2 cups/week<br>3 cups/week<br>3 cups/week<br>6.5 cups/week | 2 to 2.5 cups (4 to 5 servings) | ½ cup equivalent is:<br>• ½ cup of cut-up raw or cooked vegetable<br>• 1 cup raw leafy vegetable<br>• USDA: ½ cup vegetable juice<br>• DASH: ¾ cup vegetable juice |
| Grain group<br>• Whole grains<br>• Other grains | 6 ounce-equivalents<br>3 ounce-equivalents<br>3 ounce-equivalents | 7 to 8 ounce-equivalents<br>(7 to 8 servings) | 1 ounce-equivalent is:<br>• 1 slice bread<br>• 1 cup dry cereal<br>• ½ cup cooked rice, pasta, cereal<br>• DASH: 1 oz dry cereal (½–1¼ cup depending on cereal type—check label) |
| Meat and beans group | 5.5 ounce-equivalents | 6 ounces or less meat, poultry, fish<br><br>4 to 5 servings per week nuts, seeds, and dry beans[c] | 1 ounce-equivalent is:<br>• 1 ounce of cooked lean meats, poultry, fish<br>• 1 egg<br>• USDA: ¼ cup cooked dry beans or tofu, 1 Tbsp peanut butter, ½ oz nuts or seeds<br>• DASH: 1½ oz nuts, ½ oz seeds, ½ cup cooked dry beans |
| Milk group | 3 cups | 2 to 3 cups | 1 cup equivalent is:<br>• 1 cup low-fat/fat-free milk, yogurt<br>• 1½ oz of low-fat or fat-free natural cheese<br>• 2 oz of low-fat or fat-free processed cheese |
| Oils | 24 grams (6 tsp) | 8 to 12 grams (2 to 3 tsp) | 1 tsp equivalent is:<br>• DASH: 1 tsp soft margarine<br>• 1 Tbsp low-fat mayo<br>• 2 Tbsp light salad dressing<br>• 1 tsp vegetable oil |
| Discretionary calorie allowance<br>• Example of distribution:<br>  Solid fat[d]<br>  Added sugars | 267 calories<br><br>18 grams<br>8 tsp | <br><br><br>~2 tsp (5 Tbsp per week) | 1 Tbsp added sugar equivalent is:<br>• DASH: 1 Tbsp jelly or jam<br>• ½ oz jelly beans<br>• 8 oz lemonade |

[a] All servings are per day unless otherwise noted. USDA vegetable subgroup amounts and amounts of DASH nuts, seeds, and dry beans are per week.

[b] The 2,000-calorie USDA Food Guide is appropriate for many sedentary males 51 to 70 years of age, sedentary females 19 to 30 years of age, and for some other gender/age groups who are more physically active. See table 3 for information about gender/age/activity levels and appropriate calorie intakes. See appendixes A-2 and A-3 for more information on the food groups, amounts, and food intake patterns at other calorie levels.

[c] In the DASH Eating Plan, nuts, seeds, and dry beans are a separate food group from meat, poultry, and fish.

[d] The oils listed in this table are not considered to be part of discretionary calories because they are a major source of the vitamin E and polyunsaturated fatty acids, including the essential fatty acids, in the food pattern. In contrast, solid fats (i.e., saturated and *trans* fats) are listed separately as a source of discretionary calories.

DIETARY GUIDELINES FOR AMERICANS, 2005

**FIGURE 16-5** Comparison of the USDA Food Guide and the DASH Eating Plan for each food category with equivalent amounts for an ideal diet. From: U.S. Department of Health and Human Services and U.S. Department of Agriculture. *2015–2020 Dietary Guidelines for Americans*. 8th edition. December 2015. Available at https://health.gov/dietaryguidelines/2015/guidelines/.

**Estimated Calorie Needs per Day by Age, Gender, and Physical Activity Level.**

Estimated amounts of calories[a] needed to maintain calorie balance for various gender and age groups at three different levels of physical activity. The estimates are rounded to the nearest 200 calories for assignment to a USDA Food Pattern. An individual's calorie needs may be higher or lower than these average estimates.

| | Male | | | Female[c] | | |
|---|---|---|---|---|---|---|
| Activity level[b] | Sedentary | Moderately active | Active | Sedentary | Moderately active | Active |
| Age (years) | | | | | | |
| 2 | 1,000 | 1,000 | 1,000 | 1,000 | 1,000 | 1,000 |
| 3 | 1,200 | 1,400 | 1,400 | 1,000 | 1,200 | 1,400 |
| 4 | 1,200 | 1,400 | 1,600 | 1,200 | 1,400 | 1,400 |
| 5 | 1,200 | 1,400 | 1,600 | 1,200 | 1,400 | 1,600 |
| 6 | 1,400 | 1,600 | 1,800 | 1,200 | 1,400 | 1,600 |
| 7 | 1,400 | 1,600 | 1,800 | 1,200 | 1,600 | 1,800 |
| 8 | 1,400 | 1,600 | 2,000 | 1,400 | 1,600 | 1,800 |
| 9 | 1,600 | 1,800 | 2,000 | 1,400 | 1,600 | 1,800 |
| 10 | 1,600 | 1,800 | 2,200 | 1,400 | 1,800 | 2,000 |
| 11 | 1,800 | 2,000 | 2,200 | 1,600 | 1,800 | 2,000 |
| 12 | 1,800 | 2,200 | 2,400 | 1,600 | 2,000 | 2,200 |
| 13 | 2,000 | 2,200 | 2,600 | 1,600 | 2,000 | 2,200 |
| 14 | 2,000 | 2,400 | 2,800 | 1,800 | 2,000 | 2,400 |
| 15 | 2,200 | 2,600 | 3,000 | 1,800 | 2,000 | 2,400 |
| 16 | 2,400 | 2,800 | 3,200 | 1,800 | 2,000 | 2,400 |
| 17 | 2,400 | 2,800 | 3,200 | 1,800 | 2,000 | 2,400 |
| 18 | 2,400 | 2,800 | 3,200 | 1,800 | 2,000 | 2,400 |
| 19–20 | 2,600 | 2,800 | 3,000 | 2,000 | 2,200 | 2,400 |
| 21–25 | 2,400 | 2,800 | 3,000 | 2,000 | 2,200 | 2,400 |
| 26–30 | 2,400 | 2,600 | 3,000 | 1,800 | 2,000 | 2,400 |
| 31–35 | 2,400 | 2,600 | 3,000 | 1,800 | 2,000 | 2,200 |
| 36–40 | 2,400 | 2,600 | 2,800 | 1,800 | 2,000 | 2,200 |
| 41–45 | 2,200 | 2,600 | 2,800 | 1,800 | 2,000 | 2,200 |
| 46–50 | 2,200 | 2,400 | 2,800 | 1,800 | 2,000 | 2,200 |
| 51–55 | 2,200 | 2,400 | 2,800 | 1,600 | 1,800 | 2,200 |
| 56–60 | 2,200 | 2,400 | 2,600 | 1,600 | 1,800 | 2,200 |
| 61–65 | 2,000 | 2,400 | 2,600 | 1,600 | 1,800 | 2,000 |
| 66–70 | 2,000 | 2,200 | 2,600 | 1,600 | 1,800 | 2,000 |
| 71–75 | 2,000 | 2,200 | 2,600 | 1,600 | 1,800 | 2,000 |
| 76+ | 2,000 | 2,200 | 2,400 | 1,600 | 1,800 | 2,000 |

a. Based on Estimated Energy Requirements (EER) equations, using reference heights (average) and reference weights (healthy) for each age-gender group. For children and adolescents, reference height and weight vary. For adults, the reference man is 5 feet 10 inches tall and weighs 154 pounds. The reference woman is 5 feet 4 inches tall and weighs 126 pounds. EER equations are from the Institute of Medicine. Dietary Reference Intakes for Energy, Carbohydrate, Fiber, Fat, Fatty Acids, Cholesterol, Protein, and Amino Acids. Washington (DC): The National Academies Press; 2002.

b. Sedentary means a lifestyle that includes only the light physical activity associated with typical day-to-day life. Moderately active means a lifestyle that includes physical activity equivalent to walking about 1.5 to 3 miles per day at 3 to 4 miles per hour, in addition to the light physical activity associated with typical day-to-day life. Active means a lifestyle that includes physical activity equivalent to walking more than 3 miles per day at 3 to 4 miles per hour, in addition to the light physical activity associated with typical day-to-day life.

c. Estimates for females do not include women who are pregnant or breastfeeding.

**FIGURE 16-6** Chart of estimated calorie requirements by gender and age for three different activity levels. From: U.S. Department of Health and Human Services and U.S. Department of Agriculture. *2015–2020 Dietary Guidelines for Americans.* 8th edition. December 2015. Available at: www.cnpp.usda.gov/. Accessed May 5, 2016.

calorie requirements by gender and age for three different activity levels. Although BMI calculators are readily available online, Figure 16-7 provides a chart from which the BMI can be determined for any individual using his or her weight (in pounds) and height (in inches). Because adult BMI reference ranges don't apply to children, Figure 16-8 shows an example BMI growth chart for young boys with age percentile limits.

The publication *Your Guide to Lowering Your Blood Pressure With DASH* (USDHHS, 2006) contains details of the DASH eating plan. This plan was developed to assist with weight loss

and HTN control through nutrition and sodium restriction. Additional details about the nutritional component are found in Box 16-8. Assuming a 2,100-calorie eating plan, the DASH goals include: total fat 27% of calories, saturated fat 6% of calories, protein 18% of calories, carbohydrate 55% of calories, cholesterol 150 mg, sodium 2,300 mg (1,500 mg sodium was found to be even more effective), potassium 4,700 mg, calcium 1,250 mg, magnesium 500 mg, and fiber 30 g. Figure 16-9 shows the DASH daily servings and serving sizes for each food group.

## Adult BMI Chart

| BMI | 19 | 20 | 21 | 22 | 23 | 24 | 25 | 26 | 27 | 28 | 29 | 30 | 31 | 32 | 33 | 34 | 35 |
|-----|----|----|----|----|----|----|----|----|----|----|----|----|----|----|----|----|----|
| Height | | | | | | | Weight in Pounds | | | | | | | | | | |
| 4'10" | 91 | 96 | 100 | 105 | 110 | 115 | 119 | 124 | 129 | 134 | 138 | 143 | 148 | 153 | 158 | 162 | 167 |
| 4'11" | 94 | 99 | 104 | 109 | 114 | 119 | 124 | 128 | 133 | 138 | 143 | 148 | 153 | 158 | 163 | 168 | 173 |
| 5' | 97 | 102 | 107 | 112 | 118 | 123 | 128 | 133 | 138 | 143 | 148 | 153 | 158 | 163 | 158 | 174 | 179 |
| 5'1" | 100 | 106 | 111 | 116 | 122 | 127 | 132 | 137 | 143 | 148 | 153 | 158 | 164 | 169 | 174 | 180 | 185 |
| 5'2" | 104 | 109 | 115 | 120 | 126 | 131 | 136 | 142 | 147 | 153 | 158 | 164 | 169 | 175 | 180 | 186 | 191 |
| 5'3" | 107 | 113 | 118 | 124 | 130 | 135 | 141 | 146 | 152 | 158 | 163 | 169 | 175 | 180 | 186 | 191 | 197 |
| 5'4" | 110 | 116 | 122 | 128 | 134 | 140 | 145 | 151 | 157 | 163 | 169 | 174 | 180 | 186 | 192 | 197 | 204 |
| 5'5" | 114 | 120 | 126 | 132 | 138 | 144 | 150 | 156 | 162 | 168 | 174 | 180 | 186 | 192 | 198 | 204 | 210 |
| 5'6" | 118 | 124 | 130 | 136 | 142 | 148 | 155 | 161 | 167 | 173 | 179 | 186 | 192 | 198 | 204 | 210 | 216 |
| 5'7" | 121 | 127 | 134 | 140 | 146 | 153 | 159 | 166 | 172 | 178 | 185 | 191 | 198 | 204 | 211 | 217 | 223 |
| 5'8" | 125 | 131 | 138 | 144 | 151 | 158 | 164 | 171 | 177 | 184 | 190 | 197 | 203 | 210 | 216 | 223 | 230 |
| 5'9" | 128 | 135 | 142 | 149 | 155 | 162 | 169 | 176 | 182 | 189 | 196 | 203 | 209 | 216 | 223 | 230 | 236 |
| 5'10" | 132 | 139 | 146 | 153 | 160 | 167 | 174 | 181 | 188 | 195 | 202 | 209 | 216 | 222 | 229 | 236 | 243 |
| 5'11" | 136 | 143 | 150 | 157 | 165 | 172 | 179 | 186 | 193 | 200 | 208 | 215 | 222 | 229 | 236 | 243 | 250 |
| 6' | 140 | 147 | 154 | 162 | 169 | 177 | 184 | 191 | 199 | 206 | 213 | 221 | 228 | 235 | 242 | 250 | 258 |
| 6'1" | 144 | 151 | 159 | 166 | 174 | 182 | 189 | 197 | 204 | 212 | 219 | 227 | 235 | 242 | 250 | 257 | 265 |
| 6'2' | 148 | 155 | 163 | 171 | 179 | 186 | 194 | 202 | 210 | 218 | 225 | 233 | 241 | 249 | 256 | 264 | 272 |
| 6'3' | 152 | 160 | 168 | 176 | 184 | 192 | 200 | 208 | 216 | 224 | 232 | 240 | 248 | 256 | 264 | 272 | 279 |
| | Healthy Weight | | | | | | Overweight | | | | | Obese | | | | | |

FIGURE 16-7 A chart from which the BMI can be determined for any individual using their weight (in pounds) and height (in inches). Available at: http://health.gov/dietary guidelines/dga2005/document/images/ch3fig2.jpg. Accessed May 5, 2016.

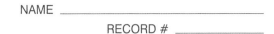

## 2 to 20 years: Boys
## Body mass index-for-age percentiles

NAME _____

RECORD # _____

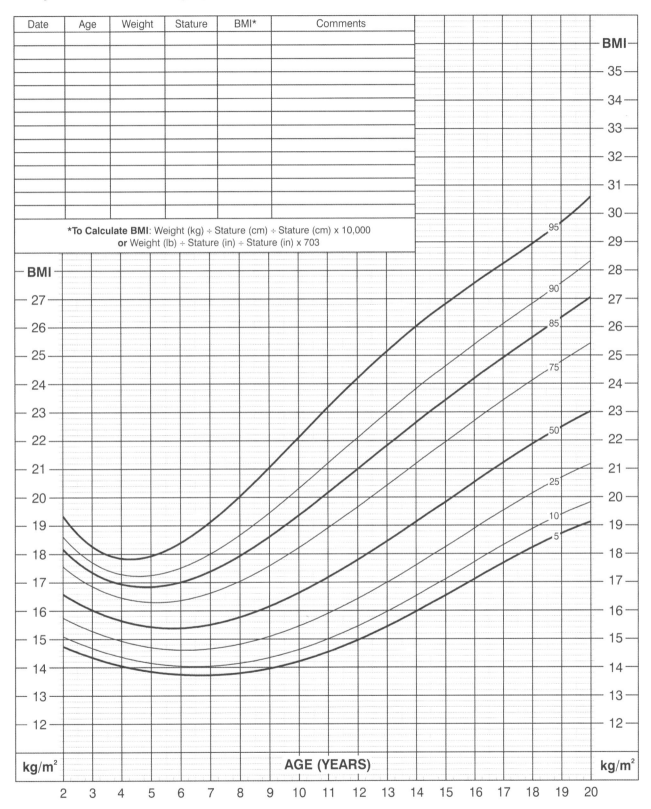

*To Calculate BMI: Weight (kg) ÷ Stature (cm) ÷ Stature (cm) x 10,000
or Weight (lb) ÷ Stature (in) ÷ Stature (in) x 703

Published May 30, 2000 (modified 10/16/00).

SOURCE: Developed by the National Center for Health Statistics in collaboration with
the National Center for Chronic Disease Prevention and Health Promotion (2000).
http://www.cdc.gov/growthcharts

SAFER · HEALTHIER · PEOPLE™

**FIGURE 16-8** An example BMI growth chart for young boys with age percentile limits. From Centers for Disease Control and Prevention, National Center for Health Statistics. Available at: www.cdc.gov/growthcharts/data/set2clinical/cj41c073.pdf. Accessed May 5, 2016.

BOX 2

# FOLLOWING THE DASH DIET

The DASH eating plan shown below is based on 2,000 calories a day. The number of daily servings in a food group may vary from those listed depending on your caloric needs. Use this chart to help you plan your menus or take it with you when you go to the store.

| FOOD GROUP | DAILY SERVINGS (except as noted) | SERVING SIZES | EXAMPLES AND NOTES | SIGNIFICANCE OF EACH FOOD GROUP TO THE DASH EATING PLAN |
|---|---|---|---|---|
| Grains & grain products | 7–8 | 1 slice bread<br>1 oz dry cereal*<br>$\frac{1}{2}$ cup cooked rice, pasta, or cereal | whole wheat bread, English muffin, pita bread, bagel, cereals, grits, oatmeal, crackers, unsalted pretzels and popcorn | major sources of energy and fiber |
| Vegetables | 4–5 | 1 cup raw leafy vegetable<br>$\frac{1}{2}$ cup cooked vegetable<br>6 oz vegetable juice | tomatoes, potatoes, carrots, green peas, squash, broccoli, turnip greens, collards, kale, spinach, artichokes, green beans, lima beans, sweet potatoes | rich sources of potassium, magnesium, and fiber |
| Fruits | 4–5 | 6 oz fruit juice<br>1 medium fruit<br>$\frac{1}{4}$ cup dried fruit<br>$\frac{1}{2}$ cup fresh, frozen, or canned fruit | apricots, bananas, dates, grapes, oranges, orange juice, grapefruit, grapefruit juice, mangoes, melons, peaches, pineapples, prunes, raisins, strawberries, tangerines | important sources of potassium, magnesium, and fiber |
| Lowfat or fat free dairy foods | 2–3 | 8 oz milk<br>1 cup yogurt<br>$1\frac{1}{2}$ oz cheese | fat free (skim) or lowfat (1%) milk, fat free or lowfat buttermilk, fat free or lowfat regular or frozen yogurt, lowfat and fat free cheese | major sources of calcium and protein |
| Meats, poultry, and fish | 2 or less | 3 oz cooked meats, poultry, or fish | select only lean; trim away visible fats; broil, roast, or boil, instead of frying; remove skin from poultry | rich sources of protein and magnesium |
| Nuts, seeds, and dry beans | 4–5 per week | $\frac{1}{3}$ cup or $1\frac{1}{2}$ oz nuts<br>2 Tbsp or $\frac{1}{2}$ oz seeds<br>$\frac{1}{2}$ cup cooked dry beans | almonds, filberts, mixed nuts, peanuts, walnuts, sunflower seeds, kidney beans, lentils, peas | rich sources of energy, magnesium, potassium, protein, and fiber |
| Fats & oils** | 2–3 | 1 tsp soft margarine<br>1 Tbsp lowfat mayonnaise<br>2 Tbsp light salad dressing<br>1 tsp vegetable oil | soft margarine, lowfat mayonnaise, light salad dressing, vegetable oil (such as olive, corn, canola, or safflower) | DASH has 27 percent of calories as fat, including that in or added to foods |
| Sweets | 5 per week | 1 Tbsp sugar<br>1 Tbsp jelly or jam<br>$\frac{1}{2}$ oz jelly beans<br>8 oz lemonade | maple syrup, sugar, jelly, jam, fruit-flavored gelatin, jelly beans, hard candy, fruit punch, sorbet, ices | sweets should be low in fat |

* Equals $\frac{1}{2}$-$1\frac{1}{4}$ cup, depending on cereal type. Check the product's nutrition label.
** Fat content changes serving counts for fats and oils: For example, 1 Tbsp of regular salad dressing equals 1 serving; 1 Tbsp of a lowfat dressing equals $\frac{1}{2}$ serving; 1 Tbsp of a fat free dressing equals 0 servings.

**FIGURE 16-9** A chart of the daily servings and serving sizes for each food group within the DASH eating plan. (Reproduced from United States Department of Health and Human Services, *Your Guide to Lowering Your Blood Pressure With DASH*, 2006.) Available at: www.nhlbi.nih.gov/files/docs/public/heart/new_dash.pdf. Accessed May 5, 2016.

## Dot, Step 3

*After your education and motivation regarding the health dangers of both smoking and obesity, Dot has decided she definitely wants to stop smoking and will try to lose weight.*

### Contemplate Clinical Decisions

1. What public-access information about smoking cessation could you share with Dot?
2. In addition to the information you share with her, it would also be beneficial for you to refer her to which type or types of health-care professionals?
3. What public-access information about weight loss could you share with Dot?
4. What are the two main aspects of intervention for weight loss?
5. Although the therapist could easily design and manage the physical activity part of the weight-loss intervention, it would probably be best to refer Dot to which other type of health-care professional?

### Polypharmacy Issues and Medication Adherence

Because rehabilitation therapists, adult and pediatric, see so many patients/clients with multiple comorbidities who are taking multiple medications, a detailed drug history that includes an assessment of polypharmacy and medication adherence is critical. Particularly in older adults, new signs and symptoms can indicate not only the onset of new physical conditions or exacerbations of known comorbidities but also adverse drug reactions, abnormal drug interactions, and drug side effects, which increase with increasing numbers of medications.

Therapists should educate patients about the recommendation regarding medication from the USDHHS *Five Steps to Safer Health Care*, listed under "Keep and bring a list of ALL the medicines you take." (Agency for Healthcare Research and Quality, *Five Steps*, 2004):

- Give your doctor and pharmacist a list of all the medicines that you take, including nonprescription medicines.
- Tell them about any drug allergies you have.
- Ask about side effects and what to avoid while taking the medicine.
- Read the label when you get your medicine, including all warnings.
- Make sure your medicine is what the doctor ordered and know how to use it.
- Ask the pharmacist about your medicine if it looks different than you expected.

The patient who maintains an accurate medication list is practicing primary prevention in the sense of preventing medical errors related to medications. Therapists should also be aware of pharmacology and potential drug interactions

particularly related to their areas of practice and the common disorders seen in that practice. Any time medication adherence problems, polypharmacy, or drug interactions are suspected, the therapist should immediately consult with, and refer the patient to, the pharmacist or physician.

### Infection

Though not part of the systems review, body temperature is another important clinical measure for therapists to implement especially when infection is suspected. Acute infection with fever (temperature >100.5°F or >38°C) is a general contraindication to exercise; however, fever associated with infection in older adults may not be as high as in younger adults because older adults may have lower basal body temperature. Thus the older individual's temperature should be taken in the evening with a lower threshold for referral for possible infection: an oral temperature of 99°F to 100°F (37.2°C to 37.7°C) with a change in function (Goodman, 2007).

### Depression

Depression is the most common adult psychiatric disorder (Goodman, 2007). It is common in older adults (Goodman, 2007; Hardage, 2007) and certainly not unexpected after neurological disorders drastically affecting function and independence. It is associated with numerous physical conditions, drugs, and somatic symptoms commonly seen in therapist practice. Signs and symptoms of clinical depression include depressed mood and **anhedonia** (an inability to enjoy pleasures in life) for ≥2 weeks; persistence of symptoms for >2 months after a loss (thus distinguishing depression from expected situational grief); significant weight change (loss or gain); sleep disturbances; restlessness; fatigue; feelings of worthlessness or guilt; decreased concentration and decision-making ability; and recurrent thoughts of suicide (Goodman, 2007). In one study, scores on the short form of the Geriatric Depression Scale (GDS) (Sheikh, 1986) identified probable depression in 24% of home health patients who were discharged from a physical therapy episode of care (Hardage, 2007).

Some individuals who present with signs and symptoms of depression may not recognize they are depressed, making screening for depression all the more important because the individual may not seek help on his or her own. Also there may be times when the therapist's type of practice setting or particular facility does not specify follow-up screening is needed for patients who present with signs and symptoms of depression or a specific instrument for follow-up screening. These decisions, then, are left to the clinician, reinforcing the concept of best practice. The short form of the GDS can be found in the appendix of Chapter 4. It has 15 items answered in a yes/no format. A score above 5 indicates probable depression and warrants referral (Sheikh, 1986).

### Osteoporosis

Screening for osteoporosis using the Simple Calculated Osteoporosis Risk Estimation (SCORE) (Lydick, 1998) or the Osteoporosis Screening Evaluation by Goodman and

Snyder (2007) is an example of secondary prevention. The SCORE is a simple questionnaire taking approximately 2 to 4 minutes to complete and is used to facilitate the identification of women likely to have low bone mineral density who would benefit from a bone mineral density test and a safe and appropriate exercise program. The use of such screening instruments can then facilitate a referral to the individual's primary care provider (e.g., physician or nurse practitioner).

### Skin Cancer

In addition to skin cancer prevention (i.e., sun protection) discussed earlier, skin cancer screening using the ABCD checklist (Wills, 2002) is an example of secondary prevention especially because many therapist interventions require the patient/client expose particular areas of the skin (including areas such as the back that patients/clients do not ordinarily visualize themselves). The ABCD checklist is simple and quick and should be used when the therapist notices a suspicious lesion. The pneumonic stands for *Asymmetry* (i.e., when bisected, one half of the lesion is not identical to the other half), *Border* (i.e., the border is uneven or ragged as opposed to smooth and straight), *Color* (i.e., the lesion is more than one shade of pigment), and *Diameter* (i.e., the diameter is greater than 6 mm). The presence of one or more of these abnormalities raises suspicion the lesion is cancerous, and the patient/client should be referred to the primary care provider.

### Stroke

Stroke is a pathology particularly illustrating how therapists can participate in primary and secondary prevention, address other dimensions of wellness, and address health issues other than the presenting problem/chief complaint. Stroke also illustrates how therapists can apply health promotion literature in these efforts.

#### Secondary Prevention of Stroke

Stroke is a serious health problem in the United States. It is the third-leading cause of death and a leading cause of disability (AHA, 2006). A key problem in the health care of people with stroke is **decision delay** on the part of the affected individual (and his or her significant others) in which people with acute stroke do not emergently seek treatment upon the initial onset of the signs and symptoms. Optimal treatment for ischemic stroke, the most common type, includes intravenous administration of tissue plasminogen activator (tPA), a thrombolytic agent to break down the thrombus. The resulting dissolution of the clot removes the occlusive cause of stroke, thereby restoring blood flow to the ischemic areas of the brain, arresting the infarction-in-progress of brain tissue, and perhaps even restoring some function depending on the extent of infarction. However, there is a narrow window of opportunity, within 3 hours of initial known onset of symptoms, in which the drug can be administered (Adams, 2007).

This medical intervention can make a tremendous difference in a range of health outcomes, including mortality and the person's subsequent level of disability. Unfortunately, most people do not receive tPA for various reasons, including

symptom onset at night (when the person is unaware of the onset of symptoms) and decision delay. Recognizing this problem, the health-care and public health communities have tried for years to convey the message that people with acute stroke should emergently seek treatment through such messages as "Stroke is a brain attack" (Scott, 2006). However the problem persists, demonstrating the need for improved stroke education programs (Alexandrov, 2007; Kleindorfer, 2006; Lacy, 2001).

Clearly then stroke is a health problem for which secondary prevention is crucial (Box 16-9). Therapists are integrally involved in the physical rehabilitation of people with stroke, constituting tertiary prevention. As the professions recognize the importance of the therapist's role in wellness, there are opportunities to contribute to health education and health promotion efforts at the levels of primary and secondary prevention. Thus secondary prevention efforts targeting stroke can be a natural progression of existing professional roles.

Many of the health education efforts in this arena include grassroots efforts such as hospital-sponsored health fairs. Therapists can easily participate in such efforts while also integrating them into their ongoing clinical practice by providing one-on-one patient/client and caregiver education. Research has shown, although recognition of signs and symptoms is critical, appropriate action is often the missing link (Giles, 2006) including not calling 911 to active emergency medical services (EMS) soon enough (Mosley, 2007; Schroeder, 2000) and not recognizing that EMS provides the best option for emergent treatment (Agyeman, 2006). Hodgson (2007) proposed three essential components of a stroke education program: consistency, simplicity, and repetition.

Broderick (2004) noted stroke education efforts for the lay public should be more focused concerning recognition of signs and symptoms and the need for emergent treatment. He suggested field-screening tests used by first responders

---

**BOX 16-9 Evidence-Based Recommendations for Primary and Secondary Prevention of Stroke**

- Secondary Prevention
  - Stroke education efforts should stress recognition and action.
  - Stroke education efforts should be consistent, simple, and repetitious.
  - Stroke support groups are an important resource.
  - Stroke education efforts should be aimed not only at those who are at risk for stroke but also their friends, family members (including children), and coworkers.
- Primary Prevention
  - Stroke education efforts should stress the myriad health benefits of physical activity, including endurance exercise.
  - Stroke education regarding optimal nutrition to avoid risk factors for atherosclerosis that can contribute to stroke.
  - Stroke education regarding control of hypertension.

could be adapted for such efforts. Specifically, he proposed the acronym FAST (*face*—numbness or weakness; *arm* and/or leg—weakness or numbness, usually on one side; *speech* difficulties; *time* to call 911 [time is critical]). This acronym can be used for public education based on the Cincinnati Prehospital Stroke Scale and the Face Arm Speech Test.

However Kleindorfer and colleagues (2007) questioned whether the use of FAST would allow the public to correctly identify as many cases of stroke as another tool, the "*suddens*" (warning signs of stroke) of the AHA (2011). The list of five "suddens" (*sudden numbness or weakness* of the face, arm or leg, especially on one side of the body; *sudden confusion,* trouble speaking or understanding; *sudden trouble seeing* in one or both eyes; *sudden trouble walking,* dizziness, loss of balance or coordination; and *sudden severe headache* with no known cause) captures more signs and symptoms but may not be as easy for the lay public to remember (Hodgson, 2007; Kleindorfer, 2007). Another education tool to enhance stroke identification is *A Simple Test for Stroke* (Overby, 2003) in which the person is asked to smile, raise both arms, and speak a simple sentence coherently. Stroke public education messages such as "Call 9-1-1 immediately if you experience symptoms! Time lost is brain lost!" (AHA, *Warning Signs*) reinforce the two components of stroke education for secondary prevention: recognition and action (Scott, 2006).

Weltermann (2000) found members of stroke support groups are knowledgeable about stroke and stated stroke support groups should be viewed as an important resource in stroke education programs. Schroeder (2000) also argued for the need for stroke education programs to stress the urgency and importance of using EMS as well as the need to target not only those at risk for stroke but also their friends and family. This recommendation for family involvement has in fact reached the level of policy recommendations (Schwamm, 2005). Wein (2000) argued large employers may be opportune gateways for stroke education programs aimed at family, caregivers, and coworkers. Some stroke education programs have targeted specific groups including children (Morgenstern, 2007; Dressman, 2002). Starting stroke support groups or participating in established stroke support groups represents another important health promotion opportunity for therapists, which can also enhance their visibility in the community and recognition as experts in the area of stroke. Therapists can also participate in primary prevention activities by educating the public about risk factors for stroke and how to decrease those risk factors.

### Physical Activity in Primary Prevention of Stroke and Other Conditions

*Healthy People 2020* (USDHHS, 2010) objectives regarding physical activity focus on increasing the proportion of adults, adolescents, and children who meet current Federal physical activity guidelines for aerobic physical activity and for muscle strengthening (PA-2–4). An objective was also set to increase the proportion of office visits that include counseling or education related to physical activity (PA-11).

The American College of Sports Medicine (ACSM) Position Statement *Exercise and Hypertension* (Pescatello, 2004) states

HTN is associated with an increased incidence of all-cause and cardiovascular disease mortality, stroke, coronary heart disease, heart failure, peripheral arterial disease, and renal insufficiency. It recommends lifestyle modification be used for the prevention, treatment, and control of HTN with exercise being an integral component. For example, blood pressure is reduced for up to 22 hours after an endurance training session with the greatest decreases among individuals with the highest baseline blood pressure. The authors state endurance exercise programs prevent the development of HTN in adults with normal BP and lower blood pressure (BP) in those with HTN and the "BP lowering effects of exercise are most pronounced in people with HTN who engage in endurance exercise with BP decreasing approximately 5 to 7 mm Hg after an isolated session (acute) or following exercise training (chronic)" (Pescatello, 2004, p. 533). Thus this document provides evidence-based recommendations for endurance exercise for the primary prevention of stroke through affecting HTN as a mediating variable.

Another document, *Quality Indicators for Screening and Prevention in Vulnerable Elders* (Gnanadesigan, 2007, p. S419), makes the following recommendation regarding physical activity in vulnerable elders (VEs):

*ALL VEs should have an assessment of their activity level (with encouragement to be active) annually **BECAUSE** physical activity plays an important role in prevention and treatment of many disabling chronic diseases in elderly people (e.g., obesity, cardiovascular disease, stroke, diabetes mellitus type 2, HTN, depression, osteoporosis, osteoarthritis, cognitive decline), and it has been shown to improve cardiovascular fitness and function and to prevent falls.*

Clearly, physical activity conveys a broad array of health benefits beyond primary prevention for stroke. An even broader recommendation is an APTA Position: *Annual Visit with a Physical Therapist* HOD P05-07-19-20 (APTA, 2007). The position states, "The American Physical Therapy Association recommends that all individuals visit a physical therapist at least annually to promote optimal health, wellness, and fitness, as well as to slow the progression of impairments, functional limitations, and disabilities." This position can be used for marketing the services of the physical therapist as providers of wellness services. The importance of enhancing physical activity among young people is supported by a variety of publications (National Center For Chronic Disease Prevention and Health Promotion, 1997; Stone, 1998; Burke, 1998; Arbeit, 1992).

In 2007, the ACSM and the AHA jointly issued two major documents with physical activity recommendations for adults, including separate guidelines for older adults. These documents can be readily applied to health promotion in geriatric physical therapy. *Physical Activity and Public Health: Updated Recommendation for Adults from the American College of Sports Medicine and the American Heart Association* (Haskell, 2007, p. 1423) makes the following primary recommendation:

*To promote and maintain health, all healthy adults aged 18 to 65 years need moderate-intensity aerobic (endurance) physical activity for a minimum of 30 minutes on 5 days each week or*

*vigorous-intensity aerobic physical activity for a minimum of 20 minutes on 3 days each week [I (A)]. Combinations of moderate- and vigorous-intensity activity can be performed to meet this recommendation [IIa (B)]. For example, a person can meet the recommendation by walking briskly for 30 minutes twice during the week and then jogging for 20 minutes on 2 other days. Moderate-intensity aerobic activity, which is generally equivalent to a brisk walk and noticeably accelerates the heart rate, can be accumulated toward the 30-minute minimum by performing bouts each lasting 10 or more minutes [I (B)]. Vigorous-intensity activity is exemplified by jogging and causes rapid breathing and a substantial increase in heart rate. In addition, every adult should perform activities that maintain or increase muscular strength and endurance a minimum of 2 days each week [IIa (A)]. Because of the dose-response relation between physical activity and health, persons who wish to further improve their personal fitness, reduce their risk for chronic diseases and disabilities or prevent unhealthy weight gain may benefit by exceeding the minimum recommended amounts of physical activity [I (A)].*

*Physical Activity and Public Health in Older Adults: Recommendation from the American College of Sports Medicine and the American Heart Association* (Nelson, 2007, p. 1439) makes recommendations specific to older adults stating, "Regular physical activity, including aerobic activity and muscle-strengthening activity, is essential for healthy aging. This preventive recommendation specifies how older adults, by engaging in each recommended type of physical activity, can reduce the risk of chronic disease, premature mortality, functional limitations, and disability." Nelson (2007, p. 1435) defines the term "older adults" as "men and women age ≥65 years and adults age 50 to 64 years with clinically significant chronic conditions and/or functional limitations." Clinical significance for a chronic condition is defined as a person's receiving (or needing to receive) regular medical care and treatment for it. Clinical significance for a functional limitation is defined as impairment in the ability to engage in physical activity. The document (Nelson, 2007, p. 1435) makes the following specific recommendations:

> ***Summary:*** *The recommendation for older adults is similar to the updated ACSM/AHA recommendation for adults but has several important differences including: the recommended intensity of aerobic activity takes into account the older adult's aerobic fitness; activities that maintain or increase flexibility are recommended; and balance exercises are recommended for older adults at risk of falls. In addition, older adults should have an activity plan for achieving recommended physical activity that integrates preventive and therapeutic recommendations. The promotion of physical activity in older adults should emphasize moderate-intensity aerobic activity, muscle-strengthening activity, reducing sedentary behavior, and risk management.*

The document goes on to make specific recommendations concerning aerobic activity, muscle-strengthening activity, benefits of greater amounts of activity, flexibility activity, balance exercise, integration of preventive and therapeutic recommendations, and the activity plan. The activity plan represents a major opportunity for therapists to use their expertise to maximize patient/client adherence. Clearly these guidelines support the role of the therapist in health promotion in geriatrics and neurology. The guidelines offer important information for the therapist and for consumers, the media, and third-party payers.

There are many simple and generic ways a therapist can encourage patients/clients and families to engage in physical activity and increase physical activity. As with any other intervention, motivation, stage of change, and practicality will affect the degree to which the individual changes the target behavior. As a simple example, a 48 year-old man might be more successful at increasing physical activity if the therapist were to suggest family recreation. Family recreation helps make physical activity part of the normal routine and offers built-in accountability and encouragement. The family can enjoy spending time together in this way and reap the health benefits; furthermore family recreation sets good habits for the rest of the family, especially children and teenagers.

Also the therapist should remind the patient all activity does not have to be strenuous; rather regular daily activities can have additive and beneficial effects. The patient could keep a diary of physical activity as a motivating mechanism and accountability structure to help initiate physical activity. Box 16-10 shows some simple tips for naturally increasing physical activity from the AHA webpage that can be encouraged for incorporation into a person's daily schedule. This public information could easily be shared with a patient/client with Internet access. Other Web-based resources are summarized in Box 16-11.

### A Systems Approach to Exercise Prescription in Neurology

In the process of developing a customized, patient/client-centered exercise and physical activity program toward optimal health, the therapist must consider how all of the body systems interact to support physical function. Table 16-12 provides a framework within which the systems can be used to organize an exercise prescription.

## Tests and Measures

The key to demonstrating and documenting both the need for and the value and results of therapy services toward health and wellness is data from reliable and valid tests and measures. Some of the more common tests and measures for screening and measuring outcomes related to health and wellness can be found in Box 16-12.

Heart rate, respiratory rate, BP, and temperature are components of the cardiovascular/pulmonary systems review, and acute infection is an absolute contraindication to exercise (ACSM, 2000). **Body mass index** (BMI) is a commonly used indicator of fitness and body composition (particularly body fat) and can easily be computed from the patient's/client's height and weight, which are recorded during the musculoskeletal systems review. Numerous online BMI calculators are available, including the CDC calculator at www.cdc.gov/

## BOX 16-10 American Heart Association Suggestions to Naturally Increase "Physical Activity in Your Daily Life"

### At Home

*It's convenient, comfortable, and safe to work out at home. It allows your children to see you being active, which sets a good example for them. You can combine exercise with other activities such as watching TV. If you buy exercise equipment, it's a one-time expense and other family members can use it. It's easy to have short bouts of activity several times a day. Try these tips:*

- Do housework yourself instead of hiring someone else to do it.
- Work in the garden or mow the grass. Using a riding mower doesn't count! Rake leaves, prune, dig, and pick up trash.
- Go out for a short walk before breakfast, after dinner, or both! Start with 5 to 10 minutes and work up to 30 minutes.
- Walk or bike to the corner store instead of driving.
- When walking, pick up the pace from leisurely to brisk. Choose a hilly route. When watching TV, sit up instead of lying on the sofa. Better yet, spend a few minutes pedaling on your stationary bicycle while watching TV. Throw away your video remote control. Instead of asking someone to bring you a drink, get up off the couch and get it yourself.
- Stand up while talking on the telephone.
- Walk the dog.
- Park farther away at the shopping mall and walk the extra distance. Wear your walking shoes and sneak in an extra lap or two around the mall.
- Stretch to reach items in high places and squat or bend to look at items at floor level.
- Keep exercise equipment repaired and use it!

### At the Office

*Most of us have sedentary jobs. Work takes up a significant part of the day. What can you do to increase your physical activity during the work-day? Why not...:*

- Brainstorm project ideas with a coworker while taking a walk.
- Stand while talking on the telephone.
- Walk down the hall to speak with someone rather than using the telephone.
- Take the stairs instead of the elevator. Or get off a few floors early and take the stairs the rest of the way.
- Walk while waiting for the plane at the airport.
- Stay at hotels with fitness centers or swimming pools and use them while on business trips.
- Take along a jump rope in your suitcase when you travel. Jump and do calisthenics in your hotel room.
- Participate in or start a recreation league at your company.
- Form a sports team to raise money for charity events.
- Join a fitness center or Y near your job. Work out before or after work to avoid rush-hour traffic or drop by for a noon workout.
- Schedule exercise time on your business calendar and treat it as any other important appointment.
- Get off the bus a few blocks early and walk the rest of the way to work or home.
- Walk around your building for a break during the workday or during lunch.
- Park a few blocks away or at the back of the lot and walk the extra distance each day.
- Take an exercise break—get up and stretch, walk around.
- Instead of snacking, take a brisk stroll.

### At Play

*Play and recreation are important for good health. Look for opportunities such as these to be active and have fun at the same time:*

- Plan family outings and vacations that include physical activity (hiking, backpacking, swimming, etc.).
- See the sights in new cities by walking, jogging, or bicycling.
- Make a date with a friend to enjoy your favorite physical activities. Do them regularly.
- Play your favorite music while exercising, something that motivates you.
- Dance with someone or by yourself. Take dancing lessons. Hit the dance floor on fast numbers instead of slow ones.
- Join a recreational club that emphasizes physical activity.
- At the beach, sit and watch the waves instead of lying flat. Better yet, get up and walk, run, or fly a kite.
- When golfing, walk instead of using a cart.
- Play singles tennis or racquetball instead of doubles.
- At a picnic, join in on badminton instead of croquet.
- At the lake, rent a rowboat instead of a canoe.

Adapted from American Heart Association website. Available at: www.americanheart.org/presenter.jhtml?identifier=2155.

---

**BOX 16-11  Physical Activity Resources for Patients Available on the Internet**

http://www.heart.org/HEARTORG/GettingHealthy/PhysicalActivity/Physical-Activity_UCM_001080_SubHomePage.jsp
- American Heart Association website includes multiple resources including Fitness Basics, Staying Motivated for Fitness, and Body Mass Index Calculator

http://www.nia.nih.gov/health/publication/exercise-physical-activity/introduction
- National Institute on Aging *Exercise & Physical Activity: Your Everyday Guide* to read online or download as a PDF

http://www.health.gov/paguidelines/guidelines/default.aspx
- 2008 Physical Activity Guidelines for Americans from USDHHS

---

**BOX 16-12  Common Tests and Measures for Outcomes Related to Health and Wellness**

**General Health**
Temperature (Goodman and Snyder, 2003)
Body mass index (BMI)

**Cardiovascular/Pulmonary System**
Borg Scale of Perceived Exertion (Borg, 1982)
6- and 12-minute Walk Tests (6MWT, 12MWT; McGavin, 1976; Butland, 1982)

**Integumentary System**
ABCD checklist for skin CA screening (Wills, 2002)

**Musculoskeletal System**
Simple Calculated Osteoporosis Risk Estimation (SCORE) (Lydick, 1998)
Osteoporosis Screening Evaluation by Goodman and Snyder (2007)

**Neuromuscular System**
Timed-Up-and-Go Test (TUG) (Podsiadlo, 1991)
Functional Reach Test (Duncan, 1990)
Tinetti Performance-oriented Mobility Assessment (POMA) (Tinetti, 1986; Tinetti and Ginter, 1988)
Short Physical Performance Battery (SPPB) (Guralnik, 1994)
Berg Balance Test (BBT) (Berg, 1993)
Fullerton Advanced Balance Scale (FAB) (Rose, 2003)
Gait Speed (Bohannon, 1997; VanSwearingen, 1998; Harada, 1995)
Dynamic Gait Index (DGI) (Shumway-Cook and Woollacott, 1995)
Functional Gait Assessment (FGA) (Wrisley, 2004)

**Communication Ability, Affect, Cognition, Language, and Learning Style**
Activities-specific Balance Confidence (ABC) Scale (Powell and Myers, 1995)
Falls Efficacy Scale (FES) (Tinetti, 1990)
Geriatric Depression Scale (GDS) (Sheikh and Yesavage, 1986)

---

| TABLE 16-12 | Factors, by Body System, the Therapist Should Consider in Exercise Prescription |
|---|---|
| **BODY SYSTEM** | **FACTORS TO CONSIDER IN EXERCISE PRESCRIPTION** |
| Cardiovascular/pulmonary system | Aerobic conditioning |
| Integumentary system | Hydration (as evidenced by skin turgor, chapping), regulation of sun exposure |
| Musculoskeletal system | Strength, flexibility, bone density |
| Neuromuscular system | Balance, coordination |
| Communication ability, affect, cognition, language, and learning style | Activity plan, physical activity through hobbies, cognitive stimulation |

---

healthyweight/assessing/bmi/index.html (CDC, *Body Mass Index*). The Borg Scale of Perceived Exertion (Borg, 1982) is a commonly used self-reported measure of exertion. The 6-minute and 12-minute walk tests (McGavin, 1976; Butland, 1982), described in Chapter 11, are commonly used evidence-based tests of exercise tolerance.

Many tests and measures for balance and **balance confidence** are available. Some are appropriate for brief screenings such as the Timed-Up-and-Go Test (Podsiadlo, 1991) and the Functional Reach Test (Duncan, 1990), and thus can be easily used at a hospital-based health fair or other venue. Balance confidence is important to assess because it can be linked to self-imposed participation restrictions (i.e., avoidance of certain tasks due to fear of falling). The Activities-specific Balance Confidence Scale (Powell, 1995) and Falls Efficacy Scale (Tinetti, 1990) measure this construct (see Chapter 9). The other tests and measures of balance—including the Tinetti Performance-oriented Mobility

Assessment (Tinetti, 1986; Tinetti and Ginter, 1988), the Short Physical Performance Battery (Guralnik, 1994), the Berg Balance Test (Berg, 1993), and the Fullerton Advanced Balance Scale (Rose, 2003)—are listed in order of appropriateness for lower-functioning to higher-functioning individuals. All of these tests are readily available and easy to learn and to administer, though some—such as the Berg Balance Test—may take more time.

Certainly some overlap exists between assessment of balance and assessment of gait especially because some tests and measures have separate sections for balance and gait. Gait speed is a good generic measure of functional mobility (see Chapter 10). Self-selected, comfortable, normal gait speed versus maximum gait speed are two ways to approach this measure, and normative values tables (Table 10-3) provide for quick evaluation of patient/client performance (Bohannon, 1997). The distances used to obtain gait data have ranged from 6 m to 20 m. Risk of recurrent falls in frail older adults has been determined using a gait speed cutoff score of 0.56 m/s (VanSwearingen, 1998). To identify individuals who would benefit from physical therapy evaluation and possible intervention, a gait speed cutoff score of 0.57 m/s has been suggested by Harada (1995). This measure has face validity for community function as gait speed is a factor in negotiating public spaces such as crosswalks. The Dynamic Gait Index (Shumway-Cook and Woollacott, 1995) (Table 10-11) is a good test of functional mobility in older adults, and the Functional Gait Assessment (Wrisley, 2004) (Table 9-6) is an upward revision of the Dynamic Gait Index to give it a higher ceiling.

## Let's Review

1. What is health promotion?

2. How can therapists incorporate health promotion into their clinical practice? How can they contribute to health promotion in other ways (i.e., other than clinical practice)?

3. What resources exist to help support therapists in their health promotion efforts?

4. How can Rimmer's model of health promotion for people with disabilities be applied to therapist practice?

5. What specific steps might you take to promote the health of your patient/client during an episode of care in an outpatient neurological rehabilitation setting? What specific steps might you take to promote the health of your patient/client upon discharge?

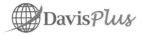 For additional resources, including Focus on Evidence tables, case study discussions, references, and glossary, please visit http://davisplus.fadavis.com

## CHAPTER SUMMARY

This chapter has centered on the therapist's role in health promotion in neurorehabilitation as a member of the health-care team. It is important to recognize other disciplines have important contributions to make and that areas of overlap occur. For instance, therapeutic recreation specialists work with people with disabilities to promote their participation in leisure activities. It is also important to recognize the great need for sharing information across disciplines. For example, therapists may benefit from health promotion literature published in nursing journals and vice versa. Recognizing the inherently transdisciplinary nature of health promotion, interprofessional dialog must take place to disseminate, synthesize, and apply the literature available and work toward a common research agenda to clearly delineate and address areas in which literature is not yet available.

Rimmer (1999) argued nutrition is a major component of the future of health promotion for people with disabilities but did not specify a particular health profession for imparting this information. Certainly team members can reinforce each other's teachings, but as always it is important to consider scope of practice and personal competence and expertise. In addition to obvious referrals (e.g., referring the patient/client who is medically unstable to a physician), it is critical to refer to other types of providers including, but not limited to, dietitians, social workers, psychologists, and nurses and advanced practice nurses (e.g., nurse practitioners, clinical nurse specialists).

Health promotion for people with disabilities is an enormous and developing topic, and many health-care professions can contribute and are contributing not only to optimal clinical care but also to wellness for this population. Therapists are part of this effort and have the expertise to expand their traditional roles in health care. Health promotion is becoming a critical component of health care as the nation is faced with the crushing social and economic burdens of lifestyle-related diseases. In *Crossing the Quality Chasm: A New Health System for the 21st Century* (Institute of Medicine, 2001, pp. 1, X), the Institute of Medicine notes:

> *Between the health care we have and the care we could have lies not just a gap, but a chasm . . . Patients, health care professionals, and policy makers are becoming all too painfully aware of the shortcomings of our current care delivery systems and the importance of finding better approaches to meeting the health care needs of all Americans. It will not be an easy road, but it will be most worthwhile.*

In helping to answer this call from the Institute of Medicine, therapists should aim for optimal health and wellness in all patients with neurological conditions for all ages across the lifespan. In many instances, this aim is easily incorporated into routine clinical practice. For example, therapists can promote adherence to HEPs by making them functional and important to the patient/client. Therapists can then take an important next step by addressing other health factors (e.g., smoking cessation for patients/clients who smoke, encouraging helmet use by patients/clients who bike for exercise, encouraging reduced sun exposure for patients/clients who live in hot, sunny climates) within their scope of practice, making referrals to other providers as appropriate. These conversations can be integrated into routine patient/client interaction throughout the episode of care and represent an important opportunity for therapists to participate in health promotion within the existing health-care paradigm. At discharge, the therapist can go the extra mile to transition the patient/client to an accessible community fitness center for ongoing physical activity for general health, rather than simply discharging the patient/client on a HEP that merely addresses one distinct health issue.

Therapists are in an ideal position in the health-care system to help patient/clients change their health behaviors. They should consider factors related to the diagnosis as well as general health status and general safety of the individual as he or she interacts with the environment and makes choices leading to his or her unique health behavior. All therapists must see themselves as change agents—professionals who motivate the patient/client toward optimal behavior change—while understanding the theories of adherence and health behavior within the context of the specific stage of change or level of planned behavior detected in the individual patient.

To this end, the chapter will help provide a framework for such interventions including screening, recognition of the need for health promotion and wellness intervention, and specific tips and guidelines for all ages that can be shared with patients/clients to optimize their health. Society as a whole, in addition to the individuals to whom we provide therapy, will benefit from the intentional focus on health and wellness, over and above the tertiary prevention, traditional therapeutic intervention attempting to remediate the primary results of the neurological pathology. As our dynamic health-care system continues to change, therapists can contribute to, support, and help shape the movement toward the wellness model of health care.

## PATIENT APPLICATION

### Mr. C

*Mr. C is a 47 year-old right-handed male who is approximately 1 month postischemic stroke in the distribution of the left middle cerebral artery with right hemiparesis. He is referred for outpatient occupational therapy, physical therapy, and speech therapy after discharge home with his wife from an inpatient rehabilitation setting. His past medical history includes hyperlipidemia, HTN, and a family history of sudden cardiac death affecting both his father and an older brother. This was his first-ever stroke.*

*Mr. and Mrs. C live in a one-story house with one step without a handrail to enter. They have three adult children who live in the area. Before Mr. C's stroke, they operated a small woodworking business. Mr. C did not engage in regular physical activity but enjoyed recreational hunting and fishing. He did not smoke or use tobacco products; however he had poor dietary habits, consuming a high-calorie high-fat diet as*

*reported by his wife, who expresses concern about the possibility Mr. C may gain weight now that his mobility is impaired.*

*Mr. C presents with significant right hemiparesis, especially of the upper extremity, which is nearly flaccid. He ambulates for short (e.g., household) distances with a hemiwalker and uses a wheelchair for community mobility. His impairments include significant expressive aphasia, but he understands and is able to follow verbal instructions. His medications include multiple antihypertensives, a statin, and an anticoagulant.*

### Contemplate Clinical Decisions

1. What should the therapist do to plan and implement a health promotion and wellness program to promote general health for Mr. C?
2. What aspects of health promotion would you implement regarding his physical activity?
   Discussion of these issues can be found in the online supplemental material.

## Acknowledgments

The authors gratefully acknowledge Meghan Miyamoto, PT, DPT, GCS, CEEAA, for her review of the manuscript.

Portions of this chapter originally appeared in an earlier form in "Health Promotion in Geriatric Physical Therapy: Applying Theoretical Foundations to Clinical Practice," an online course by the primary author for the Texas Physical Therapy Association, and are used here with permission.

## Disclaimer

This chapter includes discussion of and information on matters of law contained in statute, rule, and policy; however, it is not and should not be construed as legal advice. This discussion is for limited educational and informational purposes only. Specific facts and the application of other laws may affect the application of the laws discussed. For application of any law to any particular set of facts, you should not rely solely on this general information but should instead seek the legal advice of qualified counsel.

# Assistive Technology in Intervention: Focus on Wheelchairs, Assistive Devices, and Orthoses

Karen Y. Lunnen, PT, EdD, ▪ Renee G. Loftspring, PT, EdD

CHAPTER 17

## CHAPTER OUTLINE

## CHAPTER OBJECTIVES

Upon completion of this chapter, the learner will be able to:

1. Define "assistive device" in conceptual terms.
2. Describe federal legislation that supports access to assistive technology for individuals with disabilities.
3. Identify factors that would affect a decision about the acquisition of assistive technology in a given case scenario.
4. Provide a rationale for incorporating supported standing in the intervention plan for nonambulatory individuals.
5. Determine wheelchair (or other seating) specifications for a given case scenario.
6. Justify use of various types of assistive gait devices for particular conditions based on evidence.
7. Provide a rationale for the use of various common orthotic devices in patients of all ages with neuromuscular conditions.
8. Outline the essential components of a letter of medical necessity for assistive technology.

## ▪ Introduction

Assistive technology devices, carefully selected and used, can dramatically improve the functional status of individuals with disabilities. The Americans with Disabilities Act (ADA), Public Law (PL) 110-325, describes an individual with a disability as someone whose "important life activities are restricted as to the conditions, manner, or duration under which they can be performed in comparison to most people" (U.S. Department of Justice, 2008, Section 12102). Consistent with the broad ADA definition, the overall purpose of assistive devices is more than just enhancing physical capability. "Assistive technology should help people achieve self-determined goals and be included in all aspects of community life" (Scherer, 2002, p. 11). Assistive technology bridges the gap between impairments of body structure and function and environmental factors to allow participation in all areas of life consistent within the International Classification of Functioning, Disability, and Health (ICF) framework (World Health Organization, 2001).

The ADA was enacted in 1990 and had broad implications. However, relatively few data were available about the population of individuals with disabilities. In a major interagency initiative, the federal government conducted a two-phase data collection plan with a series of questionnaires in 1994 and 1995. The purpose of the National Health Interview Survey on Disability (NHIS-D) was "to understand disability, to develop public health policy, to produce simple prevalence estimates of selected health conditions, and to provide descriptive baseline statistics on the effects of disabilities" (Russell, 1994). The NHIS-D has not been repeated in its entirety, although a number of survey questions have been incorporated into the annual NHIS conducted by the National Center for Health Statistics (NCHS), which is part of the Centers for Disease Control and Prevention (CDC) (Ward, 2016). Specific information on the use of assistive technology has not been included.

NHIS-D results revealed that 15% of adults had great difficulty with at least one of nine functional physical activities performed without help and without use of special equipment. The functional activities included walking a quarter of a mile; climbing 10 steps without resting; standing for 2 hours; sitting for 2 hours; stooping, bending, or kneeling; reaching over the head; using the fingers to grasp or handle small objects; lifting or carrying 10 pounds; and pushing or pulling large objects (NHIS-D, 1994). The federal government has continued tracking data on disabilities, although on a more limited scale.

An estimated 75% to 90% of older community-dwelling adults use some form of assistive technology (Wolff, 2005). More people (7.4 million) use assistive technology devices to compensate for mobility impairments than for any other general type of impairment. Of those, 4.8 million use canes (single most-used device), 1.8 million use walkers, and 1.6 million use wheelchairs. The use of assistive technology devices has increased more dramatically than would be predicted by changes in population demographics (Russell, 1994). As a comparison, 6.6% of individuals aged 65 or older needed help with personal care in 1997 versus 7.2% in 2015 based on a preliminary report released by the CDC (2016).

The National Medical Expenditure Survey (LaPlante, 1992a) looked more specifically at the nature of limitations in basic life activities, which the authors categorized as (1) walking, (2) self-care (bathing, dressing, toileting, transfers, feeding oneself, and getting about the home), and (3) community and home management (household chores, handling money,

shopping, and getting about the community). Not surprisingly, the incidence of reported difficulty in basic life activities rose dramatically with each succeeding age group: 11.8% among those 65 to 74 years of age; 26.5% among those 75 to 84 years of age; and 57.6% among those 85 years and older. Activities that seemed to be most difficult were getting about the community, doing light housework, shopping, bathing, and walking. About three in four individuals with difficulty get help from others. About 5.3 million people with difficulty use special equipment, "most often walkers, canes and crutches, grab-bars and railings, a seat in the shower or tub, and wheelchairs" (LaPlante, 1992b, p. 3).

The Survey of Income and Program Participation administered by the Census Bureau estimates that 3.7 million adults aged 15 years and older have difficulty performing one or more activities of daily living (ADLs; e.g., bathing, dressing, eating, using the toilet, and transferring), and more than half of those require assistance from another person (Kennedy, 1997).

Approximately 16% of Medicare recipients are under the age of 65 and qualified because they were totally and permanently disabled. Younger Medicare beneficiaries with disabilities are more likely than the elderly to live in poverty, to be in poor health, and to experience difficulties living independently and performing basic daily tasks (Kaiser Family Foundation, 2016). Among all Medicare beneficiaries, 34% have functional impairments with limitations in one or more ADLs, and 50% have annual incomes below $23,500. Millions of people report difficulty with daily functional activities, as detailed in Table 17-1.

Assistive technology devices and services can lessen the effect of a disability on the functional abilities of millions of people. Because of the potential impact for millions of individuals with disabilities, assistive technology has received much attention from (1) the federal government in the form of legislation; (2) a wide variety of regulatory and support organizations; (3) companies that design, produce, and market assistive technology devices; (4) vendors; (5) third-party payers; and (6) health professionals.

| TABLE 17-1 | Statistics on Number of Individuals Who Reported Difficulty With Daily Functional Activities (Kraus, 1996). |
|---|---|
| **NUMBER OF INDIVIDUALS** | **DAILY FUNCTIONAL ACTIVITIES REPORTED AS DIFFICULT** |
| 17.5 million | Going up a flight of stairs without resting |
| 17.3 million | Walking a quarter mile |
| 16.2 million | Lifting or carrying something as heavy as a bag of groceries |
| 10.9 million | Hearing what is said in normal conversation |
| 9.7 million | Seeing words or letters in ordinary newsprint, even when wearing glasses or contact lenses |
| 7.8 million | Getting around outside the home |
| 5.3 million | Getting into and out of bed |
| 3.7 million | Getting around inside the home |
| 2.3 million | Having one's own speech understood |

This chapter provides an overview of assistive technology and its use across the lifespan. Proficiency in the selection, fit, and use of assistive technology is difficult to achieve. New products are continually introduced, and the policies for funding are complex and change frequently. Often evidence providing clear guidelines for decision-making is lacking. The authors' goal is to keep the content at entry level, providing a foundation of knowledge so that new practitioners can build their level of proficiency with clinical experience, mentoring, and further study. Examples of various categories of assistive technology are included in the chapter but only touch on the broad array of choices available. Assistive technology devices more specific to particular types of neurological conditions or particular functional goals are included in other chapters.

## Overview of Assistive Technology

The purpose of assistive technology is to help an individual function more effectively, efficiently, and/or safely as well as participate more fully in life roles. Appropriately used, assistive technology can inhibit increased muscle tone, inhibit abnormal movement, reduce asymmetry, improve circulation, improve bone health, improve upper extremity functioning, prevent soft tissue contractures, prevent decubiti, and enhance comfort. Assistive technology can facilitate caregiving, perhaps protecting a caregiver from a back injury or allowing the patient sufficient independence to reduce the caregiver's assistance.

Options vary from simple, commonly available, less-expensive items to technologically sophisticated and complex devices or systems. An example of a simple item is a pack of diapers used as a small "bench" seat for an infant who sits with a rounded back on the floor, perhaps because of tight hamstrings. An example of a more sophisticated device might be an elaborate environmental control system for an adult with limited function secondary to a high spinal cord injury. The impairment(s) causing the limitation in function may be temporary or permanent, and knowledge of the natural progression of the underlying condition is critical in the selection of a device. For example, a patient who has recently had a stroke and has unilateral footdrop may need immediate support to protect the foot and prevent contracture. An "off-the-shelf" orthosis may be most appropriate for immediate protection of the ankle joint in the short term, until there is a clearer picture of the amount of return the patient will gain. If this same patient is still having footdrop 2 months later, limiting an efficient, safe, gait pattern, perhaps a custom-fabricated orthosis, although expensive, is a worthwhile long-term investment.

Use of assistive technology may benefit one area of function but limit the development of long-term independent function or inhibit function in another area. A tilt-in-space, custom-designed positioning and seating system for an adult with progressive multiple sclerosis may optimize symmetrical posture for eating and tasks requiring proximal stability but limit voluntary efforts to maintain trunk control and limit access because of its size. A child may benefit from ankle-foot orthoses (AFOs) to provide stability for supported standing,

minimize the influence of hypertonic plantar flexors on gait, and prevent contractures, but the orthoses may impede creeping, an important means of independent mobility and an opportunity for improving motor control throughout the body. Therefore, it is important to determine a schedule for using assistive technology that optimizes its benefits without impeding other areas. In addition, patients and caregivers must be educated to understand the importance of such schedules. An inability to comply with a recommended schedule for whatever reason may affect the selection of equipment.

## THINK ABOUT IT 17.1

Federal legislation related to assistive technology has been referred to as civil rights legislation for people with disabilities. Why?

It is crucial that the selection of assistive technology is individualized and the patient's environment, resources, and goals are considered. As an example, the selection of an appropriate seating device for a child with disabilities must take into account the environment the child functions in and the ability and commitment of caregivers to manage the chair. When a child with spastic quadriplegia (cerebral palsy) lives in a spacious, accessible home with parents who have the resources to purchase a van, a highly customized motorized wheelchair may be optimal. The same child living in a small trailer with two active older siblings and a single mother with limited resources may not be able to use a motorized wheelchair safely and effectively in the home environment or transport the chair for community use. However the chair may be appropriate when the student is transported by a school bus and for use in a school setting.

Change must be anticipated in the selection of assistive technology. A positioning and seating system selected for a young child should have multiple adjustments so that it will "grow" with the child. A wheelchair and its positioning and seating system for an adult patient with multiple sclerosis or other neurodegenerative disorder must also have the potential to change as the patient's needs change, such as adding external supports to accommodate anticipated deterioration of strength and motor control. When the device is just a short-term assist for development of a specific skill, it might be advisable to borrow a piece of equipment or find a low-cost alternative. For instance, children with Down syndrome are often reluctant walkers and will walk sooner with a push toy than with a hand being held (Winders, 1997). Instead of using a traditional walker for extra support, they may benefit from a less-expensive, commercially available toy vacuum cleaner or shopping cart they can push.

An estimated 2.5 million people who could benefit from assistive technology cannot attain the necessary funding (LaPlante, 1992b), making cost another major consideration in purchase decisions. For example, when a supported standing device is purchased for classroom use, a highly adjustable multipurpose device might be optimal even though it is more expensive because it can be used long term with many different children. The same device might be much too costly and bulky as an alternative for a young adult who has finished growing and for whom the specific design features have been determined.

When possible, the patient should try out assistive technology so the therapist can weigh all options before finalizing recommendations for acquisition and purchase. Regardless of the amount of knowledge and experience a therapist has, it is not always possible to predict how a patient will respond to a particular device. It often takes time for a patient to adjust to something new and to understand the long-term benefit. For example, a seating system with multiple supports may initially increase spasticity and decrease function in a patient who has had a stroke. A patient may require considerable practice to maneuver a newly acquired power wheelchair with a specialized controller. Another patient may not have the cognitive ability to master a similar device regardless of the opportunities for practice.

Safety is always a consideration in the selection, use, and fit of assistive technology. Patients and/or caregivers need explicit written instructions, demonstration, and supervised practice in safely using more complex devices. It may be helpful to provide diagrams, take photographs, label parts, or color-code straps. Precautions should be carefully reviewed and may include recognizing symptoms of fatigue, inspecting for pressure areas, or practicing strategies for quickly releasing supports in the event of a seizure. Safety for the caregiver is also an important consideration so he/she does not sustain injury supporting a patient in the use of assistive technology (e.g., transferring a patient from a wheelchair to a device for supported standing).

Perhaps more difficult to ascertain but also important to consider are psychosocial issues. A well-selected assistive device often allows a patient to be more independent, to participate more actively, to feel less isolated, and to have more self-confidence. However, assistive technology can also be perceived as drawing attention to a patient's disability or as separating the patient from others socially, psychologically, and physically. Parents may opt to carry a young child with spina bifida rather than allow the child independent mobility in a wheelchair because of the perceived stigma. Even something as simple but as meaningful as a hug or a handshake can be more difficult when a patient is strapped into a wheelchair or dependent on a walker for balance.

## ■ Federal Legislation

In 1988 Congress passed PL 100-407, The Technology-Related Assistance for Individuals Act (Tech Act). The Tech Act mandated that states address policies, practices, and structures to promote access to appropriate assistive technology. The Tech Act was reauthorized in 1994, in 1998, and again in 2004 as PL 108-364, the Assistive Technology Act of 2004. The Tech Act (2004) is prefaced with the following statement: "Over 54,000,000 individuals in the United States have disabilities, with almost half experiencing severe disabilities that affect their ability to see, hear, communicate, reason,

walk, or perform other basic life functions. Disability is a natural part of the human experience and in no way diminishes the right of individuals to: (a) live independently; (b) enjoy self-determination and make choices; (c) benefit from an education; (d) pursue meaningful careers; and (e) enjoy full inclusion and integration in the economic, political, social, cultural, and education mainstream of society in the United States" (U.S. Congress, 2004). In its scope and advocacy, the Tech Act is really a civil rights act with assistive technology, a critical element in helping individuals with disabilities achieve these basic civil rights.

"Every piece of federal legislation enacted since 1988 regarding people with disabilities has explicitly referred to assistive technology devices and services" (Scherer, 2002, p. 5). PL 108-446, the Individuals with Disabilities Education Improvement Act of 2004 (IDEA), includes language similar to that in the Tech Act, ensuring that students in public education programs are provided with the assistive technology services and devices needed to function in the educational environment. The ADA ensures "reasonable accommodation" to people with disabilities to allow them to participate (U.S. Department of Justice, 2004). Often the accommodation is assistive technology that optimizes an individual's ability to function.

A number of important terms are defined in the Tech Act (2004):

a. **Assistive technology device:** ". . . any item, piece of equipment, or product system, whether acquired commercially off the shelf, modified, or customized, that is used to increase, maintain, or improve functional capabilities of individuals with disabilities." Assistive technology devices include communication devices, adaptive equipment (e.g., standers, wheelchairs), environmental control devices, adapted computers, and specialized software (H.R. 4278 Assistive Technology Act of 2004, Section 3.4)

b. **Assistive technology service:** ". . . any service that directly assists an individual with a disability in the selection, acquisition, or use of an assistive technology device" (H.R. 4278 Assistive Technology Act of 2004, Section 3.4)

Many challenges are inherent in implementing federal legislation of such broad scope. The Tech Act mandated that states address policies, practices, and structures to promote access to appropriate assistive technology. Considerable variation occurs from state to state. It is optimal (but challenging) to make services accessible, to allow individuals and families to see a variety of assistive devices, and ideally, to borrow devices to try before purchasing. Patients and caregivers often need training and ongoing support in the use of assistive technology that is also difficult for states to provide. Although IDEA mandated that states provide assistive technology devices and services, the federal government never fully funded the act, leaving significant financial burden on the states. Another challenge is that clear, objective, scientific evidence is lacking to support clinical decision-making and justify funding.

## THINK ABOUT IT 17.2

Procuring the "right" assistive technology for a patient can be a challenging process. Who are the various members of an assistive technology team, and what other resources are available to assist with the process?

In a Harris Poll conducted in 2004, respondents who identified themselves as having a disability and using at least one type of technology were asked "If you were not able to use the special equipment or assistive devices that you mentioned anymore for some reason, how would this affect your daily activities?" Thirty-five percent indicated "I would not be able to live independently or take care of myself at home." People with disabilities were asked "Is there any special equipment or type of assistive device that you currently need, but do not have?" Seventeen percent replied yes. Of those, 11% replied that they did not know where to get the equipment, and 54% replied that they could not afford it.

Day (1996) developed an interview-based tool to measure the psychosocial impact of assistive devices (PIADs) that includes 26 items in three subcategories: competence, adaptability, and self-esteem. The tool can predict whether individuals will effectively utilize assistive technology or abandon it. The tool was used in a study of 96 community-dwelling adults using mobility assistive devices (Martins, 2016). Results demonstrated generally positive impacts from assistive technology, with average subscale scores of 1.11 for competence, 1.10 for adaptability, and 0.62 for self-esteem (based on zero being no impact, 3 being maximum positive impact, and −3 being maximum negative impact). Powered wheelchairs received the highest scores, and walkers the lowest. Carver (2016) reported overall satisfaction with the extent to which mobility assistive devices supported participation for individuals with spinal cord injury and urged rehabilitation professionals to consider independence, safety, and efficiency when recommending assistive technology.

Minor and Robinson (2004) investigated barriers that prevent individuals with disabilities from benefiting from assistive technology. The authors surveyed more than 350 physiatrists and biomedical engineers and concluded that there are four key barriers: (1) continued funding challenges, (2) a lack of public awareness about potentially beneficial assistive technology, (3) a shortage of trained experts, and (4) poor collaboration among researchers, clinicians, and consumers. Kaye (2008) analyzed survey data from adult consumers of California Independent Living Centers to determine which factors limited access and use of assistive technology in this segment of the population. These factors included "lower educational attainment, racial or ethnic minority status, lower household income, later disability onset, and disability related to mental as opposed to physical or sensory functioning" (p. 194). For children with disabilities in the educational environment, barriers include lack of appropriate staff training and support, negative staff attitudes, inadequate assessment and planning processes, insufficient funding, difficulties procuring and managing equipment, and time constraints (Copley, 2004).

Environmental barriers also continue to be significant deterrents to independence. Generally improved community accessibility would decrease reliance on the use of assistive technology in many instances (Layton, 2012).

## ■ Assistive Technology Team

A team of professionals who can recognize the benefits of assistive technology for an individual, select the appropriate device(s), acquire funding, provide education, and assess outcomes is crucial. The federal mandate to provide assistive technology challenged various levels of the system regarding acquiring assistive technology and the qualifications of the professionals involved. The Rehabilitation Engineering and Assistive Technology Society of North America (RESNA) was incorporated as a 501(c)(3) organization in 1980 to support individuals with a common interest in technology and disability. Soon after incorporation, RESNA received millions of dollars in federal funding to support compliance with the Assistive Technology Act by state-level programs. RESNA has played a major role in research and development and education and advocacy. The society also took the lead in establishing standards for the qualifications and knowledge of professionals in the field of assistive technology to ensure the safe and effective provision of services and offers two national certifications (RESNA, 2015). Details can be found on the society's webpage: www.resna.org.

**Assistive Technology Professional (ATP)**—a service provider who analyzes the needs of individuals with disabilities, assists in the selection of appropriate equipment, and trains the consumer on how to properly use the equipment. Certification requires passing an examination and paying a fee.

**Seating and Mobility Specialist (SMS)**—advanced certification for those who already have ATP certification.

The concept of a certified ATP was initiated in 1996; however, ATP certification was not mandatory for nonprofessionals involved in the evaluation of a client seeking wheeled mobility, such as equipment suppliers or vendors of **durable medical equipment (DME)**, until 2008. Physical therapists, occupational therapists, and speech and language pathologists are exempt from the mandate for certification because their professional curricula include pertinent information and they are already licensed to practice. In many states, the criteria for funding assistive technology stipulate the level of professional who must be involved in various types of assistive technology decisions.

A physical therapist, occupational therapist, and/or speech and language pathologist typically takes the lead in clinical decision-making for more complex assistive technology needs (e.g., wheelchairs, orthoses, or augmentative communication devices); however, a qualified vendor should be involved as well. The therapist and/or vendor should make specific recommendations with accompanying explanations for each item only after completing a thorough evaluation and consulting with the primary funding source. Documentation, termed a **letter of medical necessity (LMN)**, details the clinical justification specific to the patient and each component being requested (e.g., armrests, leg rests, or wheels) and provides the clinical justification for funding by insurance companies or other payers. Final decisions are the right and responsibility of the patient and/or caregiver.

Knowledge in the field of assistive technology has become increasingly important with the federal mandates in the Tech Act and the inclusion of assistive technology mandates in IDEA. However, entry-level preparation is variable. Brady (2007) conducted a survey of professional education programs in the fields of occupational therapy, physical therapy, special education, and speech and language pathology. Although the survey response rate was low (15.9%), the authors reported that almost all of the programs covered assistive technology in their curricula and that respondents were generally satisfied with the amount of time devoted to the content. However, the authors concluded that "to promote contemporary practice . . ., entry-level curricula should be designed to creatively expand and enhance instruction in this growing service area" (p. 191).

Long (2008) surveyed members of the Section on Pediatrics of the American Physical Therapy Association (380 respondents) to determine the perceived adequacy of education in assistive technology, confidence levels in providing assistive technology services, and educational preferences/needs. The majority of therapists (77%) reported no training or inadequate training in legislation, regulation, and policy related to assistive technology services and lacked confidence in "assessing an individual for assistive technology services, matching or selecting a device to meet a client's needs, and evaluating the outcome of use of assistive technology services" (p. 634).

# Specific Assistive Technology and Equipment

## Orthotic Devices

### General Purpose of Orthotic Devices

An **orthosis** is "an externally applied device used to modify the structural and functional characteristics of the neuromuscular and skeletal systems" (International Society for Prosthetics and Orthotics, 2012). The term **brace** is a synonym; the term **splint** typically refers to an orthosis intended for temporary use. Depending on its design, an orthosis can serve many purposes for patients with neuromuscular disorders:

- Improving alignment
- Increasing stability at a joint or segment
- Facilitating weak muscles; inhibiting spastic muscles
- Limiting or facilitating motion
- Providing proprioceptive feedback
- Simulating an eccentric or concentric muscle contraction
- Preventing contracture or deformity (e.g., anticipating deformity on the basis of condition, maintaining

corrected position after surgery or casting, or correcting mild deformities)
- Positioning a body part for optimum function

### Design and Function of Orthotic Devices

Orthoses can be custom fabricated, custom-built from prefabricated orthoses, or purchased "off the shelf" in various sizes. Custom designs typically begin with casting the patient's extremity/body part while maintaining optimal alignment. Once dry, the cast is bivalved and removed from the patient. The orthotist then makes a positive mold of the patient's extremity/body part by filling the formed cast material with plaster.

Companies that specialize in orthotic fabrication can be valuable resources. For example, providers such as Cascade (www.cascadedafo.com) offer a "Fast Fit" alternative—especially for young children—that does not require casting. The clinician (often a physical therapist) measures the width and length of the child's foot on a sizing jig, and Cascade provides an orthosis based on these measurements. Cascade will also fabricate a custom orthosis from a molded cast impression. Many of these companies are committed to providing education in a variety of formats to improve the decision-making skills of the therapist and the quality of the measurements and mold.

Generally, the thicker the material used in an orthosis, the stiffer the product and the greater the stability and support provided. Thicker materials, however, can limit desirable movement, making the design less dynamic and creating problems with skin breakdown. Thermoplastic materials of varying thickness are most commonly used and are replacing older metal and leather devices. Additional cushioning and shock absorption may be required when using thermoplastic materials with patients who have diabetes or other conditions that increase risk for skin breakdown. Carbon graphite/acrylic resins are also used and have the advantage of being stronger than thermoplastic materials; however, modification is limited once the orthoses have been manufactured and they can be damaged by abrasion.

The cost and the time required to obtain an orthosis vary depending on the complexity of the design, the extent of customization, and the need for approval by third-party payers. Custom designs are typically fabricated by orthotists with specialized education in biomechanics and medical sciences as well as technical training. The American Academy of Orthotists and Prosthetists (www.oandp.org) has established an accreditation process and minimum educational standards as well as a certification process (with national examinations) to better ensure competency, although education and licensing requirements vary widely from state to state.

Straps secure an orthosis and are often an integral part of the design that varies with the material used, tension applied, width, and placement. It is crucial that the patient and/or caregivers are instructed in the correct application of the orthosis and strapping. Linings of various compositions (e.g., cushioned heel support) can increase the comfort and facilitate the dynamic properties of the brace. Smaller pads may be used over bony prominences to improve comfort and prevent skin breakdown. Typically, space for the pads is "built in" to the custom design of the brace. The clinician should not add pads to a tightly fitting brace in an effort to decrease pressure. Regardless of the material used, padding only increases pressure.

Orthoses for the lower extremity are always worn with socks and shoes. Socks should fit well (with no wrinkles or excess fabric that could cause pressure areas), completely cover the skin surface under the brace, and be made of a material that wicks perspiration away from the skin. Shoe selection is an important consideration because the shoe is often an integral part of the brace design and fit. Shoes must be sized to accommodate the extra bulk of the brace while not interfering with function. They should be constructed well and have a removable insole and appropriate heel height. When shoes are chosen, some special features should be avoided or must be carefully considered in the brace design so that the shoe complements the function of the brace.

An important consideration in orthosis selection is a realistic assessment of the patient and/or caregiver's willingness and ability to tolerate the "hassle factor" and actually use the device safely and appropriately. For example, when a child lives in a hot climate without air conditioning and is accustomed to going barefoot or wearing sandals, no amount of improved function will be enough to motivate wearing of a plastic brace with socks and shoes. Similarly, one must assess the motivation of an adult with a myelomeningocele to walk before spending thousands of dollars on a reciprocating gait orthosis that will require considerable effort to don and doff and may impede wheelchair function.

Typically, the patient needs to adapt to wearing the orthosis(es), which requires starting with short periods in the orthosis and gradually increasing the wearing time with close monitoring. The patient and/or caregiver must be educated about warning signs that the orthosis is not fitting properly and should check the skin frequently for areas of redness. Some redness of the skin is normal, but it should disappear within a relatively short period (Sanders, 1995).

The decision to recommend a particular type of orthosis(es) for a patient should be made with careful consideration and analysis by a team of professionals. Physical or occupational therapists are often involved in the selection, fit, and use of orthoses and, with advanced training and experience, may fabricate low-temperature molded devices from plastic materials such as Orthoplast or Aquaplast (Cusick, 1988). The physical or occupational therapist is often most involved with the functional goals for the patient and most aware of the progression of the patient's condition.

An orthosis should be the least complicated design that meets the patient's needs, recognizing that change may be needed over time. Depending on the diagnosis and prognosis, time out of the orthosis may be important so the patient has opportunities to use and strengthen weak muscle groups and not become dependent on the device. Many times, an orthosis facilitates one functional activity but limits another. For example, a patient with high lumbar level paraplegia may be ambulatory with reciprocating gait orthoses but find them

cumbersome and uncomfortable for sitting. A child may have improved lower extremity alignment for supported standing when wearing solid AFOs but find it difficult to move from sit-to-stand, squat for play, or creep on hands and knees with the devices on. The physical or occupational therapist often establishes the wearing schedule that optimizes use of the orthosis(es) to meet long-term functional goals.

The cost of custom-designed orthoses can be prohibitive. They are categorized as DME and typically require a physician prescription and extensive justification for insurance coverage. Cost is one factor in the decision-making process and may be particularly important when the device(s) will most likely be used short term or the patient will change (e.g., physical growth in a toddler or disease progression in a patient with a neurodegenerative disorder). If possible, patients will benefit from trial use of an orthosis before committing to a custom design.

### Lower Extremity Orthotic Devices

Most orthoses for the lower extremity offer varying levels of support for the foot and ankle to provide subtalar neutral alignment. This support can range from a simple double-layer, foam shoe insert, sometimes called a *foot orthosis* (first figure in Table 17-2), to progressively more medial and lateral support, ending with a supramalleolar orthosis (SMO) that captures both malleoli in the splint material (proximal strap optional) and often encases the midfoot (second figure in Table 17-2). An SMO is typically used for a child with severe pronation or supination, for example, a child with Down syndrome (Cooper, 2006; Martin, 2004). It is seldom used for adults because the height is inadequate to stabilize the longer lever arm of the adult tibia.

AFOs have a "sole" on the dorsum of the foot and varying levels of medial/lateral midfoot control. The orthosis then typically extends on the posterior aspect of the lower limb to just below the popliteal crease, approximately 10 to 15 mm distal to the head of the fibula (Knutson, 1991). The trim lines on the sole can be just distal to the toes or made of a thinner, more flexible material to allow a normal third rocker in the gait cycle (i.e., extension of the metatarsal phalangeal joints . . . which occurs during toe-off).

Increasing the thickness of the plastic and extending the coverage, as in a solid AFO, provides a very stable design but one that lacks movement and flexibility (third figure in Table 17-2). A solid AFO is typically used for patients who require ankle stability for supported standing or to maintain range of motion (ROM) but is not typically used for patients who are ambulatory. A posterior leaf spring AFO (fourth figure in Table 17-2) is made of thin, flexible plastic with trim lines posterior to the malleoli (adding to its flexibility). It allows dorsiflexion and plantar flexion, but both motions have a counteracting control moment (Brehm, 2008). The posterior leaf spring has been used to improve gait and function in a wide variety of patients with cerebral palsy (Brehm, 2008; Buckon, 2001) and in patients who have experienced a stroke (Karas, 2002; Malas, 2001). "Off-the-shelf" AFOs are usually posterior leaf spring or solid ankle designs.

**TABLE 17-2   Summary of Various Orthoses: Purpose and Construction**

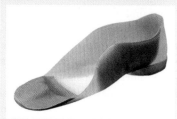

**Full contact orthosis**
Excessive pronation, metatarsus adductus

Custom-molded heel and arch; usually fairly rigid material that ends below malleoli; usually trimmed behind toes; stabilizes foot/ankle in sagittal and transverse planes

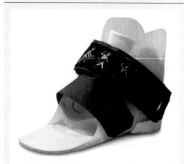

**Supramalleolar orthosis (SMO)**
Severe pronation or supination

Trimmed above malleoli; often made of flexible material; held in place with shoe

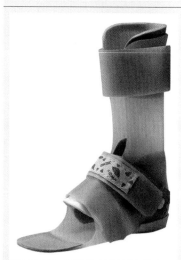

**Solid Ankle-Foot Orthosis (AFO)**
Severe hypertonia or alignment issues requiring maximum stability; maintains foot position in nonambulatory patient

Provides good support but limited mobility; recommended for nonambulatory patients; encourages knee flexion moment at initial contact to midstance; resists excessive knee flexion and ankle dorsiflexion (DF); provides medial/lateral (M/L) stability of ankle/foot

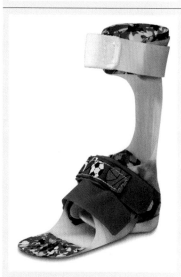

**Posterior leaf spring AFO**
Drop foot with minimal M/L instability; crouch gait; genu recurvatum

Allows DF and plantar flexion (PF) but provides a counter moment to both; flexible material trimmed anterior to malleoli with foot plate that provides M/L foot/ankle stability

| **TABLE 17-2** | **Summary of Various Orthoses: Purpose and Construction—cont'd** |
|---|---|

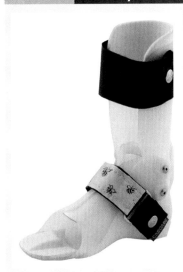

*Articulating AFO with DF assist*
Mild drop foot with M/L instability

Simulated eccentric contraction of pretibial muscle to prevent foot slap; provides good M/L stability of foot/ankle; allows DF during stance; facilitates DF during swing

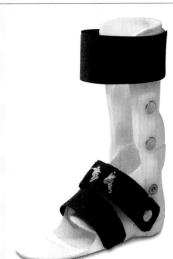

*Articulating AFO with PF stop*
Toe walking; mild to moderate genu recurvatum; moderate to severe M/L instability of foot/ankle

Allows DF and advancement of contralateral limb; provides transverse and M/L stability of foot/ankle; encourages knee flexion moment at initial contact through midstance

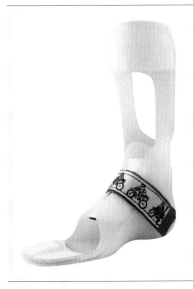

*Floor reaction AFO*
Weak quadriceps muscles without M/L knee instability; overlengthened heel cords; lower-level paraplegia associated with crouch gait

Encourages knee extension moment to prevent knee forward buckling; provides M/L stability of foot/ankle; in swing phase, allows clearance; more difficult going up hills; decreases crouch gait and keeps torso vertical and center of mass in middle of foot

*Continued*

**TABLE 17-2** | **Summary of Various Orthoses: Purpose and Construction—cont'd**

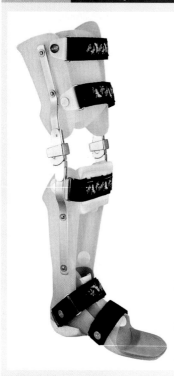

*Knee-ankle-foot orthosis*
Midlevel paraplegia; severe knee hyperextension; M/L instability at knee

AFO section provides M/L stability of foot/ankle, DF control in swing phase, ground reaction forces on knee; knee joint and thigh extension provide M/L knee support; locked knee joints provide maximal sagittal plane support; unlocks for sitting

---

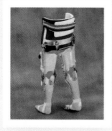

*Hip-knee-ankle-foot orthosis (HKAFO)*
*Reciprocating gait orthosis (RGO)*
Midthoracic to high lumbar paraplegia

HKAFO provides maximum support for lower extremities and lower torso
RGO is HKAFO with cable system that pairs hip flexion in one leg with hip extension in opposite leg, facilitating swing phase of gait

---

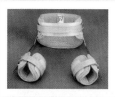

*Standing-walking and sitting hip orthosis (SWASH)*
Low to moderate adductor tone

Pelvic band and thigh cuffs with metal struts that move in elliptical path; prevents scissoring; allows for sitting; stabilizes the hip postoperatively

---

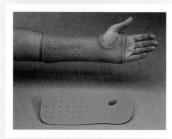

*Wrist cock-up splint*
Moderate to severe increased tone in wrist and finger flexors

Stabilizes wrist to improve function and maintain motion; allows relatively free finger and thumb motion

---

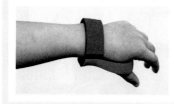

*Thumb abduction splint*
Maintaining thumb abduction with minimal interference for grasp or opportunities for tactile input

Simple construction using colorful 1/8-in.-thick neoprene straps; hook-and-loop closure system; adjustable and washable; less than $20

| **TABLE 17-2** | **Summary of Various Orthoses: Purpose and Construction—cont'd** |
|---|---|

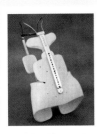

*Spinal orthosis*
Facilitation of erect spine

Custom-molded orthosis using three-point pressure system

Images 1–8 courtesy of Cascade Dafo, Inc. (http://cascadedafo.com); Images 9, 10, and 13 from Dole R, Chafetz R. *Peds Rehab Notes: Evaluation and Intervention Pocket Guide*. Philadelphia, PA: F.A. Davis Company; 2010; Image 11 courtesy of Performance Health (pattersonmedical.com); Image 12 courtesy of The Joe Cool Company (joecoolco.com).

Hinging the ankle joint permits more dynamic movement and smooths the stance phase of gait by allowing the lower limb to translate over the foot (fifth figure in Table 17-2). Allowing free ankle dorsiflexion (as in the preceding example) while preventing ankle plantar flexion can be useful in the patient who toe walks or has genu recurvatum because it encourages a knee flexion moment from the point of initial contact through midstance (sixth figure in Table 17-2). The patient must have adequate strength in the quadriceps to prevent "buckling" of the knee.

A floor reaction AFO wraps around from the medial and lateral sides, joining in an anterior position just below the patella (seventh figure in Table 17-2). Its design encourages a knee extension moment to keep the knee from buckling if the patient's quadriceps are weak or inhibits forward translation of the tibia for a patient with a crouch gait (flexion of ankles, knees, and hips). Walking on hills is very difficult in this design.

A knee-ankle-foot orthosis (KAFO) encompasses the entire lower extremity and is necessary for a patient with midlumbar paraplegia, severe knee hyperextension, or medial lateral knee instability (eighth figure in Table 17-2). The knee joint can be locked in extension for maximum stability and unlocked for sitting. A hip-knee-ankle-foot orthosis (HKAFO) includes a pelvic band and provides maximum support for the lower extremities in all three planes as well as the lower trunk. Both the knee and hip joints are hinged, and both sets of hinges can be locked or unlocked depending on the motor function desired. A reciprocating gait orthosis (RGO) is an HKAFO with an added feature (i.e., a cable system) that encourages hip flexion of the unweighted leg as the stance leg extends, facilitating the swing phase of gait. HKAFOs are typically used to support patients with paraplegia so they can stand and ambulate (ninth figure in Table 17-2).

A standing, walking, and sitting hip (SWASH) orthosis is specially designed for the individual with hypertonia in the hip adductors (10th figure in Table 17-2). It has a pelvic band and waist belt designed to prevent posterior pelvic tilt, two thigh cuffs, and bilateral metal rods connecting the pelvic band and thigh cuffs. The metal rods move in an elliptical path that facilitates abduction of the hips as they extend during the gait cycle. The SWASH orthosis can also be used postoperatively to maintain the hips in an abducted position. Embrey (2006) used surface electromyographic instrumentation to investigate whether the SWASH orthosis increases adductor muscle tone when used by children with spastic cerebral palsy and found no increase in tone during sitting, standing, or walking activities compared with children not wearing the orthosis. Additional evidence is needed, but the biomechanical principles are sound when patients are willing to wear this device.

Serial casting is an alternative for contracture management in a variety of neurological conditions and has effectively increased ROM, decreased resistance to passive stretch in spastic muscles, increased maximal torques, and reduced reflex excitability (Brouwer, 2000). More frequent cast changes (1 to 4 days compared with 5 to 7 days) resulted in comparable increases in ROM and fewer complications in a broad sample of patients with severe cerebral spasticity (Pohl, 2002). Botulinum A injections before serial casting increased ROM compared with serial casting alone in children with spastic cerebral palsy (Booth, 2003). Another option to maintain ROM in patients with neurological disorders is use of cylinder splints (typically at night) or orthoses with a spring-type mechanism that exerts a low, prolonged force over time (Skalsky, 2012).

## Upper Extremity Orthotic Devices

Upper extremity orthoses sized from extra small to extra large are available from numerous vendors at a fraction of the cost of lower extremity orthoses. Custom fabrication is possible for atypical conditions. Upper extremity orthoses are usually designed to minimize spasticity or stabilize the hand and wrist to maximize function. Common problems are a fisted hand (fingers flexed at all three joints) with the thumb strongly adducted into the palm and wrist flexion with or without ulnar deviation.

A wrist cock-up splint (11th figure in Table 17-2) helps stabilize the wrist (typically in some amount of extension) and prevent flexor contractures while still allowing finger movement and function. The splinting material is on the volar surface of the hand and forearm, with Velcro straps keeping it in place. It extends into the palm of the hand but does not interfere with flexion of the metacarpal phalangeal joints. Extending coverage to the fingertips (sometimes termed a *pan splint*) helps maintain the length of the finger flexors but does not allow function.

If thumb adduction muscle tone is severe, a splint can be made with plastic material to hold the thumb in an abducted position. Typically, these materials are bulky and prohibit functional use of the thumb. An innovative design for patients with increased thumb adductor tone is the Joe Cool splint (www.joecoolco.com). It is made of two neoprene straps; one goes around the wrist, and the other goes through the thenar web space with both ends attaching to the wrist strap (12th figure in Table 17-2). The Joe Cool splint encourages thumb abduction and promotes function of the fingers, thumb, and hand. It is comfortable, washable, colorful, and inexpensive—an excellent reminder that sometimes simple is better.

### Orthotic Devices for the Trunk

The efficacy of bracing the trunk to prevent or minimize the progression of spinal deformity (especially scoliosis) is controversial, particularly in patients who have developed spinal curvature secondary to a primary neurological diagnosis. Almost all braces for the trunk use the pelvis as a base of support while applying a three-point pressure system to counter the curve direction (last figure in Table 17-2). For idiopathic adolescent scoliosis (primary diagnosis), brace wear is typically 16 to 20 hours per day until skeletal maturity and then during sleeping hours for 1 to 2 years. Evidence on the effectiveness of bracing for idiopathic scoliosis has been mixed (Lenssinck, 2005; Richards, 2005) but a comprehensive study involving 25 institutions in the United States and Canada (Weinstein, 2013) found that bracing significantly decreased the progression of high-risk curves to the threshold for surgery with longer hours of brace wear resulting in greater benefit.

Many more factors influence decisions about trunk orthoses for patients whose spinal curvature may be just one in a long list of problems. Allowing the curve to progress results in deterioration of function, increased discomfort, and respiratory compromise. In comparison, spinal fusion is a major surgery with variable outcomes (Askin, 1997; Barsdorf, 2010. Olafsson (1999) reviewed 90 patients (24 ambulatory) with various neuromuscular diseases as well as a progressive spine deformity treated with a prefabricated, Boston-type underarm corrective brace. They concluded that the subset of the population who responded to brace treatment were ambulating patients with hypotonia and short thoracolumbar/lumbar curves less than 40 degrees. A lasting effect was not found in other types of curvature. Nevertheless, the bracing did support sitting.

Orthoses are often recommended to improve various gait parameters in patients with neurological conditions. Considerable research has been published on their efficacy. How might you evaluate the evidence to support using a specific type of orthosis with a particular neurological condition or impairment? What are some of the disparities in research studies that create challenges in developing clear-cut recommendations based on existing evidence?

## Assistive Devices for Mobility

### Positioning and Seating Systems/Wheelchairs

Many patients with neuromuscular conditions need specialized seating systems, whether wheelchairs or other types of positioning and seating equipment. Moving efficiently from the goals and functional needs of the patient and/or caregiver to acquiring a system that optimally addresses them in a cost-effective, forward-thinking manner is a complex process. The following section details the steps in this process: (1) determine the need for a wheelchair, (2) examine the patient, (3) select a positioning device and form of pressure relief, (4) determine a funding source(s), (5) document medical necessity, (6) evaluate the patient with the new wheelchair, and (7) reassess and follow up. Although these steps apply to various positioning and seating systems, the following discussion is specific to wheelchairs.

**1.** Determine the need for a wheelchair

A critical first step is to determine the unique seating needs of the patient and/or caregiver(s). This step may involve consultation with other members of the team, guided discussions with the patient/caregiver, and evaluation of the current chair as applicable. An on-site evaluation of the environment(s) where the chair will be used is recommended for all patients and is required for Medicare-eligible patients to ensure that the recommended wheelchair fits through all the doorways in the rooms and entrances the patient will be accessing and that a ramp and/or elevator is in place if necessary. The information gained will guide the remaining steps, especially the patient examination. The following questions may be relevant:

- How long will the patient be seated in the chair each day? What activities will the patient engage in while seated in the chair?
- How will the patient transfer in and out of the chair and how frequently?
- If the patient is unable to sit in the chair for a functional period, what are the reasons?
- Will the chair need to be transported? What type of vehicle (e.g., car, van, bus) is available for transport, and/or does the patient/caregiver have resources to obtain an appropriate vehicle?
- How accessible are the environments where the chair will be used (e.g., home, school, work)?
- What type of terrain will be traversed (e.g., pavement, gravel, carpet, inclines)?
- Will the patient need to pull the chair up to work surfaces (e.g., a desk or dining table)?
- Will the patient propel the chair independently, be pushed, or both?
- What safety concerns are inherent in the use of the chair? Does the patient have seizures? Will the chair be used in environments where its stability may be challenged?

- Is the patient's condition stable, or are symptoms likely to improve or to deteriorate? Is the patient likely to grow (e.g., a young child)?
- Does the patient have oxygen, intravenous therapy, or ventilator support that needs to be accommodated?

Dialogue with caregivers about their goals may reveal a need for convenience or ease getting in and out of a car, maneuverability inside and outside the home, accessibility within the patient's home environment, and direct caregiving tasks such as transfers, positioning, or feeding. In contrast, a patient's goals may relate more to cosmetics, fitting the chair under a table at a restaurant, or sitting tolerance to allow attendance at social events in and around the community or going to a family member's home for the day.

If the patient already has a wheelchair, it is important to identify the vendor, date of acquisition, payer source, and significant repairs required (and date) or recently completed and covered by insurance, as well as the patient's/caregiver's perceptions about what works well with the current seating system and what adaptations might improve function or ease of care. Selecting the "best" vendor for each patient is important and should be based on the vendor's reputation, communication skills, location, expertise, and policies/practices regarding lending equipment and offering long-term support.

**2.** Examine the patient

Components of the patient examination vary across settings, although the processes are similar. Typically, the patient is examined while supine as well as sitting with needed support (in a wheelchair or armchair or on a mat table) to gather objective data regarding muscle tone, skin integrity, posture, ROM, strength, flexibility, coordination, and balance (static and dynamic). Screening the patient's hearing, vision, and cognition is recommended before trials with powered mobility. At the same time, the therapist takes key patient measurements to determine the necessary physical dimensions of the wheelchair. Photographing the patient in his or her current wheelchair (anterior and lateral views) may aid documentation efforts for reimbursement. It is also important to assess the patient's functional abilities with the wheelchair by having him or her demonstrate a variety of tasks. For example, when a standard wheelchair is used, the following questions should be considered:

- Can the patient propel the chair? With which limb(s)? On what surface(s)? How far? At what energy cost?
- Can the patient turn the chair to the right? To the left? Around objects?
- Can the patient manage an elevator, hallway, crowds, tables, kitchen, toilet, sink, etc.? What assistance is required?
- How does the patient transfer in/out of the chair? What assistance is required?
- Does the chair increase the patient's level of independence in ADLs?

When a power wheelchair is used, additional items should be considered:

- How well is the patient able to access/manage the controller?

- Does the patient have the cognitive ability to maneuver safely and effectively?
- Does the patient or caregiver have the ability to care for the wheelchair?
- Is there a safe location for the wheelchair when not being used or when charging?
- Does the patient have a ramp, elevator, van with a lift, and other supports as needed?

Standardized measures may help to justify wheelchair acquisition as well as recommended components or features and should be included in the evaluation as appropriate. Examples include the timed up-and-go test for functional mobility, balance, gait, and safety; oxygen saturation for functional endurance; and dynamometry for grip strength. Standardized measures are covered in other chapters.

Numerous pieces of information can be included in the subjective and objective findings for a wheelchair and seating evaluation and justification. While recognizing that not all data gathered will be immediately useful, it is necessary to write a succinct yet inclusive evaluation.

### Wheelchair and Seating Evaluation and Justification Form

It is critical to decide in advance which aspects of the wheelchair and seating evaluation will be covered in a particular session and in how much detail. It is equally important to document succinctly for insurance purposes that the recommendations are clearly medically necessary for the patient. Many comprehensive forms are available to guide the examination and measurement and to document the findings. The following section summarizes information from the *Wheelchair and Seating Evaluation and Justification* form developed by the former Rehabilitation Institute of Chicago in 2006. The institute has been reorganized and is now known as the Shirley Ryan AbilityLab. The form is available upon request only.

**a.** Patient Information to include: Patient and caregiver goals and limitations that may affect care
**b.** Medical History to include: Relevant diagnosis(es), relevant surgeries, height, weight, cardiopulmonary status, and orthotics
**c.** Home Environment to include: Type of home, presence of caregivers, accessibility
**d.** Community ADLs to include: Type of vehicle and driver as well as specific requirements regarding mobility for employment, school, etc.
**e.** Functional/Sensory Processing Skills to include: Handedness and processing skills related to safe wheelchair operation
**f.** Communication to include: Verbal skills (understandability, type of aphasia, noncommunicative) and use of augmentative device (type, manufacturer/model, mounting required)
**g.** Sensation and Skin Issues to include: Sensation, skin issues/integrity, ability to perform pressure relief, pain
**h.** ADL Status (in reference to wheelchair use) to include: Dressing, eating, grooming/hygiene, meal prep, bowel/bladder management

**i.** Current Seating/Mobility to include:
  1) Mobility base, type (i.e., manufacturer, model, serial number, and year when information is available), and condition
  2) Components (e.g., seat base, cushion, back, lateral trunk supports, thigh/knee/foot support, foot strap, head support, pelvic stabilization, anterior chest/shoulder support, upper extremity support)
  3) Posture in current seating system (spine, pelvis, lower extremities, upper extremities, head)
  4) If powered mobility, mode of control (joystick, mouth stick, chin control, cheek control, head control, sip-and-puff, other)

**j.** Wheelchair Skills to include:
  1) Wheelchair parts management (e.g., operation of brakes)
  2) Transfers to/from chair, commode, bed, transportation
  3) Manual wheelchair propulsion (safety, functionality, distance)
  4) Powered mobility operation (safety, functionality, distance)
  5) Management in living environment, work, school (safety, functionality)

**k.** Mobility/Balance to include: Sitting balance, standing balance, transfers, and ambulation

**l.** Mat Evaluation to include: Posture in sitting and supine positions (positioning fixed or flexible, ROM, strength, tonal influences):
  1) Pelvic positioning (anterior/posterior tilt, obliquity, rotation)
  2) Trunk
    i. Anterior/posterior (kyphosis or lordosis)
    ii. Left/right (C curve, S curve, flexible, fixed)
    iii. Rotation (shoulders and upper trunk)
  3) Hips (position, abduction, adduction, subluxed, dislocated, neutral, windswept, ROM limitations)
  4) Knees and feet (position, ROM, limitations)
  5) Head and neck (position, ROM, control, tone, movement)
  6) Upper extremity (position, ROM, control, tone, movement)
    i. Shoulder—functional, elevated, subluxed
    ii. Scapula—depressed, protracted, retracted
    iii. Elbow—flexed, extended
    iv. Forearm—supinated, pronated
    v. Wrist and hand (presence of fisting, strength, dexterity)

**m.** Goals for Wheelchair Mobility

**n.** Goals for Seating System

**o.** Simulation Ideas

**p.** Equipment Trials to include: What was successful/unsuccessful

**3.** Select a wheelchair

The findings obtained during the patient/caregiver interview and physical examination directly influence the goals established in the plan of care. Specifying the wheelchair configuration that best serves a patient includes recognition that modifications of the standard wheelchair may be necessary. Tailoring a wheelchair to meet an individual's needs is expected, particularly when it will be the patient's primary positioning system and/or means of mobility. Obtaining accurate, complete measurements is important because wheelchair frames come in limited sizes; if a patient is between sizes, the team must decide whether to order a size larger or smaller. The decision often is made after looking at the cost to alter the frame of the wheelchair, the availability of parts, the payer's allowance, and any anticipated changes in the patient.

Clarity about the goals to be addressed with the seating equipment is important (Box 17-1). Consider asking a vendor to loan equipment for a patient trial and/or simulation before finalizing recommendations or ordering the wheelchair. Trial use of equipment may shed new light on a patient's functional abilities or confirm that a patient is not ready for the suggested equipment.

Wheelchairs can be adapted in many ways to accommodate and support the needs of patients with and without neuromotor impairments. Selecting, prescribing, and modifying adaptive seating is beyond the scope of an entry-level professional and requires consultation with an ATP and/or an experienced vendor, occupational therapist, or physical therapist. However, entry-level practitioners should be able to make basic adjustments and repairs to the wheelchair to maximize the potential benefits for the patient, recognize the need for alternatives, and know when to refer the patient to an expert.

Table 17-3 lists the main components of a wheelchair, the general specifications, and considerations that may affect positioning and functionality for the patient.

**BOX 17-1 Seating Goals**

- Accommodate fixed deformities/joint limitations
- Minimize negative influences of abnormal muscle tone
- Optimize postural alignment
- Improve posture to provide stability
- Improve head position to increase visual field and swallow
- Relieve pain to increase comfort
- Increase sitting tolerance
- Relieve pressure to prevent pressure sores
- Improve function of gastrointestinal and cardiopulmonary systems
- Improve body image
- Increase mobility
- Reduce fatigue
- Allow for growth and weight gain/changes
- Eliminate or reduce restraints
- Meet caregiver needs
- Meet transportation/vocational/school/home needs

| TABLE 17-3 | Wheelchair Components, Specifications, and Considerations | |
| --- | --- | --- |
| **COMPONENT** | **GENERAL SPECIFICATIONS** | **CONSIDERATIONS** |
| *Frame* | | |
| Size | Pediatric | Adjustable for growth of child and skill level |
| | Adult | Adjustable for weight gain/loss and skill level |
| | Bariatric | Intended for use by persons weighing 250 pounds or more |
| Type | Tilt-in-space wheelchair | Changes orientation of user when sitting while maintaining head/trunk/hip/knee angle<br>• Pressure redistribution<br>• Reduction of sheer forces<br>• Gravity assistance with positioning |
| | Recliner wheelchair | Adjustable seat-to-back angle; not meant for self-propulsion; bulky |
| *Form of propulsion* | | |
| Manual | Daily use: meets daily needs; primary mode of mobility | Propulsion options: bilateral upper extremity, bilateral lower extremity, hemi-propulsion (same-side arm and leg), unilateral upper extremity |
| | Sport: ultra-lightweight (aluminum or titanium) welded frame, no armrests, fixed yet adjustable height footrest, fixed or adjustable camber (wheel angle) | Typical weight of manual wheelchairs: 14.2 pounds (ultra-lightweight) 35 pounds (standard issue lightweight) 50 pounds (tilt-in-space) |
| | Other manual wheelchairs include power assist, transport only, heavy duty, hemi-height, and one-arm drive | |
| Powered | Intended for persons who are unable to ambulate community distances; requires independent static/dynamic sitting balance; ability to ambulate short distances with or without an assistive device | Drive options: hand (joystick); head (proximity switch or sensor, accelerometer-based); cheek (proximity switch or sensor); chin (joystick); voice (speech recognition); tongue-touch (microchip keypad); breath control (pneumatic); Lautzenhiser Drive Control (proportional control through movement of the head, hand, finger, or foot); magnetic control tongue-drive system |
| | | Typical weight of powered wheelchair: 110–300 pounds |
| | Other powered mobility (e.g., scooters) | |
| | | Considerations for manual versus powered wheelchairs include transportation options, activity tolerance, postural control, motor control, coordination, cognition, visual-perceptual status, and impairments (e.g., range of motion, strength, and tone) |
| *Frames* | | |
| Folding | Frame collapses lengthwise because of an X-brace | Remains bulky but fits in most cars and trunks; requires more energy to propel; potential to be customized/adjusted; requires more parts |

*Continued*

| TABLE 17-3 | Wheelchair Components, Specifications, and Considerations—cont'd | |
|---|---|---|
| **COMPONENT** | **GENERAL SPECIFICATIONS** | **CONSIDERATIONS** |
| Rigid | Frame is single-welded piece; back folds forward with quick-release wheels to reduce its size and weight | More energy efficient to propel because of lighter weight; fewer moving parts; limited adjustability; requires unsupported sitting balance |
| Chair height and base of support | Standard height seat bottom to ground is approximately 18.5 in. | When standard height does not match a patient's functional needs, adjustments can be made to raise or lower the seat or adjust the diameter of casters and/or wheels |
| | Hemi-height is 17 in. seat to ground | Allows patient with limited upper extremity function to propel and/or steer with leg(s) |
| | Base of support | Anterior/posterior through seat depth change; width by exchange of cross brace, style of armrest, or additional lateral inserts |
| *Wheels* | | |
| Casters (front) | Sizes typically range from 2¾ to 8¼ in. | Caster size and style affect steering, propulsion efficiency, chair stability, anterior seat height and angle, and foot clearance<br>• Smaller casters allow tighter turns<br>• Larger casters assist negotiation over uneven surfaces, higher surfaces (e.g., speed bump or pothole); may increase comfort of a ride |
| Wheels (rear) | Standard size: 24 in. | Increasing or decreasing wheel size affects propulsion efficiency, height off ground, and patient positioning (posterior seat height and angle) |
| | Spoke or MAG (plasticlike composite, forming three or more large spokes, connecting the rim to the center of the wheel)<br>• Spoke typically accepts pneumatic tires<br>• MAG accepts pneumatic or solid tires | Wheel sizes:<br>Pediatric:<br>12, 20, 22, and 24 in.<br>Adult:<br>22, 24, and 26 in. |
| Tires | Pneumatic – rubber exterior with air-filled inner tube | • Is shock absorbing<br>• Offers traction<br>• Gives smoother ride<br>• Is lightweight<br>• Is high maintenance<br>• Can puncture, requiring repair or inner tube replacement<br>• Is less durable (e.g., tread wear) |
| | Solid insert – plastic or rubber exterior with foam, rubber, or plastic inside | • Cannot become flat<br>• Is more durable<br>• Requires less maintenance<br>• Is 1.5 times heavier<br>• Provides harder ride<br>• Has less shock absorption<br>• Less traction |

| TABLE 17-3 | Wheelchair Components, Specifications, and Considerations—cont'd | |
|---|---|---|
| **COMPONENT** | **GENERAL SPECIFICATIONS** | **CONSIDERATIONS** |
| Hand rims | Purpose<br>• Reduce stress on upper extremity joints<br>• Protect digits during propulsion<br>• Reduce energy consumption with propulsion | Sizes coincide with respective tire size |
| | Natural fit | Shaped to fit a user's hand position during propulsion |
| | Chrome | Slippery; requires strong grip |
| | Composite, titanium, aluminum | |
| | Projection | For people without complete hand/wrist function (e.g., C5–C6 spinal cord injury) |
| | Plastic-coated/tubing | Plastic (textured) material intended to help maintain grip during propulsion; for persons with a weak grip |
| *Back/seat* | | |
| Sling | Standard nylon (sling) backs and nylon-covered foam (sling) seats | Not intended to provide pressure relief, postural control, or balance |
| | Off-the-shelf cushions (purchased through retail vendors) | Pressure relieving or pressure reducing; may improve or reduce postural control and balance; may influence some impairments (e.g., range of motion and tone)<br>• Quick to obtain<br>• Reduced cost<br>• Removable<br>• Less pressure protection<br>• Less support<br>• Less control of posture and tone |
| | Custom-designed cushions<br>• Can accommodate orthopedic conditions<br>• Fits any wheelchair frame<br>• Unable to modify | • Intimate fit for better control of posture, balance, and tone<br>• Pressure relief or pressure reduction built in |
| Firm | Solid seat and back | Reduces/eliminates sling effect (e.g., posterior pelvic tilt, kyphotic thoracic spine, internal rotation/adduction of humerus/femur, forward head) |
| See *Wheelchair Cushions* in this chapter for detailed information | | |
| *Armrests* | | |
| Fixed | Nonremovable for transfers; nonadjustable for height | Typical on basic wheelchairs intended for short-term use for persons without any upper body or upper extremity dysfunction |
| Removable | Lift off, swing away, or flip back | |
| Removable – nonadjustable | Removable for transfers; nonadjustable for height | May be used on a basic wheelchair intended for short-term use for persons without any upper body or upper extremity dysfunction, but who need to perform lateral transfers in and out of their wheelchair |

*Continued*

| TABLE 17-3 | Wheelchair Components, Specifications, and Considerations—cont'd | |
|---|---|---|
| **COMPONENT** | **GENERAL SPECIFICATIONS** | **CONSIDERATIONS** |
| Removable – adjustable | Removable for transfers; adjustable for height – standard | Removable for persons performing lateral transfers in and out of their wheelchair; adjustable for persons who require upper extremity support such as with a subluxed shoulder post stroke |
| Full-length | | Patient cannot get close to a desk or table; stable surface for wheelchair accessories, (e.g., a lap tray or arm trough); allows patient to push to stand using armrest |
| Desk-length | Cutout in front one-third of armrest allows wheelchair to fit under a desk or table | Not a stable surface for some wheelchair accessories (e.g., lap tray or arm trough); patient cannot push to stand from front of armrest for transfers (although cumbersome, armrest temporarily reverses for transfers) |
| *Leg rest* | | |
| Fixed | Nonremovable; 70-degree hangers (standard) | May impede transfers |
| Swing away, removable | Swings to side for removal or out of way for transfer; 60-, 70-, or 90-degree hangers available | Heavy; can get lost (misplaced) or end up out of reach for the user |
| Elevated | Swings to side for removal or out of way for transfer; 90-degree hanger elevates up to 180 degrees; adjustable calf pad | Heavy; bulky; can get lost; valuable for patients with pain or swelling of lower extremities or knee involvement |
| *Footrest* | | |
| Standard | Fixed, standard angle, non-adjustable except for height off the ground | |
| Angle adjustable foot plate | Adjustable: anterior-posterior-medial-lateral | Expensive; limited payer approval |
| Accessories for positioning | Heel loops, heel cups, or foot straps | |

Postural deviations such as pelvic obliquity and lateral trunk flexion may result from abnormal tone, contractures, or impaired sensation. Although there are many possibilities, certain postural deviations tend to be associated with particular types of neurological disorders. For example, a person who has experienced a stroke often has lateral trunk flexion and postural lean because of unilateral impairments due to hemiparesis; a person with Parkinson disease typically develops a flexed or forward posture. Table 17-4 outlines common postural deviations (beginning at the pelvis), the potential source of the deviations, and suggested interventions to address them. Although there is an emphasis on optimal sitting posture, not all patients can achieve these positions. Be mindful when modifying seating that any changes do not limit the patient's function or create musculoskeletal pain or discomfort.

## Wheelchair Cushions and Seat Backs

A carefully selected wheelchair cushion and seat back can be integral parts of the seating system and should be included in the selection and purchase of a wheelchair. Wheelchair cushions and seat backs vary according to size, style, purpose, and price (Table 17-5). Off-the-shelf cushions accommodate standard adult and pediatric wheelchairs. Cushions for some larger bariatric and smaller pediatric wheelchairs may be special orders, however. When evaluating cushions and seat backs to determine which best meet the patient's needs, the esthetics, cost, and payer source should be considered as well as the cushion's ability to distribute pressure, minimize peak pressure at bony prominences, encourage proper posture, and resist moisture (Pipkin, 2008). Seat backs not only have the potential to properly position the pelvis and improve trunk stability and comfort, but they can also influence coronal and sagittal plane alignment, affecting static and dynamic sitting balance during a functional task (May, 2004).

When available, pressure mapping can be valuable in guiding decision-making for patients who are at increased risk for skin breakdown (Figs. 17-1, 17-2, and 17-3). Pressure mapping has been reliable for assessing the effectiveness of a specific cushion in reducing maximum subcutaneous stress in

| TABLE 17-4 | Common Postural Deviations, Potential Causes, and Suggested Interventions | |
|---|---|---|
| **POSTURAL DEVIATION** | **POTENTIAL CAUSE OF DEVIATION** | **SUGGESTED INTERVENTION** |
| *Pelvis* | | |
| Posterior pelvic tilt | • Sling seat and back<br>• Foot plate too high<br>• Seat depth too long<br>• Reduced trunk support<br>• Lack of (or poorly adjusted) armrests<br>• Thoracic kyphosis<br>• Reduced lumbar extension<br>• Weak trunk extensors<br>• Anterior chest tightness<br>• Forward or flexed head<br>• Fatigue | • Firm seat back and bottom<br>• Tip (wedge) seat forward (open hip angle) or backward (depending on individual)[1]<br>• Lower foot plates<br>• Increase trunk support<br>• Adjust armrest height<br>• Replace sling with firm seat and back<br>• Increase lumbar support<br>• Increase anterior pelvic tilt<br>• Move headrest posteriorly<br>• Anchor pelvic positioner below anterior superior iliac spine, anchoring 45 degrees from the seat to secure hips<br>• Alter seat depth to 1–2 in. from popliteal crease<br>• Use knee blocks to keep pelvis from sliding forward |
| Anterior pelvic tilt | • Hip flexor tightness<br>• Fixed spinal vertebrae<br>• Lumbar support too big<br>• Excessive lumbar lordosis<br>• Reduced thoracic kyphosis<br>• Retracted shoulders<br>• Abnormal extensor tone | • Close hip angle<br>• Tip (wedge) seat posteriorly<br>• Reduce/remove lumbar support<br>• Sling seating<br>• Raise seat back<br>• Increase hip, knee, ankle flexion<br>• Place pelvic positioner above ASIS that angles up from seat to secure hips<br>• Alter seat depth to 1–2 in. from popliteal crease<br>• Reduce seat width |
| Pelvic rotation | • Seat too wide<br>• Windswept deformity<br>• Scoliosis<br>• Insufficient femur support<br>• Femoral length discrepancy | • Support bilateral femurs<br>• Deepen cushion to capture and hold pelvis<br>• Modify leg rest height |
| Pelvic obliquity | • Structural (fixed)<br>• Leg length discrepancy<br>• Muscle tightness unilaterally | • Use firm seat and back<br>• Attempt to achieve level base of support<br>• Wedge seat laterally to lengthen shortened side<br>• Use custom-molded or contoured seat or cushion to maintain midline position and/or compensate<br>• Use bolster or saddle seat to widen base of support (especially for patients with increased tone in hip adductors and internal rotators) |
| *Trunk/spine* | | |
| Cervical/thoracic kyphosis | • Poor head/trunk control<br>• Lack of upper extremity support<br>• Lack of trunk support<br>• Posterior pelvic tilt<br>• Congenital defect | • Increase head, trunk, UE support<br>• Contoured seat back<br>• Add/increase lumbar support<br>• Address anterior pelvic tilt; use harnesses, vest, chest strap, or shoulder pommel<br>• Use full or half lap tray |

*Continued*

| TABLE 17-4 | Common Postural Deviations, Potential Causes, and Suggested Interventions—cont'd | |
| --- | --- | --- |
| **POSTURAL DEVIATION** | **POTENTIAL CAUSE OF DEVIATION** | **SUGGESTED INTERVENTION** |
| Excessive lordosis | • Tight low back extensors<br>• Tight hip flexors<br>• Weak abdominals<br>• Anterior pelvic tilt | • Increase posterior pelvic tilt<br>• Place pelvic positioner above ASIS |
| Scoliosis | • Congenital defect<br>• Weak muscles<br>• Tight muscles<br>• Pelvic obliquity | • Address kyphosis, lordosis, lateral trunk support<br>• Three-point pressure system to counteract biomechanical forces generated by body, positioning, and gravity<br>• Clear lap tray (full or half)<br>• Adjust armrest height<br>• Use lateral wedge seat (lower on elongated side |
| Lateral flexion | • Weakened muscles unilaterally<br>• Tight muscles unilaterally<br>• Somatosensory/visual impairment<br>• Fatigue | See scoliosis |
| *Lower extremities (hip, femur, knee, ankle)* | | |
| Windswept deformity (one leg in external rotation and abduction, the other leg in internal rotation and adduction) | • Abnormal adductor tone<br>• Weak musculature<br>• Tight musculature<br>• Pelvic rotation<br>• Pelvic obliquity | • Improve pelvic alignment followed by spinal alignment (utilizing spinal support)<br>• Block abduction and adduction at femurs and/or knees<br>• Lengthen seat depth<br>• Use abductor/adductor wedges to promote alignment<br>• Use abduction orthoses, wedges, or pommels with function similar to bolster/saddle seats but achieved with an optional attachment<br>• Use knee blocks to prevent forward translation of the femur |
| Hip abduction or adduction | Same concepts as windswept lower extremities | • Adjustable-angle foot plates<br>• Foot loops or straps<br>• Heel loops<br>• Shoe holders/guides<br>• Wedges to align foot |
| Foot supination (adduction, inversion, and plantar flexion) | Spastic or contracted plantar flexors and invertors | If fixed, protect bony prominences and skin integrity; if flexible, consider angle adjustable foot plates to shadow individual foot positioning |
| *Upper extremity* | | |
| Abnormal flexor synergy | Increased muscle tone, weakness | Full/half lap tray<br>Arm trough |

[1]Therapists debate the effect of inclining the seat anteriorly (i.e., widening the angle between the seat and seat back) or posteriorly. Tipping the seat anteriorly opens the hip angle and is thought to shift the center of gravity forward and consequently increase lumbar lordosis, decrease thoracic kyphosis, reduce the effects of tight hamstring muscles, and decrease posterior pelvic rotation (Sochaniwskyj, 1991). The goal of a posteriorly tipped seat is to close the hip angle, increase the amount of hip flexion, and keep the pelvis back in the seat as a means of decreasing overactive hip and trunk extensors, decreasing posterior pelvic tilt, and increasing lumbar lordosis. Evidence is inconclusive (Chung, 2008; McClenaghan, 1992; Miedaner,1990; Nwaobi, 1983; Sochaniwskyj, 1991), and intersubject variability suggests that the seat angle must be determined on an individual basis (Sochaniwskyj, 1991).

| TABLE 17-5 | Wheelchair Cushions – Indications and Characteristics/Considerations |
|---|---|
| **CUSHION TYPE** | **INDICATIONS AND CHARACTERISTICS/CONSIDERATIONS** |
| Dry (air) flotation:<br>Air cells provide individual pressure adjustment; level 4 evidence supports the air cushion as producing the lowest and mean ischial tuberosity pressure and the highest area of pressure distribution (Titos, 2014) | Cushion/seat back:<br>Indications: Current or healed pressure ulcers; reduced independence with pressure relief; incontinence (cushion only); prolonged sitting; bony skeletal frame<br>Characteristics/Considerations: Moisture resistant; multiple chambers available; requires sitting balance; high maintenance; expensive; air cells can puncture/melt |
| Gel flotation | Cushion/seat back:<br>Indications: Low to moderate risk for pressure ulcers with bony frame; reduced independence with pressure relief; prolonged sitting; impaired balance; thermodysregulation<br>Characteristics/Considerations: Influences pelvic/trunk positioning; provides postural support; moisture resistant; low to moderate maintenance; expensive; can puncture/melt |
| Honeycomb | Cushion only:<br>Indications: Pressure reduction; current and healed pressure ulcers; bony frame; postural support<br>Characteristics/Considerations: Moisture resistant; minimal maintenance; moderately priced |
| Foam:<br>varies in density, memory, quality<br>• Low-density foam<br>• High-density foam | Cushion/seat back:<br>Indications: Comfort<br>Characteristics/Considerations: Inexpensive, easy to acquire; absorbs fluids and moisture; degrades over short periods; lacks memory; increases shear or friction; effectiveness related to patient size, weight, and shape; may "bottom out"; evidence lacking regarding effectiveness (Stockton, 2009)<br>Characteristics/Considerations: Pressure reduction, comfort; some moisture resistant; some adjustable, contoured; moderately priced; may absorb fluids and moisture; may degrade over short period; may not have memory; may reduce shear or friction; promotes pelvic control and balance |
| Air or gel combined with viscoelastic foam | Benefit: greater distribution of overall pressure than basic foam cushion; greater positional support with less maintenance than air flotation; not recommended for persons at high risk for skin breakdown |

a specific person (Ragan, 2002). Thus, it is clinically useful in determining how effective a particular cushion is in relieving, reducing, and/or distributing pressure over a patient's bony prominences.

**4.** Determine a funding source(s)

Before making final recommendations for a seating system for any patient, the rehabilitation team should consider whether the recommended system meets the payer's approved guidelines. The next step should include an investigation into the availability of equipment, its adaptability and/or adjustability, and the patient's/caregiver's approval.

As an example, consider two patients with the same diagnosis but different circumstances. Mr. Jones is in an acute inpatient setting, and Mr. Smith is in a long-term care setting. If Mr. Jones requires a wheelchair for 8 to 12 weeks, the physical

therapist would measure him, relay the measurements to a vendor, submit paperwork for reimbursement to the payer source, and receive the wheelchair before Mr. Jones's discharge pending approval from the payer. Because of Mr. Jones's short-term need, the payer would most likely have the patient rent the wheelchair rather than purchase it.

In contrast, if Mr. Smith needs a wheelchair for the rest of his life, the physical therapist or other member of the rehabilitation team would complete a full positioning and seating examination and complete the appropriate documentation forms (examination and LMN), requesting reimbursement for what is being recommended. Following submission of the documentation, the patient would have to wait for approval before the vendor could place an order for the equipment. Depending on the payer source (e.g., Medicaid or Medicare versus private insurance), it could take as long as 90 days

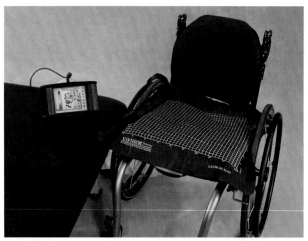

**FIGURE 17-1** Pressure mapping – wheelchair with pressure mat in place.

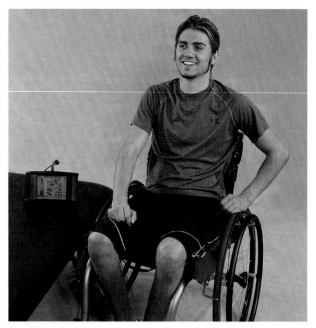

**FIGURE 17-2** Pressure mapping – patient positioned on pressure sensitive mat.

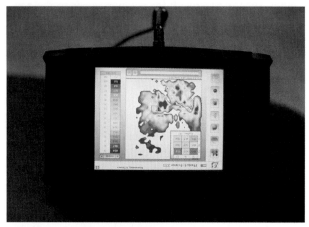

**FIGURE 17-3** Pressure mapping screen illustrating pressure distribution gradient

to receive notification about whether the request has been approved or not. In the interim, Mr. Smith would need to remain in his current wheelchair, borrow a wheelchair from the facility, or possibly receive a loaner from the vendor involved. Once the approval has been received, it could be an additional 2 to 3 weeks from the time the vendor orders the equipment until it is shipped. Adjustments to the new equipment could take an additional 1 to 4 weeks depending on the complexity of the patient's needs. Keep in mind there is never a guarantee a wheelchair will be approved because each state and insurer has its own set of rules and regulations. Each rehabilitation team member involved with positioning and seating must stay abreast of the current guidelines and regulations.

**5.** Document medical necessity

Written documentation must be prepared to justify to the payer that the recommended wheelchair addresses a medical necessity (as defined by the payer) and is cost-effective. Without convincing documentation, the payer may deny funding, so preparing a clearly written, organized, comprehensive LMN is an essential skill for a physical therapist. More details about writing an LMN are provided later in the chapter. Once the payer approves the funding, the vendor can place an order for the intended wheelchair, parts, and accessories.

**6.** Evaluate the patient with the new wheelchair

Evaluating the patient with the new seating system, a continuation of the patient examination, is the most germane step in the process because it allows the rehabilitation team to assess how effectively the chair meets the patient's/caregiver's needs and improves the patient's function. A cycle consisting of observation, modification, and trial and error assists in achieving the goals set for the patient. For example, after observing the patient's posture in the chair during a task, the team may need to modify the system to improve posture and task completion. Following the modification, the patient is observed for a few days to a week (trial and error) to assess the effects of the change. In many instances, fitting a patient for a wheelchair or seating system is achievable within two therapy sessions (e.g., when acquiring a standard wheelchair and off-the-shelf cushion for a patient with a short-term, lower extremity, weight-bearing restriction). Other patients may take weeks or months before achieving their goals because of the complexity of their problems. It is advisable to minimize initial changes or adjustments to a new system to allow the patient to adjust or respond to any altered mechanics and to encourage keeping an open mind about the changes.

A wheelchair is an integral part of a person's daily function, and purchasing a new one is similar to trying on a new pair of shoes to replace comfortable worn-out ones. Follow-up modifications may continue with each meeting until the patient and physical therapist feel the wheelchair and seating system meet the patient's/caregiver's goals. Consider as well the time of day the patient is examined and which activities the patient is asked to perform to ensure consistency. For additional information on functional wheelchair mobility, refer to Chapter 26 (related to patients with paralysis) and to Chapter 35 (as a component of seated mobility).

**7.** Reassess and follow up

Reassessment allows the physical therapist to determine the outcome(s) of the previous trial-and-error period a week, a month, or even 6 months after discontinuing a patient. By this time, it is expected that the patient, a family member, or other caregiver would have contacted the physical therapist, another member of the rehabilitation team, or the vendor if any concerns or issues have arisen. However, when there is hesitancy to speak up, no one is available to advocate for the patient, or a message intended to reach the physical therapist or rehabilitation team is "lost," an informal subjective interview can address any unnoticed issues or confirm that the seating system is meeting the intended goals and the patient is satisfied.

### Adaptive Seating Systems

Although wheelchairs are the most widely used seating systems for individuals with a disability, many other options exist, especially when self-propulsion is not a consideration. A wide variety of customizable, adjustable seating systems are available for children or adults with severe disabilities who need considerable support or for multiple populations to support functional activities (e.g., feeding/eating). Common types of seating are shown in Table 17-6.

Despite the widespread use of adaptive seating, evidence definitively supporting specific types of seating is lacking. Chung (2008) conducted a rigorous systematic review of literature published from 1980 to 2007 to answer two focused questions: (1) "What is the effect of adaptive seating on sitting posture or postural control in nonambulatory children from birth to 20 years of age with varying types and severity of CP?" and (2) "What are the effects of resultant changes in sitting posture or postural control on other aspects of functioning within the ICF model?" The authors found only 14 articles that met their criteria, ranging from levels II to V in the rating system by Sackett (2000). Similar to most research on this population, analysis of results across studies was difficult because sample sizes were small, the level of severity among participants was not classified with a validated system (e.g., Gross Motor Function Classification System-Expanded and Revised) (Palisano, 2007), the measures of postural control were not standardized, and the outcomes did not extend beyond postural control to examine the effects on function in

| TABLE 17-6 | Types of Seating Equipment | | |
|---|---|---|---|
| **ILLUSTRATION** | **TYPE OF SEATING** | **DESCRIPTION** | **PURPOSE/USE** |
| | Corner chair | Back of chair forms a 90-degree angle | Useful alternative for children with cerebral palsy who have scapular retraction and difficulty getting hands to midline because of abnormal tone |
| | Bolster chair | Seat is a large diameter bolster | Provides broad base of support and pelvic stability; especially useful for individuals with extensor synergy in legs; caution needed to ensure adequate range of motion to accommodate wide abduction |

*Continued*

| TABLE 17-6 | Types of Seating Equipment—cont'd | | |
|---|---|---|---|
| **ILLUSTRATION** | **TYPE OF SEATING** | **DESCRIPTION** | **PURPOSE/USE** |
| | Feeder seat | Molded foam seat with washable, brightly colored surface; sculpted back and pelvic indentation; slight abduction pummel; can be used with multiple bases (e.g., floor wedge, stroller, regular chair) | Accommodates many children and adults comfortably and safely for feeding; washable surface without crevices helps with clean-up |
| | Adjustable chair | Basic chair with multiple adjustments; many styles available from different vendors | Relatively economical option for environment where more than one individual might need seating; not for severely involved individuals |
| | Customized mobile seating | Seating system with myriad of options and adjustable components | Necessary for child with severe/profound disabilities who needs customized seating system |

Images 1 and 2 courtesy of Kaye Products (Kayeproducts.com); Image 3 courtesy of Performance Health (pattersonmedical.com); Image 4 courtesy of Rifton (Rifton.com); Image 5 courtesy of R82 (R82.com).

its broad interpretation (ICF model). According to their review, the authors concluded that "no single intervention has been shown to be more effective than others in improving sitting posture and/or postural control and limited evidence to suggest whether improved sitting posture and/or postural control will lead to improved functional abilities" (p. 317). It is important to recognize that their conclusions *do not* mean that adaptive seating should not be used. Confounding variables in the research included variations in population samples, types of adaptive seating, and outcome measures used. The clinical reality may be that children and adults with cerebral palsy or other complex neuromotor conditions present very differently and that seating must be customized or adapted to address the unique needs of each patient.

Rehabilitation professionals must strive to find evidence to support practice but must not lose sight of clinical judgment in selecting, adapting, and modifying adaptive seating and other types of assistive technology. Selecting reliable and valid measures for factors such as postural stability and control will add to meaningful outcomes assessment (Fife, 1991; Westcott, 1997). It is also important to consider more subjective outcomes, although many challenges are inherent in measuring outcomes such as patient satisfaction. Research and analysis by Rust (2004, 2006) and Fuhrer (2001) demonstrate the complexity of assessing assistive technology outcomes, especially the perceptions of users. A useful tool to assess patient satisfaction is the Quebec User Evaluation of Satisfaction with Assistive Technology (QUEST) by Demers (2002).

### Assistive Devices for Ambulation

The use of assistive devices for ambulation can improve balance, alleviate pain by decreasing weight-bearing, compensate for weakness or impaired motor control (in one or both legs), and increase patient confidence and sense of safety (Bateni, 2005). When the assistive device promotes greater mobility and function, the user experiences the secondary benefits of preventing osteoporosis and cardiovascular deconditioning. Long-term use of assistive devices can cause stress on the upper extremities with secondary inflammatory conditions (e.g., tendonitis, osteoarthritis, and carpal tunnel syndrome).

Ambulation with assistive devices requires considerable energy expenditure (compared with no walking), which can negatively affect performance in other areas. Franks (1991) compared the reading fluency, visuomotor accuracy, and manual dexterity of three students with lumbar level myelomeningocele when they were using a wheelchair for mobility compared with walking with crutches or a walker. The students' performance was substantially improved during weeks when they were using the wheelchair compared with weeks when they were ambulating. This does not mean walking should be abandoned, but the energy requirements should be considered when planning for equipment purchase and scheduling its use.

A high correlation exists between the use of assistive devices and increased risk of falls in older adults. The use of assistive devices may simply be an indicator of deficits in balance, functional decline, and fall risk. However, some studies suggest that ambulatory devices may interrupt balance control, compete for cognitive attention, or cause tripping among some segments of the population (Bateni, 2005; Mann, 1995a, 1995b; West, 2015; Wright, 1992).

The basic elements of selecting and fitting assistive devices for ambulation are the same for patients with neuromuscular disorders as for other populations. However, the emphasis is not on decreasing weight-bearing or unweighting, as is often true with orthopedic disorders, but to assist with balance, decrease spasticity, allow upright mobility in the home environment, and/or promote functional community mobility. With neuromuscular disorders, it is more likely that the whole body is affected, not just the lower extremities, which adds to the complexity of selecting an appropriate device. Often orthopedic disorders are short term, whereas neuromuscular disorders are more long term and may even be progressive. Determining the patient's prognosis will affect long-term goals and the choice of assistive device. Selection of a device should include these considerations:

- Reason for choosing an assistive device (e.g., unweight limb, improve balance, decrease stress on painful joints, or otherwise protect joints)
- Potential for independent function
- Medical history (e.g., diabetes, neuropathy, obesity, chronic obstructive pulmonary disease)
- Safety issues including fall risk, living environment (e.g., stairs with or without railing, clutter, type of flooring), available supports (e.g., someone to supervise or guard), mental/cognitive status, and confidence
- Energy efficiency of the device; activity tolerance of the patient
- Psychological effect or self-perception related to using an assistive device
- Ability to manage the device by a patient with known sensory and/or motor impairment
- Necessary base of support (wider if balance and postural control are compromised)
- Need for less complex motor demands (e.g., rolling versus standard walker)
- Patient's status including strength, balance, coordination, judgment, cognitive function, vision, vestibular function, physical endurance
- Patient's preference (see Table 17-7)

Ambulation devices can assist individuals with a broad range of conditions but have been particularly effective when used with certain neuromuscular conditions. Advantages and disadvantages of various types of ambulation devices are summarized in Table 17-8. Energy expenditure is an important consideration when evaluating various assistive gait devices and often must be assessed on an individual basis (Lephart, 2014). Posture-control (posterior) walkers (Fig. 17-4) are a special type of assistive device designed for children with cerebral palsy and have gained widespread use among pediatric populations with a range of disabilities and more limited use with adult populations. The walker's frame is behind the patient rather than in front, and the posterior placement has been shown to facilitate more upright posture, improve postural alignment and control, conserve energy, and improve various components of gait (Greiner, 1993; LeVangie, 1989a; LeVangie, 1989b; Logan, 1990; Mattsson, 1997; Park, 2001). Children seem to interact more readily with their peers, and both parents and children prefer posterior walkers to anterior walkers (Greiner, 1993; Mattsson,1997).

According to research by Cubo (2003), walkers (both standard and rolling) increased stability and patient confidence but significantly slowed the walking speed of patients

| TABLE 17-7 | Assistive Devices for Ambulation | |
|---|---|---|
| **DEVICE** | **ADVANTAGES** | **DISADVANTAGES** |
| Standard cane (SC) | Increased base of support (BOS) for balance<br>Can be hung on forearm when performing activities of daily living (ADL) or on back of chair when not in use | Allows least amount of upper body weight-bearing |
| Multiple leg cane (tripod or quad cane) | Provides greater BOS for balance<br>Stands alone, freeing arms for other tasks | More difficult to use than SC for some patients because all legs need to be in simultaneous contact with ground |
| Hemi-walker | Commonly used for patients with hemiplegia because it provides largest BOS/greatest stability and requires only one arm<br>Greater weight-bearing and stability than quad cane | More difficult to use on stairs than quad cane |
| Axillary crutches (ACs) | Provide greater BOS and stability than canes<br>Provide better trunk support than forearm crutches | Require considerable balance, coordination, and upper extremity (UE) strength<br>Have potential for brachial plexus injuries if misused |
| Forearm/Lofstrand crutches | Allow hands to be freed without removing crutch from arm so patient can perform UE tasks<br>Easier for patient to free self from device in event of fall | Provide less support than ACs |
| Standard walker (SW) | Most stable of all assistive devices<br>Provides up to 100% weight-bearing on UEs | Requires slower, controlled gait pattern<br>Requires significant UE strength to advance walker with each step<br>May facilitate forward flexed posture<br>Requires greater demand for attention than other ambulatory devices<br>Requires relatively complex motor task to use safely |
| Rolling walker (RW) | Good for patients who need the stability of a walker but lack UE strength, endurance, coordination, or balance required to advance an SW<br>Allows for faster gait speed<br>Encourages more normal gait pattern<br>Has lower energy demand than an SW<br>Requires less cognitive ability<br>Increases patient satisfaction | Has less stability than an SW |
| Posterior walker (PW) | Facilitates more upright posture<br>Improves postural alignment and control<br>Conserves energy<br>Decreases double stance time, increases stride length, and increases walking speed<br>Allows more direct access to work/play surfaces<br>Is preferred by both parents and children | |
| Walking pole(s) | Is beneficial as transition<br>Promotes more supinated grasp (may decrease UE tone)<br>Used well, allows smooth, rapid gait pattern | Typically requires supervision/assist for safety with children<br>Can be used by adults for fairly complex motor functions (e.g., hiking) |

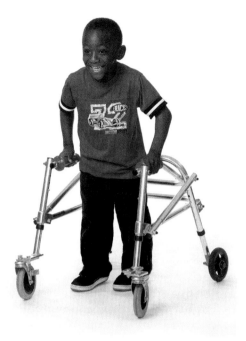

**FIGURE 17-4** Posture control (posterior) walker. *(Photo courtesy of Kay Products.)*

with Parkinson disease compared with unassisted walking; standard walkers increased the incidence of "freezing" in the same patients.

Walkers are available in sizes fitting toddlers through adults and can be adapted with a wide range of accessories:

- Wheels (either two or four)
- Forearm supports (e.g., when a patient with hemiplegia does not have sufficient hand control to use an assistive device)
- Vertical handholds that may decrease the pattern of flexor spasticity in the upper extremity by placing the forearm in more supination
- Pelvic stabilizer (bilateral pads extending out from the horizontal bar of a walker's posterior frame to facilitate midline hip position)
- Extension assist (pad on posterior frame to encourage hip extension)
- Bench for resting
- Overhead frame (for partial body weight suspension)
- Extensive options for wheel type and function (e.g., antirollback, directional wheel lock, all-terrain)
- Seating

Canes are often recommended to help patients who have experienced a stroke shift their weight toward their sound side and enhance push off during the swing phase (Kuan, 1999) while requiring less muscular effort of the erector spinae and tibialis anterior (Buurke, 2005). Because walkers usually involve use of the upper extremities, they are not the best option for patients who have experienced a stroke unless they are modified with a forearm support. Canes vary primarily by base of support size, ranging from the hemi-walker (with a very

broad base of support) to the quad/tripod cane or single (standard) cane. Patients with various levels of ambulatory assistance (from unassisted to single cane to quad cane) have found the use of a cane provides significant benefits, including decreased muscular effort, normalization of muscle activation, and improvement in gait parameters that can be measured with computerized 3-D analysis (Kuan, 1999; Laufer, 2003). In general, a wider base of support (i.e., a quad cane) provided more stability and less postural sway than a standard cane (Laufer, 2002, 2003).

Numerous factors may influence patient preference. For example, although substantially greater shoulder joint forces exist (Haubert, 2006), forearm crutches are typically used by patients with paraparesis (Melis, 1999; Ulkar, 2003), including children with myelomeningocele, because they allow greater mobility and increased velocity compared with standard crutches or walkers (Melis, 1999; Ulkar, 2003; Moore, 2001; Slavens, 2007).

### Gait Trainers

Gait trainers (Fig. 17-5) are four-wheeled devices that support patients in an upright position and allow independent mobility. Various options provide support even for individuals with multiple severe disabilities and very poor motor control. Options include a saddle seat, overhead suspension, straps (for thigh or foot) to prevent lower extremity adduction, bars to prevent the legs from crossing midline (e.g., for patients with "scissor" gait), trunk supports, forearm supports, and various wheel and base configurations.

Opinions differ among clinical practitioners about the benefits of gait trainers. Mobility is often achieved at the cost of a quality gait pattern, which may be a concern for patients who have potential for more independent gait and

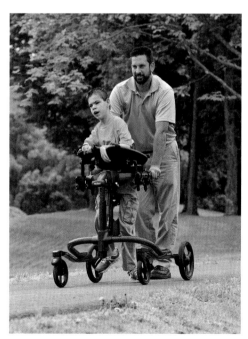

**FIGURE 17-5** Gait trainer. *(Photo courtesy of Rifton. Rifton.com)*

will need to develop postural control, symmetry, reciprocation, and other components of gait to achieve their potential. Proponents of gait trainers focus on the broad-reaching benefits of motor activity (Damiano, 2006), independent mobility, and upright positioning even when the gait pattern is poor quality.

Mobility Opportunities Via Education (MOVE) is an activity-based program for children and adults that emphasizes independence in essential motor skills of sitting, standing, and walking. MOVE's mission statement is grounded in the philosophy that "the ability to move is the first foundation stone in building personal dignity" (www.move-international.org/about). The program was initially developed to address the challenging needs of individuals with severe/profound disabilities and to enhance the quality of their life by providing them with opportunities for meaningful participation in ADLs. Gait trainers are frequently used in the MOVE curriculum to facilitate independent mobility as part of a carefully designed program promoting consistent prompts and frequent practice (Thomson, 2005).

Paleg (1997) followed 19 children (mean age of 6 years) who received 5 days of intensive therapy (20 hours) during an inpatient hospital stay with first-time exposure to gait trainers. Ninety-five percent of the children learned to walk (20 feet in a gait trainer), 58% learned to sit (erect head position for 30 seconds), and 47% learned to stand (maintain hip and knee extension while supported by hands).

### Other Mobility Devices

#### Tricycles/Bicycles

Tricycles (Fig. 17-6) come in all sizes (pediatric and adult) and with a wide variety of support options. They can promote motor control (including reciprocal motion) and increase strength while providing a fun alternative for independent mobility and non–weight-bearing exercise. Cycling may have more far-reaching benefits. Emerging evidence supports the use of forced (or augmented) exercise cycling as a promising intervention to improve motor performance and global symptoms in patients with Parkinson disease (Hindle, 2013; Ridgel, 2012, 2015; Rosenfeldt, 2015).

#### Scooters

Scooters can encourage motor control and provide mobility and sensory input in a creative manner. Large, padded scooters used individually or paired provide comfortable prone positioning for more involved patients (Fig. 17-7). Small wheeled scooters approximately 12 × 12 inches square and only a few inches high (Fig. 17-8) can be used in a variety of ways to promote motor control, increase strength, and provide vestibular input. For example, patients can be prone, supine, or sitting on the scooter; propel themselves off a wall with their feet; pull themselves using an overhead rope; spin themselves; accelerate down a ramp; or maneuver through an obstacle course. Scooters with raised handles, for which the individual stands on the scooter platform with one foot and pushes with the other for mobility, can promote coordination, reciprocal motion, unilateral weight-bearing, motor planning, and strengthening.

Carts or other types of creative mobility devices (Fig. 17-9) are available (e.g., a brightly colored "race car" design for children that is manually propelled using the wheels). Mobility options such as these are especially beneficial for the patient who has good trunk and upper extremity function but lacks functional use of the lower extremities (e.g., patients with a spinal cord injury, myelomeningocele, or spastic diplegia).

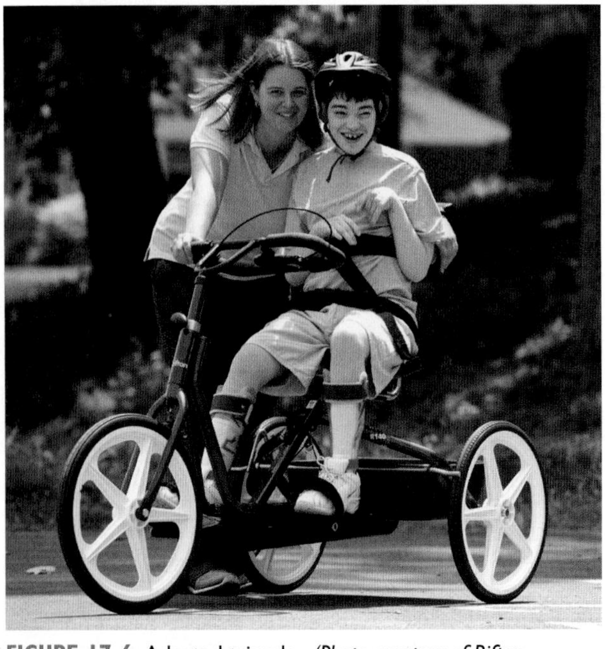

**FIGURE 17-6** Adapted tricycle. (*Photo courtesy of Rifton. Rifton.com*)

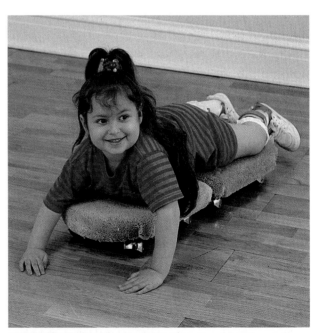

**FIGURE 17-7** Square carpeted scooter board (can be used singly or paired). (*Photo courtesy of Performance Health. pattersonmedical.com*)

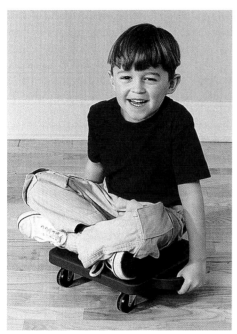

**FIGURE 17-8** Square plastic scooter *(Photo courtesy of Performance Health. pattersonmedical.com)*

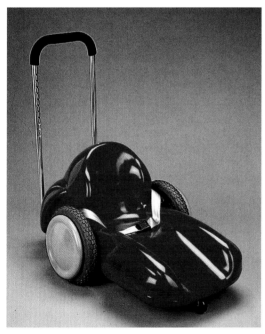

**FIGURE 17-9** Ready racer mobility for children with good upper extremity function and limited lower extremity function. *(Photo courtesy of Performance Health. pattersonmedical.com)*

## Assistive Devices to Enhance Functional Positioning

### Floor/Mat Positioning (e.g., bolsters, wedges, side-lyers)

1. Floor positioning is more common for children whose size makes moving them up and down from the floor more realistic than for adults and whose opportunities for social

interaction may be expanded by floor positioning. For example, a child with cerebral palsy who is customarily in a wheelchair would benefit from the supports that allow seating on the floor so he or she can participate in a circle group with peers. Adults may also be positioned comfortably on mats. As an example of adaptive equipment options for floor positioning, the Tumble Forms Tadpole is a portable set of vinyl-covered, molded foam shapes that connect using Velcro strips to create positioning alternatives for small children (Fig. 17-10A and 17-10B).

a. Bolsters and wedges

   i. **Bolsters** are cylindrical rolls of varying diameter and length, typically covered with a light layer of foam and vinyl or constructed of solid molded foam (e.g., Tumble Forms). Bolsters can be used (1) under a patient's chest when prone to promote upper back and head control; (2) as a "seat" for a patient to straddle with support, helping to decrease extensor tone and provide pelvic stability (Fig. 17-11); (3) as a tool to work on sit-to-stand; (4) as a moving support surface to work on balance and equilibrium reactions (front to back or side to side); or (5) as a positioning tool for a patient or a patient's extremity to facilitate optimal performance during therapeutic exercise.

   ii. **Wedges** (Fig. 17-12) come in many sizes and dimensions with and without straps and can be used under the patient's chest when prone to promote upper back and head control, to stretch hip flexors, to provide slight traction for a patient with a spinal curvature, and/or for general positioning to improve comfort or function. Typically, the height of

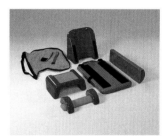

**FIGURE 17-10A** Multiuse portable positioning system (Tadpole). *(Photo courtesy of Performance Health. pattersonmedical.com)*

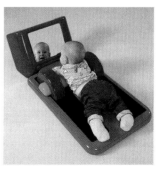

**FIGURE 17-10B** Child positioned prone in Tadpole. *(Photo courtesy of Performance Health. pattersonmedical.com)*

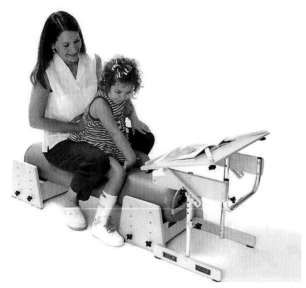

**FIGURE 17-11** Child straddling bolster raised on benches with adult behind to facilitate play. *(Photo courtesy of Kay Products.)*

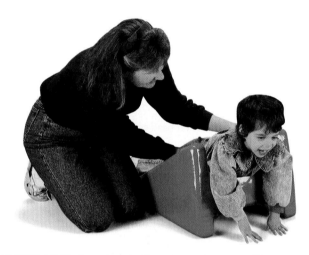

**FIGURE 17-12** Raised wedge for prone positioning. *(Photo courtesy of Performance Health. pattersonmedical.com)*

the wedge is selected so that patients can support themselves at least partially on elbows or hands. Greater inclination from prone facilitates head and upper trunk control and can be accomplished by using a large wedge to support the body and another wedge or elevated support for the arms. A patient can also be placed in an inverted position on the wedge for pulmonary (postural) drainage.

iii. Bean bags can be easily molded to provide comfortable support in reclined sitting. However, they do not encourage any active motor or postural control and can contribute to contractures and deformities, so their use should be limited.

b. Sidelying can be an excellent alternative for children or adults who have little independent mobility. The position promotes midline head position and a natural tendency for the hands to come together. It is a

neutral position for the patient who has persistent influence of tonic labyrinthine reflexes and helps to prevent aspiration. Individuals can be propped in a sidelying position with good alignment simply by using pillows or other positioners (e.g., a bolster supporting the back). Commercially made side-lyers are also available and may be a useful purchase for an individual with severe increased tone or for a classroom of children who could share the device. Of note, the patient's top leg should not be allowed to adduct (predisposing to hip dislocation) and the patient's head should be positioned so the cervical spine is in good alignment.

### Standing (e.g., standing frames, prone standers, supine standers)

Supported weight-bearing is a common intervention for children and adults who are not able to stand and/or walk independently. Varying levels of research and empirical evidence support a wide range of benefits (listed in the following section). Paleg (2013) concluded in a systematic review that moderate evidence exists to support the benefits of supported standing marked with an asterisk in the following list.

1. *Increased bone mineral density of legs and spine (Alekna, 2008; Caulton, 2004; Chad, 1999; Gudjonsdottir, 2002a; Paleg, 2013; Pin, 2007; Stuberg, 1991, 1992; Tasdemir, 2001; Thompson, 2000; Wilmhurst, 1996)
2. *Increased ROM of hip, knee, and ankle (Bohannon, 1985; Gibson, 2009; Paleg, 2013; Stuberg, 1992; Tremblay, 1990)
3. *Decreased hypertonicity of the ankle in the short term (up to 35 minutes) (Paleg, 2013; Tremblay, 1990)
4. *Improved bowel function (Dunn, 1998; Eng, 2001; Hoenig, 2001; Paleg, 2013)
5. *Facilitated optimal musculoskeletal development of the hip, knee, and ankle joints (Gudjonsdottir, 2002a; Paleg, 2013; Pountney, 2002) for children with spastic diplegia (Macias, 2005)
6. Increased ability to activate stretched muscle in the short term (Tremblay, 1990)
7. Improved head and trunk stability and control
8. Improved respiratory efficiency (improved cough, fewer infections, increased pulmonary profusion) and improved short-term ventilation in acutely ill patients (Chang, 2004)
9. Improved circulation (Eng, 2001)
10. Improved renal and bladder functions, including decreased urinary tract infections (Dunn, 1998; Eng, 2001; Paleg, 2013)
11. Pressure relief and improved skin integrity (Dunn, 1998; Eng, 2001)
12. Improved self-image, alertness, social development, and interaction with peers (Manley, 1985); improved psychological well-being (Paleg, 2013)
13. Improved gait characteristics (Salem, 2010; Zabel, 2005)

Children or adults unable to stand independently are often placed in supported standing devices to achieve one or more of the stated benefits. The time and effort required to carry out a standing program make it critical for a therapist to examine the purpose of the standing program relative to individualized goals for the patient, potential long-term benefits, and existing evidence. Many options exist for supported standing and are summarized here under general categories.

Prone stander (Fig. 17-13): A type of adjustable stander that allows nearly upright supported standing or varying degrees of forward tilt with support on the ventral surface of the body. Prone standers come with multiple options including supports for the trunk, hips, lateral aspect of the knee, and feet; a tray for upper extremity support and an accessible work/play surface; and a standard or wheeled base. Most models have sufficient adjustments and supports to allow standing even for individuals who are very severely involved. Disadvantages are that a stander cannot be used for patients with established joint contractures of the legs and that size can be prohibitive for classroom or home use.

Supine stander (Fig. 17-14): Similar to prone stander, but the individual is supine. Supine standers provide more support than other types of standers for individuals who are severely involved; if the stander can be adjusted to a horizontal position, transfers can be accomplished more easily. However, the fully supported supine position promotes little or no active motor or postural control, and a partially reclined position is not conducive to active participation and engagement.

Upright or vertical stander/standing frame (Fig. 17-15): Provides a system of trunk, hip, and knee straps to support standing in a fully upright position. Individuals with total paralysis of their legs can use standing frames; however, the frames do not safely accommodate contractures, and an individual must be able to tolerate a fully upright position and have adequate trunk control. A variation of the vertical stander is a parapodium (or similar devices), typically used by young children with myelodysplasia who swivel the stander to gain mobility. A vertical standing frame provides all the advantages

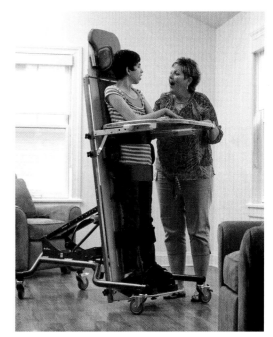

**FIGURE 17-14** Supine adult stander. *(Photo courtesy of Rifton. Rifton.com)*

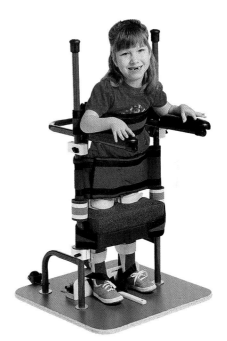

**FIGURE 17-15** Upright standing frame. *(Photo courtesy of Performance Health. pattersonmedical.com)*

of supported standing without the bulk of a prone or supine stander.

### Supine or Sit-to-Stand Devices

Placing an individual in a supported standing device can be challenging, especially when the individual is large or has very poor head and trunk control. A variety of devices can get the patient to a standing position (Figs. 17-16A, 17-16B, and 17-16C), assist with transfers (Fig. 17-17), or support the patient while ambulating (Fig. 17-18).

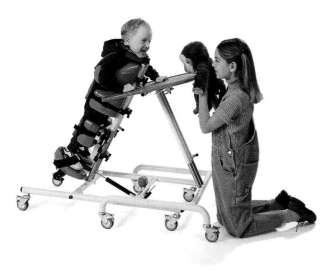

**FIGURE 17-13** Multiposition stander (adjusts supine, prone, upright; illustrated prone). *(Photo courtesy of Performance Health. pattersonmedical.com)*

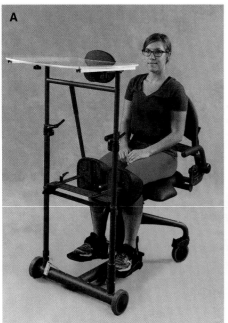
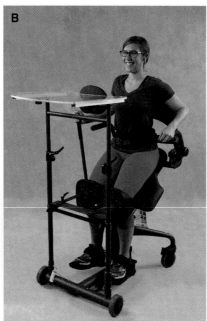
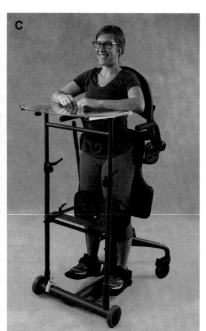

**FIGURE 17-16** ABC Sit-to-stand frame.

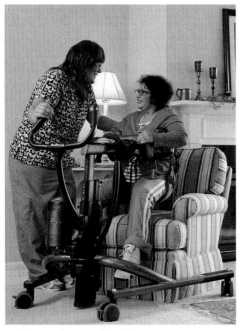

**FIGURE 17-17** Mobility and transfer device (illustrated for transfers). *(Photo courtesy of Rifton. Rifton.com)*

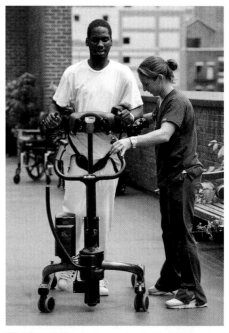

**FIGURE 17-18** Mobility and transfer device (illustrated for assisted ambulation). *(Photo courtesy of Rifton. Rifton.com)*

### Dynamic or Mobile Standers

A number of standers allow patients to propel themselves with either a power assist motor (operated by a joystick similar to a power wheelchair) or a prone stander with wheels designed for self-propulsion (Fig. 17-19). The latter is particularly beneficial for patients who have good upper extremity and trunk control (e.g., patients with a spinal cord injury, myelodysplasia, or cerebral palsy).

The term "dynamic" has been applied to at least two other designs. The Dynamic Stander by Kaye Products (Fig. 17-20)

stabilizes the legs and pelvis, allowing patients 360 degrees of movement of the upper trunk, thereby helping them to strengthen muscles, gain motor control, practice weight shift, improve balance, and learn more complex motor patterns. The amount of excursion and resistance can be adjusted to patient tolerance and ability and can be locked in a stable position when necessary (e.g., during transfers). Rigorous research to verify its efficacy is lacking, but the design incorporates sound principles of neurorehabilitation. Gudjonsdottir (2002b) reported on a motorized dynamic stander that reciprocally

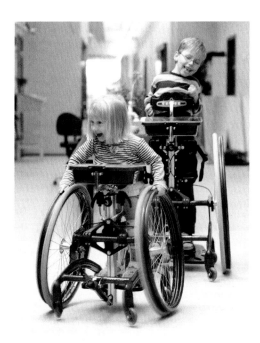

**FIGURE 17-19** Mobile stander (can be propelled by occupant). *(Photo courtesy of R82. R82.com)*

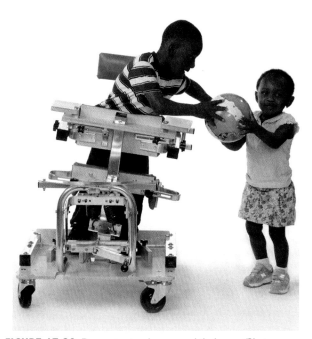

**FIGURE 17-20** Dynamic stander on mobile base. *(Photo courtesy of Kay Products.)*

shifts the patient's weight while in the stander. With a limited sample, the authors found no statistical differences in bone mineral density or behavioral variables with use of dynamic versus static standers; however, more research is needed.

Standers are available with many options, and expertise is required to select the appropriate device. When a device is purchased for a group setting (e.g., a classroom or skilled nursing facility), the range of adjustments and the ease of adjusting and cleaning them are critical because of the possibility

of multiple users. For example, the TriStander by Tumble Forms (Fig. 17-13) can be adjusted for supine, upright, or prone positioning; is made of molded foam with few crevices (i.e., is easily cleaned); is relatively easy to adjust; and comes on a wheeled base with an optional tray on a separate wheeled base.

Little solid evidence supports decisions about the type of device (e.g., prone or supine), the actual position (e.g., partially reclined or fully upright), or the optimal duration and frequency of times in the device to achieve the benefits listed. Herman (2007) found that the actual amount of weight borne in a stander is variable, and more research is needed to identify ways to maximize weight-bearing. The cost of the equipment and the challenges of placing an individual in the device are other factors to consider.

On the basis of a systematic review, Paleg (2013) developed evidence-based clinical recommendations for dosing of pediatric supported-standing programs. Researchers found strong evidence for maintaining or increasing ROM in the hamstrings (most), plantar flexors, and hip. They recommended that the individual stand at least 45 to 60 minutes daily to increase ROM. Additionally, they recommended having the individual stand in 60 degrees of bilateral hip abduction to increase abduction, placing a wedge under the forefoot to increase stretch to the plantar flexors, and use of a knee immobilizer to help distribute pressure when the hamstring muscles are tight and the individual lacks full knee extension. Standing for 30 to 45 minutes is recommended for short-term reduction in spasticity of the gastroc-soleus; thus, a possible strategy would involve having the patient stand before a therapy session.

A clinical assumption can be made that weight-bearing into the acetabulum helps deepen and form the structure, helping to prevent hip subluxation and dislocation, though evidence of this effect is mild. Paleg (2013) recommended standing daily for 60 minutes in 60 degrees of abduction for that purpose. The authors found no evidence that standing was contraindicated when one or both hips were subluxed or dislocated. Good evidence indicates that supported standing positively affects bone mineral density, and Paleg (2013) recommended standing for 60 to 90 minutes five times per week as a minimum threshold with maximum loading (i.e., with the patient as upright as possible and with minimum strapping). Although more research is needed, on the basis of existing evidence, parents/caregivers should commit to having the patient stand at least 60 minutes a day to achieve most goals.

Considerable debate surrounds recommendations for supported standing for students in the educational environment; nevertheless, it is a common intervention by pediatric physical therapists depending on the child's ambulatory status and specific needs (Taylor, 2009). It can be argued that static standing is neither inclusive (unless other children are standing for an activity) nor a functional goal (required by IDEA). Supported standing could be considered a goal-directed functional activity when it is used in preparation for a pivot transfer or supported ambulation. When rehabilitation professionals know the benefits of supported standing and recognize that a child is unlikely to stand at home after a long day at school, are there ethical issues in NOT recommending supported standing in the educational environment? More evidence is needed.

### Hygiene and Toileting

Toileting can be a stressful experience, especially for adults with severe disabilities, and may be the main reason that an individual is placed in an institution. Facilitating use of an adapted toileting system can decrease workload for caregivers, preserve the patient's dignity, and improve the patient's health (especially if catheterization and/or diaper use can be avoided). Many companies make toileting systems and commode chairs. A unique aid for personal hygiene is the Rifton Hygiene and Toileting System (Fig. 17-21), which allows even partial-weight-bearing patients to receive hygiene care or a diaper (brief) change in a more dignified upright position that improves access to clothing and skin and eliminates or reduces heavy lifting by caregivers. Bidabe (2017), founder of the MOVE curriculum, has published a toileting program based on an upright posture using the Rifton system or other types of supports.

Bureau of Labor Statistics data (2011) on high rates of musculoskeletal injuries among health-care workers have prompted standards on safe patient handling and mobility (SPHM). Overexertion injury rates for hospital workers (68 per 10,000) were twice the rate averaged across all industries (33 per 10,000), and rates for nursing home workers were more than three times the average (132 per 10,000). The greatest risk factors are manual lifting, moving, and repositioning of patients (CDC, 2014). As a result, emphasis has been placed on identifying safer ways of performing these manual tasks, typically using various assistive devices.

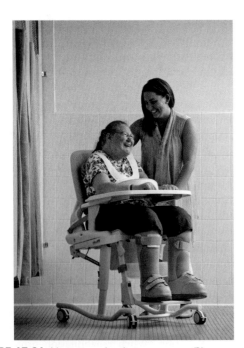

**FIGURE 17-21** Hygiene and toileting system. *(Photo courtesy of Rifton. Rifton.com)*

The American Nurses Association (2013a, 2013b) has published interprofessional national standards and an implementation guide related to SPHM for use across the care continuum. One of the comprehensive standards is specific to the selection, installation, and maintenance of technology. Many of the assistive devices previously described may complement a SPHM program, and many more are being developed, including flexible overhead suspension systems. It is important for therapists to inform themselves about various devices so they can be involved in their procurement, training, and use whether for an expansive, institution-wide SPHM program or for a particular patient.

## THINK ABOUT IT 17.3

Data on the high incidence of work-related musculoskeletal injuries among health-care workers prompted the development of safe handling and mobility standards that include the use of assistive technology. What are some of the challenges in ensuring that health-care workers utilize assistive technology safely and effectively during high-risk tasks such as lifting, moving, and repositioning patients? How might you be involved as a therapist?

### Transportation Safety (including school bus)

Safe transport of individuals with disabilities is critical but often overlooked. Discussions about transportation should be an integral part of decisions regarding technology purchases. Issues related to transportation are highly specialized and should involve a team of experienced professionals. Four major considerations are involved:

1. What type of vehicle (e.g., personal car, specially equipped van, public transport, or public school bus) is going to be used, and is the individual going to be transferred to an existing seat (preferable if the transfer can be accomplished easily and the individual has adequate postural control) or remain in the seating system?
2. Does the wheelchair meet industry standards for safety? The American National Standards Institute (ANSI) and RESNA developed design and performance criteria and test methods to assess whether a wheelchair can be safely used as a seat in a motor vehicle (RESNA, 2012). These standards are commonly referred to as WC19 (referring to Section 19 of the ANSI/RESNA *American National Standards for Wheelchairs, Volume 4: Wheelchairs and Transportation.* Features of WC19-compliant wheelchairs include tested structural integrity, four labeled securement points (optimally positioned on stable portions of the wheelchair), fewer sharp edges/hard points (which could cause injury), and gel-cell batteries (if powered).
3. Is the wheelchair safely secured using a four-point strap tie-down system or docking system that complies with applicable standards (Fig. 17-22)?
4. Is the occupant effectively restrained with a three- or five-point crash-tested system that includes pelvic

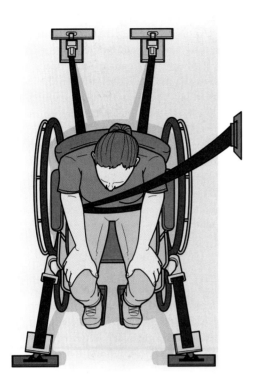

**FIGURE 17-22** Occupant and wheelchair secured for safe transport.

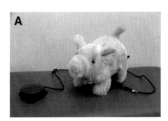
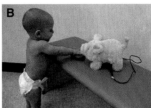

**FIGURE 17-23(A AND B)** Simple switch-activated device (toy).

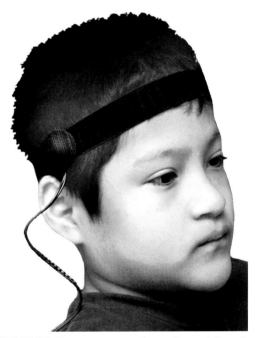

**FIGURE 17-24** Gravity-sensitive tilt switch to reinforce head control. *(Photo courtesy of Enabling Devices: Toys for Special Children; www.enablingdevices.com)*

and shoulder restraints secured to the vehicle frame (Fig. 17-22)? H-harnesses are not a safe restraint system for transportation, although they can supplement approved restraints to improve posture.

## Assistive Devices for Manual Control, Interaction, and Communication

### Switches, Controls, and Access Sites

Simple electronic switches can be used creatively for a variety of functions and are often motivating for children or adults (Figs. 17-23A and 17-23B). In its simplest design, a battery-operated toy or device is modified so that a switch is required to activate it. The activated device can range from animated stuffed animals to DVD players to vibrating cushions (or other types of sensory input). Switches can be designed to promote a variety of hand functions (e.g., pincer grasp, grip, or hand placement) or to maximize available function. Button or "jelly bean" switches in a variety of sizes and colors can be optimally placed (possibly with available mounting hardware) so that even a very light touch from an individual who is severely involved activates a response object. Tilt-sensitive switches can be fastened with a headband and used to reinforce midline head control (Fig. 17-24). Proximity switches use motion-sensitive technology to operate and can be used with individuals who have difficulty operating a switch that requires physical contact and/or sustained pressure.

Additional hardware allows the use of electronic devices (e.g., kitchen appliances such as a blender) that do not have

batteries or allows a single switch activation to activate a toy or device for a specified time (seconds or minutes) rather than requiring sustained activation by the patient. One can buy toys that are "switch-ready" and buy or fabricate cables that interrupt the battery circuitry. Learning to use switches for choices can be a starting point for contingency learning and for augmentative communication.

### Augmentative and Alternative Communication

**Augmentative and alternative communication** refers to means other than speech to send a message to another person. Augmentative communication devices supplement speech, and alternative communication devices refer to a primary means of communication for those lacking speech. Devices can be simple low-tech objects such as "Yes/No" cards at the corner of a lap tray, communication boards or notebooks, and picture wallets. High-tech devices are typically categorized according to three variables: (1) encoding method (e.g., real objects, photographs, line drawings, symbols, letters, or words); (2) access method (e.g., direct selection, pointing, or scanning); and (3) means of output (Tanchak, 1995). An iPad or similar technology can be a relatively adaptable, inexpensive alternative because of the large touch screen, voice-over feature that verbalizes text as the finger moves over the screen, and adjustable display (e.g., size of fonts or icons). Applications (apps) are available through iTunes or other online venues. Typically, the speech and language pathologist is the most knowledgeable person on the team regarding devices for augmentative or alternative communication, but a physical therapist can provide valuable input about positioning alternatives or mechanisms that will optimize motor function to operate a device.

### Computer Technology

An array of assistive technology devices is available to enable individuals with disabilities to use computers. These range from various types of keyboards to eye-pointing and voice-control activation devices. Referral to an assistive technology specialist and trial use of adaptive devices through an assistive technology resource center are typically required. A physical or occupational therapist may be valuable in optimizing a patient's position or biomechanical advantage to utilize various adaptive devices.

### Environmental Control

Environmental control units (ECUs) were introduced between the 1970s and 1980s (Dress, 1997; Palmer, 2007).

Traditionally, persons without disability have used ECUs to simplify ADLs. These devices include automatic phone dialing, lighting control, automatic timed start of a coffee maker, or remote/timed control of a television or other audiovisual media device. Depending on the input, such as voice recognition, eye gaze, switches, computer interfacing, or a combination thereof, tasks may be accomplished remotely. ECUs, more recently termed *electronic ADLs (EADLs)*, have the potential to empower a user; thus, they are paramount for persons with a physical disability who are unable to manipulate or control various devices around them. EADLs may reduce the need for personal care assistance, allow increased independent decision-making, reduce energy expenditure, improve accessibility to the environment, and improve quality of life (Boman, 2007; Craig, 2005; Little, 2010; Rigby, 2011).

Low-end EADL technology is relatively inexpensive and allows one- or two-way interaction between the receiver and source, such as a DVD player or teleconferencing. In contrast, high-end EADLs employ advanced computer technology such as virtual reality, interactive software, powered mobility, and some augmentative communication systems requiring a much larger investment. Technology also gives users varying degrees of control. *Discrete control* refers to the ability to turn a device either on or off, but *continuous control* allows adjustments such as increasing or decreasing volume or brightness. Various types of EADLs and examples of their use are summarized in Table 17-8.

When assessing the best EADL options for an individual, consider the client's goals, current functional status, ability to learn new information, vision and hearing, current positioning and seating, personal support system, future needs and payer source. As with positioning and seating, configuring and adjusting an EADL for a client may be simple, or it may require

| TABLE 17-8 | Various Types of Electronic Activities of Daily Living Technology |
|---|---|
| **TYPE OF TECHNOLOGY** | **EXAMPLES OF USE** |
| X-10 designed for home automation<br>• Plugs into a wall outlet or device (e.g., lamp or radio)<br>• Receiver communicates through house wiring | Remote control for home devices/systems such as coffee maker, lights, thermostat, security; allows discrete and continuous task control |
| Infrared—frequency range below visible light | Controller for electronics<br>Optical tracking system<br>Wireless mouse<br>Sicare light<br>• Voice recognition; operates up to 15 different infrared-run devices |
| Toggles (buttons), switches, voice control, scanning<br>• Some may allow discrete and continuous task control, others just discrete control | Augmentative communication devices<br>Computer controls |
| Motion detector | Turn indoor/outside lights on/off |
| REACH (Remote Electronic Access & Control – Hands-Free) | Touch screen computer, body movement, or voice activation controls numerous electronic devices (e.g., fan, audiovisual equipment, telephone) |

considerable time. The assistive technology team should use creativity and innovation when helping clients whose positioning and seating needs are complex and whose functional abilities and/or communication skills are more limited.

### Biofeedback

Biofeedback technology is a specialized area that can be a valuable resource; however, entry-level practitioners are not expected to be proficient. Many types of feedback can be used, including electromyographic biofeedback to decrease muscle spasm, promote relaxation, or activate weak muscles after neurological compromise; ultrasonography or computerized dynamometers to visualize muscle activation and facilitate motor control; and tilt-sensitive devices to provide feedback about head position.

### Virtual Reality Technology

Virtual reality is an emerging technology that allows a patient to interact with a simulated multisensory, multidimensional environment in real time using either standardized or individualized interventions. The therapist controls the stimulus parameters and can measure and document outcomes within a single session or over time. The technology has been used to increase compliance with breathing exercises by linking incentive spirometry to video games (Lange, 2011); using an instrumented cane on a self-paced, treadmill-based virtual reality environment with stroke patients (Perez, 2011); upper extremity rehabilitation for individuals with chronic stroke (Burdea, 2011); eye-tracking control of the virtual environment by individuals with high-functioning autism as a means of assisting attentional disengagement in a social context (Grynszpan, 2011); and various applications for children with motor impairments (Laufer, 2011). Additional research is needed to verify outcomes, but the potential applications of virtual reality technology are extensive.

### Emerging Technologies

As part of the National Robotics Initiative, the National Institutes of Health (2015) is funding three corobots, robots that work cooperatively with people. One is a four-legged walker with dual purposes: to assist ambulation (adjustable for the amount of assistance provided) and to "walk" alongside an individual carrying a load (e.g., groceries). Another is a social robot companion purported to "promote and assess curiosity and a growth mindset through various interactions."

## ■ Acquisition of Assistive Technology

### Funding Goals

Rules and regulations for state and federal agencies and private health insurance companies can be difficult to interpret and may be restrictive. It is sometimes necessary for the rehabilitation team to identify nontraditional resources to acquire assistive technology, particularly for patients with limited or no health-care coverage, as illustrated in the following examples:

- Patients who need a wheelchair for a short time or who do not need customized seating may go to the local branches of national organizations (e.g., National Multiple Sclerosis Society or Spina Bifida Association) and inquire about a wheelchair lending program or assistance with a wheelchair purchase.
- Local service or health-care organizations, charitable foundations, or assistive technology centers (created to meet federal guidelines in the Tech Act) may be able to assist a patient/resident with borrowing or purchasing a wheelchair.
- A myriad of resources can be found by searching the Internet, or family, friends, and coworkers can become involved in creative fund-raising efforts. Internet sites such as Gofundme.com that are easily linked to other social network sites, such as Facebook and Twitter, have raised billions of dollars for individuals and groups. Sometimes raising community awareness about the need for a wheelchair can result in other forms of needed assistance for the patient/caregiver(s).

## Funding Considerations

Funding considerations affect many steps in the process and many of the individuals involved. As a result of coverage limitations, some patients may not receive needed assistive technology without paying out-of-pocket fees (the amount *not* covered by insurance), which can be extremely costly. In an effort to lower costs, some manufacturers have lowered the quality of their products (which may affect function or durability) or have decreased the level of support provided. Vendors may invest considerable time with a patient who needs complex seating and yet not be able to recoup their costs if funding is denied, so they raise their fees or build in "hidden" fees.

### Reimbursement Refers to Repayment for a Necessary Expense

A payer source will not reimburse a vendor or patient for something that is not **medically necessary**. According to Medicare terminology, medically necessary refers to "health-care services or supplies needed to diagnose or treat an illness, injury, condition, disease, or its symptoms and that meet accepted standards of medicine" (Medicare.gov; https://www.medicare.gov/glossary/m.html). Cigna (n.d.) adds that anything medically necessary is ". . . not primarily for the convenience of the patient or Healthcare Provider . . ." https://www.medicare.gov/glossary/m.html (www.cigna.com/customer_care/healthcare_professional/medical/medical_necessity_definitions.html). For example, if a person can ambulate only from the bed to the bath in his/her own home but not to the kitchen, front door, or laundry room, an assistive technology device such as a wheeled walker or manual wheelchair is medically necessary so he or she can complete ADLs/IADLs. If this same person is in a nursing home, there is no medical necessity to purchase mobility equipment because the facility is responsible for providing such equipment and assisting in all care needs.

When documenting for reimbursement, one must clearly demonstrate medical necessity (most often defined by Medicare). The letter a physical therapist or member of the rehabilitation team writes is called a **letter of medical necessity** (LMN). The reviewer of an LMN will be looking for discrete evidence that the outcome sought cannot be met by any other equipment or service. The LMN is a critical document that requires time to construct. The following recommendations are integral for writing an effective LMN: (1) Make it unique to the individual (not a generic template); (2) be specific about physical presentation and abilities and write to the audience (often a layperson); (3) describe the potential of assistive technology to enhance function; (4) make a case for the selected equipment, comparing and contrasting it with similar products and being as specific as possible about observed outcomes for the patient when using the device; and (5) use research, state and federal laws/policy, and/or professional standards to justify your request (Oxender, 2015).

### Letter of Medical Necessity Guidelines

Before you start writing, preparation is key.

1. Understand the laws relating to insurance coverage.
   a. A beneficiary must prove a covered loss by submitting a claim.
   b. The insurer will either pay or deny the claim.
2. Understand the meaning of medical necessity.
   a. Insurers define the term differently.
   b. Ask the appropriate insurance company to fax or e-mail its definitions of medical necessity.
   c. Study the definition carefully and be sure to address that specific definition in your letter.
3. Compose your letter for your audience.
   a. Paint a picture of the beneficiary and create an understanding of the equipment.
   b. Use terms that can be understood by an ordinary person who has never worked in health care or heard of the equipment.

### Starting Your Letter

1. In the opening sentence, state who you are and why you are writing this LMN and use your credentials.

Sample: *My name is Susie Smith, licensed physical therapist and member of the Assistive Technology Resource Team at Franklin Skilled Nursing Facility in Greensboro, North Carolina. The purpose of this letter is to obtain financial insurance coverage for a/an* [equipment/service] *for* [patient name]. *In this letter, I have included background information on the medical and health status of* [patient name], *a description of the requested* [equipment/service], *and pertinent research-based evidence supporting its use and the specific benefits to the patient.*

2. Explain the beneficiary's condition.
   a. Discuss the effect of the condition on the patient's life, noting limitations occurring *without* the assistive technology.

Sample: *Thus far, these effects have included, but are not limited to, the following:*

- *Increased muscle spasticity in the trunk and extremities*
- *Muscle atrophy with decreased muscular girth and strength in the trunk and extremities*
- *Impaired/decreased muscular coordination (both gross and fine motor)*
- *Range-of-motion deficits at joints such as the hips, knees, ankles, shoulders, and trunk*
- *Skin sensitivity and fragility over the gluteal and lower sacral areas due to impaired independence with gross mobility tasks*
- *Impaired bowel and bladder functions with loss of volitional control*
- *Reduced pulmonary and cardiovascular functions*

   b. State the obvious: Assume insurers have not experienced a person with the disabilities you are describing.

Sample: *As a result of these limitations without the adaptive equipment/service, the patient requires additional time to . . .; requires hands-on assistance to . . .; has difficulty with . . .; has increased discomfort/pain . . ., etc.*

[patient's name] *current functional health status and abilities are as follows:*

- *Is alert, well-oriented; shows high intelligence and cognitive function*
- *Speaks and converses with others with good reciprocal comprehension*
- *Requires assistance for activities of daily living (e.g., shaving, dressing, bathing, meal preparation)*
- *Requires assistance with basic transfers from bed to wheelchair and from wheelchair to commode*
- *Is unable to ambulate with or without assistive devices*
- *Demonstrates uncoordinated movements in the trunk and extremities*
- *Is unable to propel a manual wheelchair for long distances or on uneven terrain; is able to propel inside short distances*
- *Is at risk for pressure sores, bone loss, chronic urinary tract infections, and bowel problems*
- *Has reduced respiratory and cardiovascular functions*

4. Describe the equipment/service requested.
   a. Explain how it will improve the beneficiary's function.
   b. Explain why alternatives will <u>not</u> improve the beneficiary's function.
   c. Use scientific evidence to support the explanation as much as possible.
   d. Be clear and specific.

Sample: *In an effort to improve and optimize the quality of* [patient's name] *health and reduce the risk and occurrence of further medical illness and complications,* [equipment] *is recommended.*

*An additional benefit to any associated caregivers working with this patient is that* [state the benefits].

Explain the benefits of the requested equipment in the function of various systems (e.g., cardiovascular) as well as psychological considerations, providing specific examples when possible. Discuss the functional advantages of the [equipment] for the patient in various settings (e.g., home, work, school, outdoors).

5. Explain how the equipment can decrease other expenses and is cost-effective, as appropriate.
6. Address the insurer's definition of medical necessity.
   a. Do not go overboard; state simply that the policy requires that the equipment meet certain criteria to be considered medically necessary.
   b. Provide a one-sentence explanation of how each criterion is met.
7. Make the beneficiary a real person facing a difficult adversity.
8. Enclose a copy of the prescription.
9. Enclose illustrations to supplement the text when possible (being sure to label each illustration or photograph).
   a. Download and print out pictures of the equipment from the Internet.
   b. Photograph the patient in his/her current and loaner equipment, as applicable.
10. Summarize the request, briefly highlighting the key points.

Sample: *The information previously outlined notes the many benefits of the* [equipment] *and the multiple positive effects on the various systems of the body. Being mindful of this and of* [patient's name] *current medical status, the* [equipment] *is strongly recommended as a device that will positively address many of his/her current health concerns.*

## THINK ABOUT IT 17.4

Well-written letters of medical necessity (LMNs) are essential to justify reimbursement for assistive technology devices from third-party payers. Describe at least five tips for writing a successful LMN. Companies that manufacture assistive technology devices often provide valuable resources for professionals. For example, what resources for writing an LMN to obtain a gait trainer are provided on Rifton's Web page (www.rifton.com)?

## Reimbursement Trends

The complex and ever-changing nature of our health-care system is just one of the challenges affecting a patient's ability to understand what he/she is entitled to when therapy services or assistive technology is required. The provider's ability to successfully justify funding to meet the patient's needs within the parameters of current reimbursement regulations and policy is crucial. Reimbursement trends historically have been dictated by the service delivery model (Ripat, 2005), cost of technology, training and maintenance (Ripat, 2005), efficacy (Kitchner, 2008), evidence-based research (Kitchner, 2008), and policies of the Centers for Medicare and Medicaid (CMS).

# HANDS-ON PRACTICE

1. Select an appropriate supported standing device for a particular client to meet established goals and adjust it for proper fit and alignment.
2. Compose a letter of medical necessity in consultation with a patient and caregiver(s), vendor, manufacturer, and funding source (payer).
3. Determine key features necessary on a wheelchair for a client with relatively uncomplicated needs.
4. Assess a patient in a wheelchair or other adapted seating system, making adjustments or recommendations as necessary to optimize fit and function.
5. Accurately complete the necessary measurements to determine the appropriate size of commercially available assistive technology devices for a particular patient.
6. Demonstrate and instruct others in the safe use of various devices to assist with lifting, moving, or repositioning patients.
7. Select an appropriate assistive device to support ambulation for a particular patient and demonstrate its use.

## Let's Review

1. The Technology-Related Assistance for Individuals with Disabilities Act is the major federal legislation supporting the use of assistive technology to improve the lives of people with disabilities. Which two federal legislative acts include similar provisions related to assistive technology?

2. In the Tech Act, the definition of an assistive technology device covers a broad spectrum. Can you provide examples of devices from either end of the spectrum?

**3.** The high incidence of overexertion injuries among health-care workers has focused national attention on safe patient handling and mobility standards. The greatest risk factors for injuries are manual lifting, moving, and repositioning of patients. What types of assistive technology could be used to decrease the risks associated with these tasks?

**4.** A patient arrives in your outpatient clinic with a slumped posture and posterior pelvic tilt while seated in a poorly fitted standard wheelchair. What might you want to assess and what modifications to the wheelchair might you consider to improve her seated position?

**5.** A carefully developed, well-written letter of medical necessity may make the difference in whether your patient receives needed assistive technology. What resources are available to help you?

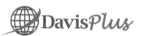 For additional resources, including Focus on Evidence tables, case study discussions, references, and glossary, please visit http://davisplus.fadavis.com

## CHAPTER SUMMARY

Assistive technology encompasses a vast array of devices and services that can promote a substantial effect on improving the function of individuals with disabilities. Research supporting clinical decision-making is expansive but of varying quality.

The effect of assistive technology devices "equates to the cost of freedom" for individuals with severe disabilities (Wallace, 1995, p. 245). Because of the potential effect of appropriately selected and fitted assistive technology devices on patients' independence, considerable federal legislation has ensured that individuals with disabilities have appropriate access. Proficiency in the application of assistive technology is a specialized professional practice, but general knowledge is essential for the entry-level practitioner so basic decisions and/or appropriate referrals can be made.

# Specific Therapeutic Intervention for Impairments of Body Structure/Body Function

## Intervention for Flaccidity and Hypotonia

Reva P. Rauk, PT, PhD, MMSc, NCS ▪ Heidi Dunfee, PT, DScPT  CHAPTER **18**

---

### CHAPTER OUTLINE

### CHAPTER OBJECTIVES

Upon completion of this chapter, the learner should be able to:

1. Describe the differences in clinical presentation between hypotonia and flaccidity.
2. Predict possible musculoskeletal problems that may be associated with hypotonia and flaccidity.
3. Describe predictors of optimal functional outcomes for individuals with hypotonia or flaccidity.
4. Explain developmental and age-related changes that may affect functional outcomes in persons with hypotonia or flaccidity.
5. Propose and plan for appropriate safety considerations in the management of hypotonia and flaccidity.
6. Choose appropriate tests and measures for a patient who displays hypotonia or flaccidity.
7. Choose appropriate supportive and protective devices for a patient who displays hypotonia or flaccidity.
8. Plan appropriate functional interventions for patients with hypotonia and flaccidity.
9. Justify appropriate use of facilitation techniques or other interventions for patients with hypotonia and flaccidity.

# ■ Introduction

*The patient is a 10 year-old with spinal muscular atrophy. This patient was born full term and weighed 6 pounds 11 ounces. At 3 months, the mother felt this child seemed "loose." What does this mean? The child was diagnosed with spinal muscular atrophy at 9 months of age. At present, she has literally no muscle tone except enough to adduct her thumb to mobilize a power wheelchair. Upon evaluation, you note the heavy, loose, floppy feeling in this child's extremities, trunk, neck, and head. This child has no functional strength in which to assist in any aspect of her mobility. Where do you begin?*

**Hypotonia** and **flaccidity**, considered variants of **muscle tone**, are impairments seen as a component of many different conditions of neuromuscular, genetic, metabolic, connective tissue, mitochondrial, or central nervous system (CNS) causes. In children, hypotonia may also be of unknown origin, termed idiopathic hypotonia or benign congenital hypotonia (BCH) (Strubhar, 2007). Muscle tone is clinically defined as the amount of tension or stiffness in a resting muscle or the amount of resistance present in a resting muscle during passive stretch (Kandel, 2013, p. 809; Hiengkaew, 2003). During passive range of motion, the limb of an individual with normal tone should feel light and move easily without resistance. With active movement, an individual with normal tone should be able to move freely and smoothly through gravity. Changes in tone, either decreased or increased from "normal," are considered atypical and are usually the result of neurological deficit. Looking beyond muscle tone within one muscle or limb, **postural tone** clinically refers to the state of muscular tension in axial musculature necessary to maintain antigravity support (Kandel, 2013, p. 936).

The terms hypotonicity and flaccidity are general with no truly objective measures available (Hunt, 2002; Leonard, 2001). Generally, hypotonia is considered to be an abnormal decrease in skeletal muscle tone, while flaccidity is considered to be the absence of muscle tone. This chapter will address hypotonia and flaccidity, from pathophysiology to examination, and present a variety of possible interventions.

## Clinical Picture of Flaccidity/Hypotonia

Flaccidity in an upper or lower extremity typically presents as a heavy floppy limb. During passive range of motion, the hypotonic limb will display diminished resistance to movement (decreased resting muscle tension) while the flaccid limb will display an absence of resistance to movement. Depending on the size of the limb (large adult versus an infant or child) the limb may actually be more difficult to move than "normal" because of the heaviness. On observation, you may see the limb in abnormal postures such as an upper extremity hanging limp alongside the body in standing or lying lifeless in a patient's lap when sitting. A lower extremity may be seen rolled out in external rotation and abduction in supine or sitting. In an infant you may see a **"frog-leg" posture** (legs flexed, externally rotated and abducted), head lag with a **pull-to-sit**, an excessively flexed spine when sitting, a **"rag-doll" posture** with ventral suspension, and on vertical suspension feeling like the infant is "slipping through your hands." With palpation, muscles will have poor definition and feel flabby or soft. Depending on the underlying condition, you may also find impaired passive range of motion (increased), joint mobility (increased laxity), sensation, proprioception, motor control, postural stability (decreased), muscle force production (decreased), coordination (decreased), deep tendon reflexes (DTR), postural reflexes, and/or the presence of **neglect** (Lesny, 1979; Martin, 2005, 2007, 2013; Schmitz, 2007). Secondary impairments may include impaired aerobic capacity and endurance (decreased activity tolerance), impaired balance, long-term changes in postural alignment, and joint instability (Martin, 2005, 2007, 2013).

## Possible Effect of Flaccidity/Hypotonia on Function

Literally all function is hampered when an extremity is flaccid or hypotonic. The possible effect on function is dependent on the severity of the hypotonia and the constellation of corresponding presentation (e.g., weakness, range of motion limitations, decreased sensation, or proprioception). Depending on the strength and sensation impairments, for example, a patient may not be able to generate enough force to lift an arm to open a door or be able to feel the arm position in space for appropriate placement on the door handle. Depending on the weakness involved, the impairments may alter an individual's ability to participate in required role activities (e.g., housekeeping, finances, car pool driving, playing, school activities, etc.). Depending on the extent of involvement, the individual may be able to learn compensatory strategies if the hypotonia and weakness become chronic, such as driving or fixing meals one-handed. A person's hobbies and leisure interests may need to be adapted to allow for participation. If a patient is unable to learn compensatory **skills** to the point of independence, the patient may need assistive or adaptive devices, environmental modification, as well as caregiver or family assistance for activities of daily living (ADL) (bathing, dressing, grooming) and other activities.

## PATIENT APPLICATION

### Patient Post-CVA

**Medical Diagnosis:** *Cerebrovascular accident (CVA)*

**Reason for Referral:** *Acute hospital neurological referral for therapy*

**History:** *John is a 56 year-old African American male with a sudden onset of a left middle cerebral artery (MCA) ischemic CVA. The medical record reveals he was at work at UPS and had initial signs of numbness and tingling in his right face, UE > LE. Upon lifting a large package, he fell to the ground where he remained unconscious. Colleagues called emergency medical services (EMS), and John was brought to the emergency room where he received tissue plasminogen activator (tPA).*

**Past Medical History:** *Type 2 Diabetes, peripheral vascular disease (PVD), hypertension (HTN)*

**Social History (per wife):** *Both John and his wife (Mary) work full time. They do not have children, and all siblings live in other parts of the United States. Even though Mary would* be able to provide care, she will be required to continue working to provide medical benefits. The couple enjoys traveling in their recreation vehicle during the summer months. John is an active bike rider, avid reader, and card player. He enjoys yard work and small machinery projects. They live in a one-story ranch style home with a two-step entrance with handrail on the right side ascending. All necessary living areas are on the main floor.

**General Status Before CVA:** John has stable diabetes with use of insulin. He has minimal numbness in his distal toes due to the PVD. He is approximately 30 pounds overweight. John also has hypertension. John was very active in his role as an UPS driver. He was independent in all ADLs and functional activities. He drove independently.

**Medications:** Diabetes: insulin (Humalog); HTN: hydrochlorothiazide

**Prior Therapies:** none

## Physical Examination
### Systems Review:

**Cardiovascular/Pulmonary:** BP 160/100; HR 72; RR 16; O₂ Sat 91%

**Integumentary:** Skin intact, slight purple discoloration of distal toes on right foot

**Neuromuscular:** Complete flaccid hemiparesis of right extremities, trunk, and face

**Musculoskeletal:** Hgt: 5'11," wt: 240; AROM WNL left side; PROM WNL right side

**Communication:** John was evaluated by speech and language pathologist and diagnosed with global aphasia affecting both motor/expressive and receptive language centers. He has a significant decrease in comprehension of spoken language and is not reliable for yes/no questions. The only automatic word this patient can speak is "yes."

**Aerobic Capacity/Endurance:** John is able to tolerate 20 to 30 minute sessions of minimal metabolic equivalents of exercise bedside in the acute hospital setting.

**Arousal, Attention, and Cognition:** John has difficulty sustaining levels of alertness for more than 30 minutes. The speech deficits challenge communication and directions for the examination and interventions. He has a right homonymous hemianopsia. At this point, John has not demonstrated any impulsive behavior or lack of judgment.

**Assistive and Adaptive Devices:** John has a hospital-issue wheelchair, 18-inch seat width, bilateral brake extensions, standard height seat, and a foam cushion.

**Range of Motion:** PROM: WNL bilaterally; AROM: WNL left side; absent right side

**Motor Function:** (as able to test due to significant communication deficits)

**Tone:** R UE: flaccid; R LE: flaccid; right facial structures drooping with drooling on the right side of mouth; in sitting, John's trunk passively flexes (severe hypotonia) and falls to the right.

**L UE/LE:** Normal tone

**Motor Control:** R UE/LE: no initiation of movement in any motion;

**L UE/LE:** Able to isolate all movements: initiate, sustain, and grade appropriately.

**Muscle Performance:** R UE/LE: 0/5; R trunk: 1/5
**L UE/LE/trunk:** 5/5

**Reflex Integrity:** R UE/LE: 1/4 (decreased but present)

**Sensory Integrity:** (Difficult to assess due to communication deficits)

**Light Touch/Sharp/Dull:** No response from John with any sensory stimuli to the R UE/LE; he is able to inconsistently respond with a facial expression when having sharp stimuli to the left side.

**Proprioception:** Unable to determine due to John's communication deficits

**Posture:** Sitting Balance/Postural Control: John requires maximal assistance ×2 to transition from supine to sidelying to sitting.

**Posture in Sitting:** Head flexed and rotated to the left; scapular depression; RUE is not utilized for any component of balance; trunk passively shortened to the right; excess passive weight-bearing on the right hip; posterior pelvic tilt; and, absent equilibrium reactions. John will fall to the right if unsupported >5 seconds.

**Gait/Locomotion/Balance:** John is unable to stand or ambulate at this time. Initial attempt at standing required maximum assistance of two people with complete control of the hip, knee, and trunk for support.

### Self-Care/Functional Skills:

**Bed Positioning/Bed Mobility:** John is unable to assist or follow commands for bed positioning and bed mobility. He attempts to use his L UE/LE to roll but is unsuccessful.

**Transfers:** Low pivot transfer (to R and L) with maximal assistance ×2 or sliding board for caregivers with limited lifting capacity.

**Bowel/Bladder:** John has a catheter and wears an adult brief.

## Contemplate Clinical Decisions

When working with patients like John with hypotonia, it is important to contemplate the continuum of care and the outcomes of function as a result of the hypotonicity and motor control status.

1. What is the distribution of supply for the L MCA? What outcomes would be expected? Does John's presentation match what you would expect? Why or why not?
2. List the risk factors and precautions present in this case in terms of management of hypotonia.
3. Describe how you would assess available passive, active assisted (facilitated), and active range of motion in a patient with hypotonia.
4. Develop a problem list of body structure impairments with resultant functional activity limitations for John.
5. Identify John's assets.
6. Describe how you would assess cognition, arousal, and judgment in a patient with global aphasia. What physical actions may help qualify this status?
7. What equipment projections do you have based on the initial case scenario?

8. Describe John's responses, posturing, and actions that may help objectively support the sensory status.
9. Can you predict possible secondary musculoskeletal problems with a patient presenting with significant hypotonia?
10. Design a plan of care to help prevent these issues from occurring in the future.
11. Consider the care of this younger patient John whose wife Mary continues to need to be in the workforce yet wants to take her husband home. How does this stroke affect their socialization, finances, home management, etc.?
12. What quality of life issues can you address?

## Safety Considerations

In early stages of the care of any patient with hypotonia, it is important to examine the laxity about each joint structure during any movement transition that includes an increased risk of traction injury. If the patient has decreased (or absent) sensory status and speech deficits, it may not be possible to vocalize any discomfort if improperly positioned, if left in a position too long so as to cause skin breakdown, if limbs are inappropriately handled or pulled on by caregivers or family members, or if limbs are left to hang unsupported. A patient may also be at risk for injury from such items as sharp objects and hot food or liquids. Due to the hypotonic state of the limb muscles, a patient is not only unable to mobilize away from a noxious stimulus but may not be able to sense the injury due to sensory deficits. The continued state of hypotonia will worsen **joint laxity** and contribute to a passive gravity-dependent range limitation, which may increase joint effusion.

Awareness of the lack of equilibrium responses is important for all caregivers. In the example of the patient case previously discussed, due to the weakened state of all right-sided musculature, John is also at high risk for falls. Due to the global aphasia, he would most likely not be able to communicate a fall to a caregiver. Safeguards must be put in place to protect John from a fall, which could significantly damage the hypotonic limbs as they would not be in a position to support his body. Table 18-1 lists possible safety considerations for individuals with hypotonia.

## ▉ Related Pathology

### Neuroanatomy of Common Pathology

The resting tone of a muscle is influenced by both the neural drive to the muscle (generated by the impulse activity of the muscle spindle 1a afferents) and the mechanical elastic properties of the muscle itself (Kandel, 2013, p. 809; Leonard, 2001). Several components or points along the length of the nervous system play a role in the control of muscle tone as illustrated in Figure 6-1: brainstem and cerebral cortex; cerebellum; basal ganglia; descending pathways; anterior horn cell; peripheral nerve; neuromuscular junction; and the muscle itself. The cerebellum helps to maintain normal muscle tone. Damage to any of these structures and interneurons may result in a decrease in muscle

| TABLE 18-1 | Safety Considerations for Hypotonia |
|---|---|
| **SAFETY CONSIDERATIONS FOR HYPOTONIA** | |
| Head/neck | • Swallowing difficulties leading to choking and aspiration<br>• Excessive flexion/extension |
| Shoulder girdle | • Joint/ligamentous laxity<br>• Careful handling to prevent damage to joint<br>• Subluxation<br>• Range of motion limitations secondary to lack of voluntary movement<br>• Pain |
| Trunk | • Balance and equilibrium reactions absent or decreased<br>• Poor breathing<br>• Poor posture control |
| Hip and knee | • Instability during transfers and gait<br>• Joint laxity leading to pain<br>• Hip subluxation or dislocation |
| Ankle/foot | • Instability during transfers and gait<br>• Joint laxity leading to pain and/or contractures |
| Overall | • If sensation is compromised: Inability to move a limb in reaction to noxious stimuli<br>• Risk for falls<br>• Joint integrity<br>• Skin breakdown due to immobility<br>• Contractures due to immobility |

tone (Bodensteiner, 2008; Crawford, 1992). Because the normal muscle tone is conveyed through the anterior horn cells and its axons, conditions such as polio or spinal muscular atrophy will cause hypotonia if only a portion of the anterior horn cells to the muscle group are damaged or flaccidity if nearly all anterior horn cells to the muscle group are damaged.

## Hypotonia/Flaccidity in Neuromuscular Diagnoses

Hypotonicity and flaccidity are impairments noted with many different conditions of neuromuscular, genetic, metabolic, connective tissue, mitochondrial, or CNS origin. Systems involved may include the voluntary and involuntary motor, sensory, and endocrine systems. Genetic disorders that are congenital may particularly affect any one of these systems with hypotonia as a resultant impairment. Charcot-Marie Tooth, a genetic demyelinating neuropathy, affects the voluntary motor system. One must consider the underlying cause of the hypotonicity and the anatomic site of the pathology when choosing a plan of care. When considering the neural drive to the muscle, is the cause of the hypotonicity of central or peripheral origin (i.e., cortex, basal ganglia, brainstem, cerebellum, descending pathways versus anterior horn cell, peripheral nerve, neuromuscular junction)? For example, muscular dystrophy is a muscle disorder of genetic origin, and spinal muscular atrophy is a genetic disorder affecting the anterior horn cell. Depending on the disorder, hypotonia may be global in nature (generally the same degree throughout the body as in Down syndrome [DS]) or present in one body area (e.g., unilateral extremity in stroke or cerebral palsy [CP]). Table 18-2 lists examples of pathologies and medical diagnoses in which hypotonia may be an impairment.

## Lifespan Influences

### Developmental Considerations

Often children with hypotonic disorders are not clearly identified until they do not achieve developmental milestones such as reaching, pulling to sit, head control, rolling, and sitting. At this time caregivers and medical personnel may identify an infant/child as "floppy," weak, clumsy, or low-toned (Jacobson, 1998). Outcomes of further examination may result in diagnoses such as CP, DS, or BCH to state a few (Jacobson, 1998). The neurological examination may identify hypotonia, decreased strength, absent or decreased DTR, exercise fatigue, and laxity about joints (Crawford, 1992). Consideration of interventions to promote postural control and gross motor

skills may be crucial to promote function and decrease negative outcomes of hypotonia (Cohen, 1998).

### Age-Related Changes

Natural aging of human systems can compromise functional activities in relation to hypotonia on many levels (Lewis, 2007). As aging occurs, muscle activation and recruitment speed is decreased, therefore causing a significant slowing of body movement. This coupled with hypotonia can present difficulties in functional tasks such as transfers, feeding, self-care, and ambulation. The human body also becomes less flexible with age and has noted soft tissue changes in muscle fibers and typically an increase in percent body fat ratios. These changes lead to a decreased ability to initiate, sustain, and grade muscle movement and manage a heavier limb due to both the actual percent body fat and also perceived weight of a hypotonic limb or trunk. Finally the recovery time for CNS healing after insult will also increase with age, which in turn may significantly limit the maximum outcomes achieved (Lewis, 2007). Age-related changes with diagnoses that include long-term hypotonia such as hemiparesis, Guillian Barré, and spinal cord injury (SCI) may include secondary issues of skin breakdown due to immobility of limbs, weight gain due to decreased endurance and decreased exercise tolerance, symptoms of complex regional pain

| TABLE 18-2 | Examples of Pathologies/Medical Diagnoses and Cause According to Anatomic Location | |
| --- | --- | --- |
| **ANATOMIC SITE** | **COMMON PATHOLOGIES/MEDICAL DIAGNOSES** | **CAUSE** |
| *Peripheral Origin* | | |
| Muscle | Congenital myopathy | Genetic |
| | Metabolic myopathy | Metabolic |
| | Muscular dystrophy | Genetic |
| | Myotonic dystrophy | Genetic |
| Neuromuscular junction | Myasthenia gravis | Autoimmune |
| | Congenital myasthenic syndromes | Genetic |
| | Botulism | Botulinum toxin (food) |
| | Eaton-Lambert syndrome | Autoimmune |
| Nerve | Charcot-Marie Tooth | Genetic |
| | Demyelinating neuropathies | Varied (infections, metabolic, immune, drugs, etc.) |
| | Acute inflammatory demyelinating polyneuropathy (AIDP), chronic inflammatory demyelinating polyneuropathy (CIDP) | Autoimmune |
| | Toxic neuropathies | Toxins |
| | Dejerine-Sottas disease | Genetic |
| | Focal nerve entrapment, compression, inflammation, ischemia | Varied (trauma, arthritis, etc.) |
| Anterior horn cell | Spinal muscular atrophy (e.g., Werdnig-Hoffmann disease) | Genetic |
| | Poliomyelitis | Viral; vaccine |
| | Arthrogryposis | Genetic |
| | Mobius syndrome | Genetic |
| | Syringomyelia | Trauma, Chiari I malformation |
| | Intrinsic cord tumor | Genetic (neurofibromatosis), unknown etiology |

*Continued*

| TABLE 18-2 | Examples of Pathologies/Medical Diagnoses and Cause According to Anatomic Location—cont'd | |
|---|---|---|
| **ANATOMIC SITE** | **COMMON PATHOLOGIES/MEDICAL DIAGNOSES** | **CAUSE** |
| *Central Origin* | | |
| Spinal cord | Tumor | Unknown etiology; genetic |
| | Epidural hematoma | Trauma |
| | Epidural abscess | Infection |
| | Transverse myelitis | Varied (idiopathic, parainfectious, immune, etc.) |
| | Tethered cord | Abnormal fetal development, trauma |
| | Traumatic spinal cord injury (SCI) | Trauma |
| | Spina bifida | Abnormal fetal development |
| Cortex, basal ganglia, cerebellum | Infarction | Ischemia of varied causes |
| | Trauma | Trauma |
| | Hemorrhage | Trauma, AV malformation, high blood pressure |
| | Tumor | Idiopathic |
| | Chromosomal disorders | Genetic |
| |    Down syndrome | |
| |    Prader-Willi Syndrome | |
| |    Noonan Syndrome | |
| | Metabolic disorders | Metabolic |
| |    Hypothyroidism | |
| |    Methemoglobinemia | |
| | Leukodystrophies | Genetic |
| | Brain dysgenesis | Abnormal development |
| | Dandy-Walker malformation | Genetic |
| | Joubert syndrome | Genetic |
| | Lissencephaly | Abnormal development |
| | Cerebral palsy | Abnormal development, perinatal hypoxia |
| | Autism spectrum disorders | Developmental disorder |
| | Sensory integration dysfunction | Developmental disorder |
| | Attention deficit disorder (ADD)/Attention deficit hyperactivity disorder (ADHD) | Developmental disorder; genetic |

(Bodensteiner, 2008; Crawford, 1992; Harris, 2008; Jacobson, 1998)

syndrome, and possibly joint subluxations or dislocations. Considerations of such possible outcomes should be addressed in the continuum of long-term management of older individuals.

## ■ Pertinent Examination/Evaluation

### Tests and Measures

A precise quantifiable measure of hypotonia is lacking. Wilson-Howle (1999) reported the use of a tone assessment scale for children with CP that includes "mild, moderate, and severe" categories of hypotonicity based on a description of both resistance to passive movement and constraints on the child's active movement (Table 18-3). Reliability and validity of the scale was not offered. Common tests used in infants to assess low tone include the pull-to-sit, the scarf sign, shoulder suspension, and vertical suspension (Table 18-3) (Bodensteiner,

2008; Malerba, 2013; Martin, 2007). The therapist observes the infant's response during each maneuver. Based on these observations alone, it is difficult to determine whether the underlying cause of the movement problem is from both hypotonia and muscle weakness or only hypotonia (Bodensteiner, 2008; Reus, 2013). Reus and colleagues (2013) developed the Infant Muscle Strength meter (IMS-meter), a method for quantifying muscle strength in infants and toddlers (ages 6 to 36 months). The test measures the maximal force an infant spontaneously uses to pull on a desirable object. Both typically developing infants and children with Prader-Willi Syndrome (PWS) were tested to determine the reliability and convergent validity of the test. Interrater reliability of the IMS-meter was good (ICC = .84), and the correlation between the IMS-meter and the Bayley Scale of Infant Development, second edition, in infants with PWS was strong ($p<.001$, r = .75). Further research is needed with other patient groups exhibiting hypotonia and muscle weakness.

**TABLE 18-3** | **Key Tests/Measures of Hypotonia**

### KEY TESTS/MEASURES OF HYPOTONIA—ADULT

| Test | Typical Test Results Seen in Hypotonia |
|---|---|
| Passive Range of Motion:<br>Assess level of resistance to passive muscle elongation and stretch | • Abnormal lack of resistance to passive movement<br>• Heaviness of the limb/body part, especially with larger sized limbs<br>• A feeling of being able to be moved too freely with increased ROM more than normal |
| Observation:<br>Observe posture in various positions and size/shape of individual muscles | • UE: May see hanging limp at the side of the body, or lying "lifeless" in lap<br>• LE: May be rolled out into external rotation when in supine or in abduction and external rotation when in sitting<br>• May see muscle wasting or atrophy; joint deformity |
| Palpation | • Muscles have poor definition<br>• Muscles feel flabby, soft |

### KEY TESTS/MEASURES OF HYPOTONIA—PEDIATRIC

| Test | Typical Test Results Seen in Hypotonia |
|---|---|
| Observation:<br>Responses to several maneuvers useful in detecting low tone:<br>• *Pull-to-sit* (with the infant in supine, grasp the hands and gently pull to sitting)<br>• *Scarf sign* (with the infant in supine, grasp one hand and pull across the chest as far as it will go without significant resistance)<br>• *Shoulder suspension* (pick up the infant holding under the arms)<br><br>• *Vertical suspension* (in prone, the infant is lifted off the surface with one hand under the chest and abdomen)<br><br><br>• *French angles factor of the INFANIB* (Ellison, 1985)<br>  • Scarf sign<br>  • Heel-to-ear (grasp infant's ankle and lift foot toward ear)<br>  • Popliteal angle (grasping legs at the knees, extend knees)<br>  • Leg abduction | • Head lag<br>  (a head lag is normal in a newborn but disappears at about 2 months of age)<br>• The elbow can be brought well beyond midline<br>  (normally the elbow can be brought to midline)<br><br>• Infant tends to slip through the therapist's hands<br>  (normally, the infant displays some head control and provides some resistance in the shoulders when being lifted)<br>• Infant hangs draped over the hand with the legs, arms, and head in a dependent position (rag doll)<br>  (normally, legs and arms will be in some flexion and will be able to maintain the head above horizontal)<br><br><br>• As previously discussed<br>• Movement results in very small angle between hip and trunk with heel at or near ear<br>• Note angle of knee flexion—see decreased knee flexion (increased extension)<br><br>• Legs abducted and externally rotated in a "frog leg" position with wide angle between legs |
| Palpation | • Muscles have poor definition<br>• Muscles feel flabby, soft |
| Passive and active movement<br>(Wilson-Howle, 1999) | −3 = Severe hypotonia<br>Active movement is characterized by:<br>  • Inability to move through gravity<br>  • Inability to cocontract proximally for stability<br>  • Apparent weakness<br>Passive movement is characterized by:<br>  • No resistance to passive movement<br>  • Full or excessive PROM<br>  • Joint hyperextensibility<br>−2 = Moderate hypotonia |

*Continued*

| TABLE 18-3 | Key Tests/Measures of Hypotonia—cont'd |
|---|---|

**KEY TESTS/MEASURES OF HYPOTONIA—PEDIATRIC**

| Test | Typical Test Results Seen in Hypotonia |
|---|---|
| | Active movement is characterized by:<br>• Decreased tone in axial and proximal muscles<br>• Ability to sustain postures is limited<br>Passive movement is characterized by:<br>• Little resistance to passive movement, especially at proximal joints<br>• Knee and ankle joint hyperextensibility when weight-bearing<br>−1 = Mild hypotonia<br>Active movement is characterized by:<br>• Decreased ability to cocontract axial muscles<br>• Delayed initiation of movement against gravity<br>• Slowed speed of postural movement adjustments<br>Passive movement is characterized by:<br>• Mild resistance to passive movement<br>• Full PROM<br>• Hand, ankle, and foot joint hyperextensibility<br>0 = Normal tone<br>+1 to +3 = Mild, moderate, and severe hypertonicity<br>IT = Intermittent tone<br>Active movement is characterized by:<br>• Occasional/unpredictable resistance to position changes, alternating between normal adjustment or a lack of resistance<br>• Difficult initiation of movement or sustaining a posture against gravity<br>• Sudden collapse of posture/position<br>Passive movement is characterized by:<br>• Unpredictable resistance to passive movement, alternating with absence of resistance |

The Modified Ashworth Scale (Gregson, 2000) is one measure commonly used to examine tone; however this measure only quantifies increased tone or hypertonicity. A score of zero on the scale is defined as "no increase in muscle tone" and equates to normal tone, not hypotonicity (refer to Chapters 6 and 19 for information on the assessment and treatment of hypertonicity). So the scale should not be used for muscles that exhibit hypotonia. The most commonly used measures to directly test hypotonia include passive range of motion, observation, and palpation (Table 18-3).

Various additional tests and measures may be used to:

■ Gain an overall picture of the individual's motor control
■ Identify the potential cause of the hypotonia (central versus peripheral source) (Table 18-4)
■ Assess impairments often seen along with hypotonia (Table 18-5)

## THINK ABOUT IT 18.1

■ What equipment would you suggest for use with John related to his hypotonia?
■ For what purpose are you using the equipment? For protection? Compensation? Remediation?
■ How does cognition play into the equipment decision process?

## Expected Outcomes and Prognostic Factors

Outcome predictions in relation to hypotonia can be challenging for both pediatric and adult populations. Attention must focus on the extent and location of the insult or lesion, the physical therapy diagnosis, the prognosis, the age of onset, and the severity of involvement to other systems. Hypotonia affects functional outcomes differently depending on its severity, the constellation of other impairments the individual may have, and the overall prognosis of the underlying disease process. The hypotonia may be more global in nature (DS) versus affecting a specific body region (stroke). It may also be a mild symptom of a comprehensive disorder such as that associated with autism, ADD/ADHD, or sensory integration disorder. Hypotonia may also be part of a progressive disorder (e.g., amyotrophic lateral sclerosis [ALS]) as well as a major impairment of a more complex problem (e.g., stroke, SCI).

Outcome analysis for the diagnosis of BCH describes recovery within the first 2 years of birth; however residual neurological symptoms noted as mild deficits included continued hypotonia, clumsy gait, speech delay, and decreased gross motor function (Strubhar, 2007). Pediatric physical therapists have identified several factors that appear to have the greatest effect on motor outcomes: primary impairments, secondary impairments, personal characteristics, and the family (Bartlett,

| TABLE 18-4 | Tests for Discerning Cause of Hypotonia (Central Versus Peripheral Origin) | |
|---|---|---|
| **TEST** | **CENTRAL** | **PERIPHERAL** |
| Muscle strength or force production (presence of weakness?) *Adult*: Manual Muscle Test (MMT) (Wadsworth, 1987) *Child*: MMT if appropriate given age; or indirect assessment of strength (e.g., lack of force generation with pull-to-sit or lack of normal resistance in shoulders during vertical suspension) *Infant Muscle Strength meter* (Reus, 2013) | Weakness is not always present with hypotonia; may have a hypotonic muscle but be strong (e.g., hypotonia caused by deep cerebellar nucleus involvement; deep tendon reflexes are diminished and the muscle feels flabby but there is no motor weakness) (Kandel, 2013) | Significant weakness (paralysis) Atrophy |
| Deep tendon reflexes | Decreased or increased | Absent |
| Postural reflexes, righting and equilibrium responses | Sluggish, slow, or absent (more often sluggish or slow, but may be absent in severe presentations of some neurological conditions, e.g., stroke, spinal cord injury) | Absent |
| Placing reactions | Sluggish or slow | Absent |
| Motor control/coordination (several tests available—see Table 18-5) | Antigravity movements-impaired | Antigravity movements-impaired to absent |

| TABLE 18-5 | Additional Tests and Measures Used in Assessing Impairments Often Seen Along With Hypotonia |
|---|---|
| **IMPAIRMENT** | **TESTS AND MEASURES (NOT A PRIORITIZED, NOR AN EXHAUSTIVE LIST)** |
| Aerobic capacity/ endurance | Blood pressure Heart rate Baseline Dyspnea Index (Mahler, 1988) Oxygen saturation—pulse oximetry Perceived exertion—Borg Scale (Dunbar, 1992) |
| Joint integrity and mobility | Joint mobility in the spine, rib cage, and limbs. Note if joint laxity is present (Beighton, 1983; Pilon, 2000) 0 = normal 1 = hypermobile • Elbow extension—passive hyperextension more than 5 degrees when shoulder flexed to 90 degrees • Knee extension—passive hyperextension to more than 10 degrees with hip slightly flexed • Thumb to wrist—passive apposition of the tip of thumb to volar aspect of forearm while shoulder and elbow flexed to 90 degrees • Fifth metacarpophalangeal extension—passive hyperextension to more than 90 degrees |
| Motor function | Motor Assessment Scale (MAS) for Stroke (Carr, 1985) Fugl-Meyer Assessment (Fugl-Meyer, 1975) Trunk Impairment Scale (Verheyden, 2004) Alberta Infant Motor Scale (Piper, 1992) Gross Motor Function Measure (Russell, 2002) Motor Assessment of Infants (Chandler, 1980) Peabody Developmental Motor Scales II (Folio, 2000) Test of Infant Motor Performance (Campbell, 1999; Finkel, 2008) |
| Pain | Numerical Rating Scale, Verbal Rating Scale, Visual Analog Scale (Berthier, 1998) |
| Reflex integrity | Postural reflexes, equilibrium, and **righting reactions** Composite Spasticity Scale (Chan, 1986) Motor Assessment of Infants (Chandler, 1980) |

*Continued*

| **TABLE 18-5**    Additional Tests and Measures Used in Assessing Impairments Often Seen Along With Hypotonia—cont'd | |
| --- | --- |
| **IMPAIRMENT** | **TESTS AND MEASURES (NOT A PRIORITIZED, NOR AN EXHAUSTIVE LIST)** |
| Sensory integrity | Light touch |
| | Sharp/dull |
| | Pressure |
| | Proprioception—appreciation of movement, direction of movement, and joint position sense |
| | Wrist Position Sense Test (Carey, 1996) |
| | Sensory integration/weighting CTSIB (Di Fabio, 1990) |
| | Rivermead Assessment of Somatosensory Performance (RASP) (Winward, 2002) |
| | Visuo-spatial neglect |
| | Bells Test (Gauthier, 1989) |
| | Rivermead Behavioral Inattention Test (RBIT) (Wilson, 1987) |
| | Bodily neglect (Bisiach, 1986) (Azouvi, 1996) |

2002). Tone and qualitative aspects of the movement disorder were listed as the top primary impairments affecting motor outcomes. Possible secondary impairments as a result of low muscle tone and joint hypermobility include patellar subluxation, hip subluxation/dislocation, and atlanto-axial subluxation for children with DS.

Prediction of motor recovery poststroke with a primary symptom of hypotonia has been reported to be associated with a poor outcome if there is a lack of voluntary motor control of the leg within the first week and no noticeable arm movements at 4 weeks (Kwakkel, 2003). Outcomes were measured at 6 months based on the Fugl-Meyer Assessment of Motor Recovery (Kwakkel, 2003). Prediction of motor recovery for individuals with SCI can be found in Chapter 26.

### PATIENT APPLICATION

*In the original case of John who has a primary symptom of hyptonia, it is crucial to prioritize the examination tests and measures to ensure the therapist will be able to quantify John's ability to mobilize in any position. Primary tests and measures should include positional assessments of range of motion, muscle tone, motor control, and sensation (to include light touch, sharp/dull, and joint proprioception). Test and measure outcomes will direct the therapist's ongoing assessment and the plan of care to identify functional goals.*

### Contemplate Clinical Decisions

1. *In this case, what specific tests and measures would you select? Why?*
2. *Can you quantify the available joint range of motion in terms of passive, active, and active assistive?*
3. *Does the state of hypotonia change when you alter John's position?*
4. *Describe muscle activation in terms of movement initiation, sustaining movement, grading movement, and terminating movement.*
5. *Based on assessment of the hypotonic status, what interventions and functional activities would be beneficial to increase muscle tone?*

6. *How do you incorporate tone-building strategies into the treatment plan when sensation is compromised?*
7. *Would you instruct John in compensation techniques? If so, when would you do so and what would they be? If not, why?*

## ■ Preparatory Intervention Specific to Flaccidity/Hypotonia

### General Approaches

#### General Therapeutic Approaches

The clinician will need to consider the patient's goals, muscle force production available in the trunk and extremities, and motor control to determine whether intervention will focus on compensation or recovery. Refer to Chapters 14 and 15 for a more detailed discussion on general approaches to management of the neurological patient/client. As described in Chapter 15, interventions may be chosen based on the patient's stage of motor control. Given the weakness and impaired motor control typically coupled with flaccidity/hypotonia, beginning at the **mobility** and/or **stability** stage of motor control may be most appropriate for a remediation focus. A patient with trace voluntary movement may benefit from **facilitation techniques** or **neuromuscular electrical stimulation** (NMES) to increase muscle activity. Several strategies for initiating muscle activity are given in subsequent sections. An individual with low tone and significant weakness who may not be able to sit independently or maintain an upper or lower extremity in a functional weight-bearing position may benefit from interventions focused on stability. Refer to Chapter 35 for trunk and sitting intervention ideas. Throughout treatment, the therapist should continue to integrate functional tasks within the environment, emphasizing the implementation of task-oriented and systems model philosophies. Some examples include requiring variability of practice by altering the environment (e.g., open versus closed, stable versus dynamic), choosing appropriate task challenge (e.g., task choice, speed, direction), and ensuring patient motivation through meaningful goal-directed activities.

Compensatory strategies may be needed for a patient at risk for injury or secondary impairments because of the hypotonia or flaccidity. Strategies may include assistive devices, wheelchairs, bracing, other equipment to support a flaccid limb or trunk, or learning to adapt without using the impaired limb. Equipment examples include the use of a sling or shoulder support for the upper extremity, an ankle foot orthosis for the lower extremity, or a wheelchair for mobility. Compensatory strategies would also include family training to prevent injury or falls such as safe transfer techniques and appropriate handling of a flaccid upper extremity. In the patient who has hypotonicity or flaccidity from an acute injury, often both compensation and remediation strategies are used during the same time period. A patient may need support for a subluxed shoulder when not in therapy or a wrist-hand splint to maintain range of motion during the night. During the day the patient may be treated with NMES (Alon, 2007) to increase motor activity.

### Equipment

Equipment is often used for support and injury prevention. A few examples of equipment are identified in Table 18-6. For more detail, refer to Chapters 17 and 33 in this text.

| TABLE 18-6 Supportive and Protective Devices | |
| --- | --- |
| **DEVICE** | **PURPOSE/BENEFITS** |
| Wrist/hand splints | Maintain range of motion<br>Prevent increased joint laxity<br>Stabilize wrist for improved mobility/function of fingers |
| **Shoulder slings**/supports<br>(Ada, 2005; Brooke, 1991; Dieruf, 2005; Williams, 1988; Zorowitz, 1995) | Prevent soft tissue stretching (capsule, ligaments)<br>Relieve pressure on neurovascular elements<br>Decrease subluxation<br>Improve shoulder and scapular alignment (if adequately addressed by sling) |
| Tabletop support<br>(May be a table, bedside table, pillow, or devices that attach to the wheelchair, i.e., full or half lap tray, arm trough) | Decrease postural asymmetries<br>Support a flaccid UE in sitting<br>Prevent shoulder subluxation<br>* Need to monitor to prevent overcorrection of a subluxation |

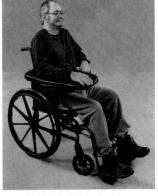
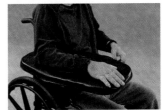
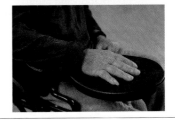

*Continued*

| TABLE 18-6 | Supportive and Protective Devices—cont'd |
| --- | --- |
| **DEVICE** | **PURPOSE/BENEFITS** |
| Lateral guard to keep the arm on lap tray or pillow | Prevent arm from falling off wheelchair lap tray or off the side of the wheelchair where the hand could get caught in the brake or wheel spokes, or elbow could get hit as the patient passes through a doorway. |
| Compression glove | Decrease edema in the dependent upper extremity |
| LE orthoses<br>Ankle-foot orthosis (AFO) or knee-ankle-foot orthosis (KAFO) if knee strength too weak to use an AFO | Provide knee and ankle support during standing and walking; provide proper alignment as a foundation for optimal bone modeling in growing infants and children<br>Prevent knee hyperextension<br>Maintain range of motion |
| Swedish knee cage | Prevent knee hyperextension |
| Abdominal binder | Trunk support in sitting<br>Decrease postural hypotension<br>Improve respiratory status |
| Gait assistive devices | Provide weight-bearing support during gait<br>Improve gait independence<br>Improve postural alignment |

## THINK ABOUT IT 18.2

- Thinking about our patient, what tests and measures were completed to give you a picture of John's hypotonia?
- What measures could have been completed to provide more objective measures and change of John's hypotonia?
- How often would you assess the tone status?

Debate in the literature exists on the positives and negatives of using shoulder supports/slings for patients with **shoulder (glenohumeral) subluxation** (Ada, 2005; Boyd, 1999; Brooke, 1991; Dieruf, 2005; Williams, 1988; Zorowitz, 1995). Subluxation is typically seen in the early stages poststroke when the patient's limb is flaccid or hypotonic. With the lack of muscle tone, poor or absent sensation and proprioception, and significant weakness, the shoulder remains reliant on the joint capsule and ligaments for support (scapular depression and downward rotation combined with humeral flexion or abduction can result in joint subluxation). Several types of shoulder supports/slings exist on the market, all claiming to reduce shoulder subluxation. According to Zorowitz (1995) and others (Ada, 2005; Brooke, 1991; Dieruf, 2005; Williams, 1988), controversy exists as to which type of sling provides the best

reduction of shoulder subluxation and even whether or not the slings are effective enough in consistently reducing the subluxation.

Traditional **single-strap hemislings** keep the arm supported in an adducted, internally rotated, and elbow-flexed position (Figure 18-1A-B). Continued use of this type of sling over a long period of time could result in limited range of motion and contractures in these positions. Having the arm held next to the body also limits the arm from any spontaneous movement or use in balance strategies as well as may increase neglect of the arm.

A **humeral cuff sling** provides support through a cuff around the humerus combined with a figure-8 harness. This support allows the arm to be free-hanging, therefore not limiting voluntary or spontaneous distal movement. Compared with the Bobath shoulder roll and the single-strap hemisling, the Roylan humeral cuff best reduced the total symmetry of the glenohumeral subluxation but did not result in complete correction (Zorowitz, 1995).

The **GivMohr sling**[1] for both adults and children use a figure-8 strap connected to two elastic straps (one anterior and one posterior) that run down the arm, cross at the dorsal

---

[1]*www.givmohrsling.com*

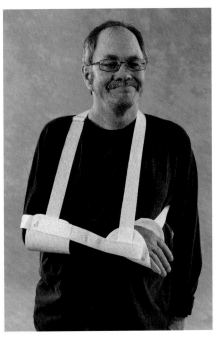

**FIGURE 18-1A** Traditional arm sling, front view.

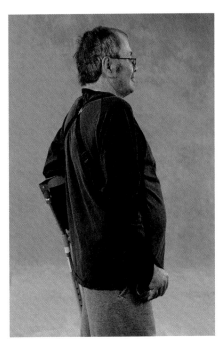

**FIGURE 18-1C** GivMohr sling.

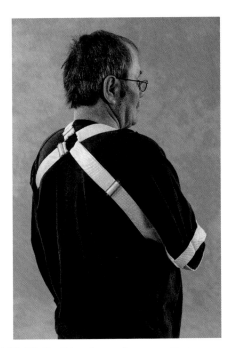

**FIGURE 18-1B** Traditional arm sling, rear view.

aspect of the wrist, and end in a palmar roll (Figure 18-1C). When fit correctly, the sling positions the shoulder in slight abduction and external rotation, the elbow in extension and the wrist in neutral.[1] This functional positioning allows for voluntary or spontaneous movement (e.g., arm swing) as well as subluxation reduction. Compared with the Roylan humeral cuff, the GivMohr sling provided the best subluxation reduction (Dieruf, 2005).

Slings or other forms of shoulder support should be used during upright activities such as standing, transfers, and gait

training when there is increased gravitational pull on the shoulder. Slings keeping the arm in an adducted internally rotated and elbow-flexed position should be used sparingly and during short bouts of upright activity due to the risks of contractures, loss of spontaneous balance control, and positioning that may possibly feed into unwanted abnormal synergy patterns.

## Therapeutic Techniques

### Positioning and Handling Considerations

Proper positioning and handling of a hypotonic extremity or trunk is essential in the management of joint integrity, mobility, and the prevention of contractures. Care must be given to identify the correct biomechanics of any given structure to then proceed to apply positioning and handling tactics ensuring the motion is not causing impingement, effusion, pain, and/or joint stress. Table 18-7 describes suggested positioning for hypotonia and flaccidity.

### Range of Motion

Management of joint integrity through passive, active assistive, and active range of motion are of utmost importance to facilitate muscle recruitment, blood flow, sensory and proprioceptive awareness, and to further prevent complications secondary to immobility and aging. All levels of range of motion intervention should focus on correct technique with careful identification of proper handling and motions available at any given joint structure. Joints should not be overstretched, pulled on by caregivers, or positioned so the patient cannot independently move the limb out of a compromised position. In a study involving patients poststroke, use of continuous passive motion (CPM) resulted in no significant differences in motor impairment, disability, pain, or tone; however CPM patients demonstrated a positive trend

| TABLE 18-7 | Suggestions for Positioning for Hypotonia and Flaccidity (De Jong, 2006) |
|---|---|
| Supine | Pillow support for UEs in a nonabnormal flexion synergistic position<br>Elevation of limbs to decrease effusion<br>Ankle support by identified system to prevent foot drop<br>Pillow support to prevent ER of LEs<br>Head, neck, trunk in midline<br>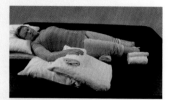 |
| Sidelying | Scapular protraction; UE ER, flexion, abduction; elbow extension; wrist neutral; forearm supination<br>LE hip neutral rotation and ABD/adduction, flexion; knee flexion; neutral ankle<br>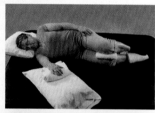<br>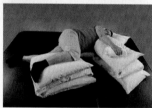 |
| Sitting | UEs supported on tabletop, wheelchair support device<br>LEs supported on leg rests and footplates with hips at 90 degrees and neutral rotation; elevated if swelling is apparent<br>(See Tabletop Supports in Table 18-6) |
| Standing | UEs supported by a sling or shoulder apparatus if necessary, including when the dependent arm position is causing pain<br>UEs supported on an elevated bedside table or standing frame |

promote, and stimulate more normal postural alignment, motor control, and functional extremity use. Key opportunities for weight-bearing must reflect the prognosis and outcomes of the identified diagnosis. For example, weight-bearing on a flaccid UE poststroke would attempt to facilitate muscle activation and functional movement. Weight-bearing on a LE postchronic complete SCI would serve a purpose of osteoporosis prevention and circulatory stimulation. Weight-bearing with proper alignment (perhaps assured with use of supramalleolar orthoses) may promote improved muscle activity and foot control by decreasing excessive joint range of motion during standing and gait in individuals with DS (Selby-Silverstein, 2001).

Interventions to promote muscle activation in upper extremities include weight-bearing on a stabilized hand. The position of the involved UE is lateral to the body in shoulder abduction, external rotation, elbow extension, wrist extension, and finger extension (Figure 18-2). Care must be taken to support each joint in the extremity to prevent hyperextension at the elbow or superior subluxation of the shoulder. Facilitation tactics can be applied to promote initiation of muscle activity (see Facilitation Techniques in the following text) and the ability to hold in a weight-bearing position.

Weight-bearing activities can be incorporated into positions such as prone on elbows, modified plantigrade, quadruped, and standing (Figure 18-3). The caregiver must identify key points of control to enhance stability around the joint, allowing for weight to pass through to the surface below and accomplish **joint approximation**.

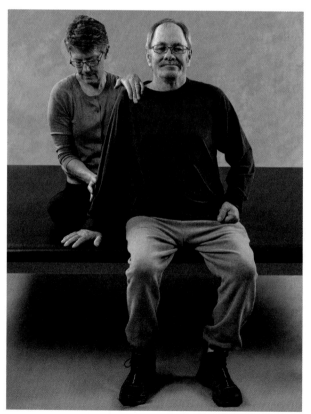

**FIGURE 18-2** Weight-bearing through impaired right upper extremity in sitting.

toward improved shoulder joint stability (*p* = .06) (Lynch, 2005). Identifying issues of pain, heterotopic bone ossification, and compromised sensory systems all play a part in the management and integration of range of motion activities.

## Weight-bearing

Integrated into positioning, handling, and range of motion techniques is the concept of **weight-bearing** to enhance,

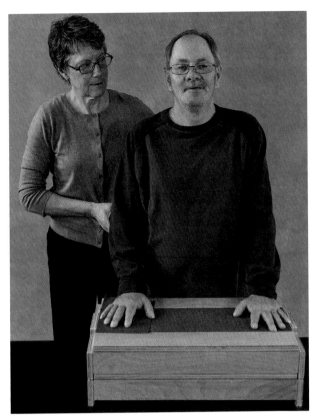

FIGURE 18-3 Weight-bearing through impaired right upper extremity in standing at a high surface.

Higher skill-set activities encourage weight-bearing on stable surfaces such as a mat or countertop and progressing to mobile surfaces such as a ball or bedside tray table. Higher-level weight-bearing activities will encourage recruitment of postural stabilizing muscles to allow for distal mobility and control.

When a patient begins to gain muscle activity, dynamic activities focusing on the progression of motor control skill can be utilized. Examples of such activities are: weight-shifting, unilateral reaching, manipulation of objects with a fixed component (e.g., elbow in weight-bearing), limb movement from a target, and holding and sustaining graded movements. Activities in this venue begin to link components of movement and enhance the refinement of isolated control. Postural control in a multitude of positions and with a variety of speeds will promote normal coordination and function. Refer to Chapter 33 for more detailed examples of specific treatment interventions for the upper extremity.

### Facilitation Techniques

Neuromuscular and sensory stimulation techniques to individual muscles or muscle groups to increase tone and muscular activity for hypotonia/flaccidity may include **quick tapping**, **quick stretch**, **vibration**, **manual contacts**, resistance, **approximation**, and **fast brushing or icing**.

#### Quick Stretch/Tapping

To facilitate a muscle contraction, the therapist can manually apply a brief quick stretch to the muscle, quickly tap, or apply vibration to the muscle belly or tendon. A quick stretch is most effective when the muscle is first placed in a lengthened position, placing the muscle spindle on stretch, therefore making it more sensitive to further stretch. A quick stretch, tapping, or vibration utilize the stretch reflex, activating the muscle spindle and Ia fiber endings, resulting in a muscle contraction (Kandel, 2013, pp. 792–809). The resultant muscle contraction is short-lived; therefore, the therapist may immediately follow with active motion or light tracking resistance.

#### Manual Contacts, Approximation, and Use of Resistance

By activating both muscle proprioceptors and tactile receptors, firm manual pressure on the skin overlying a muscle can be facilitory to the muscle underneath (Hagbarth, 1952). Joint approximation (compression of joint surfaces) activates static joint receptors to facilitate a **cocontraction** of muscles around the joint, increasing joint stability (Sullivan, 1995, p. 27; Voss, 1985, p. 294). Approximation is often applied at the shoulders or pelvis to facilitate postural stability in sitting, standing, or other weight-bearing positions.

Muscle resistance activates the Ia and II endings of the muscle spindle and Golgi tendon organs to enhance a muscle contraction (Kandel, 2013, p. 792–809; Sullivan, 1995, p. 23–25; Voss, 1985, p. 295). The resistance facilitates the agonist and its synergists while reciprocally inhibiting the antagonist. A light **tracking resistance** may be used to facilitate hypotonic muscles as giving more resistance may easily overpower the muscle. One may also consider beginning with eccentric or isometric contractions as these may be easier for the patient to complete compared with concentric contractions. Using resistance to invoke **irradiation** or **overflow** from stronger to weaker muscles is another technique used (Sullivan, 1995, p.25–26). Applying maximal resistance to a stronger muscle or muscle group may result in facilitation of a muscle contraction in weaker muscles within the same synergistic movement or in the contralateral extremity (e.g., resistance to hip flexors may facilitate ankle dorsiflexion in the same limb or resistance to ankle dorsiflexion on the right side may overflow to the left).

#### Fast Brushing or Icing

Activating tactile and thermoreceptors through brief quick strokes of the skin over a muscle with ice or with the fingertips may promote a muscle contraction (O'Sullivan, 2014; Voss, 1985, p. 312–313). The resulting muscle contraction may be small and short-lived. To increase response, immediately follow with light tracking resistance. Application of fast brushing or quick icing may potentially produce an autonomic sympathetic response and therefore should be applied with caution in patients who may present with autonomic instability or who are already in a heightened state of arousal (e.g., agitated patient following traumatic brain injury).

### Strengthening

Improving motor unit recruitment may be a goal for a patient with hypotonia when muscle activity can be facilitated. The application of resistance is the most commonly used method of strengthening to improve power and endurance. Following facilitation techniques with resistance further improves muscle contraction. A therapist can gradually increase resistance from a light tracking resistance to maximal allowable resistance while maintaining smooth coordinated movement against gravity. A therapist has several strategies of applying resistance available, including manual resistance, use of gravity and body weight, and tools such as weights, Theraband, etc.

### Shoulder Strapping/Taping

**Shoulder taping** or **strapping** has also been used as a mechanism to reduce shoulder subluxation or prevent shoulder pain in individuals poststroke, either as a stand-alone intervention or in combination with electrical stimulation (Figure 18-4). Morin (1997) looked at the efficacy of strapping in combination with a traditional hemisling to reduce shoulder subluxation in individuals poststroke. Results indicated the combination therapy significantly reduced subluxation more than each used individually. Hanger (2000) and Griffin (2006) studied the effect of strapping to prevent poststroke shoulder pain. Griffin demonstrated the strapping group developed less pain (a greater number of pain-free days) than the control group. Changes in range of motion and functional outcomes were not different between the groups. Hanger showed no significant differences in pain, range of motion, or functional outcomes. Trends were evident, however, with the treatment group developing less pain

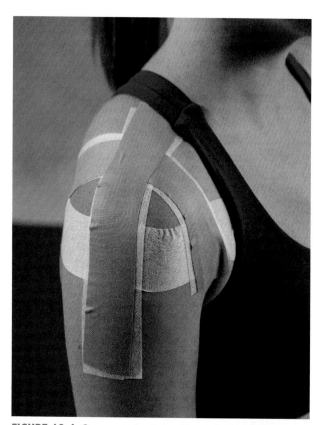

**FIGURE 18-4** One example of shoulder taping used as a mechanism to reduce shoulder subluxation and/or prevent shoulder pain.

and greater function. Peterson (2004) used a combination of taping and electrical stimulation to treat bilateral shoulder subluxation in a patient with central cord syndrome. With the combination therapy over 8 weeks, the patient's subluxation reduced from 1.5 cm (right) and 1.0 cm (left) to 0.3 cm and 0.2 cm, respectively. Refer to Griffin (2006) and Peterson (2004) for specific taping instructions.

### Neuromuscular Electrical Stimulation (NMES)

NMES delivers electrical current to specific muscles or peripheral nerves to (in the case of hypotonia or flaccidity) facilitate active muscle contraction (Albert, 1984; Modlin, 2005), improve muscle strength (Baker, 1986; Binder-Macleod, 1997; Glanz, 1996), improve joint alignment (Faghri, 1994; Linn, 1999), and prevent disuse atrophy (Bajd, 1989; Merletti, 1979). NMES is commonly used with flaccidity or hypotonia to decrease shoulder subluxation and improve upper and lower extremity function. Discussion of NMES as an adjunct to improve function is addressed in the next section.

Early research identified the supraspinatus and posterior deltoid as key muscles in reducing the inferior displacement of the humeral head in shoulder subluxation (Basmajian, 1959; Chaco, 1971). More recent evidence supports the use of electrical stimulation to the supraspinatus and posterior deltoid to prevent shoulder subluxation when initiated early poststroke in patients at risk for developing subluxation (Ada, 2002; Faghri, 1994, 1997; Koyuncu, 2010; Linn, 1999; Wang, 2000, 2002). In a systematic review of the literature, Ada (2002) identified common treatment parameters across studies. The resulting recommendation was to apply daily stimulation to individuals who scored less than a 4 on Item 6 of the Motor Assessment Scale (MAS) for Stroke (Carr, 1985) until they were able to achieve a score of 4. (Note: Item 6 on the MAS evaluates upper arm function. A score of 4 = while sitting, the patient is able to hold the arm [following therapist placement] in forward flexion to 90 degrees for 2 seconds, maintaining some external rotation and elbow extension without excessive shoulder elevation.)

Stimulation should elicit a motor contraction in the supraspinatus and posterior deltoid, at more than 30 Hz, gradually progressing from 1 to 6 hours per day. Evidence is inconclusive, however, about the benefit of using electrical stimulation in the chronic subluxed shoulder (Ada, 2002; Chae, 2005; Linn, 1999).

## ■ Intervention: Ultimately Applied in Functional Activities

### Functional Treatment

#### Functional Electrical Stimulation (FES)

**Functional electrical stimulation (FES)** applies NMES in an organized manner to promote goal-oriented movement, which enhances functional motor relearning (e.g., decreases foot drop during swing phase of gait). Electrical stimulation is also used to improve upper and lower extremity motor outcomes poststroke (Alon, 2003, 2007, 2008; Chantraine, 1999; Daly, 2000; Faghri, 1994, 1997; Popovic, 2004; Price, 2000; Sheffler, 2006;

Sullivan, 2007; Thrasher, 2008). Patients with severe motor impairment after stroke may not respond as well as patients with less impairment. Several studies using FES in patients with severe or flaccid upper extremities demonstrated improvements in volitional control and tone especially when combined with task-specific training compared with exercise without FES (Alon, 2008; Faghri, 1994, 1997; Thrasher, 2008). Individuals with less severe impairment appear to demonstrate greater functional outcomes when using FES combined with task-specific exercise (Alon, 2003, 2007; Sullivan, 2007). Similarly, Popovic (2004) studied electrical stimulation combined with intense task-specific exercise and found patients in the acute phase poststroke demonstrated greater outcomes than those in the chronic phase.

Use of electrical stimulation also improves lower extremity function and gait in individuals poststroke (Daly, 2006; Ferrante, 2008; Glanz, 1996; Kottink, 2004; Mehrholz, 2007, 2008; Robbins, 2006; Roche, 2009; Sheffler, 2006; Stevens, 2010). Meta-analyses have been conducted on the effectiveness of electrical stimulation in stroke rehabilitation (Glanz, 1996; Kottink, 2004; Mehrholz, 2007; Robbins, 2006). Mehrholz (2007) specifically reviewed the efficacy of electromechanical and robot-assisted walking for improving gait after stroke. Analysis of the eight articles meeting inclusion criteria showed patients who received electromechanical or robot-assisted gait training in combination with physical therapy were more likely to walk independently than those patients who did not receive the assisted training. Only two of the eight studies tested gait training in acute patients within 4 weeks of stroke onset, whereas the remainder ranged from 2 months to 4 years. Stroke severity among the studies ranged from a mean of 34/100 to 51/100 on the Barthel Index (a measure of an individual's independence in basic ADLs).

Robbins (2006) specifically investigated the effect of FES on increasing gait speed in individuals poststroke. Eight articles met inclusion criteria. The authors concluded FES can produce a significant increase in gait speed and can be an effective rehabilitation tool. Improvements in gait speed were seen even after the FES was removed. Only one of the eight studies included patients considered in the acute or subacute phase of less than 6 months poststroke. Stroke severity across studies was not identified. Kottink (2004) came to the same conclusions regarding gait speed and further suggested FES be used as an orthosis (e.g., using Ness L300[2] [shown in Figure 24-6] or similar device).

Glanz (1996) assessed FES in stroke rehabilitation. Muscle force production was the primary outcome measure in the four studies meeting inclusion criteria. The author concluded FES significantly improves muscle strength. More recently, Ferrante (2008) compared the use of FES-assisted cycling with standard rehabilitation. Results showed the FES-assisted cycling more effective in improving lower extremity muscle strength and sit-to-stand speeds. Because of differences among the studies included in the meta-analyses, further studies need to be undertaken to determine the optimal frequency and duration of treatment, time following stroke onset, and long-term effects.

Since 2006 several investigations have studied the use of FES as an orthosis for footdrop and/or compared FES with the use of an ankle-foot-orthosis (AFO). Sheffler (2006) compared use of electrical stimulation with an AFO and found both were comparable in improving functional ambulation poststroke. Roche (2009) and Stevens (2010) reviewed the literature regarding the use of FES as an orthosis. The authors concluded FES systems improve gait speed, decrease the physiological cost of walking, as well as improve gait symmetry and rhythmicity.

Technology has improved to allow for wireless stimulation units and implantable electrodes. Hausdorf (2008) compared a radio frequency-controlled **neuroprosthesis** on improving gait parameters in patients with chronic hemiplegia. Results showed gait asymmetry, stride time variability, and gait speed all improved significantly and supported using the device as a treatment for footdrop.

Ring (2009) compared a radio frequency-controlled neuroprosthesis with an AFO in patients with chronic hemiparesis secondary to stroke or traumatic head injury. After 8 weeks of use, stride time, swing time variability, and gait asymmetry all improved to a greater degree using the neuroprosthesis compared with the AFO. The authors concluded the neuroprosthesis more effectively managed footdrop and enhanced balance control. Laufer (2009) evaluated a group of individuals who used a neuroprosthesis for 1 year. The results supported the long-term use of the device with improved functional abilities, social reintegration, and gait speed.

The efficacy of the use of implantable stimulators or **BIONs** has recently been examined (Kottink, 2007, 2008; Weber, 2005) with mixed results. Weber (2005) compared implantable BIONs with surface electrodes and found the BION to be a practical alternative that provided more selective muscle control over surface electrodes. Kottink (2007) compared an implantable stimulator with use of an AFO and found the stimulator significantly improved gait speed over the AFO. Looking at the long-term effect of the implantable stimulator, Kottink (2008) found no functional therapeutic effect with the stimulator. Gait speed remained the same when the stimulator was turned off. The researchers did find significantly increased voluntary muscle activation of the tibialis anterior and gastroc soleus even after the stimulation was turned off, suggesting a possible plasticity effect.

FES has also enhanced gait in patients with SCI (Kim, 2004; Mirbagheri, 2002). Kim (2004) compared use of FES with an AFO and found both to be effective; however the FES resulted in increased foot clearance. Mirbagheri (2002) found FES-assisted walking helped to reduce abnormal joint stiffness. Further information on electrical stimulation in individuals with SCI can be found in Chapter 26.

### Functional Activities

The primary aim of therapeutic intervention is to improve an individual's function in daily life activities through increased use of the hypotonic limb/trunk or the ability to compensate for the impaired motor control or abnormal muscle tone that will not improve. Any of the therapeutic techniques discussed

---

[2]www.bioness.com

in the previous section can and should be used within functional tasks or activities. For example, integration of key facilitation techniques such as tapping, resistance training, and approximation are crucial components to link muscular control to function for the patient with hypotonia. During any selected functional activity, the focus of the activity should be determined and the combination of the optimal active movement of which the patient is capable with facilitation and handling techniques promoting the highest level of functional attainment should be used (e.g., if reaching is the goal, then applying distal approximation would not be helpful).

Task-specific practice is the key to motor learning and improving function; therefore, depending on available voluntary control, incorporating the hypotonic limb/trunk into daily functional tasks under a variety of environmental contexts is essential (Schmidt, 2011, p. 483). With available voluntary control, modified constraint induced therapy (mCIMT) has been found to significantly improve arm and hand function poststroke (Myint, 2008; Page, 2008, 2009; Taub, 2004). See Chapter 33 for greater detail on the use of mCIMT. Forced use of a paretic lower extremity via treadmill training may also improve lower extremity function (Dahl, 2008; Looper, 2010; Ulrich, 2008; Wu, 2007). Treadmill training is addressed

further in Chapter 37. Table 18-8 provides several ideas of possible functional activities that, depending on the severity of hypotonia, may be helpful during treatment.

## THINK ABOUT IT 18.3

- What functional activities could you include as part of your initial treatment for someone with hypotonia?
- Give examples of how you would progress functional activities with John based on his current ability.
- Are there any facilitation techniques you would consider integrating into your functional activities?

## Pediatric Considerations

Hypotonia can be an impairment associated with many neurological and nonneurological disorders in childhood: muscular (e.g., spinal muscular atrophy), genetic (e.g., DS or PWS), CNS (e.g., CP), connective tissue, and metabolic in nature (Bodensteiner, 2008). Clinical characteristics of children with hypotonia include decreased strength, hypermobile joints, increased flexibility, rounded shoulder posture, delayed motor

| TABLE 18-8 | Examples of Functional Activities for Treatment of Hypotonia |
|---|---|
| *Flaccid with no voluntary control* | • Position limb within function (e.g., placing UE/LE in a natural weight-bearing position as it would be if it were able to contribute to the function)<br>• Stabilize trunk in normal alignment (e.g., in wheelchair for eating dinner) |
| *Presence of limited voluntary control* | • Position limb in natural weight-bearing (single- and double-handed) or natural functional positions to be used as able or during constraint-induced activities: |
| Upper extremity | • Hand on countertop while brushing teeth or combing hair; hand on the arm of a chair or supporting surface during a transfer<br>• Stabilizing jar while opening with opposite hand, cereal bowl while pouring milk, or piece of paper while writing<br>• Pushing as able on elbow or hand when transitioning to sitting from sidelying<br>• Hand placed appropriately on handle of grocery cart, lawn mower, broom, or snow blower during the activity<br>• Reaching<br>• Grasp, manipulation, and release of objects; hand-off activities<br>• Ambulation with poles (horizontal in front of body, vertical) |
| Lower extremity | • Foot on floor during sitting activities such as stabilization, weight-shifting, reaching, scooting, partial standing<br>• Sit-to-stand from various seated surfaces<br>• Stepping in different directions (forward, back, side, diagonally)<br>• Transitions during function through different positions (quadruped, kneeling, half-kneeling, floor-to-stand)<br>• Placement activities on set diagrams for managing various distances and range of motion<br>• Stepping (up, down, diagonally) on various height steps and curbs<br>• Single-limb stance static and dynamic activities<br>• Balance obstacle course<br>• Body-weight supported training over ground or treadmill<br>• Ambulation over various surfaces, terrains, and in/through different environments |
| Trunk | • Incorporation of normal trunk motions to support weight-bearing during standing activities<br>• Holding of elongation and shortening for reaching, dressing, grooming, gait<br>• Rotational activities to promote control during gait, rolling, sitting |

skills, decreased activity tolerance, and a need to lean on supports. (Wilson-Howle, 1999; Westcott and Goulet, 2005; Martin, 2005, 2007, 2013; Pilon, 2000). Movement is slower and less coordinated with difficulty especially in midranges (e.g., movement within and between postures). General abnormal movement patterns include poor head control and midline orientation (infants), poor proximal stability (scapula, shoulders, pelvis, hips), poor balance between flexors and extensors, and difficulty grading muscle activity for initiating, sustaining, or terminating functional movement (Bly, 1983; Westcott, 2005; Boehme, 1990). Because postural control and movement is challenging in the context of hypotonia, these children tend to have decreased activity tolerance, poor attention and motivation, and sensory deprivation as a result of limited exploration of their environment (Martin, 2005; Boehme, 1990). Respiration may be insufficient for sustained vocalization due to rib cage instability, and oral motor problems may contribute to feeding difficulties, language delays, drooling, and limited facial expressions (Boehme, 1990). Common resulting compensatory movement strategies are identified in Table 18-9 (Bly, 1983; Boehme, 1990). With awareness of these strategies, the therapist can address and minimize them, and educate the patient.

Over the long term, if not treated, these compensatory strategies may lead to secondary complications such as preventing the development of normal extremity use, further laxities, tightness or contractures, and possible deformities. Therefore physical therapy services should be started as soon as possible with training for parents and/or other caregivers so a program can be implemented at home and/or child-care setting. Few conditions require specific medical treatment (e.g., Vitamin D for rickets or Thyroxine for hypothyroidism). Therapy is generally focused on building muscle activity and increasing postural and extremity motor control to promote optimal functional independence in sitting, standing, walking, and/or self-propulsion of a wheelchair. Interventions may include, but are not limited to: enhancing weight-bearing and extremity function, strengthening and facilitation of motor control, coordination, balance, alignment, stretching to prevent contractures, splinting/bracing to prevent spinal or postural deformities, and functional practice of daily activities. Table 18-10 includes some general intervention ideas (Bly, 1983, 1999; Boehme, 1990; Hypes, 2004).

Parents should be taught positioning/handling techniques as a means to maintain optimal range of motion (promote natural infant/child positioning commensurate with age) and facilitate head and trunk control in various positions (Kahn-D'Angel, 2006). For example, in the premature infant, positioning in side-lying or prone should include trunk flexion with a posterior pelvic tilt, neck flexion (avoid neck hyperextension), shoulder protraction, and bilateral symmetrical lower extremity flexion. Positioning in supine should place the neck in midline and provide adequate support along the trunk under the shoulders and knees. While positioned in sitting (e.g., stroller, car seats, highchairs), the child will likely need additional support for the head and trunk. Ideally positioning should promote alertness and tracking of visual and auditory cues. As the child progresses in

| TABLE 18-9 | Common Compensatory Movement Strategies |
|---|---|
| **ABNORMAL MOVEMENT** | **COMPENSATORY MOVEMENT STRATEGY** |
| Poor head control and midline orientation | Prone or sitting: May stabilize the head by elevating the shoulders and excessively hyperextending the neck (stacking) |
| Poor proximal stability—shoulders | Excessive scapular elevation, adduction, downwardly rotated, and tipped forward<br>May stabilize with arms adducted and internally rotated or with extreme scapular adduction and humeral abduction |
| Poor proximal stability—pelvis/hip | Pelvic torsion as source of postural stability can cause rotation of spine<br>Anterior pelvic tilt: May rest on anterior ligaments with resulting excessive lumbar lordosis<br>Prone, supine, or sitting: Collapse into support surface resulting in frog-legged position (extreme hip abduction and external rotation)<br>Sitting: "W" sit<br>Kneeling: Hip flexion, abduction, and external rotation with wide base of support<br>Standing/walking: Wide base of support, crouched gait or knees locked in hyperextension, weight-bearing on medial border of foot or heel border of foot |

motor ability, positioning/handling techniques should promote balance, trunk control during movements and transitions, and control in standing.

In children with hypotonia, therapists should be concerned with hip dislocation, patellar subluxation, and foot deformities (Chester, 2011; Lowes, 2005). Addressing these issues early will increase the child's potential for standing and walking. Achieving a plantigrade foot position is important not only for proper alignment and subsequent bone formation proximally but also to promote walking, to allow proper shoe fit, to facilitate positioning in sitting, and weight acceptance during transitions.

Orthoses may be considered in children with hypotonia to improve foot and lower extremity alignment during gait and prevent future deformities. Little evidence exists evaluating the effect of orthoses in children with hypotonia; however a few studies have reported improvements in gait kinematics and postural control using supramalleolar orthoses in children with DS (Kates, 2000; Grossman, 1990; Martin, 2004; Selby-Silverstein, 2001) and BCH (Bauer, 2009; Ross, 2011).

| TABLE 18-10 | Examples of General Intervention Goals/Ideas |
|---|---|
| **PROBLEM** | **EXAMPLES** |
| Child may tend to have wide base of support, sink into support surface/manual support, and fix joints, demonstrating little spontaneous movement | Promote child's active involvement; remove supports; use light, intermittent touch; wait for response to sensory input |
| Child may stabilize the head by elevating the shoulders and excessively hyperextending the neck (stacking) | Work on active chin tucking and tasks to activate neck flexors Increase normal bilateral UE use, including scapular mobility |
| Child has poor proximal stability—scapula/shoulders limiting distal control | Increase scapular stability, scapula-humeral control, and isolated UE movements Increase UE weight-bearing and weight-shifting in various positions (e.g., supported prone-on-elbows while reaching for a toy with one hand; prone over ball or bolster, arms extended out and weight-bearing, reaching for toy with one hand; sidelying on elbow, playing with toy |
| Child has poor proximal stability—pelvis/hip | Increase proximal hip stability and control in various positions, especially through lateral weight-shifting Work on dissociated LE movement (e.g., climbing, activities in ½ kneeling) Quadruped: Neutralize pelvis, lateral weight shift to one leg and lift the other (3-point) Sitting: Long sit or bench sit on bolster or tilt board (ring-sit if hamstrings too tight). Work on lateral weight-shifting the trunk with elongation on the weight-bearing side |
| Child demonstrates limited weight shift around body axis and across midline | Encourage rotation through trunk and pelvis with playful activities to either side in sitting, standing, or kneeling; may need to assist with adequate proximal stabilization through manual input or use of adaptive equipment |
| Child has limited dynamic postural control and tends to use straight plane movement transitions (e.g., moving from sitting to prone through widely abducted legs) | Discourage fixed, static positions; encourage dynamic postures and transitions; sidesitting (to either side) with transition to prone or quadruped; movement over therapy ball |

Looper (2010), on the other hand, found orthoses combined with treadmill training detrimental to gross motor skill development compared with treadmill training alone. Further research is needed.

Hypotonia is a primary impairment consistently found in children with DS. Other typical impairments include muscle weakness, delayed postural reactions, joint hyperflexibility, ligamentous laxity, foot deformities, scoliosis, and atlantoaxial instability (Shumway-Cook, 1985; Bertoti, 2008). Because of hypotonia, laxity, and decreased strength, children with DS tend to use more cocontraction, thereby decreasing degrees of movement freedom to increase stability. They also tend to "hang" on ligamentous support as a way to increase stability (Westcott, 2005). Abnormal movement patterns develop as a way to compensate for poor motor control and instability. Children with DS will often sit in a posterior pelvic tilt with a rounded slumped trunk, neck in hyperextension resting back on the shoulders, abducted hips, and extended knees (Lauteslager, 1998; Winders, 2001). Standing and walking is achieved with an anterior pelvic tilt (increased lumbar lordosis), hips externally rotated, knees hyperextended, pronated and everted feet, and arms abducted (Lauteslager, 1998; Rigoldi, 2012; Winders, 2001). If not addressed, these problems over time can cause decreased respiratory capacity in sitting, decreased use of the upper extremities, and limited trunk mobility especially during rotational components. Abnormal standing and walking patterns may lead to excessive wear on joints, including genu valgus, patellofemoral instability, pes planus, and hip instability (Chester, 2011; Lauteslager, 1998; Winders, 2001).

With practice, children with DS may be able to learn more normal movement strategies (Almeida, 1994). Therapy should be aimed at increasing strength and minimizing the development of compensatory movement patterns through emphasis on developing graded control of muscle activity, controlled movement in midranges, proximal stabilization to support distal control, and balanced use of flexors and extensors (Boehme, 1990; Winders, 1997). Examples of intervention ideas for children with DS can be found in Box 18-1 (Bly, 1999; Winders, 2001).

## BOX 18-1   Examples of Intervention Ideas Related to Hypotonia for Children With Down Syndrome

Interventions aimed at increasing strength and minimizing the development of compensatory movement patterns.

Sitting:

- Position child sitting in therapist's lap in front of therapy ball. Assist child to extend trunk with arms weight-bearing on the ball and/or playing with a toy. Through play, encourage trunk extension and rotation.
- Position child sitting across therapist's lap while therapist is in long sitting. Using hands to facilitate trunk extension, the therapist can then use legs and hands to facilitate lateral trunk weight-shifting and rotation. May integrate reaching for toys to encourage scapular-humeral movement.
- Encourage anterior and lateral pelvic weight shifts sitting on therapy ball.
- Encourage alternating LE pattern with cycling.
- Discourage W sitting.
- Discourage straight plane movement transitions (e.g., transition from sitting to prone through widely abducted legs).
- Encourage trunk rotation.

Sit-to-Stand:

- Position child straddling therapist's leg or bolster. Assist child to extend the trunk and weight shift forward to standing at a table. May also have child alongside of the table to encourage standing with trunk rotation and weight shift toward one side.

Quadruped:

- Encourage alternating LE pattern—creeping, climbing.

Standing:

- Encourage normal alignment and weight-shifting to lateral borders of the feet through handling, playing with toys at a table. May add trunk rotation.
- Marching.
- Jumping on a trampoline.

Walking:

- Encourage normal alignment and weight-shifting to lateral borders of the feet through handling, pushing rolling toys/carts, cruising around a table or toy (lateral weight shift).
- Negotiating stairs with least amount of support.

Children with BCH, also termed idiopathic hypotonia, present with generalized symmetrical hypotonia, muscle weakness, decreased reflexes, excessive passive range of motion, and joint hypermobility (Cohen, 1998; Dawson, 2004; Strubhar, 2007). Depending on the severity of the hypotonia, children may be unable to: maintain head control; maintain sitting (may fall or slide out of a chair); be unable to assume and maintain quadruped, kneeling, standing; and be unable to crawl, creep, stand, or walk (Cohen, 1998; Dawson, 2004). Abnormal postures include: prone frog-legged position; sitting with posterior pelvic tilt, rounded back, forward head (or neck in hyperextension resting on shoulders), and legs in "W" sit position; and standing and walking patterns similar to children with DS (Chester, 2011; Cohen, 1998; Dawson, 2004). Gait deviations seen in children with BCH were documented by Chester (2011). Decreased ankle plantar flexion angle and moment during stance, increased knee flexion angles during stance, decreased knee flexion moment at terminal stance, and increased hip flexion angle during loading response were significant compared with normal controls (Chester, 2011). Children with BCH did not demonstrate increased hip adduction/abduction in swing, decreased hip extension in swing, and decreased hip

flexion/extension moments all commonly seen in children with DS (Chester, 2011). Intervention ideas for children with BCH are included in Box 18-2.

Children with CP rarely are strictly hypotonic. Instead they often present with a mixture of types of tone (e.g., hypotonic trunk with extremity hypertonicity) or may have fluctuating tone (athetosis). Hypotonia in CP is more often temporary in early stages and may be a precursor to athetosis or spasticity (Wilson-Howle, 2006). Fluctuating tone is often seen in children with athetosis where muscle tone changes between hypertonicity and hypotonicity, with hypotonicity being predominant between fluctuations (Yokochi, 1989). Typical impairments seen when hypotonia is present in CP are weakness, poor postural (proximal) control, and joint hypermobility. Children show greater difficulty with movement in midranges (e.g., within positions and transitions between positions). To compensate, they tend to hold static positions by cocontracting or "fixing" proximal joints, extending joints completely, and hanging on ligaments for increased stability (Stye-Acevedo, 2008). Treatment goals and ideas presented in Table 18-10 and in Box 18-1 may be helpful for children with CP, if a child presents with problems and compensatory patterns similar to children with DS.

## BOX 18-2 Examples of Intervention Ideas for Children With Benign Congenital Hypotonia

Improving head and trunk stability:

- Positioning in midline normal alignments (key to developing motor control and providing support for feeding)
- Static and dynamic balance activities on level surfaces, tilt board, therapy ball

Improving weight-bearing:

- Wheelbarrow exercises
- Crab walk, bear walk, frog jump

Improving gross motor coordination:

- Step-ups
- Walking, hiking, swimming, pulling a wagon
- Hopping, galloping, skipping, jumping, marching
- Throwing, catching, bouncing, or kicking a ball
- Running, chasing bubbles, dancing, hopscotch
- Obstacle course, playground activities

Improving fine motor coordination:

- Writing, drawing, painting
- Fastening clothing: buttons, snaps, zippers
- Playing with playdough, silly putty, clay: roll, squeeze, twist, poke, pinch
- Cooking activities: scooping, stirring, molding, kneading, peeling, spreading, cutting, screwing and unscrewing various lids
- Legos, wind-up toys, stringing beads, Tinkertoys, K'nex, nuts and bolts, pop bubble wrap
- Pick up and release small objects with a clothspin, tweezer, tongs.
- In-hand manipulation: Picking up a group of small objects one at a time in one hand, then release one at a time into a jar

## PATIENT APPLICATION

In all patients, identification of key problems and prioritization of outcome expectations is the first essential component before development of a treatment plan of care. Based on what has previously been presented about our patient, John, here are a variety of intervention strategies that could be applied for various positions/activities, including supine, sidelying, sitting, and standing.

### Supine Interventions

The patient examination was initiated by a PROM assessment of the head/neck, UE, trunk, and LE. Facilitate John's neck rotation and visual tracking using passive movement and positioning of the head and neck, followed by verbal cuing with picture-tracking and command-following.

Protect the flaccid UE by placing your left hand under John's right scapula and facilitate upward rotation and abduction of the scapula with passive range of motion of his humerus. Using your right hand, hold John's right upper extremity in a scaption plane with external rotation and slight distraction. The support from your right hand along with stabilization of the patient's arm being held alongside your trunk combines to maintain joint integrity. John's elbow, wrist, and hand are held in extension. At any point in the PROM, incorporation of facilitation techniques such as tapping, vibration, and approximation may be utilized to encourage temporary agonist muscle activation and opportunities for practice of the intended movement.

LE facilitation is promoted by actively placing John's LEs in a hook-lying position. Stand distal to John's legs with guided weight-bearing and approximation through the knees to the feet. The patient can be asked to lift his hips in concordance with facilitation to the abdominals and the hip extensors to gain a motion of posterior pelvic tilt with hip extension and lifting. Facilitation can also occur in this position for hip rotation. Isolated facilitation of key points would place your hands so that your fingers facilitate activation of the hip abductors and your thumbs facilitate activation of the abdominals to promote this motion. Hip extension and flexion can be facilitated through active tapping, vibration, holding patterns, and isometric positions throughout the range.

### Sidelying Interventions

Facilitation of rolling can occur to either side. Key points of control are at the head/neck, abdominals, and LEs. When rolling to the affected side, John's arm should be placed in relative abduction and flexion to 90 degrees and ER to promote proper joint mobility through the transition. Weight-bearing in sidelying after a rolling strategy is conducive to sensory input through the head/neck, involved UE, trunk, pelvis, and LE. Once John is in sidelying, you may utilize techniques of hold/relax, rhythmic stabilization, alternating isometrics, and rhythmic initiation for recruitment of both agonists and antagonists. Hand placements would be on the pelvis and upper trunk in the scapular region.

### Sitting Interventions

Weight-bearing through John's right UE in supported and unsupported sitting will be an intervention to promote muscle recruitment. Sit beside John on the involved side or with one leg positioned behind his back to help stabilize the trunk. Care should be taken to note the position of the trunk and scapula before weight-bearing through the UE. The UE is placed just lateral to the hip. Hold the UE shoulder girdle in a proper position while monitoring the ability of John to hold or isolate elbow extension and flexion. From this position, facilitate weight-shifting onto the supported involved UE. John's equilibrium patterns can be assessed while performing this activity.

Weight-bearing through the lower extremities can be accomplished in sitting by positioning yourself beside or in front of John, depending on his level of sitting control. Apply approximation through the knee to the floor and facilitate partial sit-to-stand activities, scooting, weight-shifting, and single-limb support by having the noninvolved LE lift and lower.

### Standing Interventions

Weight-bearing in supported standing could be facilitated at a hemirail, windowsill, countertop, high-low mat, bedside, or parallel bars. Stand on John's involved side, applying key points of control at the trunk, pelvis, hip, and knee. Facilitate John to hold a posture and add dynamic weight-shifting, if able. This position may be altered to a modified-plantigrade posture also.

### Contemplate Clinical Decisions

1. How could you support a flaccid or hypotonic limb while applying facilitation techniques such as tapping, vibration, approximation, etc.?
2. How do you document small increments of muscle activation when an actual muscle grade improvement or achievement of a functional task is not obtained, yet progress is clearly noted?
3. At what point can you contemplate challenging John to a higher functional task even with a severely hypotonic limb? Provide the clinical reasoning for advancing a program.
4. Which muscle groups are key in postural control?
5. What orthotics or splints would you recommend to manage specific hypotonic joints? When?
6. Describe the progression of facilitation tactics, starting with a flaccid limb, then to a limb developing some motor control, and moving on to dynamic mobility.
7. List and explain compensation strategies John may employ when attempting to achieve active muscle control or move through transitions.

## Intervention: Considerations for Nontherapy Time and Discharge

### Patient and Family Education

In the complex health-care environment, the therapist must be proficient in evaluating the needs of the patient and caregiver(s) when discharged and be proactive in addressing those needs. The therapist should be aware of and able to adapt to various learning styles of both the patient and caregiver(s). Education will be most effective when a variety of instructional strategies are utilized such as demonstration, supervised practice, review, and written/verbal instruction. Patients and caregivers need ample time and opportunity to practice these management skills to be safe and confident in the next setting. Consider the sample of patient/caregiver education topics listed in Box 18-3 from which the therapist can choose.

### Activities for Home

Education with the patient, family, and caregivers of home activities needs to address function and be practical to the patient's lifestyle. Home activities should not increase the stress on the patient, family member, or caregiver. However they should be instructed with clear context as to the need to continue the home program to promote progress of function, functional safety, and prevention of negative outcomes due to hypotonia. Some sample home activities appropriate for this population are provided in Box 18-4.

---

**BOX 18-3  Sample Topics for Patient/Caregiver Education Include (but not limited to):**

- Visual, sensory, and verbal interaction to facilitate awareness of the involved side
- Bed and wheelchair positioning
- Management of the hypotonic/flaccid limb during movement transitions:
  - Supine to sidelying, to sit, to stand
  - Transfer training to a variety of surfaces
- Proper range of motion and stretching techniques for the involved UE/LE/trunk
- Nervous system mobilization techniques
- ADL training
- Application and utilization of equipment
- Skin checks
- Safety system (e.g., emergency call system such as Lifeline Medical Alert or established plan with caregivers/family)

---

**BOX 18-4  Sample Activities for Home or Home Exercise Program**

- Bed positioning and rolling
- Reaching
- Clasped hand activities
- Rolling skills to promote head righting, weight-bearing, upper, lower, and trunk dissociation and scapular movement
- Stretching of the UE and LE to maintain ROM, joint integrity, muscle structure, and nerve status
- Rolling over abducted UE to promote trunk mobility and shoulder integrity
- Weight-bearing in sitting, standing at counter, sink, windowsill, bedside
- Reaching—various object sizes and in various positions
- Sit-to-stand at countertops, bedside, table, windowsills
- Promote symmetry of motion, equal weight-bearing, neutral alignment, head righting
- Promote stretching of heel cords with symmetrical and full weight-bearing stance positions
- Promote stretching of anterior hip capsule in a full standing position
- Promote better posture with upright trunk and head control to promote improved function, breathing, visual tracking, etc.
- Transfer training/practice for functional needs
- Head turning and visual scanning to prep for awareness of environment pretransfer
- Trunk extension and flexion to promote coordination of trunk stability required in transfers
- UE-clasped hand reaching over a tabletop to promote symmetry and control of anterior trunk translation before a transfer
- Small components of sit-to-stand to promote partial weight shift forward
- Active LE placement onto objects of different heights and distances to promote judging of distance and placement of limb

# HANDS-ON PRACTICE

▮▮ **Be sure to practice the following skills from this chapter. With further practice, you should be able to:**

- Feel, assess, and handle a patient with low tone or a flaccid extremity.
- Safely position a patient with a hypotonic or flaccid upper or lower extremity in
  - Supine
  - Sidelying
  - Sitting
- Integrate task-specific weight-bearing activities in sitting, prone-on-elbows, quadruped, and standing.

- Apply quick stretch or tapping to facilitate a muscle or movement.
- Apply approximation to improve stability.
- Apply the concept of irradiation/overflow to enhance movement.
- Apply fast brushing/icing to facilitate a muscle or movement.
- Incorporate functional activities as a focus of your treatment intervention.

## Let's Review

1. Identify and list musculoskeletal diagnoses that may occur after a presentation of hypotonia. How may these musculoskeletal diagnoses relate to age, diagnoses, and prognosis?

2. When selecting tests and measures for patients with hypotonia, how will this information provide the therapist with meaningful data to direct care?

3. Compare and contrast common tests and measures utilized for patients with hypotonia and/or flaccidity.

4. How would you select facilitation techniques based on the function evaluation and reevaluation data?

5. How do age, diagnosis, and prognosis direct your care plan and patient outcome prediction?

6. In the spectrum/timeline of functional recovery posthypotonic presentation, discuss optimal and expected outcomes for various diagnoses.

7. How does positioning facilitate normal or inhibit abnormal tone presentations?

8. How does family support affect the plan of care and recommendations for home activities with patients demonstrating hypotonia?

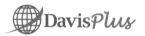 **DavisPlus**   For additional resources, including Focus on Evidence tables, case study discussions, references, and glossary, please visit http://davisplus.fadavis.com

# CHAPTER SUMMARY

## PATIENT SCENARIO

*Richard, a 52 year-old Caucasian male, is referred to inpatient rehabilitation after sustaining a T10 ASIA C SCI. Richard was checking the engine of his vehicle on a country road after a local basketball game when a drunk driver hit the car from the rear. The hood of the vehicle crushed Richard's back, causing the injury. Richard is married with five children, all of whom live at home. He is a crop farmer, and two of the oldest boys work on the farm with him. He presents with hyporeflexic paresis of bilateral lower extremities below the level of T10, diminished*

*sensation and proprioception, and loss of bowel and bladder control. Richard's goals are to return to farming and independence in all functional activities to include transfers, gait, and ADLs.*

*Two weeks postinjury, Richard demonstrates inconsistent partial initiation/activation of isolated muscles below T10. Manual muscle testing shows normal UE strength and emerging muscle strength below T10 with grades of 1+ to 2-. Sensory testing reveals slight recognition of sharp/dull and pin-prick 1/5 above knee and absent below knee. For level transfers, Richard requires a transfer board with moderate assistance of one person.*

To objectively quantify tone and strength in this case, manual muscle tests should be completed in the correct biomechanical position and tracked accordingly with clear identification of obtained range of motion and amount of applied pressure tolerated. Small increments of improved strength are crucial to justify ongoing therapy services. Documentation of tone changes using the Passive and Active Movement scale (Wilson-Howle, 1999) for hypotonicity and the Ashworth Scale for hypertonicity will offer objectivity to tone management. Tone assessments should be done daily through observation, palpation, and assessment of resistance to PROM for each joint and each joint motion below T10.

The top prioritized functional goals for Richard would include independence in all transfers and, at minimum, household ambulation. To reach his goals, therapy would focus on Richard's functional activity limitations and underlying body structure and function impairments. Specifically focusing on hypotonia, interventions beneficial for promoting increased muscle tone and strength may include but are not limited to: ROM activities in all planes in accordance with available strength; powder board (gravity-eliminated) exercises for muscles below Grade 3; use of tapping, vibration, or quick stretch to facilitate a muscle contraction; using light weights or manual resistance (e.g., PNF); FES or NMES; progressive weight-bearing activities in supine, sitting, and standing; and possible use of partial body weight-supported gait training.

Depending on recovery, Richard may require equipment for use at home. A manual lightweight wheelchair and wheelchair cushion would be recommended to facilitate mobility in/out of a vehicle and around the farm. If ambulation is chosen as a primary mode of mobility and muscle function does not completely return, a knee-ankle-foot orthosis (KAFO), ankle foot orthosis (AFO), or shoe insert (e.g., supramalleolar orthoses) may be considered depending on the level of recovery. Options for assistive gait devices include loftstrand crutches, bilateral canes, or a walker. Items such as a reacher may enhance ADLs.

As noted in the previous patient scenario, key daily functional activities may be significantly limited or impossible for the patient who has flaccid or hypotonic limb(s) and/or trunk. This chapter focused on the management of flaccidity and hypotonia. Safety considerations, examination components, evaluation, including prognostic factors and expected outcomes, and lifespan influences were discussed. Suggestions for specific interventions included proper positioning, use of weight-bearing, facilitation techniques, electrical stimulation, and strapping/taping. Patient case scenarios provided illustration for the management of flaccidity or hypotonia in individuals with different neurological diagnoses. Although available evidence was presented, evidence to support some commonly used interventions is lacking. Additional evidence on interventions for flaccidity/hypotonicity is presented in the Focus on Evidence (FOE) tables online.

# Intervention Related to Hypertonia: Spastic and Rigid

**CHAPTER 19**

Roberta Kuchler O'Shea, PT, DPT, PhD ▪ Laura White, PT, DScPT, GCS
Dennis W. Fell, PT, MD

## CHAPTER OBJECTIVES

Upon completion of this chapter, the learner should be able to:
1. Discuss the development of spasticity and rigidity.
2. Discuss the possible impact of spasticity and/or rigidity on function.
3. Identify neuromuscular diagnoses which commonly have hypertonia as a related impairment.
4. Describe the implications of surgical and pharmacological interventions for spasticity.
5. Demonstrate interventions to influence spasticity or rigidity.

## ■ Introduction

Spasticity and rigidity are the two types of hypertonia detected in individuals with neurological disorders. **Hypertonia**, also called **hypertonus**, is any increase in muscle tone (i.e., an increase in resting muscle resistance while the resting muscle is passively elongated). Among the adult population, consensus regarding accurate definitions of the different types of hypertonia has not been reached.

In 2003, several researchers gathered to create operational definitions of different types of hypertonia in children: "**Spasticity**, or **spastic hypertonia**, is defined as hypertonia in which one or both of the following signs are present: (1) resistance to externally imposed movement increases with increasing speed of stretch (i.e., velocity-dependent; Lance, 1980) and varies with the direction of movement and/or (2) resistance to externally imposed movement rises rapidly above a threshold speed or joint angle (Fig. 19-1A). **Dystonia** is defined as a movement disorder in which involuntary sustained or intermittent muscle contractions cause twisting and repetitive movements,

abnormal postures, or both. **Rigidity**, or **rigid hypertonia**, is defined as hypertonia in which all the following are true: (1) the resistance to externally imposed joint movement is present at very low and high speeds of movement, does not depend on imposed speed or angle threshold, and is usually detected throughout the available range, not just at the end ranges of movement; (2) simultaneous cocontraction of agonists and antagonists may occur, and this is reflected in an immediate resistance to a reversal of the direction of movement about a joint; (3) the limb does not tend to return toward a particular fixed posture or extreme joint angle; and (4) voluntary activity in distant muscle groups does not lead to involuntary movements about the rigid joints, although rigidity may worsen" (Sanger, 2003). In addition to the previous definition, spasticity also tends to be greater at the end of range when the muscle is on greatest stretch. Decerebrate and decorticate rigidity, defined later in this chapter and illustrated in Figure 6-15AB, could be considered the most extreme forms of spasticity as the increased tone is predominant on one side of the joint and the limbs do tend to return

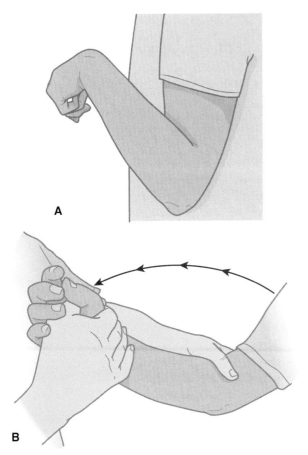

**FIGURE 19-1A & B** Diagrams comparing spasticity distribution to rigidity distribution. **A.** In spasticity, the increased resistance is found predominantly on one side of the joint and particularly toward the end of the available range. In this case, the spasticity is predominant in the elbow flexors, wrist flexors, pronators, and finger flexors, which results in this resting position. **B.** In rigidity, the increased resistance is found in both the agonist and the antagonist and is present through the range but may occur as cogwheel rigidity with repeated catches and releases through the available range.

several factors, including pathology and environmental demands. In this chapter we discuss the clinical presentation, causes of spasticity and rigidity, and various methods to at least temporarily dampen the effects and presentation of hypertonus, which may allow for more functional practice of the related muscle groups.

## Clinical Picture of Hypertonia

After CNS injury, hypertonicity tends to develop gradually over the following weeks and months (Adams, 2007; Sheean, 2009). A person with spasticity may exhibit increased tone, increased tendon reflexes, and **clonus**. Additionally each upper motor neuron pathology will present clinically in slightly different ways depending on factors such as lesion location. For example, individuals with a spinal cord injury (SCI) typically exhibit paralysis with spasms or sudden involuntary muscle contractions in addition to spasticity on both sides of the involved joints, whereas a patient after a stroke may exhibit movement synergies dominated by flexion or extension patterns combined with spasticity usually observed predominantly on one side of the joint (Adams, 2007; Ozcakir, 2007; Trompetto, 2014). A person with rigid hypertonus may have very jerky movements or no movement around a joint combined with rigid hypertonus present on both sides of the joint (Trompetto, 2014).

Although hypertonia may be associated with impairments of motor control of movement such as abnormal synergies in some patients, it is important to realize the impaired motor control is distinct from the abnormal tone. For example, spasticity in the right biceps, wrist flexors, and finger flexors (felt by the assessor during passive arm movement) is not the same as the motor control deficit observed as a flexion synergy of the upper extremity (observed when the patient actively tries to move the arm) (Phadke, 2015). The test methods are different and the related interventions are different. Hypertonus in a particular muscle group may cause difficulty with active voluntary movement of the opposing muscle group because this opposite action elongates the hypertonic muscle.

toward a particular fixed posture due to the imbalanced resting muscle tone. **Cogwheel rigidity** (Fig. 19-1B) describes the motion of a limb that catches and releases as the limb is moved passively through the available range of motion. It is commonly seen in patients with Parkinson disease.

Spasticity and rigidity are caused by damage to specific motor areas of the central nervous system (CNS). While the previous descriptions relate to observations in passive/resting muscle, the conditions can affect voluntary and involuntary movements and may significantly affect a person's activities and ability to participate in their chosen lifestyle. It is important to remember that spasticity is managed better in some patients than others. Regardless it is a lifelong issue that will affect a person's function throughout their life. In this chapter interventions for hypertonicity will be discussed with a focus on spasticity, rigidity, and dystonia.

This chapter discusses spasticity and its influence on movement. Spasticity presents in a variety of ways depending on

## THINK ABOUT IT 19.1

- How would you differentiate between weakness and lack of motor control versus lack of movement due to increased spasticity?
- What functional activities might be limited as a result of increased spasticity in the upper extremity?
- What functional activities might be enhanced by spasticity in the lower extremity?

Regardless, hypertonicity can have significant effect on a patient's body structure and independent function. A person with hypertonia is at risk for joint contractures because of decreased opportunities for the joint to move fully in the opposite direction, skin breakdown, gait abnormalities, and skeletal deformities. The secondary loss of strength may affect gait and function more than the primary hypertonia (Ross, 2007; Phadke, 2015).

## Possible Effect of Hypertonia on Function

Individuals with spasticity or rigidity may have difficulty with everyday functional skills (Haselkorn, 2005; Royal College of Physicians, 2009; Trompetto, 2014; Phadke, 2015) perhaps as the spasticity may interfere particularly with actions of opposing muscle groups that would inherently stretch the spastic muscle. Gastroc-soleus spasticity has negative effects on mobility and balance in individuals with multiple sclerosis (MS) (Sosnoff, 2011). Contraction of a muscle antagonist to a spastic muscle, particular if the contraction is rapid, may cause unwanted stretch reflex of the spastic muscle and cocontraction around the joint with negative effects on movement control (Morita, 2001; Phadke, 2015). With hypertonicity in the hands, for instance, an individual may have a decreased ability to grasp and release a utensil to self-feed or to manipulate fasteners on clothing. A person with significant spastic hypertonia may have difficulty maintaining independent sitting related to abnormal responses when the spastic muscle group is suddenly stretched by a change in position, and the person may require customized seating offering significant postural support. In some instances, particularly when spasticity is expected to be permanent and associated with a complete paralysis, particularly SCI, a patient can learn to use the influences of spasticity to achieve functional skills (Albright, 1993; Gelber, 1999; Haselkorn, 2005). For instance, a person with lower extremity spasticity related to SCI may use the increase in muscle activity to assist with attaining or maintain functional standing.

Interestingly, researchers have found decreases in strength from neurological disorders affect function more so than any associated increased spasticity (Ross, 2007). Thus although therapists may employ a variety of inhibition techniques to decrease hypertonia, it is also important to treat the underlying strength (see Chapter 22) and coordination (see Chapter 21) deficits once the hypertonia has been decreased. An **inhibition technique** is an intervention method with the purpose of minimizing some abnormal body system function, particularly a positive symptom such as hypertonicity or hypersensitivity, or trying to prevent some abnormal position, posture, or movement. By addressing both the hypertonicity and underlying related issues, the therapist also helps the client to regain functional skills and hopefully participate more fully in society. These interventions are discussed more in depth throughout this chapter.

Another way to view the potential relationship between hypertonicity and function is analyzing the results that occur after medical and surgical interventions for hypertonia. For example, improvements in functional skill can result from several specific spasticity treatments, including Botulinum toxin injections (Fehlings, 2000; Lowe, 2006; Mall, 2000) and intrathecal baclofen (ITB) (Campbell, 1995; Francisco, 2003; Ivanhoe, 2006; Meythaler, 1999;

Rawicki, 1999). If spasticity does interfere with functional use of the opposing muscle groups (Keenan, 1990) and "remaining viable motor function" (Meythaler, 1999), then techniques decreasing spasticity, even temporarily, could provide a window of time during which the person may practice more appropriate use of the opposing muscle groups in functional activities. For example, Szecsi (2009) reported that during functional electrical stimulation (FES) application during cycling, the period of short-term spasticity reduction was accompanied by greater smoothness of cycling movement, but the improvement diminished when the stimulation was terminated. Conceivably more appropriate practice and repetition of functional movement, without interference of opposing spasticity, could help to stimulate neural plasticity and optimize motor recovery (Ward, 2004).

---

**PATIENT APPLICATION**

*Anthony is a 16 year-old boy with spastic quadriplegia cerebral palsy (CP). He exhibits spastic hypertonia in all four limbs along with impaired motor control and hypotonia in his trunk. Anthony attends a private high school as a sophomore. His current goals include increasing active motion in his hands in order to operate a mixing board and computer so he can create music CDs. He would also like to ambulate indoors so he can move around his classroom and bedroom without his wheelchair.*

*Anthony lives with his parents, younger brother, and their pet dog. His house has been remodeled with an open floor plan on the main level, a first floor bedroom suite with accessible bathing area, and an elevator to allow him access to the basement recreation areas. Anthony loves country music and often writes his own lyrics and music.*

*Anthony has driven a power wheelchair since he was 3 years old. He uses an adaptive keyboard and touch screen on his phone. He does not use augmentative communication devices. He has some adaptive devices to help him with dressing. He can feed himself independently but requires assistance with food preparation and setup. He toilets independently with assistance for transfers. He can pull his clothing on with assistance.*

### Contemplate Clinical Decisions

*In treating a patient like Anthony, a therapist should consider many clinical decision-making questions. Regarding Anthony, a few such questions include:*

- *How may Anthony's spastic hypertonia affect his ability to engage in typical social activities?*
- *What additional information do you need regarding Anthony's body structure and function to explore how they will directly affect his daily functional skills?*
- *What risk factors related to hypertonia might affect Anthony's overall health and well-being?*
- *What safety concerns do you have for Anthony as well as his caregivers?*

# Related Pathology

## Anatomy and Physiology

### Neurological System

Spastic hypertonicity is most often related to damage to the CNS motor structures shaded in Figure 19-2 "Where Is It?" feature, specifically to (1) upper motor neuron cell bodies or fibers, including the primary or secondary motor cortex, the motor fibers of the corona radiata and posterior limb of the internal capsule (deep white matter of the brain), and the corticospinal tracts within the brainstem, all of which are often damaged by stroke, brain injury, MS, or brain tumors or (2) upper motor neuron descending fibers of the spinal cord, which are often damaged by SCI or MS. The descending motor pathway in the spinal cord, carrying voluntary control of limb muscles, is the lateral corticospinal tract. The ventral thalamus (Fig. 19-2) isn't directly included in this pathway but is involved in sensorimotor loops and planning for execution of movements. Rigid hypertonia is most often associated with CNS disorders or damage to the basal ganglia, particularly the substantia nigra (SN) (Fig. 19-2) as occurs in Parkinson disease. Although the SN isn't anatomically located with the basal ganglia, it has many connections throughout the CNS (brain and spinal cord), and functionally is part of the basal ganglia circuitry. Table 19-1 shows typical motor tone symptoms resulting from some of the more common CNS motor lesion locations.

### Musculoskeletal System

Hypertonicity may have a direct impact on skeletal growth and musculoskeletal deformities (Haselkorn, 2005; Trompetto, 2014). For instance, a joint may lose range of motion if the tone in the muscle is high, pulling the muscle into a shortened range. If the antagonist cannot overcome the pull from the tone of the agonist, it will become weak, overstretched, and may not be able to bring the joint through the full range of motion. In developing bones, the abnormal muscle forces can lead to skeletal deformities with abnormal bone shapes or excessive bony prominences. Typically spastic muscles tend to be weaker (i.e., have less voluntary force generation) than nonspastic muscles (Wiley, 1998; Phadke, 2015). The body may begin to rely on the spasticity to generate muscle force and neglect strength development. This lack of movement through full range may lead to joint contractures. Joint contractures may prevent a person from fully using their limbs. If a person has significant flexion contractures of the hand for instance, they may not be able to grasp and release utensils, hygiene aids, or writing utensils. If a person cannot fully extend the upper extremity, dressing will be difficult as well as reach and grasp of out of reach items. Additionally a person's balance may be affected if the arm cannot be used for support or protective balance extension. If the lower extremity is contracted, standing and walking will be diminished. Additionally depending on the ability to achieve hip and knee alignment, the patient may have difficulty sitting with a balanced posture. Often a patient with spasticity in the trunk will develop scoliosis due

## ■ WHERE IS IT?

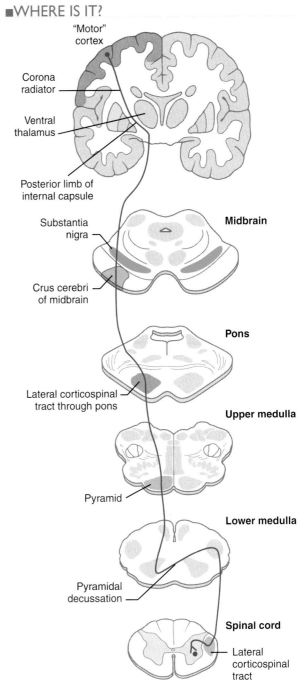

**FIGURE 19-2** This drawing highlights the major CNS locations within the brain, brainstem, and spinal cord related to muscle hypertonus. Damage to the structures shaded blue is often associated with spasticity. In the brain, the precentral gyrus is the primary motor cortex, superior frontal lobe just in front of the precentral gyrus is the premotor cortex, and the corona radiata and posterior limb of the internal capsule of the deep white matter include the corticospinal motor pathways while the ventral thalamus contains relay nuclei for motor processing from the basal ganglia and cerebellum. The corticospinal pathways continue to descend through the brainstem in the crus cerebri most anteriorly in the midbrain, through the pons and through the pyramids of the medulla, before crossing in the low medulla. After crossing, the corticospinal pathways continue to descend in the posterior aspect of the lateral funiculus of the spinal cord white matter. Damage to the SN of the basal ganglia (in green) usually results in rigidity as seen in Parkinson disease.

| TABLE 19-1 | Typical Muscle Tone Symptoms |
| --- | --- |
| **LESION LOCATIONS ASSOCIATED WITH HYPERTONICITY** | **EFFECT ON MUSCLE TONE** |
| Brainstem | • Cortical motor center loss (alpha and gamma motor neurons fire without modification) = ↑ **spastic tone**<br>• Supraspinal motor center loss (vestibular, reticular, pontine nuclei) = **severe spasticity** (often in extensor distribution) |
| Subcortical white matter (including corona radiata and internal capsule) | • Cortical motor center white matter loss (so alpha and gamma motor neurons fire without modification) = ↑ **spastic tone** |
| Primary motor cortex | • Corticospinal tract lesion allows motor neurons to fire without modification = ↑ **spastic tone** |
| Basal ganglia | • **Rigidity** |
| Cerebellum | • **Hypotonia** |

to muscle imbalances yielding asymmetrical trunk alignment. These imbalances can often lead to problems with ribcage movement and flexibility, increasing the risk of upper respiratory infections.

Muscles with long-term chronic spasticity or rigidity can develop inherent stiffness (Lieber, 2004; Sinkjær, 1994; Trompetto, 2014; Phadke, 2015) as a physical characteristic of the muscle, but this stiffness is not velocity dependent and therefore is distinct from spasticity as classically described. This stiffness has been shown to be due to changes in both muscle and nervous system (Mirbagheri, 2001).

## Hypertonia in Neuromuscular Diagnoses

Spasticity occurs in response to upper motor neuron CNS damage, including cerebral cortex cells, cerebral corticospinal pathways, and the corticospinal pathways of the spinal cord. It commonly occurs in lesions related to stroke, SCI, CP, traumatic brain injury (TBI), and MS. Although it is easily recognized, spasticity is difficult to define and measure/grade objectively, as discussed in Chapter 6. Spasticity can best be categorized as a group of positive upper motor neuron sensorimotor symptoms, including resistance to active or passive movement, exaggerated deep-tendon reflexes, and intermittent or sustained involuntary activation of muscles (Mandigo, 2006; Sheean, 2009; Trompetto, 2014; Phadke, 2015). Spasticity has been attributed to a velocity-dependent increase in the tonic stretch reflex (Mandigo, 2006; Trompetto, 2014; Phadke, 2015), but there is also some indication spasticity may be characterized more appropriately by a decrease in the stretch reflex threshold than by an increase in gain (Hui-Chan, 1993; Phadke, 2015). Currently, however, spasticity is thought

to be more related to a hypersensitivity of the reflex arc with changes occurring within the CNS, resulting in loss of descending inhibition, allowing abnormal impulses (Sheean, 2009; Phadke, 2015).

Classically spasticity tends to be velocity-dependent while rigidity is not, and the tone of dystonia fluctuates. In summary spastic hypertonia is not observable at rest but only when the stretch reflex is activated by elongation of the target muscle, and with cerebral injury is usually observed only in the agonist muscle and not the antagonist (i.e., on one side of the joint) and most distinctively at the end of the range of motion when the muscle is on maximal stretch. Rigidity is an increase in resistance/stiffness that is not velocity-dependent, found in muscles on both sides of a joint and consistently throughout the range of motion (not mostly at the end of the range), and is most commonly seen in patients with Parkinson disease.

## Lifespan Influence

Individuals with lifelong disability with related spasticity may see a greater overall effect of the chronic influences of hypertonicity. If a child's development is influenced by hypertonicity or rigidity, that child may develop atypical movement patterns and abnormal loading to particular parts of the skeleton during functional movements (Bakheit, 2010). A child may develop bunions in early adolescence from bearing weight in an asymmetrical pattern during gait. Also a child who ambulates using a walker or crutches may be at risk for overuse injuries of the shoulders. The shoulder joint was not engineered to bear a significant load during ambulation. Forces absorbed at the shoulder (if the patient is using crutches and/or a walker) may lead to impingement syndrome, bursitis, and a myriad of additional musculoskeletal pathologies.

If a patient sustains an injury after completing development, the body can still experience musculoskeletal changes from hypertonus (Trompetto, 2014). These changes will also have an effect on the musculoskeletal system, but they may not be as demonstrative or destructive to bony structures. However regardless of the timing of the injury, near birth or later in life, hypertonicity will affect the patient's body systems. Thus interventions to preserve muscle strength and joint and integumentary integrity must be implemented and continued as a permanent part of the patient's daily routine.

## ■ Pertinent Examination/Evaluation

Table 19-2 summarizes commonly used tests and measures for hypertonia. Details of the tests are described in Chapter 6.

### PATIENT APPLICATION

*Specific examination of the severity of Anthony's spasticity was documented using the Modified Ashworth Scale (MAS):*
*Upper Extremity: R biceps MAS 2; R wrist flexors MAS 2; L biceps MAS 1 +; L wrist flexors MAS 1 +.*

## TABLE 19-2   Tests and Measures for Hypertonia

| TEST/MEASURE | PURPOSE |
|---|---|
| **Modified Ashworth Scale** for spasticity (Bohannon, 1987; Price, 1991; Phadke, 2015) | • Used to rate the severity of spasticity. <br> • Six-point scale, based on magnitude of spasticity and where in the range it is detected, is detailed in Chapter 6. |
| **Dynamic electromyography** (Keenan, 1990) | • Used dynamic electromyography to assess elbow spasticity. |
| **Tardieu Scale** for spasticity (Haugh, 2006; Phadke, 2015) | • Used to rate the severity of spasticity. <br> • Designates the portion of available range that is influenced by spasticity using R1 (the first catch) and R2 (the end of available range) and compares response at slow and fast speeds. |
| **Unified Parkinson Disease Rating Scale** (Motor Examination Item for rigidity) (Fahn, 1987; Richards, 1994) | • Used to rate the severity of rigidity for five regions (neck, right upper extremity, left upper extremity, right lower extremity, left lower extremity). <br> • A five-point scale score is used (0–4) using these qualifiers: <br> 0 = rigidity is absent; <br> 1 = slight rigidity or only with muscle activation; <br> 2 = mild/moderate rigidity; <br> 3 = marked rigidity, full range of motion; <br> 4 = severe rigidity. |

_Lower Extremity:_ R quadriceps, hamstrings, and plantar flexors MAS 1; L quadriceps and plantar flexors MAS 1.

_Upper extremity motor control examination_ revealed isolated control only in L biceps through the initial 40 degrees of the range followed by flexion synergy movement through an additional ~25 degrees of the range, and L triceps through the initial 10 degrees of the range followed by extension synergy for an additional ~10 degrees of the range. All other upper extremity movements were present only in abnormal synergy combinations.

_Lower extremity motor control examination_ revealed isolated selective control through approximately the first third of available range for hip flexors, hip extensors, knee extensors, and ankle dorsiflexors and plantar flexors, bilaterally with abnormal synergies occurring with any attempted movement through further range. Motor control stability was sufficient in the hip and knee to sustain hip and knee extension in supported standing.

### Contemplate Clinical Decisions

■ What additional information do you need regarding Anthony's body structure and function that will directly affect his daily functional skills?
■ What risk factors related to hypertonia might affect Anthony's overall health and well-being the most?
■ Prioritize a problem list of functional limitations for Anthony.
■ What underlying impairments contribute to the functional limitations?
■ Write at least two appropriate goals expressing realistic functional outcomes for Anthony.
■ How might Anthony's spasticity change with changing his body position?
■ Based on your assessment, what intervention strategies would be appropriate for Anthony?

## THINK ABOUT IT 19.2

■ What would be a potential benefit of using the Tardieu scale versus the MAS?
■ How might this affect your plan of care?

## ■ Preparatory Intervention Specific to Hypertonia

### General Approaches

Before planning interventions to reduce spasticity, one should consider relevant goals for reducing spasticity. How could the reduction of hypertonus improve the patient's quality of life and functionality? When formulating goals, consider how altering spasticity (physically or pharmacologically) might enhance function, prevent contractures, increase range of motion, prevent deformity, or reduce pain. The therapist must consider these options in light of the ultimate "So what?" question. So, for example, what does it matter to the patient (in terms of improved function) if the physical therapist works to reduce spasticity or rigidity to improve range of motion?

According to Gelber (1999, p. 5), "Treatment of spasticity is generally considered when the increase in tone interferes with functional activities such as positioning, mobility, or daily cares, when it is painful, or when it leads to complications such as contractures or skin breakdown." In the clinical setting, spasticity can be addressed from several approaches, including pharmacological, surgical, positioning, and passive range of motion, manual therapeutic techniques, and equipment (Phadke, 2015). Although the therapist is not directly involved in prescribing or administering pharmacological or surgical intervention, these medical interventions certainly affect the patient's function and require the therapist to consider changes to the intervention strategy.

## Pharmacological Implications for Therapy

Typically pharmacological interventions for spasticity are coupled with therapy to reduce the influences of hypertonicity and spasticity. Also, while the medications may decrease spasticity, they also leave the patient with decreased force generation, and therefore the therapist must implement strengthening techniques, including intervention methods described in Chapter 22. Medication regime and dosages are at the discretion of the treating physician, who uses input from the therapist about the patient's clinical and functional status and the therapist's judgment about the influence of spasticity on patient function. Additionally, the physician may use input from the patient and family. In addressing spasticity a delicate balance exists between exercises, modality intervention, and pharmaceutical treatments. It is difficult, if not unrealistic, to manage hypertonicity exclusively with medication (Watanabe, 2009). As a child grows or a person becomes more active or has a change in body mass, the medication dosages will need to be adjusted.

Thus in addition to physical therapy interventions to manage spastic hypertonia, patients frequently require medications that usually have a more permanent effect in reducing the hypertonicity. Although the physician will oversee the dosing and administration of the medication, the therapist may be one of the first to notice, and should specifically observe for, changes caused by medication misdosing. Table 19-3 provides an overview of the most commonly prescribed medications and associated side effects. The evidence basis for these antispastic agents, along with the surgical dorsal rhizotomy procedure, is included at the end of the Focus on Evidence: Spasticity

| TABLE 19-3 | Commonly Prescribed Medications for Spastic Hypertonia | | | | |
|---|---|---|---|---|---|
| **MEDICATION** | **DELIVERY METHOD/ DOSAGE** | **COST** | **ACTION** | **HALF-LIFE** | **SIDE EFFECTS** |
| Baclofen Used to reduce tone. | Oral 3 times daily (see intrathecal administration of Baclofen) | Relatively inexpensive | GABA B agonist at the spinal cord level. Cleared by kidneys. | 2.5 to 4 hours | Drowsiness, weakness primarily in head/trunk, increased risk of seizures, withdrawal if stopped suddenly |
| Benzodiazepines: Diazepam (Valium) and Clonazepam (Klonopin) | Oral Diazepam: 1 to 2 times/day Clonazepam: 1 time daily | Relatively inexpensive | GABA A complex of the CNS causing presynaptic inhibition and reduction of reflexes. Metabolized in the liver. | Diazepam: 20 to 80 hours Clonazepam: 18 to 28 hours | Sedation, increased weakness and incoordination, hypotension, addiction potential, withdrawal if stopped suddenly |
| Calcium channel blockers: Dantrolene (Dantrium) Used to reduce tone associated with CP or TBI. Should not be used with acute stroke patients. | Oral 3 to 4 times per day | | Works at the calcium channel in the muscle, decreasing muscle tone, clonus, and muscle spasms. Metabolized by the liver. | 4 to 6 hours | Hepatoxicity, generalized weakness, and drowsiness |
| Imidazolenes: Tizanidine (Zanaflex) Used to treat hypertonicity associated with MS or stroke syndrome. Comparable to Baclofen. | Oral Multiple times during the day | | Alpha 2 adrenergic medications commonly used to treat hypertonicity associated with multiple sclerosis or stroke. It reduces spasms and clonus and is comparable in effect to baclofen. Metabolized by the liver. | 2.5 hours | Sedation, dizziness, cognitive effects, orthostatic hypotension, bradycardia, and dry mouth in chronic users. Hepatoxicity occurs in 5% of the users. |

| TABLE 19-3 | **Commonly Prescribed Medications for Spastic Hypertonia—cont'd** | | | | |

| MEDICATION | DELIVERY METHOD/ DOSAGE | COST | ACTION | HALF-LIFE | SIDE EFFECTS |
|---|---|---|---|---|---|
| Intrathecal baclofen (ITB) | Injectable by pump into the intrathecal space. Due to the direct delivery, smaller, more precise dosages required. | | The baclofen pump is surgically implanted under the lower abdominal fascia and delivers baclofen through a catheter into the fluid surrounding the spinal cord. | | Withdrawal, surgical risks, infection, CSF leaks, and catheter malfunction |
| Chemodenervation medications: Botulinum toxin Type A (Botox) and Type B (Myobloc), alcohol, and phenol. | Intramuscular injection. The effect should be noted within 10 to 14 days, however the peak effect occurs at 4 to 6 months. | | Type A is most frequently used in the United States. Medication used to locally treat spasticity through precise injection directly into the target muscle. | Overall effects last typically 3 to 6 months and as long as 12 months | |
| Cannabis | Orally, transcutaneous, nasal spray | Relatively inexpensive | Reduces effect of glutamate (excitatory) and enhances effect of GABA (inhibitory) neurotransmitters. | Up to 10 hours | Drowsiness, decreased balance |

Intervention Table (Table 19-6 ONL). Although readily used, little evidence is available to guide the clinical decision about which medication is best to use for specific clinical situations to increase function (Watanabe, 2009; Lapeyre, 2010).

Regarding **intrathecal baclofen** (ITB) administration, the baclofen pump is surgically implanted under the fascia of the lower abdomen and delivers baclofen through a catheter into the cerebrospinal fluid surrounding the spinal cord (Fig. 19-3A). The spinal level of the antispastic effect depends on the location/height of the tip of the catheter in the spinal canal. Due to the direct delivery, smaller dosages are required for therapeutic effect compared with oral baclofen and, therefore, the general sedation effect is less than with oral baclofen. Potential complications include pump failure and catheter malfunctions (Lynn, 2009). The pump can be programmed for dosage distribution, allowing the physician to calculate an estimated refill date. The pump alarm will sound when the medication supply is low. Typically the pump is refilled through transdermal injection into the pump reservoir every 3 to 6 months (Fig. 19-3B), and pump battery life is 5 to 7 years. The pump should be replaced every 5 to 7 years. ITB candidates include individuals with Ashworth scores of 3 to 5 in the upper and lower extremities, weight greater than 30 pounds, and older than 4 years-old. The person's spasticity must be impeding function, impeding care, causing contractures, and/or not being well controlled with oral agents. Side effects of the ITB pump include withdrawal, surgical risks, infection, cerebrospinal fluid (CSF) leaks, and catheter malfunction.

A category of medications, termed chemodenervation agents, include Botulinum toxins, alcohol, and phenol. Botulinum Toxin Type A (Botox) is used more frequently in the United States than Type B (Myobloc). Botulinum toxins are used to locally treat spasticity through precise intramuscular (IM) injection directly into the spastic muscle. The effect of the injection can be noted within 10 to 14 days of the injection. However the peak effect occurs at 4 to 6 months with overall effects lasting typically 3 to 6 months and as long as 12 months in some individuals. Botox injections should not occur more frequently than every 3 months to minimize immunity to toxin. Botox can be used in combination with oral medications or ITB. Side effects include localized muscle pain and complications if the patient is also taking anticoagulants (i.e., blood thinners). After Botox injections, the patient should continue with intensive therapy and appropriate orthotic wear.

Phenol, an alcohol, is more complicated to use than Botox. The physician delivers a small electrical impulse to localize the target nerve. This procedure is performed under sedation for children. Phenol blocks are typically used in spasticity of hip adductors or biceps. Phenol, which causes a protein denaturation at the injection site, is injected directly over a motor nerve to avoid muscle or vascular damage, which can result in painful dysesthesias/parasthesia. Thus injection sites are limited. Advantages of using phenol include longer lasting effects than Botox and its effectiveness on large muscle groups.

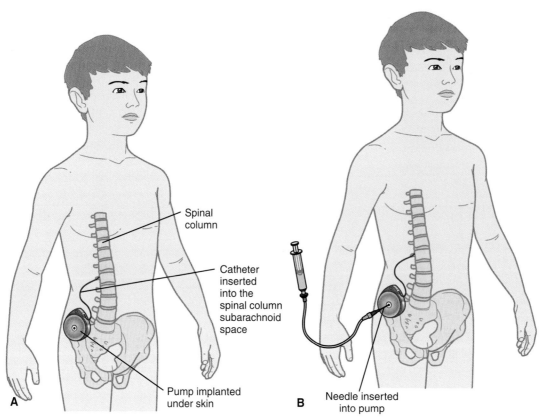

**FIGURE 19-3A & B** The baclofen pump is **A.** surgically implanted under the soft tissue of the lower abdominal wall and delivers baclofen through a catheter into the cerebrospinal fluid of the lumbar cistern. **B.** The pump can be refilled by transdermal injection into the pump reservoir.

## THINK ABOUT IT 19.3

- How would the half-life of the pharmacological drug affect your treatment session?
- What are the side effects of the medicines and the implications of these side effects for PT?
- What functional notations will you make in regards to patient performance to enhance effective decision-making for the patient's plan of care?

### Surgical Intervention

Historically the surgical techniques utilized for the management of sequelae of spastic hypertonia have included reducing tone via selective dorsal rhizotomy (SDR), baclofen pump placement, or in some cases neurosurgery to place a deep brain stimulator, or addressing the secondary orthopedic complications associated with musculoskeletal pathology underlying spasticity (Lynn, 2009). Orthopedic procedures focused on the restoration of range of motion, decreasing contractures, and the preservation of musculoskeletal function (Mandigo, 2006). Such interventions include tendon-lengthening procedures, tendon transfers, osteotomies, and arthrodesis. The primary goal of these procedures is to maintain function in lieu of succumbing to the adverse effects of spasticity (Lynn, 2009). **Tendon lengthenings** are utilized to overcome soft tissue adaptations associated with increased muscular tone in an attempt to avoid contractures; tendon transfers allow antagonist muscles to maximize function. More drastic procedures such as **osteotomies** and **arthrodesis** realign bones and help promote optimal function while slowing any further degradation of movement.

**Selective dorsal rhizotomy** (SDR) is performed to help dampen some of the sensory input associated with spastic hypertonicity. The best candidate for SDR is between 3 and 6 years-old with spastic diplegia distribution and no cognitive deficits. The patient often has sufficient strength to ambulate after the reduction of tone. SDRs are not recommended for children with significant weakness, dystonia, or athetosis (Lynn, 2009).

**Deep brain stimulation** is currently used to treat congenital dystonia or Parkinson disease. The unilateral or bilateral electrical stimulation is most often delivered through an implanted electrical stimulation unit with embedded electrodes in the areas around the thalamus (Lynn, 2009).

ITB is recommended to reduce severe spasticity in individuals with CP, TBI, stroke, SCI, or MS. Although a surgical procedure is required, the effect is pharmacological and has already been described earlier in this section. The pump, which resembles a hockey puck, is surgically placed in the lower abdominal wall under the fascia. A catheter is surgically placed from the pump across the abdominal wall and into the spinal canal to deliver the drug into the cerebral spinal fluid at the appropriate spinal level.

A combination of these neurosurgical and orthopedic surgical interventions work to reduce spasticity as well as maintain the biomechanics of the spine and extremities in individuals with CP (Lynn, 2009).

For the remaining general and specific interventions for hypertonus, a summary of evidence can be found in the Focus on Evidence: Spasticity Intervention and Focus on Evidence: Rigidity InterventionTables (Tables 19-6 and 19-7 ONL).

### Sustained Positioning and Passive Range of Motion

Several studies have noted the effectiveness of sustained positioning (Akbayrak, 2005; Fleuren, 2006) and passive range of motion (PROM) (Wu, 2006) on the reduction of hypertonicity (Adams, 2007; Mandigo, 2006; Ross, 2007; Sanger, 2003). Both stretching and PROM activities are common modes of therapeutic intervention for individuals with hypertonicity. Splinting (Kerem, 2001; Pizzi, 2005; Sheehan, 2006) and serial casting (Lannin, 2007) are also methods of providing a prolonged static stretch to spastic muscles and have been demonstrated to decrease hypertonicity and in some cases elongate shortened muscles over time. Generally, a longer duration stretch such as serial casting described in the following text may result in a longer duration of tone reduction. Similar in theory, several intervention strategies have been devised that apply a sustained stretch to a specific muscle group in an extremity. These interventions include orthotic/bracing, passive standers, as well as several adaptive seating devices described in greater detail in the Equipment section of this chapter.

Casting typically involves application of **serial casting**, a sequence of casts applied in progressively greater range over a period of several weeks (Fig. 19-4), primarily to address limited range of motion. The hypertonic muscle is placed in a position of maximal stretch and is casted in this position. The cast supplies a constant stretch to the muscle over time. The muscle fatigues and elongates. Typically the cast is changed every 2 weeks with a new casting in the new lengthened position until the desired muscle length is achieved. Immediately after completion of serial casting, an orthotic device is used to maintain the additional range of motion.

Several orthotic devices assist in controlling hypertonicity. All orthoses must be custom made to fit the client intimately. Some orthoses are made to elevate/extend the toes to reduce the lower extremity spasticity. Others may incorporate prominences in specific areas of the footplate, particularly under the first metatarsal head, to apply mild pressure to the ball of the

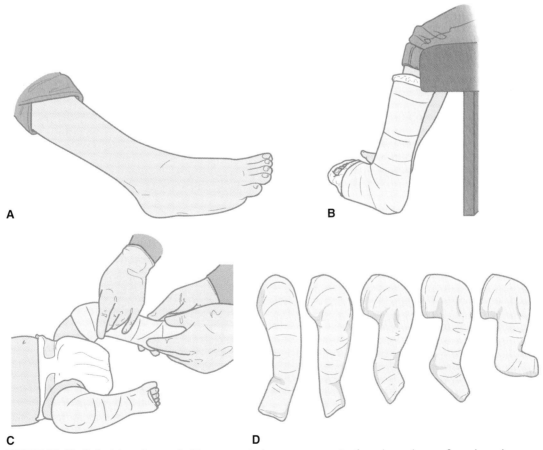

**A**    **B**

**C**    **D**

**FIGURE 19-4A–D** Serial casting, applied in progressively greater range, is often changed every 2 weeks and recast in the new maximal position to increase range of motion. The technique may also decrease spasticity. **A.** The image shows the ankle position of a person before casting. **B.** The image shows the position with cast on. **C.** The image shows casting applied bilaterally to an infant. **D.** The image shows a series of casts that were applied to progressively gain better position and decrease spasticity.

foot to decrease spasticity. All of these methods will position and maintain the joint and associated muscles in a lengthened position in attempt to gain range of motion and decrease tone. Helpful positions that may reduce spasticity include dissociation of upper and lower extremities in sitting or tall kneeling, proper weight-bearing through feet (e.g., standing with foot flat and equal weight-bearing), sidelying with flexion of the upper and lower extremity on one side, and extension of the contralateral extremities.

In addition to static stretching and positioning, more dynamic PROM interventions have been demonstrated to decrease hypertonicity. PROM may be applied either manually by a therapist or through the use of specialized equipment designed to continuously provide movement of an extremity (Wu, 2006). Chang (2007, 2013) noted improvements in spasticity as shown by a reduction in MAS scores of several subjects with SCIs after 60 minutes of continuous passive movements, thus demonstrating the value of PROM in the management of hypertonicity.

### Handling and Physical Inhibition

Several methods exist incorporating manual facilitation and inhibition to manage hypertonicity. Therapeutic handling and optimal positioning are early hallmarks of physical therapy intervention. Several intervention strategies such as Neuro-Developmental Treatment (NDT) (Bly, 1991; Butler, 2001; Kerem, 2001) and Feldenkrais (Connors, 2010) utilize intense physical cuing to attempt to reduce spasticity. NDT and Feldenkrais use gentle positioning and handling techniques to help reduce hypertonicity in an attempt to help individuals with hypertonicity maximize function. Both approaches incorporate tone-inhibiting positioning coupled with handling to achieve therapeutic goals.

### Equipment

Depending on the degree of hypertonicity, spastic or rigid; the neuroanatomic basis of the hypertonicity; and prognosis for improvement (for example, spasticity may be expected to naturally decrease over time in some patients after stroke), therapeutic techniques to temporarily reduce muscle tone may not be feasible, and the therapist may need to utilize specific equipment to help manage the effects of the hypertonicity. Table 19-4 summarizes some of the most commonly used pieces of equipment, listed by category, with a rationale for when it might be helpful.

## Therapeutic Inhibition Techniques

All techniques described in this section provide a reduction of spasticity that is temporary at best (Scanlan, 1998) but may still have a therapeutic purpose in the motor rehabilitation of an individual with neuromotor pathology. A therapist may choose to apply an inhibition technique to a spastic muscle before a mobilization or before a technique to enhance range of motion. These methods may also be useful before interventions to improve voluntary motor control of related muscle groups, particularly voluntary-controlled movement by muscles opposing the spastic muscle. In such a case, the patient may have a window of opportunity to practice motor control of muscles with which the spastic muscle normally interferes. Most of the techniques described in the following sections are applications related to interventions to alter spasticity along with available evidence. Specific techniques for rigidity are also described.

### Deep Pressure

Just as sustained positioning may temporarily decrease hypertonia, applying deep pressure to an extremity may be used

| **TABLE 19-4** | **Equipment Typically Used in Managing of Hypertonicity** | |
|---|---|---|
| **CLASSIFICATION OF EQUIPMENT** | **EXAMPLE** (SEE ILLUSTRATIONS IN CHAPTER 17) | **RATIONALE** |
| Orthotics (static and dynamic) | Ankle foot orthosis (static) | To maintain the foot in a neutral position or in slight dorsiflexion in order to disrupt the lower extremity extension synergy and provide static sustained stretch to plantar flexors, to inhibit hypertonicity of the plantar flexors. |
| | Dynamic splint | A dynamic splint may allow for some slight movement of an extremity while simultaneously providing a low load, long duration stretch to a joint, contributing to a decrease in hypertonicity. |
| Seating and positioning | Seat cushion contour | Positioning the pelvis in a posterior tilt may contribute toward a decrease in extensor tone in an individual with hypertonicity. |
| Passive stander | Supine standing frame | Standing frames provide an important element of weight-bearing to a lower extremity. Weight-bearing provides approximation to joints, which may inhibit spasticity. |

to increase joint awareness and decrease spasticity. Apply a nonnoxious-sustained compressive pressure over the longitudinal axis of the tendon of a hypertonic muscle to elicit increased activation of the golgi tendon organ (GTO). This increased activation of the GTO could help induce an elongation to the muscle, thereby reducing tone. Although clinical application of this technique is common, scientific studies are necessary to investigate the evidence-basis.

### Joint Traction

Sustained long-axis traction to a joint may provide increased joint awareness along with increased activation of joint receptors. Place one hand proximally on the extremity to provide a stabilizing force and gently distract (apply a force to pull one bone away from the other to widen the joint space) using a firm grip of your other hand applied distally. This traction force may be sustained or applied in an intermittent fashion. Contraindications for this technique include extremely hypomobile or hypermobile joints. Scientific studies are necessary to investigate the evidence-basis of this technique.

### Rhythmic Rotation

**Rhythmic rotation**, applying slow low-amplitude rhythmic rotary movements of the body/head, may provide mild repetitive input to the vestibular system and CNS, resulting in increased relaxation. The increased state of relaxation may provide some generalized dampening of both spastic and rigid muscle groups. This total-body inhibition is achieved through decreased output from the vestibulospinal reflex. By a different mechanism and for a more regional effect, you can also apply rhythmic rotation at a specific joint, such as rotation of the upper extremity alone or as body-segment rotation such as with rolling or with trunk rotation in supine (Figs. 19-5A-C) which would act through the local musculoskeletal system to cause a diagonal stretching of the related muscles, which may induce some relaxation. In addition to manual application, this type of rhythmic rotation can also be implemented actively by the patient, such as with trunk rotation exercises. In addition, as with most techniques described in this section, rhythmic rotation can be used as an isolated technique or in combination with other techniques, such as the application of long-axis traction to an upper extremity in combination to manual rhythmic rotation. Scientific studies are necessary to investigate the evidence-basis of this technique.

### Sustained Stretch

Stretching, particularly slow prolonged stretch to the spastic muscle, is supported for providing a temporary decrease in spasticity (Al-Zamil, 1995; BovendEerdt, 2008; Schmit, 2000; Selles, 2005; Yeh, 2005). A sustained stretch applied to a hypertonic muscle at a maximally elongated position provides activation of the GTO and may decrease tension and contractibility similar to the application of deep pressure. So providing a firm sustained stretch may help reduce hypertonicity in a spastic muscle. Applying a sustained stretch may have a greater effect on extensor muscles. In addition stretching a spastic muscle is often combined with or followed by

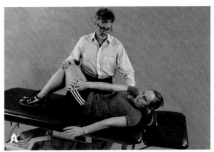
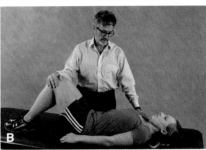
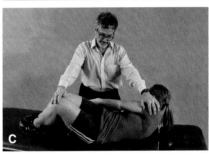

**FIGURE 19-5A–C** This photo series shows an application of passive rhythmic rotation to the trunk to stretch the trunk muscles diagonally and temporarily decrease hypertonus.

active contraction of the antagonist muscle group to provide reciprocal inhibition to the spastic muscle and may provide greater carryover. Stretching can be implemented within the direct therapy session as well as part of a patient's home program (Gallager, 2015).

### Thermal Applications: Warm or Cold

Both warm gentle heat or prolonged icing have been used to temporarily reduce tone in hypertonic spastic muscle groups. Heat is often applied clinically, including a warm therapeutic pool (see aquatic therapy section in the following text), neoprene garments, or air splint application to help provide a regional muscle relaxation in individuals to contribute to dampening of muscle tone and excitability. After a 10-minute application of warmth, the reduction in muscle tone may be sustained for as long as 30 minutes (Matsumoto, 2006).

Although 24°C (cool water) hydrotherapy has been shown to increase spasticity (Chiara, 1998), prolonged icing, such as a cold pack over a spastic muscle or immersion of the affected limb (particularly the ankle and calf muscles) into a bucket of chilled water with ice-chips, can decrease spasticity (Price, 1993) perhaps through decreasing muscle spindle activation and/or nerve conduction velocity, thereby decreasing muscle tone. Cryotherapy has also been shown to eliminate clonus with an average duration of 28 minutes (Miglietta, 1973). Generally speaking heat is better accepted by clients due to its calming effect, and heat is more comfortable than cold for most people. Contraindications for both techniques include individuals with sensory impairments, poor cognition, or intolerant diagnoses. For example, individuals with MS may have intolerance to heat, and heat may cause an increase in symptoms. If there are no contraindications present for either heat or cold, patient preference may be the deciding factor for the physical therapist to consider.

### Therapeutic Taping

**Kinesiotape** is an elastic therapeutic tape designed to mimic the qualities of human skin and might be helpful to control joint position and reduce excitability of spastic muscle fibers. If the Kinesiotape is laid perpendicular to the muscle fibers, it dampens the firing of those muscle fibers. Kinesiotaping and rigid tape can also be used to maintain the position of a joint. For instance, if a patient is exhibiting an indwelling or cortical thumb posture, rigid tape may be used to maintain the thumb in abduction and extension. Ultimately, maintaining the thumb out of the palm may help to reduce the tone in the hand. Scientific studies need to be performed to determine the effectiveness of therapeutic taping in spasticity reduction.

### Biofeedback

Biofeedback has also been investigated as a method to decrease spasticity particularly in children with spastic CP (Dursun, 2004). Biofeedback for 10 minutes per day was applied with dorsiflexor and plantar flexor activity monitored by both visual and auditory signals while the patient performed contraction of tibialis anterior and relaxation of triceps surae complex. A significant decrease in spasticity (MAS) was reported in this study for up to 3 months.

### Vibration and Sonic Pulses

At least one study has shown application of vibratory stimulation directly to spastic muscle can temporarily reduce spasticity, as measured by MAS and F-wave amplitude, for at least 30 minutes (Noma, 2009). In this study vibration was delivered at 91 Hz and 1-mm amplitude for a 5-minute duration. In clinical settings, vibration is often applied to the muscle antagonist to the spastic muscle to reduce spasticity through reciprocal inhibition. In another delivery of mechanical intervention, active "shock wave" treatment, also called extracorporeal shock wave therapy (ESWT), delivers a sequence of single sonic pulses often used in intervention for tendinopathies and has resulted in a significant decrease in spasticity (Ashworth scale) lasting for more than 4 weeks but was not sustained at 12 weeks (Manganotti, 2005). Studies have also shown that hippotherapy, details beyond the scope of this text, results in a reduction of spasticity (Lechner, 2003, 2007).

### Electrical Stimulation

Application of **electrical stimulation**, therapeutic application of electrical current to the body, has been studied as a means to temporarily reduce spasticity. In most cases motor-level stimulation, often referred to as **neuromuscular electrical stimulation (NMES)**, for spasticity is applied to the innervated antagonist muscle group with an immediate but short duration reduction in spasticity (Al-Abdulwahab, 2009; Aydin, 2005; Bakhtiary, 2008; Carmick, 1993; Dewald, 1996; Kavlak, 2005; Khalili, 2008; Santos, 2006) perhaps through reciprocal inhibition of the spastic muscle group. It may also be possible to apply NMES to the spastic muscle (Armutlu, 2003; Van der Salm, 2006), which may cause fatigue of the spastic muscle and therefore reduce spasticity temporarily (Stein, 2015). In one comparison study, NMES decreased spasticity more significantly than a program of passive stretch (King, 1996). Sensory-level electrical stimulation, in which a motor response is not elicited, may also temporarily reduce muscle spasticity (Aydin, 2005; Miller, 2007; Wang, 2000; Yan, 2009) possibly via sensory habituation of spinal pathways. A positive intervention effect to decrease spasticity has been demonstrated in a variety of neurological diagnoses, including cerebrovascular accident (Bakhtiary, 2008; King, 1996; Ng, 2007; Sonde, 2000; Wang, 2000; Yan, 2009; Stein, 2015; Ya-Yun, 2015), spastic CP (Al-Abdulwahab, 2009; Kavlak, 2005; Khalili, 2008), MS (Armutlu, 2003; Szecsi, 2009), and SCI (Aydin, 2005; Krause, 2008; Van der Salm, 2006). Specific stimulation parameters from a variety of studies are listed in the Focus on Evidence: Spasticity Intervention Table 19-6 (ONL). Parameters vary in these studies based primarily on the desired physiological response to electrical stimulation (i.e., motor or sensory). In most studies listed, a pulsed biphasic current was delivered by a portable unit designed for either motor-level stimulation of innervated muscle (i.e., NMES unit) or sensory-level stimulation for pain control (i.e., TENS unit). Table 19-5 summarizes parameters that may be used for motor-level and sensory-level electrical stimulation to decrease muscle spasticity. An additional parameter that must be considered when applying motor-level stimulation is ramp-up time. Abrupt current increases to antagonist muscles may result in an unwanted quick stretch to the spastic muscle. A subsequent increase in spasticity may occur. Ramp-up times should be adjusted between the 0 to 5 seconds available on most NMES units to ensure patient comfort and avoid a quick stretch of the spastic muscle.

As an example, application of 9 minutes of neuromuscular stimulation in surge mode (100-Hz pulse; pulse duration 0.1 ms and pulse interval 0.9 ms with alternating 4-second surge duration and 6-second rest between surge; and intensity 25% over the intensity required to create a maximum contraction) to the dorsiflexors (tibialis anterior) in individuals poststroke resulted in decreased plantar flexor spasticity as well as an increase in dorsiflexion range of motion (Bakhtiary, 2008). The spasticity-reduction effect in this study was more pronounced if combined with Bobath inhibitory techniques, including 15-minute application of passive movement of ankle joint dorsiflexion, knee joint extension, abduction, and external rotation of hip joint (Bakhtiary, 2008). Electrical stimulation applied continuously to hip abductors has decreased spasticity in hip adductor muscles (Al-Abdulwahab, 2009).

| TABLE 19-5 | Common Electrical Stimulation Parameters Used for Decreasing Spasticity | |
|---|---|---|
| | **MOTOR-LEVEL** | **SENSORY-LEVEL** |
| Waveform | Biphasic pulsed | Biphasic pulsed, amplitude-modulated alternating current (i.e., interferential current) |
| Frequency | 40 to 50 Hz | 20 to 100 Hz |
| Pulse duration | 300 to 400 μsec | 100 to 200 μsec |
| Amplitude | 20 to 60 mA Sufficient to produce a maximal but tolerable muscle contraction. | Sufficient to produce a strong but tolerable sensation with no muscle contraction. |
| Duty cycle | Variable (1:1, 4:6) | Continuous |
| Treatment time | 15 to 45 minutes per day | 15 to 60 minutes per day (although Miller, 2007, applied for 8 hours) |

(Aydin, 2005; Cheng, 2010; Mesci, 2009; Miller, 2007; Ng, 2007; Sabut, 2010; Wang, 2000; Yan, 2009)

Electrical stimulation has also been applied to acupuncture points to explore the effect on spasticity and resulted in a significant reduction of spasticity (Ng, 2007; Sonde, 2000) or a significant increase in the number of subjects with normal muscle tone (Yan, 2009).

Other novel applications of electrical stimulation have been studies with some effect on reducing spasticity. A cyclic electrical stimulation of agonist/antagonist in individuals with paralysis and spasticity from SCI demonstrated a significant reduction of the MAS after stimulation of the agonist (Van der Salm, 2006). Application of five sessions of 45-minute electrical stimulation to the skin in the area of T-12 and L-1 vertebrae also decreased spasticity in individuals with stroke (Wang, 2000).

Various electrical stimulation methods have been applied along with muscle actions—passive, voluntary, or stimulated—to decrease spasticity. When applied in children with CP, electrical stimulation to quadriceps combined with passive stretching of hamstrings has produced a significantly greater reduction in hamstring spasticity than passive stretching alone (Khalili, 2008). Functional neuromuscular electrical stimulation (FES) has been applied in individuals with complete SCI to induce cycling movements along with passive simultaneous movement by an ergometer (Krause, 2008) with biphasic rectangular pulses (pulse duration 500 μsec, frequency 20 Hz, and current 0 to 99 mA) resulting in a significant decrease in the MAS. Repeated electrical stimulation combined with volitional ankle movements also resulted in decreased ankle spasticity in subjects with stroke with improvement that further correlated with better gait symmetry and functional gait performance (Cheng, 2010). TENS applied to lower extremity acupuncture points and combined with "task specific practice" produced earlier and greater reduction in spasticity than TENS alone and also resulted in greater gait velocity (Ng, 2007). As an additional effect, neuromuscular electrical stimulation can increase sensory inputs into the CNS, which may enhance CNS plasticity for improved motor learning (Bogataj, 1995).

Reported duration of the spasticity reduction from these electrical interventions varies between the methods. After electrical stimulation to acupuncture sites in adults with hemiplegia, the improvement was observed for at least 2 weeks after the final treatment (Sonde, 2000). After application of TENS in individuals with stroke, the reduction in spasticity was sustained 4 weeks after conclusion of the intervention (Ng, 2010). In children with spastic CP, the decrease in spasticity has been observed 1 week after the stimulation (Al-Abdulwahab, 2009) and in some cases for at least 1 month after the application (Kavlak, 2005). In the FES application during cycling among individuals with MS, the significant reduction in lower extremity spasticity was recorded only short-term and not after the 2-week training period (Szecsi, 2009). Further study is needed on the clinical significance of the duration of spasticity reduction. For example, how long will the spasticity reduction allow an increase in motor control for the purposes of repetitions and practice for motor control?

### Acupuncture

**Acupuncture** is a form of Chinese alternative medicine in which fine needle tips are inserted superficially into the skin at specific predetermined locations for some therapeutic benefit. The specifics of the technique are beyond the scope of this textbook, but it has been applied in individuals with spasticity with mixed results (Fink, 2004; Wayne, 2005), including acupuncture applications in combination with strengthening exercises (Mukherjee, 2007). These studies are summarized in the Focus on Evidence: Spasticity Intervention Table 19-6 (ONL).

### Techniques Specific to Reduce Rigidity

Most of the techniques previously described have been applied specifically to alter spasticity. But several studies have investigated interventions to decrease rigidity, particularly in Parkinson disease. The details of the evidence-basis are included in the Focus on Evidence: Rigidity Intervention Table 19-7 (ONL), although the specificity of the results related to changes in rigidity could be questioned because combinations of interventions were often applied. Most studies measured the decrease in rigidity using the motor examination section of the Unified Parkinson Disease Rating Scale (UPDRS).

- Passive Stretch: Passive, slow, and prolonged stretch as previously described while the patient is at rest has also been applied in a sample with Parkinson disease and resulted in an improvement of the UPDRS motor rigidity factor (Pacchetti, 2000).
- Physical Activity and Physical Exercise: Several studies have indicated physical activity such as treadmill walking or physical exercise can temporarily reduce rigidity in the context of Parkinson disease. In one study a program of treadmill walking, 20 minutes per day, 3 days per week, for 6 weeks (with or without body weight support) resulted in an improvement of the motor examination section of the UPDRS (Toole, 2005). A physical exercise program designed to improve ROM, endurance, balance, gait, and fine motor dexterity in Parkinson disease with progression of exercise as endurance increased resulted in improvement of the UPDRS rigidity factor (Comella, 1994). In another study, a program of balance and strength training in individuals with Parkinson disease, whether PT-supervised or self-supervised, resulted in a significant improvement in the UPDRS motor subsection score (including the rigidity factor) with no significant change in the total UPDRS score (Lun, 2005). Exercise on a stationary tandem bicycle with a trainer to maintain intensity 30% greater than their voluntary exercise rate also resulted in improvement in rigidity by 41% in the intervention group (improvement in 50% of the subjects) (Ridgel, 2009).
- Aquatic Exercise in Warm Water: Individuals with Parkinson disease who do exercises to improve strength, motor control, and balance, including once a week exercise in a heated pool, have demonstrated an improvement in rigidity (Reuter, 1999).
- Stretch Exercise (from United Parkinson Foundation): An improvement, though not significant, was reported in individuals who completed 12 weeks (three times per week) of stretch exercises as provided by the United Parkinson Foundation (Palmer, 1986).
- Trager Therapy: A gentle rocking motion can be applied to the upper limbs and body, in sitting or lying, at 3 to 4 Hz and amplitude of 1 to 4 cm for 20-minute sessions as part of Trager Therapy in a sample with Parkinson disease (Duval, 2002). These specific parameters in one sample with Parkinson disease resulted in a 36% reduction of Evoked Stretch Response (ESR) in rigid muscles at 1 minute after intervention in sitting, which remained 32% lower at 11 minutes after the treatment. The administration in a supine position resulted in a 42% reduction of ESR (Duval, 2002). The authors concluded administration in a sitting position was not as efficient for a sustained effect.
- Whole Body Vibration: As a more recent intervention the application of vibratory stimulation to the whole body,

Whole Body Vibration (WBV), has been attempted for a possible effect on a variety of motor impairments. One protocol includes a series of five WBV applications of 60-second duration using mean frequency of 6 Hz and amplitude of 3 mm with a 1-minute pause between each series (Haas, 2006). This procedure resulted in a significant improvement by 16.8% in the UPDRS motor score and specifically a 24% improvement in the UPDRS rigidity score. A significant decrease in rigidity (measured by UPDRS) has also been reported after WBV administered through a physioacoustic chair (King, 2009).
- Botulinum Toxin A: Injection of Botulinum Toxin A into rigid muscles of patients with Parkinson disease, progressive supranuclear palsy, and corticobasal degeneration resulted in a decrease in rigidity in seven of the eight subjects with rigidity (Grazko, 1995). For this protocol, small muscle groups were injected at one point and larger groups at two or three points.
- Electrical Stimulation and Magnetic Pulse Stimulation: An application of low-frequency 10 to 50 Hz, max 9.9A electrical stimulation for 15 minutes twice a day resulted in amelioration of rigidity in 146 of 180 subjects, while magnetic pulse stimulation (30 minutes MPS, 15 minutes rest, 15 minutes MPS) showed an average of 32% reduction of UPDRS motor scale (Henneberg, 1998).

## Intervention: Ultimately Applied in Functional Activities

### Aquatic Therapy

Use of aquatic therapy, particularly in a warm pool, is an effective method of therapeutic exercise for individuals with hypertonicity. Therapeutic pools are typically kept at a temperature between 84°F and 94°F. At this temperature, the warmth of the pool provides a global relaxation and dampens spastic and rigid tone as previously described. A general therapeutic benefit has been demonstrated with a decrease in spasticity related to exercise in an aquatic environment (Kesiktas, 2004). The pool also provides two important factors, buoyancy and resistance. **Buoyancy** is described as an upward force expressed on an object in water that creates a floating force. Buoyancy helps create a greater degree of safety and stability when working on ambulatory activities in the water; it also helps eliminate the effects of gravity decreasing the compressive forces expressed on joints. The resistance to movement the water provides is a benefit of performing gait therapeutic exercise, more specifically, gait training in an aquatic environment. An aquatic environment provides resistance to any direction of movement and serves as an excellent strengthening tool.

### Quadruped

Transitional movements and exercises performed in the quadruped (4-point) position can be helpful in individuals with hypertonicity. Particularly in the case of extensor spasticity, the quadruped position helps induce flexion into the hips and knees, providing a prolonged stretch to the associated muscle groups. The quadruped position is important in functional mobility, particularly floor transitions. In addition maintenance of the quadruped position as a dynamic activity requires increased motor control, core strength, and balance. For younger patients, crawling may be a very age-appropriate activity to practice. Initiated in the quadruped position, crawling incorporates reciprocal agonist-antagonist muscle recruitment and motor control. This pattern of muscle contraction may help reduce spastic tone through consistent reciprocal inhibition of hypertonic muscles.

## Rolling

Rolling is a fundamental component of bed mobility. Utilization of **rhythmic initiation** and rhythmic rotation with rolling activities may help reduce hypertonicity while increasing proficiency and independence with functional mobility. While rolling may be considered a simple activity, it provides a basis for many complex transitional movements, including car transfers and pivot transfers. In addition rolling may be appropriate for all ages, depending on level of motor impairments.

## Weight-bearing Activities

Weight-bearing activities, assuring the joints are in good alignment, may also temporarily decrease hypertonus. For instance, when a person is in sitting and propping on the affected arm, the physical therapist can assist the person in side bending to the affected side to put weight through the extended spastic arm while assisting the arm to stay in an extended position. This weight-bearing, which is in essence joint approximation with compression of the joint surfaces, will reduce the hypertonicity in the arm. Similarly half kneeling can be used to improve dissociation (with opposite movements and positioning of the two limbs—one in flexion and one in extension) of the lower extremity and decrease spasticity in the lower extremities. Other beneficial weight-bearing positions include quadruped, tall kneeling, supported standing with weight through the arms on a table (modified plantigrade), and weight-bearing through legs on the floor (plantigrade standing).

Regarding the upper extremity, sometimes it is helpful to have the person ambulate while weight-bearing through the upper extremity on a table surface or on the therapist's hand during forward progression.

### Tone-Reducing Orthotics

Wearing orthotics while participating in functional weight-bearing activities has shown to decrease spasticity and improve function (Nash, 2008).

## Pediatric Considerations

Spastic hypertonia can be present in infants and children. Often children diagnosed with CP show hypotonia as neonates and then go on to develop spasticity that progressively increases as the child ages. Spasticity is also common in the context of pediatric brain injury. Depending on severity, spasticity and rigidity can affect the care of the child. Spastic tone in the lower extremities, particularly adductors for instance, can make diaper changing and general hygiene difficult. Similarly spasticity in the upper extremity flexors can bring the hand and arm into positions that also make skin care difficult, especially in the armpits, elbow creases, and palms of hands. A child with spasticity in the hands may have a tendency to maintain the hand in a fisted or closed position. Paradoxically children with spasticity in the extremities often have hypotonia in the trunk.

Developmentally children with spasticity often have difficulty acquiring the developmental motor skills, especially related to the impaired motor control that may accompany spasticity. Movement of a muscle antagonistic to the spastic muscle will cause a stretch to the spastic muscle followed by increased resistance that will limit the intended voluntary movement. These children may exhibit early development of prone skills, holding their head up early and also being able to prop on hands earlier than other children. However careful observation of these movements will reveal the child is using the influences of spasticity and not volitional motor control for these antigravity prone activities. The child is typically asymmetrical and often pushing using fisted hands. If the spasticity is bilateral, the forces of the spastic muscles may hold both lower extremities in extension with no dissociation noted. In supine, the same child may have difficulty pulling the head up off the surface and may have difficulty getting the hand to midline. Thus the child appears to be stuck in one position on the mat with the lower extremities in extension and hip internal rotation and the upper extremities in relative extension with shoulder lateral rotation. Learning to maintain their bodies in an upright orientation, sitting or standing, is often delayed and the children have difficulty using typical movement patterns to move through space. Thus reciprocal crawling and ambulation are difficult for the child and will need to be practiced in therapy. Conversely caregivers will report the child demonstrates raising the head up in prone.

### PATIENT APPLICATION

*Use the description of 16 year-old Anthony presented earlier in the chapter to answer the following questions.*

#### Contemplate Clinical Decisions

- How and why would you treat Anthony's hypertonia?
- Use principles of progression to develop three different ways to modify Anthony's activities over the next several weeks to emphasize optimal function both in the clinic and at home.
- What other treatment settings and environmental setup would you consider?
- Formulate and describe at least two additional specific treatment ideas applied within specific functions.

# ■ Intervention: Considerations for Nontherapy Time and Discharge

## Patient and Family Education

For the patient with spasticity, education is important regarding personal management of the spasticity, particularly positioning to encourage and movements to avoid during all nontherapy times at home and when out in the community. For example, teach the patient to avoid any quick movements of the affected body segment that might provide a rapid stretch to the spastic muscle group. Also instruct them to keep the affected limb in appropriate weight-bearing positions as much as possible. This will encourage optimal use of the limb and attention to the limb in natural ways. During rest, it is also important to maintain the limb in a position that keeps the spastic muscles in some degree of stretch to prevent contracture and again encourage more appropriate positioning.

## Activities for Home

Although physical intervention/therapy and pharmacological intervention are important for the patient with spasticity, the time outside of therapy is equally important. If the patient or the family can learn to position the affected body segments optimally, some effects of spasticity can be avoided. This may affect a patient differently depending if it is a child or an adult. For a child, motor development will be encouraged, and the child will benefit from more optimal practice. It is imperative the therapist teach caregivers methods for incorporating therapy techniques into the family's daily routines. Families are busy entities, and the birth of a child with a disability stresses the family further. Any treatment that can be built into regularly occurring care activities such as stretching at diaper changing time or carrying and holding the child in a way that decreases the spasticity will benefit the child and family. Thus the therapist should have a strong understanding of the patient's and family's schedules and routines from the time the patient rises in the morning to the time the patient goes to bed. For the adult patient, similar concepts prevail. Families are busy entities and spasticity-reducing activities should be embedded into everyday routines, especially dressing, eating, and leisure routines.

The therapist should also teach the patient (regardless of age) and caregivers how to look for opportunities throughout the day to embed therapeutic activities. For instance, when reading a book, watching TV, or using the computer, one's position can help to decrease spasticity. When sitting in a firm chair, the patient should always be positioned with feet flat on the floor and lower extremities in neutral position, with the trunk well supported. This can be accomplished with optimal supportive seating surfaces, maintaining the pelvis in a neutral position and allowing the legs to be slightly abducted and flexed at the hips, knees, and ankles. If the patient's feet do not reach the floor, then an elevated support should be positioned under the feet. This support could be a small footstool, a shoebox, a block of wood, thick books, or other sturdy material. If the patient has difficulty with dominant primitive reflexes such as a persistent **Asymmetrical Tonic Neck Reflex (ATNR)**, then the activity should avoid the extremes of neck rotation as much as possible as midline orientation helps to decrease the influences of the ATNR.

Gravity will also significantly influence the expression of spasticity. Gravity-eliminated or gravity-reduced positions, including the aquatic environment, may allow the patient to move more freely or gain control over his/her movements. Positioning the patient in sidelying will help to minimize the influences of gravity and allow the person to maintain reciprocal extremity positions. The lower extremities can be positioned with one leg in flexion and the other in extension to encourage dissociation and avoid the full extension pattern. In sidelying, the person may be able to use their upper extremities more efficiently as part of an activity. The patient may be able to watch TV, use the computer, read a book, or play a board game when in sidelying position.

The influences of spasticity can also be inhibited during dressing activities. While donning or doffing clothes, the extremities can be slowly stretched to gain range of movement and decrease spasticity.

Family members and caregivers should be taught beneficial positions and handling skills to help decrease spasticity. The patient should be positioned into relative flexion with dissociation of the upper extremities and lower extremities. Sidelying with one hip in flexion and the other hip in extension is a good position. For a child, spasticity may also be reduced when carrying and holding the child in a particular way. Carrying a child with legs abducted can minimize the spasticity in the lower extremities. Carrying the child facing outward with the lower extremities positioned as previously discussed is also beneficial. Additionally, by carrying the smaller child in sidelying, facing outward with the head and trunk supported and the legs positioned asymmetrically, spasticity may decrease in all extremities. In supine, individuals should be positioned with some neck flexion and the shoulders protracted to encourage midline use of the upper extremities. When in standing, an effort should be made to keep the lower extremities in neutral alignment with the trunk in extension and the upper extremities in a functional position for support or object manipulation. Long sitting will help to maintain hamstring length, however, ring/tailor sitting will provide a base of support more conducive to work on independent sitting skills. Floor sitting is easier with the younger patients than with the adult patients.

While bathing or swimming, water temperature may influence a person's muscle tone. Warmer water temperatures help to relax hypertonus and allow for easier movements. Swimming is also a gravity-eliminated activity, and a decrease in spasticity may be observed as a patient moves in the water.

## Let's Review

1. What is the clinical definition of spasticity?

2. What outcome scales are appropriate to measure spasticity?

3. Identify two interventions that will decrease spasticity.

4. Identify two interventions that may increase spasticity.

5. How would increased spasticity in the lower extremity improve a person's function?

6. Identify three ADLs that would be negatively affected by increased spasticity.

7. How might increased spasticity affect a person's overall general health?

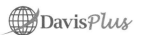 **DavisPlus**  For additional resources, including Focus on Evidence tables, case study discussions, references, and glossary, please visit http://davisplus.fadavis.com

# CHAPTER SUMMARY

### PATIENT APPLICATION

*Davis was born 12 weeks premature and lives with his mother, father, and several extended family members. He was diagnosed with spastic diplegia but did not receive any regular therapy services until he was 1 year-old. At his initial assessment Davis presented with decreased passive range with limited ankle dorsiflexion bilaterally, bilateral knee extension, and bilateral hip extension. He had Ashworth 1+ spasticity in bilateral knee extensors and bilateral ankle plantar flexors. His functional mobility pattern was commando crawling for very short distances and rolling for longer distances. When he attempts to sit independently, he falls to the side each time. He could maintain sitting with upper extremity support and could transition from kneeling to standing by pulling with his upper extremities using a symmetrical lower extremity push. When in standing, he required maximum assistance.*

*Davis' parents were taught a home exercise stretching program to start to increase functional range of motion in the lower extremities. Therapy included passive stretching, active activities, including weight shifting in four point, weight-shifting and stepping in standing, transitioning through the developmental sequence from sitting on the ground into four point, into tall kneel, into half kneel, and then standing to increase motor planning and strength. He worked on the treadmill to practice stepping and using a more typical gait pattern. Davis received intervention using a Swiss ball to work on core strengthening, ROM activities, a smaller inflatable peanut to work on trunk control in sitting, and lower extremity ROM and weight-bearing and upper extremity weight-bearing. Parent education regarding CP and parenting a child with a disability also helped Davis improve. The parents needed to follow-up at home with the stretching activities, and they also needed*

*to increase their expectations of Davis by encouraging him to be more independent and setting up the environment so Davis would get appropriate challenges throughout the day. Additionally Davis' family embedded his therapy routines into daily routines. They regularly performed range-of-motion exercises, including prolonged stretch to spastic muscle groups during dressing and diaper changes. They encouraged Davis to transition to standing every time he wanted to be picked up, and they encouraged Davis to walk as much as possible instead of being carried or rolling on the floor. The family stacked two thick books together into a small platform to rest his feet in front of a bench where Davis would sit to watch TV, color, and eat his snack. In this bench-seated position, Davis was encouraged to more easily go from sit-to-stand several times a day and then was also more motivated to walk with his walker. Davis began to ambulate with a forward wheeled walker with stand-by assist from his caregiver. He was able to learn to stand in neutral alignment and transition into and out of positions using his lower extremities.*

*Davis was referred to the developmental pediatrician, who agreed with the PT recommendation for bilateral AFOs. Davis was fitted for bilateral ankle foot orthoses to help maintain the foot in a neutral position while in standing and sitting on a bench. Davis was also considered for a pharmaceutical intervention, but the parents preferred to wait and see if therapy and the orthotics helped to decrease the tone and increase his functional ability.*

*Davis was enrolled in therapeutic horseback riding to help increase lower extremity range of motion, decrease spasticity, and improve postural responses with movement. An eclectic approach to therapy that incorporated motor and verbal facilitation, motor learning, cognitive learning, tone reduction techniques, and assistive technology assisted in helping Davis to become more independent and functional.*

Spastic hypertonia is a result of damage to motor areas of the CNS, often occurring as part of an upper motor neuron lesion. Spasticity can be observed in many neurological diagnoses, including both children and adults. The effect of spasticity on movement is variable, depending on the severity of the condition, with some individuals being dominated by spasticity and others being mildly affected. The resistance resulting from elongation of a spastic muscle is velocity-dependent with greater resistance occurring with a faster stretch. Therefore rapid limb movement in the antagonistic direction can result in expression of the spasticity, perhaps even with movement as the spastic muscle contracts. Patients with spasticity need to avoid rapid movement of the affected joints, whether active or passive. There are several ways to clinically assess and rate spasticity, including the Ashworth Scale and the Tardieu Scale. Spastic hypertonicity may be decreased with therapeutic techniques or body positioning as described in this chapter or with medications.

If the hypertonicity affects the individual's function to a significant degree or has other related impairments, medications or surgical procedures can be administered to improve function. Spasticity has been shown to be negatively correlated with antagonist muscle strength (Levin, 1994). Individuals who take antispastic drugs or who undergo spasticity-reducing surgical procedures will likely need physical therapy to then taddress the related problems that develop from or are unmasked by the medical/surgical intervention, including muscle weakness and changes in joint alignment (Brashear, 2002; Coffey, 1993; Giuliani, 1991; Koman, 1993).

A consistent home program is also beneficial in minimizing the sequelae of hypertonicity. Hypertonicity not addressed can lead to joint contractures, decreased function, and decreased quality of life. A neurologist and a physiatrist in addition to their primary care provider should follow individuals with hypertonicity. Patients should be evaluated regularly for pharmaceutical functioning, with special care taken to ensure the pharmacological goals are being met.

# Intervention for Involuntary Contractions and Movement

Jennifer Braswell Christy, PT, PhD ▪ Jeffrey M. Hoder, PT, DPT, NCS

## CHAPTER OBJECTIVES

Upon completion of this chapter, the learner should be able to:

1. Utilize evidence-based tools for adequate examination, evaluation, and treatment of patients with dyskinesia.
2. Describe the role of the basal ganglia and its connection with other neural substrates related to typical movement and dyskinesia.
3. Identify the unique impairments at all levels of the International Classification of Functioning, Disability, and Health affecting individuals with dyskinesia throughout the lifespan.

## ▪ Introduction

The purpose of this chapter is to provide information on evidence-based interventions for individuals with a variety of involuntary movement disorders. Involuntary movement disorders affect an individual's ability to control and modify movement. The movement disorders discussed in this chapter will be limited to those causing **dyskinesia** or abnormal involuntary movements arising most often from pathology within the **basal ganglia**, a group of subcortical motor-modulation nuclei. Pathological changes within the basal ganglia can also cause **bradykinesia** (slowness of movement) and rigidity (joint stiffness) as seen in patients with Parkinson disease. However the focus of this chapter is dyskinesia or involuntary movement. Due to the unique impairments seen in patients with dyskinesia, therapeutic interventions differ from those used with patients who have other movement-related impairments

such as spasticity or rigidity (described in Chapter 19), or **ataxia** (irregular inaccurate movement) (described in Chapter 21). These unique characteristics, as well as their roles in clinical decision-making, will be considered in this chapter. As you read this chapter, refer to Table 20-1 for a brief description of each dyskinesia to be addressed. Refer also to Table 20-6 for a summary of current evidence to support interventions for patients with dyskinesias with a more comprehensive table available online.

A variety of dyskinesias will be discussed, including common problems at all levels of the International Classification of Functioning, Disability, and Health (ICF) model (Steiner, 2002). Definitions for **athetosis, ballismus, chorea, choreoathetosis, dystonia, myoclonus, tics,** and **tremor** are provided in Table 20-1. Common diseases causing dyskinesias will also be discussed to include etiology, pathophysiology, and known demographic information as well as the progressive or

| TABLE 20-1 | Definitions of Dyskinesia | |
|---|---|---|
| **MOVEMENT DISORDER** | **DEFINITION/DESCRIPTION** | **TYPICAL DIAGNOSES** |
| *Tremor* (occurs at various speeds) | Tremor is the most common movement disorder. It involves involuntary, rhythmic, oscillatory movements of reciprocally innervated muscles. Tremors can occur at rest or during movement and vary in frequency. Types include: *Resting* (3 to 6 Hz), *action* or *postural* (4 to 12 Hz). Essential tremor is the most common and involves *action* tremor (Louis, 2005; Smaga, 2003). (In contrast, cerebellar tumor, ataxia, occurs only during voluntary movement, therefore terms an "intention tremor"—see Chapter 6 for examination and Chapter 21 for interventions for ataxia.) | Parkinson disease Essential tremor Multiple sclerosis |
| *Dystonia* | A persistent muscle contraction resulting in incongruous repetitive movements and distorted, unnatural positions of the body. Dystonia can be focal or generalized. (Fahn, 1998) | Focal dystonia Generalized hereditary dystonia Huntington disease Multiple sclerosis with spinal cord lesion Juvenile dystonia (Parkinson syndrome) Drug-induced dystonia Wilson disease CP AIDS |
| *Athetosis* | Comes from the Greek word meaning "unfixed" or "changeable"; Also means "without fixed position"; Slow, writhing movements typically involving the fingers, hands, toes, and tongue. Movements are purposeless and tend to flow from one to the other, spreading to muscles not normally involved in performing a volitional movement. (Yokochi, 1990) | HD Benign hereditary chorea Wilson disease Drug-induced chorea CP or stroke involving infarct to basal ganglia Subdural hematoma Syndenham chorea |
| *Chorea* | Comes from the Greek word meaning "dance"; Abrupt, involuntary, variable, and random flow of activity from one body part to another. Movements are arrhythmic, forcible, rapid, and jerky. The unpredictable nature distinguishes chorea from dystonia and tremor. (Berardelli, 1999) | |
| *Choreoathetosis* | Chorea and athetosis are often indistinguishable. A combination of the two movements typically occurs with damage or disease of the basal ganglia. Therefore, the movement can be described as choreoathetosis. | |
| *Ballismus* | Uncontrollable, violent, flailing movements of an entire limb. It is typically unilateral and might also blend with choreoathetosis. | Stroke (infarct or hemorrhage) damaging the subthalamic nucleus or surrounding structures Bilateral ballismus can result from a metabolic disease. |
| *Tics* | Also called "habit spasms." Involves sudden, rapid, recurring, non-rhythmic, stereotypical movement or vocalization. It is characterized by an irresistible urge to perform the movement and relief of tension after the movement. Motor tics typically involve the face or neck. Vocal tics involve brief grunts, coughing, howling, barking, or obscene words. (Mink, 2001; Mol Debes, 2008) | Tourette's syndrome; Typically seen in conjunction with obsessive-compulsive disorder and/or attention deficit-hyperactivity disorder |
| *Myoclonus* | Characterized by brief, sudden, and rapid asymmetrical contractions involving a group of muscles. Movements are nonrhythmic and can be focal, unilateral, or bilateral. Myoclonus can occur after seizures, with other neurological disease, or can be of unknown etiology. | Idiopathic epilepsy Myoclonic epilepsy Unknown etiology (essential myoclonus) Myoclonus due to other neurological disease |

(Blumenfeld, 2010; Cote, 1991; Samuels, 2009a, 2009b)

nonprogressive nature of the disease. Evidence-based tests and measures and intervention techniques will be presented. Cases of a patient with Huntington disease and a patient with dystonia will also be presented.

## Clinical Picture of Involuntary Movements in a Holistic Context

Patients with dyskinesia present with unique impairments and circumstances that must be considered when making clinical decisions. Depending on the client's disease, age, and severity, dyskinesia can present across a wide spectrum from a barely noticeable tic to disabling chorea. For example, a patient presenting with choreoathetosis (Table 20-1) affecting gross and fine motor function could be diagnosed with Huntington disease (see compendium of selected diagnoses at the end of this book), which is progressive in nature. However choreoathetoid movements can also be caused by nonprogressive brain insults such as cerebral palsy or stroke. Although the movement dysfunction and activity limitations appear to be similar, the clinician must consider the nature of the disease when treating the patient through his or her lifespan. The role of family members and caregivers as well as educational, occupational, and social aspects must also be considered. Environmental contexts and the effect of psychological and cognitive impairments on activities and participation should be addressed as well. Throughout this chapter, the following case of an individual diagnosed with Huntington disease will be considered:

### PATIENT APPLICATION: JD

*JD is a 43 year-old white male who was diagnosed 1 year ago with Huntington disease (HD). His father, paternal uncle, and grandfather passed away in their late 60s after also being diagnosed with HD. JD currently has symptoms, including "fidgety" legs when sitting to watch television or while relaxing. This appears to worsen with time. He has difficulty sitting still for prolonged periods of time during meetings or while attending church. JD was referred to the physical and occupational therapist by his neurologist. Additionally, he has recently begun to stumble and fall. He has full family health insurance through his employer. He is being followed in a Huntington Disease Center of Excellence every 6 months for comprehensive care.*

### Contemplate Clinical Decisions

*The case example of JD will be continued throughout the chapter. Considering what you know thus far:*

1. *What are his impairments at the body functions/body structures level?*
2. *What are his activity limitations and participation restrictions?*
3. *Can you think of any environmental barriers?*

*The answers to these questions will be made clear as the case progresses.*

## Possible Effect of Involuntary Movements on Function

The ICF model is a conceptual framework providing a systematic way to organize information around diagnoses (i.e., the disorder or disease), functioning and disability (i.e., body functions, body structures, activities, and participation), and contextual factors (i.e., environmental and personal factors) (World Health Organization, 2001). In the context of disease processes resulting in dyskinesia, impairments in *body functions* often include poor cognitive function, psychological and behavioral problems, attention deficits, and impairments in voice and speech functions in addition to movement-related impairments (e.g., choreoathetoid movement or other dyskinesia). The neurophysiologic substrate causing the dyskinesia is the impairment in *body structure* (e.g., damage to basal ganglia and thalamus, Figure 20-1). *Activity limitations* in individuals with dyskinesias might include the inability to walk or climb stairs, the inability to walk and carry objects, poor standing balance on compliant surfaces or with altered and obscured vision, or difficulty writing and manipulating small objects. *Participation restrictions* could cross many domains such as safety issues (e.g., falls, unsafe tub transfers), the inability to use transportation or drive, difficulty with basic activities of daily living (ADL; e.g., dressing, bathing, grooming), an inability to prepare meals and do household chores, difficulty caring for children, relationship problems, or an inability to participate in leisure activities or school. *Environmental barriers* greatly limit the potential of patients with dyskinesias. Patients often experience social isolation and the presence of social stigma due to the visible involuntary movements. They might have poor social support or limited physical and emotional support of family members. The physical and occupational therapist can be instrumental in breaking these barriers so each patient is able to achieve his or her full potential throughout the lifespan (World Health Organization, 2001).

## ◼ Anatomy and Physiology

Movement disorders and dyskinesias can occur in both children and adults. The following section will summarize specific anatomic regions within the brain and brainstem that contribute to dyskinesia.

### Systems Involved

Before evaluating and treating patients with dyskinesia, it is imperative that clinicians have a good understanding of the neurophysiologic reasons underlying these movement disorders. The basal ganglia play a primary role in the production of smooth coordinated movements and are often impaired in people with dyskinesia. The basal ganglia consist of five nuclei (caudate nucleus, putamen, substantia nigra, globus pallidus, and subthalamic nucleus) lying deep within the cerebrum (refer to Chapter 6 of this text for a review of the anatomy and location of the basal ganglia and related structures). The basal ganglia have no direct connection with the spinal cord

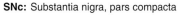

FIGURE 20-1 Schematic diagram of basal ganglia structures, connections, and neurotransmitters

| | |
|---|---|
| **SNc:** Substantia nigra, pars compacta | **D1:** Dopamine D1 receptor (for inhibition of striatum) |
| **GPe:** Globus pallidus, external segment | **D2:** Dopamine D2 receptor (for facilitation of striatum) |
| **STN:** Subthalamic nucleus | **PMRF:** Pontomedullary reticular formation |
| **GPi:** Globus pallidus, internal segment | **SupColl:** Superior colliculus |
| **SNr:** Substantia nigra, pars reticulata | **Rsp:** Reticulospinal tract |
| **VA:** Ventral anterior nucleus of the thalamus | **Vsp:** Vestibulospinal tract |
| **VL:** Ventral lateral nucleus of the thalamus | **Tsp:** Tectospinal tract |
| **MD:** Mediodorsal nucleus of the thalamus | |

but *directly* and *indirectly* influence motor pathways by way of the thalamus through connections to many areas of the frontal cortex (Figure 20-1).

The basal ganglia influence motor control through two pathways: *direct* and *indirect*. The net result of the *direct* pathway is to *facilitate* movement, and the net result of the *indirect* pathway is to *inhibit* movement. Consider an analogy to compare the movements of the body to driving a car. Consider the steering or coordination of the car to be the influence of the cerebellum and the brake and gas pedal of the car to be the influence of the basal ganglia. Both the steering and the gas/brake pedal modify the driving of the car. Once the car is in the drive position, the car will move regardless of whether or not you steer or hit the pedals. Damage to the steering or gas/brake of the car would correspond to damage to the cerebellum or basal ganglia and be considered "movement disorders" affecting the control or refinement of movement, not the ability to move.

The basal ganglia influence the initiation and continuation of movement based upon habitual learning and experience. Once an individual has become skilled at driving, the actual performance of driving becomes automatic in nature to allow for more focused attention to the environment. The basal ganglia modulate movements of the body in a similar manner. The direct pathway acts as the body's gas pedal to facilitate movement, and the indirect pathway acts as the body's brake pedal to inhibit movement. Generally this interaction is smooth and seamless, but on the occasion of basal ganglia dysfunction, movements are disrupted. Consider the taxi driver who uses both feet, one on the brake and one on the gas pedal when driving. Stopping and starting become quite abrupt with extra movements of the car thrown in. This is in essence "dyskinesia." If both pathways are working properly in conjunction with the rest of the central nervous system, the lower motor neurons receive the proper amount of facilitation and inhibition resulting in smooth coordinated movement of the limbs and postural muscles. Figure 20-1 describes the connections between the basal ganglia and other central structures as well as important neurotransmitters involved in motor control.

The basal ganglia are also involved in functions such as cognition, motivation, motor planning, working memory, oculomotor abilities, motor learning, attention, and limbic control of emotions. This occurs due to connections of the striatum (i.e., caudate and putamen) with the prefrontal cortex, orbitofrontal cortex, limbic system, and posterior parietal cortex. The mediodorsal and intralaminar nuclei of the thalamus are influenced by the basal ganglia output nuclei, and there are direct connections between thalamic nuclei and the striatum. This is the reason many disease processes involving the basal ganglia also involve cognitive, behavioral, and visual motor impairments (Draganski, 2008; Middleton, 2000, 2002; Samuels, 2009a).

## Lifespan Influence

### Developmental Considerations

Control of movement develops progressively over infancy and childhood based on development of the nervous system interacting with environmental influences (Thelen, 1994). Although most of the brain's cells are present at birth, motor skill improvement may result from new connections that develop between existing cells during infancy and early childhood and the rapid myelination occurring in the first 2 years of life. The earliest movements after birth are uncontrolled and jerky and often include unintended involuntary movement. Remember going to a parking lot and learning to drive? Basic functions like "keep the car at a constant speed and drive straight" were incredibly challenging! Many extra jerks and turns were thrown in until the skill of driving was mastered. Throughout typical infancy and childhood, motor control improves as the frequency of involuntary movements decrease. Motor coordination rapidly develops between 7 and 14 years of age. Refinement of motor control is driven by activity in the neurons of the motor cortex, including use-dependent experience of the limbs (Martin, 2005).

### Age-Related Changes Relevant to Involuntary Movement

Involuntary movement disorders become more common with aging due to age-related degenerative changes occurring within the central nervous system, particularly within the basal ganglia. The risk for development of tardive dyskinesia or slow-evolving involuntary movements frequently related to the side effect of certain medications is greater in elderly individuals compared with young adults (Goldberg, 2003; Jeste, 1999; Marshall, 2002). Other involuntary movement disorders associated with aging include spasmodic torticollis, essential non-parkinsonism tremor (Chen, 2006), and spontaneous dyskinesias, particularly blepharospasm or involuntary tight closure of the eyelids (Merrill, 2013). Movement disorders, including dystonia and hyperkinesia, also increase in the elderly from iatrogenic causes related to polypharmacy and

medications such as Metoclopramide (Reglan), an antiemetic drug (Dingli, 2007; Van Gool, 2010).

## ■ Related Pathology
### Neuroanatomy of Common Pathologies

The specific neuropathology related to the most common dyskinesias is discussed with each disease in the following section.

### Medical Diagnoses

#### Huntington Disease

HD is a severe neurodegenerative disease affecting 1 in 10,000 people (Gusella, 2007). Caused by an abnormal expansion of a gene on the short arm of chromosome 4, HD does not skip generations. A person who inherits the abnormal gene will almost always develop the disorder. Each child born to a person with HD has a 50% chance of inheriting the gene. The age at onset is generally in the third to fourth decade of life, although a juvenile form of HD is known (Cardoso, 2006). The lifespan after becoming symptomatic is typically 15 to 20 years. The characteristic dyskinesia associated with HD is chorea (derived from a Greek word for "dance-like"). Other impairments include oculomotor problems, bradykinesia, dystonia, myoclonus, tics, ataxia, **dysarthria, dysphagia,** and cognitive issues (Cardoso, 2006; Gusella, 2007; Quinn, 2002; Wheelock, 2003). Chorea begins as a subtle involuntary movement that can later progress to large, whole-body, highly visible movements. HD affects all areas of independent function to include employment, finances, social roles and activities, self-care, gait, communication, and eating (Lechich, 2008). Another common impairment is abnormal oculomotor function to include increased **saccadic latency,** the time between target movement and the onset of the first saccade toward the new target location, and an inability to generate internally triggered **saccades,** which are small sudden movements of the eyes such as when moving from one visual target to another (Berardelli, 1999; Lasker, 1997). Gait is severely impaired in individuals with HD to include slow and variable velocity and stride length and nonrhythmical cadence. Impairments of gait and postural control have been correlated with severity of the disease (Thaut, 1999). At later stages of the disease course, patients are typically bedridden, requiring assistance with ADL (Busse, 2007). Neuroanatomically in HD, striatal neurons that typically project to the globus pallidus external segment in the *indirect pathway* (Figure 20-1) are damaged, resulting in **hyperkinesis,** or too much movement. The body loses its brake pedal. With progression of HD, multiple neurotransmitters and receptors involved in basal ganglia circuits are involved to include D1 receptors within the striatum and substantia nigra. Neuronal damage is also seen in the frontal cortex (Frank, 2010). The damage to neurons in the striatum and frontal cortex, as well as observable abnormalities of gait, can be seen before noticeable symptoms begin (Kloppel, 2008; Rao, 2008). HD is typically treated with antidopaminergic and neuroleptic drugs (Table 20-2)

| TABLE 20-2 | Typical Pharmacological Treatment of Dyskinesia |
|---|---|
| **DISEASE/DYSKINESIA** | **COMMONLY USED PHARMACOLOGICAL TREATMENT** |
| Essential Tremor<br>(Louis, 2005; Zesiewicz, 2011; Schneider, 2013) | Beta-adrenergic blocker (e.g., Propranolol)<br>Anticonvulsant (e.g., Primidone)<br>BTX-A for head, hand, or voice |
| Dystonia<br>(Jankovic, 2004, 2009, 2013; Rezai, 2008) | Anticholinergic (e.g., Benzatropine)<br>Antispastic (e.g., Baclofen)<br>Muscle relaxants (e.g., Benzodiazepine)<br>Dopamine depleting (Tetrabenazine)<br>Anticonvulsant (e.g., Carbamazepine)<br>Antiparkinson (e.g., L-DOPA/Carbidopa)<br>Monoamine depleter and blocker (e.g., Reserpine)<br>BTX-A injected directly into the muscle |
| Huntington Chorea<br>(Marshall, 2004; Cardoso, 2006; Huntington<br>Study Group, 2006; Armstrong, 2012) | Neuroleptic (e.g., Haloperidol)<br>Anti-Parkinson (e.g., Amantadine)<br>Dopamine-depleting (Tetrabenazine is indicated for treatment of<br>chorea in patients with HD; Level B evidence)<br>Glutamate Blocker (Riluzole—Level B evidence)<br>*There is limited evidence that treating the chorea improves function. |
| Vascular Chorea, hemichorea, hemiballismus<br>(Mark, 2004) | Neuroleptic (e.g., Haloperidol)<br>Dopamine depleting (Tetrabenazine)<br>*The dyskinesia typically subsides without drugs. |
| Parkinson Disease<br>(Poewe, 2004; Jankovic, 2008, 2012) | Dopamine Replacement (e.g., L-DOPA/Carbidopa)<br>Dopamine Agonists (e.g., Pramipexole, Ropinirole)<br>COMT inhibitors (e.g., Entacapone)<br>Nondopaminergic (e.g., anticholinergics, amantadine)<br>Antidyskinesia drugs (e.g., Amantadine, Buspirone, Fluoxetine,<br>Propranolol, Clozapine) |
| Myoclonus<br>(Obeso, 2004) | Anticonvulsant (e.g., Clonazepam, Primidone, Sodium Valproate,<br>Piracetam) |
| Tics<br>(Shprecher, 2009) | Alpha agonists (e.g., Clonidine, Guanfacine)<br>Atypical antipsychotic (e.g., Risperidone, Clozapine)<br>Dopamine-depleting (Tetrabenazine)<br>Antiepileptic (e.g., Clonazepam) |

(Cardoso, 2006). Therefore attempts to control the extra movements are essentially making the individual with HD slower and stiffer or more parkinsonian. Parkinson disease (PD) results in damage to the direct pathway (gas pedal) resulting in overactivity of the indirect pathway or "excessive braking" of movements.

### Parkinson Disease

PD is a progressive disease affecting 1% of Americans, 0.3% of the world population, 1% of individuals aged 60 or older, and 4% to 5% of individuals aged 85 or older (Lew, 2007; Smaga, 2003). The cause of PD is unknown, although a rare form is genetic. Symptoms typically develop after age 50 and include bradykinesia, cogwheel rigidity, postural instability, and poor balance, poor coordination, depression, and cognitive issues (Lew, 2007). See Chapters 19 and 25 for discussion of interventions to address the rigidity and bradykinesia

associated with PD. The dyskinesia seen in 80% to 90% of patients with PD is resting **tremor**. The tremor typically begins distally and unilaterally in the upper extremity at a frequency of 4 to 6 Hz. Manifesting itself as flexion/extension of the elbow, supination/pronation of the forearm, or as a "pill-rolling" **tremor** of the fingers, it tends to worsen with stress and gets better with voluntary movement (Smaga, 2003). Tremor with regards to PD is accompanied by slowness of movement (bradykinesia) and/or rigidity. Resting tremor is not considered a form of hyperkinesia as it is typically seen in conjunction with bradykinesia and rigidity, which result in hypokinesia of movement. The impairments seen in PD are due to the progressive loss of dopaminergic neurons in the substantia nigra pars compacta that typically project to the striatum in the *direct* pathway (Figure 20-1) (Lew, 2007). Idiopathic PD responds to levadopa and carbidopa therapy (Table 20-2) (Blumenfeld, 2010).

## Essential Tremor

Essential tremor (ET) has a prevalence as high as 50.5/ 1,000 people over the age of 60 years. It is diagnosed clinically by the presence of visible postural tremor of the hands and forearms (Smaga, 2003) or an action tremor, which can help differentiate that of the resting tremor seen in PD. For clinical diagnosis, the tremor must be seen in at least one arm during four tasks (e.g., pouring water, using a spoon, drinking from a cup, finger to nose), and it must interfere with one activity of daily living. ET is a diagnosis of exclusion; it cannot be due to alcohol, drugs, or other neurological problems (Louis, 2000). The tremor may also involve the head and voice and can cause functional impairment as well as social embarrassment. The precise pathophysiology of ET is uncertain, but studies suggest the disease may be neurodegenerative and involve pathways between the cerebellum and basal ganglia (Louis, 2005). ET is typically treated medically with propranolol and primidone (Table 20-2), although response to medication is not optimal (Louis, 2001, 2005). Generally, 50% of those with ET can look to achieve a 50% reduction in tremor symptoms with medication. Injections of botulinum toxin type A (BTX-A) into the affected area is also an option for treatment to reduce tremors but may not correlate to improved function (Jankovic, 1996). Continuous deep brain stimulation (DBS) has been shown to be effective when pharmacological treatment is ineffective (Schuurman, 2000). DBS will be discussed in more detail later in the chapter because it is used to treat a variety of severe dyskinesia.

## Cerebral Palsy

According to the definition presented by Rosenbaum (2007), "Cerebral palsy describes a group of permanent disorders of the development of movement and posture causing activity limitations that are attributed to nonprogressive disturbances that occurred in the developing fetal or infant brain. The motor disorders of cerebral palsy are often accompanied by disturbances of sensation, perception, cognition, communication, and behavior, by epilepsy, and by secondary musculoskeletal problems." A method of classifying cerebral palsy (CP) is by the type of movement disorder (i.e., spastic, ataxic, and dyskinetic). Dyskinesia in CP is further defined by classifying the disorder as choreoathetoid or dystonic. Many children with CP have a mixed presentation of movement disorders (Rosenbaum, 2007). However 5% to 10% of children with CP have the choreoathetoid type and 70% of these cases are associated with severe perinatal complications such as hypoxic-ischemic encephalopathy or severe jaundice (Amor, 2001). MRI studies (Yokochi, 1990, 1991, 2004) showed children with choreoathetoid type of CP had damage to the ventral lateral nucleus of the thalamus and/or putamen (Figure 20-1). Periventricular areas and/or peri-Rolandic areas (i.e., cortical areas around the central sulcus) were also seen as areas of damage. The MRI studies showed spasticity only resulted if cortical areas other than the primary motor cortex were also damaged. In the choreoathetoid type of CP, oculomotor movement and sensation are typically normal. The dominant use of the left hand is common secondary to a typical presentation of damage to the left hemisphere (Yokochi, 1990). A study by Yokochi (2004) examined the movement patterns of 28 children with the choreoathetoid type of CP. Hypotonia, weakness, and difficulty moving at midjoint ranges were noted. Excessive hip flexion, posterior weight shift, and a crouched posture was the typical gait pattern observed. W-sitting and excessive trunk sway during reaching was also noted. Typical crawling patterns included crawling with excessive rotation, bunny hopping, or creeping on the back. Involuntary movements during quiet sitting were attributed to the excessive work of the muscles that must occur for stability during voluntary movements. Morris (2002) reported adults with mild athetoid CP presented with involuntary movements, clumsiness noted from a young age, and dystonia. A case report of an adult with the dystonic type of CP will be presented at the end of the chapter.

## Stroke

Dyskinesia such as hemichorea, dystonia, hemiballismus, or parkinsonism can present after hemorrhage or infarct damaging deep structures such as the thalamus, basal ganglia, and adjacent white matter. The most common cause of nongenetic chorea is stroke, although chorea only occurs in <1% of all patients with acute stroke. In patients with vascular insult to deep structures, chorea is most likely to occur in older patients (i.e., those over 75 years of age) and dystonia is more prevalent in younger patients. Hemiballismus is associated with lacunar infarct of the subthalamic nucleus (Alarcon, 2004; Cardoso, 2006).

## Movement Disorders in Children (Other Than Cerebral Palsy)

Although the clinical presentation of movement disorders in children is similar to adults, clinicians must consider the developmental stage as well as the progressive or nonprogressive nature of the dyskinesia. In a study of 684 patients, Fernandez-Alvarez (2001) examined the etiology of movement disorders in children and found the most commonly occurring disorder was tics (39%), followed by dystonia (24%), tremor (19%), mixed disorders (8%), chorea (5%), myoclonus (2%), and hypokinetic-rigid (2%).

## THINK ABOUT IT 20.1

- Return to the clinical case. Given the natural history of Huntington disease, how long would you expect JD to live?
- Describe involuntary movement disorders commonly seen with aging.
- Which basal ganglia motor control pathway is affected in Huntington disease? Parkinson disease?

## ■ Pertinent Examination/Evaluation

*Clinical Observation*: An important component of the examination is observation with description of the dyskinesia (Table 20-1). The patient should be observed at rest and during functional activities. It is often challenging to use only one term to describe a patient's involuntary movement disorder.

A patient might present with symptoms consistent with chorea, athetosis, and dystonia all at the same time. This is common in certain diagnoses such as CP, HD, and stroke. Therefore several terms might be used to describe the movement disorders. Consider the observation of the movement disorders in the continuation of the case of JD:

## PATIENT APPLICATION: JD

*The clinician notes that JD has choreoathetosis in the upper and lower extremities at rest and while walking. In sitting, he tends to keep his arms folded and legs crossed to keep from moving. This reduces his appendicular movements but enhances his axial movements. He walks with excessive rotation and weight-shifting. His feet tend to supinate during swing phase, causing him to step on his toes at initial contact rather than heel strike.*

### Contemplate Clinical Decisions

*Suggestions for clinical observations:*

1. *Describe the resting posture and abnormal movements at rest.*
2. *Observe the eyes for abnormal jerkiness at rest.*
3. *Note the patient's quality of voice during speech.*
4. *Describe the gait pattern and need for help during standing, walking, and turning.*
5. *Describe the patient's interactions with caregivers.*
   - *This will be important later when educating the patient and caregivers.*

*History, Systems Review, Tests, and Measures:* After observation, a thorough history should be obtained from the client and/or caregiver. The history provides valuable information and will guide the clinician to specific tests and measures that need to be performed in the examination. The history should include general demographics, social history, employment and work (school and play for children), growth and development to include hand dominance, living environment, general health status, social and health habits (past and present), family history, medical/surgical history, current complaints, perceived functional status and activity level, medications, other laboratory values.

## PATIENT APPLICATION: JD

*The history reveals JD is married, has two male children ages 6 and 8 years, and works as a computer programmer. When sitting at his computer workstation, he began using an ergonomic chair/kneeler about 2 years ago because of the "fidgeting" of his lower extremities. JD thought the kneeler would help him overall. Other factors regarding work include a decrease in attention to task, forgetfulness (missing meetings and deadlines), and difficulty following directions to drive to different locations to train new employees. JD verbalized these issues were related to stress and just not "paying attention." JD's work quality has not been affected in terms of evaluations. Other than the diagnosis of HD, his medical history is unremarkable. JD takes Klonapin for depression and Clozaril to control the chorea (i.e., the "fidgetiness" he describes). The diagnosis of HD was confirmed 6 years ago after genetic testing.*

*Although he has been involved in raising his children (e.g., driving children to baseball practice, assisting with bathing and dressing, assisting with homework), JD has noticed a decline in his ability to pay attention and filter distractions, especially with driving. His wife, a hairdresser, has also noticed these symptoms and has recently become concerned about the safety of their children while they are riding with their father. She also wonders if any of their children inherited the gene for HD. In addition, they both notice JD tends to stumble and lose his balance when walking on different floor surfaces within the home. He fell to the floor 2 months ago, sustaining a bruised leg and minor cut to his hand while trying to catch himself. He typically catches himself using the wall or furniture when he stumbles.*

### Contemplate Clinical Decisions

*Based on JD's history, what tests should the clinician perform as part of the systems review?*

*Following the history, a complete systems review must be completed to include screening of the following systems: cardiovascular and pulmonary, neuromuscular, musculoskeletal, and integumentary.*

The history and systems review will lead the therapist to choose appropriate tests and measures. Physical therapists may consult the *Guide to Physical Therapist Practice* (APTA, 2015) and occupational therapists may consult the *Occupational Therapy Practice Framework: Domain and Process, 2nd edition* (AOTA, 2008). Table 20-3 describes recommended tests and measures. Many of these tests (e.g., Timed Up and Go [TUG] and Berg Balance Scale) have been validated for community-dwelling elderly individuals at risk for falls and are used in studies assessing individuals with specific diseases that cause dyskinesia (e.g., ET, PD, HD). Other tests (e.g., Gross Motor Function Measure and Pediatric Evaluation of Disability Inventory) are validated for children with CP who may or may not have dyskinesias. See Section II of this text for other general tests and measures. See Table 20-4 for dyskinesia-specific scales.

## PATIENT APPLICATION: JD

*JD is 5'11" and weighs 185 lbs. His resting heart rate, blood pressure, and respiratory rate are all within normal limits. Based on JD's diagnosis, the physical therapist performed a screen of the neuromuscular system. This included testing oculomotor abilities (smooth pursuit was slightly jerky and saccades were slow and inaccurate; refer to Chapter 7 for specifics of testing), coordination (finger to nose and rapid alternating movements were impaired; Chapter 6), vestibulo-ocular reflex via head thrust (negative result; refer to Chapter 8), gross strength and range of motion (were within functional limits; refer to Chapter 6).*

### Contemplate Clinical Decisions

*Based upon the history and systems review, which tests and measures should the clinician perform and why?*

| TABLE 20-3 | Suggested Outcome Tools at the Activity/Participation Level of ICF Model | |
|---|---|---|
| **NAME OF TEST** | **METHOD OF ADMINISTRATION** | **CLINICAL MEANING** |
| Computerized Dynamic Posturography (CDP), SOT, and MCT (Salomonczyk, 2010; Medina, 2013) | Computerized dynamic posturography utilizes a dynamic force platform that has been combined with visual stimuli to determine an individual's reliance on sensory inputs (vision, somatosensory, and vestibular) to stabilize in upright standing during SOT (Sensory Organization Test) testing, and to determine reactive balance during MCT (Motor Control Test) testing. | Those with symptomatic HD demonstrated increased postural sway across all conditions. Additionally premanifest HD patients demonstrated subtle changes in postural control and sensory orientation up to 5 years before symptomatic disease onset. Premanifest HD patients did not show deficits in limits of stability, as opposed to those with symptomatic HD. |
| MiniBESTest (Jacobs, 2015) | The MiniBEST is a clinical test of balance and gait, assessing 14 items across four domains: anticipatory postural control, reactive postural control, sensory orientation, and dynamic gait. | For patients with HD, imbalance spans across multiple domains and should be comprehensively evaluated. Results significantly correlated to the UHDRS. |
| Modified Clinical Test of Sensory Interaction and Balance (MCTSIB) (Horak, 1987; Shumway-Cook, 1986; Wrisley, 2004) | The patient is timed for 30 seconds while standing in the Romberg position during four conditions: eyes open, eyes closed, on dense foam with eyes opened, and on dense foam with eyes closed. If 30 seconds are not completed, complete up to 2 more trials and take the mean score in seconds. | This test allows the clinician to discern the sensory systems that are deficient for postural control. |
| Romberg and Sharpened Romberg Test (Quinn, 2013; Steffen, 2008) | For patients with HD, the patient is timed for 30 seconds during six conditions: Romberg Eyes Opened and Closed; Sharpened Romberg Eyes Opened and Closed; Sharpened Romberg Eyes Opened and Closed with a cognitive task (i.e., counting backward by 3s). The total # of seconds is the score (max = 180). For patients with PD, conditions (Romberg and Sharpened Romberg Eyes Opened and Closed) are tested for 60 sec. | For patients with HD, the $MDC_{95}$ is 29.7 sec (premanifest); 37.43 sec (manifest); 36.27 sec (Early-Stage); 46.32 sec (Middle-Stage); and 30.93 (Late-Stage). For patients with PD, the $MDC_{95}$ was 10 and 19 sec for Romberg eyes opened and closed, and 39 and 19 sec for sharpened Romberg eyes opened and closed. |
| Timed Up and Go (TUG) (Busse, 2009; Morris, 2001; Podsiadlo, 1991; Quinn, 2013; Steffen, 2008) | The patient begins sitting in a chair. On the word "go" (or "start" for individuals with PD), the patient is timed as he/she stands and walks at a comfortable pace to a line on the floor (3 meters from the chair), then turns, walks back to the chair, and sits down. An assistive device can be used. Two trials should be completed. | <10 seconds is normal; 11–20 seconds is normal for frail elderly; ≥14 seconds is risk for falls; >20 seconds is impaired functional mobility; >30 seconds is dependent with most ADL and mobility. For patients with HD, the $MDC_{95}$ is 1.34 sec (premanifest); 2.98 sec (manifest); 2.97 sec (Early-Stage); 3.49 sec (Middle-Stage); 2.58 sec (Late-Stage). For patients with PD, the $MDC_{95}$ is 11 sec. |
| Six-Minute Walk Test (6MWT) (Quinn, 2013; Steffen, 2008) | The patient walks for a total of 6 minutes around a set course. The distance in meters is recorded. Heart rate can also be recorded. | For patients with HD, the $MDC_{95}$ in meters is 39.22 (premanifest); 86.57 (manifest); 56.6 (Early-Stage); 126.14 (Middle-Stage); and 70.65 (Late-Stage). For patients with PD, the $MDC_{95}$ is 82 meters. |
| 10 Meter Walk Test (Quinn, 2013) | The patient is timed as he/she walks at a comfortable pace across a 14-m area marked with 10 m in the middle and an additional 2 m at the beginning and end for acceleration and deceleration. Two trials should be completed and averaged for gait speed in m/s. | For patients with HD, the $MDC_{95}$ in m/s is 0.23 (premanifest); 0.34 (manifest); 0.20 (Early-Stage); 0.46 (Middle-Stage); and 0.29 (Late-Stage). |

*Continued*

| TABLE 20-3 | Suggested Outcome Tools at the Activity/Participation Level of ICF Model—cont'd | |
|---|---|---|
| **NAME OF TEST** | **METHOD OF ADMINISTRATION** | **CLINICAL MEANING** |
| Berg Balance Scale (Berg, 1992; Busse, 2009; Quinn, 2013; Shumway-Cook, 1997; Steffen, 2008) | Clinicians score 14 daily activities (e.g., sit-to-stand, reach, lean over, turn in a complete circle) using an ordinal scale of 0 (cannot perform) to 4 (normal performance). The total possible score is 56 points. | In community-dwelling older adults, a score of $\leq 36$ indicated 100% chance of falling. In individuals with HD, a score of $\leq 40$ indicated a risk of falling. For patients with HD, the $MDC_{95}$ is 1 (premanifest and early-stage); 2 (all other stages). For patients with PD, the $MDC_{95}$ is 5 points. |
| Tinetti Mobility Test (Kegelmeyer, 2007; Kloos, 2010; Quinn, 2013) | Clinicians score 16 items related to balance and gait using a criterion-referenced ordinal scale. The total score is calculated for each scale (i.e., balance and gait) and a total score out of a possibility of 28 is calculated. It takes about 5 minutes to administer. | In individuals with HD, a total score of <21 indicates risk of falls (sensitivity = 73.5%; specificity = 60%). In individuals with PD, a total score of <20 indicates risk of falls (sensitivity = 76%; specificity = 66%). For patients with HD, the $MDC_{95}$ for the total score is 1 (premanifest); 4 (manifest); 2 (Early-Stage); 3 (Middle-Stage); and 5 (Late-Stage). |
| Four-Square Step Test (Dite, 2002; Duncan, 2013; Quinn, 2013) | The patient steps over four canes positioned in squares as fast as possible in a predetermined sequence (i.e., clockwise: right, back, left; forward; then counterclockwise). One practice trial is given, two trials are timed, and the best score is recorded. Timing starts when the right foot contacts the floor in the square. | For patients with HD, the $MDC_{95}$ in seconds is 1.95 (premanifest); 15.27 (manifest); 7.94 (Early-Stage); 22.40 (Middle-Stage); and 13.02 (Late-Stage). For patients with PD, the cut-off score to distinguish fallers from nonfallers was 9.68 seconds (sensitivity = 73%; specificity = 57%). |
| Activity Balance Confidence Scale (Powell, 1995; Schepens, 2010; Steffen, 2008) | Patient rate their confidence that they will "not lose their balance or become unsteady" on a scale of 0% (not at all confident) to 100% (extremely confident) for 16 (original) or 6 (modified) hypothetical activities. | Higher scores equal greater confidence. Original version: Scores of $\geq 80\%$ indicate high functioning; 50% to 80% indicate moderate functioning; $\leq 50\%$ indicate low functioning; <67% indicates risk of falls in older adults. For patients with PD, the $MDC_{95}$ is 13%. |
| Modified Falls Efficacy Scale (MFES) (Delbaere, 2009; Edwards, 2008) | Patients rate their confidence on a scale of 1 (not confident) to 10 (completely confident). Eleven activities of daily living include indoor and outdoor use of stairs, bathtub transfers, and use of handrails. | Higher scores = greater confidence. Greater fear of falling leads to activity restrictions in community-dwelling older adults. |
| Canadian Occupational Performance Measure, 3rd edition (McColl, 2005) | A semistructured interview is administered to assess performance in 3 areas: self-care, productivity, and leisure/play. There are two rating scales (10 points) for performance and satisfaction in occupational performance areas. Problems are identified as something the patient needs, wants, or is expected to do but can't do, doesn't do, or isn't satisfied with the way he/she does. A total score is calculated. | This tool can be used to determine therapy goals and to objectively determine the extent to which goals are met. |
| Pediatric Evaluation of Disability Inventory (PEDI) (Feldman, 1990) | The PEDI is a scale that examines the functional performance and capabilities of young children ages 6 months to 7.5 years. It is made up of 197 functional skill items and 20 items of caregiver assistance. Function is assessed in three domains: self-care (use of utensils, hand washing), mobility (toilet/tub transfers), and social function (interaction with peers). The PEDI also focuses on how environment modification would benefit the individual in each of the three domains. | The PEDI is a norm-referenced tool. Standard and scaled performance scores can be obtained. |

| TABLE 20-3 | Suggested Outcome Tools at the Activity/Participation Level of ICF Model—cont'd | |
|---|---|---|
| **NAME OF TEST** | **METHOD OF ADMINISTRATION** | **CLINICAL MEANING** |
| Gross Motor Function Measure (Russell, 2000) | Criterion-referenced observational test that assesses motor function in five dimensions: (1) lying and rolling, (2) sitting, (3) crawling and kneeling, (4) standing, (5) walking, running, and jumping. Each item is scored on a 4-point scale from 0 (does not initiate) to 3 (completes) with specific descriptors for scoring items (described in the manual). | Test was designed to measure change in gross motor function over time in children with cerebral palsy ages 5 months to 16 years but is best for children 2 years and up. It takes 45 to 60 minutes to administer. It has been found to be a valid measure for conditions other than cerebral palsy. |
| Barthel Index (Collin, 1988; Quinn, 2013) | A 10-item performance-based tool to evaluate ADLs. Scores range from 0–100, 100 represents the highest score of independence. Tasks addressed are feeding, transfers, personal hygiene, locomotion, dressing, control of bowel and bladder. | This is typically completed in the inpatient setting. It is predictive of hospital length of stay and discharge status. Administration is 20 minutes if tasks are observed and 5 minutes if caregiver, patient, or health-care provider gives information. For patients with HD, the $MDC_{95}$ is 6 (manifest); 5 (Early- and Middle-Stage); and 7 (Late-Stage). |
| School Function Assessment (SFA) (Schenker, 2005) | Individuals familiar with the child's and his/her function in the school setting (teachers, therapist, parent, paraprofessionals) observe and rate children's performance of various school-related tasks. *Participation* is rated on a scale of 1 (extremely limited) to 6 (full participation). *Support* looks at adult assistance necessary to engage in specific tasks and any type of modification or adaption needed. *Activity Performance* assesses the child's ability to perform specific school-related tasks and is scored on a scale of 1 to 4. | Many professionals should participate in the completion of the tool to provide more comprehensive data for planning. The SFA takes 1.5 to 2 hours to complete. |
| Minnesota Low Vision Reading Test (MN-Read) (Legge, 1989) | The patient reads a series of sentences as they decrease in size. The clinician times the patient and notes missed words. The reading acuity, maximum reading speed, and critical print size is calculated. | Because basal ganglia disorders also may affect eye movements, this is a good test to determine whether magnification or referral to a vision specialist is needed. It is valid only if the patient has the cognitive ability to read. |
| Short Form-36 (SF-36) (Ho, 2004; Steffen, 2008) | The patient completes a 36-item questionnaire (multiple format rating scales). This scale measures quality of life; physical and mental health; and functional limitations due to ill health. | The SF-36 takes 5 to 15 minutes to complete. It is valid for individuals with HD and their caregivers. For individuals with PD, the $MDC_{95}$ is 28 for general health. |

Regardless of the cause of dyskinesia, a quantitative gait assessment is useful to determine abnormalities that could lead to falls. If available, assessments might include laboratory equipment such as motion analysis or computerized gait mat systems. However, clinicians can also measure self-paced and fast gait speeds to compare to age-appropriate normative data (Oberg, 1993). A study led by Rao (2009) determined subjects with presymptomatic HD had decreased gait velocity, shorter stride length, and increased time in double support and stance phase of gait compared with healthy controls. Gait impairments worsened with increasing disease severity. However, the TUG and Functional Reach Test did not distinguish subjects with presymptomatic HD from healthy controls

(Rao, 2009). Temporal and spatial abnormalities of gait in individuals with HD include low cadence, variable stride length and time, and variable swing and double support times (Thaut, 1999). Quinn (2013) determined the Timed Up and Go, Six-Minute Walk Test, and 10-Meter Walk Test had good test-retest reliability (ICC ≥0.86) in 75 individuals with premanifest, early, middle, and late stages of HD. The gait subscale of the Tinetti Mobility Scale had good reliability in individuals with manifest, early, and middle stages of HD (ICC ≥0.84). The Minimal Detectable Change scores (i.e., the change scores representing more than measurement error) were also provided for each outcome measure and each stage of HD (see Table 20-3 for MDC scores from this study).

| TABLE 20-4 | Dyskinesia-Specific Scales |
| --- | --- |
| **NAME OF SCALE** | **DESCRIPTION** |
| Unified **HD** Rating Scale (Huntington Study Group, 1996) | The UHDRS is a research tool that assesses several domains: motor function, cognitive function, behavioral abnormalities, independence, and functional capacity (e.g., eye movement, dysarthria, coordination, rigidity, bradykinesia, maximal dystonia of trunk, **chorea**, gait, tandem walking). It is used to quantify the severity of the symptoms of HD. To use the UHDRS, permission must be obtained from the Huntington Study Group. |
| Total Functional Capacity Scale (TFCS) (Huntington Study Group, 1996; Quinn, 2002; Shoulson, 1979) | The TFCS is a 14-point scale that measures disability and participation restrictions of life skills. The categories include occupation, activities of daily living, finances, care level, and domestic chores. |
| *Unified Dystonia Rating Scale (UDRS) (Comella, 2003) | The UDRS assessed 14 body areas. The clinician observes the patient as he/she performs prescribed activities and rates the severity (0 = no dystonia to 4 = extreme dystonia) and duration (0 = none to 4 = constant). The total score is the sum of the severity and duration scores. |
| *Global Dystonia Scale (GDS) (Comella, 2003) | The GDS rates 10 body areas using a Likert scale (0 = no dystonia in that body area, 1 = minimal, 5 = moderate, 10 = severe). Unlike the UDRS, it does not have modifying or weighting factors. Total possible score is 140. |
| Behavior Rating Scale for Tourette's Syndrome (Bagheri, 1999) | This scale rates problematic behaviors in children with Tourette's syndrome. The clinician lists symptoms to be rated, time of day that they occur, the setting in which they occur, and the severity (0 = absent to 10 = severe). It also asks to list things that improve or worsen the symptoms. |
| *Movement Disorders Society-United PD Rating Scale (MDS-UPDRS) (Goetz, 2008) | The purpose of the MDS-UPDRS is to follow the course of PD related to the following four domains: I: Nonmotor Experiences of Daily Living; II: Motor Experiences of Daily Living; III: Motor Examination; IV: Motor Complications. The scale rates 65 items across the four parts: Part I (13), Part II (13), Part III (33 scores based upon 18 items, several require assessment of each extremity), and Part IV (6). Each question is scored on a 0–4 scale, where 0 is normal and 4 is severe. The motor section specifically examines tremors. Raters are expected to complete training through the International Parkinson and Movement Disorder Society. |
| Unified Myoclonus Rating Scale (Frucht, 2002) | The patient is videotaped at rest and during various stimuli (e.g., clap hands, visual threat, tap nose, pin prick, deep tendon reflexes). The clinician watches the videotape and scores on a scale of 0–4 (based on "jerkiness") for frequency and amplitude. A questionnaire is given to the patient to determine their level of disability. Functional tests are done (e.g., writing, pouring water, using a spoon). A total score is obtained. |

*Questionnaires are owned and licensed by the International Parkinson and Movement Disorder Society. Permission and training may be required to administer this scale. Refer to www.movementdisorders.org for more information.

A study by Earhart (2009) determined individuals with ET walked slower with a lower cadence, shorter single-limb support, and longer double-limb support than healthy controls (Earhart, 2009). These subjects also had lower Activity Balance Confidence Scale and Berg Balance Test scores, shorter single-legged stance times, shorter Functional Reach Test scores, and longer TUG times than healthy controls. Therefore an assessment of postural control and balance confidence is also necessary.

Postural control can be assessed using computerized dynamic posturography (CDP) or via clinical tests such as the Modified Clinical Test for Sensory Interaction and Balance

(Table 20-3). CDP uses a force platform with the ability to provide translational and pitch plane rotational perturbations. It also uses a visual surround that moves in response to the patient's movement. The purpose is to quantitatively measure the relative contribution of the visual, somatosensory, and vestibular senses to postural control (Black, 2001). CDP tests include the sensory organization test, translational and rotational perturbations of the platform (Huttunen, 1990; Tian, 1991, 1992), and limits of stability test (Roberts-Warrior, 2000). See Chapters 9 and 30 of this text for a detailed description of the CDP. Two studies (Tian, 1991, 1992) determined individuals with HD had impairments of postural control to include increased sway during conditions that required reliance on vestibular information (i.e., eyes closed while standing on foam or on a swayed surface; eyes open with swayed visual surround and surface). The subjects with HD also had increased latency of response to translational perturbations. Quinn (2013) determined the Berg Balance Scale, Tinetti Mobility Scale (Balance Subscale), Romberg/Sharpened Romberg total time, and Four-Square Step Test had fair to good reliability (ICC ≥0.73) in individuals with HD at all stages. Minimal detectable change scores (Table 20-3) should be considered when using these clinical outcome tools (Quinn, 2013).

Balance confidence is often measured using the Activity Balance Confidence (ABC) Scale (Powell, 1995) or the Modified Falls Efficacy Scale (Edwards, 2008). The original ABC scale consists of 16 hypothetical situations for which patients rate their confidence. Patients are asked, "How confident are you that you will not lose your balance or become unsteady?" They rate their confidence on a scale of 0% (not confident) to 100% (completely confident). Examples of situations include walking around the house, standing on a chair to reach for something, and walking outside on icy sidewalks. Recently, investigators validated a six-item ABC scale with good reliability and correlated with falls better than the 16-item scale in community-dwelling older adults (Schepens, 2010). The original Falls Efficacy Scale (Tinetti, 1990) includes 10 ADL (e.g., take a bath or shower, get in and out of bed, simple shopping) and asks, "How confident are you that you can do the following activities without falling?" Patients rate each activity on a scale of 1 (very confident) to 10 (not confident at all). The modified version (Edwards, 2008) changed the scoring (i.e., 1 is now "not confident" and 10 is "very confident") and includes more challenging activities, including indoor and outdoor use of stairs with and without a handrail, getting in and out of the bathtub without falling, and sitting in and getting up from a bathtub without falling. These tests can be used to give a clinician insight into an individual's judgment as well as to determine whether or not a client is at risk for falling. It is important to note that individuals with dyskinesia and cognitive impairments might be unable to accurately complete the ABC or Falls Efficacy Scales.

## THINK ABOUT IT 20.2

Given the discussion on various tests and measures and the description of JD's case thus far, what specific tests and measures do you think would be most important to include? Why?

A multidisciplinary approach to the evaluation process should be taken. Individuals with dyskinesia may have speech-language and/or swallowing difficulty, warranting referral to a speech and language pathologist. With increased involuntary movement, clients often lose weight and will need referral to nutritionists for consultation on supplements and diet management. Disease-specific support groups exist for the support of patients and families. Physical and occupational therapists should be aware of local appropriate referrals and resources to assist patients and their families. The examination of JD now continues:

### PATIENT APPLICATION: JD

*Physical and occupational therapy tests and measures chosen for the case:*

*After JD's medical screen, the physical therapist decided to perform the 10-Meter Walk Test. A mean of two trials yielded a gait speed of 1.2 m/s, which is similar to individuals in the middle or late stages of HD (Quinn, 2013).*

*The Romberg and Sharpened Romberg Tests were done to test JD's balance. Six conditions were completed for a maximum of 30 seconds: (1) Romberg eyes opened; (2) Romberg eyes closed; (3) Sharpened Romberg eyes opened; (4) Sharpened Romberg eyes closed; (5) Sharpened Romberg eyes opened with a cognitive task of counting backward by 3s; and (6) Sharpened Romberg eyes closed with the same cognitive task (Quinn, 2013). JD's score was a total of 82.6 seconds.*

*JD completed the ABC Scale. JD obtained a score of 75% (indicating moderate level of physical functioning) and expressed little concern or insight regarding his safety and balance. However his wife's confidence in his balance was much lower, expressing a great deal of concern about his safety and judgment. Note that cognition is often impaired in individuals with HD.*

*The occupational therapist completed the Canadian Occupational Performance Measure (COPM). The COPM revealed JD was noticing decline with his ADL routines. He was slower and had to work harder to pay attention to tasks. He was easily distracted from tasks and then experienced a difficult time getting back on track. He was still independent in all areas of self-care but verbalized fear of falling in the shower. He did not currently have adaptive equipment or adaptations of any kind in the home. JD and his wife voiced they did not have medical support outside of the HD clinic.*

*Performance problems rated in terms of importance on COPM by JD and his wife:*

1. *Safety concerns in shower (performance: 3/10; satisfaction: 1/10).*
2. *Support from family and medical community (performance: 1/10; satisfaction: 1/10).*
3. *Handwriting (performance: 3/10; satisfaction: 1/10).*

*Total performance score divided by number of problems: 7/3 = 2.3.*

*Total satisfaction score divided by number of problems = 3/3 = 1.*

*Because JD had abnormal smooth pursuit and saccades, the occupational therapist also completed the MN Read test (Minnesota Low-Vision Reading Test). The MN Read is a test to determine the effect of decreasing font size on reading acuity and reading speed. In this case, the MN Read revealed normal reading speed and critical print size. Therefore the abnormal eye movements and cognitive decline did not yet affect JD's reading ability.*

*The battery of fine motor skills revealed a decline in JD's handwriting compared with a sample of his handwriting from 6 months prior. He complained of fatigue with writing, and he and his wife both recognized the decline.*

## Effect of Involuntary Movement Disorders on Caregivers

Caregiving is comprised of the caring affective component and the behavioral expression of providing care to a person. In the United States, the task of caregiving has largely shifted from the staff of skilled nursing facilities to family members or friends. Family members perform 75% to 80% of caregiving for aging individuals (Yaffe, 2008). People diagnosed with PD, Alzheimer disease, and strokes are among the largest population of individuals who require caregivers. These groups are largely represented in the caregiving literature (Yaffe, 2008). Other groups represented in the literature include persons with dementia or cognitive limitations and children with disabilities who require caregivers throughout their lifespan. The level of assistance and length of caregiving is dependent on many factors. These factors create stress and contribute to the burden of caregiving for responsible family or friends (Pearlin, 1990).

Multiple stressors exist for caregivers. For caregivers of individuals with HD, the caregiver may be a family member who is at risk for developing the disease. Also the debilitating symptoms of HD often appear at age 40, precluding the individual from contributing to the family income, creating financial stressors and burdens (Wheelock, 2003). One reported stressor can be conflicting ideas between caregivers and health-care providers. It is important for caregivers to advocate for their loved one by collaborating with and resolving conflicts between health-care providers (Hasselkus, 1998). The collaborative process is articulated in the literature as is the need for all parties to have an opportunity to discuss and understand their unique circumstances (Gitlin, 1993). When a caregiver does not perceive the freedom to ask questions, seek out information, and collaborate with others, they feel negated and more stressed. Another stressor for caregivers may come from well-intending family, friends, and associates who are attempting to help but do not regularly take part in the caregiving process. While the concerned individuals intend to be helpful, they may pose questions and suggestions that inadvertently place blame, contradict, or challenge the thoughts and intentions of the primary caregiver.

Caregivers often feel out of control and lack routine and choice when their loved ones are hospitalized or in a state of decline (Kaptein, 2007). Therefore the role of therapists should extend to the caregiver through education, support, and provision of resources so caregivers are respected and affirmed. Caregiving is hard work. Those providing care for individuals with cognitive limitations or dementia experience high emotional and physical stress. Caregivers have high rates of anxiety, stress, and burnout. Their life expectancy is reduced, and up to a third of caregivers of people with dementia are depressed (Butler, 2008). Caregivers reporting strain associated with caregiving had greater risk of mortality than non-caregiving controls (Schulz, 1999). Having resources and support makes a difference for caregivers. According to stress and coping models, caregivers who have resources and lower stress levels are less likely to experience caregiver burnout and depression (Pinquart, 2005).

Those who provide care for children over the lifetime of the child experience different challenges. Parents of children with lifelong disabilities or chronic health conditions experience a different caregiving role than do parents of children without disability or health problems. The constant attention, coordination of care, and juggling of roles can be overwhelming. As such the physical and mental health of these parents can be compromised. A study led by Raina (2005) examined relationships between various factors associated with caregiver stress, family function, and the health and behavior of the child with CP. Three significant factors were identified in this study as predictors of caregiver physical and mental well-being. These factors were child behavior, caregiving demands, and family function. The presence of child behavioral problems and decreased family functioning increased caregiving demands and contributed to poor physical and/or mental well-being. A study by Ketelaar (2008) revealed maladaptive behaviors of children with CP contributed more to parental stress than functional ability. Maladaptive behavior of the child also contributed to caregiver depression, a sense of incompetence, and relationship problems with spouses. Given the long-term effect for caregivers of children with lifelong disabilities or chronic health problems, it is necessary for occupational and physical therapists to educate caregivers on resources that will enable them to improve or maintain their own physical and mental health.

## THINK ABOUT IT 20.3

Given what you know about the stressors of caregiving:
- What questions would you ask JD's wife and JD?
- Where might you go to search out local resources for JD and his wife?
- How might your plan for patient/caregiver education change now and over time?

## PATIENT APPLICATION: JD

*JD and his wife reveal their families are supportive but distant. JD's sisters and mother visit regularly but do not like talking about his diagnosis nor any problems he or his wife are experiencing. His 30 year-old sister has four children and decided not to be tested for HD. There is an HD support group for patients and family members who meet every other month, but JD has not attended.*

## Contemplate Clinical Decisions

1. Based on the COPM evaluation results, what course of action would you take with regard to tub safety?

2. Given the functional decline of handwriting status, what intervention approach would you use with JD?

3. JD's concerns regarding his limited family and medical network are significant for anyone with a chronic health condition. What would you do (specifically) to address his and his wife's concerns in this area?

4. Dependent on the Department of Transportation laws in your state, JD may be at risk to lose his right to drive. As the occupational or physical therapist, what might be your recommendation for assessing JD's driving skills?

5. Based on the results of the TUG and Romberg/Sharpened Romberg tests, what interventions can you give JD that might help him with his balance?

6. What will you do or suggest based on the results of the ABC scale?

7. What equipment suggestions might you give him?

# ■ Preparatory Interventions Specific to Involuntary Movement Disorders

## General Approaches

Much of the current evidence for alleviating dyskinesia to improve function focuses on medical treatment of the body structure (i.e., basal ganglia and/or muscle) using drugs, DBS, or injections of botulinum toxin into the muscle (Jankovic, 1996; Rezai, 2008; Samuels, 2009a). The physical and occupational therapist, however, may be consulted to provide exercise programs, education, and strategies to improve function and participation to complement the positive results of the medical treatment (Chevrier, 2006; Kloos, 2012; Ramdharry, 2006; Tassorelli, 2006).

### Pharmacological Implications for Therapy

The first line of defense is pharmacology to include various drugs designed to change the abnormal neurochemistry in the central nervous system (Table 20-2). For treatment of cervical or focal dystonia, tremor, tics, or other movement disorders causing excessive involuntary muscle contraction, BTX-A is often injected directly into the muscle. BTX-A temporarily blocks the release of acetylcholine at the neuromuscular junction so the muscle is locally paralyzed (Evidente, 2010). The effects of BTX-A typically last from weeks to months. Some patients develop a resistance to the effects of BTX-A with repeated injections. Therefore the recommended time between injections is no shorter than 3 months (Evidente, 2003). Evidence reports central effects of BTX-A to include blocking the gamma motor neuron endings on the muscle spindle, plastic changes of the motor neuron and muscle, and retrograde transport into the central nervous system (Caleo, 2009).

### Surgical Modalities

If the dyskinesias are unresponsive to oral drugs and/or injections of BTX-A, the physician might choose to use DBS. DBS is a technique where electrodes are surgically implanted into the basal ganglia or thalamus. An implantable pulse generator or neurostimulator is also implanted superficially just below the skin and inferior to the clavicle (Rezai, 2008). The stimulation settings are programmed through a computer to interrupt the abnormal neural connections causing the dyskinesias (Albright, 2003). Brain structures typically stimulated include ventral intermediate nucleus (VIM) of the thalamus, globus pallidus internus (GPi), and subthalamic nucleus (STN) (Figure 20-1). One study described having a physical therapist present during the implantation of the DBS electrodes in 64 patients (Chevrier, 2006). The surgery took 12 hours and the patients with PD were off medications and under local anesthesia during the surgery. The therapist provided massage, stretching, and other relaxation techniques during the surgery, which reportedly reduced suffering during the surgery. Before the development of DBS, neurosurgeons performed ablation procedures of the VIM, GPi, and/or STN to relieve dyskinesias that were nonresponsive to drugs. However, DBS is now the preferred method as it does not cause long-term damage to brain structures and does not have as many complications (Rezai, 2008; Schuurman, 2000). The DBS signals can be modulated over time to minimize habituation and maximize effect.

Many studies have been done to determine the efficacy of DBS in individuals with dyskinesia. In persons with tremor due to ET, multiple sclerosis, and PD, continuous DBS of the VIM nucleus of the thalamus alleviated tremors and improved function better than thalamotomy with fewer adverse effects (Schuurman, 2000). Although DBS improves tremor, it has also been shown to cause decreased activity within the vestibular-thalamic-cortical projections and subsequently may lead to subjective disequilibrium in patients after surgery (Ceballos-Baumann, 2001; Ondo, 2006). Ondo (2006) determined patients with tremor and perceived disequilibrium due to PD and ET had overall improved sensory organization while on DBS as measured by CDP (i.e., less postural sway during various sensory conditions such as eyes closed, sway-referenced visual surround, sway-referenced surface, or a combination of these). DBS is also effective to improve symptoms in children 7 years of age and older with CP and dystonia (Albright, 2003; Marks, 2013). Newer, less-invasive surgical interventions exist via high-intensity focused ultrasound, which show promising results to address tremors in individuals with ET by temporarily ablating areas within the thalamus or basal ganglia. A study by Elias (2013) showed up to a 75% reduction in tremor after MRI-guided high-intensity focused ultrasound for a cohort of 15 patients who demonstrated medically resistant tremor. The improvements in tremor reduction seemed to positively affect overall quality of life as well (Elias, 2013; Huss, 2015).

Several case reports exist using DBS in patients with HD to alleviate choreoathetosis that was nonresponsive to medication (Fawcett, 2005; Moro, 2004). Fawcett (2005) and Moro (2004) describe the application of DBS in a 42-year-old man with HD and severe chorea who had impairments of gait, balance, speech, swallowing, and generation of saccades. While on DBS, he had improvement of self-generated saccades and improved ability to suppress unwanted saccades. Chorea, dystonia, and ability to complete ADL also improved with specific stimulation frequencies. Bonelli (2001) provides a report of a patient with confirmed HD and severe chorea who suddenly had complete cessation of chorea and improved function. Although the MRI showed caudate atrophy that was present with the chorea, it also showed bilateral degeneration of the substantia nigra coincided with the cessation of chorea. Based only on this case, the authors hypothesized it may be possible to improve chorea by performing DBS of the substantia nigra compacta. In a small study of seven patients with HD who presented with pharmacologically resistant chorea, DBS implanted in the GPi demonstrated a significant reduction in chorea in all of the patients with sustained effects over 12 months. Bradykinesia and dystonia showed a non-significant trend toward worsening partially attributed to the DBS and partially to disease progression. The authors reported "transient benefit to physical aspects of quality of life before progression of behavioral and cognitive disorders" (Gonzalez, 2014).

Although medical treatments such as oral medication, DBS, and BTX-A are typically used to reduce impairments due to dyskinesias, evidence is increasing to support the use of specific modalities and treatment techniques carried out by physical and occupational therapists.

## THINK ABOUT IT 20.4

Return to the clinical case:
- What medications is JD likely taking?
- Discuss whether (or not) you believe JD is a candidate for DBS.

## Therapeutic Techniques

When designing interventions, therapists should not only consider impairments at the body function/structures level, but also activity limitations, participation restrictions, and education of the patient and family. A qualitative study led by Quinn (2010) suggested barriers to exercise programs for individuals with HD and PD included poor cognition (e.g., inability to understand and carry out home programs), lack of information on exercise in PD and HD, safety (e.g., inability to perform challenging exercises safely due to poor balance), and location (e.g., patient preference of group exercise, gym exercise, or home program). To encourage success, therapists should set goals for each session (e.g., number of repetitions or minutes), encourage internal motivation and self-efficacy, begin exercise programs early in the disease process, include the family in the program, and keep the exercise program simple (Quinn, 2010). Evidence-basis of interventions for tremors, dystonia, and chorea is summarized in the following paragraphs and in Table 20-6.

### Interventions to Reduce Tremor

The use of **whole body vibration**, delivered to the whole body as a vibratory stimulation in one or multiple planes, has been found to benefit patients with tremor to include the resting tremor associated with PD (Haas, 2006; Jobges, 2002; King, 2009; Lee, 2008). The rationale for vibration is that the vibratory input to the muscle spindle biases information about muscle length, resulting in reduction in errors and amplitude during memory-guided movements (Feys, 2006). Other evidence-based interventions to reduce tremor include *wearing specific orthoses* (Espay, 2005; Manto, 2007; Rocon, 2007), *resistance training with weights* (Bilodeau, 2000; Sequeira, 2012; Kavanagh, 2016), *stretching and seated karate* (Palmer, 1986), *functional electrical stimulation* (Javidan, 1992; Prochazka, 1992; Zhang, 2007), *peripheral cooling of the limbs* (Cooper, 2000; Feys, 2005), *massage* (Craig, 2006; Riou, 2013), *active-assisted cycling* (Ridgel, 2012), and *bright light therapy* (Paus, 2007). Craig (2006) report a standardized method of massage called "neuromuscular therapy" is effective for patients with PD and tremor. This therapy incorporates lengthening strokes applied with moderate compression parallel to muscle groups as well as direct compression of trigger points to alleviate muscle pain and spasms. Budini (2014) found that *functional dexterity training* (three times per week for 4 weeks) significantly improved performance in patients with ET.

An alternative yet noninvasive approach to reducing resting tremor in patients with PD is the use of Transcranial Alternating Current Stimulation (TACS) and Transcranial Direct Current Stimulation (tDCS). A pilot study demonstrated TACS, applied over the motor cortex, reduced resting tremor amplitude by 50% in patients with PD (Brittain, 2013). Five days of tDCS treatment applied over the motor cortex and cerebellum has improved dyskinesias in patients with PD, Hoehn and Yahr stages 2 to 3 (Ferrucci, 2016).

### Interventions to Reduce Dystonia

Patients with dystonia present with widely varying symptomatology, distribution, and neurological cause. Therefore a thorough knowledge of each patient's medical diagnosis, classification, and prognosis is essential before designing a therapy plan (Cloud, 2010). Physical or occupational therapy is needed for exercise along with bracing to enable function and prevent secondary contractures. Evidence-basis of physical or occupational therapy interventions for patients with dystonia is limited to studies of subjects with occupational focal dystonia (e.g., musician's or writer's cramp) and cervical dystonia. Occupational dystonia occurs with intense and regular practice of a certain movement such as intensive practice on a musical instrument or repetitive typing on a keyboard or typewriter with a subsequent increase in somatotopic representation of the hand. The development of dystonia occurs when cortical representation of the digits is "smeared" or not differentiated (Byl, 2003). Evidence to improve dystonia in subjects with occupational focal dystonia includes intense sessions of specific sensory exercises and mental rehearsal (Byl, 2000, 2003; Candia, 1999, 2002).

A structured *sensorimotor training program* combined with wellness and *mental rehearsal* reportedly improved somatosensory representation of the hand (Byl, 2003) and function (Byl, 2000) in musicians with focal dystonia. For example, practice of the novel skill of *Braille reading* for 8 weeks, 30 to 60 minutes per day, improved spatial acuity and dystonia in patients with focal hand dystonia (Zeuner, 2002, 2003). *Mirror therapy* (Byl, 2000; Rosen, 2005) can also be implemented in which the dystonic hand is hidden from the patient's view by a mirror. The mirror provides a reflection of the normally functioning hand—the mirror image that looks like the dystonic hand. Mirror therapy has also been applied in individuals with arm dysfunction after stroke (Wu, 2013). As the patient moves the unaffected hand, they see a view of symmetrical movement of both hands simultaneously providing a sensory "trick" to the brain with potential to cause neural plasticity and improved motor control and UE function. An example of this is shown in Figure 25-12A and B. Other interventions to improve occupational focal dystonia include *vibration* to the abductor pollicis brevis muscle (Rosenkranz, 2008) and *immobilization of the dystonic hand for 4 to 5 weeks* (Priori, 2001). Contrary to immobilization, *constraint-induced therapy* or forced use of the dystonic hand has also been shown to improve function in patients with occupational focal dystonia (Candia, 1999, 2002) especially if the limb practices a task dissimilar to the dystonic task. Constraint-induced movement therapy combined with motor control retraining over 1 year showed an 80% reduction in abnormal movements and improvements were maintained 4 years later (Berque, 2013). Muscle fatigue has been shown to reduce dystonia transiently (i.e., for minutes) (Pesenti, 2001) possibly by decreasing the cortical area of dystonic muscle representation. *Transcutaneous electrical nerve stimulation (TENS)* to the forearm muscles may also improve writer's cramp for up to 3 weeks after treatment (Tinazzi, 2005). This improvement is attributed to remodeling the excitability of the motor cortex in individuals with writer's cramp to improve handwriting (Tinazzi, 2006). Preliminary studies also show *repetitive Transcranial Magnetic Stimulation* to the premotor cortex may improve handwriting and cortical excitability in patients with focal hand dystonia (Borich, 2009). Children with dystonia were able to reduce the amount of cocontraction when presented with visual *biofeedback* of muscle contraction (Young, 2011).

Involuntary muscle contractions with cervical dystonia cause the head to rotate or tilt in a specific direction, resulting in various forms of torticollis and laterocollis. *Sensory stimulation* to the face is one method of conservative treatment. Sensory "tricks" (often referred to within the literature as "geste antagoniste") (Poisson, 2012) can be used by touching the face or imagining the face is being touched while the patient actively turns the head to a neutral position (Schramm, 2004). Positron emission tomography during sensory tricks in subjects with cervical dystonia showed reduction of activity in the overactive supplemental motor and primary sensorimotor cortices as well as increased activation of the parietal and occipital cortices (Naumann, 2000). *Orthoses* (e.g., head and neck bracing) can be used not only to prevent contracture but also to provide the sensory feedback that will normalize the corrected position (Jankovic, 2004). One randomized controlled trial (RCT) demonstrated *active neck range of motions exercise and/or whole body relaxation* improved quality of life

and torticollis severity in patients with cervical dystonia (Boyce, 2013). In another RCT, *KinesioTape*, compared with sham tape, improved pain and temporal sensory discrimination in patients with cervical and focal hand dystonia (Pelosin, 2013).

### Interventions for Chorea (Huntington Disease)

Limited evidence exists to support physical and occupational therapy interventions specifically targeting the treatment of choreoathetosis (Busse, 2012). When the involuntary movements become violent and flailing, medication may be instituted because of the increased potential for self-injury. Possible medications include dopamine antagonists (e.g., haloperidol [Haldol] or pimozide [Orap]) but they can have troublesome side-effects, including increased risk for the development of tardive dyskinesia. Benzodiazepines such as clonazepam (Klonopin) may also be effective in decreasing the intensity of the choreiform movements. Anticonvulsant valproate sodium (Depakene) may help decrease chorea in Sydenham's chorea. When starting the medications, physical and occupational therapy are also important parts of the intervention plan particularly to address related system impairments, particularly balance dysfunction (Cardoso, 2006; Huntington Study Group, 2006; Marshall, 2004).

The rest of this section will address general interventions for patients with HD. Physical therapists can be instrumental in helping people with HD prevent falls and secondary musculoskeletal problems, obtain necessary adaptive equipment, and optimize quality of life (Quinn, 2002). A study of more than 3,000 individuals with HD indicated loss of motor function to include impaired gait, bradykinesia, and impaired tandem gait was the most predictive variable of institutionalization (Wheelock, 2003). However, physical therapy is often not utilized as a form of treatment for people with HD (Busse, 2008). A qualitative study led by Busse (2008) determined how physical therapy services were utilized for patients with HD. These investigators found an overall theme that the management of individuals with HD should be tailored to the stage of the disease. The subthemes were that therapy services are underutilized especially at the early stages; if physical therapy services are used for patients with HD, therapists tend to focus on fall prevention, problem-solving, and functional activities; and that no physical therapy outcome tools are available to measure the disease-specific impairments caused by HD. To promote exercise in patients with HD, Khalil (2012) provided 15 patients with home-exercise DVDs and found adherence in 11 of the subjects. A qualitative analysis identified barriers to exercise to include physical factors, cognitive factors, and lack of motivation. Caregiver involvement and follow up by the therapist were major factors contributing to adherence to the exercise program (Khalil, 2012). A follow-up RCT by the same author found benefits and feasibility of a structured home exercise program, including improvements in gait, balance, and levels of physical activity but not quality of life (Khalil, 2013).

When designing interventions, therapists should consider the setting in which the intervention will take place and work with the patient and family to determine the optimal setting.

If the patient is evaluated in a clinic setting such as a Huntington Disease Center of Excellence, interventions should focus on education, fall prevention, referrals to other health-care professionals, recommendations for assistive technology, and setting up a home evaluation if needed.

## PATIENT APPLICATION: JD

*Given the results of JD's evaluation, the physical therapist educated him and his wife on awareness of his environment for fall prevention. They were instructed to have night lights on in the house and to use caution in dimly lit areas and/or on compliant surfaces. JD was also instructed to slow down and stop so he can become steady after rising from sitting or after turning to change directions. He was shown how to use visual focus on a still object to regain balance when he becomes unsteady. The physical therapist also educated him by showing pictures of a rolling walker with a flip-down seat. However, JD was not willing to receive this equipment yet. The occupational therapist recommended JD receive a home visit to assess the bathroom needs for safety bars, to assess the layout of the house for safety, and to assess his driving ability.*

*Note: In the authors' experience, patients with HD and severe choreoathetosis do not use standard or two-wheel walkers very well unless the walkers are weighted down (e.g., something heavy in the basket). This is supported in a study by Kloos (2012) in which four-wheel walkers provided the most stability with improvements to temporal parameters of gait. Other devices were frequently deemed less safe and highly variable with performance (Kloos, 2012).*

*Additionally, patients tend not to do as well if the therapist or caregiver tries to "control" their base of support (e.g., using a gait belt to move their center of gravity). They prefer to walk while holding a caregiver's arm or railing and will typically progress to using a wheelchair for long distances. Some patients try to refuse to stop driving or refuse to move to assisted-living situations. This makes it very difficult for the family and caregivers.*

*JD was also referred to a local outpatient rehabilitation clinic to receive physical and occupational therapy for functional training and to instruct him in an exercise program. He and his wife were referred to a local HD support group.*

## Contemplate Clinical Decisions

*Given what you know about JD's situation:*

1. *Would you alter the functional goals you initially wrote? If so, how?*
2. *Design an appropriate exercise program for JD that includes functional training.*
3. *Given the evidence for therapy interventions, what specific strategies might you use with JD? Why?*

In the inpatient or outpatient settings, physical or occupational therapy interventions would address self-care, mobility, balance, coordination, safety, equipment needs, and discharge planning. A systematic review by Bilney (2003) contained 10 articles that were observational, case study, or expert opinion. Two of the expert opinion articles in the review addressed interventions to improve choreoathetosis, including hydrotherapy and relaxation. The other articles were limited in their description of exercise parameters and outcomes. General exercise categories included mat and chair exercises, strengthening with weighted cuffs, home exercise programs, fall prevention, task-specific practice, ball games, and breath-control exercises. One "ABA" design study showed rhythmic auditory stimulation using a metronome during slow- and fast-paced walking was found to improve gait velocity in individuals with HD (Thaut, 1999).

A case report by Quinn (2002) described a 14-week home exercise program for a 49 year-old male with HD who was concerned about recent falls and functional decline. Exercises were done five times per week and included a warm up (i.e., deep breathing, neck mobility, arm mobility, squatting, reaching × 10 repetitions); leg exercises in standing (i.e., squats, knee lifts, kicks, walking forward/back and sideways, jumping × 5 to 15 repetitions); arm exercises in standing (i.e., 10 to 15 repetitions of overhead press, arm circles, bicep curls with two-pound weights or cans, Theraband exercises of shoulder flexion/extension, and horizontal abduction); floor exercises of hamstring and inner thigh stretches (three repetitions with a 30-second hold), sit ups × 20 repetitions, straight leg raises, prone press ups, and pushups for 10 repetitions, cat/camel for 5 repetitions; and cool down (same as the warm up). In addition, the patient was instructed to do daily exercises, including single-leg stance, tandem walking, and bouncing/catching a tennis ball. A detailed instructional videotape was provided. Outcomes (SF-36, number of falls, Modified Falls Efficacy Scale, Berg Balance Scale, self-paced and fast gait speed, and Unified HD Rating Scale motor scores) all improved after the intervention (Quinn, 2002).

A study by Zinzi (2007) examined the effect of intense inpatient rehabilitation for 8 hours per day for 3 weeks in 40 subjects with early- and middle-stage HD. This was repeated three times per year, and physical outcomes as measured on Tinetti Scale and Physical Performance Test statistically improved after each session. A study by Smith (2005) examined motor learning abilities in subjects with HD and cerebellar disease using a reaching task. Unlike subjects with cerebellar disease, subjects with HD were able to adapt during reaching to demonstrate compensatory changes that positively affected subsequent movements. Similar to healthy controls, subjects with HD were also able to generalize what they learned from one direction of error to other directions. This indicates they may be able to learn new skills. The study also found responses to auditory and visual stimuli are slowed early in the disease (Smith, 2005). Leng (2003) concluded dyskinesias were not improved after a multisensory intervention or typical relaxation sessions for subjects with HD in the severe stages (i.e., profound impairment requiring total care) (Leng, 2003).

Two studies demonstrated physical therapy clinic-based interventions done twice weekly for 6 weeks significantly improved gait parameters, specifically the percentage of double support time during the gait cycle as well as balance (Bohlen, 2013; Kloos, 2013). In the study by Kloos (2013), participants played a video-based game called *Dance Dance Revolution* (Harmonix Music Systems, Inc., Cambridge, MA) where they moved their feet on a mat to the rhythm of music. Subjects in the study by Bohlen (2013) participated in a clinic-based intervention of changing positions, walking, static/dynamic balance, and motor coordination (Bohlen, 2013). Other studies examined the effect of longer bouts of PT. An RCT demonstrated that patients with HD who performed weekly supervised stationary cycling and resistance training combined with twice weekly home walking for 12 weeks tolerated the therapy well but did not statistically improve compared with the control group on measures of physical activity. (Busse, 2013). A study by Thompson et al showed that a 9-month multidisciplinary program reduced declining motor and postural stability and improved fat-free mass and strength in nine early- to middle-stage patients with HD compared with n = 11 controls. The program consisted of clinic-based therapy (5 minute warm up, 10 minutes of aerobic exercise, 40 minutes of resistance exercise, and a 5 minute cool down). The final 6 months of the program included a custom self-monitored home exercise program to be done three times per week. Adherence was better for the clinical sessions (85%) than the home program (56%) (Thompson, 2013).

### Interventions for Children with Dyskinesias

Similar to adults, children with dyskinesias require individualized physical or occupational therapy interventions depending on the specific impairments (e.g., choreoathetosis versus dystonia) (Smith, 2014). However clinicians must also consider the effect of the movement disorder on developing gross and fine motor skills. The interventions discussed in the evidence table (Table 20-6) can be used with children but must be adapted to age-specific activity and participation restrictions. A thorough orthopedic, neurological, and developmental assessment is critical so appropriate recommendations can be made. Therapists working in the school system must consider and address the effect of the involuntary movement disorder on learning ability and mobility within the learning environment. Therapists must also have a strong knowledge of the current literature and technology related to orthotic management, adaptive equipment, and dosing recommendations (Gannotti, 2014). Although practice of specific task-related activities such as walking, balance, and upper extremity activities is important, all children should be encouraged to participate in intense and regular functional activities throughout the lifespan (Damiano, 2006). These activities will most likely be done outside of the clinical setting on a playground, at school, or at a local recreational facility. The physical and occupational therapist can play an integral role in helping families to determine the best way to accomplish daily regular intense activity.

## PATIENT APPLICATION: BETTY

*A 36 year-old female patient, Betty, is diagnosed with the dystonic type of CP causing hemiplegia of the left upper and lower extremity. She has mild intellectual impairment and lives in a group home setting. Betty attends an adult day program. At rest and with activity, Betty presents with strong dystonic posturing of the left upper extremity into shoulder and elbow extension and wrist and finger flexion. Her left lower extremity is less severe but presents with plantar flexion and metatarsus adductus and generally poor control when walking. She does not wear foot orthoses. Betty has not fallen but walks slowly during various activities at the adult day center. Betty's job in the adult day program is to sort papers. However she is unable to use her dystonic arm functionally and compensates by putting the papers in her mouth, which is unacceptable (first figure). She calls her arm an "it" and states that it "does what it wants." The only functional use of her dystonic arm is to hold objects against her chest. The second figure illustrates the dystonic posturing when she walks.*

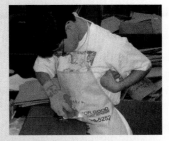

Before botulinum toxin injections and therapy, Betty was unable to use her left hand to work.

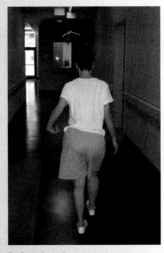

Before botulinum toxin injections and therapy, Betty walked with shoulder extension. She was unable to wear a splint because of the strong flexion of her wrist and fingers. She had internal hip rotation and difficulty achieving foot flat position in stance.

## Contemplate Clinical Decisions

1. What tests and measures would you do during the examination?
2. What medical interventions would you consider and who would you consult to provide these interventions?
3. What exercises and/or modalities would you recommend?
4. Would you recommend any equipment?

The assessment revealed the following:

1. When walking forward, backward, and side-to-side, Betty initiated stepping on the left using a toe-down and ankle-inversion pattern. She had short stance on the left and circumduction during swing phase on the left. She was unable to abduct the left leg to walk sideways.
2. When transitioning from sit-to-stand, Betty was independent but used momentum and decreased weight-shift on the left leg.
3. In quadruped, Betty was unable to put any weight on her left upper extremity. She was able to assume tall kneel but could only assume half-kneel using the right lower extremity.
4. In bimanual tasks, Betty used the left upper extremity to anchor the object and manipulated it using the right.
5. Preferred and fast gait speed were both well below published norms for Betty's age.
6. Betty was unable to tandem walk.
7. On the Modified Clinical Test of Sensory Interaction and Balance, Betty stood for 30 seconds on the floor with eyes open and closed but was unable to balance on the foam with eyes open or closed.
8. Range-of-motion assessment revealed functional limitations on the left in the shoulder extensors, elbow extensors and wrist flexors, finger flexors, and ankle plantar flexors.
9. Strength assessment of the left upper extremity was difficult due to the inability to perform individual movements. For example, when attempting to flex her shoulder, her entire arm moved into extension. Betty was able to extend her left knee, flex her left hip, and dorsiflex through partial range against gravity. She required gravity to be eliminated for active hip abduction.

Based on these results, the therapist decided to consult a physiatrist, who suggested a series of BTX-A injections to Betty's left upper and lower extremities. Five sets of injections were given 3 months apart and were complemented by exercises done three times per week and splinting. The injection schedule, muscles injected, and exercises are outlined in Table 20-5.

Betty completed a 15-month program of injections and therapeutic intervention (Figs. 20-2 and 20-3). Figures 20-4 and 20-5 demonstrate improvements in Betty's arm use and function. Betty's range of motion and active movement improved so she was now able to manipulate objects much better and could complete her work sorting papers and opening envelopes without using her mouth. She continued to lack active grasp and release but was able to use the left upper extremity for stability in weight-bearing. Betty improved her gait speed to near normal and was able to sidestep to the left without turning. She also learned to balance on foam with eyes open. Betty enjoyed her exercise sessions and complained when she was unable to exercise, stating that "it made her worse." Throughout the intervention period, the therapist constantly updated her home program so that she incorporated the exercises into her daily routine.

| TABLE 20-5 | Case Example of Injection Schedule, Muscles Injected, and Exercise Interventions for Patient with Dystonia | |
|---|---|---|
| **INJECTION NUMBER** | **MUSCLES INJECTED 3 MONTHS APART (LEFT SIDE)** | **EXERCISE INTERVENTION (3 TIMES/WEEK FOR 1 HOUR)** |
| 1 | Upper trapezius and lattisimus dorsi<br>Elbow extensors (triceps)<br>Wrist flexors (flexor carpi radialis and ulnaris)<br>Abductor and flexor pollicis longus<br>Palmaris longus<br>Flexor digitorum superficialis and profundus | 1. Massage and stretching.<br>2. Use of a resting splint to keep the wrist and fingers at neutral.<br>3. Weight-bearing activities in prone, quadruped, and sitting.<br>4. Reactions to sudden perturbations to the left (protective extension).<br>5. Isolated movements of the left UE (e.g., putting rings on a stick, picking up small objects).<br>6. Using the left UE to lift a bar above the head or push it forward with and without weights.<br>7. In standing: weight-shifting, single-leg stance, high-level gait activities (e.g., walking sideways and braiding, walking quickly, walking carrying a large object with both UEs). |
| 2 | Tibialis posterior<br>Gastrocnemius<br>Wrist flexors<br>Adductor pollicis<br>Upper latissimus | |
| 3, 4, 5 | Lower latissimus<br>Wrist flexors<br>Elbow extensors<br>Tibialis posterior<br>Gastrocnemius | |

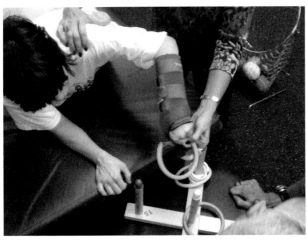

FIGURE 20-2  Betty's therapy included performing grasp release and reaching tasks in prone.

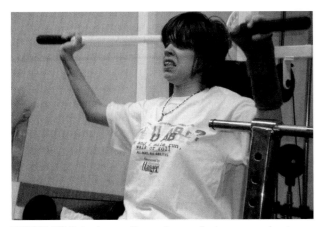

FIGURE 20-3  In therapy, Betty also worked on strengthening her shoulder muscles with weights

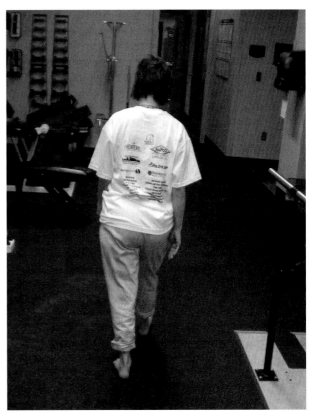

FIGURE 20-4  After injections and therapy, Betty walked with a more relaxed shoulder position and could better achieve foot flat during gait.

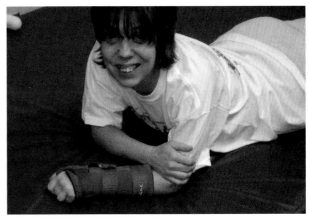

FIGURE 20-5  After injections and therapy, Betty was able to wear a resting hand splint to keep her wrist in neutral and could assume weight-bearing in prone.

## ■ Intervention: Ultimately Applied in Functional Activities

### Task-Specific Practice

If medical or therapeutic intervention decreases involuntary movements, it is essential to incorporate the improved movement ability into practice of functional activities. Task-specific practice should be a cornerstone of any intervention plan. Once the underlying movement impairment has been addressed, the individual should be encouraged to practice any skills, customized for the specific patient, from Chapters 33 through 37 that are on the patient's problem list. Orthotic devices may play a critical role in maintaining limb position so functional skills may be practiced.

### Functional Gait Practice

When dyskinesias affect the way a person walks, specific practice of gait must be emphasized in the overall intervention plan, including practice of specific components and the overall gait cycle with a progressive approximation or shaping of the normal gait cycle. For example, the choreiform movements of HD cause a tremendous negative effect on gait. The intervention for gait must include techniques from Chapter 37 to focus on increasing gait speed, increasing consistency of temporal parameters, improving consistency of stride lengths, and improving the rhythmic cadence of the continuous gait cycle.

## Pediatric Considerations

For the movement disorders occurring in childhood listed earlier in the chapter, the therapist must carefully design the physical intervention for the underlying movement disorder and the related functional activity limitations. Even more importantly, creative and interesting interventions must be planned; activities should incite engagement and motivate the child to participation. As with all interventions, therapeutic activities must be incorporated into the daily life situation.

## ■ Intervention: Considerations for Nontherapy Time and Discharge

The therapist must help the patient to find exercises and functional activities related to their dysfunction that can be performed independently outside of the therapy time and in a variety of locations (e.g., in the passenger seat of the car driving home, standing at the sink for self-care and assisting with cooking, while watching TV, in bed before nap-time or bedtime) and during each transition happening throughout the day (e.g., weight-bearing during resting postures and during transfers and sit-to-stand).

## HANDS-ON PRACTICE

- Apply a weight to your dominant wrist while eating a meal. How will this affect a tremor? Why? How does the added weight affect your posture and trunk control during the meal?
- Practice a session of mirror therapy for both an upper extremity and lower extremity dyskinesia.

- Plan a constraint-induced therapy program for an individual with right hand dystonia.
- Plan a stretching and range-of-motion program for an individual with torticollis.
- Practice using a metronome to improve gait velocity and cadence.

## Let's Review

1. Describe the role of the basal ganglia in Huntington disease compared with Parkinson disease.

2. Discuss the role the physical and occupational therapist should play in the evaluation and treatment of individuals with Huntington disease. In your discussion, consider the barriers that affect the ability of patients with HD to participate in exercise interventions.

3. Discuss three important aspects of clinical observations (what should you observe and describe) during the examination.

4. Using the Focus on Evidence Table (Table 20-6) and information from the chapter, compare and contrast evidence-based interventions. What specific intervention strategies would you suggest for individuals with:
   a. Tremor
   b. Dystonia
   c. Chorea
   d. Huntington disease—early, middle, and late in the disease process.

As always, it is the clinician's responsibility to take into consideration not only the evidence but also clinical judgment and the patient situation when choosing interventions.

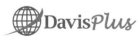 DavisPlus

For additional resources, including Focus on Evidence tables, case study discussions, references, and glossary, please visit http://davisplus.fadavis.com

# CHAPTER SUMMARY

To effectively treat individuals with dyskinesias throughout the lifespan, therapists must be aware of the neurophysiology behind movement disorders, the progressive nature of the disease, and underlying cognitive, behavioral, and motivation issues that accompany the movement dysfunction. Although high levels of evidence to support specific interventions are limited, clinicians should consider the individual patient's activity limitations and participation restrictions so an appropriate intervention program can be designed. Interventions may include dyskinesia-specific modalities as included in

Table 20-6, but should also incorporate activities to teach patients to use sensorimotor systems not affected by the disease. The evidence basis for some important interventions directed at dyskinesia is summarized in the Focus on Evidence Table 20-6 (ONL). An important component of the intervention should include education of patients and caregivers concerning the nature of the disease as well as prompt referral to disease-specific support groups and referral sources. Finally, clinicians should constantly check evidence-based databases for current tests and intervention strategies.

# Intervention for Ataxia/Incoordination

Carina Eksteen, PT, PhD • Reva P. Rauk, PT, PhD, MMSc, NCS

## CHAPTER OBJECTIVES

Upon completion of this chapter, the learner should be able to:
1. Discuss the physiology of coordinated movement.
2. Discuss the etiology, pathogenesis, and clinical presentation of ataxia/incoordination.
3. Explain the differential diagnosis between ataxia/incoordination due to a somatosensory impairment and to a cerebellar impairment.
4. Discuss the evaluation principles applicable to a patient who presents with ataxia/incoordination.
5. Discuss the principles of intervention to design an appropriate rehabilitation program for patients with cerebellar and somatosensory ataxia/incoordination.
6. Discuss precautions, monitoring, and a home program for patients with cerebellar and somatosensory ataxia/incoordination

## ■ Introduction

This chapter explains the basic anatomy and physiology of lesions known to result in ataxia/incoordination, their potential etiology, the differentiation between cerebellar and sensory ataxia/incoordination, and the rehabilitation principles for these conditions.

**Coordination**, or coordinated functional movement, is described in the coordination examination section of Chapter 6. Coordination requires precise cooperation between opposing muscle groups, related interjoint muscle groups, and interlimb muscle groups for functional activities, along with normal postural control during a volitional movement. Normal postural control depends on an anatomically intact neuromusculoskeletal system (Fig. 21-1) and intact complex interactions and cooperation between the many systems in the human body that control its biomechanical alignment and orientation within the context of environmental demands.

Ataxia/incoordination occurs as a result of either the lack/absence of sensory (in particular, proprioceptive) input from the periphery to the cerebellum, or higher sensory centers (sensory ataxia), or a lesion/disruption in the interaction among four different systems: the lower motor neurons (LMNs) in the brainstem and spinal cord, the upper motor neuron (UMN) cell bodies in the cortex and brainstem, the cerebellum, and the basal ganglia.

## Normal Motor Function

Normal coordinated, selective, voluntary and involuntary, intentional and automatic, conscious and subconscious movements are essential in a large variety of specific movement patterns (including movements of the mouth and eyes) during

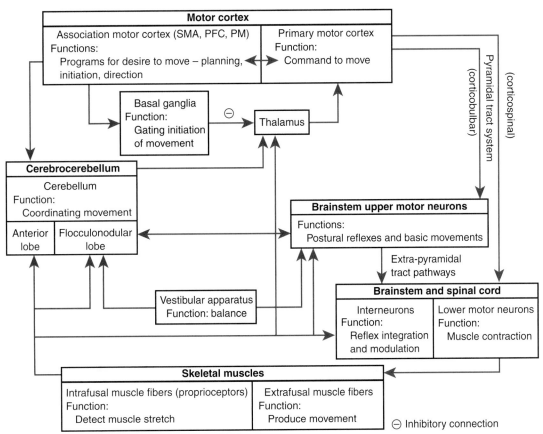

**FIGURE 21-1** Schematic representation of the circuitry involved in motor function. *(Reproduced with permission from Michael-Titus A, Revest P, Shortland P.* The Nervous System: Basic Science and Clinical Conditions. *Philadelphia, PA: Churchill Livingstone; 2007.])*

skilled activities of daily living (ADLs), recreational activities, and sporting activities. As mentioned previously, movement is controlled and coordinated through the interaction between four subsystems of the nervous system: the LMNs in the brainstem and spinal cord, the UMN cell bodies in the cortex and the brainstem, the cerebellum, and the basal ganglia (which have an inhibitory influence on the motor cortex). Both the cerebellum and the basal ganglia regulate the activity of the LMN via the UMN and the thalamus.

A simplistic but holistic understanding of the organization of the brain makes it easier to understand the sources from which ataxia or incoordination can originate and how the rehabilitation of patients with ataxia or incoordination can be planned and implemented. Figure 21-1 is a simplistic graphical representation of the systems involved in the coordination of movement.

A basic understanding of the physiology of movement coordination by the central nervous system (CNS) serves as the basis for discussing the signs and symptoms of ataxia, as well as the principles of intervention for patients with a motor coordination disorder. As shown in Fig. 21-1, the peripheral neuromusculoskeletal system both carries out the motor plan and is a major feedback system for movement controlled by the cerebrum and the cerebellum.

Optimal voluntary movement requires the dynamic combination of movement with selective motor control, coordination

between opposing muscle groups, multijoint coordination of related muscle groups, and interlimb coordination for functional movement patterns, always in the context of existing primitive and stretch reflexes. If the stretch reflex of the muscle spindle is hypersensitive or hyposensitive to stretch and contributes to impaired movement (as a result of constant increased or decreased response to the stretch reflex), the cerebellum initiates a compensatory modification of the stretch reflex.

In addition to controlling the LMNs to optimize smooth coordinated muscle contraction, the cerebellum helps regulate the *sequence of voluntary muscle contraction* through the corrective feedback mode. The corrective feedback mode is based on sensory information (from the visual, vestibular, and somatosensory systems) about a person's posture and balance and the position of his joints (limbs) via the ascending tracts (which include the spinocerebellar, cuneocerebellar, trigeminocerebellar, olivocerebellar, vestibulocerebellar, and pontocerebellar pathways) (Michael-Titus, 2007).

## The Role of the Cerebellum in Motor Learning

One of the vital functions of the cerebellum is the role it plays in motor learning.

Ito (1970) described the cerebellum as an adaptive feedforward control system that programs or models voluntary movement skills according to memory of previous sensory input and motor output. Recent evidence also indicates that motor learning can take place in the cerebellum despite disease or dysfunction (Martin, 2009). The cerebellum may play an active part in the acquisition and execution of sequential procedures of small simple programs, which can be uniquely combined to create complex motor activities. One of the "mechanisms" of relearning coordinated movement is that movement is guided by slow sensory loops through the cerebrum instead of by activation of the learned motor programs usually controlled by the cerebellum. Control of movement through the slow sensory loop in the cerebrum resembles the neurophysiological process of learning a new skill. Such movements result in incoordination and an inability to adapt to minor changes in the demands from the environment or to unusual external circumstances.

Learning new tasks (motor learning) requires repetition before the task can be completed skillfully and adapted to various demands. The cerebellum plays a vital role in neural processing, with motor adaptation also needed in order to learn through trial and error.

With cerebellar pathology, patients may need many repeated trials to adapt to changes in the conditions of a task after they have learned to perform it within one set of specific conditions. Patients with a cerebellar lesion may learn to perform a task under certain conditions and may even adapt to a change in the conditions of the task (through feedback control). But these patients may still not be able to elicit anticipatory control (feedforward control) when the condition of the task is changed to that of the original task (Morton, 2013). This further indicates the cerebellum is vital in the control of anticipatory movements during activities as well as in controlling modification of a person's response to the change in the conditions of the task (Morton, 2013). As a clinical implication of these findings, a patient with cerebellar disease not only needs many more practice sessions to learn a task but may also need to be taught alternative planning and execution of movement strategies and cognitive control (deliberate voluntary frontal lobe decision-making) and/or compensatory control of a movement.

The dentate nucleus and the cerebellar hemispheres are very active during mental rehearsal of movement (Ryding, 1993). However, patients with a lesion in the lateral region of the cerebellum have reduced capacity to act upon anticipatory cues during the execution of a pretrained task and decreased ability to form an image of the movement, which may limit mental rehearsal of the movement.

## Clinical Presentation of Ataxia/Incoordination

**Ataxia/incoordination** is characterized by the inability to perform coordinated (smooth), skilled volitional movement with an appropriate force (muscle power) and range of movement to accurately reach a target and/or to perform a fine, coordinated, skilled functional activity against the background of dynamic postural stability and control. The terms "ataxia" and "incoordination of volitional movement" are used interchangeably in the literature (Ropper, 2005). The observed signs and expressions of ataxia/incoordination are best explained as a lack of cooperation between the agonist and antagonist muscles related to the intended movement. The opposing muscles struggle against each other instead of the antagonist relaxing as the agonist muscle contracts.

Ataxia/incoordination of volitional movement (described in Chapter 6) has many distinct characteristics, which can present in a varying combination of signs depending on the area, extent, and pathology of the lesion. The clinical picture of patients with ataxia depends on the area of cerebellar pathology, the interconnections between the cerebellum and other parts of the nervous system, and/or the distribution and extent of the somatosensory feedback from the affected limbs.

Patients may therefore present clinically with varying degrees and combinations of signs and symptoms. Underlying pathologies such as multiple sclerosis (MS) or paraneoplastic cerebellar degeneration can result in unique distributions of symptoms (Perlmutter, 2003). The primary impairments exhibited may include signs of ataxia/incoordination such as **dysmetria, decomposition of movement, rebound phenomenon, dysdiadochokinesia, asthenia, intention tremor**, and **hypermetria** as defined in Chapter 6; related symptoms such as **titubation** and/or **postural tremor, dysarthria, staccato speech, nystagmus,** and control of eye movements; and when the pathology is cerebellar, associated decreased muscle tone.

## Possible Effect of Ataxia/Incoordination on Function

Coordination impairment affects the way and the degree to which a patient is able to perform functional activities with the affected limb, including performance under controlled circumstances such as in the home and work environment or during any recreational activity in which they participate, as well as in the therapy gymnasium. When the individual with ataxia attempts a movement or functional activity, the resulting function lacks precision and accuracy, often missing the target. In general, the lack of precision and accuracy is also called an "intention tremor."

Impaired coordination interferes with the ability to perform any functional skill requiring precise movement and approach to a target (such as reach and grasp, transfers, or gait). Typical functional limitations or activity limitations (World Health Organization [WHO], 2001) of individuals with ataxia include:

- Ataxic gait associated with impaired balance, affecting a patient's mobility
- Functional activities of the upper limb, such as self-care (e.g., buttoning a shirt or closing a zipper, brushing teeth), when the upper limb, head, and/or trunk are affected; effects due not only to incoordination but also to poor balance
- Poor balance as a consequence of combined primary impairments, such as changes in the control of and decrease in muscle tone, dysmetria, and rebound phenomenon, and/or as a result of primary vestibulocerebellar impairment

- Control of eye movements and gaze that affect reading and visual-temporo-spatial coordination during activities that require hand-eye and/or eye-foot coordination

## PATIENT APPLICATION I-A

*At 14 years of age, Marleen is in the ninth grade and has been diagnosed with a grade 2 astrocytoma in the brainstem. She exhibited very subtle intention tremor, but after surgery to remove the tumor, she now has pronounced titubation as well as intention tremor. The ataxia prevents her from being independent in her self-care and mobility. Marleen lives in a suburb of a large city with her parents and two siblings. Marleen is the youngest sibling in the family. Apart from her schoolwork, she paints as a hobby.*

*Brain surgery was performed to remove most of Marleen's benign tumor. After the surgery, she was treated with full ventilation in the intensive care unit for 2 weeks. The tracheostomy was removed after 2 more weeks, and she was transferred to the high care unit for 2 more weeks. She was then transferred to a general ward and after 1 week was discharged home.*

*At present, she is very weak because of the hospitalization and decreased activity for 5 weeks and presents with a general low tone, staccato speech, titubation, and severe incoordination of all four limbs but more severely on the right. She is not able to sit up independently, bathe, feed, dress, or groom herself. She is propelled in a wheelchair to the toilet by her mother and uses diapers to address bowel and bladder accidents. Her mother feeds her and takes care of her personal grooming, and her father assists with the transfers to the commode and the wheelchair.*

*Figure 21-2 provides a graphic representation of Marleen's sitting posture. Consider the following questions regarding Marleen. Some discussion of these questions is provided in the online supplemental material.*

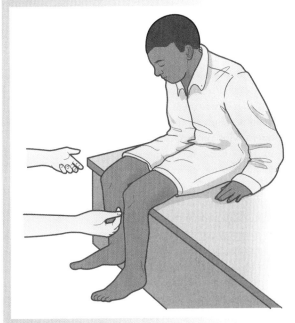

**FIGURE 21-2** Graphic presentation of Marleen's sitting posture.

### Contemplate Clinical Decisions I-A

1. *From the patient's point of view, which aspects are most important to assess?*
2. *What do you think is the most important aspect(s) to be addressed in support of Marleen's parents as her primary caregivers?*
3. *From this brief introduction to Marleen and observation of Fig. 21-2, what information would lead you to complete a more specific assessment for ataxia/incoordination?*
4. *What risk factors related to cerebellar ataxia might you want to explore given the information presented thus far?*

## ■ Functional Anatomy and Physiology Related to Ataxia/Incoordination

Understanding of the anatomy and physiology of the cerebellum, particularly the *functional organization* of the brain, spinal cord, and peripheral neuromuscular systems, is important as the basis for discussions on therapeutic interventions for patients with movement ataxia/incoordination. The cerebellum (sometimes called *the little brain*) is the most important part of the brain involved in the coordination of muscle groups during movement. Situated in the posterior-inferior fossa of the skull, it consists of three lobes: the anterior, posterior, and flocculonodular lobes. These three lobes are further divided into lobules. In contrast to the cerebrum, the cerebellum lies above the fourth ventricle.

In the horizontal plane, three areas of the cerebellum can be distinguished, namely the two lateral hemispheres and the vermis that separates them (Fig. 21-3). In the sagittal plane, three functional areas in the cerebellum can be distinguished, namely the vestibulocerebellum, spinocerebellum, and cerebrocerebellum, emphasizing the functional links with other areas of the CNS. The distinction between the three functional areas in the sagittal plane is based on the different sources or origins from which the cerebellum receives its afferent input. These three functional areas are displayed in Fig. 21-3.

Ataxia may result from damage to one or more of the following areas:

- Cerebellum
- Pathways carrying input or output from the cerebellum to other parts of the brain (vestibulocerebellum, spinocerebellum, and cerebrocerebellum)
- Afferent fibers in peripheral nerves, posterior (dorsal) nerve root, or posterior (dorsal) column disease of the spinal cord resulting in loss of/diminished proprioceptive sensation feedback/input from the peripheral parts of the body to the cerebellum or the premotor and supplementary cortex (Ropper, 2005)

The cerebellum receives input and gives output via three pairs of peduncles, namely the inferior, middle, and superior cerebellar peduncles. The inferior and middle cerebellar peduncles carry mainly *input* pathways, and the superior

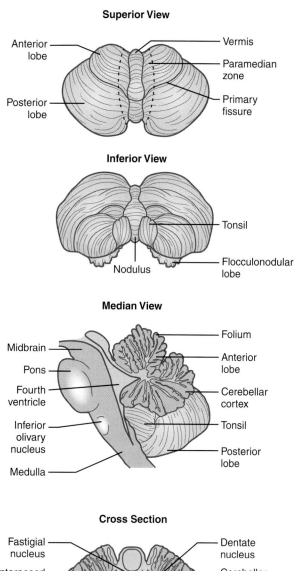

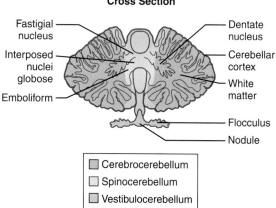

**FIGURE 21-3** General anatomical organization of the cerebellum.

cerebellar peduncles carry mainly *output* pathways. The functions of the input pathways are summarized in Table 21-1.

Each of the three subdivisions (*vestibulocerebellum, spinocerebellum,* and *cerebrocerebellum*) is associated with a pair of deep cerebellar nuclei. The deep cerebellar nuclei are associated with the flocculus and the nodule. The deep cerebellar nuclei associated with the spinocerebellum are the interposed nuclei and the fastigial nucleus, whereas the cerebrocerebellum is associated with the dentate nucleus (Fig. 21-3).

The *vestibulocerebellum* entails the most medial and hindmost (inferior) part of the cerebellum and receives information from and projects impulses (information) to the lateral vestibular nuclei and the fastigial nucleus. The lateral vestibular nuclei and the fastigial nucleus project information to the areas of the brain concerned with balance via the vestibulocerebellum-vestibular tract. The vestibulocerebellum also receives input from the semicircular canals, the utricle, and the saccule via the eighth cranial nerve and are the only nuclei within the brain to receive direct input from the Purkinje cells.

A lesion of the vestibulocerebellum therefore results in difficulty maintaining balance. Impaired balance causes difficulty with the execution of skilled or unskilled movements of the distal extremities and occurs more so in an upright position than in a horizontal position. The upright position requires the control of posture, as well as balance reactions within the "axial trunk" and simultaneously with the control of coordinated limb movement during the execution of skilled movement. The axial trunk therefore has to perform multisegmental patterns, especially during (even simple) functional activities that require limb movement, such as reaching out sideways or forward. The simultaneous control of posture and balance, with or without locomotion, and coordinated skilled movement of the limbs are characteristic of the complexity of functional activities controlled mainly by the cerebellum. A lesion of the vestibulocerebellum further results in an inability to coordinate eye movements, with movements of the head identifiable by an impaired vestibulo-ocular reflex.

To illustrate the interaction between the vestibular end organs and a lesion of the vestibulocerebellum, a simplified diagram indicating the functional organization of the vestibular system and vestibular labyrinth is given in Fig. 21-4 (Meldrum, 2004).

The vestibular nuclei are responsible for integrating impulses from the end organ (the vestibular apparatus) with impulses received from other sensory systems, as well as from the cerebellum before contributing to the control of eye movements, postural control, and the reticular formation and links with the autonomic nervous system. The clinical implication of the integration of these impulses is that patients who present with ataxia/incoordination, specifically with balance problems, gait impairment, and nystagmus, may also have an underlying vestibular impairment. Such patients most likely also present with vertigo, dizziness/light-headedness, nausea and vomiting, oscillopsia, anxiety, neck and back pain, physical deconditioning, agoraphobia, hyperventilation, and/or hearing loss/tinnitus.

The *spinocerebellum* receives information from (1) peripheral receptors (including the deep sensory receptors located in muscles, joints, and tendons) via the spinal cord and feedback input from the (2) spinal motor generators as well as from the (3) cortex regarding the motor command. The input from the spinal cord to the spinocerebellum runs via the posterior and anterior spinocerebellar tracts. The dorsal spinocerebellar tract carries accurate information regarding muscle activity. The anterior (ventral) spinocerebellar tract carries information regarding internally generated processes related to automatic

| TABLE 21-1 | Summary of the Input Pathways to the Cerebellum | | |
|---|---|---|---|
| **PATHWAY** | **ORIGIN** | **PEDUNCLE** | **FUNCTION** |
| Spinocerebellar | Clarke nucleus | Inferior cerebellar peduncle | Proprioceptive and cutaneous sensation from the trunk and legs |
| Cuneocerebellar | Accessory cuneate nucleus | Inferior cerebellar peduncle | Proprioceptive and cutaneous sensation from the arms and neck |
| Trigeminocerebellar | Trigeminal nucleus | Inferior cerebellar peduncle | Proprioceptive and cutaneous sensation from the face and jaw |
| Olivocerebellar Vestibulocerebellar Pontocerebellar | Inferior olivary nucleus Vestibular nucleus Pontine nucleus | Middle cerebellar peduncle | Motor skills learning Balance Cognitive, visual, and motor input from the cortex |

Adapted from Michael-Titus A, Revest P, Shortland P. *The Nervous System: Basic Science and Clinical Conditions.* Philadelphia, PA: Churchill Livingstone; 2007.

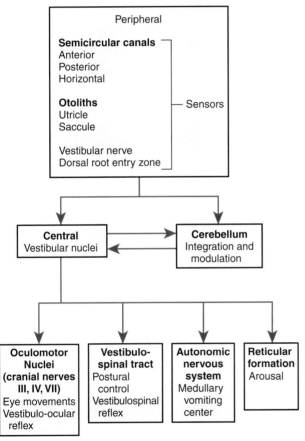

**FIGURE 21-4** Functional organization of the vestibular system. *(Adapted from Meldrum D, Walsh RM. Vestibular and balance rehabilitation. In: Stokes M, ed.* Physical Management in Neurological Rehabilitation. *Philadelphia, PA: Elsevier-Mosby; 2004:413–430.)*

rhythmic movements (e.g., walking and other centrally generated movement patterns) (Morton, 2013).

The cerebellum compares the information from the dorsal spinocerebellar tract (feedback about what actually happened) with the information received from the premotor and supplementary motor areas in the cortex (regarding the planned or intended movement); when a mismatch is present, the cerebellum acts as a compensator by sending corrective impulses via the motor thalamus to the premotor cortex. From the premotor cortex, the corrective impulses are sent via the motor pathways to the LMNs to correct the sequence and power of muscle contractions in real time. This comparison and correction of ongoing movement takes place specifically during rhythmic movement patterns and accurate voluntary movements. Functionally, it results in postural coordination as well as upper and lower limb function coordination. The lower limb coordination specifically entails the coordination of movement during gait.

The cerebellum receives more input from the lower extremities than from the upper extremities. The coordination of input from the upper and lower extremities and the trunk takes place in the medial part of the cerebellum. The anatomical areas of the cerebellum involved in coordinating the input from the upper and lower extremities as well as from the trunk are concentrated in two homunculi similar to the motor homunculus of the cerebral cortex, with disproportionately large representations for the face and hands because of the superior coordination within these areas. From the medial part of the cerebellum, pathways are projected to the motor areas of the cortex controlling proximal musculature. Posture and balance are therefore strongly influenced by lesions in the medial part of the cerebellum.

Coordination of the limbs is also controlled by the lateral spinocerebellum via the interposed nucleus and the red nucleus, which decussates on the way to the motor cortex via the thalamus. The spinocerebellum also receives input from the bulbocerebellar areas.

A lesion of the spinocerebellum causes symptoms such as hypotonia. When the interposed nucleus (which is strongly associated with ongoing movement rather than voluntary movement) is affected, the accuracy of reaching movements decreases. The *decrease in reaching movement accuracy* occurs because of impaired control of the direction, extent, force, and timing of the movement. Clinically, these signs and symptoms present as dysmetria. The lack of *movement precision* representing incoordination (ataxia) tends to present as a curved movement, especially when the movement is performed by multijoint muscles. The *impaired correction of the imprecise uncoordinated movement* in the case of an impaired spinocerebellum enhances the error in the timing and extent of the movement, which then increases the error movements even further. The increase in the error movement as the person reaches toward a target with the upper limb (hand) is called *intention tremor*. The increasing "error in movement" as the limbs are moving is also seen during gait. During gait, the error movements present as exaggerated stepping with inconsistent variability in step lengths. Exaggerated stepping during gait may be the result of excessive knee flexion.

The *cerebrocerebellum* (the largest part of the cerebellum) connects primarily with the cerebral cortex through the dentate nucleus. Afferent fibers from the pons *(cerebropontocerebellum)* are carried to the cerebellum via the middle cerebellar peduncle. The efferent fibers from the cerebellum are carried from the cerebellar cortex, synapse within the dentate nucleus, and project impulses via the superior peduncle to the contralateral thalamus and then to the frontal lobe. On their way, the efferent fibers synapse at the red nucleus (affecting the thalamic cortical connections) and the ipsilateral rubrospinal tracts. The entire tract can be called the "cerebro-ponto-dento-cerebello-dento-rubro-thalamo-cerebral" tract, indicating each nuclear mass where it synapses. At each synapse in a nuclear mass, the information being carried along the tract can be modified.

The cerebropontocerebellum is involved in the execution of complex perceptual tasks and controls the planning and execution of complex "visually guided" movements in which cognition plays a role. Examples of visually guided movements include activities requiring hand-eye coordination and the saccadic eye movements taking place during activities such as reading. The cerebropontocerebellum also controls independent limb movements.

A lesion of the *cerebropontocerebellum* (a lateral cerebellar hemisphere lesion) results in abnormal **timing of movement**; the different aspects of a movement pattern are sequenced separately instead of simultaneously into a fluent movement. The disruption of the flowing sequence of movement components that should take place simultaneously is referred to as *decomposition of movement*. Decomposition of movement is especially evident and disabling in functional hand activities such as reaching.

Melnick (2012) reported that a person with a lesion in the cerebropontocerebellum has impaired perception of timing, resulting in an inability to determine differences in the speed with which objects are moving and which objects are moving faster than others. This impairment is evident in a person's ability to solve spatial and temporal problems, as demonstrated in activities such as hitting a baseball with a bat. The involvement of the cortex in spatial and temporal problem-solving not only indicates that the cerebellum is involved in cognitive functioning but also shows that the concept of "timing of movement" can be used in more than one context.

The concept of timing of movement addresses the sequence in which the components of a movement are taking place during a functional task. For example, when a person with normal timing of movement is reaching for an object, the hand starts moving simultaneously with the proximal joints (glenohumeral and elbow joints); thus, when the object is reached, the hand is in the right position to grasp or pick it up. Concurrently, the glenohumeral and elbow joints move in synchronization with varying degrees of flexion and/or extension to position the hand in the most appropriate position in space to pick up the object.

When a person with decomposition of movement is reaching for an object, however, the movement is performed with extension of the elbow, followed by extension of the wrist, and then extension of the fingers (often excessive extension of the fingers) in preparation to grasp an object. Bastian (2000, pg 3019) describes decomposition as *subjects move the shoulder girdle while fixing the elbow, then moved the elbow while fixing the shoulder.* Bastian (1996) hypothesized that decomposition is a compensatory strategy to improve accuracy by voluntarily fixing all joints except the one performing the final action. In this example, the fingers are picking up the object. The fingers also usually perform excessive movement in order to pick up the object. The resultant effect is that decomposition reduces the interaction torque occurring at the moving joint(s) while interaction torque still occurs at the fixed joint.

Timing of movement also refers to perception of movement sequencing when solving spatial and temporal problems, for example, catching a ball moving through space by positioning the hands in the appropriate position at the right time and the right place (Morton, 2013).

## Feedback and Feedforward Control of Movement

**Feedback control** for coordination takes place when motor activities are performed outside the normal limits of stability and control. The cerebellum compares the visual, vestibular, and somatosensory feedback (from the periphery) on the basis of the current movement, with the intended/planned movement to maintain safe (dynamically stable) functional posture while performing the activity. If there is any threat to stability or failure of goal-directed movement during the activity or impaired control of the movement, impulses conveying "movement correction" are sent via the premotor and motor cortex to the LMNs controlling the sequence/timing of muscle contraction and quick reciprocal movements to prevent intention tremor, dysmetria, and decomposition of movement. The LMNs control the activity or movement on the level of the musculoskeletal system to adapt its movements to prevent a fall or optimize successful task performance. This correctional feedback takes place in response to internal (internal disturbance of equilibrium during the performance of a difficult task/action) as well as external disturbances of equilibrium (e.g., walking on a moving surface, tripping over an obstacle, or slipping while performing an activity). This process of feedback control is illustrated in Fig. 21-5A.

Regarding coordination, **feedforward control** refers to compensatory postural responses taking place in *anticipation* of a potentially destabilizing activity or an activity requiring

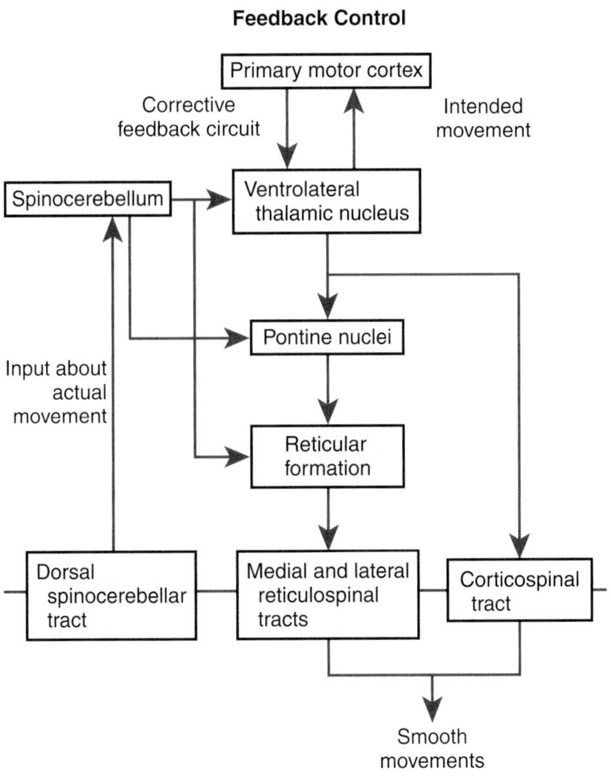

**Feedback Control**

Primary motor cortex

Corrective feedback circuit

Intended movement

Spinocerebellum → Ventrolateral thalamic nucleus

Input about actual movement

Pontine nuclei

Reticular formation

Dorsal spinocerebellar tract

Medial and lateral reticulospinal tracts

Corticospinal tract

Smooth movements

**FIGURE 21-5A** Schematic presentation of the feedback processes through which the cerebellum controls movement. *(Reproduced with permission from Michael-Titus A, Revest P, Shortland P.* The Nervous System: Basic Science and Clinical Conditions. *Philadelphia, PA: Churchill Livingstone; 2007.)*

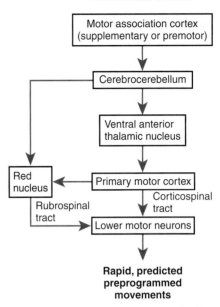

**Feedforward Control**

Motor association cortex (supplementary or premotor)

Cerebrocerebellum

Ventral anterior thalamic nucleus

Red nucleus ← Primary motor cortex

Rubrospinal tract

Corticospinal tract

Lower motor neurons

**Rapid, predicted preprogrammed movements**

**FIGURE 21-5B** Schematic presentation of the feedforward processes through which the cerebellum controls movement. *(Reproduced from with permission from Michael-Titus A, Revest P, Shortland P.* The Nervous System: Basic Science and Clinical Conditions. *Philadelphia, PA: Churchill Livingstone; 2007.)*

greater skill than the neuromuscular-skeletal system is capable of performing. The feedforward system uses previously learned skilled movement to detect errors/danger/failure in skilled movement before the movement is performed (Szklut, 2007). In the control of movement, feedforward and feedback systems interact closely: feedforward in the initiation of compensatory movement and feedback in the regulation and adaptation of movement. The process of feedforward control is illustrated in Fig. 21-5B.

The integration between feedback and feedforward responses emphasizes the importance of sensory integration (especially somatosensory, and in particular, proprioception feedback) with holistic cerebellar function to maintain coordinated, skilled movement during activities (based on the comparator-feedback and coordinator-feedforward roles of the cerebellum). The integration between the two systems therefore prevents incoordination, intention tremor, dysmetria, and decomposition of movement. A normal functioning feedback and feedforward system prevents ataxic gait.

## Lifespan Influence

### Developmental Considerations

Identifying signs of ataxia/incoordination in infants is very difficult. When an infant has ataxia, it is usually not identified until around 2 to 3 years of age or older. Ataxia/incoordination in childhood is often related to a hereditary condition. Table 21-2 summarizes the various conditions for which ataxia/incoordination is a major sign throughout the lifespan.

### Age-Related Changes Relevant to Ataxia/Incoordination

The main factors contributing to the development of age-related incoordination in older people include the decrease in muscle strength, increase in reaction time, decrease in range of motion, change in posture, and impaired postural control. Muscle strength decreases with age because of decreased muscle mass, muscle diameter, and *number* of alpha motor neurons, as well as a decrease in, or atrophy of, the slow oxidative and fast-twitch muscle fibers. The oxidative capacity of the muscles during activity or exercise also decreases and subsequently reduces the ability to produce muscle torque. Usually the more proximal muscles are more affected than the distal muscles in the trunk and both lower extremities and the muscles of the upper extremities.

The physical function a person is able to perform is closely related to his/her muscle strength and muscle power. When muscle strength decreases, functional ability also decreases. Muscle strength in the lower extremities (measured as the amount of force produced during a single maximum muscle contraction) can decrease by as much as 30% by age 70 years (Rogers, 1993) and rapidly declines after age 60 years (Bemben, 1991). Although muscle endurance can also decrease with age, it is better preserved than muscle strength.

Slowing of reaction time entails a decrease in the speed and accuracy with which activities are performed. Increased reaction time is measured as the time a stimulus is given to the

*(Text continued on page 684)*

| TABLE 21-2 | Neuromuscular Diagnoses/Conditions Presenting With Ataxia/Incoordination | |
|---|---|---|
| **MEDICAL CONDITIONS** | **CONDITION** | **OTHER CLINICAL FEATURES** |
| *Genetic conditions:* | | |
| 1. Mucopolysaccharidosis (MPS) I (A group of conditions in which lipid is stored in neurons combined with storage of polysaccharides in connective tissues. The consequence is a unique combination of neurological and skeletal abnormalities.) | Hurler disease (Hurler disease is a classic form of MPS I) | Signs and symptoms of this condition are observed toward the end of the first year of life. Mental retardation and skeletal abnormalities are characteristic. Skeletal abnormalities include dwarfism, gargoyle facies, large head with synostosis of the longitudinal suture, kyphosis, and broad hands with stubby fingers. In some forms of Hurler disease, central nervous system involvement may present. |
| 2. Partial deletion disorders (Prader-Willi syndrome [PWS] and Angelman syndrome [AS] present as a result of loss of the PWS/AS region of chromosome 15 and illustrate the effect of genomic imprinting. PWS presents when a segment of paternal chromosome 15 is absent, whereas AS presents when a segment of maternal chromosome 15 is absent or deleted. | 2.2 PWS and AS | Babies present with hypotonia, a weak cry, little spontaneous movement, areflexia, small stature, dysmorphic facies, hypoplastic genitalia, and sometimes arthrogryposis. Mental retardation becomes obvious after the first year, and obesity becomes obvious. Although muscle tone may improve, poor coordination and motor delay persist. Children walk with a broad base and are clumsy. Obesity may result in impaired breathing, which can produce sleepiness, cyanosis, cor pulmonale, and heart failure. |
| 3. Degenerative hereditary ataxia presenting in early and late childhood up to adolescence; includes most degenerative ataxia (hereditary pattern is autosomal recessive) | 3.1 Friedreich ataxia (a prototype of all forms of progressive spinocerebellar ataxic (SCA) conditions and approximately 50% of all cases of hereditary ataxia) | Signs are present when the child begins to stand and walk. Both legs are usually affected. Hands become clumsy after signs in the legs appear, followed by dysarthric speech. Musculoskeletal impairment, which may precede or follow the diagnosis, is pes cavus and kyphoscoliosis with restricted respiratory function. Cardiomyopathy is common. Degeneration occurs in the cerebellar cortex and loss of myelinated fibers is observed in the posterior column, spinocerebellar tracts, peripheral nerves, posterior roots, cells of sympathetic ganglia, and anterior horn cells at all levels of the spinal cord. Ataxic-dyskinetic syndrome appears in children when they start walking. By 4–5 years of age, the limbs show ataxia and choreoathetosis and grimacing and dysarthric speech, jerky eye movements, and slow long-latency saccades appear. The progressive disease leads to death in approximately the second decade of life. |
| | 3.2 Refsum disease (onset in late childhood, adolescence, early adulthood) 3.3 Bassen–Kornzweig syndrome (presents in late childhood and early adolescence) 3.4 Ataxia-telangiectasia | The condition manifests as a combination of retinitis pigmentosa, ataxia, and chronic polyneuropathy. Cardiomyopathy and neurogenic deafness are present in most patients. The metabolic marker of the disease is increased phytanic acid. The condition presents with weakness of the limbs with areflexia (commencing at 2 years of age) and sensory ataxia. Impaired vibration and position sense are identified when the child can cooperate in testing sensation. Cerebellar signs that present later are ataxia of gait, trunk, and the extremities; titubation of the head; |

| TABLE 21-2 | **Neuromuscular Diagnoses/Conditions Presenting With Ataxia/Incoordination—cont'd** | |
|---|---|---|
| **MEDICAL CONDITIONS** | **CONDITION** | **OTHER CLINICAL FEATURES** |
| | | dysarthria; muscle weakness; ophthalmoparesis, Babinski sign, loss of pain, and temperature. Musculoskeletal signs include pes cavus, and kyphoscoliosis may present secondary to the early onset of neuropathy. As a result, patients may not be able to stand and walk when they reach adolescence. Mental slowness occurs in some patients. The condition presents with an ataxic-dyskinetic syndrome in children who appear to be normal during the first few years of life. Gait appears to be awkward when they start walking. By the age of 4–5 years, the limbs start to be ataxic with signs of choreoathetosis, and grimacing and dysarthria present. Jerky eye movements and slow long-latency saccades and apraxia for voluntary gaze appear. Between 3 and 5 years of age, characteristic telangiectatic lesions present. The disease presents as transversely oriented subpapillary venous plexuses. It is most apparent in the outer parts of the bulbar conjunctivae, in a butterfly pattern over the ears, exposed parts of the neck, and bridge of the nose and cheeks. By 9–10 years of age, intellectual ability decreases and signs of polyneuropathy appear. Vitiligo, café-au-lait spots, loss of subcutaneous fat, and premature graying of the hair may present. Death may occur as a result of intercurrent broncho-pulmonary infection or neoplasia in the second decade of life. |
| Acute forms of cerebellar ataxia in late childhood and early adolescence are essentially nonmetabolic. Conditions that may present with a combination of upper motor neuron and cerebellar signs and symptoms and should be considered during the differential diagnosis are postinfectious encephalomyelitis, post anoxia, post meningitis, postenterovirus infections, posthyperthermic states, and drug intoxications. In cases of a pure ataxic clinical picture, postinfectious cerebillitis and tumors such as astrocytomas, hemangioblastoma, cerebellar tumors (medulla blastomas), and ganglioneuromas should be considered in the differential diagnosis (Ropper, 2005). | | |
| 4. Degenerative cerebellar ataxia in adulthood Paraneoplastic cerebellar degeneration | SCA type 6, 8, and 14 | In addition to the typical clinical signs of cerebellar ataxia, patients may present with the following clinical signs: SCA type 6 – dysarthria, nystagmus, posterior column signs SCA type 8 – sensory neuropathy and spasticity SCA type 14 – myoclonus and tremor |
| 5. Chiari (or Arnold-Chiari) deformity (malformation); classified as a developmental condition of the nervous system | Chiari types I and II entail cerebellar medullary malformation without meningomyelocele (type I) or with meningomyelocele (type II). Type III presents as a high cervical or occipitocervical meningomyelocele with cerebellar herniation. Type IV presents as cerebellar hypoplasia. | Patients have an elongated pons and medulla and a narrowed aqueduct. The displaced tissue occludes the foramen magnum. The cerebellum is displaced as if to obliterate the cisterna magna. The foramen of Luschka and foramen of Magendie open into the cervical canal. The arachnoid tissue around the herniated brainstem and cerebellum is fibrotic. All these factors contribute to the development of hydrocephalis. The spinal cord presents with a kink because the lower end of the fourth ventricle pushes the spinal cord posteriorly. Involvement of the spinal cord is usually |

*Continued*

| TABLE 21-2 | Neuromuscular Diagnoses/Conditions Presenting With Ataxia/Incoordination—cont'd |
| --- | --- |

| MEDICAL CONDITIONS | CONDITION | OTHER CLINICAL FEATURES |
| --- | --- | --- |
| | | associated with a meningomyelocele. Syringomyelia is a common finding associated with Arnold-Chiari syndrome. The developmental abnormalities that may also be present include polymicrogyria and the filum terminale extending as low as the sacrum. The posterior fossa of the cranium is small, and the foramen magnum is enlarged.<br><br>Clinical signs and symptoms vary according to the type of Chiari syndrome the patient presents with and include increased intracranial pressure, which may cause severe headaches; progressive cerebellar ataxia; progressive spastic paresis; down-beating nystagmus; and cervical syringomyelia (segmental amyotrophy, sensory loss with or without pain) (Ropper, 2005). |
| 6. Trauma (trauma to the cerebellum can occur during any phase of the lifespan) | The condition depends on the concomitant areas of the brain that are affected by the injury. | Signs and symptoms of ataxia/incoordination are often disguised in a patient with a diffuse brain injury because the effect of the hypertone due to the cortical (cerebral) injury counteracts the effect of the hypotone and incoordination due to the cerebellar lesion(s). Other signs of ataxia/incoordination that may be present are walking with a broad base and with arms in abduction, fixating with the eyes on the floor in front of the patient, high stepping gait, and impaired balance. |
| 7. Acquired disease presenting with accompanying cerebellar ataxia | 7.1 Metabolic disease (e.g., enteropathy [Celiac disease] in children and sprue in adults; hyperthermia) | The classic features are diarrhea and malabsorption. Some patients present with signs of peripheral neuropathy and sometimes progressive cerebellar ataxia, especially ataxic gait and polymyoclonus in association with gluten-sensitive enteropathy. |
| | 7.2 Cerebellar disorders associated with HIV/AIDS due to discreet cerebellar lesions resulting from opportunistic infections (e.g., toxoplasmosis and progressive multifocal leukoencephalopathy) | Patients can present with pure cerebellar signs or with a combination of cerebellar and pyramidal signs depending on the extent and localization of the lesion(s). |
| 8. Cerebellar atrophy | 8.1 Cerebellar atrophy with prominent brainstem features (sporadic and familial olivopontocerebellar atrophy) | Onset is in the fifth decade of life. The main clinical manifestation is ataxia, first in the legs followed by the arms, hands, and bulbar musculature. Extrapyramidal neuropathic signs, slow eye movements, dystonia, and vocal cord paralysis may present with the ataxia. |
| | 8.2 Cerebellar atrophy with prominent basal ganglia features | Slow, progressive ataxia starting in adolescence or early adulthood in association with hyperreflexia, extrapyramidal rigidity (parkinsonian type), dystonia, bulbar signs, distal motor weakness, and ophthalmoplegia. |
| 9. Vascular disease | Cerebellar stroke | Clinical signs of ataxia/incoordination manifest on the ipsilateral side of the lesion in the cerebellum. |

| TABLE 21-2 | Neuromuscular Diagnoses/Conditions Presenting With Ataxia/Incoordination—cont'd | |
|---|---|---|
| **MEDICAL CONDITIONS** | **CONDITION** | **OTHER CLINICAL FEATURES** |
| 10. Autoimmune disease | Multiple sclerosis | There is an unpredictable combination and course of signs and symptoms. Cerebellar and bulbar symptoms present as part of other common motor, sensory, visual, bladder and bowel, sexual, and cognitive and emotional signs and symptoms. |
| 11. Benign or malignant tumors | Cerebellar/brainstem tumors in the posterior fossa of the skull, such as medulloblastoma, astrocytoma, and secondary tumors | Tumors include any space-occupying lesions that may cause pressure on the cerebellum and pathways to and from the cerebellum. The course of the signs and symptoms of ataxia depends on how soon the tumor is diagnosed, the nature of the tumor, and the result of surgery to remove the tumor. It further depends on whether the tumor was removed completely or partially, as well as the areas of the brain affected by the surgical technique used to remove the tumor. |
| 12. Adult toxicity | Alcoholism (Wernicke-Korsakoff syndrome, which consists of Wernicke encephalopathy and Korsakoff psychosis), lack of thiamine (vitamin $B_1$), anticonvulsant drugs, and hypothyroidism | Korsakoff syndrome is associated with Wernicke encephalopathy, which is a medical emergency causing life-threatening brain disruption, confusion, staggering and stumbling, lack of coordination, and abnormal involuntary eye movements. |
| 13. Impairment of the afferent portions of peripheral nerves | 13.1 Large-fiber neuropathies, dorsal nerve roots entering the spinal cord and posterior columns of the spinal cord (dorsal column-medial lemniscal system [DM-ML] of the brainstem) | Condition involves impairment/loss of proprioceptive/somatosensory sensation conveyed to the cerebellum. Sensory ataxia can also occur when the sensory-receiving regions of the thalamus and sometimes the parietal cortex are damaged (Bastian, 1997). Loss of awareness of the sense of movement, vibration, and position below the lesion in the spinal column also occurs. Muscle power is usually retained. Deep tendon reflexes are present. Romberg sign is positive. Patients are not known to have paresthesia. Characteristic loss/impaired proprioceptive/somatosensory sensation is observed. The condition also includes loss of two-point discrimination; figure writing; detection of size, shape, weight, and texture of objects; and the ability to detect the direction and speed of a moving stimulus on the skin |
| | 13.2 Diabetic ataxia | The condition involves prominent loss of vibratory and position sense in the feet. Denervation atrophy of muscles is the main characteristic in long-standing neuropathies. Deep tendon reflexes are absent, and the Romberg sign is positive. Paresthesia ("pins and needles"), numbness, coldness, tingling, and other paresthesias (impairment of tactile, pain, and thermal sensations) are reported. Deformities of the feet are due to disproportionate muscle weakness in the pretibial and peroneal muscles. Repeated injuries and chronic subcutaneous infections may result in painless loss of digits. Trophic changes are observed. |

*Continued*

| TABLE 21-2 | Neuromuscular Diagnoses/Conditions Presenting With Ataxia/Incoordination—cont'd | |
|---|---|---|
| MEDICAL CONDITIONS | CONDITION | OTHER CLINICAL FEATURES |
| | 13.3 Sensory ataxia (tabetic syndrome) | Loss of vibratory and position sense in the feet is prominent. Muscle power is usually retained. Deep tendon reflexes are absent, and the Romberg sign is positive. Paresthesia (pins and needles), numbness, coldness, tingling, and other paresthesias (impairment of tactile, pain, and thermal sensation) are reported. Other characteristics are secondary joint deformities (Charcot joints), trophic changes, Argyll Robertson pupil, lightning pains (sharp, brief stabbing pains), and insensitive hypotonic bladder |
| 14. Age-related changes | Age-related degeneration of different areas in the brain and neuromuscular systems | Incoordination presents with aging as a result of: Decrease in muscle strength Increase in reaction time attributed to degeneration of neural conduction as well as muscle contraction Decrease in the range of movement Changes in posture Impaired postural control |

Data from Ropper AH, Brown RH. *Adam's and Victor's Principles of Neurology,* 8th edition. New York, NY: McGraw-Hill; 2005.

moment the person's response is registered. The slowing of reaction time is attributed to the degeneration taking place on the levels of neural conduction as well as the muscle contraction. The time since the movement was initiated until the time of completion of the task also increases with age. Increased time to perform a task may be more evident in older people who are physically inactive than in those who are physically active.

The decrease in joint range and spinal mobility due to biological changes in joint surfaces, degeneration in collagen fibers, dietary deficiencies, and a sedentary lifestyle is apparent. Spinal extension shows the most loss in range of movement during aging and, as such, results in a decrease in the efficiency of trunk balance reactions.

The decrease in muscle strength together with the decrease in spinal mobility leads to changes in postural alignment. The typical postural changes seen in the older person are low cervical flexion with high cervical extension (a protruding chin), thoracic kyphosis, altered lordosis, and slight hip and knee flexion. This changed posture results in a lowered center of gravity (COG) to improve postural stability. However, the decrease in joint mobility, especially spinal mobility, as well as muscle strength can contribute to decreased postural stability and increased falls in the older population.

Aging also produces changes in the neuromuscular and sensory systems (including the somatosensory, visual, and vestibular systems), multisensory deficits (including adapting senses for postural control), anticipatory postural adjustments, and cognitive aspects of postural control. Decreased functioning in these systems additionally contributes to impaired postural control. Figure 21-1 gives a holistic overview of the different levels of the musculoskeletal and neuromuscular

systems that cause incoordination when one or more of these systems are impaired because of aging.

## Ataxia/Incoordination in Neuromuscular Diagnoses

There are many causes of ataxia/incoordination. Hereditary/genetic disorders, metabolic disorders/disturbances, tumors, trauma, vascular disorders, somatosensory impairment specifically related to loss of proprioception, lesions secondary to other conditions (e.g., MS), and neuromusculoskeletal impairment due to aging can cause ataxia. Some genetic and metabolic disorders present in early or late childhood or adolescence, whereas others are not symptomatic until early adulthood. Cerebellar atrophy is a common cause of ataxic signs and symptoms in children (e.g., Friedreich ataxia) and in adults (e.g., paraneoplastic cerebellar degeneration) (Perlmutter, 2003). Genetic disorders also include skeletal malformation of the foramen magnum causing damage to the brainstem in Arnold-Chiari deformity. Toxicity and metabolic disturbances such as alcoholism, use of anticonvulsant drugs, and hypothyroidism can cause symptoms and are usually found in adults, although children exposed to toxic substances can also suffer from ataxia/incoordination.

Malignant or benign tumors in the posterior fossa can present at any age between early childhood and adulthood. Cerebellar lesions can also occur as signs and symptoms secondary to other conditions or as part of the clinical presentation in diseases such as MS. Vascular disorders found mainly in adults, particularly stroke, can also specifically affect the cerebellum.

Trauma of the cerebellum or of the efferent and afferent pathways to and from the cerebellum can also cause ataxia.

Signs of ataxia/incoordination are often disguised in a patient with a diffuse brain injury because the hypertonia due to the cortical (cerebral) injury counteracts the effect of the hypotonia and ataxia of the cerebellar lesion.

Impairment of the afferent portions of the peripheral nerves (e.g., large-fiber neuropathies, dorsal nerve root lesions, posterior column pathology) results in impaired/absent proprioceptive/somatosensory sensation in the cerebellum and can cause sensory ataxia/incoordination. Sensory ataxia can also occur when the sensory-receiving regions of the thalamus and sometimes the parietal cortex are damaged (Bastian, 1997).

Age-related changes in different levels of the brain and neuromusculoskeletal systems can contribute to ataxic symptoms. The conditions described in Table 21-2 are more common representations of ataxia/incoordination that may occur throughout the lifespan.

## Pertinent Examination/Evaluation

Examination of coordination, including specific tools, is fully discussed in Chapter 6. The clinical assessment summarized here is based on the task-oriented approach. The task-oriented approach has been referred to as the "systems approach" or the "motor control" approach to retraining functional tasks (Shumway-Cook, 2016). The basic underlying assumptions of the task-oriented approach are that (1) various systems interact to contribute to different aspects of postural control and (2) movement is organized around behavioral goals in a specific environment. This implies that in addition to stimulus/response actions, sensation contributes to the prediction and adaptation of movement control (Shumway-Cook, 2016).

The functional assessment should be planned during the interview in collaboration and active cooperation with the patient to establish the functional tasks for which he is experiencing the most problems (usually at the patient's highest functional level) as well as those performed easily. The highest functional level refers to the highest functional position the patient is able to adopt and the most skilled activity the patient is able to perform in that or any other position, for instance, standing (highest functional position) and walking with a walker (the highest skilled activity) versus sitting and reaching to the floor (e.g., picking up shoes, donning/doffing shoes, and donning/doffing trousers).

The underlying sensory, neuromotor, and cognitive systems controlling movement determine the strategies an able-bodied person uses to perform a functional task. Abnormal postural control in patients with a cerebellar or somatosensory lesion is a result of impairments within one or more of the systems controlling movement and also a compensation by the remaining systems involved in postural control. Compensatory strategies can have a negative influence on the patient's functional ability if they limit the optimization of postural control in the long term. However, when the patient uses compensatory strategies to maintain a certain level of functional ability that enhances his or her level of functioning, it may be regarded as a positive rather than negative effect on the condition, providing it does not result in muscle and short-tissue shortening and severe muscle imbalance or aggravate underlying joint pathology, such as osteoarthritis.

Examination of the patient's postural control and motor coordination during the performance of functional skills includes observation of the sensory and motor strategies used to maintain postural stability and the control of skilled movements during task performance in various contexts. According to the task-oriented approach, the assessment of a patient with ataxia/incoordination is based on identifying the individual's highest functional activity performed independently, under supervision, or with assistance. Performing the functional assessments in an environment resembling the patient's home/work/leisure environment gives the therapist a realistic picture of his functional problems on the participation level. The quality and quantity of the movement during the selected task(s) and the underlying reason(s) for the impaired quality and quantity of movement should be determined. Assessment also includes identifying the affected components of coordination and postural control (on an impairment level) leading to the development of compensatory strategies (e.g., fixation of the trunk, face, neck, or limbs/fingers/toes) to overcome the postural instability and/or incoordination (e.g., excessive use of arm and hand support, use of protective extension of the arms, protective steps with the legs, moving one joint at a time, slowing down of movement, undershooting the target). Coordination deficits may stem from a combination of a fundamental movement deficit and a compensatory strategy (Bastian, 1996).

Related outcome measures for patients with ataxia/incoordination include (on an impairment level) an assessment of the musculoskeletal system (range of motion), neuromuscular system (muscle power, gross and fine motor coordination), neuromeningeal functioning, and somatosensation (including proprioception). The examination of coordination on an impairment level is summarized in Table 21-3.

Effects on the patient's ability to adapt to disturbances in the COG (balance) and/or react in an appropriate way are best identified by the performance of the functional activities during standardized tests, such as the Scale for the Assessment and Rating of Ataxia (SARA) (Schmitz-Hubsch, 2006) and the International Cooperative Ataxia Rating Scale (ICARS) (Ilg, 2009). On an activity level, the Berg balance scale, timed up-and-go test, and 10-meter walk test are helpful for identifying impairment in activities such as standing and gait. On a participation level, suggested standardized tests include the Barthel Index, Functional Independence Measure, and Goal Attainment Score (Ilg, 2009). Details of coordination examination tests and measures (nonequilibrium coordination tests) to detect ataxia/incoordination are described as part of the motor examination in Chapter 6. Although postural control (balance) is an important role of the cerebellum, this chapter focuses on intervention to improve coordination, whereas Chapter 30 focuses on intervention to improve balance/equilibrium/postural control.

*(Text continued on page 696)*

**TABLE 21-3** Examination of Ataxia/Incoordination at the Impairment Level

| IMPAIRMENT AND DESCRIPTION | CAUSE | TEST/MEASURE | DESCRIPTION OF TEST/MEASURE | OUTCOME OF TEST/MEASURE |
|---|---|---|---|---|
| Decomposition (dyssynergia) of movement | Cerebellar lesion Somatosensory impairment | Performance of simple movements such as: Finger to nose The tested leg's heel is moved alternately with the opposite leg's knee and toe (heel to knee; heel to toe). | The shoulder is abducted to 90 degrees with the elbow extended. The patient is asked to bring the tip of the index finger to the tip of the nose. Alterations may be made in the initial starting position to observe performance from different planes of motion. Patients are positioned in supine and asked to flex the tested leg's heel to the opposite leg's knee and big toe alternately. | The patient performs the movement in a sequence of steps instead of in a single smooth movement during the activities (Schmitz, 2013). |
| | | Finger-to-therapist's finger Toe to therapist's finger | The patient and therapist sit opposite each other. The therapist's index finger is held in front of the patient. The patient is asked to touch the tip of his index finger to the therapist's index finger. The position of the therapist's finger may be altered during testing to observe the ability to change distance, direction, and force of movement. The patient is positioned in supine and instructed to touch the therapist's finger with his big toe. | Movement is irregular or appears fragmented |
| | | Finger to finger Heel on shin | Both shoulders are abducted to 90 degrees with the elbows extended. The patient is asked to bring both hands toward the midline and approximate the index fingers from opposing hands. | The patient's movement displays deficits in both the sequence and the timing of movement during the activities. |

| Impairment | Test | Procedure | Findings |
|---|---|---|---|
| *(continued)* | | The patient is positioned in supine and instructed to move the heel of the tested leg up and down the shin of the opposite leg. | Decomposition of movement is more marked during slow movements than during fast movements. |
| | Alternate nose to finger | The patient alternately touches the tip of his nose and the tip of the therapist's finger with the therapist's finger. The position of the therapist's finger may be altered during testing to observe the ability to change distance, direction, and force of movement (Schmitz, 2013). | |
| | Finger opposition | The patient touches the tip of the thumb to the tip of each finger in sequence. | Placement of the thumb on each fingertip is irregular and inaccurate. The speed of movement may gradually increase. |
| | Drawing a circle | The patient is positioned in supine/sitting and is asked to draw a circle with his finger/toe in the air. Alternatively, the patient may be asked to draw a circle with the finger on a table and his toe on the floor. | The patient draws an irregular circle with the tested limb, and the movement of the limb is characterized by decomposition. |
| **Intention tremor** | Cerebellar impairment: A deficient stability around the proximal joint (shoulder/hip) is indicated. Somatosensory impairment: The mechanism of intention tremor in patients with posterior column syndrome (somatosensory ataxia) is the corrective feedback mode of the cerebellum is impaired because the lack of incoming somatosensory and vestibular impulses from the periphery results in defective | Finger to nose, finger to finger, finger to therapist's finger; finger to finger; alternative finger to nose, alternate heel to knee, heel to toe; toe to therapist's finger; heel on shin, and drawing a circle tests. Alternatively, ask patient to reach toward an object as if he is going to take it | As described in the previous section | There is a side-to-side sway of the finger or toe as it approaches the target. The movement tends to be rhythmic, with a frequency of 3–5 Hz. If the tremor is slower, it is probably a result of the time-consuming relay of sensory input to the motor cortex needed to modulate movement when the cerebellum no longer functions effectively (Morton, 2013). The patient sways as he reaches the target (object). Intention tremor is absent at rest. |

Continued

**TABLE 21-3** **Examination of Ataxia/Incoordination at the Impairment Level—cont'd**

| IMPAIRMENT AND DESCRIPTION | CAUSE | TEST/MEASURE | DESCRIPTION OF TEST/MEASURE | OUTCOME OF TEST/MEASURE |
|---|---|---|---|---|
| | output. The output from the cerebellum via the cortex results in overcorrection or undercorrection of movement due to the lack of somatosensory and vestibular impulses received. | | | |
| Hypermetria | Cerebellar impairment Somatosensory impairment | Finger to nose, finger to therapist's finger, finger to finger; alternative nose to finger tests Alternatively, ask patient to reach toward an object as if he is going to take it | As described in the previous section | The limb (finger or toe) overshoots the target and is corrected by a series of secondary movements in which the finger or toe sways around the target before it comes to rest on the target (Ropper, 2005). |
| Postural tremor | Cerebellar impairment: Possible mechanisms of postural tremor include: Disruption of the proprioceptive feedback loops that entails a delay in the processing of sensory input or motor output due to disruption of the cerebellum's compensatory role Absence or delay in one of the sensory feedback systems as well as the spinal pathways, such as the spinal stretch reflex pathway, corticospinal pathway, and transcerebellar pathway, which can cause a noticeable oscillation of the body or the limbs Impairment of the transcerebellar pathway and/or the spinal reflex path that is ineffective in dampening the low-frequency | Postural tremor (exaggerated oscillatory movement) presents when a patient is asked to adopt and maintain a posture or maintain a limb against gravity, for instance, holding an arm in 90-degree abduction. It is elicited by a sustained posture. | | Postural tremor is characterized by tremor of the trunk and/or proximal joints (shoulder/hip). The typical frequency of postural tremor is about 3 Hz. Both the agonists and antagonists participate in causing the tremor. The characteristic postural tremor disappears when the limb is supported proximally. |

| | | | |
|---|---|---|---|
| | | | oscillation induced by the corticospinal pathway The previously described characteristics are in line with the theory that the cerebellum plays a role in the adjustment of muscle contractions over multijoint segments to produce smooth movement. |
| **Titubation** | Midline cerebellar disease (Ropper, 2005) | Observed in any position and sometimes during activities | Titubation is a rhythmic tremor mainly of the head and/or upper trunk. It is primarily present in the anteroposterior plane with a frequency of 3–4 cycles per second (Ropper, 2005). |
| **Asthenia** | The underlying mechanism of asthenia as a result of a cerebellar lesion is not clear. Bremer (cited in Morton, 2013) theorized that *asthenia is caused by a loss of cerebellar facilitation to the motor cortex, which in turn could reduce the activity of spinal motor neurons during voluntary movement.* | Performance of simple tasks Manual resistance from the therapist against holding a static posture/position against gravity Performing a movement against gravity with body weight as resistance | Patients with asthenia complain of a feeling of heaviness, excessive effort for simple tasks, and early onset of fatigue. This feeling of heaviness and excessive effort to perform simple tasks is thought to be related to the intensity of supraspinal signals required to produce a movement (Morton, 2013). |
| **Hypotonicity** | Diminished or lack of somatosensory sensation (especially in the case of a lack of proprioceptive sensation) decreases feedback to the cerebellum via the cortex. It is hypothesized that patients with somatosensory ataxia (posterior column syndrome) have decreased muscle tone (hypotonia) but *not necessarily* asthenia. | Observation of posture and sequence of components of functional movement/selective movement versus compensatory movement; ability to perform pure selective physiological movements Deep tendon reflexes (patella tendon) | Patients may be able to generate normal muscle power during a resisted movement, although not in a coordinated dynamic pattern of postural control. Cerebellar lesion: pendular movement of the free hanging lower leg Somatosensory (posterior column lesions): decreased deep tendon reflexes characteristic of hypotone. When other motor pathways in the spinal cord are affected, deep tendon reflexes may be increased. |

*Continued*

**TABLE 21-3** Examination of Ataxia/Incoordination at the Impairment Level—cont'd

| IMPAIRMENT AND DESCRIPTION | CAUSE | TEST/MEASURE | DESCRIPTION OF TEST/MEASURE | OUTCOME OF TEST/MEASURE |
|---|---|---|---|---|
| **Rebound phenomenon** | Cerebellar ataxia: impaired feedback and feedforward control of the cerebellum Somatosensory ataxia: Incomplete sensory feedback to the cerebellum results in delayed feedforward control. The cerebellum can therefore not perform the comparator and corrective processes accurately. | | Isometric contraction against elbow flexion followed by sudden release of the isometric contraction; isometric contraction against any part of the body and sudden release of the resistance A forceful movement of the limbs | Inability to stop any movement after an isometric contraction The limb/part of the limb or part of the body that was resisted suddenly moves in the opposite direction in which the resistance was applied. Inability to stop any forceful movement |
| **Dysmetria** • Loss or impairment of the direction, extent, and timing of movements (Morton, 2013) • Impaired judgment of the distance or range of a movement needed. Hypermetria is an overestimation of the requisite range of motion needed, while hypometria is the underestimation of the required range needed to reach an object or a goal. | Cerebellum lesion in the dentate nucleus; loss/impairment of anticipatory (feedforward) movements; loss of the feedforward mechanism that results in slower feedback responses Somatosensory impairment (especially loss of proprioception) | Finger-nose test; finger-to-finger test; finger-to-therapist's finger test; toe-to-therapist's-finger test; reaching for an object | Tests as described in the previous section | Different aspects of dysmetria present as: Slow onset in the development of muscle tension; reduced intensity of muscle tension Slow release of muscle tension after the task has been completed or the goal has been reached Regulation of the force of movement while maintaining a position against gravity Control of agonistic-antagonistic-agonistic muscle activity that presents as ballistic-type movements because of impaired alternating sequencing of muscle activity in the agonists and antagonists *Inability to stop a goal-directed movement in one direction* (Morton, 2013) Overshooting toward the end of a reaching task/past pointing an object; more evident in multijoint movements than in single-joint movements |

|  |  |  |  | Impaired initiation of simultaneous eye and limb movement hand-eye coordination activities |
|---|---|---|---|---|
| **Dysdiadochokinesia** | Cerebellar lesion: Dysdiadochokinesia is attributed to the inability to stop an ongoing movement due to the overlapping of antagonistic muscle activity. Inappropriate timing of muscle activity. Somatosensory impairment (especially loss of proprioception): Lack of sensory feedback from the periphery to the cerebrum and the cerebellum is incomplete, which leads to incomplete reactive feedback to the motor cortex and the lower motor neuron and results in inappropriate alternative activation of opposing muscle groups. | Inability to perform rapid alternating movements. *An attempt to abruptly reverse the direction of movement* (Morton, 2013) | Ask the patient to perform rapid alternating movements (i.e., pronation-supination of the forearm or if relevant inversion-eversion of the foot). Ask the patient to perform a rapid tapping on his knee. | Slow movement that appears to rapidly lose range and rhythm. Also described as an inability to perform alternating movements with adequate speed and accuracy. Movement that appears to be a voluntary disruption in the direction of the movement |
| **Changes in the control of muscle tone** | *Cerebellar control of muscle tone* Muscle tone is controlled by excitatory deep nuclei in the cerebellum that have an excitatory effect on the motor areas in the brain, which have an excitatory effect on the alpha and gamma motor neurons that control muscle tone during static positions as well as during activity. Cerebellar pathology results in decreased excitatory control over the alpha and gamma motor neurons and, as such, decreased muscle tone. | Quick, irregular passive movements in midrange of movement Deep tendon reflexes (DTRs) | The patient is at rest and relaxed. The therapist palpates the patient's muscles and performs quick, irregular passive movements of the upper limb and lower limbs without forcing the movement beyond the normal range. The limb is taken into a position against gravity and then *dropped from the mildly elevated position.* | Clinically, the muscles feel less firm *on palpation,* and the affected limbs feel heavy when they are moved passively. 1. The limb falls rapidly onto the supporting surface without correction (or an attempt to maintain the position). 2. When the patient is asked to hold the limb against gravity, it slowly falls toward the supporting surface or demonstrates a postural tremor. In some cases, a patient may be able to hold the limb against gravity by using |

*Continued*

**TABLE 21-3** Examination of Ataxia/Incoordination at the Impairment Level—cont'd

| IMPAIRMENT AND DESCRIPTION | CAUSE | TEST/MEASURE | DESCRIPTION OF TEST/MEASURE | OUTCOME OF TEST/MEASURE |
|---|---|---|---|---|
| | Somatosensory lesions<br>Ataxia without weakness is characteristic of a purely posterior root impairment such as tabes dorsalis, diabetic polyneuropathy, and Fisher syndrome (a variant of Guillain Barré syndrome). Patients present with hypotone without weakness (Ropper, 2005). | | | excessive cognitive concentration and by compensating for the low muscle tone with fixation (overreaction/cocontraction) of the muscles in the particular limb and/or other parts of the body.<br>Cerebellar lesions: pendular reaction to the DTR<br>Somatosensory lesions: decreased or no reflex present |
| Impaired proprioception | Dorsal column impairment in patients with posterior root or dorsal root ganglia lesions | Test vibration sense<br>Test position/movement sense in the feet/affected limb(s) | Refer to Chapter 5<br>Testing of proprioception | Refer to Chapter 5 |
| Trophic changes | Somatosensory lesions: anesthesia | Observation of the skin | | The skin is tight, shiny, and hairless; the muscle presents with atrophy; the nails become curved and rigid; subcutaneous tissue becomes thickened. |
| Paresthesia (pins and needles), numbness, coldness, tingling, or impairment of tactile, pain, and thermal sensations | Refer to Chapter 5 | Test skin sensation in dermatomes | Refer to Chapter 5 | Refer to Chapter 5 |
| Deformities of the feet due to disproportionate muscle weakness in pretibial and peroneal muscles | Denervation atrophy of motor nerves that causes muscle imbalance<br>Repetitive trauma of anaesthetized joints<br>Repeated injuries and chronic subcutaneous infections that may result in painless loss of digits | Test skin sensation (dermatomes) and myotomes<br>Observation of the skin and passive assessment of deformed joints | Refer to Chapter 5 for testing sensation and proprioception | Deformities due to muscle atrophy<br>Deformed joints resulting in Charcot arthropathy |

| | | | |
|---|---|---|---|
| **Lightning pains (sharp, brief stabbing pains)** | Probably attributed to incomplete posterior root lesions at different levels | | Refer to Chapter 5 |
| **Loss of two-point discrimination; figure writing; detection of size, shape, weight, and texture of objects; the ability to detect the direction and speed of a moving stimulus on the skin** | Refer to Chapter 5 | | Refer to Chapter 5 |
| **Argyll Robertson pupil** | Site of the lesion is unknown/unsure | Test pupil reaction to a light stimulus | Pupils are small, irregular, and unequal. Pupils fail to react to light, although they constrict on accommodation. |
| **Insensitive hypotonic bladder** | Deafferentation at the S2 and S3 spinal levels | | Insensitive hypotonic bladder with urine retention and overflow incontinence |
| **Ocular dysmetria** | Cerebellar control of the extraocular muscles. Impairment of the vestibular system or connections between these systems (Chaikin, 2007) | Patient's head is kept in a forward position and is maintained still while following the therapist's finger to move to one side, back to front, and then to the other side. | Corrective saccades occur when a patient is following an object with his eyes; when the object stops moving, the saccades continue instead of stopping with the object (Morton, 2013). (Saccades present as quick oscillatory "back-and-forth" movements of the eyes.) |
| **Gaze-evoked nystagmus** | Lack of integration of the sensory impulses, resulting in an inability to boost or sustain the output from the brainstem to stabilize the eyes during gaze (Morton, 2013) | The patient is asked to look at an object. | The patient's eyes move to the object and then drift back to the neutral position. Associated with fixation between the head, shoulder girdle, and pelvis. Associated with poor eye-hand coordination |

*Continued*

**TABLE 21-3** **Examination of Ataxia/Incoordination at the Impairment Level—cont'd**

| IMPAIRMENT AND DESCRIPTION | CAUSE | TEST/MEASURE | DESCRIPTION OF TEST/MEASURE | OUTCOME OF TEST/MEASURE |
|---|---|---|---|---|
| Independent head-eye movement | Cerebellar lesion | | The patient is asked to look at an object at his side. | The patient performs a quick head movement to the side before his eyes start moving toward the object, or the head performs a quick rotational movement within the first 30°, after which the eyes start moving (Morton, 2013). Associated with poor eye-hand coordination |
| Speech: <br> • Dysarthria <br> • Staccato speech (scanning dysarthria) | Cerebellum or its peduncles | | Listen to the way in which the patient is pronouncing his words | Slowness of speech, slurring, monotonous tone of voice <br> An unnatural separation of some syllables while others are pronounced with greater force than the patient intended; appears also as explosive speech |
| Balance and equilibrium | Lesions of the vestibulocerebellum and/or fastigial nucleus <br> Somatosensory impairment (especially loss of proprioception) | Posturograph <br> Romberg test | Standing on a posturograph <br> Functional assessment of balance during the "timed up-and-go test"; activities-specific balance confidence scale; functional reach tests; Performance Oriented Mobility Assessment (Shumway-Cook, 2016) <br> The patient is asked to stand with his feet together and his eyes open while postural stability in standing is observed. <br> The patient is then asked to stand with his eyes closed while his postural stability is observed. | Postural sway and delayed balance reactions <br> Patients with cerebellar atrophy hardly ever fall, probably because of the intact intersegmental movement between the head, trunk, and legs. <br> Fixation, which can be observed in the position of the head, the arms, and hands (e.g., pressing the thumb and second finger together in a pincer grip to create a co-contraction in the hands and aspects of the arms, forearms, and sometimes also the shoulder girdles) <br> Patient experiences balance problems more in standing and during gait than in other positions (Ropper, 2005) |

If balance is challenged in sitting, the patient fixates by keeping his trunk rigid to overcompensate for any displacement of the base of support.

Another form of compensation is double arm support and fixing the eyes on an opposite point.

The Romberg sign is positive when there is a marked discrepancy between the patient's balance with his eyes closed and with the eyes open; the patient fixes his eyes on the floor in front of him to maintain his balance.

The Romberg sign is negative when there may be only a slight difference between the patient's balance with his eyes open and with the eyes closed.

| Ataxic/uncoordinated gait | Cerebellar lesion | Observation | Cerebellar lesion: Gait is characterized by a wide base, unsteadiness, irregular steps (short step-length alternated irregularly with longer step length). |
| | Somatosensory lesion | Observation | With a bilateral cerebellar lesion, patients veer laterally to either side. Patients with a unilateral lesion usually fall to the side of the lesion. Gait is characterized by a wide base and often a slightly flexed posture. The patient "staggers and totters" in standing and walking. The stiffened legs are flung abruptly forward, and the feet are stumped onto the floor, unlike patients with cerebellar ataxia. Patients are usually unable to walk without visual cues and have great difficulty walking in the dark. |

Adapted from Morton SM, Bastian AJ. Movement dysfunction associated with cerebellar damage. In: Umphred DA. Neurological Rehabilitation, 6th edition. Philadelphia, PA: Elsevier; 2013, pp 631-652. Ropper AH, Brown RH. Adam's and Victor's Principles of Neurology, 8th edition. New York, NY: McGraw-Hill; 2005; Schmitz TJ. Examination of coordination and balance. In: O'Sullivan BS, Schmitz TJ. Physical Rehabilitation, 6th edition. Philadelphia, PA: FA Davis; 2014, pp 206-250.

Table 21-4 is a guide for differentiating between cerebellar and somatosensory ataxia, including a summary of the similarities and differences between the two conditions. Differences in the potential forms of somatosensory ataxia, specific signs and symptoms of chronic polyneuropathy, **tabetic neuritis,** and dorsal column syndrome are summarized in Table 21-5.

# THINK ABOUT IT 21.1

- How should a physical therapist assess a patient with ataxia/incoordination: Perform the impairment level assessment procedures first followed by the functional assessment, or perform the functional assessment first followed by the impairment level procedures?
- Which specific signs and symptoms assist a clinician in making a differential diagnosis between cerebellar ataxia/incoordination and somatosensory ataxia/incoordination?

## PATIENT APPLICATION I-B

Marleen is oriented in terms of date, time, and place, but she presents with staccato speech and dysarthria. She does not speak voluntarily because of the effort involved and the fact that people have difficulty understanding her (which causes her to withdraw from conversation). Because of hypotonia of the soft palate, she chokes easily and has to eat slowly. She is on a soft diet. Marleen also presents with nystagmus.

On functional and participation levels, Marleen is bedridden and cannot perform functional activities such as bridging or rolling to her side. She cannot change position from lying to sitting. When positioned in sitting at the edge of the bed, she cannot maintain the position for longer than 20 seconds without bilateral arm support. She uses fixation of the arms on the bed to stabilize, even so, she loses her balance easily. She also presents with titubation during any attempted movement in supine or sitting. If she sits supported in a chair with bilateral armrests, she can maintain the position safely. She cannot feed herself because of severe incoordination of the upper limbs and central and proximal hypotonia. Marleen has to be treated at home because of transportation barriers. Her mother dresses and feeds her. Her mother also gives maximum assistance for all position changes (Fig. 21-2).

Impairment summary: Marleen presents with asthenia, secondary muscle weakness, incoordination and intention tremor, dysmetria (**hypermetria**) of the limbs, decomposition of movement, **ocular dysmetria,** dysdiadochokinesia, titubation, and rebound phenomenon.

| **TABLE 21-4** Differential Diagnosis of Cerebellar Versus Somatosensory Ataxia/Incoordination | |
|---|---|
| **CEREBELLAR ATAXIA** | **SOMATOSENSORY ATAXIA** |
| Ataxic gait pattern is usually accompanied with signs of cerebellar **ataxia/incoordination** in the upper and/or lower limbs. When the cerebellar lesion affects both cerebellar hemispheres, titubation of the head and trunk is usually present. | Ataxic gait pattern may be associated only with fixation of the trunk, not with titubation. |
| Dizziness or vestibular impairment associated with cerebellar lesions | No dizziness |
| Decrease in muscle tone | Muscle tone can vary depending on the type of neuropathy (refer to Table 21-2). |
| Asthenia | Asthenia varies depending on the type and degree of posterior column/somatosensory impairment of sensation. |
| Decomposition of movement | Decomposition of movement |
| Rebound phenomenon | Rebound phenomenon |
| Dysmetria | Dysmetria |
| Dysdiadochokinesia | Dysdiadochokinesia |
| **Ataxia/Intention tremor** | **Ataxia/Intention tremor** |
| Gaze-evoked nystagmus | No gaze-evoked nystagmus<br>Argyll Robertson pupil |
| Balance and equilibrium impairment | Balance and equilibrium impairment |
| No somatosensory (specifically proprioception) loss | Loss of somatosensory (specifically proprioception) sensation |
| Negative Romberg test | Positive Romberg test |
| Titubation present | No titubation present |

| TABLE 21-5 | Comparison of the Signs and Symptoms of Chronic Polyneuropathy, Tabetic Syndrome, and Posterior/Dorsal Column Syndrome | | |
|---|---|---|---|
| **CHRONIC POLYNEUROPATHY (i.e., DIABETIC NEUROPATHY)** | **TABETIC SYNDROME** | **POSTERIOR/DORSAL COLUMN SYNDROME** | |
| Prominent loss of vibratory and position sense in the feet | Prominent loss of vibratory and position sense in the feet | Loss of awareness of the sense of movement, vibration, and position below the lesion in the spinal column | |
| Denervation atrophy of muscles is the main characteristic in long-standing neuropathies | Muscle power usually retained | Muscle power usually retained | |
| Absent deep tendon reflexes | Absent deep tendon reflexes | Deep tendon reflexes present | |
| Romberg sign positive | Romberg sign positive | Romberg sign positive | |
| Paresthesia (pins and needles), numbness, coldness, tingling, and other paresthesias (impairment of tactile, pain, and thermal sensations) | Paresthesia (pins and needles), numbness, coldness, tingling, and other paresthesias (impairment of tactile, pain, and thermal sensations) | Not known to have paresthesia; characteristic loss of/impaired proprioceptive/somatosensory sensation | |
| Deformities of the feet due to disproportionate muscle weakness in pretibial and peroneal muscles; repeated injuries and chronic subcutaneous infections that may result in painless loss of digits | Secondary joint deformities (Charcot joints) | - | |
|  |  | Loss of two-point discrimination; figure writing; detection of size, shape, weight, and texture of objects; the ability to detect the direction and speed of a moving stimulus on the skin | |
| Trophic changes | Trophic changes | | |
|  | Argyll Robertson pupil | - | |
|  | Lightning pains (sharp, brief stabbing pains) | | |
|  | Insensitive hypotonic bladder | | |

Data from Ropper AH, Brown RH. *Adam's and Victor's Principles of Neurology,* 8th edition. New York, NY: McGraw-Hill; 2005.

## *Contemplate Clinical Decisions 1-B*

1. *Write Marleen's functional (activity) problem list in order of priority and include underlying impairments and resulting participation restrictions.*
2. *Which outcomes measures are appropriate to implement in Marleen's case?*
3. *On which treatment approach will you base the treatment goals for Marleen?*
4. *Write appropriate goals expressing realistic functional outcomes for Marleen that will also indicate how her treatment should progress.*

## ■ **Preparatory Interventions Specific to Ataxia/Incoordination**

### General Approaches

Therapy with a general focus on motor learning approaches to enhance neural plasticity is the cornerstone of functional improvement of patients with ataxia/incoordination (Chang 2015; Ilg 2014). Although therapy is highly regarded as the main treatment of ataxia/incoordination, the literature lacks discussion regarding the scope of therapeutic intervention (Ilg, 2009). Systematic reviews by Martin (2009) and Synofzik (2014) revealed modest evidence that physical therapy has a positive effect on gait, trunk control, and activity limitations among patients with ataxia. This positive effect is ascribed to functional motor training aimed at promoting neural plasticity to treat ataxia/incoordination.

A patient's response to physiotherapeutic intervention depends on the nature of the impairment to the cerebellum as well as the areas in the cerebellum affected by the etiology of the ataxia. Rehabilitation is less successful when cerebellar structures critical for relearning of motor skills are impaired. Patients with degenerative cerebellar disease show slower functional progress than patients who sustained a cerebellar (or brainstem) stroke, underwent neurosurgery, or sustained trauma or who were diagnosed with MS (Ilg, 2010, 2014). A patient's ability to optimize function depends on the regions in the cerebellum that are spared, the process of neural adaptation, and/or the process of compensation.

The treatment approach for a patient with ataxia/incoordination should be based on the signs/symptoms and compensatory strategies he uses during functional task performance in the home, socioeconomic, and leisure environments. To adequately identify the patient's problems, a therapist should therefore have a good knowledge of basic movement science, neuroanatomy, and neurophysiology and be skilled in the observation and interpretation of his movement during the performance of functional tasks.

When assessing and treating a patient with ataxia, you should consider the following factors:

1. The ataxia may be the result of an underlying pathology, a concomitant pathology, and/or possibly comorbid conditions.

2. The patient may present with multiple signs and symptoms (e.g., asthenia, dysmetria, dysdiadochokinesia, nystagmus, rebound phenomenon) that may affect functional activities in terms of gross motor movements, precision of fine motor function, and balance. The extent to which these signs and symptoms affect the patient's function in all spheres of life should be determined and addressed so function is optimized (even if adaptations are needed to overcome the impairment(s) limiting the function).

3. The patient's movement patterns may show a combination of ataxia/incoordination and other symptoms such as choreiform movements (chorea), spasticity, stereotypical movement patterns, and muscle weakness due to nonuse because of concomitant pathology. These abnormal movement patterns need to be addressed together with the activities needed to treat the signs and symptoms of ataxia/incoordination.

4. The patient's history (duration) of the impairment and general functional and health status may influence your selection of intervention techniques and the positions in which he can be treated optimally.

5. Impaired range of motion may be due to different factors, including shortening of multijoint muscles (possibly functional tenodesis), neuromeningeal dysfunction, or joint stiffness due to long-standing dysfunction/inactivity/compensatory movement strategies. Be cognizant of the fact that the patient may be using compensatory movement strategies through substitution (refer to Chapter 26).

6. Watch out for specific compensatory movements or strategies the patient may be using that could be detrimental to the joints (in terms of degeneration) and for muscle imbalance (keeping substitution in mind).

7. Consider devices such as splints and walking aids used to compensate for specific underlying impairments to support substitution (consider the distribution of these impairments throughout the patient's body).

8. Note the patient's perceived rate of exhaustion/tiredness (often found in patients with MS who present with ataxia to a greater or lesser extent in the limbs and/or trunk) requires careful treatment planning and execution, and monitoring of their condition.

Patients with a cerebellar lesion are not always able to accommodate a variety of functional activities because of limited or delayed ability to give sustained and (un)divided attention during these tasks (Fielding, 2009; Hatzitaki, 2006). These authors have also indicated that patients with cerebellar lesions due to MS respond more slowly and take longer than normal to learn/relearn and to perform a specific task/activity. Therefore, you should work slowly and expect a slower response or slower rate of motor learning/relearning with these patients. When slower responses are identified, adapt the activities accordingly to avoid frustration and a perception of failure that may decrease (1) the patient's motivation, (2) (re-)learning of "new" tasks, and (3) functional carryover into ADLs.

The patient's insight into his personal health condition, level of anxiousness and/or depression, or cognitive impairment may cause unwillingness to participate in activities or to perform activities in the home environment to enhance functional ability. A patient who has a good understanding of his condition can overcome major functional problems and stay integrated into the community despite extensive pathology, especially when he is committed to continuing with the home program (Synofzik, 2014). Personal and/or environmental barriers or facilitating factors in the patient's environment may facilitate or limit his integration into the community (WHO, 2001).

The primary focus of functional training is to obtain central, proximal, and distal postural control, either in sequence or simultaneously. Optimization of central, proximal, and distal postural control is achieved simultaneously by choosing relevant positions in which graded weight-bearing on the limbs (or segments of limbs) can help achieve postural stabilization at central (trunk) and proximal (girdle) joints simultaneously. An example is changing position from sitting to standing by using the chair arms for support in such a way that postural control in the trunk and proximal joints is optimized.

In general, the therapist should address the underlying impairments (e.g., rebound phenomenon, dysmetria, dysdiadochokinesia, asthenia) contributing to the postural instability during functional activities, first by having the patient perform simple functional tasks within his ability (e.g., with little to no manual assistance or verbal guidance from a helper). These tasks should then be purposefully practiced during ADLs. Individuals with cerebellar or somatosensory ataxia may require many repetitions to relearn a task (Hatzitaki, 2006). Repetition of tasks using visual or auditory external cues with or without rhythm may enhance functional outcomes (Buerkers, 1995; Schmidt, 1999).

Help the patient to integrate into daily activities the improvements in coordination of physiological movements gained during rehabilitation. Preventing the use of compensatory actions (if relevant) to achieve the intended goals is also important. Strategies to perform a functional task are determined by the underlying sensory, motor (musculoskeletal as well as neuromuscular), and cognitive systems the patient can use to control his movement. Therefore, it is important to perform activities within the patient's ability because cognitive control of movement usually results in slower movement. (Fabrice, 2007).

Treatment may advance from simple functional tasks/movements (one-level tasking) to more complex movements (multilevel tasking). Complexity can also be manipulated through changing body positions (postures), the environment, or aspects of the task itself, such as integrating arm and leg movements reciprocally. Although you may progress treatment from simple to complex tasks over the course of the entire episode of care, exposing the patient to a variety of task complexities (although a smaller range of complexity) during any one session will limit cognitive fatigue that can occur from intensive concentration on movement. When treatment is progressed, activities previously performed with the patient's eyes open can be performed with the eyes closed to decrease or prevent visual fixation to compensate for lack of postural stability, coordination, or somatosensory input.

Another option is to allow the patient to perform treatment activities at a self-selected speed (which may be slower or faster than normal, without any grading control over the movement). Then either increase the speed of movement to normal speed and progress further to a faster speed but accurate movement or slow the movement down to work on slow, graded accurate movement.

Obtain postural control in symmetrical positions through weight-bearing on the limbs before performing asymmetrical limb movements in the same positions. Progress to the adoption of asymmetrical positions and obtaining segmental stability (isometric or isotonic rotational stability/mobility of the trunk and limbs) and unilateral/asymmetrical arm movements (e.g., reaching in different directions as part of functional activities with the upper extremities).

Perform movements with limited rotational trunk and limb control, such as lateral weight shifting followed by anterior-posterior weight-shifting movements in sitting or standing positions, followed by rotational weight-shifting movements in the same positions, such as unilateral reaching movement with the arms or weight shifting in stride stance. If the patient presents with titubation/hypotonia in the trunk, perform movements (such as weight shifting) in small movements (in inner ranges) and progress to larger-range movement in which the patient can manage the movement/weight shift without or with only limited (little) titubation/incoordination.

Regardless of whether the distribution of the patient's signs and symptoms are bilateral or unilateral, all activities should ultimately be performed bilaterally to ensure that the patient learns supportive as well as reactive movements (adaptive and anticipatory responses). When asthenia or hypotonia is present, activities should be performed in bilaterally symmetrical positions to achieve symmetrical stability that subsequently strengthens the patient functionally.

In patients with ataxia/incoordination due to a somatosensory impairment, it may be relevant to address the asthenia, disdiadochokinesia, and incoordination through physiologically graded movements first and then integrate improved coordinated physiological movement patterns into basic functional activities (refer to Table 21-7). In patients with cerebellar ataxia/incoordination who have problems with central and proximal instability, it may be relevant to address the instability before addressing the limb ataxia/incoordination and grading of movement, reciprocal movements, etc.

### Pharmacological Implications

Until recently, physical therapy was regarded as the primary form of intervention through which ataxia/incoordination was improved (Morton, 2009). However, pharmacotherapy for ataxia is showing promising results.

Because ataxia/incoordination often presents as a sign/symptom of other primary conditions, such as MS or paraneoplastic syndromes, medication prescribed for the primary pathology may influence the ataxia (Perlmutter, 2003). Aminopyridines not only have a beneficial effect on fatigue and gait disturbance in patients with MS but also have a beneficial effect on upper limb tremor.

The only drugs shown to be beneficial in patients with episodic ataxia type 2 are aminopyridines and acetazolamide. Acetazolamide is regarded as a first-line drug for patients with episodic ataxia type 2. However, its therapeutic use is limited because of side effects such as kidney stones (Ilg, 2014). Strupp (2011) observed that the potassium channel blocker 4-aminopyridine (4-AP) reduced the number of attacks and improved patients' quality of life. In patients with cerebellar atrophy, 4-AP reduced downbeat nystagmus and improved visual acuity, reduced postural sway, and improved motor performance (Claassen, 2013).

Schniepp (2011, 2012) observed that gait in patients with different etiologies of ataxia, such as a cerebellar stroke, multisystem atrophy, sporadic adult-onset ataxia, and downbeat nystagmus syndrome, benefited from aminopyridines. In patients with spinocerebellar ataxia (SCA) type 6, the nonselective potassium channel blocker 3,4-diaminopyridine effectively reduced downbeat nystagmus but not postural control or any other symptoms of ataxia within 1 week of administration of the drug (Kalla, 2011).

Drugs for Friedreich ataxia address the lack of mitochondrial protein frataxin, which is "involved in iron-sulfur cluster synthesis which is essential for respiratory chain and iron homeostasis," by increasing the frataxin level, reducing reactive oxygen species (ROS) through antioxidants such as coenzyme Q10, idebenone, and vitamin E to lower mitochondrial iron stores by prescribing deferiprone and to "improve energy metabolism by L-carnitine supplementation" (Ilg, 2014, pg 6). Idebenone is the most frequently used drug in patients with Friedreich ataxia (Ilg, 2014).

"Abnormal respiratory chain function and increased levels of mitochondrial iron are thought to increase levels of ROS and oxidative stress" (Ilg, 2014, pg 6). A low dosage of betamethasone (0.03 mg/kg/day) improved all patients' scores on the SARA (Brocoletti, 2011). In a randomized, placebo-controlled crossover trial, patients' scores on the ICARS improved by 30% compared with scores in the placebo group (Zannolli, 2012).

Development and testing of drugs specific for the treatment of ataxia are still in the experimental phase. Drugs such as isoniazid and carbamazepine are recommended by Armutlu

(2001), but effective outcomes require high dosages. However, the administration of long-term high dosages of these drugs is limited or prevented because of their hepatotoxic effect.

In a systematic review assessing the efficacy and tolerability of both pharmacological and nonpharmacological pleiotropic effects of riluzole treatment in patients with MS and ataxia, Mills (2007) concluded that pharmacological treatment of ataxia in MS is poorly documented and no recommendation could be made to guide the prescription of riluzole. However, Ristori (2010) riluzole to reduced neuronal hyperexcitability in patients with SCA. Further research is necessary to refine the dosage and timing of riluzole administration as well as to determine whether it can be used as disease-modifying therapy in incurable forms of cerebellar ataxia.

A study on the effects of varenicline (1 mg bid) compared with those of placebo in patients with SCA type 3 showed significant increases in SARA subscores for gait, stance, and rapid alternating movement and the timed walking test (Ilg, 2014). However, further studies are needed to determine the usefulness of varenicline in the treatment of cerebellar ataxia because of the side effects reported by patients (Ilg, 2014).

Other drugs, such as acetazolamide and amantadine, have shown promising results, but the findings should be replicated in further studies. The effect of lithium carbonate on patients with SCA is still under investigation (Ilg, 2014). Zinc sulfate supplementation together with neurorehabilitation has been shown to mildly decrease SARA subscores for gait, posture, stance, and alternating hand movements and saccadic latency in patients who presented with reduced zinc concentration in serum and cerebrospinal fluid (Ilg, 2014). Future treatment options may include stem cell therapy.

### Visuomotor Training

Patients with cerebellar lesions usually present with ocular/saccadic dysmetria, internuclear ophthalmoplegia, and fixation instability (Fielding, 2009). Visuomotor coordination is essential not only for hand-eye coordination but also for learning new tasks requiring hand-eye or foot-eye coordination, such as walking over difficult terrain. Visuomotor coordination plays a major role in the adaptation of postural reactions. Studies performed on healthy subjects indicated that mechanisms responsible for adaptive modifications in the smooth pursuit system also more generally influence processing of visuospatial information (Van Donkelaar, 1998).

Patients with cerebellar pathology are capable of substantial visuomotor learning/relearning despite their impaired motor coordination. These patients are also able to improve their performance in motor tasks requiring visuomanual coordination and the recall of irregularly shaped 2-D objects (Timmann, 1996). The role of the premotor cortex or the cortical eye fields in relearning eye-hand coordination/tracking and stepping can also contribute toward understanding and, as such, assessing and planning the effect of rehabilitation on motor function of patients with ataxia/incoordination.

Miall (2000) found that multijoint arm movements performed under visual guidance were affected in patients with cerebellar dysfunction and that visually guided movements were markedly more disrupted than movements without visual control. A possible reason for visual feedback being affected is that visual feedback processing is delayed with respect to motor commands, and the visual errors cannot be mapped directly onto the errors in the motor command that must be corrected (Miall, 1986).

Patients with MS who are diagnosed as having cerebellar ataxia often experience intention tremor and eye movement deficits. Feys (2003) examined the characteristics of intention tremor and simultaneously produced eye movements during goal-directed movements. The study participants presented with delayed onset of manual performance, slowed execution, and inaccuracy when aiming toward objects. Adding an inertial load to the limb during the performance of the activities did not affect the intention tremor. The results indicated that eye and hand movement deficits were closely related and suggested a common command structure. Impaired eye movements (e.g., visual acuity and nystagmus) are most likely to hamper accurate hand activities.

In a follow-up study, Feys (2008) found that amplitude of hand movement intention tremor during discreet movements can be enhanced by postsaccadic unsteady fixation and may lead to the development of new strategies in the management of hand tremor in individuals with MS. Physical therapy movement strategies, such as sequential execution of the saccadic eye and primary hand movement or splitting of the primary saccade into multiple saccades of smaller amplitudes, are believed to reduce hand tremor severity during reaching tasks associated with ADLs. The latter movement strategies imply that patients with MS who present with tremor have to suppress automatic movement execution while performing an activity (i.e., control their movement) by using cognitive control strategies.

On the basis of the literature, Hatzitaki (2006) concluded that patients with cerebellar lesions are compromised in learning novel sensorimotor or visuomotor recalibrations of the locomotor trajectory of postural responses to known perturbation amplitudes. They therefore designed an experiment to determine "how cerebellar dysfunction associated with multiple sclerosis affects the [patient's] ability to learn a novel visuo-postural coordination task." (Hatzitaki 2006, pg 295). Their results suggested a possible vestibular dysfunction and/or deficient integration of visual, vestibular, and somatosensory information necessary to control posture. Patients with a low score on the Expanded Disability Status Scale (EDSS) improved over the trial period, indicating learning had taken place, but at a slower rate of performance improvement and to a more limited extent than age-matched controls. Patients with a high EDSS score did not show improvement in visuomotor performance.

Despite considerable cerebellar pathology and motor learning deficits in patients with MS, there can be substantial improvement in visuomotor performance. Further research is necessary to investigate visuomotor exercises integrated into general rehabilitation programs to optimize the functional ability of patients with ataxia/incoordination during ADLs.

## The Use of Equipment During Exercise

Weighted vests and weighted ADL tools such as eating utensils and writing instruments are described in the literature as equipment that could improve function in patients with ataxia/incoordination. Gillen (1999) described an orthotic neck collar that supports head control (decreases the demand on postural control) for facilitated eating and swallowing. Wrist supports were used to externally increase wrist stability and improve hand function during finger feeding and oral care.

Other equipment to enhance a patient's independence, in the context of incoordination, during daily activities include adaptive devices such as a cutting board, adaptive devices or strategies to use the telephone, a basket with a nonskid bottom for carrying objects around, and adaptive utensils designed specifically to optimize a patient's functional ability.

Synofzik (2014) reported that exercises as part of a physiotherapy program may be complemented by video game technology (also called "exergames"), such as the commercially available Xbox. Use of exergames as part of an intervention strategy may have great advantages for patients (even for patients with neurodegenerative diseases such as SCA), especially as a long-term intervention and/or a home program, because of their highly motivating incentives. Exergames also promote interaction with rapidly changing environments, which helps patients adapt to real-world activities and promotes anticipatory reactions while they are having fun. Patients can also use exergames in the comfort of their own home, which makes it financially cost-effective in the long run. Exergames are also beneficial for children diagnosed with chronic incoordination (usually with degenerative SCA or Friedreich ataxia) because of their highly motivating effect of achieving success. It is also very relevant for patients who are wheelchair users.

Chang (2015) found that a home-based, 4-week–cycle ergometry program (15 minutes per day, 3 days per week) resulted in a significant decrease in ICARS total score in individuals with SCA. Participants' perception of improvement also changed significantly for the better. The researchers also observed spinal reflex modulation of agonist and antagonist muscles (disynaptic Ia reciprocal inhibition and D1 inhibition of the Hoffmann reflex). After 4 weeks of cycling, the SCA group demonstrated a restored capacity toward normal for modulation of the disynaptic reciprocal inhibition and the D1 inhibition, showing an adaptive spinal plasticity from training. The improvement in modulation correlated with improvements in functional performance on the ICARS.

## Therapeutic Techniques

In a systematic review, Martin (2009) concluded that motor learning is possible in spite of cerebellar damage. This suggests functional motor retraining aimed at neural plasticity is appropriate for people with cerebellar damage. The most frequently reported physical therapy techniques identified in this systematic review were proprioceptive neuromuscular facilitation (PNF), Frenkel exercises, vestibular habituation exercises, and a range of activities aimed at retraining balance.

Morton (2009) reported that although motor learning was impaired in individuals with cerebellar lesions, an intensive coordination-training program focused on balance and gait training followed by an 8-week self-directed home program resulted in improvement in participants with degenerative cerebellar ataxia. Therefore, improvements in balance and walking coordination due to motor learning are possible even in individuals with degenerative cerebellar ataxia. Similar results were reported in a group of participants with afferent ataxia (Ilg, 2009); however, in this study improvements in balance and walking coordination in individuals with afferent ataxia were not significant. According to Synofzik (2014) patients with afferent ataxia respond more slowly than patients with cerebellar ataxia probably because decreased or absent sensory input to the cerebellum limits cerebellar control over movement. Other than an intervention focus on balance and gait training, specific techniques were not mentioned. Armutlu (2001) proposed an eclectic approach to treatment using combined techniques and continually adapting to the individual's needs.

Ilg (2009, 2010, 2014) found that patients with cerebellar disease (a group of patients diagnosed with SCA type 6, Friedreich ataxia, and idiopathic cerebellar disease) who received a "coordinative physiotherapy program" for 1 hour per day, three times per week for 4 weeks, gained functional performance equivalent to 2 or more years of disease progression on the SARA scale. The coordinative physiotherapy program included progressive exercises addressing static balance, dynamic balance, trunk-limb coordination in whole-body movements, steps to prevent falling, falling strategies to prevent injury, and mobility exercises to prevent secondary complications such as contracture (see Box 21-1 for sample exercises). Patients' goal attainment scores demonstrated they were able to translate the effect of the training into important functions in daily life. Patients with afferent ataxia (somatosensory ataxia) made less progress than patients with cerebellar ataxia.

An exercise program focused on retraining whole-body coordination, posture, and gait resulted in significant improvements in individuals with mild-moderate traumatic brain injury (Ustinova, 2015). Patients completed a 20-session program of four to five sessions per week over the course of 4 to 5 weeks. Sessions initially ran for 30 to 40 minutes and were expanded to 55 to 60 minutes as the patients were able. Various coordination activities were completed in horizontal (on a mat), sitting, standing, and walking positions. Mat and sitting exercises focused on improving multisegmental coordination, sitting balance, lower extremity range of motion, movement accuracy, eye-head and eye-hand coordination, and reducing intention tremor. Standing and gait activities focused on static and dynamic balance during double- and single-limb stance and walking, agility, gait kinematics, arm-leg coordination during walking, gait initiation and termination, and walking with different bases of support. Significant improvements were seen in static and dynamic balance on the Berg balance scale, in gait on the Functional Gait Assessment, and in a decrease in ataxia symptoms on the Klockgether ataxia scale.

## BOX 21-1   Examples of Coordinative Physiotherapy Exercises

| | |
|---|---|
| Static balance | • Quadruped hold (may add proprioceptive neuromuscular facilitation [PNF] stability techniques)<br>• Quadruped hold with single upper extremity (UE) or lower extremity (LE) raise<br>• Quadruped hold with opposite UE-LE raise<br>• Quadruped hold with UE or LE on unstable surface<br>• Sitting on therapeutic ball – alternate UE-LE raises<br>• Kneeling – leaning forward/backward without hip strategy<br>• Kneeling – head turns, arm raises, throw-catch<br>• Half-kneeling – as in kneeling<br>• Modified plantigrade – with single UE or LE raise<br>• Modified plantigrade – with alternate or opposite UE/LE raises<br>• Standing – feet together, firm surface, head turns<br>• Standing – feet together, firm surface, arm raises<br>• Standing – feet together, firm surface, throw-catch<br>• Standing – feet together, compliant surface, eyes open, eyes closed<br>• Single limb stance (SLS) on stool or ball – add head turns, arm raises<br>• Tandem stance hold |
| Dynamic balance (increasing speed of movements) | • Sitting on therapeutic ball – weight shifting, throw-catch, PNF diagonal UE patterns<br>• Sitting on therapeutic ball – moving 5-lb weight in PNF UE diagonals<br>• Sitting on therapeutic ball – twist to look over shoulder<br>• Sitting on therapeutic ball – pass object behind<br>• Kneeling – weight shifting without hip strategy<br>• Kneeling – twist turns<br>• Kneeling – step forward-backward/side-side with one knee<br>• Kneeling to half-kneeling – alternate LEs<br>• Standing – weight shift to limits of stability without hip strategy<br>• Standing – reaching all directions feet together and stride stance<br>• Standing – twist turn, pass object<br>• Standing – stepping forward/backward/side/crossover<br>• Alternate foot taps on stool<br>• Standing – marching combined with alternate arm raises<br>• Squats<br>• Boxing<br>• Kick ball<br>• Kick higher target |
| Dynamic balance (during gait) | • Head turns – horizontal and vertical<br>• Step around/over obstacles<br>• Step to specific targets – clock – increasing speed<br>• Pivot turns<br>• 360 Turns<br>• Braiding<br>• Stair negotiation with and without rails<br>• Lunge forward/side, walking/stepping<br>• Jump off/on step/box<br>• Jumping jacks<br>• Walk outside on uneven ground: grass/incline |
| Treadmill or gait training | • 1.0-2.0+ mph; increasing speed as able; may modify UE support progressing to no UE support<br>Work on:<br>• Narrow base of support<br>• Even step length<br>• Even cadence – metronome<br>• Arm swing |

---

**BOX 21-1   Examples of Coordinative Physiotherapy Exercises—cont'd**

| | |
|---|---|
| | • Heel strike |
| | • Heel off with forefoot rocker |
| | Transition above to over ground |
| Trunk-limb coordination in whole-body movements | • Quadruped – raise opposite arm and leg – flex arm, leg, and trunk (curl up) – extend arm, leg, and trunk |
| | • Modified plantigrade – raise opposite arm and leg – flex arm, leg, and trunk (curl up) – extend arm, leg, and trunk |
| | • Kneeling to side-sit right to kneeling to side-sit left; repeat |
| Stepping and falling strategies | • Standing – stepping side/forward/backward/crossovers |
| | • Standing – stepping to clock |
| | • Standing – lean without hip strategy and practice stepping – all directions |
| | • Standing perturbations with patient reactive stepping strategies |
| | • Standing – reach down to touch floor and return |
| | • Standing to quadruped and return to standing |
| | • Quadruped – tuck and roll (going to floor in controlled manner) |
| | • Kneeling – tuck and roll (going to floor in controlled manner) |
| | • Half-kneeling – tuck and roll (going to floor in controlled manner) |
| | • Standing – perturbations with reactive controlled fall to floor |
| | • Walking – perturbations with reactive controlled fall to floor |
| Mobility (to prevent contracture) | • Trunk extension activities – prone, prone over wedge, bolster, or ball |
| | • Supine trunk rotation – UE and LE |
| | • Shoulder active range of motion (AROM) |
| | • Hip AROM |
| | • Check for other limitations |

Adapted and expanded from Ilg W, Bastiaan AJ, Boesch S, et al. Consensus paper: Management of degenerative cerebellar disorders. *Cerebellum.* 2014;13:248–268.

---

In the following paragraphs, the application of PNF (functional activities including balance and gait training), **Frenkel exercises, visuomotor training**, and **Cawthorne-Cooksey exercises** for patients with ataxia (and some degree of vestibular impairment) are discussed (Armutlu, 2001; Quintern, 1999). Other techniques are reported, with supporting evidence in the Focus on Evidence table for ataxia/incoordination interventions (Table 21-8 ONL).

### Proprioceptive Neuromuscular Facilitation

PNF techniques used to treat ataxia/incoordination include rhythmic initiation, combination of isotonics (agonistic reversal), isotonic reversal (slow reversal), and rhythmic stabilization (stabilizing reversal); explanations of each are presented in Chapter 15. All of these techniques address coordination between agonist and antagonist muscles during movement patterns (Adler, 2003). PNF is used as an intervention in ataxia/incoordination to achieve the following goals:

1. Enhance learning of coordinated movement through the use of verbal cueing (specifically in relation to knowledge of performance). Verbal cueing in combination with visual input to organize movement and obtain "knowledge of results" contributes to motor learning and thus optimizes coordination and postural control. Therefore,

it is important for the patient to follow the PNF movement with the eyes/head in order to see the limbs.

2. Improve coordination between antagonists and address ataxia/incoordination by implementing reciprocal or reversing movements combined with appropriate resistance to gently facilitate coordinated movement. Reciprocal or reversing movements are characteristic of goal-directed activities, and PNF can serve as the preparation for functional goal-directed movement. Special care should be taken to adapt the techniques in such a way that the concentric/eccentric muscle control characteristic of normal functional movement patterns is achieved. Reciprocal or reversing movement patterns can address ataxic/incoordination movement patterns, hypotonia in the trunk and the limbs, asthenia, dysdiadochokinesia, and decomposition of movement. When the patient has trunk hypotonia, using a compensatory strategy such as fixation or reciprocal or reversing movements with the trunk and/or limbs can contribute to central stabilization, an improvement in trunk tone, and a potential decrease in titubation.

3. Enhance the normal sequence of movement by emphasizing the distal to proximal sequencing of these patterns. Enhancing the normal sequence of movement addresses decomposition of movement.

4. Strengthen "weak" muscles ("weakness" related to hypotonia, asthenia, and/or disuse). Strengthening weak muscles in functional patterns (of the trunk and/or limbs) emphasizes proximal stability during movement of the distal segment. Strengthening and endurance should be adapted to the individual's neuromuscular and cardiovascular capacity and cognitive concentration.

5. Optimize manual contact to give exteroceptive input, which contributes to determining the direction of the movement to limit incoordination. In the case of a patient with somatosensory ataxia/incoordination, the therapist's handgrip during the performance of PNF patterns can be adapted to obtain maximal manual contact, giving as much exteroceptive input as possible. Using progressively less manual contact enables the patient to perform movements with decreasing dependence on exteroceptive input/cueing.

6. Decrease movement effort. Movement effort is an important factor to consider if it elicits or increases titubation in the trunk or limb incoordination. For example, incorporating knee flexion into the movement pattern of the lower limb may improve gait by decreasing the effort of lifting a straight leg. PNF should be performed with guiding resistance rather than maximal/optimal manual resistance because the aim is to emphasize the reciprocal functional movement patterns and avoid an increase in ataxia/incoordination, titubation, and/or rebound phenomenon that may result from excess effort. The appropriate resistance may, in fact, help to smooth out the movement and decrease the incoordination.

When using PNF, one must be careful with the application of quick stretch. Initiation of a PNF pattern or technique with a stretch reflex may increase incoordination as a result of lack of proprioceptive input (in the case of somatosensory ataxia/

incoordination) or uncontrolled regulatory output control onto the LMN (because of the cerebellum's impaired coordination of output). The stretch reflex may also be ineffective if the patient is fixating because of postural instability and should be avoided in this case. PNF can be integrated into the activities mentioned in Table 21-7 at the sections indicated in the table.

### Frenkel Coordination Exercises

Frenkel exercises (Box 21-2) were originally developed to treat lower extremity ataxia/incoordination due to a loss of proprioception that occurred as a result of posterior column impairment of the spinal cord. Since then, they have also been used to treat ataxia/incoordination as a result of MS and cerebellar lesions (Armutlu, 2001). Frenkel exercises teach the patient to use vision as the principal source of feedback in guiding the adaptation to sensory perturbations, such as loss or diminished proprioception. These authors proposed vision as the main source of information to the CNS regarding the target and hand positions, resulting in sensorimotor adaptation. Proprioception possibly plays a secondary role in sensorimotor adaptation.

Bastian (1996) also found that patients with a de-afferent lesion (resulting in somatosensory ataxia) showed great improvement in their movement performance after (1) vision of the limb at rest, (2) vision of the limb during movement, or (3) vision of the limb after movement. These results indicate that visual information may update an internal representation of the dynamic properties of the limb (Ghetz, 1995).

A patient treated with Frenkel exercises must therefore be able to see his limbs. Place the patient in a semi-Fowler (half-lying) or sitting position; or place a mirror in front of the patient if the reversed body image and movements in the mirror do not confuse him. Using the principles described for Frenkel

---

### BOX 21-2 Examples of Frenkel Exercises

| Half-lying | • Hip and knee flexion and extension of each limb, foot flat on the mat/plinth |
| --- | --- |
| | • Hip abduction and adduction of each limb with the foot flat; knee flexed; then with knee extended |
| | • Hip and knee flexion/extension of each limb, heel lifted off mat |
| | • Heel of one limb to opposite leg (toes, ankle, shin, patella) |
| | • Heel of one limb to opposite knee, sliding down crest of tibia to ankle |
| | • Hip and knee flexion and extension of both limbs, legs together |
| | • Reciprocal movements of both limbs – flexion of one leg during extension of the other |
| Sitting | • Knee extension and flexion of each limb; progress to marking time |
| | • Hip abduction and adduction |
| | • Alternate foot placing to a specific target (using floor markings or a grid in which the patient has to put his foot) |
| Standing | • Standing up and sitting down to a specific count (metronome) |
| | • Standing foot placing to a specific target (floor markings or grid) |
| | • Standing weight shifting |
| Walking | • Sideways or forward to a specific count (parallel lines or floor markings may be used as targets to control foot placement, stride length, and step width) |
| | • Turning around to a specific count (floor markings can be helpful in maintaining a stable base of support) |

exercise (i.e., start with limb movement supported on the surface and then progress to antigravity movements; encourage the patient to visually observe the limb as it moves to enhance feedback and compensation; progress from unilateral movement to bilateral symmetrical to bilateral reciprocal), you can develop a sequence of upper extremity exercises for incoordination as well.

Frenkel exercises should be performed in postures with the most stability and progress to positions that challenge the patient's stability. For example, start in the semi-Fowler or half-lying position so the patient can watch his/her limbs and progress to sitting (with the back supported or without back support), followed by progression to standing and ultimately walking. Further progression allows the patient to perform the exercises with the eyes closed.

When doing Frenkel exercises, patients are required to perform simple combined physiological movements as part of a functional activity. Initial exercises involve movements of the feet/hands while maintaining contact with the supporting surface, supported but causing slight friction on the soles of the feet/palms of the hands and forearms (increasing the exteroceptive input to the CNS regarding the movement). The friction also gives a little resistance to movement, which may increase postural tone for more coordinated movement and assists the patient in stabilizing the movement. The additional exteroceptive input, together with vision, is of major importance in this earliest phase for patients with somatosensory ataxia/incoordination.

In addition to the friction, the therapist can give manual assistance and verbal commands to help the patient adapt to performing more coordinated movements. Verbal knowledge about the results of a task provided by an observer (therapist) is a powerful source of spatial information (Buerkers, 1995; Schmidt, 1999).

Progressing Frenkel exercises includes taking away therapist assistance when the patient's coordination during the performance has improved. When coordination has improved by only using friction, the patient can be encouraged to perform an unsupported active movement, or the movement can be made more complex. When the complex movement results in increased incoordination, the friction can be added again or the patient can be assisted manually by the therapist to perform the movement. The primary intent is that repetitions of the appropriate practice results in plasticity and motor learning.

Movements should be repeated until a marked improvement is observed in the patient's coordination. The performance of a specific number of repetitions is not prescribed; the movements should be repeated until the patient's coordination has improved. A decrease in cognitive concentration and mental or physical fatigue are indications that the patient needs a rest. A sequence of progression may include the following steps: (1) taking away the therapist's assistance; (2) when the patient's coordination has improved, encouraging him to perform the free, unsupported, active movement without any friction; and (3) when coordination during the simple free active movement has improved, implementing

more complex movement (Box 21-2). Verbal cueing and rhythm can still be used to assist the patient with movement coordination. When further improvement of coordination is observed, (4) ask the patient to stop and start and change direction on command, (5) increase/decrease the range of movement, (6) change the speed of the movements, and (7) perform the movements with the eyes closed.

Movements in the semi-Fowler/half-lying position can be implemented simultaneously with simple movements in the sitting position, and if the patient can manage, also in standing position. It is not necessary to wait for the patient to master all the movements in one posture before progressing to the next posture.

Encourage the patient to concentrate mentally on controlling movement during the action. With the emphasis on cognitive movement control, patients learn through cognitive compensatory strategies to perform the movements with as much coordination as possible and improve coordination. Frenkel exercises are relevant only for patients who can manage the effort associated with visual cognitive control of coordination.

The exercises are performed at a slow comfortable speed for the patient. Rhythm (auditory cueing stimulus, such as counting out loud) can help the patient perform the exercises (simple movements) with more coordination and also help the patient's cognitive concentration on the exercises.

Verbal commands by the therapist to stop and start the movement or to change direction can be added to enhance patient concentration and challenge the patient to react to external stimuli and may serve as a variation to progress the patient's level of response. Verbal commands are a simple (low-level) way of introducing the patient to adaptation and anticipatory reactions.

A similar list of activities can be developed and adapted for the upper limbs using the principles of the Frenkel exercises and the list of activities for the lower extremities in Box 21-2. When a patient is seated on a chair with a backrest in front of a table, the friction of sliding the hand and forearm over the table and assistance by the therapist can help him compensate, together with vision for the lack of proprioceptive input in the case of somatosensory ataxia. In the case of a cerebellar lesion, visual input and repetitive guided movement (guided by the slight friction of the movement over the supporting surface and/or assistance of the therapist) have a stabilizing effect on the muscle tone in the agonistic/antagonistic muscle activity. It is advisable to select upper limb activities based on the patient's task-specific activities (ADLs) or components thereof. This type of activity enhances relearning of coordination during task-specific activities and is the approach of choice to enhance relearning of skilled movement (Gillen, 1999).

### Cawthorne-Cooksey Exercises

Cawthorne-Cooksey exercises (Cooksey, 1946) are indicated primarily for patients with impairment of the vestibular system or vestibular labyrinth impairment (Meldrum, 2004). As mentioned earlier, patients with cerebellar dysfunction may present additionally with vestibular impairment that includes the peripheral sensors (Fig. 21-4), the vestibular nuclei, or the cerebellum. Details on specific vestibular interventions are presented in Chapter 29. The purpose of Cawthorne-Cooksey exercises (Table 21-6) is to help the patient learn to compensate or, more specifically, habituate to ignore the abnormal vestibular signals.

Cawthorne-Cooksey exercises can also be implemented to prepare the patient to perform more complex visuomotor exercises as part of treatment. Impaired balance, often associated with vestibular system impairment, is treated according to the principles discussed in Table 21-7.

| TABLE 21-6 | Cawthorne-Cooksey Exercises | | | | | |
|---|---|---|---|---|---|---|
| **FOCUS OF THE EXERCISE** | **ACTIVITY** | **EXERCISE #** | **START DATE** | **ONE MONTH** | **TWO MONTHS** | **THREE MONTHS** |
| Eye movement | Movement of your eye while keeping your head still <br> (1) Up and down, then side to side following your finger | 1 | | | | |
| | (2) Focusing on your finger moving from 3 feet to 1 foot from your face | 2 | | | | |
| Head movement: eyes open | (3) Bending forward and backward | 3 | | | | |
| | (4) Turning from side to side | 4 | | | | |
| Head movement: eyes closed | (5) Bending forward and backward | 5 | | | | |
| | (6) Turning from side to side | 6 | | | | |
| Trunk movement: eyes open | Eyes and head must follow the object | | | | | |
| | (7) From standing, bend forward to pick up an object from the floor and back up to standing. | 7 | | | | |
| | (8) From standing, bend forward to pick up an object from the floor, turn to left to place the object behind, leave the object, turn to the right to pick up the object, now place the object back in front | 8 | | | | |
| | (9) From standing, drop shoulders and head sideways to left and then right | 9 | | | | |
| | (10) From standing, reach with object up into the air to left then right | 10 | | | | |
| | (11) From standing, pick up an object from the floor and reach high into the air | 11 | | | | |
| | (12) Change from sitting to standing, turn one way, sit down, stand up, turn the opposite way, sit down | 12 | | | | |
| | (13) Turning on one spot to left and right | 13 | | | | |
| Trunk movement: eyes closed | (14) From standing, bend forward to touch the floor and back to standing | 14 | | | | |
| | (15) From standing, bend forward to touch the floor, turn left to touch the chair behind, turn to right to touch the chair, back to front | 15 | | | | |

| TABLE 21-6 | Cawthorne-Cooksey Exercises—cont'd | | | | | | |
|---|---|---|---|---|---|---|---|
| FOCUS OF THE EXERCISE | ACTIVITY | EXERCISE # | START DATE | ONE MONTH | TWO MONTHS | THREE MONTHS | |
| | (16) From standing, drop shoulders and head, sideways to left and then right | 16 | | | | | |
| | (17) From standing, touch the floor, reach high into the air | 17 | | | | | |
| | (18) Change from sitting to standing, turning one way, sit down, stand up, turn opposite way, sit down | 18 | | | | | |
| | (19) Turning on spot to left and right | 19 | | | | | |
| Lying down | If possible, do not use a pillow | | | | | | |
| Lying down: eyes open | (20) Rolling head from side to side | 20 | | | | | |
| | (21) Rolling whole body from side to side | 21 | | | | | |
| | (22) Sitting up straight forward | 22 | | | | | |
| | (23) From lying, roll onto your side, sit up over the edge of the bed, lie down on the opposite side, and roll onto your back | 23 | | | | | |
| Lying down: eyes closed | (24) Rolling head from side to side | 24 | | | | | |
| | (25) Rolling whole body from side to side | 25 | | | | | |
| | (26) Sitting up straight forward | 26 | | | | | |
| | (27) From lying, roll onto your side, sit up over the edge of the bed, lie down on the opposite side, and roll onto your back. | 27 | | | | | |

During the first assessment, the patient is asked to perform each exercise five times. The patient's performance is rated on a four-point scale in which 0 = no symptoms, 1 = mild symptoms, 2 = moderate symptoms, and 3 = severe symptoms. The patient's home exercises entail the practicing of only those exercises that cause mild to moderate symptoms. Progression is based on the way the patient tolerates the effect of the exercises over time. (Adapted with permission from Meldrum D, Walsh RM. Vestibular and balance rehabilitation. In: Stokes, M, ed. *Physical Management in Neurological Rehabilitation.* Philadelphia, PA: Elsevier-Mosby; 2004:413–430.)

## ■ Intervention: Ultimately Applied in Functional Activities

### Mat Activities and Balance Training in Functional Positions

Treatment of patients with ataxia/incoordination should be started at the level of functional activity identified during the patient assessment. Table 21-7 identifies activities that may be performed with a patient who presents with ataxia/incoordination, including aspects of intervention that can be incorporated to improve coordination. Activities are described in a systematic way but in practice should be applied according to the patient's clinical and functional presentation, which may differ from patient to patient. The described sequence in Table 21-7 focuses on establishing central (trunk) stability before promoting proximal or distal control. Once trunk/proximal stability has been established, central (trunk),

proximal (shoulder and pelvic girdles), and distal (limb) control can be integrated into functional activities.

Table 21-7 further provides a guideline on how to optimize a patient's postural control in functional positions. However, it is imperative that the patient consistently integrates any gains in postural control into functional activities on a participation level to promote functional carryover into ADLs.

Repetition of tasks plays a major role in motor learning and functional carryover of treatment into ADLs. In the case of a cerebellar lesion, the patient has to relearn coordination during a skilled activity using cognitive concentration. Visual input plays a major role in exerting cognitive control over movement in order to learn adaptive and anticipatory control. Learning cognitive control over movement/skill takes place through the "long loop" of cognitive control instead of taking place in the cerebellum. Many more repetitions are therefore necessary for a patient to learn a coordinated movement (which is part of the skilled activity) through cognitive control.

*(Text continued on page 721)*

**TABLE 21-7** Mat Activities and Balance Training in Functional Positions

## OPTIMIZING POSTURAL CONTROL IN FUNCTIONAL POSITIONS

| Aim | Principle | Example of Activity in Logical Sequence | Functional Activity to Be Practiced Functionally | Precautions/Contraindications |
|---|---|---|---|---|
| 1. To prepare and teach the patient to bridge (do hip extension) in supine crook-lying position | Practice the different components of the activity (i.e., stabilization of the trunk, hip and knee flexion, hip extension concentrically and eccentrically) | | | |
| | 1.1 To enhance isometric trunk stability in a symmetrical position (trunk muscles work as stabilizers) Place the patient in symmetrical position (i.e., crook lying in supine). If incoordination in the legs or the trunk increases, stabilize the legs over a (few) pillows. | Ask the patient to breathe slowly through pursed lips to get isometric contraction of the trunk muscles. Contraction of the trunk muscles can be facilitated by placing the hand lightly over the abdomen. | | Avoid an effort that will cause an increase in titubation, facial movements, or any other compensatory strategies. Limit the number of consecutive expirations to approximately six to avoid dizziness. |
| | 1.2 Stabilization of the trunk during activities with the limbs | Place the patient in a supine crook-lying position. Ask the patient to lift both arms alternatively/simultaneously into 90-degree flexion, performing the activity with pursed lips expiration. Stabilize the shoulder girdle while performing the activity. | | The therapist guides the movement to limit incoordination and rebound reactions in the trunk and legs. Prevent fixation at neck and/or with facial movements (i.e., frowning and clenching teeth, pressing lips together/grinning). |

Patient is in supine crook-lying position with arms in slight abduction for stabilization.

Ask the patient to lift one leg at a time/both legs simultaneously (with assistance) into 90-degree hip and knee flexion. The activity can be performed with pursed lip breathing to facilitate trunk stabilization.

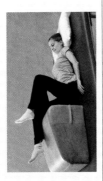

The therapist assists/guides the movement to limit incoordination and rebound reactions in the arms or trunk. Avoid fixation by performing a Valsalva maneuver.

Patient puts legs over a ball with the hips in 90-degree flexion and the lower legs resting on the ball. Patient can maintain stability/move the ball in small-range movements with or without expiration/assistance.

Avoid rebound phenomenon, titubation, increase in ataxia/ incoordination, and all previously mentioned fixation/compensatory strategies.

Ask the patient to lift one leg into 90-degree hip and knee flexion. The activity can be performed with pursed lips breathing to enhance trunk stability. This activity requires rotational stability control of the

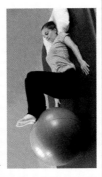

Practice the sequence of movements during the bridging activity (hip and knee flexion and hip extension). The patient may or may not assist with stabilizing her trunk by pressing on her arms.

If the patient is not ready to manage rotational trunk control, titubation of the trunk, increased intentional tremor, or rebound phenomenon may occur. Perform the activity within the patient's ability to do

*Continued*

**TABLE 21-7    Mat Activities and Balance Training in Functional Positions—cont'd**

**OPTIMIZING POSTURAL CONTROL IN FUNCTIONAL POSITIONS**

| Aim | Principle | Example of Activity in Logical Sequence | Functional Activity to Be Practiced Functionally | Precautions/Contraindications |
|---|---|---|---|---|
| | | trunk, which may be one of the limitations during bridging. 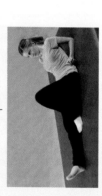 | The therapist should give just enough assistance to let her experience good quality movement. | the activity without titubation, intentional limb tremor, or rebound phenomenon occurring. |
| | 1.3 Use compensation with the eyes and cognitive concentration on performing a "smooth" movement as compensatory movement strategies to decrease ataxia). | With the patient in a half-lying/semi-Fowler position, perform hip and knee flexion by keeping the foot on the supporting surface (bed) for additional exteroceptive input through the plantar surface of the foot. The activity can also be performed in half-lying (semi-Fowler) position so that the patient can see her legs and concentrate on performing the hip and knee flexion "smoothly" and in the correct sequence. Sitting with the back supported against the bed/wall may be the best position for starting this activity. | | The friction between the foot and the supporting surface should not be so much that it causes increased incoordination/rebound phenomenon. Ensure the correct sequence of movements. Prevent unwanted compensatory strategies. |

| 1.4 To practice bridging | Supine lying: Flex the hips and knees and extend the hips to bridge. Patients should concentrate on doing a posterior tilt of the pelvis and pelvic floor contraction during the hip extension (bridging). The activity can be performed with/without pursed lips breathing. 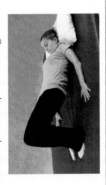 | Practice bridging in a controlled way at a speed that limits titubation, intentional tremor, or rebound phenomenon of the limbs. | Prevent/limit increase in titubation/incoordination/rebound phenomenon as well as compensatory strategies. |

When the patient is in the final stages of rehabilitation, progression can include bridging by using only one leg OR bridging with the legs/one leg on a small therapy ball. Precautions include prevention or at least limiting of titubation/incoordination/rebound phenomenon and compensatory strategies.

| 2. Rolling to one side | To obtain and implement central control in a functional activity, such as rolling to one side | Roll to one-quarter turn from supine lying by moving the shoulder girdle and pelvis forward simultaneously. Guidance by the therapist can be given against the direction of the rolling action. Repeat the activity reciprocally from sidelying toward supine and back to perform the activity bilaterally. 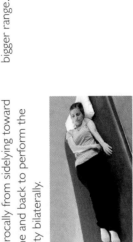 | Progression: Initiate rolling with either the pelvis or the shoulder girdle to obtain (some) rotational trunk control. Perform rolling toward prone and back to supine through a bigger range. | Limit inconsistent muscle contraction that leads to jerky movements. Prevent/limit rebound phenomenon, titubation, and/or compensatory strategies. |

Continued

**TABLE 21-7    Mat Activities and Balance Training in Functional Positions—cont'd**

**OPTIMIZING POSTURAL CONTROL IN FUNCTIONAL POSITIONS**

| Aim | Principle | Example of Activity in Logical Sequence | Functional Activity to Be Practiced Functionally | Precautions/Contraindications |
|---|---|---|---|---|
| | | | Practice actions that may include supine lying, throwing off blankets, flexing legs, bridging movement to shift sideways in bed, and rolling to the side in preparation to sit up. | |

Proprioceptive neuromuscular facilitation (PNF) with the legs and the arms can be performed at this stage. (PNF dynamic reversals of antagonists, stabilizing reversals, rhythmic stabilization, rhythmic initiation, and a combination of isotonics can be implemented.)

Frenkel exercises for the arms and/or legs in half-lying (semi-Fowler) position can also be performed at this stage.
(The principles of both PNF and Frenkel exercises are discussed in the following paragraphs.)

| Aim | Principle | Example of Activity in Logical Sequence | Functional Activity to Be Practiced Functionally | Precautions/Contraindications |
|---|---|---|---|---|
| 3. To improve sitting stability by optimizing postural reactions in sitting | Trunk stability during lateral weight shift in preparation for balance reactions and functional shifting forward and backward in sitting | Sitting symmetrically (with or without arm and feet support): Arm support can be either at the patient's side or on a table in front of her. Arm support may be necessary when the patient experiences major instability in sitting. Less arm/feet support can be used as part of the progression. | If deep pressure increases titubation or rebound phenomenon, decrease the pressure but maintain the touch to facilitate stability of the patient's trunk during the weight shift. | |

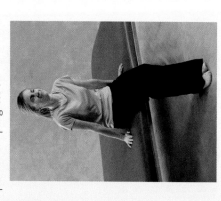

| | | |
|---|---|---|
| 4. To practice the functional task of shifting forward and backward in sitting in a plinth/bed by doing hip hitching | Careful, deep, sustained pressure on the patient's trunk can be performed to assist her in stabilizing the trunk. When the patient has achieved optimal trunk stability, perform lateral weight shift followed by anterior-posterior weight shift.<br><br>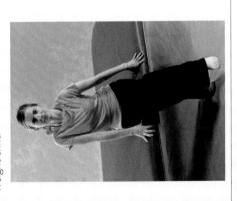<br><br>Progression:<br>Repeat the deep, sustained pressure on the trunk with the arms in various positions/asymmetrical positions. Add weight shift in asymmetrical positions as appropriate as part of the progression. | Sit independently and shift forward with unilateral pelvis elevation and anterior rotation for forward shifting and posterior rotation for backward shifting. The action can be performed on a hard surface (i.e., a plinth) or a soft surface (i.e., on the patient's bed). A soft surface is more difficult than a hard surface.<br><br>If deep pressure or the adoption of an asymmetrical position with the arms increases titubation or rebound phenomenon, decrease the pressure but maintain the touch or more symmetrical position with the arms to facilitate stability of the patient's trunk. |

*Continued*

**TABLE 21-7** Mat Activities and Balance Training in Functional Positions—cont'd

**OPTIMIZING POSTURAL CONTROL IN FUNCTIONAL POSITIONS**

| Aim | Principle | Example of Activity in Logical Sequence | Functional Activity to Be Practiced Functionally | Precautions/Contraindications |
|---|---|---|---|---|
| 5. To optimize changing position from sitting to lying | Obtain changing position by using the arms as support and to enhance eccentric control and rotational trunk control. | Assist the patient in performing eccentric arm support from sitting to sidelying, followed by lifting the legs onto the bed. Repeat the activity bilaterally. | The patient is encouraged to perform the activity independently on a hard surface as well as on her bed. | Changing position from sitting to sidelying is mechanically easier for the patient than changing position from lying to sitting. Limit titubation, rebound phenomenon, and increases in incoordination and compensatory strategies. |
| 6. To optimize changing position from lying to sitting | To optimize rotational trunk control together with eccentric and concentric control of the limbs | Assist the patient in changing position from sidelying to sitting by taking the legs off the bed and using asymmetrical arm support. Perform the activity with progressively less assistance as the patient is able to do it independently. Repeat the activity bilaterally. | Practice lying to sitting and lying down again on a hard surface as well as on the bed. | Limit titubation, rebound phenomenon, and increased incoordination due to exertion. Ensure that the patient uses appropriate righting reactions during the performance of the activity (to prevent compensatory strategies). |

| Goal | | | Precautions |
|---|---|---|---|
| 7. To optimize stability in asymmetrical positions | Optimize rotational trunk control with and without arm support as well as dynamic changing of position in sitting. | Side sitting with bilateral arm support: Careful deep sustained pressure on the patient's trunk can be performed to assist her in stabilizing the trunk and limbs. When the patient has achieved optimal trunk and limb stability, lift the less supporting arm and when possible perform weight shift by reaching toward an object. | Limit titubation, rebound phenomenon, and increased incoordination due to exertion. Ensure that the patient uses appropriate righting reactions during the performance of the activity. |
| 8. Practice changing position in sitting | With guidance to the limbs, assist the patient in changing position into side sitting to the **opposite** side. Careful, deep, sustained pressure on the patient's trunk can be performed to assist her in stabilizing the trunk and limbs. When the patient has achieved optimal trunk and limb stability, lift the less supporting arm and when possible perform weight shift by reaching diagonally toward an object with the nonsupportive hand. | Change position by moving from side sitting on one side to side sitting on the other side. Perform the changing of positions with guidance at the limbs/trunk to independence on hard and soft surfaces. | Limit titubation, rebound phenomenon, and increased incoordination due to exertion. Ensure that the patient uses appropriate postural reactions during the performance of the activity. |
| | Taking systematically more weight on the legs, perform forward weight shift in preparation for standing up. | Reaching forward with or without supporting the arms on a table or a therapy ball. | Pick up an object from the floor. Prepare for putting on socks and shoes. | Limit titubation, rebound phenomenon, and increased incoordination due to exertion. Ensure that the patient uses appropriate postural |

*Continued*

| TABLE 21-7 | Mat Activities and Balance Training in Functional Positions—cont'd | | |
|---|---|---|---|
| **OPTIMIZING POSTURAL CONTROL IN FUNCTIONAL POSITIONS** | | | |
| *Aim* | *Principle* | *Example of Activity in Logical Sequence* | *Functional Activity to Be Practiced Functionally* | *Precautions/Contraindications* |
| | | Progression would be to reach downward to the feet to pick up an object. | | reactions during the performance of the activity. |

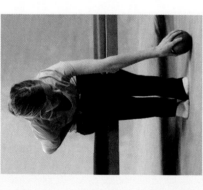

PNF techniques can be performed in sitting to optimize postural stability. Special caution should be given to prevention of aggravating titubation, ataxia/incoordination, and rebound phenomenon. Bilateral or unilateral PNF with the arms and trunk can be performed in sitting with the feet fully supported.

Frenkel exercises for the arms and/or legs in sitting with the feet fully supported can also be performed at this stage. This can be progressed to functional reaching activities during activities appropriate for the patients' self-care, household chores, socioeconomic role, etc.

Practice skilled functional activities of the upper limb in front of a table/in another appropriate environment.

Balance reactions can be practiced with the appropriate postural reactions and protective arm and leg reactions.

(The principles of PNF and Frenkel exercises are discussed in the text.)

| | | | | |
|---|---|---|---|---|
| 9. To achieve postural stability in standing | Change position from sitting to standing by using arm support, pressing down on a high surface to facilitate postural control. PRECAUTION: Standing up by pulling onto the parallel bars teaches the patient the wrong way of activating postural control during standing to sitting. | Change from sitting to standing from a high surface with a table in front of the patient for hand support in standing. Careful, deep, sustained pressure/approximation on the patient's trunk muscles and the pelvis/hip joints/upper legs to control knee extension can be performed to assist him/her in stabilizing the trunk and the hip | | If deep pressure/joint approximation increases titubation or rebound phenomenon, decrease the pressure but maintain the touch to facilitate stability of the patient's trunk/hip joints/legs to limit rebound phenomenon, and/or titubation as the trunk muscles contract/during standing. The patient should not have a surface on which she can pull herself up. |

*Continued*

joints/legs. When the patient has achieved optimal trunk stability, perform lateral weight shift followed by anterior-posterior weight shift in walk-standing.

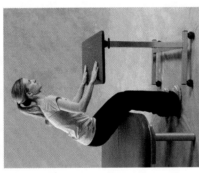 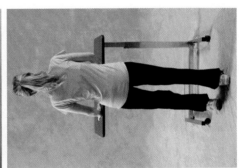

**TABLE 21-7    Mat Activities and Balance Training in Functional Positions—cont'd**

**OPTIMIZING POSTURAL CONTROL IN FUNCTIONAL POSITIONS**

| Aim | Principle | Example of Activity in Logical Sequence | Functional Activity to Be Practiced Functionally | Precautions/Contraindications |
|---|---|---|---|---|
| 10. Practice sitting to standing and standing to sitting. | Assist/facilitate postural control during changing position from standing to sitting in a symmetrical position. | Make the seating surface higher so the patient does not have to perform hip and knee flexion up to 90 degrees but only for about 30°. Sitting to standing and standing to sitting through a smaller range onto and from a higher surface decreases the effort of the activity but allows the patient to perform the activity in a more appropriate movement pattern. | Practice sitting to standing and standing to sitting. Practice sitting to standing and standing to sitting in relevant environments for the patient. Use rhythm/counting to assist the patient in performing coordinated movements. | Precautions as described in the previous section |
| 11. Prepare the patient for walking | Prepare the patient for walking by doing a lateral weight shift. Facilitate rotational trunk control further by performing weight shift in walk-standing. | Practice standing position with the arms symmetrically supported on a high surface/in parallel bars without grasping and pulling on the bars.<br><br>Standing in parallel bars is the position of choice for starting the weight shift.<br>Perform lateral weight shift by keeping the feet on the ground by | Practice marching in one spot by supporting the hands on a surface with an appropriate height. Use rhythm/counting to assist the patient in performing coordinated movements. | Precautions as described in the previous section |

lifting only the heels, progressed by lifting the feet alternately.

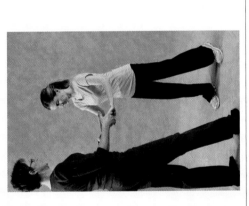

PNF to optimize the patient's postural stability in standing can be performed with the appropriate precautions as mentioned previously in sitting. Unexpected perturbation of the patient's balance in sitting or standing while reaching limits of stability. Carefully guard the patient to prevent falling. Reaching movements/activities in standing include trunk and arm movements.

Frenkel exercises in standing can also be performed at this stage. (Principles of Frenkel exercises are discussed in previous paragraphs.)

| 12. Progressing in preparing the patient for walking | Optimize postural control in standing and walking in a position that limits rotational trunk control. | Standing in a parallel bar with both hands holding onto the same bar (standing sideways in parallel bar) Initiate walking sideways while holding onto the parallel bar. Use rhythm/counting to assist the patient in performing coordinated movements. Vision can initially be used as a compensatory strategy to optimize coordination of the legs during the activity. A mirror can be used to optimize vision as a compensatory strategy if appropriate. | Practice walking sideways by pressing with the hands on a wall/holding onto furniture without grasping objects. | Precautions as described in the previous section |
| --- | --- | --- | --- | --- |
| 13. Practice walking | Optimize postural control in preparation for walking. | Assist the patient in adopting a walk-standing/step-standing position (pelvic rotation), arms symmetrically supported on a high surface/in parallel bar. Perform an anterior-posterior | Practice taking a step forward and backward. | Prevent compensatory strategies. All other precautions as described in the previous section Do not let the patient pull onto the parallel bars to prevent falling. |

*Continued*

**TABLE 21-7** Mat Activities and Balance Training in Functional Positions—cont'd

## OPTIMIZING POSTURAL CONTROL IN FUNCTIONAL POSITIONS

| Aim | Principle | Example of Activity in Logical Sequence | Functional Activity to Be Practiced Functionally | Precautions/Contraindications |
|---|---|---|---|---|
| | | weight shift by lifting only the heels/toes. Progress to lifting the feet alternately during anterior-posterior weight shift. | | Encourage the use of the trunk and protective stepping to maintain postural stability during gait. Once patients have learned to pull onto the parallel bars for stability, it is very difficult to unlearn the action, and it will limit their progress to more unstable walking aids. |
| | | Progress by walking forward and backward in the parallel bars by using rhythm/counting/vision as compensatory strategies to optimize coordination. (The principles of Frenkel exercises in standing can be performed at this stage.) | | Facilitate stability of the patient's trunk/hip joints/legs. Prevent compensatory strategies. All other precautions as described in the previous section |

The decision on how and where to start reeducation of gait and which walking aid to select depends on the patient's trunk and lower limb stability and coordination during optimizing postural stability in functional starting positions.

The most stable gait pattern that can be implemented is the four-point gait.

Progress to two-point gait with a reciprocal gait pattern with a walker that provides stability (of the arms and, as such, also the trunk) or an elbow crutch in each hand.

Further progression includes walking with a walking stick in one or both hands when the patient is relatively stable in standing.

Heavy walkers and/or weighted waist belts may decrease the presentation of ataxic gait but at the same time may increase patient fatigue (Armutlu, 2001).

Visual cues in the form of symmetrical marks on the floor that indicate an appropriate step length as well as rhythm (counting or verbal cueing to take steps) can optimize the patient's coordination and step length during gait.

Verbal feedback by the physiotherapist or caregiver; rhythm, and visual cues are still relevant even when the patient's gait has progressed to more unstable/less supportive walking aids.

Falling is very common in patients with degenerative cerebellar ataxia and often results in injuries and/or a fear of falling. Fear of falling can contribute to a decrease in the patient's mobility, leading to secondary physical impairment due to immobility, a decrease in community participation, and social isolation (van de Warrenburg, 2005).

14. Visuomotor education during functional activities enhances the equilibrium responses of patients with balance deficiencies secondary to cerebellar and vestibular ataxia, tabes dorsalis, and other somatosensory ataxias (Schulmann, 1987).

15. Balance and gait training progressed
Performing activities (step taking/walking) with eyes open and eyes closed
Walking on a line/tandem walking on a line with support and progressed to no support
Walking forward, sideways, backward and suddenly changing direction, stopping and starting movement/stepping, stepping over objects or walking around them, changing speed of walking from as fast as possible to as slow as possible
Walking on heels and toes, stair climbing, walking with turning the head (looking upward or sideways)
Unstable surfaces in sitting and standing can be used to progress balance exercises and, as such, optimize the patient's functional ability.

The main overall purpose of the mat activities and balance training in functional positions is to optimizing postural control in functional positions.

Activities should be practiced during a therapy session as well as during nontherapy sessions, as many times during the day as possible/relevant (Synofzik, 2014). Appropriate rest periods should be built into the day to prevent the perception of "overtraining" and to prevent cognitive and neuromusculoskeletal exhaustion.

Several examples of postural control implemented during functional activities in horizontal, sitting, and standing postures follow. During bridging in bed as part of shifting sideways (e.g., to change position or use a bedpan), the patient can flex the legs by keeping the feet on the bed. This provides more friction between the feet and the surface of the bed. Slight friction under the feet gives exteroceptive input, which can help the patient generate more postural control; the friction can also provide slight resistance to flexion of the knees and, as a result, provide somatosensory/proprioceptive feedback that can lead to a more coordinated movement.

When sitting at a table with the back and feet supported, the patient can reach forward toward functional objects by sliding the forearm and hand onto the table for additional exteroceptive input and slight resistance to the movement, without having to support the arm against gravity. The patient can be instructed to grasp an object and to change its position or perform an activity with it. Hard objects should be used in the beginning because patients will probably not be able to judge the firmness of the grasp needed as a result of the lack of anticipatory control. Drinking from a glass (half-filled with water/tea) can be performed initially by grasping the glass with both hands, supporting both elbows on the table, and performing elbow flexion to drink. When the patient has reached optimal functional capacity, a compensatory strategy that can be encouraged is to hold the glass/cup with both hands and press the hands together, giving additional proximal stability (compensatory fixation) while allowing function (drinking from the glass).

While sitting at a table with the back and feet supported, the patient can push his feet alternately forward with slight friction on the floor followed by lifting the foot to perform knee extension. If the patient is not ambulating and is using a wheelchair, progression would include lifting the foot in order to put it onto the footrest of the wheelchair.

To learn independent standing, the patient sits in front of a table on a chair with the back supported and the hands on the table. The action to be performed is flexion of the knees until the feet (toes) are in line with the knees. The patient then stands by using the upper extremities for support. Standing from a higher surface reduces the effort of standing and decreases the possibility of eliciting a rebound phenomenon or excessive fixation, which may contribute to learning unwanted compensatory strategies (Carr, 1998).

Functional standing can be performed in various rooms in the house (e.g., the kitchen, bathroom, or bedroom) or in a functional area in the rehabilitation center that has a stable surface the patient can hold on to while walking sideways or forward, without pulling on the surface/rail (Table 21-7). The patient should adhere to the principles learned during the previous functional session on optimizing postural control during ADLs.

## THINK ABOUT IT 21.2

- How might the sequence of the proprioceptive neuromuscular facilitation (PNF), Frenkel exercises, Cawthorne-Cooksey exercises, and mat activities and balance training differ during an intervention session in a patient with cerebellar ataxia/incoordination versus a patient with somatosensory ataxia/incoordination?
- How might PNF, Frenkel exercises, Cawthorne-Cooksey exercises, and mat activities and balance training be integrated during an intervention session?

### *General Precautions During Intervention*

Therapists should consider several precautions while treating individuals with ataxia/incoordination (Box 21-3).

## Pediatric Considerations

The principles and techniques for coordination intervention described previously apply equally to children. The therapist must find creative ways to motivate the child to participate in activities that provide meaningful, engaging practice of enhanced control/coordination. For example, **hippotherapy** (riding a horse for therapeutic purposes) is one coordination intervention technique that may be effective in children (Bertoti, 1988). Practicing coordination in midrange positions and postures first and then progressing to full-range movements may be helpful. Depending on the age and ability of the child, it may be important to ensure some form of support or external stability while the child is practicing coordination of the trunk in various postures. Working on nonskid surfaces can be very helpful. Playing with heavier (weighted) toys or objects may provide additional resistance and contribute to enhanced somatosensory feedback. In addition, a child may be intrigued by performing play or functional activities using cuff weights at the wrist or ankle or weighted tools/utensils. Theraputty or Play-Doh® can provide valuable resistance to finger and thumb movements. Most important, the therapist must find therapeutic activities that interest and excite the child, making him want to participate.

### *Monitoring the Patient's Progress*

It is important to monitor improvements in the patient's impairment (muscle strength and incoordination), functional activity, and participation level. Implementation of outcome measures on all three levels of the International Classification of Functioning, Disability and Health (ICF) is important to objectively monitor response to therapy.

Monitor spontaneous functional activities during treatments that indicate less dependence on visual input, as well as during spontaneous activities that challenge the patient's balance. Also, determine the effects on the patient's perceived experience of exertion and/or cardiovascular endurance during the intervention, as well as during general lifestyle functions (assessment on participation level).

Monitoring the patient's progress includes observing the way activities are performed during and across treatment

## BOX 21-3 Precautions During Intervention

- Limit resistance/tasks the patient performs against gravity requiring excessive effort. These activities may aggravate symptoms, such as titubation (in the case of patients with cerebellar lesions) and incoordination or rebound phenomenon (in patients with cerebellar as well as somatosensory ataxia).
- Avoid compensatory strategies while optimizing the patient's postural control; these strategies should be encouraged only when the patient has reached his optimal postural control during various tasks relevant to his prognosis.
- When the patient has decreased cardiovascular fitness, take into consideration the activity intensity and frequency to avoid overexertion, especially in patients with ataxia as part of the signs and symptoms of multiple sclerosis (Armutlu, 2001) and patients who present with asthenia. Incoordination/ataxic movements will likely increase as the patient fatigues.
- Teach patients to monitor their own perceived level of exertion. This precaution is important to empower them to adapt their functional level to activities of daily living.
- Be aware that visual and cognitive control of movement requires concentration and, as such, may cause mental fatigue. When quality of movement deteriorates because of mental or physical fatigue, the patient should rest/rehabilitation should be terminated.
- Note if eye movements are specifically emphasized during treatment; this may contribute to a temporary headache and is an indication of overexertion of the oculomotor muscles.
- Use task variability only when the patient can adapt and anticipate movements/activities. Determine the patient's motivation or willingness to learn to adapt to a variety of tasks before introducing a variety of tasks. A patient's ability to learn variations in tasks may be limited, or it may take longer to learn task variations.

sessions. Postural control of the trunk and limbs provides the patient feedback on task performance and allows the patient to know when to adapt aspects of a home program. Give special attention to the way in which the patient maintains balance. Is the patient able to maintain balance through central/proximal (postural reactions) or distal changes in postural control or protective supporting reactions? Use of the limbs to maintain postural control during activities limits the patient's functional ability to manipulate objects.

Postural trunk control severely affects the stability and control of movement at the proximal joints (glenohumeral and hip joints). The proximal joints provide the stability upon which distal joints/hands can move to accurately pick up small objects, to write, or to perform other fine motor skills with appropriately selective movement patterns. For this reason, it is important to continuously evaluate the influence of central and proximal control on the manipulation of objects (e.g., during household tasks, writing) and the performance of skilled movements with the feet (e.g., walking over uneven terrain).

Fixation in functional positions (as a compensatory strategy) may be noted in the patient's flexion posture, the position of the arms during gait (slight glenohumeral abduction and flexion), and flexion/adduction of the metacarpophalangeal joints with decreased arm swing during gait. The flexed posture may be caused secondary to the patient automatically lowering his center of mass toward the supporting surface as well as visually fixating on the floor in an attempt to stabilize the head and/or trunk.

## PATIENT APPLICATION I-C: TREATMENT PROGRESSION

*Marleen was treated according to the principles and guidelines presented in Table 21-7. Marleen's mother, her main caregiver, was with her the whole day. Therefore, she implemented the treatment principles in her ADLs to enhance the effect of the intervention.*

*By the end of the second week, Marleen could move independently from a lying to a sitting position at the edge of the bed. She could sit independently without back support and reach down to put on her shoes while holding onto the bed with one hand. She could stand up from the bed with the support of one person but did so by extending her knees into hyperextension while her trunk and hips were still flexed and before she extended her trunk and hips. (Passive and active ranges of motion at the ankle were normal and could not be a reason for the abnormal sequence of movement during standing up). She could walk with unilateral arm support provided by the therapist (Fig. 21-6).*

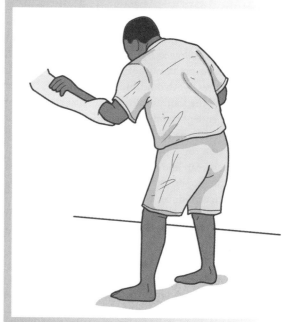

**FIGURE 21-6** Patient with cerebellar ataxia/incoordination walking with support.

*Contemplate Clinical Decisions 1-C: Treatment Progression*

1. Use the principles of progression to develop three different ways of modifying Marleen's activities to emphasize optimal function over the next several weeks.

2. What other treatment settings and environmental contexts would you consider for Marleen's treatment?

3. Formulate and describe at least two additional (different) treatment ideas that should be applied to improve Marleen's function.

## THINK ABOUT IT 21.3

### Return to Case 1C.

- Which abnormal stabilizing strategies is the patient using to stand up?
- What effects can this abnormal stabilizing strategy have on the patient's knee joints?
- How should the physical therapist limit the patient's abnormal stabilizing strategies during intervention?
- When should a physical therapist allow a patient to compensate rather than preventing abnormal stabilizing strategies?

## ■ Intervention: Considerations for Nontherapy Time and Discharge

### Activities for Home

Patients with cerebellar or somatosensory ataxia have an impaired body schema and therefore constantly overcompensate with their movements to overcome the instability or lack of awareness of where their limbs (especially the affected lower extremities) are in space. Patients with somatosensory incoordination do not have adequate and/or accurate feedback to the cerebellum to attain effective cerebellar control of movement. To enhance self-management, patients with cerebellar as well as somatosensory incoordination should be given advice and/or the opportunity to practice cognitive control over their limbs under guidance of the therapist; this will help to decrease overcompensation in the form of unwanted reactions and/or fixation of the trunk and limbs and enable more independent movement. Because of the poor body schema, patients also have impaired motor planning and therefore have

to learn to cognitively plan their movement as well as "let go" or consciously inhibit the fixation to optimize their postural control. A practical suggestion to the patient would be "to relax and start moving more slowly and think about what you are doing."

Using the Xbox kinect or the Wii balance platform (exergames) at home is fun and highly motivating for the patient and provides an effective way of improving function. Synofzik (2014) found that the more patients are involved in a home exercise program (by using the exergames), the more beneficial it is to maintain their functional capacity. Ilg (2010) found that patients who followed a "coordinative physiotherapy program" with a home program consisting of safe exercises for 1 hour per day for 1 year were able to maintain the relative functional performance they gained in the original program. Patients with progressive disease continued to progress but maintained the functional performance equivalent to 2 or more years of disease progression. Patients' goal attainment scores demonstrated that they were able to translate the effect of the training into important functions in daily life. Patients with afferent ataxia (somatosensory ataxia) made less progress than patients with cerebellar ataxia.

Another way for patients to overcome overcompensation is to consciously change their movement strategies to make them mechanically easier to perform. A good example is sitting on higher surfaces from which they have to stand up and sit down again. Higher surfaces require less muscle power and decrease incoordination. Another example is paying attention to the difference in performing a supported movement versus performing a movement in free space. Changing the environment or planning to perform tasks differently to decrease the effort required could become a helpful lifestyle strategy.

Patients with a degenerative cerebellar disease are usually discharged when they have reached a plateau in terms of their functional ability. In clinical practice, patients can periodically be readmitted to a rehabilitation program to maintain—or if possible improve—their functional ability. Improvement of ataxia depends on the extent to which patients are actively involved in a home program (Synofzik, 2014).

Consciously implementing skills learned during therapy sessions in ADLs at home/work/leisure environments enhances patients' functional ability. Having a routine of daily activity/home exercises that enhances the maintenance of functional ability and can be incorporated into the patient's lifestyle is also important (Ilg, 2009; Synofzik, 2014).

## HANDS-ON PRACTICE

Be sure to practice the following skills discussed in this chapter:

- Implementing and interpreting the outcome measures specifically related to ataxia/incoordination (i.e., the SARA and ICARS)
- PNF rhythmic initiation, combination of isotonics (agonistic reversal), isotonic reversal (slow reversal),

and rhythmic stabilization (stabilizing reversal) of the upper and lower limbs
- Frenkel exercises described in Box 21-2
- Cawthorne-Cooksey exercises described in Table 21-6
- Mat activities and balance training described in Table 21-7 and in Chapter 30

## Let's Review

1. Summarize the physiology of coordinated movement.

2. Discuss the etiology, pathogenesis, and clinical presentation of ataxia/incoordination.

3. Explain the differential diagnosis between ataxia/incoordination due to a somatosensory impairment and to a cerebellar impairment.

4. Discuss the evaluation principles that are applicable for a patient who presents with ataxia/incoordination.

5. Discuss the principles of intervention for designing an appropriate rehabilitation program for patients with cerebellar and somatosensory ataxia/incoordination.

6. Discuss the precautions, monitoring, and home program for patients with cerebellar and somatosensory ataxia/incoordination.

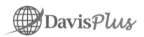 For additional resources, including Focus on Evidence tables, case study discussions, references and glossary, please visit http://davisplus.fadavis.com

## CHAPTER SUMMARY

In this chapter, the basic anatomy and physiology required to understand the etiology, pathogenesis, and clinical presentation of cerebellar and somatosensory ataxia/incoordination are discussed. The evaluation of a patient with ataxia/incoordination and its effects on impairment, activity, and participation levels is also addressed. The differential diagnoses between cerebellar and somatosensory ataxia/incoordination are summarized in Tables 21-4 and 21-5. The approach to intervention and the intervention principles are also explained.

Evidence on the positive effects of intervention in patients with cerebellar ataxia/incoordination is emerging. More research regarding physical therapy for patients with somatosensory ataxia/incoordination is necessary, but even patients with such impairment can benefit dramatically through use of unimpaired somatosensory input (neural adaptation) and compensatory strategies to improve their functional ability. A well-planned and motivational home program is beneficial for patients with cerebellar impairment.

# Interventions for Weakness in Neuromotor Disorders

Cathy C. Harro, PT, MS, NCS ▪ Kim Curbow Wilcox, PT, MS, PhD, NCS    CHAPTER 22

## CHAPTER OBJECTIVES

Upon completion of this chapter, the learner will be able to:

1. Describe factors influencing muscle force generation in healthy individuals and those with neurological conditions, including neural, structural, and mechanical factors.
2. Justify the rationale for and efficacy of strength training for persons with neurological conditions on the basis of current evidence.
3. Apply exercise science principles in the selection and prescription of strength training interventions to address weakness deficits in patients with neurological conditions.
4. Design a customized strength exercise program for specific areas of weakness in patients with neurological conditions, selecting from a variety of modes of strength training.
5. Discuss the benefits and preventive role of strength training in home- and community-based fitness programs for persons with progressive and nonprogressive neurological conditions to optimize functional abilities and improve health outcomes.

## ▪ Introduction

Strength training is a critical ingredient in physical rehabilitation for people with neuromuscular disorders because of its potential to remediate weakness deficits, prevent secondary impairments, and promote optimal health and wellness. Muscle weakness is a primary impairment in many neurological disorders and a major contributor to activity limitations and disability (Bohannon, 2007; Cameron, 2003; Kim, 2003). Strength deficits often result in limitation of an individual's functional abilities, which may require orthotics and/or assistive devices to ambulate and perform other functional tasks safely in the home or community. Excessive fatigue during activities of daily living (ADLs) and walking, related to weakness, can adversely affect community reintegration and quality

of life (Ingles 1999; White, McCoy, 2004). Current research supports the use of strength training in persons with neuromuscular disorders as an effective intervention to enhance neuromuscular function and motor recovery (Dodd, 2002; Morris, 2004; Patten, 2004; White & Dressendorfer, 2004).

Early neurorehabilitation approaches were focused on motor retraining of selective and controlled movements, with attention to quality of movement (Bobath, 1984; Howle, 2004; Sawner, 1992). Direct strengthening exercises were discouraged based on the false assumption that these types of exercises exacerbated spasticity and adversely affected motor control. Current evidence disputes this assumption, however, and provides strong support for the efficacy of strength training in persons with neurological disorders, even in the presence of spasticity (Badics, 2002; Flansbjer, 2008; Fowler, 2001; Miller, 1997). In contrast to earlier beliefs, strengthening exercises may positively affect muscle function at the structural level by reducing muscle stiffness and at the neural level by improving recruitment and timing.

Clinicians should incorporate strengthening exercises to target weak muscles for individuals with varied neurological diagnoses, including cerebral palsy (CP), stroke/cerebrovascular accident (CVA), acquired brain injury (ABI), multiple sclerosis (MS), and Parkinson disease (PD). Special considerations for exercise prescription should be given to individuals with progressive neuromuscular diseases such as amyotrophic lateral sclerosis (ALS) (Dal Bello-Haas, 2008, 2002).

For persons with neurological disorders, a customized exercise program is required to address their specific strength deficits and restore requisite motor function for daily tasks. Because of the complexity of the multisystem impairments and varied patterns of weakness in this population, skilled exercise prescription and design are critical to successful rehabilitation outcomes. Furthermore, strength training may be used in wellness programs to reduce the risk of comorbidities, prevent disuse atrophy, and slow functional decline in individuals in chronic stages of ABI or CVA, as well as for persons with progressive neurological conditions such as MS or PD. In addition to the direct strength benefits, active engagement in strengthening and aerobic exercises has been beneficial for cardiovascular, psychological, physical, and functional status, as well as to enhance bone health (Gordon, 2004; Petajan, 1996; White & Dressendorfer, 2004).

To design an individualized exercise prescription for a patient, the clinician should first complete a comprehensive physical therapy evaluation, assessing the nature, distribution, and severity of the strength deficits, and analyzing the effect of the strength impairments on the patient's functional limitations. The prognosis for potential improvements in strength and function should then be determined to prioritize areas of weakness addressed in treatment. After completing the evaluation, the therapist should design a customized strengthening intervention that takes into account the unique characteristics of the patient, such as diagnosis, age, comorbidities, functional level, balance abilities, and level of motor control recovery or stage of disease progression. Ongoing evaluation and progression of the exercise prescription is important to continually

challenge the neuromuscular system to adapt and to facilitate optimal recovery.

This chapter provides an overview of the strength deficits in persons with neuromuscular disorders, evidence that strength training effectively remediates weakness impairments and enhances overall function, and a focus on interventions for strengthening. Refer to Chapters 24 and 25 for interventions to specifically improve motor control. Primary emphasis in this chapter is on the clinical application of exercise science principles for developing strength training programs in individuals with neurological conditions and the application of therapeutic techniques and different exercise modes for strength training. Principles of exercise design and progression are demonstrated in Patient Application boxes throughout the chapter. Focus on Evidence Tables 22-20 through 22-25 (ONL) summarize the efficacy of various modes of strength training in specific neurological disorders.

## Clinical Picture of Strength and Weakness

### Force Generation in Healthy Individuals

Muscle strength can be defined as "the ability of a muscle to generate tension and control force production for the purpose of stability and mobility of the musculoskeletal system necessary for functional activities" (Harris, 2006, p. 24). Consider this simplistic definition of strength: the amount of torque that is generated during a single maximal isometric contraction (Enoka, 1994). Although this definition facilitates a clear objective measure of an individual's strength capability, the force-generation ability needed for functional skills is more complex and dynamic than this definition suggests. Functional strength is the capacity of a muscle or group of muscles to produce force necessary for initiating, maintaining, and controlling movement. Key terms related to a muscle's ability to generate tension can be found in Table 22-1.

The force-generating capability of a muscle is influenced by neural, structural, and mechanical factors. Weakness can result from deficits in a single factor or in a combination of factors. Neural factors underlying force production are related to the ability of the central nervous system (CNS) to effectively recruit and activate **motor units** (MUs), which in turn produce contraction of a group of muscle fibers. An MU encompasses

| TABLE 22-1 | Key Terms Related to Muscle Tension Generation |
|---|---|
| *Aspects of Muscle Performance Related to Force* | |
| Work | Force applied over a distance |
| Power | The rate at which work is performed (work/time or force × velocity) |
| Muscle endurance | The ability of a muscle to contract repeatedly against loads and resist fatigue over an extended time |
| *Types of Muscle Contractions* | |
| Concentric | The force developed by a muscle exceeds the magnitude of external force, resulting in shortening of the muscle |
| Isometric | The force developed by a muscle equals the magnitude of external force, resulting in no motion |
| Eccentric | The external force exceeds the force developed by a muscle, resulting in lengthening of the muscle |

an alpha motor neuron and all the muscle fibers innervated by the neuron. Disruption of descending supraspinal inputs to the alpha motor neurons or disruption of signals at the segmental spinal cord (SC) level can result in impaired MU activation and weakness. The CNS generates muscle tension by increasing the number of MUs recruited and the firing frequency and by recruiting larger MUs.

There are three types of MUs: slow, fast fatigue resistant, and fast fatigable. Table 22-2 provides descriptions of these

| TABLE 22-2 | Description of Motor Unit Classification |
|---|---|
| Slow motor unit (MU) | Composed of small axons that innervate a few small, slow, oxidative muscle fibers (type I); has a low threshold for recruitment |
| Fast fatigue-resistant MU | Composed of moderate-sized axons that innervate fast, oxidative, glycolytic muscle fibers (type IIa); has a moderate threshold for recruitment |
| Fast fatigable MU | Composed of large axons that innervate many large glycolytic muscle fibers (type IIb); has a high threshold for recruitment |

MU classifications (Harris, 2006). Figure 22-1 illustrates MU types and their respective twitch characteristics.

The normal order of MU activation is initial recruitment of the smaller slow MUs and then activation of the larger fast MUs as demand for force generation increases. This sequenced MU recruitment order is called the **size principle** (Henneman, 1965). Neural activation deficits influence one's ability to drive the MU pool and to efficiently regulate the MU firing rate (rate coding) for adequate force generation. Strength training facilitates neural adaptation, improving the efficiency of MU firing frequency, increasing MU recruitment, and activating previously inactive muscle fibers. This neural adaptation process is thought to be responsible for early (4 to 6 weeks) strength gains in healthy individuals, whereas muscle hypertrophy accounts for later (6 to 12 weeks) strength gains (Kraemer, 2000, 2013; McArdle, 2010). In neurological populations, however, improvement in neural activation plus regulation and synchronization of MU firing contribute more substantially to strength gains. These changes may reflect neural plasticity at the supraspinal or segmental spinal levels, as well as at the neuromuscular junction (Kraemer, 2013; Patten, 2004, 2013).

### Structural Factors

Structural factors underlying force production include the size and cross-sectional area (CSA) of a muscle, muscle fiber type and arrangement, and muscle fiber distribution (Kisner, 2012;

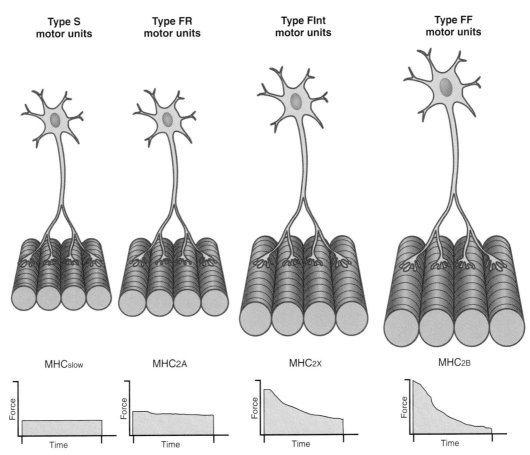

**FIGURE 22-1** Classification of motor unit types from a muscle based on histochemical profile, size, and twitch characteristics.

Soderberg, 1992). The ability of a muscle to generate tension is directly related to the size and CSA of the muscle. Larger muscles, such as quadriceps and gastrocnemius muscles, have greater tension-producing capacity than smaller muscles. During functional tasks, these larger muscles provide power for moving from sit-to-stand or walking up a flight of stairs. Strength training with progressive overloads during a 6- to 10-week period produces **muscle hypertrophy**, or increased muscle size, in both healthy and neurological populations. This muscle hypertrophy, resulting from an increase in number and size of myofibrils, improves the muscle's force-generating capacity.

Muscle fiber arrangement also influences the force-generation capability of a muscle. Short muscle fibers oriented in a pinnate or multipinnate design are angled 30 degrees up and away from the direction of force. This type of fiber orientation, found in muscles such as deltoid and gastrocnemius muscles, allows for large force production. Long muscle fibers oriented in a parallel design, such as those in sartorius or biceps femoris muscles, allow for a high rate of shortening (speed) but less force production than muscles with pinnate arrangement (see Fig. 22-2). There is functional specificity to this muscle fiber arrangement in the musculoskeletal system. Muscles that need

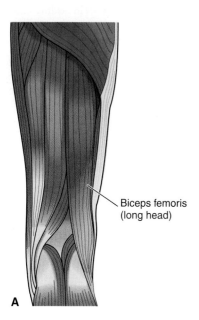

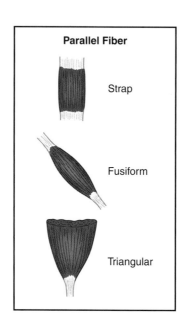

Biceps femoris
(long head)

A

**Parallel Fiber**

Strap

Fusiform

Triangular

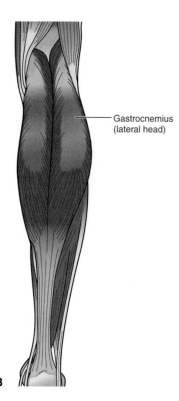

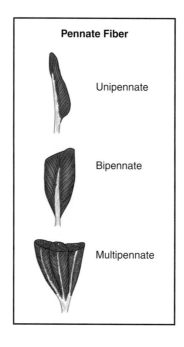

Gastrocnemius
(lateral head)

B

**Pennate Fiber**

Unipennate

Bipennate

Multipennate

**FIGURE 22-2A AND 22-2B** Skeletal muscle fiber arrangement. (A) Parallel muscle fibers as shown in the long head of a biceps femoris muscle. (B) Pennate muscle fibers as shown in the lateral belly of a gastrocnemius muscle.

to move a long lever arm quickly, such as biceps femoris for a quick knee flexion action, are usually composed of parallel muscle fiber orientations; conversely, muscles that need considerable strength to control or propel body weight, such as the *quadriceps* muscle, exhibit multipinnate fiber orientation. This functional specificity of muscle fiber type and arrangement should be considered when designing exercises for strength training.

A final structural factor influencing force generation is muscle fiber type distribution. Muscles are composed of different fiber types influenced by genetic predisposition, the muscle's function, and neural input (Astrand, 2003). Refer to Table 22-3 for a description of fiber type classification. Disuse of muscles, whether from inactivity or from loss of neural activation due to a central lesion, results in muscle atrophy and loss of both type I and type II muscle fibers. In individuals with neurological disorders, selective atrophy of type II fibers is evident, observed clinically as slowed force production and impaired ability to produce force effectively for functional tasks (Frontera, 1997; Hachisuka, 1997).

## THINK ABOUT IT 22.1

Prevention of disuse atrophy should be an important therapeutic goal in both the acute and chronic stages for clients with neuromuscular diagnoses.

- Although strengthening exercises limited to slow submaximal effort by the patient may be training only slow type I muscle fibers, building higher loads and/or speed into exercise programs is important to target type II fibers. As a clinician, pick a target muscle and describe how you can keep in mind the structural properties and functional role of the targeted muscle when prescribing strengthening exercises and intentionally build in higher loads and speeds in motor exercise.

### *Mechanical Factors*

Mechanical factors pertinent to a muscle's ability to generate force are length-tension and velocity-tension relationships. The **length-tension relationship** refers to the optimal length at which a muscle can generate maximal tension based on the binding capacity between actin and myosin molecules of the muscle fibers, according to **Starling's Law** (Astrand, 2003). Optimal length for maximal tension is near midpoint in the range of motion (ROM), whereas less force is generated when a muscle is in either the shortened or lengthened position.

In addition to muscle length, the speed of contraction affects the binding capacity of actin and myosin. The **velocity-tension relationship** refers to the inverse association between muscle tension and velocity of movement during concentric contractions. That is, as movement velocity increases, the muscle's ability to generate force decreases because actin and myosin cannot bind as efficiently during high-velocity movements (Harris, 2006). A patient may be able to slowly lift a heavy load, but the load would need to be reduced if the training goal was to

| TABLE 22-3 | Classification of Muscle Fiber Types |
|---|---|
| **MUSCLE FIBER TYPE** | **DESCRIPTION** |
| I (slow, tonic, oxidative) | Low force production<br>Sustained, repeated muscle contraction<br>Resistant to fatigue |
| II (fast, phasic)<br> IIa (fast, oxidative, glycolytic)<br> IIb (fast, phasic, glycolytic | High force production<br>Anaerobic and aerobic metabolism, fatigues slowly<br>Rapid, high-tension contraction, fatigues rapidly |

increase movement velocity. These velocity-muscle tension concepts should be considered when setting strength goals and when prescribing exercise for patients with a neurological diagnosis. Poststroke, for example, individuals have exaggerated strength impairments as movement speed demands increase (Nakumura, 1988). Training strength as opposed to muscle power (velocity dependent) requires prescription of different loads and speeds of movement.

## Effect of Weakness on Function

When an individual develops weakness, whether as a result of the typical aging process or from a neurological disorder, reduced ability to generate force has a detrimental effect on functional skill and activity. Limitations to functional activity can then contribute to decreased participation in life. For example, Mrs. Smith, now 94 years old but otherwise healthy, has decreased strength throughout her LEs and UEs, particularly in the antigravity muscles. As a result, she experiences difficulty with transfers, such as rising from the toilet or dining room chair, and it takes much more time for her to rise out of bed in the morning. She also has impaired balance reactions because of the weakness. Weight-bearing aspects of functional activities, such as climbing stairs, have become difficult and laborious. A critical threshold of adequate strength in the legs is necessary for Mrs. Smith to perform her daily functional tasks without undue fatigue. Weakness in the upper extremities (UEs) can result in difficulty with UE tasks, such as use of the arms to push during supine-to-sit transitions and functional reach or grasp activities.

## ■ Related Pathology

### Strength Impairments in Neuromuscular Diagnoses

Weakness is a primary impairment that adversely affects functional skill performance in a wide range of neurological diagnoses. Refer to Table 22-4 for an overview of neurological diagnoses classified by Neuromuscular Preferred Practice Patterns (*APTA*, 2015). In adults with nonprogressive neurological disorders affecting the CNS (*Pattern 5D*), such as stroke and TBI, strength impairments secondary to central activation

| TABLE 22-4 | Physical Therapy Preferred Practice Patterns: Neuromuscular System | | | |
|---|---|---|---|---|
| **PATTERN 5C** | **PATTERN 5D** | **PATTERN 5E** | **PATTERN 5G** | **PATTERN 5H** |
| Impaired motor function and sensory integrity associated with nonprogressive disorders of the central nervous system (CNS); congenital origin or acquired in infancy or childhood | Impaired motor function and sensory integrity associated with nonprogressive disorders of the CNS; acquired in adolescence or adulthood | Impaired motor function and sensory integrity associated with progressive disorders of the CNS | Impaired motor function and sensory integrity associated with acute or chronic polyneuropathies | Impaired motor function, peripheral nerve integrity, and sensory integrity associated with nonprogressive disorders of the spinal cord |
| • Anoxia/hypoxia<br>• Birth trauma<br>• Brain anomalies<br>• Cerebral palsy<br>• Encephalitis<br>• Hydrocephalus<br>• Infectious disease of the CNS<br>• Meningocele<br>• Neoplasm<br>• Tethered cord<br>• Traumatic brain injury | • Aneurysm<br>• Anoxia/hypoxia<br>• Stroke<br>• Infectious disease of the CNS<br>• Intracranial neurosurgery<br>• Neoplasm<br>• Seizures<br>• Traumatic brain injury | • AIDS<br>• Alcoholic ataxia<br>• Alzheimer disease<br>• Amyotrophic lateral sclerosis (ALS)<br>• Basal ganglia disorders<br>• Cerebellar disease<br>• Huntington disease<br>• Multiple sclerosis<br>• Parkinson disease<br>• Progressive muscular atrophy<br>• Seizures | • Amputation<br>• Axonal polyneuropathies<br>• ANS dysfunction<br>• Guillain-Barré syndrome<br>• Leprosy<br>• Postpolio syndrome | • Benign spinal neoplasm<br>• Complete or incomplete spinal cord injury<br>• Infectious diseases of the spinal cord (SC)<br>• SC compression<br>• Degenerative spinal joint disease<br>• Herniated disk<br>• Osteomyelitis<br>• Spondylosis |

deficits have been well documented, are directly related to the specific site and severity of the brain injury, and are correlated with functional status. Remediation of these strength deficits facilitates improved functional outcomes. In adults with progressive neurological disorders affecting the CNS (*Pattern 5E*), such as MS, PD, and ALS, a progressive decline in strength may be seen in varied muscle groups bilaterally. The decline depends on the site of neuropathology in the CNS and the duration of disease, with substantial effects on the individual's functional independence and quality of life. Individuals with neurological disorders involving the SC (*Pattern 5H*), either traumatic or degenerative, have weakness or total paralysis that correlates to the site (segmental or SC level) and the extent of SC damage (i.e., complete vs. incomplete spinal cord injury [SCI]). The extent of expected motor function recovery depends on the degree of sparing of motor pathways and neuroplasticity at the SC.

Children with nonprogressive disorders of the CNS (*Pattern 5C*), such as CP and brain anoxia/hypoxia, also have primary strength impairments that adversely affect motor development and skill acquisition (Damiano, 1998; Verschuren, 2008). Therefore, it is important to incorporate strength training into their developmental interventions.

In pathologies affecting the peripheral nervous system, such as Guillain-Barré syndrome (GBS) or polyneuropathies, weakness is the primary clinical manifestation that adversely affects function. In GBS, there is a progressive symmetrical loss of motor function that ascends from distal to proximal and may eventually involve respiratory and oral motor musculature.

The recovery phase is gradual and requires careful exercise prescription to avoid fatigue or overworking weakened, recovering muscles. Similarly, individuals with postpolio syndrome who display new-onset muscle weakness after 15+ years of stability of symptoms require skilled exercise prescription to avoid overworking already metabolically overextended motor units (Jubelt, 2004; Klein, 2002).

Clinical presentation of weakness varies across these diverse neurological diagnoses. Considering the patient's diagnosis, clinicians must carefully examine the distribution, severity, and nature of the strength deficits when developing an individualized plan of care. For example, different approaches to exercise design are required for clients with nonprogressive versus progressive neurological disorders, although both benefit from strength training. The patient's diagnosis and the time after injury or after diagnosis influence the therapeutic goals and expected outcomes related to weakness.

In addition to their primary strength impairments, individuals with neurological disorders are at risk for developing secondary strength impairments because of reduced mobility and activity levels. These secondary deficits compound the adverse effects of weakness on function, yet they can be prevented with exercise programs and patient education regarding the importance of these exercises in maintaining optimal function.

### Poststroke Weakness Impairments

The nature and distribution of poststroke strength deficits have been well documented in the literature; this information can help direct examination of strength impairments and guide decisions for designing strength interventions. Remember that the therapist needs to take care to identify whether the problem is simply force generation or an impairment of motor control, and particularly selective/isolated motor control (see Chapter 6). The distribution of weakness is primarily on the paretic side contralateral to the brain lesion; however, there is also strong evidence of mild weakness on the side ipsilateral to the lesion. On the basis of this evidence, bilateral strength training is warranted (Bohannon, 2007; Dragert, 2013; Eng, 2004; Patten, 2004).

Strength deficits are greater in the distal muscles than in the proximal muscles, since recovery is usually observed earliest in proximal muscles, and weakness can be found in the trunk muscles as well as the extremities (Adams, 1990). Flexor and extensor musculature appears to be equally affected. The degree of weakness is related to the stroke location and severity, ranging from hemiparesis (mild to moderate weakness) to hemiplegia (severe or complete loss). Poststroke weakness is reflected not just by reduced force generation, but also by slowness in force production, an excessive sense of effort, rapid onset of fatigue, and difficulty producing force effectively for specific task (Canning, 1999; Ingles, 1999; Patten, 2004). These force-generation deficits have notable effects on the performance of functional skills and consequently warrant directed intervention in stroke rehabilitation programs.

The underlying causes of poststroke weakness are primary central activation deficits, transsynaptic degeneration, and secondary changes in muscle. Damage to supraspinal pathways, particularly the corticospinal tract, results in diminished MU recruitment and regulation of MU activity. Because of this disrupted neural input, transsynaptic degeneration occurs at the spinal level, leading to motor neuron loss and altered excitability of the motor neuron pool (Eng, 2004; Landau, 2002). Refer to Table 22-5 for a summary of MU characteristics and muscle fiber changes after a stroke (Frontera, 1997; Jakobsson, 1991; McComas, 1973; Rosenfalck, 1980; Scelsi, 1984). These MU deficits are evident clinically as slow, inefficient muscle activation and difficulty regulating force output for functional tasks. When spasticity is present, altered viscoelastic and mechanical properties of paretic muscle, such as increased stiffness and overstretched sarcomeres, can also reduce force generation (Dietz, 1986; Fridén, 2003; Lamontagne, 2002).

Strength deficits are notably related to functional limitations after a stroke; hence, remediation of these deficits is important to maximize functional outcomes. Paretic lower limb strength has been significantly correlated with sit-to-stand and transfer abilities, as well as gait and stair function (Bohannon, 1990, 2007). Paretic hip flexor, knee extensor, and plantar flexor strength are strongly associated with gait function and gait recovery after a stroke (Bohannon, 1992; Nakumura, 1988; Olney, 1991; Pohl, 2002). Poststroke UE strength has been correlated with UE function and level of independence in ADLs (Boissy, 1999; Bohannon, 1992). The severity of weakness also directly relates to the need for orthotics and assistive devices for functional task performance. Energy expenditure for daily activities and walking is increased poststroke secondary to weakness and deconditioning (Ingles, 1999; Walters, 1989). A critical threshold of strength is necessary for efficient functional task performance. After a stroke, individuals often lack this requisite strength, or they may have barely sufficient strength to reach the threshold for functional capacity but lack functional reserve, resulting in rapid fatigue (Bohannon, 2007).

### Weakness Impairments in Acquired Brain Injury

The nature and distribution of strength impairments in individuals with an ABI can be widely variable depending on the sites of focal and diffuse brain injury. Strength impairments are documented in 54-58% of patients with ABI, and 82-84% recover to normal strength at one year follow-up (Brown, 2007).

Additionally, concomitant extremity factures are common following traumatic brain injury (Grotz, 2004), and compound the clinical weakness picture. The distribution of weakness following ABI may be hemiparetic in focal cortical injury or bleed, similar to that of individuals with stroke (Allison, 1999; Karman, 2003). Patients with brainstem injuries, multiple cortical injuries, bilateral cortical lesions, or diffuse axonal injury may have bilateral weakness along with other major motor control, muscle tone, and balance deficits.

The underlying cause of weakness in ABI is primarily central neural activation deficits, with impaired ability to activate MUs. However, peripheral factors may also contribute, particularly disuse atrophy. Many ABI survivors may have prolonged periods of immobility secondary to coma, medical instability, and/or fractures. These patients often present with multisystem impairments requiring extensive rehabilitation. Weakness is a key system impairment that should be targeted in a comprehensive treatment plan.

### Weakness Impairments in Multiple Sclerosis

MS is a demyelinating disorder in the CNS that can cause scattered regions of axonal degeneration and reduced or blocked nerve conduction, which may disrupt supraspinal or spinal pathways to the MU pool, resulting in weakness and muscle fatigue (Ng, 2004; Taylor, 2006). Similar to poststroke weakness, these central deficits impair MU recruitment and regulation of the MU firing rate. In addition, muscle fiber changes that are consistent with disuse atrophy can be seen (de Haan, 2000). Muscle fatigue contributes significantly to disability and reduced energy levels for daily activities in persons with MS (McDonnell, 2001; Schwid, 2002; White, McCoy, 2004; Surakka, 2004b). Individuals

| TABLE 22-5 | Poststroke Motor Unit Characteristics and Muscle Fiber Changes | |
|---|---|
| **MOTOR UNIT DEFICITS** | **MUSCLE FIBER CHANGES** |
| • Reduced number of motor units (MUs) <br> • Increased MU innervation ratios <br> • Impaired firing rate regulation | • Disuse atrophy after 4–6 weeks <br> • Type II fiber selective atrophy <br> • Increased percentage of type I fibers |

with MS reportedly have reduced and slowed force production during both isometric and isokinetic testing in lower extremity (LE) muscles (Lambert, 2001). These dynamic strength impairments directly correlate with functional limitations, including ADL skills, transfers, and gait function, and warrant directed intervention.

## Rationale for Strength Training in Persons With Neurological Disorders

Current research regarding weakness and resulting functional deficits in individuals with neuromuscular disorders provides a strong rationale for the value and potential benefits of strength training to enhance functional outcomes. Evidence supports the efficacy of strength training in patients with stroke, ABI, MS, PD, CP, and other neuromuscular diseases (MacPhail, 1995; Badics, 2002; Dal Bello-Haas, 2002, 2007; Dodd, 2002; Eng, 2004; Kjolhede, 2012; Lima, 2013; Patten, 2004; White & Dressendorfer, 2004; Schilling, 2010). Refer to Focus on Evidence Tables 22-20 through 22-24 (ONL) for details on strength training studies in stroke, MS, PD, and CP.

Strength exercise programs of at least 6 to 8 weeks in duration promote neural adaptation, thus improving recruitment and efficiency of MU activation. Moderate- to high-intensity training may also facilitate neural plasticity at the cortical, spinal, and neuromuscular levels. Research indicates that stroke and TBI survivors benefit from strength training in both the acute and chronic stages (Flansbjer, 2008; Ouellette, 2004; Patten, 2004; Weiss, 2000).

In addition to implementing strength training in acute rehabilitation, therapists should also incorporate these exercises as one component of a fitness program for community-dwelling individuals with neurological disability to maximize their functional capacity for daily activities. These fitness programs are especially needed for individuals with progressive neurological diseases, such as MS and PD (Brienesse, 2013; Dalgas, 2008; Latimer-Cheung, 2013; Lima, 2013; Petajan, 1996; White & Dressendorfer, 2004; Schilling, 2010). Strength training programs are important to prevent or reverse the unwanted effects of prolonged inactivity and to prevent comorbid medical problems such as cardiovascular disease, recurrent stroke, diabetes, obesity, and osteoporosis (Gordon, 2004). In addition, strength training has been an effective method to reduce fall risk in elderly individuals, which has implications for those with neurological comorbidities, such as PD and stroke (Hirsch, 2003; Tinetti, 1994; Toole, 2000). For individuals with progressive neuromuscular disease, such as ALS, submaximal strengthening exercises for those muscles not yet affected by the disease has been shown to prevent disuse atrophy and maximize remaining function, as well as having beneficial psychological effects (Dal Bello-Haas, 2002, 2007, 2008).

### Research Evidence for Strength Training in the Stroke Population

Strong evidence exists that resistive training is effective in improving muscle strength for both UE and LE in both acute and chronic stages after a stroke (refer to Focus on Evidence Tables 22-20 and 22-21 ONL). Five systematic reviews (Ada, 2006; Eng, 2004; Morris, 2004; Riolo, 2003; Van der Lee, 2001) provide extensive discussion and analysis of current research on strength training in the stroke population; across all studies, there were improved strength outcomes, with treatment effect sizes ranging from 1.2 to 4.5. Modes of strength training included progressive resistive exercise (PRE); circuit training; isokinetic exercise; and functional, task-specific exercises with low to high intensities. Numerous studies supported the benefit of high-intensity training (60% to 80% of maximal strength), with large strength gains reported (Flansbjer, 2008; Ouellette, 2004; Sullivan, 2007; Teixeira-Salmela, 1999; Weiss, 2000).

The efficacy of strength training in improving functional outcomes was less robust and inconsistent across studies, depending on the type of training and functional measures studied. In their systematic reviews, Eng (2004) and Van der Lee (2001) concluded that there was poor to insufficient evidence regarding the transfer effect of strength training alone on function, whereas Patten (2004) emphasized the positive training effects on function found in specific studies. Training programs that were more task specific in exercise design had better transfer to function than non-task-specific exercise (Bale, 2008; Barreca, 2004; Dean, 2000; Monger, 2002; Patten, 2013; Sullivan, 2007; Yang, 2006). In addition, strengthening programs that utilized high-intensity training demonstrated significant functional gains in gait speed and endurance (Flansbjer, 2008; Sharp, 1997; Weiss, 2000).

### Research Evidence for Strength Training in the Multiple Sclerosis Population

Exercise training combining strength and aerobic exercise is an effective intervention to improve fitness, functional capacity, and quality of life in persons with MS (Dalgas, 2009, 2010; Latimer-Cheung, 2013; Motl, 2008; Petajan, 1996; Taylor, 2006; White & Dressendorfer, 2004). Refer to Focus on Evidence Table 22-22 (ONL) for a summary of strength training studies in MS. Research provides strong evidence that resistance training significantly improves leg strength with more modest effects on arm strength, whereas transfer effects on walking function are inconclusive (Kjolhede, 2012). In a comprehensive review of research, White & Dressendorfer (2004) concluded that supervised strength training had positive effects not only on strength and function but also on psychological well-being. Documented functional gains after strength training in individuals with MS are variable across studies because of differences in exercise protocols and outcome measures; however, improved performance in ADLs, walking speed and endurance, and stair climbing and reduced self-reported levels of fatigue have been observed (Dalgas, 2010; Latimer-Cheung, 2013; White & Dressendorfer, 2004). Another important finding that was consistent across strength training studies was no increase in exacerbations owing to exercise and only minimal risk of adverse side effects.

In summary, evidence supports the effectiveness of resistive training at least twice weekly at moderate intensity, as well as task-specific training to improve strength in individuals with mild to moderate disability from MS (Broekmans, 2011; Dalgas, 2008, 2009; Dodd, 2011). Brown (2005) also provided a strong rationale and support for the role of strengthening exercises in maintaining strength capabilities and preventing functional decline in persons with moderate to severe disability from MS. Resistance training is also recommended to increase bone density because persons with MS are at increased risk for osteoporosis and fractures due to corticosteroid use and inactivity. On the basis of these multisystem benefits, resistance training is a valuable component of rehabilitation for persons with MS.

### Research Evidence for Strength Training in the Parkinson Disease Population

Trunk and LE weakness has been identified as one factor contributing to the increased fall risk and functional decline in persons with PD (Glendinning, 1997; Hirsch, 2003; Morris, 2000; Robinson, 2005). Strength training is an important component in the plan of care for persons with PD to ultimately promote optimal functional mobility, and prevent falls. Increased force generation from strength training for trunk and LE can improve dynamic balance and walking capacity in persons with PD (Brienesse, 2013; Dibble, 2006, 2006; Hirsch, 2003; Schilling, 2010; Lima, 2013; Scandalis, 2001; Toole, 2000). Refer to Focus on Evidence Table 22-24 (ONL) for a summary of strength training studies in persons with PD. Moderate-intensity resistance training is recommended two to three times weekly for 8 to 10 weeks. Scandalis (2001) demonstrated that individuals with PD had strength gains after training similar to those of healthy age-matched controls. Functional strength training using weight-bearing exercises is an effective method to strengthen LE muscles and improve functional balance in persons with PD (Hearn, 2007). Combining task-specific training with strength and aerobic exercises is recommended (Lima, 2013). Corcos (2013) reported that engagement in fitness programs, including strength training twice weekly, for 2 years resulted in a significantly better reduction in PD-related motor signs than the control group. Prescription of exercise programs for persons with PD, including strength and aerobic training, is warranted to optimize motor function and functional mobility.

### Research Evidence for Strength Training in the Cerebral Palsy Population

Children and adults with CP have multiple system impairments in motor control, sensation, perception, cognition, and communication that contribute to functional limitations and developmental delays. Reduced force production is a well-documented underlying impairment in CP that is responsive to exercise interventions. Current research provides strong support for lower extremity strength training to improve force-generation ability in children and adolescents with CP (Boyd, 2012; Damiano, 1995, 1998; McBurney, 2003; Dodd, 2002, 2003; Morton, 2005, Unger, 2006). Refer to Focus on Evidence Table 22-23 (ONL) for a summary of strength training studies in persons with CP.

Evidence regarding whether strength training results in improved gross motor function (including gait function) is inconclusive across these studies. The reader is referred to several comprehensive systematic reviews for a more detailed discussion of effects of strength training in children with CP (Darrah, 1997; Dodd, 2002; Verschuren, 2008). Overall recommendations for exercise training are submaximal progressive resistive exercise (ranging from four sets of five repetitions to three sets of eight to 10 repetitions) or functional strength training, three times weekly for at least 6 weeks' duration, to promote strength gains. Combining strength training with aerobic training and developmental function training achieves optimal functional outcomes in children with CP.

---

## PATIENT APPLICATION

*Charlie is a 21 year-old Caucasian male who sustained a severe ABI as well as right tibial and clavicular fractures secondary to a rollover motor vehicle accident. He was intubated at the scene and had a Glasgow Coma Score of 6 at hospital admission. Magnetic resonance imaging revealed focal contusions in the frontal and temporal regions, as well as diffuse axonal injury. Charlie was comatose for 25 days and remained hospitalized in an acute care setting for 5 weeks. He is now being evaluated in an inpatient rehabilitation center.*

*Charlie is a single college student majoring in business. He works part-time at a local printing company and lives with two friends in a third-story apartment in an urban setting. His medical history is unremarkable. He was not taking any medications before the accident but currently is taking phenytoin. His clavicular fracture is now well healed; however, movement restrictions are evident. He remains immobilized in a below-knee cast on his right leg with partial weight-bearing status. The cast is scheduled to be removed in 1 week.*

***Physical therapy examination findings:***
*Communication/Cognition:*

- *Charlie is alert and oriented to person, place, time, and situation; however, he has moderate impairments in short-term memory, sustained and selective attention, and executive function.*
- *He is at level VI on the Rancho Los Amigos Cognitive Function Scale. He has limited awareness of his deficits. He follows three-step commands consistently when in a quiet environment. He requires daily structure and repetition for learning new tasks.*
- *He clearly communicates his needs but has mild dysarthria.*

***Functional status:***
- *Examination findings based on the Functional Independence Measure are: Bed Mobility = 6; Transfers = 4; Wheelchair Mobility = 5; Ambulation = 4; and Stairs = 3.*
- *Charlie functions safely from a sitting position to perform his basic ADLs.*
- *He requires minimal assistance to move from sit-to-stand, with UE support and close guard for stability once in standing.*
- *His Berg balance score is 32/56 points (score indicative of increased fall risk), with inability to perform a single-limb*

stance, tandem stance, and toe taps because of partial weight-bearing status on his right leg.
- He ambulates with a single Lofstrand crutch and minimal assist on level surfaces and fatigues after 300 ft at a moderately slowed gait speed (0.5 m/s, 32% of normal speed).
- Gait pattern: Reduced right step length compared with left; asymmetrical stance times (L>R) with prolonged double-limb support. Stance phase: Left lateral trunk lean during right stance phase; strong UE crutch support; left knee hyperextension in loading response; excessive hip flexion bilaterally at stance phase. Swing phase: Excessive ankle plantar flexion with toe drag in left swing; limited left knee flexion in preswing and early swing phases.
- Charlie requires moderate assist and use of one railing on stairs and demonstrates reduced power for ascending steps, with a tendency to pull on the railing.

### Contemplate Clinical Decisions

*What potential impairments could be contributing to Charlie's functional limitations? How might centrally-based weakness be affecting his impaired standing balance and mobility skills? What objective measures would you select to assess his strength? Given his recent history of fractures, in what muscles might you expect weakness related to disuse? How will Charlie's cognitive status potentially affect the strength examination?*

## Examination of Strength Impairment and Evaluation of Effect on Function

A thorough examination of the distribution and severity of weakness is a vital component of evaluation in individuals with neuromuscular disorders. Selection and application of objective strength measures help to identify specific weakness impairments, determine the effectiveness of strength interventions, and monitor recovery. Chapter 6 describes tests and measures for strength that are appropriate in neurological populations. Manual muscle testing, a subjective but standardized judgment to quantify the force generated, must include standardized positioning and therefore cannot be completed if the person does not have isolated movements. A more objective measure of force production is the use of dynamometry to quantify the force produced. This measure can be used to document changes in force production over time and assess the effectiveness of exercise interventions.

Evaluation of the relationship between the patient's strength deficits and functional limitations assists the clinician in prioritizing the areas that need specific remediation and in developing treatment goals. For example, identification of weak power generation of plantar flexor muscles adversely affecting gait performance and the ability to ascend stairs in an elderly stroke survivor guides the clinician in designing weight-bearing exercises to improve plantar flexor strength. Weakness deficits that most directly affect functional performance should be prioritized in the treatment plan.

Strength training should be combined with task-specific functional training for optimal carryover to function. The

physical examination is a critical first step in planning directed interventions to remediate strength impairments. A comprehensive understanding of the patient's abilities, activity limitations, and underlying system impairments is needed when designing exercise interventions for individuals with neurological disorders.

### PATIENT APPLICATION

#### Part II: Examination of Strength Impairment in Charlie
*(One week after admission to inpatient rehabilitation: Note that the right LE cast has been removed with progression to full weight-bearing status.)*
**Active ROM (AROM):**
- No deficits at hips and knees bilaterally
- Ankle dorsiflexion is limited to right = 0 degrees and left = +5 degrees with knee extended
- Straight leg raise limited to right = 48 degrees, left = 65 degrees
- Right shoulder AROM limited in flexion = 152 degrees, abduction = 145 degrees, and external rotation = 34 degrees

**Muscle tone assessment:**
- Spastic hypertonicity in left quadriceps and gastrocnemius (Modified Ashworth grade = 2)
- Left wrist and finger flexors (Modified Ashworth grade = 2), evidence of spastic hypertonicity

Sensation is intact throughout the four extremities (sharp/dull, light touch, proprioception, kinesthesia).

**Manual muscle testing (MMT) for LE:**
Note: Selective motor control is evident in right LE and left hip and knee but is impaired at ankle.

- Mild proximal hip weakness bilaterally with more pronounced distal weakness
  - Hip extensors and abductors 4- / 5, bilaterally
  - Hamstrings 4 / 5, bilaterally
  - Quadriceps 4- / 5 bilaterally
  - Right dorsiflexors and evertors 3+ / 5, inversion 3 / 5, plantar flexors 3- / 5
  - Left ankle lacking selective motor control but able to isolate antigravity and take mild resistance
  - All other LE muscles 5 / 5
- Mild trunk weakness noted in abdominal muscles

**MMT for UE**
- Proximal weakness is evident in right UE
  - Right scapular stabilizers (4- / 5)
  - Shoulder abductors and external rotators 4- / 5, flexion 4 / 5
- All other UE muscles at shoulder and elbow were selective and 5 / 5 bilaterally.
- Left wrist and finger extensors show poor selective movement against gravity with flexor pattern predominance.

**Motor control demonstrates**
- Slowed movements in both LEs with impaired coordination for fast reciprocal motions
- Impaired grasp and fine motor control in left UE

*Functional strength measures:*

- *Functional test sit-to-stand: Charlie performed five repetitions of sit-to-stand without support in 32 seconds; evidence of >50% reduced from norms*
- *Rapid step-up test: With rail support, he performed 10 rapid step-ups with minimal assist in 84 seconds with left LE leading, but he was unable to perform this activity with right LE leading, which is evidence of slowed task completion compared with age-matched peers.*
- *He performed 10 partial sit-ups with arms across the chest in 110 seconds.*
- *He was unable to complete any heel raises in left single-limb stance and completed partial range in right single-limb stance and bilateral stance with UE support.*

### Contemplate Clinical Decisions

*What is Charlie's expected prognosis for recovery of strength during rehabilitation? How might remediation of these strength deficits facilitate Charlie's functional recovery? What muscles should be targeted for strength training? What modes of strength training would be most effective given the widely distributed strength deficits? Do specific muscles need isolated focus for strength training, and if so, how could you apply the specificity of training principle? What level of exercise intensity and frequency will you prescribe for Charlie's strengthening program? How will you adapt strength exercises according to Charlie's functional and balance abilities and cognitive function?*

## ■ Preparatory Interventions Specific for Weakness in Neurological Conditions

### General Approaches

A wide range of methods for strength training have been effectively applied to neurological populations. Table 22-6 classifies different modes of strength interventions. Numerous factors influence the clinician's selection of optimal mode of strength training for individuals with neurological dysfunction (refer to Box 22-1). When a patient is having difficulty initiating or generating muscle activation because of weakness, **facilitation techniques** and sensory stimulation techniques can be used to elicit and promote increased voluntary MU recruitment. Early neurorehabilitation frameworks provided theoretical constructs and treatment guidelines for use of these techniques to

enhance motor control in persons with upper motor neuron lesions, such as stroke and TBI (Bobath, 1990; Sawner, 1992; Stockmeyer, 1967; Voss, 1985). For patients who have difficulty isolating movements, strength training can be a challenge, requiring modified positions and motor facilitation techniques.

**Neuromuscular electrical stimulation (NMES)** can be applied for very weak muscles to elicit muscle activation and promote the motor recruitment needed for functional activities (De Kroon, 2002; Glanz, 1996; Nunes, 2008; Vaz, 2008). NMES is also used as an orthotic device to substitute for muscle weakness in patients with neurological conditions, with emerging technology enhancing the applicability of this tool (Alon, 2003, 2007; Dunning, 2009; Kottink, 2007; Page, 2012; Shindo, 2011).

**Electromyographic biofeedback (EMGBFB)** can be a useful adjunct for retraining activation of weak muscles by providing the patient with enhanced feedback regarding timing of muscle recruitment during task training (Glanz, 1995; Moreland, 1998; Wolf, 1983a, 1983b). The strengthening application of this modality can be improved by combining NMES with BFB, called **EMG-triggered NMES**. With this modality, the clinician adjusts the threshold of voluntary muscle activation required by the patient to trigger electrical stimulation, which then is activated to assist completion of the motion (Cauraugh, 2000, 2002; Cozean, 1988; Kraft, 1992).

With **proprioceptive neuromuscular facilitation (PNF)**, patterns and techniques can be effectively applied for strength training in persons with neurological conditions. Facilitation

---

| BOX 22-1 | Patient Factors to Consider When Selecting Strength Training Method |
|---|---|

- Diagnosis, time since diagnosis, and concomitant medical comorbidities
- Age; special consideration for children and older adults
- Severity and distribution of strength deficit
- Specific muscle groups targeted and functional goals
- Balance ability and functional level
- Motor control capabilities
- Cognitive and perceptual status
- Other system impairments that affect strength training capability and response
- Context of training and equipment available
- Interests and premorbid activity level

---

| TABLE 22-6 | Strength Training Interventions for Persons With Neurological Conditions | |
|---|---|---|
| **FOR TRAINING VERY WEAK MUSCLES** | **FOR TRAINING FUNCTIONAL MUSCLE SYNERGIES** | **FOR ISOLATED MUSCLE TRAINING** |
| • Facilitation techniques | • Task-oriented training | • Progressive resistive exercise |
| • Neuromuscular electrical stimulation (NMES) | • Proprioceptive neuromuscular facilitation | • Isokinetic equipment |
| • Electromyographic biofeedback | • Aquatic exercises | • Exercise machines |
| • Electromyographic-triggered NMES | | |

techniques, such as quick stretch and use of manual resistance, can be useful for improving motor recruitment, timing, and coordinated activation of functional motor patterns (Voss, 1985). Strength training can be designed to incorporate extremity patterns or total body patterns, applying the principle of overflow from stronger to weaker muscles. Refer to Chapter 15 for details regarding PNF patterns and techniques.

More traditional strength training approaches are also effective for neurological populations. In **progressive resistive exercise (PRE),** as originally described by Delorme (1948), a resistive load is systematically applied and progressed during training as prescribed by a specific percentage of the muscle's maximal capability. Although Delorme's original protocol proposed high-intensity training (80% of maximal ability for a single repetition, 1RM), PRE programs can incorporate low- to high-intensity training depending on the patient's age and diagnosis and the specific training goals. This exercise mode frequently focuses on a single muscle or group of muscles and straight plane movements. Types of resistance applied in PRE programs include cuff weights, free weights, weight machines, and elastic bands.

**Isokinetic exercise** is another mode of strength training commonly used in sport rehabilitation that can be effectively applied to neurological populations (Engardt, 1995; Patten, 2006; Sharp, 1997). Isokinetic exercise requires individuals to generate torque against a lever and match the preselected angular velocity (speed) of the machine, moving the limb through the ROM. This dynamic mode of exercise employs constant speed and variable muscle torque through the range.

Both isokinetic exercise and PRE programs typically use an **open chain exercise** design (Fig. 22-3A). With this type of design, proximal stabilization is applied while the distal limb segment moves freely in space against resistance. Other modes of resistance can be utilized for strength training in neurological populations, including pneumatic and hydraulic devices that provide variable resistance and **aquatic exercises** that use hydrostatic properties of water to facilitate strengthening (Broach, 2001; Chu, 2004; Ouellette, 2004; Weiss, 2000). In addition, exercise machines can be utilized for strength training with a specific exercise prescription, such as UE and LE ergometers, rowing machines, stepping and elliptical machines, and treadmills (Sullivan, 2007).

**Task-specific strength training** is a newer framework in neurorehabilitation. Initially proposed by Carr (1998), this strength-training concept utilizes functional tasks to challenge the neuromuscular and musculoskeletal systems. For example, a person participates in strength training in the context of repetitive reaching tasks, treadmill walking, or step training tasks, which also assists in improving his functional abilities. Muscles are worked in **functional synergies** rather than in isolation. In this context, some muscles work as prime movers, whereas others work as synergists or stabilizers during the task training. Unlike open chain PRE exercise, **closed chain exercise** design often works in LE muscles, such as in upright weight-bearing postures needed for function (Fig. 22-3B). In

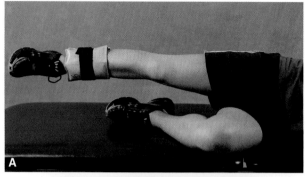

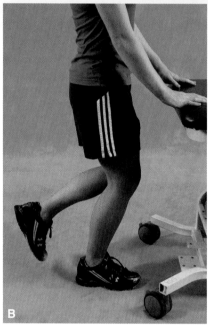

**FIGURE 22-3** Exercises for strengthening can include (A) open chain exercises such as hip abduction work against gravity with an ankle weight and (B) closed chain exercises such as single-limb partial squats.

closed chain exercises, the weight of the limb, body weight, or axial loading is the primary mode of resistance, such as partial squatting exercises that simulate a component of stand-to-sit. Strength training principles are applied to repetitive task practices by progressively amplifying the task challenge through increasing repetitions, load, or speed of movement, depending on the type of task trained. According to Carr (2003), this dynamic activity-based method of strength training has better functional specificity for training weak muscles in neurological populations, potentially yielding better functional carryover.

Current research provides emerging support for this mode of training for both UE and LE function in stroke, TBI, and MS populations (Lee, 2013; Patten, 2006; Salbach, 2004; Sullivan, 2007; Yang, 2006). Refer to Focus on Evidence Tables 22-20 through 22-22 (ONL) for details on these studies. One current example of this application is the use of body weight–supported treadmill training (BWSTT), which is a task-specific training exercise with gradual increases in strength and balance demands to enhance walking recovery (Moseley, 2005; Sullivan, 2002, 2006; Visintin, 1998).

The next section of this chapter provides an overview of exercise principles to consider in strength training design and guidelines for exercise prescription in neurological populations. The various modes of strength training discussed previously are covered in more detail, with clinical examples provided.

### Exercise Principles for Strength Training

When designing strengthening exercise programs for individuals with neurological disorders, therapists need to apply four basic principles of exercise science that lay the foundation for effective strengthening across healthy and diverse clinical populations. In the first principle, **overload**, a muscle needs to be progressively challenged in order to promote neuromuscular adaptation and produce gains in strength-generating capability. Exercise intensity sufficient to increase muscle strength is approximately 60% to 70% of the *muscle's current maximal capability for one repetition,* defined as **1RM**. High-intensity training (i.e., 80% to 100% of 1RM, six to 12 repetitions) is the most effective and efficient method to promote improved strength in healthy individuals (Harris, 2006). Several current studies provide evidence that individuals in subacute and chronic poststroke stages tolerated high-intensity training (80% of 1RM) without adverse side effects and demonstrated significant robust strength gains in the trained muscles (Flansbjer, 2008; Patten, 2006, 2013; Teixeira-Salmela, 1999; Weiss, 2000). In *Exercise Recommendations for Stroke Survivors,* the American Heart Association (AHA) prescribes moderate-intensity programs (i.e., 60% to 75% of 1RM) with higher repetitions (10 to 15 repetitions) (Gordon, 2004). Submaximal-intensity training (low, 40% to 60% of 1RM, progressing to moderate, 60% to 75% of 1RM) may be indicated early in rehabilitation training or in specific conditions. Table 22-7 summarizes specific indications for submaximal training.

## THINK ABOUT IT 22.2

Whether low, moderate, or high intensity of strength training is prescribed, overload should be individualized for each patient and applied in a progressive manner during training to continue to challenge adaptation and increased strength. Consider: What factors influence progression of exercise intensity?

The second exercise principle is **specificity of training**, which states that training effects are directly related to the type of training demands imposed on the muscle. The neuromuscular adaptation that occurs with training is specific to the *type of muscle contraction, the speed of muscle contraction, and the length of the muscle during training* (Duncan, 1989; Kisner, 2012; McArdle, 2010). For example, isometric muscle training of the quadriceps at 90 degrees promotes increased isometric strength at 90 degrees + 10 degrees (10-degree overflow) but does not necessarily transfer to improved isometric strength when the knee angle is 10 degrees or transfer to the dynamic concentric strength needed during stair climbing (Knapik, 1983). Concentric strength training on an isokinetic dynamometer at specific speeds for knee flexors and extensors improves concentric strength at those speeds (+30 degrees per second); however, there is no change in eccentric strength (Duncan, 1989; Engardt, 1995; Timm, 1987).

The clinical application of this principle of specificity of training involves designing strength exercises to match the functional demands of the trained muscle as closely as feasible, including consideration of the type and speed of muscle contraction and the muscle length. Functional goals of rehabilitation directly influence the type of strength training selected. As an illustration, a patient who is poststroke or has a TBI with weak dorsiflexors that interfere with foot clearance in gait begins the strengthening program by training the ability to recruit sufficient muscle strength for full ankle dorsiflexion against gravity (3 / 5 MMT score). The patient then progresses to increased speed of recruitment with light resistance using

| TABLE 22-7 | Indications for Submaximal Intensity Strength Training |
|---|---|
| √ | Early in exercise program to assess a patient's response to exercise and gradually build intensity |
| √ | Severely deconditioned patients who need time to build to higher intensity |
| √ | Children and older adults |
| √ | Persons with degenerative neurological diseases, such as multiple sclerosis, amyotrophic lateral sclerosis, or neuromuscular disorders, when high-intensity exercise may have adverse effects on neuromuscular function |
| √ | Persons with neurological conditions in which remyelization is in process, such as Guillain-Barré syndrome and poliomyelitis, in order to avoid overworking weakened recovering muscles |
| √ | Persons with acute conditions after musculoskeletal injuries, surgery, or immobilization due to fracture in which tissues may need protection with a gradual increase in loading stress |
| √ | Persons with osteoporosis for whom loading stress should be gradually increased |
| √ | When training goal is to improve muscle endurance |
| √ | When training goal is maintenance of strength and prevention of disuse atrophy |

the concentric and eccentric contractions necessary for gait and stair function.

A third exercise science principle commonly applied to orthopedic and sports rehabilitation that somewhat counteracts specificity of training is **cross-training**. This principle promotes prescription of a range of muscle performance demands in a strength training program, such as varied types of muscle contractions, speeds, and muscle strength and endurance components, to promote more generalized muscle capabilities. Although cross-training may be too time-intensive for inpatient rehabilitation programs, it may be appropriate for home- and fitness-based exercise programs for persons with a neurological condition.

The final exercise principle pertinent to neurological rehabilitation is **reversibility**, which refers to the potential detraining effects that can occur unless strength is maintained. In both healthy and neurologically impaired populations, the strength gains achieved from training are not sustained unless muscle activity levels using these new strength gains are continually challenged. This detraining effect can be

quite costly for individuals with neurological disabilities because strength levels can fall below the critical threshold required for functional skills. Therefore, it is important to prescribe home exercise programs or engage the individual in ongoing community-based fitness programs to maintain strength gains and challenge increased activity levels.

## Exercise Prescription for Strength Training in Neurological Populations

Exercise prescription for strength training involves making clinical decisions regarding the optimal mode of exercise and specific exercise parameters. Table 22-8 provides definitions of exercise parameters related to clinical decision-making for exercise prescription. Refer to Table 22-9 for a sample of an exercise prescription. **Exercise intensity** is determined primarily by exercise load or level of resistance; however, it is also influenced by interaction of the rate of movement and the type of muscle action required and can range from submaximal to maximal intensity. **Exercise volume** is the total exercise dose, determined by total number of repetitions (reps) and

| TABLE 22-8 | Clinical Decision-Making for Strengthening Exercise Prescription |
|---|---|
| Mode of exercise | Type of strength exercise design and resistance selected for training *Examples are isotonic progressive resistive exercise (PRE) with cuff weights or elastic bands, isokinetic training, functional training, open chain or closed chain design, use of conventional exercise machines* |
| Type of muscle contraction | Isometric, concentric, eccentric contractions |
| Exercise intensity | Effort level exerted *Influenced by exercise load/resistance, movement speed and type of contraction; in PRE calculated by percentage of 1 RM* |
| Exercise volume | Total work or exercise dose *Number of repetitions (intensity in a single training session and number of exercises per session)* |
| Rest intervals | Time allotted for recovery between sets in a single training session or between exercise sessions |
| Exercise frequency | Interval between training sessions *Number of sessions per day or per week* |
| Exercise duration | Overall length of training program |
| Exercise progression | Timing and incremental increases in repetitions, sets, or resistance during training |

(DiNubile NA. Strength training. *Clin Sports Med.* 1991;10:33–62; Kisner, 2012; Kraemer, 2004)

| TABLE 22-9 | Sample Exercise Prescription |
|---|---|
| √ | **Mode:** Progressive resistive exercise training for UE with cuff weights |
| √ | **Type of contractions:** concentric and eccentric |
| √ | **Intensity:** 60%–70% of 1RM |
| √ | **Volume:** 10–15 repetitions × two sets |
| √ | **Rest intervals:** 2 minutes between sets |
| √ | **Frequency:** 3× per week |
| √ | **Duration:** 10–12 weeks |
| √ | **Progression:** 2%–5% increase in resistance once patient can lift load 15 repetitions (two sets without fatigue for two consecutive sessions) |

sets during an exercise session. The higher the intensity of the exercise, the lower the exercise volume required, whereas higher volume (reps/sets) can be utilized when submaximal intensity (40% to 70% of 1RM) is prescribed (DiNubile, 1991; Kraemer, 2004).

**Rest intervals** are an important component of exercise sessions in persons with neurological disorders. Rest intervals are particularly vital for those who are substantially deconditioned; those with disorders involving the lower motor neurons, such as Guillain-Barré syndrome (GBS), ALS, and Post-Polio Syndrome (PPS); and those at risk for overwork weakness. In general, when the primary goal is to improve muscle strength and moderate to high intensity has been prescribed, at least 2 minutes should be provided for rest between sets to allow restoration of muscle energy sources. When the goal of training is to improve muscle endurance and low-intensity training has been prescribed, rest periods can be reduced to 1 minute or less between sets (Kraemer, 2000).

**Exercise frequency,** or number of sessions per week, should allow muscle recovery between exercise sessions. Typically, 1 day of rest between sessions is recommended for moderate- to high-intensity strength training, whereas increased frequency can be prescribed with low-intensity training. Training intervals should not exceed 1 week to prevent detraining effects.

**Exercise duration** is the overall length of the training program. A minimum of 6 weeks' duration is recommended to promote strength gains in healthy individuals and in neurological populations. In deconditioned patients, gains can be achieved in a shorter duration. Neural adaptation can be evident within several training sessions in patients with central activation deficits (Durstine, 2009; Dalgas, 2013; Fleck, 2014).

### Fatiguing Exercise

**Muscle fatigue** is the gradual reduction in force-generating ability of a muscle with repetitions of a set load (Kraemer, 2004). In healthy individuals, working a muscle to the threshold of fatigue during strength training promotes adaptation and subsequent strength gains. This guideline of working a muscle to the threshold of fatigue can be safely applied for many neurological populations, such as patients who have had a stroke or a TBI; however, a nonfatiguing strength exercise protocol is recommended in certain diagnostic groups because of the nature of the disease process. Persons with MS are particularly prone to excessive fatigue and overheating. In these patients, short bouts of low- to moderate-intensity strength training with frequent rest periods is recommended (Costello, 1996; White & Dressendorfer, 2004).

Individuals with GBS or PPS should avoid working muscles to the point of fatigue to minimize risk of **overwork weakness**, defined as a decrease in absolute strength and endurance of a muscle that is prolonged because of excessive activity (Bassile, 1996). Partially denervated muscles are at risk for overworking, which may cause further muscle damage. Signs of overwork weakness are delayed-onset muscle soreness that peaks 1 to 5 days after activity and a notable reduction in the muscle's maximal force production that gradually recovers. In individuals with GBS or PPS, overwork weakness can interfere with the ability to perform basic ADLs.

### Nonfatiguing Exercise

**Nonfatiguing exercise** involves short intervals of low- to moderate-intensity exercise (five to 10 repetitions), with frequent rests in between to recover. A 1:2 ratio of contraction to relaxation time for each exercise repetition is recommended (Agre, 1997; Jubelt, 2000; Martin, 2015). Box 22-2 provides exercise guidelines for persons with progressive neuromuscular diseases. For individuals with ALS, nonfatiguing exercise prescription should be applied for muscles not yet involved in the disease process and for those muscles with 3+ / 5 or better strength with close monitoring to avoid overworking muscles. Exercise intensity and level of resistance should be reduced as the disease progresses (Dal Bello-Haas, 2002, 2007, 2008).

### Warm-up/Cooldown

As with anyone participating in an exercise program, individuals with a neurological condition should initiate the exercise session with a warm-up and conclude it with a cool-down. Refer to Table 22-10 for recommendations.

---

**BOX 22-2 Exercise Prescription Guidelines for Persons With Progressive Neuromuscular Disease**

- Strengthen muscles not yet affected by disease process and muscles with strength grades greater than 3 +/5.
- Recommend one set of eight to 10 repetitions at submaximal effort (low intensity, 40% to 60% of 1RM)
- Structure short training sessions with long rest intervals between exercises
- Avoid heavy eccentric exercises and working to exhaustion because this has adverse effects on neuromuscular function
- Protect muscles that are severely weakened
- Monitor patient for overwork weakness; fatigue from exercises should not interfere with performance of activities of daily living and should show good recovery by next day
- Apply conservative exercise progression and reduce resistance as disease progresses

---

**TABLE 22-10 Recommendations for Warm-up and Cooldown**

| WARM-UP SUGGESTIONS | COOLDOWN SUGGESTIONS |
| --- | --- |
| 5–10 Minutes | 5–10 Minutes |
| Light exercise | Gradual reduction in activity |
| Dynamic exercise | Flexibility and stretching |
| Focus on large muscle groups | Fluid intake |

## Exercise Guidelines

Recommendations from the American Academy of Sports Medicine and the AHA recommendations for strengthening exercises in healthy adults and frail older adults or adults with cardiovascular disease are outlined in Table 22-11 (Durstine, 2009; Gordon, 2004; Pollock, 2000). According to the *American College of Sports Medicine Position Stand* (1998), in untrained healthy adults, a single set of moderate-intensity exercise is equally as effective as multiple-set programs for improving muscle strength and is more time efficient. For frail elderly individuals or adults with cardiovascular disease, initial lower-intensity exercises with slower exercise progression are recommended. The exercise guidelines recommended for stroke survivors are consistent with those proposed by the AHA for individuals with cardiovascular disease (Gordon, 2004). Current research supports the safety and efficacy of these guidelines as a starting point for strength training; however, numerous studies support higher-intensity (i.e., 60% to 80% training) as effective in subacute and chronic poststroke phases (Patten, 2007; Teixeira-Salmela, 1999). Lower-intensity training may be effective for improving muscle endurance as opposed to strength when exercise volume is increased; however, at least moderate intensity is optimal to increase strength. Cardiovascular responses to strength training should be monitored by assessment of heart rate, blood pressure level, pulse oximetry, and perceived exertion, which should not exceed the moderate level. Exercise should be stopped when the patient reports light-headedness, dizziness, chest pain or heaviness, palpitations, or excessive shortness of breath.

Exercise guidelines for persons with MS (refer to Table 22-11, "Adults With MS" column) are similar to those proposed for individuals with stroke; however, modifications may be required for exercise intensity according to the severity of the individual's condition and exercise tolerance (Dalgas, 2008, 2009; Latimer-Cheung, 2013; Mulcare, 2003; White & Dressendorfer, 2004). Progression should not be too aggressive, with adequate rest intervals provided. Closed chain exercises are an effective mode for LE training because of strong carryover to functional task demands.

Persons with MS should be educated not to exercise in warm temperatures because a rise in body temperature can worsen their symptoms. Use of a cooling vest or exercising in a cool pool (27°C to 29°C) has been reported as an effective method to control body temperature (White, 2000; White & Dressendorfer, 2004). An additional precaution for scheduling exercise sessions for persons with MS is to alternate aerobic and strength conditioning days to prevent excessive fatigue and allow adequate recovery. Therapists should monitor the effect of the exercise program on the patient's/client's daily fatigue levels using standardized self-report measures, such as the *Modified Fatigue Impact Scale* (National Multiple Sclerosis Society, 2017).

Strength exercise guidelines for children with CP are also outlined in Table 22-11. To maintain strength gains, training should continue for 10 weeks (Damiano, 1998; Dodd, 2002; O'Neil, 2006). High-intensity training should be avoided in children, and their response to exercises should be closely monitored. Through functional and play-based activities, children should be encouraged to maintain new strength gains.

## Therapeutic Techniques for Strength Training

Individualized exercise prescription for persons with neurological disorders also involves selection of the optimal mode of exercise training. In this section, the application of specific modes of exercise is discussed. Different types of resistance

| TABLE 22-11 | Recommended Exercise Guidelines for Strength Training | | | | |
|---|---|---|---|---|---|
| **EXERCISE PRESCRIPTION** | **HEALTHY OLDER ADULTS*** | **ADULT WITH CV DISEASE** | **POSTSTROKE ADULTS†** | **ADULTS WITH MS^** | **CHILDREN WITH CP**** |
| Frequency | Two or three times per week | Three times per week | Three times per week | Three times per week | Three times per week |
| Duration | 6–12 weeks | 6–12 weeks | 6–12 weeks | 6–10 weeks | 6–10 weeks |
| Intensity | 60%–80% of 1RM | 40%–60% of 1RM | 40%–60% of 1RM | 50%–60% of 1RM | 50%–65% of 1RM |
| Volume | One or two sets, 8–12 repetitions | One or two sets, 10–15 repetitions | One or two sets, 10–15 repetitions | One or two sets, 10–15 repetitions | One or two sets, 4–10 repetitions |
| Progression | 5% increase | 2%–5% increase Progress to 60%–80% of 1RM | 2%–5% increase Progress to 60%–80% of 1RM | 2%–5% increase Monitor fatigue level | 2%–5% increase Progress to 60%–70% |

*American College of Sports Medicine, 1998; Pollock, 2000; †Gordon NF, Gulanick M, Costa F, et al. Physical activity and exercise recommendations for stroke survivors: an American Heart Association scientific statement from the Council on Clinical Cardiology, Subcommittee on Exercise, Cardiac Rehabilitation, and Prevention; the Council on Cardiovascular Nursing; the Council on Nutrition, Physical Activity, and Metabolism; and the Stroke Council. *Stroke*. 2004;35:1230–1240; ^White, Dressendorfer, 2004; **Damiano DL, Abel MF. Functional outcomes of strength training in spastic cerebral palsy. *Arch Phys Med Rehabil*. 1998;79:119–125; Dodd KJ, Taylor NF, Damiano DL. A systematic review of the effectiveness of strength-training programs for people with cerebral palsy. *Arch Phys Med Rehabil*. 2002;83:1157–1164.

can be applied for strength training, including manual resistance, water resistance, use of body weights, and mechanical resistance using cuff weights, barbells, elastic bands, or exercise machines.

The advantages of using manual resistance for strength training in clients with neurological conditions are the therapist's ability to isolate the desired muscle action by the direction of applied resistance and to vary the resistance through the range according to the patient's ability to recruit the muscle. For very weak muscles, **isometric training** against manual resistance may be helpful initially to build force-generating capability at different points in the ROM. The patient is then progressed to eccentric training with controlled lowering of the limb.

Isometric training is also useful to increase strength in postural muscles that play a role in stabilizing joints. Moderate resistance should be applied to these muscles in the mid- to shortened ROM, requiring a sustained hold. Recommended duration of an isometric contraction is 4 to 10 seconds; however, the shorter the duration of contraction, the more repetitions are needed for strength gains. Caution should be taken during isometric training to monitor any breath holding or Valsalva maneuver because this can cause a major rise in the patient's systolic blood pressure.

**Eccentric training** (contraction as the muscle elongates) has greater mechanical efficiency than concentric training (contraction as the muscle shortens) because eccentric contractions require fewer MUs to generate tension. Therefore, individuals with centrally based weakness may be able to generate more force with eccentric training with less apparent effort (Clark, 2013; Duncan, 1989; Drury, 2000). Eccentric training with manual resistance or use of limb or body weight as the load is effective in early strength training after a stroke or ABI. However, high-intensity eccentric training should be avoided or used cautiously with low-intensity loads in persons with GBS, PPS, or neuromuscular disease because this mode may cause muscle damage in these patients (Costello, 1996; Dal Bello-Haas, 2002). High-intensity eccentric training in healthy individuals and in those with neurological diagnoses can cause delayed-onset muscle soreness. Hence, the patient's/client's response to this training mode should be monitored and the intensity level adjusted when soreness is reported.

**Concentric training** involves moving a load through a partial or complete ROM and should be performed slowly for 2 to 4 seconds when the goal is to improve muscle strength. When the goal is to improve muscle power, then faster speeds with lighter loads should be used. Because many functional tasks, such as stair climbing, require both concentric and eccentric contractions, it is advisable to incorporate both components in strength training. In healthy individuals, use of an eccentric contraction immediately before a concentric contraction facilitates increased force production for the concentric action. This order of muscle contraction may be a useful principle when training weak muscles in neurological conditions (Carr, 2003). The specific functional goals underlying the strength training will help guide the clinician in selecting the optimal mode of training.

## Use of Sensory Stimulation Techniques to Facilitate Muscles Activation in Very Weak Muscles

When patients have substantial weakness, with MMT scores less than 2 / 5 and ineffective central drive to activate the MU pool, neuromuscular facilitation techniques can be a useful adjunct during strength training to promote increased muscle activation. The term **facilitation** is defined as "enhanced capacity to initiate a movement response through increased neuronal activity and altered synaptic potential" (O'Sullivan, 2013, p. 490). A sensory stimulus can be applied to a single muscle or functional muscle group to enhance the patient's ability to reach a critical threshold for neuronal firing and muscle activation.

Facilitation techniques can be used as a single stimulus or in combination for an additive effect. For example, to promote muscle activation of the anterior tibialis muscle, a quick stretch can be followed by immediate resistance. This concept of simultaneous use of multiple sensory facilitation techniques, termed **spatial summation**, may be needed to enhance potential for movement response in patients with major paresis. **Temporal summation** refers to repeated use of a single stimulus in a short time to produce the desired muscle response (Stockmeyer, 1967). An example of temporal summation is the application of a series of quick stretches to facilitate movement of the hip flexors. Facilitation techniques should always be used in combination with verbal commands to the patient to encourage voluntary effort for the desired movement.

Neuromuscular facilitation techniques can be grouped by the sensory receptor system that is activated. Table 22-12 provides a list of sensory techniques used to facilitate muscle activation according to receptor classification. Most commonly used during strength training are proprioceptive facilitation techniques, including quick stretch, resistance, vibration, and joint approximation and traction. Because quick stretch activates Ia muscle spindle afferents and elicits a brief phasic response, the therapist adds light resistance to maintain the muscle contraction. The therapist initially places the weakened muscle in the gravity-eliminated plane of motion and then applies quick stretch. The quick stretch may be used with the muscle at the lengthened range or throughout points in the range to increase the strength of the contraction. Repetitive tapping to the muscle belly can also be applied to provide a quick stretch stimulus to the muscle spindle. Quick stretch is especially useful to promote

| TABLE 22-12 | Facilitation Techniques Grouped by Sensory Receptors | |
| --- | --- |
| **PROPRIOCEPTIVE INPUTS** | **EXTEROCEPTIVE INPUTS** |
| • Quick stretch | • Light touch/stroking |
| • Resistance | • Repetitive icing |
| • Vibration | • Manual contacts/pressure |
| • Joint approximation | |
| • Joint traction | |

a patient's ability to initiate movement. Resistance applied manually or with body weight in a graded manner can be an effective facilitation technique to enhance muscle contraction by activating muscle spindle (Ia, Ib) receptors and promote alpha and gamma motoneuron recruitment (Sawner, 1992; Voss, 1985).

For very weak muscles, light resistance can be employed with isometric or eccentric contractions to build muscle activation. Application of light tracking resistance to a weak concentric contraction may increase muscle activation, allowing movement through the range. As the patient gets stronger, the resistance level to single muscle or group of muscles is increased to promote optimal recruitment and overflow to the weaker muscles. Caution should be taken not to excessively overload weak muscles, which can inhibit movement or result in muscle substitution.

High frequency vibration (100 to 300 Hz) applied to the muscle belly or tendon elicits the tonic vibratory reflex, which facilitates the vibrated muscle and is inhibitory to its antagonist (Bishop, 1975). The therapist places the weak muscle in lengthened position and then vibrates the muscle belly for a duration of 10 to 60 seconds while the patient attempts to activate the targeted muscle (Fig. 22-4). Manual resistance can be added to any response to build muscle activation. Once the patient demonstrates voluntary control over the desired movement, the vibration should be removed. Vibration should not be used with infants because of their immature CNS and should be used with caution in patients with cerebellar disorders because it may have adverse effects (Umphred, 2012).

Selection of techniques to facilitate joint receptors is based on the functional role of the **target muscle** being strengthened. **Joint approximation** can be applied either manually or mechanically to facilitate postural extensors and joint stabilizers. For example, application of joint approximation through the shoulders with the patient in prone-on-elbows position may be used to strengthen scapular stabilizers. In addition, axial loading, either manually or with a backpack, can be used to enhance recruitment of postural extensors. This technique is

usually applied in closed chain or weight-bearing positions while the postural muscles are in mid- to shortened range.

In contrast, **joint traction**, a manual distraction of the limb, is used to facilitate strengthening of mobility patterns, such as UE flexion. Typically, an open chain exercise design is used with this facilitation technique in combination with light resistance.

Facilitation techniques that stimulate exteroceptive receptors and are used to strengthen very weak muscles are light touch, repetitive icing, and manual contacts. Similar to quick stretch, light touch with the fingertips, light stroking, or brief repetitive swipes with an ice cube over an area of high tactile receptivity elicits a brief phasic response, potentially enhancing a muscle's ability to activate. To illustrate, in poststroke patients with weakness of the wrist and finger extensors, the therapist may apply a series of light strokes over the forearm or dorsum of the hand while asking the patient to lift his fingers (Sawner, 1992). Another example of activating the exteroceptors is using repetitive icing over the muscle belly. Repetitive icing is applied by rubbing an ice cube with slight pressure over the hamstring muscle belly, with light stroking while the patient attempts to activate the muscle.

Manual contacts using firm, deep pressure directly over the muscle belly can facilitate enhanced muscle response and increase sensory awareness of the desired movement. This technique activates both touch and muscle receptors when the therapist adds deep stretch pressure into the muscle belly. Therapists commonly use manual contacts to provide proprioceptive and directional cues to the patient regarding the desired movement. The patient's voluntary effort to activate the muscle, along with well-timed verbal cues from the therapist when applying these facilitation techniques, is important in maximizing MU recruitment in very weak muscles.

### Neuromuscular Electrical Stimulation for Very Weak Muscles

NMES may also be an effective adjunctive tool to promote muscle strengthening in persons with centrally based weakness. In patients with severe weakness (MMT grades less than 2- / 5) NMES can facilitate muscle activation through direct stimulation to muscles and provide sensory feedback to the patient regarding the desired movement. In muscles with weak activation (MMT 2- to 3- / 5) that is not well controlled, NMES can be a muscle reeducation method to supplement the patient's voluntary efforts during functional movements and can strengthen muscle contraction (DeVahl, 1992; Packman-Braun, 1992).

NMES has the additional benefit of preventing disuse atrophy in paretic muscles during the early stages of recovery. Electrical stimulation directly activates large MUs, which individuals with centrally based weakness have difficulty recruiting. Therefore, NMES may be particularly beneficial in preventing type II fiber atrophy and promoting strength gains through large MU activation (Binder-MacLeod, 1993).

When applying NMES as a strength training intervention, the therapist needs to first select a task that promotes activation of the target muscles and then select electrode size, placement, and optimal treatment parameters for stimulation. Table 22-13

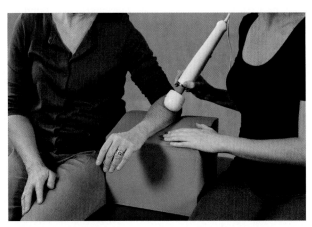

**FIGURE 22-4** Vibratory stimulation applied to the target muscle belly—wrist extensors in this case—to facilitate muscle activation while the patient attempts active movement.

| TABLE 22-13 | Guidelines for Application of Neuromuscular Electrical Stimulation in Neurological Conditions |
|---|---|
| Waveform | Symmetric preferable for large muscle groups; asymmetric for smaller muscle groups |
| Phase duration | 0.2–0.4 ms |
| Stimulation frequency | 30–35 Hz |
| Amplitude | Minimum level required to produce desired muscle contraction for task goal |
| On:off time | Depends on training goal; if using duty cycle for strengthening weak muscles, set initially at 1:5 ratio and then progress to 1:3 |
| Ramp time | 0.2–4 sec depending on task goal |
| Treatment session duration | 10–15 min; monitor for muscle fatigue |
| Treatment frequency | Two or three times per day |

provides general recommendations for treatment parameters when applying NMES in individuals with neurological conditions (Kottink, 2004; Packman-Braun, 1992; Pomeroy, 2006; Robbins, 2006). The specific activity and therapeutic goals, as well as individual patient factors, guide the therapist in selecting optimal parameters.

NMES can be applied using intramuscular electrodes or surface electrodes. One advantage of the latter is that an independent strength program can be set up for the patient with a portable NMES unit.

Recommended stimulation frequency for retraining muscle activation is 30 to 35 Hz, which is the frequency required to produce a smooth, tetanized contraction in healthy muscle. Frequencies higher than 40 Hz should be used with caution because neuromuscular fatigue is more likely (Packman-Braun, 1992). The amplitude of stimulation should match the training goal. To identify optimal amplitude for a patient, the therapist gradually increases the amplitude until a muscle contraction that satisfactorily facilitates task completion is reached. The example in Fig. 22-5 shows that the patient should attempt voluntary muscle activation within the task-specific context, simultaneous with the muscle stimulation (Sullivan, 2007).

Stimulation can be triggered with handheld or foot switches, or it can be programmed in the stimulator unit for a specific duty cycle, depending on the type of task practiced. When using a duty cycle, the therapist selects the on:off time of the stimulation, ensuring adequate rest after contraction to minimize muscle fatigue.

The strength training session can be designed for a particular number of repetitions of muscle contractions or for a set duration of the session. When using the set duration, time needs to be gradually progressed to avoid overworking the weak muscle. When muscle fatigue is a concern, the therapist may reduce the stimulation frequency, adjust the on:off cycle, or decrease the overall duration of the training session (DeVahl, 1992).

Application of NMES is contraindicated for individuals with demand-type pacemakers or epilepsy and over the lumbar or perineal region during pregnancy, cancerous regions, or carotid sinuses. NMES should be used with caution in patients with skin hypersensitivity or sensory loss and in patients with impaired ability to cognitively understand and participate

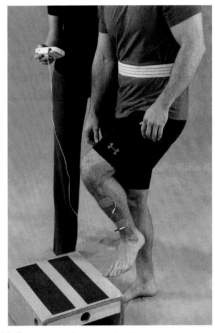

**FIGURE 22-5** As part of a strengthening program, neuromuscular stimulation can be applied to a muscle—ankle dorsiflexors in this case—while the patient attempts active (maximal patient effort) dorsiflexion during a functional stepping activity.

in training sessions. Vital signs should be monitored during initial NMES sessions in all patients, but particularly in patients with autonomic instability, such as SCI or MS, and in individuals with cardiac conditions.

A discussion of the extensive body of research on NMES applications and efficacy in the treatment of neurological conditions is beyond the scope of this chapter. The reader is referred to several excellent systematic reviews by Kottink (2004) and Robbins (2006) for LE applications and effects on walking function and by De Kroon (2002) and Pomeroy (2006) for UE applications and effects on UE function in stroke survivors.

NMES has been applied to weak dorsiflexors to address poststroke footdrop in hemiparetic gait with evidence of major gains in ankle strength and walking speed. Other studies have used multichannel NMES on paretic LE muscles (quadriceps, hamstrings, plantar flexors, and dorsiflexors) for neuromuscular and gait retraining and reported larger treatment effects than single-channel stimulation (Robbins, 2006). Although positive treatment outcomes are demonstrated in both acute and chronic poststroke phases, individuals appear to be more responsive to NMES in the acute and subacute phases of recovery (Ottawa Panel, 2006).

Numerous studies provide strong evidence that NMES applied to wrist and finger extensors is effective in improving upper limb strength, as well as improving motor recovery and functional abilities after a stroke (Alon, 2007; Chae, 1998; Kraft, 1992; Popovic, 2004; Powell, 1999). NMES has also been applied to both UEs and LEs in children with CP for neuromuscular reeducation (Carmick, 1993; Nunes, 2008; Vaz, 2008). Strength gains were noted consistently across these studies, with weak evidence of reported benefits on upper limb and walking functions. Use of NMES in children requires careful selection and modification of treatment parameters, in addition to close monitoring of the child's response to stimulation. Application of NMES during task-specific training is recommended for both children and adults to promote transfer of muscle recruitment to functional skills because motor retraining effects and functional outcomes are enhanced with this hybrid method of strength training (Hedman, 2007; Sullivan, 2004, 2007).

### Electromyographic Biofeedback as an Adjunct Tool for Training Very Weak Muscles

EMGBFB is another tool that therapists can use to enhance a patient's capability to recruit weak muscles and improve timing of activation during functional movements. Small changes in muscle activation can be detected with EMGBFB that may be difficult for the therapist to detect. The EMG signal is translated into an auditory and/or visual signal, providing augmented feedback to the patient regarding his voluntary efforts. The therapist can initially set the target threshold for muscle activation very low so that minimal activity is detected and then raise the threshold goal as the patient's ability to activate the muscle improves. Portable EMGBFB units or commercial wall units with visual screen display of the signal can be used depending on the treatment context and therapeutic goals for training. One advantage of the portable unit is the potential for the patient to use EMGBFB independently once you have trained the patient, thereby increasing the intensity of practice.

Research has demonstrated that EMGBFB is most effective when used in the context of functional training rather than isolated muscle training and when used in combination with conventional therapeutic activities (Basmajian, 1989; Binder-Macleod, 1995; Wissel, 1989). For example, training activation of the anterior tibialis muscle in the context of the swing phase of gait is more effective than training this muscle in an isolated movement.

When implementing EMGBFB as an adjunct to strength training, the therapist should first determine the therapeutic and functional goals, the target muscles, and the context for BFB training. Patients who are appropriate for EMGBFB training should be highly motivated, have adequate vision and

hearing to process the augmented EMG signal, be able to follow simple directions, and have cognitive function sufficient to understand the therapeutic goals and instructions for training (Binder-Macleod, 1995; Wolf, 1983a, 1983b).

The therapist must set three key parameters to implement EMGBFB: the gain, time constant, and target threshold (LeCraw, 1992). The gain is the extent that the EMG signal is multiplied by the amplifier. When applying EMGBFB to uptrain very weak muscles, the gain initially should be high to maximize the sensitivity to detect any muscle activation; it can then be progressively lowered during training to require more muscle activation to trigger the auditory signal. The **time constant (EMGBFB)** is the sampling frequency of the EMG signal, reflecting how often the EMG information is updated to the viewer. For portable EMGBFB units, a short time constant (0.1 second) is set for uptraining muscles needed for dynamic movements. Longer time constants (0.5 to 1.0 second) can be used for training muscles needed in static or stabilization activities. The **EMG target threshold** for uptraining weak muscles refers to the minimum amount of muscle activation needed to trigger the auditory or visual signal. This threshold is the therapeutic training goal based on a thorough initial examination of the patient's capability to activate the muscle. This threshold is progressively increased as MU recruitment improves (Basmajian, 1989). The effectiveness of an EMGBFB training session is determined by progress toward goals, such as the number of times the target threshold is reached, the length of time the muscle activation is at or above the target threshold, or effective reaching of the target threshold during functional task training.

Evidence regarding the effectiveness of EMGBFB training is primarily documented in the stroke literature, and findings are variable across studies. Many studies support EMGBFB as an effective adjunct for poststroke motor retraining to promote lower limb recovery, with gains evident in active ROM, strength, and gait function in the ankle (Moreland, 1994, 1998; Schleenbaker, 1993); however, the benefit of this tool for upper limb functional recovery is not sufficiently supported (Ottawa Panel, 2006). Other comprehensive reviews (Glanz, 1995; Woodford, 2007) provide analysis of isolated research studies that demonstrate the benefits of EMGBFB in promoting poststroke motor recovery; however, when studies were examined collectively, the results indicated insufficient evidence to support the effectiveness of EMGBFB over conventional therapy. Therefore, therapists should consider the patient's clinical presentation and therapeutic goals on a case-by-case basis to determine whether EMGBFB may be a useful adjunct for strength training.

Combining EMGBFB with electrical stimulation, called **EMG-triggered NMES**, is an alternative method to facilitate increased muscle activation and has been documented as more effective than EMGBFB alone (Cozean, 1988; Fields, 1987; Francisco, 1998). In addition, it has produced positive outcomes in UE motor function after stroke (Cozean, 1988; Franscisco, 1998; Kraft, 1992). The therapist sets the EMG target threshold that the patient tries to reach with voluntary activation. When this threshold is reached, the muscle contraction is reinforced with the onset of electrical stimulation. During training, the target threshold is progressively increased, promoting improved voluntary activation and eventually eliminating the need for NMES to trigger stronger activation. Commercial electrical stimulation units are available for clinical use to pair EMGBFB with NMES in the menu of therapeutic applications.

## THINK ABOUT IT 22.3

How would you apply neuromuscular electrical stimulation (NMES), biofeedback, or electromyographic-triggered NMES during movement retraining or functional task practice in patients poststroke or with an acquired brain injury who have limited active movement ability? What treatment effects on motor control are you expecting with the combined intervention? What is the added benefit of stimulation during task practice?

### *Progressive Resistive Exercise*

Traditionally, PRE is the most common method used for strength training across healthy, orthopedic, and neurological clinical populations. PRE has promoted neuromuscular adaptation and significant strength gains in individuals with neurological conditions (Flansbjer, 2008; Kraemer, 2004; Taylor, 2005, 2006; Weiss, 2000; White & Dressendorfer, 2004; Moreland, 2003). Neuromuscular activation levels were significantly higher during dynamic PRE than during functional exercise training (Andersen, 2006). A dose-response relationship exists between the exercise intensity in PRE training and the rate of strength gains; the higher the intensity, the greater the strength gains.

Modes of resistance that can be used for PRE are cuff weights, elastic bands, weighted bars, conventional weight machines (see Figure 22-6), and pneumatic training equipment. Guidelines for PRE prescription should include exercise intensity, volume, and frequency, as discussed earlier in this chapter (Fleck, 2014; Kraemer, 2004).

When designing PRE, the therapist identifies the specific muscle and optimal exercise to isolate this muscle or muscle group and then determines the 1RM or maximal weight that can be safely lifted through the entire ROM. Target intensity (percentage of 1RM) is then calculated to determine the starting load for exercise. An alternative method to determine the load is use of **10RM,** or the maximal load that the patient can safely lift for 10 repetitions through the entire ROM. A 10RM load is approximately 75% of a 1RM load, facilitating decision-making for exercise prescription (Kisner, 2012).

Therapists can select several exercise protocols once a patient's 10RM has been determined. (refer to Table 22-14). DeLorme's (1951) protocol is based on progressive loading across sets, allowing the muscle to warm up. In contrast, the Oxford technique utilizes a regressive progression, where the resistance is decreased across sets to account for muscle fatigue (Zinovieff, 1951). For individuals with neurological conditions, rigid application of a particular protocol is not necessary

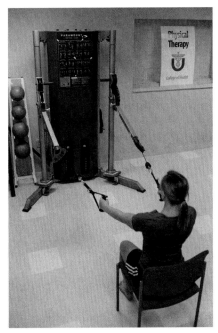

**FIGURE 22-6** Weight and pulley systems can be used for progressive resistive exercise.

| TABLE 22-14 | Exercise Protocols After Determination of 10RM | |
|---|---|---|
| | **DELORME PROTOCOL** | **OXFORD TECHNIQUE** |
| First set | 50% of 10RM | 100% of 10RM |
| Rest interval | 1–3 min | 1–3 min |
| Second set | 75% of 10RM | 75% of 10RM |
| Rest interval | 1–3 min | 1–3 min |
| Third set | 100% of 10RM | 50% of 10RM |

because research has demonstrated that variations of PRE protocols are effective in producing strength gains (Baechle, 2000; Durstine, 2009; Fleck, 2014). The protocol selected should ensure adequate overload, exercise volume, and progression and be individualized to the patient's motor control capabilities and response to training.

The patient is instructed to move at slow to moderate speed through the available range and to control eccentric lowering of the load. Patients should be instructed in proper exercise technique for production of smooth coordinated movements to avoid injury. Patients with sensory loss in the limbs may need to use visual guidance of the limb to isolate the desired motion.

Special attention should be given to provision of adequate external stabilization of the proximal limb segment for open chain PRE in order to help isolate desired motion and minimize substitution. For patients with postural instability or truncal ataxia, PRE may need to be performed in supine or in supported sitting, with manual or external stabilization of the trunk to maximize safe exercise performance. Use of free weights (barbells) may be unsafe for a patient with limb or truncal ataxia because of poor directional control and poor proximal stabilization; however, conventional exercise machines with external stabilization may be used with these patients.

PRE for strength training is advantageous once the patient has strength return of at least 3+ / 5, when he can effectively manage to move a load through the available ROM against gravity. For patients with MMT scores between 2- / 5 and 3 / 5, gravity-eliminated positions are used initially as the patient attempts to move the weight of the limb through the ROM. Use of powder boards and/or a suspension sling system to support the limb may be a helpful adjunct for strengthening exercise in gravity-eliminated positions. The external load can be progressively increased to match the estimated weight of the limb before progressing to antigravity movements.

PRE may be inappropriate for patients with major movement selectivity deficits and difficulty isolating motions. These patients may require motor retraining to isolate movements before addition of progressive loads. Therapists should observe the movement produced and be careful not to strengthen mass stereotypic movement patterns.

### Proprioceptive Neuromuscular Facilitation

A therapeutic approach that has been used extensively in both orthopedic and neurological physical therapy to improve muscle activation and coordination of functional motor patterns is PNF (Voss, 1985). Skilled application of manual resistance by the therapist is required during PNF strengthening activities to facilitate the desired muscle activation and/or movement without excessively overloading the weak muscle, which may inhibit its response. Strengthening can be performed within extremity, pelvic, or scapular patterns or total body patterns, such as weight-shifting in a quadruped or half-kneeling position. The reader is referred to Chapter 15 in this text for a detailed discussion of PNF patterns and techniques. This section provides an overview of the selection and application of these patterns and techniques for strength training in neurological conditions.

A key treatment principle underlying use of PNF patterns is strengthening functional motor patterns rather than training muscles in isolation. The therapist selects PNF patterns and techniques according to the functional roles of the target muscles and the goals of strength training. The reader is referred to several comprehensive texts for a review of PNF activities and techniques that may be useful for strength training in neurological conditions (Adler, 2007; Voss, 1985).

To strengthen muscles used for proximal stabilization, such as scapular (rhomboids), trunk (erector spinae), or pelvic stabilizers (gluteus medius), isometric muscle contractions are resisted in the mid- to shortened range or in closed chain weight-bearing postures. Selected PNF techniques for promoting stability include alternating isometrics, rhythmic stabilization, approximation, and shortened held resisted contractions. For example, to strengthen scapular and trunk stability, the therapist may apply the rhythmic stabilization technique in quadruped with manual contacts at the scapula or the pelvis. This is an example of strengthening within total patterns because synergistic muscle activation among multiple body segments is required. An example of a PNF activity using an extremity pattern for strengthening LE stabilizing muscles is application of shortened held resisted contractions during LE D1 extension pattern targeting the gluteus medius muscle. With the patient in supine or side-lying, the LE is placed in the shortened part of the range for D1 extension pattern. The therapist applies manual contacts on the proximal thigh and distal to the knee and then employs graded resistance to a series of repeated isometric contractions.

To strengthen muscles used for dynamic limb movements, such as hip flexors, dorsiflexors, or the anterior deltoid, concentric contractions are resisted through the range of movement with the distal limb segment free (open chain). Selected PNF techniques for strengthening muscle recruitment for dynamic mobility patterns include rhythmic initiation, repeated contractions, slow reversals, and timing for emphasis. For very weak muscles, application of rhythmic initiation is effective for promoting muscle recruitment because this technique progresses from passive to active assisted to resisted movement through the range.

When facilitation is needed to enhance the patient's capability to initiate movement or to recruit muscle activation at key points in the range, the technique of repeated contractions is recommended. This technique consists of a series of quick stretches, lengthening all components of the diagonal pattern, followed by light resistance through the ROM. For example, if a patient demonstrates weakness when activating the shoulder flexors, the therapist would place the limb in a lengthened position of UE D2 flexion pattern, apply a quick stretch to all components of the D2 pattern timed with the verbal command "and pull," and then provide active assistance or very light tracking resistance through the ROM (see Fig. 22-7). If the patient's motor recruitment needed facilitation at specific points in the ROM, then the therapist could add several additional quick stretches during the movement.

The advantage of utilizing PNF diagonal patterns for strength training in neurological conditions is the ability to promote overflow from stronger components in a pattern to weaker segments. For example, if a patient has very weak dorsiflexors but stronger hip flexors, the therapist could apply the PNF technique of timing for emphasis to the LE D1 flexion pattern. Overflow from the extremities to strengthen trunk musculature could be facilitated through bilateral symmetrical or asymmetrical patterns. For example, weak trunk flexors could be addressed with the UE bilateral symmetrical D2 extension pattern, using the slow reversal technique or a pulley system for resistance (see Fig. 22-8).

PNF patterns and treatment principles can be used as the basis for designing independent and home exercise programs utilizing alternate modes of resistance rather than manual resistance from the therapist. The therapist can instruct the patient in using elastic band resistance or a pulley system within a PNF extremity or combined total pattern. For example, when sitting, the patient could grasp a handle tied to an elastic band with both hands and perform a bilateral asymmetric lift pattern. This activity strengthens the UEs with simultaneous recruitment of trunk extensors and rotators. In an alternative

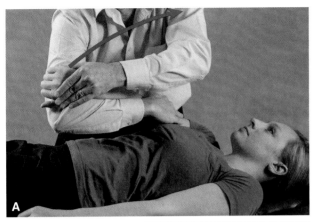
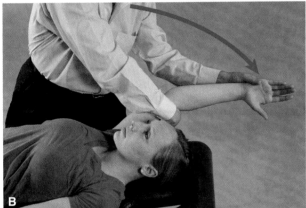

**FIGURE 22-7** Progressive resistive exercise applied in the proprioceptive neuromuscular facilitation (PNF) pattern of UE D2 flexion (A) starting position and (B) ending position. Note in the series that the limb moves through an arc of motion, and the direction of resistance must continually change throughout the movement. Additional quick stretches can be given at specific points during the movement.

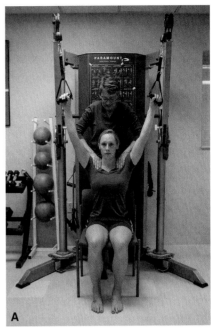
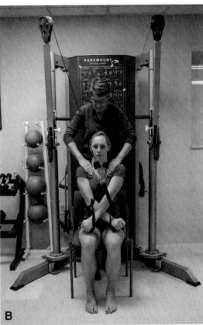

**FIGURE 22-8** The (A) start and (B) end positions using a bilateral symmetrical UE D2 extension pattern in conjunction with a pulley resistance system to add emphasis to the weak trunk flexors. A reversal of the pattern can also be utilized.

seated activity, the patient could hold a plyometric ball and perform the same lift pattern, promoting proximal upper limb and trunk strengthening. Both of these activities could be performed while the patient is on a stable surface or an unstable surface, such as a Swiss ball, or they could be done in more challenging positions, such as a tall kneel or half-kneeling, to increase the level of difficulty.

These combined multiplane movements promote full-body strengthening during which muscles work in concert for coordinated movement. In patients with distributed weakness, this type of training can address multiple areas of weakness simultaneously. When exercise is prescribed for patients with movement selectivity deficits, caution should be taken to avoid PNF patterns that reinforce the mass movement patterns, such as the D2 UE extensor pattern. Ongoing evaluation of the patient's motor response and movement quality and signs of fatigue is important during strength training utilizing PNF activities.

### Isokinetic Strength Training

Isokinetic exercise is an effective mode of dynamic strength training in which the patient is required to produce a torque with maximal or submaximal effort at a predetermined angular

velocity against a computerized isokinetic dynamometer device (see Fig. 22-9). In isokinetic training, movement velocity is constant and is determined by the therapist. Resistance or load is variable on the basis of the patient's effort and the amount of force exerted against the dynamometer arm.

One advantage of isokinetic exercise over fixed resistance exercise is that a muscle is challenged to work maximally throughout the ROM. In addition, the clinician can use this mode of exercise to challenge speed of muscle recruitment at different angular velocities, facilitating increased muscle power. Individuals who are post-CVA or who have MS have

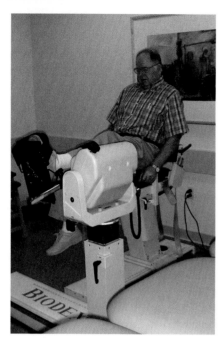

**FIGURE 22-9** Isokinetic strength training for knee musculature in a patient with Parkinson disease (equipment is Biodex System 4 Pro™).

exaggerated strength deficits at faster movement speeds, and many have difficulty generating torque at speeds greater than 90 degrees per second, which is well below limb speeds of typically functional tasks such as walking (200 to 240 degrees per second) (Chen, 1987; Kisner, 2012; Lambert, 2001; Nakumura, 1988). To address the goal of improving muscle power, clinicians can design isokinetic training that requires a patient to exercise across the velocity spectrum (Moreau, 2013), beginning with one or two sets of eight to 10 repetitions at 30, 60, or 90 degrees per second and gradually progressing to increased speeds (one or two sets at 90, 120, or 180 degrees per second) (Davies, 1992). Patten (2007) demonstrated the effectiveness of this type of speed training for the LE in an individual poststroke and documented robust gains in strength and power, as well as improved gait speed.

Isokinetic strength training can be designed to work unidirectionally or with reciprocal motions and to work in the concentric or eccentric mode of exercise. Clinical decisions regarding the appropriate exercise mode for training should be made on the basis of the target muscle and its functional role, applying the specificity of the training principle. Although both modes of isokinetic exercise have been effective for strengthening in persons after a stroke, there is evidence that the eccentric mode produces slightly larger gains and carryover to both concentric and eccentric motor actions (Clark, 2013; Engardt, 1995).

The therapist may opt to begin isokinetic training with unidirectional exercise for patients with imbalance of antagonistic activation or those with substantial spasticity in antagonists to the target muscle. The target muscle can be trained concentrically and eccentrically within each repetition. Progression to reciprocal motions is recommended to

promote improved motor control for functional activities. Because of the high intensity of isokinetic exercise, it is important to include a 5-minute warm-up before the exercise and an opportunity for several submaximal practice trials at selected speeds before maximal effort training. During initial training sessions, vital signs should be monitored to assess the patient's cardiovascular response to this intense exercise. Several researchers documented that persons in subacute and chronic poststroke stages tolerated this high-intensity training without adverse effects (Kim, 2001; Patten, 2006, 2007; Sharp, 1997). The therapist should also watch carefully for signs of fatigue, noting when the torque output drops to 50% of initial values, and provide adequate rest (longer than 1 minute) between sets.

Isokinetic training has the motivational advantage of providing online visual feedback of the torque produced during ROM for the patient. These quantitative torque data are also useful for the therapist to objectively document progress during training.

The majority of studies that examined isokinetic training in persons poststroke trained the LE, mainly knee flexion and extension, in concentric and eccentric modes and reported significant strength gains with transfer effect to gait function (Clark, 2013; Engardt, 1995; Kim, 2001; Sharp, 1997). Few studies have examined the application of isokinetic training for UE strengthening poststroke. Patten (2006, 2013) demonstrated that combined isokinetic strength training and task-specific training in persons 6 to 18 months after a stroke was superior to either training program alone for improving UE strength, power, and functional skills.

Some disadvantages of isokinetic strength training are outlined in Box 22-3. Despite the inherent limitations of isokinetic training, this dynamic mode of strength training provides high-intensity exercise for target muscles that is effective for promoting overload and neural adaptation for central-based weakness. This exercise option is especially beneficial for improving muscle power and ability to generate force at increased movement speeds.

## Aquatic Exercise for Strength Training

Aquatic exercise is an appropriate mode of strengthening for patients with neurological conditions that can be used in both acute and chronic phases of recovery. Aquatic activities may

---

**BOX 22-3 Disadvantages of Isokinetic Training**

- Isolated muscle strengthening as opposed to functional motor patterns
- Typically, training of only single-plane motions
- Sufficient minimal strength (greater than 3 +/5) and selective motor control required to generate torque on the machine
- The time required to set up, position, and align joint and calibrate the machine
- The expense and lack of portability of equipment

be a patient's initial introduction to rehabilitation or may supplement land-based therapy throughout the rehabilitation process. Regardless, aquatic exercise should be an adjunct to land-based therapy, with the ultimate goal of achieving land-based goals. Once the patient can perform the activities on land, water-based therapy may no longer be necessary. The reader is referred to Chapter 15 and additional resources for further discussion of aquatic rehabilitation, including the basic hydrodynamic principles and the physiological effects of immersion.

The advantages of aquatic strength training for patients with neurological deficits are numerous. The hydrodynamic principles of water allow the patient to improve strength and functional abilities in a supported environment, with reduced LE weight-bearing. Because of the buoyancy of water, this environment allows earlier weight-bearing, upright positioning, and functional activities, such as walking and stair climbing. Depending on the patient's position and the devices used, water can support, assist, or resist movement and balance reactions. The level of difficulty of an activity is increased by increasing the speed of the movement, increasing the surface area of the moving part, or increasing the water depth. Movement of the water and a warm water temperature can assist in reducing pain (Whitlatch, 1996), anxiety, and spasticity, thus increasing ease of movement. Conversely, a cooler water temperature serves to stimulate patient response. Water temperature may substantially affect patients with MS; the National Multiple Sclerosis Society recommends water temperatures lower than 85°F (National Multiple Sclerosis Society, 2015).

Because of the characteristics of water, functional activities may initially be easier to perform in this environment than on land. With appropriate modifications, the patient may practice sitting and standing balance activities, sit-to-stand, and walking in a supported environment. For example, a patient with LE weakness may be able to stand and progress to ambulation in chest-deep water earlier than in waist-deep water and much earlier than he could on land. A patient experiencing UE weakness may be able to participate in a buoyancy-assisted strengthening program that would not be possible on land.

In addition to facilitating functional activities, the principles of water may be used to resist or assist the patient's movement for strengthening. For example, with the patient sitting in chest-deep water, turbulence and viscosity provide resistance to knee extension while turbulence, viscosity, and buoyancy provide resistance to flexion with increased speed of movement.

Aquatic exercise has also been beneficial in improving the physical condition of healthy older adults (Poyhonen, 2002; Takeshima, 2002; Whitlatch, 1996). Although research is limited, the benefits of aquatic exercise appear to extend to those with neurological diagnoses, including people with MS. Studies indicate that people living with stroke (Noh, 2008), brain injury (Driver, 2004), or MS (Pariser, 2006) may experience various gains from participating in a water-based program, including improved cardiovascular fitness

(Chu, 2004), gait speed (Teixeira-Salmela, 2001; Chu, 2004), LE strength (Chu, 2004), and ROM (Driver, 2004). Studies of persons with MS also support aquatic therapy as a positive intervention to improve gross motor function (Broach, 2001), as well as self-reported quality of life and fatigue status (Kargarfard, 2012; Roehrs, 2004). Results related to strength measures vary; however, Broach (2003) reported that individuals with MS maintained or improved strength after a water-based exercise program.

The limited studies available on the effects of aquatic exercise in children with CP demonstrate a trend toward positive outcomes (Blohm, 2011), including improved LE strength, gait velocity (Thorpe, 2005), functional status (Dorval, 1996), and respiratory status (Hutzler, 1998). Additional evidence in children with CP shows improvements in standing balance, walking, running, and jumping skills, as well as timed up-and-go scores (Thorpe, 2005) after aquatic intervention. Water-based exercise may also benefit adults with CP in the areas of ROM, pain (Vogtle, 1998), walking ability, balance, and strength (Thorpe, 2000).

Although working in the pool may benefit a patient, detrimental effects must also be considered. Buoyancy may hinder progress because of reduced weight-bearing and proprioceptive input. The patient may experience more difficulty moving in the water, especially if he has a high ratio of adipose tissue to lean muscle mass. For some patients, movement of the water may be disconcerting, resulting in a feeling of dizziness or nausea. For others, chemicals used in the pool environment may affect breathing or burn the eyes. Although aquatic therapy can be a valuable adjunct to land-based therapy, it is not appropriate for all patients. Refer to a limited list of precautions and contraindications for aquatic exercise in Tables 22-15 and 22-16.

### Use of Exercise Machines for Strength Training

Therapists can choose from a wide variety of exercise machines designed for strength training when developing programs for patients with neurological diagnosis. Some factors to consider in making this selection are mode of strength exercise, target muscles, patient characteristics, independent or therapist-directed programs, the setting in which the exercise will be performed, and the availability and cost of the equipment.

For clinic-based exercise programs, multiexercise pulley systems can be used from different patient positions, such as supported sitting in a wheelchair, tall kneeling, or standing.

| TABLE 22-15 | Partial List of Precautions for Aquatic Therapy | |
|---|---|
| • Lack of a gag reflex | • Colostomy/G-tube |
| • Diabetes | • Serial casting |
| • Homeostatic abnormalities | • Hypertension |
| • Controlled seizures | • Superficial wounds |
| • Breathing difficulty | • Fear of water |
| • Autonomic dysreflexia | • Limited water safety skills |
| • Nasogastric tube | • Chemical hypersensitivity |

| TABLE 22-16 | Partial List of Contraindications for Aquatic Therapy | |
|---|---|
| • Open wounds | • Uncontrolled agitation |
| • Infections (urinary tract infection, skin rash, respiratory infection) | • Isolation precautions |
| • Fever | • Continuous nasal oxygen |
| • Bladder incontinence | • IV or indwelling catheter |
| • Bowel incontinence | • Incompatibility with facility infection control procedures |
| • Tracheostomy | • Uncontrolled seizures |
| • Uncontrolled blood pressure | • Unstable fractures |
| • Casts due to fractures | |

Therapists can design strength training for UEs and LEs using single-plane or multiplane motions with newer pulley systems (Fig. 22-8). When patients lack sufficient grasp ability, mitts can be used to secure hands on the handles. For closed chain LE strength training, the Total Gym® system can be used. This system employs a glide board and allows the patient to perform single or bilateral LE exercises, such as squats and heel raises, with some degree of the body unweighted in semireclined to upright positions. As the patient's LE strength progresses, weights can be added for resistance in this system.

In clinical and fitness-based gym settings, weight-cable machines, hydraulic or pneumatic machines that provide variable resistance through ROM, can be effective choices if the patient has sufficient prerequisite strength and motor control to lift/push loads against gravity. These machines often incorporate bilateral UE or LE exercise demands, such as inclined press and rowing exercises. Typically, the user is required to transfer to a seat on the machine. Patients with balance problems or motor control deficits may need additional stabilization when using these machines. Most machines are designed for single-plane movement to isolate muscles; however, newer models incorporate multiplane motion, which promotes more functional movement patterns (e.g., Cybex Fitness, LifeCycle, Nautilus fitness units). When prescribing strength exercise using these machines, the therapist needs to instruct the patient on proper setup if exercising independently and teach safety and proper exercise form to prevent injury.

Other exercise machines typically used for aerobic training can be applied for strength training in neurological populations. LE ergometry, both in upright or semireclined models, can be beneficial for strengthening hip and knee extensors and promoting bilateral LE exercise effects. Therapists should design ergometry exercise programs with sufficient load to challenge muscle strength without undue cardiovascular fatigue and provide specific exercise parameters for level of resistance and pedal rate (average revolutions per minute [RPM]). To challenge muscle power, speed intervals (30 to 60 seconds) can be prescribed with lighter resistance and high RPM

(greater than 90). When the patient has insufficient motor control to keep the foot on the pedal, foot straps can provide stability. Thigh or leg straps can also be used to control legs more proximally (see Fig. 22-10).

Similar exercise programs can be designed using UE ergometers with close monitoring of muscular fatigue. Other exercise machines that can have cross-training effects for both strengthening and aerobic function include stepping machines, such as StairMaster(tm) or NuStep(tm), rowing machines, elliptical trainers, and cross-country ski machines. For application to neurological populations, the therapist needs to consider the minimum requirements in postural control, motor control, and coordination for these exercise options.

Finally, treadmill training with or without body weight support (BWS), as discussed earlier in the functional strength training section of this chapter, can be an effective tool for strength training. Exercise parameters considered for strength training with a treadmill are speed, incline, and duration of training, as well as use of rails for support. In all options, cardiovascular response to exercise needs to be closely monitored, and use of a target heart rate zone or Borg's *Perceived Exertion Scale* is recommended to ensure a safe range of exercise performance (Borg, 1982). Because of the complex multisystem impairments in neurological populations, a customized exercise prescription as described in earlier sections of this chapter is recommended with use of these exercise machines for strength training.

## ■ Weakness Intervention: Ultimately Applied in Functional Activities

### Functional Task-Oriented Strength Training

Impaired motor control in neurological conditions is frequently a multifaceted problem, as weakness, movement selectivity deficits, impaired timing, and coordination all may

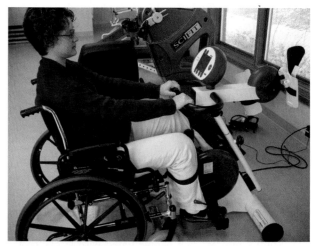

**FIGURE 22-10** Lower extremity seated exercise cycle (MotoMed™ model) with adapted strapping to stabilize feet and legs on pedals and control leg position for an individual with neurological deficits.

contribute to movement dysfunction. Designing a strength training program utilizing functional motor activities addresses multiple system impairments and promotes transfer to functional skills. In addition, task-specific strength training facilitates activity-dependent neuroplasticity, potentially enhancing neurological recovery (Fisher, 2001; Liepert, 2001; Nelles, 2001). The principles of strength intervention described earlier can be applied to all of the functional tasks covered in Chapters 33 to 37.

According to Carr (2003), strength training should be task specific and geared toward movements that are characteristic of required functional tasks. For example, practicing repetitive step-up activities to a single stair or platform not only strengthens LE extensors but also transfers to improved power generation for stair climbing (see Fig. 22-11). Exercise prescription for this activity can be applied by having the patient practice the maximum number of steps that can be performed with good control until fatigue is evident, then resting and repeating a second set. This exercise can be progressed by increasing the number of repetitions in each set or increasing the step height. For LE strength training, numerous closed chain task-oriented activities can be prescribed to improve a patient's requisite strength for transfers, walking, and stairs. Refer to Table 22-17 for a partial list of LE functional strengthening exercises.

Individualized exercise prescription is required for functional strength training. Task design may need to be modified to meet the strength and balance capabilities of the patient. For example, during sit-to-stand training, a raised seat may initially be needed for a patient with weak LE extensors. A counter or table placed in front of the patient for UE support once he is

| TABLE 22-17 | Lower Extremity Functional Strengthening Exercises |
|---|---|
| Sit-to-stands (and eccentric stand-to-sit) | Forward step-down |
| Partial standing squats | Forward step-ups |
| Toe touches to block/step of varied heights | Lateral step-ups |
| Heel raises and toe raises | Marching |
| Lateral leg kicks | Ergometry cycling |
| Posterior leg kicks | Treadmill training |

upright may be beneficial when balance is unsteady. This activity can be progressed by reducing seat height, removing UE support, or increasing exercise volume (repetitions/sets). The therapist should observe the patient's movement quality carefully to determine whether any compensatory or substitutive movements are used and to note evidence of fatigue. The overload principle for strength training should be applied to these functional exercises to facilitate optimal strength gains (Barreca, 2004; Canning, 2003; Monger, 2002). Practicing a few repetitions of sit-to-stand will not necessarily translate to improved strength if the individual is not challenged beyond his current strength level.

### Lower Extremity Functional Activities

Research supports the effectiveness of LE functional strength training on improved strength and functional mobility in persons with stroke, ABI, and MS (Dean, 2000; Lee, 2013; Salbach, 2004; Yang, 2006). Refer to Focus on Evidence Tables 22-20, 22-21, and 22-22 (ONL) for details on these studies.

Treadmill training with and without BWS is an example of task-specific training that places activity-specific strength demands on LEs (Sullivan, 2002, 2007; Visintin, 1998). BWSTT has produced higher strength gains and improvements in walking measures than either resisted cycling or control groups (Sullivan, 2007). Higher-intensity and increased speeds of treadmill training produced more robust walking outcomes (Lamontagne, 2004; Pohl, 2002). The reader is referred to Chapter 37 regarding ambulation training for further details on treadmill training. Collectively, this research supports the efficacy of task-specific strength training for LE function.

### Upper Extremity Functional Activities

Functional strength training concepts can be applied to UE and trunk weakness as well. Training on reaching tasks beyond arm's length requiring UE and dynamic trunk movements has improved trunk strength and reaching ability (Dean, 1997; Thielman, 2004). Other examples of functional trunk exercises that require trunk stabilization are repetitive practice of moving from sidelying to sitting and dynamic bilateral UE tasks against a load, such as lifting, pushing, and pulling. Examples of functional strengthening activities for the upper limb are open chain activities, such as varied reaching tasks with progression from supported to unsupported

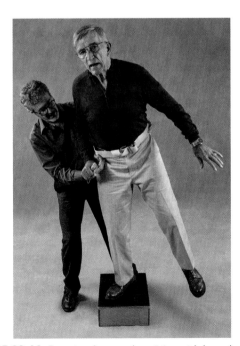

**FIGURE 22-11** Functional strength training with lateral step-up activity. A patient can practice repetitive step-up actions to a stool, single stair, or platform to strengthen the LE antigravity muscles and prepare for the task-specific functional activity of stair climbing.

upper limb, no load to progressively increased load (see Fig. 22-12), bimanual to unimanual task demands, and increased height and distance of reaching.

Rather than working muscles in isolation, these task-oriented activities work the muscles in functional synergies. One advantage of this mode of strength training is that activities can be designed to address both strength and motor control deficits to improve timing and coordination of functional movement patterns. However, the severity of selective motor control impairments can be a constraint to task design for this type of strength training. Meaningful task-specific training for UE motion promotes more superior motor recovery than training isolated motions (Carr, 2003; Patten, 2006, 2013; Trombly, 1986; vanVliet, 1995). The robust motor and functional gains achieved after constraint-induced movement therapy after a stroke may be partially due to systematic, progressive demands on upper limb strength and motor control, as well as the high intensity of training (Winstein, 2004; Wolf, 2002, 2006).

## Considerations for Nontherapy Time and Discharge

In the acute care and rehabilitation settings, a patient generally spends a portion of his day engaged in supervised therapeutic activities. The actual time of the supervised activities varies widely depending on the patient's medical status and needs. The remainder of the patient's day may be consumed by nontherapeutic activities. Because of the decline in length of hospital stay, it is imperative that therapists efficiently use available time to prepare the patient for discharge to home or another environment in the continuum of care.

Refer to Tables 22-18 and 22-19 for patient-specific variables and teaching variables that should be considered when developing an exercise program for nontherapy time or home use. Research indicates that older individuals are less adherent with exercise and medication programs than their younger counterparts are for a variety of reasons (Burton, 1999; Conn, 1998; Forkan, 2006; King, 2002; Melillo, 1996; Resnick, 2001). Often, barriers such as lack of interest, poor health, weather, and low expectations rather than motivation influence adherence with an exercise program (Forkan, 2006). According to Forkan (2006), 90% of older adults discharged from the hospital environment reported receiving a home exercise program, but only 53% continued the program, regardless of the time since discharge. Although adherence may be limited, home programs have been effective in the treatment of a variety of conditions (Shimizu, 2002), including PD (Lun, 2005), stroke (Duncan, 1998) and CP (Wang, 2013), and are important in preventing a decline in strength and function in persons with neurological conditions.

## Activities for Home: Strength Training

When an exercise program is developed for patients to use during nontherapy time or at home, it is important to prioritize activities according to the needs of the patient to facilitate adherence. Therapists should focus on activities that provide the greatest benefit to the patient and can be efficiently performed

| TABLE 22-18 | Patient Variables to Consider in Home Program Development |
|---|---|
| √ | Prioritized assessment of patient's needs |
| √ | Learning style |
| √ | Cognitive/perceptual status |
| √ | Age and previous activity level |
| √ | Hearing/visual status |
| √ | Educational level |
| √ | Readiness to learn |
| √ | Motivation to learn |
| √ | Available assistance |
| √ | Cultural beliefs |

| TABLE 22-19 | Teaching Variables to Consider in Home Program Development |
|---|---|
| √ | Content and prioritization of home program |
| √ | Teaching environment |
| √ | Teaching method |
| √ | Teaching sequence |
| √ | Evaluation of teaching effectiveness |
| √ | Customizing teaching methods |

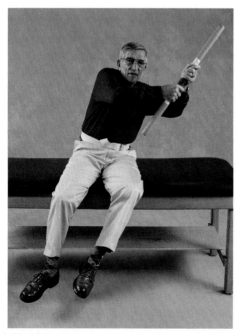

**FIGURE 22-12** Functional strength training with trunk stabilization and an external load.

during daily activities. Integrating a task-oriented approach may be an efficient and effective means of strength training while also working on functional activity. For example, a gait training program was effective in improving gait speed and walking distance after stroke (van de Port, 2007).

Therapeutic strengthening activities used in the clinic can be modified for hospital room or home use. For example, when the goal of the program is LE strengthening, the patient can use an elastic band to resist straight-plane or diagonal movements of the LE while in a stable sitting position in a chair or wheelchair. Task-specific strength training can be prescribed and incorporated into daily activities, such as repetitive sit-to-stand while standing at the sink during grooming tasks or standing at the kitchen counter to make a sandwich. By incorporating strengthening activities into the patient's daily routine, carryover may be enhanced and the patient may more readily understand the benefit of the activities.

## PATIENT APPLICATION PART III: EXAMPLES OF STRENGTH INTERVENTIONS FOR CHARLIE

### Application of PNF Activities to Strengthen Total-Body Functional Patterns

- With Charlie in a sitting position, the therapist may facilitate the bilateral asymmetrical lift pattern using the right UE as the lead arm both to address UE proximal shoulder weakness and to promote overflow to the trunk musculature. The slow reversal technique with appropriate manual resistance applied throughout the available ROM may increase strength and control of movement.

- Scapular stabilization, trunk weakness, and proximal LE weakness may be addressed with Charlie in quadruped. The therapist first performs rhythmic stabilization with manual contacts at the pelvis, building stability in the position. The level of difficulty can be increased by asking Charlie to perform the LE D1 extension pattern with left LE while the therapist applies rhythmic initiation with one manual contact at the contralateral pelvis and one contact on the left proximal posterolateral thigh. This activity promotes strengthening of proximal hip muscles bilaterally, as well as increasing stabilization demands on the trunk and UEs.

- Finally, to address distal right ankle weakness and promote overflow from stronger proximal muscles, the therapist facilitates the LE D1 flexion or LE D2 flexion pattern using timing for emphasis technique, with manual contacts on the proximal thigh and distal foot/ankle. Manual resistance is graded to the patient's ability to recruit muscles, and quick stretch is used to facilitate enhanced recruitment of ankle muscles. The right ankle dorsiflexors may be initially facilitated with Charlie supine and then progressed to standing with a short step forward or a small step-up to a stair.

### Application of Aquatic Rehabilitation for Strength Training

- Aquatic therapy is an appropriate adjunct to land-based strength training and may assist in Charlie's return to community activities. After removal of the right LE cast, Charlie meets the criteria for aquatic therapy.

- Sample strengthening activities to address LE weakness include movements against the resistance of buoyancy, either with or without additional resistance.

- As an illustration, right hip abductor weakness may be addressed with Charlie in standing with UE support and application of a flotation device to his ankle to add resistance to concentric contractions through the range of movement.

- Water walking in progressively shallower depths using correct form and facilitation as needed serves to improve gait pattern as well as strength.

### Application of Functional Task-Oriented Strength Training

- A series of closed chain exercises with light UE support and close guard as needed for balance are appropriate interventions to strengthen LE musculature.

- Sample activities include
  - Sets of sit-to-stand from chair height that he can perform without physical assistance;
  - Partial squats with return to stand to simulate stand-to-sit while standing at the countertop for support;
  - Repeated step-ups forward and lateral to a step with rail support, emphasizing proper form and control;
  - Bilateral heel raises from the floor in bilateral stance position, then with left LE placed in forward step position to increase demands on right plantar flexor muscles;
  - Examples of open chain functional exercises for LE in supported standing, such as practicing clearing obstacles of varied heights with the right foot or placing the foot on platform steps of increasing height.

### Application of PRE and Exercise Machines for Strength Training

- Use of the Total Gym® system may be beneficial after a LE cast has been removed to strengthen LE extensor musculature, with gradual progression of body weight resistance and external load.

- For generalized LE strengthening as Charlie progresses in his recovery, he could perform upright cycle ergometer training with moderate resistance and a target RPM of 60 to 80 and a rating of perceived exertion ranging from 11 to 13. If he is too deconditioned to perform 10 to 15 minutes of continuous cycling, the therapist could structure several short bouts (5 minutes) of light- to moderate-intensity cycling followed by adequate rest periods (3 to 5 minutes) between bouts.

- Another combined aerobic and strength training option is the Airdyne® Stationary Bicycle with use of a mitt for left-hand grip to promote both UE and LE training.

- For strengthening proximal scapular and shoulder muscles, a traditional PRE program could be designed using cuff weights or weight circuit exercise machines, such as bilateral rower, chest press, and incline press. A mitt may be needed to assist with stabilization of the left hand for grip to the handle.

- Because of his cognitive status, Charlie needs supervision for safe use of this equipment and verbal cueing for proper technique.

### Application of Home Exercise Program

- At this point in Charlie's rehabilitation, he should participate in strengthening and functional activities throughout the day to reinforce therapy activities. On the basis of his progress, these additional activities may be modified for incorporation into his home exercise program at discharge from the rehabilitation setting.
- For continued strengthening of the UEs and LEs and trunk, the therapist may recommend exercises with elastic band resistance, which Charlie can perform independently.
- Charlie could also perform bilateral large arc UE motions, such as overhead lifts and bilateral PNF patterns, with the use of a weighted plyometric ball for resistance. Initially, these strengthening exercises may be performed while sitting on a stable chair, with progression to standing.
- For continued functional strengthening after discharge, Charlie may participate in a walking program that includes inclines and progressive increases in distance and speed or negotiating steps and stairs.
- A community-based exercise program such as aquatic exercise or circuit weight training may also be beneficial in maintaining or improving strength and function, as well as providing interaction with others in a more social environment.

# HANDS-ON PRACTICE

The student should gain the following practical skills from reading and applying concepts in this chapter to her clinical practice:

1. Distinguish the design and purpose of an exercise prescription for strength training to improve **muscle endurance, muscle strength,** versus **muscle power.**
2. Identify the role of strength training in a physical therapy plan of care for individuals with various non-progressive and progressive neurological diagnoses.
3. Apply exercise science principles of **overload, specificity** of training, **cross-training,** and **reversibility** when designing and progressing strengthening exercises in patients with neurological conditions.
4. Select an appropriate **exercise mode** and individualize the **exercise prescription** according to the patient's/client's neurological diagnosis, time postinjury for nonprogressive diagnoses or disease severity for progressive diagnoses, functional level, and movement abilities.
5. Design a **preventive strength training program** for individuals with chronic neurological disability living in the community as one component of their wellness-based fitness program.
6. Select and apply therapeutic interventions for enhancing muscle recruitment and strength in **very weak muscles** (less than 2+ / 5) in patients with neurological conditions.
7. Prescribe a **progressive resistive exercise** for targeted weak muscles in persons with varied neurological diagnoses, including prescription of exercise intensity, frequency, durations, volume, and progression.
8. Identify when a **nonfatiguing protocol** in strength exercise prescription is indicated in specific neurological diagnoses, and apply these principles in exercise design.
9. Design **functional strengthening exercises** according to a patient's/client's functional level, applying exercise prescription and progression concepts in persons with neurological diagnoses.
10. Determine the appropriate mode of strength training (isometric, eccentric, or concentric) on the basis of the functional role of the target muscle(s) and the degree of muscle weakness.
11. Apply **neuromuscular electrical stimulation** to target muscles and determine appropriate parameters for strength training in persons with major weakness from neurological conditions.
12. Apply the principles of **aquatic exercise** for strength training in persons with neurological diagnoses, with appropriate identification of contraindications and precautions for aquatic therapy.
13. Select an appropriate mode of strength training and design a **home exercise prescription** for patients/clients with neurological conditions.

## Let's Review

1. What role and potential benefits does strength training have in the physical therapy plan of care for individuals with neurological conditions (nonprogressive and progressive diagnoses)?
2. What factors (neural, structural, mechanical) influence the force-generating capacity of a muscle?
3. How does a physical therapist design progressive resistive exercise prescription for improving **muscle endurance versus muscle power** in patients with weakness?
4. What **exercise science principles** should be applied in strength training design and progression for improving strength in individuals with neurological diagnoses?

5. Describe varied **modes of strength training** that the physical therapist can utilize according to the individual patient's/client's diagnosis, clinical presentation, and distribution of weakness.

6. What key **exercise prescription variables** must the physical therapist consider in clinical decision-making regarding design of a strength training program?

7. What therapeutic interventions could the physical therapist apply for enhancing muscle recruitment and strength training in patients with neurological conditions who have **severe weakness** and limited ability to activate target muscles?

8. In which types of neurological diagnoses or conditions is a **nonfatiguing exercise protocol** indicated, and what are key elements of this protocol?

9. When **aquatic exercise** is used for strength training in patients with neurological conditions, how can the physical therapist progress the resistance or level of difficulty of the exercise?

10. Describe exercise design and progression-applying concepts of **functional strengthening exercises**. What are the potential benefits of this type of strength training in patients with neurological conditions?

---

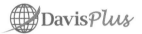 **DavisPlus**  For additional resources, including Focus on Evidence tables, case study discussions, references and glossary, please visit http://davisplus.fadavis.com

## CHAPTER SUMMARY

The purposes of this chapter are (1) to provide a clinician's insight into the physiological basis of weakness in neurological disorders and (2) to provide a rationale and guidelines for strength training programs at all phases of the continuum of care to address both centrally based muscle activation deficits and reverse or prevent the effects of inactivity and disuse atrophy. Weakness is a primary contributor to functional limitations for persons with neurological conditions. Remediation of these strength deficits has direct effects on improved functional outcomes in persons with nonprogressive disorders of the CNS, including stroke, TBI, and CP. When combined with aerobic training using a health promotion framework, strength training effectively optimizes functional abilities and improves quality of life in persons with progressive disorders of the CNS, such as PD or MS.

The exercise principles for strength training provided in this chapter should guide the therapist in designing an individualized exercise prescription for persons with neurological conditions, including application of the overload principle, specificity of training, systematic exercise progression, and reversibility of training. Customized exercise prescription requires that the therapist make clinical decisions regarding exercise intensity, volume, frequency, and duration, as well as optimal mode of strength training, for each patient.

A wide range of therapeutic techniques and modes of strength training are available to the therapist when designing exercise programs. For individuals with very weak muscles and difficulty voluntarily activating these muscles, sensory stimulation techniques, NMES, EMGBFB, or EMG-triggered NMES can facilitate the increased motor recruitment and timing needed for functional movement patterns. PNF patterns, activities, and techniques can also improve muscle recruitment required for functional motor patterns. Moderate-to high-intensity training using traditional PRE or isokinetic exercise is an effective mode to target specific isolated muscles or muscle groups. Functional strength training utilizes task-specific activities to progressively challenge muscle recruitment within functional motor synergies and promotes optimal transfer of strength training to functional skills. As a result, this approach has excellent application for patients with multisystem neurological impairments.

For clinic-based, community-based, or home-based strength training programs, the therapist can select from a wide range of exercise modes and machines. Selection is based on consideration of the patient's specific strength impairments and goals, functional capabilities, and limitations, as well as individual preferences. Therapists should prescribe home or community-based exercise programs at discharge for patients who are completing their rehabilitation phase, as well as for those individuals with neurological disability who are living in the community. The purpose of these exercise programs is to prevent detraining effects and a decline in functional abilities due to deconditioning. All individuals with neurological disorders should be educated about basic fitness principles, including the role of ongoing strength and aerobic training for health maintenance and disease prevention.

# Intervention for Limited Passive Range of Motion

## CHAPTER 23

Patricia Kluding, PT, PhD ▪ Blair P. Saale, PT, DPT, NCS

## CHAPTER OBJECTIVES

Upon completion of this chapter, the learner should be able to:

1. Summarize the factors that contribute to loss of passive range of motion (PROM) in people with neuromuscular pathology and injury.
2. Utilize range of motion (ROM) examination data and evaluation from a patient case to obtain information that drives clinical intervention decisions.
3. Identify situations in which it is appropriate to provide a ROM intervention to improve function.
4. Describe evidence for implementation of a variety of ROM interventions.
5. Apply principles of ROM intervention to a patient case.

## ▪ Introduction

Normal movements of the body are fluid and occur with exquisite motor control. Sometimes this normal movement can be restricted by limitations of the bony joint surfaces or of the soft tissue structures at the joint. Range of motion (ROM), the degree to which excursion can take place at a particular joint, is commonly decreased in individuals with neuromuscular impairments. These limitations are of concern because they restrict movement options even when motor control is not impaired and can contribute to pain, loss of function, or altered appearance. For example, the shoulder joint provides us with a wide range of movement options in all planes of motion, but pathological changes that decrease shoulder flexion can cause a multitude of functional impairments, including difficulty reaching overhead to retrieve objects and performing upper body dressing tasks.

Active range of motion (AROM) refers to the ability of a person to use muscle contractions to move a body segment through the motion available at the joint. This ability is primarily an indication of motor strength and motor control and may vary depending on the position of the body segment and the effects of gravity. AROM is an important part of the physical examination, but AROM deficits cannot be reported in isolation. An observed deficit in AROM requires further testing to determine the cause of the restriction, such as limitations of the bony joint surfaces, decreased soft tissue extensibility at the joint, pain, impaired motor control, or muscular weakness.

This chapter focuses on physical interventions for limited **passive range of motion (PROM)** due to bony joint surface deformities or restrictions in soft tissue extensibility.

**PROM** refers to movements at a joint caused by an external force when a person is fully relaxed, such as when a physical therapist moves a body segment. This motion can be limited by pain, bony joint surface deformities, or restriction of soft tissue extensibility. PROM at a joint that is limited by tightness of a muscle, joint capsule, or other soft tissue is referred to as a **contracture** (Halar, 1978). There are two types of contractures: muscle contractures and joint contractures. **Muscle contractures** are specifically due to shortened muscles, and **joint contractures** are due to joint capsular tightness. These differences may be difficult to discern in the typical clinical setting. Passive **stiffness** can be felt as resistance to stretch. This resistance may occur even in midrange and when a person is relaxed and not actively contracting the opposing muscle groups to generate resistance.

## THINK ABOUT IT 23.1

During your evaluation, you notice that your patient has limited active range of motion (AROM) at the elbow. She is able to actively flex her elbow only from 0 to 15 degrees but has 0 to 135 degrees passive range of motion. Is this a problem with the bony surface or soft tissue extensibility? What else do you need to examine to determine the cause of the AROM deficit?

Central nervous system (CNS) pathology can cause a variety of motor and sensory impairments that contribute to the development of joint contractures. People who experience a spinal cord injury (SCI), brain trauma, or stroke most commonly have contractures in the hip, ankle, shoulder, and elbow (Chung, 2004; Diong, 2012; Fergusson, 2006; Kwah, 2012; Singer, 2004; Yarkony, 1987). Contractures also occur in children with CNS pathology, with a high incidence of lower extremity contractures reported in children with cerebral palsy (CP) (Svehlík, 2010; Wren, 2004), Duchenne muscular dystrophy (DMD) (Gaudreault, 2009), spina bifida (Snela, 2000; Verhoef, 2004), and spinal muscular atrophy (SMA) (Fujak, 2011; Wang, 2004).

We follow two patient examples throughout this chapter: a young adult with CP and an elderly woman with Parkinson disease (PD). Possible answers to the discussion questions for each case are provided in the supplemental material available online.

## Clinical Picture of Passive Range of Motion in a Holistic Context

Adequate PROM at each related joint is critical to any voluntary movement, but it is only one part of the total human system that must work together to generate smooth, controlled movement. This is the basis for all functional activity and participation. For example, a joint must have adequate ROM to achieve a desired movement. The brain must engage to send a signal to the spinal cord to activate enough alpha motor neurons to generate adequate muscle force for the movement. The CNS instantaneously and continually adjusts the plan of all muscles involved, including timing and intensity, to produce the motor control that makes our movements refined and regulated. Cognition must drive the decision and motivation

to move. Each of these pieces is critical for the execution of a voluntary task.

## Potential Effect of Contracture on Function

Deficits of PROM, documented in the physical examination, can directly or indirectly contribute to functional problems. For example, there appears to be a direct link between limited ankle mobility in the elderly and the ability to respond to a balance perturbation (Gehlsen, 1990; Mecagni, 2000). ROM loss can lead to secondary complications that exacerbate the primary impairments (Gajdosik, 2002). Patients with CNS pathology may have concurrent deficits in strength, sensation, and other components of motor control, making the relationship between PROM loss and functional activities challenging to discern.

A gain in PROM alone does not necessarily result in improved function. As a result, goals focusing solely on regaining full PROM are not typically suitable for rehabilitation unless it is meaningful to the patient or unless PROM limitations result in pain, abnormal posture, functional deficits, or difficulty with self-care tasks. In these situations, it is appropriate to address PROM deficits when setting goals with your patient.

Specific PROM deficits cause very specific problems in certain functional activities. A plantar flexion contracture at the ankle prevents heel-strike at initial contact, limits forward progression of the tibia during the stance phase of gait, and causes a foot-drag or toe catching on the floor during the swing phase of gait. A knee flexion contracture prevents full knee extension during the stance phase of gait and prevents symmetry in standing activities. A hip flexion contracture and the resulting lack of full hip extension in a patient with paraplegia from SCI prevents the individual from being able to fully stand or to ambulate with a bilateral swing-through pattern. Contractures in the fingers and wrist prevent manipulation and grasp activities. An elbow flexion contracture prevents upper extremity weight-bearing.

The relationship between ROM and function is further complicated in situations in which restricted ROM is actually beneficial for function. Individuals with tetraplegia are often advised to avoid stretching out their wrist and finger flexors to promote a more functional tenodesis grasp (see Chapter 26), and tightness of the low back may promote sitting balance and greater ease of movement during transfers for these patients. In contrast, excessive ROM at a joint is desirable to compensate for other deficits in some situations, such as the need for hamstring hypermobility in individuals with paraplegia or tetraplegia. Hamstring ROM of 110 to 120 degrees allows these patients to attain a long-sitting position important for dressing, bed mobility, and floor transfers.

### PATIENT APPLICATION: CEREBRAL PALSY

*Danny is an 18 year-old man with spastic diplegic CP. He has also been diagnosed with attention-deficit hyperactivity disorder and scoliosis (at age 12 years), but his remaining medical history is unremarkable.*

*Danny is at Gross Motor Function Classification System (GMFCS) level II (Palisano, 2007); he is able to ambulate independently over flat surfaces without an assistive device, but he requires support from a railing or a hand-hold assist on stairs and falls frequently when walking over uneven ground. He wore bilateral ankle-foot orthotics as a child but has refused to wear them for the last 3 years. He prefers to wear high-top sneakers instead. He has received botulinum toxin A injections for plantar flexor hypertonicity.*

*Danny lives with his parents and older sister and attends a public high school. He has two periods per day of "life skills" classes and is mainstreamed for the rest of his classes. Danny works out daily in the school fitness center and is very active in his church youth group and other extracurricular activities. His goals after graduation are to live in a supervised apartment and find a job that he enjoys.*

## Contemplate Clinical Decisions: Cerebral Palsy

- *What are Danny's risk factors for limitations in PROM?*
- *What body segments would you examine for possible PROM limitations?*
- *What potential PROM limitations do you think are most important from the patient's perception of his dysfunction?*

### PATIENT APPLICATION: PARKINSON DISEASE

*Mrs. B is a 73 year-old female who was diagnosed with PD 2 years ago. Her medical history is significant for emphysema (she is no longer smoking) and seizure disorder. She also reports chronic right knee pain and swelling. Her medications are Sinemet and Lodosin for PD and Depacote for seizures.*

*Mrs. B lives with her daughter and son-in-law; the daughter is available to provide assistance throughout the day and night. Mrs. B's chief complaints are difficulty with standing and walking and frequent loss of balance. She requires assistance from her daughter for all mobility tasks. The patient's and family's goals include her being able to walk and get into/out of bed independently.*

## Contemplate Clinical Decisions: Parkinson Disease

- *What are Mrs. B's risk factors for limitations in PROM?*
- *What body segments would you examine for possible PROM limitations?*
- *What potential PROM limitations do you think are most important from the perspective of the patient and her family?*

## ■ Anatomy and Physiology

### Systems Involved

Limitations in passive movement in adult or pediatric patients with neurological pathology may be caused by many complex factors. When a body part is moved in a relaxed subject, passive resistance is encountered from three potential sources: (1) the inertia of the limb, (2) a stretch reflex that may cause a muscle contraction opposing the movement, and (3) viscoelastic properties of the muscle, connective tissue, and joint capsule that may resist movement. Although these factors are relevant for anyone with or without neuromuscular disease, they can lead to pathological levels of increased stiffness and contractures in individuals with neuromuscular disorders.

### Limb Inertia

The inertia of a limb produces initial resistance to any passive movement. In physics, Newton's first law of motion deals with the concept of inertia: An object in a state of rest remains at rest unless acted upon by an external force. A phenomenon called *thixotropy* in the muscles may contribute even more resistance to the movement of a joint (Vattanasilp, 2000). Muscle behaves as a thixotropic substance because increased stiffness is demonstrated when it has not been moved recently, with decreased resistance to movement after being stretched or moved. A thixotropic response has been demonstrated in the calf muscles of people after a stroke and in healthy controls (Vattanasilp, 2000). It appears that either prolonged or cyclic stretching can decrease muscle stiffness in people with a stroke (Bressel, 2002; Gao, 2011), which illustrates that interventions aimed at improving PROM may affect the thixotropic response.

### Neural Factors

A lesion of the CNS may cause stretch reflex hyperactivity and hypertonia (specifically **spasticity**), which substantially influences muscle stiffness (de Gooijer-van de Groep, 2013, 2016; Given, 1995; Sinkjaer, 1994; Vattanasilp, 2000). Spasticity is a **neural factor** that can lead to higher levels of stiffness, thus contributing to contracture. **Nonneural factors** are also known to increase the resistance of limb movement and contribute to the development of contractures; these are discussed in the next section.

Spastic hypertonia and hyperreflexia, found in patients with CNS pathology, are due to a lowered threshold of alpha motor neuron activation. The type Ia afferents from the muscle spindle are preferentially activated by a high-velocity, low-amplitude stretch and results in monosynaptic excitation of the alpha motor neuron, as illustrated in Fig. 23-1. Because of the lowered threshold, the alpha motor neuron is closer to depolarization, and a relatively small input (i.e., stretch) can result in a muscle contraction that has higher-than-normal amplitude.

Sinkjaer (1994) defined "**reflex stiffness**" as the component of total joint stiffness mediated by stretch reflex mechanisms. Spasticity is most evident when assessed at rest. There is some controversy over how much it influences active movement or function (Burne, 2005). Examination for disorders of muscle tone and other motor dysfunction is covered in detail in Chapter 6. Chapter 18 describes intervention for flaccidity and hypotonia, whereas Chapter 19 describes interventions for spastic and rigid hypertonia.

The increase in resting muscle tone due to spasticity can result in a sustained posture that eventually leads to a more permanent, fixed contracture. The patient in the photograph (Fig. 23-2) had

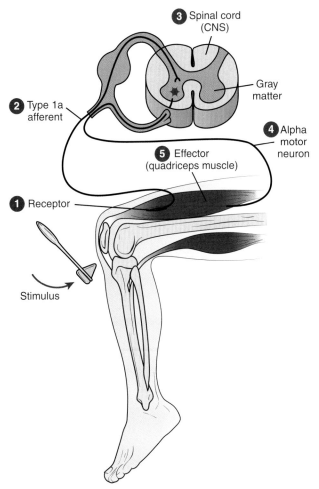

**FIGURE 23-1** Illustration of a stretch reflex pathway. Type Ia afferents in the muscle spindle are activated by a high-velocity, low-amplitude stretch, which results in monosynaptic excitation of the alpha motor neurons.

a stroke that affected the right side of his body. His natural resting posture is illustrated in Fig. 23-2. Over time, this patient will develop increased resistance to stretch of the flexor muscles from both spasticity and connective tissue tightness.

### Nonneural Factors

Passive mobility of skeletal joints may be limited by tightness in one of the many principal structures that surround the joint. These structures are classified as either contractile or noncontractile. **Contractile** elements, which include the muscle with its in-series tendons and attachments, can contribute to stiffness via the neural mechanisms discussed previously or because of the tightness of these structures. **Noncontractile** elements include the ligaments, joint capsule, and bones. Tendons and ligaments are viscoelastic structures composed primarily of collagen. The collagen molecules form cross-links to create microfibrils, which aggregate to form bundles (Carlstedt, 1989). Nonneural contributions to joint stiffness include greater amounts of intramuscular connective tissue, a greater percentage of slow-twitch muscle fibers, and a greater cross-section of muscle area at the ankle than at the elbow (Given, 1995). Factors such as pathology, immobilization,

and aging that can alter the biomechanical properties of these structures are discussed in the following sections.

It may be very difficult to distinguish between contractile and noncontractile tissues when stiffness is felt with movement of a body part. Cyriax (1982) proposed a classification scheme to distinguish capsular from noncapsular patterns of restriction unique to each joint, with capsular patterns observed with irritation of the entire synovial membrane or joint capsule, as with degenerative joint disease or arthritis. However, this classification system is controversial and has not been consistently supported by research (Klässbo, 2003). People with CNS pathology may experience changes in the mechanical properties of muscle and connective tissue, as well as changes from loss of strength or the aging process.

Careful manipulation of movement velocity can be used to distinguish neural versus nonneural contributions to stiffness, as slow passive movements minimize the influence of the velocity-dependent stretch reflex associated with spasticity (i.e., the neural factor) and identify resistance due to intrinsic muscular properties. This may be done in the research laboratory using electromyography (EMG) to identify the velocity threshold that elicits muscle activity. The Modified Tardieu Scale is an example of a scale used clinically to make the distinction between neural and nonneural stiffness by comparing muscle reaction and ROM at three velocities: V1 is as slow as possible to minimize the stretch reflex, V2 is the speed of the segment falling under gravity, and V3 is as fast as possible (Fosang, 2003).

It appears that biomechanical or nonneural changes can contribute substantially to the amount of stiffness felt at the joint (even at very slow velocities of stretch), over and above the influence of spasticity or hyperactive stretch reflexes (de Gooijer-van de Groep, 2013, 2016; Patrick, 2006). These adaptive muscle and connective tissue changes occur relatively rapidly after onset of brain lesions, such as a stroke, and seem to be at least partially responsible for the clinical impression of hypertonia.

## THINK ABOUT IT 23.2

You are working with a patient who was recently diagnosed with a right stroke, resulting in left hemiparesis. What neural and nonneural factors could affect range of motion in this patient? How can you distinguish between the two?

### Effect of Immobilization

Patients with CNS pathology may not actively move their limbs as often or as far as people without pathology. This can be due to impaired functional mobility, impaired motor control, or impaired strength. The frequent use of splints and orthotics in this population further compounds this "immobilization." For a patient with a neuromuscular disorder, wearing an upper extremity sling (Fig. 23-3) to provide support at the shoulder has the unintended effect of reinforcing an already flexed and fixed posture. Immobilization resulting from decreased motor function and restricted limb motion can lead to further mechanical changes and joint contracture, setting up a vicious cycle.

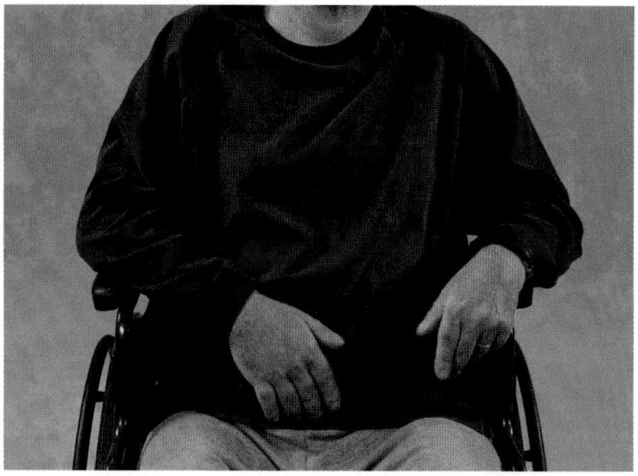

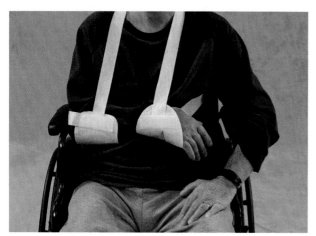

**FIGURE 23-2** A person with stroke in a natural resting posture with upper extremity in flexed position. This posture is partially due to higher resting muscle tone, which can eventually lead to a permanent, fixed contracture if it is not addressed.

**FIGURE 23-3** The same person with stroke wearing a resting shoulder sling that negatively reinforces the flexed and internally-rotated position.

A study of the time course for the development of wrist contractures after a stroke found that subjects without functional use of the hand were more likely to develop wrist flexion contractures within 6 to 8 weeks after the stroke (Pandyan, 2003). In another study, children with CP who had the ability to walk had fewer lower extremity contractures than children without walking ability (Hagglund, 2005).

In rats, immobilization increased the rate of collagen synthesis, with fibers laid down in a random orientation (Amiel, 1982; Gillette, 1996). A review of animal and human studies revealed several other relevant changes in synovial joints with prolonged immobilization (Akeson, 1987). Ligament fibrils were disorganized, and adhesions developed between connective tissue surfaces. These adhesions, as well as the random insertion of new collagen fibers in the joint and joint capsule, also increased joint stiffness.

This disordered deposition of fibrils impedes flexibility in the normally extensible joint capsule and results in a joint contracture. Although this process occurs over a matter of weeks, it may take months for a patient to recover.

### Heterotopic Ossification

**Heterotopic ossification (HO)** refers to the formation of bone (or ossification) within soft tissues outside normal bone and joint structures. This occurs most often in muscle. The presence of bone outside the joint can certainly cause limited ROM and pain with movement. The etiology of HO is unclear, but it is relatively common in the affected part of the body in people with an SCI. HO has an incidence of up to approximately 50% in this population (van Kuijk, 2002). It can also occur after a traumatic brain injury (TBI), severe burns, surgery such as total hip replacement, or joint trauma. HO can be managed surgically or pharmacologically (Banovac, 2004). There is controversy regarding treatment because of the high recurrence rates. More details on HO are included in the SCI outline of the Compendium of Neuromuscular Disorders at the end of the book.

## Lifespan Influence

### Developmental Considerations

Contractures may develop during childhood with neuromuscular diseases such as CP, DMD, spina bifida, and SMA (Fujak, 2011; Gaudreault, 2009; Snela, 2000; Svehlík, 2010; Verhoef, 2004; Wang, 2004; Wren, 2004). In a growing child, a muscle that is already in a shortened state from a neuromuscular condition combined with increasing bone length will accentuate the problem of limited ROM. These types of contractures appear to worsen with increasing age (Broughton, 1993; Hägglund, 2011). DMD involves damage to muscle tissue and replacement with fatty and fibrotic tissue that further accelerates muscle contracture.

Studies of the natural history of contractures in children are complicated by the introduction of new surgical and non-surgical approaches that emphasize early identification and management (Hagglund, 2005). As children grow into adulthood, these contractures may worsen and contribute to the development of pain, musculoskeletal deformities such as scoliosis, arthritis, overuse syndromes, and nerve entrapments (Gajdosik, 2002).

### Age-Related Changes Relevant to Limitations in PROM

Loss of passive joint ROM in the elderly may be due to the combined effect of changes that occur as part of the aging process, lack of mobility, and pain (Offenbächer, 2014). In the ankle, PROM was decreased secondary to a shortened calf musculotendinous unit. This was possibly due to the decreased number of sarcomeres or motor units or decreased muscle mass that occurs with age (Gajdosik, 1999).

## ■ Related Pathology

### Neuroanatomy of Common Pathologies

In the context of neuromuscular disorders, it is important to know that contractures almost always occur as secondary impairments (i.e., contractures are not a primary result of a nervous system injury and typically occur sometime later). Lesions to areas that contain upper motor neurons (e.g., the cerebral motor cortex, subcortical white matter of the corona radiata and internal capsule, and corticospinal tracts passing through the brainstem and spinal cord) result in paralysis and spasticity. Spasticity tends to pull the joint in one direction while the accompanying paralysis prevents active movement out of that stereotyped position. This imbalance promotes the development of contractures.

In contrast, lower motor neuron lesions to the anterior horn cells of the spinal cord or the motor fibers of peripheral nerves can cause profound paralysis of a specific body segment with either hypotonia or flaccidity, depending on how many motor units of the muscle are affected. This type of paralysis leaves the limb susceptible to the force of gravity, with the limb staying mostly in a gravity-dependent position. Without the ability to actively move out of this position, the patient is at major risk for contracture development.

## Medical Diagnoses

Common cerebral pathologies associated with deficits in PROM from damage to the upper motor neurons include stroke, traumatic and anoxic brain injury, cerebral tumors, CP, and encephalopathy. Degenerative disorders, such as multiple sclerosis, amyotrophic lateral sclerosis (ALS), Friedreich ataxia, PD, and progressive bulbar palsies, also commonly have associated PROM limitations. Common diagnoses that affect the spinal cord include SCIs, spina bifida, transverse myelitis, and syringomyelia. Genetic conditions associated with low muscle tone frequently cause limited PROM unless stretching programs are instituted. These disorders include Down syndrome, muscular dystrophy, Angelman syndrome, SMA, and neurofibromatosis. Diagnoses with notable loss of lower motor neurons or motor units include Guillain-Barré syndrome, polio, postpolio, and muscular dystrophy. Any neuromuscular condition in which movement is impaired and the limb does not regularly move through the full range places the individual at risk for limited PROM.

## ■ Pertinent Examination/Evaluation

Review the information on examination techniques for PROM in Chapter 6. Revisit the descriptions of Danny and Mrs. B presented earlier and consider the following discussion questions.

### Contemplate Clinical Decisions: Cerebral Palsy

■ Given Danny's medical history and age, which of the following contributing factors may be relevant to his limitations in PROM: limb inertia, neural factors, nonneural factors, immobilization, HO, and/or development and aging issues?
■ Using the information in Chapter 6, describe how you would specifically examine and document PROM of the relevant body segments.

■ With this patient's multisystem involvement, how would you prioritize your physical therapy examination so that it is completed in less than 60 minutes?
■ Develop a list of Danny's functional limitations and identify those that may be directly or indirectly related to expected limitations in PROM.

### Contemplate Clinical Decisions: Parkinson Disease

■ Given Mrs. B's medical history and age, which of the following factors may be contributing to her limitations in PROM: limb inertia, neural factors, nonneural factors, immobilization, HO, and/or development and aging issues?
■ Using the information in Chapter 6, describe how you would specifically examine and document PROM of the relevant body segments.
■ With this patient's multisystem involvement, how would you prioritize your physical therapy examination so that it is completed in less than 60 minutes?
■ Develop a list of Mrs. B's functional limitations and identify those that may be directly or indirectly related to expected limitations in PROM.

## ■ Preparatory Interventions Specific to Range of Motion Limitations
### General Approaches

In general, intervention to improve PROM involves providing some form of stretch to the shortened tissues. The stretch must be applied slowly and sustained for optimal effect. Once PROM has been regained, it is essential to incorporate exercises and activities at home with the patient and caregivers to maintain and utilize the additional ROM. It is particularly important to identify home exercises and activities that easily fit into the established daily routine and that regularly stress the tissue that is prone to shortening.

Interestingly, the PROM measurement techniques used in an examination (see Chapter 6) are also used as a stretching intervention for each muscle group. The main differences are that during examination a goniometer is used for accurate angle measurement, and during intervention, clinicians may rely more heavily on visual and tactile assessments. Therapists can visually assess PROM gains while feeling tension in the soft tissue being stretched. Goniometers are still needed when reassessing ROM gains after intervention strategies.

### Pharmacological Implications for Therapy and Surgical Intervention

Pharmacological intervention is not a common approach for management of ROM limitations; however, it may be useful with some focal forms of joint contractures such as Dupuytren contracture of the fingers. In these patients, collagenase clostridium histolyticum, an enzyme that breaks down collagen, is injected into the contracted collagen cord as an outpatient alternative to surgical fasciectomy (Hurst, 2009). Enzyme activation takes approximately 24 hours. The patient has a manipulation followed by intensive physical therapy.

This intervention has significantly reduced contractures (Hurst, 2009). Gilpin (2010) demonstrated a significantly greater increase in ROM with collagenase compared with placebo. In one 8-year follow-up study, 72 of 80 patients who received the enzymatic fasciotomy experienced reduction of the joint contracture to within 0 to 5 degrees of normal with high patient satisfaction (Watt, 2010). In one systematic review, the recurrence rate after collagenase ranged from 10% to 31%, with significantly less recurrence after collagenase injection than after needle aponeurotomy or open partial fasciectomy (p = 0.001) (Chen, 2011). Less severe involvement than before the initial collagenase injection was also reported (Watt, 2010). There are no reports of collagenase use in other joints or other neuromuscular conditions that cause ROM restrictions.

If physical therapeutic measures alone are not successful in restoring or maintaining functional ROM, other medical management techniques may be utilized. Medical management in conditions such as CP and DMD often includes surgical "release" or tendon lengthening procedures (tenotomies). Various techniques have been described in the literature (Katz, 2000; Yoshimoto, 2005), but recurrence is common. Physical function may also deteriorate after surgery if the contracture is a useful adaptation and not a primary cause of the functional deficit.

Surgical lengthening procedures are most commonly performed on the hamstrings (Damron, 1991, 1993; Temelli, 2009) and on the plantar flexors (Chen, 2009; Manzur, 1992; Stricker, 1998) for knee flexion contractures and crouched gait. Surgical lengthening of the Achilles tendon has also been used in patients who have diabetic neuropathy and plantar flexion contractures to increase motion at the ankle and to reduce stress on the forefoot. This can help prevent skin breakdown or promote healing of neuropathic ulcers in this population (Armstrong, 1999; Mueller, 2003).

Contractures that are complicated by the presence of HO may be managed by surgical resection of the extraneous bony tissue. This procedure is controversial because of the frequency of recurrence after surgery. When surgical resection is performed, the timing of HO surgery varies by diagnosis. HO surgery is performed after approximately 6 months in people with joint trauma, after 1 year in patients with SCI, and after 1.5 years in people with a TBI (Garland, 1991).

In diagnoses such as CP, an increased focus on prevention of contractures appears to decrease the incidence of these surgical lengthening procedures (Hagglund, 2005). Even after surgical procedures to lengthen the muscle, physical therapy is an essential component of optimal recovery and rehabilitation. Therapists can help patients learn to use and maintain the additional range. These physical therapeutic techniques are explained throughout the rest of this chapter.

## Therapeutic Techniques

### Stretching

Stretching refers to the application of sustained tension in order to increase the extensibility of connective tissue. People who are at risk for developing ROM limitations as a result of immobility, age, abnormal muscle tone, or specific neuromuscular pathology may benefit from stretching to prevent contracture or injury. Stretching may also be used to prevent worsening of a contracture.

Viscous deformation is a short-lived increase in ROM in response to stretching. This simple mechanical response reverses when the stretch is removed (Harvey, 2002). A more long-term response occurs when there are actual structural adaptations in the tissue as a result of the stretch. To promote structural adaptation during stretch, perform slow, prolonged stretches. Generally, avoid high-velocity stretches because they may cause tearing of soft tissue. High-velocity stretches given with a light force (low amplitude) activate the type Ia afferent pathway of the muscle spindle, which causes a reflexive muscle contraction (illustrated in Fig. 23-1). This contraction, similar to that observed when tapping a tendon with a reflex hammer, is the opposite of what is typically intended when applying a stretch. Also, individuals with CNS pathology can have hyperreflexia, which accentuates the problem. This lowered reflex threshold means that even stretches applied at a very slow velocity may trigger a muscle contraction.

Although stretching is the most common clinical approach to addressing limited PROM, research on the effectiveness of stretching is challenging to apply because of the wide variation in stretching techniques, positions, and dosages tested. There are also major methodological flaws in much of the literature. A systematic review that included a meta-analysis of similar studies concluded that regular stretching of healthy tissues over several days produced improved ROM when tested more than 1 day later (Harvey, 2002). Another study found that a single 30-second bout of stretching was more effective than longer stretches and that repeated shorter-duration stretches were also effective (Decoster, 2005). The total duration of stretch may be most important, with greater ROM increases found in sessions that lasted at least 15 minutes (Radford, 2006).

The Focus on Evidence table (Table 23-3 ONL) provides detailed information on research studies investigating the effect of stretching on preventing or reducing contracture in people with neurological disability. The levels of evidence are indicated for each study according to accepted criteria (Centre for Evidence-Based Medicine, 2009).

One way to assess the effectiveness of a treatment designed to prevent contracture is to examine patients who are likely to develop a contracture. This was done in several studies of people who recently had a stroke and had little or no arm movement. Although these patients were expected to develop a contracture in their shoulder or hand because of neural and nonneural risk factors, it appears that daily positioning for 30 minutes in a sustained stretch position prevented the development of contracture (Ada, 2005; de Jong, 2006).

Adherence with this type of program may be an issue because of patient discomfort (Turton, 2005). The stretch position recommended by these studies for the upper extremity after stroke is illustrated in Fig. 23-4.

Only two randomized controlled trials have investigated the use of stretch to reduce a contracture. Both studies investigated stretching of ankle contractures in individuals with an SCI; stretch was not effective when applied for 30 minutes daily over 4 weeks (Harvey, 2000), but it was marginally effective when applied in two 10-minute sessions daily over 6 months (Harvey, 2009). Several uncontrolled cohort studies and case reports reported variable results on the effectiveness of PROM or sustained stretching to reduce a contracture that was already present in people with CP (Cadenhead, 2002), a TBI (Linan, 2001; Singer, 2004), and stroke (Bressel, 2002; Selles, 2005). It appears likely that a more aggressive technique may be required to overcome a contracture that has already developed.

In summary, teach positioning in a prolonged stretch (daily for 30-minute periods over several weeks) to maintain full PROM in patients who are at risk for contracture. Incorporate the positioning into the patient's daily routine, and modify the position when pain is present to further enhance compliance. For example, encourage stretch positioning while watching a 30-minute game show on television for distraction. The research is not conclusive on whether stretching is effective for patients with an established contracture. Therefore, incorporating stretches into functional training activities could be more appropriate than spending time on stretching activities by themselves. For example, patients can stretch the upper extremity while reaching for an object or putting on a shirt or stretch the trunk and lower extremity while bending over to reach an object on the floor. Other interventions should be explored for people with established contractures that are limiting specific functional activities or causing pain.

### Splinting

Static or dynamic **splints** may be used to provide a prolonged stretch over many hours. Static splints can be custom-made for comfort and to avoid pressure points. They are especially appropriate when there is a structural deformity or existing contracture. Dynamic splints provide the option of applying varied levels of stretching force to the joint, typically starting with smaller levels of force and gradually building up tolerance for higher levels of force and for longer times. It is more challenging to make custom dynamic splints, and there are many options that are commercially available. You should clearly specify the intended schedule for application of the splint. Consider what schedule will have the least effect on the patient's physical activity. Often, splints that are large, heavy, and bulky are applied only at night (during sleep) or during specific rest periods. These are not typically recommended during periods of physical activity or home exercise.

Hand splints are often used to prevent or treat contracture, especially in individuals without active functional use of the hand. The purpose of the hand splint is typically to prevent adaptive shortening of muscles and connective tissue and to potentially inhibit grasp reflexes. However, research has questioned the effectiveness of hand splints in people with a stroke or brain injury and contractures. Two randomized controlled trials of hand splints found no benefit from a static, palmar resting splint worn at night in individuals with recent stroke or brain injury (Lannin, 2003, 2007). In both trials, no meaningful differences in ROM were found in the group that wore the splints compared with controls. In fact, splinting may actually decrease functional use of the upper extremity and increase reports of upper extremity pain (Lannin, 2003).

A recently developed, purely mechanical dynamic hand orthosis, the SaeboFlex(tm) (Fig. 23-5), is designed to position the hand and wrist in extension using spring tension to allow functional grasp and release practice after a stroke. The early research on this device (included in FOE Table 23-3 under the "dynamic splints" category) focused on changes in AROM and function after use for 6 hours a day for 1 to 2 weeks (Butler, 2006; Farrell, 2007). The SaeboStretch™ (Fig. 23-6) provides a low-load, long-duration stretch to improve ROM in the wrist and fingers. It remains to be seen whether long-term improvements in PROM will be found in the fingers and wrist of patients who use these devices.

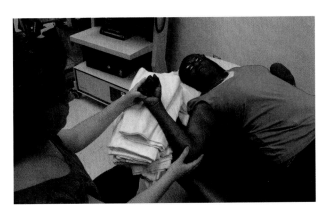

**FIGURE 23-4** Photograph of sustained stretch posture for the upper extremity in an individual at risk for flexion and internal rotation contractures after a stroke.

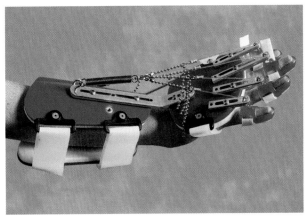

**FIGURE 23-5** The SaeboFlex™ dynamic hand orthotic, which uses spring tension to pull the wrist and fingers into extension to allow practice of reach and grasp, helping to maintain PROM.

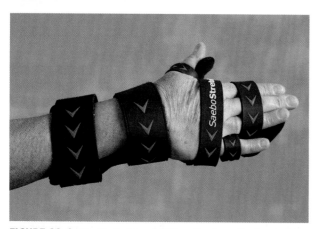

**FIGURE 23-6** The SaeboStretch™ hand/wrist orthotic provides a low-load, long-duration stretch and may maintain and improve joint PROM.

Most studies of dynamic splints have involved uncontrolled cohorts or case reports, with a wide range of splint-wearing times (daily wear ranged from 1 to 23 hours, and duration of the studies ranged from 10 days to 6 months). Most studies did report improved PROM in patients who wore the splint; however, the only randomized controlled trial on this topic did not find increased knee ROM in elderly nursing home residents after they wore a dynamic splint for 1 to 3 hours per night (Steffen, 1995).

The studies on dynamic and static splints do not indicate a robust effect for prevention or treatment of contractures. The routine use of hand splints in the clinic for stroke patients should be questioned because of the wide variety of intervention protocols. Additional controlled studies are needed to explore the use of dynamic splints for different types of patients. The use of dynamic splints for prolonged periods with or without functional task practice would seem to be a valid approach to address contractures.

### Serial Casting

**Serial casting** is a form of prolonged stretch delivered through the use of successive plaster or fiberglass casts that stretch the joint structures into a more normal position over time. With this technique, the joint or joints are immobilized in a cast at the end of the available range in a position that provides a comfortable stretch. Typically, the therapist removes and reapplies the cast weekly in the newly gained position (see Fig. 19-4), gradually increasing the ROM. This process is repeated until the ROM goal has been met or no further changes are observed. To maintain the ROM gained from serial casting, the final cast can be cut into a bivalve cast that can be worn on a long-term basis as either a resting splint or a night splint.

General indications for serial casting include treatment of an established contracture with or without concurrent spasticity. The application of serial casts to provide a constant, sustained stretch has generally been effective in increasing ROM in individuals with a TBI (Moseley, 1997, 2008; Pohl, 2002, 2003; Singer, 2003) and CP (Cottalorda, 2000; Kay, 2004; Westberry, 2006). A systematic review of upper extremity

casting concluded that after casting, subjects with CP had improved upper limb movement and subjects with a TBI had short-term improvement in PROM (Lannin, 2007).

It is important to consider the relatively high risk of adverse events with the application of a serial casting program. Complication rates have been as high as 20% (Pohl, 2003). In one study, physical therapists reported that adverse events were 15 times more frequent in patients after casting than in a control group who did not receive casting treatment (Lannin, 2007).

Common adverse events caused by the cast include skin irritation and breakdown, pain, swelling, numbness, and nerve impingement. General contraindications to the use of casting include medical instability, open wounds, skin infection, and cellulitis. Caution should be used in individuals with impaired sensation, cognition, or communication.

Although serial casting may be effective in improving ROM for the short term, this intervention should be applied selectively. A great deal of skill is required on the part of the physical therapist to place the body part in the appropriate position for cast application and to minimize the risk of adverse events. As with all interventions to increase PROM, it is essential to follow up the intervention with activities that incorporate the newly gained ROM and prevent further loss of movement.

### Joint Mobilization

Joint **mobilizations**, or passive movements of the articular surfaces, are indicated for mechanical joint dysfunction in which accessory motion is restricted because of a hypomobile joint capsule. Accessory movements occur within a joint and surrounding soft tissues and are necessary for normal ROM. To indicate whether there is restriction in the noncontractile elements of the joint (e.g., the joint capsule, ligaments), the amount of joint play can be determined manually.

Kaltenborn (1999) identified three grades of joint mobilization force that apply to all populations. Grade I or II manual traction, or gliding up to 50% of the available joint play motion, may be used to assess joint play as noted previously and may be applied first as a trial treatment to determine the patient's response to the technique. Grade III mobilizations, moving one bone on the other to the end of available joint play motion, stretch the tissues crossing the joint. The stretch should be maintained for at least 1 minute, and the treatments should be continued as long as improvement in joint play is noted after the mobilization stretch (Kaltenborn, 1999).

The use of mobilizations has been generally recommended to treat shoulder capsular dysfunction and other ROM deficits in children with CNS dysfunction (Cochrane, 1987; Harris, 1991). However, research supporting the use of joint mobilizations, even for people without CNS pathology, is somewhat limited. Ankle joint mobilizations have increased joint ROM and improved gait performance in people with acute ankle sprains (Green, 2001) and increased PROM after 10 sessions of ankle and foot mobilizations in a small group of patients with diabetic neuropathy (Dijs, 2000). Two small studies found that ankle joint mobilizations improved PROM at the ankle in people with a stroke (Kluding, 2004, 2008).

However, no subjects in either study demonstrated significant changes in sit-to-stand or gait kinematics despite improvements in passive motion at the ankle. In these studies, mobilizations were provided to the proximal and distal tibia-fibula articulations and the talocrural joint for 5 minutes per session. The technique described in these studies is illustrated in Figure 23-7.

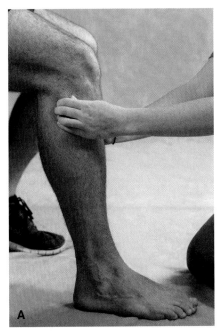

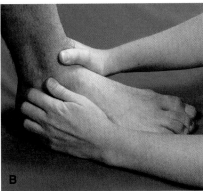

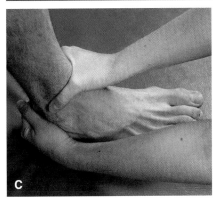

**FIGURE 23-7** Therapist's hand placement and patient positioning for distal lower extremity joint mobilizations. (A) Proximal tibia-fibula mobilization. (B) Distal tibia-fibula mobilization. (C) Talocrural mobilization.

## Heat Modalities

Increasing the temperature of soft tissues through heating modalities has several effects that may increase PROM. These effects include increased tissue extensibility, pain relief, blood flow, and general body relaxation. Superficial heat modalities, such as a hot pack heated in a hydrocollator, generally heat the skin and subcutaneous tissues approximately 1 cm deep (Robertson, 2005). The primary benefit of superficial heat is pain relief and relaxation, as the increased temperature reaches the majority of skin nerve fibers but not deeper tissues that may be limiting ROM.

To increase tissue extensibility of deeper tissues, such as muscle, ligaments, and joint capsules, a deeper modality is required. Deep heating can be delivered by either therapeutic ultrasound or short-wave diathermy. Both of these modalities are effective at increasing the temperature of tissues 3 cm deep by approximately 4°C (Draper, 1995, 1999). Deep heating modalities, applied with or without stretching, appear to improve PROM in healthy subjects (Knight, 2001; Robertson, 2005).

Although heat may be effective at improving ROM, very limited research is available on the use of heat modalities in people with CNS pathology. One study used hot packs on the upper extremity of people with stroke as a sensory input which was associated with improved active ROM into wrist extension, as well as sensation and motor recovery, compared with a control group (Chen, 2005). Changes in PROM were not assessed. However, heat modalities should be used with caution in people with CNS pathology because impaired sensation, communication, and cognition can increase risk for injury from skin burns. Further, people with multiple sclerosis may experience increased fatigue with heat applications (Schwid, 2003).

## Referral for Surgical Release

The therapist must recognize that surgical lengthening of the tendons, as explained earlier in this chapter, may be indicated when there is a long-standing contracture that does not improve with the standard physical interventions described previously. In such cases, refer the patient to a physician, who will confirm the need for intervention and determine the procedure to be performed. For example, lengthening of the Achilles or hamstring tendons may be necessary to improve function in some children or adults with CP.

Physical therapy is always indicated after surgical release to promote function (see Chapters 33 through 37) and increase strength (Chapter 22) in newly gained ROM, as well as to prevent recurrence of the contracture. The techniques for prevention and treatment of contractures previously reviewed in this section are appropriate for these patients.

## THINK ABOUT IT 23.3

Why do you think increased range of motion from surgical release does not automatically result in increased function? What other underlying impairments may play a role in function in these patients?

# ■ Intervention: Ultimately Applied in Functional Activities

As PROM is regained through the techniques described previously, the therapist must ultimately apply the newly gained range to the functional activities that were previously limited, as well as to other activities that stretch the tissue at risk for shortening. In fact, it seems reasonable that if functional tasks that utilize the full extent of range are implemented on a regular basis, they will help to maintain the PROM. Therefore, seek and incorporate specific functional activities that naturally stretch the joint in question, considering the factors described earlier that contribute to PROM loss. Positions and postures in the lengthened portion of the range should be intentionally built into the daily routine to provide more prolonged static stretch.

In addition to the functional intervention activities described in Chapters 33 to 37, Table 23-1 lists a variety of functional activities that target planar movements at specific joints to either increase or maintain PROM.

## Pediatric Considerations

When ROM becomes limited in a pediatric patient, the caregiver must take a major role in recovering the functional range, in addition to the skilled intervention provided by the therapist. The parent is often required to provide home stretching and positioning activities. When developing these home exercises and activities, always try to incorporate them into the usual home routine. For example, if hip adductors are tight, encourage the parent to provide manual stretch to the adductor muscles during each diaper change. Also, certain positions that are a common part of pediatric movement patterns can be incorporated in the therapy session or at home to increase or maintain ROM. The prone position and prone-on-elbows position are excellent options to stretch into hip extension.

Working with pediatric patients requires special creativity, even in designing simple activities to increase and maintain ROM in those at risk. For example, to encourage additional dorsiflexion in a child with shortened plantar flexors or in children with idiopathic toe-walking, you can implement practice ambulation with swim fins or flippers to add a new dimension of motivation (especially if the therapist is also walking around wearing a pair of swim fins).

### PATIENT APPLICATION

*Revisit the descriptions of Danny and Mrs. B presented earlier in this chapter, along with their problem lists, risk factors for contractures, and potential PROM limitations. Review possible interventions for these limitations in Danny's case and develop*

| TABLE 23-1 | Examples of Functional Activities to Increase/Maintain Passive Range of Motion (PROM) |
|---|---|
| **COMMON PROM LIMITATION TO ADDRESS** | **EXAMPLES OF FUNCTIONAL ACTIVITIES TO INCLUDE IN INTERVENTION** |
| Short plantar flexors | • Walking up ramps/inclines<br>• Walking down stairs |
| Short hamstrings | • Riding a bicycle (emphasizing knee extension during hip flexion)<br>• Activities in long-sitting position (if possible) |
| Short hip flexors | • Lying in prone position (may need to start with a pillow under the pelvis if hip flexors are short) and raising the trunk off the surface, with posterior pelvic tilt, into hip extension<br>• In a kneeling position with one knee in a forward position and with upper extremity support, lunging toward the forward leg to bring the trailing leg into actual hip extension (keeping the pelvis as posteriorly tilted as possible) |
| Short wrist flexors | • Plantigrade position with open palm, upper extremity weight-bearing (with wrist extension) on a waist-high table surface<br>• Using an open palm and the maximal force the patient can generate to push a surface directly in front of the patient |
| Short elbow flexors | • Plantigrade position with upper extremity, open palm weight-bearing on a waist-high table surface, with full elbow extension<br>• Quadruped position with full elbow extension |
| Short shoulder adductors | • While facing sideways in standing, reaching up to get a plate out of the kitchen cabinet<br>• Reaching overhead and behind the back and to the back of neck and then toward the opposite scapula |
| Short shoulder internal rotators | • While keeping the elbow adjacent to the trunk and the elbow flexed so the hand rests on a table, moving the hand laterally to retrieve an object from a tabletop<br>• Supporting a long object overhead with a bilateral grasp (holding a banner/sign or a fluorescent light tube) |

*a treatment plan. More information follows about Mrs. B; review this information and answer the clinical decision-making questions.*

*Mrs. B demonstrates extremity strength rated good or 4/5 overall. PROM limitations are noted in the upper trunk (maintained in flexion), the bilateral shoulders, and the right knee: Her shoulder flexion is 0 to 120 degrees, shoulder abduction is 0 to 90 degrees, and right knee extension is −5 degrees. When sitting, she is able to reach 13 in. forward and 4 in. to either side, but she easily loses her balance in the backward direction. She requires contact guarding for sit-to-stand and is able to stand for 30 seconds with supervision before becoming short of breath. She is able to ambulate 5 ft with a rolling walker and contact guarding; she maintains her right knee slightly flexed throughout the stance and tends to lose her balance toward that side.*

### Contemplate Clinical Decisions

- *What are the functional implications of improving PROM in the upper trunk, shoulders, and/or right knee?*
- *How would your treatment address Mrs. B's secondary diagnosis of emphysema?*
- *Which intervention(s) for limited PROM discussed in this chapter would be most appropriate for Mrs. B?*
- *If you wanted to give the patient and her daughter a home program of exercises for focusing on PROM after this first visit, what would you include?*
- *Recall that the patient's and family's goals include being able to walk and get her into/out of bed independently. What is Mrs. B's prognosis for achieving these goals?*

## ■ Intervention: Considerations for Nontherapy Time and Discharge

Several interventions discussed in this chapter are appropriate only for skilled physical and occupational therapists to administer during therapy sessions with the patient, such as aggressive passive stretching, design and initial application of a splint, serial casting, joint mobilization, or deep heat modalities. However, involvement of the patient and family in home activities outside of therapy time and after discharge is often essential to provide sustained and prolonged stretch with sufficient frequency to increase or maintain functional PROM. It is also important to encourage the patient to assume positions that place the at-risk tissues on stretch and increase and maintain extensibility throughout the day during all nontherapy times (e.g., in the car, in the home, or during community activities).

## Aspects of Patient and Family Education

As previously mentioned, the patient and family should be actively involved in selecting activities for home that are functional, fit easily into their routine, and provide a stretch to the body parts that need motion to prevent contracture. It is imperative that the patient and caregivers understand why certain muscles and soft tissue are at risk for adaptive shortening and why these activities are important. This understanding may help increase adherence to the home exercise program. Use of a daily checklist with pictures or "exercise calendars" can serve as reminders and help monitor adherence initially.

## Activities for Home

Table 23-1 provides several examples of activities that could be modified for home exercise programs to provide a PROM stretch to specific body parts. The following general activities are supported by the research reviewed in this chapter and are appropriate for application in the home after instruction and education by the therapist:

- Position patient daily in a sustained stretch position with a 30-minute timer.
- Incorporate stretches into functional activities (e.g., while dressing, feeding, bathing, crawling/creeping, cruising, standing, and stepping).
- When a dynamic or static splint is indicated, provide a detailed schedule to promote wearing of the splint during rest periods so functional use of body part is not compromised.

# HANDS-ON PRACTICE

The student should gain the following practical skills from reading and applying concepts in this chapter to his/her clinical practice:

- Developing appropriate treatment sequences for patients who are at risk for contracture development
- Developing appropriate treatment sequences for patients who have an existing contracture
- Performing appropriate stretching techniques to increase passive range of motion

- Educating a patient on an appropriate schedule for wearing a splint for contracture prevention
- Applying heat modalities to address passive range of motion limitations
- Designing and educating a patient on an appropriate home exercise program for passive range of motion limitations

## Let's Review

1. What are the key differences between AROM and PROM? What structures/tissues result in PROM limitation? How does this influence how you treat PROM deficits?

2. What is the relationship between decreased PROM and function? What types of PROM deficits may result in functional limitations?

3. How can spasticity and decreased strength contribute to PROM deficits? What types of interventions can you use to prevent contractures in these patients?

4. Describe the interventions typically used to address a PROM limitation. When would you need to refer the patient back to the physician?

5. What types of functional activities can be used to increase/maintain PROM? Which muscles/motion does each activity address?

6. What components of intervention would you incorporate into patient training/education for use of nontherapy time and home exercises?

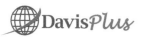 **DavisPlus** For additional resources, including Focus on Evidence tables, case study discussions, references and glossary, please visit http://davisplus.fadavis.com

## CHAPTER SUMMARY

Many factors may contribute to limited PROM. Although they may overlap in an individual patient, it is important to identify the factors that are most important to each patient through customized examination and intervention. This allows the therapist to design and implement the most appropriate intervention strategy for that individual. Table 23-2 summarizes application of the intervention techniques described in this chapter. The strongest evidence exists for the use of daily positioning to *prevent* a contracture and serial casting to *reduce* an established contracture that is resistant to manual stretching. The evidence summarized in the online Focus on Evidence Table 23-3 is promising but not conclusive regarding less-invasive treatments of established contractures, such as stretching, splinting, joint mobilizations, and heat modalities. When therapists use these options with their patients, they should carefully monitor their effectiveness to determine the course of continued treatments. Referral for surgical release may be indicated when a long-standing contracture does not respond to treatment and is limiting function.

In addition, patients and caregivers must be involved in home activities outside of therapy time and after discharge to increase or maintain functional PROM. Identify activities that are meaningful and easy to incorporate in a daily routine for improved patient adherence.

| TABLE 23-2 | Summary of Principles in Interventions for Restricted Range of Motion |
|---|---|
| **INTERVENTION** | **PRINCIPLES AND ACTIVITIES*** |
| Stretching to address contracture | • Administer a slow-velocity, low-amplitude manual stretch (avoiding the reflexive effects of spastic hypertonus) in bouts of at least 30 seconds for a 15-minute session.<br>• Provide support/stabilization to the proximal segment using hand placement or a supportive surface while moving the distal segment. If the patient is supine, provide a comfortable pillow under the head; if sitting, provide a comfortable chair.<br>• Hold the stretch at the point where pain is tolerable for the patient. Gradually increase pressure if tolerated.<br>• If the patient is nervous, empower him to tell you when he has had enough and needs a rest.<br>• Encourage the patient to relax. Use calming words and tone of voice; monitor the patient's breathing to encourage deep and regular breaths. Dim the lights, especially if the patient is supine and looking toward the ceiling. |

| TABLE 23-2 | Summary of Principles in Interventions for Restricted Range of Motion—cont'd |
|---|---|
| **INTERVENTION** | **PRINCIPLES AND ACTIVITIES** |
| Stretching to prevent contracture | • Teach the patient static positioning in a prolonged stretch in natural positions and activities (daily for 30-minute periods over several weeks) to maintain full passive range of motion (PROM); find ways to incorporate this in the daily routine.<br>• See splinting also in the following section. |
| Splinting | • Use static or dynamic splints, with the purpose of administering a low-load, long-duration stretch (longer than the manual stretch that a therapist can provide).<br>• Apply the splint during periods of rest, including nighttime, if the patient will wear the splint at this time. This will avoid interference with functional activity, as the splinting material is often very heavy. |
| Serial casting | • Cast the limb at the end of the available range to provide a comfortable stretch.<br>• About weekly, recast at the new stretch point (additional range is gained each time).<br>• When the goal is reached (or no further change is needed), bivalve the final cast to be used as a resting or night splint for long-term maintenance. |
| Joint mobilization | • Maintain grade I, II, or III mobilizations for 1–5 minutes per session.<br>• Continue until no further improvement in joint play is noted after mobilization. |
| Heat modalities | • Apply deep-heating physical agents (therapeutic ultrasound or short-wave diathermy) to increase the temperature of tissues up to 3 cm below the surface, which may improve PROM (demonstrated in healthy subjects) (Knight, 2001; Robertson, 2005). |

*Additional details and rationales can be found within the text.

# Therapeutic Intervention for Impaired Motor Control—Stability

Deborah Nervik Chamberlain, PT, DPT, MHS, DHS, PCS
Monica Diamond, PT, MS, NCS, C/NDT ▪ Megan Danzl, PT, DPT, PhD, NCS
Dennis W. Fell, PT, MD

CHAPTER 24

## CHAPTER OBJECTIVES

Upon completion of this chapter, the learner should be able to:
1. Describe clinical examples of impaired motor control-stability.
2. Develop and implement patient-centered therapeutic interventions to improve stability aspects of motor control.
3. Develop and implement functional interventions that include opportunities to apply joint or segment stability in the context of essential functional activities.

## Introduction

*Since his stroke 6 months ago, Mr. Simon has had obvious problems with his left arm and leg, particularly with stabilizing the knee joint during weight-bearing. His left knee snaps back into locked extension during left midstance weight-bearing (right swing) of gait 100% of the time. Another patient, Mrs. Desonier, had a stroke that affected primarily her left upper extremity, leaving her with a dense hemiplegia with complete paralysis. She has developed major, painful left shoulder subluxation and cannot stabilize the shoulder joint because of lack of motor control of the rotator cuff muscles. Both patients demonstrate the same underlying impairment, lack of motor control-stability, but in different body joints. Once the problem has been identified, what therapeutic options are available for these patients?*

As described in Chapter 6, motor control includes aspects of precise neuromotor control for both stability and movement. **Motor control-stability** is the aspect of motor control that allows a joint or body segment to be stable at a time when movement is not supposed to occur there (often a different part of the body is supposed to move at that same time). Such stability requires coordination between the neuromotor and the musculoskeletal systems. In this chapter, the terms "motor control-stability," "stability motor control," and **"neuromotor stability"** are used interchangeably, which implies that the instability is related to problems in the way the brain controls movement and not to disruptions of a capsule, ligament, or tendon. Impairments in joint or body segment stability due to lack of motor control can be seen in patients with a wide variety of neurological diseases across the lifespan and in most peripheral joints, the trunk, and the neck segment. The term "body segment" refers to a part of

| TABLE 24-1 | Examples of Joint or Body Segment Instability Commonly Related to Neuromuscular Disorders |
|---|---|
| **JOINT OR BODY SEGMENT** | **EXAMPLE OF INSTABILITY** |
| Shoulder | Subluxation |
| Scapula | Scapulothoracic winging |
| Wrist/hand | Inability to grasp |
| Lumbopelvic area | Trunk instability |
| Hip | Trendelenburg |
| Knee | Genu recurvatum or knee collapse into flexion |
| Ankle | Footdrop or medial/lateral wobble |

## THINK ABOUT IT 24.1

What functional activities and activities of daily living might be difficult in the context of each of the examples of instability given in Table 24-1?

the body that may include more than one joint, such as the trunk, whereas "joint" is limited to one joint, such as the knee. Common examples of joint or body segment instability related to musculoskeletal disorders are summarized in Table 24-1.

**Joint stability** is "the result of the integration of articular geometry, soft tissue restraints, and the loads applied to the joint" from weight-bearing and muscle action (Williams, 2001, p. 546). The dynamic interactions described between muscle forces in all the muscles that surround the target joint and gravitational forces, especially during weight-bearing activity, produce motor control-stability. When something is stable, it is said to be firmly established, steady in purpose, constant and durable, and resistant to change (*Merriam-Webster Dictionary*, 1997).

Dynamic **coactivation** or **cocontraction**, particularly of opposing muscle groups, is inherent in motor control-stability at a joint, as surrounding muscle groups contract simultaneously in a graded manner to prevent joint movement in available directions. Motor control-stability is distinct from postural stability, a term used to refer to balance and equilibrium, as further described in Chapter 30. When there is a complete lack of ability to activate muscles to stabilize a joint, the term "paralysis" is applied. Paralysis-related interventions are discussed in Chapter 26.

**Motor control**, the neural regulation of motor behavior, is an integral component in achieving and maintaining dynamic joint stability. As described in Chapter 6, motor control-movement allows an individual to initiate and cease movements, vary movement velocity, produce movements in small ranges of motion, and produce isolated movements. Motor control-stability includes the ability to voluntarily contract and relax muscles or muscle groups to stabilize particular joints or body segments during functional activities or phases of functional activities that are weight-bearing or require stable joints.

## BOX 24-1  Common Musculoskeletal Impairments Causing Joint Instability That Are Not Motor Control Issues

Decreased range of motion (ROM) or lack of flexibility, especially if preventing stable alignment
Joint disease or injury
Ligament or joint capsule laxity or injury
Increased ROM (hypermobility)
Muscle weakness

Although decreased joint stability may be due in some cases to impairments in the musculoskeletal system (see Box 24-1), the focus of this chapter is on motor control for joint or segment stability mediated through nervous system control (Table 24-1).

## Clinical Picture of Motor Control-Stability in a Holistic Context

Clearly, joints that are stabilized by adequate motor control, which is crucial to both static posture and dynamic mobility, are very important for function. Joint stability is the foundation of purposeful and functional movements. Any posture, position, or activity that requires holding the body up against gravity (including, but not limited to, prone on elbows; crawling/creeping; supported sitting; unsupported sitting; quadruped; kneeling; half-kneeling; standing; ambulation; negotiating stairs, curbs, or ramps; and propping on upper extremities in any position) requires the muscles of supporting joints or body segments to cocontract to prevent joint movement so the body can be supported.

## Possible Effect of Impaired Motor Control-Stability on Function

Independence in weight-bearing, closed chain positions within one's environment is difficult or impossible without neuromotor stability at supporting joints. Even functional open chain movements of one part of the body require other parts to stabilize. For instance, a patient who has sustained a stroke or a child with cerebral palsy may lack joint stability at the knee because of poor coactivation of agonists and antagonists in the stance phase, preventing independent standing. Decreased joint stability in movement may be seen in poor coactivation of agonists and antagonists at the elbow in a child with athetosis, causing involuntary over- or undershooting when reaching for objects. A lack of proximal stability in the scapula contributes to impaired distal movement of the hand, as seen in adults with a stroke or brain injury or in children with hypotonia or developmental coordination disorder, which causes difficulty with handwriting skills. Impaired motor control-stability in the lower extremity negatively affects ambulation; possible manifestations include biomechanical, locked extension of the knee in midstance, medial/lateral wobble of the ankle in midstance, or an inability to stabilize the ankle in neutral/slight dorsiflexion as the leg moves through swing phase.

Dynamic joint stability provides the individual with the ability to not only be appropriately stable when needed for function but also to release and grade muscle activation when a joint or segment of the body needs to move. Although joints or body segments can be excessively stable (e.g., Parkinson disease) or excessively mobile (e.g., related to hypotonia), this chapter focuses primarily on the problem of joint or segment instability.

## PATIENT APPLICATION: INTRODUCTION

*Richard B. is a 48 year-old man who has returned 1 year after his stroke for additional physical therapy because of new activity limitations. He demonstrated progress through inpatient and outpatient rehabilitation, including the ability to transition from using a walker to a cane. He is now walking without a device; however, he reports that he is not pleased with his walking because it is slow and fatiguing. He states, "I still drag my right foot sometimes. I don't trust my knee to hold me up, and my walking is too slow." At the initial examination, Richard's gait is noticeably asymmetrical and slow. He is observed to trip as he turns to sit, but recovers.*

*As you escort Richard to the treatment area to continue the examination, the clinic scheduler reminds you that Richard's insurance company requires prior authorization for therapy visits after the initial visit on the basis of the results of his evaluation. She also reminds you that he is scheduled for an occupational therapy evaluation after your physical therapy (PT) session.*

### Contemplate Clinical Decisions

- *On the basis of what you have observed so far, what questions might you ask the patient at this point to obtain additional relevant information?*
- *In addition to gait, what other functional activities will you assess?*
- *What are your initial thoughts regarding which tests and measures will provide the most relevant and useful information for formulating patient-centered goals and an appropriate/effective plan of care?*
- *Which body systems need further examination? What are possible causes for Richard's right foot drag, slow gait, and knee instability? So that you can complete the examination, evaluation, and treatment plan in your 1-hour session, which systems do you anticipate examining in detail and which do you think need to be screened only?*
- *What are your early thoughts on possible goals and functional outcomes, frequency of treatment, and number of sessions for an outpatient episode of care for this patient?*

## Anatomy and Physiology

Joint instability due to lack of motor control may be related to a number of lesions in the neuromotor system (see Table 24-2) that lead to easily recognized impairments

| TABLE 24-2 | Location of Nervous System Lesions That Impair Motor Control-Stability |
|---|---|
| **STRUCTURE (ANATOMICAL AREA)** | **DEFICIT CAUSED BY LESION IN THE STRUCTURE** |
| Primary motor area of cerebral cortex | Impaired voluntary/conscious movement |
| Premotor area of cerebral cortex | Impaired motor planning (apraxia) |
| Motor association area of cerebral cortex | Impaired cognitive planning of movement |
| Putamen of the basal ganglia | Decreased initiation of movement |
| Caudate of the basal ganglia | Decreased inhibition of movement |
| Globus pallidus of the basal ganglia | Decreased facilitation of movement |
| Posterior lobe of the cerebellum | Ataxia, dysmetria (inability to judge distance), intention tremors, adiadochokinesia (inability to perform rapidly alternating movements), dyssynergia (inability to move segments together smoothly) |
| Anterior lobe of the cerebellum | Increased extensor tone |
| Flocculonodular lobe of the cerebellum | Uncoordinated trunk movements, decreased balance |

and activity limitations (Gutman, 2008). The study of motor control and brain circuitry is beyond the scope of this text. Some basic understanding is necessary, however, and a brief review is provided here.

At the most basic level of understanding, execution of voluntary motor control of joint position and movement begins in the primary motor area of the cerebral cortex as the brain sends signals through the corticospinal tracts to activate specific muscles. Many other areas of the brain, including the cerebellum and the basal ganglia, activate to assist in achieving the desired outcome of smooth, accurate, regulated, controlled movement and posture. These structures have direct connections to the motor cortex to modulate motor output, as well as connections and influences on each other (Gutman, 2008).

The cerebellum receives input from the vestibular nuclei, spinal cord (through the spinocerebellar tracts), and cerebral hemispheres. It processes the input and sends out signals to refine movement by adjusting muscle contraction and joint position, which leads to improved motor control. Lesions to the cerebellum can cause problems with coordination of movement and body equilibrium, but the focus of cerebellar problems in this chapter relates to maintaining postural alignment and proximal stability (Gutman, 2008).

The basal ganglia also play a crucial role in motor control. The primary motor and premotor areas of the cortex send signals to the basal ganglia, which send signals sequentially to the subthalamus, reticular formation, substantia nigra, and ventrolateral nucleus of the thalamus and ultimately back to the primary motor cortex and premotor cortex to either inhibit or facilitate movement. Lesions in the basal ganglia can lead to difficulty initiating, continuing, and stopping movement, as well as stiffness and involuntary and unwanted movements. These movement deficits decrease the ability to control joint position (Gutman, 2008).

Mechanoreceptors in muscle spindles and joints send signals to the brain through the medial lemniscal system, including the fasciculus gracilis and fasciculus cuneatus tracts. These sensory receptors in the muscles and joints assist with joint stability by providing: (1) joint position sense or proprioception (awareness of static position) and (2) joint movement sense or kinesthesia (awareness of magnitude, velocity, and direction of movement).

## Lifespan Influence

Stability created by cocontraction from precise neuromotor control is obviously not present at birth but improves through the developmental process. The newborn infant cannot control the neck muscles, even for simple tasks such as keeping the head upright when the body is supported upright on the parent's chest or maintaining the head in midline while lying supine. Gradually, through motor control-stability, the neonate gains skills to maintain head position against gravity. The neonate's inability to prop or support on the arms is gradually replaced by the ability to cocontract at the shoulder and elbow to allow arm support during the prone-on-elbows position and ultimately propped sitting and standing with upper extremity (UE) support.

In the earliest efforts to stand, a toddler is unable to sustain a cocontracted, partially flexed knee in stance, as observed by irregular "bouncing" in stance as the knee joint suddenly drops into excessive flexion followed by a recovery with some active extension. After practice and repetitions, and perhaps additional myelination, the child gains exquisite control of the knee muscles to allow dynamic control of knee position while playing in a standing position and throughout the stance phase of gait.

As the aging process occurs in late adulthood, the decline in sensory and motor neurons and slowing of nerve conduction velocity and central processing may contribute to impaired motor control-stability. In addition to these age-related system changes, certain neurological disorders such as stroke or cerebral vascular accident (CVA), peripheral neuropathy, and cerebral tumors become more prevalent in the geriatric population and are associated with proximal instability or weight-bearing instability.

## ■ Related Pathology

Some of the more common neuromuscular disorders that result in decreased motor control-stability include cerebral pathology (CVA, traumatic and anoxic brain injury, cerebral tumors, cerebral palsy), spinal cord pathology (incomplete spinal cord injuries, spina bifida), degenerative disorders (multiple sclerosis, amyotrophic lateral sclerosis, Friedreich's ataxia, progressive bulbar palsies), genetic conditions with low muscle tone (Down syndrome, Angelman syndrome, spinal muscular atrophy, neurofibromatosis), and conditions with major loss of lower motor neurons or motor units (Guillain-Barré, polio, postpolio syndrome, muscular dystrophy).

## ■ Pertinent Examination and Evaluation

Clarifying the cause of apparent instability at an individual joint or body segment in a patient can be an evaluation challenging for the clinician and is often more complex than it initially appears. The therapist's initial observations, and often the patient or family's verbal description of the problem, may draw attention to a specific body segment (e.g., "My knee snaps back when I walk" or "My elbow won't hold when I lean on my arm"). The challenge for the clinician is to evaluate this symptom of "instability" with a global or holistic perspective, as well as detailed consideration of specific influences on the body segment in question. The temptation exists for the therapist to become focused on a single segment that can be addressed via specific exercises or therapeutic adjuncts. Although it is appropriate to identify specific problems, the skilled clinician will thoroughly evaluate the interrelationships among all body segments and among all impairments, as well as between impairments and function, to view the patient as a whole, not just as an "unstable knee."

## Examination of Motor Control-Stability

A patient often has many coexisting activity limitations and underlying impairments with pathology of the neuromotor system, which makes determination of the optimal plan of care a challenge. The key to determining the best treatment lies in the therapist's ability to (1) identify the limitations in function, (2) determine the specific underlying impairments, and (3) prioritize the problems in an effective plan of care. This is certainly true for the individual with neuromotor instability related to impaired motor control.

To provide a basis for prioritizing, the therapist chooses examination tools that are appropriate for the specific medical diagnosis, patient history, and setting (e.g., intensive care unit, acute rehabilitation unit, school district, home, or outpatient clinic). Specific tests of motor control described in Chapter 6 may be used to measure impairments, guided by the therapist's hypotheses regarding underlying or related causes of the activity limitations. For example, patients with neuromotor system pathology often demonstrate joint instability with primary or secondary range of motion (ROM) impairments. Although specific ROM testing may provide detailed information, it may not be necessary or appropriate to conduct a formal comprehensive ROM examination, given the need to prioritize and use available time effectively. Screening within a functional task may be adequate. Similarly, completing a

---

**BOX 24-2  Questions and Considerations for Examination of Deficits in Motor Control-Stability**

**Function**

- How does the instability observed at a specific joint or body segment affect function?
- Does the instability hinder the patient in achieving functional activity goals? For example, does the segmental instability threaten balance in certain functional postures?
- Is the instability associated with pain?
- Is the same type of instability apparent in other activities (e.g., standing at the sink to wash hands, as well as during walking)?
- Will function improve if the patient can gain control of this segment?

**Movement**

- What specific postural and movement components occur with this observed instability, and what else occurs in the rest of the body at the time of the instability? For example, in the gait cycle, does **knee hyperextension (genu recurvatum)** or **locked knee extension** occur? What are the other segments of the body doing at this time?
- Are there influences above and below the impaired segment that could be causing or contributing to the problem? The following factors might be involved:
  - Trunk flexion and a forward head position may develop as a result of walking with a cane or walker. Biomechanically, this may result in a posterior position of the pelvis on the affected side, creating a force that produces or contributes to knee hyperextension.
  - The individual may lack control in multiple planes above and below the unstable segment. For example, movement in the sagittal and frontal planes may be easier for the therapist to observe, whereas the effects of complex patterns of rotational control that contribute to the stability of segments may require more effort and concentration to evaluate. Knee hyperextension may result from unbalanced activation of medial versus lateral hamstrings or of muscles that control internal and external tibial rotation. The unbalanced rotational forces can hinder controlling and grading of knee flexion and extension and may be more easily examined during a hands-on assessment of muscle activation during a functional activity.

**Specific Body Systems**

- Could a sensory deficit be contributing to the instability? The patient may be unaware of the instability, with the lack of awareness contributing to the lack of control. This screening observation indicates the need for a detailed examination of sensation.
- Are there specific muscle length or strength deficits related to this specific joint or body segment that should be specifically examined?
- Is the observed abnormal motor pattern consistent, intermittent, or increasingly obvious across attempts? Joint instability that increases with longer periods of practice or activity could be associated with impaired cardiovascular or muscular endurance, whereas other patterns may be related to a neuromotor timing problem.

---

manual muscle test for strength in all major muscle groups is probably not appropriate for a very weak and deconditioned patient in the intensive care unit who has segment instability with muscle weakness as a possible contributor. The clinician should critically select functional outcome measures to determine the effect of the joint or segment instability on function.

The examination must be comprehensive and specific enough to detect and document the impairments that contribute to the instability. Questions and considerations to guide the examination are provided in Box 24-2. The therapist can use these questions and considerations to formulate hypotheses regarding the relationship of the impairments effecting a specific joint segment to the patient's functional movement in a broader context. This active thought process should continue through the examination and evaluation.

## PATIENT APPLICATION – EXAMINATION

*As you walk back to the clinic with Richard B, you observe his gait pattern, particularly the instability of his right knee. You ask questions regarding his history and function and obtain the following subjective information:*

**Medical and Social:**

- *Richard takes medication for hypertension and has a history of stomach ulcer.*
- *He does not know if his stroke was ischemic or hemorrhagic.*
- *He lives with his significant other in a second-floor apartment in a downtown neighborhood.*
- *He can access community activities and shopping by cab (via subsidized services to disabled individuals), and he no longer needs van/wheelchair transportation.*
- *He previously worked at a variety of jobs and is currently receiving disability. He is in the process of applying for a volunteer position with the American Heart Association.*
- *He must walk short distances in the community, and he is concerned because he walks "too slow" and feels it makes him a "target" for attack or robbery.*

**Function**

- *Richard reports that he can walk slowly for one block before he becomes fatigued and needs to sit down to rest.*
- *He goes up and down stairs with supervision from his friend and a railing (to and from his second-floor apartment), using a "step-to" pattern he learned during rehabilitation. When*

questioned, he states that he has not encountered stairs without a railing but does not think he would be able to ascend stairs without a railing.

- He occasionally takes his cane along when in the community, usually when the weather is bad.
- Richard has partial functional use of his right upper extremity, but he reports that it feels stiff and moves slowly. His right hand is his dominant hand, but he has learned to use his left hand for many functions previously done by the right.
- Richard has not fallen recently. His last fall was shortly after discharge from inpatient rehabilitation and occurred when he was attempting to turn and reach for an item while standing.
- He previously used a prefabricated **ankle-foot orthosis** (AFO) but stopped using it several months ago because he did not think it was helping him.

## Observation:

The following information was gained by observation of Richard B. as he moved around the clinic, performing functional activities as requested:

- Richard walks slowly without a device or AFO, but he drags his right foot five times during the 100-ft walk on the way to the PT gym. The toe drag causes a disruption to his gait rhythm, but he is able to maintain his balance.
- Gait pattern observations:
  - The trunk is in extension, and the upper body is posterior to the pelvis throughout the gait cycle.
  - Overall, his body looks "inactive," although head, trunk, and upper extremities are relatively symmetrical (with the exception of less arm swing on the right than on the left).
  - The pelvis is rotated posteriorly on the right throughout the gait cycle, but it worsens in late right stance and during initiation of swing on the right.
  - Hip motion on the right appears limited to about 50% of normal motion in flexion and extension, and excessive motion of the pelvis is observed (rotation and anterior/posterior tilt) at points in the gait cycle when hip motion is insufficient.
  - Initial contact on the right usually occurs with the foot flat or occasionally with the heel as initial contact and is accompanied by excessive hip and knee flexion.
  - Throughout early to mid right stance, there is excessive hip and knee flexion.
  - During late right stance, Richard demonstrates right knee–locked hyperextension 7/10 steps, or he keeps the right knee excessively flexed in 2/10 steps.
  - During late right swing, Richard's right leg demonstrates knee extension that is too slow and insufficient to position the right heel correctly for heel strike.
  - Step length is inconsistent, with the left step usually shorter than the right step.

## Tests and Measures:

Several tests were performed to obtain objective information to justify the treatment (to the insurance provider) and to show change at the end of the episode of care. Outcome measures were chosen on the basis of Richard's goals and initial observation of his functional limitations.

- Medium speed self-selected gait velocity – 0.32 m/s
- 6-minute walk test – 748 ft
- Berg Balance Scale score – 51/56 (Blum, 2008)
- Dynamic Gait Index – 21/24
- Number of instances of right foot drag in 100 ft – five

## Impairments:
*Musculoskeletal System*

- Passive right ankle dorsiflexion only to neutral and tight at end range
- Right hamstring tighter than the left but within functional range
- Passive motion of right hip slightly restricted (particularly in combined hip extension with abduction) but functional
- At this point in the examination, musculoskeletal system impairments only screened, not measured specifically, to use evaluation session time efficiently; also during the screening, musculoskeletal system impairments did not appear to be major contributors to Richard's subjective and objectively observed functional limitations

*Sensory-Perceptual System*

- Richard wears glasses for reading.
- No obvious inattention (right-sided neglect) is noted.
- Because Richard appears alert and has fairly good cognition, sensation is screened by asking him whether he thinks sensation on the right arm is the same as on the left and the same for his leg. He reports that he thinks it is the same. In addition, when asked, Richard replies that he can feel his foot drag.

*Cardiopulmonary system*

- Richard reports, "You're making me work really hard" and asks for several breaks during the evaluation session.

*Neuromotor system*

- Richard demonstrates active and isolated control through approximately three-quarter to full range in his right upper and lower extremity muscle groups (no deficits observed on the left). He is able to hold against minimal resistance in most movements, although not consistently throughout the available range of motion or in all positions.
- Richard demonstrates unbalanced muscle activity in the trunk in most activities, using extension strongly and recruiting abdominals on a more intermittent basis.
- Speed of movement is decreased in the right extremities, and he reports a feeling of "stiffness" throughout the right side.
- Although Richard demonstrates active motion at all joints, he demonstrates limited ability to completely isolate motion and requires verbal or manual cues to prevent compensatory movements. Specifically, he cannot actively flex his right hip past 90 degrees in sitting. He can actively straighten his right knee to only −20 degrees of extension in sitting, and he can actively dorsiflex his right ankle to neutral, although slowly.

## Contemplate Clinical Decisions

- What other activity limitations might Richard demonstrate or report? How might his participation in life and in social and recreational activities be limited?
- Suggest one specific impairment in the sensory system and one in the musculoskeletal system that might contribute to Richard's activity limitations.
- Describe three possible neuromotor system impairments that could contribute to Richard's knee instability during gait.
- Describe another potentially "unstable" segment of the body that could contribute to Richard's observed and reported gait limitations.
- At this point, what do you consider possible functional outcome goals for Richard?
- Using the information on tests and measures in Chapter 6, discuss the significance of the functional outcome measures indicated previously. How might this information be incorporated into both the evaluation and treatment planning processes?
- What other information will you need in order to complete your evaluation and establish a prognosis and plan of care?

## Evaluation of Motor Control-Stability

The astute clinician synthesizes the results of the examination in order to determine the relationship and relevance of an observed instability of a specific body segment or joint to the functional ability of the individual as a whole. A number of questions must be considered, including the following:

- How significant is the problem in the segment or joint in relation to the individual's overall function? Does this instability directly limit function, or are other factors more significant?
- What are the importance and influence of other impairments, activity limitations, participation restrictions, and contextual factors? For example, a patient may be able to walk safely when thinking about the strategies he has learned to control his knee and ankle, but at school, when distracted by social interactions with friends and the need to negotiate environmental challenges, he experiences frequent falls because his knee buckles or his ankle is unstable (medial/lateral wobble).
- What are the contributing roles of other parts of the body, the relationships among body systems, and the relationship between primary and secondary impairments? For example, a patient may develop instability and lack of segmental control in one part of the body to compensate for another segment that is too tight or stiff. A common example is an individual who has limited mobility at the glenohumeral joint and then develops a hypermobile scapula through active or passive attempts to achieve a position with the arm over the head. For another example, an individual recovering from a stroke may use excessive mobility of the lumbar spine to substitute for limited mobility and control at the hip.
- What considerations regarding time frame must be taken into account when determining interventions to address

this individual's segmental instability? For example, an individual receiving several hours of therapy each day in inpatient rehabilitation may be able to devote more therapy time to specific underlying problem areas and still have more time to work on whole body movements and functional activities than a person who attends outpatient therapy twice a week.

The therapist examines and evaluates the patient with the goal of prioritizing and addressing impairments that most limit function and can cause secondary impairments. In the case of joint or body segment instability from impaired motor control, the therapist must identify specific factors that contribute to the instability in order to design effective treatment strategies to address them and facilitate a change in function.

## PATIENT APPLICATION: EVALUATION

Richard has functional limitations, including some that pose safety risks (e.g., may cause tripping and falling). Impairments that underlie the functional loss include (1) motor control deficits such as the inability to adequately control and sustain dynamic coactivation at the ankle, knee, and possibly the hip on the right, especially in weight-bearing and (2) an overall inability to maintain adequate activation at multiple segments of the body at once, including the trunk. He demonstrates limitations in quickly activating muscles and quickly switching activation from one group of muscles to another. His ability to sustain muscle activity also appears limited throughout the right side.

Several mild musculoskeletal limitations are noted, specifically his limited ROM in ankle dorsiflexion and in hip motions. Decreased muscle length is noted in the right hamstrings. Because these limitations are asymmetrical and Richard has reported no other pertinent history, it is hypothesized that the musculoskeletal impairments are secondary and thus require remediation of the primary neuromotor impairments to achieve sustained improvement.

## Contemplate Clinical Decisions

- Write a long-term functional goal for ambulation for Richard.
- How long do you think it will take to achieve this goal, assuming you see him twice a week for 45 minutes each session?
- What other functional activities might you address in your functional goals?
- How might you use safety as a consideration in justifying treatment?
- Because Richard is also scheduled for an occupational therapy evaluation, what functional limitations and underlying impairments might you discuss with the occupational therapist to ensure that your goals in addressing Richard's impairments do not overlap?
- Describe a treatment strategy for use in the clinic to remediate Richard's neuromotor system impairments. Explain how your strategy will address specific aspects of his motor control-stability deficit.
- Describe one home exercise program (HEP) activity you can teach Richard to increase carryover of your intervention.

# ■ Preparatory Interventions Specific to Impaired Motor Control-Stability

## General Approaches

Current and customized clinical decision-making regarding intervention requires avoidance of "doing things the way we've always done them." This may seem complex or daunting, especially for the novice therapist. Dorothy Voss, in her American Physical Therapy Association Mary McMillan Lecture, reminded us of Hellenbrandt's words, "The unquestioned acceptance of traditional methods is one of the ills from which physical therapy education suffers" (Voss, 1982). An **evidence-based practice (EBP)** approach for intervention clinical decision-making, as discussed in Chapters 1 and 2, enables contemporary practice and includes integrating the best available research from the literature *with* the clinician's clinical experience and patient values (Sackett, 2000). When evaluating the evidence, look for links between improvement in impairments and functional outcomes. For instance, does improved ROM merely increase flexibility without leading to improved function or new skill acquisition?

Before choosing to implement an intervention that is customized for the patient's specific problems, self-evaluate your ability to perform the intervention to ensure competent and safe execution. This entails adequate training and experience in the particular intervention. In addition, determine whether the intervention matches the patient's values and goals. An intervention will fail if you do not have the skill to execute the intervention or if the patient is not in agreement and does not adhere. For example, if you decide to use electrical stimulation (ES) with a patient after attending a vendor in-service on the modality, but you have not had proper training or practice with the device, it may fail to produce positive results. In addition, if you think an AFO is the best way to treat ankle instability in the sagittal plane but the patient adamantly refuses bracing for cosmetic reasons and will not wear an AFO, the orthosis is the wrong choice for intervention (i.e., unless the patient can be convinced of its value).

When considering which approach or intervention to use to treat decreased motor control-stability, determine whether the goal is (1) for the patient to achieve improved or independent volitional motor control (remediation of the impairment), (2) for the adjunct equipment to provide external support for constant control of the joint instability (compensation for the impairment), or (3) a combination of remediation and compensation. To make this decision, consider the patient's diagnosis and prognosis, the patient's stage of rehabilitation, and whether the neurological disease process is acute, chronic, progressive, or unknown. In addition, it is helpful to know the type, duration, and frequency of interventions the patient has experienced in the past.

The choice of intervention philosophy (remediation versus compensation), however, is not one that is decided "all or none" or "once and for all"; rather, it is initially determined and then modified on an ongoing basis as the intervention progresses. For example, a patient with a recent stroke may initially require an AFO at all times to provide medial-lateral ankle stability while learning to walk, but she may wear the AFO intermittently and for shorter periods as recovery progresses.

Finally, in beginning an intervention focused on gaining joint stability through improved motor control, ensure there are no barriers to achieving the stated goals, including decreased joint mobility, muscle length, strength, or sensory awareness. For instance, if the patient is unable to maintain a neutral position of his knee in stance because of tight gastrocsoleus muscles, those muscles should be stretched before or while working on control of the knee in stance. If the patient is unable to achieve and hold a joint in a stable position because of a strength deficit, attempting to strengthen the muscles surrounding the joint may be appropriate. A patient's lack of normal sensory awareness (e.g., tactile, proprioceptive) may affect his ability to adjust joint position and may lead to joint instability. In this case, preparatory or simultaneous interventions for underlying impairments include treatment of the sensory system (refer to Chapter 27).

### Integrated Approach

Exclusive use of a single approach or intervention is never appropriate. Instead, therapists must use critical thinking and EBP to determine which approach or intervention to use with a specific patient. Intervention often becomes a blend of many approaches. This section includes a brief review of the main therapeutic approaches for addressing motor control instability, followed by information on specific techniques that can be combined with therapeutic approaches.

The Neuro-Developmental Treatment (NDT) approach, originally conceived for the management and treatment of adults and children with neuropathology, has developed over time as a result of new scientific information and knowledge gained from clinical experience (Howle, 2002). The NDT approach has been described as a problem-solving approach as opposed to a specific technique (Graham, 2009). When using this approach to treat joint or segment neuromotor instability, the therapist utilizes the individual's functional abilities and limitations to systematically assess for related effective and ineffective components of joint or segment instability. The therapist's ability to analyze movement and to use this information to determine the interrelationship among various impairments leads to the creation of an individualized treatment plan for neurologically based instability upon which specific treatment strategies are developed. The strategies frequently include handling that is systematically progressed (gradual withdrawal of manual assistance or support) to address multiple impairments and movement problems simultaneously to achieve a functional goal.

Difficulty with control of a particular body segment may be addressed with a treatment strategy addressing several impairments and body segments at once. However, strategies that isolate the specific body segment may be helpful initially to remediate impairments and facilitate control in one area of the body. This newly gained control can then be incorporated, often with graded therapeutic handling, into movements and functional activities involving the whole body. Chapter 15 provides additional information on the NDT approach.

Proprioceptive neuromuscular facilitation (PNF) was developed to help patients learn how to move more effectively to improve function. Improvement in function is accomplished using 10 basic concepts: manual contacts, body position and body mechanics, stretch, manual resistance, irradiation (overflow), joint facilitation, timing of movement, patterns of movement, visual cues, and verbal input (Martin, 2007). Joint approximation (see Fig. 24-1AB) is one technique used in PNF (as well as other treatment approaches) to facilitate cocontraction/coactivation and enhance motor control for joint stability. When PNF was used with patients with hemiparesis, it improved not only pelvic stability but also gait function (Wang, 1994). Chapter 15 provides an in-depth discussion of the PNF approach.

Motor development and motor learning, previously described in Chapter 14, are separate but interrelated entities discussed below as contributors to motor control-stability. In the healthy individual, the integration of these elements results in smooth and coordinated movement and muscular stability.

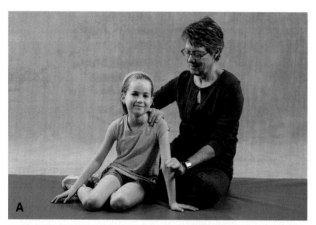

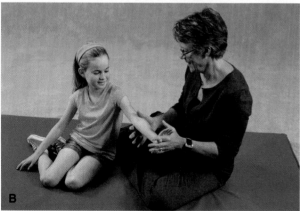

**FIGURE 24-1** (A) Approximation through upper extremity weight-bearing is assisted by the therapist, giving pressure through the shoulder and downward toward the weight-bearing open hand while supporting extension at the elbow. Joint stability is facilitated as the muscles around the shoulder, elbow, and wrist joints cocontract. (B) Approximation through the upper extremity in a non–weight-bearing position. With the arm straight (elbow in full extension), give pressure through the open hand toward the shoulder, making sure the elbow maintains 0 degrees of extension.

**Motor development** varies greatly from person to person and occurs throughout the lifespan as motor skills are gained and then decay in the closing years of life. From an ecological perspective, many different systems are involved in motor development, motor learning, and motor control. According to Newell's Model (Haywood, 2009), these systems are both internal (individual constraints of body systems, cognition, and emotion) and external (environmental and task constraints). Joints form, develop, and then may deteriorate across the lifespan. The young child may struggle with joint/segment instability that is "developmental" because of immature structures or lack of time and experience in weight-bearing positions, whereas the elderly may struggle with insufficient support or asymmetry due to arthritis, faulty posture, stiffness, weakness, or other medical, social, and emotional factors. When neurological conditions are added to the equation, the challenge of achieving or maintaining motor control-stability is greatly increased. Problems with joint or segment stability can impede a patient's ability to achieve developmental milestones and can diminish the quality of these skills, particularly ones involving weight-bearing. Likewise, a patient learning or relearning motor skills may have limited success because of instability in key joints.

Ultimately, all interventions to improve motor control-stability, regardless of the specific approach utilized, must emphasize motor learning (see Chapter 14) of the specific motor control through task-specific multiple repetitions for feedback. Essential elements in **motor learning** include sensing the desire or need to move, making the decision to move, and then putting the motor plan into action. When working to gain motor control-stability through this learning process, one can choose from numerous guidelines (see Table 24-3). Feedback can be given during a movement as knowledge of performance ("How am I doing?") as well as knowledge of results after the movement ("How did I do?") (Effgen, 2005). Refer to Chapter 14 for more details on motor learning strategies.

| TABLE 24-3 | Guidelines for Motor Skill Attainment |
|---|---|
| Use lots of practice and repetition |
| Make practice motivating |
| Determine a specific focus of activity |
| Change the tasks as needed to meet an appropriate level of difficulty |
| Schedule practice at different times and places to generalize the skill |
| Change the environment as needed to allow for success |
| Monitor and facilitate the psychosocial environment for patient comfort |
| Provide varying amounts and types of feedback |

Adapted from Effgen S. *Meeting the Physical Therapy Needs of Children.* Philadelphia, PA: F. A. Davis; 2004.

## Equipment

When a patient has decreased joint or segment stability as a result of impaired motor control-stability, it is often necessary to provide external support or bracing for the affected part in the early stages of recovery or when the deficit is permanent with no expected recovery of function. As discussed in Chapter 17, a variety of splints and braces may be applied. Later in this chapter, taping, pressure garments, functional electrical stimulation (FES), and biofeedback units are discussed as potential interventions.

## Specific Therapeutic Techniques

Emerging evidence provides direction for choosing techniques and adjuncts to treat joint or segment instability. An adjunct is a tool or element that supports or is incorporated into the therapy plan but is not usually used alone. The adjuncts described in this section are frequently used in combination with therapeutic exercise or one of the integrated approaches (e.g., NDT, PNF, motor learning). Adjuncts for treating joint or segment instability include biofeedback, ES, FES, taping/strapping, splinting/bracing, pressure garments, and body weight-support ambulation training (BWSAT). Optimal patient engagement and effort, sufficient repetitions, and appropriate feedback are essential for motor learning and relatively permanent long-term improvements in motor behavior through specific techniques and adjuncts. Evidence for the techniques and adjuncts described is summarized in the Focus on Evidence (FOE) table available online.

Therapists utilize various types of exercises and activities to improve motor control for joint stability. The purpose of these exercises is to produce coordinated and graded cocontraction/coactivation of muscles around a joint to allow the joint to remain steady when movement is not wanted and to maintain the appropriate amount of coactivation in agonists and antagonists for graded control when movement is desired.

### Resistance Exercise

Resistance exercise can improve motor control-stability at joints or segments. Patella instability can improve with isokinetic exercise (Hazneci, 2005), whereas scapular stability can improve with progressive resistance exercise (McNeely, 2004).

PNF techniques that target joint stability through manual resistance, include alternating isometrics (including rhythmic stabilization), slow reversal, and slow reversal hold. These are particularly useful for motor control-stability impairments because they incorporate contractions of both agonists and antagonists, creating a stable, cocontracted joint or segment. In **alternating isometrics** (see Fig. 24-2AB), resistance is used through specific hand placements on key body parts to facilitate isometric contraction of agonist muscles on one side of the joint or body segment followed by facilitation of antagonistic muscles on the other side of the joint or body segment. Facilitation is given in verbal commands ("Don't let me move you; hold still") and by manual contact (touching or resisting the muscles you want to contract).

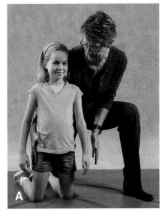

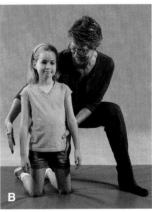

**FIGURE 24-2** Proprioceptive neuromuscular facilitation–alternating isometrics in a child that focus on increasing pelvic/trunk stability. (A) With your hand on the right hip, tell the child, "Don't let me move you" while you apply pressure laterally, maintaining just enough pressure so the child holds the position (isometric contraction). (B) Alternate your contact to the left side and give resistance in the opposite direction, again telling the child, "Don't let me move you."

In **rhythmic stabilization** (Fig. 24-3AB), facilitation and resistance are given alternately to agonists then to antagonists while the patient holds a body position to promote cocontraction around the joint. Resistance is increased or decreased depending on the patient's ability to "hold" and keep the joint or segment from moving.

The **slow reversal** technique varies from this by facilitating controlled movement (with joint stability at related segments) through a desired range in one direction followed by facilitation of the antagonist, with a reversal of the pattern creating a series of active contractions with successive movement in each direction. **Slow reversal hold** is similar to slow reversal, but a cocontraction "hold" is facilitated at the end range of movement (Martin, 2007).

For all these techniques, manual contact and application of resistance is thought to provide internal feedback in the muscle and joint receptors, helping the patient to sense the position of the joint (e.g., amount of flexion, extension), which facilitates keeping the joint in stable and anatomically correct positions during movement.

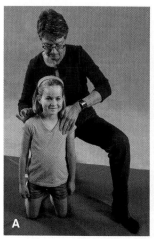
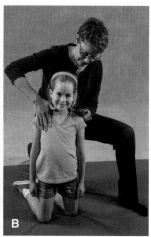

**FIGURE 24-3** Proprioceptive neuromuscular facilitation–rhythmic stabilization that focuses on trunk stability in a child. (A) Place one hand on the anterior trunk/shoulder area of the patient and the other hand on the posterior trunk/shoulder area on the opposite side. In this example, ask the patient to "turn to the right" while you resist each movement. This will cause cocontraction around the segment and train trunk stability. (B) Repeat these steps, but switch hand placements and ask the patient to "turn to the left."

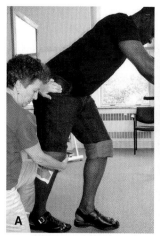
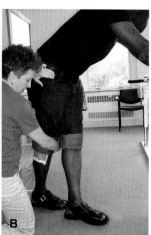

**FIGURE 24-4** (A) Neuro-Developmental Treatment (NDT) strategy to address Richard B.'s difficulty with isolated control of the right knee while also addressing other motor control and musculoskeletal impairments. (B) To modify the same NDT strategy, the change in direction of the left step adds more demand on the right lower extremity, including the need to control rotational components.

PNF can increase quadriceps and hamstring strength and joint position sense in patients with patellar instability (Hazneci, 2005). In one study, PNF did not improve gait velocity after 4 weeks of neuromuscular exercise (Coughlan, 2007). Additional research is needed to provide guidelines for proprioceptive interventions in patients with neuromotor pathology.

### Stance Weight-Bearing Exercise

Figure 24-4AB demonstrates one way the NDT approach might be used in weight-bearing therapeutic exercise in stance to remediate a problem with stability control at the right knee. Because many factors contribute to this problem, however, the most significant or limiting factors should be addressed first. Attempts to treat every issue simultaneously may lead to limited improvement in any one area. This may result in little change in function because resources (treatment) are spread too thinly. Addressing only one problematic area in isolation, however, may result in lack of carryover if the ability of the segment is not retrained in the context of overall function.

The treatment shown in Figure 24-4A was designed to address motor control difficulty in the case of patient Richard B., with easily identifiable right hemiplegia. He does not sustain and control activation of multiple body segments at once. The design of the intervention emphasizes facilitation of isolated and graded control in end ranges of knee extension. Because this activity demands activation in lengthened ranges of the gastrocsoleus and hamstring muscles, you can concurrently address the secondary musculoskeletal impairments in these areas, making optimal use of treatment time.

The **modified plantigrade position** combines stance (with lower extremity weight-bearing primarily on the right) with a slight forward incline of the body and bilateral UE support; it can be used with a verbal cue of "Push with your arms, tuck your chin, and push your body away from the bar." This results in coactivation of trunk muscles, with increased activity of the trunk flexors to improve proximal control, instead of Richard's typical pattern of using primarily trunk extension for trunk stability and control.

Using the closed chain position allows you to control the number of segments and amount of motion at these segments more easily. Then you can cue and facilitate correct alignment and motion of lower body segments to optimize conditions for muscle activation. Facilitation and directional guidance for correct rotation of the tibia and femur and correct alignment of proximal segments over the right foot should be provided during graded and controlled knee flexion/extension. The tape on the posterior aspect of the knee provides "extra hands" and sensory feedback to allow the patient to move into full knee extension without hyperextension so he can practice control of knee stability in that position.

## THINK ABOUT IT 24.2

Stand up and assume a modified plantigrade position. What different activities and exercises can you complete in this position? What joints/segments require motor control-stability to complete these activities/exercises?

### Postural Exercise

Postural exercises, including lumbar stabilization exercises, may be implemented to increase trunk stability and improve patient outcomes. The primary goal of lumbar stabilization programs is to teach the patient to achieve, control, and maintain a neutral spinal position with a healthy amount of lumbar extension when at rest and during all upright postures, movement activities, and transfers, including sit-to-stand. The program involves strengthening of abdominals and improving motor control of the trunk (maintaining and coordinating the amount of tension in both agonist and antagonist muscle groups to keep the trunk stable and cocontracted). Spinal stability can improve with instruction (Brown, 2006) and lumbar bracing exercises (Grenier, 2007).

Verbal, visual, and tactile input can be used to teach the patient the concept of spinal control. Instruct the patient to "Bring your belly button to your spine," demonstrate spinal neutral, and give hands-on feedback while the patient attempts the exercise. Use a mirror so the patient can see what appropriate spinal posture looks like for self-correction. Many patients with neurological pathology have difficulty with this task because of poor neuromotor control of the trunk musculature. If left untreated, poor trunk stability can lead to decreased function, pain, and injury, making this an important area to address.

Most published evidence regarding postural exercises involves healthy subjects or subjects without neurological pathology, limiting generalization of results to patients with neurological diagnoses. However, this evidence can be a useful starting point to determine which exercises and positions to try initially based on which muscles you want your patient to activate. For example, McGill (2009) described the core muscles that fire in three different exercises and optimal exercise progression in healthy subjects.

### Biofeedback

**Biofeedback** is an intervention that helps patients gain or regain control over bodily processes. There are several types of biofeedback, including thermal feedback (feedback from skin temperature), neurofeedback (feedback from an electroencephalogram [EEG] measuring brain activity), and electromyographic (EMG) feedback, an intervention for reeducating muscles. EMG biofeedback is discussed here because it is the main form used by therapists, particularly for motor reeducation, and can help patients learn to control key areas of neuromotor instability.

EMG biofeedback can decrease muscle tension, spasm, and overuse and can increase contraction for strengthening purposes. This motor learning tool works because EMG signals from surface electrodes over a muscle produce an audio or visual signal to alert the patient about the status of activity in that particular muscle group. When the patient sees or hears the signal, he can practice control over the contraction in response to the signal, either attempting to increase the signal when the goal is to increase muscle contraction or attempting to decrease the signal when the goal is to decrease motor activity. The EMG sensors detect the force of the contraction so the patient can repeatedly contract the muscle while using the auditory and/or visual feedback until he reaches the desired amount of contraction (see Fig. 24-5 for an example of quadriceps biofeedback).

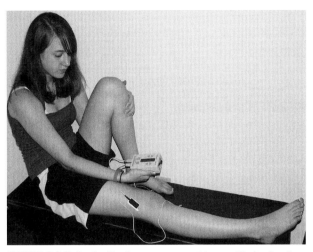

**FIGURE 24-5** Biofeedback setup to provide specific feedback on quadriceps activation on the affected side.

Through this motor learning process, the patient can potentially improve motor control-stability, practicing the grading on and grading off of muscle activity with the key muscles surrounding a joint. Biofeedback may complement or enhance other motor control interventions in the plan of care and is appropriate for individuals of any age who can respond to auditory or visual feedback and for a variety of diagnoses. Biofeedback has no reported side effects.

Evidence to support the use of biofeedback is emerging. Biofeedback has promoted greater stability, resulting in improved gait (Morris, 1992), improved head stability (Cattaneo, 2005), improved neck stability (Bolek, 2007), and improved ankle strength (Moreland, 1998). Biofeedback also improved function in patients after a stroke (Jonsdottir, 2007; Woodford, 2007). As a clinician deciding whether to use biofeedback, consider whether research supports its use with the population or diagnosis that presents to you. In practice, keep these key points in mind:

1. Use biofeedback in functional situations (real-life tasks) and not for isolated or nonpurposeful practice of muscle contraction (Huang, 2006).
2. Employ motor learning strategies while using biofeedback (encouraging optimal patient effort and engagement for appropriate functional practice, varied and frequent practice, practice in real-life environments, targeted/focused/purposeful practice, repetition, knowledge of performance, knowledge of results, and patient motivation).
3. Improved functional outcome is the goal, which requires success in both timing of and intensity of contractions to achieve the desired task.
4. Work from patient-directed goals because the patient's desire to accomplish a specific skill will motivate her to learn how to use the biofeedback unit.
5. Given the variety of unit types, choose a biofeedback device on the basis of patient/therapist comfort and skill in using it, cost, sophistication of the device, and

features of the auditory/visual monitor. The therapist will need time and practice using the machine before patient use.

6. Many patient trials and practice sessions are needed to achieve progress or reach goals.

### Electrical Stimulation

ES, a form of electrotherapy, is an important treatment option to improve motor control. For motor learning purposes, incorporate ES with patient voluntary motor activation and include practice, repetitions, and feedback. ES is especially appropriate for addressing impaired motor control-stability that is isolated to a specific segment or muscle group and warrants direct focused attention.

The use of ES to assist motor recovery in individuals with a neuromotor system diagnosis has a long history (Liberson, 1961). Use of ES is supported in a variety of diagnoses, including stroke (Alon, 2002), spinal cord injury (Alon, 2003), cerebral palsy (Elbaum, 2008), and multiple sclerosis (Armutlu, 2003; Kent-Braun, 1996; Popovic, 2009). Reported outcomes include improved function and remediation of impairments such as spasticity, pain, weakness, and impaired motor control. Additional benefits of ES include minimizing disuse atrophy, increasing local blood circulation, and maintaining or increasing ROM, especially during early stages of recovery from a diagnosis such as stroke.

## THINK ABOUT IT 24.3

Electrical stimulation with patient voluntary motor activation can improve motor control-stability at a specific joint or segment.

- Is electrical motor stimulation appropriate for Richard B.? Why or why not?
- Where would you place the electrodes and what parameters would you select?

Several different types of ES are currently used. Low-intensity ES results in sensory stimulation without muscle contraction (transcutaneous electrical nerve stimulation or **TENS**). TENS can decrease spasticity (Armutlu, 2003) and improve gait speed and muscle strength after a stroke (Teasell, 2016).

ES used at a higher intensity to produce muscle contractions for reeducation or strengthening is known as **neuromuscular electrical stimulation (NMES)**; when it is used to supplement a functional activity, it is known as FES. NMES is typically used in combination with other therapeutic interventions, such as therapeutic exercise and splinting (Kraft, 1992), an AFO for ambulation (Dutta, 2008; Kim, 2004), partial body weight support (Lindquist, 2007), Botox (Baricich, 2008), and biofeedback (Pomeroy, 2006). Evidence for the use of NMES is not sufficiently robust to draw conclusions about the effectiveness of neuromuscular retraining in individuals after a stroke because of variations in variables studied, such as type

of stroke, intensity, type of ES, and dosage (Pomeroy, 2006). Use of FES with gait retraining to improve hemiplegic gait has been supported; in addition, evidence for the effectiveness of ES used as compensation or as a neuroprosthesis (Popovic, 2002) outweighs that for reeducation with the goal of improved function once the stimulation has been removed. More research on the degree of patient engagement, voluntary effort, and practice with ES is needed.

Attempts have been made to further define and standardize situations in which ES is most beneficial for improving impairments and patient-centered functional outcomes. Examples include recent studies designed to determine best stimulation parameters, such as frequency and duration (Gorgey, 2008), and studies to assess the effectiveness of ES with or without concurrent use of Botox and other adjuncts (Munin, 2010). Long-term carryover of the effects of ES is unknown and requires consideration when making treatment decisions.

Newer devices have been designed to overcome the barriers typically encountered with older models. These advances enable more consistent electrode placement, improved ease of application and use by the patient, and improved selection of optimal stimulation patterns (see Fig. 24-6 and Fig. 24-7). Implantable nerve stimulators (Kottink, 2008) and the use of fine wire electrodes for percutaneous nerve stimulation may make ES more convenient and tolerable, with fewer noxious electrical sensations because the current does not have to penetrate the skin and subcutaneous layers. The recent development of more sophisticated systems, with additional studies investigating their efficacy, may also assist with insurance coverage for ES units.

Clinically, ES is most often provided to a single group of muscles (e.g., ankle dorsiflexors) or to opposing muscle groups in an alternating pattern of stimulation at a particular joint (e.g., wrist flexors and extensors). In an individual with locked knee extension in midstance, try applying ES to the gastrocs

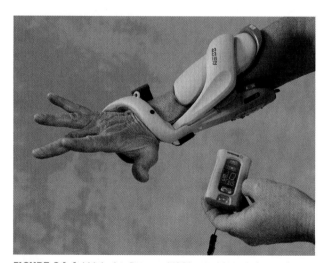

**FIGURE 24-6** With this Bioness H200 unit, electrical stimulation activates wrist and finger extensors in an individual recovering from a stroke.

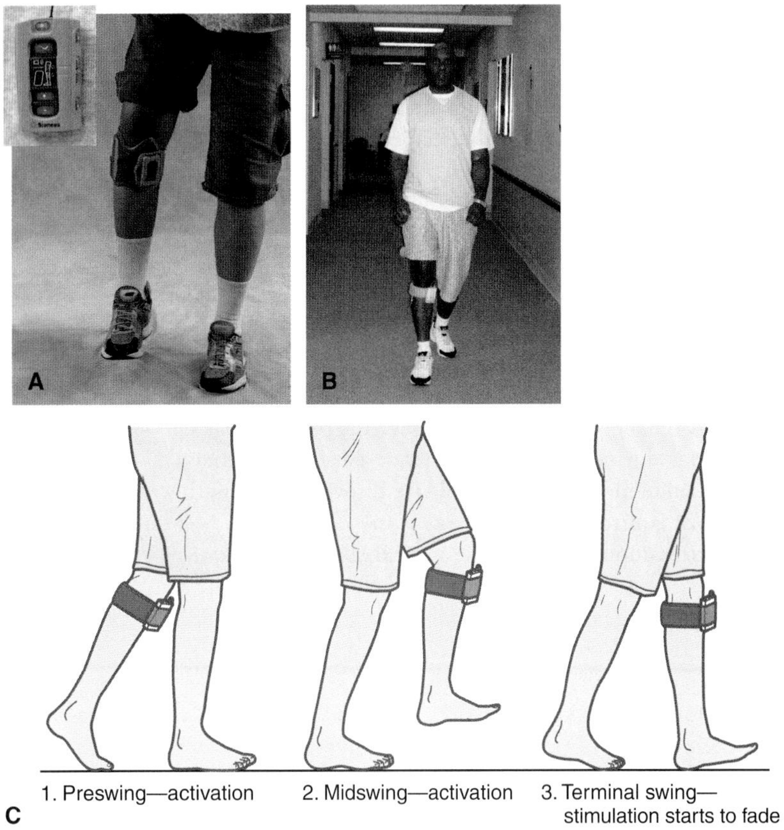

**FIGURE 24-7** These lower extremity systems use functional electrical stimulation to facilitate dorsiflexion at appropriate times in the gait cycle and was used on a trial basis in the clinic to assess the potential benefit of long-term use for this patient. (A) This Bioness L300 device (photo inset shows the remote control on a lanyard) uses a heel pressure sensor to activate dorsiflexors when the foot is not weight-bearing (i.e., swing-phase). (B) The WalkAide device uses an inclinometer in the unit at the knee to activate dorsiflexors when the tibia starts to incline forward. (C) The WalkAide device assists dorsiflexion in this patient. The electrical stimulation with both devices is customizable, ramps on in preswing, remains active in midswing, and starts to fade at terminal swing when the foot is approaching the ground.

1. Preswing—activation    2. Midswing—activation    3. Terminal swing—stimulation starts to fade

with activation during stance, using a heel switch on the opposite foot. When activated by stance on the opposite foot, the gastrocs brings the knee forward with slight knee flexion, preventing the locked extension and providing the individual with opportunities to practice coactivation around the partially flexed knee.

Electrode placement options for shoulder subluxation vary and include the supraspinatus and posterior deltoid (Wang, 2000), middle deltoid (Kobayashi, 1999), and long head of the biceps (Manigandan, 2014). Devices are available to provide stimulation to muscle groups over several body segments at once, including an orthosis that combines ES over several UE segments (Alon, 2003) and various devices that use ES to assist with walking (Tong, 2006). These devices are not yet widely available for clinic use, however. Other potential uses include application of FES early in poststroke recovery to reduce or prevent (Linn, 1999) shoulder subluxation and shoulder pain (Koyuncu, 2010), or to help stabilize the ankle.

Evaluate and carefully interpret results of research on ES, because a reduction in impairment does not necessarily result in improved function. For example, improving the position of the shoulder is not strongly correlated with improved motor control, improved function, or a decrease in pain. Also, use of a device that provides stability externally at a joint via continuous ES may limit opportunities for the individual to gain motor control through motor learning because opportunities for volitional movements

with repetitions and feedback are rare (because of the orthotic/supportive effect of the stimulation). Consider implementing intentional periods of practice without ES to watch for recent changes in muscle function, and schedule a planned withdrawal of ES.

Numerous factors should be considered in clinical decision-making and determining whether to use ES with a particular patient. ES should generally not be used with an individual with a demand-type cardiac pacemaker or defibrillator, over a malignancy, or over other acute problems such as a fracture. Consider and attempt to address potential discomfort to the patient. When the patient is unable to understand the purpose of the treatment but would benefit from ES and appears to tolerate it well, provide education to caregivers, if appropriate, regarding the purpose and use of the technique. If the unit is to be used at home, provide and evaluate the effectiveness of patient and caregiver education to facilitate follow-through with treatment and adherence to safety precautions. If the stimulation is to be used in conjunction with the patient's active attempts to move, adequate cognition and communication are required.

Practical considerations include the cost and availability of the equipment if used in the clinic and funding for the equipment if used at home. As a therapist contemplating the use of ES in a treatment plan, prioritize the need for treatment of a specific segment versus the need to devote time and resources to other segments or to the interaction and coordination of body segments working together.

As is true of any treatment adjunct, ES should be part of a comprehensive treatment plan that has specific and measurable functional outcomes and is reevaluated on an ongoing basis. Clearly anticipate the effect on impaired motor control-stability and the relationship to anticipated functional outcomes. For example, you might decide to use FES to increase strength and provide reeducation of ankle dorsiflexors and everters during gait training early in a patient's recovery from a stroke. The anticipated long-term result might be improved activation of muscles at the ankle joint to allow the patient to eventually walk functionally without an AFO or ES. The reason for using ES is pivotal in treatment plan decisions. In this case, you might use the FES unit during gait training and have the patient wear it for periods during the day to stimulate passive- or active-assisted ankle movements to facilitate recovery of strength and motor control.

As an example, consider the individual with a chronic disability from CVA who has impaired motor control-stability at the ankle, such that the ankle cannot be maintained in neutral to slight dorsiflexion during the swing phase. Therefore, dropfoot occurs during the swing phase with toe drag. The treatment plan for this patient might include FES as a substitute for an AFO (i.e., as compensation for lack of active control rather than for reeducation). With this patient, initially address application and problem-solving to facilitate optimal results with the device. Subsequent treatment sessions could focus primarily on gait training and fine-tuning of settings to assist the individual in achieving functional gait goals, such as improved gait speed, safety, or independence using the device. Some FES systems for ankle dorsiflexion, such as the Bioness L300 Foot Drop System (Figure 24-7A) by Bioness (http://www.bioness.com/Products/L300_for_Foot_Drop.php), use foot switches that trigger stimulation to the affected dorsiflexors any time the foot of the impaired leg is not in contact with the floor (swing phase). In contrast, other FES ankle systems such as the WalkAide System (Figs. 24-7B and 24-7C) by Innovative Neurotronics (http://www.walkaide.com/EN-US/Pages/default.aspx) are activated by inclinometers and accelerometers strapped on or near the affected knee that initiate stimulation as soon as the tibia inclines forward (Fig. 24-7B). Parameters can usually be adjusted, including ramp-up time and duration of stimulation.

In a patient with little or no movement in the affected UE after a stroke, the use of ES to maintain muscle length and prevent atrophy in the wrist extensors may require a different treatment plan. The protocol for an ES unit would be developed by the therapist in conjunction with the patient, and the patient could follow through independently, wearing the unit while performing activities for one or several sessions each day when not in therapy. Short-term impairment-related goals for direct PT intervention are reeducation of trunk control, remediation of perceptual deficits, and facilitation of coordination and integration of motor control-stability between body segments. As the patient improves and can incorporate a greater number of body segments into treatment activities, the UE can be involved. The goals of ES are to maintain muscle length and mobility and prevent atrophy during the early recovery period, when the emphasis of direct intervention is on proximal control.

### Taping/Strapping

Taping is a therapeutic adjunct commonly used by therapists to treat patients with orthopedic and sports injuries and musculoskeletal diagnoses. The frequency of descriptions of taping in the neurological population is increasing (Morin, 1997; Peterson, 2004; Yasukawa, 2006). Taping effectively addresses both primary impairments in the neuromotor or sensory-perceptual systems and impairments in the musculoskeletal system (which are often secondary).

There are two primary types of tape, nonelastic (e.g., Leukotape® P) and elastic (e.g., Kinesio®Tape). Indications for the two types are similar, although the tapes provide input to the patient in different ways. Regarding the type of input the tape provides to the patient's system, think of nonelastic tape as "yelling" a command at a patient and elastic tape as "nagging" or "suggesting." In general, nonelastic tape is more appropriate when strong or sustained input is needed. Depending on the body part treated, elastic tape can be used in various configurations such as an "I," "X," "Y," or forked shape to provide gentle but persistent input (Kase, 2003). In addition, application of elastic tape differs depending on how the therapist is using the "rebound" characteristic (e.g., applying the tape to pull from a muscle's insertion to origin for facilitation of a weak or inactive muscle or applying the stretch so that the tape pulls the tissues toward a muscle's insertion to relieve excessive tension and stress on a painful area).

Taping may directly treat an impairment (e.g., to relieve pain through realignment and support of an unstable shoulder as shown in Fig. 24-8ABC) or provide "extra hands" to address one of many problematic impairments in a patient with complex, multisystem limitations (e.g., preventing excessive knee hyperextension so the therapist can attend to more proximal components during gait training, as shown in Fig. 24-9). You may use taping to provide indirect intervention, as in taping to help facilitate the activity of scapular stabilizers so that the patient's hand can be used more effectively during a functional task. The creative therapist may use taping to assist with problem-solving and treatment planning, such as assisting dorsiflexion to evaluate whether an AFO would be beneficial (Fig. 24-10 and Fig. 24-11), taping the wrist to maintain a more optimal position while fabricating a splint, or taping the ankle for stability and prevention of skin irritation while awaiting delivery of an AFO (Fig. 24-12AB). Enhanced carryover of treatment goals is achieved by "sending the therapist's hands home with the patient" through carefully applied tape, and by instructing a family member or caregiver to reapply the tape to improve the effectiveness of home activities.

Contraindications to the use of taping include an allergy to adhesives or to latex (if the tape contains latex) and an inability to understand safe wearing and removal instructions

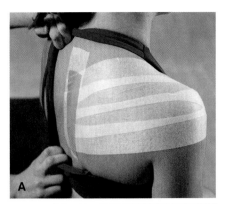

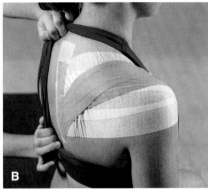

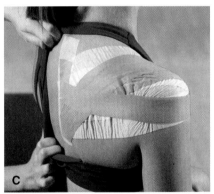

**FIGURE 24-8** (A) Initial steps of taping to improve alignment and increase stability in an individual receiving rehabilitation for a recent stroke. Protective tape is applied to the area, followed by an anchor of nonelastic tape to the spine on the opposite side. (B) Tape is applied to assist with scapular upward rotation, depression, and adduction and to better align the scapula on the rib cage. (C) Tape is used to position the head of the humerus back into alignment with the repositioned glenoid fossa.

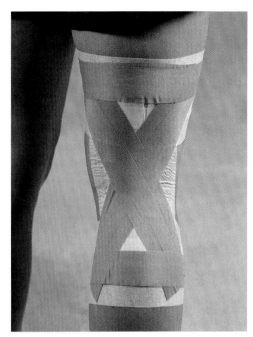

**FIGURE 24-9** Nonelastic tape is used to prevent knee hyperextension, helping the patient to relearn motor control through enhanced sensory feedback.

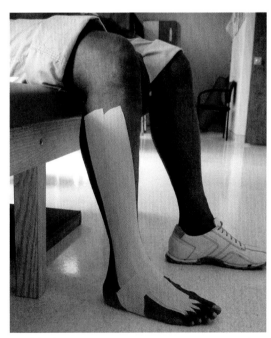

**FIGURE 24-10** Elastic tape is applied to assist the dorsiflexors and everters. The tape is worn for several days to assist with reeducation, and in this patient's case, to assist with decision-making regarding use of a more permanent adjunct, such as an ankle-foot orthosis to assist with foot clearance during gait.

(and no caregiver who can be educated to monitor safe wearing and removal).

As with decisions regarding any adjunct, effective use of therapy time is a primary consideration with taping. The potential carryover of the tape's effect when the patient is not with the therapist must be balanced with the time required for the therapist to apply the tape or teach the family/caregiver to apply it and to provide the necessary education.

Although evidence of the effectiveness of either type of taping is limited, several resources describe general clinical considerations for taping (Jaraczewska, 2006; Kase, 2003)

and others document its use in a case study or with a specific population (Host, 1995). One pilot study with children demonstrated improved UE and hand function as a result of treatment with Kinesio®Tape (Footer, 2006) and another showed increased hip extension during gait using gluteal taping in subjects with chronic stroke (Kilbreath, 2006).

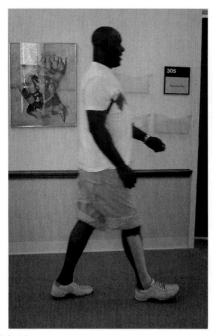

**FIGURE 24-11** Richard demonstrates improved gait with elastic tape facilitating ankle dorsiflexion. Improvements include increased right terminal knee extension, increased dorsiflexion, and initial contact on the right with the heel instead of the entire foot. Be sure to emphasize patient voluntary engagement in motor control while the taping provides assistance.

### Splinting/Bracing

An individual with lack of motor control-stability at a particular body segment may benefit from external support, especially when the degree of instability poses a safety issue or when no improvement is expected. The support influences or provides mechanical stability during movement (see examples in Fig. 24-13), enhances sensory feedback on a short- or long-term basis, or maintains or regains musculoskeletal components such as muscle length and joint alignment. Table 24-4 summarizes uses of some of these adjuncts. Further descriptions of many supportive adjuncts can be found in Chapter 17.

The therapist should consider the following critical questions regarding adjuncts to improve joint or segmental control:

- During which functions is the support needed? For example, a patient may no longer require use of an AFO for short walks but may be instructed to use it for ambulation of longer distances to prevent excessive repetition of compensatory movements that lead to secondary impairments.
- How much support is needed (e.g., choosing between elastic and nonelastic tape to support and reeducate scapular stabilizers)?
- Is support needed on a long-term basis to compensate for a lack of control or on a short-term basis with an emphasis on reeducation while waiting for recovery?
- In actual use, does the adjunct function as expected?

Once the therapist has a "best guess" regarding whether to use an external support or adjunct and has decided which type would be most effective, the hypothesis is tested during actual use of the device or intervention. The clinician continues to evaluate and modify use of the device as needed or considers alternatives.

Finally, many supports and adjuncts, including lapboards and slings, enhance passive alignment of the body part and support for parts that lack active movement. Although this is important, excessive attention to passive positioning may limit the time for addressing activation and reeducation of individual body segments and may encourage static inactive postures. Also, keep in mind several main drawbacks of external bracing in a population with neuromuscular dysfunction (especially if recovery of function is possible). A

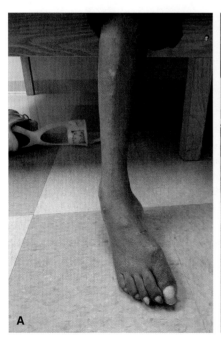

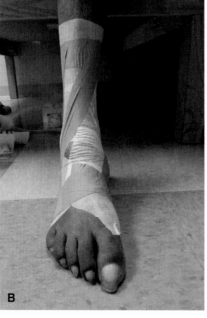

**FIGURE 24-12** (A) The ankle at the initial evaluation of a patient with stroke who reported pressure from her current ankle-foot orthosis (AFO). (B) Taping was applied to support the patient's ankle while arrangements were made to obtain an AFO that was more effective for her. Additional benefits of the taping were that the faulty position of her ankle was corrected and the structures were stretched so that casting for the new AFO could be done with the ankle in better alignment.

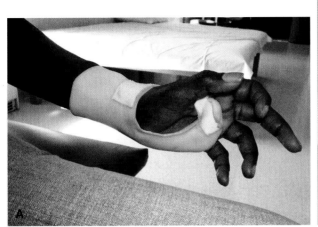
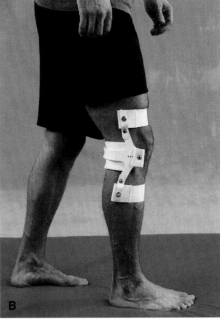

**FIGURE 24-13** (A) This custom-fabricated wrist splint was designed to address a motor control impairment at the wrist and hand. The patient needed to learn to stabilize the wrist while moving her fingers instead of using incorrect timing and sequencing with flexion of the wrist to initiate movement of the fingers. The splint initially enclosed her thumb to provide firm input and realign the carpal bones for correct wrist and thumb movement. The splint was later modified to allow the patient to use the thumb control that she gained and continue to provide a gentle but consistent reminder for dynamic wrist extension stability during function. (B) Use of a Swedish knee cage during gait permits knee flexion during swing phase. The cage also limits excessive knee and biomechanical locked knee extensions during the single-limb stance phase, allowing the patient to experience/practice control of the knee extensors while the brace provides support.

| TABLE 24-4 | Support Adjuncts and Their Indications and Uses Among Patients With Impaired Motor Control-Stability |
|---|---|
| **ADJUNCT** | **INDICATIONS AND USE** |
| Taping (see Figs. 24-8ABC and 24-9) | See the detailed description in earlier section. |
| Casting | This technique is often used with individuals recovering from brain injury and other diagnoses. The goal of casting is to prevent or remediate secondary impairments in the musculoskeletal system and possibly limit the strengthening of undesirable patterns due to involuntary muscle activity. Casting is often used for individuals with increased tone who may not be able to participate in reeducation activities to learn segmental control. The literature reports little consistency in or consensus regarding the use of casting in practice. Few studies included a comparison with a control condition such as no stretch. |
| Orthotics, (ankle-foot orthosis [AFO], knee/ankle/foot orthosis [KAFO], and more) | Many types of orthoses are available, and their features vary (see Chapter 17). An orthosis can provide static positioning, assist with movement, or allow free movement in one direction or plane but not the other. The therapist often works in conjunction with the orthotist to explore options that address specific patient problems and best meet the patient's needs. For example, a custom-molded AFO can prevent ankle wobble when the patient has medial-lateral subtalar neuromotor instability, correct footdrop in swing phase, and maintain the ankle in some degree of dorsiflexion for efficiency in gait. |
| Swedish knee cage (see Fig. 24-13B) | This support permits knee flexion but limits excessive knee extension and is marketed for orthotic management of genu recurvatum. Clinical limitations may occur when forces or biomechanics of the body overcome the control provided by the device. Carefully assess the overall effect of the device on the whole body, not just its effect at the knee. |

*Continued*

| TABLE 24-4 | Support Adjuncts and Their Indications and Uses Among Patients With Impaired Motor Control-Stability—cont'd | |
|---|---|
| **ADJUNCT** | **INDICATIONS AND USE** |
| Heel lift | A heel lift may assist with knee flexion, compensate for knee flexion contracture, or lessen the effort required to achieve swing of the affected lower extremity when used on the stronger leg. Use with caution and assess the possible and actual alterations in alignment of the body, both short and long term, because the heel lift may introduce asymmetry with undesirable consequences. |
| Splint | A splint is used to position a joint, usually for protection, or to maintain or regain muscle length or joint alignment. For example, a splint may be worn at night to maintain carpal alignment and muscle length at the wrist, or it may be worn during the day to provide feedback for reeducation. An ankle stirrup splint may be used to prevent excessive inversion during gait. |
| Air splint | These inflatable plastic cuff splints provide support and pressure on arms, legs, hands, or feet. The splint is applied to the patient's limb and then inflated. During inflation, the soft inner layer molds exactly to the limb, providing all-over, even pressure when inflation is complete. Air splints can be used to stabilize a body part during treatment, freeing the therapist's hands to assist with other areas, or air splints can be used for passive positioning or in conjunction with a home program. The amount of support provided by the air splint is adjusted by adding air or allowing air to escape. For example, for a patient with genu recurvatum, using an air splint at the knee and progressively lowering the inflation across sessions allows the patient to progressively practice more control over knee neuromotor stability. |
| Sling | For the neurological patient, a sling is primarily a passive support for a shoulder with inadequate muscle control; this protects the shoulder from excessive stretch from gravity's pull when the patient is upright. Studies suggest that use of a sling can prevent subluxation, but findings are inconclusive regarding the most effective sling. Evidence regarding use of a sling to affect pain or functional outcome is inconclusive. |
| Lapboard, lap tray, or arm trough | A lapboard provides some support to the shoulder and upper extremity in an individual who lacks active movement in the limb. Different styles of lapboards and supports are available, and there are benefits and limitations to each. A full lapboard may provide good support but may restrict the patient's movement. Half lapboards are less supportive, but they may allow the individual more independence in setting up for a transfer. Clear models can be used to encourage awareness of the lower extremities, which are otherwise hidden below the lapboard. An arm trough is less restrictive during transfers in and out of the chair, but its position along the arm of the chair may be uncomfortable for an individual who has lost external rotation range in the shoulder. Achieving good shoulder alignment while using a lapboard can be difficult, and an emphasis on alignment may discourage the movement and repositioning that normally occur in a seated individual. |

brace or orthotic that consistently and completely supports the joint without neuromotor stability may decrease the activation of the muscles surrounding the joint. From a motor learning standpoint, the muscles do not have to try to work because the brace is doing all the work. Although a brace enhances safety and may improve current performance of some functional skills (because of the external support), it offers little opportunity for practice and feedback, and motor control-stability may not improve. For example, the person wearing an AFO has few opportunities to practice active use of ankle dorsiflexors. A focus on activation and control of individual muscle groups, as discussed later in this

chapter, increases the chances of improving the individual's ability to function.

### Pressure Garments

**Pressure garments**, tight-fitting elastic clothing that contours to the body, are external supports that provide some degree of stability to a joint when the patient does not have internal neuromotor stability from ligaments or voluntary muscle activity. These garments may be temporary adjuncts until the patient is able to stabilize without the help of the garment, or they may be necessary for indefinite periods when the prognosis includes little to no expected return of voluntary joint control. Several types of pressure garments are available. The more common ones are the Stabilizing Pressure Input Orthosis (SPIO™), Benik systems, Hip Helpers®, and TheraTogs™.

Manufacturers of these devices state that their effectiveness is due to sensory feedback (primarily proprioceptive) and physical pressure, which together improve stability and increase function. Numerous case reports and studies have documented their effectiveness in providing stability and improving functional status (Blair, 1995; Hylton, 1997; Marcus, 2001; Nicholson, 2001; Paleg, 1999). However, most of these studies were observational rather than randomized controlled trials. Although before and after videos can demonstrate fairly dramatic improvement with the use of pressure garments, more research with larger samples, use of controls, and use of validated outcome measures to determine long-term benefits is needed.

SPIO™ garments (see Fig. 24-14) include vests, shirts, pants, unitards, and gloves that provide support to a variety of joints including the spine, hips, knees, shoulders, elbows, and hands. According to www.spioworks.com, "SPIO™ garments are made from a Lycra®-like blend material that provides deep pressure through compression to improve positional limb and body awareness, core muscle and joint stabilization, and increased precision of muscle activation and movement."

Benik garments are made of neoprene, which gives the patient more external support than Lycra but may be less comfortable because of its increased stiffness. Neoprene garments are also less "breathable," thus retaining more heat than Lycra garments. Benik pediatric systems include knee/wrist/elbow/trunk/shoulder supports, universal wraps, and shorts; adult systems include knee/wrist/elbow/shoulder/lumbar supports, toe/ankle/calf/thigh/groin supports, shorts, and athletic garments.

Hip Helpers® are inexpensive shorts (about $15.00) made from nylon and Lycra fabric that children with excessive hip mobility can wear to decrease hip abduction and thereby improve posture and stability (Nicholson, 2001). They can be ordered online by the therapist or parent at www.hiphelpers.com.

TheraTogs™, developed by a physical therapist, Beverly Cusick, are garment systems consisting of pieces made of nylon and spandex with foam backing that provide support and sensory input to specific body segments. TheraTogs come in six product configurations and size ranges from infant to adult. Strapping can be attached to the garments externally and configured to address a variety of alignment and motor control problems (Flanagan, 2009). Figure 24-15AB illustrates the use

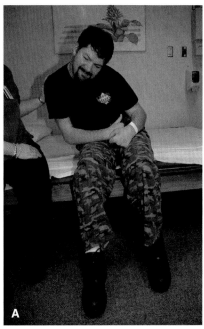

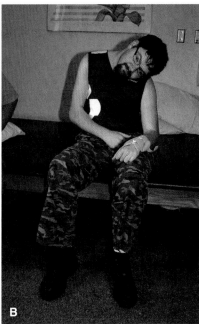

**FIGURE 24-15** (A) Sitting posture of a young man before application of TheraTogs™ (therapist is assisting with balance). (B) Sitting posture of the same young man with TheraTogs™ applied. He is able to sit briefly without physical support.

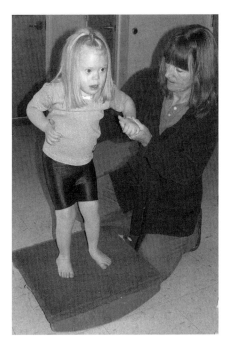

**FIGURE 24-14** SPIO™ Hip Helpers® pelvic support pressure garment.

of TheraTogs to improve trunk stability and upright sitting posture in a young adult.

In practice, use clinical decision-making to recommend the most appropriate pressure garment. The choice of garment depends on the degree of support needed, the type and characteristics of material desired, the cost, the ease of use of the garment (by both the therapist and the patient), the targeted joint/body segment, and the skill/knowledge/experience of the therapist in using the garment. Interventions with use of pressure garments include instructions in donning and doffing, performing and practicing specific functional tasks with the garment on, evaluating the benefit of the garment (Is there a change in function using the garment?), and deciding when and if the patient is ready to be weaned from the garment as she gains voluntary motor control over the targeted instability. Pressure garments are measured and ordered by therapists per manufacturer's guidelines.

### Body-Weight Support Ambulation Training

BWSAT is sometimes called **body-weight support treadmill training (BWSTT)**. Body-weight support systems are used over ground or on a treadmill. They have grown in popularity and success over the last decade as a treatment not only to assist ambulation but also to address instability of the weight-bearing joints of the lower extremities, and provide opportunities for the patient to practice and learn control and not just have the device provide control. Locomotion training is introduced in Chapter 15, with more specific functional intervention applications described in Chapter 37.

These systems provide the patient with a more independent and functional form of standing and walking, particularly early in the rehabilitation process. The body-weight support allows individuals to practice graded lower extremity control of stability and movement during ambulation as they progressively support more and more of their own body-weight throughout the rehabilitation process. The harness system provides balance support for the patient in an upright anti-gravity position and prevents falling, thus freeing the therapist for hand use to guide and facilitate proper trunk and lower extremity alignment and movement. When the weight-bearing effort of the patient is decreased through unweighting by the harness system, the patient can focus more on practicing and learning cocontraction and stability at key weight-bearing lower extremity joints and controlled grading of movement.

Consider this clinical scenario: A person with hemiparesis may have instability causing the affected knee to either buckle into flexion or snap into locked knee extension in midstance of gait on the affected side (during single limb support) because of impaired motor control-stability. When the knee lacks neuromotor control stability for appropriate cocontraction, the knee may move into a locked extension position in an attempt to biomechanically stabilize the knee. This thrust into extension that occurs in midstance is referred to as "genu recurvatum" when the knee actually snaps into a hyperextension position. BWSAT intervention allows this individual to repetitively practice the weight-bearing aspects of ambulation that require motor control-stability while the system relieves the patient of up to 40% of body weight. The therapist can then progressively withdraw the body weight support as the individual regains motor control-stability of the hip, knee, and ankle.

BWSAT may also be helpful to address motor control movement during ambulation (see Chapter 25) and motor coordination (see Chapter 26). A more detailed description of BWSAT and the evidence supporting its use are provided in Chapter 37, which focuses on functional interventions for ambulation.

## ■ Intervention: Ultimately Applied in Functional Activities

Intervention for decreased motor control-stability cannot stop at treatment focused only on gaining neuromotor stability at one segment but must optimally be progressed to multisegment (whole body) control, leading directly to improved overall functional activity and participation for the patient. Patient goals and functional outcomes must always provide the underlying guidance for any intervention. Interventions should be progressed from simple to complex functional tasks, which can occur in several ways. The demand or difficulty of a task can increase as the variables of speed, distance, and force are increased.

To think about progression, consider your patient with traumatic brain injury who is working on gaining motor control-stability in the shoulder. Exercises could include UE closed chain, weight-bearing positions (listed in order of increased difficulty: modified plantigrade, propped sitting, prone on elbows, prone on extended arms, or quadruped) focusing on coactivation around the scapulothoracic and glenohumeral joints and using taping as an external support. Next, progress from treating the impairment of shoulder instability as an isolated, single joint problem to working on an open chain functional task such as reaching for a cup in a cupboard. In this activity, the patient must not only use more than one joint to complete the movement but must also focus on an activity (not just isolated muscle control) that requires stability at the scapula/shoulder during the movement task. Design a practice structure that requires graded stability in a variety of movements and transitions with varying demands. Repetition is key to motor learning. Feedback, both external and internal (as discussed earlier), is essential as the patient goes through the learning process.

Examples of functional treatments related to motor control-stability are described in following sections. Chapters 33 to 37 provide more specific details on functional interventions in specific activities, including enhancement of motor control-stability in these tasks.

### Functional Activities

Functional mobility and the ability to transition from one position to another with control are important to patients of all ages and medical diagnoses. For patients with joint stability problems, controlled transitional movements with weight-bearing components are especially challenging. The patient must be able to complete the transitional movement and learn to perform with good quality, maintaining good alignment and stability in related segments.

Emphasize safety in both usual and unpredictable situations (e.g., sit-to/from-stand with control from a stable chair as well as safe recovery when the unstable lawn chair or rocker suddenly tips). Incorporate tasks and environmental setups that require the patient to stop, reverse, or continue movement, as appropriate for the task and environmental considerations. The use of a variety of positions and transitions provides opportunities for the patient to develop mobility and stability of many segments as well as coordination of multiple body segments. Select specific activities, described in following sections, according to functional goals and the specific impairments to be addressed. Patients can practice rolling, supine-to-sit, sit-to-stand transition, cruising in stance, and finally walking, as these are typical aspects of daily activity for everyone that require neuromotor stability, especially in weight-bearing joints.

For physically able adults and children, the transitions and mobility of creeping, kneeling, and floor-to-stand through half-kneeling can be progressively included to improve function (e.g., reaching for shoes that someone has kicked under the bed) and address specific impairments. While the patient performs these tasks, the therapist can help her maintain good segment control at the affected joints (see the examples that follow).

### Transitioning Between Supine and Sitting, Including Quadruped

Individuals achieve a sitting position in a variety of ways depending on the starting position, the surface, the reason for moving into sitting, and other factors. Many people get into a sitting position from lying down by rolling to their side and then pushing into sitting using their UEs. Some may transition directly into sitting by flexing at the hips, whereas others (primarily children) rise into sitting by getting onto all fours and pushing back into sitting. This functional transition, which could occur multiple times a day depending on patient age, is a good activity for helping the patient learn motor control-stability throughout the movement, especially stability of the trunk and pelvis.

**Quadruped position**, sometimes called "hands and knees" or "all fours," can be a very useful functional position for therapeutic intervention activities because it requires neuromotor stability at the trunk and in proximal girdle segments (shoulder and pelvis/hip) as well as the elbow, wrist, and knee. Moving from supine-to-sit (see Fig. 24-16ABCD) may also

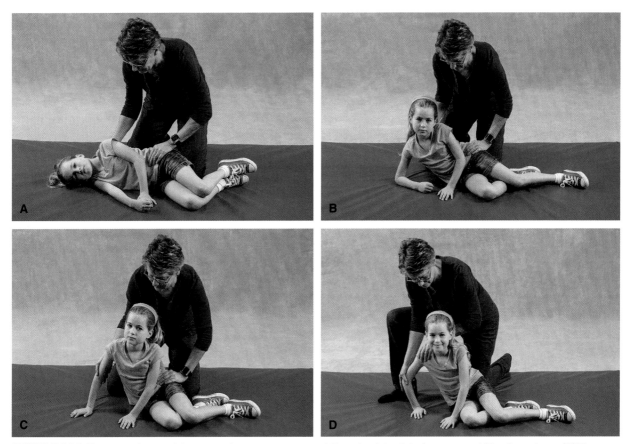

FIGURE 24-16 Transition from sidelying to side-sitting on a mat while maintaining joint/segment stability throughout. (A) To begin assisting the child to come into sitting from sidelying, put one hand on the child's pelvis and one on the opposite shoulder, facilitating an upward weight shift while the child laterally flexes the trunk. This facilitates trunk, shoulder, and elbow stability. (B) Next, shift your weight while moving with the child, helping her to weight-bear on her elbow. (C) Continue laterally flexing the trunk and bringing the elbow into full extension. Assist the elbow in maintaining extension without overextending, looking for cocontraction (stability) at both the shoulder and the elbow. (D) Finally, have the patient practice lowering the trunk slowly toward side-lying on the mat or table (eccentric contraction of elbow extensors) while maintaining control.

improve stability by focusing on lateral trunk flexion and rotation of the trunk and stability of the head on the trunk (neck stability). This movement can also be used to facilitate gradations of UE control by going from forearm weight-bearing to extended arm weight-bearing; this is coordinated with lateral trunk flexion for weight shift toward the UE when lying down or toward the hips when coming to sit.

### Transitioning Between Sit and Stand (Rise-to-Stand and Eccentric Lowering)

Once the patient can attain a sitting position, skilled movement from sit-to-stand and the return to sitting, which requires additional segment stability in the trunk and lower extremities, must be achieved. This task, described in greater detail in Chapter 36, is achieved by leaning the trunk forward from sitting, which creates an anterior weight shift to the feet, followed by a lower extremity, extensor concentric push into the standing position (see Fig. 24-17ABC). Trunk stability is needed throughout the transition (without trunk flexion), along with dynamic stability of the hip, knee, and ankle. Depending on their age and ability, some patients also need to use their arms to push themselves into the upright position.

Before beginning the sit-to-stand transfer, the patient who is relearning sit-to-stand may benefit from optimal preparation, including attaining appropriate upright trunk posture in sitting. This consists of bilateral/symmetrical weight-bearing through the pelvis; an erect spine, head, and trunk in midline; and feet flat on the floor with knees flexed beyond 90 degrees.

Assess sit-to-stand without arm use first; if the patient is unable, then assess sit-to-stand with UE use. From a power and safety standpoint, determine first whether the UEs are needed to push up from the sitting surface or arms of a chair, and do not allow the patient to use the arms if they are not needed. The knee can be particularly difficult to manage in the transition from a midflexed position to full extension. Often, patients do not stop at 0 degrees of extension but snap back into knee hyperextension or biomechanically lock the knee in a fully extended position because of lack of control or inability to judge where the end position is.

When the patient is lowering back to the sitting position, the extensor muscles must eccentrically contract to control the descent, and dynamic joint stability is needed to coordinate timing and sequencing of movements in the trunk and lower extremity joints. To increase the difficulty of this task, lower the height of the seating surface and decrease the percentage of arm support. To increase the challenge even more, ask the patient to hold something, such as a full glass of water, while completing the transition. Use of this activity in treatment might include assessing the functional need for the transition (e.g., getting out of a soft bed, getting up from a toilet with no rails available), incorporating other abilities or limitations such as the ability or inability to use one or both UEs to assist.

Facilitate graded control during rising from sitting and during lowering, with variations at points in the transition to address specific joint/segment motor control limitations. For example, for the individual who cannot control stability of the

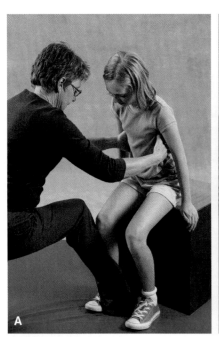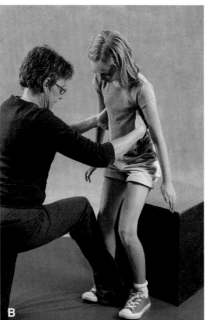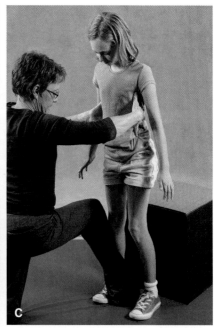

**FIGURE 24-17** Transition from sit-to-stand with focus on motor control-stability of the knee. (A) Ask the patient to lean forward from the edge of the bench with the feet flat on the floor. Stand or kneel at the patient's right side, bracing your knee near/against the patient's affected knee for support as needed. Continually assess the situation and be prepared to supplement the patient's control at the knee. (B) Assist the patient in shifting her weight in a forward lean by placing your arms around the trunk as she leans forward and stands up slowly, helping to shift weight onto the right leg with continued support of the right knee as needed to prevent it from buckling. (C) Once the patient is standing, check the knee for position and stability (to ensure that it is not buckling or hyperextending). Then slowly, eccentrically, lower the patient back to the bench.

ankle to keep the tibia forward over the foot for balance during the sit-to-stand transition, you could facilitate the patient's ability to come partway up, then ask the patient to weight shift slightly to the side and sit; this lateral shift requires sustained but dynamic ankle control to maintain balance during the weight shift. Means of progressing the activity include decreasing the amount of facilitation, changing the direction, adding a movement component such as rotation, or using the transition for a function such as partially standing to adjust clothing or to obtain something that is just out of reach in sitting.

### Transitioning Between Stand and Squat

For many patients, transitioning from a standing position to a squat or partial squat is an everyday occurrence that requires neuromotor stability of the trunk and pelvis and dynamic stability of the hip, knee, and ankle. Repeated performance of this functional activity with therapist input can be an appropriate intervention with variety for improving motor control-stability in lower extremity joints.

The therapist needs to initially guard against buckling of lower extremity weight-bearing joints and provide support for balance while lower extremity joint stability is challenged. This can be done as the therapist has the patient complete repetitions of squats, progressively increasing the demand for lower extremity joint stability by progressing to deeper range squats, squatting while holding progressively heavier objects (such as lowering an object to the floor), and squatting with the feet on two different surfaces or levels and progressively placing greater weight-bearing demand on the affected lower limb (see Fig. 24-18AB).

### Complex Functional Activities

Eventually, the patient should be progressed to activities that incorporate the whole body and teach integrated control of all body segments, including stability with mobility. Complex functional activities integrating the whole body, such as ambulation, stair ascent, and walking to and getting into the car, require control of multiple segments, not just a knee or an ankle. These activities include multiple transitions of a single joint between stability and movement functions. Repetition of these functional activities (versus isolated exercises or tasks), although difficult, ensures transfer of learning and generalization into real-life, everyday tasks for true benefit to the patient. For example, it is important to incorporate practice of weight-bearing in stance (lateral weight shift with a partially flexed knee) and gait (with a partially flexed knee) during functional activities, with an emphasis on avoiding biomechanical locking of the knee in extension.

In addition to functional mobility skills (transfer, gait), neuromotor stability at specific joints is required for many other activities that occur throughout a typical day. Object manipulation, including reaching, lifting, carrying, and releasing, requires motor control at numerous body segments, with motor control-stability required in the hand and wrist for grasp and grip. When deficits of muscular stability interfere with function, therapy must include training and teaching at specific body segments where instability interferes with the given function.

As a therapist, you must make decisions regarding choice of activity, feedback, manual facilitation, and progression of an activity based on assessment of the patient's performance, not only in terms of functional accomplishment (Is the patient able to stand up?) but also in terms of the quality and effectiveness of the movement components and the potential effects of using these patterns on a regular basis. This assessment leads to ongoing revision of the treatment plan. As the patient gains control and can maintain segment stability in static postures, progress her to more challenging activities. You can increase the difficulty of a task (Fell, 2004) by decreasing the support provided to the patient, narrowing the base of support in weight-bearing postures, and varying the direction and distance

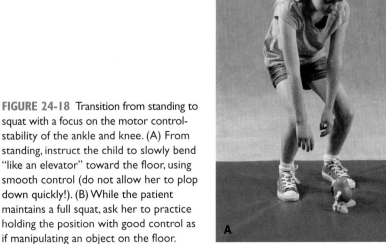
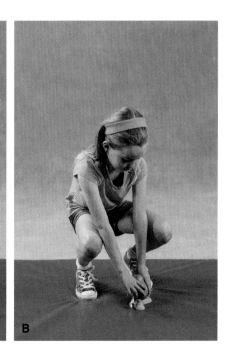

**FIGURE 24-18** Transition from standing to squat with a focus on the motor control-stability of the ankle and knee. (A) From standing, instruct the child to slowly bend "like an elevator" toward the floor, using smooth control (do not allow her to plop down quickly!). (B) While the patient maintains a full squat, ask her to practice holding the position with good control as if manipulating an object on the floor.

of weight shifting. In standing, progression can also include more activities in single-limb stance. When increasing the difficulty of an activity, pay careful attention to the quality of control the patient demonstrates and gradually progress the activity. If the patient begins to lose control at the affected segment, give feedback to facilitate learning of neuromotor stability in the functional skill.

### Adjustments to the Environment

To facilitate motor control-stability, adjustments can be made to the physical environment, equipment used, and task design. As you work with the patient to improve segment stability in the functional skills described previously, there are many ways you can manipulate aspects of the environment; these adjustments can address the patient's current ability while advancing her to activities that increase the challenge or progress the demand as improvement is noted (Fell, 2004). For example, changing gait assistive devices or ambulation surfaces provides "opportunities" for selecting different patterns of movement and motor control to achieve lower extremity neuromotor stability in a variety of contexts.

Consider biomechanical influences on the ability to stabilize a specific joint in functional activities. The patient who lacks neuromotor stability (control) at a joint, especially when the joint is involved in weight-bearing, often resorts to artificial stability gained through alternative biomechanical positioning. For example, some individuals lack motor control to stabilize the affected knee in an extended position in weight-bearing using coactivation/cocontraction (with the

normal, very slight flexion of the knee). Through unbalanced extension moments, they may snap the knee back into a mechanically locked position of knee extension (genu recurvatum if hyperextended) in order to safely bear weight through the limb and maintain extension. Long-term use of the joint in this way can damage the joint.

When planning intervention, design practice in a functional posture that prevents the mechanical compensation from taking place. In the case described, your intervention might include practicing lower extremity weight-bearing while you or an AFO keep the patient's tibia forward in some degree of dorsiflexion; this prevents full knee extension and provides opportunities to simultaneously practice neuromotor stability of the knee through cocontraction of knee flexors and knee extensors.

For techniques that allow practice of motor control-stability at the knee, review Table 24-5, which summarizes intervention activities in standing and ambulation. From a motor learning standpoint, it is very important to couple these biomechanical adjustments with opportunities to volitionally experience and practice holding the target joint in a stable cocontracted position in progressively demanding environmental contexts.

Biomechanically, posterior rotation and retraction of the pelvis on the affected side, which is sometimes seen on the affected side in individuals with hemiparesis, makes locked knee extension more likely. Training the patient to reposition the pelvis in a more neutral position, possibly through emphasis on restoring stability between the lower trunk/pelvis and the upper trunk, may decrease the likelihood of abnormal locked knee extension.

| TABLE 24-5 | **Examples of Interventions for Locked Knee Extension in Stance From Impaired Motor Control-Stability** | |
|---|---|
| Intervention for patients with lower-level function | • Half-bridging on the affected side to activate the hip extensors and rotate the affected side of the pelvis forward using hip extension, abduction, and external rotation while keeping the foot on the surface (incorporates dynamic coactivation of knee flexors and extensors to stabilize the knee position over the foot while activating hip muscles that control the position of the hip over the knee and foot; also reeducates stability at the knee combined with mobility at the hip)<br>• Partial sit-to-stand to help the individual learn to control dynamic stability at the ankle as the body moves over the foot |
| Intervention focused at the ankle | • Ambulation with an ankle-foot orthosis, positioned in slight dorsiflexion to keep the tibia inclined forward |
| Intervention focused at the knee | • Repetitive practice of a shallow-squat activity with varying amounts of demand on the affected lower extremity, progressing to eccentric and concentric focus and incorporating functional actions such as reaching to the floor |
| Intervention focused at the hip | • Facilitation and reeducation of forward weight-shift of the body with hip-extension during midstance to late stance |
| Intervention to adjust the environment of ambulation | • Single-leg stance activities to increase the challenge on the affected leg<br>• Body-weight support ambulation training to allow progressive practice of knee coactivation/stability without the need to support full body weight<br>• Backward walking, a more novel form of ambulation, to encourage coactivation of knee flexors and extensors while the weight-bearing hip is moving from extension toward flexion<br>• Ambulation without an assistive device to create greater demand and to change the sensory input through the LE |

Adapted from Diamond M. A question of flexion: Preventing knee hyperextension in the adult. *Neuro-Dev Treat Assoc NDTA Network.* 2005;12(6):16–22.

Another example of biomechanical constraints to consider is the effect of limited dorsiflexion range in one ankle. If the tibia cannot move forward during stance because of limited passive dorsiflexion, the knee will be forced into extension as the upper body continues to translate forward through stance phase. In this case, adequate ROM must be restored to the affected ankle to allow normal cocontraction around the knee. For the patient with genu recurvatum who requires an AFO to support dorsiflexion in midswing or to provide medial/lateral ankle stability in stance phase, adjusting the posterior stop of the AFO to rest in greater dorsiflexion may inhibit full knee extension; this may also facilitate more balanced coactivation to improve stability control of the knee through the gait cycle.

## Pediatric Considerations

In addition to the general pediatric principles described in Chapter 15, certain pediatric diagnoses require special focus on joint neuromotor stability. In children with Down syndrome, generalized low muscle tone and weakness in addition to joint laxity can contribute to instability in any joint or body segment. Hypotonia in proximal muscle groups in children with Down syndrome contributes to substantial neuromotor instability and may affect function, mobility, and motor skill. For instance, when a child with Down syndrome is walking on uneven surfaces and unexpected perturbations occur, the hip musculature may not respond quickly enough to provide stability; in this case, the hip is more likely to give way, and the child is more likely to fall. Or when a child who lacks hip control (i.e, to provide stability) attempts to kick a ball—a move that requires one-legged balance and cocontraction at the hip—success in completing the task will be limited. In a child with cerebral palsy, a lack of neuromotor segment stability and increased muscle tone can occur. The child with decreased selective control and abnormal synergies at the ankle, who attempts to step down off a curb but lacks the ability to hold the foot/ankle in a flat and stable position, is at risk for ankle injury or falling. Figure 24-19 illustrates a pediatric therapeutic activity for a home setting, including **family-centered**

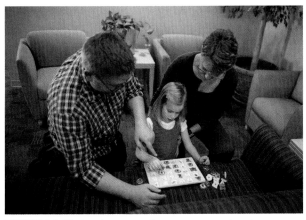

**FIGURE 24-19** Family-centered care in a natural environment (home-based intervention) while working on stability of the trunk segment.

care in a **natural environment,** with a therapeutic focus on trunk and UE stability in a kneeling position. The interventions described in this chapter may be implemented to improve stability in these cases.

Although this chapter focuses on impaired motor control-stability, musculoskeletal impairments can also affect joint stability. Children with Down syndrome have generalized joint laxity, and 10% to 20% of these children have instability at the atlantoaxial junction (C1-C2) (Pueschel, 1981), increasing the risk for subluxation and spinal cord compression. Symptoms of spinal cord involvement include sensory deficits, increased muscle weakness, bowel and/or bladder dysfunction, gait changes, neck pain or torticollis, and motor incoordination. To determine whether atlantoaxial instability (AAI) is present, ask during the initial examination if a radiograph has previously ruled out the instability.

Controversy exists as to whether radiography should be a part of routine medical care for these children. The American Academy of Pediatrics does not recommend routine films, whereas many other experts in the field and the Special Olympics Organization do (American Academy of Pediatrics, 1995; Cohen, 1998; Pueschel, 1998). Despite this controversy, therapists should educate families on the possible presence and significance of AAI and avoid hyperextension or flexion of the neck, tumbling activities, or contact sports until medically cleared.

Children with developmental dysplasia of the hip (DDH) can have pathological hip instability, either subluxation or dislocation. Because DDH is associated with numerous neurological pathologies, therapists should routinely monitor for the presence or absence of this instability and refer the child to an orthopedist when the condition is suspected. Signs of DDH include asymmetry of hip ROM, decreased hip abduction ROM, leg length discrepancy, and asymmetrical thigh skin folds. Conservative management of DDH includes bracing, exercise, and positioning. When this is ineffective, surgery may be necessary to reduce the hip.

### Contemplate Clinical Decisions

*Richard B.'s insurance provider has authorized 1 month of twice-weekly therapy visits, and an additional month was subsequently requested and approved. Using the knowledge gained through this chapter, describe the specific aspects of intervention you would incorporate into his treatment plan to improve motor control-stability in his right lower extremity.*

## ■ Intervention: Considerations for Nontherapy Time and Discharge

The therapist can maximize the benefits achieved by the patient during therapy visits by designing a HEP or a customized plan of home activities that targets the impaired neuromotor stability of specific joints or body segments. The home program is a definite component of every plan of care and is reviewed and upgraded or modified as needed during therapy visits to achieve optimal patient improvement (see Chapter 1). Include exercises or activities in the HEP that the patient is comfortable doing and can do effectively without therapist supervision or caregiver assistance. Optimally, select activities that fit into the individual's daily schedule. The list of exercises/activities should not be exhaustive or so complicated that the patient becomes discouraged and does not follow through. Depending on the needs and the age of the patient, family members may be involved in assisting with activities to improve joint or segment neuromotor stability.

In addition to specific exercises, the patient needs to be aware of correct posture and positioning while at home to maintain proper alignment and enhance stability. Faulty posture can lead to asymmetry in muscle length or abnormal joint range, which can affect strength and neuromotor stability. Secondary impairments (e.g., decreased flexibility, increased joint ROM, weakness) that result from poor positioning can unnecessarily delay improvements in motor control.

## Aspects of Patient and Family Education

When adjuncts to therapy are provided for home use (e.g., splints, braces, pressure garments, and home FES or biofeedback units), it is critical to spend time during therapy reviewing and explaining their use and educating the patient on ways to reduce risks or potential harm involved in the activity. Emphasize safety, particularly regarding unstable joints! In the case of motor control-stability deficits of a particular joint, postural instability and falling from joint collapse are potential risks any time the unstable joint is placed in a weight-bearing posture or activity. Demonstration, visual and written materials, and patient practice are several ways to ensure that the adjunct is used correctly.

Before allowing a patient to take equipment home, make sure it can be used safely, including understanding the setup, use, precautions, and potential adverse effects. Therapists need to help patients not only improve their function but also prevent injury or secondary impairments by ensuring that they can manage every aspect of their HEP, including use of adjuncts, with the help of their family members or caregivers as appropriate.

For some patients, such as those with increased tone in an antagonistic muscle, the use of Botulinum toxin (Botox) or other tone-modifying medications may be beneficial and has implications for patient education. The roles of the therapist regarding tone-modifying medications are to (1) educate patients and caregivers, (2) refer patients to a primary care physician or specialist when medication or Botox may be beneficial, (3) recommend specific muscles to inject, (4) evaluate the effectiveness of the medication to improve function and (5) provide a follow-up report to the physician along with recommendations for the next Botox treatment or continuation of medication.

An understanding of Botox is necessary to fulfill these roles. If joint instability is compromised because one muscle group is contracting too strongly (e.g., because of spasticity), a Botox injection in the overactive muscle may help restore the balance of forces around the joint, allowing the opposing muscle to strengthen and aiding in muscle reeducation and increased stability. Botox works by inhibiting the neurotransmitter acetylcholine to decrease muscle contraction. The effects of a Botox injection last for about 3 to 4 months. Research regarding effectiveness is inconclusive (http://www.nlm.nih.gov/medlineplus/botox.html). In relation to stroke, there is strong evidence that treatment with Botox reduced lower-limb spasticity; however, there is conflicting evidence on whether functional outcomes improved (Foley, 2009).

## Activities for Home

For the patient with instability of a joint or body segment due to impaired neuromotor control, the home activity program should incorporate opportunities for progressive practice of body support and cocontraction at the target joint in a variety of positions. Early in the rehabilitation, before focusing on practicing these home activities, institute home exercises to improve neural activation and increase strength or force production (Chapter 22) as a foundation for motor control-stability. Create a home program that includes weight-bearing activities in multiple body positions, with weight-bearing through the target joint. Progressively increase the weight-bearing demand as the patient gradually gains control.

### PATIENT APPLICATION – SUMMARY AND OUTCOMES

During the 2 months he was seen, Richard demonstrated the following functional improvements:

- His 6-minute walk distance improved from 748 to 931 ft.
- His Dynamic Gait Index improved from 21/24 to 22/24.
- His Berg Balance Scale score improved from 51/56 to 53/56.
- At discharge, right locked knee extension during gait occurred in 3/10 steps (compared with 7/10 steps initially), and no collapsing into flexion was observed. Richard also reported that he felt more confident in weight-bearing through the right leg.
- During a 100-ft walk, Richard demonstrated one instance of foot drag (compared with five initially), although he still reports increased frequency of foot drag when he is fatigued.

The therapist hypothesized that Richard's difficulty with segmental control was strongly related to his overall low level of muscle activation and difficulty sustaining activity in multiple areas at once. The HEP (with an emphasis on sustained activities with an increasing number of repetitions for increased endurance) was a critical component and was emphasized to Richard throughout the PT sessions.

Richard continues to demonstrate inconsistency in his gait pattern. The use of adjuncts (especially taping of the right ankle, which he can leave on for several days at a time) did result in reported and demonstrated improvements in function. The patient's previous prefabricated AFO was reassessed, but it was very flexible and unable to maintain the desired ankle position during function. As plans were made to obtain an AFO that Richard can use for safer ambulation of longer distances, it was determined that his Veteran's Administration benefits (which he had not mentioned earlier in treatment) might cover the cost of an ES unit to assist dorsiflexion. Richard is very interested in *this option and has participated in trials of two units as part of an assessment of the benefits of various adjuncts for his functional gait limitation.*

*As the treatment series ends, summary reports (verbal and written) are provided to the U.S. Department of Veterans Affairs for follow-up, outlining the results of the assessment, the treatment Richard has received, and a summary of his functional*

*limitations and impairments (in the opinion of the treating therapist). The therapist recommends that Richard would benefit from an ES unit and provides the basis for the recommendation. A custom AFO with adequate control to assist Richard's dorsiflexion during gait is recommended as the second-best option if he is unable to obtain the ES unit. The therapist also requests that Richard be reminded to continue with his HEP.*

# HANDS-ON PRACTICE

Be sure to practice the following skills from this chapter. With further practice, you should be able to:

- Use PNF techniques (e.g., joint approximation, alternating isometrics, rhythmic stabilization, slow reversal, slow reversal hold) to promote motor control-stability at a joint or segment
- Apply the NDT approach with a patient who has hemiparesis in stance weight-bearing using a modified plantigrade position (Fig. 24-4AB)
- Instruct/guide/assist a patient in a lumbar stabilization program for postural exercise
- Apply tape to a shoulder to improve alignment (Fig. 24-8ABC), to a knee to prevent hyperextension (Fig. 24-9), and to an ankle to assist dorsiflexors and everters (Fig. 24-10)
- Instruct/guide/assist a patient in repositioning the pelvis in a more neutral position in sitting and standing

- Instruct/guide/assist a patient through controlled transitional movements with weight-bearing components including:
  - Half-bridging on the affected side
  - Rolling
  - Supine-to/from-sit
  - Sidelying-to/from-sit
  - Sit-to/from-stand
  - Quadruped, creeping
  - Kneeling
  - Floor-to-stand through half-kneeling
  - Stand-to/from-squat
  - Cruising in stance
  - Walking (forward and backward)
  - Stair ascent and descent

## Let's Review

1. What is motor control-stability?

2. What are common manifestations of instability at the shoulder, scapula, wrist/hand, lumbopelvic area, hip, knee, and ankle?

3. What nervous system structure lesions can impair motor-control stability and why?

4. Compare and contrast NDT, PNF, and motor learning approaches to improve motor control-stability.

5. Describe the mechanism of action of biofeedback and why it may be a useful adjunct to improve motor control-stability.

6. Among the following therapeutic adjuncts, explain why you would choose each to improve motor control-stability at a patient's ankle: biofeedback, ES, taping/strapping, splinting/bracing?

7. Describe common deficits in motor control-stability associated with Down syndrome and DDH.

8. What principles would you emphasize when designing a home program and providing patient/caregiver education to improve motor control-stability?

9. What evidence supports interventions that improve motor control-stability?

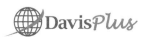 For additional resources, including Focus on Evidence tables, case study discussions, references and glossary, please visit http://davisplus.fadavis.com

## CHAPTER SUMMARY

The impairment of joint instability due to a lack of motor control is a problem that affects many individuals with neurological pathology. The inability of a group of muscles to cocontract/coactivate around a joint can lead to functional limitations of activity along with pain, dysfunction, and injury. Although instability may occur at only one segment, the impairment can affect one side of the body or the whole body, complicating the performance of daily activities.

Fortunately, therapists have numerous choices for intervention in their "tool bag," including therapeutic exercise, taping and strapping, biofeedback, ES, FES, pressure garments, and the practice of functional activities. Integration of these techniques and adjuncts with therapy approaches (e.g., NDT, PNF,

constraint-induced therapy, motor learning) forms the basis of intervention for joint or body segment instability. Because research supporting many of these interventions is limited, however, therapists are encouraged to add to the base of knowledge by completing studies that validate their current practice and to be diligent in using standardized functional outcome measures to support their treatment decisions.

Evidence regarding interventions for motor control-stability is summarized in Table 24-6 (Online). To facilitate critical thinking and decision-making, use the best evidence available, as well as clinical experience and patient values, when choosing appropriate interventions for each patient.

# Intervention for Impaired Motor Control—Movement

David M. Morris, PT, PhD, FAPTA ▪ Laura K. Vogtle, PhD, OTR/L, FAOTA
Blair P. Saale, PT, DPT, NCS ▪ Dennis W. Fell, PT, MD

CHAPTER **25**

## CHAPTER OBJECTIVES

Upon completion of this chapter, the learner should be able to:
1. Identify elements of skilled motor control-movement and body systems responsible for motor control-movement.
2. Describe selected impairments of motor control-movement including problems with timing, scaling, activation, and sequencing.
3. Describe common neuromuscular disorders associated with motor control-movement impairments.
4. Discuss the principles behind and evidence for selected therapeutic interventions for improving impaired motor control-movement.

## ▪ Introduction

***Martha Jones*** *is a 75 year-old African American female who experienced a cerebrovascular accident (CVA) 3 months ago. She reports that earlier on the day of the stroke she was dizzy and numb on her left side. These symptoms progressed until she was completely paralyzed on her left side. At that time, her husband called 911, and she was transported by ambulance to the emergency department at a local hospital. Magnetic resonance imaging confirmed that she had a thrombotic clot of the middle cerebral artery in the right cerebral hemisphere.*

The repertoire of everyday human movement ranges from simple reflex reactions to complex, preplanned, volitional actions. Movement characteristics, such as speed, variability, and the need for accuracy, vary as movement complexity increases. However, even simple tasks can be complicated because of the many motor and sensory parameters that must be controlled by the central nervous system (CNS). To optimize efficiency, functional movements are performed with a goal in mind. The success or failure of that movement goal is often determined by its context and the environment in which it is performed. For example, walking is a common lower extremity movement task. Walking is considered successful when one can get from one place to another in a reasonable time frame, with minimal energy costs and without tripping or falling. In most situations, the lower extremity movements involved with walking are rhythmical and do not require conscious effort to complete the task. However, walking in other situations, such as over an icy surface, may require a great deal of conscious effort.

To be optimally functional, humans are required to quickly and effectively generate movements in ways that are extremely flexible and adaptable. **Motor control**, as defined in Chapter 6, is the process by which the brain organizes and regulates actions of the muscular and skeletal systems, including movement and dynamic postural adjustments of a joint or body segment. Occupational therapists and physical therapists have been referred to as "applied motor control physiologists" because their professional duties are directed toward examination and intervention to restore functional movements (Brooks, 1986). Therefore, understanding how the CNS initiates and modifies functional movement is essential for their success.

Neuromuscular disorders can result in primary or secondary movement control impairments that negatively influence one's success with functional movement. Chapter 24 discusses therapeutic interventions to address impairment of motor control-stability. In this chapter, interventions that influence the movement aspects of motor control, a frequent focus of therapeutic rehabilitation, are examined. As described in Chapter 6, **motor control for movement** (**MC-movement**), also called **movement control**, includes all aspects of motor control related to muscles as they are creating movement (e.g., planning, initiating, sustaining, and efficiently and accurately controlling movement) with a goal of creating isolated or selective movement that appears smooth and regulated. More specifically, disorders of movement activation, sequencing, timing, and scaling are explored. To address these issues, we explore the prerequisites to skilled movement control, common disorders leading to impaired movement control, examination of abnormal movement control, selected interventions for improving movement control after a neuromuscular disorder, and evidence supporting the use of selected movement control impairment intervention strategies.

## Normal Motor Control-Movement

One must first understand the mechanisms underlying normal movement to understand the management of neuromuscular impairments. Skilled movement can be described as emerging from the interaction of three factors: the individual, the task, and the environment (Shumway-Cook, 2007). Considered from the *individual* perspective, movement emerges from cooperative efforts among the many brain structures and processes discussed later in this chapter. These brain processes can be further subdivided into sensory perception, cognition, and action. *Perception* involves deriving meaning from multiple sensory impressions related to movement. For example, the ability to accurately determine the body's position in space

is critical to motor control. *Cognitive* processes include aspects of attention, motivation, and emotion. The description of movement *action* is derived from the context of performing a particular task (e.g., walking up a hill or reaching overhead). Each specific action is characterized by the movement output from the CNS to the muscles in order to perform the task and is modified, as needed, by sensory and cognitive feedback. Most actions require precise coordination between numerous muscles and joints, leading to what Bernstein (1967) referred to as the process of mastering the redundant degrees of freedom of the moving organism.

Considering movement from the *task* perspective involves categorizing movement on the basis of its inherent characteristics. This can be done by characterizing the attributes of the task itself, by looking at the base of support and how it moves during a task, by classifying the role of the extremity movement during a task, and by defining the role of the environment during task performance. For example, tasks that are categorized as **discrete** have a distinct beginning and end (e.g., throwing a ball). Several discrete tasks performed together are **serial** tasks (e.g., performing a stand pivot transfer or putting on a shirt). Many activities of daily living (ADLs) are categorized as serial tasks. Alternatively, tasks can be **continuous**. Continuous tasks have no recognizable beginning or end. Tasks such as walking and running are continuous, with endpoints that are not inherent characteristics of the task but are arbitrarily determined by the performer.

Using a task perspective, movements can also be classified according to whether the performer's base of support is still, which is classified as a **stability** task, or is in motion, as in a **mobility** task. Stability tasks are inherently less complex than mobility tasks. Upper extremity movement increases the complexity of the task. These **manipulation** tasks are more complex because they require the performer to do two things at once: manipulate an object while stabilizing or moving the body. When two hands are manipulating different objects simultaneously, the intricacy of the task increases exponentially. The accuracy and speed required from one or both upper extremities directly influence the complexity of the manipulation task. When speed is increased, it is more difficult to be accurate with a task, a phenomenon known as Fitt's Law (Fitts, 1954).

Finally, tasks can be classified according to the interaction requirements imposed by the environment. **Open** movement tasks are performed in constantly changing environments and require performers to constantly monitor their movements and rapidly alter them as the environment demands. On the other hand, **closed** movement tasks are performed in relatively fixed environments and are characterized by patterns of movement that are fixed and vary minimally from trial to trial. Because they lack the fluidity and complexity of open movements, closed movement tasks are less complex, with lower information processing and attention demands.

The characteristics of open versus closed environments, stability versus mobility tasks, and manipulation tasks are incorporated into Gentile's (2000) comprehensive taxonomy of movement tasks described in Chapter 14. This taxonomy can be used to evaluate a patient's functional capabilities (i.e., to systematically identify task characteristics that are problematic for the patient) and to design intervention activities for task retraining (i.e., systematically increase the complexity of task characteristics).

Although we can speculate about the many factors influencing the execution of functional movement, the exact way the CNS responds to these task and environmental demands to produce functional movements are still not completely understood. Many motor control theories have been proposed to explain this phenomenon (Gordon, 2000; Horak, 1990; Shumway-Cook, 2007). Selected motor control theories are addressed elsewhere in this text. It is important to note that no single motor control theory is universally accepted, and each theory has shortcomings for fully explaining the complex phenomenon of movement control. Common to most contemporary views on the topic are two conceptual models for controlling voluntary movement: closed loop and open loop systems of motor control.

## THINK ABOUT IT 25.1

1. You are teaching a patient to walk with a quad cane in a busy rehabilitation gym. Other therapists and patients are walking all around you. What type of tasks are you asking this patient to accomplish (e.g., closed or open; simple or complex)?

2. How can you further characterize this task according to its attributes, stability requirements, and manipulation requirements?

The CNS can control movement through a **closed loop system** by using input from the sensory system as movement is executed. In these closed loop systems, input about the individual's movement goal is provided to an internal reference mechanism. The reference mechanism then compares how closely the actual and desired movements are matched within the context of the environment to determine movement error. Plans to reduce movement errors are made at the executive level. Finally, if needed, input is provided to movement effectors in an attempt to refine the movement as it takes place. Feedback available during the movement comes from various sensory receptors and is traditionally classified into three categories. Least important for movement is *interoceptor* feedback, which tells us about the state of our internal organs. More critical is sensory input received about the movement of objects in our environment from *exteroceptors* and information received about our own movements from the body's *proprioceptors.*

An example of a closed loop system is threading a needle. The dominant hand grips the thread while the nondominant hand holds the needle. One uses sensory feedback from vision and proprioception (from the hand and wrist) to guide successful movements. If the thread is passed to the right of the needle hole, one's vision perceives the change, and signals are sent to the movement effectors to correct the mistake by moving the thread to the left. The processes of error detection and correction occur simultaneously during the task.

The CNS also controls movement with an **open loop control system.** This open loop control of voluntary movement is needed with shorter duration movements that do not have sufficient time to receive and respond to peripheral feedback. This type of control is also needed when the body must prepare ahead of the voluntary movement (e.g., the leg muscles must contract to provide a preparatory postural response before a heavy object is lifted). Instead of being triggered by a response to feedback, open loop mechanisms rely on past experiences for which the CNS has learned the best way, or at least a reasonable way, to execute the movement. Also, open loop systems take advantage of a variety of preprogrammed movement control mechanisms that greatly influence movement without feedback. These range from local viscoelastic and reflexive muscle properties to more complex mechanisms, such as the central pattern generators (CPGs) discussed later in this chapter.

An example of an open loop mechanism is a tennis serve. The tennis player has an existing movement plan for executing a tennis serve that was developed through completing multiple repetitions of a tennis serve. The player uses vision to determine whether the serve was successful and remembers the force required from the muscles and the position of their joints. Instead of making an ongoing correction, the outcome and feeling of that movement are compared with those of past movements, and corrections are made for the next movement.

## Abnormal Motor Control-Movement

The term *impairment* is defined as a loss or abnormality of psychological, physiological, or anatomical structure or function. Like other impairments, movement control impairments can be classified as **signs** (i.e., objective findings that can be determined by the therapist's physical examination) or **symptoms** (i.e., subjective complaints coming from the patient that may not be observable by the therapist). Neuromuscular signs and symptoms can also be described as **positive,** or as an increase in abnormal behaviors that can typically be controlled or inhibited by the CNS and not normally observed (e.g., hyperactive reflexes, hypertonus). Conversely, these signs and symptoms can be **negative,** or characterized by a reduction or loss of normal activity (e.g., paresis, hypotonia, incoordination). Finally, neuromuscular signs and symptoms can be classified as primary or secondary impairments. **Primary impairments** are the direct result of an abnormality in the CNS. For example, a spinal cord injury leads to a primary impairment of limb paralysis and sensory deficits, among others. **Secondary impairments** do not result directly from a CNS lesion but from the primary impairment. For example, the primary impairment of paralysis results in loss of motion, which in turn can result in the development of secondary impairments such as soft tissue restrictions in muscles and joints. In this chapter, we address abnormal signs of movement control resulting from neuromuscular disorders that can be classified as either positive or negative, sometimes simultaneously.

We also examine both primary and secondary effects of CNS disorders.

## Activation and Sequencing Problems

Functional movement requires precise recruitment of the muscles needed for an action (i.e., agonist muscles) and relaxation of those muscles that are not needed or that may even interfere with the movement (i.e., antagonist muscles). When groups of muscles are functionally coupled to move together, they are referred to as moving in **synergy**. The timing and sequencing of these coupled movements determines whether the synergies are successful. **Abnormal synergies** (also called *mass patterns*) are commonly seen after a neuromuscular disorder. These abnormal synergistic movements often lack fractionation, or the ability to move intended muscles without recruiting unwanted activity from other muscles. They frequently have obvious positive neurological signs such as muscle hyperactivity. Abnormal synergies may also manifest with less apparent and negative signs, such as muscle weakness.

Abnormal synergy patterns are often described as stereotypical (i.e., characteristically repeated) and obligatory (i.e., movement outside the pattern is frequently impossible). Stereotypical abnormal synergies associated with stroke have been described (Brunnstrom, 1970; Duncan, 1987). For example, an upper extremity flexor synergy usually occurs in association with volitional upper extremity elevation, with antigravity movement, or with an intended flexion motion. The upper extremity flexion synergy is observed as a combination of scapular retraction and elevation, shoulder abduction and external rotation, elbow flexion, forearm supination, and wrist and finger flexion. The most common lower extremity abnormal synergy is an extensor synergy. It is most often observed during a lower extremity extension action, such as the swing phase of gait, and is characterized by hip extension, adduction, and internal rotation; knee extension; ankle plantar flexion and inversion; and plantar flexion of the toes.

Recently, some movement scientists have suggested that synergistic movement may not be a maladaptive, primary sign of neuromuscular impairment but rather an adaptive response to ensure better flexibility and stable performance with motor tasks (Latash, 2006). The motor control model titled the Uncontrolled Manifold Hypothesis (Scholz, 1999) suggests that some stereotypical movement patterns may be important to a successful functional outcome for persons with neuromuscular disorders.

**Coactivation** at inappropriate times during intended movement is a specific type of movement sequencing problem in which agonist and antagonist muscles fire simultaneously and prevent functional movement through the intended range of motion. Coactivation is cited as one of the four major movement impairments in children with cerebral palsy (CP) (Crenna, 1998). Although commonly seen after a neuromuscular disorder, coactivation is also characteristic of neurologically intact individuals during the early stages of learning a skilled movement task. Healthy infants and children use coactivation in the early stages of postural stability development. As such, it is unclear whether coactivation is a primary impairment resulting from neuromuscular dysfunction or a primitive, unrefined, and normal form of movement coordination.

Normal coordinated synergistic movement is characterized by synchronized firing of muscles in the synergy group to allow smooth excursion of the moving body part. When the synchrony of muscle contractions is disturbed (e.g., one or more muscles fire out of sequence), the resulting movement has **impaired interjoint coordination** requiring intervention (see Chapter 23). Studies report a variety of interjoint coordination impairments associated with CNS pathology. For example, patients with cerebellar pathology have been observed with **decomposition** of large movements, or breaking them down into sequential movements at a single joint, to compensate for an impaired ability to coordinate multijoint movement synergies (Bastian, 1996). Persons with hemiparesis after a stroke have demonstrated disturbed sequencing of arm movement trajectories characterized by movement at one joint followed by delayed movement at a related joint, rather than a more normal interjoint coordinated manner of reaching (Levin, 1996).

## Timing Problems

To achieve a functional outcome, movement must be timed appropriately with regard to its initiation (reaction time), execution (movement time), and termination (termination time). **Reaction time** begins when an individual decides to move, and it ends when the intended movement is actually initiated. A variety of factors can hinder reaction time: (1) generating inadequate muscle force; (2) generating muscle force too slowly; (3) lacking motivation to move; and (4) lacking the ability to stabilize proximal portions of the body before moving more distal body parts. Cognitive factors, including difficulty recalling a movement plan, can also interfere with reaction time.

**Movement time** is the time between initiation and completion of a task. Movement time is particularly important with open tasks, for which task completion requires successful interaction with moving objects in the environment. Impaired movement time has been reported with a variety of neuromuscular disorders including stroke, Parkinson disease (PD), CP, and cerebellar dysfunction.

Impaired **termination**, or the stopping of movement, leads to difficulty with stopping and/or changing the direction of a movement. Difficulty with terminating movement can result from the inability to control forces in the agonist muscle at the end of a movement. Termination impairment can also result from inadequate timing and/or force generation in the antagonistic muscle, leading to the inability to stop the movement. Termination problems are common with cerebellar disorders and can manifest as an inability to perform rapidly alternating movements and/or as an involuntary rebound, as seen when resistance is given to an extremity muscle that is contracting isometrically.

## Scaling Problems

Movement *scaling problems* result in misjudging (over- or underestimating) the force required to move a body part through its intended range of motion. **Dysmetria** is defined as the inability to scale movement forces appropriately to task requirements. Two types of dysmetria are commonly observed: *hypometria* and *hypermetria*. Hypometria is a negative sign characterized by undershooting or underestimating the required force and falling short of a target. Hypermetria is a positive sign characterized by overshooting or overestimating the force required and moving past the target. Persons with cerebellar disorders commonly exhibit hypermetria, whereas persons with PD often exhibit hypometria.

Scheets (2007) proposed movement system diagnoses for persons with neuromuscular disorders largely on the basis of systematic observations over many years. Of the nine diagnostic categories described, four are most relevant to the movement control impairments discussed in this chapter: movement pattern coordination deficit, fractionated movement deficit, hypermetria, and hypokinesia.

## PATIENT APPLICATION

*Here is some more information on Mrs. Jones, who was introduced at the beginning of the chapter.*

*After her stroke, Mrs. Jones was admitted to the acute care hospital for 8 days, was transferred to the rehabilitation center for 2 weeks, and then was discharged home with her husband, where she has been receiving home health services. She can walk with minimal assistance for short distances (i.e., 25 ft at a time) using a wide-based quad cane and an ankle-foot orthotic (AFO). Otherwise, she uses a hemi-wheelchair around the house.*

*When asked to describe her movement problems, Mrs. Jones states that she "cannot control her arm and leg." For example, when she tries to lift her arm at her shoulder to reach for something, her elbow bends instead of extending and her hand makes a fist instead of extending her fingers. She reports similar problems with walking; when she tries to step forward, she says, her knee tightens and her ankle points down and turns inward.*

### Contemplate Clinical Decisions

*Consider these questions related to Mrs. Jones.*

1. *How would you describe the movement impairments reported by Mrs. Jones (using terminology presented earlier in this chapter)?*

2. *Considering the movement impairments described previously, what positive and negative signs and symptoms would you expect to be present?*

3. *What activity limitations do you think might be negatively affected by these movement impairments?*

## ■ Anatomy and Physiology

Ghez (1985) described movement control as coming from four system levels within the CNS, arranged hierarchically from the most basic to the most complex (see Fig. 25-1). The first level is the spinal cord, which controls simple, reflexive, and often automatic movement mechanisms. The second level is the brainstem and includes the related basal ganglia and

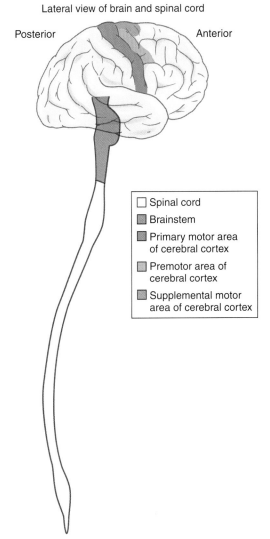

Lateral view of brain and spinal cord

Posterior    Anterior

- ☐ Spinal cord
- ■ Brainstem
- ■ Primary motor area of cerebral cortex
- ☐ Premotor area of cerebral cortex
- ■ Supplemental motor area of cerebral cortex

**FIGURE 25-1** Four hierarchical system levels of movement control in the central nervous system are the spinal cord, brainstem, primary motor cortex, and premotor/supplementary cortex of the cerebrum.

cerebellum. This second level serves as an important relay center and interacts with both ascending sensory input and descending motor output. The third level is the primary motor area of the cerebral cortex, where motor commands originate. The fourth and most complex level comprises the premotor and supplemental motor areas of the cerebral cortex, which are responsible for analyzing the movement environment and selecting an appropriate course of motor actions to achieve a functional end. The following section examines each level in greater detail.

The first level of movement control, the spinal cord, deals with the relatively simple relationships between sensory input and motor output for localized areas of the body. The spinal cord is involved with the initial reception of sensory input, which contributes to posture and movement. The motor neurons of the spinal cord are also referred to as the final common pathway because it is here that the last processing takes place before muscle activation occurs. Sensory input contributing to posture and movement enters the spinal cord through the dorsal horn and can connect directly to alpha motor neurons in the ventral horn to make up the monosynaptic reflex (see Fig. 25-2). This afferent input can also send impulses to other ventral horn motor neurons and travel up or down several segments in the spinal column, exerting an influence on other levels of the spinal cord. The columns are functionally arranged, with the medial portion exerting control over the trunk muscles and the lateral portion controlling limb movements. The ventral aspect of the column controls muscles that extend joints, and the dorsal aspect of the columns controls muscles that flex joints.

Interneurons between the dorsal and ventral horns travel up and down in the white matter of the spinal cord, exerting an influence over motor program execution. Interneurons located in the spinal cord have demonstrated the ability to execute simple flexion and extension movements without input from higher centers in the CNS. These CPGs are activated during automatic movements that do not require conscious effort, such as walking, swimming, and chewing food. Descending commands from higher levels of the CNS exert control over more complex movements requiring conscious effort.

When midlevels of movement control are discussed, it is important to address the brainstem and three related infracortical structures: the cerebellum (Fig. 25-3A), the basal ganglia, and the thalamus (see Fig. 25-3B). These structures have both direct and indirect connections with higher levels of motor control. The basal ganglia do not directly connect with the lower centers (spinal cord). Instead, they connect with the cerebral cortex by way of the thalamus. The basal ganglia are a collection of five CNS nuclei: substantia nigra, caudate nucleus, putamen, and globus pallidus internus and externus. The caudate nucleus and putamen are also referred to as the striatum. Regulation of movement from the striatum occurs through a series of complex loops between the basal ganglia, thalamus, and cerebral cortex.

There are several theories regarding basal ganglia neurophysiology; however, the exact role of the basal ganglia over movement is not completely understood. Some studies suggest the basal ganglia are more active during complex movements requiring greater cognitive processing and therefore are important for motor learning (Mushiake, 1993).

The cerebellum plays a crucial role in adjusting the output of the major descending motor systems of the brain. Although

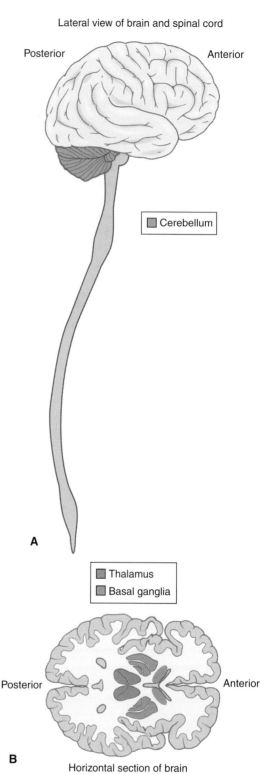

Lateral view of brain and spinal cord

Posterior     Anterior

☐ Cerebellum

A

☐ Thalamus
☐ Basal ganglia

Posterior     Anterior

**B**
Horizontal section of brain

**FIGURE 25-3** Three main subcortical motor structures that interact with and support the cerebral motor cortex. (A) The cerebellum shown in a lateral view of cerebrum and spinal cord. (B) The basal ganglia (i.e., the caudate, putamen, and globus pallidus) and the thalamus are shown in a horizontal brain section.

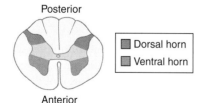

Posterior

☐ Dorsal horn
☐ Ventral horn

Anterior
Horizontal section of spinal cord

**FIGURE 25-2** Afferent and efferent components of the spinal cord that comprise the monosynaptic reflex loop supporting voluntary movement.

important to motor learning, the cerebellum is more important for ongoing monitoring of movement during execution and fine-tuning of the motor program. According to its surface appearance, the cerebellum has three lobes: the flocculonodular, anterior, and posterior lobes. Functionally, however, the cerebellum is better described along the medial-to-lateral dimension. Along this dimension, the cerebellum has three major functional parts: the vermis, intermediate hemisphere, and lateral hemisphere. The vermis and intermediate hemisphere make up the spinocerebellum. Primarily responsible for monitoring motor programs, the spinocerebellum sends output signals to the red nuclei of the midbrain and motor cortex. The lateral hemisphere is also called the cerebrocerebellum. This region is believed to be responsible for motor program planning, timing, and initiation. The cerebrocerebellum also sends output signals to the red nucleus and cerebral cortex. Contreras-Vidal (1997) suggested that the cerebellum modulates movement velocity and force through antagonist muscle activation and is critical in providing feedback during relatively slow movements. As limb movement speeds increase, however, the cerebellum has limited ability to provide feedback control, and feed-forward mechanisms become more important.

The thalamus is a major processing center in the brain. It receives sensory information from ascending tracts of the spinal cord as well as from other parts of the brain, including the basal ganglia and cerebellum. Different nuclei within the thalamus are dedicated to specific types of input and in turn relay information to specific areas in the cerebral cortex. A lesion in the thalamus can result in severe sensory and motor impairments.

The next level of movement control is the primary motor area of the cerebral cortex (see Fig. 25-1). Located in the frontal lobe, this area interacts with sensory processing areas in the parietal lobe as well as the basal ganglia and cerebellum to identify movements we wish to make, establish a plan to accomplish those movements, and then execute the movement plan. The primary motor area is believed to be associated more with voluntary, skilled movements and less with automatic, reflexive movements. Specific areas of the primary motor cortex are dedicated to activities involving specific body parts and are often illustrated in neurology texts in pictures of the motor homunculus. Body parts used more often and/or that require the most detailed control (e.g., the mouth and hand) are generally most highly represented in this motor map.

The primary motor cortex sends impulses down projections to the corticospinal tract and makes excitatory monosynaptic and polysynaptic connections with alpha motor neurons and gamma motor neurons, respectively, throughout the spinal cord. The corticospinal tract fibers descend ipsilaterally from the cerebral cortex through the internal capsule, midbrain, and medulla. Near the junction of the medulla and spinal cord, 90% of the fibers cross and form the lateral corticospinal tract of the spinal cord. The remaining 10% continue uncrossed as the anterior corticospinal tract.

The highest CNS movement control level includes the premotor and supplementary motor areas of the cerebral cortex (see Fig. 25-1). These areas are believed to be involved with the preparatory phase of self-paced, internally generated, complex movements. Both the premotor and supplementary motor areas project to the primary motor area. However, the two areas receive distinct input from different parts of the thalamus and other cortical areas and are believed to have different functions. Musiake (1991) reported that both areas were involved in the performance of a sequential task. However, neurons in the premotor area were more active during sequential tasks that were visually guided. The supplementary motor area was more active when the sequence was remembered and self-initiated.

**Neural plasticity** is the nervous system's ability to alter its structure in response to environmental diversity and purposeful repetition/activity (Kolb, 2008) and is the primary mechanism of recovery after CNS injury. Although the term is used commonly in neurorehabilitation, it is difficult to define and is used to describe a wide range of change processes at many levels of the nervous system, from molecular to behavioral. Most all experiences have the potential to alter the brain, and plastic changes can either be positive (enhancing functional ability) or negative (reducing functional ability).

In persons with neuromuscular disorders, the primary brain injury or initial event that led to nervous system injury (e.g., stroke, traumatic brain injury [TBI]) can typically be identified. However, the extent of the total brain injury is not the result of that single event. Instead, the initial event is followed by a cascade of cellular events that extend the brain injury. This secondary brain injury sometimes extends into areas of the nervous system that are remote to the area of initial injury. A variety of physiological mechanisms account for spreading the injury, including neuron degeneration, diaschisis, edema, and denervation sensitivity (Shumway-Cook, 2006). Further, when patients with neuromuscular disorders cease to use a body part, nervous tissue previously dedicated to participating in its use can be recruited (or reorganized) to participate in the function of another body part, making recovery of function even more difficult (Nudo, 2007).

Although factors outside the CNS (muscle fiber type, tissue flexibility) can influence movement control impairments, there appears to be a direct relationship between negative neural plastic changes and the degree of movement control impairment observed (Kolb, 2008; Nudo, 2005). Therefore, interventions directed at improving movement control impairments must incorporate strategies to inhibit negative neural plasticity and promote positive neural plasticity. Generally, the CNS has three ways to compensate for negative neural plastic changes: (1) reorganization of the remaining neuronal networks, (2) development of novel networks, and (3) regeneration of the lost tissue.

It is believed that most recovery processes take place in the acute phase of recovery. However, recovery is possible even many years after an injury. The exact processes behind neural plasticity are not completely understood. Still, most neuroscientists agree on several guiding principles for promoting neural plasticity. First, neural plasticity is behavior specific. When improved hand function is desired, training should emphasize hand use. Second, permanent neural plastic changes require extensive and concentrated practice of training tasks. Third, training tasks used to promote neural plasticity must cognitively engage the patient; rote actions requiring no cognitive input do not likely promote plastic changes. Fourth, training tasks should be interesting specifically to the patient to increase motivation and ensure continued practice attempts and enhanced cognitive drive. Finally, the complexity of training tasks should be systematically and incrementally increased as the participant's skills improve.

Although each of the interventions addressed in the following sections approaches neural plasticity differently, they all work to promote it in one way or another. Kleim (2008) conducted an extensive review of animal studies of neural plasticity and summarized strategies to promote such processes. From this review, they identified 10 principles of training for promoting activity-dependent neural plasticity (summarized in Table 14-2).

## THINK ABOUT IT 25.2

1. How can a physical therapist utilize the principles to enhance neuroplasticity when designing an intervention for movement control in a patient with a neurological diagnosis?
2. What key components should be included (see Chapter 14)?

## ■ Related Pathology

A variety of neural disorders result in problems with movement aspects of motor control. More details on each of these medical diagnoses can be found in the compendium of medical diagnoses at the end of the book.

### Stroke

A stroke is a sudden, devastating vascular event that results in destruction of surrounding brain tissues. When the stroke occurs in one of the cerebral hemispheres, subsequent movement deficits are most prominent on the contralateral side of the body. However, less severe movement deficits are also present in the ipsilateral extremities. Ipsilateral movement deficits occur because the hemispheres are connected and do not work in isolation.

Movement-related impairments associated with stroke include abnormal muscle tone, abnormal reflexes, muscle weakness, decreased endurance, and abnormal postural adjustments. Movement control impairments associated with stroke that are most relevant to this chapter include abnormal movement synergies, incorrect timing of components within a movement pattern, and poor interjoint coordination. Problems with incorrect timing of movements common in stroke include increased reaction time, movement time, and time needed to stop a movement. Stroke occurring in the cerebellum and basal ganglia commonly results in scaling problems.

## Traumatic Brain Injury

TBI is caused by external forces acting on and damaging brain tissue. The movement control impairments resulting from TBI vary by location and the extent of the injury. Disorders of muscle activation, sequencing, and timing have been documented as a result of TBI. Ataxia is another common movement control deficit resulting from TBI. Motor ataxia can result from a focal injury to the cerebellum as well as from a diffuse axonal injury involving the cerebellum.

## Parkinson Disease

PD is a chronic, progressive nervous system disorder affecting primarily the basal ganglia and characterized by rigidity, bradykinesia, tremor, and balance dysfunction. The rigidity seen with PD is characterized by increased resistance to passive muscle stretch that is uniform (not velocity dependent), often leading to the development of contractures and postural deformities. The tremor associated with PD is an involuntary rhythmic movement seen at rest, is most noticeable in the hands and wrists, and is pronounced immediately after movement.

Functionally, PD can lead to significant gait and balance deficits. Persons with PD often exhibit a festinating gait pattern characterized by short, shuffling steps and reduced arm swing. This gait instability can be anteropulsive (in a forward direction) or retropulsive (in a backward direction). Freezing of gait (FOG) is also commonly seen with PD and is defined as a transient halt in motor activity while attempting to walk. (Nutt, 2011) identified five types of FOG: (1) start hesitation, (2) turn hesitation, (3) hesitation in tight quarters, (4) destination-hesitation, when a person freezes as he approaches a target, and (5) open space hesitation. Clinically, two distinct categories of PD have been identified: one with dominant symptoms of postural instability and gait disturbances and the other dominated by tremor. Typically, persons with tremor-dominant PD exhibit few problems with gait and postural instability.

Many different motor control problems occur in PD. First, PD disturbs movement timing. Initiation of movement and termination of movement are delayed in PD. Second, hypometric movements associated with PD occur because of decreased force generation. The patient with PD is often unaware that his movements are hypometric; therefore, the therapist must first draw attention clinically to the decreased amplitude of movements before correcting them.

## Cerebral Palsy

CP is defined as a group of permanent disorders in the development of movement and posture that cause activity limitation and are attributed to nonprogressive disturbances that occurred in the developing fetal or infant brain. Movement disorders in CP are complex and include lack of anticipatory and postural control; delayed muscle and balance response to environmental shifts; muscle weakness; problems with modulation of sensory inputs to match changes in task and environmental demands; inability to match sensory information with experience, memory and specific tasks; difficulty with graded control resulting from balanced interactions between muscle agonists and antagonists; and temporal control of movement events (Duff, 2003; Eliasson, 1995, 2000; Gordon, 1999a, 1999b, 2003; Lesny, 1993; Yekutiel, 1994). These impairments are distributed over various body areas (hemiplegia, diplegia, quadriplegia) and can be mild, moderate, or severe. It should be noted that almost all existing movement studies in CP have been carried out in children, not adults.

## Multiple Sclerosis

MS is a chronic multifocal neurological disease characterized by demyelination of the CNS white matter and is best known for exacerbations and remissions of symptoms found in **relapsing-remitting MS**. Initial symptoms of MS vary considerably; the same symptoms may be present in a range of neurological diseases, which can make accurate diagnosis difficult (Polman, 2005). Motor impairments include spasticity, muscle weakness, balance impairments, inefficient movement, tremors, and motor control deficits including incoordination, loss of selective control, and inaccurate targeting.

## ■ Pertinent Examination/Evaluation of Movement Control Impairment

Examination is a comprehensive screening and specific testing process occurring early in the patient/client and therapist encounter; clinical decision-making includes diagnostic classification and/or referral to another practitioner when appropriate (APTA, 2017). The selection of specific examination procedures and the depth of exploration depend on a variety of patient/client factors, including the severity of the problem, stage of recovery, phase of rehabilitation, and psychosocial factors. The examination consists of three components: the patient/client history, systems review, and use of tests and measures. In the following sections, each component is addressed as it relates to the examination of movement control impairment.

## History

The history is systematically obtained in a variety of ways including reading the patient/client chart or record, interviewing the patient and/or family/caregivers, and consulting with another practitioner (APTA, 2017). This history should address both past and current data related to the request for patient/client rehabilitation services. Data typically explored are listed in Box 25-1. Although all of these data are important, certain categories may be more relevant for persons with movement control impairments. For example, exploration of the chief complaint is particularly relevant. This should include the motor control impairments the patient perceives as particularly problematic and the functional deficits resulting from them. In addition, it is helpful to ascertain which therapeutic interventions have been attempted and their level of success. Current medications can provide significant insights

---

**BOX 25-1  Types of Data Generated From a Patient/Client History**

- General demographics
- Social history
- Employment/work (job/school/play)
- Growth and development
- Living environment
- General health status (self-report, family report, caregiver report)
- Social/health habits (past and current)
- Family history
- Medical/surgical history
- Current conditions(s)/chief complaint(s)
- Functional status and activity level
- Medications
- Other clinical tests

---

into side effects/adverse drug reactions that may be improving or worsening movement control impairment. Functional status, activity level, living environment, and employment/work issues should be thoroughly explored because these are most likely profoundly influenced by the motor control impairment.

## Systems Review

The systems review is a brief or limited exploration of the patient's/client's anatomical and physiological status in all body systems (cardiovascular/pulmonary, integumentary, musculoskeletal, and neuromuscular), regardless of whether they are directly related to the primary medical diagnosis (in this case, the neuromuscular system). All of these systems warrant review because many patients with neuromuscular dysfunction and resulting motor control impairment are also physically inactive, which can lead to musculoskeletal adaptations, cardiovascular/pulmonary deconditioning, and/or poor circulation. Also, motor control impairment is often accompanied by sensory alterations that require thorough screening of the integumentary system. Comorbid conditions commonly associated with neuromuscular dysfunction (e.g., hypertension, diabetes, cardiac dysfunction) can also negatively influence all body systems.

## Tests and Measures

Data gathered from the history and systems review assist the rehabilitation therapist in determining the patient's/client's needs and generating diagnostic hypotheses. The therapist must then select and utilize appropriate tests and measures to systematically gather data to support, refute, or elaborate upon these hypotheses. The therapist should select only those tests and measures that (1) confirm or reject a hypothesis about the factors contributing to a less-than-optimal level of patient/client function; (2) support the therapist's clinical judgments about appropriate interventions, anticipated goals, and expected outcomes; (3) are appropriate for the setting on the basis of time and equipment restraints; and (4) are appropriate for the patient's current level of function and/or cognition.

Twenty-four categories of tests and measures are commonly used in physical rehabilitation (see Box 25-2). The tests and

measures in the Motor Function category (i.e., motor control and motor learning) are most relevant to the examination of movement control impairments. Per the Guide to Physical Therapist Practice (2017), these tests measure the patient's ability to skillfully and efficiently assume, maintain, modify, and control voluntary postures and movement patterns. Selected tests and measures that reflect motor control-movement are included in Table 25-1. However, movement control impairment also profoundly influences other categories of function and tests and measures. For example, tests of self-care and home management should be considered in almost all cases. Self-care management is the ability to perform ADLs, and home management is the ability to perform the more complex instrumental ADLs.

## BOX 25-2 Guide Categories for Tests and Measures

Aerobic capacity/endurance
Anthropometric characteristics
Arousal, attention, and cognition
Assistive and adaptive devices
Circulation (arterial, venous, lymphatic)
Cranial and peripheral nerve integrity
Environmental, home, and work (job/school/play) barriers
Ergonomics and body mechanics
Gait, locomotion, and balance
Integumentary integrity
Joint integrity and mobility
Motor function (motor control and motor learning)
Muscle performance (including strength, power, and endurance)
Neuromotor development and sensory integration
Orthotic, protective, and supportive devices
Pain
Posture
Prosthetic requirements
Range of motion (including muscle length)
Reflex integrity
Self-care and home management (including activities of daily living and instrumental activities of daily living)
Sensory integrity
Ventilation and respiration/gas exchange
Work (job/school/play), community, and leisure integration or reintegration (including instrumental activities of daily living)

## PATIENT APPLICATION

*Consider the following examination data when answering questions about Mrs. Jones (introduced earlier in this chapter):*

*Mrs. Jones lives with her husband, who is also retired, in a split-level home with three bedrooms and two bathrooms. Mrs. Jones and her husband share the master bedroom on the top level. The house has five steps to the front door. Mrs. Jones has been confined to the lower level of the home because the stairs to the top level are very difficult for her to manage. She reports that she has essentially lost use of her left arm. The couple has two married daughters who live within 30 minutes of their home.*

*Mrs. Jones is a retired elementary school teacher and is active in her church and community (she was neighborhood president). Her hobbies include gardening and singing in the church choir.*

*Mrs. Jones has a history of hypertension and hyperlipidemia and smoked one to two packs of cigarettes each day until she quit at the age of 60 years. During the initial examination, Mr. Jones expresses concern about the fact that his wife has been "down" and says he hears her crying on occasion.*

| TABLE 25-1 | Selected Tests of Movement Control Issues Associated With Neuromuscular Dysfunction | |
|---|---|---|
| **NAME OF TEST** | **DESCRIPTION** | **CLINIMETRIC PROPERTIES** |
| Wolf Motor Function Test (WMFT) | The test consists of 17 items, two of which involve strength measures and 15 of which involve timed performances on various functional tasks. The first half of the test involves simple limb movements, primarily of the proximal musculature; the second half of the test involves tasks performed in a life situation using the distal musculature. Performance time (up to 120 seconds), strength (for lifting and handgrip), and quality of motor function (6-point scale of functional ability) are assessed. | Shown to have test-retest reliability, intrarater reliability, and construct validity (Ang, 2006; Morris, 2001; Wolf, 2001, 2005; Whitall, 2006) |
| Action Research Arm Test (ARAT) | The test consists of 19 items divided into four categories (grasp, grip, pinch, and gross movement), with each item graded on a 4-point ordinal scale (0 = can perform no | Shown to have test-retest reliability, intrarater reliability and validity (Lyle, 1981; Van de Lee, 2001) |

| TABLE 25-1 | Selected Tests of Movement Control Issues Associated With Neuromuscular Dysfunction—cont'd | |
|---|---|---|
| **NAME OF TEST** | **DESCRIPTION** | **CLINIMETRIC PROPERTIES** |
| | part of the test, 1 = performs test partially, 2 = completes test but takes abnormally long time or has great difficulty, and 3 = performs test normally. The test is hierarchically arranged from least to most difficult tasks so that it can be stopped when a task cannot be performed. | |
| Jebsen-Taylor Test of Hand Function | The test consists of seven timed subtests: writing, card turning, picking up small items, simulated feeding, stacking checkers, picking up light cans, and picking up heavy cans. It requires that both hands be tested (nondominant hand tested first) and takes 10–15 minutes to administer. | Shown to have high test-retest reliability except for writing task (Stern, 1992), construct validity (Lynch, 1989); norms established for adults (Jebsen, 1969) and children (Taylor, 1973) |
| Nine-Hole Peg Test | Test is a therapist-scored, patient-completed measure of manual dexterity. Patient places nine pegs in nine holes in a square board as quickly as possible. The result can be measured as the number of seconds to place all pegs, the number of pegs placed in 50 seconds, or the number of seconds to place each peg. | Shown to have test-retest reliability and construct validity (Heller, 1987; Mathiowetz, 1985); adult norms are available (Mathiowetz, 1985) |
| Rivermead Motor Assessment (RMA) | The test consists of three sections: gross function (13 items), leg and trunk (10 items), and arm (15 items). A score of 1 is given when the participant can perform the item, and a score of 0 is given when she cannot. Participants are given three attempts at each item, and the best attempt is scored. The items are hierarchically arranged, and the test is stopped when a 0 is assigned to three consecutive items. | Shown to have test-retest reliability, intrarater reliability (Lincoln, 1979), criterion validity (Endres, 1990), and construct validity (Collin, 1990) |
| Berg Balance Scale (BBS) | This 14-item scale was designed to measure balance in the older adult in a clinical setting. Scoring is achieved with a 5-point ordinal scale, ranging from 0–4; 0 indicates the lowest level of function and 4 the highest level of function. The test takes 5–20 minutes to administer, and scores are interpreted as 41–56 = low fall risk; 21–40 = medium fall risk; and 0–20 = high fall risk. | Shown to have intrarater reliability (Berg, 1995) and construct validity (Berg, 1992; Tyson, 2004) |
| Six-Minute Walk Test (6MWT) | | Shown to have test-retest reliability, criterion validity, and construct validity (Eng, 2004; Flansbjer, 2005; Fulk, 2008) |
| Motor Activity Log (MAL) | The MAL is a semistructured interview during which respondents are asked to rate how much and how well they use their more affected arm for 30 activities of daily living (ADLs) in the home over a specified period. The MAL is administered independently to the patient and an informant. The tasks include brushing the teeth, buttoning a shirt or blouse, and eating with a fork or spoon. For each item, the participant must report how often and how well (on 6-point scales) each activity was performed during a specified period. Primarily useful for hemiplegia. | Shown to have test-retest reliability and construct validity (Uswatte, 2006) |
| Stroke Impact Scale (SIS) | The SIS is a stroke-specific, self-report, health status measure. It was designed to assess multidimensional stroke outcomes, including strength, hand function, ADLs/instrumental ADLs, mobility, communication, emotion, memory and thinking, and participation. The SIS can be used in both clinical and research settings. | Shown to have test-retest reliability and concurrent and construct validity (Duncan, 1999, 2001, 2003) |

# Preparatory Interventions for Motor Control-Movement Impairment

Several different techniques can be used as preparatory activities in the treatment of motor control impairments (i.e., in preparation for functional interventions). These techniques help the patient experience success in improving motor control, with the ultimate goal of enhancing motor control during functional activities. Task characteristics such as complexity, environment, and timing can be manipulated to grade an exercise appropriately for the patient and progress it as they improve. Tasks that require use of a single joint are easier to control initially than tasks requiring control of multiple joints. Midrange tasks may also be easier to control initially than large-excursion or full-range tasks. As the patient improves, stability, timing, and directional changes can add task complexity. During task performance, the goal is controlled movement with appropriate speed, timing, and direction. These same challenges can be applied to the completion of functional tasks (as discussed in the next section). Other options for preparatory interventions to address motor control impairments include, but are not limited to, the use of proprioceptive neuromuscular facilitation (PNF), neurodevelopmental technique (NDT), constraint-induced movement therapy (CI therapy), neuromuscular electrical stimulation (NMES), motor relearning techniques, and technology.

## Proprioceptive Neuromuscular Facilitation

PNF, described in Chapter 15, is one approach to improving motor control. "Slow reversal" is a technique that provides opportunities for the patient to practice alternating concentric control between antagonistic muscle groups against resistance, including during functional tasks. The "combination of isotonics" technique, which employs alternating concentric and eccentric contractions of the target muscle group, can be useful for working on motor control impairments. Eccentric contractions can be particularly useful for practicing motor control because of the novel experience of controlling movement. "Repeated isotonic" contractions may be helpful for improving initiation of movement in a target muscle in conditions such as stroke and PD. Timing, direction, range, and speed can also be manipulated during PNF to focus on underlying motor control deficits. Please refer to Chapter 15 for additional details on this technique.

## Neurodevelopmental Treatment (Bobath) Intervention

In the United States and United Kingdom, one of the most common clinical approaches to therapeutic management of neurological conditions, particularly stroke, CP, and other acquired brain injuries, is **NDT**, also known as the **Bobath approach** (Lennon, 2001; Natarajan, 2008), described in Chapter 15. The Bobath approach was based on a hierarchical concept of the CNS and proximal-to-distal developmental motor theory. They originally hypothesized that primitive reflexes limited the evolution of the motor system to more advanced postural responses and control, and the initial intervention strategies were aimed at limiting these reflexes using "reflex inhibiting" postures. Managing spasticity was another element of early Bobath therapy, in which the client was basically a passive participant in periods of tone intervention aimed at "normalizing" muscle tone.

The theoretical premises underlying NDT have changed considerably since its inception, partly because of changes by the Bobaths and others, as well as evolving understanding of the CNS, neural plasticity, and motor learning (Bly, 1994; Bobath, 1984; Howle, 1999). More recently the NDT approach is described as a problem solving approach to the assessment and treatment of individuals with disturbances of function, movement, and tone due to a lesion in the central nervous system (Raine, 2006). As the focus in rehabilitation moved away from impairment-based interventions and toward functional outcomes, the Bobaths acknowledged the importance of goal-oriented treatment (Bobath, 1984). Treatment became an active interaction between the client and clinician, with tone management rather than alteration as a treatment concern; achievement of dynamic postural and limb control for carrying out specific motor outcomes was the aim of therapy. Using the Delphi technique and experts in the Bobath approach, Raine (2007) determined that the aim of treatment is to optimize postural and movement strategies to improve efficiency. Practice of functional activity goals within Bobath interventions is important to the success of treatment as well.

Although the goals of the Bobath approach are clear, the processes therapists undertake to achieve them are not uniform or standardized. Paci (2003) noted that the lack of a clear definition and standardized approach to NDT intervention is a significant methodological concern for research on the approach. Although efforts to update the approach with current understanding of the CNS, motor learning and motor control approaches, and new concepts of intervention are laudable, efficacy studies of the approach remain complicated because of lack of standardization. Four recent systematic reviews have focused on or included studies of Bobath interventions and outcomes (Anttila, 2008; Kollen, 2009; Luke, 2004; Paci, 2003). The overall conclusion from these reviews is that although the Bobath approach did not produce better outcomes, methodological flaws of the studies limit the ability to make sound conclusions. The studies overall failed to indicate whether therapists were in fact trained to use the approach or to describe the intervention procedures in enough detail to determine what was provided to participants. Instrumentation and outcome measures varied significantly across trials, as did body areas and aspects of function addressed (upper limb, lower limb, gait, ADLs). Two randomized controlled trials (RCTs) are summarized in the next paragraphs to demonstrate these difficulties.

Platz (2005) carried out a multicenter RCT comparing Bobath therapy with Arm BASIS training. The two interventions were added to standard rehabilitation interventions. Three rehabilitation centers in Germany recruited a sample of 62 participants who had experienced a stroke within the preceding 3 weeks to 6 months and had severe arm impairments. The participants were randomly assigned to one of three groups: no augmented rehabilitation, Bobath-augmented rehabilitation, and Arm BASIS–augmented rehabilitation. Twenty augmented sessions were delivered over a 4-week period for 45 minutes per session. Therapeutic interventions were described in advance. A Bobath manual, which was developed before the study by a senior Bobath-trained therapist, emphasized control of muscle tone and active arm recruitment in functional motor activities carried out in various positions. The Arm BASIS protocol was designed to train active movement in the upper limb in three stages: isolated movement without postural control, isolated movement with postural control, and selective complex motions with postural control. The Fugl-Meyer assessment was used as the primary outcome measure, with the Action Research Arm Test (ARAT) as a secondary outcome measure.

Results demonstrated that although augmented therapy did not result in significant change, a statistically significant difference in favor of Arm BASIS training ($F$[1, 55] = 4.28; $p$ = .043) was found on the Fugl-Meyer arm motor scores but not on the ARAT. No change in function or sensory scores was observed. Cointerventions in this study (standard physical therapy, occupational therapy, speech), as well as the issue of maturation effects (i.e., given the timing of the intervention), bring the study outcomes into question.

van Vliet (2005) used a RCT design to assess whether Bobath therapy or movement science–based intervention was more effective with persons who had a stroke. One hundred twenty participants were randomly assigned within 2 weeks of their stroke to one of the interventions. Different physiotherapists, assisted by physical therapist assistants, provided each intervention per guidelines developed before the study. Specific descriptions of these interventions were not provided. Instruments used to assess outcomes included the primary outcome measures, the Rivermead Motor Assessment, and the Motor Assessment Scale (MAS). Secondary outcome measures included the Barthel Index, the 10-hole peg test, the 6-minute walk test, the Modified Ashworth Scale, the Nottingham Sensory Assessment, and the Extended Activities of Daily Living Scale. Outcomes were collected at 1, 3, and 6 months by a data collector blinded to group assignment.

There were no significant differences on any outcome measure at any data point over time. At 6 months, participants in the Bobath group had statistically significant improvements

in the supine-to-sitting section of the MAS, whereas at 1 month, participants in the movement science intervention were significantly more likely to go out socially as measured by the Extended Activities of Daily Living Scale and to bathe more independently (assessed on the Barthel Index). As in the first study presented, maturation effects of the sample are a concern. In addition, neither intervention is described in this article, raising questions as to what treatments the participants did, in fact, receive.

The broad clinical acceptance of the Bobath, or NDT, approach and the lack of research support for the intervention illustrate the wide gap between clinical practice and research. The quality of existing evidence, discussed in Chapter 15, is not strong enough to compare this approach with other interventions. However, no other treatments have been found to be superior to the Bobath approach.

Future research should explore which treatment options optimize outcomes for patients according to degree of neurological impairment. To improve movement control and enhance isolated/selective control, clinical applications of NDT could include manual guidance and facilitation of the affected limb or body segment through specific activities, with an intentional and gradual withdrawal of guidance/facilitation as the patient gains more control of the movement. NDT also incorporates motor learning principles with a progressive withdrawal of feedback.

## Constraint-Induced Movement Therapy

**Constraint-induced movement therapy,** or **CI therapy,** involves a variety of intervention components to increase use of a more-impaired extremity both in the research laboratory/clinic and, most importantly, in the home setting (Morris, 2007; Taub, 1993, 1999). The CI therapy protocol originated in basic research exploring the influence of the surgical abolition of sensation on movement in monkeys. This series of deafferentation studies led Taub (1977, 1980) to propose a behavioral mechanism, **learned nonuse,** in which a growing dependence on the nonaffected limb, with a learned lack of use of the affected limb, can interfere with recovery of function of an impaired extremity after a neurological insult. More recently, a linked but separate mechanism called use-dependent brain plasticity was proposed as a contributor to positive outcomes from CI therapy (Mark, 2006).

CI therapy is a "therapeutic package" consisting of several components. Some of these intervention elements have been employed in previous neurorehabilitation approaches, but usually as individual procedures performed at reduced intensity compared with CI therapy protocol. The main novel components of CI therapy are (1) the introduction of several techniques designed to promote transfer of the therapeutic gains achieved in the clinic/laboratory to the home environment and (2) the combination of these treatment components and their application in a prescribed, integrated, and systematic manner for many hours a day for 2 or 3 consecutive weeks (depending on the severity of the initial deficit). The goal is to induce a patient to use a more-impaired extremity.

Although CI therapy has evolved and undergone modification over the last 2 decades, most of the original treatment elements remain part of the standard procedure. The present CI therapy protocol consists of three main elements with multiple components and subcomponents: (1) repetitive, task-oriented movement training of the more-impaired upper extremity (UE) for several hours a day for 10 or 15 consecutive weekdays, depending on the severity of the initial deficit (shaping and task practice are the movement training techniques used most frequently in the CI therapy protocol); (2) applying a "transfer package" of adherence-enhancing behavioral methods designed to transfer gains made in the research laboratory or clinical setting to the patient's real-world environment; and (3) inducing the patient to use the more-impaired UE during waking hours over the course of treatment, usually by restraining the less-impaired UE. Morris (2007) described the CI therapy protocol in detail. The component and subcomponent strategies of CI therapy are listed in Box 25-3 and are described in the following sections.

### Repetitive, Task-Oriented Training

On each weekday during the intervention period, participants receive training for several hours under the supervision of an interventionist. The original CI Therapy protocol called for 6 hours per day for this training, but more recent studies indicate a shorter daily training period (i.e., 3 hours per day) is also effective for certain groups of patients (Dettmers, 2005; Page, 2008). Two distinct movement-training techniques are employed as patients practice functional task activities: shaping and task practice.

---

**BOX 25-3 Components and Subcomponent of the Constraint-Induced Therapy Protocol**

1. Repetitive, task-oriented training
   a. Shaping
   b. Task practice
2. Adherence-enhancing behavioral strategies (i.e., transfer package)
   a. Daily administration of the Motor Activity Log (MAL)
   b. Home diary
   c. Problem-solving to overcome apparent barriers to use of the more affected upper extremity (UE) in a real-world situation
   d. Behavioral contract
   e. Caregiver contract
   f. Home skill assignment
   g. Home practice
   h. Daily schedule
   i. Weekly phone calls for the first month after treatment to administer the MAL and problem solve
3. Constraining use of the more-affected UE
   a. Mitt restraint
   b. Any method that continually reminds the participant to use the more-affected UE

---

**Shaping** is based on the principles of behavioral training (Taub, 1999). In this approach, a motor or behavioral objective is introduced in small steps by "successive approximations." For example, the task can be made more difficult by changing the requirements for successful completion (e.g., speed of performance, distance traveled, and height of the step). Each functional activity is practiced for a set of ten 30-second trials, and explicit feedback is provided regarding the participant's performance immediately after each trial. When the level of difficulty of a shaping task is increased, the progression parameter selected for change should relate to the participant's movement problems. For example, if the participant's most significant movement deficits involve thumb and finger flexion and adduction (i.e., making a pincer grasp) and an object-flipping task is used, the difficulty is increased by making the object progressively smaller. Conversely, if the movement problem involves thumb and finger extension and abduction (i.e., releasing a pincer grasp), the difficulty of the task is increased by making the object progressively larger.

As the participant's performance improves, the shaping task is made progressively more difficult. The increase in difficulty should still allow the participant to accomplish the task, but should require effort. This ensures achievement of a given objective that might not be attainable if several large increments in motor performance were required. Another advantage of this approach is that it avoids excessive participant frustration and ensures continued motivation to engage in the training.

At the end of each activity, feedback is given in an objective form/measure that allows the patient to compare the current performance with previous performances (see examples in Table 25-2). For example, "You completed the action 15 times within 30 seconds, compared with your previous maximum of 11 times in 30 seconds."

Figure 25-4A shows a patient engaged in an upper-extremity shaping task as part of the CI therapy protocol. The patient in Fig. 25-4B is performing a shaping task for movement control of the involved right lower extremity that involves stepping to the "Xs" sequentially in forward, sideways, and backward directions; the pattern is repeated for the maximum number of steps that can be completed in, for example, 30 seconds. Table 25-2 includes examples of lower extremity shaping tasks.

**Task practice** is another less structured, repetitive, task-oriented training procedure. It involves functionally based activities performed continuously for 15 to 20 minutes (e.g., wrapping a present, writing). The tasks are not set up as individual trials of discrete movements that are measured each time. In successive periods of task practice, the parameters of the activity, such as spatial requirements or duration, can be changed to require more demanding control of limb segments for task completion. Global feedback about overall performance is provided at the end of the 15- to 20-minute period. Figure 25-5 shows a patient engaged in a task practice activity as part of the CI therapy protocol.

Training tasks are selected for each patient while considering (1) specific joint movements exhibiting the most

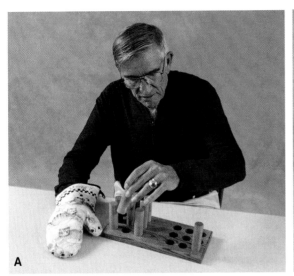
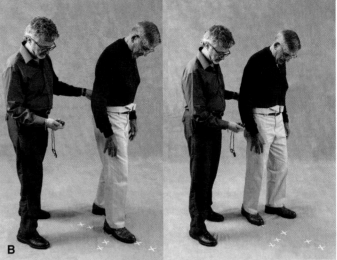

**FIGURE 25-4** Two examples of shaping tasks. (A) A patient is engaged in a peg-placement task with the involved upper extremity; the success of the task is measured by the time taken and the accuracy. (B) Two positions used as a patient performs shaping with the involved lower extremity during stepping to Xs taped to the floor. Starting with the toe on the center X (i.e., Start), he steps forward to the closest X and then back to the start position, steps to the right X and back to start, steps backward to the X and back to the start, and then repeats the pattern. Improvement over time can be measured by the number of cycles the patient can complete in 30 seconds or how many seconds it takes to complete three or four cycles as determined by the therapist.

| TABLE 25-2 | Examples of Lower Extremity Shaping Tasks |
|---|---|
| Step to the Xs (with the affected or unaffected leg)* | Description: Place one foot at X targets forward, to the side, and then to the back; trials of stepping with the unaffected leg emphasize weight-bearing and motor control stability in the affected leg, and trials of stepping with the affected leg emphasize selective movement control in the affected leg.<br>*Emphasizes hip flexion, abduction, and extension; knee control/stability on the stationary leg |
| | Shaping progression for stepping with affected lower extremity: Increase the distance of stepping, decrease assist device/UE support, and decrease ankle orthotic.<br>Shaping progression for stepping with less-affected lower extremity: Increase the distance of stepping, decrease assistive device/UE support, use knee angle monitor as feedback to alarm when the knee gets too close to full extension (locked knee-extension or genu recurvatum). |
| | Feedback: Number of cycles completed in a given time period (e.g., 20 or 30 seconds), number of knee monitor alarms as a percentage of total steps |
| Dorsiflexion | Description: The patient is standing, with upper extremity support if needed. A weight on a string is hung from the countertop edge or standard walker so the weight is suspended above the toes of the affected lower extremity. Place the weight at a height where the patient can dorsiflex to touch the weight, but not easily. Instruct the patient to lift the foot, without hip or knee flexion, to touch the weight as many times as she can within 20 (or 30) seconds.<br>*Emphasizes isolated ankle dorsiflexion without abnormal synergy and improved timing of movement |
| | Shaping progression: Increase the height of the target, progress to alternate/bilateral ankle dorsiflexion, decrease upper extremity support. |
| | Feedback: Number of cycles completed in a given time period (20 or 30 seconds), increasing percentage of success at reaching the target with isolated dorsiflexion |

*Continued*

| TABLE 25-2 | Examples of Lower Extremity Shaping Tasks—cont'd |
|---|---|
| Step to the stool | Description: Place foot on a stool and then back to the floor, continuing for time period (can do separate trial with each leg). <br> *Emphasizes hip flexion, knee flexion, ankle dorsiflexion in step leg; knee control/stability on supporting leg |
| | Shaping progression: Increase height of stool, less assistive device use, less orthotic use, knee angle monitor for feedback to achieve knee flexion during step or to inhibit knee hyperextension |
| | Feedback: Number of cycles in a specified time period (20 or 30 seconds), number of knee monitor alarms |
| Sit-to-stand | Description: From a chair, the patient rises to stand and returns to sitting and is instructed to bear weight on the involved leg. <br> *Emphasizes weight shift to more involved leg, hip/knee/ankle control, hip extension, knee extension |
| | Shaping progression: Decrease seat height, decrease assistive device use, decrease orthotic use, eliminate upper extremity support, limb-load monitor to indicate when more involved lower extremity bears the desired amount of weight. |
| | Feedback: Number of cycles in specified time period (20 or 30 seconds), number of times the monitor indicates desired weight-bearing (negative or positive) |
| Picking up objects | Description: From standing, the patient picks up a lightweight object (cone?) from a low surface and places it on a higher surface. <br> *Emphasizes wt shift to more involved leg, hip/knee/ankle control, hip extension, knee extension |
| | Shaping progression: Increase height of higher surface, decrease height of lower surface, decrease assistive device and orthotic support, limb-load monitor to indicate when more involved lower extremity bears desired amount of weight. |
| | Feedback: Amount of time required to pick up and place a certain number of cones or number of cones that can be picked up and placed in a specified time; number of times the monitor indicates desired weight-bearing (negative or positive) |

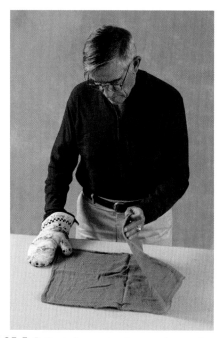

FIGURE 25-5 Patient demonstrating a task-practice activity, folding a towel using the involved upper extremity only.

pronounced deficits, (2) the joint movements therapists believe have the greatest potential for improvement, and (3) patient preference among tasks with similar potential for producing specific improvement. Frequent rest intervals are provided throughout the training day. Intensity of training (i.e., the number of trials/hour [shaping] or the amount of time spent on each training procedure [task practice]), is recorded.

With conventional CI therapy protocol, facilitation is rarely used to influence quality of movement during training. When poor quality of movement (e.g., compensatory movement) is observed during the performance of a shaping or task activity, the therapist coaches the patient on strategies to improve the quality of the movement and/or adjusts the difficulty level of the task. Easier tasks require less effort and make a compensatory movement strategy for task completion less likely.

### Adherence-Enhancing Behavioral Methods to Increase Transfer to the Life Situation (Transfer Package)

One of the overriding goals of CI therapy is to transfer gains made in the research or clinical setting to the participant's real-world environment (e.g., home and community settings).

To achieve this goal, a set of techniques, summarized in Table 25-3 and referred to as a "**transfer package**," is used to hold the patient accountable for adherence to the requirements of the therapy. In this way, the patient takes responsibility for self-improvement. The participant must actively engage in and adhere to the intervention without constant supervision from a therapist, especially in the life situation when the therapist is not present. Attention is directed toward using the more-impaired UE during functional tasks, obtaining appropriate assistance from caregivers if available (i.e., assistance to prevent patients from struggling excessively, but allowing them to try as many tasks by themselves as feasible), and wearing the mitt as much as possible (when it is safe to do so).

Many individual intervention principles have successfully enhanced adherence to exercise and physical function-oriented behaviors. Four are most relevant to and utilized in the adherence-enhancing behavioral components of CI therapy: monitoring, problem-solving, behavioral contracting, and social support. A detailed description of the transfer package subcomponents is beyond the scope of this chapter. Readers interested in learning more should read resources from the Taub research group (Morris, 2007; Taub, 2013).

### Constraining Use of the Less-Impaired UE

The most commonly applied CI therapy treatment protocol incorporates use of a restraint device (either a sling or protective safety mitt) on the less-impaired UE to prevent patients from succumbing to the strong urge to use that UE during most or all functional activities, even when the therapist is present. The protective safety mitt, which eliminates the ability to use the fingers, is preferred for restraint because it prevents functional use of the less-impaired UE for most purposes while still allowing protective extension of that UE in case of falling, reciprocal arm swing in ambulation, and use of the arm to maintain balance. Patients are taught to put on and take off the mitt (or sling) independently. They decide with the therapist when use of the mitt or sling is feasible and safe. The goal for mitt use in patients with mild/moderate motor deficits is 90% of waking hours. This so-called "forced use" is arguably the most visible element of the intervention in the rehabilitation community and is frequently and mistakenly described as synonymous with "CI therapy." However, Taub (1999) has clarified that there is nothing magical about use of a sling, protective safety mitt, or other restraining device on the less-affected UE as long as the more-impaired UE is exclusively engaged in repeated practice. "Constraint," as used in the name of the therapy, does not refer only to the application of a physical restraint, such as a mitt; it also indicates a constraint of opportunity to use the more-impaired UE for functional activities (Taub, 1999). As such, any strategy that encourages exclusive use of the more-impaired UE is viewed as a "constraining" component of the treatment package. For example, shaping was meant to constitute a very important constraint on behavior; either the participant succeeds at the task, or he is not rewarded (e.g., by praise or knowledge of improvement).

Preliminary findings indicate a significant treatment effect using CI therapy without the physical restraint component (Sterr, 2002). Likewise, similar findings were obtained with a small group of participants (n = 9) when a CI therapy protocol without physical restraint was employed (Uswatte, 2005). However, the latter study suggested that this group experienced a larger decrement at 2-year follow-up testing than groups that used physical restraint. Use of the mitt also minimized the need for the therapist or caregiver to keep reminding the patient to limit use of the less-impaired UE during the intervention period.

| TABLE 25-3 | Additional Techniques Employed in Constraint-Induced Movement Therapy to Facilitate Transfer of Gains From the Therapeutic Setting to the Home | |
|---|---|---|
| **TECHNIQUE** | **DESCRIPTION** | |
| Behavioral contract | At the outset of treatment, the therapist negotiates a contract with the participant and caregiver, if one is available, in which they agree that the participant will wear the restraint device for up to 90% of waking hours (whenever it is safe) and use the more-impaired arm as much as possible outside the laboratory. Specific activities during which the participant can practice using the more-impaired arm are discussed and written down. | |
| Daily home diary | During treatment, the participant catalogs how much he has worn the restraint device and used the more-affected arm for the activities specified in the behavioral contract. The diary is kept for the part of the day spent outside the laboratory and is reviewed each morning with the therapist. | |
| Home practice exercises | During treatment, participants are asked to spend 15–30 minutes at home daily performing specific upper extremity tasks repetitively with the more-affected arm. The tasks typically employ commonly available materials (e.g., stacking Styrofoam cups). Toward the end of treatment, an individualized post-treatment home practice program consisting of similar tasks is drawn up. Participants are encouraged to do these tasks for 30 minutes daily after the 2-week treatment period. | |
| Problem-solving | During treatment and four weekly phone contacts after treatment, the therapist helps the participant think through any barriers to using the more-impaired arm. For example, if a patient is concerned about spilling liquid from a glass, the therapist can suggest filling the glass only halfway. | |

Over the last 20 years, a substantial body of evidence has accumulated to support the efficacy of CI therapy for hemiparesis after chronic stroke, defined as 1 or more years after injury (Taub, 2006a). Evidence of efficacy includes results from an initial small RCT of CI therapy in individuals with UE hemiparesis secondary to chronic stroke (Taub, 1993), a larger placebo-controlled trial in individuals of the same chronicity and level of impairment (Taub, 2006b), and a number of other studies (Kunkel, 1999; Miltner, 1999; Sterr, 2002). A large multisite RCT was also conducted in individuals with UE hemiparesis in the subacute phase of recovery (i.e., 3 to 9 months' poststroke) (Winstein, 2003; Wolf, 2006, 2007).

The signature CI therapy protocol that included 6 hours of task-oriented training daily for consecutive days over a 2-week period has been modified and incorporates fewer hours of supervised training and a distributed schedule of three times each week for 10 weeks (Dettmers, 2005; Page, 2008). The modified protocol yielded similar positive results.

Recent findings from Taub's laboratory explain why the modified protocol may be as effective as the more intense protocol (Gauthier, 2008). In a "factors" study, the investigators used different combinations of the three protocol components with different groups of participants. Results demonstrated that when the transfer package was eliminated from the protocol, participants experienced a much reduced treatment effect. This finding suggests that the transfer package (i.e., behavioral management elements focused on increasing use of the more-affected extremity at home and in the community) may be more important to treatment outcomes than the amount and schedule of therapist-supervised task-oriented training.

Taub (2006a) also developed an automated training device (the Autocite) that includes eight shaping tasks and reduces the intensity of the therapist supervision required. Studies with the Autocite suggest that substituting the device with therapist supervision yielded similar results. It is important to note that recent innovations that reduce the amount of therapist supervision during task-oriented training do not diminish the need for a licensed professional when CI therapy interventions are delivered. The skilled therapist is still needed for the movement/task analysis, safety monitoring, problem-solving, and patient/client education aspects of executing the transfer package. More research examining these issues is needed.

CI therapy has also been applied to adults recovering from other neuromuscular disorders, including TBI (Shaw, 2005) and MS (Mark, 2008). The approach has also successfully improved UE use in children with CP and after hemispherectomy (DeLuca, 2003, 2004, 2007). Altogether, more than 200 studies on the clinical effects of CI therapy have been published, all with positive results. Several systematic reviews concerning CI therapy have also been published (Corbetta, 2010, 2015; Sitori, 2010). These reviews indicate that the studies analyzed had mixed results. However, it should be noted that some of the studies in the reviews failed to use all components of the signature CI therapy protocol. Further, the component most often omitted was the transfer package, which is thought to be the most influential for optimal outcomes.

Research with CI therapy suggests that improvements are realized in motor control impairments as well as in functional use. However, functional use is typically the most significant improvement realized (Taub, 2006a). Still, studies using laboratory motor function tests (e.g., the Wolf Motor Function Test (WMFT), Fugl Meyer Assessment (FMA), and ARAT) suggest quality of movement improved with CI therapy. Lin (2007) found that participants in a CI therapy protocol demonstrated more efficient reaching and grasping movements compared with participants who received an equivalent intensity of traditional rehabilitation. Further, a growing number of reports have described positive neural plastic changes accompanying improved movement and functional gains after CI therapy (Gauthier, 2008; Mark, 2006).

Although CI therapy has been well researched and has demonstrated excellent outcomes for patients with chronic stroke, the method has some potential drawbacks. The intensive schedule of 6 hours of therapy per day may not be feasible in many clinical settings and has related reimbursement issues. Evidence of the effectiveness of a modified CI therapy program in acute stroke populations is only preliminary, with a shorter dosing of supervised intervention (Page, 2005). CI therapy also has quite strict inclusion and exclusion criteria. Inclusion criteria for upper extremity studies commonly are (1) active extension of 10 degrees in any joint of two fingers, 10 degrees of wrist extension, and 10 degrees of thumb abduction and (2) a score of 22 or higher on the Mini-Mental State Examination and/or the ability to follow three-step directions (Blanton, 2008). Exclusion criteria for lower extremity CI therapy include the patient's need for an assistive device for safe ambulation. This well-defined and focused sample substantially limits the evidence-based generalizability of CI therapy to patients who do not meet these criteria.

## Neuromuscular Electrical Stimulation

NMES, or the stimulation of an innervated muscle, can be delivered as functional electrical stimulation, providing a useful movement by stimulating a muscle deprived of nervous control. As early as 1961, Lieberson proposed using NMES to improve gait in patients with hemiparesis. With surface or implanted electrodes, NMES can be used to completely activate the muscle or simply enhance its function by stimulating motor nerves. The lower motor neuron must be intact to induce muscle contractions in target muscles. And from a motor learning standpoint, it is essential that the patient volitionally engage with the stimulation provided by NMES. Repetitive electrical stimulation is believed to elicit lasting changes in corticospinal excitability, possibly as a result of coactivating motor and sensory fibers (Knash, 2003).

Several types of electrical stimulator devices are available; however, many of these devices were developed for one specific treatment purpose or to restore a single bodily function, which limits the versatility of any one stimulator (Povovich, 2001). Recently, more versatile devices have been developed. Newer stimulators have radio frequency communication between the sensors and the stimulating device (Fisekovic, 2007).

The therapeutic benefits of NMES may occur through both central and peripheral nervous system factors. The CNS is believed to be positively influenced by NMES. Movement generated from the stimulation helps to generate cortical reorganization and positive neuronal plasticity (Liepert, 2000). Peripheral benefits may include improvements in muscle strength, increased flexibility, and reduced spasticity (Rushton, 2003).

NMES can be used for a variety of functional tasks including ambulation, UE performance of ADLs, and control of respiration and bladder function. To date, NMES has been used most extensively for neurorehabilitation with persons recovering from a stroke and spinal cord injury (SCI). Specific applications have been proposed and preliminarily investigated, including two common broad applications: an NMES-based neuroprosthetic device to enhance functional activity while the device is worn and NMES for repetitive-movement training to produce motor relearning and a more permanent return to function without the use of electrical stimulation. Both applications are addressed next.

### NMES as a Neuroprosthesis

Upper limb neuroprostheses have been used to provide grasp and release function for individuals with SCI, primarily at the C5 and C6 level, and for persons with some retained proximal movement function. Peckham (2001) successfully used implanted NMES neuroprostheses to reduce impairments and activity limitations in 50 participants with C5 or C6 SCI. Positive results from this multicenter trial were observed after treatment and throughout a 4-year postimplant period (Wuolle, 2003). In similar participants, NMES neuroprostheses have successfully enhanced overall UE use for additional muscles, including the triceps (Bryden, 2000), pronator quadratus (Lemay 1996), and finger intrinsics (Lauer, 1999).

A limited number of studies, all with small sample sizes, have described use of NMES-based UE neuroprostheses with persons recovering from a stroke (Alon, 1998, 2002; Merletti, 1975; Rebersek, 1973). These studies used surface electrodes and reported success limited to a small number of selected functional tasks. The investigators cited increased hypertonia as a major obstacle to successfully using NMES-based UE neuroprostheses to improve function after stroke. Chae (2003) recommended NMES-based UE neuroprosthesis systems for stroke recovery, including features that (1) facilitate bilateral tasks, (2) provide proximal and distal control, (3) are miniaturized to avoid interfering with ambulation, (4) utilize control paradigms that produce effortless movements of the impaired UE without compromising the function of the less-affected UE, and (5) reduce spasticity by "turning off" over-active muscles as well as stimulating weak muscles.

### Lower Limb Neuroprostheses

Pioneering work from the 1970s and 1980s using NMES-based neuroprostheses to restore standing and walking in persons with complete and incomplete SCI continues to evolve today (Bajd, 1982; Kralj, 1989). Superficial electrodes are used with these systems, and standing is achieved by simultaneous activation of the quadriceps muscle groups in both legs. The swing phase of walking is initiated by maintaining stimulation to the quadriceps muscles of one leg while electrically facilitating a flexor withdrawal response in the swing leg (Kim, 1976; Veltink, 1992). The swing phase is completed by activation of the knee extensors of the swing leg while the reflex remains active. This results in hip flexion. When extensor muscle tone interferes with dorsiflexion, the addition of a peroneal nerve stimulator can help inhibit the plantar flexor/extensor muscle tone (Bajd, 1999). Systems that stimulate the hip abductors, hamstrings, and trunk extensors have also been reported (Granat, 1993), and implanted systems have been produced (Kobetic, 1994). However, these systems activate individual muscles instead of reflex patterns.

Hybrid systems that combine various bracing and NMES components have also been developed (Solomonow, 1992). The Louisiana State University Reciprocating Gait Orthosis (RGO) is one example that has demonstrated long-standing and functional use by system recipients, with RGOs used by 41% for walking (Franceschini, 1997) and 66% for exercise (Solomonow, 1997). The locked brace provides support and allows periods of discontinued stimulation, thus preventing NMES-induced muscle fatigue. The bracing component also protects insensate body parts and osteoporotic extremities during weight-bearing. Hybrid NMES systems with a medial-linkage knee-ankle-foot orthosis (Shimada, 2006), an energy storage orthosis (Durfee, 2005), and a more energy-efficient and cosmetically accepted hip-knee-ankle orthosis has been developed (Middleton, 1997; Saitoh, 1996). Although showing great promise with lower limb use for short distances, these NMES-based neuroprostheses are not currently a complete alternative to wheelchair use because of their high metabolic energy demands (Sheffler, 2006).

NMES-based neuroprotheses with superficial electrodes have been successfully used to facilitate ankle dorsiflexion during gait in persons recovering from a stroke (Burridge, 1997; Lieberson, 1961). However, such units may be infrequently used clinically in the United States. Recent evidence for superiority to AFOs and U.S. Food and Drug Administration (FDA) approval of three peroneal nerve stimulators may increase use of these devices (Sheffler, 2006). The Bioness L300 is FDA approved to address footdrop, and the L300 Plus system includes additional stimulation for quadriceps to support knee extension. Implantable NMES-based neuroprostheses have also been developed (Kljajic, 1992; Weber, 2004). However, problems with their use, including need for reimplantation, have been reported.

### Upper Limb Motor Relearning

A large amount of evidence indicates that goal-oriented, active, repetitive movement training leads to both neuroplastic changes and skill acquisition. As such, it is reasonable to expect that NMES-based repetitive movement can achieve these changes when active patient engagement in the stimulated movement is emphasized. These activities should be goal oriented, require cognitive effort, and become progressively more difficult as the participant's skill improves, all accepted principles for improving skill and neural plastic changes.

Most of the literature concerning NMES for motor relearning addresses application in persons with hemiparesis from a stroke. Three types of electrical stimulation are available for this purpose: cyclic NMES used to activate paretic muscles at a set duty cycle for a preset duration (people using this form of NMES are relatively passive participants of the stimulation), electromyography (EMG) or biofeedback-mediated electrical stimulation applied to participants who are able to partially activate paretic muscles but lack sufficient activation to use them functionally, and NMES as a neuroprosthesis during repetitive task practice (RTP) (see Fig. 25-6). Cyclic NMES systems were shown to be effective for improving motor impairments in patients in both acute and chronic phases of recovery from a stroke (Chae, 1998; Powell, 1999; Rosewilliam, 2012; Sonde, 1998, 2000; Sullivan, 2004; Wong, 1999). However, patients in the chronic phase of recovery did not experience enduring improvements at the motor impairment level.

Only one study completed with acute stroke subjects demonstrated improvements at the activity limitation level (Chae, 1998). Studies using EMG biofeedback or EMG-triggered NMES also demonstrated improvements in motor impairments immediately after treatment (Cauraugh, 2000, 2002; Francisco, 1998; Kimberley, 2004; Kraft, 1992). However, only one of these studies demonstrated long-lasting improvements in motor impairment (Kraft, 1992). Two of the studies did reveal improvements in activity limitations (Francisco, 1998; Kimberley, 2004).

Studies in which the primary objective was to examine the use of NMES-based UE neuroprostheses also demonstrated improved motor impairments and activity limitations after

the unit was removed (Alon, 2003; Popovic, 2007). An RCT examining the use of NMES along with usual care for motor retraining in the early phase of recovery from stroke is currently under way (Fletcher-Smith, 2016).

### Lower Limb Motor Relearning

Numerous case studies have reported the effects of NMES applied to the peroneal nerve during gait for motor relearning after stroke (Kljajic, 1992; Taylor, 1999). Positive effects have included improved ambulation, more normal EMG activation patterns, and decreased cocontraction of antagonist muscles. However, no blinded RCTs have examined this approach. Others have demonstrated positive effects from using cyclic NMES (Levin, 1992; Merletti, 1978; Yan, 2005) and EMG-triggered NMES (Cozean, 1988; Fields, 1987) for isolated ankle dorsiflexion. In addition, Burridge (1997) demonstrated positive motor learning effects with a peroneal nerve NMES-based neuroprosthesis.

Several studies have reported positive motor learning effects with multichannel NMES systems for stimulating additional movements with ankle dorsiflexion (Bogataj, 1989, 1995; Daly, 2000; Stanic, 1978). Systems used in these studies stimulated a variety of muscles throughout the lower limb, including the ankle eversion and plantar flexion; knee flexion and extension; and hip flexion, extension, and abduction.

Two other studies, stimulating different muscle groups, demonstrated superior results with a multichannel NMES system to conventional therapy (Bogataj, 1995) and receiving no NMES (Daly, 2000). Daly (2006) has conducted an RCT of a multichannel NMES system for this purpose. Although findings are promising, these investigators reported challenges with multichannel systems, including reduced muscle selectivity, poor reliability with stimulation, and pain from sensory stimulation.

In summary, although methodological limitations have been reported, growing evidence indicates that various forms of NMES are beneficial for improving movement control impairments for persons with SCI and stroke. Although it appears that NMES-based neuroprostheses are more effective than cyclic and EMG- or biofeedback-triggered NMES, no direct comparison studies support this claim. Continued work is needed to improve the technology of NMES systems and to investigate their use in persons with other neuromuscular disorders.

## Technology Approaches to Neurorehabilitation

Health care has been evolving in the United States, with particular changes noted over the last 40 to 50 years. Patient outcomes are no longer measured by mortality, morbidity, and/or impairments, but by functional change. The concern in both acute and rehabilitation settings is effectiveness and efficiency of interventions at the lowest cost. As documented throughout this chapter, current evidence supports intensive practice of meaningful tasks as efficacious in promoting better outcomes for patients undergoing neurorehabilitation. In

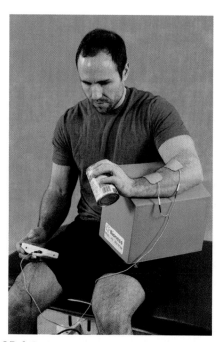

**FIGURE 25-6** Patient using a hand switch to activate neuromuscular electrical stimulation on upper extremity muscles, grasping and lifting a can during repetitive task practice.

addition, it has been recommended that the requirements of such tasks incorporate ongoing challenges to the client to be effective (Van Peppen, 2004). Although occupational and physical therapists incorporate these elements into their interventions, increasing concerns about cost containment for both inpatient and outpatient services affect choices regarding patient care. Technological advances have the potential to augment rehabilitation by incorporating meaningful tasks, providing intensive practice, and presenting challenging interventions to persons in rehabilitation settings. To this end, engineers, in conjunction with occupational and physical therapists, are exploring alternative rehabilitation technologies that can provide intensive task practice, collect accurate data on performance in real time, and offer motivating tasks independent of therapists. Two such rehabilitation technologies, robotics and virtual reality (VR), are discussed in the next paragraphs.

## Robotics

In the rehabilitation context, **robotics** is the field of mechanical devices with electronic, computerized control systems designed to perform human functions. "Formerly their use was almost exclusive to industry, however certain human functions now can be controlled through bioelectronic (bionic) devices such as automatic insulin pumps, and other prostheses" (Kwakkel, 2008). Robotic technologies have been under development since 1978, with much of the early work accomplished within the Veterans Administration (VA) system (Burgar, 2000). Robotics can be used to replace function and to improve recovery by providing intensive and repetitive practice. Sufficient intensity and repetition enhance neural plasticity. Although much of this early development highlighted the use of robotics to support ADLs, the 1990s saw the expansion of robotic study into therapeutic use (Burgar, 2000; Fasoli, 2004). The role of these systems, or **haptic robots**, is to sense user movements, use the resulting information to plan subsequent motion, and provide force feedback to the user (Brewer, 2007). This discussion addresses only those robotic devices used in the rehabilitation process rather than bioelectronic devices used for functional activity, as discussed previously in this chapter. Although most studies have focused on the diagnosis of stroke, limited studies have also been carried out on persons with a SCI.

The scope of the robotic field is evolving rapidly, as demonstrated by the variety of systems available and the scale of options within these systems. Some robots facilitate reaching; examples include the Mirror Image Movement Enabler (MIME) (Lum, 2006) and the Assisted Rehabilitation and Measurement (ARM) Guide (Kahn, 2006). Passive movement of participants' arms, a sort of manual guidance, can be carried out by some robotic systems, including the GENTLE/s, MIME, and REHABROB, whereas active-assisted movement is the output of systems such as the MIT-Manus and InMotion2. Rehabilitation incorporating bilateral upper limb activity during intervention after stroke has been proposed and implemented in studies (McCombe, 2008). The MIME enables

the user to mirror motions carried out by the nonaffected limb with the impaired upper limb. Although most devices are aimed at developing proximal or gross motor movements in the upper limb, some emerging robotic technologies are beginning to address movements in the forearm, wrist, and hand. A particular strength of this technology is its use across the spectrum of impairments found in stroke, from severe to mild limitations. Robotics is also used for rehabilitation in the lower limb (Hornby, 2005).

Motor learning theory was used in the design of robotics. However, Brewer (2007) suggested that there has been a limited application of these theories to date. The primary theoretical emphasis has been a massed practice approach. Other promising paradigms that have yet to be incorporated into robotic technology include **implicit learning** (unconscious learning strategies) and **error magnification** (resistance to moving in the desired direction) approaches.

Studies have shown that robotics improved impairments associated with neurological injury, such as weakness, range limitations, and neuromuscular incoordination. However, changes in functional outcome have not been consistently demonstrated (Brewer, 2007; Kwakkel, 2008). Robotics has demonstrated greater short-term improvements in active joint movement and reaching than conventional therapy. However, participants undergoing conventional therapy have similar results over a longer time frame (Lum, 2002, 2006). Robotic devices can facilitate massed practice for extended duration with programming and provide consistent resistance and feedback to the patient, without requiring 1:1 therapist attention. They can also be customized to fit the patient's needs. Outcomes can be accurately and consistently measured in a cost-effective manner.

Kwakkel (2008) described five robotic devices studied in RCTs to support rehabilitation interventions (Box 25-4). An RCT was completed more recently with robotic-assisted therapy at the wrist and hand (Kutner, 2010). Other devices have also been included in quasi-experimental designs.

In the following paragraphs, three recent studies incorporating robotic technology into stroke rehabilitation are discussed in detail. In the first study, a robot was used in combination with repetitive massed practice. The next two studies describe "next steps" in the evolution of **robotic** use in the rehabilitation

---

**BOX 25-4 Five Robotic Devices to Support Motor Rehabilitation**

MIME robot

MIT-MANUS robot

ARM-GUIDE robot

InMotion Shoulder-Elbow robot

Bi-Manu-Track robot

Kwakkel G, Kollen BJ, Krebs HI. Effects of robot-assisted therapy on upper limb recovery after stroke: A systematic review. *Neurorehabil Neural Repair.* 2007;22:111–120.

process. The second study describes robotics used in a purposeful task meaningful to persons after a stroke. The third study describes the engagement of occupational and physical therapists in designing a robotic device that meets their needs in a clinical setting.

Most robotic devices are used with the proximal aspect of the upper limb. Using an RCT design, Kutner (2010) used a distal robot, the Hand Mentor (HM), in combination with a RTP intervention and compared outcomes with those obtained with repetitive massed practice alone (see Fig. 25-7). Seven participants completed the repetitive practice only arm of the study, whereas 10 completed the combined intervention (HM and RTP). Sixty hours of RTP were compared with a combined 30 hours of RTP plus 30 hours of HM intervention. HM was designed to improve active motion at the wrist and fingers. The primary outcome measure was quality of life as measured by the Stroke Impact Scale. Data were collected before intervention, immediately after intervention, and 2 months after intervention. Significant changes in mood and social participation were observed in the RTP group after intervention as well as improvement in stroke recovery at follow-up.

Both interventions resulted in a statistically significant change in ADLs between the preintervention and the postintervention periods and with hand function from the postintervention measurement to the follow-up period. The combined intervention demonstrated a significant change in stroke recovery at the postintervention period and at follow-up. Not all changes met the criterion for clinically significant differences. This study suggested that the robot-assisted RTP therapy resulted in outcomes similar to those with RTP alone, providing support for integration of robots in the clinical setting.

In a pilot study, Johnson (2005) used a robotic device that simulated the CI therapy principle of constraining the unaffected arm during a driving simulation task. Rather than using a mitt or glove to restrain the unaffected arm, the steering wheel of the driving simulator "stiffened" when the unaffected arm was used. The aim of the study was to see if such a system increased use of the affected arm in persons who had had a stroke. A control group of four adults without a stroke was compared with eight adults with a stroke, equally distributed among right-sided and left-sided impairments; "cueing" via steering wheel resistance in the control group was incorporated on the dominant arm to encourage use of the nondominant arm in the driving simulator. Unilateral and bilateral driving sequences were evaluated using the same moving road sequence, with defined tasks (e.g., turning) under both forced cue and no forced cue situations. EMG recordings were collected on seven muscles in the elbow, shoulder, and forearm.

As expected, study outcomes demonstrated that persons without a stroke had significantly better muscle activity in their nondominant arm. For both groups, there was a significant interaction between movement direction and forced-cue versus no forced-cue conditions. Both groups used the studied arms better in the forced-cue condition, but only when the steering wheel was turned in an against-gravity direction. There were no significant changes in muscle activity for either group in gravity-eliminated directions. The effect of postural changes as a substitute for arm activity was also evaluated. Three participants with hemiplegia demonstrated increased postural movements. However, these increases did not appear to explain the increase in upper limb muscle activity.

The use of a meaningful task that incorporated bilateral arm activity (driving) in conjunction with a robotic device simulating constraint of the unimpaired arm demonstrated increases in muscle activity in the impaired arm. EMG data were collected to assess changes in arm movement. The study demonstrated some of the potential for robotics. Intensive practice of meaningful tasks with parameters of the task controlled by the robot encouraged clinical change.

Lam (2008) described an interactive design process with occupational and physical therapists that resulted in a prototype system for upper limb rehabilitation. This system can generate subtle cues to enhance reaching activity for persons after stroke without restraint. The resulting system has four primary components: It emulates weight-bearing. It contains postural sensors to detect atypical posture used during use. It uses an elbow stimulation device that can cue the elbow during use. It utilizes a computer interface that provides feedback during use. The system left the user's hand free, and the cueing consisted of gentle vibration at the elbow to facilitate extended reaching. The shoulder movements available in the system included a wide range of motion so activities other than reaching could be performed. A virtual environment was added using a computer screen to motivate patients.

The pilot study for this prototype was carried out with eight therapists as subjects, four occupational therapists and four physical therapists (Lam, 2008). This was done for safety reasons and to provide evaluation of the system for the designers. The outcomes generated many comments for improving the device. There were consistent complaints about the elbow vibration unit: The support system of the robotic device was

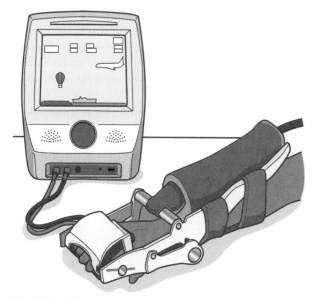

**FIGURE 25-7** The Hand Mentor robotic system and its components.

too high and might preclude its use in patients using wheelchairs. The software on the computer interface needed more development to be stimulating to potential patients. In conclusion, the authors described how therapist feedback would be used in the development of the next iteration of the system.

The results from Lam (2008) demonstrate the importance of the engineer/therapist partnership when robotic devices are designed for clinical use. This discussion is continued in the VR section of this chapter, where such partnerships are supported by the engineering community so that systems will augment the rehabilitation process effectively.

In summary, robotic devices have improved motor outcomes in persons after stroke through intensity of practice and type and duration of intervention. Movement can be controlled more precisely with a robotic device than by therapists, as demonstrated by Johnson (2005). Robotic devices can add incentives through use of motivating activities, such as computer or video games and virtual environments (Brewer, 2007; Fasoli, 2004). Providing immediate feedback on progress has increased client satisfaction as well. A particular benefit of robotic systems is their ability to be tailored to the unique needs of the individual.

A 2012 systematic review of robot-assisted therapy concluded that no difference existed between "intensive" conventional therapy and robotic-assisted training in terms of patient outcomes (Norouzi-Gheidari, 2012). However, the authors also concluded that for certain groups of patients, robot-assisted training along with conventional therapy showed great promise. Challenges to the use of robotics in rehabilitation settings include patient preferences for human intervention, the high cost of these devices, and resistance on the part of service providers (i.e., therapists and physicians) (Brewer, 2007; Fasoli, 2004). As newer systems that can be used in a variety of contexts become available, their benefits should help overcome some of these concerns.

## ■ Intervention Ultimately Applied in Functional Activities

As mentioned previously, the goal of motor control intervention is to ultimately improve motor control to optimize patient function. Techniques such as NDT, NMES, CI therapy with task-specific practice, and robotics can be progressed for use during functional activities. Other interventional strategies can also be used to address functional deficits resulting from motor control impairments. These include upper and lower extremity activity, locomotor training, and VR systems.

### Upper Extremity Functional Activity

All the "preparatory interventions" and "upper limb motor relearning" activities described in the previous sections can be applied to almost any upper extremity functional task. It is important to intentionally progress toward patient engagement in movement, with application in real functional activities, and personal control of that movement by systematically challenging the patient. Another goal is to increase

dependence on intrinsic feedback from within the patient versus extrinsic feedback from the therapist.

Another option to improve movement control during early rehabilitation, when the patient is relearning control of movement, is to incorporate equipment to assist the movement. One option for use with the upper extremities is a dynamic hand orthosis. An example is the SaeboFlex® orthosis (see Fig. 23-4), which provides mechanical assistance to voluntary wrist/finger extension movements.

For patients who can flex/grasp but not extend, the **SaeboFlex orthosis** is custom fitted and uses an extension spring system to mechanically open the hand and extend the wrist. From this position, the patient can grasp objects by voluntarily flexing the fingers. When the patient relaxes, the orthosis applies mechanical force to open the hand and extend the wrist again. Even during this passive extension movement, the patient can use motor imagery to "practice" opening the hand or contribute to the extension movement in whatever capacity she can. This allows higher repetitions of the task-specific practice of opening and closing the hand. The SaeboFlex also allows use of the hand at home, contributing to increased use throughout the day (increasing the number of repetitions of use), and may help motivate the patient to use the extremity outside therapy time.

A 2-week intervention was associated with improvements in motor control (17% reduction in WMFT time and 17% improvement in UE Fugl-Meyer score) at 3-month follow-up in a 44 year-old with chronic stroke (Butler, 2006). Individuals with stroke (n = 13) who participated in 5 days of training (6 hours per day), including SaeboFlex, exercises and functional electrical stimulation, demonstrated improved movement at the shoulder and elbow and wrist extension but no improvement in wrist flexion and finger movement; in contrast, Fugl-Meyer and Motor Assessment Scale scores both improved significantly (Farrell, 2007).

In another study, 12 days of SaeboFlex intervention was associated with significant improvement in mean ARAT score and clinically significant improvements in the upper limb Motricity Index (Stuck, 2012).

Dynamic hand orthoses may also contain a component to address elbow function. A related orthosis that can address upper extremity motor control-movement is the SaeboReach, which is ideal for patients who lack control of both elbow extension and hand-opening. The **SaeboReach** consists of the SaeboFlex orthosis plus an above-elbow component; thus, the device can mechanically assist elbow extension for functional reach during grasp and release activities and provide opportunities for higher repetitions of elbow flexion movement.

When you choose an orthotic, select one that allows the patient to work the muscle group that is supported by the orthotic. The goal is to induce positive neuroplastic changes to support motor control improvement. Ideally, such orthotics should not be used simply to assist passive movement on the patient's part. The patient must be instructed to work the muscle group that is being supported by the orthotic (e.g., the patient wearing an AFO should be encouraged to actively and intentionally initiate and contract the dorsiflexors). This active participation is necessary for motor learning and to drive positive neuroplastic changes within the CNS.

## Lower Extremity Functional Activity

Motor control-movement impairments result in a variety of functional deficits during activities involving the lower extremities. These deficits include difficulty moving the lower extremities for bed mobility, transfers, and gait. Many of the general techniques and approaches discussed in the preparatory intervention section can be applied to these lower extremity activities. Manipulating the variables of timing, speed, direction, degrees of freedom, range of motion, and stability requirements during the activity allows the therapist to develop a program that intentionally progresses interventions in a challenging and optimal way. For example, a patient may have difficulty with lower extremity motor control, complicating performance of efficient and effective sit-to-stand transfers. This task can be made easier for initial learning by starting from a higher surface height (decreasing range and work), by adjusting the surface (a solid surface is easier to move from than a soft/compliant surface), or by adjusting any of the variables addressed in the preparatory section. The sit-to-stand transfer can be made more difficult by systematically adjusting variables to optimally challenge motor control in the task.

You can also utilize the principles behind the PNF technique of combination of isotonics to address motor control deficits. By adding starts and stops during the transfer, the patient must switch between various contraction types in a coordinated manner. For example, you can instruct the patient to begin the stand-to-sit transfer. Then ask her to halt in midrange on your command and finally return to standing. This works on the motor system's ability to control concentric, isometric, and eccentric contractions during a functional activity and to transition between contraction types in a coordinated manner. These same techniques can be applied to the other movements performed by the lower extremities during functional activities.

## Locomotor Training

Locomotor training (LT) is a physiologically based approach to gait rehabilitation incorporating intrinsic mechanisms of the spinal cord that respond to specific afferent input to produce stepping motions (Barbeau, 1991, 2003a, 2003b; Behrman, 2000, 2005, 2006; Beres-Jones, 2004; Dietz, 1995; Dobkin, 1995; Field-Fote, 2002; Harkema, 1997; Stewart, 1991; Visintin, 1989; Werning, 1995). The concept is introduced in Chapter 15, with more specific functional applications given in Chapter 37.

The approach developed from basic research demonstrating that cats with complete spinal cord transections were capable of responding to intense walking training (Barbeau, 1987; de Leon, 1998; Lovely, 1986). Despite the absence of supraspinal output, the cats were capable of generating stepping responses when provided with truncal support, manually assisted loading, and the sensory signals initiated by a moving treadmill. This observation led to the belief that the spinal

cord has an intrinsic capacity to integrate afferent input, interpret it, and respond with an appropriate motor output. This ability is believed to be possible through a network of spinal interneurons referred to as **central pattern generators** (CPGs) (Forssberg, 1979).

The second line of evidence driving LT comes from research exploring specific afferent input to the neurological control of walking (Dietz, 2000; Van de Crommert, 1998). These studies suggest specific sensory cues are critical to the control of reciprocal stepping. For example, several lines of research indicate proprioceptive input coming from a stretch to the hip flexor muscles is important for initiating the swing phase of gait (Sherrington, 1910). Therefore, sufficient hip extension in the terminal stance phase of the gait cycle is critical for effective reciprocal stepping. Also, extensor loads relayed by the Golgi tendon organs (Ib) in the ankle extensor muscles are believed to be important for stimulating appropriate muscle activation patterns needed during the stance-to-swing phase of gait (Dietz, 2000; Van de Crommert, 1998). As such, the level of loading through the legs during gait is critical to reciprocal stepping. Therefore, guidelines for LT maximize loading the legs instead of the arms (i.e., as with use of a walker) during gait training.

According to Behrman (2000, pg. 689), the sensory cues listed as critical to inducing stepping are "(1) generating stepping speeds approximating normal walking speeds (0.75–1.25 m/s); (2) providing the maximum sustainable load on the stance limb; (3) maintaining an upright and extended trunk and head; (4) approximating normal hip, knee, and ankle kinematics for walking; (5) synchronizing timing of extension of the hip in stance and unloading of the contralateral limb; (6) avoiding weight bearing on the arms and facilitating reciprocal arm swing; (7) facilitating symmetrical interlimb coordination; and (8) minimizing sensory stimulation that would conflict with sensory information associated with locomotion (e.g., stimulation of extensor afferents during swing and flexor afferents during stance)."

Although it is critical for propulsion, reciprocal stepping alone is insufficient for controlled walking. Two additional mechanisms, balance (upright and dynamic equilibrium) and adaptability (the ability of the individual to respond to the demands of the environment and to meet her own behavioral goals), are also needed for functional walking behavior (Barbeau, 2003a; Behrman, 2006;). Research surrounding the control of balance and adaptability serves as the basis for LT intervention principles. On the basis of these findings, Behrman (2005) proposed a clinical decision-making algorithm that can be applied to LT for persons with an incomplete SCI (see Figs. 25-8 and 25-9).

LT protocols have been developed for persons with either complete or incomplete injuries of the spinal cord. For the purposes of this chapter, only LT protocols for persons with incomplete SCI are described. Specific guidelines for LT have been provided for two major categories of interventions: body-weight support treadmill training as shown in Fig. 25-10 and progression of the intervention to overground gait and balance skills. Subcomponents within these categories include specific guidelines for environmental adaptations (e.g., amount of

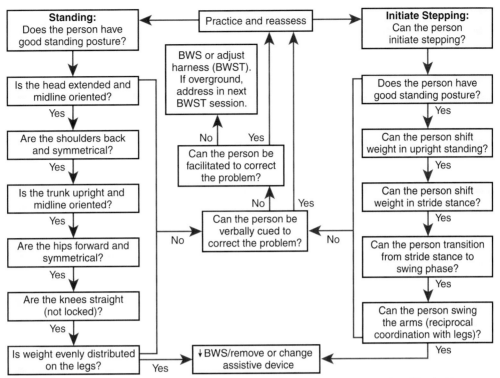

**FIGURE 25-8** Decision-making algorithm for standing and step initiation progression. *(Used with permission from Behrman AL, Lawless-Dixon AR, Davis SB, et al. Locomotor training progression and outcomes after incomplete spinal cord injury. Phys Ther. 2005;85:1356–1371.)*

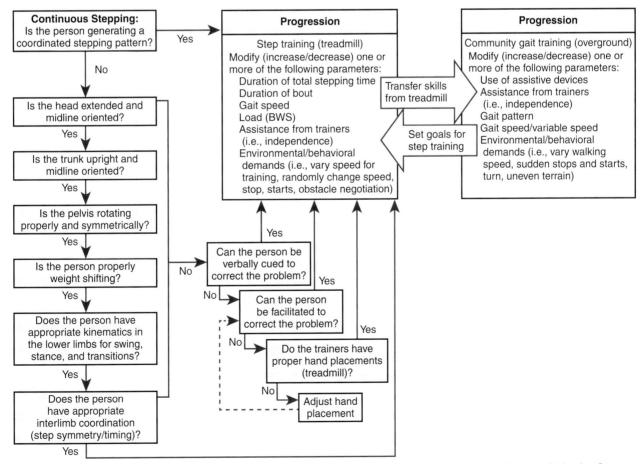

**FIGURE 25-9** Decision-making algorithm for continuous stepping progression. *(Used with permission from Behrman AL, Lawless-Dixon AR, Davis SB, et al. Locomotor training progression and outcomes after incomplete spinal cord injury. Phys Ther. 2005;85:1356–1371.)*

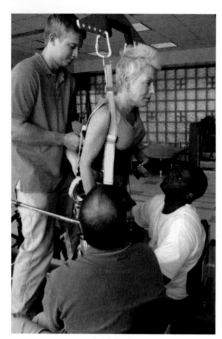

**FIGURE 25-10** An individual ambulating on a treadmill during body weight support ambulation training.

weight-bearing experienced by the participant, treadmill speed, equipment used, obstacles introduced), manual assistance provided (amount and location of facilitating input from trainers), and verbal cueing provided. In addition, overground training can be further subdivided into clinic and community gait and balance training components.

LT has been investigated with a variety of patient populations. Barbeau (1987) first used a body weight support system in conjunction with a treadmill for gait training with seven participants with SCI. The intervention significantly increased the participants' self-selected, maximal walking speed and demonstrated that the approach was safe. Wernig (1992) observed similar findings and reported that four of eight participants gained the ability to walk overground despite the absence of voluntary limb movement at rest. These findings support the hypothesis that LT provides a stimulus capable for producing walking. In a larger LT study including participants in the acute and chronic phases of recovery from SCI, both groups demonstrated significant improvement in ambulation (Werning, 1992). These investigators also demonstrated greater improvements in acute-phase participants than in another group of participants receiving conventional therapy during the acute stage of recovery (Werning, 1992).

Behrman (2000) expanded the evidence for LT with a series of case studies. Of significance, these case studies provided a more uniform and detailed protocol for carrying out the LT intervention than previous publications. These same LT intervention principles were used in a multisite RCT in persons in the acute phase of recovery from SCI (Dobkin, 2006). This trial did not show differences between the experimental group (LT) and control group (traditional rehabilitation) However, methodological challenges were reported, and both groups included a high percentage of independent posttreatment ambulators (Dobkin, 2006).

A recent retrospective study suggested that providing LT for persons with an SCI in a hospital-based setting with one trained physical therapist, two technicians, and one well-trained volunteer was not only effective but was also financially feasible (Morrison, 2007). A Cochrane Database review exploring studies using LT alone and in combination with other interventions in persons with an SCI concluded that the approach has promise but conclusive evidence is still lacking (Mehrholz, 2012).

At least 20 clinical studies have examined the efficacy of LT for persons recovering from a stroke (Mosely, 2003). Recent publications report improved gait speed following LT compared with participants receiving conventional therapy (Ada, 2003; Eich, 2004; Patterson, 2008.) reported that the motor gains observed in their participants included significant changes in cortical reorganization as evidenced by functional magnetic resonance imaging. A multicenter RCT of LT for persons in the acute phase of recovery from stroke, the Locomotor Experience Applied Post Stroke (LEAPS) trial, concluded that LT was effective in improving walking function (Duncan, 2007; Nadeau, 2013). However, the locomotor intervention was not superior to a more traditional, impairment-based strength and balance program. Preliminary evidence has also supported use of LT for children with CP (Day, 2004; Richards, 1997; Schindl, 2000) and cerebral hemispherectomy (de Bode, 2007). It has also shown promise in adults with MS (Geisser, 2015) and adults with certain classes of PD (Rose, 2013).

Similar to CI therapy, LT appears to have greater influence on functional improvement than on improvement in movement control impairment. For example, Behrman (2005) reported dramatic improvements in ambulation with relatively little improvement in isolated movement control in persons with an incomplete SCI. However, several studies of LT for persons recovering from stroke have demonstrated significant improvements in the quality of movement (Eich, 2004; Patterson, 2008).

## Virtual Reality

One of the emerging rehabilitation technologies showing significant promise for those with movement disorders of the CNS is **VR**, defined as an advanced form of computer technology used in the remediation of cognitive and motor impairments and function (Lam, 2006). VR systems are designed to simulate real-world environments in **virtual environments** where users perceive themselves as engaging in tasks and activities they would carry out in everyday life (Deutsch, 2007). The degree of immersion in the virtual world is called **presence,** which is dependent on the integration of multisensory inputs in the virtual environment (Henderson, 2007). Most systems incorporate visual and auditory inputs, and some involve haptic or sensory inputs as well.

In an RCT, Yang (2008) augmented treadmill training for persons with strokes using 3-D VR with widescreen visual enhancement, auditory cues, and changes in acceleration on the treadmill. Nine participants were assigned to treadmill only training, and 11 received VR-augmented treadmill training. All participants received nine sessions over a 3-week period consisting of three 20-minute sessions three times a week. Participants in the VR-augmented training demonstrated significant improvements in walking speed, community walking time, and walking ability in community activities as measured by the walking ability questionnaire (WAQ). Persons in the control group demonstrated changes in community walking time alone in the immediate postintervention data collection period. Follow-up studies showed persons who participated in the VR-augmented treadmill training could walk significantly faster after treatment in both community and clinic tests, as well as demonstrating significantly higher WAQ scores (Yang, 2008).

A systematic review by Henderson (2007) on the outcomes of upper limb motor recovery using VR concluded that although existing evidence was limited, the results were encouraging and supported further study of the VR approach.

Systems are designated as either immersive or nonimmersive VR, depending on the technology utilized. **Immersive systems** use large-screen projection, head-mounted displays, and cave systems in which the environment is projected onto a concave surface to create the sense of presence or immersion (see Fig. 25-11). Virtual environments may also include video capture systems in which the user views self or an **avatar** (representation of the limb) in the scene on a computer screen as if watching a television program (Deutsch, 2007). **Nonimmersive VR** may use a computer screen controlled with a mouse or other device.

Broeren (2008) used computer games in a community activity center to see if they improved upper limb use. Outcomes demonstrated improvements in motor skills, but these changes did not translate into real-life activities.

Given that the use of VR in rehabilitation is a young evolving field, existing studies have incorporated a wide range of newly developed technologies, including immersive and nonimmersive systems. The literature can be confusing if one does not have some idea of the technologies available under the auspices of VR.

This technology has been used mostly with stroke but has been studied in other diagnoses, such as autism, intellectual impairments, and CP. Concerns regarding the ability of persons with cognitive impairments to interact with VR systems have been minimized by the success of pertinent studies (Lotan, 2009; Standen, 2005; Yalon-Chamovitz, 2008). A review by Standen (2005) summarized existing studies of VR interventions in persons with cognitive impairments. They concluded that VR provided a safe and effective intervention, with skills learned in studies transferring to real-world environments.

The focus of various intervention environments include ADLs (grocery shopping, baking, driving, using public transportation, crossing the street), cognitive function, social skills,

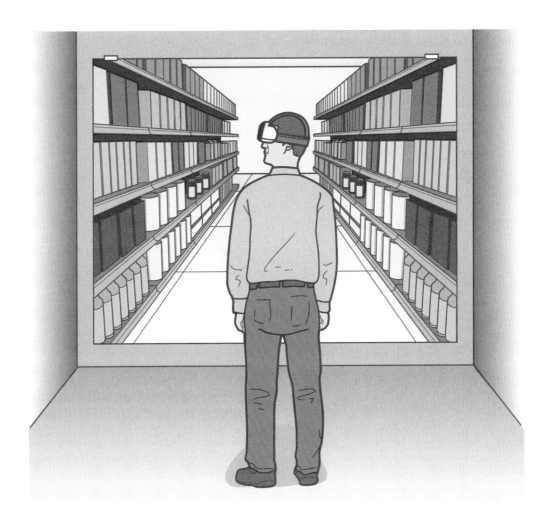

**FIGURE 25-11** A virtual reality setup of a virtual grocery store.

leisure skills, physical fitness, and improved motor impairment in both upper and lower limbs (Crosbie, 2007; Erren-Wolters, 2007; Lam, 2006; Lotan, 2008; Kizony, 2010). To date, the results of such studies have been encouraging and suggest that VR can improve function, motor and cognitive skills, driving skills, leisure, and physical fitness across a range of settings (home, hospital, telerehabilitation, and community centers).

Although the versatility of VR technology offers a realm of opportunities to the rehabilitation field, many studies have incorporated motor learning principles into programs. Deutsch (2004) emphasized the importance of motor learning theory in the development of VR technology hardware and software and discussed how **knowledge of performance (KP)** and **knowledge of results (KR)** were integrated into VR systems to encourage learning and promote motivation. This includes descriptions of how regular KP and KR were incorporated into newly developed VR systems.

VR provides skill training in an enriched environment designed to promote behavioral changes and sensorimotor plasticity at the neural and behavioral levels by using intense repetitive practice (Nudo, 1996, 1998). Intense repetitive practice is a key element of CI, robotic therapies, and VR; however, VR may sustain motivation to a greater extent and is more flexible in the contexts in which it is used. These characteristics meet the guiding principles discussed earlier in this chapter to promote neural plasticity, such as behavior specificity, extensive and concentrated practice of training tasks, cognitive engagement of the participant, and provision of interesting and important activities for participant motivation.

The benefits of VR are that it is customizable, enjoyable (Piron, 2008; Yalon-Chamovitz, 2008), motivating, and meaningful to the patient when the tasks or activities are incorporated into the technology. Challenges of using such systems include the attitudes of clinicians and users, cost, safety, and feasibility (Henderson, 2007). There are side effects associated with the technology, including sweating, nausea, disorientation, headaches, and balance disturbances. Such disturbances are attributable to the large difference between the processing speed for incoming stimuli in the sensory system and a corresponding but slower autonomic regulation (Kiryu, 2007). More healthy adults than users who have had a stroke have reported side effects (Crosbie, 2007). A 2015 review of VR studies involving participants after a stroke suggested that VR interventions may have a positive effect on balance and gait recovery, especially when combined with conventional therapy (Cavalcanti, 2013; Luque-Moreno, 2015). As this new technology continues to evolve, larger and more controlled studies will be needed to support its use in clinical and nonclinical settings. Based on the evidence to date, VR appears to hold exciting possibilities for the rehabilitation field.

## Mirror Therapy

Mirror therapy involves the practice of functional limb movement of the nonparetic side while observing the reflection of this movement in a mirror. The view in the mirror makes it appear as if the paretic side is moving. The technique could be related to motor imagery because the paretic limb does not

actually have to move, or it could be considered a low-tech means of VR that allows the brain to "observe" normal movement of the paretic limb. The mirror is placed in front of the chest for upper extremity therapy or between the legs for lower extremity therapy, with the mirror surface facing the nonparetic limb. The nonparetic limb is typically moved for approximately 30 minutes of activity while the patient looks in the mirror and observes what appears to be normal movement of the paretic limb.

Patients using mirror therapy to address ankle dorsiflexion movement showed significant improvement in selective motor control compared with control groups (Sutbeyaz, 2007). Application of mirror therapy to the upper extremity has also demonstrated greater improvement in Brunnstrom stage (more selective control) than controls not receiving mirror therapy (Yavuzer, 2008). Thirty minutes of mirror therapy was also associated with improvements on the upper extremity scale of the Fugl-Meyer assessment, with improvements in useful grasp and reach during the ARAT (Dohle, 2009). See Fig. 25-12A for mirror box therapy for UE movement control and Fig. 25-12B for mirror therapy for LE movement control of the affected side.

## THINK ABOUT IT 25.3

1. When a patient has difficulty with motor control that causes difficulty in performing reaching tasks of the upper extremity, how can you modify the characteristics of the task to focus on motor control?
2. How can you progress this activity as the patient improves?
3. What other techniques can you utilize to improve motor control of this task?

## Pediatric Considerations

Regardless of patient age, interventions to improve selective movement control should focus on optimizing the number of repetitions (massed practice) of normal movement in appropriate doses to enhance neural plasticity. Activities must be naturally motivating, a point that is extremely important when working with children. The goal is to create the desire to move in specific ways and to complete multiple repetitions of the action. For example, practice touching a specific target with the hand could be accomplished by using a motivational pressure switch that incorporates light or sound when the location is touched.

## ■ Intervention Considerations for Nontherapy Time and Discharge

Improvements in movement control impairment are not realized quickly. It has become increasingly evident that permanent changes in movement control require intensive task practice. Most likely, this intensive practice promotes the positive neural plasticity needed for improved movement skills. To achieve this intensity of practice, therapists must ensure that their patients continue therapeutic activities well beyond

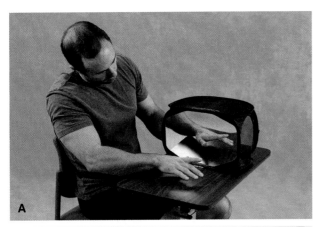

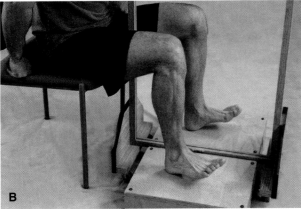

**FIGURE 25-12** Activities using mirror therapy for practice of movement control. (A) With use of a mirror box, the affected upper extremity is placed inside the box, and the less-affected limb is placed outside the box, adjacent to the mirror surface. As the patient moves the less-affected arm, he visualizes and imagines moving the affected arm—and in the mirror it appears to move normally. Using the mirror, he gets visual feedback indicating that the affected limb is moving more normally. (B) A lower extremity movement using a mirror on wheels. The mirror is rolled up between the patient's legs while he is seated, with the mirror surface facing the less-affected leg. As the patient moves the nonparetic leg, the view in the mirror appears to be the affected leg moving normally.

the time spent under their supervision. Many rehabilitation scientists recognize this need, and many contemporary rehabilitation approaches include structured strategies to ensure independent movement practice to supplement therapist-supervised sessions. For example, the transfer package component of CI

therapy is primarily directed at ensuring concentrated and safe use of the hemiparetic extremity in the patient's home and community settings. When this transfer package is removed from the treatment protocol, improvements are substantially reduced. This suggests that a systematic approach to enhancing adherence to continued practice is extremely important (Gauthier, 2008).

Several factors are necessary for ensuring effective independent practice of movement. First, safety issues should be addressed. This discussion must include activities that, when practiced independently, pose a risk for injury. Second, the patient should be educated about desirable and undesirable movement patterns. Practice and coaching during supervised therapy sessions can be helpful for developing the patient's ability to problem solve through movement challenges (e.g., selecting feasible movement skills for practice, using adaptive equipment, emphasizing movement patterns in need of practice). Finally, whenever possible, caregivers should be enlisted to assist with movement task practice outside the clinical setting. Caregivers should be educated on the goals of movement practice as well as when to assist and not assist the patient during these sessions.

---

### PATIENT APPLICATION

*Consider the following information from the tests and measures portion of Mrs. Jones's examination and address the clinical questions presented.*

*Mrs. Jones was referred to an outpatient rehabilitation clinic in her community for therapy. Standardized tests and measures used in her examination included the ARAT, Motor Activity Log (MAL), and the Berg balance scale (BBS). Her ARAT total score was 3 (she could perform only two items in the gross movement section of the test). Her mean score on the MAL was 0.5 on a 5-point scale. Her total score on the BBS was 8.*

---

### Contemplate Clinical Decisions

1. *Consider the interventions presented in the preceding section of this chapter. What are the expected benefits and challenges posed for each approach as potential therapeutic interventions for Mrs. Jones?*
2. *How can Mrs. Jones's therapists ensure her adherence to therapeutic activities away from the clinic?*
3. *What newer rehabilitation technologies do you believe Mrs. Jones would benefit from? Why?*

---

# HANDS-ON PRACTICE

Be sure to practice the following skills described in this chapter. With further practice, you should be able to perform:

- Manual guidance of movement with feedback
- Task-oriented training with shaping
- Constraining of the less-impaired limb

- NMES, including appropriate parameters
- Donning of appropriate orthotics
- LT
- VR setup
- Mirror therapy: UE and LE

## Let's Review

1. What key task characteristics must the physical therapist consider when categorizing movement, and how might these variables be manipulated to change the complexity of a task?

2. What types of deficits would you expect to see in a patient with abnormal motor control-movement, and how would you describe them?

3. Describe the impairments and functional limitations you would expect to see with damage to each system level of the CNS that plays a role in motor control (i.e., spinal cord, brainstem, primary motor area, and premotor/supplemental motor areas). How is this influenced by patient diagnosis?

4. When designing an intervention for a patient with a neurological diagnosis, what neuroplasticity principles should be incorporated to induce positive neuroplastic changes?

5. What key components should be included in the examination/evaluation of a patient with motor control deficits? What tests/measures are appropriate to include?

6. Describe the use of NDT, CI Therapy, NMES, robotics, VR, and mirror training to improve movement control. Do these interventions follow the guidelines for promotion of positive neuroplastic changes in the CNS? What are the pros/cons for their incorporation into physical therapy clinical practice?

7. How can the therapist incorporate functional activity training into the treatment design? Why is this important in treating motor control impairments?

8. What are the components of the CI Therapy transfer package, and how can these ideas be included in patient training/education for activity during nontherapy time and home exercises?

9. What strategies should be used to ensure independent movement practice as a supplement to therapist supervised sessions? How can the physical therapist ensure the safety and effectiveness of these supplemental programs?

---

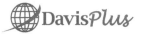 **DavisPlus**    For additional resources, including Focus on Evidence tables, case study discussions, references and glossary, please visit http://davisplus.fadavis.com

---

## CHAPTER SUMMARY

Functional movement can vary from relatively simple and automatic actions to highly complex motions requiring a great deal of planning and monitoring throughout execution. A wide range of movement impairments is possible after a neurological disorder. The specific impairments observed will depend, at least partially, on the part or parts of the CNS most influenced by the disease. The resulting movement impairment can have profoundly negative effects on a patient's functional ability and independence. Rehabilitation professionals have become more optimistic in recent years about a patient's ability to improve performance of functional movements. A variety of evidence-based therapeutic interventions have been effective for inducing positive changes in the CNS (i.e., neural plasticity) and

improvements in control of movement. It is widely accepted that to effectively promote positive neuroplastic changes, interventions must motivate the patient to actively engage in concentrated bouts of motor practice specific to the movements that need improvement. Although numerous approaches have been proposed and described in this chapter, some of them are more clinically feasible and more widely used than others.

The Focus on Evidence (FOE) table summarizing the most important evidence related to interventions for impaired motor control-movement and selective control is provided in its entirety in the online resources for Chapter 25. Further research and technological advances are expected to improve the clinical applicability of these approaches in the years to come.

# Therapeutic Interventions for Complete Paralysis

Aaron B. Rindflesch, PT, PhD, NCS
Martha Freeman Somers, MS, DPT ▪ Dennis W. Fell, PT, MD

## CHAPTER OUTLINE

## CHAPTER OBJECTIVES

Upon completion of this chapter, the learner should be able to:

1. Summarize the anatomy and physiology of typical causes of complete paralysis.
2. List and describe the related pathologies that often accompany complete paralysis.
3. Describe compensatory movement strategies and therapeutic techniques used with individuals with complete paralysis.
4. Describe typical interventions used with individuals with complete paralysis and apply them to a case.
5. Summarize special considerations for interventions used with individuals with complete paralysis.

## ▨ Introduction

This chapter focuses on interventions that address **complete paralysis** of a specific muscle, muscle group, or body region. This condition is most commonly the result of damage to the corticospinal system, the portion of the nervous system carrying voluntary motor commands from the motor cortex to the neurons innervating the skeletal muscles of the limbs and trunk. In this chapter, *complete paralysis* refers to a total and permanent loss of voluntary motor function in at least one region of the body. This loss most frequently results from interruption of motor commands to the extremities and trunk, as

occurs globally with a complete spinal cord injury (SCI) or, in some cases, in more specific regions after an incomplete SCI. Complete paralysis of an individual muscle or small groups of muscles can also result from a nerve root or peripheral nerve injury, depending on the severity of injury.

Damage to the corticospinal system can be attributed to many pathologies, including trauma, infection, compression, and ischemia. The most common example, as illustrated throughout this chapter, is damage to the corticospinal system from an SCI. An SCI can occur in a variety of traumatic and nontraumatic ways. Common traumatic causes are motor vehicle crashes, falls, violence, and sports accidents

(National Spinal Cord Injury Statistical Center [NSCISC], 2017). Common nontraumatic causes include spinal stenosis and neoplasm (McKinley, 1999b, NSCISC 2016).

## Normal Function

In a normally functioning nervous system, motor control is achieved with a complex interplay between central and peripheral structures. In the corticospinal system, motor commands travel in tracts descending from the cerebral cortex through the midbrain, pons, medulla, and spinal cord to synapse in the cord directly on both alpha motor neurons and interneurons (Fix, 2005). The interneurons in turn synapse with alpha motor neurons at the same level of the cord, at nearby levels, and at distant levels (Haines, 2007; Lundy-Ekman, 2007). The axons of the alpha motor neurons exit the spinal cord and travel peripherally through the spinal nerves, often through plexuses, then through named peripheral nerves to the skeletal muscles (Crossman, 2000). Each alpha motor neuron innervates a number of fibers, called a *motor unit*, within a single muscle (Kiernan, 2005). Alpha motor neurons are the "final common pathway" for motor behavior; all voluntary and involuntary motor commands to skeletal muscles travel through these neurons (Kandel, 2000).

## Clinical Picture of Complete Paralysis in a Holistic Context

When complete paralysis results from damage to the spinal cord, the extent of motor function deficits depends on the location of the damage; rostrally located lesions result in more profound loss of motor function than do caudal lesions. Not all damage to the spinal cord results in total loss of voluntary motor function below the lesion. Damage is most often incomplete (NSCISC, 2017), with some preservation of sensory function, voluntary motor function, or both in areas of the body innervated by portions of the cord caudal to the lesion.

Complete spinal cord damage in the cervical region or in the first thoracic segment results in **tetraplegia** (formerly called *quadriplegia*), with loss of voluntary control in some or all upper extremity muscles, as well as loss of all voluntary function in the trunk and lower extremities. Complete lesions in the remainder of the thoracic region of the cord or in lower segments result in **paraplegia**, with preservation of all upper extremity function but loss of voluntary motor function in the lower extremities and in those portions of the trunk innervated at or caudal to the level of the lesion. Complete lumbar and sacral lesions cause paralysis in lower extremity muscles innervated at and/or caudal to the level of the lesion.

The functional effect of complete paralysis resulting from damage to the spinal cord depends largely on the **neurological level of injury**, and more specifically the **motor level** (i.e., the most caudal key muscle/myotome that has a muscle strength of 3/5 or above while the segment above is normal [5/5], as determined by examination) (American Spinal Injury Association [ASIA], 2015; Burns, 2001; Consortium for Spinal Cord Medicine [CSCM], 1999; Daverat, 1995; Lazar, 1989;

van Middendorp, 2009, 2011; Zorner, 2010). For further definitions of neurological level of injury and motor level, refer to ASIA (2015).

At one extreme, people with high cervical, complete cross-sectional lesions require a ventilator to breathe and are unable to perform any functional activities independently when first injured because of the profound extent of complete motor loss. During the course of rehabilitation, they can typically learn to control power wheelchairs and use environmental control units and computers, but they remain dependent in all other functional tasks unless **neurological recovery** (or **neurological return**) occurs. At the other extreme, people with complete cross-sectional lesions lower in the cord (i.e., low lumbar or sacral lesions) are most likely to gain independence—though not necessarily normal movement—in most if not all functional tasks during the course of rehabilitation because more muscle groups retain at least some degree of function.

Spinal cord damage is not limited to paralysis in the trunk and limb musculature. Concomitant impairments include sensory deficits, abnormal muscle tone, altered cardiovascular functioning, impaired breathing and coughing, sphincter paralysis and altered autonomic function in the bowel and bladder, changes in genital functioning, decreased blood pressure, and impaired thermoregulation. SCIs can also cause numerous secondary conditions, including autonomic dysreflexia, deep vein thromboses, gastrointestinal hemorrhage, **heterotopic ossification**, joint contractures, osteoporosis and fractures, pain, pressure injuries (pressure ulcers), pulmonary embolism, respiratory complications (atelectasis, pneumonia, respiratory insufficiency), stress ulcers, and urinary tract complications (infections, kidney and bladder stones, hydronephrosis, renal failure) (Alander, 1997; Anson, 1996; Campagnolo, 2002a; Charlifue, 1999; Chen, 1999; CSCM, 2008; Johnson, 1998; Levi, 1995a; McKinley, 1999a; Siddall, 2001; Wuermser, 2007). **Autonomic dysreflexia** is a potentially life-threatening syndrome, particularly in individuals with an SCI at or above the T6 level, with uncontrolled sympathetic nervous system discharge below the level of the lesion (high blood pressure) and parasympathetic response above the level of the lesion (Krassioukov, 2009).

Most SCI complications can be prevented—or at least minimized—with proper care and preventive measures (Anson, 1996; Campagnolo, 2002a; Chen, 1999; McKinley, 1999a). However, care and preventive measures are beyond the scope of this chapter. The reader is referred to the CSCM documents (1998a, 1998b, 1999, 2001, 2005a, 2005b, 2006, 2008, 2010, 2014, 2016).

## Possible Effect of Paralysis on Function

Complete paralysis can obviously have a profound effect on a person's ability to move the body in space and to stabilize affected joints and body segments in order to perform motor tasks involved in self-care, other activities of daily living, and performance of home- and family-related tasks. These decreased physical abilities can alter participation in home, work, school, and community activities. In sum, complete paralysis can hinder the performance of physical tasks and activities inherent in the performance of role expectations in virtually every area of a person's life, resulting in disability. The problem can be compounded by societal attitudes about people with disabling conditions—attitudes held by others and by the person with complete paralysis (Fichtenbaum, 2002; Tunks, 1986).

In the end, the potential for disability is great. However, the disabling effect of complete paralysis can be mitigated through the acquisition of compensatory movement skills and assistive equipment during rehabilitation, as well as strategies aimed at enhancing psychological and social adaptation. This chapter focuses on important compensatory movement skills after complete paralysis. For details of assistive and adaptive equipment to provide external joint stability for persons with neurological injury, see Chapter 17.

## PATIENT APPLICATION

*Mr. Johnson, a 21 year-old male, was recently involved in a motor vehicle crash in which he was an unbelted driver. He was ejected from the vehicle in the crash, fracturing and dislocating his vertebrae at the fifth and sixth cervical levels. Before undergoing surgical stabilization of his cervical spine, he was clinically assessed using the standardized physical examination in the International Standards for Neurological Classification of Spinal Cord Injury (ISNCSCI; ASIA, 2015). His neurological level of injury was determined to be C6 and is complete, defined in the standards as the absence of motor and sensory function in the lowest sacral segment of the spinal cord. The first through sixth cervical segments remain intact.*

*Before the crash, he worked as a laborer in the home construction trade.*

### Contemplate Clinical Decisions

- *What do you think is most important from the patient's perception of his dysfunction?*
- *On which activities or social roles will his rehabilitation need to focus?*

## ■ Anatomy and Physiology of Complete Paralysis

### Spinal Cord Anatomy

The spinal cord begins caudal to the medulla, extending from just above the foramen magnum to the level of the L1 or L2 vertebra (the spinal canal below L1/L2 contains only cerebrospinal fluid and loose nerve roots—the cauda equina). The cord is segmentally organized, consisting of eight cervical, 12 thoracic, five lumbar, five sacral, and one coccygeal segments and corresponding pairs of spinal nerves. In the thoracic region and below, nerves exit through the intervertebral foramen immediately caudal to the vertebra with the corresponding

name and number. In the cervical region, spinal nerves exit through the intervertebral foramen immediately superior to the vertebra with the corresponding name and number, with the exception of C8, which exits below the C8 vertebra.

Seen in cross section, the cord includes an H-shaped central area of gray matter that contains the cell bodies of neurons, small projection fibers, and glial cells. The gray matter includes dorsal (posterior) and ventral (anterior) horns (Fig. 26-1). Neurons in the dorsal horns receive sensory input from the periphery. The ventral horns contain the cell bodies of motor neurons innervating the skeletal muscles. The gray matter in the T1 through L2 or L3 and the S2 through S4 segments of the cord also includes the cell bodies of preganglionic autonomic neurons (Crossman, 2000; Haines, 2007; Kiernan, 2005; Lundy-Ekman, 2007), located in an intermediate zone between the dorsal and ventral horns.

The gray matter in the spinal cord is surrounded by white matter, the reverse of the organization of the cerebral cortex. The white matter contains ascending and descending tracts carrying sensory information to—and motor commands from—the brain. The most important tracts that contribute to motor control and conscious sensory perception are pictured in Fig. 26-2. The tracts are functionally organized; different sensory and motor functions are carried in each tract (Fix, 2005; Haines, 2007). Table 26-1 summarizes the motor and sensory tracts of the spinal cord and the functions they convey.

Two additional features of the tracts within the spinal cord are worth mentioning here because they affect the presentation of injury. First, the tracts differ in regard to the side of the body they innervate: Some tracts are located in the spinal cord ipsilateral to the side of the body that they innervate (i.e., they do not cross the midline in the cord), some lie on the contralateral side of the body (i.e., they cross the midline at some

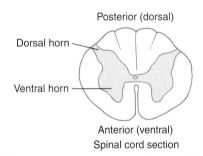

**FIGURE 26-1** Schematic cross section of the spinal cord.

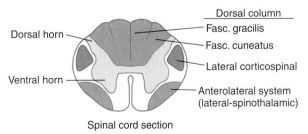

**FIGURE 26-2** Important ascending and descending fiber tracts in the spinal cord. Ascending tracts are shown on the left.

| TABLE 26-1 | Motor and Sensory Tracts of the Spinal Cord | |
|---|---|---|
| TRACT | CROSSING/DECUSSATION | FUNCTION |
| *Major Motor Tracts (Descending)* | | |
| Lateral corticospinal | Medulla | Voluntary movement of limbs |
| Anterior corticospinal | Spinal cord | Voluntary movement of axial muscles |
| Rubrospinal | Midbrain (ventral tegmental decussation) | Voluntary movement of primarily flexors in the limbs |
| Vestibulospinal | Does not cross | Trunk and limb extensors for posture and balance (involuntary) |
| Reticulospinal | Most do not cross | Posture, balance, modulation of reflexes, complements corticospinal (involuntary) |
| *Major Sensory Tracts (Ascending)* | | |
| Dorsal column (fasciculus gracilis and cuneatus) | Medulla | Proprioception, vibration, deep touch, and discriminative touch |
| Spinocerebellar | Dorsal spinocerebellar does not cross; ventral spinocerebellar crosses in the spinal cord | Unconscious proprioception from the trunk and extremities |
| Spinothalamic, spinoreticular, and spinotectal | Spinal cord; typically crosses within one or two segments | Pain, temperature, and crude touch |

point), and some carry fibers that innervate both sides of the body (Table 26-1). Second, many of the tracts have a somatotopic organization: Fibers terminating in more rostral segments of the cord lie closer to the gray matter than do fibers terminating more caudally. Figure 26-3 illustrates the spatial arrangement of fibers innervating the cervical, thoracic, lumbar, and sacral portions of the body.

The clinical significance of these two features, ipsilateral versus contralateral innervation and somatotopic organization, becomes apparent when a person sustains partial damage to a segment of the spinal cord. The result is incomplete paralysis and/or incomplete loss of sensory function. Stated conversely, some neurological functions can be preserved because of these unique features.

In addition to containing the tracts that communicate with the brain, the white matter houses ascending and descending nerve fibers that interconnect different levels of the spinal cord. These fibers form a thin layer lying just peripheral to the gray matter (Crossman, 2000).

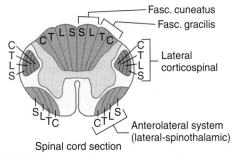

FIGURE 26-3 Somatotopic organization of the spinal cord.

**Upper motor neuron (UMN) lesions** result from damage to the motor aspects of the cerebral cortex, subcortical white matter (corona radiata or internal capsule), brainstem, or white matter motor tracts of the spinal cord and cause a syndrome of weakness, decreased motor control, spasticity, and increased spinal reflexes. An injury to the white matter of any segment of the spinal cord can result in these UMN signs, along with sensory loss at and most likely below the level of the lesion. Depending on the extent of the injury, complete paralysis can result in the muscles innervated by that segment. Because of the cephalocaudal organization of the spinal cord, when a complete cross-sectional injury occurs to an individual segment, the areas of the body innervated by the segments caudal to the complete injury of the spinal cord also exhibit paralysis.

## Nerve Roots and Peripheral Nerves

Each segment of the spinal cord gives rise to pairs of dorsal and ventral nerve roots, one dorsal and one ventral root on each side per cord segment. Dorsal roots contain the axons of sensory (**afferent**) neurons. Ventral roots contain the axons of motor (**efferent**) neurons. On each side of the cord, the dorsal and ventral nerve roots combine at each spinal level to form a spinal nerve that exits the spinal canal through the intervertebral foramen for that side (Crossman, 2000; Fix, 2005). Each spinal nerve innervates specific muscles (the myotome for that level) and specific areas of the skin (the dermatome for that level).

Upon exiting the spinal canal, the spinal nerves arising from the C5 through T1 segments of the spinal cord join to form the brachial plexus. Within the brachial plexus, the nerve fibers associated with different cord segments intermingle and redistribute before passing into the peripheral nerves that innervate the shoulder girdle and upper extremities. Spinal nerves arising from the T12 through S4 segments of the cord join to form the lumbosacral plexus (also referred to as the lumbar and sacral plexuses), where they intermingle and redistribute before passing into the peripheral nerves that innervate the pelvic girdle and lower extremities (Crossman, 2000; Martini, 2005). Spinal nerves arising from the T2 through T12 segments of the cord do not pass through a plexus en route to the periphery and primarily innervate structures of the trunk (Martini, 2005).

A **lower motor neuron (LMN) lesion** refers to damage to the anterior horn cells of the spinal cord, motor neurons of the brainstem, or motor portions of peripheral nerves; it causes a syndrome of symptoms including motor weakness and decreased or absent muscle tone and reflexes. Injury to the gray matter of the spinal cord, a single ventral nerve root, spinal nerve, plexus, or named peripheral nerve causes unilateral weakness, a loss of sensation, and a decrease in spinal reflexes. The extent of the neural lesion dictates the severity of the weakness, loss of sensation, or decrease in reflexes. A complete injury in the peripheral nervous system results in local weakness that is unilateral, unlike the bilateral symptoms of a complete injury in the central nervous system spinal cord. In addition, the peripheral nervous system is capable of some regeneration depending on the extent of the lesion, so paralysis may not be permanent.

## Excitation/Inhibition of Alpha Motor Neurons

In the central nervous system, every neuron typically receives input from several other neurons (presynaptic neurons), each of which either facilitates or inhibits the activity of the postsynaptic neuron. If the postsynaptic neuron receives more inhibitory input than excitatory input at a given time, the net effect is inhibition: the postsynaptic neuron will not generate an action potential. If the neuron receives more excitation than inhibition and if the net effect is enough to depolarize the neuron to threshold, the neuron will fire.

Active motion of the limbs and trunk occurs as a result of firing of alpha motor neurons in the ventral horns of the spinal cord. These neurons receive input from a variety of other neurons, including those carrying input from the cerebral cortex and brainstem. The descending input from the supraspinal structures, which includes both excitation and inhibition, is necessary for refinement of voluntary movement and maintenance of balance and posture.

Although supraspinal input is essential for normal motor control, spinal-level circuitry also plays an important role. Alpha motor neurons receive input from sensory neurons that innervate muscle spindles (Iyer, 1999). This input is important in the regulation of muscle force during motor tasks. Some control and coordination of normal movement also occurs through the activity of interneurons. These neurons, which can be either excitatory or inhibitory, provide connections within a single level of the cord as well as communication between multiple levels. The activity of interneurons is influenced by input from sensory neurons innervating the muscle spindles, Golgi tendon organs, and skin, as well as by input from neurons in descending tracts carrying motor commands from the brain. Interneurons in turn influence the activity of alpha motor neurons, contributing to muscle force regulation and reflexive coordination of the activity of different muscle groups (Kiernan, 2005).

In summary, the activity of a given motor neuron is influenced both by descending input from the brain and by spinal-level circuitry. Whether a particular alpha motor neuron fires at a given time depends on the combined effect of all of the inhibitory and excitatory input from supraspinal and spinal sources converging on the neuron at that time.

## Lifespan Influence

### Developmental Considerations

Early in the course of nervous system formation in the developing embryo, the cells that will eventually form the nervous system consist of a layer of cells called the *neural plate* or *neuroectoderm*. The lateral aspects of the neural plate elevate, thicken, move medially, and fuse to form the neural tube, which eventually develops into the spinal cord and brain. Neural tube formation begins in the middle region of the neural plate and proceeds rostrally and caudally toward the two ends. The neural tube remains open at its ends for a short time, but it eventually closes during normal embryonic development. When the caudal aspect of the neural tube fails to close, the result is spina bifida (Cabana, 1999). Spina bifida results in varying degrees of motor and sensory deficits and can cause complete paralysis, depending on the extent of the neural tube defect.

During the formation of the neural tube, cells in the neural plate also form an adjacent structure called the *neural crest*. The neural crest eventually develops into the peripheral nervous system. Cranial and spinal sensory ganglia may originate from other embryonic tissues (Cabana, 1999).

### Age-Related Changes Relevant to Complete Paralysis

Trauma, the most frequent cause of SCI and thus the most frequent cause of complete paralysis, occurs most frequently in young males between the ages of 16 and 30 years (Nobunaga, 1999; NSCISC, 2016, 2017). The average age at injury has steadily risen in recent years. Since the 1970s, the average age of injury has risen from 29 years to 42 years (NSCISC, 2017). The cause traumatic spinal cord damage varies with age; people who are older at the time of injury are more likely to be injured in falls or from medical or surgical causes and are less likely to be injured in acts of violence or sporting activities (McGlinchey-Berroth, 1995; Nobunaga, 1999; NSCISC, 2016, 2017). Younger individuals are more likely to be injured as a result of violence or vehicular crashes (NSCISC, 2016, 2017).

One explanation for the prevalence of spinal cord damage in older individuals after a fall is preexisting cervical spine osteoarthritis. Osteoarthritis can cause narrowing of the spinal canal, decreasing the space that allows movement and increasing the risk of cord damage during a fall. In older individuals, even minimal trauma can result in an SCI (McKinley, 1999a). For example, 56% of older people who sustained SCIs in falls did so in falls down stairs or from a sitting or standing position, whereas 83% of younger people with fall-related SCIs fell from a greater height, such as from a building (McGlinchey-Berroth, 1995).

Neurological damage and outcomes also differ depending on the age of the individual. Cervical injuries are more prevalent among older people who sustain cord injuries, as are neurologically incomplete injuries (McGlinchey-Berroth, 1995; Nobunaga, 1999; NSCISC, 2016, 2017). Among people with paralysis resulting from an SCI, those who are younger typically have better outcomes. Advanced age at time of injury is associated with high rates of medical complications (Alander, 1997; Chen, 1999; McKinley, 1999a) and mortality (DeVivo, 1992, 1999).

The higher rates of morbidity and mortality in older individuals most likely result, at least in part, from a higher incidence of premorbid pathologies such as cardiovascular disease and diabetes. In addition, numerous physical changes associated with normal aging are particularly problematic when coupled with damage to the spinal cord. For example, normal aging is associated with reductions in muscle strength and endurance, bone mass, cardiac output, vital capacity, and skin thickness and elasticity (Bottomley, 2003; Waters, 2001). All these systems are negatively affected by spinal cord damage. The combination of the sequelae of spinal cord damage with normal age-related changes appears to increase vulnerability to medical and orthopedic complications. Simply stated, older individuals usually do not possess as much reserve in these systems. Damage to the spinal cord, an injury presenting a significant challenge to many of the body's systems, rapidly depletes any existing reserve, more easily resulting in impairment and ultimately death.

Advanced age at the time of an SCI is also associated with decreased functional outcomes (Alander, 1997; Penrod, 1990; Roth, 1990). Poorer functional outcomes are thought to result from the interaction between age-related changes and the physical demands of rehabilitation and functional activities after an SCI. Reductions in respiratory reserve, endurance, and muscle strength significantly affect functional status. Pathologies and impairments such as arthritis, rotator cuff tears, and carpal tunnel syndrome are likely to interfere with use of the upper extremities in the performance of transfers, wheelchair propulsion, and ambulation with an assistive device. With the exception of ambulation with assistive devices, these are activities that an individual with complete paralysis of the lower extremities will need in order to resume functional independence.

Although greater age at injury is associated with more medical problems, some orthopedic complications of injury are more common in younger people. Injury at an earlier age has been associated with a higher prevalence of spinal deformity (Levi, 1995b) and greater severity of spinal deformity (Bergstrom, 1999). The development of spinal deformity appears to be a greater risk when the injury occurs before the individual reaches skeletal maturity (Vogel, 1997). In addition, hip contractures, subluxations, and dislocations are common in people who were injured as children (Vogel, 1997).

An SCI also shortens life expectancy, though the amount of decrease depends on the level of injury and the ability to survive the first year after injury (NSCISC, 2016, 2017). For example, a 20 year-old without an SCI has a life expectancy of 59.6 additional years. In contrast, a 20 year-old who sustains an SCI resulting in paraplegia and survives the first 24 hours has a life expectancy of approximately 45.9 additional years; this drops to 40.3 additional years for a 20 year-old with low tetraplegia and to 34 additional years for a 20 year-old with high tetraplegia (NSCISC, 2017). When a person sustains an SCI at any level at age 20 years and is ventilator dependent after 1 year of recovery, life expectancy is approximately 18.1 additional years.

Surviving the first year after an SCI increases additional life expectancy at all levels of injury, though not equivalent to the number of years expected without an SCI. On average, surviving the first year after injury increases life expectancy by 1 to 5 years beyond the life expectancy of individuals who survive the first 24 hours. Even when survival during the first year after an SCI is factored in, life expectancy for those with paraplegia or tetraplegia and for those with ventilator dependency is just 14% to 78% of that for persons without an SCI, with paraplegia being closest to the norm (NSCISC, 2016, 2017).

### Aging With a Spinal Cord Injury

Life expectancy after an SCI is increasing, a major change compared with SCI statistics 6 to 7 decades ago. Life expectancy after an SCI used to be stated in months rather than years, and living longer than 2 years after an SCI was rare. Most persons with an SCI acquired septic infections or renal failure, which contributed to their death. A commonly reported early reference to SCI, written approximately 5000 years ago by an Egyptian physician, stated that the condition was "an ailment not to be treated." At the time, persons with sudden paralysis and sensory loss simply died soon after injury. Today, persons with an SCI receive better initial care and advanced medical management, though there is still much to discover and to perfect. Living longer after an SCI has raised new issues related to aging with the injury.

The demands on the body after an SCI are numerous. To function, persons must use the upper extremities for weight-bearing, straining the joints of the upper extremities. The paralyzed lower extremities and lower trunk no longer have normal neural or muscular function, resulting in osteopenia and risk of fracture. Contractures can easily develop from long-term sitting with limited mobility. Limited cardiovascular exercise in the years after an SCI can lead to cardiovascular disease.

When secondary conditions, such as osteopenia, contracture, and cardiovascular deconditioning, are combined with normal age-associated changes (discussed previously), the threshold for effects on functional abilities is lowered, making complications more likely. When a reduction in bone mass is combined with SCI-induced osteopenia, a lower extremity or spinal fracture is more likely. When a reduction in skin thickness and elasticity is combined with the relentlessly excessive skin pressures associated with long-term sitting, a pressure injury becomes more likely. When an age-associated decrease in cardiac output is combined with an all-too-common decrease in cardiovascular activity, cardiovascular disease is more likely. When a reduction in vital capacity is combined with a greater likelihood of being sedentary after an SCI, respiratory dysfunction and infection become more likely.

Aging with an SCI lowers the threshold for pathology affecting function. Indeed, it is common for a person with an SCI to have a history free of pressure injuries, only to acquire one 20 to 25 years after injury, despite no significant changes in seating system, functional activities, or sitting time. The risk of pressure injury development is stable over the first 10 years after the injury but increases as soon as 15 years after (Chen, 2005), most likely because the threshold for effect has been lowered by normal age-associated changes.

# ■ Related Pathology
## Complete Spinal Cord Injury

The anatomic feature of the spinal cord most relevant to understanding complete paralysis is its cephalocaudal organization. The axons of neurons carrying motor commands from the brain to the body descend in the spinal cord and terminate at cord levels specific to the structures they innervate. For example, neurons carrying motor commands to the upper extremities terminate in the cervical cord segments (brachial plexus). Those carrying motor commands to the trunk terminate in the thoracic and lumbar segments, and those carrying motor commands to the lower extremities terminate in the lumbar and sacral segments (lumbosacral plexus) of the spinal cord. The cord at any given level contains the tracts carrying motor and sensory information between the brain and all segments of the cord located below that level. Thus, the cervical portion of the spinal cord contains ascending and descending tracts innervating the upper extremities, trunk, and lower extremities. Areas of the cord caudal to the cervical region do not contain neurons innervating the upper extremities because these neurons terminate (i.e., they exit to the upper extremities) at those higher cord levels.

In this chapter, a *complete SCI* refers to a lesion in which the cross section of one or more spinal cord segments is completely damaged, preventing afferent or efferent impulses from traveling through it. This differs from the definition of complete SCI found in the international standards (ASIA, 2015). To facilitate understanding, this chapter uses the term "cross-sectionally complete" to indicate complete damage at a specific segmental level. A cross-sectionally **complete spinal cord injury** interrupts the communication between the brain and all structures innervated at and below the level of the lesion. The

resulting impairments include loss of voluntary motor function, abnormal muscle tone, sensory loss, disrupted autonomic function, impaired breathing and coughing, and bladder and bowel incontinence. Secondary complications, such as osteoporosis and heterotopic ossification, are numerous.

### Loss of Voluntary Motor Function

With a cross-sectionally complete SCI, voluntary motor function is typically normal above the level of the lesion and absent in areas innervated by lower cord levels. Table 26-2 presents the ISNCSCI key muscles associated with the different levels of the spinal cord.

In an SCI, muscles in a transitional area, which are often innervated at or just below the neurological level of injury, display impaired strength (less than 5/5 in a manual muscle test) but not absent strength. For example, an individual with complete C6 tetraplegia (**ASIA Impairment Scale** A) could have manual muscle test results of 5/5 in the elbow flexors, 4/5 in the radial wrist extensors, 1/5 in the triceps, and 0/5 in all muscles innervated below that point. With complete injuries, cord levels below the neurological level of injury that retain partial motor or sensory function are termed the "**zone of partial preservation.**" In this example, the zone of partial preservation includes the C7 level.

Cross-sectionally complete spinal cord injuries can also result in a region of asymmetrical muscle strength close to the level of the lesion. For example, an individual with L3 paraplegia could have quadriceps strength of 4/5 on the left and 3/5 on the right and anterior tibialis strength of 2/5 on the left and 0/5 on the right.

### Abnormal Muscle Tone

Damage to the spinal cord can cause elevated muscle tone, flaccid paralysis, or both. The cause of spasticity after a nervous system lesion is not fully understood at this time (Priebe, 2002). Elevated muscle tone is thought to result from damage to the descending tracts in the cord and presents as spasticity,

| **TABLE 26-2** | ISNCSCI Key Muscles Associated With the Different Levels of the Spinal Cord |
|---|---|
| **SEGMENTAL LEVEL** | **MUSCLE GROUP** |
| C5 | Elbow flexors |
| C6 | Wrist extensors |
| C7 | Elbow extensors |
| C8 | Long finger flexors |
| T1 | Fifth finger abductors |
| L2 | Hip flexors |
| L3 | Knee extensors |
| L4 | Ankle dorsiflexors |
| L5 | Long toe extensors |
| S1 | Ankle plantar flexors |

muscle spasms, clonus, and increased deep tendon reflexes (DTRs) in muscles innervated by segments caudal to the lesion, which are released from cerebral control. This cluster of signs, accompanied by weakness and loss of sensation, indicates a UMN lesion. (In contrast to the spasticity of cerebral injuries, which are accompanied by movements characterized by abnormal synergies, a complete SCI results in spasticity accompanied by complete paralysis, or absence of voluntary movement.) Elevated muscle tone is more prevalent in people with cervical and upper thoracic lesions and in people with incomplete lesions (Little, 1999; Maynard, 1990). Because incomplete lesions are most common after a traumatic SCI (NSCISC, 2017), most persons with an SCI do experience spasticity.

Flaccidity, an absence of muscle tone, presents with absent DTRs and absent reflexive responses (resistance) to passive stretch. Flaccid paralysis is typical of an LMN lesion and occurs frequently with lesions of the conus medullaris, cauda equina, or peripheral nerves (Maynard, 1990; Siegel, 2006). People with lesions higher in the spinal cord can also have flaccid paralysis of muscles innervated by segments at the level of the neurological lesion because of damage to the gray matter of the anterior horn cells and/or nerve roots, particularly when broad sections of the spinal cord are affected. These same individuals may also experience spasticity below the level of the lesion, where the anterior horn cells and nerve roots are more likely to be intact, along with the intact spinal reflex loop of the spinal cord (Berman, 1996).

### Sensory Impairments

A cross-sectionally complete SCI, in which the cross section of the spinal cord is completely damaged at one or more segmental levels, causes a loss of all sensory modalities in areas of the body innervated below and/or at the level of the lesion. As is true with motor function, a transitional area is often innervated at or just below the neurological level of injury and displays impaired, but not entirely absent, sensation. This impairment can be in the form of either diminished sensory ability or hyperesthesia. Unfortunately, pain, may emanate from partially intact segments or manifest as neurogenic pain, affecting 65% of those with an SCI (Siddall, 2001).

### Disruption of Autonomic Function

The spinal cord is also integral to the autonomic nervous system, which is involved in the regulation of many of the body's involuntary functions. The autonomic system includes two divisions, the sympathetic and parasympathetic systems. Supraspinal control of both the sympathetic and parasympathetic systems involves structures in the brainstem. In the sympathetic system, these supraspinal structures communicate with preganglionic cells in the thoracic and upper lumbar regions of the spinal cord (T1 to L2 or L3). All sympathetic outflow arises from these cells. Preganglionic cells of the parasympathetic system are located in two areas: the brain and the sacral (S2 to S4) region of the spinal cord. The cranial portion of the parasympathetic system provides outflow to structures in the head, thorax, and abdomen. The

sacral parasympathetic preganglionic cells innervate pelvic structures, including the urinary system, lower colon, anal sphincter, and genital/reproductive system.

Normal autonomic control involves balanced and coordinated functioning of the sympathetic and parasympathetic systems. A complete SCI disrupts descending input from the brain to the preganglionic autonomic cells located in the cord caudal to the lesion. Damage to the preganglionic cells in the cord also disrupts the spinal-level autonomic reflexes controlled by these cells. The autonomic effects of an SCI depend on the location of the lesion relative to the thoracolumbar and sacral areas of the cord. Cervical and upper thoracic injuries (generally those above the T6 neurological level) impair the body's ability to respond appropriately to a sympathetic surge from a noxious stimulus, resulting in sympathetic dominance below the level of the lesion but parasympathetic dominance above, a condition called *autonomic dysreflexia* (Campagnolo, 2002b), as defined earlier. These individuals experience the occurrence of hypertension combined with bradycardia and headache, sweating, and flushing of the skin above the lesion. Persons with low thoracic or lumbar injuries generally do not experience this imbalance.

### Impairment of Breathing and Coughing

Breathing involves the action of a variety of muscles innervated by different levels of the spinal cord. The most important muscle involved in inhalation is the diaphragm, which is innervated by the C3, C4, and C5 segments. Other muscles that participate in inhalation include the intercostal muscles (T1 to T11 innervation) and a variety of accessory muscles (supraspinal, cervical, and thoracic innervation). Abdominal muscles (T6 to L1 innervation) contribute to inhalation by supporting the diaphragm in an optimal position for function (Lanig, 2000; Martini, 2005; Somers, 2010.

Exhalation during quiet breathing occurs as a result of passive recoil of the rib cage and diaphragm. Eccentric contraction of the diaphragm slows the rate of air leaving the lungs during quiet exhalation. Forced exhalation, as occurs with coughing or during exercise, primarily involves contraction of the abdominals. Additional muscles supporting forced exhalation include the intercostals, quadratus lumborum (T12 to L4 innervation), and serratus posterior inferior (T9 to T12 innervation) (Frownfelter, 2006; Lanig, 2000; Martini, 2005).

The effects of spinal cord damage on breathing and coughing ability depend on the neurological level of injury. The severity of impairment ranges from total loss of breathing and coughing ability in people with high cervical lesions to no impairment of breathing or coughing in people with lumbar or sacral lesions (Lanig, 2000; Winslow, 2003; Zimmer, 2007). Individuals with complete injuries above C3 experience paralysis of the primary muscle of inspiration, the diaphragm. As a result, these individuals are dependent on mechanical ventilation for all breathing.

Following the international standards of ASIA, designation of a neurological level of injury implies sparing of that level and damage to the levels below (ASIA, 2015). Individuals with neurological level of injury at C3 or C4 have partial innervation of the diaphragm and may not require mechanical ventilation during at least a portion of a 24-hour period. For individuals with neurological level of injury at C5 and below, the primary inspiratory muscle is fully innervated, but accessory muscles and muscles used during forced expiration may be impaired. Combined with postural changes (i.e., the inability to maintain an upright posture), respiratory reserve, tidal volume, and the ability to clear respiratory secretions all decrease. Respiratory complications are among the most common causes of death after an SCI (NSCISC, 2016). Therefore, respiratory management techniques are vital for the person with an SCI (CSCM, 2005b). A complete description of respiratory management is outside the scope of this chapter.

### Bladder and Bowel Incontinence

Neurological control of bladder function normally involves sacral (S2 to S4) parasympathetic reflexes and supraspinal control. A complete SCI disrupts the communication between the brain and the sacral cord, causing loss of voluntary bladder control (Benevento, 2002). Subsequent bladder function will depend on the integrity of the sacral reflex arc. If it is intact, the bladder will empty reflexively each time it reaches a critical level of fullness. If sacral function is impaired, the bladder will remain flaccid, and high volumes of urine can accumulate without reflexive emptying.

Neurological control of bowel function normally involves a combination of autonomic reflexes, enteric reflexes (i.e., the gastrointestinal tract has its own primitive nervous system, which contributes to the control of peristalsis and evacuation), and supraspinal control. A cross-sectionally complete SCI disrupts the communication between the brain and the sacral cord, causing a loss of voluntary bowel control. Similar to bladder function after spinal cord damage, bowel movements can occur reflexively when the sacral reflex arc remains intact. When the sacral reflex arc is disrupted, reflex evacuation will not occur.

Individuals with a cross-sectionally complete SCI need to manage bowel and bladder function differently than those without an SCI. Most often, intermittent catheterization four to six times per day is used for bladder management, especially for those with a spastic bladder (Benevento, 2002). Bowel management programs typically include digital stimulation of the rectum with use of suppositories. Bowel and bladder management techniques are crucial to prevent a variety of secondary conditions, including infections, kidney damage, chronic constipation, and skin breakdown, and minimize peer-rejection and other negative aspects of the social environment (CSCM, 1998b, 2006).

For more information, refer to other texts specifically on SCI management, including specific descriptions of bowel and bladder management techniques.

## Neurological Return

Resumption of motor or sensory function that was absent after an SCI is called *neurological recovery* or *neurological return*. Most return occurs during the first year after injury (Ditunno, 1992; Waters, 1994a, 1994b), with the speed of recovery being greatest during the first 6 months (Ditunno, 1992). After that point, the rate of motor and sensory improvement is more likely to be slow, and the extent of additional return is likely to decrease. By 12 to 18 months after injury, most individuals have reached a plateau, and additional neurological recovery is most often limited (Burns, 2001). However, neurological return has been reported as late as 5 or more years after an SCI (Piepmeier, 1988).

The extent of neurological return occurring after an SCI is highly variable. Some individuals do not regain any motor or sensory function. Others experience minimal return, regaining sensation only, anal sphincter control but no use of any trunk or limb muscles, or minimal voluntary motor function in a small number of muscles. At the other extreme, a few individuals regain normal sensation and full use of their musculature. The degree of neurological return that an individual experiences certainly depends on the cross-sectional extent and location of damage to the spinal cord.

Immediately after an SCI, it is impossible to determine exactly how much return will occur. The following factors have been associated with an improved prognosis for major motor return: an incomplete injury (Burns, 2001); preservation of motor or sensory function below the lesion at hospital admission after the injury (Ditunno, 1995; Mange, 1990), 72 hours after injury (Burns, 2001; Wu, 1992), or 1 month after injury (Burns, 2001; Waters, 1995); and preservation of pinprick sensation in the sacral region or the extremities (Waters, 1994b). Neurological return is also more likely when the SCI was the result of a fall as opposed to other etiologies (Nobunaga, 1999).

In general, lack of neurological return in the days immediately after an SCI usually results in a poorer long-term prognosis for return. Eighty percent to 90% of complete injuries at 1 week after injury remain complete (CSCM, 1999).

## Incomplete Spinal Cord Injury

Not all SCIs cause complete paralysis; approximately 66% of traumatic injuries are **incomplete SCIs** (NSCISC, 2017) with only partial damage of the spinal cord at the level of the lesion. With partial damage, some communication remains between the brain and areas of the body innervated by cord levels caudal to the lesion. The cross-sectional spatial organization of the spinal cord (Fig. 26-3) is relevant to understanding the impairments that result from an incomplete SCI. The motor and sensory impairments resulting from an incomplete injury depend on the cross-sectional location of the cord damage. Table 26-3 presents the motor and sensory impairments typical of three incomplete SCI syndromes.

In addition to causing sensory and voluntary motor deficits, incomplete SCI can cause many of the impairments and secondary complications associated with complete SCIs (described earlier in this chapter). The severity of the impairments varies with the extent and level of the lesion. In general, the greater the cross-sectional area of damage, the greater the effects of the injury at that level and potentially caudal to that level.

| TABLE 26-3 | Incomplete Spinal Cord Injury Syndromes |
|---|---|

| SYNDROME | IMAGE | SYMPTOMS (DAMAGED STRUCTURES) |
|---|---|---|
| Central cord syndrome | 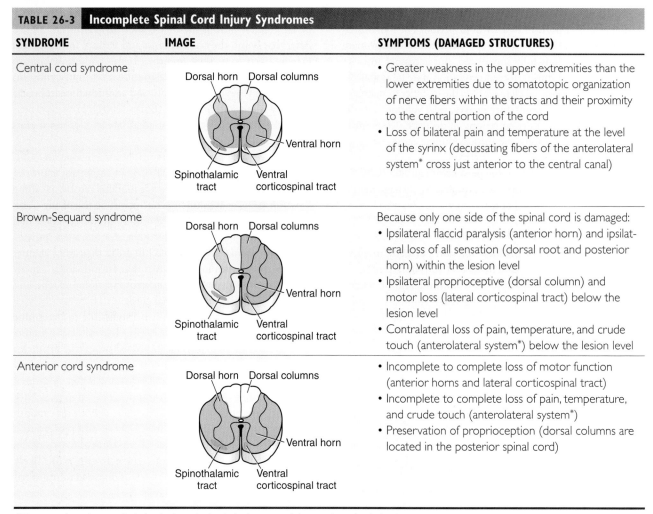 | • Greater weakness in the upper extremities than the lower extremities due to somatotopic organization of nerve fibers within the tracts and their proximity to the central portion of the cord<br>• Loss of bilateral pain and temperature at the level of the syrinx (decussating fibers of the anterolateral system* cross just anterior to the central canal) |
| Brown-Sequard syndrome | | Because only one side of the spinal cord is damaged:<br>• Ipsilateral flaccid paralysis (anterior horn) and ipsilateral loss of all sensation (dorsal root and posterior horn) within the lesion level<br>• Ipsilateral proprioceptive (dorsal column) and motor loss (lateral corticospinal tract) below the lesion level<br>• Contralateral loss of pain, temperature, and crude touch (anterolateral system*) below the lesion level |
| Anterior cord syndrome | | • Incomplete to complete loss of motor function (anterior horns and lateral corticospinal tract)<br>• Incomplete to complete loss of pain, temperature, and crude touch (anterolateral system*)<br>• Preservation of proprioception (dorsal columns are located in the posterior spinal cord) |

*The anterolateral system includes the lateral spinothalamic tract and the anterior spinothalamic tract.

## Spinal Shock

Immediately after spinal cord damage, spinal-level reflexes are absent or depressed below the level of injury (Atkinson, 1996; Ditunno, 2004). This cessation or depression of reflexes, called **spinal shock**, can occur with complete or incomplete lesions (Ko, 1999). Spinal shock typically begins to resolve within a few days after the spinal cord is injured (Ko,1999), but it can take months to resolve completely (Little, 1999). Resolution of spinal shock is heralded by the return of reflexive functioning in portions of the body innervated below the lesion. When the cord injury is incomplete, the individual also experiences a resumption of sensation, voluntary motor function, or both as spinal shock resolves. With a complete SCI, the resolution of spinal shock is indicated by the appearance of spinal reflexes and UMN signs below the level of the lesion.

## Peripheral Nerve Injury

Paralysis can also be caused by damage to the peripheral nervous system, with injury occurring at any point between the nerve root and the distal end of a peripheral nerve. Complete bilateral paralysis does not occur with a single peripheral neuropathy. In a peripheral nerve injury, motor and sensory functions are lost in the muscles and dermatomes innervated by the injured nerve or nerves. Peripheral nerve injuries result in an LMN injury and differ from spinal cord damage in several ways (Smith, 2003; Stockert, 2007):

1. Because the axons of neurons associated with different cord segments intermingle and redistribute between the spinal cord and the peripheral nerves, the patterns of motor and sensory impairments resulting from peripheral nerve damage are quite different from those caused by spinal cord damage. However, damage to nerve roots or the cauda equina result in motor and sensory impairments consistent with segmental innervation.
2. Peripheral nerve injuries cause impairments on one side of the body and typically in one limb rather than in multiple extremities and the trunk.
3. Peripheral nerve injuries are not associated with the global physiological changes that result from spinal cord damage because they do not interfere with the autonomic system's control of the cardiovascular system and viscera.
4. Damaged peripheral nerves can regenerate, depending on the severity of the injury. Peripheral nerve injuries

involving the outer coverings of the nerve (i.e., the endoneurium and myelin) are more likely to recover function than an injury involving the outer coverings and the internal axon. Regardless, the prognosis for return of strength and sensation in affected areas is greater after a peripheral nerve injury than after an SCI because of the ability to regenerate.

5. Peripheral nerve injuries disrupt the reflex arc, resulting in hypotonia or flaccidity. SCIs that leave the reflex arc intact lead to hypertonia or spasticity.

6. Complex regional pain syndrome (CRPS), formerly referred to as *reflex sympathetic dystrophy,* is thought to represent a reflex neurogenic inflammation in which the sympathetic nervous system is hyperactive. Patients with CRPS experience burning pain, hyperalgesia, edema, and trophic skin changes in the affected area.

Complete bilateral paralysis cannot occur with a single peripheral neuropathy. However, **polyneuropathy,** a condition with simultaneous functional disruption of many nerves, can cause complete bilateral paralysis when the damage is extensive enough. Interventions may be similar to those for complete paralysis resulting from an SCI, as described in this chapter. For interventions after a single peripheral nerve injury, see Chapter 22.

## Other Medical Causes of Complete Paralysis

### Nontraumatic SCI

Spinal cord damage can result from a variety of causes. In the United States, SCIs occur most frequently as a result of motor vehicle crashes, followed by falls, acts of violence, recreational sporting activities, and other causes (NSCISC, 2016, 2017). Although most spinal cord damage occurs as a result of trauma, it can also result from infection, spinal stenosis, vascular accident, surgery, tumors, transverse myelitis, or syringomyelia (McKinley, 1999b, 2001; New, 2002). Medical diagnoses include anterior cord syndrome, central cord syndrome, and Brown-Séquard syndrome described in Table 26-3.

### Peripheral Nerve Injury

Traumatic injury to peripheral nerves caused by compression, tension, or ischemia can be categorized according to the classic work of Sneddon (1943) and later modified by Sunderland (1978). **Neurapraxia** is the mildest injury, involving demyelination of the nerve while the axon remains intact. In neurapraxia, the muscle may be weak or paralyzed, but atrophy is not expected and regeneration or remyelination is probable in the absence of other disease. **Axonotmesis** is more severe, with injury to the axon while the outer coverings of the nerve—the myelin and endoneurium—remain intact. In this injury, the axon undergoes Wallerian degeneration before regeneration occurs. Weakness or paralysis is expected with atrophy of the muscle. In the absence of disease, the axon may grow back but may not always grow to replicate the original axon. **Neurotmesis** is the most severe peripheral nerve injury in which the axon is severed and the connective tissue coverings are disrupted. Again, in the absence of

disease, regeneration is possible in neurotmesis but not as likely or as effective as in neurapraxia or axonotmesis. Complete paralysis from an injury to multiple peripheral nerves may result in functional limitations similar to those caused by an SCI. Individuals with neurotmesis are not likely to experience neurological recovery and may need training in compensatory movements for permanent losses, as described later in this chapter.

### Other Diagnoses/Conditions Resulting in Complete Paralysis

Other pathologies can result in complete paralysis, including those involving the peripheral and central nervous system. Guillain-Barré syndrome was originally described by and named for the French neurologists who published case reports describing a syndrome of flaccid paralysis and areflexia (Burns, 2008). It has many variants, including acute inflammatory demyelinating polyneuropathy and chronic inflammatory demyelinating polyneuropathy, and is thought to result from an autoimmune reaction. Flaccid paralysis can be permanent, though the likelihood of permanency is related to the severity and chronicity of the disease. Polio, a viral infection of the anterior horn cells in the spinal cord, results in cell death and permanent flaccid paralysis of the muscles innervated by the neurological segment when all motor units to that muscle are destroyed (Smith, 2003). Other peripheral nervous system lesions that can result in complete paralysis include Charcot-Marie-Tooth disease, diabetic neuropathy, and critical illness polyneuropathy. All these causes of total paralysis result in symptoms consistent with an LMN lesion: areflexia, flaccid paralysis, and muscular atrophy. Rehabilitation of complete paralysis from any of these pathologies is similar, assuming the paralysis is stable and nonprogressive.

In the central nervous system, severe stroke—either in the brain or brainstem—can result in complete paralysis when the corticospinal tract is damaged. Again, the principles of rehabilitation are similar and are reviewed later in this chapter. An exception is a stroke in the brain, which causes hemiplegia, not paraplegia or tetraplegia. Interventions for hemiplegia are the subjects of other chapters in this text.

Another cause of complete paralysis is amyotrophic lateral sclerosis (ALS), a degenerative motor neuron disease that typically results in mixed features of UMN and LMN lesions. Death from the most common form of ALS typically occurs 2 to 5 years after diagnosis (Fuller, 2003). Because of the degenerative and progressive nature of the disease, principles of management for ALS are different from those described for complete paralysis in this chapter.

## ■ Pertinent Examination/Evaluation

Examination is the first step in the development of an appropriate physical therapy plan of care. During the examination, the patient's history is acquired, a systems review is performed, and specific tests and measures are administered as indicated by the history and the findings of the systems review (American Physical Therapy Association [APTA], 2014). After the examination is complete, the results are evaluated, a diagnosis and prognosis are established, and a plan of care specific to the patient is determined. The plan of care includes goals collaboratively established with the patient. For patients with complete paralysis related to an SCI, the standardized *ISNCSCI* examination (ASIA, 2015; NSCISC, 2017), explained in Chapters 5 and 6 (see Fig. 5-11), is performed. Further information on SCIs can be found in the SCI diagnosis outline in the online (ONL) compendium.

## Primary Tests and Measures

Table 26-4 lists the primary tests and measures that may be included in the examination of a patient with complete paralysis. Detailed descriptions of tests and measures for sensory, musculoskeletal, balance, and functional status are provided in Chapters 3 through 13. The systematic examination in the *ISNCSCI* (see Fig. 5-11) should be performed in addition to the examination areas included in Table 26-4. The ISNCSCI examination is standardized and allows the patient's neurological injury and prognosis to be compared with outcomes data compiled by the NSCISC (ASIA, 2015; NSCISC, 2016, 2017). Examples of specific tests and measures conducted with persons with complete paralysis resulting from an SCI include the Functional Independence Measure, the Walking Index for Spinal Cord Injury, the Spinal Cord Independence Measure, the Spinal Cord Injury Functional Ambulation Inventory, and the Wheelchair Skills Test (WST) (Alm, 2008; ANPT, 2013; Curtis, 1995; Ditunno, 2005; Kirby, 2016; Marino, 2005).

## Goals and Expected Outcomes

Throughout the process of the examination and evaluation, focus should remain on the central question of physical therapy: What is the relationships between the patient's impairments and functional limitations (APTA, 2014)? The therapist should help the patient discern which impairments interfere with his functional abilities and which of these functional limitations can be ameliorated or remediated through therapeutic interventions.

When setting goals as part of the plan of care, the therapist should keep in mind the outcomes that the patient can be reasonably expected to achieve (prognosis), taking into account the impairments and other relevant factors identified during the examination. When working with a patient with an SCI, the therapist needs to at least determine a rudimentary prognosis based on initial examination using the *ISNCSCI* examination. General prognostic rules need to be remembered, as discussed in Table 2-1, and the following principle specific for SCI should be considered: Injuries complete at 1 week are likely to remain complete. Most neurological recovery in incomplete injury will take place in the first 6 months after an SCI. For peripheral nerve injuries, recovery depends on the extent of the initial injury. A person with an injury that spares the axon is more likely to experience regeneration than a person with a transection injury of the nerve. For persons with complete paralysis resulting from diseases such as Guillain-Barré syndrome, these prognostic rules may not apply.

Table 26-5 presents the functional outcomes typical for people with complete SCIs at different levels. These outcomes

| TABLE 26-4 | Commonly Used Tests and Measures in Complete Paralysis From a Spinal Cord Injury |
|---|---|
| **CLINICAL TEST OR MEASURE** | **CLINICAL REASONING OR INFORMATION PROVIDED** |
| Hoffman sign and/or Babinski test | Helps determine the presence of upper motor neuron lesion |
| Dermatome testing | Provides sensory distribution of lesion and can help determine sensory level |
| Myotome testing | Provides motor distribution of lesion and can help determine motor level |
| Beevor sign | Indicates weakness of the lower abdominal muscles if the navel moves toward the head while the neck is flexed. |
| Reflex testing | Helps determine presence of reflex arc, including afferent and efferent components, at specific segmental levels |
| Muscle tone | Provides information regarding resting state of the muscle and potential effect of muscle tone on movement |
| Range of motion | Provides information to determine utility of joint for functional activities |
| Skin integrity | Indicates if skin is intact (vital for individuals with complete paralysis to detect and manage pressure injury) |
| Breathing and coughing | Evaluates ability to breathe and cough (an important functional skill to minimize respiratory complications) |
| Functional skills:<br>  Mat and bed skills<br>  Transfers<br>  Wheelchair skills<br>  Ambulation/walking<br>  Instruction of others | Determines need for improvement, compensation, or development to prepare the individual for maximized functional independence after injury and defines the starting point for functional activity interventions; examples of specific tests and measures appropriate for use with persons with complete paralysis resulting from spinal cord injury include the Functional Independence Measure (FIM), the Walking Index for Spinal Cord Injury (WISCI), the Spinal Cord Independence Measure (SCIM), the Spinal Cord Injury Functional Ambulation Inventory (SCI-FAI), and the Wheelchair Skills Test (WST) |

| TABLE 26-5 | **Expected Functional Outcomes After Complete Spinal Cord Injury** | | | | |
|---|---|---|---|---|---|
| **NEUROLOGICAL LEVEL OF INJURY** | **MUSCLES INTACT** | **BED MOBILITY** | **TRANSFERS** | **WHEELCHAIR MOBILITY** | **STANDING AND/OR AMBULATION** |
| C1–C3 | Sternocleidomastoid; cervical paraspinal; neck accessory | Total assist | Total assist | **Power:** Independent with adapted drive[1] **Manual:** Total assist | None, though tilt table may be used |
| C4 | As in C3 plus upper trapezius; diaphragm | Total assist | Total assist | **Power:** As in C3 **Manual:** Total assist | None, though tilt table may be used |
| C5 | As in C4 plus deltoid, biceps, brachialis, brachioradialis, rhomboids, partial serratus anterior | Some assist (using power bed functions and/or side rails) | Total assist | **Power:** Independent with adapted arm drive control **Manual:** Some independence on level surfaces[2] | No functional ambulation, though standing frame or tilt table may be used |
| C6 | As in C5 plus extensor carpi radialis longus and brevis, serratus anterior, latissimus dorsi | Some assist (using power bed functions and/or side rails); may use full to king standard bed | **Level:** some assist to independent **Uneven:** Some assist to total assist | **Power:** Independent with standard arm drive **Manual:** Independent indoors; some assist outdoors[2] | No functional ambulation, though standing frame or tilt table may be used |
| C7–C8 | As in C6 plus pectoralis, triceps, pronator quadratus, extensor carpi ulnaris, flexor carpi radialis, finger flexors, abductor pollicis, some lumbricals | Independent to some assist (full power bed or full to king standard bed) | **Level:** Independent **Uneven:** Independent to some assist | **Manual:** Independent indoors and on level outdoor surfaces; some assist with uneven surfaces | No functional ambulation, though standing frame or standing wheelchair may be used |
| T1–T9 | As in C7–C8 plus hand and thumb intrinsics, intercostals, erector spinae | Independent (full to king standard bed) | Independent (may use sliding board) | Independent with lightweight manual wheelchair | Typically not functional ambulation, though standing frame or standing wheelchair may be used |
| T10–L1 | As in T1–T9 plus abdominals | Independent (full to king standard bed) | Independent | Independent indoors and outdoors | Independent in standing with frame OR walker with knee-ankle-foot orthoses; may ambulate functionally with some assist to independent |
| L2–S5 | As in T10–L1 plus fully intact abdominals and partially to fully intact LE | Independent | Independent | Independent | Independent (may use orthoses and/or gait aid) |

[1]Head, mouth, chin, or breath control drive mechanisms are most typical. Can also control power seat functions, such as tilt-in-space, to allow independence in pressure relief.

[2]Ultra-lightweight, rigid-framed, or folding wheelchair with handrim adaptations and cambered wheels.

Based on Consortium for Spinal Cord Medicine. Outcomes following traumatic spinal cord injury: clinical practice guidelines for health-care professionals. Available at: http://www.pve.org/publications/clinical-practic-guidelines. Published 1999. Accessed June 17, 2017.

reflect the functional status most individuals eventually achieve during or after rehabilitation. A given individual may have outcomes either worse or better than those listed depending on a variety of factors. Research has shown the following factors are associated with lower functional outcomes: advanced age, pressure injuries, spasticity, pain, and limitations in range of motion (Alander, 1997; Daverat, 1995; Penrod, 1990; Roth, 1990; Yarkony, 1995).

## PATIENT APPLICATION

*Mr. Johnson was transferred to the operating room of the hospital, where a posterior cervical fusion was performed on the last three cervical vertebrae. During the next 3 days, he had several postoperative complications, including a deep vein thrombosis. After 3 days of recovery, a consult for rehabilitation services was ordered.*

### Sensory Integrity

*Mr. Johnson does not have intact sensation or motor function in the lowest sacral segments. Your evaluation reveals he has abnormal light touch sensation, abnormal sharp/dull discrimination, abnormal deep pressure sensation, and abnormal proprioception in the dermatomes in the ulnar side of his hands and forearms and throughout his trunk and lower extremities. You perform the ISNCSCI examination, for which he scores a "zero" on the sensory tests of the key sensory points in these areas. The tests reveal that his sensation is normal on the key sensory points on the radial side of his hands and forearms as well as on the lateral portion of his upper arm, shoulder, neck, and head.*

### Motor Function and Muscle Performance

*Your testing reveals absent strength (zero on a 0 to 5 scale) in all lower extremity myotomes and key muscles. He has a very weak cough, nearly absent, and cannot participate in strength testing of the trunk muscles. In fact, he asks you to help him with an assisted cough during your examination. Due to orthopedic precautions prohibiting the application of resistance to the proximal upper extremity, strength testing was completed through active functional movement. Upper extremity strength appears to be fair to good strength in the deltoids and scapular elevators, as well as in the elbow flexors and wrist extensors; however, postsurgical neck pain limits his ability to perform a maximum voluntary contraction in these muscles. He has absent strength in his finger and wrist flexors, his elbow extensors, and all hand intrinsic muscles. He has very poor endurance of all intact muscles.*

### Range of Motion

*He displays passive range of motion within normal limits in all upper extremity joints, though his fingers and wrists are beginning to show end-range tightness. You cannot test his spinal joints, due to spinal precautions (cervical range of motion not appropriate). He has passive range of motion within normal limits in his hips and knees. He has bilateral passive ankle movement of 15 degrees dorsiflexion to 0-30 degrees plantarflexion.*

### Reflex Integrity

*You note absent L3 (patellar tendon) and S1 (Achilles tendon) DTRs. The C5 (biceps) DTR is normal, and the C6 (brachioradialis) and C7 (triceps) DTRs are hypoactive but present. He scores a zero on the Modified Ashworth Scale (MAS) in the lower extremities and fingers. DTRs are absent in the lower extremities. You rate his muscle tone as normal in the proximal upper extremities, moderately hypotonic in the distal upper extremities, and flaccid in the lower extremities.*

### Mental Functions

*You note that Mr. Johnson can participate in conversation, is alert and oriented to person, time, and place, and can recall events that have happened since his motor-vehicle accident. He does not remember the accident from his direct experience. Various family members and medical professionals have told him about it, and he can accurately recite those details. You recall that he was unconscious for a short time immediately after the accident.*

### Circulation

*Mr. Johnson has adequate tissue perfusion in his extremities.*

### Gait

*Mr. Johnson is not able to walk at this time. He also cannot rise from supine-to-sit and cannot sit independently at the edge of the bed. He tells you during your evaluation that he desperately wants to walk again but is concerned he may not be able to. Mr. Johnson has not yet been out of bed.*

### Integumentary Integrity

*Mr. Johnson has a 2-cm grade II sacral pressure injury and bilateral grade I calcaneal pressure injuries. Otherwise, his surgical incision is intact and healing well. He has no other skin issues.*

### Self-Care and Domestic Life

***Bed mobility, transfers and activities of daily living*** *have not yet been assessed.*

### Pain

*Mr. Johnson complains of lingering neck pain, especially after sitting with the head of the bed elevated for prolonged periods.*

### Environmental, Home, and Work Barriers

*Mr. Johnson is a laborer in the home construction trades. He tells you he would like to return to work after he starts to walk again.*

## Contemplate Clinical Decisions

- *What functional limitations does Mr. Johnson currently face?*
- *What are his impairments?*
- *What is the neurological level of injury?*
- *What are the functional expectations for Mr. Johnson, assuming his injury remains complete?*
- *Write at least two appropriate functional long-term goals for Mr. Johnson's plan of care.*

# ◾ Preparatory Interventions Specific to Complete Paralysis

## General Approaches

In the presence of complete and permanent paralysis, the goal of functional rehabilitation is compensation or substitution training rather than neural adaptation to the injury. When an individual has lost the use of a group of muscles and function in those muscles is not expected to return, he or she must learn new ways to perform functional tasks to maximize independence.

Individuals with complete paralysis may use the following strategies to maximize their functional independence: compensatory movement strategies, strengthening of spared/innervated musculature, development and preservation of range of motion, use of equipment, and application of a variety of preventive measures to avoid secondary impairments and pathologies. The following sections refer specifically to functional rehabilitation after a complete SCI as an example of bilateral loss of voluntary motor function with *permanent, complete* paralysis of groups of muscles. Box 26-1 describes the differences in therapeutic approach for individuals who have incomplete SCIs or less extensive loss of motor function, such as with neurapraxia or axonotmesis. Motor rehabilitation after a peripheral nerve injury, which focuses on strengthening affected muscles, is described in Chapter 22. Rehabilitation for individuals with extensive polyneuropathy causing complete paralysis may be similar to rehabilitation for individuals after an SCI.

### Pharmacological Implications

People who sustain an SCI typically take a number of medications during the acute stage after injury, during rehabilitation, and in the years that follow. Medication certainly contributes to the extensive costs incurred by a person with an SCI (NSCISC, 2016). One medication that has received a good deal of attention is methylprednisolone, a corticosteroid anti-inflammatory drug. This drug, given in high doses within the first 8 hours after injury, became the standard of care in much of the world after research demonstrated patients receiving it during this time window had significantly improved motor and sensory outcomes (Bracken, 2001; Miller, 2008; Sayer, 2006); controlling inflammation in the acute phase may help to prevent ongoing damage as the spinal cord swells within the fixed bony space of the spinal canal. In recent years, however, the efficacy, safety, and functional effects of methylprednisolone have been questioned (Hurlbert, 2008; Miller, 2008). A number of other medications have been investigated, though none have been definitively beneficial in large clinical trials (Baptiste, 2006; Dumont, 2001).

Individuals with an SCI may take additional medications, in part because of the multiple medical and musculoskeletal problems associated with damage to the spinal cord. Drugs are also commonly used for spasticity control, blood clot prevention (heparin, dicoumarol), pain management, enhancement of bowel or bladder function, treatment of infections, and enhancement of penile erections. A complete listing of these medications is beyond the scope of this chapter.

### Development of Compensatory Movement Strategies

When an individual loses the use of a large number of muscles, typical/normal movement patterns are no longer an option. To function independently, the patient must learn to use the remaining musculature, supplemented by equipment and technology, to perform tasks previously accomplished using

---

### ◼ BOX 26-1   Potential Therapeutic Approaches for Incomplete Paralysis

**Neural Adaptation**

Individuals with an incomplete spinal cord injury—an injury with some motor and/or sensory function present in the lowest sacral segments—as well as individuals with less severe peripheral nerve injury (i.e., neurapraxia or axonotmesis) should participate in activities that drive changes in the structure and function of the nervous system (see Chapters 24 and 25). Repetitive, attended practice of functional activities has had a positive effect on neural plasticity. Repetition is needed in the practice of desired functional activities. A strong desire and work ethic on the part of the patient is also needed.

Create functional activities that are goal directed, repetitive, progressed in difficulty, increased in variety and depth, spaced over time, and rewarded and complimented with feedback on accuracy (Umphred, 2007). Avoid compensation or substitution to the extent possible with the individual's motor function.

**Impairment-Based Training**

Focus is on increasing function in affected muscles, especially muscles used in the desired functional activity. A number of treatment strategies can be used for strengthening (see Chapter 22) and optimizing flexibility (Chapter 23), such as resistance training, active-assisted range of motion, stretching, and electrical stimulation.

**Body-Weight Supported Treadmill Training (BWSTT)**

Using an overhead transom connected to an abdominal and/or pelvic harness to deload the body allows a person with weakness of the lower extremities to participate in multiple repetitions of the movements necessary for walking (see Chapters 15 and 37). BWSTT is supported by the literature for use in treating incomplete spinal cord injuries (Behrman, 2005).

now paralyzed muscles. In these cases, three compensatory movement strategies are employed to help accomplish many functional skills: muscle substitution, momentum, and use of the head-hips relationship. Therapists typically teach and intentionally practice these movement strategies in physical therapy. Strategies for practice during rehabilitation are presented later in this chapter.

### Muscle Substitution

**Muscle substitution** involves using an alternative muscle to compensate for other muscles that are weak or nonfunctional.

*Substitution by Synergist.* One type of muscle substitution is likely familiar to most readers: substitution by synergists. In this type of muscle substitution, muscles that are synergists of weak or nonfunctional muscles work to accomplish the motor task normally performed by the impaired muscle. For example, the tensor fascia lata can substitute for a weak or absent gluteus medius in hip abduction. Unfortunately, for people with complete paralysis from an SCI, there is often not a functioning synergist available to perform the substitution because the neurological damage affecting one muscle is likely to also affect its synergists. In the absence of functioning synergists, people with complete paralysis can use gravity, passive structures, or closed chain mechanics to perform muscle substitutions for many tasks.

*Substitution Using Gravity.* Some motions can be performed by moving the joint into a position and allowing gravity to cause the desired motion. For example, a person who lacks functioning triceps can reach out as shown in Fig. 26-4AB by flexing or abducting the externally rotated shoulder. In this case, gravity extends the elbow. The forearm must be supinated and the shoulder externally rotated enough to place the forearm in a position that allows gravity to pull the elbow toward extension. The biceps must relax (or contract eccentrically) to allow this motion to occur.

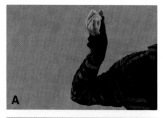
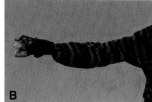

**FIGURE 26-4** Substitution using gravity. (A and B) An individual lacking triceps action is sitting on a mat, leaning on the left arm. In this externally rotated position with forearm supination (right arm), flexion or abduction of the shoulder will result in extension of the elbow.

*Substitution Using Tension in Passive Structures.* Using this type of muscle substitution, a person actively moves a joint into a position, creating passive tension in muscles that are not innervated. The **tenodesis grasp** is the best example of this movement strategy. Used by people who lack active finger flexion but do have active wrist extension (C6 or C7 tetraplegia), a tenodesis grasp is accomplished by extending the wrist. Wrist extension puts tension on the long finger flexors, causing the fingers to flex (Fig. 26-5).

*Substitution Using Closed Chain Mechanics.* This type of muscle substitution is accomplished by stabilizing the distal end of an extremity on an object and using proximal musculature to move an intermediate joint. (Fig. 26-6AB). People with C5 or C6 tetraplegia, who lack functioning triceps, can use this strategy to extend their elbows (Harvey, 1999; Marciello, 1995). This involves bearing weight on the palm and using the anterior deltoid and clavicular pectoralis major to flex or adduct the shoulder, depending on the position of the upper extremity. The same strategy can be used to maintain elbow extension or stabilize a flexed elbow (i.e., prevent additional flexion) while propping on the arm, (Gefen, 1997; Harvey, 1999); it can also be used in one or both arms at once.

### Angular Momentum

**Momentum** is the tendency of an object to continue moving once it has been set in motion. People with complete paralysis also use momentum for a variety of functional tasks. Both linear and angular momentum can be exploited to enhance compensatory function in this population.

Linear momentum is the tendency of an object to move in a straight line once it is moving and is proportional to the object's velocity and mass. This physical property can be helpful for negotiating curbs in a wheelchair. If the wheelchair is moving with enough velocity when it reaches the curb and if the chair is positioned correctly, with caster wheels elevated, its tendency to continue moving forward (momentum) will assist in the wheel's curb ascent.

Angular momentum is the tendency of an object to continue rotation about an axis. The angular momentum of an object is equal to the sum of the angular momenta of all of its parts. Thus, the angular momentum of a person is equal to the sum of the angular momenta of all the person's body parts.

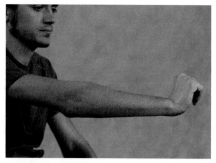

**FIGURE 26-5** Substitution using tension in passive structures. Tenodesis grasp used by people with C6 and C7 tetraplegia. Fingers close upon wrist extension.

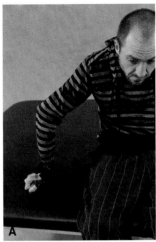

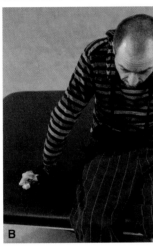

**FIGURE 26-6** Substitution using closed chain mechanics. (A) With the right hand in weight-bearing, when the humerus is adducted, the proximal forearm also moves medially. (B) This results in elbow extension.

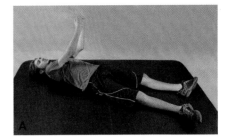

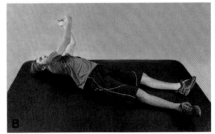

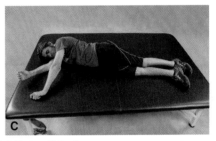

**FIGURE 26-7** (A–C) Rolling supine to prone using upper extremity momentum without equipment.

The angular momentum of each part is proportional to its velocity, mass, and moment arm. (The moment arm is the distance of the part from the axis of rotation.) One example of this strategy is throwing the head and arms to roll from supine. This method of rolling, used by people who are unable to roll using trunk and leg musculature, involves repeatedly throwing the head and arms right and left (Fig. 26-7ABC). Throwing the arms and head in this manner creates angular momentum and, if done with adequate speed and appropriate timing and with the arms positioned correctly, causes the lower (paralyzed) portions of the body to roll from supine.

### Head-Hips Relationship

The third compensatory movement strategy, use of the head-hips relationship, involves moving the head in one direction to move the buttocks in the opposite direction. To use this strategy, a person pivots on his or her arms, using the shoulders as a fulcrum. Transfers are a good example of the use of the head-hips relationship. To transfer from a bed to a wheelchair, teach the person who lacks lower extremity function to pivot on his arms, moving the head down and away from

the wheelchair, to lift and move the buttocks toward the wheelchair.

### Strengthening of Innervated Musculature

When a substantial number of muscles are paralyzed, the muscles retaining function are needed to compensate for the loss. Upper extremity muscular strength and endurance are needed to walk, transfer, propel a wheelchair, stabilize the trunk in sitting, and perform countless functional tasks that previously were performed by muscles in the legs and trunk.

Strengthening of spared/innervated musculature is an important component of functional rehabilitation for people with complete paralysis. It is essential to realize that even muscles of the trunk and upper body that test 5/5 on manual muscle test grades can be strengthened, as is true for individuals without neurologic injury. Therefore, for documentation of improvement in strength after intervention, it is best to record initial strength in spared muscles using dynamometry instead of manual muscle testing. Build strength in muscles used in compensatory movements to enhance the individual's capacity to perform those movements. For example, strengthen the anterior deltoids and clavicular pectoralis major to enhance the capacity for elbow extension in a closed chain position in a person who lacks functioning triceps. This ability to extend the elbows and stabilize them in extension can make functional tasks, such as transfers, possible.

In recent years, attention has been directed toward developing balanced strength in the shoulder and scapular musculature. This has been a response to growing awareness that shoulder pain is a common late-developing sequela of an SCI, presumably because of the high stresses placed on the shoulders during the performance of functional tasks (CSCM, 2005a; Sie, 1992). Strength imbalances around the shoulder and shoulder girdle may contribute to the problem by placing the glenohumeral joint in disadvantageous positions during the performance of functional tasks, increasing the trauma to local tissues (Nyland, 2000). These strength imbalances can result from repeated daily use of muscles such as shoulder flexors, horizontal adductors, and scapular abductors during functional tasks. Thus, a strengthening program should include the shoulder's rotators and scapular stabilizers to create more balanced muscle strength around the shoulder and scapula, in turn creating more normal shoulder biomechanics and causing less trauma and pain (CSCM, 2005a; Curtis, 1999b; Figoni, 1997; Kirshblum, 1997).

### Development and Preservation of Range of Motion

In addition to requiring adequate muscle strength, compensatory movements require adequate—sometimes extensive—joint range of motion and muscle flexibility. Normal range of motion makes many functional tasks easier, whereas severe or even moderate limitations can seriously impede function. For example, elbow flexion contractures can interfere with a person's ability to independently support himself on extended upper extremities during a seated transfer as described previously.

In some activities, greater-than-normal flexibility is beneficial. The hamstrings are a good example; for the patient with an SCI, highly flexible hamstrings make a variety of tasks, such as dressing or floor-to-wheelchair transfers, more feasible by allowing a hands-free, long-sitting position without an overly flexed spine. However, when hamstrings are too flexible, (i.e., allowing 130 degrees of straight-leg raise or more) they do not provide the passive tension necessary to prevent a forward collapse of the pelvis and trunk during long sitting.

Finally, mild limitations of range of motion can be helpful in some situations with complete paralysis. The best example of a beneficial range-of-motion limitation is mild contracture of the long finger flexors. Tightness/contracture of the long finger flexors allows functional tenodesis grasp in individuals who lack active finger flexion but do have active wrist extension (Harvey, 1996). One focus of rehabilitation is to obtain the desired passive range of motion—not too much, not too little.

The importance of range-of-motion exercises in functional rehabilitation programs becomes more evident when one considers that people with complete paralysis are prone to developing joint contractures. In addition to the paralysis and decreased movement, muscle imbalance around joints contributes to this problem. For example, people with C5 or C6 tetraplegia tend to develop elbow flexion contractures owing to the combination of strong elbow flexors and absent or very weak triceps. These individuals are not able to actively extend

the elbows and, as a result, may rarely get an end-range stretch into extension during the typical day. Another contributing factor is chronic positioning. Examples of contractures from chronic positioning include plantar flexion contractures developed during prolonged bedrest (or long-term wheelchair use in which the feet are not properly supported on the footplates) and hip flexion contractures resulting from chronic wheelchair use (i.e., a seated position with hips at 90 degrees).

As with strength imbalances, range limitations are possible contributors to the development of chronic shoulder pain in individuals with an SCI. Flexibility exercises to preserve or restore normal glenohumeral and scapulothoracic motions may help prevent or ameliorate this problem (Ballinger, 2000; Hart, 1998; Kirshblum, 1997).

### THINK ABOUT IT 26.1

- Return to the case.
  - Without intervention, which undesirable contractures will Mr. Johnson most likely develop?
  - List at least two desirable contractures Mr. Johnson could develop to compensate for paralyzed muscles.

### Use of Equipment to Compensate

People with complete paralysis require proper equipment for functional enhancement, physical health, and prevention of secondary sequelae. In the context of complete paralysis, equipment is required to do what the impaired muscles can no longer do, particularly provide stability around joints that no longer have inherent neuromotor stability. Equipment selection and procurement are vital components of rehabilitation, especially when complete paralysis and other neurological deficits are expected to be permanent.

Table 26-6 summarizes the typical equipment needs for people with various spinal cord levels of injury. Keep in mind, however, that numerous factors—in addition to motor function—influence the highly individualized process of equipment selection, perhaps none greater than available funding and reimbursement. Specific information regarding equipment selection, including wheelchairs, cushions, orthoses, and assistive devices for individuals with neuromuscular disorders such as complete paralysis, is presented in Chapter 17.

### Therapeutic Techniques

When planning interventions for an individual with complete paralysis, such as Mr. Johnson in the scenario used throughout this chapter, keep in mind the specific physical skills he needs to acquire during rehabilitation to maximize independence. Each functional activity has basic requirements for strength, range-of-motion, and movement abilities. These requirements are not the same for all functional tasks. An example is wheeled mobility: The physical movements used to propel a manual wheelchair are very different from those used to drive

| **TABLE 26-6** | **Summary of Equipment Typically Used by Individuals With Complete Spinal Cord Injury** |
| --- | --- |
| **NEUROLOGICAL LEVEL OF INJURY** | **SUMMARY OF EQUIPMENT TYPICALLY USED** |
| C1–C3 | Ventilator, suctioning equipment, battery backup for ventilator<br>Padded, rolling, reclining shower/commode chair<br>Powered hospital bed<br>Mechanical transfer device<br>Power wheelchair with power recline, power tilt-in-space, and power elevating leg rests as well as ventilator tray and positioning equipment<br>Pressure-distributing mattress<br>Pressure-distributing wheelchair cushion<br>Environmental control unit<br>Computer<br>Adaptive communication devices<br>Attendant-operated van with lift, tie-downs, etc. |
| C4 | Similar equipment needs as in C1–C3<br>Possibility of being ventilator free<br>May not need adaptive communication devices |
| C5 | Ventilator and suctioning equipment usually not needed |
| C6 | Padded, rolling shower/commode chair OR padded transfer tub bench with commode cutout<br>Powered hospital bed<br>Pressure-distributing mattress<br>Transfer board and/or mechanical transfer device<br>Power wheelchair with power recline, power tilt-in-space, and power elevating leg rests<br>May used lightweight or ultra-lightweight manual wheelchair with handrim modifications<br>C6 may use manual wheelchair more than power wheelchair on level surfaces<br>Hand splints<br>Adaptive eating, dressing, and grooming devices<br>Computer<br>Adaptive communication devices for page turning, writing, button pushing<br>Highly specialized modified van with lift |
| C7–C8 | Padded tub bench with commode cutout or shower commode chair<br>Powered hospital bed OR full to king standard bed<br>Pressure-distributing mattress or overlay<br>Transfer board<br>Manual lightweight or ultra-lightweight wheelchair<br>Pressure distributing wheelchair cushion<br>May use standing frame<br>Adaptive eating, dressing, grooming, bathing, and communication devices as needed<br>May use modified van |
| T1–T9 | Elevated padded toilet seat or padded tub bench with commode cutout |
| T10–L1 | Full to king standard bed |
| L2–S5 | Pressure-distributing mattress or overlay<br>May use transfer board to preserve upper extremities<br>Manual lightweight or ultra-lightweight wheelchair<br>Pressure-distributing wheelchair cushion<br>Handheld shower<br>Standing frame<br>Hand controls in vehicle<br>T10-S5 may also use reciprocating-gait-orthoses/knee-ankle-foot orthoses/ankle-foot orthoses and forearm crutches or walker |

Adapted from Consortium for Spinal Cord Medicine. Outcomes following traumatic spinal cord injury: clinical practice guidelines for health-care professionals. Available at: http://www.pve.org/publications/clinical-practic-guidelines. Published 1999. Accessed June 17, 2017.

a power wheelchair. Moreover, the movements required to drive a power wheelchair depend on the type of input device used. Movements to propel a manual wheelchair are similar to those used to propel a power-assist manual wheelchair, but the force needed differs. Thus, the interventions appropriate for independent wheeled mobility depend on the type of wheelchair the patient uses.

Think about the specific functional skills your patient is working to achieve and ask yourself key questions. Which movement strategies will he use to come to sitting, perform even transfers, or propel a wheelchair? Which functions are absolutely essential? Which functions are nice to have or may be used only occasionally? Which functions are possible but not advisable to perform on a regular basis because of the risk of injury, such as negotiating stairs in a seated position without a wheelchair or performing a floor-to-wheelchair transfer? Which architectural barriers are anticipated for the individual, and how will they be negotiated? How is the individual's home laid out, and which barriers must be overcome? Is walking a goal?

Taking into consideration the specific strength, range-of-motion, and skill requirements of all the functional tasks the patient needs to learn, design the therapeutic program to enhance individual performance as needed in each area. For individuals with complete paralysis, all functional activities involve a balance between doing the activity independently, gaining or maintaining strength and conditioning as a result of doing the activity, ensuring efficiency when doing the

activity, matching the amount of assistance available to the person, and considering the number of other functional activities to be performed during the day.

### Strengthening Exercises

There is relatively little research on strength training for spared muscle groups in individuals with complete paralysis, especially in the acute stage of rehabilitation (Nash, 2002, 2005). Strengthening activities in rehabilitation depend on the individual muscle groups remaining innervated as well as the anticipated functional activities to be performed; they are also essential in compensating for areas of permanent complete paralysis.

Once you have determined which of the patient's muscle groups have priority in the strengthening program, design exercises appropriate for the individual's current status. Depending on a muscle's strength, appropriate exercises can involve multiangle isometric contractions (e.g., various resisted shoulder isometric exercises typically performed in sitting), movement in a gravity-eliminated plane (e.g., shoulder abduction "snow angel" exercises performed in supine for the shoulders), or resisted movement against gravity (e.g., use of free weights or pulleys). Resistance can be provided using weights, therapeutic elastic bands, manual resistance, exercise machines, or the weight of the patient's body in either open-chain or closed-chain exercises. Table 26-7 summarizes the muscles you should consider emphasizing in strengthening programs for people with complete paralysis due to an SCI according to the level of injury. Keep in mind, however, that patients

| **TABLE 26-7** | **Summary of Muscle Groups to Be Strengthened in Acute Rehabilitation of Complete Paralysis** |
|---|---|
| **NEUROLOGICAL LEVEL OF INJURY** | **MUSCLE GROUPS TO BE STRENGTHENED** |
| C1–C3 C4 | • Cervical flexors, extensors, and rotators to help prepare individual for use of head in operating wheelchair, postural support, or in lifting head during transfers<br>• At C3 or C4, diaphragmatic strengthening to increase respiratory function |
| C5 | • Glenohumeral abductors and elbow flexors for use of upper extremity in feeding, grooming, dressing, and wheelchair propulsion<br>• Scapular stabilizers for use in stabilizing upper extremity during functional activities |
| C6 | In addition to C5 muscles:<br>• Glenohumeral extensors and horizontal adductors for stability during transfers when upper extremity is weight-bearing<br>• Scapular protractors for use in moving trunk during transfers when upper extremity is weight-bearing<br>• Wrist extensors for use of hand in functional activities associated with tenodesis grasp |
| C7–C8 | In addition to C6 muscles:<br>• Elbow extensors for use in nearly all mobility and stability activities of the upper extremity<br>• Wrist and finger flexors (C8) for use in nearly all activities of daily living |
| T1–T9 | • Fully intact upper extremities: strengthening of all major muscle groups of the upper extremities to promote their use in weight-bearing activities, such as wheelchair propulsion and transfers |
| T10–L1 | In addition to T1–T9 muscles:<br>• Abdominal muscle strengthening to improve trunk stability and the ability to lift the pelvis during transfers, reducing the need for a transfer board |
| L2–S5 | • Select lower extremity muscular strengthening for use in standing and ambulation; hip flexor and knee extensor strength important for use of ankle-foot orthosis versus knee-ankle-foot orthosis |

have different strength requirements depending on the specific movement skills they will use to function.

Consistent with recommendations from the literature, two primary aspects are involved in strength training: overloading the muscle group and specificity of training, meaning exercises incorporated into a strengthening program should mimic the anticipated function (Kisner, 2007). Strength training with a mean intensity of 60% of a one-repetition maximum elicits maximal gains in untrained individuals, whereas 80% is most effective in those who are trained (Rhea, 2003). On the basis of this information, the amount of resistance is gradually increased during typical rehabilitation. After the desired strength has been achieved, ongoing maintenance of training is recommended. The desired amount of strength can be tested by having the individual perform the appropriate functional task (e.g., a lateral transfer or floor-to-wheelchair transfer) while assessing the amount of assistance needed and the quality of movement achieved.

## THINK ABOUT IT 26.2

- Return to the case.
    - Which muscle groups should be initially targeted in a rehabilitation program for Mr. Johnson?

### Range-of-Motion and Stretching Exercises

As discussed earlier in this chapter, each functional task requires a specific amount of range of motion and flexibility. As a rule, normal range of motion and flexibility are considered functional in complete paralysis. However, sometimes greater-than-normal flexibility is required, whereas mild contracture can be beneficial in some joints in other situations. Table 26-8 summarizes typical range-of-motion requirements for individuals with complete paralysis resulting from an SCI.

| TABLE 26-8 | Typical Range of Motion Requirements for Functional Activities After Complete Paralysis Caused by Spinal Cord Injury | |
|---|---|---|
| **JOINT(S)** | **REQUIRED RANGE OF MOTION** | **FUNCTIONAL APPLICATION** |
| Cervical | Full active range of motion within any limits imposed by surgery | Assists with bed/mat activities such as rolling, transfers, upper body dressing, head/hips relationship |
| Low back | Some contracture beneficial for cervical and upper thoracic injuries. Normal AROM for low thoracic and lumbar injuries | Assists with bed/mat activities such as rolling, transfers, upper body dressing, head/hips relationship. Some contracture beneficial to keep spine stable during transfers |
| Shoulders | Flexion 165–180 degrees. Extension 30–60 degrees. External rotation 80–90 degrees | Flexion to assist with overhead activities. Extension to allow wheelchair push-ups, assuming standing with walker and knee-ankle-foot orthoses, wheelchair↔floor transfers. External rotation to allow wrapping of UE around wheelchair push handle in sitting and supine-to-sit with some methods |
| Elbows | Full extension | Allows weight-bearing with reduced triceps work compared with a slightly flexed elbow position; essential for C6 or C5 injuries |
| Forearms | Full pronation and supination | Allows manipulation of hand in C6 injuries; needed for placement of hand during transfers and many activities of daily living |
| Wrists | Full flexion and extension | Extension needed for tenodesis grasp and for hand placement during transfers; C6 may not have full flexion because of tenodesis |
| Fingers | In C6 and C7, mild contracture of long finger flexors | Allows tenodesis grasp (C6 and C7) |
| Hips | Full flexion, extension, and external rotation | Full flexion allows long-sitting position with minimal spinal flexion. External rotation needed for manipulation of lower extremities during transfers and dressing. Extension needed for standing and/or gait in paraplegia |
| Knees | Full extension. Flexion to at least 90 degrees | Full extension allows proper positioning during long sitting. Flexion to at least 90 degrees allows proper positioning of feet on typical rigid-framed wheelchair |
| Hamstrings | 100- to 110-degree straight-leg raise | Allows long sitting for use in dressing, bed mobility, transfers, wheelchair↔floor transfers, and floor↔standing for ambulators |
| Ankles | At least 10 degrees of dorsiflexion | Needed for ambulation and for proper foot placement on footrests of wheelchair. |

Adapted from Somers, Martha Freeman, Spinal Cord Injury: Functional Rehabilitation, 3rd Ed, © 2010. Reprinted by permission of Pearson Education, Inc. New York, New York.

Design your patient's program to achieve the appropriate flexibility for his functional requirements but also encourage joint stability when needed. Although short-term functional gains are important, long-term joint health should also be considered. Individuals who sit in a wheelchair for most functional activities, as opposed to standing for those activities, are at risk of developing contractures in hip flexion, knee flexion, and ankle plantar flexion. Prolonged sitting also promotes excessive posterior pelvic rotation and spinal flexion. Care should be taken to prevent contracture in these motions, especially when promoted by spasticity. Shoulder joints are particularly important, as previous studies have shown 59% of individuals with tetraplegia and 41% of individuals with paraplegia experienced shoulder pain (Sie, 1992). Make sure your patient performs daily range-of-motion exercises. Design the rehabilitation program so range of motion becomes a habit to be carried over at home.

Appropriate flexibility most likely involves performing passive range of motion to preserve range in some areas while stretching to increase it in others. Chapter 23 describes therapeutic interventions for preserving or increasing range of motion. When mild tightness in the low back or long finger flexors are likely to be functionally beneficial, avoid placing these tissues on stretch. Proper hand placement and positioning during transfers are essential. For example, in a patient with an SCI at the C6 or C7 level, maintaining proximal and distal interphalangeal joint flexion during transfers (by weight-bearing on a palm with flexed fingers) is important to preserve a tenodesis grasp (see Fig. 26-8AB).

## ◼ Intervention: Ultimately Applied in Functional Activities

Therapeutic exercise alone does not enhance the functional independence of patients with complete paralysis; physical therapy interventions must also address the development of new movement abilities related to specific functions. This section describes functional movement activities that can help your patients develop basic movement skills. These basic skills can be useful in performing a variety of functional tasks, even in the compensatory ways often required for individuals with complete paralysis. Remember, however, that each exercise is appropriate only for patients who have the potential to use the skill functionally, safely, and efficiently and who are not yet adept in the skill.

Functional training should be initiated in the plan of care as soon as possible, provided the patient is ready to participate. Early functional training can have great psychological benefits and further motivate the patient. Confidence can be built, and acquisition of functional skills and independence can foster acceptance of the injury. Rehabilitation of complete paralysis may be the most difficult task an individual can undertake.

Common barriers to participation in therapeutic functional activities include orthopedic precautions on the spine

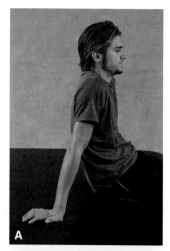

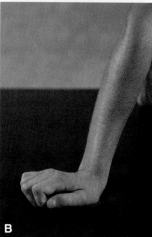

**FIGURE 26-8** Preservation of the tenodesis grasp. (A) Extension of the wrist and interphalangeal joints in combination can impair the potential for tenodesis grasp by overstretching the long finger flexors. (B) Flexion of the interphalangeal joints when the wrist is extended preserves the tenodesis grasp.

or extremities, the presence of an orthosis limiting movement, skin breakdown, blood pressure regulation issues, brain injury, and psychological adaptation to the injury that limits new learning and/or motivation. A list of precautions and prevention measures during functional rehabilitation follows this section.

## Functional Training Principles

### Postural Progression

When functional training is performed, several strategies can facilitate the acquisition of new skills. There should be a logical progression to the postures or body positions needed to perform the functional task. For example, an individual with new C6 complete tetraplegia should not immediately progress to long sitting during functional rehabilitation. Easier, less taxing, positions should be tried and mastered first, such as rolling or supported short sitting. Generally, the following order of positions for functional tasks is used: supine, sidelying, supported short sitting, supported long sitting, unsupported long sitting, unsupported short sitting, and passive standing. The sequence can be varied depending on patient needs or capability. For example, functional practice in sidelying may well precede practice in supine, and rolling practice may start in side-lying instead of supine. In addition, some postures may be contraindicated, depending on the neurological level of the lesion. For example, a person with a high, cross-sectional complete cervical SCI would not likely achieve unsupported postures.

### Task Analysis

Complex functional tasks should be broken down into smaller parts (part-practice) to allow easier mastery. For example, before a person with complete paralysis learns to transfer, he should learn to perform weight shifts in sitting and learn the head-hips relationship and how it can assist transfers. During rehabilitation sessions, practice should be conducted first on the smaller tasks. When mastery occurs or when the patient demonstrates some controlled mobility, the task can be combined with other smaller tasks into the larger functional task. Viewed this way, functional rehabilitation involves a process of collaborative exploration of movement strategies that occurs between the therapist and the patient. Therapists need to know how to break down each functional task into smaller movements as well as how to teach each movement or skill. Indeed, some see rehabilitation after a nervous system injury as largely a teaching and learning process (Umphred, 2007).

For a clinical example of the application of these principles of task analysis, see Box 26-2.

### Task Complexity

Plan for success with the patient while ensuring that the tasks are difficult yet doable. Patients learning new tasks may be fearful: regarding the injury, recovery, the effect of the injury on loved ones, or about returning home and caring for themselves. Encourage the patient to accept challenges. Reward the patient for each success. Progress the activities from easiest to difficult to ensure that the patient continues to succeed (Fell, 2004). For example, if the patient has never transferred into or out of a wheelchair from a seated position, consider performing the first transfer while providing more assistance than necessary and verbalizing the expectation that eventually the patient will do as much of the activity as possible. Then break down the movements necessary for a seated transfer. Teach the movements to the patient and have the patient practice during rehabilitation sessions.

### Environment

Gradually progress the complexity of the environment in which the task is practiced or performed. For the patient with paralysis, start with an easier environment; next, progress to a more difficult environment and then to one ultimately similar to the patient's home. An example is using a rehabilitation mat versus using a standard bed to practice rolling or supine-to-sit. A rehabilitation mat is firmer and allows the patient to move with less hindrance, whereas a standard bed is softer and may require more strength and skill to perform the task. The same can be said for using side rails on a bed and eventually practicing without the use of side rails, assuming the patient will not have side rails on the bed at home.

Another example is considering how the patient needs to move against gravity. Level transfers, with the height of the wheelchair identical to the height of the mat or bed, are easier to perform than transfers in which the destination object is higher than the original location. Thus, you could also start training for the individual with an SCI by asking for a transfer to a destination object slightly lower than the original location, allowing gravity to help the transfer, increasing the chances for success in the early stages of rehabilitation.

## Rolling

For a person with complete paralysis, rolling is a basic skill used to progress to sitting, performing activities of daily living (e.g., dressing), and simply turning in bed for pressure relief. To perform this functional movement, the patient must have adequate strength and range of motion in the shoulders. Elbow extensor strength is not required but certainly makes the task easier to perform.

### Supine-to-Prone With Equipment

When an individual with complete paralysis lacks sufficient strength or range of motion to independently roll without

---

**BOX 26-2  Applying the Principles of Task Analysis**

You are assigned as the primary physical therapist for Mr. Smith, a 35 year-old male recently injured at the T12 neurological level. His injury is complete. He is medically stable and is an inpatient at your rehabilitation unit. He can sit upright in a wheelchair for up to 3 hours without significant orthostatic hypotension. Thus far, he has been transferred dependently.

In your session, you transfer him from his wheelchair to the rehabilitation mat, where you perform lower extremity passive range of motion and extended hamstring stretching, attempting to achieve the eventual 110 degrees of straight-leg raise required for optimum long sitting. Mr. Smith has not yet learned how to transfer, roll, or transition from supine to sitting.

Mr. Smith needs to learn how to transfer himself in order to go home in a few weeks.

What do you need to teach him regarding transfers, rolling, and position transitions? In what order would you go about teaching him?

equipment, he may use equipment to assist. The most common equipment for this purpose is a looped strap, a bed side rail, and a wheelchair parked next to the bed. The use of a wheelchair is preferred over the other examples because the wheelchair will most likely be parked next to the bed anyway and does not require purchase or maintenance of any special equipment. Figure 26-9AB demonstrates use of a looped strap.

An individual with complete paralysis of the lower body who does not possess hand function can first position the arm in the loop, under the bed side rail, or under the wheelchair armrest or pushrim with a supinated forearm. The person then uses the elbow, shoulder flexors, and/or shoulder horizontal adduction to pull, in effect rolling the trunk toward the equipment. Simultaneously, the person should right the head and swing it and the opposite arm toward the equipment, increasing momentum. The person should continue moving the opposite arm toward the equipment and use the arm on the equipment to complete the roll.

### Supine-to-Prone Without Equipment

The patient should move the arms back and forth to the right and left to generate momentum in the direction in which the roll will take place. To do this, the patient swings his arms with gradually increasing force and distance, adding head righting and head and trunk movement to the swing in the direction to be rolled when possible. A horizontal movement of the arms (i.e., in the plane of the shoulders) is possible for those with innervated triceps. For those without innervated triceps, a hip-to-shoulder movement should be attempted (i.e., when rolling to the right, begin movement at the left hip, moving the arms toward the right shoulder) to prevent uncontrolled elbow flexion during which the forearms or hands may hit the patient's face (see Fig. 26-7ABC).

### Assuming Prone-on-Elbows

Prone-on-elbows is also an important basic skill for the individual with complete paralysis from an SCI. This position can be used to move in bed, as a transition between supine and sitting, or to simply provide a stretch to the spine and hips. From supine, the individual should roll as described previously. Once in the sidelying position, the patient may be pulled to prone by gravity; however, it is important for the person to have the arms strategically placed so not to end up pinned underneath the trunk. The shoulder and elbow of both arms should be flexed. As the patient moves toward the prone position, the elbow of the lower arm should be pushed down into the mat using the posterior deltoid. With enough strength and practice, this movement allows the trunk to move forward over the elbow. The person can then tuck his chin to assist the movement.

To complete the movement to prone-on-elbows, the free arm should be forcefully swung forward, protracting the scapula, until the forearm contacts the surface. After contact with the surface, the elbow can then be pushed into the mat similarly to the first elbow, pulling the trunk over the arms. The patient should then attempt to protract the shoulders, completing the movement to prone-on-elbows. Figures 26-10A-C depict an alternate strategy whereby the individual begins in prone with shoulders in 90 degrees' abduction and elbows in 90 degrees' flexion. The individual begins to shift weight side-to-side while progressively adducting the shoulders until the prone-on-elbows position is achieved.

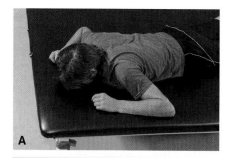

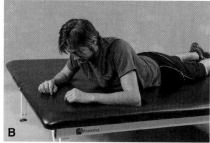

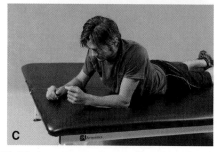

FIGURE 26-10 Assuming prone-on-elbows position from prone, shoulders abducted. (A) Starting position. (B) Partway up. (C) Weight shifting and moving the unweighted arm medially.

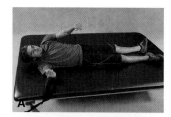

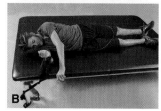

FIGURE 26-9 (A and B) Rolling supine to prone with equipment.

The therapist can assist in any of these movements by gently moving the patient's body or extremities to obtain momentum. This movement is particularly difficult for persons with C5 or C6 injuries. Equipment such as a wheelchair or a loop ladder may be helpful for this person.

## Transition to Sitting

For any person with complete paralysis, sitting is obviously an essential position to ensure function. Transitioning to sitting is a major component of the rehabilitation process. The individual with complete paralysis may have several problems associated with this transition: orthostatic hypotension, difficulty breathing, insufficient strength, or impaired range of motion and balance. A potential problem that may be overlooked is the patient's anxiety associated with sitting. Again, design the rehabilitation program to maximize the probability of success. Tolerance to upright sitting can be developed using a reclining wheelchair, starting with the patient in the wheelchair with the legrests elevated and the backrest fully reclined. As the patient's blood pressure allows, he can be moved gradually and incrementally into positions with the torso more upright and the legs more dependent. Lower extremity compressive garments or wraps and an elastic abdominal binder can be used to increase peripheral resistance. As the patient's tolerance to sitting allows, the time in sitting can be increased.

These activities may be passive for the patient. Assuming sitting is an active part of rehabilitation. As with other functional movements, the therapist should break the task of active transition to sitting into small components sequenced logically.

### Assuming Sitting With Equipment

As described with rolling, assumption of a sitting position can be assisted with a loop ladder, bed side rails, or a wheelchair positioned at the bedside. The loop ladder may be attached to the frame at the foot of the bed. Starting in supine, the individual should hook a forearm in the loop ladder and pull. Pulling should force the person to one side, and the individual should put the "pulling" elbow in a weight-bearing position. After weight-bearing, the individual should reach forward with the free arm, hooking the loop with the forearm, and pulling the body into a "sidelying-on-elbows" position. From that point, it may be possible to hook the forearm around the thighs, position the arm closest to the loop ladder in a supinated, elbow-extended position, and pull to long sitting (see Figs. 26-11ABC).

The higher the neurological level of injury, the more likely the individual will need to use equipment or assistance to actively assume sitting. For the individual injured at C5 or C6, use of equipment is typical. Above C5, this task is not possible. Below C6, the lower the injury, the easier it is to perform. At C5 or C6, the individual may also need head and neck movements to help transfer the required center of mass and achieve the long-sitting position.

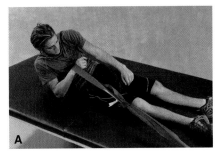

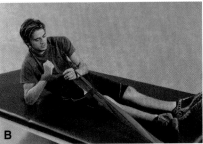

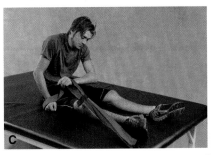

**FIGURE 26-11** Coming to sitting using a loop ladder. The starting position is supine. (A) The upper trunk is lifted by pulling on the loop and driving the supporting elbow into the mat. (B) The other hand assists by pulling on the next loop. (C) Both arms pull on the loop ladder up to long sitting.

### Assuming Sitting Without Equipment

With functioning elbow extensors (i.e., C7 and lower neurologic level of injury), this movement is much easier. An individual with complete paralysis and functioning C5, C6, and C7 myotomes—including functioning triceps—may be able to transition to sitting directly from supine by pushing extended arms into the mat or by rolling side to side until it is possible to extend the arms behind the back to push to long-sitting, one arm at a time. An alternative movement strategy involves the patient putting his hands in the front pants pockets to assist in pulling forward (Figs. 26-12ABCD). Active use of abdominals greatly assists this movement, so persons with lower injuries have much less difficulty.

With normally innervated upper extremities and active abdominals, the individual with an SCI may transition from supine to sit much like a person without an SCI: rolling to the side, moving lower extremities off the mat or bed to the floor, then using the upper extremities to push to a sitting position. The primary difference is in moving the legs to the floor: The person with an SCI needs to use the upper extremities to move the lower extremities. If unable to do so from a sidelying position, the patient may first push up into long-sitting and then move the legs off the bed.

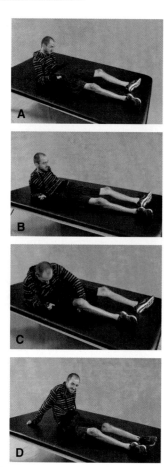

**FIGURE 26-12** Coming to sitting without equipment. The starting position is supine. (A) Hands are placed in pockets as a distal point of stability. The upper trunk is lifted by flexing the elbows and driving the supporting elbows into the mat. (B) Through weight shifting, the elbows are positioned under the shoulders, achieving a supine-on-elbows position. (C) Weight is shifted onto the right elbow, and the left arm is hooked under the right knee to pull up into (D) long sitting.

Without functioning elbow extensors, the individual will likely need to roll and throw the arms in a pendulum-like manner, as described in the section on rolling. Once in the prone-on-elbows position, the individual can "walk" the elbows toward the hips, moving the trunk laterally toward the lower extremities. The individual should then hook his legs with the top forearm. The individual should pull with the arm hooked around the legs and move his head in this direction while walking the trunk closer to the body with the weight-bearing upper extremity. He can then internally rotate the shoulder of the weight-bearing upper extremity to plant the palm on the mat. By pushing with this supporting upper extremity, and pulling on his lower extremities, he can transition to long sitting. The individual needs sufficient hamstring flexibility and hip and shoulder passive range of motion to perform this functional movement.

As with other movements, the therapist can assist anywhere in the process to support the person's body or limbs or can assist with momentum allowing the movement (see Figs. 26-13A–H). This movement is very difficult and can take weeks to learn and execute. This is a task where part-practice would be appropriate as well as working on the skill in reverse. For a patient who lacks functioning elbow extensors, equipment will likely be needed to assume sitting.

## Long sitting

Long sitting is an important position for the individual with complete paralysis. When it is properly executed, the individual can long-sit, relying on the passive tension of the hamstrings to maintain an upright, balanced position, provided the hamstrings are not overstretched. Depending on the amount of trunk control and balance, this position can reduce or eliminate the need for upper extremity support in sitting, freeing the upper extremities to perform functional tasks such as applying socks, tying shoes, or donning a shirt. To maintain

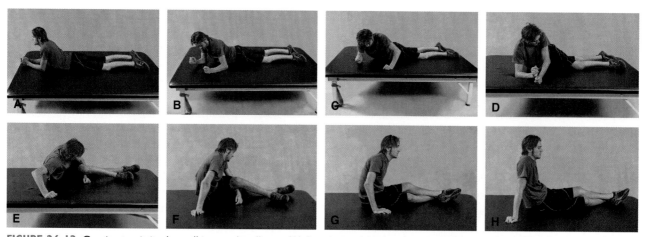

**FIGURE 26-13** Coming to sitting by walking on the elbows. (A) Starting position: prone-on-elbows. (B and C) The elbows are walked to the side until the trunk does not laterally flex any farther. (D) The pelvis is rolled from prone toward sidelying, and the elbows/hands are walked toward the legs. (E) An arm is hooked around the thigh(s). (F) The supporting arm is walked toward the legs. (G) The palm is planted on the mat, and the body is rocked into position over the legs. (H) The torso is pushed to upright and long sitting.

this position, the individual must have 100 to 110 degrees of straight-leg raise and passive tightness of the lower spine to reduce the chances he will sit in the circle-sit position, noted by a flexed spine with externally rotated hips and flexed knees.

The therapist must ensure that the individual with an SCI is trained properly to this point. Adequate passive range of motion, including hamstring length, is needed to allow long sitting. For individuals with inadequate hamstring length, allowing a circle-sit position will avoid having to sit with excessive posterior pelvic tilt and spinal flexion. Over-stretching the lower back can in turn interfere with functional independence.

### Leg Management

Leg management is essential for the person with complete paralysis of the lower extremities. Individuals with flaccid paralysis of the lower extremities may need to work harder than those with spasticity to minimize injury during positioning or movement. Figure 26-14 illustrates proper long sitting. The person should use the contralateral arm to move the leg while weight-bearing on the ipsilateral arm, leaning away from the leg being moved to facilitate the movement (see Fig. 26-13F).

## Short Sitting

During rehabilitation, the short-sitting position is the position from which transfers will eventually be performed. Short sitting eliminates the support of tension in the hamstrings that is present in the long-sitting position, though it makes the position much more unstable for the person with complete tetraplegia or high paraplegia involving the trunk. Learning and executing short-sitting takes time to develop balance and arm positioning (see Fig. 26-15).

### Forward, Backward, and Side Movements

In the short-sitting position, the patient is on the mat with the therapist in front or behind him to guard and assist while the patient moves his trunk forward, backward, or to the side. Many therapists prefer to be in front of the patient because it is easier to guard and prevent forward falls. Also, many patients feel less frightened during early practice if the therapist is in front. The patient practices balancing and moving the trunk away from and toward upright by using the head and upper extremity positioning. This skill is practiced often during inpatient

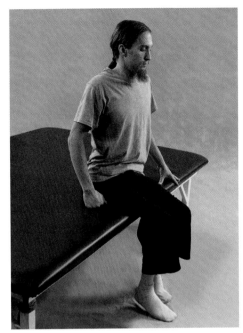

**FIGURE 26-15** Proper short-sitting position.

rehabilitation until the individual can assume and maintain the short-sitting position without assistance, maintaining both static and dynamic sitting balance using compensatory movements.

### Push-Ups

Blocks can be used on the mat, or push-ups can take place in the wheelchair or in a chair positioned in the parallel bars (see Figs. 26-16ABCD). For the individual with innervated elbow extensors, active elbow extensions can be done in this position for strengthening and to challenge balance. For the individual who lacks elbow extensors, the upper extremities can be positioned with the hands on the mat with supinated wrists (to allow the elbow to biomechanically lock), fully extended elbows, and elevated shoulders; the individual can then practice shoulder depressions and protractions in an attempt to lift the body.

## Transfers

For the person with complete paralysis, an important goal of inpatient rehabilitation is often to improve the ability to transfer, especially with independence. Many methods of transferring can be used depending on the amount of active movement preserved in the upper extremities. The amount of active trunk control also determines the type of transfer that can be performed. Simply stated, an individual with full active control of the upper extremities and trunk should be able to perform a seated transfer without assistive devices or assistance, barring any comorbidity. An individual with even partial paralysis of the upper extremities may need an assistive device or assistance to perform the transfer or may perform the transfer with an alternative movement strategy. Again, the process of teaching the individual with complete paralysis to transfer should be broken down into smaller tasks. The first task is movement in the wheelchair.

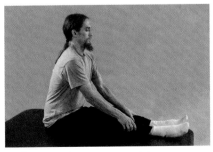

**FIGURE 26-14** Proper long-sitting position.

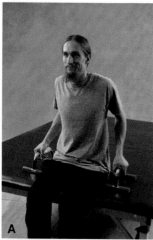

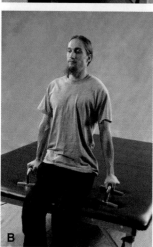

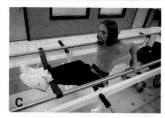

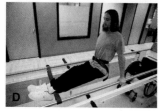

**FIGURE 26-16** Push-ups. (A and B) Push-ups using standard push-up blocks. (C and D) More advanced training: dips in the parallel bars with legs supported.

## Stability and Movement in the Wheelchair

To transfer out of a wheelchair, the patient needs a combination of stability and mobility. Stability is needed to remain upright while placing a transfer board (when used), removing an armrest, or applying a brake. Mobility is needed to shift to the side enough to place the transfer board, to lean forward enough to unload the buttocks, or to move forward in the seat to prepare for the transfer.

One method for supporting and stabilizing the trunk in the wheelchair is to hook one arm behind a push handle as shown in Figs. 26-17ABC. Also, the individual who can extend his elbow using triceps or muscle substitution can push on a thigh or the wheelchair seat or armrest to provide stability. Either strategy can also be used when leaning to the side.

To lean forward in the wheelchair, the individual can pull on any stable anterior structure of the wheelchair, such as the locked armrest or front rigging. The patient can also push on the posterior portion of the armrest or wheel to lean or push forward to the desired position. Do not underestimate the difficulty or possible anxiety involved in leaning forward for the person with an SCI. Most SCI levels cause paralysis of the hip extensors because of their primarily sacral innervation. Depending on the level of injury, the individual may also lack the low back extensors needed to prevent falling forward. If the person had active hip extensors and low back extensors sufficient to prevent falling forward, he would probably not need a wheelchair. He would most likely have enough strength to walk.

To facilitate the forward lean, individuals with an SCI often need to be encouraged and supported. Kneel or sit in front of the patient who is sitting in the wheelchair and teach the patient how to push or pull the trunk forward (pushing is often more efficient). Encourage the patient to use the hands or elbows on the anterior thighs for support after the lean forward. Teach the patient how to transition back to upright sitting by pushing on the thighs or an anterior component of the wheelchair, such as the front rigging or armrest. Ensure that the patient is comfortable with this transition and skilled at returning to upright sitting before teaching him to scoot the pelvis forward or move the legs in preparation for the transfer. Patients who cannot perform a forward lean efficiently typically cannot perform a transfer well. The forward lean moves the center of mass forward so it is positioned over the thighs. This unloads weight from the buttocks and pelvis, making them easier to move in the transfer.

Another important preparatory skill for a safe transfer is properly positioning the wheelchair. The wheelchair should be positioned at roughly a 30-degree angle toward the mat or bed. Brakes should be applied and footrests removed or repositioned if applicable. The patient may place one or both feet on the floor or footrests. Positioning the wheelchair at a 30-degree angle allows the front corner of the wheelchair seat to be closest to the mat or bed, decreasing the distance traveled during the transfer. After the individual with an SCI has learned to lean forward, applying the brakes can be practiced. Leg management needed to swing away the footrests of the wheelchair is discussed next.

## Moving Forward and Leg Management in the Wheelchair

After the forward lean has been learned, the next steps are managing the legs and moving the center of mass forward in the chair in preparation for transfer. Both of these steps involve managing the lower extremities. To successfully swing away the footrests on the wheelchair (or move the feet off a

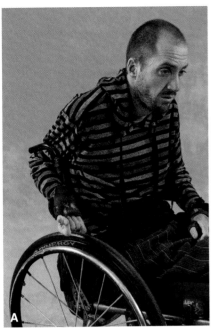
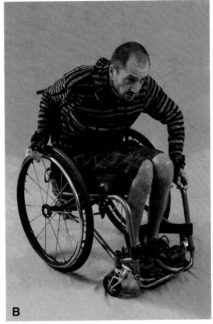
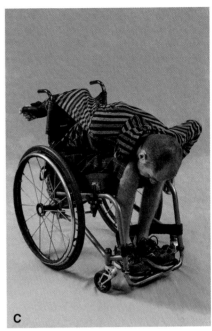

**FIGURE 26-17** Arm positions for stabilizing the trunk in a wheelchair. (A) Sitting upright with the arm wrapped around the wheelchair push handle. (B) Slight forward lean. (C) Pronounced forward lean.

rigid wheelchair with a solid footplate), the feet must be lifted one at a time off the footrest. To do this, the individual with an SCI can place his hand under the opposite thigh (of the leg to be lifted), place the elbow of the same arm on the ipsilateral thigh, and lean away from the leg being moved. With enough lift and lateral trunk movement, the individual should be able to free the foot from the footrest. This foot can be crossed over the opposite foot. The individual can then reach down—using the forward leaning strategy described earlier or by hooking an arm around the push handle of the wheelchair back—and swing away the footrest. Repeat to remove the other foot.

After the feet are on the floor, the individual must move the pelvis forward in the wheelchair. Translating forward allows two essential components of the transfer to take place if needed: placement of the transfer board and ensuring the transfer takes place on the front edge of the seat. Transferring with the pelvis starting from the back portion of the seat of a manual wheelchair will most likely result in the buttocks contacting the wheel during the transfer. This is dangerous for the individual with an SCI. Not only will contact with the wheel impede the progress of the transfer, but it could also result in skin trauma exacerbated by sensory deficits. A commonly used strategy to translate the pelvis forward is a twisting upper-trunk motion combined with hooking one arm around a push handle. The hooked arm should be on the side toward which the individual is twisting the upper trunk. The individual should move his head in the same direction, pulling the opposite buttock forward (see Fig. 26-18). The other side should then be done, alternating back and forth until the buttocks are in the correct position for the transfer.

For a safe transfer, the feet should be flat on the floor (or footrest), the wheelchair should be placed at a 25- to 30-degree

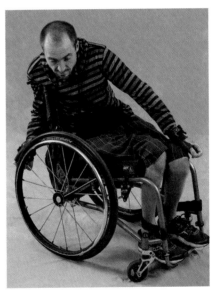

**FIGURE 26-18** Moving the buttocks out in the wheelchair seat. The person twists the head and upper torso to the right and back to move the buttocks forward and to the left.

angle to the bed or mat, the brakes should be engaged, and the armrest should be removed from the side on which the transfer will take place.

### Placing and Removing the Transfer Board

Placing the transfer board can be a very difficult maneuver; the individual with complete paralysis may feel that he needs one arm to support the body, one arm to lift the leg, and a third arm to place the board. To properly place the board, the individual should grasp the end or side of the board, and pull until the closer end is under the proximal thigh and buttocks.

The individual may need to move the board back and forth to ensure proper placement. Leaning away from the board will make this process easier. With impaired hand function, the individual can pull using the forearm or the back of the hand. When neither of these movements is possible, the individual will not likely be able to independently place the board.

### Even Transfers With Equipment

A transfer board can serve as a bridge for a transfer between the wheelchair and the object the individual is transferring toward. This bridge can be used in two ways: for sliding or for interim rests when multiple steps are used along the way during the transfer. Sliding on the board should be done with extreme caution, and the board should be placed carefully because skin shearing will occur during a transfer. To maintain skin integrity, it is recommended that individuals with complete paralysis use a transfer board and multiple steps rather than sliding (Somers, 2010).

After ensuring proper and safe placement of the board, the individual should use the head-hips relationship described earlier in this chapter to move the buttocks toward the ultimate transfer location. The leading hand should be initially placed on the edge of the board, not under it, to ensure that the board does not move during the first portion of the transfer. The hand on the wheelchair side may be placed on the armrest or seat base of the wheelchair, provided the cushion has a firm spot for pushing.

The movement toward the object does not have to be completed in one step. Rather, the individual can perform smaller, shorter lifts and/or slides in an effort to make the transfer as safe as possible (see Figs. 26-19ABC). If the individual performs a movement that is too large or is done too quickly for his current level of skill, control or balance is often lost, making the transfer less safe.

### Even Transfers (Level Surface) Without Equipment

To perform a level transfer without a transfer board, an individual with complete paralysis should have active elbow extensors. Elbow extensors allow active extension of the elbows during the transfer, increasing the likelihood of actively lifting of the pelvis off the surface and replacing the need for sliding with the lifting action. (Active trunk musculature also greatly assists this transfer.) This transfer method is superior for protecting skin integrity, decreasing the chances of skin trauma during the transfer. A transfer without equipment should be done as described previously, but the individual will likely have to use one movement from the chair to the transfer object rather than the multiple movements used with the transfer board (Figs. 26-20AB). Even for individuals who will transfer without a board, use of the board should be taught initially. As skill and strength increase, the individual may reduce dependence on the board until he no longer needs it to transfer safely. He may continue to use the board for some transfers, however, to reduce the damaging forces on his upper extremities.

Attention is drawn to two important items. First, the ratio of arm length to trunk length can determine whether a person with complete paralysis can master an even transfer without a board. For an individual with shorter arms than trunk, lifting the pelvis will be difficult. For an individual with arms longer than the trunk, extending the elbows to end range will facilitate a lift of the pelvis. Second, the individual with complete paralysis should be taught to protect his wrists and hands during the transfer. He should avoid placing the wrists in full extension if possible. This can be accomplished by using a handgrip if available, or by allowing the fingers to drape over the edge of the transfer surface. (CSCM, 2005a) (see Figs. 26-19ABC). Long-term use of the wrists in an extended position during transfers may promote carpal tunnel syndrome.

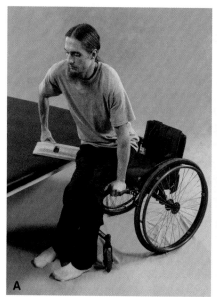 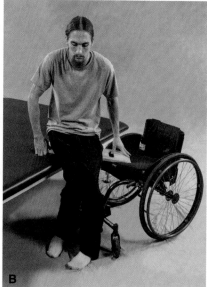 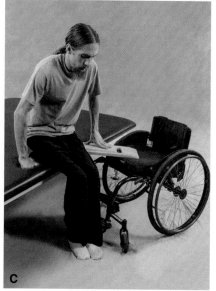

**FIGURE 26-19** Even transfers with equipment. (A) Initial positioning of the transfer board and first side scoot. (B) Middle of transfer. (C) End of transfer after which the transfer board can be removed.

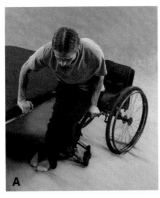

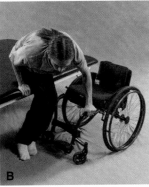

**FIGURE 26-20** Even transfer without equipment. (A) Starting position. (B) Head thrown down and away from the bed to lift the buttocks up and toward the bed.

## Basic Wheelchairs Skills

Wheelchair skills are imperative for the person with complete paralysis, particularly those who are full-time wheelchair users. Starting with the patient's first out-of-bed session, it is critical that the patient's skin is protected whenever the patient sits in a wheelchair. This protection involves pressure reliefs every 15 to 30 minutes, and use of an appropriate wheelchair and pressure-relieving cushion. For a review of appropriate wheelchairs and cushions for individuals with complete paralysis, see Chapter 17.

Several skills must be mastered by the manual wheelchair user, including pressure relief (by sitting push-ups or weight shifts), forward propulsion, turning, and negotiating curbs, inclines, and declines. As with other functional movements, these skills should be taught in a simple-to-complex fashion. Thus, push-ups, weight shifts, and forward propulsion should probably be taught first. The basic skills of push-ups, weight shifts, and forward propulsion are described here.

### Push-Up

To perform a seated push-up, the individual should grasp the armrests or wheels (with the brakes applied) and extend the elbows while leaning forward slightly. The forward lean unloads weight from the ischial tuberosities of the pelvis, making it easier to lift. Balance is difficult, though, particularly after the pelvis has cleared the seat. To ensure stability, many individuals with an SCI initially choose not to lean forward or are fearful of it. You should encourage the forward lean. Keeping

the back against the wheelchair backrest during the push-up results in the center of mass being positioned over the pelvis, making the lift more difficult. This also increases the force on each shoulder, perhaps the most important joint to keep healthy after an SCI (CSCM, 2005a).

### Forward Lean

When the individual with an SCI lacks functioning elbow extensors, has existing upper extremity joint pathology, is too heavy for the amount of upper extremity strength possessed, has arms that are significantly shorter than the trunk, or wishes to reduce damaging forces on the upper extremities, a forward lean may be used instead of the seated push-up for pressure relief. Leaning forward until the chest rests on the thighs can allow enough weight shift to unload the ischial tuberosities, reducing the chances of developing a pressure injury (see Fig. 26-17C). Leaning forward, particularly diagonally forward, has resulted in adequate pressure redistribution (Eksteen, 2006). Leaning forward is also necessary to prepare for a transfer out of the wheelchair.

The wheelchair push-up and forward lean while seated are important skills to help prevent a pressure injury in the individual with an SCI. Pressure injury prevalence in the SCI population ranges from 20% to 66% (Langemo, 1990). Although frequency may vary, most recommend a pressure relief—such as a push-up or forward lean—every 15 to 30 minutes (CSCM, 2014; National Pressure Ulcer Advisory Panel [NPUAP], 2007). The US Department of Health and Human Services (HHS; 1992) advises performing a push-up every 15 minutes while in a wheelchair, holding the push-up for up to 60 seconds to help prevent a pressure injury. Unfortunately, most wheelchair users do not achieve the recommendations. One study found 20.8% of wheelchair users moved once per hour, whereas 54.7% moved less than once per hour (Stockton, 2002). Even with the best equipment (i.e., a properly fitted skin-protecting and positioning wheelchair cushion, a wheelchair configured to the individual, and for individuals with mid-to-upper cervical lesions, power seat functions), the individual with an SCI must still perform regular weight shifts.

Educating the person with an SCI about the importance of regular weight shifts and pressure injury prevention is crucial. There are many barriers to learning among persons with an SCI, including unawareness of the lifelong risk of developing a pressure injury (Schubart, 2008). You should ensure that the person with an SCI understands the risk and preventive measures early on as part of a comprehensive rehabilitation program. Pictures of pressure injuries are readily available to help these individuals learn to recognize skin lesions (NPUAP, 2008).

### Wheelchair Propulsion

Teaching a person with an SCI to propel the wheelchair, including turning it, should be done only after he has tolerated sitting with minimal or no complications (e.g., orthostatic hypotension). The person with an SCI must also be stable in the wheelchair. Stability can be accomplished using seating principles that are beyond the scope of this chapter.

Individuals with an SCI may use a manual wheelchair or a power wheelchair, depending on the level of their injury. A manual wheelchair with power-assisted pushrims may also be used. This wheelchair requires the user to manually propel it but engages motors in the wheels to assist each active push stroke. Power wheelchair propulsion usually takes place via a joystick mounted on the right- or left-side armrest of the wheelchair. The individual with a C5 or lower neurologic level of injury should be able to mobilize the power wheelchair with a hand-operated joystick, though the joystick may need adaptation for those individuals without good hand function. Individuals with injuries above C5 need alternative controls, such as a head array (controlled by neck motion) or a sip-and-puff system (controlled by airflow generated by the patient's respiratory system).

Basic manual wheelchair propulsion should be taught early in the rehabilitation program. The manual wheelchair should be configured to provide optimum biomechanics for the user to minimize long-term shoulder problems (CSCM, 2005a). It should be customizable, meaning the axle can be moved so it is positioned under the shoulder and results in an elbow angle between 100 and 120 degrees when the hand is on the pushrim at top-dead center. It should be lightweight, reducing the amount of weight the wheelchair user must propel with each push stroke. It must be high strength, remaining intact under heavy use conditions such as outdoor propulsion. Loose axles, hubs, or other moving parts (e.g., cross brace) decrease the efficiency of wheelchair propulsion.

A manual wheelchair can be propelled by several methods. Because repetitive upper extremity movements can lead to shoulder, elbow, and wrist pathologies, manual wheelchair users need to be educated about optimal biomechanical principles (CSCM, 2005a). First, the person with an SCI should use long, smooth strokes that limit high impacts on the pushrim. Teach the user to place his hands well back on the wheelchair pushrims when beginning the stroke, then pushing forward using elbow extension combined with shoulder adduction, external rotation, and flexion. The long push stroke minimizes the number of repetitions to propel the wheelchair.

Second, teach the user to keep his hands low (keeping them below the pushrim) after finishing each push stroke, to optimally prepare for the next stroke. This phase of propulsion is often referred to as the *recovery phase* (Boninger, 2002). Four distinct patterns of recovery have been named: arc, semicircular, single-looping over, and double-looping over. Although the single-looping over method of recovery is most commonly used by individuals with paraplegia, the semicircular recovery method is recommended because it results in fewer push strokes, more time spent in the push phase (also reducing repetitions), and less angular joint velocity and acceleration (Boninger, 2002; CSCM, 2005a). A depiction of the desired push stroke is included in Figs. 26-21ABC.

In patients without functioning elbow extensors and active finger flexors, you should critically evaluate the need for a manual wheelchair compared with a power wheelchair. With this degree of arm impairment, the individual will have difficulty propelling a manual wheelchair on nonlevel surfaces, even with the optimum configuration. If a manual wheelchair is used, several adaptations should be made to maximize efficiency or propulsion. The person's anterior deltoids are used to extend the elbows while he is pushing the pushrims forward. In this phase, the user should externally rotate the shoulders and extend the wrists. The thenar or hypothenar eminence of the hand should contact the pushrim if the individual cannot actively grasp. The user should wear gloves with a palmar surface that provides friction with the pushrim,

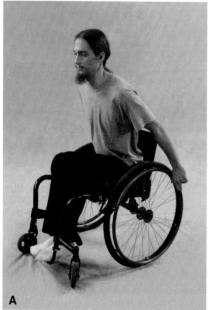 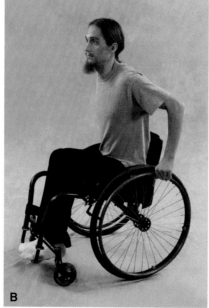 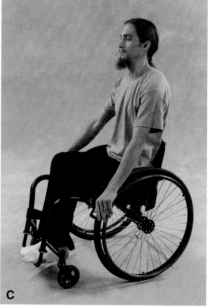

**FIGURE 26-21** (A–C) The recommended propulsion pattern is shown, after which the hands would complete the circle down, back, and up to the original starting position in (A).

which should have a covering promoting friction with the glove. The remaining biomechanics should be similar to those recommended previously. A semicircular recovery pattern should be used, though the individual will not likely obtain an arc as wide as that of an individual with normal upper extremity function.

Successfully executing turns in the wheelchair requires practice. Using more force on the right pushrim than on the left results in a turn to the left. Holding the left pushrim (or pulling backward) while advancing the right results in a sharper turn. The person with an SCI should practice maneuvering around obstacles during rehabilitation. Cones or chairs are commonly used for practice. The rehabilitation facility typically has open hallways and/or a gym that allows errors during practice without damaging the user, wheelchair, or environment. Because homes and apartments are rarely as spacious, the user needs to master turning during the rehabilitation program.

## THINK ABOUT IT 26.3

- Return to the case.
  - How would you justify Mr. Johnson's need for a power wheelchair? List three potential benefits of using a power wheelchair over a manual wheelchair for Mr. Johnson.

## Advanced Skills

Advanced wheelchair skills, such as negotiating curbs and inclines, are essential for the manual wheelchair user in the community. For the therapist, the most comprehensive tool for evaluating manual wheelchair skills is the WST (Kirby, 2002, 2004; Mountain, 2004) discussed in Chapter 10, Fig. 10-10. This assessment covers basic skills, such as applying brakes and removing armrests, which can also be used as wheelchair activities in the treatment session; it also includes more advanced skills. Advanced skills included in the WST version 4.1 are listed in Box 26-3 and can serve as a framework for practicing advanced wheelchair activities.

Practicing a **wheelie**, lifting the front casters off the ground and balancing the chair on two wheels only, is an appropriate place to start when teaching the most difficult advanced skills such as ascending or descending a curb (see Fig. 26-22). While supporting the user's wheelchair, you should instruct the patient in this skill by tilting the wheelchair backward until a balance point is reached, then asking the patient to push forward and backward on the wheels slightly to experience movement and boundaries of balance. The therapist can stand behind the chair to provide support at the push handles or may hold on to a gait belt attached to the lower rear frame of the chair. Ask the patient to keep light pressure on the pushrims; the user's tendency when performing this skill is to use a tight grip on the pushrims, making maneuvering more difficult. If the person with an SCI is able, have him move his head and neck forward during the wheelie. This helps maintain the center of mass within the base of support of the wheelchair.

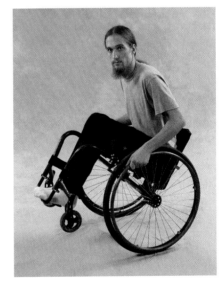

**FIGURE 26-22** Patient demonstrating a wheelie.

After the person with an SCI is comfortable in the wheelie position, you should gradually decrease your support of the wheelchair. You can then gradually decrease your support by removing your hands from the push handles but remaining behind the wheelchair to "catch" it if the user falls backward out of control. The patient should also practice lifting the casters to assume the wheelie position, and practice propelling the wheelchair with the casters lifted.

If you wish to provide a safe environment for independent practice assuming and maintaining a static wheelie position, you could use a set of straps looped around the push handles and secured to an anchor in the ceiling or an overhead grid. The straps should have enough slack in them when the wheelchair is on four wheels to allow the wheelie to be performed. The straps should not have so much slack that they allow the wheelchair to completely tip backward when on two wheels.

After the wheelie is mastered, the person with an SCI can learn to ascend and descend curbs. You should use a support position similar to that of the wheelie when teaching these skills. Start with a 2-inch curb and progress the height to the user's skill level. As a reference, many curbs in the community are at least 5 to 6 inches in height. When ascending, the user should go forward, performing a wheelie to rest the front casters on the curb. The rear wheels should then be propelled forward until they contact the curb. After contact, the user should lean forward, move his hands rearward on the pushrims, and then propel forward, lifting the wheelchair over the curb onto the elevated surface.

Descending a curb can be done forward or backward. When done backward, the user should lean forward as far as possible, pushing the rear wheels backward until they slowly *and symmetrically* descend the curb onto the lower surface. The casters can then be brought down by performing a wheelie or by turning the wheelchair sharply to one side. The backward strategy may not be safe for curbs taller than 4 inches. When going down a curb forward, the preferred method for curbs taller than 4 inches involves performing a wheelie, then descending the curb in the wheelie position, making sure the wheelchair lands on the lower surface rear wheels first. If the user contacts the front casters first on the lower surface, he may bottom out and be ejected from the wheelchair.

## Gait Training

Most persons with an SCI initially prefer to walk when asked how they would like to get around. After the individual sees or experiences how difficult walking is after complete paralysis with neurologic level of injury at or above L3 or L4, and how efficient wheelchair propulsion can be, he usually changes preference toward wheelchair mobility.

Walking can be beneficial, though, for individuals with complete paralysis, but not without costs. The primary benefits of walking after complete paralysis are decreased spasticity, exercise and the benefits of exercise, and an improved psyche. There are many costs. Persons with complete paralysis, even in only part of the legs, may require bracing to walk. The bracing may disrupt skin integrity. The person with complete paralysis will rely on upper extremity weight-bearing via a gait aid, putting tremendous strain on the shoulder joints. Shoulders are already in peril because of the increased demands on them from transfers and wheelchair propulsion.

A person who has complete paralysis of the lower extremities but wants to walk will most likely need bilateral knee-ankle-foot orthoses (KAFOs) and a gait aid such as a standard walker or Lofstrand crutches. If the KAFOs are not secured together, the user will not be able to control frontal plane movements of the lower extremities (such as excessive

adduction or abduction). Individuals with lower thoracic injuries and lumbar injuries are the best candidates for walking because they possess some trunk control and have full upper extremity control. Because of the high energy requirements for walking, however, most will use wheelchairs for functional mobility.

Before walking, a patient must learn how to balance and manage losses of balance in their KAFOs. This training is typically done first in the parallel bars (Figure 26-23AB). In this population, walking is typically done with knees locked in full extension within the KAFOs and using a swing-to or swing-through strategy in which the legs are advanced forward simultaneously by the action of trunk flexors and hip flexors if present, either to the gait aid or through (i.e., past) the gait aid, respectively. When the feet land, the person with a complete SCI walking with KAFOs must quickly move the pelvis forward so that his center of gravity falls posterior to the hips. This creates an extension moment at the hips, needed to prevent jack-knifing (rapid and uncontrolled forward trunk flexion at the hips) in the absence of innervated hip extensors.

In a **swing-to gait pattern** the individual swings the legs forward together/symmetrically until the feet make contact

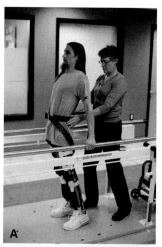

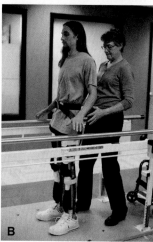

**FIGURE 26-23** (A and B) Learning to balance with knee-ankle-foot orthoses in parallel bars.

with the ground between the crutches, to "swing-to" the crutches (or walker) and not past (Fig. 26-24ABC). This position is inherently less stable than the "swing-through" pattern. Figures 26-25A–F illustrate a bilateral **"swing-through" gait pattern** using Lofstrand crutches. When walking with KAFOs is taught, many skills need to be mastered, including donning/doffing orthoses (see Fig. 26-26), balanced standing, rising from sitting, descending to sit, and of course, falling safely.

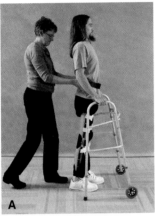

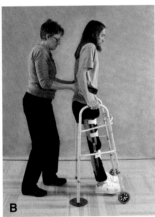

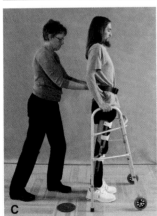

**FIGURE 26-24** Swing-to gait pattern with knee-ankle-foot orthoses and front-wheeled walker. (A) Balanced standing posture. (B) Walker advanced, pelvis and legs lifted, torso and legs swing forward as a pendulum, and heels strike. (C) Balanced standing posture regained by lifting head, retracting scapulae, and pushing on walker to push pelvis forward.

Energy expenditure for those who walk with bilateral KAFOs is 226% of normal (Waters, 1999). Persons who walk with KAFOs and a gait aid load 79% of their body weight through the upper limbs and walk at only 0.32 m/s. Any interruption of a flat surface—a dip or rise in the floor, a threshold, or an object on the floor—can easily cause the person to fall. Because the costs are so great and can permanently affect the functional abilities of the person with an SCI, you should ensure that the individual understands all costs, risks, and benefits before beginning a gait training program. In the rehabilitation environment where time is at a premium, other skills, such as transfers and basic wheelchair skills, should be accomplished and mastered before gait training for the person with complete paralysis who is not expected to experience neurological recovery.

Another gait training option for persons with complete paralysis is robotic assistance (Esquenazi, 2012a; Krebs, 2012). Locomotor training with robotic assistance has been shown to be safe (Zeilig, 2012) and to improve walking function in individuals after an SCI (Tefertiller, 2011). The ReWalk system has been shown to improve gait distance and velocity (Esquenazi, 2012b) (Fig. 26-27). Other positive effects of using robotic assistance have been reported, such as improvements in pain, bowel and bladder function, and spasticity (Esquenazi, 2012b).

## PATIENT APPLICATION

*Mr. Johnson, described earlier in this chapter, experienced an injury to his spinal cord resulting in C6 AIS-A tetraplegia. He has complete paralysis of the muscles below the zone of partial preservation. During his stay in the intensive care unit, he successfully sat in the hospital bed with the head of the bed raised 50 degrees. He was mobilized from the bed to a wheelchair that fully reclines, then sat in the chair in progressively more upright positions, up to 30 minutes two or three times a day. Elastic wraps were needed on his lower extremities, and an elastic abdominal wrap was also needed to minimize orthostatic hypotension in sitting.*

*Mr. Johnson has now transitioned to your inpatient rehabilitation facility. You need to create a plan of care for him that considers his level of injury and prognosis. He is not expected to experience further neurological return.*

## Contemplate Clinical Decisions

- *Which muscles would you target in a strengthening program designed for Mr. Johnson? Why?*
- *Which joints require normal range of motion given his level of injury? Which joints require more than normal range of motion? In which joints would you want to promote some contracture?*
- *What equipment is important for him?*
- *Which functional activities does he need to learn and master? In what order would you teach the functional activities? How would you break down each activity to allow for better learning?*
- *Given Mr. Johnson's level of injury, which wheelchair skills are important for him? How do you expect him to perform pressure relief maneuvers? How should he propel a manual wheelchair?*

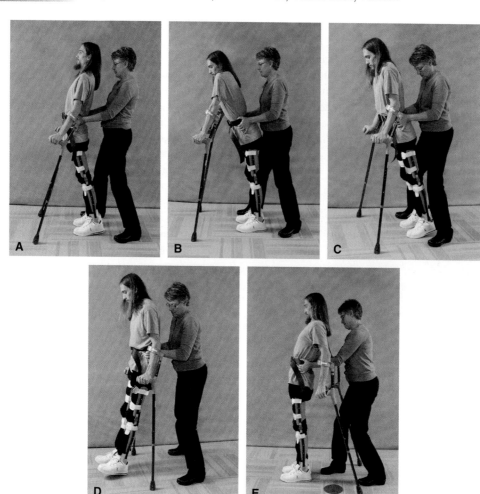

**FIGURE 26-25** Swing-through gait with knee-ankle-foot orthoses and Lofstrand crutches. (A) Balanced standing posture. (B) Crutches advanced. (C) Lifting the pelvis and legs by extending the elbows, depressing and protracting the scapulae, and tucking the head. (D) Once lifted, the torso and legs swing forward as a pendulum. (E) Balanced standing posture regained by lifting the head, retracting the scapulae, and pushing on the crutches to push the pelvis forward.

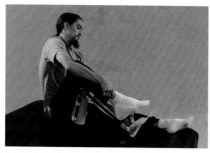

**FIGURE 26-26** Donning a knee-ankle-foot orthosis in long sitting on a mat.

# ■ Special Considerations for Interventions

## Medical and Orthopedic Precautions

Individuals with complete paralysis from an SCI are vulnerable to a number of physical complications. Many of these complications are relevant to physical therapy; therapists must

take measures to avoid causing harm during therapy and must recognize and respond appropriately when problems develop. Therapists should also be prepared for questions from patients regarding pathophysiology or management.

### Spine Precautions

When paralysis is the result of trauma to the spine, there is likely to be a period after the injury during which the vertebral column is unstable and healing. During this time, take extreme care to avoid stress to the injured area, because motion at the site of injury can cause additional neurological or musculoskeletal damage. The degree of vertebral instability present and the length of time it continues are determined by the nature of the injury, surgical procedures, and orthotic stabilization.

When working with a patient during the first several months after a traumatic SCI, strictly adhere to the spine precautions prescribed by the patient's physician. Spine precautions may include restriction to bed, log-rolling when turning in bed, use of a spinal orthosis when out of bed, use of a spinal

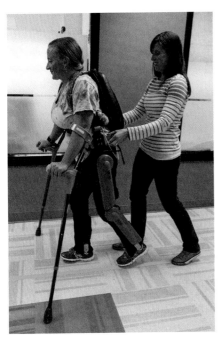

**FIGURE 26-27** A patient with T10 paraplegia practices with the ReWalk system.

orthosis at all times, lifting restrictions, avoidance of pillows under the head, or avoidance of trunk flexion or rotation or hip flexion with the knee extended. When no spinal restrictions are specified, obtain clarification before performing any procedures or placing the patient in any positions that could cause motion of the spine. Until the patient has been cleared for unrestricted activity, consult with the physician before initiating any new activities that could place stress on the spine.

Precautions specific to therapeutic exercise are worth mentioning here. These precautions are commonly observed but may not always be evidence based. When the cervical spine is unstable, take care to avoid strong contraction of the shoulder musculature and perform passive shoulder motions gently. Also, avoid abduction or flexion past 90 degrees as long as the cervical spine remains unstable. In a similar manner, exercise caution in the presence of an unstable lumbar spine. Avoid strong contraction of the hip musculature, perform hip range-of-motion exercises gently, avoid flexion past 90 degrees, and perform passive straight-leg raises only within a range that does not cause any vertebral motion.

### Fracture Prevention

After an SCI, calcium and collagen are rapidly lost from the bones below the lesion. Osteoporosis develops in the extremities innervated caudal to the lesion, causing an increased risk of fracture (Szollar, 1998). Fractures due to osteoporosis are more frequent in people with the following characteristics: motor complete injury, paraplegia, white race, extended time since injury, and female sex (Levi, 1995b).

When an individual has osteoporosis, avoid activities that place excessive stress on the affected bones. In particular, use caution during therapeutic exercise and electrical stimulation, as well as during any activities or positions that could cause

force to be applied to the osteoporotic bones. An example of such a position is prone-lying when the person has both osteoporosis in the femurs and hip flexion contractures. A person with complete paralysis may have weakened bones even if he does not have a declared diagnosis of osteoporosis. Regardless of diagnosis, this condition is likely to be present in the extremities caudal to the lesion, particularly if substantial time has passed since the spinal cord was damaged. Individuals with an SCI experience extensive loss of bone mineral density even during the first 6 months after injury (Shields, 2002).

### Skin Precautions

Pressure injuries are a common complication after an SCI because of the combined effects of sensory impairment, reduced mobility, changes in peripheral circulation, and reduction of skin collagen content (Mawson, 1993; Salzberg, 1998). When a person has a complete SCI, the vulnerability to pressure injuries begins at the time of injury and continues for the duration of the person's life. Pressure injuries are preventable, but their prevention requires virtually constant vigilance.

Prolonged unrelieved pressure is the most common cause of pressure injuries after an SCI (Ditunno, 1994). Standard precautions to avoid skin damage from prolonged unrelieved pressure include repositioning (turning) at least every 2 hours when in bed, and pressure relief every 15 to 30 minutes when sitting (CSCM, 2014; NPUAP, 2007). Additional preventive measures in physical therapy include avoidance of shear forces, friction, blunt trauma, and prolonged exposure to moisture; skin inspection; provision of appropriate wheelchair and cushion; and education and training of patients and their caregivers (Arnold, 2003; CSCM, 2014; Somers, 2010).

### Orthostatic Hypotension

Orthostatic hypotension is a drop in blood pressure brought on by assumption of an upright (sitting or standing) posture. Symptoms include light-headedness, dizziness, loss of vision, ringing in the ears, nausea, and loss of consciousness (Illman, 2000; Nobunaga, 1998). Orthostatic hypotension is common during the acute phase after a cervical or upper thoracic injury, resulting from the disruption of autonomic control of the peripheral vasculature. It typically resolves within a few weeks of injury (Naso, 1992). Sometimes medications such as midodrine can be used to elevate blood pressure and reduce orthostatic hypotension.

Orthostatic hypotensive episodes frequently occur during physical therapy sessions, as physical therapists are involved in early mobilization out of bed, in upright positions (Illman, 2000). To help minimize this problem, make sure the patient is wearing compressive stockings or elastic wraps and an abdominal binder to increase peripheral resistance. Initiate out-of-bed activities in a reclining wheelchair with the backrest at least partially reclined and the leg rests fully elevated. As the patient tolerates it, *gradually* move the backrest to more upright positions and lower the leg rests. Each change in backrest or leg rest position should be small. Allow the patient to adjust to the change in position before making another adjustment. If an individual has difficulty tolerating the progressively upright positions (i.e., develops symptoms of orthostatic hypotension), try adjusting the backrest alone and then adjust the leg rests after the patient has had time to accommodate to the more upright trunk position. Throughout the session, monitor the patient for signs and symptoms of orthostatic hypotension. When they occur, simply elevate the leg rests, lower the backrest, or both. Symptoms are likely to subside in the reclined position.

### Autonomic Dysreflexia

Autonomic dysreflexia is an exaggerated sympathetic response brought on by a noxious stimulus in an area innervated caudal to the spinal cord lesion. The hallmark of autonomic dysreflexia is a pronounced elevation in blood pressure level. Additional signs and symptoms frequently occurring with autonomic dysreflexia include a severe pounding headache, flushing and sweating above the lesion, bradycardia, piloerection, changes in vision, nasal congestion, anxiety, chest pain, and cardiac arrhythmia. Autonomic dysreflexia most typically occurs in people with a neurological level of injury of T6 or higher, but it has been reported at lower levels (CSCM, 2001).

Complications of autonomic dysreflexia include retinal or subarachnoid hemorrhage, seizures, coma, and death (Campagnolo, 2002b). Because serious harm can result from autonomic dysreflexia, it is imperative to recognize and respond quickly and appropriately when it occurs. If you are working with a patient who has a neurological level of injury at or above T6, you should suspect autonomic dysreflexia if he or she exhibits any of its signs or symptoms. If the patient is lying down, assist him into a short-sitting position. Short sitting places the lower extremities below the heart, encouraging orthostatic hypotension, which should reduce a blood pressure level that may be dangerously high, especially in the brain, in the person experiencing dysreflexia. You should monitor the patient's blood pressure level and if possible eliminate the source of the noxious stimulus that elicited the dysreflexic response (CSCM, 2001). Examples of noxious stimuli you can eliminate include hamstring stretching, constricting clothing, or bladder distention due to urinary catheter tubing occluded by a kink or an overextended urine collection bag.

However, the source of the noxious stimulus may be something a physical therapist cannot address. The patient may require catheterization, for example, or need to have a bowel impaction removed. The patient may also have a urinary tract infection. If your attempts to identify and eliminate the source of the patient's dysreflexic response do not result in the patient's blood pressure level returning to normal, you must ensure that he or she quickly receives emergency care from appropriate medical professionals.

## Overuse Syndromes

Individuals with complete paralysis frequently develop overuse syndromes in their upper extremities. Common problems experienced by individuals with a long-standing SCI include pain, degenerative joint changes, shoulder impingement, rotator cuff pathologies, tendinitis, and carpal tunnel syndrome

(Curtis, 1999a, 1999b; Gellman, 1988; Lal, 1998; Noreau, 2000; Sie, 1992; Silfverskiold, 1991). Upper extremity pain and degenerative changes are thought to develop as a result of cumulative trauma from repeatedly and chronically placed stresses on the upper extremities of these individuals while they perform functional activities such as transfers and manual wheelchair propulsion (Gellman, 1988; Noreau, 2000; Silfverskiold, 1991). Muscle imbalances are likely contributing factors, particularly in individuals with tetraplegia (Powers, 1994; Silfverskiold, 1991). Overuse syndromes are of particular concern because they can interfere with functional independence and community integration.

The existence of overuse syndromes following an SCI is well documented. Strategies for their prevention have been developed (CSCM, 2005a). In an effort to reduce your patients' risk of developing upper extremity problems over time, you should consider implementing the following measures:

1. During training, select strategies for accomplishing functional tasks that are less stressful on the upper extremities (Boninger, 1999; Sie, 1992).
2. Instruct patients in energy conservation and pacing of activities (Boninger, 1999; Sie, 1992).
3. Encourage patients to maintain their ideal body weight because added weight increases the strain placed on the upper extremities during functional activities (Boninger, 1999).
4. When ordering wheelchairs, consider the long-term orthopedic effects of manual wheelchair propulsion. A power (Boninger, 1999; Sie, 1992) or power-assist (Cooper, 2001) wheelchair may be appropriate in some cases to reduce demands on the upper extremities.
5. For patients who use manual wheelchairs, prescribe and adjust their wheelchairs to minimize cumulative upper extremity trauma. Beneficial features in a manual wheelchair include ultralight weight (Boninger, 1999), rear wheel axles positioned to minimize upper extremity forces (Boninger, 2000), and back height and seating systems that optimize posture and thereby promote normal scapular position and shoulder mechanics (Kirshblum, 1997).
6. Use therapeutic exercise to develop muscle endurance (Pentland, 1994a, 1994b) and balanced strength and flexibility in the shoulder girdles. More normal biomechanics may result, reducing stress on the shoulders (Ballinger, 2000; Kirshblum, 1997).
7. Educate your patients about overuse injuries. Encourage them to seek treatment when symptoms first occur, to avoid the development of chronic problems (Noreau, 2000).

## Preservation of Beneficial Tightness

The precautions presented in this section, aimed at preserving beneficial tightness, are required for a different purpose: maximizing functional potential. Mild tightness in the low back and long finger flexors can be functionally beneficial for some individuals with complete paralysis as described earlier in this chapter. To preserve this beneficial tightness, you should avoid placing these tissues on stretch and should instruct the patient and family to do the same.

Mild tightness in the long finger flexors is beneficial for individuals who use a tenodesis grasp (described earlier in the chapter; see Figs. 26-5 and 26-8) to hold and manipulate objects. People with C6 or C7 tetraplegia lack innervation to their finger flexors, but they can flex their fingers biomechanically by extending their wrists actively. Mild tightness in their long-finger flexors can enhance their capacity to grasp objects using this tenodesis action. Overstretching these muscles results in a loss of tenodesis action. People with C5 tetraplegia can also benefit from mild tightness in the long finger flexors because this tightness can enhance their ability to use their fingers to hook objects. Moreover, during the first year after injury, many individuals with C5 tetraplegia experience motor return in their wrist extensors and therefore can develop the capacity to use a tenodesis grasp.

The following precaution applies to all individuals with C5, C6, or C7 tetraplegia: Avoid simultaneous wrist and finger extension. Keep this precaution in mind whenever you perform passive range-of-motion exercises, practice activities with the patient involving weight-bearing on the palms, or educate the patient or family about exercise or functional skills.

Mild tightness in the low back can be functionally beneficial for individuals who lack innervation to their trunk musculature. This tightness makes it possible for motions of the head and arms to effect motion in the lower body by placing tension on the soft tissues of the back. This movement strategy is used during activities such as rolling in bed or transferring to and from a wheelchair. The following measures will prevent overstretching of the low back:

1. Avoid long sitting when hamstring tightness prevents passive straight-leg raise of at least 100 degrees.
2. When stretching the hamstrings, ensure that the stretching force is applied to the hamstrings and not to the low back. The simplest way to do this is to stabilize the patient's pelvis and lumbar spine by positioning him in supine and stabilizing the contralateral hip in extension whenever performing passive hamstring stretching.
3. Avoid prolonged sitting with the pelvis in posterior tilt.

# ■ Intervention: Considerations for Nontherapy Time and Discharge
## Aspects of Patient and Family Education

Numerous preventable secondary pathologies and impairments are associated with complete paralysis resulting from an SCI. Many of these problems can be profoundly detrimental to the individual's physical health, functional capabilities, and capacity to participate in family and community activities. Moreover, a person who has a complete SCI will remain vulnerable to these secondary conditions for the duration of his life.

You can help patients optimize their future health by providing appropriate education and training. Table 26-9 summarizes the areas of knowledge and physical skills you should address in physical therapy for individuals with complete paralysis. Although other members of the rehabilitation team usually address additional health-related topics such as bowel and bladder management, medication use, safety and sexuality after an SCI, the therapist needs good working knowledge of all these topics. Patients will ask, and the therapist needs to be prepared to respond appropriately. As is true with all aspects of rehabilitation, the education and training you provide to each patient should be tailored to his unique abilities, goals, and needs.

Ideally, the patient will learn to perform the physical skills involved in health maintenance. Individuals who do not have the potential to acquire these skills should learn how to instruct and supervise others as they provide the needed assistance. For example, a person with high tetraplegia should practice verbally directing an attendant in how to position him properly in a wheelchair. All patients should learn to self-direct

| TABLE 26-9 | Teaching Components in a Typical Physical Therapy Rehabilitation Program for the Individual With Complete Paralysis |
|---|---|
| **TOPIC** | **GENERAL GOAL FOR PATIENT EDUCATION** |
| Neurological level of injury | Understand basic anatomy of spinal cord, neurological level of injury, and functional expectations so individual can perform or direct care |
| Skin management | Know causes of skin breakdown and how to prevent, detect, and manage it; understand pressure reliefs, positioning, posture, equipment, and skin care as they affect skin integrity |
| Secondary complications | Know and follow spinal precautions, if present; know how to manage and/or prevent secondary complications such as hypotension, autonomic dysreflexia, respiratory complications, genitourinary complications, gastrointestinal disturbances, and pain |
| Transfers | Know transfer techniques and typical options: bed, chair, wheelchair, toilet, tub/shower, floor, and car |
| Mobility | Know types of wheelchairs that are appropriate and how to maintain, propel, and use them on level and nonlevel surfaces |
| Accessibility | Know home design modifications typically needed for individuals with complete paralysis |
| Equipment | Understand how to use, maintain, and/or apply equipment such as braces or functional aides |

their care in case a caregiver cannot be present or the caregiver has not been previously trained in the care being provided.

## Activities for Home

Individuals with complete paralysis should be encouraged to carry through principles and activities of rehabilitation in the home setting. A home exercise program is a must for the individual to maintain the strength, range of motion, and skills needed to perform the difficult functional activities in complete paralysis. The exercise program should consist of range of motion, strengthening, and functional practice of the activities learned in rehabilitation.

Of course, a typical range-of-motion program for the individual with complete paralysis depends on the level of injury. For the individual with paraplegia, the lower extremities need to be stretched to maintain the desired 100 to 110 degrees of straight-leg raise needed for long sitting. This can be accomplished by using the long-sitting position during functional activities. Hips do not often get extended in functional positions, so to maintain joint health, oftentimes patients use the prone-on-elbows position or use a standing frame that allows passive weight-bearing with relative hip extension.

Upper extremities also need regular range of motion in addition to movements during functional activities. The shoulder joint was not designed to have the combination of mobility and stability that it repetitively needs during movements of the person with complete paralysis, such as rolling to prone-on-elbows or a transfer from wheelchair to floor. Thus, the individual with complete paralysis should perform a daily shoulder range-of-motion program that encourages shoulder external rotation and retraction and upward rotation of the scapula (CSCM, 2005a). For the person who lacks triceps activation, maintenance of end-range elbow extension is also vital. This can be accomplished using gravity with supinated forearms in an antigravity position. An elbow flexion contracture for the person with complete paralysis who lacks triceps function may prevent upper extremity weight-bearing functional activities.

Maintenance of strength in the upper extremities should not be underestimated. It is typically not enough to simply perform the functional activities of daily living, such as transfers and wheelchair propulsion. The shoulder joint in particular needs regular strengthening to ensure it can handle the demands placed on it (CSCM, 2005a). Rotator cuff and scapular stabilizer strengthening (e.g., by using a resistance band or pulley system) must occur. Exercises such as these should take place two to three days per week.

Finally, regular performance of functional activities is essential to maintaining an individual's abilities from both practice and therapeutic standpoints. Continued practice of the skill will help the individual maintain it. Performing the skill helps to keep the individual's muscles strong enough and the range of motion adequate to complete the task. Patients are encouraged to live by the adage "If you don't use it, you lose it."

## Considerations for a Healthy Active Lifestyle

Individuals with a recent-onset SCI resulting in complete paralysis live in an era when life expectancy is creeping closer to that of individuals without an SCI (NSCISC, 2016, 2017). Efforts must be made during rehabilitation to prepare the person with an SCI for life-long health. Efforts must also be made to minimize the secondary complications of SCI (see sections on secondary complications and aging with SCI). Teach the patient to protect the shoulders, elbows, and wrists (CSCM, 2005a), prevent pressure injuries (CSCM, 2014), and pay close attention to posture so osteopenia or osteoporosis does not result in vertebral damage and permanent postural changes. Teach the individual to minimize unwanted contractures, as in the hip flexors, knee flexors, and ankle plantar flexors, by performing daily range-of-motion and stretching exercises.

Physical health also involves regular cardiovascular exercise. All individuals should get 30 minutes or more of moderate-intensity exercise at least 5 days per week or at least 20 minutes of vigorous-intensity exercise at least 3 days per week (Haskell, 2007; HHS, 2010). Outside of manual wheelchair propulsion, obtaining prolonged moderate- to vigorous-intensity exercise is difficult for the person with an SCI. Upper extremity ergometers can provide cardiovascular exercise, but the person with an SCI will be repetitively using the arms, an action that can lead to earlier upper extremity joint dysfunction. Bicycles with electrical stimulation provide some hope. Walking with KAFOs and a gait aid may also be possible, particularly for those with thoracic or lumbar lesions. When cardiovascular exercise is difficult to obtain, nutrition must be closely monitored to minimize weight gain after an SCI.

## HANDS-ON PRACTICE

Be sure to review the skills covered in this chapter. With further practice, you should be able to teach and/or assist the patient in performing the following skills:
- Rolling supine-to-prone with or without equipment
- Moving from prone to prone-on-elbows
- Moving from prone-on-elbows to long sitting with or without equipment

- Maintaining the long- or short-sitting position
- Performing a seated push-up and/or forward lean
- Performing level or nonlevel transfers with or without equipment
- Propelling a manual wheelchair
- Basic gait training with complete paralysis of the lower extremities

## Let's Review

1. Summarize the anatomy and physiology of the typical causes of complete paralysis.

2. List and describe the pathologies that often accompany complete paralysis.

3. Describe compensatory movement strategies and therapeutic techniques used with individuals with complete paralysis.
   a. Rolling
   b. Achieving long sitting
   c. Performing a seated push-up
   d. Performing a transfer to or from the wheelchair, with or without equipment
   e. Propelling a manual wheelchair
   f. Gait training with complete paralysis of the lower extremities

4. Describe typical interventions used with individuals with complete paralysis and apply them to a case.

5. Summarize special considerations for interventions used with individuals with complete paralysis.

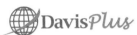 For additional resources, including Focus on Evidence tables, case study discussions, references and glossary, please visit http://davisplus.fadavis.com

## CHAPTER SUMMARY

This chapter describes therapeutic interventions for the person with complete paralysis along with the typical anatomy, secondary conditions, precautions, and home-going considerations. The Focus on Evidence (FOE) tables, available online, summarize important data regarding interventions for focal/regional paralysis, such as Erb palsy, Bell palsy, and peripheral neuropathy paralysis (Table 26-10 ONL), and complete paralysis of broader regions associated with an SCI (Table 26-11 ONL). Individuals with complete paralysis experience extensive loss of function but can learn alternative strategies to compensate for this loss. Considerations for use of these interventions by the therapist are also presented. The patient and therapist need time and tenacity to learn and teach the functional movements described in this chapter. Before beginning functional training, the therapist should ensure that the patient has adequate range of motion, strength, and medical stability to begin practicing the task.

---

*Note: Small portions of Martha Freeman Somer's text, Spinal Cord Injury: Functional Rehabilitation, 3rd Ed (© 2010), appear in this chapter with permission of the publisher, Pearson Education, Inc., New York, New York.*

## CHAPTER 27

# Intervention for Sensory Impairment

### Deborah Nervik Chamberlain, PT, DPT, MHS, DHS, PCS
### Dennis W. Fell, PT, MD

**CHAPTER OBJECTIVES**

Upon completion of this chapter, the learner should be able to:

1. Distinguish between normal and abnormal sensory functions.
2. Describe the mechanisms of common pathologies related to sensory impairment.
3. Recognize common signs and symptoms of sensory impairment.
4. Formulate functional patient-centered goals based on results of an examination.
5. Design an appropriate plan of care for sensory impairments.
6. Choose sensory interventions using current research and evidence-based practice.

## ■ Introduction to Sensory Impairment

*Imagine a warm summer day, and you are sitting on your front porch, quietly rocking in a wicker chair with your bare feet. You feel the breeze blow across you while you sip on a glass of iced tea. Out of nowhere, a tiny mouse runs across your feet, causing you to leap out of your seat and spill the icy tea all over yourself. Without having to think about it, your sensory system works instantly and automatically to take in, process, organize, and plan a response to the myriad sensory events that just took place. In an instant, sensory receptors in your joints, skin, and head alerted the central nervous system to process and respond to the numerous temperature, touch, movement, and pressure stimuli.*

The human body possesses numerous sensory systems that function both independently and in conjunction with each other. The mechanisms determining how they work are different, yet they all share the overall goal of helping the person be aware of and react to internal (body) and external (environment) stimulations in a functional and purposeful manner. The sensory systems can be categorized as **somatosensory** (tactile and proprioceptive), vestibular, and other special senses such as vision, hearing, taste, and smell. Impairments in tactile, **proprioceptive**, and vestibular systems are the sensory dysfunctions covered in this chapter. The reader is also referred to Chapters 7 and 29 for additional information on vestibular, visual, olfactory, taste, and auditory impairments.

### Normal Sensory Function

According to the *Guide to Physical Therapist Practice (Guide)*, **sensory integrity** is the accuracy of cortical sensory processing, to include **proprioception**, vibration sense, **stereognosis**, and cutaneous sense (American Physical Therapy Association [APTA], 2015b). Sensory processing is defined by the *Guide* as the ability to integrate movement-related information that is derived from the environment (APTA, 2015b). It involves taking in, processing, organizing, and planning a motor response to sensory stimuli. In normal, healthy individuals, this response is an automatic, efficient, and effective occurrence. Perhaps an overlooked, taken for granted event, it occurs continually throughout the day for every person. When disease or injury does not permit the sensory system to function smoothly, automatically, completely, or efficiently, however, it suddenly gains our attention.

## THINK ABOUT IT 27.1

How might movement-related symptoms present differently in an individual depending on whether the dysfunction is in the afferent input, the processing/organizing of sensory information, or the motor response?

## Clinical Picture of Sensory Impairment and Its Effect on Function

The various types of sensory impairments caused by pathology can disrupt virtually all motor activities in one's life, including mobility, activities of daily living (ADLs), recreation, and vocational tasks, thereby leading to functional limitation and potential disability. Both children and adults are affected. In a study of children with and without sensory dysfunction, as determined by the Sensory Profile evaluation tool (Dunn, 1999), White (2007) discovered that children with sensory dysfunction had lower motor performance scores on the *Assessment of Motor and Process Skills* (Fisher, 2014).

Sensory impairments can be categorized as **hyposensitivity** (low response) or **hypersensitivity** (high response). Hyposensitivity includes **anesthesia** (total loss of sensation), partial or poor (low) registration of sensation, reduced sensory discrimination, and/or **sensory neglect**. Hypersensitivity includes **sensory defensiveness**, **sensory avoidance**, and **paresthesia** (altered or painful sensation). Both hyposensitivity and hypersensitivity can result in poor motor skills, decreased posture and balance, and problems with motor learning. Sensory impairments may lead individuals to either seek increased sensory input or to avoid it.

Both hyposensitivity and hypersensitivity can also lead to safety and health concerns by increasing the risk of injury or secondary impairment. A lack of sensation, poor sensory awareness, or decreased sensation does not allow a person to protect his/her skin from injury from extreme temperature or sharp surfaces or know when to shift weight to provide pressure relief and prevent skin breakdown. When hypersensitivity or paresthesia is present, inefficient or inappropriate reactions to sensory input may cause a person to ignore or misinterpret important sensory information, leading to injury. For example, when a patient has hypersensitivity to touch, she may interpret an unexpected touch (e.g., someone brushing up against her in a hallway) as a noxious stimulus and lash out by hitting or pushing that person away. This chronic irritation or discomfort can create difficulties in social, work, or play situations, thereby decreasing quality of life.

### PATIENT APPLICATION: CASE INTRODUCTION

Sammie is an 8 year-old boy who sustained a traumatic head injury (TBI) in a motor vehicle accident 6 months ago. The damage to his right cerebral hemisphere resulted in left hemiparesis. After 1 month in intensive care and 4 months in a rehabilitation center, he is now at home with his family and ready to return to school. He has progressed to walking independently for short distances, but he continues to trip or bump into things and fatigues quickly. He often appears unaware of his left side and does not like it when people touch his left hand or leg. Sammie is scheduled to begin outpatient physical therapy next week to continue his recovery.

According to the Guide to Physical Therapist Practice, the preferred practice pattern for this diagnosis is 5C Impaired Motor Function and Sensory Integrity Associated with Nonprogressive Disorders of the Central Nervous System—Congenital Origin or Acquired in Infancy or Childhood (APTA, 2015a).

### Contemplate Clinical Decisions: Initial Questions

Given Sammie's case as described:

- From this brief introduction, what further information about his medical history do you need in order to proceed?
- What family and social information is important to know?
- What environmental constraints at home and at school may be important to consider?
- What else do you need to know about Sammie's functional level?
- What consultation needs to occur with the school district?
- What are Sammie's goals? His family's goals?
- Why is it important to have the discharge summary from the rehabilitation center?

## ■ Anatomy and Physiology

### Sensory Systems

**Sensation** is defined as neural activity that results from a stimulus that activates a sensory receptor and then travels along sensory nerve pathways to the brain (Haywood, 2009). **Perception** is defined as a multistage process in which the brain selects, processes, organizes, and integrates information received from the senses (Haywood, 2009). From these two definitions, we see that sensory processing involves the peripheral and central nervous systems, beginning with the sensory receptor. Before discussing examination or intervention for sensory dysfunction, a brief review is needed to look at the three sensory systems covered in this chapter: tactile, vestibular and proprioceptive.

The tactile sensory system serves dual purposes: protection and discrimination. **Mechanoreceptors** in the skin (tactile receptors including Meissner's corpuscles, Pacinian corpuscles, Merkel's disks, and Ruffini's corpuscles) respond to touch and can distinguish the different textures, contours, sizes, shapes, and localization of touch. Our sense of touch allows us to distinguish if things are sharp or dull or if they are hot or cold, which protects us from injury. It informs our body about pressure against our skin, which is important in preventing skin breakdown. It allows us to know the qualities of the things we touch so we can precisely manipulate objects and use our fine motor skills for work, play, and ADLs.

The vestibular system is a complex sensory system serving many purposes, such as regulating muscle tone and coordination; maintaining balance and equilibrium; assisting in ocular-motor control; maintaining the head in an upright, vertical position; and affecting arousal and attention levels. Three main vestibular sensory receptors are located in the inner ear: the semicircular canals, the saccule, and the utricle. The semicircular canals register speed, force, and direction of head rotation. They respond to angular acceleration and deceleration (rotation) as well as to linear acceleration and deceleration (moving forward). The saccule and utricle are sensitive to the force of gravity and changes in head position. Through numerous pathways and connections throughout the nervous system, these receptors respond to input by adjusting body position and movement (Guttman, 2008) (see Fig. 5-2, Fig. 5-3, and Table 5-1 for details). Functional correlations to a working vestibular system are good balance, tone, coordination, and response to movement leading to appropriate posture, mobility, and gross motor skills necessary for daily living and life skills.

The proprioceptive system provides perception of movement and position of the body in space. It interprets the rate and timing of movement, the amount of force exerted by the muscles, how much and how fast a muscle is stretched, and the relation of the body in space and the body parts to each other. Efficient motor planning, praxis, fine and gross motor skills, mobility, and ADLs are all dependent on a functioning proprioceptive system.

Proprioceptive receptors are located in the muscles, tendons, and joints. **Muscle spindles**, located in skeletal muscles, provide the body with information on the length, tension, and load on the muscle. **Golgi tendon organs**, located in the tendons, detect the amount of tension in the tendon of a contracting muscle. Joint receptors are found in the connective tissue of a joint capsule and respond to mechanical deformation in the capsule and ligaments. As with the vestibular system, once a receptor detects a signal, numerous pathways and connections course throughout the nervous system (see Fig. 5-2, Fig. 5-3, and Table 5-1 for details).

The visual and vestibular systems are also important in balance and assist a person in maintaining/adjusting the position in space. They should be considered when patients have difficulty with proprioception.

**Sensory thresholds** are important in understanding how each system functions. How much input does it take to activate the sensory receptors and fire the system? Some patients' sensory systems are hypoactive, needing a lot of input to fire (high threshold), and some patients' sensory systems are hypersensitive, having a low threshold for firing, and may be overly reactive to very little sensory input. Depending on the health or status of the system, a different amount of energy is required before a stimulus registers (threshold).

## Lifespan Influence: Developmental and Age-Related Changes

Growth, development, and function of the sensory system begin in utero and mature throughout childhood. When an infant is born, tactile sensation is present, but fine discrimination develops over time. Evidence that an infant possesses touch sensation is the presence of the rooting reaction. When the side of the baby's face is touched, the baby reacts by turning toward the source of touch. Proprioception and vestibular sensation are also present at birth but mature over time. Babies respond to deep pressure, proprioceptive input, and vestibular input when they stop crying and calm down when wrapped up, cuddled, and rocked. In contrast, they wake up and become more alert and active when quickly bounced. Over the first few years of life, maturation and sensory refinement occur because of the combination of rapid brain growth (increases in neurons and synaptic formation), myelination, and the child's numerous movement and sensory experiences. Normal maturation of neural systems allows the child to rely more on kinesthetic feedback than on visual feedback. **Tactile discrimination** improves along with fine motor skills. The vestibular system is challenged and strengthened as gross motor skills progress.

Many factors affect how the sensory system changes over the lifespan, and these vary greatly from person to person. In general, however, it appears the senses of touch, **kinesthesia**, and proprioception deteriorate with age, which may be due to fewer numbers of receptors as well as less efficient functioning (Shaffer, 2007). Clinically, fewer sensory receptors in the joints have been associated with decreased proprioception, particularly in the lower extremities, which may have a direct effect on balance and mobility (Shaffer, 2007). Fewer cutaneous sensory receptors have also been associated with decreased vibration, two-point discrimination, and monofilament testing. Less efficiency may be due to decreased nerve conduction velocities with age (Dyck, 1972; Evans, 1992; Horch, 1992) along with increased somatosensory thresholds (Dorfman, 1979). This results in some older people showing a longer reaction time to **sensory stimulation**, as well as requiring more sensory input to get the same reaction as younger people. For instance, when touching a hot surface, an older person may not sense the temperature unless it is very hot and may not feel the heat until several seconds after first touching the surface. Age-related decreases in sensory functioning can lead to secondary impairments with motor and functional implications. In the case just described, when a patient's ability to sense a hot surface is impaired, she may be badly burned, causing tissue destruction, limited use of the body part, and inability to function in her usual capacity.

## ■ Related Pathology
### Neuroanatomy of Common Pathologies With Sensory Deficits

Injury, disease, and abnormal growth or development can occur in any of the structures of the body's complex sensory systems, including the sensory receptors (tactile, joint, or muscle spindle; see Fig. 5-1), the primary somatosensory cortex (see Fig. 5-2), and sensory pathways that carry information from the receptors through the spinal cord and brainstem to the brain cortex. The primary conscious sensory pathways (lateral spinothalamic, anterior spinothalamic, and dorsal columns) are shown in Figure 5-3. The altered body system structure results in altered sensory function, as described in Chapter 5.

Patients who experience hyposensitivity may have little or no response to a painful or noxious stimulus. Thus, falling and bumping the head does not lead to a negative reaction, and bruises and cuts do not register or are not seen as painful. A decreased ability to discriminate touch or textures leads to astereognosis, or the inability to distinguish characteristics of an object by touching it. For example, a person with astereognosis is unable to distinguish between a nickel and a dime without looking at the coins. In extreme situations, **sensory neglect** may be present, in which a patient totally ignores or is unaware of part of the body. A patient with a hyposensitivity in the vestibular system may have little interest in movement or no response to movement.

Individuals with decreased proprioception have decreased knowledge or awareness of their body in space, which can affect their balance and increase their fall risk. Many patients with sensory loss after a stoke experience poor balance and a higher incidence of falls (Tyson, 2006; Yates, 2002). Mobility and gross motor skills are also affected, and in many cases, motor recovery is slower in individuals with sensory impairment (Reding, 1988). Hyposensitivity in any system may cause a person to seek out additional or extra sensory input in an effort to reach a threshold and register the stimulus. Decreased discrimination or processing in any system also prevents the patient from deriving meaningful information from her senses, which may affect learning and lead to serious functional limitations and increased disability.

In contrast, the patient with hypersensitivity may avoid sensory input or have an overreaction to it. Sensory defensiveness (negative reaction to sensory input) may manifest as **tactile defensiveness** (intense dislike of textures or touch) or **gravitational insecurity** (fear or dislike of movement). Either scenario results in abnormal use of sensory systems and thus decreases function and motor outcomes.

## Medical Diagnoses

Common diagnoses in patients with sensory impairment include stroke, multiple sclerosis, cerebral palsy (CP), spinal cord injury (SCI), TBI, peripheral nerve injury, sensory integrative disorder, and autism. Patients with these diagnoses may experience a loss of sensation (partial or complete), oversensitivity to sensory input, or abnormal and uncomfortable sensations (e.g., pain, burning, tingling, numbness). Some people may experience a combination of hyposensitivity and hypersensitivity symptoms. Depending on the diagnosis, patients may have temporary, progressive, or permanent sensory impairment. Knowing the cause of impairment will help guide the therapist's expectations, determination of prognosis, and anticipated outcomes (Table 27-1).

**TABLE 27-1   Sensory Impairment and Prognosis in Neurological Diagnoses**

| MEDICAL DIAGNOSIS | SENSORY IMPAIRMENT | PROGNOSIS |
|---|---|---|
| Cerebrovascular accident (stroke) | Total or partial sensory loss, sensory neglect, and/or hypersensitivity | Varied; some sensory return expected |
| Cerebral palsy | Hyposensitivity, hypersensitivity, or a combination | Nonprogressive; may improve with therapy |
| Traumatic brain injury | Hyposensation, hypersensation, paresthesia, or a combination of all | Sensory abilities change over time as part of recovery; may progress from hyposensitivity (during coma) to hypersensitivity and irritation to more normalized sensation; some deficits may be permanent |
| Peripheral vascular disease | Decreased sensation and pain or paresthesia | May worsen as disease progresses; may improve with therapy |
| Multiple sclerosis | Loss of sensation, altered sensation: tingling, numbness, and/or painful paresthesia | Progressive demyelination; symptoms come and go but get worse over time; may respond to treatment |
| Autism | **Sensory integrative dysfunction**; may have hyposensitivity and/or hypersensitivity | May improve over time or with therapy; nonprogressive |
| Spinal cord injury | Partial or total loss of sensation depending on level and type of injury | Permanent damage; will need compensatory strategies to prevent secondary impairments |
| Peripheral nerve injury | Partial or total loss of sensation (and motor function); reflective of the level and type of injury | Partial or full recovery occurs over time; may respond to therapy |

## THINK ABOUT IT 27.2

Would a child who has never experienced normal sensory input have different manifestation of symptoms and a different prognosis than an individual who developed sensory impairments of either a progressive or permanent nature in adulthood?

in movement/facial or body reaction/grimace/eye opening should be noted as a response to sensory input even when the patient does not verbally describe the perceived sensation. Clear documentation of sensory findings is critical for physical therapy evaluation, diagnosis and prognosis, program planning, and progress. Once the sensory examination is complete, it is time to think about setting goals and planning treatment.

## ■ Pertinent Examination/Evaluation

Before treatment decisions can be made for sensory impairment, a thorough and complete examination and evaluation of the sensory system must be performed. On the basis of the patient history and systems review, the need for specific tests and measures should become apparent. Most often, when concerns about a sensory system arise during an initial screening, the sensory integrity of the tactile, proprioceptive, and vestibular systems is fully examined. Specific tests will depend on the age of the patient, the presenting symptoms, the availability of the test, and the skill of the therapist. For example, Eeles (2013) conducted a systematic review of assessments of sensory function within the first 2 years of life and identified three that they would recommend. For example, the *Test of Sensory Functions in Infants* (DeGangi, 1989), is only appropriate for children age 4 to 18 months of age, and could not be used for children not in that age group. Two parent-report measures for infants and young children from birth to 3 years of age are the *Sensory Rating Scale for Infants and Young Children* (Provost, 1994) and the *Infant/Toddler Sensory Profile* (Dunn, 2002). Examples of assessments for adults include the Adolescent/ Adult Sensory Profile (Brown, 2002) and the *Adult Sensory Interview* (ADULTS-SI) (Kinnealey, 1999).

Some tests require therapist certification for administration, such as the *Sensory Integration and Praxis Tests* (Ayres, 1989), whereas others are diagnosis specific, such as the American Spinal Injury Association (ASIA, 2016) *International Standards for Neurological Classification of Spinal Cord Injury* for sensory functioning and the Fugl-Meyer Assessment of sensorimotor function after stroke (Fugl-Meyer, 1975). Some tests may require a certain level of cognitive and communicative ability from the patient, which is important to consider when choosing a tool. A screening tool such as the Sensory Profile (Dunn, 1999) is a good choice because it encompasses products for different ages (infant/toddler and adolescent/adult) and circumstances (e.g., school companion). Family members or caregivers can also complete the Sensory Profile to provide information on the patient's sensory processing and its effects on daily functioning. Complete details concerning sensory examination and testing for pain, temperature, light touch, vibration, stereognosis, two-point discrimination, and proprioception can be found in Chapter 5. Examination of vestibular function is covered in Chapter 8.

Often, sensory testing comes down to the therapist's skilled observation of the patient's response to sensory stimuli, especially for patients who are very young, nonverbal, or cognitively impaired. For example, touch or pinprick to an area resulting

### PATIENT APPLICATION: EXAMINATION/ EVALUATION

*A complete history and systems review is completed along with appropriate tests and measures as part of Sammie's initial outpatient visit. Sammie has a strong family support system and adequate health insurance. His mother works part-time as a nurse, and his father works as a police officer. Sammie is an only child who is in the second grade.*

*Before the motor vehicle accident, Sammie was healthy and developing typically and was a good student. His family's main goal is that he can reintegrate into school, play with his friends, and do well academically. He can communicate normally but is experiencing some mild social and cognitive impairments, including a short attention span, frequent temper tantrums, and short-term memory loss.*

*Range of motion (ROM) measurements and manual muscle testing reveal that Sammie's range and strength are decreased on his left side, with more distal than proximal involvement. Right-side measurements are within normal limits. His modified Ashworth scale (Bohannon, 1987) score for muscle tone in his ankle, hand, and shoulder is 2 (more marked increase in muscle tone through most of the ROM, but the affected joint is easily moved). His endurance is normal, and he can be physically active for an hour without fatigue. All his vital signs (heart rate, respiratory rate, blood pressure) are within normal limits. Sensory testing reveals he has hypersensitivity to movement (demonstrating gravitational insecurity) and tactile defensiveness on his left side. He also demonstrates a left-sided neglect (i.e., he appears to be unaware of the left side of his body).*

*Functionally, Sammie can walk independently on level and uneven surfaces including stairs, but he requires an ankle-foot orthosis (AFO) for support on his left foot and tends to drag his leg forward, with decreased weight-bearing on the left compared with the right. He does not use his left arm or hand unless prompted, but he can lift his arm 90 degrees independently and flex and extend his elbow fully; however, he keeps his hand in a fisted position most of the time. He has a dynamic hand splint to assist with a more functional open hand and extended wrist position. The neglect and hemiparesis of the left side make it difficult for Sammie to complete common age-appropriate bilateral activities such as pushing, pulling, or carrying large objects; throwing and catching a ball; pulling his pants up with two hands; crawling and climbing on playground structures; and various bimanual fine motor activities. It also affects his ability to read and write because these skills require crossing the midline from left to right. Reaching/moving across the midline of the body with either hand or visually scanning with head movement from side to side entails crossing this midline.*

# Preparatory Intervention Specific to Sensory Impairment

Impairment-focused intervention for sensory dysfunction entails a combination of facilitating sensory recovery and compensating for impairments, applied early in rehab and in preparation for a focus on functional improvement. The choice of interventions focusing on recovery or compensation often depends on the patient's diagnosis and medical status and may change over time depending on her progress. When providing sensory interventions, it is important to pay close attention to the patient's responses and to read both verbal and nonverbal cues closely. Because sensory processing is both an internal and an external experience, only patients can truly describe the degree to which they perceive the sensation and how the intervention may be resulting in improvement

As with any intervention, but particularly with sensory intervention, patients should never be forced to continue treatment, and their desire to proceed slowly should be respected because sensory input may be uncomfortable or difficult to process. "More" is not always "better." Providing too much sensory input may result in a rebound effect later (Bundy, 2002). As much as possible, sensory interventions should be integrated into patients' normal daily routines and tasks instead of added randomly out of context. This makes the sensory stimulation more meaningful and functional.

In the history and examination process, key questions should be asked and answered concerning the patient's normal daily sensory experiences and what issues are affecting function or safety. A hypothesis as to the nature and reasoning behind the sensory issues should be made before deciding on a specific intervention. Once an appropriate intervention has been chosen, it should focus on improved skills and functional outcomes, not just a impact at the impairment level.

Therapists have the ability and privilege to affect and change the sensory systems of the patients they work with and to help them achieve their goals through various therapeutic strategies. Sensory intervention not only leads to improvements at the impairment and functional levels but may also affect brain plasticity. Providing cutaneous, muscle, and/or articular input through various sensory interventions activates both sensory and motor cortices for up to an hour, providing opportunities for retraining/relearning of both sensory and motor systems (Dobkin, 2003).

Physical therapists use a variety of interventions to treat sensory impairment. These interventions should be evidence based: a blend of current research evidence, the therapist's clinical judgment, and individual patient values. Unfortunately, randomized controlled trials sometimes lack definitive, specified interventions. Case studies and case reports may be available, but anecdotal information is often widespread. One must be cautious about using interventions with limited evidence in clinical decision-making. Fortunately, published research in this area is growing (Sullivan, 2008).

When providing sensory interventions, remember to also address underlying or comorbid impairments, such as weakness, tightness, and endurance, because they also affect progress and outcomes. A holistic view of the patient is mandatory because all systems affect others. In addition, decisions regarding appropriate interventions depend on where the therapy will be done; some environments, such as homes or schools, may not have the necessary space or equipment. Furthermore, not all therapists are trained in specific interventions or have the required equipment. Above all, when making clinical decisions about interventions, consider the family's/patient's needs and goals, with a focus on functional and meaningful outcomes.

## General Approaches: Recovery Versus Compensation

A variety of treatment approaches are used for sensory impairment. Each approach is built on one of two assumptions: The nervous system has the capacity to reorganize and recover to some extent because of neuroplasticity, or the system is irreparably damaged and needs intervention to compensate for lost function. Treatment approaches can be categorized as interventions for hyposensitivity, hypersensitivity, and paresthesia. Although different intervention approaches are discussed in subsequent sections, it is important to remember that no single approach has been proven to be the most effective or most appropriate; thus, an integrated approach to therapy should be based on patient examination and the therapist's evaluation and clinical decision-making. In addition, when providing any type of sensory intervention, therapists should offer consistent feedback on sensory performance/understanding and choose activities that are meaningful to the patient to aid in learning.

## Specific Therapeutic Techniques

### Hyposensitivity

#### Sensory Integration Therapy

**Sensory integration therapy** (SIT) involves activities that are meaningful to the patient and includes enhanced sensations (tactile, vestibular, and proprioceptive) and active participation that elicit adaptive motor responses (Bundy, 2002). SIT was developed by Jean Ayres in the 1970s to treat sensory impairments that she hypothesized were often present in children with learning disabilities; the therapy is now used with individuals who have a variety of neurological diagnoses, including sensory impairments. Ayres (1972) postulated that "**sensory integration** is the neurological process that organizes sensation from one's own body and from the environment and makes it possible to use the body effectively within the environment" (p. 11)

Occupational therapists have led the way in developing and using SIT; however, physical therapists with training are also using the technique. Full certification in SIT is required in order to administer the main assessment tool, the *Southern California Sensory Integration Test* (SCSIT) (Ayres, 1989); however, SIT intervention strategies can be used by therapists without certification.

Evidence supporting the use of SIT is increasing; however, it is still limited because of the lack of randomized controlled trials and inconclusive results in many studies. In some cases, SIT has improved sensory functioning as measured by increased scores on the SCSIT in children with CP (Bumin, 2001), learning disabilities, and sensory integrative dysfunction (Humphries, 1990). Because of increasing awareness and use of SIT by occupational and physical therapists, along with emerging research, the American Academy of Pediatrics released a policy statement supporting the therapy as part of a comprehensive plan of care for the patient. The policy statement includes the following recommendations: (1) Specific goals should be developed; (2) progress should be monitored; and (3) if progress is not seen by a certain time, a new intervention should be considered (American Academy of Pediatrics, 2012).

For individuals with hyposensitivity, consistent participation in specific sensory modalities (an integral component to sensory integration) may lower the sensory threshold required for neuron firing and processing, leading to improved motor outcomes. White (2007) found a significant correlation between motor difficulty and atypical sensory processing. For individuals with decreased tactile awareness, activities rich in tactile qualities help to increase registration and processing. Different textures are recommended (e.g., hard, soft, scratchy, smooth, bumpy, silky). For children, activities may include playing with a container of dry rice and beans (e.g., pouring contents from cup to cup or hiding/finding objects), playing at sand and water tables, and exploring toys with different textures. For adults, this may include manipulating objects with different textures, washing with a washcloth, and using therapeutic putty.

For individuals with decreased proprioceptive awareness, activities providing deep pressure input to joint and muscle sensory receptors are recommended. Activities that stimulate vestibular input include swinging the child from suspended equipment (Fig. 27-1), jumping on a trampoline (Fig. 27-2) or on the floor, bouncing on a therapy ball, the rotary experience of sitting on a Sit 'n Spin (Fig. 27-3), weight-bearing on arms (e.g., maneuvering in quadruped), and pushing/pulling heavy objects.

Participation in these sensory activities cannot be random and without purpose; SIT does not provide sensory stimulation alone. Meaningful, adaptive, functional activities must be part of the sensory intervention. The sensory activities must not be completely passive (e.g., the therapist rubbing textures on the skin or bouncing the child on a ball) but must involve

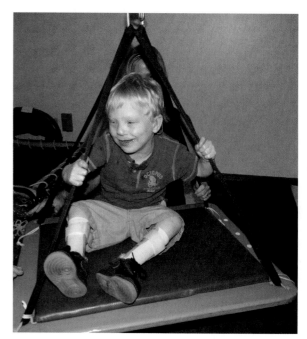

**FIGURE 27-1** A child on suspended equipment (platform swing) that provides vestibular input: linear and/or rotary.

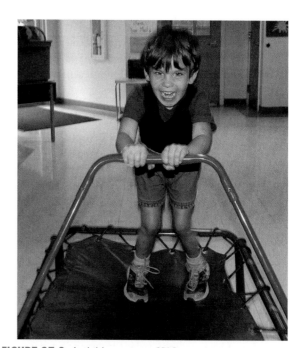

**FIGURE 27-2** A child wearing a SPIO compression vest on a trampoline, providing vestibular and proprioceptive inputs.

active patient participation. Both children and adults have ample opportunities throughout the typical day to participate in functional tasks that include sensory components. Additional suggestions are described in Table 27-2 and relate to Figure 27-4, Figure 27-5, and Figure 27-6, with appropriate suggestions in various sensory modalities.

During treatment, the therapist manipulates the intensity, duration, and location of the sensory input according to the patient's reactions and tolerance. As hyposensitivity improves, the patient needs less sensory input and less time to respond to sensory exposure, which would be reflected in improved sensory testing scores. Careful documentation of the parameters of the sensory input, the response, progress toward goals, and effects on daily function are essential components of SIT intervention.

## THINK ABOUT IT 27.3

The Individuals with Disabilities Education Act requires that schools use programs, curricula, and practices based on scientifically based research "to the extent practicable." What challenges might this pose for a therapist wanting to include sensory integration therapy as part of a child's individualized education program?

"**Sensory diets,**" a common therapeutic strategy in SIT, are often recommended for patients with both hyposensitivity and hypersensitivity problems to help with daily sensory issues (Wilbarger, 1991). These "diets" were designed to simulate nutritional diets, with the idea that people need a certain

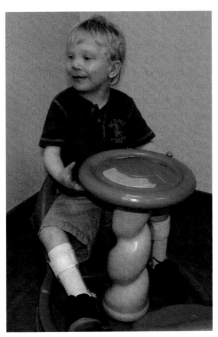

**FIGURE 27-3** A child on a Sit 'n Spin that provides rotary vestibular input.

| **TABLE 27-2** | **Daily Activities and Therapeutic Interventions to Provide Sensory Input** | | |
|---|---|---|---|
| **PROPRIOCEPTIVE** | **VESTIBULAR** | **TACTILE** | **ORAL-MOTOR** |
| • Lifting objects<br>• Pushing objects<br>• Pulling objects<br>• Carrying objects<br>• Sweeping or vacuuming<br>• Shoveling<br>• Pushing a lawn mower<br>• Washing a table or mirror<br>• Using a weighted vest or blanket<br>• Theraband exercise<br>• Wall or floor push-ups<br>• Hugs<br>• Joint compressions<br>• Squeezing a stress ball<br>• "Resistive" toys or activities such as opening or closing a jar, playing with Legos or pop beads, hammering, or pounding<br>• Jumping or hopping<br>• Wheelbarrow walk<br>• Compression garments<br>• Vibrators | • Swinging on a swing or suspended equipment (Fig. 27-1)<br>• Power walks<br>• Sit 'n Spin or other spinning activities (Fig. 27-3)<br>• Jumping in place or on a mini-trampoline (Fig. 27-2)<br>• Jumping jacks<br>• Stretching and moving up and down<br>• Rocking in a rocking chair<br>• Dancing<br>• Bouncing or rolling on a therapy ball<br>• Log rolling<br>• Somersaults<br>• Weight shifting on a rocker board<br>• Bike riding<br>• Swimming<br>• Skating<br>• Skiing or snowboarding<br>• Gymnastics<br>• Moving on a scooter board (Fig. 27-4)<br>• Going down a slide<br>• Rides at amusement park | • Squeezing, kneading, rolling dough, Play-Doh, or therapy putty<br>• Exploration in "tactile" bins such as containers of beans and rice<br>• Washing dishes<br>• Playing in shaving cream<br>• Finger painting<br>• Water activities<br>• "Sensory" toys or objects such as Koosh balls, different textured objects— bumpy, hard, soft, scratchy, silky, etc. (Fig. 27-5)<br>• Walking barefoot in sand<br>• Rubbing lotion on hands and feet<br>• Brushing (Fig. 27-6) | • Chewy foods such as granola bars, dried fruit, Slim Jims, gummy bears<br>• Crunchy foods such as carrots, apples, graham crackers<br>• Sour foods such as lemons, pickles, WARHEADS candy<br>• Oral-motor activities such as chewing on straws, blowing bubbles, blowing into musical instruments<br>• Oral-motor exercises: imitate facial movements<br>• Chewing on a rubber chewy tube (special therapy tubing) |

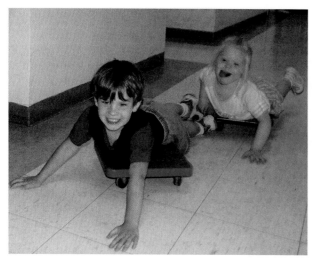

**FIGURE 27-4** Children on scooter boards that provide proprioceptive and vestibular inputs (linear).

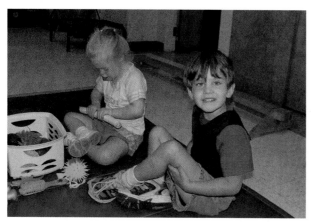

**FIGURE 27-5** Children exploring different textures with their hands to provide enriched tactile input.

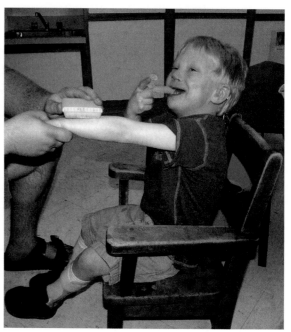

**FIGURE 27-6** A child participating in a brushing program to decrease tactile defensiveness while using a chew tube to provide oral-motor input.

amount of food (i.e., sensory input) to keep them healthy and functioning well. When individuals get hungry, they need to eat or they may become distracted, grumpy, or uncomfortable. Some people with sensory dysfunction may feel and act this way until they are "fed" sensory input. In a sensory diet, planned and scheduled sensory activities are developed by the therapist and carried out by the patient (and family as needed) to adjust her awareness/arousal level.

For patients with hyposensation, alerting activities are recommended to "wake up" their body. These may include light/unexpected/quick touch, bright and visually stimulating media, oral-motor input with foods that have strong flavors or require work to chew, and/or bouncing or quick movements. Some examples of sensory diet activities for children can be found at sensorysmarts.com/sensory-diet.pdf.. Once again, careful and consistent documentation of the parameters of the sensory input, the response, progress toward goals, and effects on daily function are essential components of sensory diets.

## Functional Training and Motor Learning

Patients with pure sensory stroke have shown improvement in not only motor control but also sensory awareness when participating in functional training and motor learning exercises (Montagnana, 2003); this finding provides evidence that sensory function can also improve with physical rehabilitation interventions, perhaps as a result of neural plasticity. Functional training can include any ADL such as dressing, bathing, or grooming along with functional activities such as transfers, mobility, work, and household tasks. When traditional strengthening and endurance exercises were combined with repeated practice of ADLs along with functional work training, patients demonstrated improved tactile discrimination, joint position sense, pressure sensation, and fine motor skills (Montagnana, 2003). Although this intervention did not specifically target the sensory system through sensory input or training, it was successful in making meaningful changes in sensory outcomes.

Sensory and motor connections are obvious. One cannot remove sensory input when completing motor tasks such as daily activities or participating in exercise programs. As we move and complete tasks, sensory recruitment and activation of tactile, proprioceptive, and vestibular systems occur without us realizing or targeting them. Thus, although they are described as functional training, the same activities can also be considered sensory interventions.

Exercise training may provide some preventive benefits as well. In one study, patients with diabetes who participated in an exercise program of brisk treadmill walking for 4 hours per week over 4 year, were significantly less likely to develop peripheral nerve disease with sensory neuropathy (Balducci, 2006). A walking program, especially with the added demand of walking a pet (see Fig. 27-7), is an excellent wellness and health activity incorporated into any therapy program; for people at risk for peripheral nerve damage and with a potential for sensory loss, it can also help prevent impairment. As individuals participate in functional training and physical exercise, the effect on the sensory system should be monitored.

### Intermittent Pneumatic Compression

Intermittent pneumatic compression (IPC) is commonly used by therapists to prevent deep vein thrombosis (Woolson, 1996) and to treat lymphedema (Szuba, 2002). Intermittent compression of an extremity is achieved by the mechanical pumping of a sleeve wrapped around the extremity, which alternately fills and empties with air to assist with circulation and movement of fluid. It has also been effective for treating decreased sensation in certain patients. In a randomized controlled study, 10 cycles of 3-minute IPC, with a peak of 40 mm Hg, was used on the involved hemiparetic upper extremity of 11 patients after a stroke combined with neuro-developmental therapy (NDT); a control group of 12 patients received NDT and a sham shortwave treatment. Tactile and kinesthetic sensations and stereognosis improved in both groups; however, the improvement in the experimental group was significantly higher than that of the control group (Cambier, 2003).

For patients with restless leg syndrome, use of IPC at 40 mm Hg for 1 hour a day significantly alleviated unpleasant sensory sensitivity, making it an option for treatment (Lettieri, 2009). As research on the effects of IPC accelerates, more specific parameters can be developed to guide physical therapists in this intervention.

### Thermal Modalities

Thermal modalities as an effective intervention for hyposensitivity are increasingly supported by evidence. Chen (2005) demonstrated that application of alternating cold and hot modalities positively affected sensory functioning in some patients after a stroke, with improvement in tactile sensation

based on Semmes-Weinstein monofilament scores (Kumar, 1995).

To use this intervention (Chen, 2005), first do a trial on the nonaffected side by asking the patient to describe the sensation of a hot pack or cold pack as either hot or cold. After this, place the hot pack on the affected side for 15 seconds followed a 30-second rest period for a total of 10 trials. Follow this with the application of a cold pack for 30 seconds followed by a 30-second rest period for a total of 10 trials. Reassess the patient's sensations to determine training effect and changes in sensory awareness. This treatment should be done daily for several weeks to determine its effectiveness. Application of ice alone (without use of heat) as in short, repeated ice immersions of an extremity with decreased sensation (5 seconds in ice followed by 45 seconds of rest) has not been effective (Bohls, 2005). Immersing the extremity in hot water (105.8°F) for 10 minutes may be an effective technique to decrease spasticity (Matsumoto, 2006).

Thermal modalities are inexpensive and easily reproduced and should be considered as part of a comprehensive program. However, caution is advised when applying thermal modalities to young children and the elderly because their skin is particularly sensitive.

### Sensory Retraining

**Sensory retraining** includes active exercises to improve localizing, thus increasing awareness and interpretation of sensory input. Sensory retraining often begins with sensory stimulation, using a variety of textures and movements to facilitate awareness of sensory input and increase patient alertness and attention, as well as passive movement (Phillips, 2007; Phillips, 2010). For example, to increase proprioception, begin by occluding the patient's vision, flexing the index finger of the extremity with sensory loss, and then having the patient try to replicate the finger position on the nonaffected side. If the patient is unable to match the position without using vision, you can repeat the activity while allowing visual observation while copying the position. Repeated practice could improve sensory functioning.

To enforce use of stereognosis in sensory intervention (see Fig. 27-8), give the patient various sizes, shapes, and textures of objects to explore and identify with the eyes open. Then instruct the patient to repeat the process with the eyes closed to improve the ability to recognize objects by touch. Children often like these activities, especially when done in a playful or competitive manner. This "forced use" of impaired sensory systems is similar to the theory used in constraint-induced movement—removing the stronger component and forcing the weaker component to activate and strengthen.

Although therapists may use this approach, evidence is sparse (Schabrun, 2009). Most studies examining this technique included small sample sizes and were of lower methodological quality. In one study, a small group of three patients underwent an intense 2-week program of sensory reeducation that included explaining what sensation is and why it is important, followed by practice in localizing and discriminating different textures. The study targeted foot sensation in patients

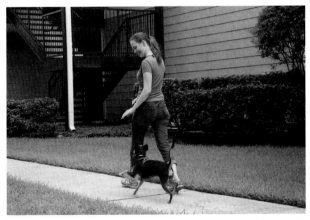

**FIGURE 27-7** An adult walking her dog, an example of functional training and physical activity in a natural environment that affect sensation and sensory processing.

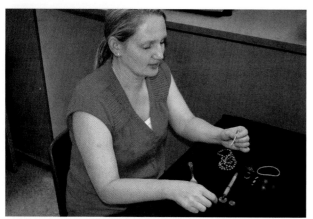

**FIGURE 27-8** An adult participating in sensory retraining through stereognosis, with tactile exploration of familiar objects (i.e., a paper clip, fork, Mardi Gras beads, pen, coins, rubber band).

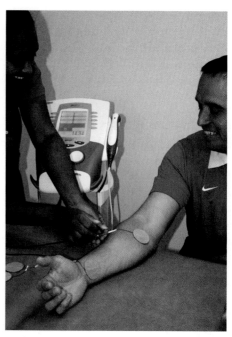

**FIGURE 27-9** A therapist works with a patient using electrical stimulation as part of the sensory intervention program.

after a stroke to see if sensation improved and if it affected balance and function. Two of the three patients demonstrated a significant change in tactile sensation, but none showed a change in proprioception. All patients demonstrated a trend toward improved single leg balance (Hiller, 2006). In a single-case report, a patient demonstrated improved tactile sensation after a stroke but did not show significant changes in proprioception (Carey, 1993). One group of patients with sensory loss after a stroke received sensory retraining daily for 2 weeks; they demonstrated improvements in motor functioning but mixed results regarding changes in sensation (Lynch, 2007).

### Electrophysical Agents

Various types of electrical stimulation (e-Stim) (see Fig. 27-9) have been used to treat patients with decreased sensation. Often, e-Stim is done in conjunction with or in addition to other forms of treatment, usually therapeutic exercise or functional training. The most significant outcomes have been seen with this combined approach (Sullivan, 2008). Activity in the sensorimotor cortex increased with use of afferent e-Stim in some cases. With increased neuronal activity and thus increased recruitment of sensory pathways, increased motor performance may be possible (Golaszewski, 2004).

Sensory ability may improve in patients with stroke with application of neuromuscular e-Stim (NMES) and/or sensory amplitude e-Stim (Sullivan, 2004, 2007) and combined with NDT (Yelnik, 2008) or task-specific training (Carey, 2005). Daily e-Stim ranging from 15 minutes to 2 hours directed at the area of sensory impairment may improve sensory awareness and motor functioning (Sullivan, 2007). Portable transcutaneous electrical nerve stimulation (TENS) and NMES units can be used to provide electrical input, making this a convenient home-based intervention (Sullivan, 2004, 2007; Yozbatiran, 2006) (Fig. 27-9). When cutaneous e-Stim was performed along with sensory retraining exercises, improvement was also seen (Dannenbaum, 1988). e-Stim as an adjunct to motor skill and functional training has shown benefits for patients with SCI as well (Beekhulzen, 2008). Even without additional forms of intervention, e-Stim may be effective for some patients

(Peurala, 2002). The use of TENS and functional training promotes activity in both sensory and motor cortices, improving patient outcomes. Significant improvements in spasticity, strength, and gait speed were seen in patients with a stroke when TENS was applied daily for 60 minutes followed by 60 minutes of functional training that included a variety of weight-bearing and gait activities (Ng, 2007).

Electrical or mechanical "noise" stimulation has been explored as an intervention to improve sensory function (Dhruv, 2002; Liu, 2002). Liu (2002) found that use of mechanical tactile noise enhanced sensory ability in a sample of healthy older adults as well as in individuals with central or peripheral nerve damage from a stroke or diabetes and concluded that "noise-based techniques and devices may prove useful in overcoming age- and disease-related losses in sensorimotor function" (p. 171) Electrical noise tactile stimulation also significantly increased fine-touch sensitivity in a sample of older adults (Dhruv, 2002).

### Monochromatic Infrared Photo Energy

Several studies showed that monochromatic infrared energy (MIRE) may be effective in improving sensation in patients with diabetic peripheral neuropathy. MIRE is theorized to improve sensation because of increased dilation of the veins, leading to improved circulation and nerve function. When MIRE was used in a home program (see Fig. 27-10AB), not only did sensation improve, as evidenced by Semmes-Weinstein monofilament scores, but patients also experienced a decrease in formation of new wounds compared to that expected in individuals with diabetic peripheral neuropathy (Powell, 2004). When reexamined a year later, these same patients had maintained the positive results (Powell, 2006). Similar improvements in sensation were seen in other studies (Clifft, 2005; Leonard, 2004; Jianping, 2005).

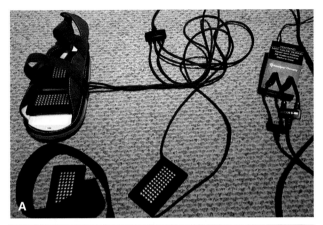
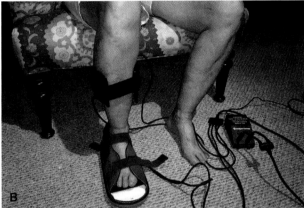

**FIGURE 27-10AB** Monochromatic infrared energy (MIRE). (A) Up close and (B) applied as part of a home intervention program to improve sensation in peripheral neuropathy.

When daily MIRE treatments were combined with balance training, neuromuscular reeducation, strength training, and stretching exercises, sensation improved and the incidence of falls decreased (Kochman, 2004). In a study of more than 2,000 patients with peripheral neuropathy and associated sensory impairment, more than 50% experienced complete resolution of loss of protective sensation and 67% reduction in pain when using MIRE for 1 hour each day (Harkless, 2006). In a review of medical records of more than 1,000 patients who received MIRE, 71% reported improved sensation, with many experiencing complete resolution of sensory impairment (DeLellis, 2005).

Application and use of MIRE were similar in these studies but were individualized according to needs. Flexible MIRE pads were placed on the skin surrounding the area to be treated. The pads emitted photo energy in the near-infrared spectrum, pulsed on a 50% on/off cycle for 30 to 40 minutes. The treatment was done on a daily basis or two to three times a week for 1 to 2 months. Most of the studies reported sensory improvement in protective sensation only, with no changes in proprioception. However, one study did report a change in temperature sensation as well (Jie, 2005). Despite the variability in clinical practice and a lack of rigor in some studies, these emerging findings make MIRE another potential choice for sensory intervention.

## Compensatory Strategies

Compensatory strategies (i.e., altering or adjusting the sensory environment) to accommodate hyper- or hyposensitivity may be necessary in certain situations. When sensory loss is not expected to return or when other sensory interventions have yielded minimal results, compensating for hyposensitivity may best help to meet functional goals and prevent injury. This compensation may involve a combination of altering the environment, educating the patient, and/or using adaptive equipment.

With the loss of sensation, the patient is at risk of injury in the home or work environment and may not be aware of the damage. Home and work inspections can reveal potential sources of injury, which can be rectified before an injury occurs, similar to baby-proofing a home with young children. Examples of potential hazards include sharp corners on furniture or counters, exposed radiators, wood stoves not surrounded by a fence/gate, and high water temperatures. Patient education may include instructing the individual to inspect the area of insensate skin for signs of injury and inspect the environment for dangers such as hot stoves or flames and sharp items such as knives or scissors. Weight-shifting activities/exercises to prevent skin breakdown should also be included in the education plan because a patient without sensation does not feel the need to shift her weight.

Use of assistive devices for mobility (e.g., canes, walkers) because of decreased awareness and function in the lower extremities allows the patient to be independent and functional despite sensory loss. Orthotics such as an AFO may give stability and improve function in a lower extremity that lacks sensation. Other examples of assistive technology/equipment designed to augment a deficient sensory system include chair cushions filled with gel or air, which provide proprioceptive input as well as protection from skin breakdown for insensate areas. Proprioception can also be increased through use of compression garments, as described in Chapter 24 and shown in Figure 24-14, Fig. 24-15, and Figure 27-11, or weighted vests or blankets.

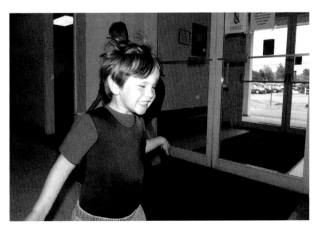

**FIGURE 27-11** A child wearing a SPIO compression vest for additional sensory input during a play activity.

## Hypersensitivity

### Sensory Integration Therapy

As described earlier, SIT is an intervention strategy based on the work of Ayres that may be appropriate for treating both hyposensitivity and hypersensitivity. Engagement in planned, controlled, and specific sensory activities on a regular basis may improve tolerance to sensory input, which may decrease sensory defensiveness (hypersensitivity), improve motor functioning, and enhance quality of life (Pfeiffer, 2003; Urwin, 2005). In a study of 15 adults with sensory defensiveness as determined by the Adult Sensory Questionnaire and the Adult Sensory Interview (Kinnealey, 1999), individualized programs of daily tactile, proprioceptive, and vestibular activities (of patient choice and therapist direction) were developed and used independently by patients for 1 month. At the end of the month, the patients' levels of sensory defensiveness and anxiety had decreased. No control group was used in this study (Pfeiffer, 2003).

In SIT, the amount and type of sensory input depend on the patient's level of hypersensitivity or defensiveness and the specific sensory modality that is impaired. Tactile, proprioceptive, and and/or vestibular senses may be involved, as well as auditory, visual, and olfactory systems. Tactile defensiveness is characterized by an adverse overreaction to everyday common touch or textures. Unexpected or light touch and objects with varied textures are particularly difficult, often making it hard for patients to participate in typical daily activities, such as dressing, working, or playing with different materials, or being touched by others. Specific examples include being bothered or distracted by labels on clothes; overreacting to being bumped or the unexpected touch by a classmate, coworker, or family member; having difficulty washing dishes; or being uncomfortable walking barefoot in the sand.

A therapist working with someone with tactile defensiveness should use firm touch and always tell the patient before touching her. A patient with hypersensitivity to vestibular input may experience gravitational insecurity or intolerance to movement related to dysfunction in the otolithic organs and/or semicircular canals. Signs of vestibular hypersensitivity include vertigo, nausea, vomiting, sweating, pallor, avoidance of movement, or motion sickness. The therapist needs to be aware of these reactions and progress the patient slowly through therapy as she becomes accustomed to movement activities and her tolerance improves. One may learn to accommodate to the perceived noxious stimulus by gradual and planned exposure; a learned acceptance or habituation of sensory input is the intended goal.

Activities and tasks for hypersensitivity are often similar to those used for hyposensitivity, but the time spent participating is often different, with a gradual increase in tolerance (and thus time) as therapy progresses in patients who are hypersensitive. In patients with decreased registration or sensation, a negative reaction is not seen; thus, tolerance is usually greater, with more time spent engaging in the activity. Table 27-3 lists examples of intervention for sensory defensiveness.

Like the patient with hyposensitivity, the patient with hypersensitivity may benefit from a sensory diet to help decrease overreactions to sensory input. Activities may focus on calming sensory stimuli and enhanced organization of the system to facilitate lower levels of anxiety and an appropriate level of alertness. They include tactile, proprioceptive, and vestibular input that is firm, predictable, smooth, and rhythmic. Environmental sensory input (visual, auditory, olfactory) should be bland and minimal. Accurate and clear documentation must be used to monitor progress and to change the sensory input as the patient's response or function changes.

### Brushing Program

The Wilbarger Brushing Protocol, which is a component of many sensory integration programs, is used to decrease tactile defensiveness (Wilbarger, 1991, 2002). Despite lack of research verifying its efficacy, this program has been used extensively by occupational and physical therapists to treat hypersensitivity to tactile input. This method uses a surgical brush to provide deep touch pressure and joint compressions to provide proprioceptive input in as a method to decrease the hypersensitivity to tactile input. It is performed by firmly brushing the arm/leg

| TABLE 27-3 | Interventions for Sensory Defensiveness | | |
|---|---|---|---|
| **SENSORY DYSFUNCTION** | **TREATMENT** | **RESPONSES** | **COMMENTS** |
| Tactile defensiveness (hyperreaction to touch or textures) | Planned vestibular-proprioceptive input, increased exposure to tactile input as tolerated, Wilbarger brushing program | Gradually improved tolerance to touch and textures; patient may do better in a quiet, controlled environment to begin with | Best if patient provides input to himself to self-monitor tolerance |
| Gravitational insecurity (hyperreaction to changes in head position or base of support) | Controlled linear vestibular and proprioceptive input Progress from maximum support to minimum support and from predictable to less predictable | Patients perceive small movements as large ones; will need lots of encouragement to feel safe and engender trust | Progress slowly; begin with patient's feet touching the ground or prone activities; backward movement is more difficult and should be used cautiously |

(going into the direction of the hair) several times in a consistent rhythmic manner (Fig. 27-12), followed by joint compressions to all joints in the extremity. The program is initially done six or more times a day for 2 weeks; it is then tapered off and used as needed as a maintenance program (Wilbarger, 2002). Positive outcomes have included decreased sensory defensiveness and anxiety and improved behavior (Stagnitti, 1999).

### Vibration

Vibration may help decrease hypersensitivity to tactile stimulation by providing artificial proprioception. When vibration was performed at 80 Hz for 10 minutes, mean tactile thresholds increased for a short time in healthy volunteers compared with a control group. The effect did not last longer than 10 minutes (Hochreiter, 1983). Caution must be taken when using this intervention because the powerful effects after vibration may negatively affect some individuals. Because individuals react differently to vibration, careful trial and error may be necessary to determine reactions and outcomes.

### Compensatory Strategies

People experiencing sensory overload or hypersensitivity need help and guidance to learn how to live with the impairment while they are recovering or when the impairment is not expected to improve. One way to decrease discomfort or anxiety over sensory input is to modify the environment. When the patient is overly sensitive to noise or visual stimulation, a quiet room with little clutter is advised. When the patient has tactile defensiveness, simple things such as removing tags from clothing or avoiding brushing up to people may ward off feelings of discomfort. Daily deep pressure/proprioception assists with organizing and calming the nervous system. Equipment providing external compression, such as weighted vests, weighted blankets, and compression garments (e.g., SPIO, Benik, and TheraTogs), may help. Teaching the patient ways to monitor her own sensory needs and appropriately accommodate is essential. "How Does Your Engine Run?" is one program teaching these concepts of awareness and self-regulation (Williams, 1996). Empowering individuals

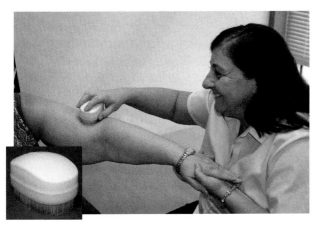

**FIGURE 27-12** A therapist using a brushing program with an adult patient.

to manage their own health will lead to improved quality of life and functional independence.

### Paresthesia

**Paresthesia** is a sensory impairment that does not fit clearly into either hyposensitivity or hypersensitivity categories because it has qualities of both. A patient experiencing paresthesia has altered and uncomfortable sensations, including numbness, tingling, stinging, burning, or pain. This abnormal and often painful condition can lead to chronic pain, causing great discomfort and affecting function and quality of life. Several interventions are used to treat this disabling condition, often with mixed results. Brief explanations of some of these interventions follow; however, the reader is referred to Chapter 28 for a detailed, in-depth description of pain impairments and interventions.

### Electrophysical Agents

E-Stim, percutaneous electrical nerve stimulation (PENS), transcutaneous electrostimulation, and TENS are modalities that decrease the symptoms associated with painful paresthesia (Armstrong, 1997; Hamza, 2000; Kesler, 1988; Kumar, 1997; Wilder, 1992). Patients with painful diabetic neuropathy receiving pulsed, direct current e-Stim daily for a month experienced a dramatic decrease in pain at the end of treatment, with only a minimal increase in symptoms noted at 1 month after treatment (Armstrong, 1997).

With PENS, acupuncture-like needles are placed percutaneously to stimulate peripheral sensory nerves and then are electrically stimulated to provide analgesia to the area of neuropathic pain. It has had short-term success at alleviating acute and chronic pain syndromes. In addition to the decrease in pain, patients experienced improved sleeping patterns and increased physical activity during treatment. However, lasting effects of treatment have not been reported (Hamza, 2000).

During transcutaneous electrostimulation, percutaneous electrodes are placed around painful areas and a biphasic waveform produces nonfatiguing muscle contractions. This method was effective in decreasing symptoms in a group of adults with painful peripheral neuropathy following 1 month of treatment. Symptoms however, began to return 1 month later (Kumar, 1997).

### Other

As described previously, MIRE is a recently developed modality to treat impaired sensation. The intervention also effectively helps with paresthesia and pain arising from peripheral neuropathy (Volkert, 2006). In a multisite study of MIRE delivered with the Anodyne Therapy System, 272 patients with peripheral nerve pain and diminished sensation received 30- to 60-minute treatments to the lower extremities with four separate diode-containing pads per limb three times per week (Volkert, 2006). These patients also received traditional therapy, such as stretching, strengthening, balance exercise, and neuromuscular reeducation. Significant decreases in pain, increases in sensation, and improvements in balance were observed. The study did not have a control group, and it is unclear which intervention was responsible for the improvements. Other preliminary studies cited similar improvements (DeLellis, 2005; Kochman, 2002; Leonard, 2004; Prendergast, 2004). Decreasing or eliminating debilitating pain would improve patients' quality of life and ability to complete daily activities. More research on MIRE is needed.

# Intervention: Ultimately Applied in Functional Activities

## Adult and Pediatric Considerations

When considering the functional implications of abnormal sensory processing in children and adults, you need to think only about what they do in a typical day. Both children and adults need to eat, wash, dress, and undress every day. These activities involve movement and interacting with different textures. Sensory impairments affect tolerance to or awareness of everyday exposure to textures and movement related to different foods and clothing, as well as various tasks such as washing and brushing hair, brushing teeth, and even cutting fingernails.

Children and adults differ in how they spend time during the day, with children most often playing or attending school and adults working or spending the day at home or in the community. For all of these environments, the sensory experiences to which the patient must accommodate should be examined in order to plan effective strategies for success. For example, for individuals with decreased sensation, environmental safety measures may include lowering the highest allowable temperature of the water heater or covering/padding sharp/pointed edges of counters and furniture. For patients with hypersensitivity, the environment can be adjusted to decrease sensory stimulation, and a special quiet place can be created to alleviate overstimulation.

When choosing sensory activities, consider age-appropriate equipment and activities. For instance, children are much more interested in and motivated to participate in climbing and movement on suspended equipment than are adults. They are also more likely than adults to play in sand and at water tables as a tactile activity. For an adult, age-appropriate tactile input may be achieved through kneading dough or using sandpaper to make a project. In addition, adults are more likely to feel comfortable receiving movement input from rocking in a chair or riding a bike. Depending on the physical status of the adult, it may be a long time since she felt comfortable lying prone, being in quadruped or kneeling, or even getting up and down from the floor. These are all considerations in determining a plan of care.

## PATIENT APPLICATION: INTERVENTION

On the basis of the results of the examination, Sammie, his family, and the therapist agree on the following goals:

- Decrease hypersensitivity to movement to allow play with peers at school, on the playground, and in physical education class without fear or overreaction.

- Decrease tactile defensiveness of the left side to enable more exploration of sensory experiences and use of the left side without adverse reaction.
- Decrease neglect of the left side of the body to allow more consistent and voluntary use in unilateral and bilateral activities.
- Increase strength of the left extremities to allow more functional use in recreational and daily activities.

Therapy is initiated twice weekly, including the following interventions (and rationales):

- To decrease hypersensitivity to movement and gradually increase Sammie's tolerance, exposure to a variety of movement experiences is provided, including use of suspended equipment, therapy balls, and a mini-trampoline.
- To decrease tactile defensiveness, firm pressure and deep proprioceptive input are given, including rub/towel down of the left arm and leg throughout the day at normal grooming and dressing times and play and exploration with a variety of textures (e.g., Play-Doh, sand table, and tactile toys). Gradually increased tolerance to different textures is facilitated by (assisted) exploration of different textures as well as progressing from firm and predictable tactile inputs to lighter, less predictable inputs.
- To decrease neglect/increase sensory awareness and use of the left side, sensory-level electrical stimulation is provided, as well as introduction of a variety of tactile modalities. Toys and materials are placed on Sammie's left side to encourage visual attention to the left. Practice of two-handed activities, such as throwing and catching a ball, are performed with therapist assistance as needed (firm pressure, no unexpected or light touch). Use of a mirror to increase visual attention to the left side is included to increase total body awareness.
- To increase the strength of the left arm and leg, a combination of strengthening exercises, gross and fine motor functional activities, and motor-level electrical stimulation is used.

In addition to direct physical therapy intervention, Sammie's plan of care includes consultation with his local school district to begin transition planning for his return to school.

## Contemplate Clinical Decisions: Intervention

Introduction of sensory input was gradual and was based on Sammie's acceptance of input. It was important for Sammie to feel a sense of control in his therapy and to feel safe, as both his hyposensitivity and hypersensitivity often make him anxious and frustrated.

Based on this,

- How could you progress movement activities from rolling on a mat to swinging on suspended equipment?
- How could you deal with refusal of hand-over-hand assistance in facilitating use of the left hand?
- What sensory systems (other than tactile or proprioceptive) could be tapped to increase awareness of the left side?

■ At this point, what equipment might be helpful to add to
Sammie's plan of care?

■ How could the environment be modified to facilitate progress
or compensate for decreased sensory processing?

## ▓ Intervention: Considerations for Nontherapy Time and Discharge

### Patient and Family Education

During nontherapy times and after discharge, primary areas
of focus for any client with sensory impairment, regardless
of age or diagnosis, are risk reduction and injury prevention.
Patients and their families/caregivers should be fully aware
of the extent of sensory impairment and how this can affect
safety and the potential for secondary impairment. As discussed earlier in the chapter, both hyposensation and hypersensation of the sensory system can cause lack of awareness
or atypical response to sensory input, thus leading to injury
and/or decreased function. For instance, with loss of sensation due to an SCI, the person is not aware of the need
to shift her weight to relieve pressure after being in one
position for an extended time, which can lead to skin breakdown. When tactile defensiveness is severe, a person may
overreact to unexpected touch and move quickly/unsafely
away from the source of input, sustaining an injury. To prevent these types of injuries, patient and family education is
critical.

Home, work, and school environments should be assessed
and modified to create safe surroundings. Reminding the patient
and family about the importance of skin inspection is another
key to preventing secondary impairment. If the patient uses
equipment or assistive devices, their proper use and maintenance
should be reviewed. Both written and pictorial instructions
should be given.

At discharge, patients may be ready to discontinue use of
adaptive equipment or the home exercise program (HEP), or
they may be encouraged to continue with them for maintenance of sensory functioning. They should be instructed to
inform their primary care physician when changes occur in
sensory functioning in the future, which may indicate the
need for further therapy intervention.

### Activities for a Home Exercise Program

Completing a HEP obviously depends on the individual's
needs and the plan of care. When appropriate, a HEP is often
helpful to continue improvements or preventing regression.
HEPs should be clearly detailed and reviewed with both the
family and the patient. Patients and families/caregivers
should confirm understanding of the program by demonstrating techniques in the presence of the therapist when possible
so adjustments can be given as needed. As stated previously,
both written and pictorial instructions should be given.
Activities/techniques to carry over into an HEP include
providing sensory input throughout the day (sensory diet),
sensory retraining, and use of prescribed modalities.

## HANDS-ON PRACTICE

1. The focus of intervention for sensory impairment may
be based on recovery or compensation.
2. Interventions can be targeted for hyposensitivity,
hypersensitivity, or paresthesia.
3. An individual who is hyposensitive to sensory input
may benefit from sensory integration therapy: meaningful therapeutic activities characterized by enhanced
sensation (tactile, vestibular, and proprioceptive)
involving active participation and adaptive interaction.
4. For tactile input, examples include:
   a. For children, manually exploring items in a container of dry rice or small beans or exploring toys
   with different textures
   b. For adults, manipulating objects with different
   textures or washing with a textured washcloth
5. For proprioceptive input, examples include jumping
(on a trampoline or other surface), bouncing on a
therapy ball, weight-bearing on arms (e.g., maneuvering in quadruped or imitating various animal species),
and pushing/pulling heavy objects.
6. Sensory diet activities may involve the following
categories: listening/auditory, looking/vision, smell/
taste/oral, touch/deep pressure, and movement/
proprioception (Biel, 2008).
7. Functional training and motor learning exercises may
improve motor control as well as sensory awareness.
8. In patients who have experienced a stroke, daily
intermittent pneumatic compression (ICP) on hemiparetic upper extremities, with 10 cycles of 3 minutes
(90 seconds of inflation followed by 90 seconds of
deflation) and a peak of 40 mm Hg, may be beneficial.
9. ICP can be applied for restless leg syndrome, using
40 mm Hg for 1 hour a day to decrease unpleasant
sensitivity.
10. For hyposensitivity after a stroke, alternate hot and cold
thermal modalities daily for several weeks: 10 trials of
a hot pack on the affected side for 15 seconds then
30 seconds of rest. Follow this with 10 trials of a cold
pack for 30 seconds with a 30-second rest.
11. Sensory retraining involves exercises to improve localizing, increasing awareness to and interpretation of
sensory input; it often begins with sensory stimulation
and active and passive movements targeted to the type
of impaired sensation (e.g., stereognosis or proprioception), followed by repeated practice.
12. Electrophysical agents can improve sensory function
in patients after a stroke; outcomes improve when
electrical stimulation is used in conjunction with

*Continued*

# HANDS-ON PRACTICE—cont'd

neurodevelopmental therapy or task-specific training. Daily electrical stimulation ranging from 15 minutes to 2 hours may improve sensory awareness and motor function.

13. Electrical or mechanical "noise" stimulation has enhanced sensory abilities in older adults, both healthy populations as well as those with sensory impairment secondary to diabetes or stroke.

14. Monochromatic infrared energy (MIRE) may improve sensory function and decrease pain in patients with peripheral neuropathy secondary to diabetes. Flexible MIRE pads are placed on the skin surrounding the area to be treated. The pads emit photo energy in the near-infrared spectrum, pulsed on a 50% on/off cycle for 30 to 40 minutes. The treatment is done daily or two to three times a week for 1 to 2 months.

15. The Wilbarger Brushing Protocol reportedly decreases tactile defensiveness by using a surgical brush to provide deep touch/pressure input to the arms and legs followed by joint compressions to the ankles, knees, hips, wrists, elbows, shoulders, toes, and fingers. The program is initially done six or more times a day for 2 weeks and then is tapered off and used as needed for maintenance.

## Let's Review

1. What types of interventions are available for hyposensation?

2. What types of interventions are available for hypersensation?

3. In addition to improved sensation, what patient outcomes to sensory intervention have been noted in the literature?

4. What is monochromatic infrared energy (MIRE) therapy, and how and why does it affect sensation?

5. What types of electrical stimulation (and devices) can be used as interventions for sensory impairment?

6. What neurological conditions can involve impaired sensation?

7. What is the difference between recovery and compensation? Why might one be chosen over the other?

8. Explain the purpose of a sensory diet and give an example.

9. What is the rationale behind the Wilbarger brushing program, and how is it done?

10. What is intermittent pneumatic compression, and how does it help individuals with sensory impairment?

11. How do physical exercise and functional task training affect the sensory system and patient outcomes?

12. What is important to consider when using thermomodalities with young children and the elderly?

13. What research in sensory intervention is still needed?

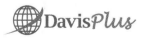 For additional resources, including Focus on Evidence tables, case study discussions, references and glossary, please visit http://davisplus.fadavis.com

## CHAPTER SUMMARY

*Sammie* *was seen twice weekly in outpatient therapy for 3 months and was discharged for transition to school-based physical therapy services. At the time of his discharge, Sammie had made good progress toward his goals and was able to not only tolerate but also enjoy a variety of movement activities, both in therapy and at school with his friends on the playground. With less fear of movement, he can now relax enough to participate more actively in therapy and demonstrate increased balance and gross motor skills. Sammie is also less tactilely defensive and can accept more sensory input without overreacting. He is also aware of and able to compensate for hypersensitivity by avoiding certain activities.*

Sensory impairment is caused by various insults to the nervous system that may limit activity and, in many cases, lead to functional disability. Impairments range from mild to severe and temporary to permanent. Intervention for sensory impairment is as varied as its causes and must be highly individualized for each patient. Most often, a combination of interventions is used. Although evidence supporting many of these sensory interventions is emerging (see Chapter 27 Focus on Evidence (FOE) tables (ONL) in online resources for evidence supporting interventions for hypersensitivity and hyposensitivity), the research is still somewhat limited, and additional evidence is needed. Some of the most promising interventions are sensory integration, sensory retraining, e-Stim modalities, and MIRE.

# Interventions for Chronic Pain

CHAPTER **28**

Jason Boyd Hardage, PT, DPT, DScPT ▪ Francisco X. Barrios, PhD
Marisa L. Suarez, MS, OTR/L, SWC ▪ Amy Barnes, MSOT, OTR/L, SWC

## CHAPTER OBJECTIVES

Upon completing this chapter, the learner will be able to:

1. Define, compare, and contrast acute pain and chronic pain.
2. Identify medical diagnoses in neurology that often produce chronic pain.
3. Describe the pathophysiology of chronic pain, including central sensitization.
4. Describe challenges to the optimal management of chronic pain.
5. Describe the assessment of chronic pain and related areas and give examples of specific instruments that are used.
6. Describe the functional restoration approach.
7. Describe the roles of the psychologist and the therapist in the functional restoration approach.
8. State examples of disease-specific considerations in the management of chronic pain.
9. Describe how shoulder-hand syndrome is best managed.
10. Describe Moseley's work in complex regional pain syndrome type 1.
11. Identify other medical diagnoses to which Moseley's work is applicable, and describe the implications for therapist management of chronic pain.

## ▪ Introduction

*You have seen this before in your outpatient neurology clinic: Your 72 year-old patient, Mr. Simons, had a cerebrovascular accident 1 month ago and had been exhibiting some motor recovery in his affected arm. Now he has developed intense pain throughout the arm, down to the hand, and the arm is extremely sensitive to touch. He also has developed edema. His wife tells you that he has quit trying to move the arm. What will you do? This chapter will equip you to develop a plan for intervention for this and other pain syndromes.*

**Pain,** particularly chronic pain, is commonly observed in occupational and physical therapy practice in those with neurologic conditions. It creates a challenging clinical problem requiring interdisciplinary (i.e., collaborative) treatment for optimal outcomes. We will see that the experience of pain includes not only the sensation but also the subjective awareness/perception and response to the unpleasant sensory experience, with profoundly detrimental effects on the individual's functional activity and participation.

# Foundational Concepts

## What Is Chronic Pain?

Chronic pain is a complicated phenomenon. Consider two definitions of "pain":

- A disturbed sensation that causes suffering or distress (American Physical Therapy Association [APTA], 2015).
- An unpleasant sensory and emotional experience associated with actual or potential tissue damage or described in terms of such damage (International Association for the Study of Pain [IASP], 1994).

Inherent in these definitions is the concept that pain involves both physical (sensory) and psychological (affective) components. As such, pain is always subjective—a symptom rather than a sign (IASP, 1994). However, **pain behavior** can be an accompanying sign—and chronic pain itself can be considered a disease (World Health Organization [WHO], 2006). Pain behavior is defined as "[v]erbal or nonverbal actions understood by observers to indicate a person may be experiencing pain and suffering. These actions may include audible complaints, facial expressions, abnormal postures or gait, use of prosthetic devices, avoidance of activities, overt expressions, and verbal or nonverbal complaints of pain, distress, and suffering" (Turk, 2001b, p. 17). Signs and symptoms of chronic pain include immobility and consequent wasting of muscles and joints; immune system suppression leading to increased susceptibility to disease; disturbed sleep; poor appetite and nutrition; dependence on medication; overdependence on family and other caregivers; overuse and inappropriate use of health-care providers and systems; poor job performance or disability; social isolation, including isolation from family; anxiety and fear; and bitterness, frustration, depression, and suicide (WHO, 2006).

## Classification

There are many ways to classify pain, and the classifications can overlap. Pain can be characterized by the underlying mechanism (e.g., mechanical pain, inflammatory pain, ischemic pain, referred pain), the region of the body (e.g., abdominal pain, shoulder pain), and the underlying medical diagnosis (e.g., arthritis pain, cancer pain). Often pain is characterized temporally as either acute or chronic (Fig. 28-1). **Acute pain** is defined as having a sudden onset, commonly declining over a short time (i.e., days, hours, minutes) after injury to the body, and generally disappearing when that injury heals. It is often, but not always, associated with signs of autonomic nervous system activity such as tachycardia, hypertension, diaphoresis, mydriasis, and pallor (APS Glossary). In contrast, **chronic pain** is generally considered to be pain that lasts more than 6 months, is ongoing, is caused by non–life-threatening causes, has not responded to current available treatment methods, and may continue for the remainder of the person's life (Wall, 1999). This type of chronic pain is also termed *chronic nonmalignant pain* to differentiate it from pain due to cancer.

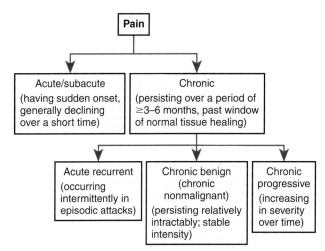

**FIGURE 28-1  A Taxonomy of Pain by Time.** Examples of acute recurrent pain include migraine headache and trigeminal neuralgia. Examples of chronic benign (chronic nonmalignant) pain include chronic low back pain and fibromyalgia syndrome. Examples of chronic progressive pain include cancer (also termed *malignant pain*) and rheumatoid arthritis (after Taylor, 2006).

Similarly, Bonica (1953) noted that chronic pain persists after the expected period of tissue healing and that the demarcation between acute and chronic pain may be made at 3 months with respect to nonmalignant pain in clinical practice (IASP, 1994). The IASP further states that in research, the demarcation between acute pain and chronic pain may be made at 6 months. Turk (2001b) indicated that such distinctions are in fact arbitrary.

Chronic pain may be further categorized as acute recurrent, chronic benign, and chronic progressive. *Acute recurrent pain* is intermittent and acute in character but chronic in the sense that the condition persists for longer than 6 months (e.g., migraine headache, trigeminal neuralgia). *Chronic benign pain* lasts for more than 6 months and is relatively **intractable** (e.g., chronic low back pain [LBP], myofascial pain syndrome). *Chronic progressive pain* lasts for more than 6 months and increases in severity over time (e.g., rheumatoid arthritis, cancer) (Taylor, 2006). Differences between acute and chronic pain are presented in Table 28-1.

Another term associated with chronic pain is *chronic widespread pain*. Although there is not a standardized definition for chronic widespread pain, it generally refers to pain involving multiple regions of the body, as in fibromyalgia syndrome (FMS) (Cieza, 2004).

## Chronic Pain in Neurology

Pain can also be classified by origin in the sensory system (i.e., nociceptive pain) or resulting from damage to the nervous system (i.e., **neuropathic pain**; Fig. 28-2). We commonly think of pain as arising from the sensory system, but it can also result from damage to the nervous system. This distinction, in turn, paves the way for our discussion of chronic pain in neurology (Fig. 28-3).

| TABLE 28-1  Major Differences Between Acute and Chronic Pain | |
| --- | --- |
| **ACUTE PAIN** | **CHRONIC PAIN** |
| Pain is a symptom | Pain is a disease |
| Well-defined time of onset | Time of onset sometimes well defined |
| Pathology is often identifiable | Pathology may not be identifiable |
| Objective signs of autonomic nervous system activity | Dysregulation of autonomic nervous system activity |
| Response to tissue injury | Response to peripheral and/or central changes in somatosensory pathways |
| Has a biological function | Unknown biological function |
| Often relieved by treatment directed at pain | Does not respond to treatment directed at pain |
| Usually responsive to medication | Less responsive to medication |
| Associated with anxiety | Associated with anxiety, depression, helplessness, hopelessness, weight changes, loss of libido |
| Primarily involves the individual | Involves the individual, family, social network, lifestyle |
| Responds to biomedical approach | May respond to biopsychosocial approach |
| Impairment/functional limitation | Functional limitation/disability |

Used with permission from Wolff MS. *Chronic Pain: Assessment of Physical Therapists' Knowledge and Attitudes* [thesis]. Boston, MA: Massachusetts General Hospital Institute of Health Professions; 1989.

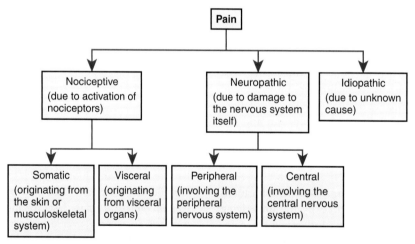

FIGURE 28-2  **A Taxonomy of Pain by System of Origin.** Nociceptors are primary sensory neurons for pain. Examples of peripheral neuropathic pain include painful diabetic neuropathy, acute herpes zoster, postherpetic neuralgia, chemotherapy-induced neuropathy, and stump pain after amputation. Examples of central neuropathic pain include central poststroke pain, central pain in patients with multiple sclerosis, and central pain due to damage to the spinal cord (*myelopathic pain,* which may involve the nerve roots) from intrinsic causes (e.g., multiple sclerosis, acute transverse myelitis, neurotoxins) or extrinsic causes (e.g., spinal cord injury, compression due to tumors, compression due to infections). Phantom limb pain after amputation is also classified as central neuropathic pain (after WHO, 2006).

Pain can be a direct or an indirect consequence of a neurological disorder, and either way, it can complicate the disability associated with the neurological disorder. Pain is associated with neurological disorders in three ways: as neuropathic pain resulting from diseases of, infections of, or injuries to the central and peripheral nervous system; as musculoskeletal pain secondary to neurological disorders; and as **complex regional pain syndrome** (CRPS), which involves both the somatic and autonomic nervous systems (WHO, 2006). The term **radiculopathy** refers to any disease of a nerve root and is often associated with radicular pain (i.e., pain that radiates or is felt in a place distant from the actual site of injury).

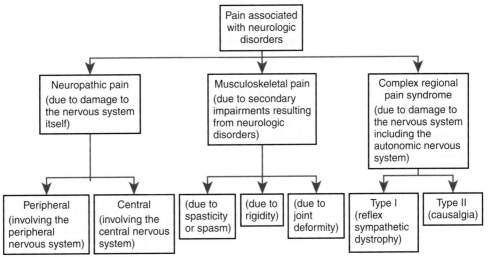

**FIGURE 28-3** **A Taxonomy of Pain Associated With Neurological Disorders.** In developed countries, the main causes of painful spasticity are stroke, demyelinating diseases such as multiple sclerosis, and spinal cord injuries, whereas painful rigidity is typically seen in Parkinson disease and dystonia. An example of musculoskeletal pain due to joint deformity is adhesive capsulitis after stroke. Other causes of joint deformity include neuropathies and infections. Pain associated with neurological disorders also includes headache and facial pain (after WHO, 2006).

Neuropathic pain is difficult to treat (Rasmussen, 2004). It has many characteristics including sensitized nociceptors, allodynia, hyperalgesia, abnormal temporal summation, and extraterritorial spread. Neuropathic pain can be *spontaneous pain* (pain that is stimulus independent) or **evoked pain** (pain that is stimulus dependent). Qualities or the nature of spontaneous pain includes a constant burning sensation (a common presentation); intermittent shooting, lancinating sensations; electric shocklike sensations; and **dysesthesias** (abnormal and unpleasant sensations). Stimulus-dependent pain can be caused by mechanical, thermal, and chemical stimuli. **Allodynia**, pain due to stimuli that are not normally painful, and **hyperalgesia**, a heightened pain response to stimuli that are normally painful, fall under this category. Mechanical allodynia is further classified as dynamic (brush evoked) or static (pressure evoked) (Cruccu, 2004).

Neuropathic pain is particularly characterized by abnormal temporal summation, cold and brush allodynia, and abnormal temperature sensation (Rasmussen, 2004). In addition, it is often accompanied by marked emotional changes, especially depression, and disability in activities of daily living (ADLs) (WHO, 2006) and instrumental activities of daily living (IADLs).

### Prevalence

Chronic pain is surprisingly prevalent, representing a major public health burden. Estimates vary widely (e.g., 11.5% to 55.2%; Harstall, 2003) depending on such factors as the definition and criteria used. However, one review estimated the prevalence of severe chronic pain in the general adult population is 11% (Harstall, 2003), whereas another report estimated 9% of the adult population in the United States suffers from moderate to severe chronic nonmalignant pain (Roper Starch Worldwide, 1999). According to the WHO, chronic pain affects approximately 5% to 33% of people in both developed and developing countries and is associated with anxiety and depression (as cited in Gureje, 1998). Similarly, Breivik (2006) found chronic pain of moderate to severe intensity affects 19% of adults in 15 European countries and Israel, with only 2% being treated by pain specialists, 40% reporting dissatisfaction with their pain management, and 21% reporting they have been diagnosed with depression. The authors noted that people with chronic pain often suspect their physicians do not consider the pain to be a problem. From these and other studies, the WHO (2006) has concluded that the prevalence rate for chronic pain is 18% to 20% in the general adult population in developed countries. However, the WHO (2006) also noted that these studies do not provide much information about pain associated with neurological disorders in particular.

There is agreement, however, that neuropathic pain has a high prevalence (Cruccu, 2004; WHO, 2006). **Neuropathy** is a general term referring to any disease or dysfunction of a peripheral nerve or nerves, including **mononeuropathy** (disease or dysfunction of a single nerve) and polyneuropathy (disease or dysfunction of multiple nerves). In terms of peripheral neuropathic pain, diabetic neuropathy occurs in approximately 45% to 75% of patients with diabetes mellitus; of these, approximately 10% develop painful diabetic neuropathy. Also, in approximately 9% to 14% of patients with herpes zoster, acute pain persists as chronic pain (postherpetic neuralgia) after the healing of the rash (WHO, 2006). Peripheral neuropathic pain occurs in approximately 2% of people with multiple sclerosis (MS) (Österberg, 2005).

In terms of central neuropathic pain, approximately two-thirds of people with a spinal cord injury have chronic pain from all causes, including neuropathic pain (Finnerup, 2004). In contrast, central pain occurs in approximately 8% of people during the first year after a stroke; of these, 63% experience central pain during the first month after a stroke (Andersen, 1995). Andersen (1995) also noted that the incidence of central neuropathic pain after stroke (i.e., 8%) is similar to the incidence of phantom limb pain (PLP) in people with amputation and **central pain** in people with a spinal cord injury. Approximately 58% of people with MS have chronic pain, and approximately 28% of people with MS have central neuropathic pain (Österberg, 2005).

Acute neuropathic pain (e.g., peripheral nerve injuries during surgery) is a risk factor for chronic pain; therefore, prompt treatment of acute neuropathic pain is important. In short, many people suffer from chronic pain resulting from diseases of the nervous system or trauma to the nervous system, including damage to peripheral nerves during surgery (WHO, 2006).

### Treatment Barriers

Chronic pain is as complex as it is prevalent, involving such factors as sex differences (Harstall, 2003), culture and ethnicity differences (Lasch, 2002; Morris, 2001), and disparities in health-care access (Green, 2004). (For a review of racial and ethnic disparities in pain, see Anderson, 2009.) Despite the prevalence of chronic pain and in part because of its complexities, there are numerous obstacles its treatment:

- People with pain are not aware they can ask for pain treatment (APS Advocacy).
- There are a limited number of specialized facilities for pain treatment (WHO, 2006).
- Some groups, including older adults, women, and members of racial and ethnic minorities, are more likely to be undertreated for pain than others (APS Advocacy).
- People with pain who have been treated often have negative experiences during their interactions with the health-care system. The Task Force on Guidelines for Desirable Characteristics for Pain Treatment Facilities of the IASP stated: "We should remember that the etiologies of chronic pain are not well understood; medical treatments have already failed many of these patients..." (Loeser, 1991). Many people have experienced learned helplessness and hopelessness as a result, often leading to decreased engagement in the management of pain and ultimately decreased daily functioning and participation (Frischenschlager, 2002).
- Many health-care professionals have little or no training in pain management (APS Advocacy; Moseley, 2003b; WHO, 2006) and underestimate patients' ability to understand current information about the neurophysiology of pain (Moseley, 2003b).
- FMS is particularly frustrating to physicians, other types of health-care professionals, and patients alike (Ablin, 2008).

## THINK ABOUT IT 28.1

Many patients with chronic pain will come to your clinic already frustrated with the care they have received from other providers. Think about why that is and how this may inform your care.

### Interdisciplinary Approach

Because pain is subjective, there is a complex interplay between physical variables (e.g., the initial physiological basis of the pain, other physical impairments caused by the pain such as difficulty sleeping) and psychological variables. Psychological variables include cognition (e.g., **catastrophizing, coping**), **affect** (e.g., **depression,** anxiety), and behavior (e.g., physical inactivity, social isolation, learned nonuse, fear-avoidance). This interplay is reciprocal, meaning the physical and psychological variables interact in a cascade of events and result in the patient's ultimate level of disability. For example, when a patient decreases participation in physical activity as a response to pain, he is more likely to gradually suffer from the secondary physical complication of general deconditioning (i.e., decreases in musculoskeletal, neuromuscular, and cardiovascular/pulmonary performance), which itself has negative consequences for the patient's physical and psychosocial functioning. Thus, both the physical and the psychological variables must be addressed. Clinical psychologists are integral members of the treatment team, in part because depression is common in people with chronic pain and the presence of depression is associated with an increased experience and decreased tolerance of pain (WHO, 2006). Consequently, the therapist's role involves not only providing patient-related instruction and procedural interventions but also coordinating and communicating with other treatment team members and recommending referrals as appropriate.

The guidelines for Pain Treatment Services put forth by the IASP (2009) stated that the diagnosis and treatment of chronic pain is so complex that multiple skills and knowledge are required, necessitating a multidisciplinary approach regardless of etiology. (We prefer the term "interdisciplinary" because the term "multidisciplinary" does not necessarily imply collaboration.) In addition to a physician, the team may include psychologists, nurses, physical therapists, occupational therapists, social workers, vocational counselors, and others as shown in Figure 28-4. Pain treatment services are also defined on the basis of available clinical services and research activities (Table 28-2).

Of note, within the chronic pain field, there are many possible subdivisions of chronic pain based not only on etiology and pathophysiology, but also on specialization of the health-care practitioners who typically treat it. Physicians who treat patients with chronic pain include family practice physicians, internists, rheumatologists, anesthesiologists, endocrinologists, psychiatrists, and physical medicine and rehabilitation specialists. Similarly, occupational and physical therapists who treat patients with chronic pain include orthopedic specialists—who may treat patients with arthritis, spine pathology, and on-the-job work-related musculoskeletal injury—and neurological specialists—who may treat patients with stroke, a spinal cord injury, or MS. Therapists who specialize in other areas, such as ergonomics, women's health, geriatrics, and pediatrics, also treat patients with chronic pain depending on their areas of expertise.

Classifications based on the specialization of the health-care provider are not always clear, however. For instance, shoulder pathology (an orthopedic concern) is a possible long-term problem in people with a spinal cord injury (a neurological condition). Also, although many conditions causing

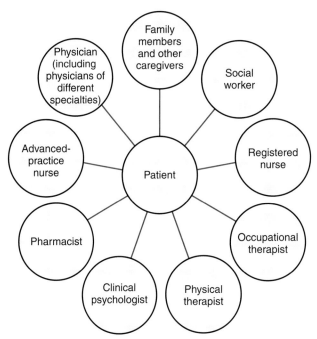

**FIGURE 28-4 An Interdisciplinary Model of Patient-Centered Care for Patients With Chronic Pain.** Types of physicians who may be involved in the treatment of patients with chronic pain include, but are not limited to, family practice physicians, internists, rheumatologists, anesthesiologists, endocrinologists, psychiatrists, and physical medicine and rehabilitation specialists. Not all patients receive all the services represented here, and other types of health-care providers not represented here may be involved as well (e.g., physician assistants, rehabilitation counselors).

chronic pain are classified as musculoskeletal, this classification can obscure important neuromuscular considerations. The pathophysiology of FMS, although not well understood, is thought to involve four regulatory systems: (1) the hypothalamic-pituitary-adrenal axis, (2) the autonomic nervous system, (3) the reproductive hormone axis, and (4) the immune system, suggesting a neuroendocrine etiology (Goodman, 2003, p. 184). Indeed, the overall constellation of clinical manifestations—including muscle pain (myalgia) and tender points, visual problems, mental and physical fatigue, sleep disturbance/morning fatigue, global anxiety, cognitive problems (e.g., issues with memory, problem-solving, insight, executive function), **paresthesias,** neutrally mediated hypotension, and depression—argues for a neuromuscular, rather than a musculoskeletal, classification. This is an important consideration because "the diagnostic label indicates the primary dysfunctions toward which the physical therapist directs interventions" (APTA, 2015). In addition, the expertise of a physical therapist who largely practices within the musculoskeletal arena may differ from that of a physical therapist who practices primarily within the neuromuscular area. For instance, it is conceivable that the neurological specialist has particular sensitivity to issues of balance, cognition, and multisystem involvement.

Similarly, an occupational therapist who follows the *Occupational Therapy Practice Framework* (OTPF), 2nd edition (Roley, 2008) would ultimately address the performance patterns (i.e., habits, routines, rituals, and roles) in a person with chronic pain but may focus only on those typically addressed within his specialty. For example, an occupational therapist specializing in physical disabilities may address body

| TABLE 28-2 | Definitions of Pain Treatment Facilities |
|---|---|
| **TERM** | **DESCRIPTION** |
| Pain treatment facility | A generic term used to describe all forms of pain treatment facilities without regard to personnel involved or types of patients served. Pain unit is a synonym for pain treatment facility. |
| Multidisciplinary pain center | An organization of health-care professionals and basic scientists that includes research, teaching, and patient care related to acute and chronic pain. This is the largest and most complex of the pain treatment facilities and ideally exists as a component of a medical school or teaching hospital. Clinical programs must be supervised by an appropriately trained and licensed clinical director; a wide array of health-care specialists is required, such as physicians, psychologists, nurses, physical therapists, occupational therapists, vocational counselors, social workers, and other specialized health-care providers. The disciplines of health-care providers are a function of the variety of patients seen and the health-care resources of the community. The members of the treatment team must communicate with each other on a regular basis, both about specific patients and about overall development. Health-care services in a multidisciplinary pain clinic must be integrated and based upon multidisciplinary assessment and management of the patient. Inpatient and outpatient programs are offered in these facilities. |
| Multidisciplinary pain clinic | A health-care delivery facility staffed by physicians of different specialties and other nonphysician health-care providers who specialize in the diagnosis and management of patients with chronic pain. This type of facility differs from a multidisciplinary pain center only because it does not include research and teaching activities in its regular programs. A multidisciplinary pain clinic may have diagnostic and treatment facilities that are outpatient, inpatient, or both. |
| Pain clinic | A health-care delivery facility focusing on the diagnosis and management of patients with chronic pain. A pain clinic may specialize in specific diagnoses or in pain related to a specific region of the body. A pain clinic may be large or small, but it should never be a label for an isolated solo practitioner. A single physician functioning |

*Continued*

| TABLE 28-2 | Definitions of Pain Treatment Facilities—cont'd |
| --- | --- |
| **TERM** | **DESCRIPTION** |
| | within a complex health-care institution that offers appropriate consultative and therapeutic services could qualify as a pain clinic if patients with chronic pain are suitably assessed and managed. The absence of interdisciplinary assessment and management distinguishes this type of facility from a multidisciplinary pain center or clinic. Pain clinics can, and should be encouraged to, carry out research, but it is not a required characteristic of this type of facility. |
| Modality-oriented clinic | This is a health-care facility that offers a specific type of treatment and does not provide comprehensive assessment or management. Examples include nerve block clinics, transcutaneous nerve stimulation clinics, acupuncture clinics, and biofeedback clinics. Such a facility may have one or more health-care providers with different professional training; because of its limited treatment and the lack of an integrated, comprehensive approach, it does not qualify for the term "multidisciplinary." |

Loeser JD; IASP Task Force Committee Pain Clinic Guidelines.
Desirable characteristics for pain treatment facilities: Report of the IASP task force. In: Bond MR, Charlton JE, Woolf CJ, eds. *Proceedings of the Sixth World Congress on Pain.* Seattle, WA: International Association for the Study of Pain; 1991:411–415.
IASP. Pain Treatment Services, Available at: https://www.iasp-pain.org/Education/Content.aspx?ItemNumber=1381. Accessed July 11, 2017.

mechanics and energy conservation pertaining to a patient's habits during daily routines, whereas an occupational therapist specializing in mental health may address habitual coping strategies and behaviors in response to pain and stressors within the person's daily life. Certainly, individual therapists can have skills in more than one area of practice; however, at times therapists should refer to or consult with not only other types of health-care providers but also other therapists depending on their area of specialization.

Scope of practice also warrants consideration. There is considerable overlap between the occupational therapy and physical therapy professions, such that therapists have the expertise to treat many of the same patient populations. Indeed, occupational and physical therapists often work collaboratively, and at times the choice of which professional addresses which aspects of any given patient's care is somewhat arbitrary or is a matter of convention, convenience, or both. Different policy documents may disagree on the specific roles of the occupational therapist and physical therapist; however, for our purposes, we simply note the importance of working collaboratively and always remaining within one's scope of practice as delineated by state practice acts and other relevant documents. We use the inclusive term *therapist* in this chapter to denote both occupational and physical therapists.

## THINK ABOUT IT 28.2

Although there can be overlap in the scope of practice among occupational therapists, physical therapists, and psychologists, it is ideal to have all three disciplines represented on the interdisciplinary team. How many patients with chronic pain do you believe have access to interdisciplinary pain centers and clinics according to the International Association for the Study of Pain definitions? How can you help address this need when you practice in a clinic that does not meet these definitions?

### Physical Rehabilitation Treatment Approaches

The Curriculum Outline on Pain for Occupational Therapy and Physical Therapy of the IASP ad hoc Subcommittee for Occupational Therapy/Physical Therapy Curriculum (IASP, n.d.) recommends the following therapeutic objectives for the treatment of patients with chronic pain:

- Reduction of pain and associated disability
- Promotion of optimal function and participation in everyday living
- Enabling meaningful family and social relationships

To accomplish these objectives, the subcommittee recommends the following elements:

- Person-centered care
- Promotion of health and well-being through prevention of pain and disability resulting from pain
- A holistic and collaborative view of the needs of the patient with pain
- Recognition of the numerous misconceptions about pain and people with pain and the ability to refute and challenge this misinformation
- Family education

A broad treatment approach to chronic pain is the functional restoration approach. The term "functional restoration" was introduced in the 1980s and refers to an approach that focuses on restoring function rather than eliminating pain, which is often not a realistic goal (Mayer, 1985, 1986, 1988). The central premise is that people with chronic pain benefit from a combination of psychological interventions (to improve their coping abilities and readiness for change) and engagement in structured, progressive physical activity (to overcome the effects of musculoskeletal and cardiovascular/pulmonary deconditioning due to the inactivity of chronic pain). Although the functional restoration approach was initially developed for people with chronic LBP, it can be regarded as a general approach to managing chronic benign (i.e., nonmalignant) pain, regardless of its location or the underlying disease process. Further discussion of the roles of the occupational therapist, physical therapist, and psychologist follow later in the chapter.

### Physical Activity Considerations

Although physical activity is just one component of the functional restoration approach, this component requires special considerations in patients/clients with neurological conditions. When there are no medical contraindications or precautions for physical activity, the functional restoration approach is used to decrease deconditioning and other complications attributable to the inactivity of chronic pain, thus optimizing function and decreasing disability. However, as we will see, this approach may need to be modified as a result of disease-specific considerations.

The functional restoration approach can be modified for patients who have disease-specific considerations for physical activity. For instance, patients with FMS and MS often experience not only chronic pain but also debilitating fatigue as part of the disease process; for them, excessive physical activity can exacerbate both pain and fatigue, requiring calibration of the activity. In conditions such as postpolio syndrome and Guillain-Barré syndrome, overwork is contraindicated because it may exacerbate not only the symptoms but also the disease process. In other conditions, such as painful diabetic neuropathy and chemotherapy-induced neuropathy, there are at least two types of disease-specific considerations: activity precautions (e.g., the importance of wearing appropriate footwear) in the insensate individual and activity precautions due to complications of diabetes and cancer (which can vary considerably from one individual to another). Of course, in any patient, there may be activity contraindications and precautions due to comorbidities. In general, a modified functional restoration approach can be useful for patients for whom the primary goal is to decrease deconditioning and other secondary complications attributable to the inactivity of chronic pain.

Depending on the disease and the individual, however, decreasing deconditioning and other complications attributable to inactivity may not be the primary goal. For instance, patients with MS and postpolio syndrome typically have myriad impairments that also need to be addressed (e.g., neurologically mediated muscle weakness). In these cases, it may be more helpful to conceptualize therapist management in terms of disease-specific approaches rather than the functional restoration approach—though functional restoration may still be the ultimate goal. Also, in conditions such as poststroke shoulder pain (PSSP), CRPS, and PLP, remediation of chronic pain may be a reasonable goal, and there may be specific treatment recommendations based on the medical diagnosis. Further complicating the picture, there may be multiple causes of chronic pain in the same individual, some of which are more amenable to remediation than others.

In cases of neuropathic pain, relatively few physical rehabilitation techniques are useful for treating the pain itself, so functional restoration may be the therapist's primary goal. In contrast, pain management (e.g., through pharmacological means) is typically the primary goal of the physician. On the other hand, when musculoskeletal pain is a secondary impairment of neurological disorders, physical rehabilitation techniques can help prevent, remediate, or limit its effects.

In sum, disease-specific considerations may necessitate modifications to the functional restoration approach. They might broaden the focus, or they may dictate a different approach altogether. Unlike chronic pain of musculoskeletal origin (e.g., chronic LBP), chronic pain in individuals with neurologic conditions is not typically the basis for physical rehabilitation services; rather, chronic pain is one impairment among many that the therapist manages and addresses simultaneously. The functional restoration approach, whether pure or modified, is probably most helpful when the inactivity of chronic pain is the primary basis for the involvement of physical rehabilitation services.

Smart (2006) described a mechanisms-based clinical reasoning approach for five categories of pain: (1) nociceptive, (2) peripheral neurogenic, (3) central, (4) autonomic/sympathetic, and (5) cognitive-affective. This approach, which is largely congruent with the WHO (2006) classification of pain, may be useful to the clinician in determining the origin of pain and the corresponding treatment approach.

The purpose of this chapter is to introduce the topic of chronic pain in neurology and illustrate how one might work with health-care providers of other disciplines. In particular, we wish to emphasize the interrelatedness of occupational, physical, and psychological rehabilitation efforts. For additional information, see the list of resources at the end of the chapter.

## Clinical Picture of Chronic Pain in a Holistic Context

As we have seen, acute pain is a mechanism designed to protect against or limit the degree of tissue damage. Chronic pain is generally considered to be pain that has no physiological benefit and thus serves no purpose. It persists long after the initial tissue damage has healed (WHO, 2006).

Chronic pain affects all domains of a person's life. According to the OTPF (Roley, 2008), these domains represent the areas of **occupation**, including ADLs (e.g., self-care, sexual activity, functional mobility), IADLs (e.g., childcare, home management, cooking, financial management, community mobility), rest and sleep, education, work, play, leisure, and social participation. In the *Guide* (APTA, 2015), these domains comprise self-care, home management, work (job/school/play), community, and leisure roles.

When considering a holistic context, it is important to compare and contrast the biopsychosocial and biomedical models. In 1977, Engel used the term "biopsychosocial model" to describe the incorporation of psychosocial variables in health and illness, in contrast with the traditional biomedical model, which was dominant in health care at that time. The biomedical model explained illness according to biological factors, emphasized disease over health, and was based on reductionism (i.e., the belief that illness is best understood and treated at the molecular level) and mind-body dualism (i.e., the belief that biological and psychological and social processes are unrelated to and do not interact with one another in the development and treatment of illness) (Engel, 1977).

The biopsychosocial model, on the other hand, considers interactions between biological, psychological, and social factors; emphasizes health and illness; and is based on systems theory (Engel, 1977, 1980; Schwartz, 1982). The biopsychosocial model is well suited for the study of chronic pain because it posits that psychological and social factors mediate the effects of chronic pain on the patient's life. Thus, it can account for variability in patients' responses to living with chronic pain. For example, experienced clinicians often see patients with similar pain profiles but very different levels of subsequent disability.

## Possible Effect of Chronic Pain on Function

Chronic pain can lead to life-changing disability. To discuss disability, we need to use a disablement/enablement model (see Chapter 1 for further discussion). The *Guide* (APTA, 2015) is informed by the International Classification of Functioning, Disability, and Health (ICF) (see Fig. 1-1 and the bottom of Fig. 1-3). The biopsychosocial model relates well to the ICF framework, which incorporates the elements of the earlier models but makes two major changes: (1) It considers the effects of environmental and personal factors, and (2) it links all components of the model with bidirectional arrows to show the oftentimes reciprocal interplay between them. (An example of reciprocal interplay is as follows: nonadherence—a personal factor—to the medical management regimen for diabetes mellitus can result in worsening of the disease.)

Chronic pain and its associated impairments can lead to significant functional limitations and disability (conceptualized as activity limitations and participation restrictions in the ICF model); as mentioned, however, two people with the same constellation of active pathology and impairment may have very different functional limitations and disability. The explicit consideration of environmental and personal factors gives clinicians additional opportunities to buffer the effects of chronic pain on the patient's life and fits well with the functional restoration approach.

### PATIENT APPLICATION

*Mrs. Q. is a 35 year-old female who is referred for outpatient therapy with a medical diagnosis of FMS. During her initial examination and evaluation, Mrs. Q. reports that she has been experiencing the gradual onset of chronic widespread pain and fatigue since a motor vehicle accident 2 years ago. The pain has progressed to the point that she has had to reduce her hours at work and needs her mother's help to care for her two young children because her husband works long hours with frequent travel. She tearfully mentions that her family relationships have become strained because she has struggled to cope with sleep and appetite disturbances. She adds, "I can't seem to please my children or my husband. I just feel worthless."*

### Contemplate Clinical Decisions

- *How does this patient's initial clinical presentation relate to the International Classification of Functioning, Disability, and Health model?*
- *Assuming you are working in a general outpatient setting, what resources are needed to provide this patient with appropriate care?*
- *What referrals would you consider making for this patient?*
- *From this brief introduction to the patient, what information would you want to gain during the examination and evaluation?*
- *What risk factors might you want to explore given the information presented thus far?*
- *For occupational therapists: What areas of occupation appear to be affected given the information presented?*
- *For physical therapists: What domains other than physical function might you consider during the examination and evaluation?*

## ■ Anatomy and Physiology

### Systems Involved

Conceptually, sensory receptors in the periphery (i.e., **nociceptors**) give rise to the sensory component of pain. These sensory receptors detect stimuli and send their input through the peripheral nervous system to the spinal cord; from there, it is conducted via the lateral spinothalamic tract to the thalamus and then cortical representation in the sensory cortex for the perception of pain. This perception of pain is then integrated with other brain centers for the cognitive, affective, and behavioral components of pain. **Nociception** refers to the sensation that occurs when a stimulus activates peripheral nerve fibers that carry pain and the afferent input is perceived as pain. Neuropathic pain is caused by a lesion of the nervous system—either the peripheral nervous system or the central nervous system.

In general, the etiology of chronic pain is poorly understood. However, our understanding of the biological bases of chronic pain is gradually increasing. In 1965, Melzack proposed the gate theory of pain, in which active inhibitory input from large fibers in the periphery or from the brainstem centrally modulates pain transmission in the dorsal horns of the spinal cord; conversely, loss of these inhibitory mechanisms (e.g., through nerve injury) results in the loss of this modulation (i.e., the loss of the ability to close the pain gate). Woolf (1983, 2007) discovered the phenomenon of central sensitization, a manifestation of activity-dependent synaptic plasticity whereby dorsal horn neurons become hypersensitive to pain in response to high levels of nociceptor input; this causes secondary hyperalgesia, abnormally large receptive fields (giving rise to heightened pain sensitivity adjacent to an area of injury), and tactile allodynia.

More recently, the pain neuromatrix theory (Melzack, 2001, 2005) has extended our understanding of pain; this theory holds that pain is a multidimensional experience produced by characteristic neurosignature patterns of nerve impulses generated by a widely distributed neural network—the "body-self neuromatrix." The theory attempts to explain why chronic pain can persist in the absence of identifiable pathology and why psychological and physical stress exacerbates chronic pain. Thus, it continues the evolution from the biomedical model to the biopsychosocial model because it accounts for variability in people's experience of pain.

Of note, research into the biological processes of pain continues to elucidate the biology behind it. May (2008) suggested that people with chronic pain have a characteristic neurosignature of activity in the brain structures that regulates the experience and anticipation of pain as a consequence of frequent nociceptive input. Such neuroplastic changes are reversible. Considering the neuromatrix theory, Moseley (2003a) proposed using desensitization and graded activation of components of the pain neuromatrix to manage chronic pain, described later in the chapter. Interestingly, emerging evidence indicates that the immune system, along with nerve trauma, is an important contributor to peripheral neuropathic pain (Watkins, 2004). It is also important to recognize that certain medical diagnoses have multifactorial etiologies. For example, FMS is thought to involve central nervous system sensitization, an external insult, and a genetic component (Ablin, 2008).

Sullivan (2008), a noted pain expert, described another model called the biopsychomotor conceptualization of pain. Sullivan's model addresses both the gate control theory and the pain neuromatrix theory while adding a behavioral dimension via communicative pain behaviors, protective pain behaviors, and social response behaviors, the latter representing the response of other people to the person in pain. As such, this model is arguably more complete than its predecessors and certainly is consistent with the biopsychosocial model of health and illness.

Although conceptual models such as the pain neuromatrix theory are complex, especially for entry-level therapists, they are consistent with the explosion of neuroscience research on neuroplasticity. As such, they not only highlight the complex nature of chronic pain but also offer new mechanism-based approaches with more options for conservative treatment and corresponding roles for therapists—roles that are well defined, standardized, and evidence based. These new directions are explored later in the chapter.

## Lifespan Influence

Cognitive status is one consideration with implications across the lifespan. Patients with cognitive limitations—either due to normal developmental issues or to pathology—require special attention during assessment. For instance, a variety of instruments based on pain behaviors are available and can be chosen based on an individual's cognitive status, such as instruments based on the pictorial presentation of faces versus visual or verbal analog scales. (For an in-depth review, please see Turk, 2001a)

### Developmental Considerations

In the past, neonates' nervous systems were not thought to be developed enough for the perception of pain. As a result,

invasive procedures such as circumcision were performed without anesthesia. However, this supposition has been disproved, and the need to provide neonates with appropriate **analgesia** is now understood (Menon, 2008). The APS has published a relevant position statement titled "The Assessment and Management of Acute Pain in Infants, Children, and Adolescents" (APS, 2001).

### Age-Related Changes Relevant to Chronic Pain

The accumulation of pathologies in older adults raises at least two age-related considerations. First, these pathologies may decrease their sensitivity to pain (e.g., peripheral hypoalgesia due to diabetic neuropathy, hemihypoalgesia due to stroke), increasing their risk for injury. However, the pathologies may also cause pain (e.g., painful diabetic neuropathy, shoulder-hand syndrome in stroke). Thus, the same type of pathology can have opposite effects in different people.

## ■ Related Pathology

### Neuroanatomy of Common Pathologies

As always, the question in neurology is "Where is the lesion?" As discussed previously, pain is associated with neurological disorders in three ways: as neuropathic pain, as secondary musculoskeletal pain, and as CRPS. Neuropathic pain can be peripheral or central, whereas CRPS involves both the somatic and autonomic nervous systems (WHO, 2006). Figures 5-2 and 5-3 illustrate the "Where is it?" query for pain perception, including the postcentral gyrus and thalamus—particularly the ventral posteriormedial nucleus and ventral posteriorlateral nucleus. The posterior horn of the spinal cord and the anterolateral system/lateral spinothalamic tract of the spinal cord (but not the posterior column) are especially important for conveying pain sensation.

### Medical Diagnoses

Many neurological conditions (or conditions with neurological components) can cause chronic pain, including stroke, traumatic spinal cord injury, traumatic brain injury, MS, amyotrophic lateral sclerosis, peripheral neuropathy from diabetes mellitus or other causes, CRPS, **neuralgia**, FMS, and amputation leading to PLP.

## ■ Pertinent Examination and Evaluation

When pain types and underlying disease processes are evaluated, it is important to remember that any given patient's pain may be comprised of multiple sub-types of pain (WHO, 2006). Equally important, pain occurs in the context of the whole person, necessitating not only a neurological examination (Cruccu, 2004) but also a systems review (APTA, 2015). Evaluations of psychosocial and environmental factors related to the person's perception of pain and the effects of pain on level of occupational performance are also crucial (Engel, 2003).

Essentials of the sensory examination related to pain assessment are described in Chapter 5. The process of examination and evaluation begins with the history and includes assessment of the intensity, quality, and temporal and physical characteristics of the pain (APTA, 2015). Numerous general pain assessment forms are available (e.g., Fig. 5-12 in Chapter 5),

and the characteristics of pain in the individual should be further delineated using tests and measures with both objective and self-report measures (Table 28-3).

Objective measures include a detailed clinical examination of sensory function for patients with neuropathic pain; although this is simple to perform, it is very important. Touch and

| TABLE 28-3 | Selected Methods and Instruments for Assessing Pain and Related Domains | | |
|---|---|---|---|
| DOMAIN | METHODS AND INSTRUMENTS | SELF-REPORT (S), PERFORMANCE-BASED (P), OR MIXED (M) METHOD OR INSTRUMENT | GENERIC (G) OR DISEASE-SPECIFIC (D) METHOD OR INSTRUMENT |
| *Pain* | | | |
| Location | Body chart | S | G |
| Intensity | VAS, NRS, VRS, Faces, MPQ, SF-MPQ | S | G |
| Sensory components (quality) | VRS, MPQ, SF-MPQ | S | G |
| Affective components (unpleasantness) | VRS, MPQ, SF-MPQ | | |
| Evaluative component | VRS, MPQ | S | G |
| Temporal characteristics | Pain diary, VRS, MPQ | S | G |
| Pain behavior | Clinician observation | P | G |
| Neuropathic characteristics | LANSS | M | G |
| | S-LANSS, NPS, PQAS | S | G |
| Sensory function | Cotton wool (touch) | P | G |
| | 128-Hz tuning fork (vibration) | | |
| | Toothpick (pinprick sense [i.e., sharp pain]) | | |
| | Metal thermorollers (cold and warmth) | | |
| *Sleep* | | | |
| | VAS, NRS, VRS | S | G |
| *Mood* | | | |
| | BDI | S | G |
| *Functional Status* | | | |
| | SIP | S | G |
| | PSFS | S | G |
| | FIM | P | G |
| | FCE | P | G |
| | 6MWT, 12MWT | P | G |
| | FGA | P | G |
| | ODI | S | G |
| | COPM | S | G |
| | Worker Role Interview | S | G |
| | Barthel Index | P | G |
| | AM-PAC™ | P | G |

| TABLE 28-3 | Selected Methods and Instruments for Assessing Pain and Related Domains—cont'd | | |
|---|---|---|---|
| **DOMAIN** | **METHODS AND INSTRUMENTS** | **SELF-REPORT (S), PERFORMANCE-BASED (P), OR MIXED (M) METHOD OR INSTRUMENT** | **GENERIC (G) OR DISEASE-SPECIFIC (D) METHOD OR INSTRUMENT** |
| *Quality of Life* | | | |
| | SF-36 | S | G |
| | FIQ | S | D |
| | QOLS | S | G |

Abbreviations: AM-PAC™ = Activity Measure for Post-Acute Care™; BDI = Beck Depression Inventory; COPM = Canadian Occupational Performance Measure; FCE = functional capacity evaluation; FGA = Functional Gait Assessment; FIM = Functional Independence Measure; FIQ = Fibromyalgia Impact Questionnaire; LANSS = Leeds Assessment of Neuropathic Symptoms and Signs; MPQ = McGill Pain Questionnaire; NPS = Neuropathic Pain Scale; NRS = numerical rating scale; ODI = Oswestry Disability Index; PQAS = Pain Quality Assessment Scale; PSFS = Patient-Specific Functional Scale; QOLS = Quality of Life Scale; SF-36 = Medical Outcomes Study–Short Form 36; SF-MPQ = Short-Form McGill Pain Questionnaire; SIP = Sickness Impact Profile; S-LANSS = Self-Administered Leeds Assessment of Neuropathic Symptoms and Signs; VAS = visual analog scale; VRS = verbal rating scale; 6MWT = 6-Minute Walk Test; 12MWT = 12-Minute Walk Test.

vibration, which are carried on A-$\beta$ fibers, are assessed using a piece of cotton wool and a 128-Hz tuning fork, respectively. Pinprick sense (i.e., sharp pain), which is carried on A-$\delta$ fibers, is assessed using a wooden cocktail stick (i.e., a toothpick). Thermal sense for cold (which is carried on A-$\delta$ fibers) and warmth (which is carried on C fibers) is assessed using cold and warm objects (e.g., metal thermorollers).

Throughout sensory testing, any abnormalities in intensity, quality, and temporal and spatial characteristics should be noted. Sensory testing ideally occurs at the end of the neurological examination because patients with chronic pain are likely to experience sensory testing as unpleasant (Cruccu, 2004). This timing not only allows the therapist to develop initial rapport with the patient, but it also ensures that the patient gives his history and otherwise participates to the best of his ability throughout most of the initial visit.

Self-report measures include pain quality and intensity scales (see Chapter 5). As Cruccu (2004) indicated, simple scales include the visual analog scale (VAS), numerical rating scale (NRS), and verbal rating scale (VRS). The VAS is one of the oldest, easiest, and most-validated pain measures. Among numerical scales, the 11-point Likert scale (0 = no pain; 10 = worst possible pain) has been most widely used in recent studies of neuropathic pain. Verbal scales consist of spoken descriptors that can be used for multiple assessment, including intensity and unpleasantness. The McGill Pain Questionnaire (Melzack, 1975; see Chapter 5) and its short form (Melzack, 1987) are the most frequently used self-report measures for pain and yield information about both sensory and affective components of pain. The European Federation of Neurological Societies Panel on Neuropathic Pain recommended that the intensity and unpleasantness of pain be rated separately and that the scale for intensity be used also for separate ratings of the patient's pain components, whether spontaneous or evoked (Cruccu, 2004). Faces scales can be used when there are language barriers because of age (i.e., in children and older adults) or with patients for whom English

is not the first language. Other assessment tools include pain drawings (i.e., body charts), diaries for tracking temporal variations in pain, and the clinician's notation of pain behavior. The clinician should also consider factors that can affect the patient's clinical presentation, including sex and ethnic and cultural backgrounds (WHO, 2006).

Another useful tool is the Patient-Specific Functional Scale (Stratford, 1995), which asks the patient to identify up to five important activities that he is having difficulty performing or has been unable to perform since the onset of a painful condition (see Fig. 28-5). The tool uses an 11-point NRS to score each of the tasks, with 0 indicating "unable to perform activity" and 10 indicating "able to perform activity at same level as before injury or problem." According to Moseley (2008b), this tool is repeatable, is sensitive to change, and has been used across multiple chronic pain conditions, including complex regional pain syndrome type 1 (CRPS1) and PLP; it has the distinct advantage of maximizing sensitivity (i.e., the ability to detect a change in function) because the patient self-selects up to five important tasks that he finds especially difficult. However, because the tasks vary from patient to patient, comparison with data obtained from generic tools is difficult. Although this limitation has implications for research, the advantages of the scale make it useful overall in clinical practice.

An additional tool that can assist with goal setting and evaluating areas of perceived impaired occupational performance is the Canadian Occupational Performance Measure (Law, 1990). This tool is similar to the Patient-Specific Functional Scale in that it encourages patients to identify five activities with which they are experiencing difficulty. However, it also assesses the importance of these activities to the patient, the patient's perceived performance ability, and the patient's satisfaction with his current level of performance using a 10-point NRS for each category. This tool can be used as a baseline measure to assist with goal setting and to assess changes in the patient's self-perception of chronic pain after intervention.

CLINICIAN TO READ AND FILL IN BELOW: Complete at the end of the history and prior to physical examination.

**Initial assessment:**

I am going to ask you to identify up to three important activities that you are unable to do or are having difficulty with as a result of your _____ problem. Today, are there any activities that you are unable to do or having difficulty with because of your _____ problem? (Clinician: show scale to patient and have the patient rate each activity.)

**Follow-up assessments:**

When I assessed you on (state previous assessment date) you told me that you had difficulty with (read all activities from list at a time). Today, do you still have difficulty with: (read and have patient score every item in the list)?

**PATIENT-SPECIFIC ACTIVITY SCORING SCHEME (Point to one number):**

0   1   2   3   4   5   6   7   8   9   10

Unable to
perform activity.

Able to perform
activity at same
level as before
injury or problem.

| Activity | Initial | | | | | | |
|----------|---------|--|--|--|--|--|--|
| 1 | | | | | | | |
| 2 | | | | | | | |
| 3 | | | | | | | |
| 4 | | | | | | | |
| 5 | | | | | | | |
| Additional | | | | | | | |
| Additional | | | | | | | |

(Date and score)

**FIGURE 28-5 Patient-Specific Functional Scale** *Reprinted with permission from: Stratford PW, Gill C, Westaway M, Binkley JM. Assessing disability and change on individual patients: A report of a patient-specific measure. Physiother Can. 1995;47: 258–263. © Stratford, 1995.*

Other self-report measures of functional status include the Oswestry Disability Index (Fairbank, 1980) and the Worker Role Interview (Biernacki, 1993). The Worker Role Interview is used to identify psychosocial and environmental factors influencing an individual's ability to return to work. This information can be beneficial when considering a patient's self-perception and beliefs regarding his functional limitations and capacity to return to work (Paquette, 2008).

Because patients' perceptions of their function may differ from their actual performance, self-report measures of function such as the Sickness Impact Profile (Bergner, 1981) and performance-based instruments (Harding, 1998; Lee, 2001) are also useful. Performance-based instruments include generic measures of functional status, such as the Functional Independence Measure (Keith, 1987), the Barthel Index (Mahoney, 1965), and the Activity Measure for Post-Acute Care™ (Haley, 2004). Other performance-based instruments include functional capacity evaluations that measure an individual's safe maximum physical abilities for industrial job–related tasks (either preemployment or postinjury) and physical performance batteries that were developed for people with chronic pain. (For a brief review of the latter, see Harding, 1998.)

Tests of functional exercise capacity, such as the 6-minute and 12-minute walk tests (Butland, 1982; McGavin, 1976),

also fall into this category, as do clinical measures of balance such as the Functional Gait Assessment (Wrisley, 2004). Clinical measures of balance are important to consider in neurological populations; indeed, research suggests that balance impairments may be a feature of chronic pain syndromes such as FMS (Jones, 2009).

Multiple tools are useful for measuring neuropathic pain. The Leeds Assessment of Neuropathic Symptoms and Signs (Bennett, 2001) is a clinician-administered assessment providing both subjective and objective data to distinguish patients with and without neuropathic pain (Jensen, 2006a). It is also available in a self-report version, the Self-Report Leeds Assessment of Neuropathic Symptoms and Signs (Bennett, 2005). Another tool for measuring neuropathic pain is the Neuropathic Pain Scale (Galer, 1997). This scale (Fig. 28-6) is also available as an appendix to the original reference and has been used in clinical research (e.g., Moseley, 2004b, 2005b) on CRPS1. Jensen (2006a) concluded that the Neuropathic Pain Scale is the best outcome measure; however, she predicted that another instrument in development at that time, the Pain Quality Assessment Scale (Jensen, 2006b) would be even more helpful because it captures additional descriptors of neuropathic pain.

The European Federation of Neurological Societies Panel on Neuropathic Pain recommended use of the simplest scales

Appendix

## NEUROPATHY PAIN SCALE

*Instructions:* There are several different aspects of pain which we are interested in measuring: pain **sharpness**, **heat/cold**, **dullness**, **intensity**, overall **unpleasantness**, and **surface vs. deep pain**.

The distinction between these aspects of pain might be clearer if you think of taste. For example, people might agree on how *sweet* a piece of pie might be (the *intensity* of the sweetness), but some might enjoy it more if it were sweeter while others might prefer it to be less sweet. Similarly, people can judge the loudness of music and agree on what is more quiet and what is louder, but disagree on how it makes them feel. Some people prefer quiet music and some prefer it more loud. In short, the *intensity* of a sensation is not the same as how it makes you feel. A sound might be unpleasant and still be quiet (think of someone grating their fingernails along a chalkboard). A sound can be quiet and "dull" or loud and "dull."

Pain is the same. Many people are able to tell the difference between many aspects of their pain: for example, *how much* it hurts and *how unpleasant* or annoying it is. Although often the intensity of pain has a strong influence on how unpleasant the experience of pain is, some people are able to experience more pain than others before they feel very bad about it.

There are scales for measuring different aspects of pain. For one patient, a pain might feel extremely hot, but not at all dull, while another patient may not experience any heat, but feel like their pain is very dull. We expect you to rate very high on some of the scales below and very low on others. We want you to use the measures that follow to tell us exactly what you experience.

---

1. Please use the scale below to tell us how **intense** your pain is. Place an "X" through the number that best describes the intensity of your pain.

No pain | 0 | 1 | 2 | 3 | 4 | 5 | 6 | 7 | 8 | 9 | 10 | The most **intense** pain sensation imaginable

---

2. Please use the scale below to tell us how **sharp** your pain is. Words used to describe "sharp" feelings include "like a knife," "like a spike," "jabbing" or "like jolts."

Not sharp | 0 | 1 | 2 | 3 | 4 | 5 | 6 | 7 | 8 | 9 | 10 | The most **sharp** sensation imaginable ("like a knife")

---

3. Please use the scale below to tell us how **hot** your pain is. Words used to describe very hot pain include "burning" and "on fire."

Not hot | 0 | 1 | 2 | 3 | 4 | 5 | 6 | 7 | 8 | 9 | 10 | The most **hot** sensation imaginable ( "on fire")

---

4. Please use the scale below to tell us how **dull** your pain is. Words used to describe very dull pain include "like a dull toothache," "dull pain," "aching" and "like a bruise."

Not dull | 0 | 1 | 2 | 3 | 4 | 5 | 6 | 7 | 8 | 9 | 10 | The most **dull** sensation imaginable

---

5. Please use the scale below to tell us how **cold** your pain is. Words used to describe very cold pain include "like ice" and "freezing."

Not cold | 0 | 1 | 2 | 3 | 4 | 5 | 6 | 7 | 8 | 9 | 10 | The most **cold** sensation imaginable ("freezing")

---

6. Please use the scale below to tell us how **sensitive** your skin is to light touch or clothing. Words used to describe sensitive skin include "like sunburned skin" and "raw skin."

Not sensitive | 0 | 1 | 2 | 3 | 4 | 5 | 6 | 7 | 8 | 9 | 10 | The most **sensitive** sensation imaginable ("raw skin")

---

7. Please use the scale below to tell us how **itchy** your pain is. Words used to describe itchy pain include "like poison oak" and "like a mosquito bite."

Not itchy | 0 | 1 | 2 | 3 | 4 | 5 | 6 | 7 | 8 | 9 | 10 | The most **itchy** sensation imaginable

---

8. Which of the following best describes the **time** quality of your pain? Please check only one answer.

❏ I feel a background pain <u>all of the time</u> and occasional flare-ups (break-through pain) <u>some of the time</u>.
　Describe the background pain:_____
　Describe the flare-up (break-through) pain:_____
❏ I feel a single type of pain <u>all the time</u>. Describe this pain:_____
❏ I feel a single type of pain only <u>sometimes</u>. Other times, I am pain free.
　Describe this occasional pain:_____

---

9. Now that you have told us the different physical aspects of your pain, the different types of sensations, we want you to tell us overall how **unpleasant** your pain is to you. Words used to describe very unpleasant pain include "miserable" and "intolerable." Remember, pain can have a low intensity, but still feel extremely unpleasant, and some kinds of pain can have a high intensity but be very tolerable. With this scale, please tell us how **unpleasant** your pain feels.

Not unpleasant | 0 | 1 | 2 | 3 | 4 | 5 | 6 | 7 | 8 | 9 | 10 | The most **unpleasant** sensation imaginable ("intolerable")

---

10. Lastly, we want you to give us an estimate of the severity of your <u>deep</u> versus <u>surface</u> pain. We want you to rate each location of pain separately. We realize that it can be difficult to make these estimates, and most likely it will be a "best guess," but please give us your best estimate.

HOW INTENSE IS YOUR *DEEP* PAIN?

No **deep** pain | 0 | 1 | 2 | 3 | 4 | 5 | 6 | 7 | 8 | 9 | 10 | The most **intense deep** pain sensation imaginable

HOW INTENSE IS YOUR *SURFACE* PAIN?

No **surface** pain | 0 | 1 | 2 | 3 | 4 | 5 | 6 | 7 | 8 | 9 | 10 | The most **intense surface** pain sensation imaginable

---

**FIGURE 28-6 Neuropathic Pain Scale** *From: Galer BS, Jensen MP. Development and preliminary validation of a pain measure specific to neuropathic pain: The Neuropathic Pain Scale. Neurology. 1997;48:332–338. Used with permission from Wolters Kluwer Health.*

and **quality-of-life** (QoL) measures in both clinical practice and controlled trials. It further recommended that relevant research studies include the assessment of sleep, mood, functional capacity, and QoL as secondary endpoints in addition to pain reduction as the primary endpoint. Examples of assessment tools in these domains include the VAS, NRS, or VRS for sleep; the Beck Depression Inventory (Beck, 1961); the Sickness Impact Profile (Bergner, 1981) for functional status; and the Medical Outcomes Study–Short Form 36 (SF-36) (Ware, 1992) and Quality of Life Scale (Flanagan, 1978; reviewed by Burckhardt, 2003) for QoL (Cruccu, 2004).

We recommend that the interdisciplinary team includes such assessments in routine clinical practice as well, recognizing that generic QoL measures are mostly epidemiological tools intended to measure change in large populations rather than in individuals (Wittink, 2008). However, generic QoL measures such as the SF-36 can be combined with disease-specific measures such as the Fibromyalgia Impact Questionnaire (Burckhardt, 1991) to maximize the information available to the interdisciplinary team for treatment planning (Wittink, 2008).

## THINK ABOUT IT 28.3

Among the occupational therapists, physical therapists, and psychologists at your clinic, who do you think would administer each of these tests and measures? Are there tests and measures that could be administered by multiple disciplines?

For treatment planning, the therapist should also ask what types of activities the patient enjoys and must perform for work. Furthermore, the therapist should incorporate other tests and measures not related to chronic pain as appropriate to the medical diagnosis and the patient's clinical presentation. Finally, it is also important to screen for pain-related red flags and changes in chronic pain that may indicate the presence of new, as-yet-undiagnosed problems (e.g., cancer). Box 28-1 lists some prognostic factors that may help determine expected outcomes.

### PATIENT APPLICATION

*Mrs. Q. uses a body chart to indicate multiple areas of pain consistent with her medical diagnosis of FMS, which by definition is a syndrome of chronic widespread pain. She also uses an NRS (0 to 10 scale) to give the following pain ratings: current = 6; worst in the past 24 hours = 8; best in the past 24 hours = 5. Sensory testing reveals both allodynia and hyperalgesia, with accompanying pain behavior, including flinching and grimacing. Mrs. Q. also completes multiple outcome measures across several domains: the Neuropathic Pain Scale, McGill Pain Questionnaire, Patient-Specific Functional Scale, 6-Minute Walk Test, Functional Gait Assessment, NRS (for sleep), Beck Depression Inventory, Sickness Impact Profile, SF-36, and Fibromyalgia Impact Questionnaire.*

### BOX 28-1  Positive Prognostic Factors That May Be Helpful to Determine Expected Outcomes

↑ Levels of physical activity
↑ Sleep and appetite
↑ Participation in leisure activities
↑ Interpersonal relationships
↑ Optimism/optimistic attributional style
↑ **Self-efficacy**
↑ Internal locus of control
↑ Cognitive flexibility (i.e., the belief that there is more than one way to do things)
↑ Educational level
↑ Socioeconomic status
↑ History of exercise
↓ Emotional distress
↓ Social conflict
↓ Use of medications
↓ Utilization of health-care services in general
Participation in vocational rehabilitation as appropriate

### Contemplate Clinical Decisions

- *How might the patient's pain behaviors affect treatment?*
- *What general treatment approach might you choose for Mrs. Q.?*
- *What exercises and other activities might you prescribe?*
- *How will you measure and monitor Mrs. Q.'s progress?*
- *What prognostic factors are relevant to her case?*

## ◼ Preparatory Intervention Specific to Chronic Pain

In the early steps of therapy to address chronic pain, the therapist first tries approaches or specific techniques to address the impairment itself, perhaps through changing the physiology of this system as described in the following sections.

### General Approaches

Treatment options for chronic pain include pharmacological, interventional (e.g., nerve blocks), physical, and psychological therapies. When pain is part of a primary condition, such as MS, then treatment for that pain will be one component of the overall treatment for that condition (WHO, 2006). Considerable evidence supports the effectiveness of multidisciplinary treatment of chronic nonmalignant pain (Scascighini, 2008b). According to Scascighini (2008a), "(h)igh-quality randomized controlled trials indicate that multidisciplinary pain programs represent the best therapeutic option for the management of patients with complaints associated with complex chronic pain." Similar conclusions have been reached for other conditions as well, including chronic LBP (Guzmán, 2002), work-related back and neck pain (Schonstein, 2003), and FMS (Burckhardt, 2005; Häuser, 2009a). Even when strong research support is lacking for specific patient populations (e.g., patients with CRPS) (Daly, 2009), there are still calls for a multidisciplinary approach (Harden, 2006a; Kirby, 2009).

It is important to recognize that the terms "biopsychosocial approach" and "functional restoration approach" may be used as synonyms for "multidisciplinary approach," reflecting the high degree of overlap of these concepts. The inclusion of cognitive-behavioral therapy (CBT) and physical rehabilitation is often inherent in the terms.

## Pharmacological Implications for Therapy

Because of the complexity of pain syndromes, numerous pharmacological agents are used in their management, including opioid analgesics, NSAIDs, and medications to treat painful muscle spasms and spasticity. These agents are usually prescribed by physicians and other primary care providers such as nurse practitioners in a stepwise fashion according to the **WHO analgesic ladder.** Indeed, pharmacological treatment constitutes a major component of overall medical management.

According to Rasmussen (2004), antidepressants and anticonvulsants are most commonly used to treat neuropathic pain. For patients with FMS, antidepressants, anticonvulsants, tramadol (Ultram), a tramadol/acetaminophen combination (Ultracet), and the muscle relaxant cyclobenzaprine (Flexeril) have been effective (Chakrabarty, 2007). For patients with painful diabetic neuropathy or postherpetic neuralgia, the combination of gabapentin (an anticonvulsant) and nortriptyline (a tricyclic antidepressant) was more efficacious with respect to pain intensity and pain-related sleep disturbance than either drug alone (Gilron, 2009).

Regardless of the pharmacological agents used, the patient, physicians, and other members of the interdisciplinary team must work closely together to ensure that the agents chosen are effective in controlling the patient's pain, that the patient tolerates the agents without objectionable side effects, and that the patient adheres to the medication regimen. Thus, it is important that the therapist regularly assesses the patient's pain and side effects and refers the patient back to the medical management team as needed.

## Psychological Interventions for Pain Syndromes

From the psychologist's perspective, comprehensive pain management should be based on three goals: (1) to help the therapist gain familiarity with the psychologist's role as part of the interdisciplinary pain management team, (2) to help the therapist appreciate the interrelatedness of physical and psychological factors in chronic pain, and (3) to teach the therapist how to reinforce the psychologist's patient/family education efforts—or personally address this area. Although occupational therapists frequently use psychological interventions in practice (Roley, 2008), this is an emerging area of practice for physical therapists. There is a small but important body of literature on the use of psychological interventions by physical therapists, which can be helpful when the patient does not have access to an occupational therapist or psychologist.

This literature is presented in the section on therapeutic techniques.

*Background.* The use of psychological interventions with chronic pain syndromes such as FMS is well established (Rossy, 1999). The rationale can be found in the gate theory of pain (Melzack, 1965), which shifted conceptualization of pain away from a purely sensory phenomenon and toward a multivariate model that assigned great importance to cognitive and affective variables. This view received further support from Engel (1977), who used the term "biopsychosocial model" (as opposed to the traditional biomedical model, which was dominant in health care up to that time) to describe the incorporation of psychosocial variables in health and illness.

Fordyce (1976) was one of the first psychologists to use behavioral principles in the treatment of people with pain. In view of the difficulty inherent in measuring pain, he proposed that psychologists concentrate on the objective, measurable concomitants of pain, which he termed "pain behaviors" or "operants." According to Fordyce, pain behaviors (e.g., verbal complaints, moaning, grimacing, exhibiting distorted gait, holding the affected area) are subject to the same environmental contingencies as other behaviors and thus can be rewarded (to increase the probability of their recurrence), ignored, or punished (to decrease the probability of their recurrence). A behavioral program that selectively reinforces wellness behavior (e.g., activity, social interaction) and discourages illness behavior may then improve QoL and decrease disability.

During the 1980s, psychologists focused more on the role of cognitive and emotional factors in the development and treatment of many clinical conditions, and pain was no exception (Holzman, 1986a; Turk, 1983). These newer approaches to pain management emphasized self-management and focused on assessment and modification of the beliefs, perceptions, emotions, and interpersonal relationships of people with pain as a critical part of rehabilitation (Gatchel, 1999). These techniques are described more fully in the next section.

## Psychological Assessment in Chronic Pain

Psychologists have devoted considerable effort to assessing the psychosocial components of chronic pain conditions. As you might expect, much of this effort has focused on determining the location, intensity, and properties of the pain experience. The McGill Pain Questionnaire (Melzack, 1975) is a frequently used assessment instrument; however, many other scales and questionnaires have been developed (Jensen, 2001).

Other self-report measures assess different aspects of chronic pain. The Sickness Impact Profile (Bergner, 1981) is a psychometrically sophisticated instrument that provides a comprehensive picture of current functioning by asking about the effects of pain on work, sleep, leisure activities, and physical mobility, among other areas, and generating corresponding impairment indices. The West Haven-Yale Multidimensional Pain Inventory (Kerns, 1985) addresses not only pain severity and impairment but also equally important dimensions such as perceived control, responses to pain from significant others, and affective distress.

The effect of emotional states on pain is well-documented (Gatchel, 2007) and is discussed more fully in the section on treatment. However, considerable attention has been devoted to assessing emotional distress either through comprehensive personality inventories such as the Minnesota Multiphasic Personality Inventory-2 (Hathaway, 1989) and Symptom Checklist-90 (DeRogatis, 1983) or through brief focused measures such as the Pain Distress Inventory (Osman, 2003), Pain Anxiety Symptoms Scale (McCracken, 1992), and Pain Catastrophizing Scale (Sullivan, 1995). Alternatively, there has been considerable interest in assessing individuals' naturally occurring attempts to cope with pain, including the Coping Strategies Questionnaire (Rosenstiel, 1983) and Pain Stages of Change Questionnaire (Kerns, 1997).

Psychophysiological assessment of chronic pain is another method used by psychologists (Flor, 1993). Given the assumed relationship between many pain syndromes and muscle spasms (Zimmerman, 1993), interest in electromyographic assessment has grown (Flor, 2001a). Investigators have focused on resting electromyographic levels, which are sometimes elevated in people with pain (Flor, 1989), stress reactivity (Turk, 1999), and abnormal movement patterns that are sometimes observed in people with pain (Cassisi, 1999).

## Psychological Interventions in Chronic Pain

CBT is the psychological treatment of choice for chronic pain syndromes including FMS (Gatchel, 2007). Bradley (1996) outlined the basic assumptions of CBT. For example, people are viewed as active processors of information; their behavior is influenced by thoughts, emotions, and physiological processes, which in turn affect behavior. As a logical consequence, for effective treatment of pain syndromes, these dimensions must be assessed, and each patient should be involved as an active participant in treatment.

Central to an understanding of the role of CBT in pain management is its emphasis upon observable behavior and function. Gatchel (1996) indicated that an emphasis on subjective pain reports or psychological disorders is not effective. To be effective, pain rehabilitation must emphasize functional restoration over pain relief. However, given the high level of demoralization, helplessness, and negative mood often observed in people with chronic pain (Turk, 1989), mobilizing and motivating them to implement positive lifestyle changes is challenging.

Bradley (1996) identified four essential components of CBT interventions for chronic pain: (1) education, (2) skills acquisition, (3) cognitive and behavioral rehearsal, and (4) generalization/maintenance. These interventions have been used successfully to treat chronic pain (Barrios, 1990) and will now be described in detail.

*Patient Education.* Although insufficient by itself, patient education is necessary for successful intervention. People with pain most likely subscribe to an outmoded biomedical model of pain (Engel, 1977), which leads them to view pain as a purely sensory event. According to this view, cognitive,

emotional, and behavioral components of pain are irrelevant, if they are considered at all. Although this model is popular with many health-care providers, it is insufficient for managing pain. It is essential to give people with pain information that is consistent with a biopsychosocial model and its treatment implications. Among these implications is the influence of moods, emotions, beliefs, and interpersonal behavior on pain and vice versa. People with pain should be exposed to basic behavioral principles (Whaley, 1971) so they are aware of the correlation between pain and psychosocial events and can perceive their pain severity as something that is not totally beyond their control. Because uncontrollable events are perceived as more stressful than controllable events (Thompson, 1981), such a revelation is likely therapeutic in itself.

During the education phase, teach patients other essential information as well, including the difference between hurt and harm, making them more likely to adhere to physical activity quota programs. Also, expose the patient to the functional restoration model (Mayer, 1988), with its emphasis on functional behavior rather than pain relief. Although pain relief may occur as activity levels increase, tell patients not to expect total pain relief after treatment. However, lead them to expect a significant improvement in mood and **QoL** as impairment decreases.

*Skill Acquisition.* *Skill acquisition* begins when the individual with pain expresses understanding of and willingness to try a functional restoration approach. For patients who are resistant to this reconceptualization, Jensen (1996) described additional motivation enhancement strategies. Cognitive and behavioral skills are equally critical for treatment success.

Among *cognitive skills,* goal setting, reconceptualization, and self-instructional training are used frequently. **Goal setting** is a collaborative process in which the patient identifies personally relevant treatment goals and the professional provides feedback about the degree to which the goals themselves, or the level at which they are likely to be performed, are realistic (Holzman, 1986b). People with pain may cling to premorbid levels of performance as their only acceptable criterion of success, although their physical limitations may make a return to baseline impossible. Failure to meet their performance expectations on a regular basis is likely to contribute to the high prevalence of depression in people with chronic pain (Gatchel, 2007).

**Reconceptualization** builds on the information provided during the education phase. Actively teach skills that are designed to counteract the most common cognitive distortions or irrational beliefs manifested by people with pain (e.g., all-or-none thinking, selective perception, catastrophizing) (Gil, 1990; Keefe, 1989). **Self-instructional training** (Meichenbaum, 1977) is based on the premise that teaching people how to engage in effective coping statements (i.e., self-talk) not only keeps them focused on the task at hand but also replaces dysfunctional self-talk (e.g., "I cannot do this"; "It is going to hurt too much.").

*Behavioral skills* taught to people with chronic pain include pacing, problem-solving, relaxation, and social training

(Barrios, 1990; Fedoravicius, 1986). **Pacing skills training** represents application of the realistic goal setting mentioned previously. Teach your patients to "work smarter, not harder" by breaking up large tasks into smaller, more manageable components. For example, instead of suggesting that patients clean the entire house or mow the entire lawn at once, teach them to complete a part of the task and take frequent breaks; when the task is sufficiently large, completing it over several days can be proposed as an option.

Problem-solving is another skill that should be taught to the patient to increase the likelihood of successfully meeting goals. Examples include modifying tasks, utilizing accommodations, mobilizing social support, and restructuring the environment in ways that allow household chores or work tasks to be accomplished without inducing a pain flare-up. **Relaxation training** (Bernstein, 1973) is a self-management strategy to reduce muscle tension, which aggravates pain, and increase patients' awareness of the importance of taking breaks rather than spending all of their time meeting others' needs and demands.

Finally, **social skills training** is a critical but often-overlooked component of CBT in chronic pain. This component includes assertion training (e.g., expressing needs clearly, refusing unreasonable requests from others), active listening (e.g., "What I hear you saying is…"), and expression of feelings (e.g., "When you do…, it makes me feel…"). Many people with chronic pain, as well as others in the general population, are deficient in these areas. Although this deficiency may not have been a major problem before the onset of the pain, many people with pain find that family, friends, and coworkers do not usually appreciate the chronic nature of their pain. Thus, unless they communicate their limitations more effectively when others expect them to resume normal activities at a premorbid level, interpersonal conflict, increased pain flare-ups, or both can result.

*Cognitive and Behavioral Rehearsal.* Once these skills have been taught, they should be regularly implemented in the person's natural environment. For this reason, *cognitive and behavioral rehearsal* is used. Homework assignments are given by the occupational therapist, psychologist, or both, and the outcome of these assignments is discussed in subsequent meetings. The purposes of these assignments include (1) enhancing the person's awareness of factors that increase or decrease pain, (2) increasing the person's ability to identify others' adaptive and maladaptive responses to his pain, (3) increasing the person's physical activity, and (4) providing reinforcement for activity that is incompatible with pain behavior (Turk, 1983).

*Maintenance of Therapeutic Gains.* The effectiveness of CBT in managing chronic pain is well documented. As with most other conditions that have a major behavioral component, however, *maintenance* of therapeutic gains is an ongoing challenge. The concept of relapse prevention was originally developed for the treatment of addictive disorders (Marlatt, 2005). The general principles, however, are easily adapted for chronic pain. In their simplest form, they identify the

abstinence violation effect, a negative emotional state that follows a lapse, as a predictor of full-blown relapse to pre-treatment behaviors. Teach patients to identify high-risk situations, develop a set of coping skills for dealing with them (e.g., modifying the environment, changing self-talk, increasing assertiveness), and engage in lifestyle rebalancing, which is the addition of other healthy life changes (e.g., diet, exercise, smoking cessation) as preventive strategies. There is evidence for the efficacy of these interventions in chronic pain (Keefe, 1993).

## Therapeutic Techniques

Now that we have seen some of the tools that are used to manage chronic pain, let us look at how they are implemented and identify areas of overlap and distinction among the roles of the occupational therapist, physical therapist, and psychologist.

### *Psychological Interventions*

Both occupational therapists and psychologists employ psychological interventions (including CBT) as a fundamental component of their practice, and they therefore work closely together. According to the OTPF, "Engagement in occupation as the focus of occupational therapy intervention involves addressing both subjective (emotional and psychological) and objective (physically observable) aspects of performance. Occupational therapy practitioners understand engagement from this dual and holistic perspective and address all aspects of performance when providing interventions" (Roley, 2008, p. 628). In an ideal scenario in which the interdisciplinary model is fully realized, the clinical psychologist introduces concepts and the occupational therapist then promotes application of this education to daily life. Psychological interventions initiated, reinforced, or both by occupational therapists include goal setting, communication and social skills, relaxation, biofeedback, energy conservation and pacing, sleep hygiene, and distraction.

Research conducted by van Huet et al. (2012) suggests that a patient's acceptance and readiness to change is crucial to successful intervention and proposes two models: agentic (active) and victimic (passive) approaches to conceptualizing chronic pain. Agentic themes included having valued roles, good social support, and acceptance and readiness for change; setting goals; pacing; relaxing; and using CBT. Victimic themes included losing valued roles, being severely depressed, receiving compensation, lacking social support, being fearful, looking for a cure, not knowing what to expect, being unable to set goals, being unable to use strategies, and using CBT to "meet a force with a force" (Huet, 2012, p. 61).

This research suggests that a patient's narrative type (i.e., agentic or victimic) may influence his acceptance and readiness to change, thereby affecting the ability to apply the education to his daily life. The occupational therapist should continue to assess a patient's narrative type throughout the intervention process. Polkinghorne (1996) asserted that occupational therapists can work toward changing a patient's narrative type from victimic to agentic with engagement in meaningful occupations while promoting transformation toward a more agentic identity.

Physical therapists can also integrate CBT into their practice, either to reinforce the work of the occupational therapist and psychologist or to address psychological variables such as cognition and behavior when the patient does not have access to an occupational therapist or psychologist. Supporting the assertion that CBT is a discipline-neutral approach, the Curriculum Outline on Pain for Occupational Therapy and Physical Therapy of the IASP ad hoc Subcommittee for Occupational Therapy/Physical Therapy Curriculum (IASP, n.d.) stated that therapists may use cognitive-behavioral strategies and supportive and educational approaches to reduce pain and improve function and quality of life.

One example of how physical therapists can incorporate CBT is the Progressive Goal Attainment Program (PGAP), a standardized psychosocial intervention program administered by rehabilitation professionals including occupational therapists and occupational health nurses (Sullivan, 2006). The PGAP was designed to promote daily involvement in goal-directed physical activity and eventual return to work by targeting three psychosocial barriers to the rehabilitation process: pain catastrophizing, fear of movement or reinjury, and perceived disability. The main components of the PGAP are (1) receiving education and reassurance, (2) maintaining an activity log, (3) developing an activity schedule, (4) participating in a walking program, (5) increasing activity involvement, and (6) overcoming psychological obstacles to activity involvement. According to one study, the addition of the PGAP to a functional restoration–based physical therapy program improved the return-to-work rate in patients with whiplash injuries (Sullivan, 2006). Although this study involved participants with a particular musculoskeletal diagnosis, the model is applicable to chronic pain in general.

Another study examined the long-term effects of physical therapy that was CBT based versus exercise based for persistent musculoskeletal pain (Åsenlöf, 2009). Patients in the CBT-based treatment group reported lower levels of pain-related disability than patients in the exercise-based treatment group at 2-year follow-up. Patients in the exercise-based treatment group also had higher levels of fear of movement and injury or reinjury than patients in the CBT-based treatment group.

Although only a minority of physical therapists use CBT techniques in managing chronic pain in older adults (Beissner, 2009), there is substantial interest in using these techniques in clinical practice. Consistent with the results of the survey conducted in this study, physical therapists can incorporate the most-often-used CBT techniques: those that are most directly related to increasing physical activity, including activity pacing and pleasurable activity scheduling. Interestingly, the most frequently reported barrier by far to the use of CBT was insufficient knowledge about CBT techniques (Beissner, 2009).

As awareness of and interest in CBT grows among physical therapists, it seems both likely and desirable that use of these techniques will increase, especially because many patients simply do not have access to interdisciplinary care.

## Functional Restoration

Consistent with the guidance of the OTPF, the *Guide,* and the IASP, major areas of the functional restoration approach include patient/family education, goal setting, and physical activity. *Patient/family education* includes the pathophysiology of chronic pain (e.g., secondary deconditioning), the pathophysiology of any underlying disease process, the overall goals of the functional restoration approach, specific goals that are both meaningful and realistic, and a prescription for physical activity, including exercise.

It is important to review the patient's medical diagnosis and offer pertinent information about concepts such as central sensitization (Burckhardt, 2005). Many patients find a thorough explanation of their pain to be therapeutic in itself, as they are reassured that their health-care providers take their concerns seriously—in essence, that their providers believe them. Moseley (2003b) found that both clinicians and patients can understand current information about the neurophysiology of pain, but that clinicians underestimate patients' ability to understand that same material. Moseley (2004a) advocated that the neurophysiology of pain be a component of patient education and found in a follow-up study that such education improved **pain cognition** and physical performance in patients with chronic LBP. Changes in pain cognition (e.g., teaching that "hurt does not equal harm") after a single educational session have been associated with immediate changes in physical performance, again in patients with chronic LBP (Moseley, 2004a, c). Among patients with FMS, fear of pain resulting from increased activity was prevalent; thus management should include education to address patient fears to reduce disability and rates of nonadherence and attrition from outcome studies (Turk, 2004).

In terms of the overall *goals* of the functional restoration approach, the patient must be taught that the initial aim may not be pain relief but improved function and that initial attempts to gradually increase physical activity may result in transient increases in pain. Therefore, it is critical that the patient learns to set realistic goals for therapy. Developing initial rapport with patients and using excellent communication skills is helpful because many patients with chronic pain have encountered obstacles to effective treatment in the health-care system.

Although there are areas of overlap and opportunities for each discipline to reinforce the work of the others (indeed, doing so is key to an interdisciplinary program), there are role distinctions as well. With respect to the role of the occupational therapist, the OTPF states that "[t]he defining contribution of occupational therapy is the application of core values, knowledge, and skills to assist clients to engage in everyday activities or occupations that they want and need to do in a manner that supports health and participation" (Roley, 2008, p. 626). The occupational therapist assesses the patient's goals as they relate to occupational performance and helps the patient set his own realistic, achievable goals to promote a more agentic identity (Polkinghorne, 1996). The occupational therapist then employs a client-centered approach to address the identified goals. Within a functional restoration approach, occupational therapy includes therapeutic exercise, education (e.g., body mechanics, energy conservation, sleep hygiene), graded functional activity (e.g., activity tolerance, graduated return to work, use of adaptive methods and equipment), environmental modifications (e.g., ergonomics, joint protection principles), and cognitive-behavioral strategies (e.g., positive reinforcement, the challenging negative cognitive distortions) (Snodgrass, 2011).

Physical therapists tend to focus on safe titration of physical activity for function, health, and fitness. In many ways, the functional restoration approach is highly compatible with the language and concepts of the *Guide:* "Physical therapy is a dynamic profession with an established theoretical and scientific base and widespread clinical applications in the restoration, maintenance, and promotion of optimal physical function" (APTA, 2015, p1). In terms of prevention and the promotion of health, wellness, and fitness in the context of disablement, treating patients with chronic pain falls under the category of tertiary prevention: "limiting the degree of disability and promoting rehabilitation and restoration of function in patients with chronic and irreversible diseases" (APTA, 2015, p1).

Physical therapists help patients (1) achieve and restore optimal functional capacity; (2) minimize impairments, functional limitations, and disabilities related to congenital and acquired conditions; (3) maintain health (thereby preventing further deterioration or future illness); and (4) create appropriate environmental adaptations to enhance independent function (APTA, 2015). People with chronic pain need intervention in the areas of fitness, including physical performance (e.g., decreased ability to tolerate strength training because of pain, limited participation in leisure sports because of pain) and health and wellness (e.g., limited information about living with pain) (APTA, 2015).

The prescription for *physical activity* including exercise is critical as many people with chronic pain resort to inactivity as a misguided attempt to manage their condition, thus contributing to a downward spiral of secondary deconditioning that in turn further limits their functional capacity. For example, compared to patients with rheumatoid arthritis, patients with FMS are similarly disabled and limited in their physical activity as measured by self-report and objective activity monitor, respectively, demonstrating measurable disability and activity limitations (Raftery, 2009). Many programs address this area of concern by first attempting to change patients' pain cognition by teaching patients axioms such as "hurt does not equal harm" and "motion is lotion." Fear of physical activity must be challenged before the patient is ready to change his or her behavior.

Next, formulate a prescription for physical activity (e.g., strengthening, stretching, and aerobic exercise) using evidence-based guidelines when they are available. For example, the APS provides recommendations for exercise in people with FMS (Burckhardt, 2005) (see Table 28-4). Individualize the

| **TABLE 28-4** | **American Pain Society Recommendations for Exercise in People With Fibromyalgia Syndrome** |
|---|---|
| **NUMBER** | **RECOMMENDATION** |
| 1. | "Encourage and support people with FMS to perform moderately intense aerobic exercise (60–75% of age-adjusted maximal heart rate [210 minus the person's age]) 2–3 times per week. In individuals who are deconditioned, this rate can be achieved with very low levels of exercise." |
| 2. | "Advise people with FMS to avoid exercise-induced pain by stretching to the point of slight resistance, not to the point of pain. This is especially important in a subgroup of individuals who have joint hypermobility." |
| 3. | "Begin exercise programs for people with FMS at a level just below their capacity, and progress in frequency, duration, or intensity as their levels of fitness and strength rise. Exercise progression should be slow and gradual, or participants will experience a marked, exercise-induced exacerbation of pain that may lead to discontinuation of the exercise program." |
| 4. | "Encourage people with FMS to perform muscle-strengthening exercise 2 times per week." |
| 5. | "Encourage ongoing exercise to maintain exercise-induced gains." |

Abbreviation: FMS = fibromyalgia syndrome.
From: Burckhardt CS, Goldenberg D, Crofford L, et al. *Guideline for the Management of Fibromyalgia Syndrome Pain in Adults and Children* [APS Clinical Practice Guidelines Series, No. 4]. Glenview, IL: American Pain Society; 2005.

prescription on the basis of the underlying disease process (e.g., MS); the patient's particular constellation of impairments and functional limitations, such as balance and gait issues (which can differ even in patients with the same medical diagnosis); and the patient's medical history (e.g., prior athletic injuries). Address other goals of education related to physical activity by teaching the patient basic body mechanics, including back safety, any activity precautions, the incorporation of adapted methods as needed, and an emphasis on pacing.

Pacing of physical activity is often included because some patients engage in a cycle of overactivity when they are feeling better, followed by inactivity because of debilitating pain, fatigue, or both from overexertion. The deconditioning of chronic inactivity contributes to this cycle; the result is that the individual functions at or near the maximal capacity for ADLs and IADLs (Harding, 1998) and is unable to participate in more demanding tasks.

### Maintenance and Relapse Management

An important component of any rehabilitation program is adherence, particularly adherence to the discharge program for maintenance and relapse prevention regarding pain. **Adherence** is the condition of an individual being empowered to act after an episode of health education (e.g., advice or a home program from a health professional, often developed with input from the patient/client) by adopting a healthy behavior. Although adherence denotes a more patient-centered approach, which is consistent with the biopsychosocial model, the term **compliance** denotes a more authoritarian approach in which an individual follows a health-care provider's advice because of her authority, consistent with the biomedical model. Adherence is a complex topic with a large body of literature. As discussed earlier, the psychologist addresses maintenance during CBT, and the therapist and psychologist should coordinate to reinforce each other's teachings directed at adherence.

Patients with chronic pain have demonstrated losses in the domains of disability and depression 1 year after participating in interdisciplinary pain management programs (Jensen, 2007). The association between psychological variables (pain beliefs, catastrophizing, and coping) and outcomes (pain and functioning) was studied in patients with chronic pain who had received multidisciplinary care, and researchers found that at 12-month follow-up patients had levels of pain similar to levels immediately after treatment. However, there was an association between the psychological variables and increased disability and depression (Jensen, 2007). These negative outcomes were associated with a dominant sense of being disabled by pain; increased catastrophizing; increased use of resting, guarding, and asking for assistance in response to pain; and decreased perceived control over pain. This work, as well as the observation that people with one type of chronic pain are vulnerable to other types (Croft, 2007), suggests the need for periodic aftercare to enhance maintenance after discharge from interdisciplinary pain management programs.

For the therapist, the adherence-enhancing behavioral strategies of constraint-induced movement therapy (CI therapy), termed the "transfer package," may be applied to patients with chronic pain. As with the therapeutic package of CI therapy, the transfer package is notable for the combination of elements and strong, repetitive emphasis that patients receive rather than the individual elements of the program. The transfer package in CI therapy consists of a behavioral contract to maximize patient buy-in, the Motor Activity Log to monitor arm use, home practice exercises, and problem-solving with a therapist to address and overcome perceived barriers to the therapeutic plan (for a complete description, see Morris [2006]). Even the use of a training diary as a stand-alone intervention for pain management has increased adherence to a home program in patients with CRPS1, with an effect magnitude of approximately 8% (Moseley, 2006a). (Interestingly, in this study Moseley also found patients tended to overestimate their adherence to a home program by approximately 10%!)

### Livengood's "Beginning at the End" Model

Livengood (2004) developed a model of patient-centered, interdisciplinary care she termed "beginning at the end" (Table 28-5). This model incorporates patient/family education, goal setting, and physical activity, but begins by the patient, medical practitioner, and other team members asking the patient to describe how life would be different with no pain or less pain. Then, each provider relates his or her discipline

| TABLE 28-5 | Livengood's "Beginning at the End" Model | | | |
|---|---|---|---|---|
| | **AWARENESS** | **AGREEMENT** | **ADOPTION** | **ADHERENCE** |
| Patient | Treatment begins with the end: Patients describe their interests and goals to practitioners. | Patients acknowledge their agreement with medical, psychological, and physical therapy regimens through verbal or written agreements. | Patients adopt and continually apply medical, psychological, and physical therapy treatment regimens. | Patients adhere to a personalized, multidisciplinary regimen to meet their goals. Motivation draws upon the value assigned to goals identified at the beginning of treatment. |
| Medical practitioner | Practitioner asks patients how their lives would be different with no pain or less pain and presents available medical treatments to help them meet their goals. | Patient and provider agree on a treatment plan (e.g., dosage and frequency for prescribed medications, exercise regimens, and medical procedures). | During follow-up, regimens and functional goals are modified and titrated. Invasive procedures and implantable devices may be considered. | Patients adhere to the treatment strategy, do not take shortcuts or easy paths that favor short-term goals at the expense of long-term benefits, and communicate with the psychologist, occupational therapist, and physical therapist. |

| **TABLE 28-5** | **Livengood's "Beginning at the End" Model—cont'd** | | | |
|---|---|---|---|---|
| | **AWARENESS** | **AGREEMENT** | **ADOPTION** | **ADHERENCE** |
| Psychologist | Psychologist asks patients how their lives would be different with no pain or less pain and educates patients about psychological interventions (e.g., behavioral, cognitive-behavioral therapy) relevant to their goal. | Patient and psychologist jointly select types of therapy that will help the patient meet his goal (e.g., behavioral therapy, cognitive-behavioral therapy, biofeedback, sleep education). | The patient adopts changes in behavior and thought processes through daily use of behavioral and cognitive-behavioral skills. On subsequent visits, additional skills are taught until the patient incorporates them into daily life. | Patient's desired goal is kept in mind at each session. Adheres to chronic pain intervention, resisting the temptation to provide therapy for ancillary issues (e.g., divorce counseling). When appropriate, the patient is referred for marital therapy, etc. Communication with other team members is maintained. |
| Occupational therapist | Therapist asks patients how their lives would be different with no pain or less pain, works with patients to identify occupational performance problem areas, and educates patients on the role of the occupational therapist and interventions relevant to these areas. | Patient and occupational therapist jointly construct achievable, measurable goals as realistic steps toward broader overarching goals and select types of interventions that will help the patient meet his goals (e.g., energy conservation, sleep hygiene, relaxation techniques, body mechanics). | Patient adopts changes in behavior and body mechanics through daily use of activity analysis and task modification, using skills taught by the occupational therapist. On subsequent visits, the occupational therapist assists the patient in progressing toward goals, promoting increased awareness and understanding of gradation of activity within the patient's habits, roles, and routines. | The therapist encourages the patient to continue to establish achievable and measurable goals, progressing toward broader overarching goals. Patients adhere to chronic pain intervention, promoting increased participation in daily activity. Therapist communicates with team members regarding patient's progress and continued goal setting. |
| Physical therapist | Therapist asks patients how their lives would be different with no pain or less pain, instructs patients on range-of-motion and strengthening exercises that build strength and endurance needed to meet and maintain goals, and may alert patients to movements that impede progress or worsen pain. | Patient and therapist agree on a physical therapy regimen. The therapist emphasizes the rationale for exercises to reach specific goals. Agreement is made (e.g., on the number of repetitions per set and number of sets per day). Agreement is also reached regarding appropriate action if exercises or increased activity contributes to increased pain. | Patients incorporate physical therapy into their daily activity. On subsequent visits, the therapist introduces additional exercises that the patient adopts into his daily life. The patient is then discharged to an independent home program. | The therapist encourages the patient to reach goals despite possible temporary increases in pain and updates other providers as to patient's progress. |

From: Livengood, JM. Pain education: Molding the trainee-patient dialogue. *Pain: Clin Updates.* 2004;XII(3):1–4. Adapted and used with permission from the International Association for the Study of Pain.

to the patient's goals. You could incorporate this model into your practice setting by drawing out the patient's perspective of his or her final goal and then relate your plan of care to the patient's carefully designed goals. This model is a useful way to conceptualize treatment progression through stages Livengood termed (1) "awareness," (2) "agreement," (3) "adoption," and (4) "adherence" while broadly delineating roles within the treatment team.

### Broadening the Interdisciplinary Team

In keeping with the interdisciplinary approach, it is essential to communicate and coordinate with other members of the health-care team (e.g., regarding the effectiveness of the patient's current pain medication regimen and the patient's progress across other domains) and consider the need for referrals as appropriate, including referrals to facilitate psychosocial support (WHO, 2006) and for complementary and alternative medicine. In fact, the APS recommends the provider actively ask the patient with FMS about complementary and alternative medicine and facilitate other types of clinician-assisted treatments for pain relief (Burckhardt, 2005).

### Equipment

Equipment applicable to chronic pain can be divided into several categories. Obviously, some equipment is necessary for conducting interventions targeted at improving pain and function (e.g., the mirror box for Moseley's graded motor imagery, described later in this chapter). Some patients may benefit from the use of equipment for task modification (e.g., ergonomic considerations, energy conservation); this includes reachers, jar openers, dressing aids, and sock aids to avoid portions of the range that are more painful or to avoid painful force production. Finally, a patient may also require equipment (e.g., orthotics, assistive devices for ambulation) to address other impairments resulting from a primary condition such as stroke.

### Electrophysical Agents

*Interventions for administration of electrical or physical energy* may also be employed. One of the most prominent is **transcutaneous electrical nerve stimulation (TENS)**, the administration of electrical current produced by an electronic device to stimulate the nerves for a therapeutic effect. It is important to consider agents such as TENS because of their widespread use. TENS is an easy-to-use analgesic modality, but its effectiveness in the treatment of chronic pain is inconclusive. Early reports suggested TENS helped some patients with peripheral neuropathic pain but was of limited benefit in patients with central neuropathic pain (Hansson, 1994). Evidence is insufficient to draw any conclusions about its effectiveness for treating chronic pain in adults (Carroll, 2000). For example, in a review of the effectiveness of TENS as an isolated modality for treating chronic LBP, Khadilkar (2005) found only two randomized controlled trials that met the eligibility criteria for the review, and their results were conflicting. Of note, the authors did not review the use of TENS as part of a multidisciplinary approach.

A recent meta-analysis of electrical nerve stimulation (both transcutaneous and percutaneous) for treating chronic musculoskeletal pain found it was effective and that previous inconclusive results may have been due to studies with inadequate statistical power (Johnson, 2007). However, a prospective, randomized, placebo-controlled trial comparing high-frequency TENS with sham TENS in patients with chronic pain found no differences in effects on pain intensity (Oosterhof, 2008). A review of PLP treatment in older adults recommended a trial of TENS for each patient on the basis of a small number of studies that used the device on the residual limb, the contralateral limb, and the ear (Baron, 1998). In summary, although TENs may provide some benefits, definitive evidence regarding its use in patients with chronic pain remains elusive.

### Disease-specific Considerations

Although functional restoration represents a useful general approach to the management of chronic pain, there are numerous neurologic conditions with disease-specific considerations. A discussion of all of them is beyond the scope of this chapter; however, we give examples for stroke, CRPS, and PLP. As we will see, these three medical diagnoses share common neurophysiological mechanisms that indicate exciting new directions in treatment and are supported by emerging research.

#### Stroke

Causes of poststroke discomfort include joint pain from spasticity, immobility, muscle weakness, headache, centrally mediated pain, and shoulder pain. Pain assessment in this population should include use of the 0 to 10 scale and determination of likely etiology (i.e., musculoskeletal or neuropathic); location; quality, quantity, duration, and intensity; and aggravating and relieving factors. Lower doses of centrally acting analgesics are recommended to decrease the risk of undesirable cognitive side effects (Duncan, 2005).

PSSP is common. Although estimates of the incidence vary, it is thought to affect approximately 70% of patients with stroke (Bender, 2001; Bohannon, 1986; Van Ouwenaller, 1986) and is associated with reduced QoL (Chae, 2007). The many underlying causes include adhesive capsulitis (which occurs in approximately 5% to 8% of people with stroke; WHO, 2006), traction/compression neuropathy, CRPS1, shoulder trauma, bursitis/tendonitis, rotator cuff tear, and heterotrophic ossification (Duncan, 2005). Other authors have postulated that sources of shoulder pain include associated muscles as well as altered sensitivity (Bender, 2001). The possible contribution of glenohumeral subluxation to PSSP remains controversial (Bender, 2001; Duncan, 2005).

CRPS1, also called *shoulder-hand syndrome* in patients with stroke, is a secondary complication of cerebral damage. Estimates of the incidence of shoulder-hand syndrome vary widely, reflecting both the lack of uniform diagnostic criteria and the symptom overlap with hemiplegia in patients who do not have shoulder-hand syndrome (Pertoldi, 2005). A reported frequency of shoulder-hand syndrome of 27% (with major risk factors of subluxation, paresis of the shoulder girdle, moderate spasticity, and deficits in confrontation visual field testing indicating hemianopsia, visual neglect, or both) was reduced to 8% with early education of patients, family, and staff aimed at decreasing shoulder trauma; this suggests that shoulder-hand syndrome is largely preventable by avoiding trauma to the affected shoulder (Braus, 1994). (See the next section on CRPS.)

PSSP can impede recovery through two mechanisms: The painful joint limits the person's ability to use the affected upper extremity (e.g., with an assistive device for ambulation, for completing daily self-care tasks) and may also mask improvement in motor function (Duncan, 2005). The American Heart Association has endorsed the following recommendations for addressing PSSP (Duncan, 2005):

1. Prevention
   - Surface electrical stimulation to improve the external rotation passive range of motion of the shoulder, possibly due to decreased glenohumeral subluxation (Price, 2000)
   - Shoulder strapping
   - Staff education to prevent trauma to the hemiplegic shoulder
2. Avoidance of the use of overhead pulleys, which encourage uncontrolled abduction and are strongly associated with the development of PSSP (Kumar, 1990)
3. Treatment
   - Steroid injections/medication: Intra-articular injections of triamcinolone have significantly affected pain (Dekker, 1997).
   - Shoulder strapping: Strapping may delay the onset of acute PSSP (Ancliffe, 1992), although a larger study (Hanger, 2000) found no significant reduction in pain while noting a trend toward less pain in 6 weeks.
   - Improved range of motion through stretching and mobilization techniques focusing on external rotation and abduction to prevent adhesive capsulitis and shoulder-hand syndrome: Bohannon (1986) found that of five variables—patient age, time since onset of hemiplegia, external rotation range of motion of the shoulder, spasticity, and weakness—external rotation range of motion related most significantly to the occurrence of PSSP.
   - Modalities including ice, heat, soft tissue massage, and mobilization: These modalities are commonly used, though no evidence supports their efficacy in PSSP.
   - Functional electrical stimulation
   - Strengthening
   - Shoulder positioning protocols: These were not shown to reduce PSSP (Dean, 2000); however, as noted previously, protecting the affected upper extremity from trauma has reduced the frequency of shoulder-hand syndrome.

It is important to note that not all of these American Heart Association–endorsed practice guidelines for adults with stroke are supported by evidence, reflecting the limitations of the existing literature.

Bender (2001) provided general recommendations for addressing PSSP that include maintaining joint alignment and integrity and preventing shortening or lengthening of surrounding soft tissues. The following recommendations are included:

- Appropriate positioning into abduction, external rotation, and flexion to prevent excessive internal rotation and adduction, both when seated using an external support for the affected upper extremity (a trough attached to the chair armrest) and through careful positioning in bed (using pillows)
- Daily static position stretches (as described by Dean [2000])
- Motor retraining
- Strapping of the scapula to maintain postural tone and symmetry
- Avoidance of shoulder slings because of a lack of evidence that they are effective in reducing subluxation

Bender (2001) concluded that the application of functional electrical stimulation in motor retraining requires more evidence.

Ada (2005) found insufficient evidence on whether slings and wheelchair attachments prevent subluxation or decrease PSSP, although there is evidence that shoulder strapping delays the onset—but not the severity—of pain. Interestingly, neither Duncan (2005) nor Bender (2001) recommended the use of TENS in the treatment of PSSP. Price (2000) concluded there was insufficient evidence to either recommend or discourage routine use of TENS in PSSP.

## Complex Regional Pain Syndrome

CRPS is a potentially devastating chronic pain condition affecting a lower or upper limb. CRPS is a set of disorders involving the nervous system, including the autonomic nervous system (WHO, 2006). Although the etiology is still unclear, this condition, is often—but not always—preceded by a peripheral trauma such as a nerve injury or a central event such as a stroke or spinal cord injury which can render the limb exquisitely painful, leading to a vicious cycle of guarding and immobility (Echternach, 1996). This, in turn, may contribute to long-term changes that are characteristic of the condition, including muscle atrophy, osteoporosis, and joint contractures. Less commonly, there may not be a known cause (Pertoldi, 2005).

There is ongoing debate and lack of agreement as to terminology and diagnostic criteria for CRPS, leading to difficulty discussing the condition in the literature and hampering research efforts (Harden, 2007). However, the IASP has defined two types: CRPS1 and CRPS type 2 (CRPS2). The IASP introduced these terms in 1994, replacing the terms **reflex sympathetic dystrophy** and **causalgia,** respectively. CRPS1 develops after a minor injury to or fracture of the involved limb. In CRPS2, the trigger is damage to a peripheral nerve. In CRPS1, there is no known nerve damage, so the development of the condition is unexpected. In both types, there is an exaggerated physiological response, such that the severity and duration of the symptoms are greater than typically expected given the nature of the initial injury.

Signs and symptoms in the affected limb include **spontaneous pain** (pain that is stimulus-independent), *allodynia* (pain due to stimuli that are not normally painful), and *hyperalgesia* (a heightened pain response to stimuli that are normally painful); motor dysfunction; autonomic changes (e.g., edema, vasomotor dysfunction, sudomotor dysfunction); and later trophic changes (i.e., changes in the nutrition, health, and appearance of the tissues of the affected limb).

CRPS is typically a chronic, intractable condition, and it is associated with significant psychological and psychiatric involvement (WHO, 2006) as affected individuals grapple with an excruciatingly painful extremity that ultimately becomes essentially nonfunctional (Echternach, 1996). Early diagnosis and treatment is therefore thought to be crucial.

Management of CRPS includes a variety of medical interventions such as pharmacological treatments, regional anesthesia techniques (e.g., sympathetic blocks, somatic blocks), neuromodulation (e.g., spinal cord stimulation, intrathecal analgesia), and sympathectomy, as well as conservative treatments including occupational therapy, physical therapy, and psychotherapy in a multidisciplinary approach (Pertoldi, 2005). The traditional approach in occupational therapy and physical therapy is one of functional restoration and includes systematic desensitization and progressive physical activity involving the affected limb. This progressive physical activity is a stress-loading program that includes scrubbing and carrying activities to promote weight-bearing on the involved upper extremity (Harden, 2006a, 2006b).

When shoulder-hand syndrome is considered, it is easy to see why the emphasis is on prevention: Patients who have experienced a stroke may have limited ability to participate in movement-based therapy. However, many authors (Daly, 2009; Pertoldi, 2005) note a dearth of evidence to support traditional management of CRPS. In fact, in a systematic review of physical therapy management of the syndrome, Daly (2009) concluded there was no evidence to support the traditional approach (i.e., stress loading) still recommended in clinical guidelines (e.g., Harden, 2006a). However, there was evidence (good to very good quality level II evidence, meaning the evidence comes from at least one well-designed randomized controlled trial) to support a new approach called *graded motor imagery*, described in a following section.

### Phantom Limb Pain

Although clinically challenging, treatment of PLP provides the fascinating opportunity to apply the latest research and expert opinion on neuroplasticity to the treatment of chronic pain. A review article (Halbert, 2002) concluded there was little high-quality evidence to guide clinical treatment of PLP in either the acute or chronic phase, particularly for conservative interventions within the scope of practice for therapists. The article cites Katz (1991), suggesting that auricular TENS reduces PLP, but a trial examining peripherally applied TENS (Lundeberg, 1985) was inconclusive because of the large dropout rate. Similarly, a review by Flor (2002) noted a limited role for therapists in the management of PLP, finding evidence to support primarily pharmacological treatment.

However, Flor did identify emerging evidence supporting the use of sensory discrimination training and mirror therapy—modalities that have been researched further since this review was published.

### New Directions

G. Lorimer Moseley, a leading researcher in novel treatment approaches consistent with the pain neuromatrix theory, has helped delineate a profile of characteristics that accompany chronic pain, including body image distortions, decreased limb laterality recognition, and decreased tactile acuity. For example, Moseley (2005a) found that people with CRPS perceive the affected limb to be of larger size than it actually is. Also, as reviewed by Moseley (2009), people with CRPS often present with findings characteristic of hemispatial neglect, including difficulty identifying a pictured limb as a left limb or a right limb when the pictured limb corresponds to the individual's affected side. These associated characteristics implicate the central mechanisms underlying chronic pain.

In a watershed paper, Moseley and colleagues (Acerra, 2007) proposed that although stroke, CRPS1, and PLP are distinct conditions, they share common central mechanisms and thus may respond to common interventions, including mirror therapy and motor imagery, CI therapy, and sensory discrimination training. Although these three conditions originate from different mechanisms (cortical damage, peripheral trauma, and deafferentation, respectively), their clinical presentations are similar, and they lead to common patterns of cortical reorganization whereby cortical representation of the affected limb in the primary somatosensory cortex is diminished. This loss of cortical representation is correlated with the presence and degree of pain in CRPS1 and PLP. Interventions aimed at countering this loss of cortical representation by inducing positive neuroplastic changes may therefore decrease pain in all three conditions, possibly by providing the types and amount of input needed to influence cortical representation (Acerra, 2007).

Emerging evidence supports all three types of interventions in the treatment of chronic pain (Acerra, 2007), and CI therapy is already well established in the treatment of hemiparesis (Morris, 2006). Although more research is needed to strengthen the available evidence and provide more specific treatment protocols, this trend toward a mechanisms-based treatment approach (as opposed to approaches aimed at peripheral symptoms) in the literature is an exciting advancement in the evidence-based treatment of chronic pain. Furthermore, it defines an important role for therapists, as these approaches are within their respective scope of practice.

As described by Acerra (2007), mirror therapy consists of bilateral limb movements. During these movements, the affected limb is hidden with an interposed mirror facing the unaffected limb so the patient views only the unaffected limb and its mirror image (which appears as if it is the affected limb). Mirror therapy is a component of graded motor imagery (www.gradedmotorimagery.com) that has been successfully used to treat people with CRPS1, resulting in decreased pain and disability and increased function (Moseley, 2004b, 2005b,

2006b). Graded motor imagery involves three procedures applied in sequence (i.e., the proper order of the procedures is needed) for 2 weeks each: (1) recognition of limb laterality (i.e., identifying a limb as being a left limb or a right limb); (2) imagined limb movements; and (3) mirror movements.

In Moseley's (2004b, 2005b, 2006b) protocol, limb laterality training was performed by presenting pictures of hands on a monitor before a seated patient and having the patient identify the hand as being a left hand or a right hand by pressing a button as quickly as possible. Thus, emphasis was on both accuracy and speed. Patients used a notebook computer and were instructed to perform the task (consisting of 56 pictures) three times each waking hour for a total of approximately 10 minutes of training per hour. For imagined hand movement training, 28 pictures of hands ipsilateral to the patient's affected hand were presented to the patient, who was instructed three times to actively imagine moving his own hand to adopt the position shown in the picture. The emphasis for this task was on accuracy, not speed. Patients were instructed to perform the task three times each waking hour for a total of approximately 15 minutes of training per hour.

Finally, for mirror movements training, patients placed both hands into a cardboard mirror box consisting of two compartments (300 x 300 x 300 mm each) separated by a vertical mirror. The equipment was arranged so that the affected hand was concealed behind the mirror; emphasis was placed on the patient watching the reflection of the unaffected hand in the mirror while moving both hands to match the position of paper copies of pictures of hands modeling less-complex movements. Unlike the imagined hand movements training, the pictures in the mirror movements training were contralateral to the patient's affected hand. Patients were instructed to perform the task slowly and smoothly with both hands five to 10 times each waking hour for a total of approximately 10 minutes of training per hour. Patients were instructed to stop if they experienced increased pain either during or immediately after the movements. After the intervention, the patients experienced decreased pain (by approximately 20 points on the Neuropathic Pain Scale) and swelling that were maintained for at least 6 weeks, and 50% of patients no longer met diagnostic criteria for CRPS1 at 6 weeks (Moseley, 2004b).

At least two systematic reviews (Cossins, 2013; Daly, 2008) have found strong evidence (based on a small number of randomized controlled trials) for the efficacy of graded motor imagery in the treatment of CRPS. Although there is emerging evidence for graded motor imagery, the mechanisms underlying its effectiveness are still being elucidated. Moseley speculated that because the treatment effect depended on the order of training, the underlying mechanism was sequential activation of cortical sensory and motor networks to overcome the altered cortical representation of the affected body part (Acerra, 2007). Mirror therapy increases excitability of the ipsilateral primary motor cortex, and researchers have postulated that mirror neurons play a role in the effectiveness of motor imagery (Acerra, 2007). For a review of mirror therapy that includes the work of other researchers, see Moseley (2008a) and Ramachandran (2005).

Noting that high-dose repetitive practice leads to documented increases in cortical representation and sensory and motor performance in healthy participants as well as people with stroke, Moseley recommended the use of CI therapy in patients with CRPS1 because the disorder is associated with generalized disuse, similar to stroke (Acerra, 2007).

Citing an important study in patients with PLP, (Flor, 2001b) also recommended the use of sensory discrimination training for the treatment of chronic pain in stroke, CRPS1, and PLP because chronic pain is often associated with decreased tactile acuity. Sensory discrimination training entails discriminating the type and location of stimuli applied to the skin. In the Flor (2001) study, patients with chronic PLP participated in 90-minute sessions daily for 10 days over a period of 2 weeks during which they received short-duration, high-frequency, nonpainful electrical stimulation to the residual limb and were instructed to discriminate the frequency or location of each stimulus. Patients demonstrated reduced PLP intensity (by approximately 60%), normalized organization of the primary somatosensory cortex, and correlations between both of these findings and improved sensory discrimination ability as evidenced by better two-point discrimination thresholds (Flor, 2001).

Similarly, Moseley (2008b) found that tactile discrimination, but not tactile stimulation alone, reduced chronic pain and the two-point discrimination threshold in people with CRPS1. In this study, it was not enough that participants merely receive tactile stimulation (i.e., as a passive modality); to improve, they needed to actively attend to the stimulation by attempting to discriminate the type (specifically, the diameter) and location of tactile stimuli. This finding is consistent with contemporary neuroscience literature on the critical elements needed for the acquisition of skilled movement, including active participation and information processing. **Active participation** refers to the fact that the participant actively attends to and participates in the activity—not that he is a passive recipient. **Information processing** specifies that the participant have sufficient cognitive ability to use available information for problem-solving. For an excellent review, see Callahan (2006).

Moseley (2008b) also cited evidence that attention to tactile input or a behavioral objective that is associated with the input was critical for reorganization of the primary somatosensory cortex and that such attention improved tactile performance.

Moseley's (2008b) protocol involved the use of two cork probes of different diameters (2 and 11 mm) that were each mounted atop a spring-loaded cartridge to allow standardization of the pressure applied to participants' skin. (For the home program, participants were given a wine cork and pen lid to use instead of the cork probes.) A digital photograph was taken of the participant's hand, and this photograph was placed in the participant's view while his affected hand was kept hidden behind a screen. The photograph was marked at five locations that were spaced on the basis of the results of prior two-point discrimination testing using a caliper. Stimulation was applied with randomization of both the probe diameter and the location, and the participant responded by identifying the location using the photograph and the probe diameter. Stimuli were applied every 15 seconds for three 6-minute sets of 24 stimuli, with a 3-minute rest period between sets for a total of 72 stimuli in 24 minutes. This procedure was repeated each weekday for 11 to 17 days and was randomly allocated for each participant; participants were also instructed to perform one home session daily with the aid of a caregiver who was trained by the clinic staff. Two-point discrimination testing was performed every other clinic day to allow adjustment of the tactile stimulation locations as needed as the participants' two-point discrimination improved.

This protocol (Moseley, 2008b) yielded improvements in pain, as measured by a VAS, and in the two-point discrimination threshold, as measured in millimeters using a caliper, as well as in function, as measured by a task-specific NRS. The mean (95% confidence interval) effect size for pain as measured by the VAS was 27 mm, and for two-point discrimination, it was 5.7 mm; of critical importance, these gains were maintained at 3-month follow-up testing.

In summary, the interventions espoused by Moseley and colleagues are both effective and practical, and graded motor imagery is potentially applicable to multiple patient populations. As you can see, although these interventions are based on mounting research evidence, they are quite different from the traditional stress-loading (i.e., scrubbing-and-carrying) approach used for the treatment of CRPS1. As health care continues to move toward evidence-based practice, clinicians will be increasingly called upon to justify the intervention approaches they choose.

On the other hand, in many ways, the evidence base is still a work in progress (as always) and has limitations. For instance, there is limited evidence to guide the management of multilimb CRPS (e.g., when an individual has CRPS affecting both upper extremities), and at least one report suggests it may be difficult to translate Moseley's complex graded motor imagery research protocol into clinical practice (Johnson, 2012). (Note: Since the Johnson study was published, Moseley (2012a) published a resource for clinical implementation, *The Graded Motor Imagery Handbook.*)

Interestingly, Moseley's work involves a large treatment dose (e.g., performing graded motor imagery training tasks every waking hour, performing sensory discrimination training tasks both in the clinic and at home daily), similar to CI therapy and consistent with the neuroscience literature on the large amount of task practice needed to induce neuroplastic changes. As with graded motor imagery, there appears to be potential for application of CI therapy to a growing pool of patient populations, including those with chronic pain. Moseley and colleagues (Acerra, 2007) proposed that CI therapy could be effective in CRPS1, and one might speculate that CI therapy might be applied after graded motor imagery for optimal effect. For further review of novel therapies targeting cortical representations in the treatment of chronic pain, see Moseley (2012b) and Pollard (2013).

For a personal account of living with CRPS, see the website for the National Center on Health, Physical Activity, and Disability: www.ncpad.org/176/1321/Complex-Regional-Pain-Syndrome--Beating-the-Unbeatable.

# ■ Intervention: Ultimately Applied in Functional Activities

## Functional Treatment

As we have seen, the goal of functional restoration and other approaches is to improve function in a variety of ways. Functional restoration must include overcoming deconditioning to improve functional exercise capacity, improving ability to perform ADLs, and returning to work or meaningful activities/participation. A progressive increase in the quantity of functional activity is an essential component of the intervention for pain. The aquatic environment can also be a great place to practice functional activities for this population (Assis, 2006) because the water provides a very gentle and broadly consistent tactile pressure over the affected body segment, along with gentle resistance to functional movements. Educating patients to set realistic, functional goals; to pace their physical activity; and to increase their physical activity is a central concept in the functional restoration approach. All of the functional treatment activities described in Chapters 33 to 37 are appropriate as the intervention plan of care for pain progresses.

## Pediatric Considerations

The APS's (2012) position statement "Assessment and Management of Children with Chronic Pain" echoes the call for a multidisciplinary approach for complex or refractory chronic pain, especially for pediatric patients, who should be referred to pediatric pain programs when possible. It also calls for increased research into pain specifically in children, noting that in the absence of such research, findings in adults are often applied to children. In an excellent review article on chronic pain in children, Clinch (2009) noted some well-validated assessment instruments designed for use in children as well as instruments to measure the effect of the child's pain on his parents/caregivers. For an excellent resource list for pain in children, see Finley (2005). Interestingly, a report on the management of CRPS in pediatric patients (Wilder, 2006) stated that physical therapy is the treatment of choice for this patient population, referencing work by Sherry (1999) that demonstrated high cure rates with intensive physical therapy (up to 6 hours per day) as the sole intervention.

**PATIENT APPLICATION**

Mary P. is a 12 year-old female who is referred for outpatient therapy with a medical diagnosis of CRPS1 of the left lower extremity. During the initial examination and evaluation, her parents report the onset of pain after a minor injury to her left lower extremity approximately 2 months ago. The pain has progressed to the point that Mary uses crutches for ambulation and is having *difficulty with functional mobility at school (particularly making class changes on time). She reports decreased tolerance to warm environments and lately can tolerate wearing only shorts rather than long pants. She presents with signs of allodynia and autonomic dysfunction in the affected extremity.*

### Contemplate Clinical Decisions

- *How does this patient's initial clinical presentation relate to the International Classification of Functioning, Disability, and Health model?*
- *Based on the available evidence, what treatment approach would you choose for this patient?*
- *What is the ideal treatment setting for this patient?*
- *What if the family lived in a rural setting and did not have access to such a program?*
- *Assuming you are working in a general outpatient setting, what resources are needed to provide this patient with appropriate care?*
- *What referrals would you consider making for this patient?*
- *From this brief introduction to the patient, what information would you want to obtain during the examination, and how would you decide which assessment instruments to use?*
- *Other than physical function, which domains might you consider during the examination?*

## ■ Intervention: Considerations for Nontherapy Time and Discharge

As we have seen, a home program is a critical component of the functional restoration approach; this includes use of a physical activity chart or diary for helping patients meet their goals for physical activity while learning how to pace their physical activity appropriately. Patient education is another critical component and may be reinforced with written materials and referrals for support groups and Internet-based resources. Discharge planning should emphasize long-term management, including relapse management, with the therapist preparing the patient for the possibility of future pain flare-ups due to occasional overactivity or other causes while prospectively problem-solving how to cope with such relapses. These relapses should be seen as occasional temporary setbacks rather than catastrophic indicators that the pain management plan has failed (Harding, 1998).

## Aspects of Patient and Family Education

As previously described, interdisciplinary patient and family education is foundational to the functional restoration approach; this includes information about the pathophysiology of chronic pain and any underlying disease processes, the deleterious effects of secondary deconditioning, the need to set realistic goals for chronic pain management with a focus on improving function rather than eliminating pain, the need to set realistic targets for physical activity, the need to learn and practice appropriate coping strategies (both for self-management and the management of social relationships), and the need to learn skills for relapse management. Patient buy-in and active participation in the pain management program are indispensable.

## Activities for Home

Although the therapist's treatment plan may incorporate home- or community-based exercise, the larger picture is the return to optimal physical function both in the home (e.g., ADLs) and in the community (e.g., participation in social events, participation in leisure events, and return to work/play). Thus, engagement in physical activity and meaningful occupations at home is arguably the major focus of the functional restoration approach.

## HANDS-ON PRACTICE

Here are some important skills in the therapeutic management of chronic pain:
- Administering and interpreting tests and measures across many domains, including pain, physical function (including balance), social function, sleep, and cognitive factors
- Providing patient and family education
- Designing a structured program of lifestyle changes and helping the patient overcome barriers to implementing it
- Using cognitive-behavioral therapy
- Prescribing physical activity, including exercise
- Using particular modalities, including electrophysical agents
- Using particular approaches, such as graded motor imagery, constraint-induced therapy, and tactile discrimination training
- Implementing interdisciplinary communication and coordination

## Let's Review

1. How is pain classified? How is chronic pain different from acute pain?

2. Why does the management of chronic pain necessitate an interdisciplinary approach?

3. What types of providers comprise this interdisciplinary team, and what does each type of provider contribute?

4. What tests and measures are useful in this patient population? Why?

5. What is the functional restoration approach, and how can it be modified to address disease-specific considerations?

6. What is the evidence basis for traditional management of complex regional pain syndrome?

7. What is the evidence basis for graded motor imagery, constraint-induced therapy, and other novel therapies?

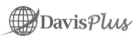 For additional resources, including Focus on Evidence tables, case study discussions, references and glossary, please visit http://davisplus.fadavis.com

## CHAPTER SUMMARY

Chronic pain by itself can be considered a disease because, by definition, it persists after the expected time frame for completion of tissue healing and thus serves no identifiable biological purpose. Chronic pain can result from inadequately treated acute pain due to changes in central nervous system function, or it can be a feature of neurological disease. However it begins, chronic pain becomes a negative spiral that radically changes all domains of a person's life.

As we have seen, much of the therapist's management of chronic pain hinges on conceptual bases for practice, with the functional restoration approach being a useful model in neurology. The focus is therefore on the therapist's contributions to a functional restoration program, with the realization that people with chronic pain present with a wide variety of activity limitations and participation restrictions, necessitating a highly individualized approach. As part of this individualized approach, the examination and evaluation should encompass an array of tests and measures across a number of domains, including not only pain but also physical function (including balance), social function, sleep, and cognitive variables.

For intervention, the therapist must be proficient in designing a structured program of lifestyle changes and helping the patient overcome barriers to implementing it, necessitating skills in psychological interventions including CBT, prescription of physical activity including exercise, and health education (see Chapter 16). When appropriate, the therapist should also use particular modalities, including electrophysical agents,

and particular approaches, such as graded motor imagery, CI therapy, and tactile discrimination training. Skills in patient and family education are critical, as is interdisciplinary communication and coordination.

A recent report (Feigin, 2013) found that the global burden of stroke is increasing, highlighting the urgent need for more research on chronic pain of neurological origin and more education and training for health-care providers who serve patients with chronic pain (WHO, 2006). This research, education, and training should emphasize intervention strategies and approaches that enhance neural plasticity to promote restoration of more normal cortical representation. Indeed, the management of chronic pain is an area of health care with room for tremendous improvement because patients/clients often do not receive interdisciplinary care, and evidence to support some traditional treatment approaches is lacking. However, there is currently an explosion of research in this area, signaling both new hope and new challenges for the future as emerging evidence becomes available for translation into widespread clinical practice.

In an editorial on Moseley's (2006b) study on graded motor imagery for chronic pain, Birklein (2006) stated that "[t]he Moseley study opens the door for a new era of physiotherapy of chronic pain." Taken as a whole, the work of this pioneering physiotherapist and prolific researcher promises to give therapists effective new tools that are evidence based, marking an exciting advance in the conservative management of chronic pain in neurology.

## ■ Acknowledgments

The authors gratefully acknowledge Meghan Miyamoto, PT, DPT, and Kathi Tomsky, FNP, MSN, MHS, for their review of the manuscript.

## RESOURCES

### Professional Associations

- American Pain Society (APS) (http://americanpainsociety.org)
  - American Pain Society Ethical Principles for Pain-Related Clinical Practice
- International Association for the Study of Pain (IASP) (www.iasp-pain.org)
  - Clinical updates available under "Publications" tab
  - Special Interest Group on Neuropathic Pain (www.neupsig.org)
- National Fibromyalgia Association (www.fmaware.org)
- Pain Management Special Interest Group, Orthopaedic Section, American Physical Therapy Association (www.orthopt.org)
- Reflex Sympathetic Dystrophy Syndrome Association (www.rsds.org)

### Websites

- National Center on Health, Physical Activity, and Disability (www.ncpad.org)
- Neuro Orthopaedic Institute (www.noigroup.com and www.gradedmotorimagery.com)

### Journals

- *J Pain* (American Pain Society)
- *Pain* (International Association for the Study of Pain)
- *Pain Med* (American Academy of Pain Medicine)

### Texts

- Gatchel RJ, Turk DC. *Psychosocial Factors in Pain: Critical Perspectives.* New York, NY: Guilford Press; 1999.

- Loeser JD, Butler SH, Chapman CR, Turk DC. *Bonica's Management of Pain,* 3rd edition. Philadelphia, PA: Lippincott Williams & Wilkins; 2001.
- Thorn BE. *Cognitive Therapy for Chronic Pain: A Step-by-Step Guide.* New York, NY: Guilford Press; 2004.
- Turk DC, Gatchel RJ. *Psychological Approaches to Pain Management: A Practitioner's Handbook,* 2nd edition. New York, NY: Guilford Press; 2002.
- Turk DC, Melzack R. *Handbook of Pain Assessment,* 2nd edition. New York, NY: Guilford Press; 2001.
- Wittink H, Hoskins Michel T. *Chronic Pain Management for Physical Therapists,* 2nd edition. Boston, MA: Butterworth Heinemann; 2002.

### Other Print Resources

- Butler DS, Moseley GL. *Explain Pain,* 2nd edition. Adelaide, Australia: Noigroup Publications; 2013.
- Moseley GL. *Painful Yarns: Metaphors & Stories to Help Understand the Biology of Pain,* 2nd edition. Minneapolis, MN: OPTP; 2011.
- Moseley GL, Butler DS, Beames TB, Giles TJ. *The Graded Motor Imagery Handbook.* Adelaide, Australia: Noigroup Publications; 2012.
- World Health Organization. Neurologic disorders: A public health approach. In: *Neurologic Disorders: Public Health Challenges.* Geneva, Switzerland: WHO Press; 2006. Available at: http://www.who.int/mental_health/neurology/neurodiso/en/index.html. Accessed October 17, 2013.

# Intervention for Vestibular Impairment

Denise Gobert, PT, MEd, PhD, NCS, CEEAA
Heather Mattingly, PT, MS ▪ Bridgett Wallace, PT, DPT
Holly Cauthen, PT, DPT ▪ Dennis W. Fell, PT, MD

CHAPTER **29**

## CHAPTER OBJECTIVES

Upon completion of this chapter, the learner should be able to:

1. Identify the primary anatomical structures involved with vestibular-related pathology.
2. Recognize impairments associated with a vestibular dysfunction.
3. Identify mechanisms of recovery from a vestibular dysfunction.
4. Identify indications for vestibular rehabilitation therapy.
5. Design general treatment strategies for vestibular rehabilitation, incorporating associated principles.
6. Design treatment strategies for stable unilateral versus bilateral vestibular hypofunction.
7. Design treatment strategies for benign paroxysmal positional vertigo.
8. Predict expected patient outcomes for given treatment strategies.

## Introduction to Vestibular Interventions

Persons with vestibular disorders exhibit symptoms primarily relating to motion sensitivity, **gaze stability** (i.e., the ability to visually fixate on a target during brief, rapid head movements), and postural stability, which were introduced in Chapter 8, Examination and Evaluation of Vestibular Function. In most cases, everyday activities (e.g., walking, going to the grocery store) help promote compensation for vestibular impairments even when the individual is not involved in a vestibular rehabilitation program. The compensatory process requires that sensory input be coordinated with motor activity. Therefore, optimal intervention strategies require both motor learning of exercises and matching of sensory input. The goal of vestibular rehabilitation therapists is to optimize patient recovery by addressing gaze stability, motion sensitivity, and postural stability deficits through customized therapeutic exercise and patient education.

In addition to postural instability, patients may report movement-related impairments (see details in Chapter 8) including **dizziness** (i.e., a nonspecific sense of unsteadiness in which a person feels as if she may fall), **vertigo** (i.e., a subjective illusion of rotary movement, or "spinning"; the person feels as if the room is spinning or she is spinning in the room), **oscillopsia** (i.e., a false illusion of movement or "oscillation" of the environment or objects in the environment), fatigue, and/or audiological symptoms. Audiological symptoms may include tinnitus (i.e., the perception of "ringing in the ears" in the absence of a true environmental sound), aural fullness/pressure, hearing loss, and/or sensitivity to sounds. Vestibular symptoms, particularly with benign paroxysmal positional vertigo (BPPV), usually include vertigo (i.e., room spinning) and nystagmus elicited with position changes (e.g., lying down, rolling over in bed, looking up). **Nystagmus** is involuntary, rhythmic, rapid eye movements often associated with vestibular or cerebellar pathology.

Because the vestibular system is highly integrated with the visual system, it is imperative to examine both systems to more confidently identify the etiologies of the symptoms and to apply the most appropriate plan of care/interventions. The vestibular examination is discussed in detail in Chapter 8. In this chapter, we briefly review the primary reflexes of the inner ear because most treatment strategies are based on impairments in this area.

The vestibular system influences two very important reflex functions that help to maintain gaze and postural control and contribute to the perception of movement in space. The **vestibulo-ocular reflex (VOR)** provides gaze stability in response to head movement and related changing stimuli in the visual surroundings. With the VOR, a movement of the head in any direction results in conjugate movement of both eyes in the opposite direction but with equal amplitude (i.e., same degree of movement) so the eyes stay fixed on the visual target. After a perturbation, vestibular input from the **vestibular spinal reflex (VSR)** controls muscular responses to support coordination and postural control during activities of daily living (ADLs) and all functional skills. These responses are known as balance strategies, or the appropriate and timely use of ankle, hip, and stepping strategies, as described in Chapter 9.

## Possible Effect of Vestibular Impairment on Function

Balance is essential for individuals to move about their environment and successfully carry out daily activities. Vestibular dysfunction often causes unsteadiness as a result of poor sensory organization. In most cases, sensory analysis reveals normal use of somatosensory and visual cues with abnormal use of vestibular cues to maintain balance. Central systems are normally found to be intact. Positional changes, busy visual environments, dim or dark environments, and riding as a passenger in the car often exacerbate symptoms of dizziness and unsteadiness, increasing the risk for falls (Asprella, 2012). Common functional and participation limitations that can result from vestibular impairment include difficulty walking in the dark or on uneven surfaces, walking with a wider base of support, or avoidance of busy places such as grocery stores and shopping malls. Individuals with vestibular dysfunction typically limit their head movements to minimize symptoms, which can lead to secondary problems such as neck stiffness and/or pain.

The literature suggests less than 40% of the adult population reports dizziness to their physician, with an estimated 85% of these symptoms due to vestibular dysfunction when central findings are not present (Bloom, 1989). Also of concern is the psychological effect of disruption in ADLs due to vestibular disorders. Delayed and/or inaccurate diagnosis with delayed or lack of referral for treatment can result in depression, anxiety, fear, and other psychological problems.

Numerous treatment options exist to manage vestibular disorders. In this chapter, we discuss **vestibular rehabilitation therapy (VRT)**, including therapeutic approaches, exercises, and activities to restore vestibular function when possible, remediate function when necessary, and restore optimal functional activity. Specific repositioning maneuvers to remove dislodged or adhered debris in one or more of the semicircular canals along with various exercises to decrease the severity of symptoms are explained. VRT is a successful exercise-based approach that has grown in popularity over the last decade, although the concept dates back to the 1940s when Cawthorne, an otolaryngologist, and Cooksey, a physiotherapist, developed the "Cawthorne-Cooksey" protocol of exercises to decrease dizziness (Cawthorne, 1946), which are still in use (Enticott, 2005; Giray, 2009). In the 1980s, early publications of treatment protocols and research on the efficacy of VRT for patients with vestibular dysfunction appeared (Brandt, 1980).

**BPPV** is the most common cause of vertigo, characterized by the episodic (paroxysmal), subjective sense of spinning, which is typically triggered by head movements, including lying down, rolling over in bed, looking up, and bending over. The vertigo, with a 20- to 30-second latency before nystagmus begins, is usually brief (<60 seconds) and can be accompanied by nausea and unsteadiness. However, there are strategies commonly used by patients to help manage symptoms. For instance, one might try keeping the room cool, or use cold moist cloths or cold packs to help minimize nausea.

### PATIENT APPLICATION

*Joan is a 36 year-old female who presents to the clinic with dizziness and unsteadiness. She reports the sudden onset of severe vertigo 4 weeks ago. Joan describes the initial onset as "the room spinning," which lasted for 4 to 5 hours. The vertigo was accompanied by nausea and vomiting. Joan's husband drove her to the emergency department (ED), where she underwent extensive testing and received IV fluids for dehydration. Her imaging studies, cardiac tests, and blood work results were normal. Joan was discharged from the ED with the diagnosis of "vertigo" and was given a prescription for meclizine and phenergan. She was also encouraged to follow up with her primary care physician (PCP) and/or schedule an appointment with an ear, nose, and throat (ENT) physician. Joan saw her PCP and was referred to an ENT because of ongoing dizziness and unsteadiness. She underwent vestibular diagnostic testing including electronystagmography (ENG). The caloric testing portion of the ENG revealed a 38% left vestibular weakness. The remainder of her ENG results were essentially normal, as were her audiogram results. Joan was given "some exercises," which she describes as lying down quickly on one side then the other. However, she stopped the exercises because they "only made it worse," and she continues to have symptoms. Additional symptoms include fatigue, concentration problems, "wooziness," and some nausea.*

*Before the onset of these symptoms, the patient worked full-time as an accountant and exercised three to four times a week. However, she has returned to work only on a part-time basis because of her ongoing symptoms. Joan has a medical history of allergies and hypothyroidism controlled by over-the-counter medications and Synthroid, respectively.*

## Contemplate Clinical Decisions

1. To facilitate diagnosis, what questions about Joan's history are important to ask?
2. What specific information do you want to know regarding Joan's dizziness?
3. What effects might Joan's medications have on her symptoms?
4. What effect might the antihistamine or sedative medication have on Joan's recovery?
5. What additional physical therapy tests and measures may be appropriate for Joan?
6. What therapeutic interventions may be appropriate for Joan?
7. Given Joan's history, what do you expect for optimal treatment response? Why?
8. To encourage adherence, what patient education is appropriate?

## ■ Related Pathology

### Neuroanatomy of Common Pathologies

The vestibular system is composed of two primary neural subsystems: the peripheral vestibular and central vestibular systems. For protection, these systems are housed within the bony structures of the temporal skull region; however, they are easily susceptible to injury as a result of aging, trauma, or disease processes. The **peripheral vestibular system** is composed of three semicircular canals and two otolith organs that detect angular and linear acceleration, respectively. Specifically, the three **semicircular canals** (posterior, anterior, and horizontal) are fluid-filled loops in the inner ear, and the two **otoliths** (utricle and saccule) house otoconia within the otolithic membrane. **Otoconia** are small, sandlike, calcium carbonite crystals that are normally present in the utricle and saccule but can become dislodged, causing positional vertigo. Together with the central neural circuitry, these vestibular organs comprise the vestibular system, which provides information about forces created by gravity and those generated by our movements. In so doing, it provides information about orientation in space, maintains gaze stability for focusing on the surrounding environment, and generates appropriate postural reflexes for balance. Therefore, disorders of the vestibular system can disrupt functional movement with incorrect information about body orientation in space, resulting in visual instability and loss of balance control. For further information regarding the anatomy of the peripheral and **central vestibular systems**, refer to Chapter 8.

## Vestibular-Related Function Across the Lifespan

Although the vestibular system plays an important role in postural control and balance throughout the lifespan, research indicates the normal human system undergoes a gradual decrease in function over time as the body ages. Research indicates a progressive loss in vestibular function each year after the age of 40 years (Ishiyama, 2009).

### Developmental Considerations

The vestibular system is functional at birth and, in fact, is the first sensory system to develop in utero (Jeffery, 2004; Nandi, 2008). The physical structure is developed by the end of the second month in utero and neural connections in the sixth month, with functionality present in the eighth to ninth month. Although functional at birth, the system requires time to mature. Gradual modulation continues until maturity, when a child reaches 10 to 14 years of age.

### Age-Related Changes

Age-related changes in the vestibular system have been well documented. On a cellular level, otolith demineralization is the earliest change seen (Ross, 1976). The number of utricle and saccule otoconia has substantially decreased when the elderly are compared with the young (Ishiyama, 2009; Serrador, 2009; Walther, 2007). Degeneration is seen in individuals over 50 years of age, progressing in severity with advancing age. Hair cell degeneration and loss also occur after age 50 (Ishiyama, 2009; Walther, 2007). Hair cell density in the utricle seems to be spared (21% decrease) compared with density in the saccule (24% decrease) and cristae (40% decrease) in individuals over 70 years of age (Ishiyama, 2009).

Impaired vestibular function manifests as a decline in the VOR in individuals over 55 years of age (Ishiyama, 2009; Walther, 2007). Changes in the VOR include prolonged latencies, reduced catch-up saccades, and smaller amplitude responses. With aging, declines in VOR function may contribute to changes in gait and balance because of the inability to maintain gaze stability during functional mobility. Decreases in **vestibular evoked myogenic potential (VEMP)**, a test of the neurophysiological response of the utricle and saccule to a specific kinematic or motion stimulus, are also seen with advancing age, or possibly due to BPPV in some individuals (Ishiyama, 2009). Serrador (2009) examined both **otolith counterrolling** and **ocular counterrolling (OCR)**, the reflexive conjugate rotational movement of the eyes rotating opposite to the direction of head tilt and balance, in healthy individuals aged 21 to 93 years. Results showed a linear decrease in OCR with increasing age, especially in females compared with males. A strong relationship between declining OCR and increasing mediolateral sway with the eyes closed while on a stable surface was also reported. Compared with nonfallers, fallers were found to have greater mediolateral sway and decreased OCR. These findings suggest that decreased OCR may increase fall risk (Serrador, 2009).

Both cellular and functional age-related changes seen in the vestibular system likely play a role in gait and balance changes with increasing age. Therapists should therefore include vestibular screening in patients who demonstrate gait and balance deficits. Therapists should also keep in mind, however, that numerous studies have shown that age does not significantly affect the outcomes of VRT, although recovery may take longer (Whitney, 2002).

## Vestibular Impairment in Neuromuscular Diagnoses

Deficits in gaze stability, motion sensitivity, and postural stability can result from impairments in the peripheral and/or central vestibular system. Vestibular impairment can be associated with several neuromuscular diagnoses or conditions. Table 29-1 identifies common medical diagnoses associated with peripheral and central vestibular impairments in adults and children, along with the type of vestibular dysfunction.

## ■ Pertinent Examination/Evaluation

Chapter 8 discusses the selection of appropriate clinical tests and measures to identify vestibular dysfunction. In addition, Chapter 8 discusses more sophisticated technology, such as **videonystagmography** or **ENG** testing, that provides specific measurement of eye movements, including nystagmus, using video or electrodes respectively, during caloric, positional, or visual tracking tests.

## ■ Preparatory Interventions Specific to Vestibular Impairment

### Mechanisms of Recovery

To plan effective interventions for vestibular impairments, the therapist must first understand the primary mechanisms leading to recovery. Mechanisms of recovery vary according to the severity of the vestibular dysfunction. Some individuals

### TABLE 29-1  Common Medical Diagnoses Associated With Vestibular Impairment

#### ADULT

| Peripheral (3/4 of all Etiologies) | Type of Vestibular Dysfunction* |
| --- | --- |
| Benign paroxysmal positional vertigo | Structural |
| Uncompensated Ménière's disease | Fluctuating or hypofunction; progressive |
| Vestibular neuronitis | Reduced/hypofunction |
| Labyrinthitis | Reduced/hypofunction |
| Perilymphatic fistula/superior canal dehiscence | Fluctuating |
| Acoustic neuroma | Reduced/hypofunction |
| Age-related degeneration/drug-related ototoxicity | Reduced/hypofunction; unilateral or bilateral loss |
| Central (1/4 of all Etiologies) | |
| Medullary or cerebrovascular occlusion | Hypofunction or distorted (depends on location of lesion) |
| Brain trauma with white fiber damage or cerebellar pathology | Hypofunction or distorted (depends on location of lesion) |
| Migraine | Fluctuating |
| Neurodegenerative disease (e.g., multiple sclerosis) | Hypofunction or distorted (depends on location of lesion) |
| Tumors in posterior fossa | Reduced/hypofunction |
| **PEDIATRIC** | |
| Migraine | Fluctuating |
| Benign paroxysmal positional vertigo of childhood | Structural or hypofunction |
| Otitis media | Reduced/hypofunction |
| Trauma | Reduced/hypofunction |
| Congenital vestibular failure | Hypofunction |
| Usher syndrome type 3 | Progressive hypofunction |
| Alstrom syndrome | Progressive hypofunction |
| Refsum disease | Progressive hypofunction |
| Wolfram disease | Progressive hypofunction |

*(Black, 1986).

have spontaneous recovery, which results in a rebalancing of tonic activity within the vestibular nuclei (at the cellular level). Individuals whose systems do not spontaneously recover may require further intervention through a VRT program. Three primary mechanisms of recovery have been described: (1) adaptation, (2) substitution, and (3) habituation (Herdman, 2014). **Vestibular adaptation** is a recovery mechanism for the VOR; it allows the vestibular system to make long-term improvements in how it responds to input to capitalize on remaining capabilities. **Substitution** is the use of other strategies to replace the lost function; it is therefore not classified as a true mechanism of recovery. After vestibular damage with bilateral VOR loss, such strategies may include increased reliance on the **cervical-ocular reflex** (Kasai, 1978), in which neck position, through feedback from neck proprioception, can cause stereotypic eye movements. Other substitution strategies include increased reliance on visual and somatosensory inputs with loss of the VSR (balance strategies).

**Habituation exercises** are defined as exercises in which the provoking position or stimulus is repeated until the person no longer has symptoms (Herdman, 2014; Telian, 1990). The approach is based on the concept that repeated exposure to a stimulus decreases the brain's pathological response to that stimulus (Banfield, 2000). Refer to the section on therapeutic habitation exercises for motion sensitivity for specific techniques. When recovery is not possible through these techniques, **compensation**—interventions that encourage complex brain changes to allow cerebral adjustments to the altered sensory input and abolish the perception of vestibular symptoms—may be required for functional mobility with decreased symptoms. For example, visual focus can be used to perform activities such as rolling, sitting up, or turning while walking.

Introduced in the 1980s, adaptation exercises produce long-term improvement of the vestibular system's ability to stabilize vision with head movement. Adaptation involves combining head movement and visual input to modify the VOR gain. **Gain** is a ratio used to describe the relationship of eye movement to head movement or eye movement to target movement. As mentioned earlier, the VOR is a reflexive movement that stabilizes vision during head movement by producing head and eye movements in opposite directions, therefore keeping an image in the center of the visual field. VOR gain is defined as the change in the eye angle divided by the change in the head angle. Ideally, VOR gain should equal 1 or very close to it. When the gain is impaired, **retinal slip**, or movement of the visual image on the retina during head movement, occurs. This slip causes the visual image to become blurry or jump with optokinetic eye movements.

During these treatments, you should inform the patient that you are trying to create these error signals but that too much error will increase symptoms and impede progress. The patient may report these changes even when the therapist does not observe the slip. The best way to induce adaptation is to produce an error signal that the central nervous system tries to correct by modifying the gain of the VOR; the best way to accomplish this is by incorporating visual stimuli with head movement (Herdman, 2014). Vestibular adaptation can be

induced with periods of stimulation as short as 1 to 2 minutes (Herdman, 2014; Shepard, 1995). For example, one adaptation exercise could be to ask the patient to maintain visual focus on a business card held at arm's length and then perform gentle but quick head movements from side to side and up-and-down while maintaining visual focus on a discrete target (a single word or letter) on the card.

Repeated exposure to retinal slip during gaze stabilization exercises allows for vestibular adaptation. During the time the brain is trying to correct the error signal, the patient may experience symptoms; however, it is important that the patient continue with the exercise for the full minute without stopping. The velocity and amplitude of the head movement should stress the system, but not to the point where the visual target becomes unfocused (Leigh, 2015).

Studies have shown that gradually increasing retinal slip errors was more effective than producing large errors (Schubert, 2010). As the system begins to adapt, the exercises can be performed under more demanding situations (e.g., from sitting to standing to walking, incorporating busier visual backgrounds). In addition, the duration can slowly be increased to 2 minutes. Because normal head movements occur at various frequencies, exercises should be performed over a range of frequencies to optimize the effects of adaptation (Leigh, 2015; Topuz, 2004). See the section on therapeutic adaptation exercises for gaze stability for detailed techniques.

## Indications for Treatment

Several indications for treatment of vestibular disorders exist. One crucial component of a successful treatment program is identifying the underlying etiology and pathology of the disorder. In this chapter, we discuss indications for treatment based on selected diagnostic categories. Table 29-2 identifies typical functional deficits and recovery mechanisms for each of the vestibular rehabilitation categories.

**Stable unilateral deficit:** Individuals with this diagnosis are good candidates for VRT based on adaptation. Common disorders include status-post acute **vestibular neuritis/labyrinthitis** (an inner ear infection), vestibular surgery (e.g., acoustic neuroma or ablation), and/or inactive Ménière's disease (Szturm, 1994).

**Stable bilateral deficit:** Individuals with this diagnosis may have reduced losses or complete losses bilaterally. Treatment focuses on habituation and substitution, especially the use of visual and somatosensory inputs. The most common cause of bilateral vestibular loss is exposure to aminoglycoside antibiotics and certain chemotherapy drugs.

**Unstable unilateral** or **bilateral deficit:** Individuals with this diagnosis are typically not good candidates for VRT, and the priority is to stabilize through pharmaceutical intervention, lifestyle changes, and/or rest. In some cases, surgical options are necessary.

**Central vestibular deficit:** A number of neurological disorders may result in dizziness and/or vestibular disorders, including stroke, head trauma, multiple sclerosis, and migraine.

| TABLE 29-2 | Common Vestibular Rehabilitation Categories and Recovery Strategies | |
|---|---|---|
| | **FUNCTIONAL DEFICITS** | **MECHANISM OF RECOVERY** |
| Vestibulo-ocular reflex (VOR)—static | Differences in vestibular tonic firing rates in response to stimuli | Rebalancing of tonic activity (or spontaneous recovery if acute) |
| VOR disturbance—dynamic | Abnormalities in gain or timing of eyes relative to head movements | Vestibular adaptation—recalibration of neural response based on altered firing rates. CNS habituation—progressive decline in the response to a given stimulus |
| Vestibular spinal reflex (VSR) disturbance—sensory disorganization | Misuse of sensory feedback (visual, vestibular, or somatosensory) for postural control | Specific sensory organization exercises for balance while availability and accuracy of sensory input is systematically varied |
| VSR disturbance—motor disorganization | Underlying musculoskeletal or neuro-muscular impairment | Specific motor organization exercises to improve coordination of muscle responses to static and dynamic activities |
| Complete vestibular loss | Minimal or no vestibular feedback for postural control | Substitution with alternative strategies |

**Nonvestibular deficit:** One of the more common non-vestibular balance disorders is peripheral neuropathy. Because of the nature of sensory loss, treatment focuses on maximizing use of remaining peripheral cues (e.g., visual and vestibular) as well as general strengthening, conditioning, and fall prevention strategies. Therapists should also be aware of the high correlation between vestibular disorders and migraines, which can cause vertigo, nausea, unsteadiness, and tinnitus. The similarity of symptoms makes it a challenge to identify their underlying cause. In addition, a number of studies have shown a high incidence of migraines in persons with Ménière's disease (Cha, 2007; Neff, 2012; Radtke, 2002). Researchers have also found by comparison, a higher incidence of BPPV in people with migraines (Ishiyama, 2000). Anxiety and/or panic disorders are commonly associated with vestibular disorders, and when deemed appropriate, vestibular rehabilitation combined with behavior modification has been beneficial, similar to exposure therapy with types of phobias (Shepard, 1995).

Additional disorders commonly seen by vestibular therapists include **mal de débarquement syndrome (MdDS)** and **persistent postural-perceptual dizziness (PPPD)**. MdDS is a rare disorder that causes a feeling of rocking or swaying that is worse when still and is improved, if not alleviated, during movement. Rotational (or spinning) vertigo is typically not associated with MdDS and most commonly occurs after prolonged cruise, car, and/or train travel, predominantly affecting middle-aged women. Van Ombergen (2016b) described a set of criteria for the diagnosis of MdDS: (1) chronic rocking/swaying dizziness after prolonged passive motion or exposure to virtual reality; (2) symptoms lasting for at least 1 month; (3) normal vestibular and audiological test results; (4) normal imaging of the brain; and (5) no symptoms associated with another diagnosis. Currently, there is no cure for MdDS, and it is often managed with medication and vestibular rehabilitation.

PPPD was first described in 1996 by Brandt, and was called phobic postural vertigo (PPV). The primary symptoms include persistent postural dizziness without rotational vertigo that is worse when upright and exacerbated by busy environments, illness, and/or stressful events. As with MdDS, there is no other identifiable cause of the person's symptoms. Staab (2012) expanded on the PPV syndrome and renamed it chronic subjective dizziness (CSD). Unlike MdDS symptoms, CSD symptoms include exacerbation by movement but no identifiable vestibular or visual impairment to explain the dizziness.

An international panel of experts increased research into PPV/CSD and in 2014 reached a consensus regarding key symptoms that define the diagnosis. This syndrome became known as persistent postural-perceptual dizziness (PPPD), which was to be added to the *International Classification of Diseases (ICD-11)* in 2017 by the World Health Organization. The current diagnostic criteria include (1) normal imaging and other laboratory test results; (2) primary symptoms of dizziness/unsteadiness that have been present for 3 months or more; (3) fluctuating symptoms that depend on triggers (vestibular event, other illness, and/or psychiatric event); and (4) symptom provocation related to body position and typically most severe when standing/walking and often absent when lying down. The most common treatments for PPPD include medication, vestibular rehabilitation for behavioral modification, and counseling.

## General Intervention Techniques

Once a patient has been examined and VRT is indicated, the program should begin as soon as possible—within 2 to 3 days of onset of vestibular loss. In the acute phase, exercises are typically brief and have minimal distress or sensory distractions (e.g., done in a quiet room with good lighting and minimal visual stimulus). To optimize the use of graded sensory inputs, the patient often begins with a VOR adaptation exercise, habituation exercises, and balance-retraining exercises, which are described fully later in this chapter. The VRT program should be patient centered and problem oriented. This requires a thorough understanding of the patient's history, underlying etiology, impairments, and prognosis. Thus, the VRT program is customized to the patient's subjective complaints and examination results.

The need for VRT specific exercises was first introduced in the 1940s by Cawthorne-Cooksey for patients with a unilateral vestibular lesion (UVL) and postconcussion symptoms. Patients who used these exercises had a faster and more complete recovery than patients who were sedentary (Cooksey, 1946). Since the introduction of the Cawthorne-Cooksey exercises, research has expanded for patients with both vestibular dysfunction and traumatic brain injury (Motin, 2005; Ribeiro, 2005; Scherer, 2009). An ever-growing body of knowledge is now accessible to clinicians and to patients, resulting in better outcomes through a more patient-specific care plan.

As noted by several authors, the primary components of a VRT program include gaze stabilization through slow VOR exercises and postural stability through VSR exercises (Braswell, 2004; Schubert, 2006, 2008a). Additional conditioning and strengthening activities are often required, and when indicated, repositioning maneuvers for BPPV are performed. These activities are used for patients classified as stable unilateral hypofunction.

### Therapeutic Adaptation Exercises for Gaze Stability

Adaptation is the most appropriate approach in patients with reduced vestibular function (e.g., unilateral loss), whereas substitution is used as first-line treatment when there is no remaining vestibular function (e.g., bilateral loss). Gaze stability exercises involve head turning in the horizontal and vertical planes for 1 minute while staring at a target held at eye level. The exercises are performed in both sitting and standing positions four to five times per day (Enticott, 2005). In healthy individuals, head movements generally range from 2 to 6 Hz or 70 to 120 degrees per second for activities such as walking, driving, and running (Pozzo, 1990).

Interventions can consist of visual-motor exercises based on the plane of movement for the object or the head. Head movements can include "**pitch**" movements (neck movements to nod the head up-and-down about the x-axis) as shown in Fig. 29-1A; "**yaw**" movements as shown in Fig. 29-1B (neck rotation to turn the head side to side, right and left about the y-axis); or diagonal/oblique movements as shown in Fig. 29-1C. Functionally, these head movements are incorporated with entire body movements such as walking, resulting in visual-motor exercises.

Treatment sessions for unilateral hypofunction, along with the daily home exercise program described later in the chapter, can occur one to three times per week for a minimum of 45 minutes each time. An average of 10 weeks may be required for bilateral vestibular hypofunction; the average is 2 to 3 weeks

in acute or subacute unilateral vestibular hypofunction without significant comorbidities or 4 to 6 weeks for chronic vestibular hypofunction (Hall, 2016a). The length of intervention often depends on patient adherence to the home exercise program. Variations in the speed of head or target movements, the complexity of the background, foot placement, and the font size of targets to increase the level of difficulty are discussed later (Braswell, 2004).

Gaze stabilization exercises comprise a specific set of adaptation and substitution exercises that address impaired gain of the VOR and are progressed as described here. These exercises involve visual fixation during head movements (Herdman, 2014). Traditionally, adaptation exercises are implemented first and include the following exercises: VOR X1 viewing (referred to as "times one viewing") and VOR X2 viewing (referred to as "times two viewing"). Substitution exercises are implemented around week two of vestibular rehabilitation and include active eye-head movements between two targets and remembered targets (Herdman, 2013).

The designations VOR X1 and VOR X2 exercises (Fig. 29-2) describe the number of components (head and/or target) that are moving during the exercise, but specifically refer to the gain (difference between amplitude of eye movement and corresponding head movement) during the activity: "X1" involves movement of the head alone and gain of 1 (amplitude of eye movement equals head movement), whereas "X2" involves movement of the head and target in equal and opposite directions and gain of 2 (amplitude of eye movement is twice that of head movement). During these exercises, the patient is instructed to keep the eyes focused on a target while moving the head. If glasses are normally worn for impaired visual acuity, the patient is instructed to perform these exercises wearing glasses, but the target should stay within the central vision and not go outside the frame of the glasses.

To start, the exercises are performed in a quiet environment, with a solid neutral background, in a position of minimal postural challenge (i.e., sitting or standing on a firm surface with a wide base of support). As the patient becomes more proficient with the exercises, the therapist will observe increasing duration of the exercise, increasing speed of movement with no visible or reported retinal slip, and/or a decrease in symptoms. The exercises can then be advanced to include a visually disturbing, busily patterned, optokinetic background; use of open environments; varying distances from the target; or more challenging postural positions, such as standing with a progressively decreasing base of support (e.g., progressing from a wide stance to a tandem stance, as demonstrated in Fig. 29-1D).

During **VOR X1 viewing exercises** (Fig. 29-2A), the target should remain stable while the patient moves the head in a horizontal or vertical direction (or much less frequently in an oblique direction). Typically, the target is a small letter written on a sticky note or a word printed on a business card. The target should be small enough so that it is a challenge to keep it in focus. Larger targets are generally used with patients challenged by impaired static visual acuity. Herdman (2013) recommends varying the distance from arm's length to 6 to 10 feet from the target. Instruct the patient to hold the letter at arm's

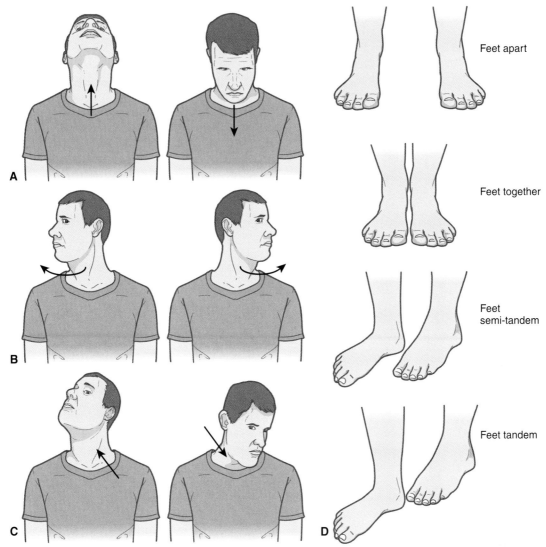

**FIGURE 29-1** Head movements for vestibulo-ocular reflex adaptation exercises can include (A) pitch movements, nodding the head up and down; (B) yaw movements, turning the head right and left; and (C) rarely diagonal head movements. It is imperative that the patient maintain gaze on the visual target at all times during adaptation exercises. Progression of adaptation exercises can also (D) progressively involve decreasing the base of support as the patient is able, from a wide stance to a narrow stance to a semitandem stance, to a full-tandem stance.

length, and/or place a sticky note at eye level on a neutral wall at that distance. The patient should keep her eyes fixed on the target, with horizontal and vertical head turns performed as fast as possible while keeping the letter/word in focus.

Because the patient may start to experience symptoms (i.e., blurry vision, dizziness, nausea, unsteadiness) during testing, it is important to forewarn her that this is normal and that the symptoms should subside relatively quickly with termination of the exercises. It is also important to ask the patient to perform the exercise just within the range she can tolerate (provoking symptoms but keeping the target in focus) in order to facilitate improvement in the VOR gain.

In the context of acute or subacute vestibular hypofunction, instruct the patient to complete 1- to 2-minute intervals of these gaze stabilization exercises a minimum of three times per day for a total of 12 minutes per day or more, or at least

20 minutes per day for chronic vestibular hypofunction (Hall, 2016a). The frequency of the VOR X1 exercise should gradually increase as the patient is able, with a goal of reaching 2 Hz or faster. Several guidelines that integrate adaptation exercises have been suggested for developing an exercise program for the patient with unilateral peripheral loss; these are summarized in Box 29-1 (Herdman, 2014; Hall, 2016).

Substitution exercises should be implemented after VOR X1 viewing in week two of vestibular rehabilitation. **Active eye-head movements between two targets** is the first substitution exercise incorporated in the plan of care. Place two targets (e.g., large dots drawn on two business cards) on a neutral wall at nose level. The two targets should be placed close enough that the patient is never required to use peripheral vision to focus on them. Starting with the head turned toward one target and the eyes focused on the same target, instruct the patient to first

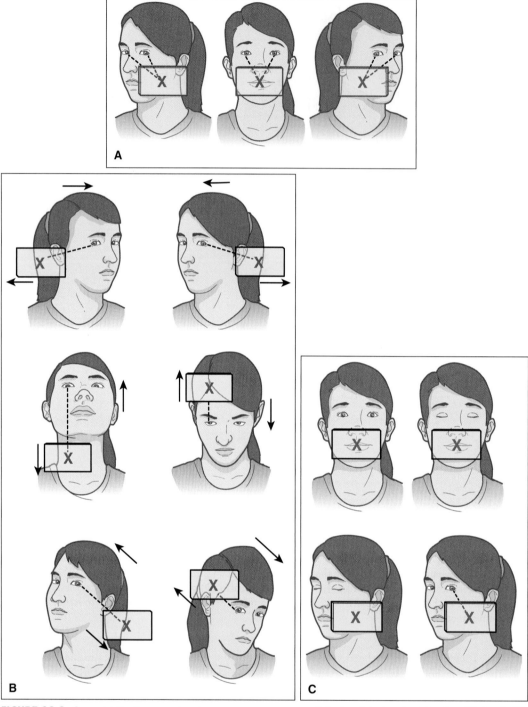

**FIGURE 29-2** Gaze stabilization exercises incorporate movements of the head during visual fixation. (A) For "X1" viewing, the patient moves the head back and forth in a horizontal, vertical, or oblique direction while maintaining visual fixation on a fixed target at shoulder height. (B) For "X2" viewing, the head moves in these same planes while the target moves in the opposite direction requiring eye movement through twice the distance. (C) The final progression is imaginary fixation, starting with the patient staring at a stationary target, then closing the eyes (see top row) and then, as shown on the bottom row, moving the head in one direction, and then opening the eyes to see if visual gaze has remained focused on the stationary target throughout the movement.

move the eyes to the second target (without head movement) and then move the head to the second target. Repeat this sequence in the opposite direction, and then repeat the cycle. It is essential that the patient understand that the eyes never move at the same time as the head.

Once the patient can perform VOR X1 exercises for 2-minute intervals with a minimal increase in symptoms, she may be ready to progress to VOR X2 exercises. The **VOR X2 viewing** exercises (Fig. 29-2B) are performed in the same fashion as the VOR X1 exercises, except the head

## BOX 29-1 Exercise Guidelines for Individuals With Unilateral Peripheral Vestibular Loss

- **Utilize exercises that produce an "error" signal:** The patient performs eye and head coordination exercises that stimulate the vestibule-ocular reflex (VOR) as shown in Fig. 29-2B during the movements of Fig. 29-1 (e.g., fixating on an object during a head movement). This results in an error message, or "retinal slip," due to vestibular dysfunction. This retinal slip results in the eyes lagging behind the head at a ratio that is greater than normal. Through repetition, the central nervous system tries to correct the error messages by increasing the VOR gain. Such exercises can be performed in various planes and speeds because recovery is context specific.

- **Provide a prolonged stimulus:** Although adaptation can occur within 1 to 2 minutes of vestibular stimulation, it is important to inform the patient that such exercises can increase symptoms, and encourage the patient to continue without stopping for 1- to 2-minute intervals.

- **Integrate context-specific VOR exercises:** To maximize recovery, exercises must facilitate the vestibular system in a variety of ways. For instance, vestibular adaptation is frequency dependent (>2 Hz or 120 bpm). Thus, greater VOR gain occurs at the speed of the exercise. Because normal movement occurs across several frequency ranges and different planes, exercises should be performed at various speeds and with the head in different planes.

- **Focus on the task at hand:** VOR function can be improved even in the dark if the patient just imagines focusing on a target during head movement. Although this VOR is not as meaningful as a VOR achieved when vision is utilized, it emphasizes the importance of focusing on the task with minimal distraction, especially in earlier phases.

- **Customize the program:** Customizing the vestibular rehabilitation therapy program to the patient is critical. Exercises should include an understanding of the underlying etiology, should address the impairments identified in the evaluation and examination, and should be coordinated with the patient/family. As noted earlier, the program will most likely entail specific sensory organization exercises, VOR exercises, and general conditioning/strengthening (Herdman, 2014).

and the target are moving in opposite directions during the exercise. Therefore, to perform VOR X2 exercises, instruct the patient to start by holding the target at shoulder height and an arm's length away with the eyes fixed on it. Have the patient move the target in one direction while moving the head in the opposite direction at the same pace and maintaining visual fixation on the target. For example, if the patient moves the target left, she will turn the head to the right while maintaining the eyes on the target. Instruct the patient to then repetitively move the head and the target in opposite directions but at equal speeds. To learn to coordinate the movement, the patient may have to start slowly and gradually increase the speed. The patient should again work just inside symptom-tolerance level while maintaining focus on

the target. This exercise is also prescribed at 1- to 2-minute intervals to be completed three times per day.

After tolerating VOR X2 viewing for up to 2 minutes without an increase in symptoms, the patient may be progressed to **remembered targets** using a stationary target (Fig. 29-2C). During this exercise, instruct the patient to focus on an imaginary target, then close her eyes and turn her head in a horizontal, vertical, or oblique direction while maintaining visual focus on the imaginary target for 1 to 2 minutes. Once the patient stops the head turns, instruct her to open her eyes and see if they have remained focused on the imaginary target. This technique is thought to facilitate the use of cervical inputs or to strengthen the cortical coordination of head and eye movements in order to strengthen gaze stability (Herdman, 2014).

For patients who are unable to tolerate gaze stability exercises because of severe impairments, ocular exercises may be required before X1 viewing exercises are initiated. These can include **smooth pursuit eye movements** and volitional continuous eye movements focused on a moving target, as well as vertical or horizontal eye movements to track slowly moving targets without head movement. All exercises are performed no longer than 1 minute each in both sitting and standing positions three times per day. Components of the oculomotor examination described in Chapter 8 may also be used as interventions, including smooth pursuit, saccadic movements, and convergence. These exercises are generally used with dizziness associated with a central lesion. Once again, dynamic balance activities such as ambulation can be included to increase exercise complexity (Gill-Body, 2000; Herdman, 2014).

### Therapeutic Habituation Exercises for Motion Sensitivity

Habituation is another intervention strategy that is often inappropriately interchanged with adaptation (Norre, 1980). Habituation differs from adaptation in that it is defined by a long-term reduction in neurological response to a noxious stimulus (Shepard, 1996). Thus, repeating movements that provoke symptoms can decrease a patient's symptomatic response to the movement stimulus. This approach has been used to treat position- and/or movement-related dizziness (Shepard, 1996).

During habituation exercises, movements are performed slowly at first, and then the speed of movement is gradually increased as the patient tolerates the increased stimulation. During habituation exercises, the patient should experience an increase in symptoms during the movements, but the increase in symptoms should subside within a fairly short time after terminating the movement.

As described earlier in the chapter, Cawthorne-Cooksey exercises were some of the first exercises developed to address vestibular impairments, and they are also the first exercises developed for habituation (Herdman, 2014). **Cawthorne-Cooksey exercises** incorporate eye-head movements and begin in sitting position, progressing to standing, then walking (Cooksey 1946). The original protocol was standardized and was typically performed in a group setting. Although the exercises are still used today, they are usually customized to the patient's needs. Optokinetic stimuli, including movements with complex backgrounds, can also be utilized as a UVL compensatory strategy to decrease sensitivity to visual disturbance (Pavlou, 2004, 2010, 2013; Van Ombergen, 2016a).

The Motion Sensitivity Quotient Test (Shepard, 1995) is a commonly used assessment to determine symptomatic positions for patients with unilateral peripheral vestibular loss. As a result, this tool may help determine positions to include in an individualized habituation exercise program. Movements within this tool include moving between sitting and supine, between left and right **Dix–Hallpike positions** (in which the patient rapidly lies back from long-sitting to a horizontal position with the head hanging over the edge of the plinth and with 45-degree neck rotation and ~20-degree neck extension), and returning to sitting. Proposed guidelines for developing a habituation exercise program can be found in Box 29-2 (Herdman, 2014).

### Therapeutic Combination Exercises for Postural Stability

Sometimes patients do not respond to a single exercise strategy alone. In such cases, the therapist may use a customized combination of exercises according to patient response. This often includes integration of balance-retraining activities with head turns or other positional changes to stimulate the vestibular system. Box 29-3 summarizes the general guidelines and considerations for vestibular rehabilitation exercises.

---

**BOX 29-2  Guidelines for Developing a Habituation Exercise Program**

- Choose up to four movements that cause the patient to have symptoms during testing. The patient is to perform these movements two or three times twice a day.
- The patient should perform movements quickly enough and through a full enough range of motion to produce mild to moderate symptoms using the Motion Sensitivity Test (0% = no symptoms to 100% = severe symptoms); mild to moderate symptoms equate to 11% to 30% (Akin, 2003).
- Increase the speed, intensity, and environmental demands as habituation to the movements occurs.
- Allow the patient to rest after each movement until symptoms resolve. The symptoms should resolve within 1 minute of stopping the movement or within 15 to 30 minutes of cessation of all exercises.
- Inform the patient that it may take up to 4 weeks before the symptoms decrease. Exercises are typically performed for at least 2 months. After the 2-month mark, exercises are typically reduced to once per day.
- Use caution with older adults. Movements that cause this population to rise quickly should be avoided. Habituation is not for everyone. Precautions include orthostatic hypotension and intolerance (severe autonomic reactions such as severe dizziness, sweating, or changes in blood pressure) in response to sensory stimulation (Herdman 2014).

---

**BOX 29-3  Summary of General Principles for Vestibular Rehabilitation**

- Intervention should begin as soon as possible.
- Adaptation is enhanced when the exercises are customized to the individual and performed under supervision.
- Exercises should be brief in nature but repeated throughout the day (e.g., vestibulo-ocular reflex exercises for 1 to 2 minutes).
- Inform the patient that the exercises may increase the symptoms and encourage the patient to work through the symptoms. Patients are often quite frightened about this; thus, the therapist must have a good rapport with the patient and understand this anxiety. There may be times when the exercises are modified and perhaps discontinued.
- Although frequency and duration of visits will vary, it is common to see patients with a unilateral vestibular lesion twice a week over 6 weeks. A bilateral loss, however, often requires months of therapy and an ongoing home program.
- General conditioning activities are often a component of a vestibular rehabilitation program—both the treatment session and home program.
- Patient education regarding vestibular disorders is a critical component of a successful treatment program. This patient population is often misunderstood, and establishing clear communication is essential.

---

### General Pharmacological Implications for Therapy

Therapists must know how specific medications may aid or hinder patient response to vestibular rehabilitation interventions. Common medical treatments include antihistamines, neurosuppressants, diuretics, and antibiotics. In the case of an acute peripheral vestibular lesion, such as from a viral or ischemic neurolabyrinthitis, recovery typically takes a matter of weeks (Leigh, 2015). Medications such as prednisone may improve recovery, especially when hearing loss is present. Antiviral medications are a debatable option that is still being explored (Strupp, 2004).

Medications are usually sedative by nature and should be used sparingly to treat symptoms of vertigo. Prolonged use can have deleterious effects, which retard central compensation or response to rehabilitation exercises (Herdman, 2014; Strupp, 2004). Usually patients are encouraged to increase activities as soon as possible to facilitate recovery. Failure to do so can limit full recovery. Clinical trials are currently aimed at finding medications that promote vestibular compensation (Horn, 1997, 2009; Leigh, 2015). Table 29-3 summarizes the common medications used for vestibular-related disorders and patient indications.

### Psychotherapy and Vestibular Rehabilitation

In special cases, a patient may have symptoms related to **somatoform dizziness,** a persistent subjective dizziness that is chronic and is caused by psychological factors. Somatoform dizziness

| TABLE 29-3 | Common Medications Used for Vestibular Deficits | |
|---|---|---|
| **MEDICATION/DRUG CLASS** | | **INDICATION** |
| *Vestibular Suppressants* | | |
| Meclizine (Antivert)/ antihistamine-anticholinergic | | Used in the acute phase of vestibular dysfunction to reduce motion sickness and nausea/vomiting |
| Dimenhydrinate (Dramamine)/ antihistamine-anticholinergic | | |
| Diazepam (Valium)/ benzodiazepine | | |
| Lorazepam (Ativan)/ benzodiazepine | | |
| Clonazepam (Klonopin)/ benzodiazepine | | |
| *Steroids* | | |
| Prednisone | | Reduces inflammation secondary to infection |
| *Antivirals* | | |
| Acyclovir (Zovirax) Valacyclovir (Valtrex) | | Reduce inflammation/ viral infection |
| *Antibiotics* | | |
| Amoxicillin | | Reduces inflammation/ bacterial infection |
| *Antiemetics* | | |
| Droperidol (Inapsine)/ antidopaminergic | | Reduces nausea and vomiting |
| Promethazine (Phenergan)/ antihistamine | | |
| Prochlorperazine (Compazine)/ Phenothiazine | | |
| Ondansetron (Zophren)/ serotonin 5-HT$_3$ receptor antagonist | | |
| *IV fluids* | | Dehydration |

(Baloh, 2011).

is usually considered late in the differential diagnosis process, if at all. The difficulty with this disorder is that patients have often previously consulted several specialists, such as an ENT physician, neurologist, or internist, who may not be as familiar with somatoform dizziness as the vestibular rehabilitation specialist is. Because patients present with dizziness as the chief complaint, a logical approach is usually taken, including specific avoidance behavior or a diagnosis that vegetative symptoms are associated with organically caused dizziness.

With persistent symptoms of dizziness, the patient tends to graduate to conditions of somatoform dizziness, which is chronic and frequently associated with severe impairment in ADLs, even early retirement and increased health-care expenses.

Somatoform dizziness lasting longer than 12 weeks and severe impairment of quality of life should initiate interdisciplinary diagnostics, including medical and ophthalmological, differential neurological or neuro-otologic, and psychosomatic diagnostics. Treatment is indicated primarily by clinical presentation and includes aspects of psychotherapy. When the disorder is diagnosed as being mild and of short duration, a focused outpatient rehabilitation program can be successful. When the condition is considered severe, pharmacotherapy is the treatment of choice (Herdman, 2014; Meli, 2007).

## THINK ABOUT IT 29.1

- When are adaptation exercises indicated for vestibular rehabilitation?
- When are habituation exercises indicated for vestibular rehabilitation?
- How can a combined therapy approach that includes postural stability benefit the progression of the plan of care?
- When might an interdisciplinary team be consulted to address vestibular-related impairments?

## Specific Therapeutic Techniques

### Benign Paroxysmal Positional Vertigo

BPPV, classified as a stable unilateral variant lesion, is the most common type of peripheral vestibular disorder and accounts for 20% to 30% of all patients seen for vertigo (Michel, 2009). BPPV occurs in adults at a variety of ages but is more common among older adults and accounts for 160,000 new cases of dizziness each year (Eaton, 2003; Froehling, 1991; Hansson, 2005). The clinical presentation of BPPV is typically classic—both subjectively and objectively.

BPPV is a mechanical problem of the inner ear and was first described in 1921 (Bárány, 1921; Hansson, 2005). Dix (1952) established more specific testing in 1952, which led to the standard "Dix-Hallpike" test used today. The originators further defined BPPV nystagmus and identified two key characteristics: (1) the latency, 20 to 30 seconds, before onset of nystagmus and vertigo in the supine position and (2) the reversal of nystagmus during the return to the sitting portion of the Dix-Hallpike. The diagnosis of BPPV is often indicated by the patient's subjective report alone, with objective testing providing confirmation. The standard Dix-Hallpike maneuver has a reported sensitivity of 79% and a specificity of 75%. whereas the sidelying test is also supported with a sensitivity of 90% and a specificity of 75% (Halker, 2008). For more information on techniques for positional testing, refer to Chapter 8, Examination/Evaluation of the Vestibular System. Table 29-4 provides essential guidelines for interpreting the results of Dix-Hallpike testing to differentiate posterior from anterior canal BPPV according to the characteristics of the nystagmus (Herdman, 1994).

Patients with BPPV can be treated most often with canalith (particle) repositioning maneuvers, as described later in this

| TABLE 29-4 | Nystagmus Characteristics Associated With Anterior Versus Posterior Canal and Horizontal Canal Benign Paroxysmal Positional Vertigo | |
|---|---|---|
| **CANAL** | **DIX-HALLPIKE TEST** | **REVERSAL PHASE UPON RETURN TO SITTING** |
| Right posterior* | Up-beating Right torsional | Down-beating Left torsional |
| Left posterior* | Up-beating Left torsional | Down-beating Right torsional |
| Right anterior* | Down-beating Right torsional | Up-beating Left torsional |
| Left anterior* | Down-beating Left torsional | Up-beating Right torsional |
| **CANAL** | **ROLL TEST** | **NOTE** |
| Horizontal canalithiasis | Geotropic and <60 seconds | *The side of strongest nystagmus/symptoms is the affected side* |
| Horizontal cupulolithiasis | Ageotropic and >60 seconds | *The side of weakest nystagmus/symptoms is the affected side* |

*Wait at least 30 seconds for latency period before claiming no symptoms.
For posterior and anterior canal canalithiasis, nystagmus lasts <60 seconds; for cupulolithiasis, nystagmus lasts >60 seconds.
Adapted from Herdman, 1994.

chapter. Several effective strategies can be customized to the patient's history and symptoms. In some cases, patients can even learn to perform these maneuvers independently as part of a home program (Radtke, 2004) or in addition to direct intervention by the therapist, although this should be done with caution because of the increased complication rate (Tanimoto, 2005).

In the past, common home recommendations included the use of a cervical collar, daily repetition of the Brandt-Daroff exercises described later, and prolonged periods of sleeping in an upright position, although these strategies have not been validated in the literature and are no longer recommended as standard care (Brandt, 1994; Helminski, 2005; Moon, 2005; Cakir, 2006; Devaiah, 2010). In addition, debate continues as to whether or not mastoid vibration during the maneuvers is beneficial for management of cupulolithiasis (Hain, 2000; Macias, 2004; Motamed, 2004). Repeated maneuvers in a single session, however, may be more effective in most cases (Gordon, 2004). In fact, patients without positional symptoms, such as those with multiple sclerosis, have responded favorably to particle repositioning procedures (Dewey, 2003).

### What Causes BPPV?

The causes of BPPV are often considered "idiopathic," or occurring for no known reason. However, BPPV is more common after head trauma, an illness (e.g., inner ear infection), or ischemia of the anterior vestibular artery (Froehling, 1991). BPPV is also common in the older adult population simply as a result of degenerative changes of the inner ear (Agrawal, 2009). Some resources suggest that up to 50% of all dizziness in older people is due to BPPV (Bloom, 1989). As noted earlier, persons with migraines also have a higher incidence of BPPV than nonmigraine sufferers.

Baloh (1987) following 240 cases presenting with BPPV first described support for two mechanisms: (1) canalithiasis

(otoconia are abnormally present but free-floating in the canal) and (2) cupulolithiasis (particles are abnormally adherent to the cupula of the crista ampullaris) as described in Chapter 8. Given the possible difficulty in properly diagnosing BPPV, it becomes ever more important to use differential diagnostic strategies for peripheral versus central pathology. Therefore, causes of central vertigo should be ruled out when symptoms vary from the traditional presentation. Oculomotor abnormalities such as sustained nystagmus not suppressed by visual fixation can be a sign of a central lesion. This can be indicative of possible ischemia of the pontomedullary brainstem or another part of the central vestibular neural pathway. In addition, cerebellar lesions can be associated with dizziness in supine positions with the head rotated to either side and in extension. A pure down-beating nystagmus in any position may indicate an infratentorial disorder related to a vascular insult such as Arnold-Chiari malformation, stroke, or subdural hematoma. Nystagmus has also been documented with progressive forms of multiple sclerotic lesions in this area (Leigh, 2015). Episodic dizziness that worsens with position changes can also be associated with the aura of migraine (Roberts, 2006a). The sections in this chapter discussing therapeutic adaptation exercises for gaze stability and therapeutic habitation exercises for motion sensitivity describe treatment techniques to address central vestibular conditions.

Complaints of slight dizziness do not always indicate pathology and may simply indicate a typical response from otolithic organs being put in a position/angle not typical of daily activity. However, symptoms of dizziness mentioned in the foregoing section describe conditions where symptoms disrupt or prevent continued common daily activities.

### Therapeutic Interventions for BPPV

Once the BPPV has been confirmed and diagnosed as canalithiasis or cupulolithiasis in the posterior, anterior,

| TABLE 29-5 | Canal-Specific Intervention Recommendations by Type of BPPV | |
|---|---|---|
| **CANAL** | **CANALITHIASIS** | **CUPULOLITHIASIS** |
| Posterior | • CRM* (modified Epley maneuver)<br>• Liberatory (Semont maneuver)<br>• Brandt-Daroff exercises | • Liberatory* (Semont maneuver)<br>• CRM (modified Epley maneuver) *with mastoid vibration in resistant cases*<br>• Brandt-Daroff |
| Anterior | • CRM* (modified Epley maneuver) | • Liberatory (Semont)<br>• Brandt-Daroff |
| Horizontal | • Barbecue roll*<br>• Appiani or Gufoni to the unaffected side<br>• Forced prolonged positioning (FPP) | • Casani (modified Semont) or Gufoni to the affected side)<br>• FPP |

*Preferred method listed first. CRM = canalith repositioning maneuver.

and/or horizontal canal, the patient can be treated accordingly (Gold, 2014). If the history does not show a clearly suspected canal, testing for posterior canal using the Dix-Hallpike should be done first because this canal is most commonly involved. If the patient is asymptomatic with this test and no nystagmus is observed, the clinician can keep the patient in supine and proceed with the roll test (Herdman, 1993). Refer to Chapter 8 for more details regarding examination techniques and diagnostic criteria for BPPV.

The three main categories of intervention for BPPV are canalith (particle) repositioning maneuvers (CRMs/PRMs), liberatory maneuvers, and when resistant, Brandt-Daroff exercises as a last resort. The most common CRM for posterior and anterior canalithiasis, known as the Epley maneuver, was first introduced by John Epley, MD, in 1979. Since its inception, it has been modified to the current repositioning maneuver described in the next section (Epley, 1992). Table 29-5 summarizes guidelines for the treatment of BPPV (Herdman, 1994). The following sections discuss specific interventions for BPPV by involved canal and type (canalithiasis vs. cupulolithiasis).

*Intervention for Posterior Canal BPPV.* The current **Epley maneuver** (Fig. 29-3) is the most widely used and accepted maneuver for posterior canal canalithiasis–type BPPV. Recent literature supports no clinical difference between the effectiveness of the Epley maneuver and that of the Semont maneuver in treating posterior canal BPPV; when canal conversions with the two maneuvers were compared, four of 51 patients converted to a geotropic horizontal canal–type BPPV after the Epley, whereas none of the 51 who received the Semont converted to geotropic horizontal canal BPPV (Anagnostou, 2015).

This chapter focuses on the most widely used CRM, the Epley maneuver (Fig. 29-3): Start the patient in a long-sitting position. To ensure that the patient is positioned the precise distance from the edge of the mat (i.e., when the patient lies back, the head and neck are off the table, and she is able to move into neck extension), use a pillow to determine the distance from the mat surface to the top of the shoulders and position the pelvis this distance from the edge. Start the maneuver by quickly moving the patient into the Dix-Hallpike head-down position (supine position with the head rotated 45 degrees toward the affected side, and the neck extended 30 degrees beyond the horizontal plane). Have the patient hold this position until the nystagmus or vertigo stops. Rotate the patient's head to the opposite side with the neck remaining in extension. Ask the patient to hold this position for 30 seconds. Nystagmus is typically not observed in this position unless there is horizontal and/or multiple canal involvement. From here, assist the patient onto the uninvolved side with the head remaining in 45-degree rotation so she is looking toward the floor and her chin is tucked. Again, the position is held until the nystagmus and symptoms stop. Instruct the patient to bring her legs off the table and slowly return to sitting, with the head maintained in a rotated position toward the unaffected side and tilted downward. Maintain at least one hand on the patient's shoulder because she may experience some vertigo upon returning to the sitting position.

Once the CRM is completed and the patient returns to sitting, have her hold onto the side of the table for safety, and remain at her side. It is also important to observe for eye movement at this time. If the clinician observes a rotary transient nystagmus in the opposite direction of the original Dix-Hallpike, some of the otoconia may have fallen back into the canal (Herdman, 2014). If the clinician observes

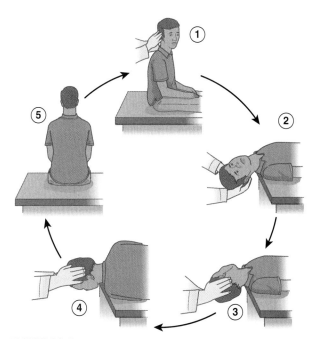

**FIGURE 29-3** The Epley maneuver shown for right posterior canalithiasis benign paroxysmal positional vertigo.

horizontal nystagmus during the maneuver, it is assumed the otoconia were transitioned into the horizontal canal during the maneuver (Lempert, 1996; Molina, 2007) or the patient may have multiple canal involvement. This does not commonly occur, but the clinician must be prepared. Patients commonly have nausea and may become very ill. The intervention may then require a CRM for the horizontal canal. Again, this does not occur often but is possible when BPPV is treated, especially in persons with head trauma who may have involvement of multiple canals.

Clinicians vary on how to proceed after a CRM (Prokopakis, 2005). Some clinicians proceed with home instruction and reexamine the patient in 3 to 5 days, whereas others repeat the testing (and CRM if needed) within the same treatment session. Often, these decisions are based on the patient's tolerance of the intervention. Hughes (2015) reported that symptoms resolved after one maneuver in 47% of patients, after two maneuvers in 16%, and after three maneuvers in 21%. The authors of this chapter repeat testing and treatment within the same session (up to five CRMs if needed) until the BPPV has resolved only when the patient can tolerate repeated maneuvers. Home instruction after the CRM is then provided to the patient, including an educational handout on the condition of BPPV.

Once treatment for BPPV is complete, past recommendations have included activity restrictions for 1 to 2 days to increase the likelihood of the otoconia adhering back into the macula. Activity restrictions vary among clinicians and are not required, but examples include:

- Avoid lying flat; maintain an elevation of at least 45 degrees
- Avoid certain head movements, such as cervical flexion or extension
- Avoid lying on the involved side

The use of postural restrictions has been debated in recently published literature. Fife (2008) took an in-depth look at the literature. Serious consideration was given to the level of research performed in the studies. Two class I studies and three class II studies showed benefits from the CRM with and without the use of postural restrictions. The studies were not designed to look specifically at whether postural restrictions played a role in the success of the CRM. Several class IV studies showed no added benefits from the use of postural restrictions. Fife (2008) concluded there was insufficient evidence (based on the methodology and class level of the studies) to support or rebuke the use of postural restrictions after CRM.

Another study looked retrospectively at patient outcomes after CRM and the use of postural restrictions, according to the length of the restriction (McGinnis, 2009). This group came to the same basic conclusion as Fife (2008), stating that the extent of the effects of postural restrictions on patient outcomes is uncertain. The group suggested that maintaining upright posture for 24 hours (as opposed to 48 hours) could produce favorable outcomes, but it also recommended that future randomized controlled studies should compare treatment outcomes of patients using postural restrictions for 24 hours with those not using restrictions (Cakir, 2006; McGinnis, 2009).

The **Semont (or liberatory) maneuver** (Fig. 29-4) developed by Semont (1988) has been effective for the correction of posterior canal cupulolithiasis BPPV, although it is thought to be more difficult for the patient to tolerate (Cohen, 2007). The patient initially sits up on the edge of the treatment table. Continuing with the example of the affected right posterior canal, the patient's head is turned 45 degrees to the left. The patient is moved into right sidelying, keeping the head turned so she is looking at the ceiling. Although there is no consensus regarding time spent in each position, Semont (1988) initially recommended that the patient remain in this position for 2 to 3 minutes and then rapidly move in an upward arc through the sitting position and down to left sidelying with the head maintained in 45 degrees of rotation to the left. This final position has the patient looking downward toward the treatment table because the left neck rotation is maintained throughout the maneuver. The patient should stay in this final position for an additional 2 to 3 minutes; the initial recommendation of 5 minutes is no longer standard (Brandt, 2013; Leigh, 2015). Nystagmus and vertigo may occur in each sidelying position because this treatment is very similar to the sidelying test. The patient is then brought back into the original sitting position.

A variety of clinical recommendations have been proposed for the Semont, including at least 45 seconds between the two movements and angles of 20 degrees or more below horizontal (Obrist, 2016). Other suggested modifications include staying in each position 4 minutes (Herdman, 1993), maintaining the patient in the provoking positions for around 1 minute (Tusa, 2005), and holding the initial sidelying position for 2 minutes and the final position for 3 minutes (Levrat, 2003). Typically, the same postural restrictions given after CRM are given after treatment with the Semont maneuver (Gans, 2002). Overall, studies have shown the Semont maneuver is successful in one or two visits, but the studies are not mentioned in the BPPV practice guidelines (Bhattacharyya, 2008, 2017).

**Brandt-Daroff exercises** (Fig. 29-5), developed by Brandt (1980) before BPPV repositioning techniques, are considered habituation exercises and should be used by the clinician as a last resort for BPPV, when repositioning is ineffective. This is especially important because CRM has been found to have a >80% success rate in one or two office

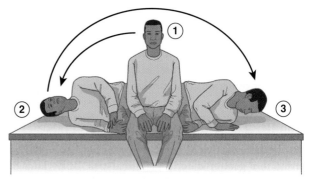

**FIGURE 29-4** The Semont (liberatory) maneuver shown for right posterior canal cupulolithiasis with the head turned to the nonaffected side as the patient lies down for step 2.

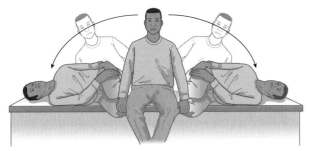

**FIGURE 29-5** Brandt-Daroff exercises for habituation.

visits (Helminski, 2010). The Brandt-Daroff procedure is similar to the Semont maneuver, but the patient is required to repeatedly move into the provoking position and stops in the middle to rest and change head positions. To begin, position the patient sitting at the edge of the treatment table with the head rotated 45 degrees *away* from the affected ear, and then ask the patient to close both eyes and lie down on the affected side (for the example of right BPPV, the patient now turns the head 45 degrees to the left and then rapidly goes into right sidelying). Ask the patient to maintain neck rotation for 30 seconds or until the vertigo resolves, and then assist the patient back to the sitting position with the head in neutral and wait approximately 30 seconds. Finally, ask the patient to rotate *toward* the affected ear and lie down to the unaffected side (in the example, rotate the head to the right and then lie down to the left side.). Hold this position for 30 seconds or until the symptoms resolve, and then instruct the patient to return to sitting. Maintain this position for 30 seconds or until symptoms resolve, and then ask the patient to return to sitting. The patient then repeats the entire maneuver multiple times to help desensitize the system to the provoking movements. The patient is instructed to continue this activity as part of a home program until the vertigo diminishes.

Originally, it was recommended that this sequence be repeated every 3 hours until experiencing 2 consecutive days without vertigo (Roberts, 2006a). More common clinical practice, however, involves asking the patient to perform 10 to 15 repetitions three times a day. A recent study found that 80.5% of patients had a negative Dix-Hallpike 1 week after the CRM compared with only 25% after Brandt-Daroff exercises (Amor-Dorado, 2012).

*Interventions for Anterior Canal BPPV.* Initially, a "reverse Epley" was recommended for anterior canalithiasis BPPV. For instance, when the clinician suspected right anterior canal BPPV, the Epley maneuver was performed in the sequence for the left posterior canal. However, this proposed treatment is not clearly understood, and when the anatomical position of the anterior canal is considered, it does not appear to be effective. More recently, the literature has focused on other approaches, one of which is to treat the anterior canal the same as the posterior canal (Waleem, 2008). Thus, when considering the case study, the clinician would repeat the Epley maneuver for the right anterior canal in the same series

previously discussed for the right posterior canal. Research has shown high success rates with this approach, although the sample sizes have been small (Jackson, 2007; Lopez-Escamez, 2005).

An alternative approach for anterior canalithiasis is to ask the patient to start in a sitting position and rotate the head to the unaffected side. As related in the case study in this chapter, the clinician asks the patient to turn the head 45 degrees to the left. With the head held in rotation, the patient is assisted into the supine position with the head extended 30 to 45 degrees off the end of the table. The therapist holds the patient in this position for 2 minutes and then assists the patient's head into 0-degree extension but keeps the rotation and holds for 1 minute. The therapist continues to support the patient's head, and then assists her in returning to the seated position with the neck rotated 0 degrees with 30 degrees of extension. Kim (2005) found that symptoms resolved after two treatments in 80% of patients treated with this technique and 96.7% with more than two treatments.

Yacovino (2009) modified this approach by starting the patient in a sitting position but without head rotation; the patient was then assisted into the supine position with the head extended 30 degrees. The patient's head was supported and maintained in this position for 30 seconds, and then the patient's neck was quickly flexed into a chin-to-chest position. This position was held for 30 seconds, and then the patient was assisted back to the sitting position while the neck remained in flexion for an additional 30 seconds. Yacovino (2009) found that symptoms resolved in 84.6% of patients after one treatment and 100% of patients after two treatments.

Treatment of the anterior canal (Casani, 2011a) remains controversial and is not addressed in the BPPV guidelines. Success rates have been high, as noted previously, but the sample sizes have been small. In addition, in the modified Epley approaches, the published studies lacked a control group. Posttreatment instructions for patients vary among clinicians, but as previously noted, the authors of this chapter support the 48-hour precautions.

Anterior canal cupulolithiasis is rare, and the research is sparse. Initially, the Semont maneuver was proposed but with the head turned to the affected side, which is opposite to the treatment of posterior cupulolithiasis. For example, if the anterior canal of the right ear is affected, ask the patient to turn the head 45 degrees to the right, and then move her quickly from sitting on the edge of the table into right sidelying. After 1 minute, quickly transition the patient from right sidelying to left sidelying, with the head still turned 45 degrees to the right. The position is held for 1 minute, and then the patient slowly moves back into a sitting position.

Jackson (2007) discussed performing the CRM as described previously but added mastoid vibration or performance of the Semont maneuver followed by the CRM. Brandt-Daroff exercises which were not canal specific were performed as described for the posterior canal. Again, the lack of evidence specific to the anterior canal makes it difficult to suggest a specific approach, although the treatment can be similar to approaches described earlier.

*Interventions for Horizontal Canal BPPV.* As discussed in Chapter 8 and summarized in Table 29-4, the roll test for the horizontal canal more commonly elicits geotropic (toward the ground) nystagmus and is most often associated with horizontal canalithiasis, for which the barbeque roll is used. Ageotropic (away from the ground) nystagmus, sometimes referred to as *apogeotropic nystagmus*, is associated with cupulolithiasis in the long arm or canalithiasis in the short (anterior) arm of the horizontal canal. The following treatment approaches have been described in the literature for ageotropic nystagmus.

When the patient is diagnosed with horizontal canal BPPV, the treatment approach differs from that of the posterior or anterior canal. Historically, the treatment for horizontal canal BPPV is called the **horizontal roll or barbecue roll (or Lempert maneuver)** (Fig. 29-6) for horizontal canalithiasis (Asprella, 2005; Tirelli, 2004). To begin this maneuver, position the patient in supine with the neck flexed 20 to 30 degrees and rotated 90 degrees toward the involved side so that the affected ear is parallel with the table (toward the right for our patient example with right-sided horizontal canal BPPV). Hold the patient in this position for 30 to 60 seconds or until the nystagmus stops. When the patient has limited cervical

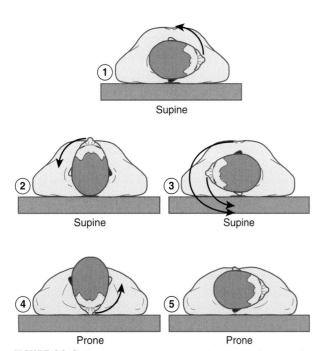

**FIGURE 29-6** The horizontal roll and barbecue roll (Lempert) techniques shown for right-sided horizontal canalithiasis. In these diagrams, patient's affected ear (right) is shown in red. (A) Start with the head turned 90 degrees toward the lesion (right) side with the nose pointing to the side. (B) Turn the head 90 degrees toward the opposite side so the nose is pointing up. (C) Turn the head 90 degrees toward the unaffected side, with the nose pointing toward the unaffected side (180 degrees from position A). (D) Turn the head 90 degrees and the body 180 degrees toward the unaffected ear to end in the supine position with the nose pointing down (ending 240 degrees from position A). (E) Finally, turn the nose and body toward the unaffected ear, returning to the start position.

range of motion, the clinician can start the patient in right sidelying (versus the supine position with right neck rotation). Once the nystagmus and symptoms have resolved, slowly roll the patient's head 90 degrees toward the uninvolved side, ending in a centered position, facing up. This position is held for 30 to 60 seconds or until the symptoms resolve. Then continue to roll the patient's head 90 degrees toward the unaffected ear so the affected ear is now facing up toward the ceiling. The position is again held for about 30 to 60 seconds or until the symptoms resolve. Next, instruct the patient to roll the head and body in the same direction, toward the uninvolved side, resulting in the patient now facing the floor (in the prone position or in the prone-on-elbow position) with the neck slightly flexed. In the stated patient example, the clinician is moving the patient in a counterclockwise position (away from the right ear). This last position is also held for about 30 to 60 seconds or until the symptoms resolve; then the patient is slowly rotated back into the original starting position. Hold this position for 30 to 60 seconds or until the symptoms resolve. While remaining in close contact with the patient, ask her to return to a sitting position, keeping the head level or slightly pitched down about 20 to 30 degrees.

A more recent intervention for horizontal canalithiasis was described by Appiani (2001) and Gufoni (1998), and the literature labels this technique either the **Appiani maneuver** or the **Gufoni maneuver to the unaffected side** for the anterior, or short arm, of the horizontal canal.

As shown in Fig. 29-7, start the Appiani or Gufoni procedure with the patient centered on a treatment table, sitting at the edge. Bring the patient down toward the unaffected ear (to left sidelying in the example of right horizontal canalithiasis), and ask her to remain in this sidelying position for 2 minutes. Then turn the head down 45 degrees toward the unaffected side so the patient is facedown (toward the left in our patient example), and again hold this position for 2 minutes. Finally, bring the patient back into the sitting position (Mandalà, 2013).

A variant of the Appiani or Gufoni maneuver specifically for *horizontal canal cupulolithiasis* is a modified Semont maneuver termed the **Casani maneuver** (Casani, 2002, 2011b) or **Gufoni to the affected side,** shown in Fig. 29-8 (van den Broek, 2014). Start with the patient sitting on the edge of the table with the head maintained in the neutral position but supported with the clinician's hands. Ask the patient to *quickly* lie down on the affected side (toward the right side for our patient example), and immediately rotate the patient's neck 45 degrees to the affected side (right in this example) while maintaining support of the head, ending in a nose-down position. Hold this position for 2 to 3 minutes and then return the patient to the seated position. Finally, return the head to neutral.

Research supporting the Casani maneuver is limited, and there is less evidence of accuracy in identifying which ear is involved with horizontal BPPV than with posterior canal BPPV. Typically, the affected ear for horizontal canalithiasis is identified as being the side or position that evokes the strongest response (see Table 29-4). However, the position that

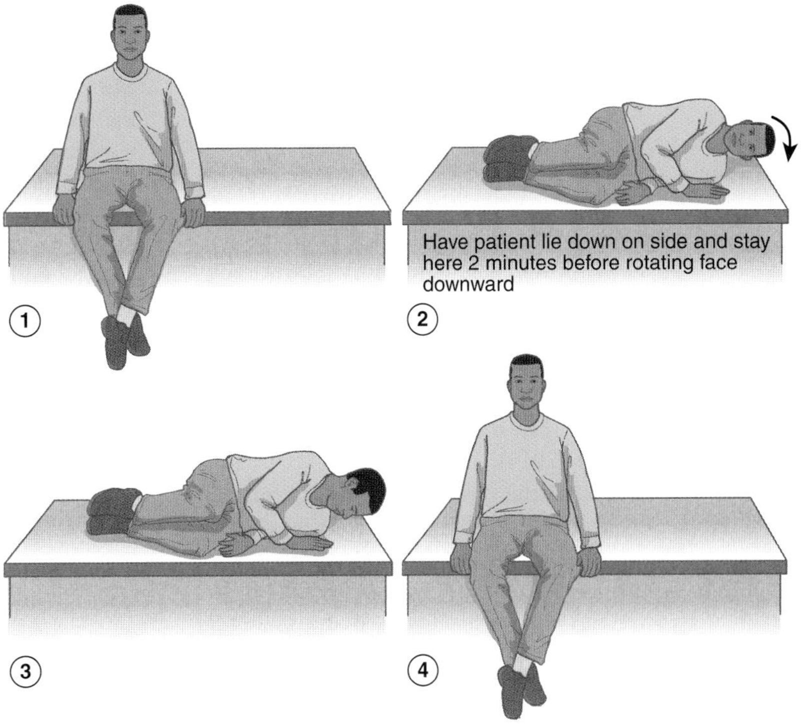

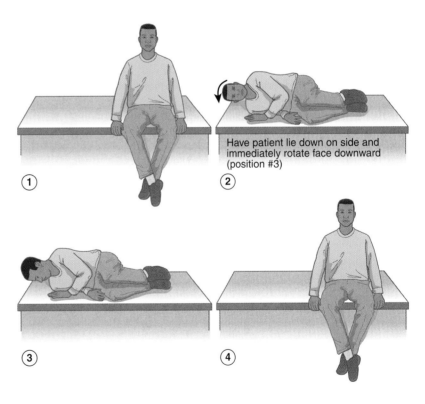

**FIGURE 29-7** The Appiani maneuver (Gufoni to the unaffected side) shown for right-sided horizontal canalithiasis. (1) Start in a sitting position on the edge of a mat, head neutral, nose forward. (2) Move into sidelying toward the unaffected ear, head neutral with the nose forward, and hold for 2 minutes. (3) Then in sidelying, quickly turn the head 45 degrees toward the unaffected side with the face down and hold for 2 minutes. (4) Return to sitting on the edge with the head still turned 45 degrees toward the unaffected side, the nose away from the side of the lesion, finally turning the head toward neutral with the nose forward.

Have patient lie down on side and stay here 2 minutes before rotating face downward

**FIGURE 29-8** The Casani maneuver (Gufoni to the affected side) shown for right-sided horizontal canal cupulolithiasis. (1) Start in a sitting position on the edge of the mat with the head neutral and nose forward. (2) Quickly move into sidelying toward the affected side, with the head neutral and the nose forward. (3) *Immediately*, you quickly turn the head 45 degrees toward the affected side with the nose down and hold the position for 2 minutes. (4) Return to sitting on the edge with the head still rotated 45 degrees and the nose toward the lesioned side, finally turning the head back to neutral with the nose forward.

Have patient lie down on side and immediately rotate face downward (position #3)

provokes the least amount of nystagmus might be considered the affected ear when ageotropic nystagmus is present, in cupulolithiasis. Another special circumstance might be when a patient has posterior canal BPPV on the right side, the contralateral ear might also have horizontal canal involvement. When treatment for one side is not effective within a reasonable time, treating the opposite side is recommended.

Regardless, special consideration should be taken with any repositioning procedure involving the horizontal canals because this type of BPPV can cause very intense symptoms relative to those involving the anterior or posterior canals.

**Forced prolonged positioning** is another technique for treating horizontal canal BPPV, especially when the patient is unable to perform the positions necessary for a barbecue roll maneuver, as in the elderly and obese (Chiou, 2005; Gufoni, 1998). A patient with horizontal canalithiasis should be instructed to (1) lie down on the affected side for 30 to 60 seconds, (2) roll to supine, (3) roll onto the unaffected side, and (4) remain in this position for 12 hours (Vannucchi, 1997). As imagined, this is not a widely used technique, but it has been effective in this population (Crevits, 2004; Han, 2006) and particularly in combination with the barbeque roll intervention (Casani, 2002). Comparisons of forced prolonged positioning with Gufoni and barbeque roll maneuvers in the treatment of horizontal canal BPPV have revealed similar nonsignificant success rates (i.e., 76% for prolonged positioning and 89% for Gufoni); however, each maneuver was more successful than the barbeque roll (i.e., success rate of 38%) after one application (Maranhão, 2015).

Table 29-5 prioritizes the various interventions for each canal involvement and type of BPPV (canalithiasis vs. cupulolithiasis). Helminski (2010) analyzed the research for BPPV, looking at the quality and methodology of the studies. The CRM received a level A recommendation from the researchers as an effective tool for the treatment of posterior canal BPPV. The liberatory (Semont) maneuver is proposed next as possibly effective, receiving a level C recommendation on the basis of the quality and methodology of the research. To date, the Brandt-Daroff exercises have been the least effective self-administered treatment according to the available evidence (Helminski, 2010). Considering the level of the studies analyzed for the horizontal and anterior canal treatments (class IV studies), the proposed techniques appear to be moderately effective (Hansson, 2007).

Once a patient's BPPV has resolved, either as a result of spontaneous recovery or from treatment by an experienced clinician, the patient may continue to complain of residual balance problems. In this case, traditional physical therapy balance rehabilitation is appropriate. Exercise techniques should focus on existing impairments in the balance, musculoskeletal, and neuromuscular systems.

Surgery is rarely used to treat BPPV but may be necessary and is performed by an ENT physician—typically an otologist or neurotologist.

## THINK ABOUT IT 29.2

- When are canalith repositioning maneuvers indicated for benign paroxysmal positional vertigo (BPPV) in vestibular rehabilitation?
- How will you differentiate between anterior, posterior, and horizontal canal BPPV? How will your interventions differ on the basis of the involved canal and canalithiasis versus cupulolithiasis?
- What type of patient education and postintervention instructions will you provide your patient after completion of the different techniques?
  - Canalith repositioning (Epley maneuver)
  - Liberatory maneuver
  - Brandt-Daroff
  - Barbeque roll or modified Gufoni

## Summary Pearls for BPPV

BPPV is a common disorder that can cause vertigo, dizziness, and nausea as a result of misplaced particles in one or more of the semicircular canals; nevertheless, there is a high rate of resolution of symptoms in one or two office visits. However, the clinician should also be aware of the possibility of recurrence. There is a 15% recurrence rate in the first year after treatment, and by 5 years, the incidence rate increases to 50% (Hain, 2000; Nunez, 2000). Postural instability may also be associated with BPPV, as well as other symptoms that suggest additional pathology. Thus, comprehensive examination and evaluation are recommended for all patients with classic BPPV symptoms.

A final recommendation, especially for clinicians who are in a vestibular rehabilitation setting, is the use of advanced technology. For example, performing positional testing with technology is preferred for obtaining the most accurate diagnosis, especially in confirming which canal(s) may be involved and for differential diagnosis of nystagmus (e.g., an acute vestibular lesion and/or central nervous system pathology) (Strupp, 1998). Additional diagnostic assessments may include positional testing using infrared video goggles; this test has the greatest accuracy for observing the components of nystagmus, which are often difficult to observe without magnification (Herdman, 2007). Frenzel lenses can also be used and are cost-effective for the clinician when viewing nystagmus. ENG is often considered the "gold standard" for diagnosing vestibular dysfunction, but it may not adequately record the torsional component of the nystagmus found with BPPV (Molina, 2007). Of course, BPPV is often diagnosed accurately without any technology, relying merely on the clinical observation of the tester.

Although BPPV can occur by itself, it is commonly seen with other inner ear disorders. Therefore, additional balance and hearing tests can provide comprehensive information about underlying causes of BPPV. Underlying pathology is a concern when the patient has additional symptoms, such as tinnitus, hearing loss, recurring spells of vertigo, postural instability, and/or additional neurological findings.

## PATIENT APPLICATION

*Susan is a 76 year-old female who presents to the clinic with a chief complaint of "dizziness." When asked to clarify her symptoms, she states, "Two weeks ago, the room began spinning in the middle of the night when I rolled onto my right side in bed." Since that time, Susan reports experiencing brief episodes of vertigo (approximately 15 seconds) when she tilts her head to look upward and when she bends forward to tie her shoes. She denies gross instability between episodes of vertigo, but she reports feeling "off-balance." After her initial episode of vertigo, she was seen by her PCP. Her physician ruled out vertigo due to central nervous system pathology.*

## Contemplate Clinical Decisions

1. *On the basis of Susan's subjective reporting, what working hypothesis have you developed relating to a physical therapy diagnosis?*

2. *What further questions are important to ask Susan?*

3. *What physical therapy tests and measures would be most appropriate in your examination of Susan?*

4. *What goals would be appropriate for this patient?*

5. *What intervention(s) do you anticipate as part of your plan of care?*

6. *What patient education will be important for this patient?*

### Equipment to Supplement Vestibular Rehabilitation

New advances in interactive computer technology provide a virtual reality (VR) environment featuring a progression of sensorimotor challenges. Technologies that augment sensory feedback using tactile or vibratory feedback systems are also available. However, additional clinical trials are necessary to document the role of these new technologies in the evidence-based treatment of vestibular-related impairments (Bromwich, 2008; Clement, 2007).

Several computerized devices have been developed to assist in positioning patients for the vestibular examination, evaluation, differential diagnosis, and treatment of BPPV, including the analysis of different types of nystagmus. The Epley Omniax chair (Vesticon, Portland, OR), shown in Fig. 29-9, is a multiaxis rotary chair that can position the patient securely while also stabilizing the head relative to the body, moving the patient—and most importantly the head—in space with great ease. This chair can rotate the patient 360 degrees in any plane in order to place the head in the required position relative to gravity. The computer system helps to document and analyze nystagmus, providing the clinician with advanced information for differential diagnosis. The clinician then programs the computer to move the patient through the treatment maneuver specific for her type of BPPV.

Another computerized positioning device is the TRV Chair by Interacoustics (www.interacoustics.com) (Fig. 29-10). The chair is ideally balanced, and its support mechanisms allow the examiner to easily move the patient in three dimensions and hold the patient in any position for vestibular intervention (Cauthen, 2016), in conjunction with the analysis of nystagmus via infrared goggles for a detailed examination of the vestibular system. The TRV Chair allows 360-degree rotational movement in the precise plane of each semicircular canal. During analysis and treatment, the patient remains in a seated position. With the TRV Chair, rehabilitation of patients with BPPV includes maneuvers such as the Epley, Semont, and barbeque rolls. The effectiveness of these maneuvers can be enhanced by adding kinetic energy; this is done by driving the main arm of the chair against a hydraulic stop, which can generate sufficient force to free small otoconia. The TRV Chair may substantially improve treatment efficacy and decrease the number of treatment sessions for successful repositioning compared with traditional canalith repositioning procedures (Tan, 2014).

VR is another area with growing applications for vestibular rehabilitation. Sensitivity to visual phenomena can be extremely debilitating for a patient with vestibular dysfunction. Everyday activities such as grocery shopping, riding as a passenger in the car, and walking on busy carpeting can become intolerable. In recent years, VRT has attempted to recreate busy visual stimuli in the clinic using technology and computer systems such as Wii Balance, a disco ball, and optokinetic exercises that can be found on YouTube or downloaded as smartphone/tablet apps. In 2014, Google created a VR device called Google

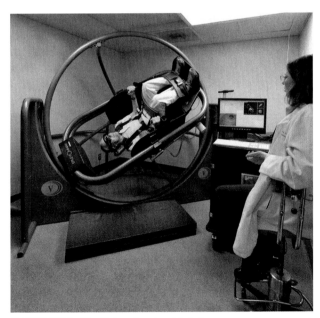

**FIGURE 29-9** The Epley Omniax Chair is a computer-operated, patient positioning system (i.e., the patient is strapped securely in the multiaxial chair) that facilitates standardized positional testing; used with video nystagmography to improve diagnosis and enhance direct intervention for benign paroxysmal positional vertigo by recreating the repositioning techniques that are specific for the patient's diagnosis.

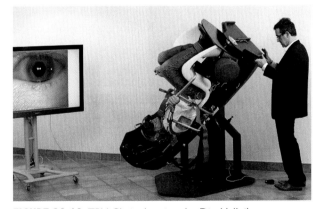

**FIGURE 29-10** TRV Chair showing the Dix-Hallpike maneuver for the right posterior canal. The TRV Chair enhances diagnosis of benign paroxysmal positional vertigo, simplifies and increases the effectiveness of treatment, and is particularly useful for those unable to be repositioned manually. *(Photo courtesy of Interacoustics, http://www.interacoustics.com/trv-chair)*

VR (https://vr.google.com/) that allows patients to experience 3-D activities visually, such as riding a roller coaster and walking through Paris. Samsung Gear VR is a similar device . Although these systems are considered "gaming devices" for entertainment, they provide an inexpensive and fun way to expose patients to uncomfortable stimuli and, in turn, decrease sensitivity to visual disturbances (Cauthen, 2016).

# ■ Intervention: Ultimately Applied in Functional Activities

The primary goal of any rehabilitation program is to improve the patient's functional abilities during daily activities and enhance overall quality of life. Therefore, vestibular rehabilitation should address patient-specific functional tasks related to activity limitations and participation restrictions identified during the initial examination. And obviously, a patient with vestibular dysfunction needs to receive interventions focused on improving balance (see Chapter 30) in a variety of functional tasks (see Chapters 33 through 37).

## Functional Interventions

Functional outcomes can be assessed according to specific categories, including basic or advanced functional mobility or patient-specific higher skills required for work or leisure activities (Borello-France, 1999, 2002). A clinician may integrate the following functional activities into interventions to address limitations identified during the evaluation.

### Basic Mobility Skills

When the goal is decreasing the influence of abnormal vestibular responses, basic mobility skills to practice include bed mobility (e.g., rolling, supine to sit) discussed in Chapter 34, functional transfers (e.g., bathroom maneuvers, chair transfers) discussed in Chapter 35, and gait (e.g., on even surfaces or in small spaces) discussed in Chapter 37. Limitations of basic mobility skills may be identified from patient responses to the Motion Sensitivity Quotient or by observing the patient performing these functional skills. The therapist may instruct the patient to practice the tasks that are challenging or that provoke symptoms on the basis of the patient's presentation.

### Advanced Mobility Skills

Advanced mobility skills may include gait over uneven terrain (i.e., grass vs. gravel), climbing skills (i.e., stairs or ladders), and mobility with changes of body postures (i.e., crawling or hopping). Practice of these advanced mobility skills may be integrated to improve functional mobility and decrease the risk of falls. As a progression to the plan of care, adaptation exercises can be integrated into these functional mobility skills as appropriate to continue vestibular-specific activities.

### Specialty Skills

Specialty mobility skills include driving, running, working in high places, reading or computer work, or special occupations such as military service (Cohen, 2003b; Hamish, 2009; Scherer,

2009). When a patient identifies a need to return to performing these skills, activities that simulate them will be beneficial in the plan of care. Partial-task practice of these skills or education on shorter duration of these activities may also gradually progress the patient toward completion of the whole task.

## THINK ABOUT IT 29.3

- Why is it important to understand the activity limitations and participation restrictions of your patients with vestibular involvement?
- How can functional tasks be integrated into the intervention plan for a patient with vestibular involvement?

## Pediatric Considerations

According to recent studies, there is a 20% incidence of BPPV in pediatric patients who present with balance problems, dizziness, oscillopsia, or vertigo (Batson, 2004; Rine, 2016). Children with sensorineural hearing loss have documented deficits in dynamic visual acuity (Braswell, 2001). Therefore, a complete vestibular assessment is crucial before attempting rehabilitative treatments in this population (Rine, 2016). Treatment of BPPV in children is similar to that of adults, but with special considerations. Treatment strategies should emphasize adaptation, habituation, and/or substitution as described in earlier sections of this chapter. However, the intervention should also include developmental postures because of the high incidence of associated motor impairments and delayed development of the visual or somatosensory feedback for balance and coordination (Rajendran, 2012; Wiener-Vacher, 2008, 2012). The disruption of normal vestibular function may dramatically interfere with both static and dynamic postural control, especially when the child is younger than 6 years old, which is before typical adult balance skills develop (Rine, 2014). In fact, benign paroxysmal positional vertigo of childhood is a condition specific to children younger than 6 years and is characterized by symptoms that are not always related to position or movement. The child may experience acute bouts of vertigo or vomiting despite having normal hearing and without nystagmus or tinnitus. Symptoms are commonly misdiagnosed as the flu; however, symptoms do recur periodically to interfere with ADLs. Affected children respond well to targeted rehabilitation.

### PATIENT APPLICATION

*Patrick is a well-developed 5 year-old male who has just started kindergarten. His parents report that he fell on the playground 2 weeks ago with no evident injuries; however, he complains of problems seeing the chalkboard at school. He has been falling a lot recently during play. When questioned about why he is falling, he states that he feels worse in the morning when he gets out of bed, and his stomach feels funny sometimes, so he refuses to eat breakfast. His parents report that recent doctor visits and laboratory tests revealed no problems.*

- *Patient treatment plan and follow-up*

*An appropriate canalith repositioning procedure may be helpful. Therapeutic exercises could include visual tracking of favorite toys while the patient assumes static and dynamic postures to promote gaze stability, balance, and movement activities for age-appropriate play activities. A 6-week program including gaze stability exercises, 20 minutes per session, three times per week could improve motor scores (Braswell, 2006; Rine, 2004).*

- *Considerations for development of a patient-specific treatment plan*

  *Problems list:*

1. *Age (<6 years), developing balance system*
2. *Recent fall at school associated with onset of symptoms*
3. *Problems with visual gaze stability (difficulty with chalkboard at school)*
4. *Increased symptoms upon rising from bed in the morning, sometimes severe enough to cause nausea*
5. *Evidence of impaired balance and coordination with recent falls*

### Contemplate Clinical Decisions

*Based on Patrick's symptoms and his parents' report, what working hypothesis have you developed related to a physical therapy diagnosis?*

1. *What additional questions are important to ask Patrick and his parents?*
2. *What physical therapy tests and measures would be most appropriate in your examination?*
3. *What age-appropriate goals might be set for this patient?*
4. *What intervention(s) would you anticipate as part of your plan of care?*
5. *What self-care education will be important for this patient and his parents?*

## ◾ Intervention: Considerations for Nontherapy Time and Discharge

The focus of VRT is to provide not only symptom relief during treatment sessions but also patient education on self-management and improvement of life skills for better function.

## Patient and Family Education

Patient education is crucial to any rehabilitation program because patients should learn how to practice prescribed exercise routines on their own for ongoing improvement and maintenance of any gains realized. In addition, it may be helpful to instruct family members or caregivers in special symptom management techniques to ensure proper patient care at home.

In the context of vestibular impairment, patient education regarding expectations and symptom management is particularly important, with a home program that integrates vestibular techniques. For example, home exercise programs that include adaptation and habituation exercises may exacerbate symptoms for a short time. If patients are not aware of this possibility, they may perceive that the program is having a negative effect on the recovery process. On the other hand, patients should be educated about when to terminate exercises to avoid overstimulation of the vestibular system

## Activities for Home

Possible home activities include adaptation exercises, habituation exercises, or a combination that includes functional tasks specific to the patient's activity limitations or participation restrictions. Patients may also benefit from integration of balance exercises at home, performed in a safe manner, to improve postural instability. To progress the patient toward individual goals, mobility activities can also be integrated in a variety of home environments, with supervision for safety. For example, the patient may be instructed to practice turning in tight spaces while carrying the groceries or laundry or going up or down stairs at home with a family member to ensure safety.

### PATIENT APPLICATION

*Missy is a 53 year-old female who presents to the clinic with dizziness and decreased balance. She reports feeling very unsteady. She was sick 2 months ago with a bacterial infection for which she received gentamicin. She saw her PCP, who ruled out any central neurological deficit. Results of magnetic resonance imaging of her brain were normal. Missy's medications include levothyroxine, meclizine, multiple vitamins with iron, and vitamin $D_3$. Missy's goals are to return to her previously active lifestyle, especially walking with her dogs daily for 3 to 5 miles.*

*A physical examination reveals normal range of motion; she has 5/5 strength in bilateral extremities; her extraocular movements show full motion with no nystagmus; results of the Romberg test are negative; and her timed up-and-go rate is 13.2 seconds. Missy ambulates without an assistive device but displays ataxia. Her gait is wide-based with three episodes of balance loss within 100 ft. Missy can self-catch with use of her upper extremities on near objects. Further testing reveals corrective saccades with head thrust to both left and right and normal visual acuity that is decreased with head movement. On clinical test for sensory integration and balance testing, Missy shows increased sway on foam, and she was unable to maintain her balance on foam with her eyes closed.*

*Given Missy's history, the therapist refers her to an otolaryngologist who completes rotary chair and caloric testing, posturography, and VEMPs. Caloric testing shows absent responses bilaterally. Rotary chair testing revealed no eye movements at frequencies <0.5 Hz and only a few beats of nystagmus with deceleration from 90 degrees per second constant velocity. On posturography, Missy demonstrates excessive sway on situation 5 (moving platform with eyes closed) and is unable to maintain her balance on situation 6 (altered platform with inaccurate visual cues). VEMPs show reduced responses bilaterally. Differential diagnosis: bilateral vestibular dysfunction secondary to ototoxicity. Missy returns to therapy for vestibular rehabilitation.*

## Contemplate Clinical Decisions

*What additional information do you need to know to better individualize Missy's plan of care?*

1. *What is the prognosis for recovery in this case?*
2. *Based on this case, what vestibular rehabilitation techniques would you integrate in the treatment of Missy's condition?*
3. *What patient education do you anticipate integrating into your therapy sessions?*

### PATIENT APPLICATION CONTINUED

*Vestibular rehabilitation for Missy includes gaze stabilization exercises, starting with VOR X1 exercises. Missy completes three sets of 1-minute intervals of VOR X1 exercises in horizontal and vertical directions while standing. Missy can perform the exercises with a slight increase in her symptoms, which resolve with rest breaks. She is instructed to perform these exercises at home in the standing position. Missy is educated on the*

*importance of pushing into her symptoms of dizziness during the exercises but to stop before they became too severe. The symptoms should resolve within 30 minutes of the exercises. When symptoms do not resolve in 30 minutes, it indicates that she has overworked the system and may want to do a little less next time.*

*During the physical therapy intervention, Missy is asked to perform balance training activities that integrate various surfaces, such as walking on foam or walking outdoors on a grassy surface while performing horizontal or vertical head turns. Missy is introduced to habituation exercises by asking her to repeatedly transition into and out of the supine position five times in each direction, as this position change is the one most likely to provoke her dizziness. Missy is instructed to wait for her symptoms to resolve before the next repetition of the supine-to-sit sequence. Missy is educated on integrating this therapeutic activity of repeated supine-to/from-sit transitions at home by performing two or three repetitions twice per day.*

# HANDS-ON PRACTICE

After completion of this chapter and with further practice, you should be able to perform the following vestibular rehabilitation intervention techniques:

- Adaptation exercises
  - VOR X1 and VOR X2 viewing exercises
- Substitution/compensation exercises
  - Active eye-head movements between two targets
  - Remembered targets
  - Cawthorne-Cooksey exercises
- Habituation exercises
  - Brandt-Daroff exercises
  - Use of provoking positions/movements to develop individualized exercises

- Canalith repositioning maneuvers
  - Epley maneuver
  - Semont liberatory maneuver
  - Barbecue roll (Lempert maneuver)
  - Appiani (or Gufoni toward the unaffected side) maneuver
  - Casani (or Gufoni toward the affected side) maneuver

## Let's Review

1. How will you determine which patients are appropriate for vestibular rehabilitation therapy?

2. What specific interventions are appropriate for addressing vestibular hypofunction resulting in issues with gaze stability? How do these system-targeted interventions impact expected recovery?

3. What specific interventions are appropriate for addressing vestibular impairments related to motion sensitivity? How might systems-targeted interventions impact expected movement tolerance?

4. What specific interventions are appropriate for addressing benign paroxysmal positional vertigo? How will you decide which maneuver to apply to your patient?

5. How do activity limitations and participation restrictions affect your treatment plan for patients with vestibular impairments?

**6.** How do you progress your patient's intervention plan, and how do you know when your patient is ready to be progressed?

**7.** What are key components related to patient education for those undergoing vestibular rehabilitation therapy?

**8.** How might you have to modify your intervention for a pediatric patient?

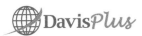 For additional resources, including Focus on Evidence tables, case study discussions, references, and glossary, please visit http://davisplus.fadavis.com

## CHAPTER SUMMARY

Intervention for vestibular impairment should include treatment strategies based on the concepts of adaptation, substitution, and habituation, particularly when the patient has peripheral vestibular hypofunction (unilateral or bilateral). Interventions for BPPV include specific canalith repositioning procedures, most commonly the Epley maneuver for posterior and anterior canal canalithiasis. With all vestibular impairments, it is essential to assess and address gaze stabilization and vestibular-related postural instability and their effects on functional activities. While this chapter presents the basics of vestibular rehabilitation, there are courses that present advanced vestibular rehabiliation reasoning and techniques.

The Focus on Evidence (FOE) tables with evidence supporting vestibular rehabilitation (Vestibular Hypofunction in Table 29-6 and BPPV in Table 29-7 ONL), including all major studies that contribute to the evidence base, can be found in the online resources that will be made available to readers.

## CHAPTER OBJECTIVES

Upon completion of this chapter, the learner should be able to:
1. Recognize and describe the pathophysiology of balance impairment including the influence of aging.
2. Design a balance intervention plan that is customized for a specific patient and his stage of disease or recovery.
3. Design a balance intervention plan that addresses identified underlying impairments of body structure/body function.
4. Implement a balance intervention plan including intentional progressive demand through advancing functional activities.

## ▰ Introduction

*Fawn*, age 17 years, was very athletic and active in her school before the accident. She now has a medical diagnosis of traumatic brain injury. She was the passenger in a motor vehicle accident and was not wearing her seat belt when her friend, the driver of the car, ran a stop sign. Her side of the car was hit by a city bus going 45 miles per hour. She was thrown from the car, sustained a closed head injury, and was unconscious for 3 days with an initial Glasgow Coma Scale (GCS) score of 7. Computed tomography scans revealed a subdural hematoma in the left parietal area, with cerebral contusions and scattered subarachnoid hemorrhages over the posterior aspects of the frontal lobe and the anterior aspects of the parietal lobe on the left, and focal hemorrhagic lesions of the deep cerebral white matter (corona radiata and internal capsule) on the left and the anterior surface of the brainstem on the left, particularly the cerebral peduncle, pons, and pyramids. With this damage, motor impairments are certain, with expected decreases in Fawn's balance.

**Balance,** as described in more detail in Chapter 9, is the ability to maintain physical **equilibrium** or *stability* in an upright posture; it is pervasive across higher human physical functioning. **Postural control,** a related term, is defined by Horak (1987, p.1881) as "the ability to maintain equilibrium in a gravitational environment." Upright balance can also be described using terms from the field of physics: A stable object is physically in *equilibrium,* with balanced interactions between all parts and the environment. With the upright human body, balance occurs by avoiding leaning too far forward, too far back, or too far to either side, with balanced use of lower extremity muscles to maintain the body over the points of support. Balance or postural control is an essential part of every upright skill we perform. We depend on balance to keep the body upright during a wide variety of functional tasks, ranging from simple, quiet standing to standing against extreme external disturbances. Whether sitting or standing, balance can be observed in every social setting. The postural adjustments used to maintain balance range from the nearly imperceptible to the extremely obvious.

The term *balance* can describe a process/action or a state or outcome. The concept of balance is sometimes described using other terms. **Postural balance** and **postural control** are more general terms describing balance aimed at maintaining an upright posture. *Equilibrium reaction* is a term used particularly for balance during the developmental process, which involves the ability to balance in upright. Humans generally begin to acquire balance through integrated action of sensory and motor systems as part of normal development in the first year of life.

When the systems involved in balance are intact, humans can maintain an upright posture across a continuum of external challenges during static activities, such as reading a favorite book while quietly sitting or standing still without disturbance to avoid getting bumped by an overzealous shopper at the department store clearance sale. We also respond to drastic postural perturbations and unexpected external forces, such as being tackled on the football field. Remarkably, much of this central nervous system processing takes place very quickly and at a subconscious level.

Because balance is a critical component of all upright functional tasks, impaired balance usually interferes with function. When deficits occur in the ability to maintain balance, the risk of falling increases. As an individual becomes aware of his increased personal risk, the level of activity is purposefully decreased, with fewer risks taken. The overall decreased mobility leads to decreased strength, endurance, and neuromuscular control. This in turn results in disability because the individual is unable to complete certain life roles. For example, a patient may be unable to maintain balance in ambulation after a brain injury because of impaired lower extremity motor control. This can lead to immobility that decreases muscle strength and endurance. All of these factors impair his ability to walk. He cannot maintain his job and requires assistance for much of his self-care and transfers. For the individual, the resulting increased safety risk and fear of falling become major concerns, necessitating comprehensive examination and individualized therapeutic intervention with education.

## Clinical Picture of Balance Impairment

Clinically, patients with balance impairment often compensate for functional limitations by using assistive devices to increase stability, especially in ambulation. Among elders, better performance on balance tests is associated with greater independence in mobility and activities of daily living (ADLs) (Era, 1997).

Depending on the severity of the dysfunction, a person with decreased balance may have difficulty performing any of the following functional tasks: maintaining upright sitting posture; scooting while in a sitting position; reaching from a sitting position; completing transitional movements such as sit-to-stand or transfers; maintaining static standing without external disturbance; reaching from standing; squatting to lift an object from the floor; or ambulating on level surfaces, uneven surfaces, or up and down stairs. In children, balance is also commonly required in quadruped, kneeling, and half-kneeling. As a result of functional limitations in any of these activities, a person may be unable to fulfill one or more life roles and may become disabled.

Just as the aforementioned skills can be categorized as static or dynamic, the balance components contributing to each can be categorized as static balance or dynamic balance, as defined in Chapter 9. Both static and dynamic balance can be assessed using a variety of objective measures (see Chapter 9), including force-platform data, depending on whether the person intends to stay still in the posture or intends to move.

For the patient with a balance impairment, the therapist has several overarching objectives: (1) to educate the patient regarding safety and fall prevention, (2) to maximally remediate or correct identified impairments through skilled intervention, (3) to help the patient gain and learn compensatory strategies when remediation cannot be completed, (4) to improve the patient's confidence in his balance abilities, and (5) to return the patient to ADLs and recreational activities that were impaired by the balance dysfunction. Initially, the focus is usually on the first two tasks. In conditions with more permanent impairment (e.g., a complete spinal cord injury or other trauma for which improvement is unlikely), the focus shifts to alternative strategies, patterns, or assistive devices.

The potential to enhance and improve balance abilities exists even in people without impairments or limitations, especially through environmental manipulation and practice (i.e., consider the tightrope walker). This same principle is seen when healthy individuals regularly go to the gym and increase their strength beyond what is considered "normal." Regarding balance, Crotts (1996) used a single-leg stance modification of the Clinical Test of Sensory Interaction in Balance (CTSIB) to show that "under sensory challenged conditions, professional dancers were better able to maintain their postures upright against gravity" (p.12) than was the common nondancer. The elderly also have the ability to enhance and improve both strength and balance with specific training (Granacher, 2011; Hess, 2005; Holviala, 2014). They also have the ability to improve balance with static balance training (Jacobson, 2011).

## Safety Concerns

Instability is inherent and should be expected when impaired balance is part of a patient's problem list. Consequently, when evaluating the performance of the patient's balance systems and during any balance intervention, the therapist must have safety uppermost in mind. This attention to safety is particularly essential during intervention for balance impairment because the therapist will have to stress the impaired systems and place optimal demands on the patient's whole body through use of challenging, unstable, and precarious positions. Proper guarding techniques should be utilized at all times. Safety is maintained by using a gait belt or safety harness, working in or near parallel bars or hemi-bars, and working near a stable plinth or even near a wall; this can maximize patient safety and ensure the therapist's ability to safely help patients recover when they "lose" their balance.

The therapist should also be wearing sensible, flat, non-slip shoes and keep a wide base of support (BOS), avoiding transitional positions such as a single-limb stance. For example, a therapist who balances on one leg during a balance activity while pushing an obstacle out of the way with the other foot has diminished the ability to respond if the patient loses balance. This ultimately places the patient in jeopardy.

Although it is essential to give the patient sufficient support for safety, overguarding, support, and guidance are detrimental from a motor learning standpoint. Safety is always the first priority, and the therapist should err on the side of caution in terms of external support. The amount of upper extremity support should be decreased during these activities to progressively increase demand on the sensory and motor systems involved in balance. Practice with decreased upper extremity support gives the patient opportunities to use and integrate the systems, especially those related to the lower extremities.

## PATIENT APPLICATION

*Fawn was hospitalized for 6 weeks, including the intensive care stay, and required ventilator support for just 1 week. She was bedbound for 2 weeks before the physician ordered physical and occupational therapy evaluations for ADL training, transfers, mobility, and sitting balance. The hospitalization was followed by 6 weeks of inpatient rehabilitation therapy. The therapy focused on Fawn's primary balance impairment, which limited her transfer, ambulation, endurance, and ADL self-care abilities. She made dramatic improvements. Now that she is home with her parents, she is referred to you for home health therapy.*

*During your examination, Fawn is generally cheerful in her interactions with you. Despite the obvious asymmetry of her body, with a droopy right face and decreased movements of the right extremities, she is able to verbally communicate with you. Her speech is slurred and laborious. As she gets to know you, she shares that her greatest concerns are what her peers think about her appearance and the way she walks. She is a senior in high school, and she will barely be able to finish all of her classes this school year. She tells you she dreads the graduation ceremony 6 months from now because of how awkward it will be walking across the stage in front of everyone. She still trips so easily, and she realizes how stilted and "off" her walking looks to others. Yet deep inside, she dreams of being able to walk up and grab her diploma in her own hands. She has been working very hard to achieve this goal. When you ask what is most important to her, including her personal goals, she replies, "I will graduate this year, and I want to have good enough balance to be able to walk across the stage at my graduation without a cane and without tripping."*

### Contemplate Clinical Decisions

- What effect does Fawn's current cognitive level (GCS of 7) have on her balance and mobility?
- What implications do Fawn's medical diagnosis, acuity, and severity have in this initial stage of clinical decision-making, especially related to prognosis? Is continued recovery expected? Upon what do you base these conclusions?
- Identify other family, support, and home/social issues that have implications for her rehabilitation.
- What does her stated personal goal tell you about her priorities and motivation? Do you think her personal goal is achievable?
- List five ways you could enhance the patient-therapist relationship and model open communication with Fawn at this stage.
- How will her motivation contribute to her outcomes?

## ■ Anatomy and Physiology of Balance
### Systems Involved in Balance

While using the information in this chapter to formulate an intervention plan for balance, the therapist must realize that maintaining equilibrium is one of the most complex system interactions we will encounter when addressing human function. It is also essential to realize that although balance is not a function in and of itself, it is required for every functional activity and task. Balance dysfunction is a complex impairment that depends on the interaction of multiple sensory and motor systems, as described in Chapter 9.

Interventions can be developed to purposefully manipulate the inextricable interactions between the person, the environment, and the task. The three components of postural control as described by Horak (1987) are (1) biomechanical components (center of pressure [COP]; Fig. 30-1) and limits of stability (Fig. 30-2); (2) sensory components (somatosensory, visual, vestibular); and (3) motor components (the motor responses to maintain balance, including ankle, hip, and stepping strategies). Horak (2009) further expanded those subsets with the Balance Evaluating Systems Test (BESTest), which has six components: Biomechanical Constraints, Limits of Stability, Anticipatory Postural Adjustments, Postural Responses, Sensory Orientation, and Stability in Gait. These components are described in detail in Chapter 9 and must be considered carefully while developing the balance intervention plan.

The three levels of complex motor interactions, or three balance strategies have been described and categorized as **ankle strategy**, **hip strategy**, and **stepping strategy**, all described in detail in Chapter 9 (Horak, 1986; Nashner, 1976, 1985, 1990). From an intervention standpoint, the "strategy" model is a helpful framework, but universal application may be limited because the strategies were studied only in one plane and with EMG on selected muscles. Individuals often use a combination of strategies instead of an isolated ankle or hip strategy to respond to postural perturbations (Chvatal, 2011). The direction and timing of the movement of our center of mass (COM), not the direction of the perturbation, dictates which strategy one chooses

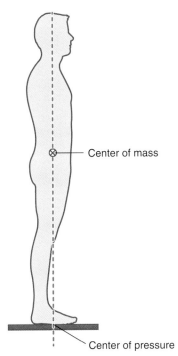

**FIGURE 30-1** Drawing of center of mass (COM) and center of pressure (COP) relationship to the standing body position: The point on the floor where a gravitational line falls directly from the COM is considered the COP.

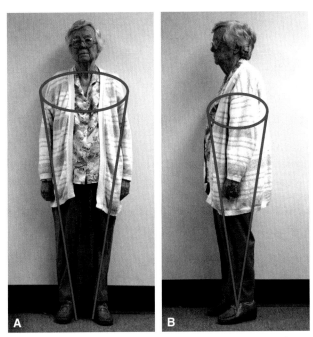

**FIGURE 30-2AB** Photograph of a patient with cone-shaped representation of the limits of stability (LOS) overdrawn, including anterior and lateral views, showing the degree to which a person can sway without loss of balance.

(Chvatal, 2011). The balance strategy we choose also depends on the position of our body. For example, a patient will respond with a different strategy if he loses his balance in a single-limb stance position versus a squatting position (Torres-Oviedo, 2010). Therefore, since real life dictates the need for humans to

catch their balance in a variety of positions, the therapist should train balance reactions in various positions (Torres-Oviedo, 2010).

Several researchers have suggested that postural control is a flexible process dependent on morphological and task constraints (Keshner, 1990). Horak (1997) concluded that balance is "not based on a fixed set of equilibrium reflexes but on a flexible, functional motor skill that can adapt with training and experience" (p. 517). This observation has profound implications for the therapist intervening to improve functional balance. Although it is important to understand and recognize the typical strategies of balance reactions described previously, one must realize that there is more than just the ankle strategy, hip strategy, and stepping strategy. More importantly, these motor skills apparently can be enhanced and learned through intervention and practice (Horak, 1997). It is, however, possible that overlearning can actually inhibit adaptation (Keshner, 1990). Excessive emphasis on one pattern of response—practicing one strategy over and over—can create a situation where the patient is so comfortable with the one response that he is less able to adapt and use a response that is more appropriate to the situation.

## THINK ABOUT IT 30.1

- Based on the information provided previously, what exercises could you provide for postural responses using perturbations of balance? How would you position the patient?
- How could you provide perturbations to the patient's body? How could you provide perturbations to the surface upon which he is standing?
- How could you complete these tasks statically and dynamically? How could the patient safely carry over these exercises at home?

## Lifespan Effects

### Developmental Considerations

Balance reactions begin to be acquired as part of normal development during the first year of life. The first upright equilibrium reactions to develop are those in the sitting position, easily observed when the child is seated on an equilibrium board with mild perturbation. With tilting, an initial curvature of the spine is observed, with concavity toward the elevated side and abduction of the extremities on the same side, both probably attempting weight shift "uphill." The same response can be observed by gently nudging a child during quiet sitting on a stable surface and watching for the same trunk and extremity reactions. Children first begin to exhibit some degree of distinctive order to motor response in sitting between 4 and 5 months of age (Hartbourne, 1987). Independent, unsupported sitting is usually demonstrated by 6 months of age. Dynamic sitting equilibrium first occurs between 7 and 8 months of age. Equilibrium reactions in quadruped position, essential for creeping, begin between 9 and 12 months of age. Equilibrium reactions in standing develop last and may be initially observed at around 12 to 21 months of age.

**Protective extension** reactions are related to equilibrium reactions. When an individual is sufficiently displaced and unable to recover balance, the appropriate arm or leg is abducted or extended outward to reset and broaden the BOS and prevent falling (see Fig. 30-3). Protective extension therefore widens the BOS to encompass the new COM location. Lower extremity protective extension is analogous to the stepping strategy described earlier as a motor aspect of balance. Protective extension serves as a safety feature to protect the individual in instances when balance is lost, allowing stability to be regained even when the COM has moved well outside the BOS. Protective extension reactions develop first in the upper extremities: sideways at 7 months, and backward by 9 to 10 months. Lower extremity protective extension reactions in standing can be seen by 15 to 18 months of age.

### Aging Considerations

A well-documented decline in balance occurs progressively as part of the usual aging process (Bohannon, 1984; Briggs, 1989; Kollegger, 1992; Thelen, 1997). This decline in balance has been associated with a major increase in the incidence of falling and injury in the elderly (MacRae, 1992; Shumway-Cook, 1997a) and after stroke (Teasell, 2002). Exercise can improve balance and decrease falls (Shumway-Cook, 1997b). Specific changes in the visual, vestibular, somatosensory, and musculoskeletal systems that occur with aging contribute to the observed balance decline (Craik, 1993; Tideiksaar, 1986), and is associated with age-related changes in "feet-in-place" responses as well as "profound age-related impairments in the control of compensatory stepping movements" (Maki, 1996, p. 635). Another study suggests that older adults are more dependent on the sensory systems, as 50% of an elderly group lost their balance with a reduction of visual and ankle/foot inputs compared with only 10% of younger subjects (Wolson, 1993). An increase in reaction times has also been demonstrated with aging (Birren, 1979; Stelmach, 1985). For appropriate balance reactions, it appears that when a balance correction does not occur within 800 milliseconds, a fall is extremely likely (Jones, 1992).

Age-related impairment of balance can be related to deficits in any portion of the tripartite sensory system, interruption of central nervous system integration and perception, or impairment of the motor output systems. Loss of neurons in these systems is known to accelerate with age. Based on Rothstein's (1986, 2003) hypothesis-based algorithm for clinicians, effective clinical decision-making toward patient-centered intervention requires the therapist to formulate an educated guess as to the underlying impairments. This again emphasizes the extreme importance of a valid and reliable assessment before initiating treatment.

## ■ Related Pathology
### Neuroanatomy of Common Pathologies

Balance deficit is among the most common impairments observed in the neuromuscular rehabilitation population. Remember that the balance system operates on the basis of information inputted from at least three sensory systems, with central processing in the brainstem and cerebral structures and output through the neuromotor systems. Therefore, lesions in diverse anatomical structures related to any of these can cause balance dysfunction. Balance deficits may accompany anatomical lesions in many different central nervous system locations, as summarized in Fig. 9-6 and explained in the following section.

Anatomical lesions in the sensory or motor system or central nervous system processing centers may result in balance impairment. Balance dysfunction is most commonly associated with lesions in the brainstem, cerebellum, motor or sensory cortex, sensory organs (i.e., vestibular system, pacinian corpuscle), or any of the motor or sensory pathways of the spinal cord connecting these essential areas. Lesions to the brainstem may disrupt vestibular structures or pathways or cerebellar pathways. Central or peripheral vestibular pathology (fully discussed in Chapter 29) impairs balance because of the lost ability to accurately monitor position and movement of the head in space. Some types of vestibular pathology result in information that conflicts with other sensory information, increasing the risk for balance loss. Cerebellar lesions in the cerebellar cortex, deep cerebellar nuclei, or cerebellar pathways of the brainstem may be associated with balance impairment because cerebellar processing of subconscious proprioception is lost. Lesions to the somatosensory cortex or sensory pathways interfere with optimal balance because the nervous system is forced to respond to incomplete or erroneous information

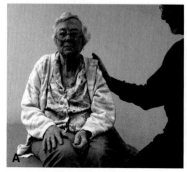
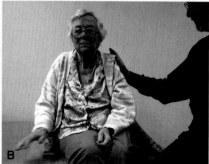
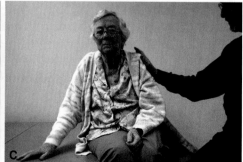

**FIGURE 30-3ABC** Series of photographs showing a patient in sitting and protective extension of the upper extremity in a lateral direction to prevent falling.

about the body's position in relation to the environment. Lesions to the motor cortex or pathways are associated with impaired balance because of the inability to program or carry out specific motor responses.

## Medical Diagnoses

Table 30-1 summarizes common neuromuscular medical diagnoses for which balance impairment may appear on the problem list. Balance impairment is a common feature of most neuromuscular diagnoses seen by therapists for rehabilitation. Cerebrovascular accident or stroke (ischemic or hemorrhagic) and traumatic or anoxic brain injury are among the most common neurological diagnoses associated with balance impairment in adults, especially when the motor cortex, brainstem, cerebellum, or vestibular system is involved. In fact, balance dysfunction is one of the most common impairments associated with traumatic brain injury (Newton, 1990). This may occur because the intracranial structures listed in the previous section are so intimately related to the inner table of the skull and therefore are more susceptible to force-induced trauma. Also, traumatic brain injuries are typically diffuse, so damage to a variety of structures is common. Even in patients without clear neurological signs, deficits in both static and dynamic balance have been documented after a traumatic brain injury, specifically a >50% increase in anterior-posterior sway and lateral sway and a 20% decrease in weight-shifting speed, as measured by force-platform COP amplitude and velocity (Geurts, 1996). A study of 105 patients with hemiparesis concluded that those with left hemiparesis were more likely to have difficulty with independent sitting than patients with right hemiparesis (Bohannon, 1986).

One specific mechanism of imbalance in standing found in some patients with hemiplegia from cerebral injury has been described as the "**pusher syndrome**," also called **ipsilateral pushing** (Pedersen, 1996), lateral **retropulsion** (Bohannon, 1998), and **contraversive pushing** (Karnath, 2003). This syndrome, which is also discussed in Chapter 31, is most likely an expression of perceptual dysfunction. The pusher syndrome is clinically observed in standing as strong extensor activity of the nonaffected lower limb, with hemineglect of the affected side, resulting in severe postural imbalance. As a result, the patient "pushes" or leans toward the affected side but without antigravity activation of the affected side. Pedersen (1996) found the pusher syndrome in 10% of a patient sample and reported that the syndrome was associated with a 3.6-week prolongation of treatment duration, most likely because of postural instability in reaching the same goals as subjects without pusher syndrome.

Traumatic spinal cord injuries may result in incomplete or complete paraplegia or tetraplegia. Because of the permanent nature of the lower extremity deficits in paraplegia and lower and upper extremity deficits in quadriplegia, sitting balance becomes a priority, especially in the functionally important long-sitting position. In patients with incomplete paraplegia and quadriplegia who have potential for functional ambulation with bracing, modified standing balance (i.e., with orthotics and assistive devices) must be learned and incorporated into standing and walking.

Recall that a certain amount of deterioration in balance is ultimately expected as individuals approach the end of the lifespan. When age-related dysfunction is combined with neuromuscular pathology, the incidence of which increases with aging, an especially profound balance deficit can occur. For example, if an 80 year-old man who already has age-related visual and vestibular deficits and muscle weakness has a stroke, the resulting balance deficit will likely be more severe than that associated with a comparable anatomic lesion in a younger individual. The younger individual also has greater potential for recovery and therefore a better outcome with balance training. Comorbidity in the aging population has

| **TABLE 30-1** | **Neuromuscular Medical Diagnoses That Commonly Include Balance Deficit** |
|---|---|
| **CATEGORY** | **DIAGNOSES** |
| Vascular disease | Cerebrovascular accident; intracranial hematoma |
| Trauma | Traumatic brain injury; traumatic spinal cord injury (complete and incomplete); traumatic peripheral nerve injury |
| Tumors | Intracranial tumors, especially cerebellar/brainstem with vestibular involvement; neurofibromatosis; spinal cord tumors |
| Infectious/toxic/inflammatory disease | Viral encephalitis; meningitis; neonatal TORCH infections; lead toxicity (encephalopathy); transverse myelitis; acute inflammatory demyelinating polyneuropathy (Guillain-Barré syndrome); chronic inflammatory demyelinating polyneuropathy |
| Degenerative disease | Parkinson disease (stages III–V) (Smithson, 1998); Alzheimer disease; multiple sclerosis; Friedreich ataxia; syringomyelia; amyotrophic lateral sclerosis |
| Neuropathy | Peripheral neuropathy (diabetes or other metabolic disease); Charcot-Marie-Tooth disease |
| Developmental/genetic disorder | Down syndrome; cerebral palsy (spastic, athetoid, ataxic); developmental coordination disorder; spina bifida; seizure disorder; muscular dystrophy; attention-deficit hyperactivity disorder |

TORCH = common neonatal infections: toxoplasmosis, others, rubella, cytomegalovirus, herpes simplex.

profound implications for therapeutic interventions addressing balance impairment.

## Pertinent Examination/Evaluation

Tests/measures of sensory and motor systems that have implications for balance are presented in Chapters 5 and 6, respectively. Examination methods and objective measures of functional balance are described in Chapter 9, including static and dynamic balance in both sitting and standing positions. Ultimately, the therapist must identify functional limitations that result from balance impairment and the safety risks that follow. Clinical reasoning to determine the underlying impairments that contribute to the balance deficits allows optimal treatment planning to maximize functional outcome (Rothstein, 2003). The clinician can also use the BESTest to determine which balance subsystems are involved (Horak, 2009). Many of the examination methods provide data for determining optimal treatment and comparison with future measures to monitor improvement. Documenting positive changes is essential in describing and quantifying improvement in follow-up assessment and discharge planning and for purposes of communicating with third-party payers. Table 30-2 summarizes objective examination methods for balance.

### PATIENT APPLICATION: "MORE ON OUR PATIENT"

With a big smile (more so on the left), Fawn walks out of the house onto her front porch using a quad cane to meet you. Her speech impairment is obvious to you, her words slightly dysarthric and slurred.

As for her mental status, Fawn is alert and impulsive, frequently responding to situations without thinking through all the consequences. She is oriented to person and place but not time, and her cognitive processing is slow in problem-solving, even answering simple questions. Her four errors on the 10 Mini-Mental Status Examination items categorize her as having "mild intellectual impairment." Her nonverbal interaction and comments are often inappropriate, especially toward male personnel.

Tests and measures:

- Cranial nerves: With the exception of the drooping right corner of her mouth, Fawn's cranial nerves are without deficits. Her facial sensation is intact.
- Sensation: Sensations throughout the rest of the body are without deficit for pinprick and light touch. Joint position sense is intact in all extremities.
- Range of motion (ROM): Passive range is without limitations except for R ankle dorsiflexion, which is limited to −5 degrees.
- Muscle tone: Spasticity, graded Ashworth 1, was detected in the R UE (shoulder internal rotators) and R elbow flexors and wrist flexors. The R hip and knee extensors are both graded as Ashworth 1 + spastic hypertonia, and the R ankle plantar flexors are graded as 2 on the Ashworth scale.
- Muscle strength: Manual muscle testing reveals G+ to N throughout the L UE and L LE and G− for R shoulder flexors and extensors but was not performed in R UE or R LE

secondary to the lack of isolated movement and presence of synergies.

- Motor function: Normal isolated movement is performed in all L UE and L LE muscle groups. In the R UE, Fawn is able to perform isolated shoulder flexion and extension through the full range. Active isolated elbow movement is limited to the occurrence of abnormal synergies, allowing isolated elbow extension through only ~1/4 range and isolated elbow flexion through only ~3/4 range. Overhead reaching occurs only through an abnormal synergistic flexion pattern. In the R LE, abnormal synergies interfere with isolated hip and knee flexion in sitting, allowing isolated movement through only 1/2 range for each group. Hip and knee extensions are isolated for only the first 1/4 range.
- Coordination: Mild ataxia is noted in R extremity active movements and interferes with functional tasks of the R UE and LE.
- Vestibular: Fawn reports no dizziness, spinning, or lightheadedness during movement of the head, including rotation and sitting up from lying, turning, or bending down to pick something up from sitting or from standing. There is no observed nystagmus or abnormal responses to vestibulo-ocular reflex (VOR) testing or positional provocation testing.
- Functional status: Fawn is now independent with mat mobility, both horizontal and in sitting. Level surface transfers via modified stand-and-pivot is accomplished with Min A and the hemi-walker. Sit-to-stand requires Mod A x1, not for the power of the lift but for balance and safety. Fawn ambulates a distance of 25 feet on level surfaces using a hemi-walker and requiring Mod A x1 for balance. Her gait velocity at self-selected medium speed is 0.19 m per second (0.62 ft/sec). Obvious gait deviations include inability to obtain neutral dorsiflexion of the R ankle during the R swing phase, for which she compensates by greater hip and knee flexion. Self-induced balance errors in the R LE during ambulation are not corrected until they are excessive and require a steppage strategy on >50% of occasions. Static standing balance is graded as F. Dynamic standing balance is graded as P. "Functional Reach" measure is 8 inches, timed up-and-go measure for a 3-meter distance is 40 seconds, and she has a score of 12/24 on the Dynamic Gait Index.

### Contemplate Clinical Decisions:

- As you begin to develop your treatment plan for Fawn, which aspects of limited function would you rate as most important for improvement?
- Using the aforementioned evaluation information and a comparison with normative values from the examination chapters of Section II, develop a prioritized problem list for functional limitations of activity for Fawn.
- Because the focus of this chapter is therapy for balance impairment, alongside the Functional Problem List enumerate the organ/system impairments identified in the evaluation that could contribute to Fawn's balance disturbance.
- On the basis of Fawn's medical diagnosis, progress to date, and status, summarize her general prognosis for further improvement in balance and her rehabilitation potential.
- Formulate three functional goals to guide development of a treatment plan for Fawn.

| TABLE 30-2 | Balance Assessment Methods Summarized From Chapter 9 |
|---|---|
| **ASPECT OF BALANCE TESTED** | **SPECIFIC EXAMINATION METHOD (SEE CHAPTER 9 FOR DETAILS)** |
| Static and dynamic sitting, static and dynamic standing | • Grading/scales<br>• Performance-based assessment |
| Dynamic sitting | • Modified (Sitting) Functional Reach Test<br>• Stability in Sitting Test |
| Static standing | • Maximal Load Test<br>• Clinical Test of Sensory Interaction in Balance (CTSIB) (focus on sensory systems utilized)<br>• Sensory Organization Test (like CTSIB, focus on sensory systems utilized but performed with posturography)<br>• Single-limb stance<br>• Computerized posturography (force-platform center of pressure excursion) |
| Dynamic standing | • Gait velocity<br>• Timed up and go test (TUG)<br>• Step test<br>• Functional Reach Test; Multidirectional Reach Test (a reflection of limits of stability (LOS)<br>• Hierarchical Assessment of Balance and Mobility (HABAM)<br>• Computerized posturography (force-platform LOS)<br>• Obstacle course<br>• Four-Square Step Test<br>• Walking within a 4-in.-wide path<br>• Dynamic Gait Index; Functional Gait Assessment |
| Static and dynamic standing | • Berg Balance Scale<br>• Performance-Oriented Mobility Assessment (POMA) – Tinetti<br>• Balance Evaluation System Test (BESTest) |
| Balance self-confidence | • Activities-Specific Balance Confidence (ABC) scales<br>• Balance Efficacy Scale<br>• Falls Efficacy Scale |

# ■ Preparatory Intervention Specific to Balance Impairment

## General Approaches

General approaches to therapy include the principles and broad treatment processes that apply to all specific treatment activities. The approaches described in this section can be used to guide the development and application of the specific treatment techniques and functional treatment activities described later.

To design intervention for impaired balance, clinical decision-making requires consideration of several questions: Have certain interventions for balance impairment been effective in clinical scenarios with individuals similar to my patient? Can the effectiveness of the therapy be assumed with some confidence in similar populations? When approaches and techniques are compared, has one been superior to all others? Is there an optimal dosing for these therapies?

Too often, the answers to these questions are not clear. Although interventions for balance impairment have more supportive evidence than other areas of neurological physical therapy, most of the research has involved elderly patients, with fewer studies using patients with neuromuscular

disorders. Potential for improvement of balance has even been demonstrated in a normal, healthy sample, for whom balance surpassed what is considered normal after practice of certain strategies, skills, and techniques (Crotts, 1996). At least in principle, this builds a case for balance improvement in elders with balance impairment and possibly in patients with neuromuscular disorders who have a measurable balance deficit. This is especially relevant in the context of expected neural plasticity and the ability of the central nervous system to reorganize itself and establish new connections with repetitive task-oriented practice. Through evaluation and assessment, the therapist can provide individualized therapeutic intervention.

Treatment to improve balance is a consideration in rehabilitation for most patients with acute or subacute conditions of either neurological or orthopedic origin. In an acute care setting, Bohannon (1999) found half of elderly patients referred for physical therapy were unable to maintain standing, feet apart or together, and all lost balance in the posterior direction. In a sample of 52 acute rehabilitation patients, both balance rated on an ordinal scale and Functional Independence Measure (FIM) scores increased significantly ($p < 0.0001$) between initial and final assessments (mean interval of 17.5 days) (Bohannon, 1995). In a study of elderly individuals in a residential care facility who had impaired balance and difficulty performing at least one functional activity, improvement in balance was documented after 1 month of physical therapy and was maintained through an additional 1-month follow-up, whereas gait speed did not statistically improve (Harada, 1995). This may indicate that a longer duration of treatment is required to show improvement in gait velocity.

With the importance of intervention for balance deficit in the rehabilitation process established, we present the guiding principles that apply to specific treatment activities.

### Address Underlying Impairments

In a complicated multisystem impairment such as balance dysfunction, underlying or contributing impairments and possible contributory factors must be identified and addressed (Campbell, 1997; Horak, 1990, 1997; LaBan, 1998; Rothstein, 2003). On the basis of the individual examination, the therapist addresses the impairments hypothesized as contributing to the balance impairment. For example, lower extremity weakness has been discussed as a primary contributor to decreased balance with increased risk of falling (Brill, 1999; Campbell, 1997; Chandler, 1998; Johnston, 1998; Verfaillie, 1997). When a regional lower extremity weakness is identified in the patient with impaired balance, the appropriate muscle group(s) should be strengthened. Treatments to specifically address weakness are discussed in Chapter 22. When the identified cause is restricted mobility at a joint (i.e., the ankle) that prevents adequate motor response, the ROM limitations must be improved (Badke, 1990; Schenkman, 1990), as discussed in Chapter 23. When vestibular dysfunction is identified as an underlying cause of postural instability, therapy specifically related to the vestibular impairment must be given, as detailed in Chapter 29.

Once the therapist improves or corrects the primary contributor to balance dysfunction, he must bring these improvements back into function. In the aforementioned patient with lower extremity weakness and impaired motor control as primary contributors to imbalance, the patient uses his newfound strength gains in tasks that were difficult or impossible to complete before therapy.

Because pusher syndrome and its associated balance dysfunction are related to perceptual deficits, specific interventions for this form of balance impairment are discussed in Chapter 31. Intervention for other underlying impairments related to balance impairment, including ataxia, impaired motor control, and sensory deficits, are found in other chapters in Section III. Often, contributing environmental factors such as poor lighting, loose floor rugs, medications, or the need for home modifications should be addressed, primarily through patient education and environmental modifications, as discussed in later sections.

### Manipulate the Environment to Alter Contributing Systems

Once it was understood that maintaining balance is a multiple-system process, certain principles of treatment emerged.

In general, the therapist must choose a task or therapeutic activity and then manipulate the environment to alter the contributing systems, especially the sensory components or the environmental context. For example, even elderly patients without clinical evidence of neurological disease who practice repeated trials of activity with imposed limited visual input have improved their balance and adapted to challenging balance conditions (Judge, 1995). Judge attributed this effect to adaptation of other systems because vision was systematically limited. Presumably, the improved ability is related to increased abilities in other systems because of the increased demand placed on them and increased opportunities for practice at using these systems during the intervention. This also emphasizes the importance of repetition and repeated practice of challenging functional balance activities in the process of retraining balance abilities.

Shumway-Cook (1986) pointed out the importance of interaction of the sensory systems in balance. Balance examination, described in Chapter 9, helps determine which underlying systems are impaired and are contributing to balance deficits. The CTSIB, as described in Chapter 9, is useful in determining the underlying sensory impairments that contribute to balance impairment (Shumway-Cook, 1986). For example, a person with vestibular loss tends to have increased sway or even loss of balance in CTSIB conditions 5 and 6, with combined visual and surface challenges. The BESTest also helps determine the affected balance subsystem (Horak, 2009). Once you have identified the dysfunctional component system or systems that are interfering with normal balance, you must then address them specifically in your treatment plan.

To improve the patient's balance, you should challenge and stress the system that is dysfunctional, with repetitions of practice using the impaired underlying system. Disadvantage or eliminate the intact, functioning systems (described in detail in the next paragraph) to place greater demands on the dysfunctional system with potential opportunities for central nervous system reorganization and motor learning. For example, a patient may be "visually dependent," with overdependence on visual input for postural control, perhaps related to vestibular deficits. In this patient, the initial treatment strategy may include disturbing or eliminating visual input to promote practice using other sensory systems to determine appropriate balance strategies in a controlled environment. Because of the induced instability, it is essential to appropriately guard the patient during such activities.

Possible methods to disadvantage each sensory system are summarized in Table 30-3. The vestibular system is the most difficult to disadvantage and is best accomplished by creating environmental situations where the vision and vestibular systems provide conflicting information. As the therapist, you can treat balance disturbance by disadvantaging the sensory systems, such as blindfolding the patient during various upright positions and simple activities in preparation for more functional activities. A developmental progression may be followed as an overall, general treatment framework, including progression through quadruped, kneeling, half-kneeling, sitting, or standing, with variations such as narrowing the BOS as the patient is able.

| TABLE 30-3 | Techniques to Disadvantage the Sensory Systems Involved in Balance |
|---|---|
| **SENSORY SYSTEM** | **TECHNIQUES TO STRESS THIS SYSTEM*** |
| Vision | • Have the patient walk in a dimly lit room.<br>• Have the patient wear distortion glasses or alternatively use safety glasses coated with Vaseline or covered with layers of crumpled, plastic cling wrap (kitchen wrap).<br>• Have the patient walk with eyes closed (intermittently or fully).<br>• Eliminate vision with use of a blindfold.<br>• Impose nonfunctional, nonrhythmic eye movements during functional tasks.<br>• Use a force platform with a surround that provides inaccurate visual feedback. |
| Somatosensory | • Have the patient stand on an unstable surface such as an equilibrium board or rocker board.<br>• Have the patient stand on an unstable surface such as a BAPS board.<br>• Have the patient stand on an unstable/pliable surface such as a thick foam mat.<br>• Have the patient stand on an unstable, elastic surface such as a trampoline.<br>• Have the patient walk in a grassy area outdoors (grass clumps, ground divots). |
| Vestibular | • Enforce unusual static head positions during functional tasks.<br>• Enforce unusual head movements or body turns during functional tasks. |

*Obviously, it is very important to take appropriate safety precautions to prevent falls when you put the patient in these demanding activities. This may include proper guarding, application of a gait belt, and/or use of a safety harness system.

However, depending on the patient's needs, the progression need not be strictly followed. This treatment progression allows the therapist to assess and ensure patient safety and confidence in one position before progressing to a more advanced, less stable posture with a narrower BOS. Sensory limitations can be applied in both static and dynamic activities.

### Enhance Cardiopulmonary Conditioning

Physical exercise, conditioning, and endurance training have been associated with improved balance among elderly individuals (Buchner, 1997; Era, 1997), perhaps because each provides natural challenges to balance abilities. Cardiopulmonary conditioning has thus been proposed to prevent balance loss or address balance deficits, perhaps because conditioning activities tend to be very active and involve quick movements and adjustments to self-induced perturbations. At least one study concluded that good balance contributes to enhanced performance of functional mobility and ADL functions (Era, 1997). Details of treatment activities that improve cardiopulmonary fitness are discussed in Chapter 35.

As part of the focus on a patient's overall health status, most treatment plans incorporate endurance activities for health promotion in the individual. Conditioning and endurance activities often involve active, rhythmic movements in upright postures, with movement of the COM toward and temporarily beyond the limits of stability. In a randomized controlled trial, walking and aerobic movement activities after supervised exercises three times a week for 3 months were superior to stationary cycling in improving balance measures and therefore decreasing fall risk in an elderly population (Buchner, 1997). This difference might be explained by the fact that both walking and aerobics take place in an upright posture, whereas cycling is done in a sitting position. The improved balance remained significant only in the aerobic movement group after 3 months of self-directed exercise of any

type. Overall, the authors concluded that walking seems to be most useful for fall prevention because it improved at least one measure of all major outcomes (endurance, strength, gait, balance, health status) (Buchner, 1997). These activities, including aerobic treadmill training, may treat balance impairment as well as improve cardiopulmonary status in patients with neuromuscular disorders (Smith, 2000).

### Encourage Mental Practice

Mental practice is thought to improve physical performance in individuals, from athletes to rehabilitation patients. Ideokinetic facilitation was originally described as imagined movement with the potential to change posture and neuromuscular patterning (Sweigard, 1974). Mental practice, which has been used experimentally, involves utilizing idealized visual and kinesthetic mental imaging (Fansler, 1985). Mental practice of a physical task, specifically balance reactions, improved motor performance in an elderly population (Fansler, 1985). Further study of such applications in patients with postural instability is needed to clarify its value in the clinical setting, especially in combination with or in preparation for actual practice.

One possible application could be mental practice of a balance task before the initial psychomotor practice of a functional activity. For example, you could tell the patient to close his eyes and use mental practice several times to "visualize yourself standing on your right leg only, with the left foot up in the air behind you, while you reach for something from the back of the cabinet shelf." To implement variety in practice with repetitions, you could follow this activity with actual motor practice of the same or similar tasks. Mental practice of functional balance tasks can also be part of the home activity program, especially for those postures or positions that place the patient at risk for falling when performed independently. This is also an effective time management skill in the inpatient rehabilitation environment, where it is common to treat two patients at one time. While you are working with one patient, the other patient can practice mental imagery while resting. Evidence supports this approach (Driskell, 1994). Use of virtual reality also has potential. In particular, a virtual cycling system that combines virtual reality technology with a bicycle (Kim, 1999) and locomotor virtual systems (Deutsch, 2004; Whitney, 2006; You, 2005) can improve postural balance control.

### Withdraw Assistance Gradually

An essential principle in the treatment of impaired balance is that the therapist must initially provide as much support and assistance as necessary to ensure safety and success! At the same time, from the standpoint of intervention using movement control principles, support and assistance must be progressively withdrawn from the patient, enforcing a gradual increase in demand on the systems involved (Fell, 2004). This withdrawal allows the person to practice the necessary balance strategies. These two seemingly paradoxical principles must be appropriately applied in each patient. For example, with body-weight support ambulation training, no demand is placed on the patient's balance systems during phases with high levels of body-weight support; without progression to decreasing percentages of body-weight support, lower limb control in ambulation may improve, but the patient does not have opportunities to practice balance strategies and reactions.

The therapist's assistance can also be gradually withdrawn over time. The therapist may start with proximal support and progress to more distal points of contact with less support being given, as shown in Fig. 30-4. Proximal support may be given at the hips when the patient has adequate trunk control or at the shoulders when additional input and support are needed for trunk control.

As support is changed to a more distal location, greater requirements are placed on the patient's postural control. For example, while facing the patient, have him rest his forearm and hands on your forearm. The patient can also grip your upper arm just above the elbow. The therapist has additional control in this position because the patient's elbows are resting in the therapist's hands. Ultimately, the patient may be asked to perform a standing balance activity with only fingertip contact on the therapist's palm. These positions allow the therapist to monitor the amount of upper extremity support utilized during standing functional balance activities. A gradual withdrawal of assistance from the therapist ensures that the patient has increasing opportunities to practice using sensory and motor systems to carry out balance reactions.

The neurodevelopmental treatment (NDT) perspective, the principles of which are discussed in Chapter 14, encourages progressive withdrawal of assistance leading to optimal independence. In this approach, compensatory strategies, including excessive dependence on external support, are avoided unless the impairment cannot be improved or safety is a concern. In the early stages, the therapist provides as much assistance as needed to ensure practice of normal movement patterns. Specific application of the NDT approach to balance treatment includes functional balance activities practiced with the least amount of upper extremity support necessary, ultimately progressing to no assistance when possible. Within this approach, facilitation of optimal alignment of body segments and efficient movement patterns occur either by direct tactile contact over muscles that need to be activated or by manual guidance of a particular movement. The facilitation is especially important for the stability of the trunk and lower extremity weight-bearing segments and the experience and practice of smooth, controlled movements for balance reactions. The facilitation is most important in early rehabilitation before functional balance activities are performed because normal alignment of a body segment promotes more normal movement patterns and responses.

### Decrease Dependence on Assistive Devices and Orthotics

Handheld gait assistive devices, including the cane, hemiwalker, or walker, are essential for the safety of some patients with balance impairment and increased risk of falling. In these

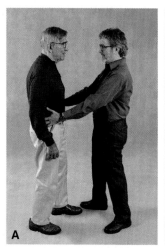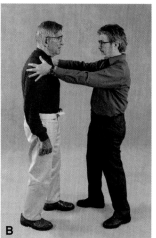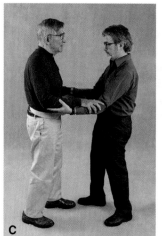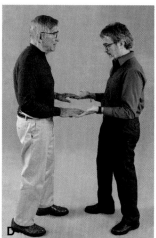

**FIGURE 30-4ABCD** Series of photographs showing a patient in standing and the therapist's progressive withdrawal of support during an upright dynamic stepping activity: at hips or shoulders early in rehabilitation and at forearms and ultimately fingertip support in later rehabilitation.

patients, the assistive device specifically widens the BOS to increase stability, with occasional use allowing the arms to function in postural support. In comparison, in the typical orthopedic patient, assistive devices are used primarily as consistent weight-bearing devices.

In neuromuscular disorders, you should watch for a natural tendency in many patients to excessively use the assistive device for upper extremity weight-bearing to compensate for lower extremity weakness or incoordination. Such use should be viewed as temporary in all patients with a prognosis of further recovery. In this instance, the focus should be on gradual weaning from the assistive device. Through patient education, you should discourage physical or emotional dependence on the assistive device, perhaps even discussing the possibility of future function without the device, particularly in patients you anticipate will not need support on a permanent basis.

Assistive devices are also recommended to enhance patient safety. However, use of assistive devices most likely changes biomechanical and sensory constraints for posture (Horak, 1997; Jeka, 1997). For example, an assistive device increases the BOS and therefore increases stability. However, patients using a unilateral assistive device have greater weight shift toward the assistive device and decreased ability to shift away from it (Milezarek, 1993).

From the outset of rehabilitation, the therapist should emphasize the role of the assistive device to the patient. After cerebral pathology, assistive devices are used to augment stability rather than for weight-bearing. Discourage your patient from "pushing through the assistive device," unless lower extremity weakness, profound ataxia, or lack of motor control severely interferes with the ability of the lower extremities to support the person. Rather, encourage him to purposefully work toward simply resting his hands on the device, not "squeezing" it, and ultimately to have just finger contact with the assistive device to ensure that minimal weight-bearing is taking place through the walker or cane.

Orthotics, as discussed in detail in Chapter 17, can help support specific joints. The ankle-foot orthosis (AFO), the most common orthotic, supports the ankle in optimal alignment, especially when there is unstable footdrop (LaBan, 1998). The AFO enhances foot clearance in the swing phase of gait and therefore minimizes self-induced perturbations that otherwise occur in midswing from the toe catching on the floor. AFOs can also improve balance by supporting proper ankle position during the stance phase, enhancing the contributions of the more affected lower extremity to balance strategies.

### An Integrated Approach

Currently, treatment for balance impairment is broad and integrated, as no specific intervention strategies have shown superiority over others. The treatment plan should specifically address abnormal or absent balance strategies, motor and sensory components of the balance system, and ultimately application to functional activities. The effectiveness of an individualized multidimensional exercise program addressing

specific impairments in the individual was demonstrated in a quasi-experimental study on adults older than 65 years with a history of falling (Shumway-Cook, 1997b, p. 49). In that study, mobility training focused on "improving stability during a variety of gait tasks, including unperturbed gait, perturbed gait, transfers, and stair climbing."

In a dual case study led by Gill-Body (1997), rehabilitation of balance was described for two patients with cerebellar dysfunction. A variety of preparatory impairment-based interventions as well as functional treatment activities were outlined for each patient. Details are described further in the remainder of the chapter. Table 30-4 lists the activities of an integrated treatment approach for one of these patients with cerebellar dysfunction, with a rationale for each activity as stated by the investigators.

An integrated program of balance retraining activities has also been described in two elderly patients with disequilibrium (Asher, 1997). A summary of the treatment activities and rationale for each is included in Table 30-5. A comprehensive, patient-centered treatment plan addressing balance impairment in the context of neuromuscular disorders most likely includes a collection of the specific interventions and activities described on the remaining pages of this chapter. The therapist should carefully select components of the treatment plan according to the impairments and functional limitations identified in the examination and evaluation process.

## Therapeutic Techniques

*Therapeutic techniques* are defined in this text as rehabilitation treatments or specific therapeutic methods and activities most often used to correct or address a specific impairment. Techniques specific to a particular impairment are usually performed as a preparatory intervention before the performance of related functional tasks. They are not often applied in a functional activity, at least initially. The treatment should clearly contribute to and prepare the patient for performing the functional activity with a hypothesized link that is clearly identified in the clinical decision-making. In the case of balance, therapeutic techniques include activities to disadvantage certain components of the balance system. These activities place greater demand on and enhance practice opportunities for the dysfunctional system, as well as alter resulting environmental situations and cues.

### Light Touch Contact

After a series of studies, Jeka (1997) suggested that use of light touch contact at the fingertip or through a cane can reduce postural sway both in subjects without balance impairment and in those with vestibular dysfunction. Clinically, we frequently observe patients with balance disturbance using light contact with surrounding surfaces as they walk along, including walls and even light contact with the arm of spouse or the person with whom they are walking. This is sometimes referred to as "furniture walking." Jeka reported that the recorded force levels at the point of contact were inadequate to serve as a true physical support for the body and that measured force did not increase

| TABLE 30-4 | Balance Rehabilitation Treatment Program and Its Rationale for Patients With Resected Cerebellar Tumor |
|---|---|

| RATIONALE | TREATMENT ACTIVITY |
|---|---|
| **Phase 1** | |
| • Promote use of VOR and COR for gaze stability | Visual fixation, EO, stationary target, slow head movements |
| • Promote use of saccadic eye movements for gaze stability | Active eye and head movements between two stationary targets |
| • Promote VOR cancellation | EO, moving target with head movement, self-selected speed |
| • Improve ability to use somatosensory and vestibular inputs for postural control | Static stance, EO and EC, feet together, arms close to body, head movements |
| • Improve ability to use vestibular and visual inputs for postural control | Static stance on foam surface, EC intermittently, feet 2.54–5.08 cm (1–2 in.) apart |
| • Improve postural control using all sensory inputs | Gait with narrowed base of support, EO, wide turns to right and left |
| • Improve postural control using visual and vestibular inputs | March in place, EO, on firm and foam surfaces, prolonged pauses in unilateral stance |
| **Phase 2** | |
| • Promote use of VOR and COR for gaze stability | Visual fixation, EO, stationary and moving targets, slow and fast speeds, simple static background; imaginary visual fixation, EC |
| • Promote use of saccadic eye movements for gaze stability | Active eye and head movements between two targets, slow and fast speeds, EO, moving target with head movement, fast and slow speeds |
| • Promote VOR cancellation | |
| • Improve ability to use somatosensory and vestibular inputs for postural control | Semitandem stance, EO and EC, arms crossed |
| • Improve ability to use vestibular inputs for postural control | Stance on foam, EC intermittently, feet 2.54–5.08 cm apart |
| • Improve postural control using visual and vestibular inputs | Gait with EO with sharp 180 degree turns to the right and left, firm and padded surfaces |
| • Improve postural control using vestibular and somatosensory inputs | March in place, EC, prolonged pauses in unilateral stance |
| • Improve postural control using all sensory inputs | Walking sideways and backward; standing EO and EC, heel touches forward, toe touches backward |
| • Improve postural control with head moving using all sensory inputs | Gait with EO, normal base of support, slow head movements |
| **Phase 3** | |
| • Promote use of VOR and COR for gaze stability | Visual fixation, EO, stationary and moving targets, various speeds, complex static and dynamic backgrounds; imaginary visual fixation, EC |
| • Promote use of saccadic eye movements for gaze stability | Active eye and head movements between two targets, various speeds |
| • Promote VOR cancellation | EO, moving target with head movement, various speeds, complex static and dynamic backgrounds |
| • Improve ability to use somatosensory and vestibular inputs for postural control | Semitandem stance with EC continuously, and with EO on firm and padded surfaces |
| • Improve postural control using vestibular and somatosensory inputs | Gait with EC with base of support progressively narrowed, firm and padded surfaces; march in place slowly, EO and EC on firm and foam surfaces |
| • Improve postural control using visual and vestibular inputs | Gait with EO, rapid sharp turns to right and left, firm and padded surfaces |
| • Improve postural control when head is moving using all sensory inputs | Gait with normal base of support, EO, fast head movements |
| • Improve postural control using all sensory inputs | Braiding; active practice of ankle sway movements; bending and reaching activities |

COR = cerebro-ocular reflex, EC = eyes closed, EO = eyes open, VOR = vestibulo-ocular reflex.

Reprinted with permission, Gill-Body KM, Popat RA, Parker SW, Krebs DE. Rehabilitation of balance in two patients with cerebellar dysfunction. *Phys Ther.* 1997;77(5):534–552.

| TABLE 30-5 | Balance Retraining Activities and Rationale for Their Use |
|---|---|
| **TREATMENT ACTIVITY** | **RATIONALE** |
| • Rolling around bolster by pushing with feet | Improve single limb stance impacting gait stride and ability to climb stairs |
| • Ascend/descend 1- to 8-in. platforms with and without | Improve single limb stance rails |
| • Stand on firm surface with eyes closed | Improve ability to use vestibular and somatosensory information for balance |
| • Stand on compliant surface with eyes open | Improve ability to use vestibular and visual information for balance |
| • Stand on compliant surface with eyes closed | Improve ability to use vestibular information for balance |
| • Postural sway biofeedback | Improve awareness and control of center of mass |
| • Walk on level compliant surfaces | Improve ability to use vestibular information in dynamic balance activities |
| • Walk on uneven compliant surfaces | Improve dynamic balance while receiving conflicting visual information |
| • Walking combined with head movements | Improve ability to process vestibular information during dynamic balance activity |
| • Playing catch with and without taking steps | Improve balance reactions during dynamic activity |
| • Chair rise from a variety of heights | Improve ability to shift weight over new base of support |

(Reprinted with permission from Asher A. Disequilibrium in the elderly: Two case studies. *Neurol Rep.* 1997;21(1):11–16.)

during sway toward the point of contact. However, the therapist should realize that even light contact with a countertop can completely change postural responses (Schiepatti, 1995). One possible implication of light touch contact is that it provides additional sensory input from the environment, rather than simply additional support. This strategy may prove useful during functional treatment activities to support progressive withdrawal of external assistance.

You can incorporate this technique in a treatment session by allowing the patient to make light touch contact with your hand, perhaps using the fingertips, during the functional activities listed later in this chapter and ultimately in all home activities. This position also allows you to subjectively monitor the degree to which the patient is using or not using a surface for weight-bearing contact. In patients who have sufficient lower extremity control to make the activity safe, this technique can be applied in the home program by encouraging fingertip contact with an assistive device or a countertop. As stated previously, the patient should remove the contact as soon as possible. The patient can try removing contact for a few seconds at a time and gradually increasing the time without light touch contact as he feels comfortable.

### Visual Fixation and Head Movement

Eye movements and visual fixation have been implicated in balance impairment. Tracking of eye movements, performed by the patient, has reportedly had a negative effect on balance, suggesting that instructing patients to fixate visually on a nonmoving object may aid stability (Schulmann, 1987). Use of visual fixation and eye and head movement activities to enhance gaze stability and VOR influence has been reported in a cerebellar dysfunction case study (Gill-Body, 1997). Visual fixation on stationary and moving targets during slow head movements and eventually application during complex static and dynamic situations may promote use of vestibulo-ocular

and cervico-ocular reflexes for gaze stability. Active eye and head movements at increasing speeds between two stationary targets may promote use of saccadic eye movements for gaze stability. Use of a moving target, eyes open, with head movement can promote VOR cancellation.

These activities were incorporated along with standing balance and gait activities in a comprehensive treatment plan described in a case study. Both subjects from this study demonstrated improvements in postural stability and function along with self-reported improvements in their perception of disequilibrium (Gill-Body, 1997).

### Throwing and Catching Activities

Balance reactions are commonly required during functional tasks that include throwing and catching objects. According to a group of studies on dynamic balance intervention, training included interlimb coordination as well as coordination between lower extremity and upper body movements (Woollacott, 1997). In addition, this activity requires dual processing, which is more difficult than single processing. The therapist can throw a ball or beanbag to the patient who is seated or standing (Asher, 1997; Francese, 1997) or bat an inflated balloon back and forth to begin eliciting dynamic movements (of the trunk when sitting or of the legs and trunk when standing) and equilibrium reactions. Use of a balloon in such activities requires graded force production and reaction times that do not have to be as fast as with a heavier object such as a ball, a beanbag, or even a weighted medicine ball. Depending on the extent of the patient's deficit, you may need an assistant to throw the ball while you guard or assist the patient directly, facilitating certain trunk and leg components. A program utilizing beanbags, beach balls, and a Velcro ball and mitt while music played in the background resulted in a significant increase in balance in individuals with Alzheimer disease compared with controls (Francese, 1997).

Throwing and catching activities encourage anticipatory and predictive postural control and give the patient opportunities to practice and improve such reactions, making them more automatic. You can progress this activity by introducing variable forces, variable trajectories, and trajectories that require the patient to reach beyond his core, eventually throwing even beyond the limits of the patient's reach, requiring him to appropriately respond with greater amplitude of movement.

### Static Activities on Unstable Surfaces

Static activities can be carried out on unstable surfaces such as outdoor grassy areas, thick compliant foam, rocker boards, equilibrium boards, inflatable disks, a BAPS board, a BOSU ball, or a physioball and then progress to dynamic movement on these surfaces. For sitting balance, you can start with the patient sitting on a large therapeutic ball with external support (only as necessary) from the therapist. The ball, being inherently unstable, introduces greater challenge to the patient's static sitting balance, especially when perturbations are added.

While the patient is sitting on the ball, ask him to use his legs to dynamically roll the ball forward and backward, starting with small ranges of movement. You can later progress to lateral movements and then even diagonal and circular patterns with ever-increasing excursions of ball movement. As patients advance, these same principles can be applied to the other types of unstable surfaces listed previously and to standing activities on the aforementioned unstable surfaces, standing with one foot on an unstable physioball and eventually a single-leg stance on these unstable surfaces.

## THINK ABOUT IT 30.2

- How do you determine when it is appropriate to progress the patient from a static to a dynamic activity?
- How do you determine when it is appropriate to progress a patient from an easier unstable surface, such as a rocker board, to a more challenging unstable surface, such as a BOSU ball?

### Training the Strategies

As previously described, the strategies for maintaining equilibrium in stance include ankle, hip, and stepping strategies or a combination of the activities described previously. They are often abnormal or absent after neuromuscular pathologies and should be evaluated and then addressed when there is a deficit. According to a series of studies, these automatic responses to external perturbations were described as "quick, coordinated, multisegmental strategies responsible for maintaining equilibrium" (Horak, 1997, p. 518). Horak concluded that these balance strategies become more efficient and effective with practice, particularly repeated exposure to perturbations or destabilizing stimuli. The patient must practice these strategies in the context of postural perturbation to have effective carryover into function. The therapist induces a postural perturbation, and the patient responds with the appropriate recovery mechanism (Mansfield, 2015). Because of the potentially

destabilizing nature of these activities, proper safety precautions, such as guarding techniques and/or use of a harness, should be utilized to keep the patient safe. This supports the repetitions and practice of these strategies as part of the treatment plan.

Underlying impairments that contribute to abnormal strategies, such as "prolonged latencies, poor coordination, inadequate force, or inability to adapt postural responses," need to be identified and then addressed in the treatment program (Horak, 1997, p. 530). Finally, regarding functional carryover, Horak concluded that "characterization of equilibrium responses to postural perturbations does not necessarily allow for the prediction of how a patient will perform functionally in activities of daily living, although it may allow for the prediction of how well the patient will respond to similar situations such as reacting to surface perturbations induced by accelerations and decelerations of a bus or subway train, a jostle in a crowd, or a pull by a pet on a leash" (p. 530).

From the NDT perspective, discussed in Chapter 15, the motor aspects of balance reactions or strategies may be learned by practicing tasks that require balance combined with initial manual guidance of the movement pattern. Such facilitation of appropriate motor synergies through manual guidance allow the patient to experience the appropriate movement pattern early in rehabilitation. The location and purpose of hand placements in NDT, **key points of control**, or hand contacts include the hips, knees, or feet, depending on which strategy you are trying to facilitate. As the patient gains skill through repetitions, progressive demand and optimal practice can be maintained with a gradual withdrawal of guidance or assistance from the therapist, as discussed earlier.

The patient may also be taught an additional strategy, the suspensory strategy, which can be employed during any uncertain or technically challenging situation. As part of the suspensory strategy, the patient may flex the lower extremities to intentionally lower the whole body with the center mass closer to the BOS and the floor. From a physical standpoint, this enhances the stability of the system and also minimizes the risk of injury when the person does fall.

Proprioceptive neuromuscular facilitation (PNF) techniques, explored in detail in Chapter 15, may be useful to retrain and strengthen specific components of motor strategies of balance because lower extremity strengthening programs have been associated with improved balance (Brouwer, 2003; Cao, 2007; Duncan, 1998; Goodwin, 2008). PNF most commonly strengthens through the principle of appropriate resistance, defined as the maximal amount of resistance one can give during an isotonic contraction that still allows maintenance of a smooth, controlled, coordinated contraction. Therefore, as the patient gets stronger, you increase the amount of resistance to the maximal point at which smooth movement still occurs. For balance intervention, appropriate resistance of the PNF diagonal patterns in the lower extremity is progressive and includes the desired lower extremity motions of the target strategy. For example, the pattern of flexion, adduction, and external rotation of the lower extremity D1 diagonal can strengthen the active ankle dorsiflexion needed to shift body weight forward.

### Single-Leg Support Activities With a Ball

In standing, the patient can put one foot up on a plastic or paper cup, cone, or large therapeutic ball to begin simulating a single-leg stance; this activity has been discussed by several authors as part of intervention for balance impairment (Asher, 1997; Davies, 1990). Although this setup is not purely functional, there are occasions when individuals need to balance on one leg while performing a functional task, such as an overhead reach to the shelf. While standing in front of the patient, you can allow him to support himself with hands or forearms on your forearms, and you can give direct facilitation at the pelvis and hips when needed. Reductions in the amount of assistance can take place by eventually requesting hand-in-hand contact and ultimately fingertip contact or no contact. In this position, you can also monitor the degree of upper extremity support the patient is using. This activity can also be progressed by using progressively larger therapeutic balls as the patient improves. Once the patient is standing with one foot on a ball, start by asking him to maintain this position with minimal shifts or movement. This position requires static balance, weight-bearing, and stability at the ankle of the stance leg, or the leg in contact with the ground.

Dynamic balance is trained by asking the patient to roll the ball using the foot that is on the ball. The ball is rolled backward (Fig. 30-5A) and forward (Fig. 30-5B), then side to side before progressing to rolling the ball around in circles on the floor. These activities require dynamic balance in the stance ankle during the active movement of the other leg. The therapist can provide support at the upper extremities initially but gradually withdraw that support as the patient improves. Repeat the series of activities using the opposite foot, so each lower extremity gets practice being the support leg. Although this activity is not purely functional, it may be good preparation for the balance required in the stance phase of gait and dynamic functional activities; these require that a single-leg stance be prolonged, including the single-limb support phase of stair-climbing. On such devices, dynamic movements in single-leg support are very challenging, even for people with near-normal balance.

Although no studies have addressed single-leg stance activities in balance treatment for populations with neuromuscular disorders, several sources reported use of single-leg stance activities in the treatment of balance deficits associated with lower extremity orthopedic conditions, namely chronic anterior cruciate ligament insufficiency and unilateral inversion injury of the ankle (Goldie, 1994; Zatterstrom, 1994). Single-leg stance practice, incorporated with mental practice in the elderly, has already been discussed (Fansler, 1985).

### Tai Chi

Tai chi is a widely practiced Chinese martial art. It has long been used in China as an exercise among elderly citizens (Ross, 1998; Wolf, 1997a,b). Tai chi is used in the United States more commonly as an exercise form, especially to improve balance and awareness of one's own body. The graceful movements are performed slowly and rhythmically, flowing from one position to the next, incorporating movement at all

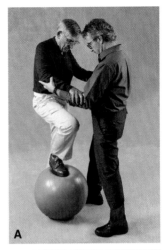

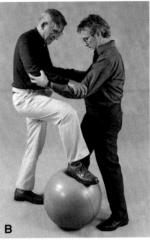

**FIGURE 30-5AB** Dynamic stance activities with a patient in single-leg support. With the non–weight-bearing foot on a therapeutic ball, the patient rolls the ball backward and forward with the other foot, placing balance demands on the weight-bearing foot.

body joints and engaging the full concentration of the mind (Plummer, 1982). The sequential postures and movements of a tai chi routine include carefully controlled rotational movements of the body. Simultaneously, there is a progressive narrowing of the BOS, even to single-leg support postures, placing obvious demands on the balance systems, even to the casual observer. The 108 forms have been reduced to 10 that can be used clinically. An illustration of these 10 forms of tai chi is available at http://www.archives-pmr.org/article/S0003-9993(97)90206-9/pdf (Wolf, 1997b). The exact directions for the 10 forms are given in Box 30-1 (Wolf, 1997b). Clinically, you can demonstrate these to your patient and incorporate the exercises into the program of home activities. It is recommended that tai chi not be viewed as the only exercise form for a patient; to be most effective, it should be considered part of a comprehensive falls management strategy (Skelton, 1999).

In clinical application, Wolf (1997b) identified seven therapeutic elements to be applied within the 10 forms: "(1) Continuous, slow movement may be slightly increased once mastered. (2) Small to larger degrees of motion are

## BOX 30-1    Directions and Therapeutic Elements for Learning 10 Forms of Tai Chi

### FORM 1. Directions

(1) Stand upright with feet shoulder-width apart, toes pointing forward, arms hanging naturally at sides. Look straight ahead (1A).

(2) Raise arms slowly forward to shoulder level, palms down. The hands do not go above the shoulders and the elbows are held in (1B & 1C).

(3) Bend knees as you press palms down gently, with elbows dropping toward knees. Look straight ahead (1D).

### FORM 1. Therapeutic Elements 3, 4

This "warmup" form begins with nonstressful bilateral stance where all thoughts other than those about movement clear the head. Attention is directed to relaxing all muscles except those of the legs—the feet are to "stick to the ground." As movement begins, concentration is directed to move all four extremities at the same constant speed that begins and ends concomitantly in the arms and legs.

### FORM 2. Directions

The body is turned slightly to the left, with left foot at 9 o'clock for a left bow stance. The left forearm and back of hand are at shoulder level, while right hand is at the side of right hip, palm down. Look at left forearm (2A). Turn torso slightly to left (9 o'clock) while extending left hand forward, palm down. Turn torso slightly right while pulling both hands down past abdomen, until right hand is extended sideways at shoulder level, palm up, and left forearm is across chest, palm turned inward. Shift weight onto right leg. Look at right hand (2B).

### FORM 2. Therapeutic Elements 1–7

The trunk and head rotate while both feet remain on floor. The arms move in asymmetrical positions so that the center of mass is extended further from left to right due to arm positions. The trunk and head are kept erect so that rotation is around a central axis. The body weight is predominantly on a flexed leg for greater balance and strength mechanism.

### FORM 3. Directions

Look straight ahead, face 9 o'clock with weight on left leg in a bow stance and hands forward at shoulder height in a pushing position (3A). Turn both palms downward as right hand passes over left wrist, moves forward, then to the right until it is on the same level with left hand. Separate hands shoulder-width apart, and draw them back to the front of abdomen, palms facing obliquely downward. At the same time, sit back and shift weight onto right leg, slightly bent, raising toes of left foot. Look straight ahead (3B; 3C).

### FORM 3. Therapeutic Elements 1–4; 7

The body center of mass moves diagonally, more posteriorly than other forms with a decreased base of support from only heel contact of the left leg, demanding greater balance and strength than the previous form. The trunk rotation is decreased and the arm movement is symmetrical.

### FORM 4. Directions

Turn torso to left (10–11 o'clock), shifting weight to left leg. Move left hand in a curve past face with palm turned slowly leftward, while right hand moves up to the front of left shoulder with palm turned obliquely inward. As right hand moves upward, right foot and left foot are parallel and 10–20 cm apart. Look at right hand (4A). Turn torso gradually to right (1–2 o'clock), shifting weight onto right leg. At the same time, move right hand continuously to right past face, palm turned slowly outward, while left hand moves in a curve past abdomen up to shoulder level with palm turned slowly obliquely inward (4B; 4C).

### FORM 4. Therapeutic Elements 1–7

While the legs are symmetrical, weight is shifted laterally. The arms are asymmetrical, the trunk and head rotate with arm movement. Both knees are flexed, and weight shifts to the leg on the side to which the arms are moving.

### FORM 5. Directions

Turn torso slightly to the right, moving right hand down in a curve past abdomen and then upward to shoulder level, palm up and arm slightly bent. Turn left palm up and place toes of left foot on floor. Eyes first look to the right as body turns in that direction, and then to look at left hand (5A; 5B).

### FORM 5. Therapeutic Elements 1–7

Again, there is a smaller base of support with the majority of the weight on one extremity. The arm on the weight-bearing side is curved back into shoulder extension. The movement is completed on the right leg and then reversed and completed on the left leg. Again the trunk rotates at the end of the movement.

## BOX 30-1 Directions and Therapeutic Elements for Learning 10 Forms of Tai Chi—cont'd

### FORM 6. Directions
Hold torso erect and keep chest relaxed. Move arms in a curve without stretching them when you separate hands. Use waist as the axis in body turns. The movements in taking a bow stance and separating hands must be smooth and synchronized in tempo. Place front foot slowly in position, heel coming down first. The knee of front leg should not go beyond toes while rear leg should be straightened, forming 45° with the ground. There should be a transverse distance of 10–30 cm between heels. Face 9 o'clock in final position.

### FORM 6. Therapeutic Elements 1–7
Hand assumes a position of holding a ball initially. Movements in the form are diagonals and rotations of the trunk and head. Movements slide back and forth, in and out of 6A and 6B, then position is reversed for right and left.

### FORM 7. Directions
Turn torso to the right (11 o'clock) as right hand circles up to ear level with arm slightly bent and palm facing obliquely upward, while left hand moves to the front of the right part of the chest, palm facing obliquely downward. Look at right hand (7A).

Turn torso to the left (9 o'clock) as left foot takes a step in that direction for a left bow stance. At the same time, right hand draws leftward past right ear and following body turn, pushes forward at nose level, with palm facing forward, while left hand circles around left knee to stop beside left hip, palm down. Look at fingers of right hand (7B; 7C).

### FORM 7. Therapeutic Elements 1–7
This form begins in the position of 7A, but with both feet flat on the floor. They remain on the floor throughout the exercise. Move in and out of the positions 7A, B, C, A, B, C, then reverse right-left positions.

### FORM 8. Directions
Continue to move hands in a downward-inward-upward curve until wrists come in front of chest, with right hand in front and both palms turned inward. At the same time, draw right foot to the side of left foot, toes on floor. Look forward (8A). Separate hands, turning torso slightly to 8 o'clock and extending both arms sideways at shoulder level with elbows slightly bent and palms turned outward. At the same time, raise right knee and thrust foot gradually toward 10 o'clock. Look at right hand (8B; 8C).

### FORM 8. Therapeutic Element 1–7
With the elderly, the kick is only a small part of their available range. The form is utilized for kicking with both dorsiflexion and plantar flexion of the foot. Forms 8 and 9 are the most stressful for maintaining balance due to the small base of support and the extreme movement of the kicking leg. However, forms are done continuously with slow movements and a strong degree of concentration. The range for the kick is not extreme in the elderly.

### FORM 9. Directions
Shift weight onto right leg, and draw left foot to the side of right foot, toes on floor. At the same time, move both hands in a downward-inward-upward curve until wrists cross in front of chest, with left hand in front and both palms facing inward. Look forward to the left (9A; 9B).

Separate hands, extending both arms sideways at shoulder level, elbows slightly bent and palms facing outward. Meanwhile, raise left knee and thrust foot gradually toward 4 o'clock. Look at left hand (9C; 9D).

### FORM 9. Therapeutic Elements 1–7
The same as form 8, but right and left are reversed.

### FORM 10. Directions
Turn palms forward and downward while lowering both hands gradually to the side of hips. Look straight ahead (10A, 10B; 10C).

### FORM 10. Therapeutic Elements
This is a warm-down form like Form 1 and constitutes both a physical and mental ending of the exercise.

(Reprinted with permission from Wolf 1997b.)

undertaken, depending on the ROM and strength characteristics of the individual. (3) Progressive flexion of the knees is performed to varying degrees with 70% of body weight generally on one leg, then shifting to the other leg so that most of lower extremity muscle strengthening would be expected during loading onto that limb. (4) Straight and extended head and trunk positioning is developed, a prerequisite for promoting a less flexed posture. Consequently, rigorous attention is needed to prevent leaning of the trunk or protrusion of the sacrum. (5) Trunk, head, and extremity rotation is emphasized in all but the first and last exercise forms. Movements are done in circles, especially in the upper extremities, and require a strong rotational component. The eyes often follow the hand movements, thus promoting head and trunk rotation through eye movements. (6) Symmetrical and diagonal arm and lower extremity movements are used as a major part of the selected forms, not only to promote arm swing in gait but also to increase trunk rotation around the waist. (7) Constant shifting to and from the right and left legs emphasizes progressively more displacement of body mass (Forms 2 to 9) to develop skill at ultimately achieving unilateral weight and balance through self-awareness of limitations in postural stability," (p. 888-9)

Tse (1992, p. 297) proposed that the practice of tai chi promotes postural control for the following reasons:

1. "All Tai Chi movements are circular, slow, continuous, even and smooth. Patterns of movement flow from one to the next. The slow, even tempo facilitates a sensory awareness of the speed, force, trajectory, and execution of movement throughout the exercise.
2. Because movements are well controlled, all unnecessary exertion is avoided, and only sufficient effort is used to overcome gravity (Plummer, 1982). Muscle coordination instead of rigid cocontraction can, therefore, be promoted.
3. Throughout the exercises, the body is constantly shifted from one foot to the other. This is likely to facilitate improvement of dynamic standing balance.
4. Throughout the exercises, different parts of the body take turns in playing the role of stabilizer and mover, allowing smooth movements to be executed without compromising the balance and stability of the body. This relationship between the firmly held position (postural stabilization) and the moving part (focal movement) of the body has been the focus of postural control in many studies."

Positive clinical effects of tai chi, including improved balance (Li, 2012), have been suggested in elderly and neurologically impaired samples (Hain, 1999; Ross, 1999; Tse, 1992; Wolf, 1996;). Details of related studies can be found in the online (ONL) Focus on Evidence table. Further research is needed regarding the effectiveness of tai chi among populations with specific neurological disorders. In such patients, the principles of progressively narrowing the BOS over time, eventually to a single-leg stance if possible, combined with body and trunk rotation through greater ranges and reciprocal movements of the arms may be of value in improving balance deficits.

### Force-Platform Biofeedback

Training of balance may also be accomplished utilizing biofeedback from a computerized system that monitors and displays force-platform data regarding movement of the COP (see Fig. 30-6). Nichols (1997) discussed the use of force-platform biofeedback to retrain balance after stroke. She suggested that it is especially useful in the rehabilitation of patients with postural asymmetry or diminished limits of stability. While standing on the force platform, the patient monitors his position and movement subjectively through internal sensory feedback and objective feedback about sway provided through the monitor screen (Srivastava, 2009). The patient

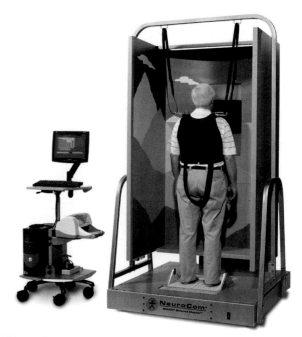

**FIGURE 30-6** A patient standing on a computerized force-platform system, the NeuroCom® Smart Balance Master® system, including a dynamic surface and moving visual surround with visual computer feedback regarding center of pressure movement. *(Courtesy of NeuroCom.)*

can use this augmented information to make accurate adjustments. Such biofeedback can be used to train static stance or steadiness and dynamic stance, also called *movement*.

Training static stance is accomplished by giving the patient visual feedback on a monitor screen regarding location of his COP, represented by a cursor in relation to a shaded central target area, during a task that requires maintenance of a stable stance. The patient gets almost immediate feedback regarding body sway and whether correctional movements are appropriate in direction and amplitude. After the trial, the patient is given specific feedback regarding the distance and direction of excursion of the COM over a specific period.

Training for symmetry in stance is carried out by asking the patient to keep the cursor in the center of the computer screen, depicted by a vertical line, while in a quiet stance. Symmetry training can also involve visual information in the form of graphical displays of two columns that represent the percentage of body weight on each foot, with a goal of equalizing the two.

Training protocols also address dynamic postural stability. This is most often accomplished with activities that require active weight shift to selected targets displayed on the screen at the extreme right, left, and front-back (see Fig. 30-7A) and circumferential targets at the periphery of the limits of stability, as shown in Fig. 30-7B. The designated target changes on a specific schedule from the center target to one of the peripheral targets and then back to the center, then out to the next peripheral target, back to the center, and continuing this pattern around the periphery. The patient can visually see how accurately he gets to the desired target as he moves.

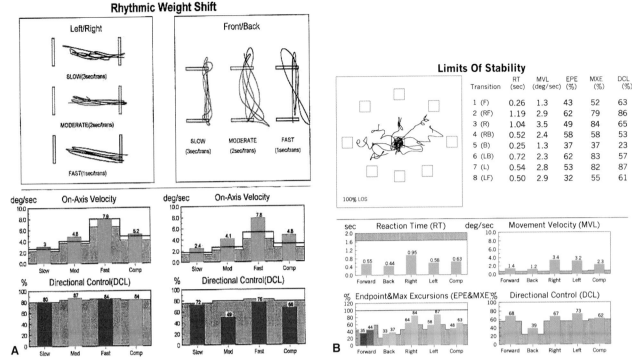

**FIGURE 30-7AB** Computer monitor views (excursion of center of pressure and relative weight-bearing for each side) for force-platform training activities. (A) Dynamic balance activity for left-right weight shift (this individual is able to shift to the right but is not able to shift adequately toward the left target) and front-back weight shift (these front-back weight shifts also show that the subject has most weight on the right side because he is able to shift forward and backward). (B) Dynamic balance activity to improve limits of stability with circumferential targets at the periphery toward which the subject shifts, with visual feedback as shown in these images. *(Courtesy of NeuroCom.)*

There are many commercially available force-platform systems, though the cost is comparatively very high, often too high for smaller facilities. A growing body of evidence supports the effectiveness of feedback through force-platform systems, including studies with subjects who have a neuromuscular disease. Significant improvement in static standing symmetry has been shown in hemiparetic adults after force-platform training for stance symmetry (Winstein, 1989). Regarding specificity of training, Winstein noted that although there was increased symmetry in stance, there was no significant association with increased symmetry in ambulation. In a study that included subjects with hemiplegia, postural sway biofeedback was shown to have a greater effect in reducing sway than conventional physical therapy intervention (Shumway-Cook, 1988). Details of this method can be found in the online (ONL) Focus on Evidence table.

For clinics that cannot afford a force-plate system, the Nintendo Wii Balance Board has been effective in poststroke intervention (Cheok, 2015), with the game Wii Fit demonstrating excellent test-retest reliability for COP excursion and validity concurrent with that of laboratory-grade force plates (Clark, 2010. Limitations of the Wii system include the inability to detect rapid, high-force movements (jumping and running) and to assess horizontal forces (Clark, 2010).

### Aquatic Therapy

The beneficial effects of the aquatic environment have been applied throughout much of recorded history. Recently, more attention has been paid to the physical therapeutic effects of treatment activities in a pool setting as part of the rehabilitation process. For balance impairment, several of the physical properties of water can enhance training in a pool. First, the body is buoyant in water because it has a lower density relative to the water. This can be accentuated by use of appropriate flotation devices and by using deeper depths of water. Because the center of buoyancy in humans is between the T2 and T4 vertebral levels, standing in deep water above these vertebral levels provides a degree of natural support to the trunk in upright postures, whether sitting or standing, with a greater effect as the water level deepens. Buoyancy also allows more time for the patient to react to COM changes as part of balance training. The hydrostatic pressure of water also contributes to this stability, with a steady external force applied toward the body from all directions.

The aquatic environment has been described as a "low-risk environment" for balance intervention because of the reduced fear of falling and thus reduced anxiety (Lord, 1993; Skelton, 1999). Part of the reduced fear of falling and enhanced feeling of safety is related to the support from water buoyancy and the extra time afforded for balance reactions. You must, however, consider and ensure the safety of the patient with balance impairment both in the pool, at poolside, and during entry into and exit from the water.

Several treatment techniques can be utilized in the aquatic environment as interventions for balance impairment. Turbulence can be generated by moving an object or body part under the water and to apply perturbations while the patient is maintaining an upright posture in the training of balance strategies. Morris (1997) discussed specific aquatic solutions for balance dysfunction and suggested aquatic stretching and strengthening techniques in the pool to correct these underlying deficits. In addition, the Watsu, Bad Ragaz Ring, and Halliwick methods are proposed to improve balance in patients with neuromuscular pathology. These methods are described in the aquatic unit of Chapter 14.

Approximations of functional activities performed in the pool have been described as part of an aquatic program for balance, with improvement noted among a group of elderly independent ambulators (Simmons, 1996). Details of the evidence basis of this treatment are presented in the summary chart at the end of this chapter. In the following activities, 10 repetitions of each standing task and four repetitions of 6.1-meter distance (pool width) for walking tasks were completed:

- Walking forward and backward
- Walking backward while high-stepping
- Marching forward and backward with knees bent
- Walking forward and backward with knees straight
- Side stepping without crossing the legs
- Side stepping with crossing of the legs
- Heel-to-toe walking forward and backward
- Marching in place
- Standing partial squats
- Toe raises
- Heel raises
- Kicking in a diagonal direction
- Kicking in cardinal planes of motion
- Twisting

In addition to the activities described by Simmons (1996), the patient can perform functional activities such as seated scooting on an underwater bench or stool, seated reaching while on an underwater bench or stool, the sit-to-stand transition (Fig. 30-8A), and stepping on steps, up and down (Fig. 30-8B).

### Vestibular Rehabilitation

Because vestibular dysfunction is a common underlying impairment related to balance deficits, intervention should target specific vestibular problems identified in the examination. A full description of vestibular rehabilitation is provided in Chapter 29.

## ■ Intervention: Ultimately Applied in Functional Activities

Functional treatments for balance deficits are categorized as static sitting activities, dynamic sitting activities, static standing activities, and dynamic standing activities. Balance in quadruped, kneeling, and high-/tall-kneeling is also considered functional, especially in the pediatric population. Individuals at risk of falling also need good balance in quadruped and high-kneeling positions to return to a chair. In addition to the functional balance interventions described in the

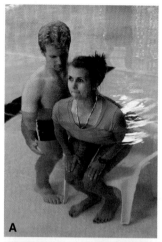

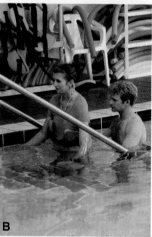

**FIGURE 30-8AB** A patient in the pool, with assistance of the therapist. (A) Performing sit-to-stand with partial support of the buoyancy of the water. (B) Taking steps up the pool stairs.

remainder of this chapter, examples of specific functions are described in Chapters 34 through 37. In all of these functional treatment activities, the safety of the patient must be considered as the first and minimal goal to achieve, eventually progressing beyond just "safe" to functional!

## Static Sitting Balance

### Posture Education

Static sitting activities are the simplest for patients to perform. They are often a good starting point for the treatment plan, especially in acute care and early rehabilitation. Proximal stability is necessary for distal mobility. The patient is first educated in proper sitting posture and alignment of the trunk, including mild lumbar spine extension with slight anterior tilt of the pelvis; scapular retraction pulling the shoulders up and back, which facilitates proper position of the thoracic spine; an upright cervical spine with slight cervical extension; and slight chin tuck. This position can be easily facilitated as the therapist sits on a physioball, which is placed to support the patient's low back (Fig. 30-9). In patients with poor control, guidance or manual facilitation may be required to achieve this optimal position.

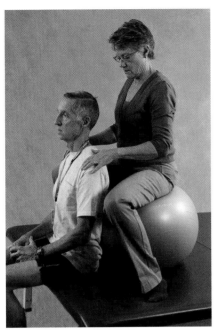

FIGURE 30-9 Therapist is sitting on a physioball behind the patient, who is short-sitting on the edge of the mat. The therapist can manually assist or create perturbation at the upper trunk while the stabilized physioball provides support at the trunk/low back.

A good position, especially for a patient with hemiplegia or hemiparesis, is to sit sideways on the involved side (Fig. 30-10). In this position, you can support the patient with your leg if he requires minimum to moderate assistance. When the patient requires maximum assistance, you can use one upper extremity. In this position, at least one of your arms is free to use for another task, such as holding an object up for reaching. Perceptual deficits may need to be addressed at this point (see Chapter 31). Once the desired

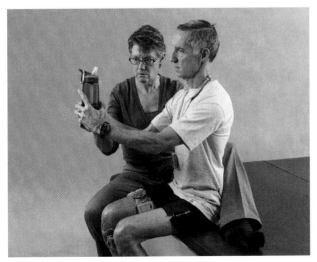

FIGURE 30-10 Therapist is sitting at the patient's side, oriented perpendicular to the patient and with one leg extended behind the patient, which the therapist can use, in addition to the arms, to support the patient.

position has been attained, the patient is asked to maintain upright sitting on firm and pliable surfaces and later to tolerate externally imposed displacement or perturbation while on these surfaces.

### Static Sitting on an Unstable Surface

You can ask your patient to maintain upright, midline sitting while seated on an unstable surface such as an equilibrium board, inflatable disc, or therapeutic ball (Fig. 30-11). The functionally related activity would be sitting on the seat of a moving car or bus that is starting and stopping. When the bus stops suddenly, the individual must make rapid adjustments to stay upright. As the patient improves, this can be progressed to asking the patient to sit on the ball with one leg crossed over the other so that only one foot at a time is in contact with the floor. In this condition, the patient must not only control the appropriate trunk reactions for sitting equilibrium but also must control the position of the ball.

## Dynamic Sitting Balance

### Progressive Trunk Control

Encourage progressive increase in trunk control for dynamic sitting balance by adding more and more challenges to sitting tasks over time. This may also be achieved by progressively moving the points of assistance lower on the trunk, requiring control of additional trunk segments. One specific application was examined in a pediatric population with cerebral palsy (Butler, 1998). "Targeted training" uses equipment to eliminate movement of the segments directly beneath the trunk joints that have been targeted for training. Padded supports and strapping are used to control positioning of the spine below the targeted vertebral joints, including hip and knee positioning to keep the lower spine in a neutral position (see Fig. 30-12). The uppermost support can be adjusted downward as the child gains control at the initial target levels. This allows the child to practice control of the specific target joint during external disturbances, including a rocking base to the equipment, with all segments below the target joints supported by the equipment. Thus, the child can learn control of only one or two joints at a time. As the child learns to control the target joints, the equipment is adjusted to support lower segments and allows practice at controlling additional vertebral-level segments. Over the period of intervention, "full control of the whole vertebral column can be gained in stages" (Butler, 1998, p. 282). Evidence supported use of this method among six children with cerebral palsy, with a demonstrated increase in both trunk control and function in all six children (Butler, 1998).

This same concept can be used in adults, with the therapist guarding from the side and the therapist's leg behind the patient supporting the trunk (Fig. 30-13A). You can move your leg, which is supporting the patient's trunk, lower on the patient's back (Fig. 30-13B) as he needs less assistance, allowing him to control more spinal segments.

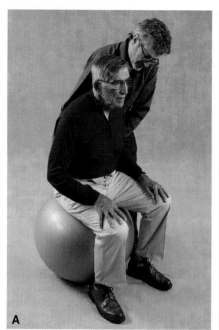
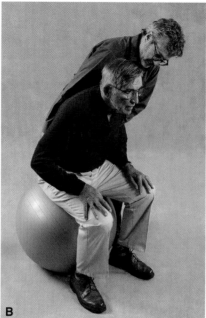
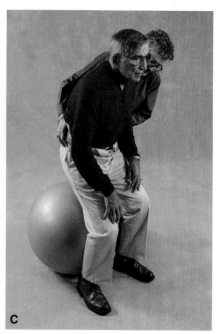

**FIGURE 30-11** A series of photos showing a patient sitting on a therapeutic ball, guarded by the therapist while actively rolling the therapeutic ball forward and backward and performing sit-to-stand from the ball.

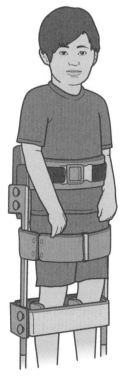

**FIGURE 30-12** A pediatric patient supported by the equipment for "targeted training" of the trunk for sitting balance training. As the child gains trunk control in sitting, the uppermost support can be adjusted downward so the child can practice greater trunk control.

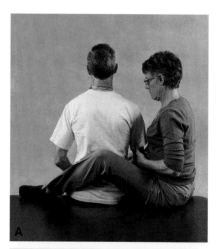

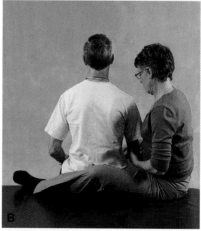

**FIGURE 30-13AB** Therapist guarding the patient from the side (A) using the leg to support the trunk and (B) with the leg positioned lower on the patient's back when the patient requires less assistance.

## Functional Weight-Shift and Reach While Sitting

The simplest functional task for dynamic sitting is weight shift anteroposteriorly, mediolaterally, and ultimately in all directions. Ask the patient to shift as he would in a theater to view the stage around the person with the big hairdo sitting in front of him. The magnitude of weight shift can be progressively increased as the patient improves, including rapid changes in the direction of weight shift.

The most obvious functional task in dynamic sitting is reaching and grasping an object using trunk movement. Have the patient practice the reach in all directions of movement, including the full periphery, as well as reaching to a variety of surface heights. Reaching down as if picking something up from the floor while sitting should also be included, with variety in the pattern of repetitions. These activities focus mainly on the patient mastering anticipatory postural control in sitting.

## Weight-Shift and Reach While Sitting on an Unstable Surface

Finally, the dynamic sitting activities described above can be carried out while sitting on an unstable surface or during disturbance of the other components of balance. Internal perturbations, such as sudden movement of one's own limbs, and external perturbations, including nudges or sudden disturbances from the therapist, should eventually be incorporated into the treatment activity and increased in magnitude as the patient improves. Both types of perturbations are encountered by individuals daily and can be incorporated into a progressive intervention plan, probably starting with mild internal perturbations (simply lifting the hand off the lap) and later progressing to moderate internal perturbations (reaching for an object) and mild external perturbations (gentle nudge to the trunk), and ultimately to moderate/more extreme internal and external perturbations when possible (stair-climbing and bumping, as with a fellow department store shopper).

These activities focus mainly on the patient mastering reactive postural control in sitting. It is important to incorporate both anticipatory and reactive postural control activities in sitting balance tasks because the patient will use both, often at the same time, in real life.

**Hippotherapy**, application of horseback riding for therapeutic effects, has improved kinematics and functional performance of human movement (Park, 2013). In a case presentation of two children with cerebral palsy, functional mobility improved (Haehl, 1999).

## Static Standing Balance

### Static Stance Progression

Static standing activities are commonly used in rehabilitation settings and are reported in the literature. For example, Gill-Body (1997) reported a progression of stance activities in three phases:

1. Phase 1: Start with static stance on a firm surface, with eyes open and eyes closed, feet together, and arms close to the body while moving the head. Also included in this phase is static stance on a foam surface with eyes closed intermittently and feet 1 to 2 inches apart.

2. Phase 2: **Semitandem** stance on firm surface, eyes open and eyes closed, is performed with arms crossed. (Semitandem stance is a posture in which the feet are not side by side, but one foot is placed more forward—step length in front of the other.) Stance on foam, with eyes closed intermittently and feet 1 to 2 inches apart, is also included in this phase.

3. Phase 3: Semitandem stance on a firm surface is progressed to eyes closed continuously, and with eyes open on firm and compliant surfaces.

A general progression of static stance activities starts with performance on a flat, stable surface, with progression to pliable surfaces, such as foam mats, and eventually unstable, movable surfaces, such as an equilibrium board, BOSU ball, or BAPS board. You can add additional challenges to these activities by eliminating or disturbing vision, progressively narrowing the BOS, eventually including tandem stance and even single-leg stance, adding a dual task (cognitive and/or physical), and applying unexpected, mild perturbations during which the patient must maintain the static standing position.

## Upper Extremity Activities While Standing

Performing upper extremity tasks while standing creates self-induced perturbations to which the patient must respond. This gives the patient opportunities to practice balance strategies and maintain the static upright posture. Some clinics have rings to move across a plastic tube arc or cones to move on the opposite side as preliminary, prefunctional activities.

A single-subject design was used to examine an intervention program for balance impairment for patients with hemiplegia (Wu, 1996). The intervention program consisted of two standing activities and results suggested a trend toward improved balance (Wu, 1996). Sanding at a standing table and playing a beanbag game while standing were done for 30 min each day. Even the beanbag task can be viewed as a functional activity (e.g., in the grandfather whose primary rehabilitation goal is to play throw and catch games with his grandchildren). Regardless, the activities simulate myriad standing activities in which use of the upper extremities challenges one's own balance.

As your patient moves toward true functional activities, ask him to move canned goods from one side across the midline while standing or to wash windows or mirrors while standing (see Fig. 30-14), or creatively incorporate your patient's favorite hobby (crochet, woodworking, cooking, workbench activities, etc.) into a standing protocol, especially as a home activity. More challenging lower extremity support conditions can be added to these tasks as well. The more variability you can integrate into your practice, the better. Real-life activities force a patient to reach for many different objects, all with different shapes, sizes, and weights. Therefore, the patient should practice reaching for as many objects as possible to simulate real-life tasks.

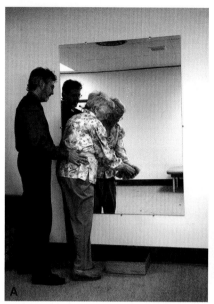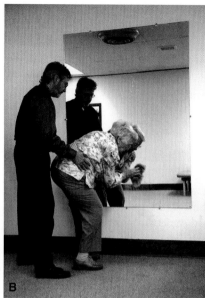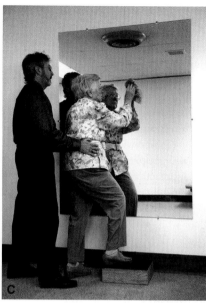

**FIGURE 30-14ABC** A patient washes a mirror while standing for functional balance training, including (A) reaching at arm level, (B) reaching down in a partial squat, and (C) washing with the right foot on a higher surface to bias weight-bearing to the left foot.

### Resistive Exercise in Standing

Activities that apply resistance to the lower extremities or to the whole body may be useful for increasing strength and applying perturbations for practice of appropriate balance reactions. One resistance training program that improved balance in older adults included three self-paced, resistive activities after a 3-min warm-up of walking at a normal pace (Rooks, 1997):

- Stair-climbing exercise: Three sets of ascending and descending a flight of 14 stairs were performed with a weighted nylon skin-diving belt around the waist for added resistance, with a 1- to 2-min rest period between sets. A 0.91-kilogram (2-pound) weight was added to the belt when the subject felt he could handle the additional weight.
- Resisted knee extension: While the patient was seated, knee extensions were performed (one leg at a time) using equipment that provided accommodating resistance via a brake system; the resistance increased as the subject exerted more effort, allowing him to moderate the resistance repetition by repetition. A verbal cadence of 2 seconds for the concentric phase and 4 seconds for the eccentric phase were used to guide the repetitions, with rest periods between the three sets of eight repetitions.
- Standing plantar flexion: Standing with both hands placed on the wall for stability and toes approximately 12 inches from the wall, the person lifted up on the toes for a 1-second concentric contraction and a 2-second eccentric contraction. Three sets of 15 repetitions were performed using body weight as resistance.

Others have suggested use of Theraband™ or rubber tubing for resistance training in the geriatric and neurological populations (Duncan, 1997; Topp, 1993). Specific isolated movements that contribute to normal balance synergies can be strengthened by applying the principles of resistance with the knowledge of movement direction for specific muscles.

The relationship between resisted exercise and balance improvement has also been explored. A dynamic strength training program with six upper body and six lower body resistance exercises has been described for older adults (Topp, 1993). This program included three sessions of strength training using elastic tubing per week for 12 weeks. Posttest measures for the exercise group revealed some enhanced balance, whereas some balance measures did not improve. There were more obvious and consistent increases in lower extremity strength measures, which supports the case for specificity in training and practice. Clinical application could include strengthening of hip extensors, flexors, abductors, and adductors; knee flexors and extensors; and ankle plantar flexors and dorsiflexors.

Resistive tubing or bands of stretchable rubber material such as Theraband™ can also be used to generate perturbation simultaneously with the stretching exercises. For example, as the patient performs hip extension exercises in standing, he will spend a portion of his time in single-limb stance. With each movement into resisted extension, the stretched, resistive material creates a momentary perturbation or disturbance, requiring a response from the patient. Each time the hip swings into the end range of hip extension, the elastic material will suddenly pull the leg back into flexion, necessitating an ankle, hip, or stepping strategy from the leg that is in contact with the floor.

"Therabalance," an innovative, easy-to-construct balance intervention, also uses resistive bands in almost any treatment setting (Studor, 1998). Studor conceived the use of Therabalance, which uses two pieces of stretchable banding forming an "X" that crosses the front of the patient from under the axilla bilaterally (see Fig. 30-15). The patient stands with his back to the wall or to a closed door, and the ends of the therapy banding are attached to metal eyes that are screwed into the wall or door facing. The value of this setup is that patients are free to experience and practice balance reactions and moving within the limits of stability without the use of arms for support, even for light touch contact. It also frees the therapist from direct contact with the patient, allowing the therapist the freedom to step back and observe the patient from a variety of angles and to provide more challenging cognitive stimulation simultaneously with the balance task as the patient improves. Care must be taken to ensure patient safety, especially because patients may lean too far forward. Studor (1998) reported that "most patients have to lean forward (without any type of stepping or hip strategy) to about 35 degrees from vertical before the harness cannot support them."

Therabalance has been used in patients with standing balance impairment, related to CVA, brain injury, ataxia, Parkinson's disease, and multiple sclerosis, with even broader use possible, including home programs (see the "Home" section that follows) (Studor, 1998). No clinical trials have been reported on this method.

## Dynamic Standing Balance

### Preambulation Weight Shift

As a preparatory activity addressing body structure/body function, weight shift in standing involves part-task training toward ambulation and specifically prepares for the functional dynamic balance required for independent ambulation. Weight shifts are often performed initially in a lateral direction with parallel stance, with feet beside each other (Fig. 30-16A) because it is often simpler to perform and may feel safer because of foot placement. Considering the principle of specificity of training, it is important to progress as early as possible to a semitandem or diagonal stance (Fig. 30-16B) because diagonal weight shift is more commonly part of mobility tasks. Lateral weight shift is functional for tasks such as standing at the kitchen counter and shifting laterally to retrieve a box from the side cabinet, but not for ambulation. You can progress later to a semitandem stance with one foot placed further forward than the other, which more closely approximates the weight shift that accompanies ambulation and other dynamic balance tasks.

When the patient is unable to independently produce a full weight shift, you can manually guide the weight shift to the

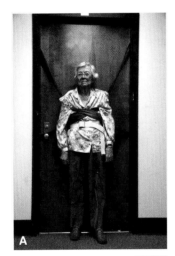

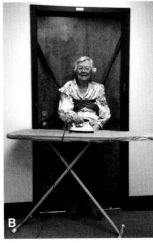

**FIGURE 30-15AB** Patient in Therabalance setup in a residential setting (A) in front of a doorway and (B) incorporating the functional activity of ironing.

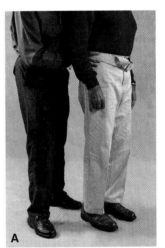

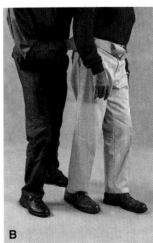

**FIGURE 30-16AB** Foot positions for balance and pre-gait activities: (A) parallel stance and (B) semitandem or diagonal stance.

full extent. This is probably best accomplished with hand contacts at the pelvis to encourage pelvic movement that shifts the entire trunk as a unit. Your patient may try to initiate weight shift by leaning the upper trunk, a very common, abnormal, compensatory method observed in patients with cerebral pathology. In a patient with potential for appropriate movement, the therapist should manually prevent and discourage practicing of abnormal, inefficient, and compensatory movement patterns. Instead, encourage sufficient opportunities to practice optimal, efficient movement patterns.

Progressing the difficulty of the task can start with gradually increasing the weight-shift amplitude. Several forms of feedback may be helpful. Shumway-Cook (2007) suggested using a flashlight attached to the trunk, allowing the light beam to move across a wall as a reflection of patient weight shift (a laser pointer may provide a more specific location). Clinically, more objective and useful feedback regarding the weight shift or sway can be given using a small retractable tape measure. The tape measure case is taped to the wall while the end of the tape is pinned to the patient's clothes at the waist (see Fig. 30-17A). This method can be used for

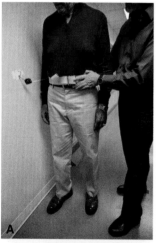

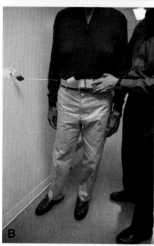

**FIGURE 30-17AB** Patient using a retractable tape measure for feedback regarding weight shift amplitude. (A) The patient shifts close to the wall. (B) The patient is shown during weight shift away from the wall.

weight shift in any direction: patient facing the wall for anterior-posterior weight shift, patient diagonal to the wall for diagonal shift, and patient with side to the wall for lateral shift (Fig. 30-17B). This is an inexpensive way to provide objective feedback to the patient regarding the degree and magnitude of weight shift.

Video games, such as the Wii Fit or Kinect system, also provide objective feedback to the patient regarding the degree and magnitude of weight shift, although they are a little more expensive than the above-mentioned tools (Szturm, 2011).

Once weight shift is sufficient to completely unload one leg, you can ask the patient to pick up the unweighted foot momentarily. Then, to enhance the patient's understanding and allow experience of the task, you may want to give a trial with weight shift to the less-affected side and lifting of the affected foot. Over several sessions, have the patient gradually increase the time that the foot is suspended in the air. Repeat the activity with weight shift to the more-affected leg and lifting of the opposite leg. Further progression may include lifting the leg progressively higher with progressively longer holds in single-leg stance, weight shifting on a pliable surface (e.g., foam), and obviously decreasing external support.

Another treatment approach to encourage weight shifting and balance on one lower extremity is to change the support surface for the less-involved lower extremity. This makes the patient rely and put more weight on the involved lower extremity. This treatment approach is quite useful in the patient with hemiparesis. For example, a patient with right-sided hemiparesis may exhibit difficulty in balance and/or neuromuscular control with the right lower extremity. You could start with the patient standing with the right lower extremity on the ground and the left lower extremity on a step or stool. This forces the patient to bear more weight on the right lower extremity. As the patient progresses, you can lessen the weight-bearing through the left lower extremity and thus increase the right lower extremity weight-bearing by having him place the left lower extremity onto a cup or cone, foam disc, or small ball.

### Dynamic, Symmetrical Stance Activities With Upper Extremity Support

For dynamic balance activities in standing, bilateral and symmetrical standing is a simple place to start with patients in the rehabilitation process. In early activities, upper extremity support will likely be necessary, either from the therapist or with a stable surface or assistive device. You should guard the patient properly at all times and/or use a safety harness.

Start dynamic training with symmetrical activities, such as very shallow squats with an early emphasis on symmetry, and progress to asymmetric squatting, which is a functional part of lifting small objects from the floor. To give the patient visual feedback in terms of the degree of symmetry, it may be helpful for him to face a mirror. You can place a piece of tape vertically and instruct the patient to align the tape on the mirror with the image of their body. From a balance standpoint, asymmetric squatting emphasizes the leg with greater weight-bearing (i.e., the leg closest to the COP). An added benefit of such an activity is that lower extremity extensor strength is also trained and in a functional position. The patient may hold onto parallel bars or use the edge of a tall plinth for upper extremity support. Keep in mind that upper extremity support should be progressively withdrawn as soon as possible to train the trunk and lower extremities, rather than the upper extremities, as postural muscles.

Dynamic stance activities can also be practiced on unstable surfaces, always with support from the therapist or a safety harness during initial attempts, for experience in responding to environmental perturbations. Unstable surfaces for dynamic stance, listed from least to most challenging, could be a foam pad, a single-axis equilibrium board, and finally a BAPS board, BOSU ball, or inflatable disk that moves along multiple axes (see Fig. 30-18AB). Single-axis equilibrium boards with auditory feedback that is initiated by contact switches on either end of the board are also commercially available. This system has been described and its effectiveness demonstrated (Nordt, 1999).

Clinically, you can use the single-axis equilibrium board with lateral movement or have the patient facing the plane of

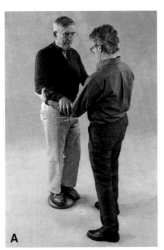

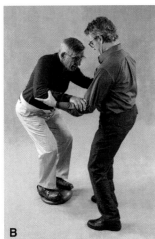

**FIGURE 30-18AB**  Patient (A) standing on an inflatable disk and (B) performing a shallow squat activity. This type of unstable surface can be used to challenge balance during the functional activity.

motion in a semitandem stance to practice a forward weight shift and balance, which more closely approximates ambulation. In each case, it is often helpful to have the patient emphasize decelerating the movement using muscles in the downside leg on a weight-bearing, flexed knee while shifting the trunk and center of gravity in the upward direction to maintain balance.

Do not forget that early balance activities on moving surfaces most likely require external support, a safety harness, or therapist assistance, which is gradually withdrawn over time. Speed of movement and unexpected disturbances can also increase as the patient improves. When patients get to higher functional levels, you can ask them for momentary and eventually longer trials of single leg stance on the unstable surface using the affected leg.

### Ambulation, Narrowed Base, and Variations

The ultimate dynamic standing activity for most of our patients is ambulation. Almost every rehabilitation patient who cannot walk reports as a personal goal "I want to be able to walk again." After beginning with simple, forward "normal" walking, the BOS in gait can be varied, and then adjustments to various sensory, step, and directional variables may be incorporated to train balance. You may start with the relatively mild restriction of requesting a narrower BOS to the more highly restrictive heel-to-toe or tandem walking (Gill-Body, 1997; Verfaillie, 1997); walking over a thick foam surface or over a variety of surface textures in series; and decreasing visual input (i.e., a dim room, eyes closed if you guard them).

Gill-Body (1997) described the following progression for gait activities:

1. Phase 1: Gait with a narrowed BOS with eyes open and wide turns to the right and to the left; with eyes open, marching in place on firm and foam surfaces with prolonged pauses in unilateral stance
2. Phase 2: Gait with eyes open with sharp 180-degree turns to the right and left on firm and padded surfaces; marching in place with eyes closed and prolonged pauses in unilateral stance and gait with eyes open and a normal BOS accompanied by slow head movements
3. Phase 3: Three gait activities:
    - Gait with eyes closed and BOS progressively narrowed on firm and padded surfaces, marching in place slowly with eyes open and eyes closed on firm and foam surfaces
    - Gait with eyes open and rapid sharp turns to the right and left on firm and padded surfaces
    - Gait with a normal BOS, with eyes open during fast head movements

Woollacott (1997) suggested brisk walking as part of the treatment plan to address decreased balance because it appears that fast and powerful muscle activity generation is helpful for effective and efficient reactive balance control.

For patients to return to safe community mobility, they must be able to walk on an uneven surface. One way to clinically simulate this is to place canes or other objects underneath a mat and have the patient walk across the mat. The canes simulate the cracks and bumps in the sidewalk. This forces the patient to work on anticipatory postural control as he visually scans for the bumps and prepares his body for perturbation and on reactive postural control as he responds to destabilization induced by stepping on the cane. The therapist can name this exercise affectionately after the city in which they are practicing (e.g., the "New Orleans Sidewalk Exercise").

Attempts to enhance safety in dynamic standing balance training have included devices that increase external support. The overhead harness and trolley system has enhanced patient safety in the examination and treatment of both balance and motor control in gait (Harburn, 1993). Similar devices are now commercially available (see Fig. 30-19), including treadmills with overhead harness systems attached or freely moving frames that move around with the patient and support him from overhead (Seif-Naraghi, 1999).

When such devices, including body-weight support ambulation training, are overused or used on a prolonged basis without progression to more independent ambulation, they may have unwanted effects on balance because they seemingly decrease demand on the balance system and opportunities to practice balance strategies. Therefore, use of body-weight support systems should be gradually tapered from the standpoint of balance training.

### Variable Step Patterns

Variations in walking patterns can also be used in balance intervention. Not only is this a functional task, but patients also need to step in a variety of directions when using a stepping strategy for recovery from a balance loss. This activity is especially important in older adults who tend to rely more on a hip or stepping strategy than an ankle strategy to regain balance

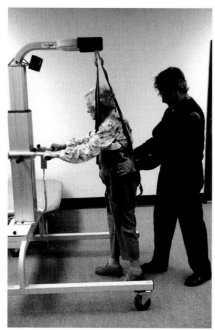

**FIGURE 30-19** A patient supported by an overhead harness attached to a rolling frame during ambulation.

(Shumway-Cook, 2007). *Side-stepping* is one commonly used example in the literature (Gill-Body, 1997; Verfaillie, 1997) that occurs with the feet staying parallel and always in appropriate right-left relation. In this activity, many patients turn their trunk diagonally, partially facing the direction of movement. For optimal demand, stress the importance of good trunk alignment and upright trunk posture, with the patient facing perpendicular to the direction of the side stepping.

Braiding, also called braid-walking or crossover stepping, has been used clinically to address balance impairment (Gill-Body, 1997; Verfaillie, 1997). Also sometimes called "grapevining," or "karaoke," **braid-walking**, or **braiding**, is a more advanced form of stepping sideways with several variations, all involving stepping across the stance foot (Fig. 30-20).

When teaching a patient braiding, you should start with a consistent pattern, especially when there is a cognitive deficit. For the early trials, step consistently across in front of the leg or across behind the leg (see Fig. 30-20A). Remember that the trailing foot is always the one that crosses. That is, if a person is braiding to the left, he will probably start with a left step laterally with the left foot. Then the right foot will step across, either in front or behind the stance leg, to the left side of the left foot. The left foot simply steps around to the left again to start the series over again. A common mistake patients make when completing this activity is turning the hips to the side instead of keeping them pointed forward, so watch the patient's hips closely during this activity. You can progress the intervention, eventually alternating a step across the front with a step across the back, and then repeat this alternating pattern (see Fig. 30-20ABCD). Have your patient step to the right for a series of steps and then step to the left. This activity may be started in parallel bars early on for enhanced safety and stability as the patient is learning the movement pattern.

Upper extremity support can be given manually from the front, as described before, if necessary. You can provide the support dynamically as the patient performs braiding or side stepping, either with the patient's hands on your forearms or shoulders (remind the patient this is NOT for weight-bearing) or with your hands at the patient's hips.

Backward walking was reported in a case study as a part of a balance impairment treatment program in patients with cerebellar dysfunction (Gill-Body, 1997). Backward walking may be helpful as a component of treatment because it minimizes visual input. Some may reject backward walking because they view it as nonfunctional, but we must back ourselves out of tight spaces when we are unable to turn around to leave, back up to sit in a chair, or step backward as part of opening a door.

## THINK ABOUT IT 30.3

- What is different about steps taken under anticipatory postural control versus steps taken as a reaction to a destabilizing stimulus or balance perturbation?
- Clinically, how can you incorporate stepping in a variety of directions for anticipatory postural control and as a reaction to a balance perturbation?

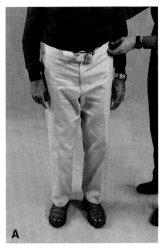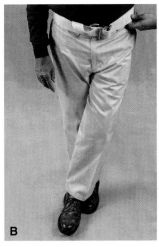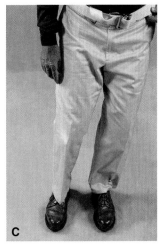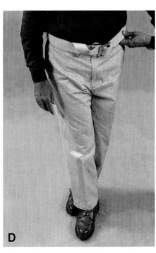

**FIGURE 30-20ABCD** Braid-walking technique. (A) The patient starts in normal stance with the feet parallel. (B) Sideways stepping is initiated by the trailing foot (left foot in this example) crossing over in front of the stance leg; (C) the patient then uncrosses the legs by stepping behind with the original stance foot and (D) crossing the legs again by crossing over in back of the stance leg, and then uncrossing back to starting parallel position. The therapist supports the patient as needed. Greater challenge occurs through this pattern of alternating between (B) stepping in front with the left leg and (D) stepping behind with the left leg.

## Practice Components of Balance and Gait

Gill-Body (1997) suggested active practice of specific components of balance in gait as a treatment activity. Standing with eyes open and eyes closed during heel touches forward and toe touches backward may improve postural control in a functional activity through use of all sensory systems. This may be viewed as part-task training of ambulation with a focus on practicing balance, especially of the stance limb. These authors also used active practice of ankle sway movements as treatment.

## Intentional Creative Movement in Stance

Creative dance and a movement exploration program have been proposed for treating balance impairment in children with cognitive deficits (Boswell, 1991). Young or older patients can be encouraged to participate in dance, gymnastics, aquatic exercise, golf, and other creative, skilled movement activities to enhance balance. Tai chi, discussed earlier in this chapter, fits in this category because the emphasis is on self-awareness and quality of movement. Creative movement such as dance, gymnastics, or tai chi are most effective when they were an integral part of the patient's life before the onset of dysfunction, enhancing motivation to be regularly involved in the activity. We should encourage our patients to get back into an active lifestyle, with emphasis on prior activities in which they are naturally motivated to participate, particularly those that stress quality of movement and skill in movement.

## Practice of Functional Transitions

Repetitions of functional transitional movements that require balance are an excellent way to retrain balance in function. Repetition of level surface and uneven surface transfers allows the patient to experience the appropriate pattern of movement and focus on perception of the movement. When necessary, the patient can initially compensate for deficit components in an atmosphere of safety created by the therapist's presence, assistance, and preparatory setup.

The sit-to-stand transition is also a good activity in which to practice balance. This transition is one in which patients often feel anxious because the BOS changes from one of very stable anteroposterior depth, encompassing feet and buttocks, to a greatly diminished anteroposterior depth (the length of the person's foot). Because the weight is shifting forward away from the seating surface during this change of BOS, a highly unstable situation occurs. As a result, many patients need extra verbal reassurance and greater assistance, especially in the early attempts. As the patient progresses, these activities can be performed while he is constrained, by lowering the surface, softening the surface, and/or altering the setup to require more weight-bearing and balance from one particular leg. This may be done by placing the foot you wish to disadvantage either out of normal lower extremity alignment (slightly off to the side), further forward than the other foot, or up on a short stool or using a combination of these (see Fig. 30-21A, B).

## Bending and Reaching Activities

Bending and reaching activities in standing, a common functional task, are often incorporated into balance treatment (Gill-Body, 1997). These skills require significant upright postural control and often place the patient in a more precarious position than simple ambulation. These functional skills incorporate components of many of the previously described activities and may be practiced to enhance motor learning. You can make these activities obviously functional by having the patient stoop to pick up an object such as a rolled-up newspaper, a key chain, or a can of green beans. The patient can place additional demand on the balance system by bending and reaching while the feet are on two different surface heights, with the affected leg on the lower surface (Fig. 30-21C), by standing on an

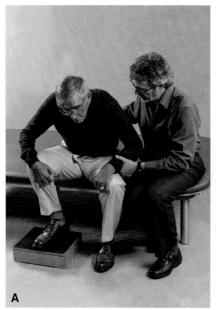
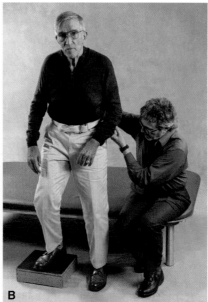
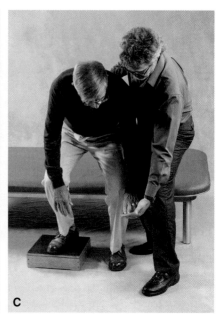

**FIGURE 30-21ABC** During a functional transition such as sit-to-stand, (A and B) placing the less-affected foot on a higher surface places greater demand on the affected limb. (C) Bending down to reach for a lower object can also be performed with the less-affected foot on a higher surface.

unstable surface, or for greater challenge by bending and reaching in single-leg-stance.

### Climbing Stairs

Stair-climbing for balance impairment (Lee, 2014) is a very advanced form of ambulation because in addition to forward progression, there is work against gravity to lift the body at each new level. An early form of stair training to address balance impairment can include stepping up on and down from a platform 1 to 8 inches high with the minimum amount of assistance or support required to focus on increased single-limb stance (see Fig. 30-22AB) (Asher, 1997). Stair-climbing with weights has been included as part of an overall balance treatment with positive results (Rooks, 1997). Stair-climbing is also challenging because substantial time is spent in single-leg support during which the COM continually moves forward and up while ascending or forward and down while descending.

You can incorporate balance training both up and down stairs with progressively less assistance being offered. You can start by allowing the patient to use the handrail and later allowing only touch of the handrail without major weight-bearing through the upper extremities. Finally, you can ask the patient to walk up and down stairs with no upper extremity contact and ultimately even with added nudges or perturbations. Remember, when you add perturbations, careful guarding is necessary to ensure patient safety.

### Obstacle Course

Obstacle courses are a common intervention for balance impairment in clinical settings, but their validity or effectiveness has not been investigated. One course design consisting of

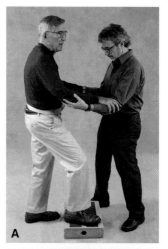

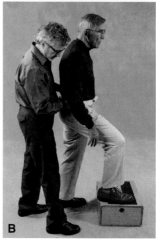

**FIGURE 30-22AB** A patient stepping up and down (A) from a 4-inch platform step and (B) from an 8-inch platform step.

12 simulated functional tasks is suggested as a treatment for balance impairment in function (Means, 1996). The 12 stations are as follows:

- Four different surfaces to walk across (sand, pine bark chips, artificial turf, and deep pile carpeting)
- Two graded surfaces to walk on (up and down ramps)
- Two commercial stairs (one with eight shallow steps and 7.6-centimeter riser height and one with four standard steps and 15.2-centimeter riser height)
- Four functional tasks and maneuvers (opening a closed door; arising from a soft, armless chair; walking a slalom course between a straight line of eight plastic cones spaced 61 centimeters apart; and stepping over three parallel cylindrical foam bolsters that are 10.2, 15.2, and 20.3 centimeters in circumference

In addition to tackling these obstacles, the patient steps over small boxes (shoe box size), reaches down to pick up objects from the floor, kicks or moves an object out of the way, walks around a chair, squats to step under a tension rod placed in a doorway, or walks on a foam surface. In addition to withdrawing assistance over time, you can progressively request increased speed for a discrete set of obstacles as a constraint to increase performance time.

A person's adequate balance in a functional task can worsen while he is performing a cognitive or physical task along with the primary functional task (e.g., trying to complete a conversation while walking). For intervention, dual task activities such as a cognitive task along with a mobility task can be incorporated, as discussed in Chapter 37. This task also works on scanning, which is a useful intervention for patients with inattention or a visual field cut (see Chapters 7 and 31). You can also incorporate picking up objects off the floor by having the patient clean up the obstacle course. There is much room here for creativity from the therapist, with a focus on tailoring the obstacles to real-life events and situations in the patient's life. Gentile's (1987) taxonomy of a task, as discussed in Chapter 14, can also guide progression of this intervention, including object manipulation.

## Pediatric Considerations

The principles, techniques, and activities previously described for balance are also applicable in a pediatric setting. Often, the techniques and activities must be adapted, as discussed previously, with a focus on motivating the child and ensuring that the activities are age appropriate. A survey of American Physical Therapy Association Pediatric Section members from across the United States revealed that respondents used a combination of functional and more traditional treatment activities to address balance dysfunction in children and most often identified with the NDT approach encouraging functional activity (Westcott, 1998). In addition to functional activities in sitting and standing, balance in quadruped and kneeling is an essential ability in normal development. These postures are developmentally appropriate as balance treatment activities for children.

### Quadruped Activities

If improving balance in quadruped and creeping (forward mobility in a quadruped position) is a general objective of therapy, the child is often placed in quadruped position, i.e., hands and knees, during a treatment session. When the child needs additional support in this position early in rehabilitation, a small bolster or pillow can be placed under the trunk, providing partially stable trunk support (see Fig. 30-23A). As the child's abilities progress, the trunk can be supported using a small ball (see Fig. 30-23B), which is a more unstable support surface than the bolster, and ultimately progressing to no support at all.

A more dynamic aspect of quadruped function involves creeping across the room. When sufficient external support is given by the therapist, the child may begin to experiment with the weight shift and sway that can take place in quadruped by rocking forward, sideways to each side, and diagonally in each direction, an activity that is often observed in children just before the first attempts at creeping. Later, you can make the activity more challenging and begin to approximate components of creeping by using toys and other environmental stimuli to encourage an upper body–weight shift, with lifting of the unweighted arm for a reach task or for repositioning of the arm for forward progression of creeping.

### Kneeling and Half-Kneeling Activities

You could start balance activities in kneeling as static postural activities with some degree of upper extremity weight-bearing allows, depending on the patient's impairments and their severity. The child can play while kneeling at a bench, with toys for play on the bench, which limits weight-bearing use

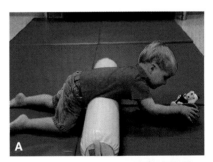

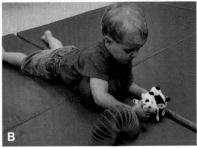

**FIGURE 30-23AB** A child (A) with significant trunk support by a bolster to allow practice and experience with static balance and (B) with trunk supported by a small ball, which requires more control from the child. Even greater demand would be required if the child was in quadruped.

of at least one arm. You can create a more challenging task by having the child kneel with hands supported at chest height on a therapeutic ball or an unstable surface (see Fig. 30-24). Make sure you progress to placing the objects outside of the comfortable reach of the child, making the child really reach and shift the body weight. Static balance in kneeling should ultimately progress to tall-kneeling play (hips in extension) and activities with single upper limb support and eventually no upper extremity support. Additional challenges can be added by changing the density and stability of the kneeling surface, including foam, equilibrium, or wobble board.

Dynamic activities in kneeling should include weight shift in tall-kneeling with upper extremity reach for objects and the accompanying body-weight shift as a functional adjunct. Set up the environment with motivating visual cues to encourage reach and weight shift in forward, diagonal, and sideways directions. To further challenge balance in kneeling, transitional movements can be incorporated into the treatment session, including quadruped to and from kneeling and kneeling to and from half-kneeling (see Chapter 34). These functional transitions include the challenge of a changing BOS.

---

### PATIENT APPLICATION: "MORE ON OUR PATIENT"

Consider Fawn's clinical situation further, including the expected progression of her functional abilities. Use the following questions to guide development of a patient-centered treatment plan, including activities you would use to work toward functional outcomes.

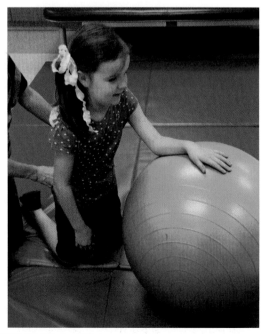

**FIGURE 30-24** A child practicing balance in supported tall-kneeling with upper extremity support on an unstable therapeutic ball.

---

### Contemplate Clinical Decisions

- Use the information and activities presented in this chapter to design four specific treatment activities to improve Fawn's balance, given her functional limitations and underlying impairments. Focus on balance in standing postures. Be sure to specify the amount and location of assistance you would allow from external sources and that you would provide.
- Specify the rationale for choosing each component of the activities you designed.

---

## ■ Intervention: Considerations for Nontherapy Time and Discharge

### Aspects of Patient and Family Education

In counseling the patient with balance impairment, an attitude of safety should be emphasized, especially regarding the activities he will perform at home, the amount of assistance he will use, and whether a family member or caregiver should be present. Too often, a patient has such a strong desire to get better that he takes excessive risks, placing himself in jeopardy and increasing the risk of falling. The therapist should encourage optimal activity at home with the least amount of assistance required to be safe and should help the patient understand these parameters before giving home activities. Also, it may be helpful to delineate the possible consequences of falling, particularly fractures of the wrist, hip, or ankle; contusions of muscles or skin; brain injury; and heightened fear of subsequent falls.

A health promotion focus for individuals with balance deficit involves preventing falls by addressing contributing factors from internal and external environments (Tideiksaar, 1986; Tinetti, 1994). Box 30-2 summarizes helpful ideas for patients for correcting frequent problems.

### Activities for Home

At the therapist's discretion, the patient may practice many of the aforementioned balance activities at home, especially those that fit into the daily routine. Carefully consider and clearly communicate with the family when the selected activities will require assistance or supervision from a family member or other caregiver. Family members need to be instructed in how to give optimal support without creating dependency.

The patient may be able to perform some of these activities at home if he has sufficient support. For example, the patient may grasp or at least rest the hands on a stable surface, such as the back of a sofa, a stable table, or a countertop. For extra stability in a home setting, some patients can do these activities standing with their back to a corner of the wall or with their hands resting on the back of a kitchen chair in front of them for upper extremity support. For early rehabilitation activities (i.e., before confidence has developed), this setup may provide a measure of security to the patient, promoting a feeling of being enveloped by the wall and chair. The Therabalance setup (Studor, 1998) described earlier in this chapter also increases a sense of security relative to balance activities in free

---

**BOX 30-2  Ideas to Prevent Falls in Patients at Risk**

- Suggest use of a night-light to illuminate hallways and bathrooms at night because falls often occur when getting up to use the restroom at night.
- Advise patients to take extra caution with slippery surfaces and obstacles, including furniture and electrical cords across walk spaces.
- Recommend a formal eye examination to ensure that vision is corrected with appropriate lenses.
- Encourage patients to discard loose floor rugs, which can be frequent sources of slipping or tripping on a turned-up edge, and replace them with carpeting or larger, flat, nonskid rugs.
- Encourage appropriate footwear, properly fitted to enhance a solid base of support.
- Provide education/referral regarding use of sedative-hypnotic agents (Tinetti, 1994).
- Recommend safer furniture (height and stability) and possible installation of grab bars in the bathroom and handrails on stairs (Tinetti, 1994).
- Recommend analysis of current medications for potential effect on balance.

---

space and may be suitable in a home activity program for patients with a normal stepping strategy.

An important part of home intervention is education of the patient and family or other caregivers. Overall, there should be a strong emphasis on ensuring safety during the activities, not taking risks, and taking rest breaks when the lower extremities become fatigued. As you educate the patient regarding balance, emphasize the importance of weaning himself over time from the use of upper extremity support while transferring the workload and requirements for balance to the lower extremities. Again, plant a seed in the patient's mind to help him think toward the future, when less support and assistance will be needed, and encourage small movement toward that goal each day.

Because patients with poor balance are at great risk for falling, patients should also be educated to avoid common environmental contributors to falls, such as slippery surfaces, loose rugs, poor lighting, obstacles, and alcoholism (Robbins, 1989). In addition to balance training, strengthening, and flexibility, guidelines for therapists working with older people who have fallen include teaching the patient how to rise from the floor (to avoid a "long lie" in case the patient does fall and coping skills such as summoning help and keeping warm while on the floor) (Simpson, 1998).

## A Sample Home Exercise Program

A patient who is 7 months post-CVA has regained sufficient motor control of the right lower extremity to ambulate with a quad cane for 75 feet with the assistance of only one person, mostly to prevent rare loss of balance (only one episode on stairs during 50 minutes of activities) and safety. The following activities represent home activities at one point along the progression toward optimal improvement (or this could be a home program for our patient Fawn).

- The patient stands with the hands resting on a stable support (back of couch, countertop, etc.) and with a symmetrical stance and performs shallow squats (Fig. 30-25A) using both legs equally for the concentric and eccentric work of lowering and raising the body. This activity can be progressed by changing foot position, with the less-affected

leg placed more laterally out of alignment, placing more weight-bearing demand on the more affected leg.
- The patient stands with hands resting on a stable surface as previously described, in a parallel or semitandem stance and practices repetitions of weight shift from one foot to the other (Fig. 30-25B). The patient should make sure the weight shift occurs with the trunk moving as a unit, not just the shoulders and not just the pelvis.
- Working toward a prolonged single-leg stance at the end of a weight shift in the previous activity, the patient can lift the unweighted foot just an inch or so from the floor and try to hold it up, even if just momentarily (Fig. 30-25C). Weight shift should be emphasized as an essential preliminary step before lifting the foot. The patient should also be reminded to use the least amount of arm/fingertip support needed and to expect that the amount needed will decrease week by week.
- Hopping on one foot
- Hopping from one foot to the other
- Walking at a faster pace than usual

### PATIENT APPLICATION: "MORE ON OUR PATIENT"

*After 5 months of intervention, Fawn has now progressed to ambulation with a cane and can even do so independently on flat grassy areas. She reports that she still finds herself pushing or "leaning" on the cane more often than she wants. When walking without the cane, she catches her toe on the tile floor approximately every other step. She has 4 weeks until graduation!*

### Contemplate Clinical Decisions

- *For each treatment activity previously developed, specify how you would progress that activity over time to reflect improvements in Fawn's status.*
- *Discuss your discharge plans for Fawn, including the home activity program she should carry out after discharge.*
- *Consider health promotion and wellness aspects of a discharge plan that may have ongoing positive effects on her balance, as well as her self-esteem, overall health, and safety.*

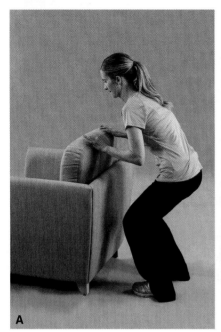
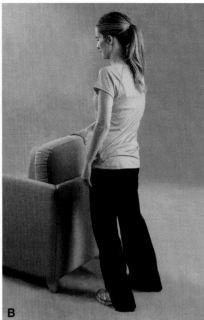
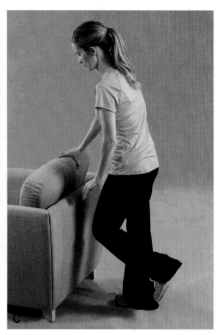

**FIGURE 30-25ABC** Home exercise program using a large, stable piece of furniture for upper extremity support. (A) Patient performing symmetric shallow squats. (B) Patient performing weight shifts in stance with an upper extremity reach at the extreme of the weight shift. (C) Patient lifting one foot off the floor momentarily.

### PATIENT APPLICATION: OUTCOME FOR FAWN:

*Fawn is ultimately able to meet her personal goal. She graduates, is able to walk up the stage stairs without a cane, walk across the stage, and shake the school principal's hand as she receives her diploma. Although the therapist still observes*

*obvious asymmetry in her gait pattern, Fawn has relearned a more normal gait pattern that allows sufficient foot clearance so that she rarely trips now, even on uneven outdoor terrain.*

- *Her gait velocity at a self-selected medium pace has increased to 0.65 m/sec (2.13 ft/sec), and the timed up-and-go test score (3 meters) improved to 9.7 seconds.*

## HANDS-ON PRACTICE

■ **After reading the chapter, you should be able to perform these hands-on skills:**

- Guarding during static and dynamic balance interventions
- Incorporation of visual fixation and head movements during dynamic activities
- Dynamic functional activities, including throwing and catching
- Facilitation of static and dynamic activities on an unstable surface

- Activities to train the strategies (ankle strategy, hip strategy, stepping strategy)
- Use of a therapy ball to work toward single-leg support activities
- Incorporation of tai chi actions to challenge balance
- Use of biofeedback (including force platform)
- Hands-on facilitation of appropriate postures or movements

## Let's Review

1. Describe therapeutic interventions that focus on underlying impairments in patients with identified proprioceptive deficits in the lower extremity, visual impairment, or vestibular impairment.

2. In the general progression of therapeutic interventions for balance impairment, why is it important to incorporate activities on unstable surfaces? Provide some examples of how this can be done.

3. If you want to provide feedback to the patient about weight shift, but you do not have a force platform, what are other ways to provide this feedback?

4. Describe a series of functional activities that place a progressive demand on balance systems during static and dynamic sitting.

5. Describe a series of functional activities that place a progressive demand on balance systems during static and dynamic standing.

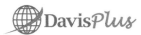 For additional resources, including case study discussions, please visit http://davisplus.fadavis.com

## CHAPTER SUMMARY

Balance impairment is one of the more complex rehabilitation body structure/body function diagnoses and is also very widespread among patients with neuromuscular disorders. The therapist must have a comprehensive understanding of the underlying sensory, central processing, and motor systems that contribute to maintaining an upright position against gravity and against external perturbations, as discussed in this chapter and Chapter 9 (Balance Examination). Table 30-6 online (ONL) summarizes some of the important research studies that form the evidence basis for balance intervention. The treatment plan must first address the underlying impairments of body structure/body function identified during the examination and evaluation that are hypothesized to contribute to the balance deficits.

This chapter describes an array of intervention techniques that target components of impaired balance. Other chapters of Section IV describe intervention techniques specific for the impairments that contribute to decreased balance, including interventions related to involuntary contractions (Chapter 20), coordination (Chapter 21), weakness (Chapter 22), ROM (Chapter 23), motor control (Chapters 24 and 25), sensory impairment (Chapter 27), vestibular impairment (Chapter 29), and cognition (Chapter 31). As these underlying impairments are addressed in treatment and show improvement, the intervention should begin to focus more exclusively on function, working toward improved functional outcomes, particularly improved balance in each functional skill that is a problem for the patient and especially skills that are a priority for the patient. The latter part of this chapter describes function-based treatment activities for balance, supplemented by the functional interventions of Chapters 34 to 37; suggestions for progression of each activity's parameters as the patient improves are also included.

# Overcoming Challenges of Impaired Perception, Cognition, and Communication (Aphasia or Dysarthria)

Jane Mertz Garcia, PhD, CCC-SLP ▪ Beth Cardell, PhD, OTR/L
Dennis W. Fell, PT, MD ▪ Jill Champley, PhD, CCC-SLP

CHAPTER **31**

## CHAPTER OBJECTIVES

Upon completion of this chapter, the learner should be able to:

1. List and describe characteristics of cognitive disorders, perceptual impairments, aphasia, and dysarthria.
2. Infer the effects of communication deficits on clinical intervention for physical impairments and the ability to meet therapeutic goals.
3. Identify ways to promote successful communication with patients with neurological disorders.

## ■ Introduction: Becoming an Effective Partner in Communication

Although the focus of this textbook is on the physical impairments (characteristics, evaluation, and intervention) of people with neurological conditions, the reality is that many of these individuals present with related disorders that are outside the scope of physical therapy (PT) and occupational therapy (OT) practice and create unique challenges in service delivery by the therapist. Speech-language pathologists (SLPs) evaluate and diagnose disorders of communication and design intervention programs to enhance the communication abilities of many of the patients described in this textbook. Various medical professionals, including

SLPs, PTs, and OTs, address cognitive and perceptual deficits in some manner. Knowledge and skills related to definitive communication interventions are not the focus of this chapter; instead, the emphasis is on strategies that promote functional communication and optimize cognitive abilities and perceptual skills in patients to enhance clinical intervention for physical impairments. As a result, the focus and goals for this chapter are much different from those of other therapeutic intervention chapters and include strategies and tips rather than specific communication or language interventions.

A critical aspect of this chapter is understanding the importance of interacting effectively with patients with communicative impairments. Communication is broadly defined as the exchange of ideas using both verbal and non-verbal modes. Successful communication includes accurate "**encoding**" of messages by the speaker (sender) and "**decoding**" of messages by the listener (receiver). Communication supports enhanced interpersonal exchanges and patients' participation in activities of daily living (ADLs). In addition, effective use of communication strategies adds to a patient's sense of competence and accomplishment (Simmons-Mackie, 2013). Well-prepared health-care providers contribute to patients' overall quality of care by accommodating their communication needs and recognizing factors in the environment that affect clinical exchanges.

Like most healthy adults, health-care professionals successfully apply the processes of **communication** (speaking, listening, gesturing, reading, and writing) in an effortless manner each day. In contrast, patients with communication impairments may be overwhelmed by routine aspects of clinical interactions such as asking them to describe their level of discomfort with an exercise or directing them to "lock the wheelchair brakes." Imagine the frustration of patients who are unable to verbally express their pain or who struggle to comprehend a simple request.

You are apt to hear the expression that "no two brain injuries are alike," which certainly applies to the unique characteristics of patients who are communicatively impaired. It is important to keep in mind that the disorders described in subsequent sections are quite different from one another (e.g., dysarthria vs. aphasia), and there are various profiles within a particular type (e.g., a number of people with aphasia speak telegraphically in sentences of two to three words, whereas others speak continuously in long sentences composed of many errant words). In addition, some people present with more than one communication deficit, which may be complicated by other concerns such as impaired swallowing (**dysphagia**). Swallowing disorders affect people across the lifespan and have numerous causes such as TBI, stroke, cerebral palsy, and Parkinson disease. Because a discussion of dysphagia is beyond the scope of this chapter, you are encouraged to view public resources available through the American-Speech-Language Hearing Association (http://www.asha.org/public/) to learn more about the disorder.

The strategies offered in this chapter provide general considerations for promoting successful communication between the therapist and patient and are not intended to represent an exhaustive listing. Some suggestions will most likely be more helpful than others. It is always important to consult with members of a patient's treatment team, especially the SLP, to verify each communication diagnosis and the appropriateness of specific strategies. In addition, many patients have preexisting vision or hearing impairments that can affect the success of a therapy program. It is important to know if a patient has glasses, hearing aids, or hearing loss and how to appropriately accommodate these issues in conversation exchanges.

## THINK ABOUT IT 31.1

- Speech-language pathologists help children and adults who have difficulty with communication and/or swallowing. Learn more about their roles and responsibilities at http://www.asha.org/policy/SP2016-00343.
- Describe how person-first language is a simple but important way to be sensitive to others.

## ■ Foundation Skills: Cognitive Processes and Perceptual Abilities

### Functional Implications

**Perceptual** ability, or **perception**, is essential to understanding sensory stimuli encountered throughout the day can affect decisions made and actions taken, and can be impaired in patients with neurological conditions. Perceptual skills must be intact to ensure daily choices that are safe and appropriate. Knowing when to take a step up, how far to reach, and where to locate an item on a cluttered desk all depend on perceptual skills. Deficits in perceptual skills have been a major factor in decreased independence in ADLs and mobility after stroke (Nys, 2007). Disruptions in cognitive function and/or perceptual deficits are due to a multitude of causes, including TBI (McKenna, 2006), stroke (particularly right hemisphere damage) (Barker-Collo, 2010; Vossel, 2013), and degenerative conditions (Gitlin, 2005).

Proper perception of sensory input is heavily related to other **cognitive processes** and systems (e.g., attention, memory, organization, and executive function). The combination of all of these skills provide the foundation for effective clinical interactions. Cognitive impairments affect communication and conversation exchanges in a number of important ways. For example, a patient's distractibility, inability to remember, and/or inability to extract main ideas while listening may result in unsafe decisions during structured motor tasks (e.g., transfers) or independent ADLs (e.g., safely crossing the street). In addition, more complex motor activities and execution of difficult motor tasks increase demands on specific processes such as attention (Tappan, 2002). Cognitive deficits are also considered a risk factor for mobility concerns, including falls (Harris, 2005; Hyndman, 2003; Muir, 2012).

The severity of cognitive impairments varies from patient to patient, with a corresponding variance in their effect on safe function. Some patients are disoriented to aspects of person, time, place, and purpose (e.g., knowing what happened and why they are in therapy) (Hux, 2011). Another factor affecting function is **attention** and type of attention impairment (Table 31-1) (Murray, 2006). For example, some patients do not *selectively* attend to spoken instructions, becoming easily distracted by nearby conversations and noises, or do not *focus* or *sustain* attention to task at an adequate level of vigilance (Gillen, 2009). For others, the challenge is to

| TABLE 31-1 | Types of Attention and Corresponding Functional Deficit |
| --- | --- |
| **TYPE OF ATTENTION** | **FUNCTIONAL PRESENTATION OF DEFICIT** |
| Selective | Easily distracted by any activity in the environment; responds to background noise; difficulty attending to therapist's directions while in a crowded therapy clinic |
| Sustained | Difficulty with details; stops a task midway; stops doing exercises after six repetitions when asked to do 15 |
| Divided | Unable to do two things at one time: complete dressing and answer questions about weekend plans |
| Alternating | Unable to return to original task if interrupted: during cooking activity, therapist stops patient to correct use of mobility device; patient requires cue to resume cooking task |

*divide* their attention across multiple stimuli (McDowd, 2007; Tappan, 2002). For example, a patient may not notice a change in pavement elevation (e.g., walking off curb) because of focused attention on approaching traffic.

Deficits in perceptual skills are often seen in conjunction with other cognitive impairments and can affect the therapeutic process in many ways. Visuospatial impairments (Table 31-2)

can affect a patient's abilities to safely judge distances during transfers or accurately avoid items in crowded surroundings during ambulation.

Rehabilitation outcomes can be substantially affected by the attention deficit known as unilateral **neglect**. Unilateral neglect is characterized as the failure to respond to stimuli presented to the side of the body or environment opposite a

| TABLE 31-2 | Definitions and Common Presentations of Visual Perceptual Skills | |
| --- | --- | --- |
| **VISUOSPATIAL SKILL AND DEFINITION** | **FUNCTIONAL USE OF A SKILL** | **FUNCTIONAL PRESENTATION OF A DEFICIT** |
| Depth perception: ability to judge distance between objects or between objects and self | Walking over uneven ground; managing stairs; reaching for a cup; transferring between surfaces | May overshoot (knock over cup) or undershoot (grab empty space); stumbling when unable to predict dips in the grass |
| Figure ground: distinguishing objects in the foreground from pattern in the background | Finding an object in a cluttered drawer; locating a white washcloth on a white bedsheet; picking a friend out of a crowd | Difficulty identifying an object across the room; unable to distinguish the brake on the wheelchair from the rest of the chrome |
| Spatial relations: ability to interpret where objects are in space and how they relate to self and to other objects | Assembling an item from written directions; positioning self and items for proper use; understanding terms: under, over, next to, behind, etc. | Difficulty with aligning self and wheelchair for transfers; unable to follow verbal directions; appears confused by directional terms |
| Right/left discrimination: Ability to understand and apply concepts of right and left Personal: left and right as they relate to own body parts Extrapersonal: how left and right are interpreted in the environment | Following driving directions; donning clothing correctly | Difficulty following verbal or written directions; dons clothing improperly |
| Form constancy: ability to identify objects represented in different views or when only a portion is visible | Recognizing scissors in a cup when only the handle is seen; identifying own car from the rear | Unable to identify common objects unless seen in their entirety; reports losing items frequently |
| Topographical orientation: ability to find familiar or new routes | Use of environmental cues to orient to current location; ability to return to original destination or to follow maps or directions | Difficulty finding way from patient room to treatment gym; routinely turns incorrect direction when leaving room |

Árnadóttir G. *The Brain and Behavior: Assessing Cortical Dysfunction Through Activities of Daily Living.* St. Louis, MO: Mosby; 1990.
Árnadóttir G. Impact of neurobehavioral deficits on activities of daily living. In: Gillen G, Burkhardt A, eds. *Stroke Rehabilitation: A Function-based Approach,* 2nd edition. St. Louis, MO: Elsevier/Mosby; 2004.
Zoltan B. *Vision, Perception and Cognition: A Manual for the Evaluation and Treatment of the Adult With Acquired Brain Injury,* 4th edition. Thorofare, NJ: SLACK; 2007.

brain lesion (Heilman, 1985). It is most often seen with right hemisphere damage, which causes left-sided unilateral neglect (Gillen, 2011; Swan, 2001). Patients with neglect often have greater functional deficits (Vossel, 2013) and progress through rehabilitation at a slower pace (Barker-Collo, 2010; Buxbaum, 2004) than individuals who do not experience neglect. Figure 31-1 illustrates a typical representation of left-sided neglect during a clock drawing assessment.

This deficit is referred to by many different names, including inattention, unilateral spatial neglect, hemi-inattention, and personal or extrapersonal neglect. Inattention is often used to indicate a less severe form of neglect. The terms *body/personal neglect* and *spatial/extrapersonal neglect* are often used to describe the types of information the patient is neglecting. Personal neglect includes parts of the patient's body, seen most often as neglect of the patient's left arm. This patient might

dress only the right arm when donning a cardigan sweater or attempt to transfer from supine to sitting without assisting the hemiplegic leg over the side of the bed. A patient with extrapersonal neglect may not attend to environmental space beyond the body. For example, the patient may not eat food off the left side of the plate or may be unable to locate items placed on the left portion of the bedside table.

**Hemianopsia** and **anosognosia** are terms frequently confused with unilateral neglect. Hemianopsia refers to visual fields cuts, whereas anosognosia is generally used to describe decreased awareness of paralysis (Gillen, 2009). Although it is possible for a patient to have visual field cuts, perceptual deficits, and denial of paralysis after a stroke, these are three distinct deficits, and the terms should not be used interchangeably. Table 31-3 includes pertinent questions to help screen the characteristics of neglect from those associated with visual field cuts (hemianopsia).

**Memory loss** and impairment of higher-level thought processes are common, especially in neurological conditions such as TBI. Although patients with TBI typically remember much of the distant past (**remote memories**), more recently acquired memories are vulnerable to loss (Murray, 2006). A patient may not recall therapy instructions from one day to the next or during one treatment session. Because memory terms are sometimes defined differently (e.g., there is not a universal definition for short-term memory), documenting the length of time a patient is able to remember specific information is more descriptive and clinically relevant than the use of a specific memory term and allows various team members to understand the patient's performance level. **Prospective memory** deficits typically emerge in everyday living situations when patients do not remember to execute an intended action (e.g., return for a follow-up outpatient therapy session) (Sohlberg, 2001).

Higher-level processes related to problem-solving, critical thinking, and **executive functioning** also affect patient safety

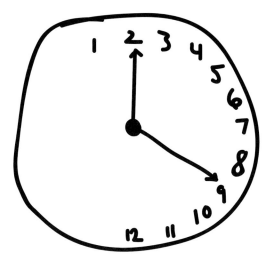

**FIGURE 31-1** Characteristic clock drawing by a patient who presents with visual neglect.

| TABLE 31-3 | Screening Questions to Assist in Differentiating Hemianopsia From Neglect | | |
|---|---|---|---|
| **DOES THE PATIENT** | | **HEMIANOPSIA/ VISUAL FIELD CUT** | **NEGLECT** |
| Complain of having difficulty seeing items or state the inability to find things? | | Yes | No |
| Miss details in one visual field? | | Yes | Yes |
| Locate lost items once cued to the location? | | Yes | No |
| Attempt to make eye contact during conversations, regardless of where the therapist stands? | | Yes | No |
| Spontaneously use both upper extremities when needed for a task? | | Yes | No |
| Spontaneously compensate for loss of vision by turning head? | | Yes | No |
| Walk/propel into things on one side without noticing? | | No | Yes |
| Lose track of limbs, letting them fall off footrests or table without repositioning? | | No | Yes |
| Seem to forget position of affected hand and drop or spill items? | | No | Yes |

Corben L, Unsworth C. Evaluation and intervention with unilateral neglect. In: Unsworth C, ed. *Cognitive and Perceptual Dysfunction: A Clinical Reasoning Approach to Evaluation and Intervention.* Philadelphia, PA: F.A. Davis; 1999.

Gillen G. *Stroke Rehabilitation: A Function-Based Approach.* St. Louis, MO: Elsevier/Mosby; 2011.

Warren M. Evaluation and treatment of visual deficits following brain injury. In: Pendleton HM, Schultz-Krohn W. eds. *Pedretti's Occupational Therapy: Practice Skills for Physical Dysfunction,* 6th edition. St. Louis, MO: Elsevier Health Sciences; 2006:532–572.

(Hux, 2011; Myers, 2005). For example, these patients may not identify hazards in their immediate environment or develop safe solutions to a problem because of poor thought organization, poor sequencing, and inflexible thinking (Sohlberg, 2001; Studer, 2007).

Changes in cognitive processes, along with other factors, contribute to impaired social communication, resulting in inappropriate behaviors and social responses to a situation (Hux, 2011; Myers, 2005; Willis, 2003; Ylvisaker, 2005; Yody, 2000). For example, inattentive patients may appear disinterested or have a tendency to ramble or quickly change the topic of conversation without warning, which may worsen in a noisier, distracting physical environment. Impaired **recent memory** may cause some to repeat parts of conversations or forget the topic and switch to a new one prematurely. It also is difficult to interact with patients who interrupt or make inappropriate comments because they are not reading the cues of the situation and are not inferring appropriate consequences. Other patients have a tendency to "ramble," which may simply be a sign of impaired thought organization and the inability to extract main ideas. In this situation, a simple request, such as "Tell me how it went getting in and out of the car with your wife," may elicit a series of detailed (arbitrarily sequenced) statements. The patient's response may or may not relate to the objective of the request, which was to learn about the patient's use of strategies in ADLs. The combination of these behaviors may reflect a patient who seems unmotivated, noncompliant, or purposely disruptive to her plan of care, when it actually reflects the effects of cognitive impairments on social effectiveness (Ylvisaker, 2005).

## Strategies to Enhance Interactions

This section offers general ideas to enhance clinical interactions, keeping in mind that the dynamics of an injury (e.g., the blunt trauma of TBI) often affects multiple aspects of a patient's cognitive system and areas of communication (Hux, 2011). For example, some patients with central nervous system involvement experience language deficits such as word-finding difficulty. In addition, about one-third of individuals who experience a TBI are diagnosed with dysarthria of speech (Sarno, 1986; Theodoros, 2001). The following strategies target perceptual and cognitive concerns, even though patients may benefit from a combination of approaches given their overall profile of communication strengths and weaknesses.

### Structure and Routine

Promote success by structuring clinical interactions for the patient who is cognitively impaired (Box 31-1). Consistent wording and use of nonverbal communication add redundancy to a message, which is especially important when interacting with a child or adult who is inattentive or has difficulty remembering (Murray, 2006). Additional verbal or tactile cues may increase attention during completion of motor tasks (Tappan, 2002).

Some patients benefit from structured interactions that promote learning and memory of new behaviors through **procedural memory**, which may be relatively spared with some brain injuries (Sohlberg, 2001). This method of instruction emphasizes learning to develop new habits through practice (performance-based memory for skills and action patterns). An example is developing a specific procedure for transferring from the bed to the wheelchair. The goal is to eliminate the patient's potential for error by breaking the task into its component parts, modeling target behavior, and fading prompts with success; the "errorless" learning approach provides systematic and repeated practice of discrete steps that contribute to success even for patients with severely impaired **declarative memory** (Clare, 2008; Evans, 2000; Sohlberg, 2005).

Disrupted attention may contribute to confusion and disorientation, which also is accompanied by agitation in some patients (Tittle, 2011). These patients become safety risks because of their restlessness and unpredictable behavior. In addition, it is difficult to target therapy objectives with patients who attend for only brief periods. There are a number of treatment strategies for patients who are confused and possibly agitated (Rothke, 1998; Willis, 2003; Ylvisaker, 2003). Key themes in this situation are to provide maximum continuity and consistency while maintaining a calm demeanor (Box 31-2). Confronting the

---

### BOX 31-1 Strategies to Structure Clinical Communication Interactions

Altering the Presentation of Information for Patients With Attention Deficits

- Establish and maintain eye contact with your patient before presenting directions.
- Offer instructions in small chunks.
- Slow the rate of presentation by asking the patient to repeat (in their own words) or demonstrate understanding of instructions before providing additional information.
- When family is present or when you are participating in a cotreatment, avoid interruptions and designate one person to do all of the instructing.
- Incorporate short breaks into treatments that involve a high level of attention in order to manage fatigue.
- Avoid interrupting the patient in the middle of a task. Limit unnecessary conversations.
- Stop the patient to provide additional information during natural breaks between steps.

Gillen G. *Cognitive and Perceptual Rehabilitation: Optimizing Function.* St. Louis, MO: Elsevier/Mosby; 2009.
Sohlberg MM, Mateer CA. *Cognitive Rehabilitation: An Integrative Neuropsychological Approach.* New York, NY: Guilford; 2001.
Zoltan B. *Vision, Perception and Cognition: A Manual for the Evaluation and Treatment of the Adult With Acquired Brain Injury,* 4th edition. Thorofare, NJ: SLACK; 2007.

---

**BOX 31-2 Interaction Strategies for Patients With Cognitive Impairment Who Are Confused and Irritable**

- Model calm, quiet, and confident behavior to the patient in your speech and actions. Be sure that your nonverbal and verbal communications convey the same information.
- Avoid surprises. Limit any changes because dullness and repetition are appropriate at this time. Group interactions (e.g., several visitors at one time) may serve to "overload" the person and increase confusion and agitation.
- Do not confront the patient's confusion or inappropriate behavior. Doing so may only increase agitation. It is better to simply change the subject.
- When your patient seems obsessed with unproductive thoughts or behaviors, try to *redirect* the person's attention to a different topic. Confused individuals are prone to suggestion; thus, simply getting the person's attention to another topic or activity often moves the focus away from disturbing or confusing subjects.
- Provide your patient with continuity in your personal interactions, and also be sure your reactions to difficult situations are consistent with those of other team members.
- Do not shout. Speak in a normal tone of voice. Speaking louder or with a "stern" voice may only increase the person's agitation or frustration.
- Minimize distractions because a person with a brain injury may have difficulty concentrating. When possible, interact with the person one-to-one in a quiet room.
- Keep it simple. Try something less demanding that promotes some degree of success. Allowing your patient to "walk off" excessive restlessness may effectively decrease agitation.

Rothke SE, Berquist TF, Schmidt M, Landre NA, Speizman R. *Behavioral Management Strategies for Working With Persons With Brain Injury: A Manual*, 2nd edition. Chicago, IL: Rehabilitation Institute of Chicago; 1998.

Willis TJ, LaVigna GW. The safe management of physical aggression using multi-element positive practices in community settings. *J Head Trauma Rehabil.* 2003;18:75–87.

Yody BB, Schaub C, Conway J, Peters S, Strauss D, Helsinger S. Applied behavior management and acquired brain injury: Approaches and assessment. *J Head Trauma Rehabil.* 2000;15:1041–1060.

---

patient's agitated behavior simply worsens the situation; instead, redirect the patient's attention to a different topic, away from the situation or source of frustration. Most important, do not leave the patient unattended and do not take the agitated behavior and verbal or physical aggression personally. It simply reflects the patient's brain injury.

## Environmental Modifications

A nondistracting physical environment is typically recommended for patients with cognitive deficits (Box 31-3). Examples of environmental modifications include limiting physical obstacles and clutter in a therapy area to help a patient selectively attend to a task while minimizing demands on her divided attention (Cicerone, 2002; Gillen, 2011; Tappan, 2002). Eliminating other sources of distraction, such as the noise of a television or toys not being used as part of intervention (Gillen, 2011), while optimizing visual cues through room lighting and reducing sources of glare also helps patients attend (Murray, 2006). Figure 31-2 provides a contrast of cluttered versus visually organized therapeutic environments.

Organization of patients' physical space reduces their cognitive load (Sohlberg, 2001). Physically locate important information (e.g., orientation charts, safety reminders) to take advantage of the patient's typical viewing level whether standing or sitting in a wheelchair. Consistent and routine placement of objects (e.g., quad cane) in the patient's physical environment is another type of memory aid (Parente, 2003). For example, storing adaptive equipment in the same, accessible physical location may contribute to the regularity of its

---

**BOX 31-3 Environmental Modifications to Limit Opportunities for Distraction**

- Remove unnecessary stimuli: Turn off the television, close the door, or pull the curtains.
- Conduct therapy in the patient's room or in a quiet treatment area whenever possible.
- When treatment must take place in a busy therapy clinic, turn the patient away from the visual stimulus of other people.
- Keep the treatment environment organized by putting away any irrelevant therapy tools between patients.
- Suggest that the patient wear earplugs or headphones to reduce noise.

Cicerone KD, Langenbahn DM, Braden C, et al. Evidence-based cognitive rehabilitation: Updated review of the literature from 2003 through 2008. *Arch Phys Med Rehab.* 2011;92:519–530.

Gillen G. *Stroke Rehabilitation: A Function-Based Approach.* St. Louis, MO: Elsevier/Mosby; 2011.

Sohlberg MM, Mateer CA. *Cognitive Rehabilitation: An Integrative Neuropsychological Approach.* New York, NY: Guilford; 2001.

Zoltan B. *Vision, Perception and Cognition: A Manual for the Evaluation and Treatment of the Adult With Acquired Brain Injury,* 4th edition. Thorofare, NJ: SLACK; 2007.

---

use because the constant location becomes a predictable visual reminder and part of the patient's habit and routine.

## External Aids and Compensatory Strategies

Many patients benefit from external strategies that enhance orientation, memory, organization, and problem-solving

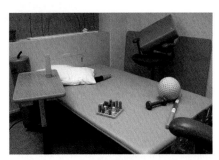

Cluttered

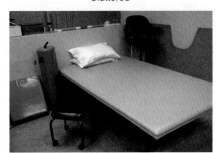

Uncluttered

**FIGURE 31-2** Contrast of a cluttered versus an uncluttered (visually organized) therapeutic environment.

(Table 31-4). Some aids are a natural part of the surrounding environment, such as clocks, calendars, daily schedules, and name tags worn by health-care providers. These strategies provide patients with a constant source of information to help their orientation (Gillen, 2011).

Clinical interventions for impaired memory and executive function often incorporate external aids, such as an organizer, visual schedule, or memory log for ADLs (Fig. 31-3). Always consult with team members regarding the function of these aids because some patients lack awareness about their use and/or need assistance with execution (e.g., verbal cues to write down important information). Patients also may benefit from other strategies, including written sequences in checklist form, reminder notes in high-visibility locations, and electronic aids such as digital voice recorders for verbal notes or watches and cellular phones with programmed alarms and reminders (Cicerone, 2011; Gillen, 2011; Parente, 2003). Portable electronic devices such as smartphones and personal digital assistants reportedly help patients with aspects of their memory, planning, and organization in everyday living tasks, such as executing a daily schedule, recalling nonroutine appointments, and completing clinical assignments (programmed "to-do" lists) (DePompei, 2008; O'Neil-Pirozzi, 2004).

| TABLE 31-4 | Therapeutic Strategies to Use With Patients Who Have Memory Impairment |
|---|---|
| **STRATEGY** | **EXAMPLES** |
| Give information in small chunks. | "First I need you to stand up" (wait for action). "Now, using your walker, take a few steps" (wait for action). "Let's walk to the kitchen." |
| Establish a routine with the patient while teaching new information. | Use the same words each time you run through the steps to prepare for a transfer. |
| Use real-life activities to teach a patient new concepts. | Teach the patient how to use hip precautions while she is transferring out of bed. |
| Store frequently used items in the same location each day. | Always place hearing aids in the same area each night while preparing for bed. |
| Ask the patient to paraphrase the information you have reviewed in the session. | "How would you summarize what we did in therapy today?" |
| Use multiple modalities when presenting information. | "The first exercise is..." "Copy the same movement I am doing." "Here is a picture of someone doing this exercise.'" "I have written directions so you can complete these at home." |
| Relate the information to the patient's life with specific examples (how this will help, why this is important). | "Completing these exercises will help you feel more confident while picking up your daughter." "It is important to lock your brakes so your family can feel safe leaving you home alone." |
| Use external supports. | Record information in a notepad; utilize a personal digital assistant, smartphone, alarm, voice recorder, or calendar. |

Gillen G. *Cognitive and Perceptual Rehabilitation: Optimizing Function.* St. Louis, MO: Elsevier/Mosby; 2009.
Green BS, Stevens KM, Wolfe TD. *Mild Traumatic Brain Injury: A Therapy and Resource Manual.* San Diego, CA: Singular; 1997.
Parente R, Kolakowsky-Hayner S, Krug K. Retraining working memory after traumatic brain injury. *Neurorehabilitation.* 1999;13(3):157–163.
Zoltan B. *Vision, Perception and Cognition: A Manual for the Evaluation and Treatment of the Adult With Acquired Brain Injury,* 4th edition. Thorofare, NJ: SLACK; 2007.

| Today's date is: *August 27, 2017* | |
|---|---|
| 7:30–8:00 am | Get up |
| 8:30 am | Breakfast  *Toast & peanut butter* |
| 9:00 am | Morning group  *Found out it might rain* |
| 9:30 am | Speech therapy  *Updated my memory log* |
| 10:00 am | Break  *Watched TV in the break room* |
| 10:30 am | Occupational therapy  *Worked on my hand-eye* |
| 11:00 am | Physical therapy  *Walked 50 feet by myself! YEA* |
| 11:30 am | Break  ~~Later?~~ *rested* |
| 12:00 pm | Lunch  *Sandwich was awful- good chips* |
| 12:30 pm | Speech therapy  *Had to problem solve stuff* |
| 1:00 pm | Rest period  *Took a nap... snooze!* |
| 1:30 pm | *snooze* |
| 2:00 pm | Counselor  *Talked about what I do next* |
| 2:30 pm | Recreational therapy  *Played cards - won* |
| 3:00 pm | Physical therapy  *Walked up and down stairs* |
| 3:30 pm | Occupational therapy  *Worked with money - count it* |
| 4:00 pm | Wrap up group  *My friend Jim had a bad day* |
| 4:30 pm | Break  *Listened to music* |
| 5:00 pm | Dinner  *hamburger was good* |
| 5:30 pm | |
| 6:00 pm | Free time  *watched TV* |
| 6:30 pm | *Mom & Dad came to see me!* |
| 7:00 pm | Snack  *Choc chip cookies* |
| 9:00–9:30 pm | ~~watched~~ *went to bed* |

**FIGURE 31-3** Sample log for enhancing memory of daily events.

### Strategies for Perceptual Deficits Including Unilateral Neglect

Empirical evidence supports compensatory strategies and environment/task adaptation, rather than a remedial approach, as the best interventions for perceptual disorders (Árnadóttir, 2004; Gillen, 2011; Walker, 2004). Some general treatment strategies are useful regardless of the type of impairment (Box 31-4). For example, when possible, patients benefit from training in the use of general strategies during routine daily tasks in natural environments (Gillen, 2011; Walker, 2004). Simple environmental modifications can increase safety and independence when coupled with patient and family training (Gitlin, 2005). Instructing the patient and family on how to adapt the environment increases the generalization of skills to the patient's home upon discharge.

Although neglect can have major effects on the functional status of a patient, the evidence supporting interventions needs further development. The literature suggests the overall goal of intervention should be to increase awareness of the deficit by using verbal, visual, and tactile feedback to "show" the patient the neglected information (Swan, 2001; Tham, 2001) (see Box 31-5).

**Scanning training** is widely used to teach the patient with neglect a more effective visual scanning pattern (Cicerone, 2011; Gillen, 2011). This training includes compensating with exaggerated body movements and use of perceptual anchors. Examples of exaggerated body movements include rotating the patient's trunk (or chair) to the left and/or teaching the patient to overexaggerate head movements during scanning. The patient is instructed to continually turn toward the left until the perceptual anchor (usually a brightly colored object) can be located. Although scanning training has been successful with patients, it is often difficult to generalize to all environments and is most successful when used with specific training during functional tasks (Gillen, 2009; Pambakian, 2005; Parton, 2004).

Another technique supported by research is the lighthouse strategy, which combines scanning training with visual imagery as an effective intervention for unilateral neglect (Niemeier, 2001). During the training, the therapist instructs the patient to scan the environment by moving the head and eyes like a lighthouse scanning the horizon. The therapist demonstrates this by scanning slowly, horizontally, moving the chin from the tip of the right shoulder to the tip of the left shoulder. The patient is asked to copy this movement while the therapist provides verbal and tactile cues (e.g., lightly tapping the left shoulder).

Several studies have shown limb activation can increase attention to the left side (Cicerone, 2011; Frassinetti, 2001; Reinhart, 2012; Robertson, 1993, 1998). This approach is based on the idea that even small activation of left body parts in the neglected hemispace improves unilateral neglect. The patient is asked to participate in a scanning activity while engaging the left upper extremity in active movement. For

---

### BOX 31-4  Five Strategies for Patients With Visuospatial Deficits

Compensatory Strategies

- Direct the patient in using tactile cues when judging distances during reaching, transfers, and ambulation activities.
- Allow time for adjustment when transitioning between light sources (inside to outside, bright to dim).
- Adjust language so directional terms have clear, functional meaning: "Turn toward the window" versus "Turn right."
- Assist in increasing the patient's awareness by discussing the effects of deficits and possible areas for caution.
- Suggest the patient use polarized sunglasses to decrease glare.
- Sit parallel to the person so there is no confusion regarding direction or space.

Environmental Modifications and Task Adaptations

- Decrease visual and tactile clutter so the patient has less information to process.
- Use contrasting colors to assist the patient in locating objects or being able to determine where one surface ends and the next begins. Red, orange, and yellow are generally easier to see than blues and greens. Examples include:
  - Taping the edge of the top step
  - Putting tape on the handle of the patient's quad cane
  - Putting drops of blue dye in the bath water to increase contrast
  - Using a placemat of contrasting color under a plate on the table
- Ensure that work spaces have sufficient lighting.
- Label important surfaces with tactile cues by adhering the hooked side of a hook-and-loop fastener to a surface.
- Recommend installation of secure handrails on steps.
- Organize the patient's environment so common items are kept in the same location.
- Use landmarks as a way of giving directions (e.g., a picture on the wall, an information desk).
- Present common objects directly in front of the patient with the most distinctive characteristic of the object facing her.

Gillen G. *Stroke Rehabilitation: A Function-Based Approach.* St. Louis, MO: Elsevier/Mosby; 2011.

Gitlin LN, Corcoran MA. Examples of environmental strategies for targeted management areas. In: Gitlin LN, Corcoran MA, eds. *Occupational Therapy and Dementia Care.* Bethesda, MD: AOTA Press; 2005.

Zoltan B. *Vision, Perception and Cognition: A Manual for the Evaluation and Treatment of the Adult With Acquired Brain Injury,* 4th edition. Thorofare, NJ: SLACK; 2007.

---

### BOX 31-5  Strategies to Maximize Interactions When Treating Patients With Unilateral Neglect (Left-sided)

- Improve comprehension of information by having the patient read along using his/her index finger as a guide.
- During transfers and mobility, cue the patient to locate and safely position the left limbs before movement.
- Anchor the left side of the patient's environment by placement of a brightly colored item or border. Ask the patient to look to the left until the border is seen.
- Utilize functional, meaningful activities when addressing issues of neglect. This assists in generalization of skills.
- Conduct therapeutic activities in natural settings.
- Improve the patient's awareness of deficits by providing direct feedback during activities.

Corben L, Unsworth C. Evaluation and intervention with unilateral neglect. In: Unsworth C, ed. *Cognitive and Perceptual Dysfunction: A Clinical Reasoning Approach to Evaluation and Intervention.* Philadelphia, PA: F.A. Davis; 1999.

Gillen G. *Cognitive and Perceptual Rehabilitation: Optimizing Function.* St. Louis, MO: Elsevier/Mosby; 2009.

Zoltan B. *Vision, Perception and Cognition: A Manual for the Evaluation and Treatment of the Adult With Acquired Brain Injury,* 4th edition. Thorofare, NJ: SLACK; 2007.

---

example, the patient completes a cancellation task while tapping her fingers on her left hand or while moving the left arm through range-of-motion exercises. One obvious issue with this intervention is the fact that many patients with unilateral neglect also experience hemiplegia. Although more research is needed, one study had encouraging results for this population, demonstrating that even passive movement of the hemiplegic arm decreased neglect as evidenced by improved scanning performance (Frassinetti, 2001).

There are two different approaches for interacting with a patient who has unilateral neglect—one that challenges and one

that assists. Depending on the patient, the activity, and the outcome you hope to achieve, you can use one approach or a combination of both. Each method is achieved by adapting the presentation of stimuli. When the patient is having difficulty attending to information presented on the left, you can present all information from the right in order to increase appropriate responses, decrease frustration, and ensure safety. This includes standing to the right of the patient when instructing, rearranging furniture so important items are located on the right, and/or placing written materials to the right of midline. When the patient is responding well to cueing and is ready for additional challenges, you can present information closer to the left side. This can be done gradually by addressing the patient from the left, moving frequently used items slightly past midline, and involving the patient in simple bilateral tasks. Regardless of the approach, before leaving the patient, be sure her call light and telephone are located where she can easily operate them. Consider the following case and clinical questions, with discussion answers provided in the online resources.

## PATIENT APPLICATION: CASE I

*Tim Miller is the 16 year-old survivor of a motor vehicle accident, in which he sustained a brain injury as well as a number of orthopedic injuries. He was in an acute care hospital for 2 weeks and was transferred to your rehabilitation center. His behavior was incoherent and combative for the first 2 days, reflecting his level of confusion and agitation. He continues to experience some confusion and agitation in specific situations, although this has substantially improved. Other concerns in cognitive functioning include poor attention (easily distracted), significant memory loss for events since the injury, and a high safety risk due to limited awareness and insight into his injuries.*

### Contemplate Clinical Decisions

*Problem-solve the following situations and select the most appropriate response to optimize communication.*

1. *You walk into Tim's room to find that he is very upset with the physical therapist assistant (PTA) who is attempting to change his leg splint. Tim is becoming increasingly agitated and attempting to kick the PTA. Identify an intervention strategy for this situation.*
   A. *Quickly grab Tim and remind him the PTA is only trying to help.*
   B. *Redirect Tim's attention to his nearby family photos while the PTA finishes the task.*
   C. *Find two other assistants to help hold Tim down in order to change the splint.*
2. *Tim brings his memory log to each therapy session but never writes anything down. You should:*
   A. *Guide Tim in writing down important points or make notes for him when he is unable to do so.*
   B. *Not worry about him bringing the log to therapy until he is able to use it more effectively.*
   C. *Set aside a few minutes at the end of therapy and ask him to write a summary of the session.*
3. *Tim has made steady improvement and is now ready to navigate natural obstacles in his environment, including changes in elevation (one or two steps). Given his current cognitive status (tendency to become distracted and diminished awareness), which factor(s) should be considered in your method of instruction?*
   A. *Develop a written checklist to help Tim with his sequence of motor movements.*
   B. *Provide models and break the task into small steps with repeated practice.*
   C. *Both A and B are reasonable considerations.*

## ■ Aphasia (With Possible Apraxia of Speech)

### Functional Implications

**Aphasia** is described as a "language disorder resulting from damage to brain areas that subserve the formulation and understanding of language and its components (i.e., semantic, phonological, morphological, and syntactic knowledge" (Helm-Estabrooks, 2014, p. 27), which is very different from the challenges posed by cognitive and/or perceptual impairments (McNeil, 2011). Aphasia is an acquired impairment in a patient's language system and is *not* considered a disorder of thought or a memory disorder (Helm-Estabrooks, 2014).

Language symbols form the basis of any conversation exchange, which means patients with aphasia often struggle to say the word they have in mind, to comprehend what is said, to read and write, and to use gestural communication. Aphasia typically affects all these modes of communication to a greater or lesser extent (Hallowell, 2008). For example, it may be quite difficult to explain an important modification in an exercise regimen and feel comfortable that the patient understands it. Furthermore, a patient with aphasia may have a multitude of questions about her plan of care but not have the language skills to express them. In essence, aphasia affects most (if not all) aspects of everyday communication exchanges. It also influences rehabilitation outcomes for some (Gialanella, 2011).

The language characteristics of patients with aphasia broadly represent some degree of difficulty in receptive and/or expressive language, varying in severity with mild to profound consequences. **Receptive aphasia** means that a patient is experiencing some type of difficulty understanding language. For example, some patients experience errors in syntax (i.e., applying rules for word order and sentence forms) (Hanne, 2011; Patterson 2008). What seems like a simple request to a patient (e.g., "Before you stand up, lock your wheelchair brakes") is quite difficult for many to comprehend because of its syntactic complexity (i.e., the sentence involves components that must be reordered and quickly processed to accurately interpret it).

Other patients experience semantic errors in listening, which cause misinterpretation of a word or sentence (e.g., the patient reaches for the foot pedal rather than the wheelchair brake in response to a spoken direction) (Morris, 2012; Patterson, 2008). One way to conceptualize this type of difficulty is to imagine interacting with a person who is speaking a foreign language. Although some words make sense because of other communication cues (e.g., facial expression, gestures, and intonation), most of the words are not recognizable and, as a result, are easily misinterpreted.

The expressive deficits resulting from aphasia vary as well. It is common for people with aphasia to have some degree of word-finding difficulty, which is described as anomia (Helm-Estabrooks, 2014). Imagine the frustration of knowing what you want to say but being unable to say it. The "tip of the tongue" phenomenon that typical communicators encounter occasionally is one that a patient with aphasia experiences quite frequently. Some patients learn compensation strategies, such as saying "I can think it, but I can't say it" to clarify their knowledge of the word when unable to verbally express it. Other patients with aphasia produce an overabundance of words while conversing, including frequent substitutions (**paraphasias**) that range from semantically related errors (e.g., "table" instead of "chair") to words that sound made up or from a different language (e.g., "nesse" for "chair") (Helm-Estabrooks, 2014).

**Wernicke's aphasia** is a type of receptive aphasia in which patients use an overabundance of words while speaking. People with Wernicke's aphasia speak smoothly and without effort; however, their speech is filled with numerous erroneous word substitutions. In describing a recent trip to the mall, a patient with Wernicke's aphasia might say, *"Like I said, you go get it by the area table by the door area in the nisses. Well, it's something like that thing you do when you go there and get it done."* The comprehension ability of these patients is quite impaired for both spoken information and written content (Brookshire, 2007).

**Apraxia of speech** coexists with some forms of **expressive aphasia** because the centers for motor planning are associated with the anterior regions of the left hemisphere (Duffy, 2013). Verbal apraxia typically results in an effortful speech pattern with numerous articulation errors, especially for words with difficult sound sequences (e.g., <u>str</u>aight) or more than one syllable (e.g., ambulation). Patients who experience apraxia and aphasia together typically struggle with verbal expression, often speaking in short sentences that are agrammatic in their structure, with a reduced number and type of spoken words (Helm-Estabrooks, 2014).

**Broca's aphasia** is a common type of expressive aphasia. Patients with this condition tend to speak "telegraphically" (i.e., use content words such as nouns and verbs) and omit other parts of speech (e.g., articles and prepositions). For example, in describing a family outing to the movies, a patient with Broca's aphasia might say, *"Well...wife...and son...movie...on the day... eat popcorn...good...lots of fun."* In patients with Broca's aphasia, the ability to comprehend what they hear (spoken information) and read (print material) is typically better than their ability to speak or express themselves in writing (Brookshire, 2007).

## Strategies to Maximize Communication With Patients With Aphasia

A first step in interacting effectively with a person who has aphasia is valuing the importance of the communication relationship. Effective communication partners "treat the person with aphasia as a trustworthy, competent, interesting, and sincere person" (Simmons-Mackie, 1999, p. 817). A common mistake of beginning health-care professionals is assuming that patients with aphasia are confused when they incorrectly respond to questions about their orientation to time or place. Most such patients are not confused or disoriented, they are simply unable to say the correct words due to impaired language (aphasia). The patient may understand the question but not have the word-finding skills to verbally answer. To others, a spoken question may sound like a foreign language, making it difficult to respond accurately.

Patients with aphasia often take advantage of their preserved strengths (e.g., cognitive and social skills) to communicate successfully, reflecting their inherent competence as a communicator (Kagan, 1995, 2001). Health-care professionals acknowledge this competence through positive communication behaviors, such as being respectful and responding in a sensitive and encouraging manner (Purdy, 2005).

With this in mind, the strategies that follow are grouped by suggestions to enhance the patient's comprehension and/or expression of a message. As always, confer with the SLP to verify strategies that will be most beneficial for a particular patient.

### Considerations for Message Comprehension

Modifying communication patterns enhances patients' comprehension (Kagan, 1995, 2001; Marshall, 2004; Purdy, 2005; Simmons-Mackie, 1999). Optimize communication by learning to "adapt, adjust, and accommodate" to the needs of the patient (Box 31-6). First, evaluate your typical pattern of speaking and

---

**BOX 31-6 Strategies to Maximize Comprehension of Patients With Aphasia**

Adapt your <u>Communication</u>
- Slow down and "chunk" information into meaningful parts—this allows your patient more time to process what you say and take advantage of other speech cues.
- Alert your patient to listen—hand signals and verbal cues prime the auditory system to focus on what you are going to say.
- Inform your patient about a change in topic or task—it reduces attention demands on your patient.

Adjust How You Say It
- State it succinctly and specifically—break multistep directions into parts for your patient to implement one segment at a time.
- Avoid complex sentence forms—use straightforward language that is easy to comprehend.

Accommodate Impaired Auditory Comprehension
- Take advantage of natural cues that provide visual information—manually demonstrate or show the patient your request to provide additional contextual information. Supplement what you say with other modes; other visual input including written words, drawings, or related props may enhance understanding.

consider ways to *adapt* your communication style for patients who may not comprehend well. A simple but important modification is to slow down in order to enhance the patient's ability to process what you say. A natural means to achieve this is to insert short pauses at normal syntactic boundaries that help "chunk" information into meaningful units (e.g., "Your right side is improving…and helping your walking"). Slowing down naturally helps maintain a typical rhythm and intonation while speaking, contributing to some patients' understanding.

Many patients with aphasia also experience difficulty with aspects of attention (Helm-Estabrooks, 2014). Simple alerting cues prime the auditory system to listen (e.g., "get ready" or say the patient's name paired with a hand signal); also, keep the focus on one topic at a time and alert the patient to any change in activity (e.g., "We're done with that…Let's work on a different exercise") (Marshall, 2004). Remember that the typical environment for service delivery (PT exercise area) is often noisy and distracting, which adds another layer of complexity to the patient's ability to comprehend.

It also is important to *adjust* what you say to patients with comprehension challenges. Although it is natural to speak in long and complex sentences, these message forms are very difficult for people with aphasia to comprehend. Be sure to interact in an adult manner, but adjust the message content to reflect wording that is direct and to the point, reducing syntactic complexity and message length (Marshall, 2004). A direction such as "You're going to stand up, but move your foot pedals out of the way after you lock your wheelchair brakes" is multifaceted and stated in a complex manner. State the direction specifically, one part at a time, and in the sequence of its completion (e.g., "Lock your brakes"… "Move your foot pedals"… "Stand up slowly").

You can *accommodate* a patient's impaired comprehension by capitalizing on other modes to supplement the auditory message. Because much of communication is nonverbal (as much as 93% of face-to-face interactions; Moore, 2010), position yourself where the patient can see you while talking. This allows the patient to take advantage of natural cues such as facial expressions and illustrative gestures to enhance functional comprehension, which is especially important for patients with poor receptive skills (Rose, 2001, 2008). Other considerations include combining more than one mode of communication (e.g., supplement what is said by also writing down key points) and incorporating props, such as manually demonstrating (showing) the direction along with its verbal description (Lasker, 2007; Purdy, 2005).

## THINK ABOUT IT 31.2

- An important consideration in creating a positive communication environment is your attitude as a therapist. Discuss how your attitude can have a positive effect.
- Give examples of how you can adapt your communication style, adjust what you say, and make accommodations to enhance communication interactions.

### Promoting Message Expression

It is equally important to be sensitive to the expressive challenges of aphasia, ensuring opportunities for patients to convey their questions, thoughts, and feelings. Effective communication partners are flexible and consider "other styles of interaction even when the alternative is not entirely successful" (Simmons-Mackie, 1999, p. 815). Although some patients have strategies, they may need prompting and encouragement to apply them during conversation. For example, a patient who cannot say "yes" or "no" may accurately express it with a thumb up or thumb down gesture. Patients with aphasia augment their expression in many positive ways, including gestures that "show you" and communication notebooks with written text, calendars, photos, rating scales, and maps that indicate topics and convey specific needs (Garrett, 2013; Sekine, 2013) (Fig. 31-4). Other patients have the ability to draw (e.g., quad cane) as a means to express a concern (e.g., "Can I walk with this?"). Drawing minimizes demands on areas of language (speaking and spelling) that are impaired by aphasia (Helm-Estabrooks, 2014; Lyon, 1995). Always give patients extra time to formulate and express an answer with any method of communication (Purdy, 2005).

The type of question or way in which it is posed also affects a patient's ability to successfully respond. Everyday questions (e.g., "What's going on?" or "What have you been doing today?") require language proficiency in word finding and sentence construction, making it difficult for a patient with expressive aphasia to answer. In addition, the open-ended nature of the question complicates anticipating the patient's response, which only adds to her frustration if she is unable to respond in a manner that is understandable. As a general rule of thumb, ask closed-ended questions to enhance the patient's expressive skills as well as your ability to verify and confirm (Kagan, 1995). Patients with severe aphasia also may benefit from yes/no responses and associated head nods tagged to the end of these (e.g., "Did the heat treatment help your shoulder pain…yes or no?") (Garrett, 2013). Some patients are able to better express opinions in a conversational exchange when the questions are combined with spoken/and or written choices (e.g., "Does it feel better when you raise it or lower it?"). In this example, the patient may be able to vocalize, use facial expressions, or gesture in a way that conveys the first or second choice (Garrett, 2013).

You also help a patient's expression by learning strategies that resolve communication breakdowns (i.e., situations in which the patient is attempting to convey something but you are not sure what). Closed-ended questions organized in a "20 questions" format may work in this situation. The basic idea is to first identify the broad topic and then apply clarification questions with yes/no answers that continually narrow to the specific information the patient is attempting to express (Fig. 31-5). It is easier to predict what the patient is communicating when you know the topic. This strategy

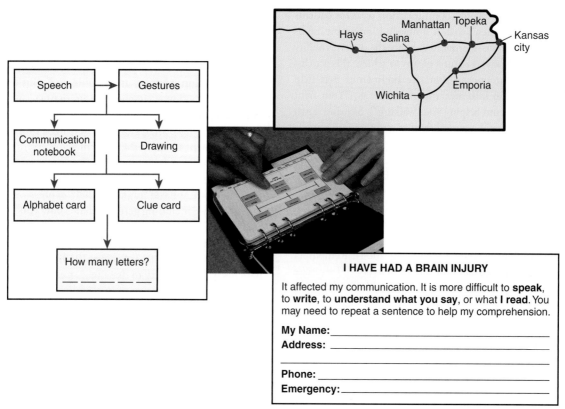

**FIGURE 31-4** Using alternative modes to promote message expression for people with aphasia.

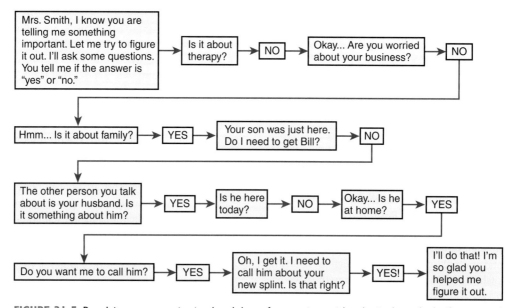

**FIGURE 31-5** Resolving a communication breakdown for a patient with aphasia through clarification and verification of the topic.

of clarification and verification may work in some but not all situations. For example, you may narrow the topic somewhat but not understand the specifics, as in the case of a patient who successfully describes where she lives but is unable to express the exact address. In this event, summarize to the point you understood (e.g., "I see...you live close to our medical center; it takes only a few minutes to drive here") to help achieve closure in a manner that is considered face-saving for both you and your patient (Simmons-Mackie, 1999).

## THINK ABOUT IT 31.3

- Discuss how being an attentive listener can assist you in understanding and clarifying messages, including "listening" to nonverbal cues.
- Discuss how allowing extra time for your patient to find the right word or organize thoughts is helpful.
- If you do not understand a patient, should you pretend to understand her even if you really do not know what she said? Why or why not?

## PATIENT APPLICATION: CASE 2

*Mrs. Smith, a 68 year-old female, is a new admission into the rehabilitation unit at your center. She experienced a left hemisphere stroke a few days earlier. The SLP reports at your first team meeting that Mrs. Smith presents with both receptive and expressive aphasia; she follows one-part directions with 90% accuracy and two-part directions with approximately 40% accuracy. You conducted your initial evaluation with Mrs. Smith during your morning and afternoon sessions. Immediately, it became clear that the severity of her aphasia complicated your assessment of her right-side paresis and her preexisting back pain. Although she sometimes uttered words such as "okay" and "that's it," Mrs. Smith appeared frustrated by her inability to explain her back pain and ask questions about her right-side involvement.*

### Contemplate Clinical Decisions

*Problem-solve the following situations and select the most appropriate response to optimize communication.*

1. *Mrs. Smith has physician's orders for heat packs and exercises for her lower back each day. This requires specific instructions for positioning her on the PT mat, lying on her left side. Which of the following is the best way to word your directions to help Mrs. Smith understand what to do?*
   - A. *"I want you to lie down and then roll to your left side."*
   - B. *"You're going to be on your left; I need you to lie down first."*
   - C. *"Mrs. Smith, you need to lie down...Okay...now, roll to your left."*
2. *Mrs. Smith has made steady improvement in her physical recovery over the last week. In fact, you are ready to explore adaptive equipment for ambulation, including her safe use of a quad cane. Although you adapt and adjust how you speak, you are concerned that Mrs. Smith does not fully understand your verbal directions for sequencing her motor movements. Appropriate accommodations for this situation include which of the following?*
   - A. *Manually illustrating your directions with the quad cane*
   - B. *Writing down key parts as you verbally explain them*
   - C. *Both A and B are reasonable accommodations.*
3. *Mrs. Smith also seems to converse with you mostly in telegraphic sentences, such as "Hot... pack... ready to go." You recently modified her ankle-foot orthosis (AFO) because of her physical improvement. Today, she seems particularly frustrated with it, but you are not sure why. You know her concerns relate to pain and discomfort, but you are less confident about the specifics. The more frustrated she becomes in attempting to tell you, the more difficulty she has in communicating (i.e., repeating "Darn it...darn it!"). To help Mrs. Smith express herself, you should consider:*
   - A. *Alerting her to listen and saying "Take your time and tell me what's happening with your AFO."*
   - B. *Asking her to "show you" where it hurts and/or asking questions with written choices about her pain.*
   - C. *Telling her that you understand as a strategy to help calm her down.*

# ■ Dysarthria of Speech

## Functional Implications

**Dysarthria** is defined as a "neurogenic motor speech impairment that is characterized by slow, weak, imprecise, and/or uncoordinated movements of the speech musculature" (Yorkston, 2010, p. 4). It is the result of neurological injury to the central or peripheral nervous system, including developmental conditions (e.g., cerebral palsy) and etiologies such as stroke, TBI, and disease processes (e.g., Parkinson disease, multiple sclerosis, amyotrophic lateral sclerosis). Dysarthria is a motor speech disorder affecting movement and control of movement while speaking, including appropriate use of respiration (breath support), phonation (voice), velopharyngeal control (amount of nasal resonance), and articulatory control of the lips, tongue, and jaw for accurate sound production. Some or all of these components may be affected because of possible weakness, spasticity, incoordination, changes in muscle tone, and/or involuntary movements (Duffy, 2013).

A patient's inability to execute neuromuscular control can range in severity from quite mild differences to a profound range of impairment that renders speech nonfunctional. Some patients may simply sound less natural because the timing and rhythm of speech are different. For example, the patient's production of "I went to therapy" (appropriate stress on the first syllable) may sound like "I went to therapy" (resulting in an unnatural production of the word that draws negative attention because it sounds "odd").

Other patients may have substantially impaired speech intelligibility, meaning their speech is difficult to understand. Although the sentence structure and word choices are accurate, the spoken message may sound slurred, distorted, or indistinct, with parts of words within the sentence less distinguishable. In more severe forms of intelligibility impairment in which even less of the message is discernible, patients may use low-tech (e.g., communication or picture boards) or high-tech systems (e.g., electronic communication devices) to enhance their interactions (Beukelman, 2013). It is important to consult with the patient's SLP to understand the purpose of the communication aid and how it functions so you can help the patient apply it effectively during conversation.

Although a general perception of dysarthria is that the person does not speak clearly, the specific speech and voice characteristics are quite variable, affected by the underlying neuropathology and type of motor system involvement (Duffy, 2013; Kim, 2011). The voice quality of a patient with dysarthria can range along a continuum from breathiness (airy sounding) to a voice quality that is especially harsh and strained (word productions sound very effortful). Some patients with dysarthria speak too rapidly, whereas others talk very slowly with noticeable pauses between each word. A person may sound as if she "talks through her nose" or "runs out of air," making a moderate length sentence like "It feels stiff when I move my arm up and down" difficult for you to understand. In addition, the overall melody of a sentence may have too little variation (monopitch) or too much variation (abrupt changes in pitch or loudness). Again, the goal is not to diagnose or differentiate characteristics but to know that speech and voice features vary greatly from one patient to another.

## Strategies to Maximize Understanding of Dysarthric Speech

As a listener, you integrate information from multiple sources in your perception of speech. This is particularly important when speech is less intelligible, which is the case for many patients with dysarthria. Although some of the suggested strategies help clarify communication, most emphasize the concept of optimizing other sources of information to help you distinguish words and understand the spoken message (Frankoff, 2011; Hanson, 2013; Vogel, 2001). These strategies are grouped into three areas: setting the stage with a positive communication environment, building your awareness of message cues, and learning to use clarifying techniques when the spoken words are not understandable. These strategies are described in the sections that follow and are illustrated in a flowchart (Fig. 31-6).

### Set the Stage for Effective Communication

An effective communication partner always considers the immediate environment (lighting, noise, distance, and situation) and its possible effects when interacting with a person who is dysarthric (Frankoff, 2011; Yorkston, 2010). A well-lit environment is important in order to take advantage of the patient's facial cues while she is speaking, which may enhance your comprehension of the spoken message (Garcia, 2004). A positive environment also is one in which extraneous noise is minimized and noise sources are controlled. For example, you may provide clinical services in the patient's room, which includes common sources of background noise, such as the television and radio. Turn them off whenever possible. Sometimes, the noise source cannot be eliminated, as when several patient/therapist pairs are in a PT exercise area. The best solution in this situation is to move away from the primary source of noise, perhaps toward a corner or more private location in a large space.

Minimizing noise is particularly important when speech is hard to understand, especially because it may be very difficult for your patient to modulate loudness and attempts to talk louder may be quite fatiguing (Dykstra, 2013; Yorkston, 2004). Along this line, it may be difficult for a patient to speak loudly enough to communicate to you at a distance, which may be the distance from one end of the parallel bars to the other or from the patient's bed to the doorway several feet away. An effective communication partner decreases the distance to optimize a verbal exchange while minimizing the speaking effort of the patient.

In addition to factors that relate to the physical environment, another consideration is the situation or special circumstance surrounding a conversation. For example, when providing clinical services to a patient who is mentally or physically fatigued or simply not feeling well, you may perceive a change in neuromuscular control of speech as well (i.e., the patient may speak with less clarity.) Try to avoid important conversations at these times; this includes asking the patient to self-evaluate progress when the responses may affect your clinical decision-making. In both children and adults, posture is another factor that affects neuromuscular control while speaking (Yorkston, 2010). For example, you may help your patient improve respiratory support for speech through simple postural adjustments with a sitting position, making speech easier to understand.

### Build Awareness of Message Cues

Many natural cues are integrated within communication, and building awareness of these factors contributes to the successful exchange of information. In addition to watching facial cues, be attentive to other aspects of a patient's nonverbal communication. For example, a child or adult's use of hand gestures while speaking to illustrate or describe what is said provides content information to supplement your understanding of less intelligible speech (Garcia, 1998, 2000, 2004). Patients with dysarthria may be able to incorporate other types of communication cues to clarify the message (e.g., writing it down, spelling it on a letter board, or drawing a key concept). For example, some patients use an alphabet board and point to the first letter of each word while they say it (Fig. 31-7). This type of message cue (i.e., showing the first letter of the word) greatly enhances your understanding of dysarthric speech (Hanson, 2013; Hustad, 2005).

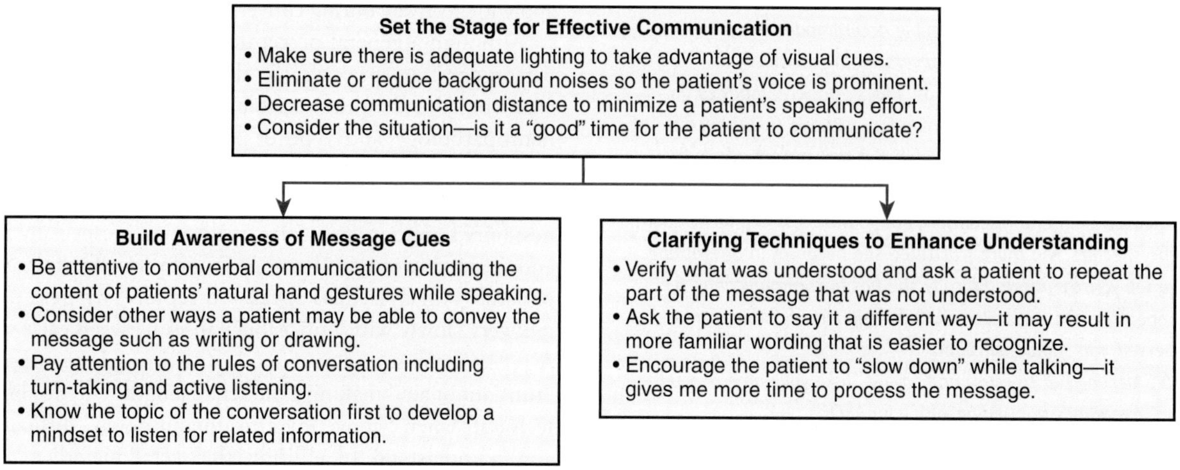

---

**Set the Stage for Effective Communication**
- Make sure there is adequate lighting to take advantage of visual cues.
- Eliminate or reduce background noises so the patient's voice is prominent.
- Decrease communication distance to minimize a patient's speaking effort.
- Consider the situation—is it a "good" time for the patient to communicate?

**Build Awareness of Message Cues**
- Be attentive to nonverbal communication including the content of patients' natural hand gestures while speaking.
- Consider other ways a patient may be able to convey the message such as writing or drawing.
- Pay attention to the rules of conversation including turn-taking and active listening.
- Know the topic of the conversation first to develop a mindset to listen for related information.

**Clarifying Techniques to Enhance Understanding**
- Verify what was understood and ask a patient to repeat the part of the message that was not understood.
- Ask the patient to say it a different way—it may result in more familiar wording that is easier to recognize.
- Encourage the patient to "slow down" while talking—it gives me more time to process the message.

**FIGURE 31-6** Flowchart of strategies to optimize communication with patients with dysarthria.

| I'll point to the first letter of each word as I say it. | | | | | | |
|---|---|---|---|---|---|---|
| Please repeat each word right after I say it—that way I'll know that you understood me. | | | | | | |
| A | B | C | D | E | F | You misunderstood |
| G | H | I | J | K | L | I'll repeat it |
| M | N | O | P | Q | R | I'll spell that word |
| S | T | U | V | W | X | End of sentence |
| Y | Z | Space | | Delete | | New topic/idea |

**FIGURE 31-7** Sample communication system for a person who has severe dysarthria.

A typical message exchange involves at least two participants who take turns speaking *and* listening. Be sure you always provide an opportunity for your patient to speak and you take a turn at being an active listener. This is especially important because the patient's speaking rate may be much slower than yours, making it difficult to signify a "start" and to tell when the "turn" is complete.

In addition, it is imperative to verify the topic of the conversation first because it helps you develop a mindset for more accurate understanding of the words and sentences that follow (Hanson, 2004; Hustad, 2001). A simple strategy is to encourage the patient to always start with the main idea (e.g., "It's something about my arm."). Then, she can say the specific concern or point (e.g., "I feel stiffness moving it back and forth"). Others may be able to reference a visual image such as sharing a digital photograph of an event to clarify the topic (Hanson, 2013).

### Clarifying Techniques to Enhance Understanding

Be honest with patients and ask for clarification when you do not understand what they are saying. A simple request to repeat a part of the message may be appropriate. When this is the case, be sure to state the portion you *understood* so the patient does not have to restate the entire message. If the message is still unclear, ask the patient to "say it a different way" (i.e., rephrase it), which might result in the patient choosing more common (i.e., recognizable) words. For example, a patient's request to "close it when you leave" may not be clear; restated in a different way (e.g., "Shut the door behind you") is a familiar request that may be more recognizable.

Subtle differences in word choice that convey more predictable content helps listeners understand patients with moderate to severely impaired intelligibility of speech (Garcia, 1998; Hustad, 2005). Overall, most patients with dysarthria are easier to understand when they talk in complete sentences, which means that the understandable words help you distinguish words that are less clear (i.e., you can fill in the blanks from what you understood). The opposite pattern is true for patients who are profoundly impaired (Hanson, 2004). In that situation, it may be most effective to ask the patient if there is one "key" or main word that sums up the message.

Another clarifying strategy that helps some patients with dysarthria is to slow their rate of speech. Although it already seems slow, it may be too fast for the patient's neuromuscular control (Yorkston, 2010). Saying the message at a slower rate may help some patients coordinate or execute the various speech movements more effectively, resulting in improved speech intelligibility. A slower speech rate also gives you more time to decode the message, which may enhance listening accuracy and understanding (Yorkston, 2010).

## PATIENT APPLICATION: CASE 3

*Mr. Jones, a 72 year-old male, recently fractured a hip and was transferred to the orthopedic unit of your medical facility. His history also indicates a diagnosis of Parkinson disease 7 years ago. In fact, his recent fall most likely resulted from declining balance and stability in gross motor skills. There also is a report from the SLP, which includes the following summary: "Mr. Jones presents with moderate to severe dysarthria of speech, characterized by a soft voice, occasional short rushes of speech with imprecise articulation, and overall monotonicity of pitch and loudness." Problem-solve the following situations and select the most appropriate response to optimize communication.*

### Contemplate Clinical Decisions – Case 3

1. *You enter the patient's room to begin your clinical intervention. One of your first considerations for communication is to:*
   A. *Strike up a conversation with Mr. Jones about his family to become familiar with his pattern of speech.*
   B. *Suggest that he write down answers in order to minimize his efforts at speaking.*
   C. *Be sure there is adequate lighting to take advantage of visual cues and turn down the volume on the television.*
2. *Mr. Jones begins to explain his concerns about pain and discomfort, but you are not certain about the entirety of his message. You are confident that he said "I feel a lot of pain," but you do not understood the remaining part of his sentence (his explanation of where it is located). Which of the following responses is reasonable in this situation?*
   A. *"Mr. Jones, I did not understand your entire sentence. I know you said that you have pain. I did not understand the last part. Could you please repeat that part of your sentence?"*
   B. *"Mr. Jones, I know you are really tired today, but you need to talk loudly. I'm having a hard time hearing you because of the noisy people walking down the hallway."*
   C. *"Mr. Jones, that sounds reasonable. We'll try to fix it while you're here."*
3. *After discussing the pain in his hip, Mr. Jones begins talking about something else. Unfortunately, you do not know what he is trying to tell you. Which of the following message cues is important for this situation?*
   A. *Determine the topic of his conversation to develop a mindset for the information that follows.*
   B. *Interrupt Mr. Jones and ask him a question about a different topic.*
   C. *This is not a good time for Mr. Jones. Try to conclude your interaction as quickly as possible.*

## Let's Review

1. What are the different ways we communicate with one another? Now, think about how an impairment in one of these aspects of communication can interfere with or influence your clinical interactions with a patient.

2. How is your clinical expertise important to the speech-language pathologist's ability to evaluate and treat patients who present with physical involvement?

3. When adults have conditions that affect communication, it is important to maintain "adultlike" interactions. What does this mean? Why is this important?

4. What is an important distinction (contrast) in the verbal communication skills of a person with aphasia versus a person with dysarthria?

5. What memory or organizational strategies do you apply during your daily work or study?

6. Having a patient's attention is important. Why is this important for the person with aphasia? What is another rationale for its importance to people with a cognitive impairment?

7. Select one or two tasks that you consider routine aspects of most clinical interactions. Now think about two or three ways to improve your explanation of these tasks for a person with aphasia (e.g., how to transfer from one location to another).

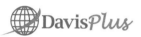 **DavisPlus**   For additional resources, including case study discussions, please visit http://davisplus.fadavis.com

## CHAPTER SUMMARY

You are an important "partner" in patients' ability to effectively convey their feelings and needs, as well as in seeking information about their physical impairments and for their plan of care. This chapter provides you with a foundation for understanding the consequences of cognitive disorders, impaired perceptual skills, aphasia, and dysarthria and how these disorders affect the therapeutic environment. The strategies offered in this chapter are meant to promote successful communication and enhance clinical intervention for physical impairments. Always collaborate with other members of the patient's treatment team to identify the most appropriate and effective strategies for your patient.

# Intervention for Cardiovascular and Pulmonary Impairments in Neurological Populations

Marilyn MacKay-Lyons, BSc(PT), MSc(PT), PhD ▪ Blair P. Saale, PT, DPT, NCS

CHAPTER 32

## CHAPTER OBJECTIVES

Upon completion of this chapter, the learner should be able to:

1. Explain basic physiological principles underlying cardiovascular and pulmonary functions related to exercise metabolism.
2. Discuss factors contributing to and possible mechanisms involved in reduced exercise capacity in populations with neurological conditions.
3. Discuss possible mechanisms underlying reductions in exercise capacity in people with neurological conditions.
4. Identify potential benefits of cardiovascular fitness training in populations with neurological conditions.
5. Design exercise programs to improve the cardiovascular health and fitness of people with neurological conditions.

## ▪ Introduction

*After a dramatic exacerbation of her multiple sclerosis 1 month ago, Mrs. Mack is just beginning to experience some motor recovery. During this time of reduced physical activity, she reports frustration that her stamina and endurance have decreased from levels before the exacerbation. The physical therapist notes that Mrs. Mack's resting heart rate is high; in addition, she experiences shortness of breath and her heart rate increases dramatically during physical activity.*

*With patients such as Mrs. Mack, it is essential to provide physical rehabilitation interventions that improve their cardiovascular/pulmonary status. This also applies to individuals with neuromuscular diagnoses, who may have primary or secondary impairments of cardiovascular/pulmonary function, as discussed in this chapter.*

The importance of effective functioning of the cardiovascular and pulmonary systems to good health is irrefutable. Nevertheless, the cardiopulmonary health and fitness of individuals with neurological disabilities have long been overshadowed by a preoccupation with the neuromuscular system. Traditionally, recovery in neurological populations was attributed almost exclusively to improved functioning of the neuromuscular system; consequentially, most interventions were directed at enhancing the capacity of that system. This "single-system" approach seemed rational, given the obvious limitations imposed by neurological impairments (e.g., muscle weakness, changes in muscle tone, and sensory-perceptual disturbances). However, traditional approaches have not optimized functional independence, leading therapists to seek more effective, multisystem approaches to neurorehabilitation. With this broader perspective came a greater emphasis on the cardiovascular system and, to a lesser extent, the pulmonary system.

It has become standard practice in some neurorehabilitation facilities to engage patients in aerobic training to enhance their daily function and quality of life. However, challenges remain in improving cardiopulmonary health and fitness in neurological populations. Fitness in these populations is affected by a host of interacting factors, such as the location and extent of the neurological lesion, presence of comorbidities (particularly cardiovascular disease and diabetes), lifestyle habits, and premorbid activity level. Some of these factors can be modified, whereas other factors, such as age and severity of the neurological condition, are nonmodifiable and therefore limit the potential for cardiopulmonary adaptations to training. Moreover, establishing baseline fitness levels and monitoring responses to training in individuals with compromised motor and postural control are not easy tasks. Thus, it is vitally important for rehabilitation professionals to understand the fundamental aspects of fitness assessment and training protocols and the principles upon which they are based.

This chapter begins with a brief overview of normal cardiovascular and pulmonary functions in relation to exercise metabolism, with emphasis on the terminology needed to understand the underlying physiological principles. Evidence of cardiopulmonary fitness levels in children and adults with neurological disabilities is summarized, followed by a description of factors contributing to the deconditioned state. Possible mechanisms responsible for reduced exercise capacity are then reviewed. Adaptive responses to aerobic training in neurological populations are discussed, and a wide range of potential benefits from these responses are presented. The chapter closes with a summary of factors for consideration when designing exercise programs to improve cardiopulmonary health and fitness in neurorehabilitation.

## ■ Cardiovascular and Pulmonary Functions Related to Exercise Metabolism

The human body at rest consumes approximately 3.5 mL/kg/min of oxygen ($O_2$) or one **metabolic equivalent of task** (MET) (Jette, 1990), with skeletal muscle activity accounting for about the same proportion of total energy expenditure as the

brain (less than 20% each) (Zauner, 2002). In the resting state, contractions of the heart and breathing can be sustained indefinitely because these activities occur well below the **critical power** of the muscles, defined as the maximal rate of work that can be endured indefinitely (Clingeleffer, 1994). Above the critical power, the capacity of the aerobic process to supply energy for muscle contraction is exceeded; thus, energy must also be supplied by the anaerobic glycolytic system (Fig. 32-1) (Conley, 2001).

The point at which the rate of glycolysis exceeds oxidative phosphorylation is called the **anaerobic threshold** (the exercise intensity at which lactic acid starts to accumulate in the bloodstream, approximating the ventilatory threshold or lactate threshold) (Wasserman, 2005). At the threshold, pyruvic acid is converted to lactic acid, which completely dissociates to lactate and hydrogen ions, causing a rise in blood lactate level and a fall in intramuscular pH value. Exercise-induced muscular fatigue is due in part to the exponential accumulation of lactate and the drop in intramuscular pH value, with negative effects on the actinomyosin turnover rate, enzyme activities, and excitation-contraction coupling.

During exercise, the neuromuscular, cardiovascular, and pulmonary systems interact in response to the metabolic demands of contracting muscles and the by-products of increased energy metabolism occurring within the active skeletal, cardiac, and respiratory muscles. The capacity to withstand the physiological stresses of prolonged exercise is referred to as **cardiorespiratory fitness** or **exercise capacity**. Increased metabolism relies on (1) the capacity of the respiratory and circulatory systems to transport $O_2$ to the tissues, which is influenced to a large extent by central factors, particularly cardiac output, and (2) $O_2$ utilization by the metabolically active tissues to convert chemical potential energy to mechanical energy (determined by peripheral factors, namely arteriovenous $O_2$ difference) (Conley, 2001). **Cardiac output** is the amount of blood pumped by the heart (**stroke volume**) each minute; in other words, it is the product of stroke volume and heart rate [cardiac output (L/min) = stroke volume (L) × heart rate (bpm)]. Early in exercise, stroke volume plateaus, with further increases in cardiac output achieved by a proportional increase in heart rate (Hartley,

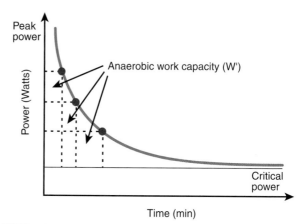

**FIGURE 32-1** Graph showing the relationship between critical power and anaerobic work capacity.

1969). **Arteriovenous $O_2$ difference** ($AVO_2$ difference), the difference in $O_2$ content between arterial and mixed venous blood, reflects the ability of skeletal muscle tissue to extract $O_2$ from the muscle capillary blood and to use $O_2$ in the mitochondria. **Oxygen consumption** ($VO_2$), the product of cardiac output and $AVO_2$ difference, increases almost linearly with workload because of both increased $O_2$ transport to and $O_2$ utilization by the tissues (Rowell, 1974). The highest $O_2$ intake an individual can attain during physical work is termed **maximal oxygen consumption** ($VO_2max$) (Wasserman, 2005). $VO_2max$ can be expressed in *absolute* terms (L $O_2$/min) or in *relative* terms (mL $O_2$/kg of body weight/min). Because a true $VO_2max$ is often difficult to achieve in both **deconditioned** individuals and individuals with neurological impairments, **peak oxygen consumption** ($VO_2peak$) is a more accurate term to use (Howley, 1995).

Blood pressure is the product of cardiac output and **total peripheral resistance** (or systemic vascular resistance). **Systolic blood pressure** ($BP_{sys}$) increases markedly during exercise, whereas **diastolic blood pressure** ($BP_{dias}$) remains unchanged or lowers slightly, thereby moderating increases in **mean arterial pressure** (MAP); $MAP = BP_{dias} + (BP_{sys} - BP_{dias})/3$ (Wasserman, 2005). $BP_{dias}$ varies minimally (plus or minus 10mm Hg) because endothelial-regulated changes in vascular tone cause redistribution of blood flow to the working muscles, decreasing total peripheral resistance (Hillegass, 2011). Vasodilation is mediated mainly by metabolites (e.g., carbon dioxide, hydrogen ions, nitric oxide, potassium ions, adenosine) acting on the vascular smooth muscle of the arterioles, whereas vasoconstriction occurs in tissue with low metabolic demand (Saltin, 1985). Blood flow to working muscles can increase to 20 times or more of flow in the resting state, whereas blood flow to other vascular beds (e.g., renal and splanchnic beds) is unchanged or decreases through active vasoconstriction primarily from increased sympathetic discharge (Saltin, 1985; DeTurk, 2011). **Cerebral autoregulation,** the intrinsic ability of cerebral vessels to maintain a relatively constant, steady-state blood flow, ensures stability of regional and total cerebral blood flow and $O_2$ delivery over a wide range of blood pressures (Busija, 1984; Hellstrom, 1996; Madsen, 1993). During exercise, vasoconstriction (mediated by sympathetic nervous system) shunts blood away from skin, inactive skeletal muscle and renal/splanchnic circulation; vasodilation causes an increase in blood flow to vital organs and working muscle, as much as a 25% increase from resting levels in the brain and heart (DeTurk, 2011).

The respiratory system does not typically limit cardiorespiratory fitness in able-bodied individuals because healthy lungs have a large reserve (Keteyian, 2006). Nevertheless, respiration plays a vital role in blood oxygenation at rest and during exercise. As much as 10% of $VO_2max$ is required at maximal workloads to support the mechanical work of the diaphragm, accessory inspiratory muscles, and abdominal muscles (Clausen, 1977). During low-intensity exercise, ventilation increases mainly by increases in **tidal volume** (VT), the volume of air expired with each breath); during more intense exercise, **respiratory rate** (RR), the number of breaths per minute, rises with little additional increase in VT (Wasserman, 1999). As exercise intensity increases, the volume of air expired in 1 minute, or **minute ventilation** (VE) [$VE = VT \times RR$], increases to remove $CO_2$ and regulate pH balance. A useful indicator of the respiratory response to exercise is the **ventilatory efficiency,** the ratio of VE to carbon dioxide; this ratio should be under 35 at peak exercise (Sun, 2002).

## ■ Cardiovascular and Pulmonary Impairments in People With Neurological Conditions

Many individuals with neurological disabilities are deconditioned, as reflected in abnormally low $VO_2peak$ values (Table 32-1). Mechanisms underlying the unfit state are variable and multifactorial; the nature, severity, location, and chronicity of the neurological condition contribute to the variability. For example, for people with multiple sclerosis (MS), each 1-point increase on the Expanded Disability Status Scale (Kurtz, 1983) is associated with a decrease in $VO_2peak$ of about 2 mL/kg/min (Romberg, 2004). Using the figures presented in Table 32-1, people with tetraplegia have approximately half the exercise capacity of those with paraplegia (mean $VO_2peak$ of 13 mL/kg/min and 23 mL/kg/min, respectively) because of diminished muscle mass and adrenergic dysfunction. Figure 32-2 illustrates the complexity of interactions of primary (direct) and secondary (indirect) effects of the neurological condition as well as personal and environmental factors on cardiovascular, neuromuscular, and respiratory impairments, and how these complex interactions influence cardiorespiratory health and fitness, independence and quality of life. The sections that follow describe these effects in detail.

### Cardiovascular Impairments

Cardiovascular complications are the leading cause of death in persons with stroke (Matsumoto, 1973), spinal cord injury (SCI) (Kennedy, 1986), and MS (Sadovnick, 1991). Various combinations of primary and secondary as well as central and peripheral factors underlie the cardiovascular impairments typically associated with neurological conditions. Examples of impaired primary central factors include disruption of the sympathetic cardiac drive after an SCI and interruption in the connections with the cardiovascular center in the medulla oblongata resulting from traumatic brain injury (TBI) or stroke. In addition, reductions in stroke volume can be secondary to impaired myocardial function and increased venous pooling. Peripheral changes accompanying unloading of muscles through inactivity and lack of weight-bearing include decreases in oxidative enzymes, mitochondria, and capillary density (Whipp, 1994) as well as inhibition of protein synthesis, leading to muscle atrophy and weakness (Biolo, 2005).

In many instances, impaired cardiac function is due to coexisting cardiovascular comorbidities. A good example is stroke. After a stroke, approximately 75% of patients have

**TABLE 32-1    Exercise Capacity in Common Neurological Conditions**

| DIAGNOSIS | REFERENCE | TIME SINCE ONSET, yr | # OF Pts | SEX M:F | AGE, yr MEAN ± SD | TEST MODALITY | VO$_2$peak, mL/kg/min MEAN ± SD | VO$_2$peak,% OF NORMAL |
|---|---|---|---|---|---|---|---|---|
| Cerebral palsy | (Unnithan, 2007) | NA | 7 | 2:5 | 16 ± 1 | Arm ergometer | 17.5 ± 4 | NR |
| | (Maltais, 2005) | NA | 11 | 7:4 | 10–16 | Treadmill | 34.0 ± 9 | NR |
| | (Tobimatsu, 1998) | NA | 12 | 12:0 | 21 + | Arm ergometer | 25.6 ± 3 | 87% |
| Charcot-Marie-Tooth disease | (El Mhandi, 2008) | NR | 8 | 8:0 | 33 ± 9 | Bike ergometer | 36.4 ± 5 | NR |
| Down syndrome | (Varela, 2001) | N/A | 16 | 16:0 | 21 ± 3 | Treadmill | 31.8 ± 5 | NR |
| | (Millar, 1993) | N/A | 14 | 11:3 | 18 ± 3 | Treadmill | 26.7 ± 7 | NR |
| Guillain-Barré syndrome | (Garssen, 2004) | 0.5–15 | 20* | 6:14 | 22–66 | Bike ergometer | 25.0 ± 8 | 76 |
| | (Pitetti, 1993) | 3 | 1 | 1:0 | 57 | Arm-leg ergometer | 27 | NR |
| Multiple sclerosis | (Schulz, 2004) | NR | 28 | 9:19 | 39 ± 10 | Cycle ergometer | 31.0 ± 7 | NR |
| | (Mostert, 2002) | 12 ± 8 | 26 | 21:5 | 45 ± 8 | Cycle ergometer | 22.5 | 70 |
| | (Petajan, 1996) | 7 ± 1 | 46 | 15:31 | 40 ± 2 | Arm-leg ergometer | 25.2 ± 1 | 79 |
| | (Ponichtera-Mulcare, 1995) | 3 ± 5 | 10 | 4:6 | 39 ± 6 | Arm-leg ergometer | 39.0 ± 8 | 87 |
| Parkinson disease | (Bergen, 2002) | ~8 | 8 | NR | 60 ± 8 | Cycle ergometer | 17.7 | NR |
| | (Stanley, 1999) | 9 ± 4 | 20 | 13:7 | 64 ± 7 | Cycle ergometer | 22.0 ± 7 | 100 |
| | (Canning, 1997) | 6 ± 3 | 16 | 13:3 | 54 ± 5 | Cycle ergometer | 27.6 ± 5 | 93 |
| Postpoliomyelitis | (Oncu, 2009) | 25 ± 9 | 28 | 12:16 | 42 ± 8 | Treadmill | 19.0 ± 5 | NR |
| | (Willén, 1999) | 46 ± 3 | 32 | 16:16 | 50 ± 10 | Cycle ergometer | 20.5 ± 7 | 74 |
| | (Stanghelle, 1993) | 11 ± 8 | 68 | 23:45 | 53 ± 11 | Cycle ergometer (n = 37) | 23.1 ± 5 | 63 |
| | | | | | | Arm ergometer (n = 31) | 15.3 ± 5 | 65 |
| | (Kriz, 1992) | 11–45 | 20 | 10:10 | 43 ± 6 | Cycle ergometer | 17.7 ± 6 | 73 |
| Spina bifida | (de Groot, 2008a) | NA | 23 | 13:11 | 10 ± 3 | Treadmill | 33.1 | NR |
| | (Widman, 2007) | NA | 37 | 19:18 | 16 ± 2 | Arm ergometer | 17.3 ± 6 | NR |
| Spinal cord injury: paraplegia | (Widman, 2007) | 5.1 ± 4.2 | 19 | 10:9 | 16 ± 3 | Arm ergometer | 16.9 ± 6 | NR |
| | (Haisma, 2006) | 0.3 ± 0.2 | 110 | 83:27 | 41 ± 15 | W/C ergometer | 14.7 ± 5 | NR |
| | (El-Sayed, 2005) | 0.3 ± 0.1 | 6 | 5:1 | 29 ± 14 | W/C ergometer | 17.3 (estimated) | NR |

| Category | Study | | N | | Age | Modality | $VO_2peak$ | % normal |
|---|---|---|---|---|---|---|---|---|
| | (Jacobs, 2002b) | 7 ± 5 | 6 | 6:0 | 36 ± 10 | Arm ergometer | 23.7 ± 3 | NR |
| | (Price, 1999) | 21 ± 8 | 9 | 9:0 | 30 ± 7 | Arm ergometer | 30.5 ± 8 | 71 |
| | (Lin, 1993) | 0.5 | 39 | 39:0 | 30 ± 1 | Arm ergometer | 19.4 ± 1 | 69 |
| | (Paré, 1993) | >3 | 46 | 46:0 | 33 ± 9 | W/C ergometer | 23.9 ± 5 | NR |
| | (Coutts, 1983) | >0.5 | 13 | NR | 29 ± 4 | Arm ergometer | 29.4 ± 10 | NR |
| Spinal cord injury: tetraplegia | (Haisma, 2006) | 0.3 ± 0.2 | 75 | 56:19 | 39 ± 13 | W/C ergometer | 12.1 ± 4 | NR |
| | (Coutts, 1983) | >0.5 | 8 | NR | 29.3 ± 4 | Arm ergometer | 16.1 ± 3 | NR |
| | (DiCarlo, 1988) | 7 ± 6 | 8 | 8:0 | 24 ± 4 | Arm ergometer | 12.1 ± 1 | NR |
| Stroke <6 mo | (Tang, 2009b) | 0.05 ± 0.01 | 36 | 22:14 | 65 ± 3 | Semirecumbent ergometer | 11.4 ± 0.6 | NR |
| | (Tang, 2006b) | 0.05 ± 0.01 | 35 | 19:16 | 66 ± 3 | Semirecumbent ergometer | 10.7 ± 2 | NR |
| | (Kelly, 2003) | 0.08 ± 0.03 | 17 | 13:4 | 61 ± 16 | Semirecumbent ergometer | 14.7 ± 4 | 51 |
| | (Duncan, 2003) | 0.2 ± 0.01 | 100 | 56:44 | 70 ± 10 | Cycle ergometer | 11.4 ± 3 | NR |
| | (MacKay-Lyons, 2002b) | 0.07 ± 0.02 | 29 | 22:7 | 65 ± 14 | Treadmill | 14.4 ± 5 | 61 |
| | (da Cunha Filho, 2001) | 0.04 ± 0.02 | 12 | 12:0 | 59 ± 10 | Cycle ergometer | 8.3 ± 2 | NR |
| | (Bachynski-Cole, 1985) | 0.3 ± 0.2 | 8 | 8:0 | 52 ± 10 | Cycle ergometer | 16.1 ± 4 | NR |
| Stroke >6 mo | (Lee, 2008 ) | 4.8 ± 4.5 | 48 | 28:20 | 63 ± 9 | Cycle ergometer | 14.4 ± 3 | NR |
| | (Pang, 2005) | >1.0 | 63 | 37:26 | 65 ± 9 | Cycle ergometer | 22.0 ± 5 | NR |
| | (Dobrovolny, 2003) | 3.0 | 53 | 44:9 | 64 ± 8 | Treadmill | 14.7 ± 3.9 | NR |
| | (Ryan, 2000) | >0.5 | 26 | 22:4 | 66 ± 9 | Treadmill | 15.6 ± 4 | NR |
| | (Fujitani, 1999) | 0.9 | 30 | 30:0 | 54 | Cycle ergometer | 17.7 ± 4 | NR |
| | (Potempa, 1995) | >0.5 | 42 | 23:19 | 56 ± 12 | Cycle ergometer | 15.8 ± 5 | NR |
| Traumatic brain injury | (Mossberg, 2007) | 0.8 ± 0.8 | 13 | NR | 32 ± 8 | Treadmill | 27.0 ± 5 | 76 |
| | (Bhambhani, 2003) | 1.4 ± 1.4 | 36 | 22:8 | 32 ± 10 | Cycle ergometer | 22.3 ± 9 | 65 |
| | (Mossberg, 2002) | 2 ± 4 | 40 | 29:11 | 33 ± 11 | Treadmill | 23.5 ± 7 | NR |
| | (Jankowski, 1990) | NR | 14 | | 29 ± 2 | Treadmill | 31.3 ± 9 | 67 |

GBS = Guillain-Barré syndrome; NA = not applicable; NR = not reported; VO₂peak = peak oxygen consumption; VO₂peak % normal = peak oxygen consumption expressed as a percentage of normative values; Pts = patients; W/C = wheelchair.

*Includes 4 patients with chronic inflammatory demyelinating polyneuropathy.

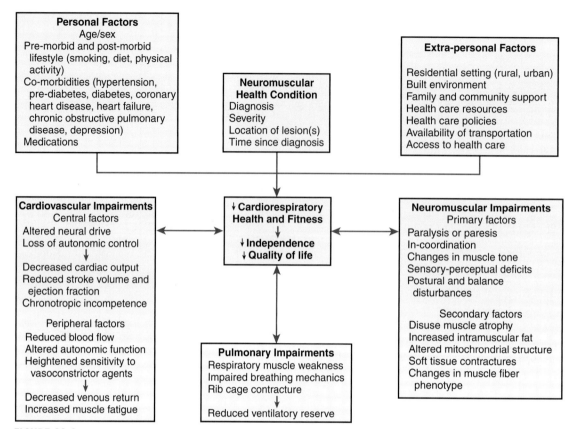

**Personal Factors**
Age/sex
Pre-morbid and post-morbid lifestyle (smoking, diet, physical activity)
Co-morbidities (hypertension, pre-diabetes, diabetes, coronary heart disease, heart failure, chronic obstructive pulmonary disease, depression)
Medications

**Neuromuscular Health Condition**
Diagnosis
Severity
Location of lesion(s)
Time since diagnosis

**Extra-personal Factors**
Residential setting (rural, urban)
Built environment
Family and community support
Health care resources
Health care policies
Availability of transportation
Access to health care

**Cardiovascular Impairments**
Central factors
Altered neural drive
Loss of autonomic control
↓
Decreased cardiac output
Reduced stroke volume and ejection fraction
Chronotropic incompetence

Peripheral factors
Reduced blood flow
Altered autonomic function
Heightened sensitivity to vasoconstrictor agents
↓
Decreased venous return
Increased muscle fatigue

**↓ Cardiorespiratory Health and Fitness**
**↓ Independence**
**↓ Quality of life**

**Pulmonary Impairments**
Respiratory muscle weakness
Impaired breathing mechanics
Rib cage contracture
↓
Reduced ventilatory reserve

**Neuromuscular Impairments**
Primary factors
Paralysis or paresis
In-coordination
Changes in muscle tone
Sensory-perceptual deficits
Postural and balance disturbances

Secondary factors
Disuse muscle atrophy
Increased intramuscular fat
Altered mitochrondrial structure
Soft tissue contractures
Changes in muscle fiber phenotype

**FIGURE 32-2** Model illustrating the complexity of the interactions contributing to reduced cardiorespiratory fitness characteristics of people after a stroke.

underlying cardiovascular dysfunction (Roth, 1993), and most have atherosclerotic lesions throughout the vascular system (Wolf, 1999).

Two principal mechanisms help explain reductions in aerobic capacity in the presence of cardiac dysfunction: reductions in ejection fraction and stroke volume (Clausen, 1973) and **chronotropic incompetence**—the inability of the pacemaking center in the right atrium, the **sinoatrial node**, to respond to the metabolic demands of exercise by increasing heart rate (Camm, 1996).

## THINK ABOUT IT 32.1

How does knowledge that 75% of individuals poststroke have underlying cardiovascular dysfunction influence your choice of interventions? How do you anticipate the stroke will affect their physical fitness? Why?

Peripheral factors contributing to reduced cardiovascular fitness include reduced blood flow, which compromises $O_2$ transport and energy production in the working muscles (Camm, 1996). Decreases in flow observed in acute anterior poliomyelitis appear to be related to histochemical and morphological changes in the vascular network itself (Kozak, 1968). In the case of stroke, both resting blood flow and postischemic reactive hyperemic blood flow were lower (~36% reduction) in the paretic lower extremity (Billinger, 2009;

Ivey, 2005). These reductions are possibly due to a combination of altered autonomic function (Herbaut, 1990), heightened sensitivity to endogenous vasoconstrictor agents (Bevan, 1993), and changes in muscle fiber composition in the paretic limb (Landin, 1977). In addition, poststroke reductions in arterial diameter have been reported despite near normal (i.e., above 0.90) mean ankle brachial index values (Billinger, 2009).

After an SCI, autonomic reflex activity and sympathetic vasomotor outflow can become impaired (Coutts, 1983; Glaser, 1986). As a result, reductions in venous return and stroke volume (**circulatory hypokinesis**) ensue, impairing delivery of $O_2$ and nutrients to and removal of metabolites from exercising muscles, which in turn intensifies muscle fatigue (Davis, 1988).

People with paraplegia may exhibit an exaggerated heart rate response when exercising to compensate for reduced stroke volume. Adrenergic dysfunction accompanying lesions above the T1 sympathetic outflow prevent this compensatory mechanism (Lewis, 2007).

## Neuromuscular Impairments

For most individuals with neurological conditions, the existence of neuromuscular impairments can confound physiological responses to exercise. Although the deconditioned state of able-bodied individuals is largely due to metabolic inefficiencies, people with neurological conditions are further challenged by biomechanical inefficiencies and related increases in energy expenditure resulting from neuromuscular impairments. The interplay of metabolic and biomechanical inefficiencies lowers cardiopulmonary health and fitness relative to that of an individual with an intact nervous system.

Primary effects of upper motor neuron damage that complicate responses to exercise include paresis, incoordination, abnormal muscle tone, sensory-perceptual disorders, and disturbed postural and balance control. Paresis reduces the pool of motor units available for recruitment during physical work (Dietz, 1986); for example, upward of 50% of motor units are not functioning after stroke (McComas, 1973). The subsequent reduction in metabolically active tissue lowers the oxidative potential (Landin, 1977). Hypertonia in extremity muscles restricts venous return and lactate clearance, thus contributing to increased muscle fatigability and reduced exercise capacity (Unnithan, 1998). In addition, high levels of **cocontraction** (i.e., simultaneous contraction of agonist and antagonist muscle groups), as seen in children with cerebral palsy (CP), may induce early fatigue of skeletal muscle, which in turn increases the energy cost of walking and reduces $VO_2peak$ (Bar-Or, 1986; Unnithan, 1998). Indeed, children with CP experience undue fatigue at walking speeds that would be considered slow for individuals who are able-bodied (Unnithan, 1998).

Secondary changes in skeletal muscles also contribute to deconditioning and impaired exercise response. Contrary to traditional belief, disuse muscle atrophy can occur after upper motor neuron lesions (Hafer-Macko, 2008). Lean mass of both thighs and self-selected walking speed were independent predictors of reduced fitness ($VO_2peak$) and accounted for 61% of the observed variance in $VO_2peak$ in 26 people in the chronic phase after stroke (Ryan, 2000). Other examples of secondary changes in skeletal muscle associated with reductions in $VO_2peak$ were increased intramuscular fat (Ryan, 2002), altered mitochondrial structure, (Landin, 1977), and decreased concentration of oxidative enzymes, particularly succinate dehydrogenase (Saltin, 1975).

In addition, muscle fiber type distribution can influence cardiovascular fitness. Skeletal muscles are composed of fibers that express different **myosin heavy chain** (MHC) **isoforms**. Slow (type I) MHC isoform fibers have higher oxidative function, are more fatigue resistant, and are more sensitive to insulin-mediated glucose uptake; fast (type II) MHC fibers are recruited for more powerful movements, are more reliant on anaerobic or glycolytic means of energy production, fatigue rapidly, and are less sensitive to the action of insulin (Daugaard, 2001). Thus, a shift in **phenotype** from type I to type II muscle fibers may reduce insulin sensitivity and oxidative capacity (Kernan, 2003), thereby increasing use of anaerobic processes in working muscles during dynamic exercise (DeDeyne, 2004; Huey, 2001). Elevated proportions of type II fibers have been found in the vastus lateralis of hemiparetic lower extremities (DeDeyne, 2004) in contrast to the relatively equal quantities of slow and fast MHC isoforms found in the same muscle of nondisabled individuals (Landin, 1977).

## Pulmonary Impairments

As in able-bodied people, pulmonary impairment is usually not the limiting factor in the ability of patients with neurological conditions to respond to exercise. For example, exercise capacity tends to be in the normal or near-normal range (Canning, 1997; Stanley, 1999) in patients with mild to moderate Parkinson disease despite substantial weakness of the respiratory muscles (Haas, 2004) and a reported 87% incidence of obstructive pulmonary dysfunction (Neu, 1967). Nevertheless, **ventilatory reserve**, the difference between maximal available ventilation and ventilation during exercise (Clark, 1969), is often decreased in persons with neurological conditions either as a direct complication of the pulmonary pathology (e.g., impaired breathing mechanics, muscle weakness) or secondary to cardiovascular dysfunction (e.g., congestive heart failure), comorbidities (e.g., chronic obstructive pulmonary disease), or lifestyle factors (e.g., physical inactivity, smoking habits) (Vingerhoets, 1994; Wiercisiewski, 1998; Howard, 1992; Mutluay, 2005).

Impairments associated with various neurological conditions can cause respiratory compromise. Reduced breathing efficiency resulting from respiratory muscle spasticity has been implicated in reduced exercise capacity in children with CP (Unnithan, 1998). Pulmonary impairment after a stroke is often modest and typically occurs in the hyperacute phase (Rowat, 2007) as a direct consequence of the stroke (e.g., brainstem stroke) or secondary to other factors (e.g., cardiovascular dysfunction, unhealthy lifestyle, aspiration pneumonia). **Respiratory insufficiency**, manifested by low pulmonary diffusing capacity, decreased lung volume, and ventilation-perfusion mismatching, may contribute to the overwhelming fatigue often associated with stroke (Haas, 1967). Expiratory dysfunction after stroke or other neurological conditions is related to the extent of motor impairment (e.g., hemi-abdominal muscle weakness), whereas inspiratory limitations are more often related to rib cage contracture (Fugl-Meyer, 1983). Diaphragmatic excursion of people with hemiplegia or tetraplegia may be restricted, and chest wall excursion may be depressed and paradoxical (Fugl-Meyer, 1984; Vingerhoets, 1994).

## Personal and Extrapersonal Factors

In all likelihood, many neurological patients experience *premorbid* (i.e., before occurrence of the disease) reductions in cardiorespiratory health. In support of this supposition, low aerobic capacity (Kurl, 2003) and conditions such as diabetes or **prediabetes** (i.e., impaired fasting glucose level or impaired glucose tolerance) that accelerate atherosclerosis have been identified as independent risk factors for primary stroke (Kernan, 2004). Indeed, a substantial percentage of people who experience a stroke were known to be hypertensive before stroke onset (Semplicini, 2003), and those with high $BP_{sys}$ or $BP_{dias}$ at the time of acute stroke are at 1.5- to 5-fold increased risk of dying or dependency compared with their normotensive counterparts (Willmot, 2004). Within the general population, an inverse relationship exists between cardiorespiratory fitness and eventual mortality from stroke, independent of body mass index, hypertension, diabetes mellitus, family history of cardiac disease, cigarette smoking, and alcohol consumption (Lee, 2002).

Negative lifestyle choices such as smoking, unhealthy diet, and physical inactivity impair exercise capacity (Huie, 1996). Smoking elicits acute increases in heart rate, myocardial contractility, and myocardial oxygen demand, which lead to atherosclerosis and increased risk of acute cardiovascular events over time (Rempher, 2006). Within the stroke population, smokers have double the risk of death (equivalent of a 7-year reduction in lifespan) compared with nonsmokers and ex-smokers (Myint, 2006).

The relationship between cardiovascular disease and dietary habits is currently under study in a major international initiative (Danesh, 2007). Obesity predisposes an individual to several other cardiovascular risk factors, including impaired glucose tolerance and type 2 diabetes, hypertension, and dyslipidemia (Pérez, 2007). Abdominal obesity, an early marker of atherosclerotic disease, has been independently associated with an increased risk of primary ischemic stroke (Lu, 2006; Walker, 1996). Overweight individuals age 11-21 years of age with spinal cord dysfunction are more likely to have reduced cardiovascular fitness than their normal-weight counterparts (Widman, 2007).

The link between physical activity and cardiopulmonary health and fitness is well known (Hu, 2004; Inoue, 2008; Ketelhut, 2004; Laughlin, 2004). Physical inactivity (and concomitant reductions in exercise capacity) is an independent risk factor for cardiovascular disease (Fletcher, 1992). In contrast, premorbid physical activity has had a positive effect on stroke severity and long-term outcomes (Krarup, 2008).

Physical impairments (e.g., paralysis, muscle weakness) associated with neurological conditions and related comorbidities restrict mobility and physical activity. A 2000 study reported that 56% of American adults with disabilities did not engage in any leisure-time physical activity compared with 36% of adults without disability (U.S. Department of Health and Human Services, 2000). In fact, people who have sustained an SCI have been classified as the most sedentary members of society (Dearwater, 1985), spending at little as 2% of their waking hours engaged in leisure-time physical activity (Latimer, 2006). Low physical activity in youth with chronic disabilities (including CP and SCI) has been correlated with increased cardiovascular risk factors, including hypertension and dyslipidemia (Morris, 2008). In the case of MS, exercise-induced elevations in body temperature and heightened fatigability serve as disincentives to activity (Ng, 1997). As a consequence of spending as much as 50% of the day resting in bed (Bernhardt, 2004), patients in the early poststroke period are at risk of rapid decreases in aerobic capacity (Convertino, 1982; Saltin, 1968; Winstein, 2016). In addition, a sedentary lifestyle is a key factor leading to insulin resistance (Knowler, 2002).

Other personal factors influencing exercise capacity include age and sex of the individual. Age is discussed in the lifespan section. Differences between the male and female response to dynamic exercise, both physiological and functional, have been reported for most of the major determinants of exercise capacity (Sheel, 2004). In terms of sex, $VO_2max$ values in women are approximately 77% of values in men after adjustments for body weight and activity level (Bruce, 1973). Older men and women respond to maximal exercise in a similar manner, with older women tending to have lower $BP_{sys}$ than men during maximal exercise (Fleg, 1995). Racial differences in terms of exercise capacity have not been well studied; no differences were found in the degree of physical deconditioning between 66 black and 52 white stroke survivors (Hinson, 2007).

Little attention has been paid to the relative contributions of personal and extrapersonal factors in mediating physical activity and cardiopulmonary fitness in neurological populations. Extrapersonal factors encompass residential setting (e.g., urban, rural), family and community support, the built environment (e.g., sidewalks, parks, walking trails), and governmental policies related to health-care resources, access to health care, and public transportation. Focus groups conducted with people with chronic disabilities, as well as with architects, fitness/recreation professionals, city planners, and park district managers underlined the inherent inaccessibility of both natural and built environments (Rimmer, 2004).

Researchers identified the need for an ecological model of biological, behavioral, and environmental factors related to physical activity in populations with disabilities (Rimmer, 2004). Initiatives sponsored by programs such as the Active Living by Design attempted to address this need by adopting a comprehensive ecological framework (Bors, 2009). This framework identifies and breaks down barriers to physical activity (e.g., lack of opportunities and built environments) by establishing multidisciplinary community partnerships (Bors, 2009). Although challenging to implement, this model has been successful in creating community change and an environment that supports active lifestyles (Bors, 2009). However, more research is warranted regarding the effect of these programs on populations with disabilities.

In summary, numerous interacting factors contribute to the low cardiopulmonary fitness levels seen in many populations with neurological conditions (see Fig. 32-1). Neuromuscular and respiratory impairments are superimposed on fitness levels already compromised by comorbid cardiovascular disease and premorbid health- and lifestyle-related declines in exercise capacity. Paresis and subsequent reduction in lean muscle mass, changes in muscle fiber phenotype, and increased reliance on anaerobic processes for energy production increase the metabolic costs of physical activity. In turn, cardiac reserves available for meaningful daily activities are limited, which negatively affects fatigability and quality of life. Societal barriers to activity that are beyond the control of the individual intensify the problem. The convergence of these influences facilitates an even more sedentary lifestyle, which further diminishes cardiopulmonary fitness.

## THINK ABOUT IT 32.2

What factors contribute to poor cardiopulmonary fitness in patients with neurological diagnoses? What aspects can be changed to help promote mobility and fitness in this population?

## ■ Lifespan Influences on Cardiac and Pulmonary Impairments

Aerobic capacity is known to decline with age. The Baltimore Longitudinal Study of Aging, which followed 375 women and 435 men ages 21-87 years of age, found that the rate of decline in aerobic capacity, as measured by peak $VO_2$ was 3-6% per 10 years in the 20's and 30's and 20% per 10 years in the 70's and beyond (Fleg, 2005; Ades, 2005). The study also found the rate of decline was larger in men than women from the 40's onward and occurred independent of muscle mass or physical activity habits. The rate of decline can be cut in half when physical activity and body composition are maintained at healthy levels during senescence (Jackson, 1995).

Gradual reductions in $VO_2$max are due to both decreased $O_2$-transporting and utilization capacity associated with cardiac, respiratory, and muscular changes (Fig. 32-3). *Central cardiac changes,* including increased myocardial stiffness and decreased left ventricular contractility, are primarily responsible for the two hallmarks of cardiovascular aging: reduction in ejection fraction and decline in maximal heart rate ($HR_{max}$) of 6 to 10 beats per minute per decade (Ogawa, 1992; Stratton, 1994). In addition, total peripheral resistance, and hence blood pressure, is higher during maximal exercise in older adults than in young adults (Fleg, 1995). *Peripheral changes* during the aging process that lower the oxidative capacity of the working muscles include alterations in skeletal muscle microcirculation, mitochondrial structure and distribution, and oxidative enzyme activity (Coggan, 1992), as well as **sarcopenia** (age-related loss of skeletal muscle) due to reduced number and size of fibers, particularly type II fibers (Jackson, 1995).

After peaking between 20 and 30 years of age, pulmonary function gradually declines. Age-related pulmonary deficiencies are due in part to restricted compliance of the lungs secondary to decreased elastic recoil of lung tissue and calcification and stiffening of the cartilaginous articulations of the ribs, progressive weakness of inspiratory and expiratory muscles, structural restrictions including progressive kyphosis, and decreased ability to clear mucus from the lungs (Frontera, 1986; Lowery, 2013). Reduced elastic recoil leads to enlargement of the thorax (barrel-shaped appearance) and flattening of the diaphragm, which in turn increases the work of breathing. In addition, airway patency, particularly during forced voluntary breathing, is less well maintained in the aged lung (Zaugg, 2000).

Age-related changes in cardiovascular, respiratory, and neuromuscular systems limit the capacity to respond to the metabolic demands imposed by prolonged physical activity and reduce the threshold for physical fatigue. Despite gradual loss of aerobic capacity with increasing age, able-bodied people retain adequate reserves for daily activities. In contrast, for people aging with a neurological impairment, this loss can reduce an already compromised reserve and threaten further loss of functional independence. Individuals with CP or other developmental disabilities are particularly disadvantaged because incomplete development of their musculoskeletal and cardiorespiratory systems at the time of neurological insult accelerates the aging process (Damiano, 2006). In the case of people who have an SCI, the risk of both cardiac and respiratory complications increases substantially with age (Hitzig, 2008).

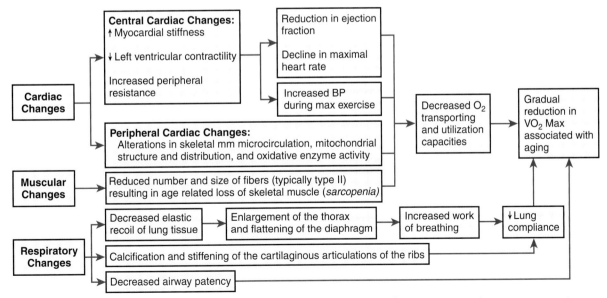

**FIGURE 32-3** Age-related cardiac, muscular, and respiratory changes and their influence on maximal oxygen consumption ($VO_2$max).

# Functional Implications of Low Cardiorespiratory Fitness in Neurological Populations

For people with neurological involvement, the implications of poor cardiorespiratory fitness can be substantial. One of the most profound consequences is reduced functional independence. Although people without physical disability use only a small fraction of the reserve capacity of the cardiovascular and respiratory systems for the metabolic challenges of physical activity (Westerterp, 2004), individuals with neurological impairments typically have low fitness levels that compromise their physiological reserve (Macko, 2001).

Low cardiorespiratory fitness is also associated with increased risk for future vascular events, including a second stroke, acute coronary syndrome (i.e., unstable angina and myocardial infarction), and heart failure (Blair, 1996). Such secondary events can contribute substantially to the overall personal and economic burden of the primary neurological condition. For instance, recurrent strokes have higher fatality rates than primary strokes, and for those who survive a second stroke, a large proportion will experience long-term disability and institutionalization (Hankey, 2002). The effect of reduced exercise capacity on daily function is best illustrated using a case study.

## PATIENT APPLICATION

*Mr. A is a 64 year-old male with long-standing coronary artery disease who had a lacunar stroke 18 days before admission to a rehabilitation center. His exercise capacity was 4.5 METs (15.6 mL of $O_2$/kg/min) or about 60% of the normative value for his age, sex, stature, and activity level. To put a MET level of 4.5 into perspective, consider the following points: (1) A peak MET of less than 84% of normal is considered pathological (Wasserman, 2005); (2) the combination of coronary artery disease (CAD) and a peak MET of less than 6 METs (21 mL/kg/min) places an individual such as Mr. A in the high mortality group (Morris, 1991); and (3) about 5.7 METs (20 mL/kg/min) is the level needed for independent living (Cress, 2003).*

*Assuming the metabolic demands of activities of daily living are about 3 to 5 METs (10.5 to 17.5 mL of $O_2$/kg/min) (Ainsworth, 2000), Mr. A requires 55% to 67% of his exercise capacity (2.5 to 3 METS) to accomplish certain daily tasks (e.g., brushing his teeth, tidying his room) and about 100% of his capacity (4.5 METS) to do other tasks (e.g., washing windows, mopping), leaving insufficient capacity to do more physically demanding work (e.g., snow shoveling, digging). These figures are conservative, given that the metabolic demands of performing household chores after a stroke can be almost double the normative metabolic demand values (Bjuro, 1975). In contrast, Mr. A's able-bodied friend Mr. Z has a peak MET level of 7.5 (26.4 mL of $O_2$/kg/min) and therefore requires only 40% to 67% of his exercise capacity to accomplish the same tasks.*

*The relative metabolic demands on Mr. A make performance of basic daily tasks unsustainable for an extended time and*

*provide little reserve for other activities. Moreover, assuming an anaerobic threshold of about 60% of $VO_2$peak, Mr. A meets this threshold at 2.7 METs, compared with 4.5 METs for Mr. Z. Although Mr. Z can perform daily activities using aerobic metabolism, Mr. A relies on activation of anaerobic pathways for basic activities. Therefore, in his daily life, Mr. A experiences an exponential build-up of lactate, leading to rapid exhaustion and inability to function effectively without assistance.*

*Excessive fatigability and lack of functional independence has had a negative effect on Mr. A's perceived self-efficacy and quality of life. For example, despite regaining good motor control of his involved upper and lower extremities, Mr. A cannot walk to Mr. Z's house, an activity he performed three or more times per week before his stroke.*

### Contemplate Clinical Decisions

1. How might you link Mr. A's cardiopulmonary symptoms with activities that were important to him before his stroke to increase his awareness and eventually his compliance with an exercise program?
2. From this brief introduction to Mr. A, which information would lead you to undertake a more specific examination of his cardiopulmonary impairments?
3. Given the information presented thus far, what risk factors related to Mr. A's cardiopulmonary impairments would you want to explore?

# Measurement of Cardiorespiratory Health and Fitness

Cardiopulmonary fitness can be measured using maximal or submaximal tests, which are described in detail in Chapter 11. Cardiopulmonary fitness tests specifically adapted for neurological populations are outlined in Table 32-2. Standard safety guidelines apply, regardless of which test is used. Contraindications to testing are listed in Table 32-3. Pretraining tests to screen for cardiac disease should include electrocardiogram monitoring by qualified personnel. All fitness tests should be preceded by a 3- to 5-minute warm-up at a metabolic rate that is approximately twice that of resting level (i.e., 2 METs) to prevent premature and excessive local muscle fatigue (American College of Sports Medicine, 2010). Similarly, testing should be followed with a 3- to 5-minute cooldown to support venous return and prevent pooling of blood in the peripheral vasculature and a subsequent drop in diastolic pressure. Monitoring of blood pressure before, during, and after testing is an important safety consideration.

## Maximal Tests of Cardiorespiratory Fitness

$VO_2$max is generally considered the definitive index of fitness, or "gold standard" (Foster, 1996). $VO_2$max is a stable and reproducible variable, with repeated measurements varying only 2% to 4% in nondisabled adults (Taylor, 1955) and an

| TABLE 32-2 | Measures of Cardiopulmonary Fitness Adapted for Neurological Populations |
| --- | --- |
| **TEST** | **DESCRIPTION** |
| Body weight– supported treadmill test (MacKay-Lyons, 2002b) | *General description:* Symptom-limited maximal treadmill test<br>*Health condition studied:* Stroke (mean of 26 days after stroke)<br>*Protocol:* 15% of body weight is supported during the test; 2 stages beginning with walking at self-selected speed and 0% treadmill grade for 2 minutes, followed by a 2.5% increase in grade every 2 minutes until an incline of 10% is reached; thereafter, a 0.05-m/sec increase in speed every 2 minutes until test termination.<br>*Test-retest reliability:* $ICC_{3,1} = 0.94$ for $VO_2$peak and $ICC_{3,1} = 0.93$ for peak heart rate<br>*Validity:* 86.4% ± 11% of age-predicted maximal heart rate achieved using this protocol |
| Semirecumbent cycle ergometry (Tang, 2006b) | *General description:* Symptom-limited maximal semirecumbent cycle ergometry exercise test<br>*Health condition studied:* Stroke (mean of 17.6 days after stroke)<br>*Protocol:* Ramp protocol included a 2-minute warm-up at 10 W at a target cadence of 50 rpm, followed by progressive 5 W increases in work rate every minute<br>*Test-retest reliability:* ICC = 0.50 for $VO_2$peak and 0.74 for peak heart rate<br>*Validity:* 9% of participants reached a peak heart rate within 10 bpm of the age-predicted maximal heart rate |
| Recumbent stepper (Billinger, 2008) | *General description:* Modified exercise test using a total-body recumbent stepper (mTBRS-XT) in individuals after stroke.<br>*Health condition studied:* Stroke (mean of 40.1 months after stroke)<br>*Protocol:* 2-minute stages at a stepping cadence of 80 steps/min with an initial resistance of 25 W, which was increased at each stage until test termination<br>*Test-retest reliability:* $ICC_{3,1} = 0.94$ for $VO_2$peak, 0.93 for peak heart rate<br>*Validity:* Correlation between mTBRS-XT and cycle ergometry for $VO_2$peak, $r = 0.91$; peak heart rate, $r = 0.89$ |
| Combined upper and lower limb ergometer (Hill, 2005) | *General description:* Symptom-limited maximal test using combined upper and lower limb ergometer<br>*Health condition studied:* Stroke (mean of 7.3 weeks after stroke)<br>*Protocol:* 3-minute stages at a cycling cadence of 30–40 revolutions/min with resistance increased at each stage until test termination (resistance applied was not reported)<br>*Test-retest reliability:* Not reported<br>*Validity:* 75% ± 11% of age-predicted maximal heart rate achieved using this protocol |
| Modified Shuttle Test (MST) (Hassett, 2007) | *General description:* Symptom-limited incremental walking test<br>*Neurological conditions studied:* Traumatic brain injury<br>*Protocol:* Walking between two cones (20 meters apart) to volitional fatigue; modifications to original test included adding lower levels of automated pacing to accommodate slower walking speeds<br>*Test-retest reliability:* Not reported<br>*Validity:* Correlation between MST $VO_2$peak and treadmill test $VO_2$peak, $r = 0.96$; correlation between MST peak heart rate and treadmill test peak heart rate, $r = 0.80$ |
| 6-Minute walk test (6MWT) (Eng, 2004; van Hedel, 2005) | *General description:* Submaximal walking test<br>*Health condition studied:* Stroke (Eng, 2004); SCI (van Hedel, 2005)<br>*Protocol:* Walking at self-selected speed for 6 minutes, inclusive of rest intervals<br>*Test-retest reliability:* $ICC_{2,1}$ for $VO_2 = 0.96$; $ICC_{2,1}$ for distance covered = 0.99 (Eng 2004); distance covered with a 7-day interval varied by 20.5 ± 27 meters (van Hedel, 2005)<br>*Validity:* Correlation between 6MWT $VO_2$ and $VO_2$peak, $r = -0.66$; between 6MWT distance and $VO_2$peak, $r = -0.37$; between heart rate at end of 6MWT and $VO_2$peak, $r = -0.18$ (Eng, 2004)<br>*Special notes:* Wu (2003) suggested that a single 6MWT may be adequate in the rehabilitation setting provided that modest learning effects are considered when interpreting the results. |
| 6-Minute arm test (6MAT) (Hol, 2007) | *General description:* Submaximal arm ergometer test<br>*Health condition studied:* SCI (mean of 12 years after injury)<br>*Protocol:* Arm cranking for 6 minutes at a power output to elicit a steady-state heart rate of 60%–70% of age-predicted maximum heart rate (for patients with low-level paraplegia) or a rating of 11–15 on the Borg RPE scale4–20 (for subjects with tetraplegia or high-level paraplegia)<br>*Test-retest reliability:* $ICC_{2,1}$ for steady-state $VO_2 = 0.81$, for heart rate = 0.90<br>*Validity:* Correlation between $VO_2$peak and 6MAT $VO_2$, $r = 0.92$ |

*Continued*

| TABLE 32-2 | Measures of Cardiopulmonary Fitness Adapted for Neurological Populations—cont'd |
|---|---|
| **TEST** | **DESCRIPTION** |
| 6-Minute wheel test (6MWhT) (MacKay-Lyons, unpublished data) | *General description:* Submaximal wheelchair test<br>*Neurological conditions studied:* SCI (mean of 13.7 years after injury)<br>*Protocol:* Propelling wheelchair for 6 minutes (inclusive of rest breaks) with distance covered as the main variable<br>*Test-retest reliability:* Not reported<br>*Validity:* Correlation between 6MWhT steady-state $VO_2$ and $VO_2$peak, $r = 0.80$; between 6MWhT steady-state $VO_2$ and 6MAT steady-state $VO_2$, $r = 0.88$ |

ICC = intraclass correlation coefficient; RPE = rating of perceived exertion; SCI = spinal cord injury; $VO_2$peak = peak oxygen consumption.

| TABLE 32-3 | Contraindications to Exercise Testing and Training. |
|---|---|
| **HEALTH CONDITION** | **ABSOLUTE CONTRAINDICATION** |
| Myocardial infarction (MI) | Recent or complicated MI with ejection fraction <30% |
| Angina | Unstable angina or not controlled with medication/intervention |
| Heart surgery | Recent coronary artery bypass surgery; valve replacement/repair |
| Aortic stenosis | Severe or symptomatic stenosis |
| Pulmonary embolus or pulmonary infarction | Acute pulmonary embolus or pulmonary infarction |
| Myocarditis/pericarditis | Suspected or known acute myocarditis or pericarditis |
| Dissecting aneurysm | Suspected or known dissecting aneurysm |
| Systemic infection | Acute systemic infection accompanied by fever, body aches, or swollen lymph glands |
| Ventricular dysrhythmia | Ventricular dysrhythmia that cannot be controlled with medication |
| Atrial dysrhythmia | Uncontrolled atrial dysrhythmia that compromises cardiac function |
| Heart failure | Acute or uncontrolled heart failure |
| Valvular heart disease | Symptomatic or moderate stenotic valvular heart disease |
| Electrolyte abnormalities | Hypo- or hyperkalemia or hypomagnesemia |
| Hypertension (arterial) | Resting $BP_{sys}$ >200 mm Hg and/or resting $BP_{dias}$ >110mm Hg |
| Dysrhythmia | Tachydysrhythmia (>120 bpm) or bradydysrhythmia |
| Resting ST-segment displacement | >2-mm displacement in more than one lead (excluding chronic bundle branch block) |
| Arteriovenous block | Symptomatic or high-degree arteriovenous block without pacemaker |
| Shortness of breath at rest | Unknown etiology or decompensated congestive heart failure |
| Carotid stenosis | Severe stenosis |
| Large-vessel intracranial stenosis | Severe stenosis |
| Thrombophlebitis/intracardiac thrombi | Untreated thrombophlebitis/intracardiac thrombi |
| Peripheral arterial disease | Symptomatic such that it prevents exercise |
| Mental impairment | Impairment that leads to inability to exercise adequately |
| Pacemaker | Fixed-rate pacemaker |
| Chronic infectious disease | Mononucleosis, hepatitis, AIDS |
| Metabolic disease | Uncontrolled diabetes with resting blood glucose level >400 mg/dL, thyrotoxicosis, myxoedema |
| Orthostatic hypotension | >20 mm Hg drop with symptoms |
| Dizziness | Severe motion-induced dizziness/vertigo |
| Arthritis/musculoskeletal disorder | Severe pain on weight-bearing or inability to exercise |
| Neuromuscular disorder | Neuromuscular disorders that are exacerbated by exercise |

Note: Relative contraindications can be superseded when the benefits outweigh the risks of exercising. In such cases, caution and low-level endpoints should be used, particularly when the individual is symptomatic at rest.
Adapted from (American College of Sports Medicine. *ACSM's Guidelines for Exercise Testing and Prescription.* 7th ed. Philadelphia, PA: Lippincott Williams & Wilkins, 2006; American College of Sports Medicine. *ACSM's Guidelines for Exercise Testing and Prescription.* 8th ed. Philadelphia, PA: Lippincott Williams & Wilkins, 2010.)

intraclass correlation coefficient of 0.93 reported in patients after a stroke (Eng, 2004). The reproducibility (in terms of Spearman rank correlation) in children with CP is 0.72 to 0.84 compared with 0.90 in able-bodied children (van den Berg-Emons, 1996).

Accurate determination of VO$_2$max requires recruitment of at least 50% of total muscle mass (Rowell, 1974) and thorough familiarization with the testing procedure (Hoofwijk, 1995). The optimal duration of a maximal test is 8 to 12 minutes, with termination occurring when the subject is (1) no longer able to generate the required power, (2) limited by symptoms, or (3) unable to continue safely (Jones, 1997), making it difficult to complete in patients with neurological dysfunction. Exercise intensity is increased in a continuous, progressive manner (i.e., ramp or step protocol) or less commonly in a discontinuous, progressive manner (i.e., with rests between stages).

Peak intensity and total exercise time are not reliable indicators of maximal effort because they depend on the test protocol (Revill, 2002). Instead, VO$_2$max is indicated by attainment of a plateau in VO$_2$ beyond which there is change of less than 100 mL/min; further increases in workload depend solely on anaerobic metabolism (Jones, 1997). In contrast, VO$_2$peak criteria include attainment of the age-predicted maximal heart rate, ratio of expired carbon dioxide to O$_2$ (referred to as the **respiratory exchange ratio**) in excess of 1.15, VE greater than the predicted maximal voluntary ventilation, VT greater than 90% of the inspiratory capacity, and obvious patient exhaustion (American Thoracic Society/ American College of Chest Physicians, 2003).

Selection of mode of exercise (e.g., treadmill walking, cycling, stepping, arm cranking, arm-leg ergometry) should take the patient's functional abilities and needs into consideration. The mode affects VO$_2$max values, with the treadmill eliciting the greatest metabolic response. Bike ergometry yields 85% to 90% and arm ergometry 70% of the VO$_2$max achieved with a treadmill (Rowell, 1974). In addition, muscles activated on the treadmill most closely resemble the mobility pattern used by most patients (i.e., walking). In patients with neuromuscular conditions, however, impaired motor and postural control may preclude the use of standard treadmill testing protocols. An exercise protocol using a body weight– support system permits safe and valid exercise testing early after stroke (MacKay-Lyons, 2001).

For individuals with an SCI, wheelchair treadmills are more functional than arm-crank ergometry. Furthermore, arm cranking engages a smaller muscle mass, thereby limiting the reduction in total peripheral resistance and increasing the blood pressure response.

Peak heart rate achieved during a maximal exercise test can be used to estimate VO$_2$peak because of the linear relationship between VO$_2$ and heart rate. However, although VO$_2$ is relatively impervious to testing conditions, heart rate is markedly affected by stresses such as dehydration and changes in body temperature, thus limiting the accuracy of the estimation (Rowell, 1974). In fact, discrepancies between estimated and measured VO$_2$max in individuals with low exercise capacity can be as high as 25% (Davies, 1968).

Further, because there is considerable variability in HR$_{max}$ among healthy individuals, percentage of predicted HR$_{max}$ (HR$_{max}$ = 220 – age) is not a robust measure of exercise capacity (Robergs, 2002).

## Submaximal Tests of Cardiopulmonary Fitness

As detailed in Chapter 11, submaximal exercise tests may be more appropriate than maximal tests for clinical testing in neurorehabilitation because they are more readily available, administration is less expensive, and patients are subjected to lower risk of adverse events. Testing protocols, such as the Åstrand-Ryhming Nomogram (Åstrand, 1954), estimate VO$_2$max from heart rate measurements taken at a fixed work rate or test duration at a given power output on a cycle ergometer or at a given grade and speed on a treadmill. However, it should be noted that the accuracy of the estimations has not been validated in special populations, including patients with neurological conditions. In addition, the heart rate response at a specific submaximal workload can be affected by testing mode; work performed by the upper extremities (e.g., arm ergometer) generally elicits higher heart rate responses than lower extremity work. According to Davies (1968), using heart rate at a fixed submaximal load as an indicator of cardiovascular fitness is only 75% accurate.

An advantage of the 6-minute walk test (6MWT) (see Table 32-2) is that the patient tends to walk at a constant speed at a pace near his critical power; thus, VO$_2$ is in a steady-state condition for most of the test. Further, predictive equations permit assessment of the distance covered relative to normative values (Dean, 2001). However, the weak correlations, at least in the stroke population, between distance walked and VO$_2$peak, as well as the weak association between heart rate at the end of the 6MWT and VO$_2$peak and the reliance on the ambulation status, limit this clinical test as a measure of cardiovascular fitness (Eng, 2004; Tang, 2006a).

## Vascular Risk Assessment

Many people with neurological impairments are at risk of further vascular morbidity. For instance, approximately 20% to 25% of people who have experienced a stroke will have a second stroke or other cardiovascular incident in the ensuing 3 years (Burn 1994; Warlow, 1992). Goldberg (1988) maintained that prevention of stroke recurrence is a critical, albeit underaddressed, goal of stroke rehabilitation. Thus, risk assessment should be a part of the neurological evaluation.

**Metabolic syndrome** (also known as insulin resistance syndrome, syndrome X, or dysmetabolic syndrome) is a constellation of metabolic abnormalities that interact to accelerate the progression of atherosclerosis and increase the risk of developing cardiovascular or cerebrovascular disease (Gami, 2007). In other words, metabolic syndrome has the predictive quality of distinguishing patients at high risk for future vascular events (Vlek, 2008). As a composite risk assessment, this syndrome has been defined using various criteria; Table 32-4

| TABLE 32-4 | Components of Metabolic Syndrome Using the International Diabetic Federation Definition |
| --- | --- |
| **COMPONENT** | **PARAMETERS** |
| Obesity | Waist circumference >102 cm in males, >88 cm in females |
| *Plus any 2 of the following:* | |
| • Hypertension | $BP_{sys}$ >130 mm Hg or $BP_{dias}$ >85 mm Hg OR treatment of previously diagnosed hypertension |
| • Hypertriglyceridemia | Serum triglyceride level >1.7 mmol/L (150 mg/dL) |
| • Low high-density lipoprotein cholesterol (HDL-C) level | Serum HDL-C <1.03 mmol/L (40 mg/dL) in men, <1.29 mmol/L (50 mg/dL) in women OR specific treatment for these lipid abnormalities |
| • Insulin resistance | Fasting serum glucose level of ≥5.6 mmol/L (100 mg/dL) OR previously diagnosed type 2 diabetes |

(Alberti K, Zimmet P, Shaw J. Metabolic syndrome: A new world-wide definition: A consensus statement from the International Diabetes Federation. *Diabet Med.* 2006;23:469–480.)

outlines the definition adopted by the International Diabetes Federation (IDF) (Alberti, 2006). The incidence of metabolic syndrome in neurological populations is high. A retrospective study reported that 60.5% of 200 patients in stroke rehabilitation met the criteria for the syndrome (MacKay-Lyons, 2009).

## PATIENT APPLICATION

*For an example of a clinical assessment of cardiovascular fitness, we return to the case of Mr. A, who was introduced earlier in this chapter. From Mr. A's perspective, his main concern since his stroke is his fatigability; for example, he scored 26 of 32 on the Daily Fatigue Impact Scale (Fisk, 2002). This presentation is consistent with a report that 40% of patients who have experienced a stroke rate fatigue among the worst symptoms of the disorder (Ingles, 1999). Moreover, poststroke fatigue has been an independent predictor of decreased functional independence, institutionalization, and mortality (Glader, 2002). Indeed, excessive fatigue prevented Mr. A from completing not only his daily household chores but also his most valued social activity—walking 0.5 kilometer to visit his friend.*

*It is very likely that poor cardiovascular fitness contributed to Mr. A's fatigue. As previously mentioned, his results on a laboratory-based maximal test of fitness yielded a relative*

$VO_2$peak of 15.6 mL of $O_2$/kg/min (4.5 METs), which is considered poor for his sex and age. Similarly, his performance on a more clinically based submaximal test of walking endurance, the 6MWT, was abnormally low, covering a total distance of 216 meters (about 40% of the predicted normative value) unaided but with standby supervision. With an overground walking speed of 0.56 meters per second, which is about 44% of the normative value, (Öberg, 1993), Mr. A is classified as a "most-limited community ambulator" (Perry, 1995). Thus, both measures precluded Mr. A from meeting the criteria for effective outdoor ambulation, namely the ability to walk 500 meters continuously (Hill, 1997) and walking speed enabling safe crossing of streets (i.e., 71 cm/sec for slowest walk signals to 138 cm/sec for fastest signals) (Robinett, 1988).

To assess Mr. A's risk of further vascular events, the components of metabolic syndrome as defined by the IDF (see Table 32-4) were examined. Although his lipid profile was within the desired range, Mr. A met the following criteria for metabolic syndrome: (1) waist circumference was 109 centimeters, (2) resting blood pressure was 170/82 mm Hg, and (3) his fasting serum glucose level was 7.8 mmol/L.

## Contemplate Clinical Decisions

1. Develop a list of Mr. A's functional limitations.
2. List the underlying impairments possibly contributing to each of these functional limitations.
3. Prioritize Mr. A's concerns.
4. Write at least two appropriate long-term goals expressing realistic functional outcomes for Mr. A. Include all components of the goal.

## ■ Interventions to Improve Cardiorespiratory Fitness in Neurological Populations

The challenges of achieving and maintaining cardiovascular fitness in most patients with chronic neurological disabilities are nontrivial. Secondary impairments (e.g., disuse muscle atrophy, contracture formation, fatigue) superimposed on primary impairments (e.g., paralysis, muscle tone changes, postural and sensory-perceptual disturbances) elevate the physical demands of everyday life, lessening the energy reserves people with an intact neuromuscular system can access for fitness training. On the other hand, it is well accepted that improved physical conditioning can reduce secondary impairments. Thus, it is imperative that cardiovascular fitness training be given a high priority in neurorehabilitation. In 2006, Damiano called for a paradigm shift in management of CP toward "a more focused and proactive approach to promoting activity through more active training protocols, lifestyle modifications, and mobility-enhancing devices" (p. 1534).

Cardiovascular fitness or exercise capacity can be improved through either progressive physical activity or aerobic exercise.

**Physical activity** refers to bodily movement produced by skeletal muscle contractions that occurs either in brief bursts of low to high intensity or in long, sustained periods of lower intensity depending on the type of activity and the fitness level and that substantially increases energy expenditure (U.S. Department of Health and Human Services, 1996). Physical activities include lifting weights, walking in the neighborhood, or playing sports. **Aerobic exercise** is structured and repetitive physical activity performed for extended periods and at sufficient intensity to elicit long-term adaptations. Examples of aerobic activities include brisk walking, ergometry, jogging, biking, dancing, and swimming. Most of the evidence regarding the effects of fitness training in neurological populations has been derived from aerobic exercise studies.

## Effects of Cardiorespiratory Fitness Training in Neurological Populations

### Increased Exercise Capacity

Trainability of youth and adults with neurological disabilities has been demonstrated in several studies conducted over the past decade, as indicated in FOE Table 32-7 (ONL). One review focusing on adolescents with chronic disabilities (including those with CP, SB, and SCI) (Morris, 2008) and another focusing on children with CP (Verschuren, 2008) concluded that cardiovascular training can yield positive effects on aerobic capacity, even in children with severe disabilities (Pang, 2006). The authors of a Cochrane Database review (Saunders, 2016) concluded cardiorespiratory training and to a lesser extent mixed training involving walking within post-stroke rehabilitation programs can reduce disability, improve speed and tolerance of walking and possibly improve balance. They found insufficient evidence to support the use of resistance training. Pang (2006) concluded that sufficient evidence existed to support the use of aerobic training in people with mild and moderate stroke, and Marsden (2013) concluded that interventions with an aerobic component can improve cardiorespiratory fitness after a stroke and should be considered as part of routine care. A Cochrane Database systematic review on the effect of exercise in MS showed strong evidence in favor of exercise therapy compared with no exercise therapy for improving exercise tolerance (Rietberg, 2004). The main conclusion reached in two separate reviews on SCIs was that despite considerable variation in study results, the physical capacity of people with either paraplegia or tetraplegia could be enhanced through exercise training (Valent, 2007; Warburton, 2007). In contrast, a Cochrane Database review was inconclusive regarding the effects of fitness training for cardiorespiratory conditioning in individuals after a TBI (Hassett, 2008). The results of one small study involving three patients with Parkinson disease (Schenkman, 2008) and two small studies involving patients with Guillain-Barré syndrome suggest positive effects (Pitetti, 1993; Bussman, 2007) (Table 32-7, ONL).

The magnitude of training-induced increases in $VO_2$peak reported for healthy, sedentary adults (Samitz, 1991) and cardiac rehabilitation participants (Franklin, 1978; Mertens, 1996) is about 15%. The mean improvement in $VO_2$peak in cited training studies was 23% for post-SCI trials, 14% for trials of people less than 6 months after a stroke, and 12% in trials of people more than 6 months after a stroke. The extent of change was influenced by factors such as variations in neurological condition, severity, and baseline fitness (the most deconditioned subjects attained the largest increments in exercise capacity [Saltin, 1969]), differences in mode and intensity of training, and disparities in levels of adherence to the exercise protocol.

Proposed mechanisms for training-induced improvements in exercise capacity in populations with neurologic conditions have been based primarily on extrapolation from studies involving populations without disability. A principal contributing factor is increased maximal cardiac output (Hartley, 1969) resulting from greater stroke volume, which in turn is secondary to enhanced myocardial contractility (Clausen, 1977). Maximal heart rate, the other factor determining $VO_2$max, remains unchanged with training. Despite higher cardiac output with training, mean arterial pressure is not elevated because of improved venous return and dampening of the sympathetically induced vasoconstriction in the nonworking muscles (Clausen, 1977). In the periphery, larger $AVO_2$ differences within the active muscles result from increases in capillary density (Saltin, 1985), size and number of mitochondria, myoglobin levels, and metabolic enzymes (e.g., succinate dehydrogenase, cytochrome oxidase) (Whipp, 1994).

Within neurological populations, it is unknown whether improved exercise capacity is largely due to central or peripheral mechanisms. However, for patients with CAD, increases in $VO_2$max are more highly correlated with central than with peripheral adaptations (Fergueson, 1982).

### Increased Cardiac Efficiency

The reduction in heart rate at a fixed submaximal workload resulting from cardiovascular training is explained by various mechanisms: elevation in total blood volume (Wilmore, 1996), increase in vagal activity, reduction in sympathetic-adrenergic drive, and reduction in resting heart rate (Casaburi, 1994). Although blood pressure at a given submaximal workload usually remains unchanged with training, the **rate-pressure product** ($BP_{sys} \times$ heart rate) decreases (Ogawa, 1992). A reduction in rate-pressure product is indicative of improved cardiac efficiency (e.g., reduced myocardial $VO_2$ demand, increased maximal coronary blood flow) (Nelson, 1974).

### Reduced Respiratory Effort

Training-induced improvements in fitness levels result in delays in the demand for increased anaerobic metabolism, which in turn reduces VE and respiratory effort at a given submaximal workload (Casaburi, 1994). The converse is also a possibility—improved pulmonary function in people with MS, gained through targeted expiratory (Chiara, 2006) and inspiratory (Fry, 2007) muscle training, may increase tolerance for exercise training. Short-term improvements in respiratory muscle function and exercise capacity have been demonstrated in patients with stroke and SCI after respiratory muscle training (Postma, 2014; Sutbeyaz, 2010). Inspiratory and expiratory muscle strength training has also improved respiratory muscle strength in individuals with slowly progressive neuromuscular disease (Aslan, 2014).

## Reduction in Vascular Risk Factors

Through its positive influences on cardiac and respiratory efficiency, energy balance, and body weight, aerobic training is effective in improving vascular risk factors, including blood pressure (Jolliffe, 2001), glycemic control in type 2 diabetes (Thomas, 2006), and lipid profile (particularly total cholesterol, low-density lipoproteins, and triglyceride levels) (Jolliffe, 2001). Evidence of risk factor reduction in neurological populations is beginning to emerge. A systematic review concluded that exercise training after an SCI appeared to be an effective intervention for reducing the risk for cardiovascular disease and comorbidities (e.g., type 2 diabetes, hypertension, obesity) because of beneficial effects on glucose homeostasis, lipid lipoprotein profiles, and cardiovascular fitness (Warburton, 2007). However, the authors noted a lack of evidence as to whether these training-induced effects translated into reduced incidence of cardiovascular disease and premature mortality in the SCI population (Warburton, 2007).

A 15-week training program for patients with MS resulted in decreases in skinfold thickness, triglyceride levels, and very low–density lipoprotein levels as well as improvements in depression and fatigue (Petajan, 1996). Treadmill exercise training over a 6-month period reduced insulin resistance in patients after a stroke (Ivey, 2007). A 10-week cardiac rehabilitation program for nonacute ischemic stroke was associated with greater improvements in cardiac risk score compared with usual care (Lennon, 2008). The effects of exercise on risk factor reduction in Parkinson disease have not been investigated despite the fact that 50% to 80% of people with the disease have impaired glucose tolerance (Ristow, 2004).

## Improved Motor Function and Mobility

Improved gross motor function in children with CP was reported after participation in an 8-month circuit-training program (Verschuren, 2007) and a 12-week aerobic interval and strength training program (Unnithan, 2007). Luft (2008) provided preliminary evidence that training-induced gains in walking ability after stroke (da Cunha Filho, 2002; Pohl, 2002) may be explained by neuroplastic mechanisms involving cerebellum-midbrain circuits. It is important to note that spasticity is not aggravated during aerobic training (Saunders, 2004; Smith, 1999; Teixeira-Salmela, 1999). In fact, evidence

from studies of spinal cats (Coté, 2003) and humans after an SCI (Trimble, 1998) indicates that treadmill training may reduce spasticity by improving stretch reflex modulation.

## Decreased Fatigability

Cardiorespiratory intervention has had variable effects on fatigue in the neurological population. An 8-week, hospital-based, training study in patients with postpoliomyelitis was associated with reduced fatigue (Oncu, 2009). In contrast, a training study involving patients with Guillain-Barré syndrome demonstrated no effect on fatigue (Bussman, 2007). A systematic review (Rietberg, 2004) reported no evidence of a modulating effect of exercise on pathological fatigue in patients with MS. Although a single-cohort study found no change in fatigue levels after 12 sessions of treadmill walking (Newman, 2007), a randomized controlled trial showed a reduction in fatigue after 12 weeks of aerobic exercise (McCullagh, 2008). For patients with Charcot-Marie-Tooth disease, who also experience undue fatigue, a 24-week interval training program resulted in decreased body fatigue but not skeletal muscle fatigue (El Mhandi, 2008). These results indicate cardiorespiratory intervention may positively influence patient fatigue in many neurological diagnoses. Further research in this area is warranted.

## Enhanced Emotional Well-Being

Increased exercise capacity has been associated with enhanced mental well-being (i.e., reduced anxiety and depression) in people with cardiac disease (Jolliffe, 2001; Lewin, 1992); moderate evidence was also found for improving mood in MS (Rietberg, 2004). In a meta-analysis, exercise appeared to have a positive effect on depressive symptoms of stroke in both the subacute and chronic stages of recovery with higher intensity exercise protocols more effective than lower intensity protocols (Eng, 2014). Depressive symptoms were reduced immediately after the exercise program but not retained in subsequent followup (Eng, 2014). A stroke trial comparing a 10-week cardiac rehabilitation program with usual care showed greater improvements in depressive symptoms in the rehabilitation group (Lennon, 2008; Winstein, 2016). In agreement, a clinical trial of a 6-month community-based group exercise program for stroke survivors found the exercise group had an average 4.4-point increase on the Hamilton Rating Scale for Depression (Hamilton, 1980), whereas the control group demonstrated no change (Stuart, 2009). Saunders, et al. (2016) concluded in a Cochrane Systematic Review that data was insufficient to determine the effects of physical fitness training on mood, including depression, in patients with stroke.

## Improved Neuroplasticity

Attention is directed toward better understanding of the influences of exercise on the central nervous system. Animal studies have demonstrated favorable effects of aerobic training on neural function through modulation of synaptic plasticity that underlies neuroprotective and neuroadaptive processes (Dishman, 2006). Brain-derived neurotrophic factor (BDNF) affects neural function and neuroplasticity by facilitating long-term potentiation, a long-lasting increase in the strength of connection between two neurons that are repeatedly activated together, and by promoting dendritic growth and remodeling (Mang, 2013). Voluntary exercise can increase levels of BDNF and other growth factors, stimulate neurogenesis, increase resistance to brain insult, and improve learning and mental performance (Cotman, 2002). In a rodent stroke model, treadmill exercise enhanced gene expression for BDNF with a corresponding reduction in brain infarct volume (Ang, 2003). Similarly, exercise attenuated the effects of TBI, again in a rodent model, through a BDNF-mediated mechanism (Griesbach, 2004). Aerobic exercise promotes BDNF production in individuals after stroke and has implications for pairing aerobic exercise and functional training to promote neuroplasticity (Mang, 2013) (Fig. 32-4). These neuroplastic responses appear to be dose dependent (Tong, 2001).

## Improved Memory and Cognition

Neuroplastic responses also have implications for memory and cognition. For example, learning and memory were enhanced in rats after 1 week of voluntary wheel running (Van Praag, 1999), possibly through upregulation of BDNF or other growth factors (Neeper, 1996). Evidence of a causal relationship between exercise training and improved cognition has been reported in older adults without known cognitive impairment (Angevaren, 2008; Colcombe, 2003) and in people with cardiovascular disease (Gunstad, 2005). Quaney (2009)

provided preliminary evidence on the effects of exercise training on cognitive executive function and motor learning in chronic stroke survivors. After an 8-week cycle ergometry exercise program, significant improvements were found in measures of information processing and complex motor learning tasks. Gordon (1998) speculated that the improved cognitive function observed in individuals who exercised regularly after a TBI (Novack, 2000) may be attributed to exercise-induced increases in BDNF or other growth factors. Saunders, et al. (2016) concluded there was insufficient data to draw conclusions on the effect of physical fitness training on cognitive function in stroke patients.

## Improved Health-Related Quality of Life

Studies have reported improved quality of life for people with CP (Verschuren, 2007) and MS (Petajan, 1996) after participation in exercise programs. A cross-sectional cohort study found people with MS who exercised regularly had better social and role functioning than their less active counterparts (Turner, 2009). Both hospital- and home-based aerobic exercise programs can enhance the quality of life of people with postpolio syndrome (Oncu, 2009). Several systematic reviews of fitness trials involving people after a stroke were inconclusive regarding beneficial effects on quality of life because of lack of data (Meek, 2003; Saunders, 2016; van de Port, 2007). However, evidence of improved quality of life has been reported in individual studies involving people in the subacute phase after a stroke (Langhammer, 2008; Studenski, 2005).

Figure 32-5 provides examples of how quality of life can be improved with cardiorespiratory fitness.

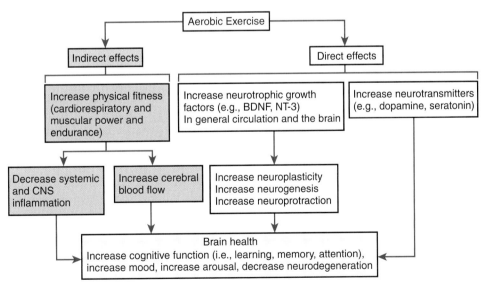

FIGURE 32-4 Examples of indirect and direct pathways for positive effects of aerobic exercise on the brain. (Adapted from Mang CS, Campbell KL, Warming T, et al. Promoting neuroplasticity for motor rehabilitation after stroke: Considering the effects of aerobic exercise and genetic variation of brain-derived neurotrophic factor. Phys Ther. 2013;93(12):1707–1716.)

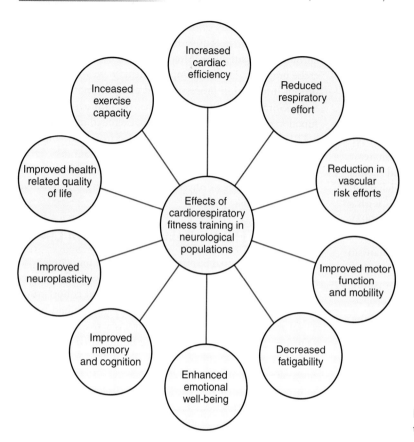

**FIGURE 32-5** Effects of cardiorespiratory fitness training in neurological populations.

## Exercise Prescription for Cardiovascular Fitness

Guidelines for prescribing cardiovascular fitness and physical activity programs for people with neurological impairments have been based largely on protocols designed for nondisabled populations (American College of Sports Medicine, 2010). Nonetheless, recent studies involving specific neurological populations have begun to inform exercise prescription in neurorehabilitation.

### Initiation of Training

The optimal time to initiate aerobic training after onset of a neurological condition is unknown. Most of the training studies in Table 32-7 (ONL) involved participants in the chronic stage of their condition, although some trials safely recruited people in the subacute period. One systematic review and meta-analysis concluded that stroke survivors may benefit from cardiovascular exercise during subacute stages to improve peak $O_2$ uptake and walking distance (Stoller, 2012). Low-intensity ergometer aerobic training may be feasible and effective in patients who are early after stroke or are more severely impaired (Wang, 2014), although further research is needed regarding aerobic exercise early in the acute phase after stroke and in severely affected individuals.

Macko (1997b) raised the possibility that if training is introduced in the acute period when cerebral autoregulation is most likely to be compromised, adverse vascular responses

(e.g., hypotension, dysrhythmia) may impede perfusion of ischemic brain tissue. Concerns about early training are tempered by knowledge that in the first month after an ischemic stroke, the peri-infarct cortex is in a state of heightened plasticity (e.g., axonal sprouting and neurogenesis) that mediates functional recovery (Carmichael, 2006).

### Exercise Setting

The patient's medical status, level of mobility, and social support system should be considered when selecting the exercise setting. When training high-risk individuals, such as patients with major cardiac comorbidities, immediate access to emergency medical equipment and trained personnel is critical during training sessions, and the adverse event protocol should be rehearsed at regular intervals. For lower-risk individuals, supervised community- (Eng, 2003) or home-based (Duncan, 2003) aerobic exercise programs may be a safe and effective option. However, a disadvantage of home-based programs is the lack of appropriate equipment, most importantly, emergency medical equipment (Duncan, 2005). Oncu (2009) reported reduced fatigue and improved quality of life but no change in $VO_2$peak in postpolio patients who trained in either the hospital or at home. Poststroke patients who engaged in either an unsupervised home-based program or a supervised, facility-based program achieved similar gains in exercise capacity (Hassett, 2009).

Particular attention should be paid to the training environment. Thermal dysregulation is common in patients with neurological impairments, particularly MS (Ponichtera-Mulcare,

1993) and higher levels of SCI, because of loss of vasomotor and sudomotor responses (Price, 1999). Thus, careful control of ambient temperature and provision of fans, spray bottles, towels, and a water cooler are recommended. A water bottle with volumetric indicators is useful to monitor hydration before exercise and rehydration after exercise. The training facility should be wheelchair accessible, with adequate space to permit transfer to/from exercise equipment.

## Scheduling of Exercise Sessions

Training sessions should be scheduled with the convenience of the participants in mind. When fatigue is a concern, training should be scheduled for morning hours, when circadian body temperature is lowest. For certain patient groups, including people with Parkinson disease, timing of medication to optimize performance during training is an important consideration.

## Preparation for Exercise

Exercise participants should be advised to wear comfortable clothing and supportive footwear and to avoid eating 2 hours before training. Emptying the bowel and bladder before training is particularly important for people with an SCI above T6 to reduce the risk of **autonomic dysreflexia**, or loss of central autonomic control resulting in reflex adrenergic responses (e.g., extreme hypertension, intense headaches, profuse sweating) to noxious stimuli, such as a full bladder.

## Session Frequency

Optimal training requires three to five sessions per week, although fitness can improve with twice-weekly sessions (American College of Sports Medicine, 2010). Very deconditioned individuals may benefit from multiple brief exercise sessions daily.

## Session Duration

Moderate exercise for at least 30 minutes on most days of the week is recommended, but the benefits are apparent even for light to moderate exercise, such as walking (Kelley, 2001;

Winstein, 2016). A minimum of 20 minutes of exercise within the training target zone is required to elicit a training effect (American College of Sports Medicine, 2016). For very deconditioned individuals, exercise may be delivered in 5-minute "bouts," with rest periods between bouts. Two additional 5-minute periods are required for an active warm-up and cooldown; hence, the minimal time required to complete a training session is 30 minutes.

## Timing of Aerobic Exercise Within Treatment Sessions

Because aerobic exercise influences BDNF and other neural factors, timing of aerobic exercise within treatment sessions can be used to promote positive neuroplasticity. Mang (2013) suggested that aerobic exercise be used to increase BDNF levels before functional training to prime motor rehabilitation in poststroke patients (Fig. 32-6). Continued research is needed to determine optimal training parameters for promotion of positive neuroplasticity (Ploughman, 2015).

## Exercise Mode

Selection of training mode depends mainly on the motor status of the individual and the equipment available. Traditional modes of aerobic exercise include arm, leg, and arm-leg ergometers. Arm ergometers, which activate a smaller portion of total muscle mass than the other types of ergometers, are effective for training patients with tetraplegia (DiCarlo, 1988). Other modes include water-based exercises, bicycles, treadmills, body weight–supported treadmills, brisk walking, and other repetitive and structured physical activity performed for appropriate duration and intensity to elicit long-term adaptations.

In recent years, alternative approaches have been introduced to overcome limitations to exercise training imposed by neurological damage, including balance impairments and paresis. Within the stroke population, water-based exercise has had demonstrable benefit in improving cardiovascular fitness (Chu, 2004) as well as in dealing with the challenges of

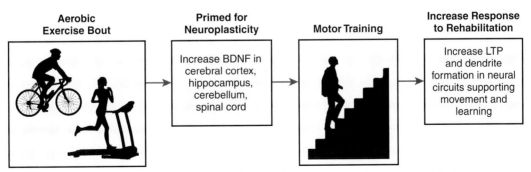

**FIGURE 32-6** Use of aerobic exercise to prime the central nervous system for neuroplasticity to support motor rehabilitation after a stroke. *(Adapted from Mang CS, Campbell KL, Warming T, et al. Promoting neuroplasticity for motor rehabilitation after stroke: Considering the effects of aerobic exercise and genetic variation of brain-derived neurotrophic factor. Phys Ther. 2013;93(12):1707–1716.)* BDNF = brain-derived neurotrophic factor; LTP = long-term potentiation.

living with stroke (Huijbregts, 2008). Body weight–supported treadmill training (BWSTT), originally introduced to facilitate early gait retraining (Barbeau, 2003), has been used successfully for aerobic training early after stroke (da Cunha Filho, 2001). The addition of BWSTT in treatment sessions after a stroke has improved cardiovascular fitness and walking endurance (Mackay-Lyons, 2013). Training at higher speeds on the treadmill may lead to greater step length on the involved side and greater improvements on the 6MWT (Lee, 2015). Using electrical stimulation of lower extremity muscles to augment voluntary muscle contraction of upper extremity muscles has been effective for aerobic training in people after an SCI (Wheeler, 2002). Another novel approach has been the use of virtual reality as an adjunct to fitness training. For example, a virtual reality recumbent ergometer appeared to enhance attention to the task of exercising in patients after a TBI (Grealy, 1999).

Many different forms of exercise can be used alone or in combination to promote aerobic conditioning when performed at the correct intensity and duration. Combined strengthening and aerobic training for people with type 2 diabetes was more effective than aerobic training alone in improving $VO_2peak$, walking endurance, and lipid profile (Lambers, 2008). The combination of aerobic and strengthening exercise also improved fitness outcomes in people after a stroke (Teixeira-Salmela, 1999). Circuit training involving resistance exercises and arm cranking not only improved fitness levels but also reduced shoulder pain in people after an SCI (Nash, 2007). It is important to monitor the cardiopulmonary system during exercise to ensure optimal training parameters.

## Exercise Intensity

Intensity of exercise is of foremost concern because it dictates the level of metabolic stress to which the participant is exposed and is the most important factor in ensuring an adequate and safe dosage to elicit a training effect. In recent years, knowledge regarding exercise prescription specific to neurological populations has increased. Higher exercises intensities yield greater functional benefits after stroke (Pohl, 2002) and more pronounced improvements in lipid profile after an SCI (de Groot, 2003). Dose-dependent effects on blood pressure and total cholesterol levels have also been noted after stroke, with better results attained with moderate-intensity, shorter duration (30 minutes) training than with low-intensity, longer duration (60 minutes) exercise (Rimmer, 2009).

Initial exercise intensity and progression must be individualized. Deconditioned individuals can benefit from intensities as low as 55% to 64% of $HR_{max}$ or 40% of **heart rate reserve** (HRR); $HRR = HR_{max}$ – resting heart rate (American College of Sports Medicine, 2010). However, a 2002 meta-analysis by Swain concluded that for very unfit patients, intensities as low as 30% of reserve can be effective. Continuous heart rate monitoring and periodic blood pressure readings are recommended. Evidence suggests that music, properly timed to rhythmic motor events such as walking or cycling,

potentiates muscle activation and may be beneficial in pacing movement (McIntosh, 1997; Rossignol, 1976).

For some neurological populations, heart rate is not an accurate indicator of exercise intensity. For example, people with tetraplegia (above T1–L2 sympathetic nerve outflow) exhibit a blunted heart rate response during exercise, with heart rate often peaking at around 125 beats per minute (Nash, 1995). In contrast, individuals with midthoracic lesions may have excessive heart rates at rest and during exercise, possibly because of adrenergic overactivity to compensate for reduced stroke volume secondary to pooling of blood in the lower extremities and reduced venous return.

Simple proxy measures of exercise intensity have been introduced, of which the rate of perceived exertion (RPE) is most commonly used (Borg, 1982). The RPE range associated with physiological adaptation to exercise is 12 to 16 on the Borg category scale (that rates exercise intensity from 6-20) or 4-6 on the Borg category-ratio scale modified for dyspnea (0 to 10 rating of perceived respiratory effort) (American College of Sports Medicine, 2016). Goode (1998) reported that the point of "hearing your breath" while exercising also occurs at or near the ventilatory threshold.

Another proxy measure of intensity is the **Talk Test**: The participant should be able to talk while exercising, but if he can sing, the intensity should be increased. If the participant cannot talk, the intensity should be decreased. Foster (2008) confirmed that the exercise intensity at the ventilatory threshold coincides with the last intensity at which a subject can comfortably speak. Relationships among RPE, Talk Test, and more physiological measures of intensity are outlined in Table 32-5.

A recently introduced proxy measure is the **Count Talk Test** (CTT), which measures how high the person at rest can count aloud without taking a second breath, starting with "one, one-thousand; two, one thousand..." (Norman, 2008). The percentage of resting CTT during exercise has strongly correlated with percentage of HRR, $VO_2$ reserve, and RPE, with 50% of CTT corresponding to moderate intensity exercise (Norman, 2008).

Neurorehabilitation clinicians should note, however, that the validity of these proxy measures of intensity have not been validated in neurological populations. Indeed, a lack of association between RPE and both heart rate and $VO_2$ has been reported in patients with an SCI (Lewis, 2007). Table 32-6 summarizes applications of exercise prescription for cardiovascular fitness.

## THINK ABOUT IT 32.3

What should you consider when prescribing aerobic exercise for the following patients: a patient with a 5-year history of Parkinson disease, a patient status postacute stroke, and a patient with a 10-year history of spinal cord injury? How would you determine location, timing, initiation, setting, mode, frequency, and intensity? What other information would you need to obtain?

**TABLE 32-5  Rating of Perceived Exertion**

| CLINICAL TESTS | | | | RELATIVE INTENSITY | | |
| --- | --- | --- | --- | --- | --- | --- |
| Borg Scale | | | Talk Test | % Max HR | % HR Reserve | % VO₂max |
| 1–10 | 6–20 | Description | | | | |
| 1 | 6 | No exertion at all | | | | |
|  | 6.5 | | | | | |
|  | 7 | Extremely light | Very easy – you can sing or converse with no effort | <35 | <20 | <30 |
| 2 | 8 | | | | | |
|  | 9 | Very light | | | | |
| 3 | 9.5 | | Easy – you can converse with almost no effort | 35–54 | 20–39 | 30–46 |
|  | 10 | | | | | |
| 4 | 11 | Fairly light | Moderately easy – you can converse comfortably with little effort | | | |
|  | 12 | | | | | |
| 5 | 12.5 | | Moderate – conversation requires some effort | 55–69 | 40–59 | 46–79 |
|  | 13 | Somewhat hard | | | | |
| 6 | 14 | | Moderately hard –conversation requires quite a bit of effort | 70–89 | 60–84 | 80–84 |
|  | 15 | Hard (heavy) | | | | |
| 7 | 15.5 | | Difficult – can talk but must stop talking to catch breath – conversation requires quite a bit of effort | | | |
|  | 16 | | | | | |
| 8 | 17 | Very hard | Very difficult – conversation requires maximum effort | ≥90 | ≥85 | ≥85 |
|  | 18 | | | | | |
| 9 | 18.5 | | Approaching extreme – difficult to breath | | | |
|  | 19 | Extremely hard | | | | |
| 10 | 20 | Maximum exertion | Extreme effort – cannot continue | 100 | 100 | 100 |

HR = heart rate; VO₂max = maximal oxygen consumption.
Used with permission from J. Eng.

**TABLE 32-6  Overview of Exercise Prescription for Cardiovascular Fitness**

| | |
| --- | --- |
| Initiation of training | • Optimal time is unknown<br>• Most research in chronic phase although may be beneficial in subacute and acute phases (Carmichael, 2006; Stoller, 2012; Wang, 2014) |
| Exercise setting | • Considerations for medical status, level of mobility, and social support<br>• Considerations for equipment needs<br>• Considerations for environment |
| Scheduling of exercise sessions | • Considerations for patient convenience<br>• Considerations for fatigue |
| Preparation for exercise | • Comfortable clothing and footwear<br>• Empty bowel and bladder (especially with a spinal cord injury above T6) |
| Session frequency | • Optimal training: Three to five sessions per week but can improve with twice weekly sessions (American College of Sports Medicine, 2010) |
| Session duration | • Moderate exercise for at least 30 minutes on most days of the weak but benefits even with light to moderate exercise (Kelley, 2001; Winstein, 2016)<br>  • Minimum of 20 minutes of exercise within training target zone necessary for training effect with 5-minute warm-up and 5-minute cooldown (American College of Sports Medicine, 2010)<br>• Can deliver exercise in 5-minute bouts with rest periods in very deconditioned individuals |

Continued

| TABLE 32-6 | Overview of Exercise Prescription for Cardiovascular Fitness—cont'd |
|---|---|
| Timing of aerobic exercise within treatment sessions | • Can potentially be used before functional training to help prime neurological system for positive neuroplasticity by increasing circulating levels of BDNF (Mang, 2013) |
| Exercise mode | • Dependent on motor status of the individual and equipment availability |
| Exercise intensity | • Increased intensity results in greater functional poststroke benefits (Pohl, 2002)<br>• Deconditioned individuals can benefit from intensities as low as 55%–64% of maximal heart rate or 40% of heart rate reserve (American College of Sports Medicine, 2010)<br>• For very unfit patients, intensities as low as 30% of heart rate reserve may be effective (Swain, 2002)<br>• Continuous monitoring of blood pressure and heart rate are recommended<br>• Heart rate may not be an accurate indicator of exercise intensity in some patients, so measures such as rating of perceived exertion, the Talk Test, and the Count Talk Test may be useful for choosing appropriate intensity (Borg, 1982; Foster, 2008; Nash, 1995; Norman, 2008) |

BDNF = brain-derived neurotrophic factor.

## Long-Term Engagement in Aerobic Exercise

It has long been recognized that benefits of training decline notably without ongoing participation in physical activity (Bruce, 1973). Thus, sustained behavioral change must be the ultimate goal of any fitness program. In fact, behavioral modifications may be as potent as antihypertensive and cholesterol-lowering agents in secondary prevention of stroke (Myint, 2006). Nonetheless, for many people with or without neurological impairments, establishing and maintaining a fitness regimen can be difficult. Discouragingly, one study revealed that 39% of 691 patients failed to adhere to the exercise regimen prescribed by their physical therapist (Sluijs, 1993). Further, a recent study found that more than 75% of community-dwelling people after a stroke were not in a state of readiness to incorporate exercise into their lifestyle (Garner, 2005; Lennon, 2008).

Some individuals are reluctant to engage in physical activity because of concerns about their symptoms. For example, people with Parkinson disease who experience excessive fatigue tend to avoid exercise for fear of increasing their fatigue level (Fertl, 1993). Similarly, people with MS often avoid physical activity in an attempt to minimize fatigue and prevent elevations in body temperature (Ng, 1997). Consistent with this observation, less than 30% of 2,995 people with MS claimed to endorse any form of exercise (Turner, 2009), and the overall rate of exercise adherence in one training study involving patients with MS was only 65% (Mostert, 2002).

It is important to consider aerobic and physical activity that is meaningful and enjoyable to the individual patient. Strategies to improve overall physical activity during nontreatment time or after discharge include pedometers, accelerometers, or other activity monitors. These devices may be a feasible way to give objective feedback and motivate patients with chronic stroke to increase their physical activity level (Sullivan, 2014). Another way to improve physical activity in patients with neurological disorders is the use of virtual reality or gaming systems. Wii, PlayStation 2, or other gaming systems may provide motivation and opportunities for increased activity levels in neurological populations (Laufer, 2014; Meldrum, 2012; Saposnik, 2010; Taylor, 2011). Neuroprostheses and robotic exoskeletons are

being explored for patients with an SCI, stroke, or other neurological diagnosis to potentially increase activity (Proffitt, 2015). Another way to increase physical activity is to encourage group exercise classes or specialized programs dedicated to patients with mobility disorders in individuals who can safely participate. For example, some communities have adaptable sports programs for children and adults with disabilities, such as wheelchair basketball, adapted baseball, water aerobics, and therapeutic horseback riding.

Neurorehabilitation clinicians who understand the theoretical frameworks underlying adherence behavior (Sirur, 2009) can optimize patient compliance by designing exercise programs to fit their patients' level of function and social and environmental contexts. A systematic review of strategies to increase adherence in cardiac rehabilitation supported the use of educational sessions, spousal/family involvement, flexible and convenient scheduling of sessions, ongoing positive reinforcement and enjoyment (e.g., motivational letters, pamphlets, conversations), and self-management aids (e.g., self-report diets, activity logs, individualized goal setting) (Beswick, 2005). Additional strategies include gradually progressing exercise intensity, establishing regularity of training sessions, minimizing the risk of muscular soreness, exercising in groups, and when feasible, offering assistance with transportation and childcare. Considering sedentary time over the day and focusing on increasing light-intensity activity over the course of the whole day are also beneficial (Manns, 2012). These strategies should take into consideration personal (e.g., sex, level of disability), social, cultural, and environmental (e.g., facility accessibility) factors that influence participant engagement and adherence to physical activity and exercise (Morris, 2009).

### PATIENT APPLICATION

*Mr. A spent 43 days as an inpatient and participated in physical therapy sessions scheduled each weekday for a mean duration of 63 minutes per session. The main objectives of physical therapy were to improve his lower extremity motor control, postural control, locomotor ability, and cardiopulmonary fitness. Occupational* therapy sessions, also 5 days per week, focused on upper extremity motor control and functional activities. Approximately 60% of each physical therapy session was devoted to activities in standing, including BWSTT, overground walking, and active exercises (balance retraining, sit-to-stand practice and resisted calf raises, hamstring curls, and hip abduction). Another 20% of each session was devoted to active exercises in lying and sitting (e.g., bridging, abdominal curls, resisted straight-leg raises and quadriceps exercises, and upper extremity exercises). In the remaining 20% of the session, Mr. A was metabolically inactive (e.g., rested, was educated or counseled by the physical therapist, and received passive range-of-motion intervention).

The BWSTT component of Mr. A's intervention progressed from two or three bouts of 5 minutes' duration to a single 30-minute bout by the time of discharge, with a 3- to 5-minute warm-up and cooldown. Body-weight support was gradually reduced from an initial level of 35% to 10% as his walking pattern and exercise capacity improved. Similarly, treadmill speed was gradually progressed from a baseline of 1.4 km/h (39 cm/sec) to 2.7 km/h (75 cm/sec), with a corresponding increase in mean heart rate from 32% to 67% of HRR. During training, his $RPE_{0-10}$ was maintained between 4 and 6.

Mr. A's discharge destination was his sister's single-story home because his balance instability prevented safe negotiation of the stairs to his second-floor apartment. At the time of discharge, his relative $VO_2$peak improved 16% (to 18.1 mL of $O_2$/kg/min or 5.2 METs, which is about 70% of normative value). This change was reflected in his reduced score on the Daily Fatigue Impact Scale (to 18 out of 32). The distance covered in the 6MWT increased 19% (to 289 meters, or 53.5% of normative value), and standby supervision was no longer required. His gain of 73 meters exceeded the substantial change estimates of 47 to 49 meters reported for the 6MWT (Perera, 2006). Overground walking speed increased 22%, to 68 cm/sec, thus improving Mr. A's ambulatory classification to a "least-limited community ambulator" (Perry, 1995). The 22-cm/sec gain in speed surpassed that deemed necessary for a most substantial change (i.e., 9 to 14 cm/sec) (Perera, 2006). In terms of Mr. A's vascular risk assessment, his waist circumference changed marginally from 109 to 107 cm, his resting blood pressure level improved from 170/82 mm Hg to 154/80 mm Hg, and his fasting serum glucose value decreased from 7.8 mmol/L to 6.7 mmol/L.

Despite substantive gains in Mr. A's clinical presentation, further rehabilitation as an outpatient was warranted for the following reasons: (1) His exercise capacity (18.1 mL/kg/min or 5.2 METs) remained in the pathological range (i.e., less than 84% of predicted) and fell short of the 5.7 METs (20 mL/kg/min) needed for independent living; (2) his walking tolerance and speed were less than that needed for effective community ambulation; and (3) he continued to meet the criteria for metabolic syndrome.

## Contemplate Clinical Decisions

1. Use the principles of progression to develop three different modifications of the patient's activities to emphasize optimal function over the next several weeks, both in the clinic and at home.

2. What other treatment settings and environmental setups would you consider for Mr. A?

3. Formulate and describe at least two additional treatment ideas applied to specific functions that are meaningful for Mr. A.

## PATIENT APPLICATION: HOME EXERCISE PROGRAM

At the time of discharge, Mr. A returned for outpatient physical therapy three times per week. To augment his therapy, he was given a home program involving a few task-oriented exercises that addressed two of his main functional goals. After completing warm-up exercises of ankle pumping in sitting and marching on the spot, Mr. A was instructed to perform the following program:

### Goal #1: To return to living full-time in his second-floor apartment

Main limiting factors: Poor balance control and reduced eccentric control of plantar flexors, precluding independent and safe ascent and descent of stairs.
Time required: 5 minutes
Examples of exercises:

1. Heel rises: Standing on left leg with light fingertip support on back of chair. Controlled lifting and lowering of left heel, 10 times. Repeat on right leg.
2. Partial squats: Standing on left leg with light fingertip support on back of chair. Controlled bending and straightening of the left knee, 10 times. Repeat on right leg.
3. Step-ups: Standing facing a single step with the left side close to a wall. Place left foot and then right foot on step. Lower left foot and then right foot, backward to starting position, 10 times. Repeat beginning with right foot. Use wall for support as needed.

### Goal #2: Three times a week, to walk 0.5 kilometer without sitting to rest in order to visit his friend

Main limiting factor: Poor balance control and cardiovascular fitness contributing to excessive fatigue and restricted walking tolerance.
Time required: 15 minutes
Examples of exercises:

1. Walking while bouncing a ball.
2. Stepping over lines on the floor, progressing to stepping over objects.
3. Carrying objects of various sizes and weights back and forth from two baskets 7.5 meters apart, one placed on the floor and the other placed on an overhead shelf 7.5 meters away.
4. Tandem walking: Standing with the left side close to a wall. Step left foot in front of right foot to form a straight line. Step right foot in front of left foot. Continue in this manner for 5 meters. Use wall for support as needed.
5. Walking on foam: Standing facing a foam exercise mat, with left side close to a wall. Walk back and forth on foam mat three times. Use wall for support as needed.

## Let's Review

1. What basic physiological principles underlie cardiovascular and pulmonary functions related to exercise metabolism?

2. What factors contribute to poor cardiopulmonary fitness in patients with neuromuscular impairments? How can you address some of these in your physical therapy or occupational therapy practice?

3. What are the benefits of including interventions directed at cardiovascular fitness in the neurological population?

4. How would you design an exercise program to promote cardiovascular health and fitness in individuals with neurological diagnoses? What should you consider regarding individual patient diagnoses such as multiple sclerosis, stroke, spinal cord injury, Parkinson disease, and cerebral palsy?

5. What specific activities may be appropriate in patients with poor cardiovascular fitness?

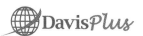 **DavisPlus**    For additional resources, including Focus on Evidence tables, case study discussions, references, and glossary, please visit http://davisplus.fadavis.com

## CHAPTER SUMMARY

Integration of cardiopulmonary physiology, assessment procedures, and interventions to ensure a holistic, multisystem approach to neurorehabilitation is becoming the standard of care. Primary and musculoskeletal limitations, as well as underlying personal and extrapersonal factors, combine with cardiopulmonary deficiencies to adversely influence both exercise capacity and muscular efficiency. Without effective monitoring and intervention, these interactions can have profoundly negative consequences on mobility, energy costs,

and quality of life. There is growing evidence that despite typically poor cardiopulmonary fitness at their initial presentation, children and adults with neurological impairments can respond to exercise training in essentially the same manner as individuals without impairments. Although the principles and techniques for cardiovascular-pulmonary interventions are discussed in the chapter, the online Focus on Evidence (FOE) Table (Table 32-8 ONL) summarizes some of the more important evidence supporting these interventions.

# Specific Functional Intervention to Improve Activity/Participation

## Functional Activity Intervention in Upper Extremity Tasks

Rebecca I. Estes, PhD, OTR, CAPS ▪ Donna A. Wooster, PhD, OTR/L
Tracy O'Connor, OTD, OTR/L

CHAPTER 33

---

## CHAPTER 26

**CHAPTER OUTLINE**

CHAPTER OBJECTIVES

INTRODUCTION
  Typical Characteristics and Patterns of Movement in the Upper Extremity
  Clinical Picture of Upper Extremity Activity in a Holistic Context
  Possible Impairments Underlying Abnormal Upper Extremity Tasks

Safety Considerations
Lifespan Influence on Upper Extremity Use
Pertinent Examination/Evaluation

FUNCTIONAL INTERVENTIONS FOR UPPER EXTREMITY TASKS
  General Approaches
  Therapeutic Functional Activities
  Pediatric Considerations for Intervention

CONSIDERATIONS FOR NONTHERAPY TIME AND DISCHARGE
  Aspects of Patient and Family Education
  Activities for Nontherapy Time
  Illustrated Sample Home Exercise Program

CHAPTER SUMMARY

REFERENCES (ONL)

---

**CHAPTER OBJECTIVES**

Upon completion of this chapter, the learner should be able to:
1. Identify the effects of neurologically based illness or injury on the functional repertoire of the hand and arm related to the performance of daily tasks and engagement in life activities.
2. Identify examinations, evaluations, and interventions at the basic function and skill levels for an upper extremity affected by neurologically based illness or injury.
3. Choose appropriate evidence-based examinations, evaluations, and interventions at the occupational performance skill level for an upper extremity affected by neurologically based illness or injury.
4. List the typical clinical pictures of neurological impairment characteristics of the hand and upper extremity, including impairments underlying abnormal neurological function, safety considerations, and lifespan influence.

## ▧ Introduction

***Dana***, *a 58 year-old musician, had a right hemisphere cerebrovascular accident. She tells you that her "left arm feels tight and stiff, and it is difficult to move. I can't do anything!" You observe that all left upper extremity movements are in the form of abnormal synergies with no isolated movements. In addition to other body function impairments, you detect spasticity in the left upper extremity.*

*Because the patient has identified left upper extremity tasks as a priority problem, you will need to further explore all underlying impairments potentially contributing to the movement dysfunction, the specifics of the muscle tone examination, and precisely how each upper extremity function has been affected. We will learn more about Dana as the chapter progresses.*

This morning, you may have pushed the snooze button on your alarm clock, reached for the blankets, and plumped your pillow for an extra minute of "shut-eye." Or perhaps you threw back the covers, ran your hands through your hair, and faced the new day. As you prepared for the day, you ran a familiar upper extremity (UE) obstacle course that included manipulation and navigation of small items, such as a razor; toothpaste, shampoo, creams, or pill bottle caps; slippery soaps and lotions; tubes, pencils, and brushes for makeup; and buttons, zippers, ties, snaps, and Velcro for closures—not to mention remote controls and microwave buttons. You successfully met many challenges just to get ready for the day. Depending on the education, work, leisure, or other tasks scheduled in your day, you then carried out additional unique sets of coordinated hand and arm tasks. For the most part, all of these were accomplished with ease owing to the dexterity, coordination, and control of your hands and UEs.

**Upper extremity (UE)**, a term generally used to describe all the muscular, skeletal, nervous, and soft tissues of the shoulder, arm, forearm, and hand, is inadequate for describing the importance of this portion of the anatomy in the performance of **occupations** or **activities of daily living**; these actions, which people engage in throughout their life, give them meaning and include care of their body, home, and family, as well as work, education, and leisure activities. When use of the UEs is lost as a result of illness or injury, all aspects of the performance of daily tasks are significantly affected and, therefore, the level of engagement in life is impaired. The therapist providing services for clients with UE injury must conduct appropriate examination, evaluation, and intervention to adequately address the deficits. Examination, evaluation, and intervention is completed at both the body function and skill level and the occupational performance level. This chapter begins with an overview of typical characteristics of the hand and UE, clinical impairments that underlie abnormal activity/function in neurological disorders, safety considerations, and the lifespan influence on UE function. After a review of related tests and measures, the chapter presents a range of intervention activities to restore the

functional use of the UE. Cases interspersed throughout the chapter and in the online resources illustrate some of these key concepts.

## Typical Characteristics and Patterns of Movement in the Upper Extremity

An understanding of functional movement patterns is essential to the evaluation and treatment of UE dysfunction. Skilled, independent UE use begins with the ability to stabilize proximally, particularly the trunk, without UE propping. This facilitates the free use of the UEs for related functional tasks. The typical development of reach and grasp skills across childhood is described in Table 33-1.

Normally developing children in transition may use one hand to prop themselves up while manipulating or reaching for a toy with the other hand. However, individuals of any age who lack adequate postural stability in sitting or standing are hampered in their ability to use the UEs to interact with objects in the environment, especially tasks requiring bilateral UE or hand use. Studies on the biomechanics of sitting, conducted for ergonomic analysis and investigation of risk of injury, have shown that the number of joints and potential movements available in a seated position influence the amount of stability experienced (Hendriks, 2006), that there is a risk for injury when pushing and pulling tasks are done in an unstable seated posture (Lee, 2008), and that multidirectional aspects of seated stability should be measured during reaching and leaning tasks in the rehabilitation of individuals with poor sitting balance and in the design and application of seating systems (Kerr, 2002; Tanaka, 2010; Wu, 2016).

In the normal adult, the arm and hand work as one unit, but in a tremendous variety of patterns, to **reach** (i.e., to stretch or extend the arm to touch or obtain objects) and then manipulate items in the environment (see Fig. 33-1). Initially,

| TABLE 33-1 | Normal Development of Reach and Grasp Skills | | |
|---|---|---|---|
| | **REACH** | **GRASP/BIMANUAL SKILLS** | **RELEASE** |
| Infants | *5–6 Months* <br> • Supported sitting/ independent sitting <br> • Visually guided reach with accuracy <br> • Bilateral (two-handed) skills <br> • Hand-to-hand transfers <br> *9–10 Months* <br> • Prone/quadruped <br> • Forearm weight-bearing and cradling toys in hand <br> • Weight-bear one arm, reach with other | *Birth–2 Months* <br> Traction and grasp reflex when object inserted in ulnar side of hand <br> *3–5 Months* <br> Grasp reflex with object inserted in radial side of hand <br> Reach with unilateral approach <br> *6–9 Months* <br> Radial palmar grasp (6 months) <br> Radial digital grasp (8 months) <br> Crude raking grasp <br> *9–12 Months* <br> Slight wrist extension and forearm supination achieved <br> Three-jaw chuck grasp <br> Scissor or lateral pinch <br> Pincher grasp | Unintentional release <br> Intentional release against surface <br> Release with elbow extended |

| TABLE 33-1 | Normal Development of Reach and Grasp Skills—cont'd | | |
|---|---|---|---|
| | **REACH** | **GRASP/BIMANUAL SKILLS** | **RELEASE** |
| Toddlers | *18 Months–2 Years*<br>Bimanual skills with stability and mobility, one hand holds, other manipulates<br>Stabilize proximal arm/hand for controlled release (up to 18 months)<br>Controlled release (2 years) | *1–1.5 Years*<br>Palmar supinate grasp on crayons<br>*2–3 Years*<br>Digital pronate grasp | Release with elbow flexed<br>Release into larger containers<br>Release into smaller containers |
| Preschoolers | Reach with precision<br>Reach across midline<br>Reach and visually track slowly moving objects | *3½–4 Years*<br>Static tripod grasp<br>*4½–6 Years*<br>Dynamic tripod grasp<br>Grip strength improves throughout preschool years | Two-handed activities (one holds, the other manipulates)<br>Increased hand grip strength<br>Hand preference or handedness (usually established by age 4 years)<br>Fasteners: zip, snap, large buttons<br>Release continues to improve with steadiness, dexterity, precision, and speed |
| Elementary age | Improved reaching accuracy, including racket sports | In-hand manipulation skills<br>Established hand dominance<br>Dynamic tripod grasp on pencil<br>Increased strength for grip and pincher grasp<br>Precision of isolated finger movements | Precision release |

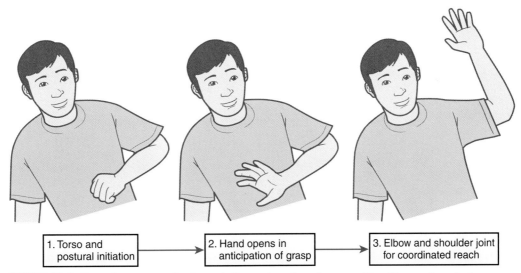

| 1. Torso and postural initiation | → | 2. Hand opens in anticipation of grasp | → | 3. Elbow and shoulder joint for coordinated reach |
|---|---|---|---|---|

**FIGURE 33-1** Flow of movement. A schematic illustration of trunk, arm, and hand interactions during an upper extremity functional task, including the trunk's role in stability and posture, the hand's preparation (opening) for grasp, and the coordinated movement of the elbow and shoulder to place the hand in the correct location.

the hand opens at the start of the reach in preparation for **grasp**, (i.e., the action of the hand and fingers to embrace and/or clasp an object). More specifically, **grip** refers to the strength of the hold on an object.

All reaching tasks begin at the torso and include postural adjustments based on the demands of the activity. The central initiation of orientation to reach is followed almost simultaneously by the extension of the hand, opening in anticipation of grasp and working as one unit with the arm to reach, grasp, and manipulate items (Oztop, 2010; Weiss, 1998). The interaction of the humerus and scapula during normal reach is well established. The humerus and scapula work together in approximately a 2:1 ratio; for every 2 degrees of movement of the humerus, the scapula moves 1 degree (Cailliet, 1980; Miyashita, 2010; Romeo, 1998). For example, when the shoulder flexes to 120 degrees, the humerus normally moves 80 degrees, and the scapula contributes 40 degrees of the overall motion. In addition, achieving 180 degrees of shoulder flexion requires recruitment of thoracic

and lumbar extensors. Without this normal ratio of movement, dysfunctional movement and compensatory strategies develop, and pain and injury may result.

## THINK ABOUT IT 33.1

Functional use of the upper extremity (UE), especially for the client with neurological dysfunction, is more complex than a reductionist view of measures of each joint's range or strength. UE assessment of use must consider performance of the patterns of movement that underlie function.

Normal hand skill components, such as grasp, in-hand manipulation, and handedness, are essential for manipulation of objects in the environment. Once mature grasps have developed, the demands of an activity determine how a person will grip the object to complete a task successfully. Grasp is an integral part of UE functioning. Table 33-2 lists types of

| TABLE 33-2 | Types of Grasps With Description/Definition |
|---|---|
| **HAND GRASP PATTERNS** | |
| Spherical grasp 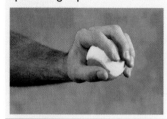 | A type of grasp in which the hand contours to a spherical shape, cupping the thenar and hypothenar eminences with varying degrees of finger flexion (e.g., holding a tennis ball) |
| Hook grasp 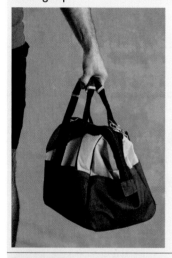 | A type of grip in which the hand assumes a hooklike appearance formed by flexed fingers without thumb involvement, usually a static nature for a period of time (e.g., gripping a suitcase handle or carrying a bucket by the handle) |
| Power grasp 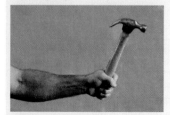 | A type of hand function that involves most digits when large forces are required (e.g., using a hammer or lifting up a chair/furniture) |

| TABLE 33-2 | Types of Grasps With Description/Definition—cont'd |
|---|---|
| **HAND GRASP PATTERNS** | |
| Cylindrical grasp 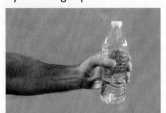 | A type of power grip in which the entire palmar surface of the hand grasps around a cylindrical-shaped object (e.g., holding a glass/cup or a handrail) |
| *Finger Grasp Patterns* | |
| Three-jaw chuck 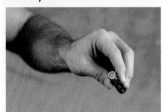 | A prehension (finger) grasp pattern formed with the thumb, index finger, and middle finger (e.g., holding a short paintbrush/pencil or picking up an egg) |
| Lateral pinch 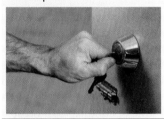 | A finger grasp in which the thumb pad opposes the middle phalanx of the index finger (e.g., holding a key to place it in a lock or zipping/unzipping pants) |
| Tip-to-tip pinch; "pincer grasp" 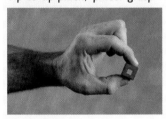 | A finger grasp with opposition between the tips of the thumb and index finger (e.g., picking up an M&M or flipping a light switch) |

grasp with definition/description, including those using the hand and fingers and those using only the fingers. The figures in Table 33-2 illustrate types of grasp in mature patterns during functional use.

The **functional position** for the wrist and hand is generally described as the wrist in slight extension, the hand in slight ulnar deviation, and the digits all slightly flexed with the thumb in opposition to the second and third digits (Coppard, 2008). The position and movement of the wrist is very important to consider during hand use, especially during performance of grasp and release activities. Wrist extension facilitates grasp as a result of activated wrist extensors creating a pull on the extrinsic flexor tendons, especially when the long flexors are shortened, causing the fingers to move into gross flexion (see Fig. 26-5). When the wrist is flexed, the fingers are released from tension and move into extension, facilitating release. In patients who are unable to voluntarily activate long finger flexors but can actively extend the wrist (i.e., spinal cord injury C6 complete), **tenodesis** allows the active wrist extension action to cause passive closure of the hand, creating some grasp force (see Chapter 26).

## Clinical Picture of Upper Extremity Activity in a Holistic Context

*Dana*, our 58 year-old musician, shares during the initial interview that she plays in an orchestra as her primary income. She also teaches saxophone to budding musicians in her home and performs onstage as a singer for secondary income.

In clinical evaluation and intervention, the UE must be viewed holistically because it is involved in the daily performance of whole-body occupations and tasks. Patient/client factors, such as the underlying physical, cognitive, and psychosocial aspects of a person, reflect a more unique view of the individual (American Occupational Therapy Association [AOTA], 2008). For Dana, the patient with a cerebrovascular accident (CVA) introduced at the beginning of this chapter, factors of concern are the severity of spastic tone and lack of voluntary control in the left UE and hand (recall her primary complaint of "*My left arm feels tight and stiff, and it is difficult to move. I can't do anything!*"). The therapist needs to assess how that affects functional use of the involved extremity. Performance skills include the ability to move around in and interact with objects in the environment (motor skills); the ability to organize, direct, and alter actions involved with completing a task (process skills); and the ability to share personal intentions and needs and interact in a social context (communication/interaction skills) (AOTA, 2008). Evaluating these performance skills allows the therapist to take a step back and look holistically at the process aspect of functional movement. Dana presented with motor skill deficits, such as a lack of controlled, isolated finger movements to play the saxophone and decreased smooth, coordinated flow of movement in the performance of her actions on stage.

## THINK ABOUT IT 33.2

Playing the saxophone is a whole-body task. The effect of upper extremity involvement is mentioned here; however, holistically, what effects would trunk and lower extremity involvement after a cerebrovascular accident have on playing the saxophone?

Interrelated with motor performance are patient factors such as visual and sensory functions. These must also be considered by the therapist for an integrated perspective of UE function. Vision is an important component for both children and adults when performing or learning UE motor skills. For children, vision is necessary for skills ranging from basic reaching to more refined movements, such as stringing beads, cutting, coloring, and completing puzzles. Vision is also an integral part of adult advanced hand manipulation skills and is unique to important tasks in work, leisure, and other daily activities. Sensory discriminatory functions of the hands also play an important role in the performance and development of fine motor skills (Kägi, 2010). At around 2½ years of age, children can identify common objects by touch alone, and 5 year-olds can recognize unfamiliar objects by touch alone (Brushnell, 1998). These skills continue to develop and become further refined throughout adolescence (Shiah, 2011; Stillwell, 1995). Deficits in sensory functions, even when motor control is unimpaired, can lead to major hand function problems (Pehoski, 2006). Additional information on the importance of sensory function may be found in Chapters 5 and 27.

## THINK ABOUT IT 33.3

Review your knowledge of sequelae of neurological insult. Is there a need to assess and potentially intervene for vision and sensory deficits for our saxophone-playing musician, Dana?

An occupation encompasses not just employment but all aspects that "occupy" a person's time and life, including activities of daily living, instrumental activities of daily living, education, work, play, leisure, and social participation (AOTA, 2008). The deficits in Dana's UE, resulting from her CVA, probably affect her ability to perform most of her occupations, from bilateral self-care tasks to work activities of performance onstage and playing and teaching the saxophone. To truly be holistic, the therapist must have an integrated perspective of UE use in all the occupations a patient engages in. An integrated perspective incorporates knowledge of underlying patient factors, aspects of performance skills, and the influence of the context of the activity as well as the performance patterns (habits, roles, and routines) of the occupations of the patient.

## Possible Impairments Underlying Abnormal Upper Extremity Tasks

The UE impairments and abnormalities discussed in this section are grouped into categories of common impairments related to the neurological disorders explored in this text. The following categories of symptoms are discussed as they relate to UE function: decreased sensation, paresis and paralysis and resulting contractures, hypertonicity including spasticity and resulting contractures, impaired motor control, hypotonicity, increased pain and complex regional pain syndrome, and decreased joint stability resulting in poor posture. Table 33-3 provides a detailed description of each impairment as it relates to abnormal movement, posturing, performance of occupations, and precautions.

Additional motor performance skills of the UE affected by neurological insult include inability to establish **hand dominance**, difficulty isolating movements, poorly coordinated movements, and unilateral UE use (i.e., nonuse of the affected side). A lack of established handedness by age 6 is considered an indicator of neuromaturational delay (Bishop, 1990). Annett (1998) conducted extensive research in this area and established handedness categories to describe handedness status: right or left handedness, unestablished handedness, mixed handedness, switched handedness, pathological handedness, and ambidexterity. Each category has unique performance components, tasks, and skills that are developmental in nature.

A patient with difficulty isolating movements usually exhibits more immature or primitive motor patterns. Extension or flexion synergies may be seen when the patient attempts to perform discrete reach, grasp, or release. More mature combination movements are often difficult or impossible, such as reaching using shoulder flexion combined with elbow extension or flexion, wrist extension combined with finger flexion, or elbow flexion combined with finger extension.

Poor coordination and control of motor actions is commonly seen in patients with neurological conditions. Patients who have increased muscle tone may have associated poor motor control, with the difficulty of overcoming the dysfunctional synergy

| TABLE 33-3 | Common Neurologic Impairment and Effects on Upper Extremity Function | | | |
| --- | --- | --- | --- | --- |
| **COMMON NEUROLOGICAL IMPAIRMENT** | **ABNORMAL MOVEMENT** | **ABNORMAL POSTURING** | **PERFORMANCE OF OCCUPATION** | **PRECAUTIONS** |
| Decreased sensation | May experience difficulty with upper extremity control as well as a decreased awareness of the environment | May occur when protective posturing is used | Decrease in safe, independent completion of occupations | Compensatory techniques are required for safe performance of tasks; education is needed on injury risks associated with decreased sensation |
| Paresis and paralysis | Decreased or absent voluntary movement and skilled control | Contractures may develop as a result of immobility, limiting full range of motion | Decreased skill and independent performance of occupations | Decreased external application of movement through the range of motion resulting in immobility and contractures |
| Hypertonicity | Spastic or rigid hypertonus can limit active movement of the antagonistic muscles; hypertonus and spasm can result in local pain | Increased severity places patient at risk for contractures, such as fisting of the hand with tight finger flexors with or without indwelling thumb | Decreased ability to independently complete basic activities of daily living, instrumental activities of daily living, work, and leisure tasks | Major concern is hygiene of the hand because skin-to-skin contact can lead to excess moisture accumulation, skin breakdown, and possible fungal infections |
| Impaired motor control/ impaired selective control | Abnormal synergies, either flexor or extensor pattern; decreased control and inability to isolate movement; difficulty alternating movements | Unintended components of abnormal synergies can result in abnormal postures | Decreased ability to complete basic movements and tasks with efficiency | Unintended movement components can cause problems, such as touching an unintended button or touching a surface that should be avoided |
| Hypotonicity of the upper extremity/ hand | Exaggerated joint range and decreased joint stability; although mobility is not impaired, may have excessive range of motion, particularly the elbows; significant hypotonicity associated with weakness and difficulty holding and maintaining grasp, especially with resistance | Often can gain stability only at the extreme end of the joint range; often presents with less definition of the thenar and hypothenar eminences | Tasks are performed with weak and slow movements | Be careful to guard joints at the end range, during weight-bearing, and during any distraction movements |
| Pain and Chronic Regional Pain Syndrome | May result in restricted range of motion, muscular atrophy | Protective posturing of the involved limb is common; resistance to use or movement may lead to contractures | Experiences limitations in performance of all occupations (avoidance), with pain being the primary limiting factor | Experiences pain, edema, and vascular instability |

*Continued*

| TABLE 33-3 | Common Neurologic Impairments and Effects on Upper Extremity Function—cont'd |
| --- | --- |

| COMMON NEUROLOGICAL IMPAIRMENT | ABNORMAL MOVEMENT | ABNORMAL POSTURING | PERFORMANCE OF OCCUPATION | PRECAUTIONS |
| --- | --- | --- | --- | --- |
| Decreased joint stability and/or muscle weakness resulting in poor posture control | Must work to hold oneself upright against gravity, limiting overall motion in reach and eliminating one hand for bilateral tasks when propping | Use of propping with upper extremities as compensatory support for poor postural stability; may seek compensatory stability by holding the head up with the hands while elbows rest on a table surface; when asked to assume a hands-and-knees position, patient with low tone in the shoulders often presents with scapular winging | Decreased stability reduces ability to maximize interaction with the environment and perform occupations effectively | Reaching tasks may cause postural instability, resulting in the need to use one hand to support balance and avoid falls |

patterns mentioned previously. Figure 33-2 illustrates some abnormal UE posturing related to hypertonia. Patients with decreased muscle tone may demonstrate poor control resulting from lack of joint stability or muscle weakness. Unilateral use of the UE results when the inability to use one UE is so compromised that it is not functional and activities are performed in one-handed adaptations. A variety of hand deformities related to contractures from neurological disorders can occur, particularly in the nonsplinted hand of individuals with abnormal movement and muscle imbalances (see Fig. 33-3).

## Safety Considerations

Safety is the number one priority for all patients and clients, regardless of the activity being implemented. It is essential to be aware of certain safety considerations (see Box 33-1 for examples) any time impairments result in abnormal functional use of the UE. For example, impaired sensation can lead to injury from either decreased awareness of pain or temperature or decreased protective response (e.g., lack of awareness of a burn when touching a hot stove); it is imperative to educate the patient about skin protection methods and frequent scanning of the environment for potential injury.

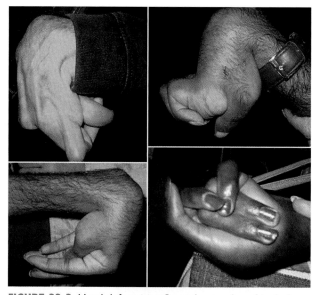

FIGURE 33-3 Hand deformities. Several examples of typical hand deformities with contracture in nonsplinted adults with cerebral palsy.

## Lifespan Influence on Upper Extremity Use

When examining possible impairment in arm and hand skills throughout the lifespan, one must recognize many systems affect development and skill performance, as discussed earlier in the chapter. Components of motor development and control, neurological organization and function, sensory function (most notably vision and touch), cognitive development and integrity, environmental factors, cultural context, and caregiving practices (Exner, 2005) affect arm and hand skill development. Truly, movement emerges through an interaction of the performer, the task, and the environment (Shumway-Cook, 2007).

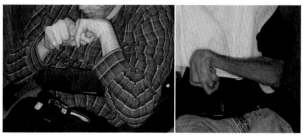

FIGURE 33-2 Upper extremity posturing, which is typical with severe hypertonicity.

---

### BOX 33-1  Safety Considerations

1. When there is impaired sensation, teach compensatory techniques, such as visual vigilance and inspection. For example, look in the silverware drawer before inserting the hand to retrieve an item. There may be a sharp knife with a blade pointing up or an object that is unexpected.
   - Look at the affected arm while moving or placing it. Avoid placing or using the affected upper extremity (UE) near or on objects/equipment with moving parts.
   - Always test water temperature with the unaffected UE before submerging the affected arm.
2. When there is poor antigravity postural control, provide stability with extra trunk supports as needed to allow greater use of both hands together.
3. When there is poor endurance, the patient needs to learn to "chunk" the activity into easier parts and do the more difficult/demanding parts first, when energy levels are higher, and the easier, less-demanding parts later, when energy levels are lower.
   - Begin by sitting more than standing during tasks and increase standing as task appropriate and as tolerated.
   - To reduce effort during standing or sitting, rest the elbows on the tabletop when it does not interfere with task performance.
   - To reduce effortful dynamic reach, minimize overhead reaching by placing items on shelves and countertops between head and hip heights.
4. When there is pain, the patient needs to identify contributing factors aggravating the pain, learn to incorporate alternative strategies to minimize the pain, and take appropriate medications before more painful tasks.
5. Involve caregivers in safety issues. Discuss with the family safety concerns due to decreased or absent sensation, poor postural control, decreased endurance, and/or pain.

---

## Neonatal and Childhood Considerations

Although aspects of typical motor development are discussed in Chapter 13, this section focuses on UE and hand skills. UE and hand skill development occurs through the interaction of many systems. Development of functional hand skills can be divided into three stages (see Table 33-4). Influencing factors have been well established and include infant size, growth, biomechanical attributes, neurological maturation, perceptual abilities, sensation, and cognition (Gordon, 1997; Manoel, 1998; Thelen, 1987, 1995). The sensory systems most influencing UE development are vision, tactile sensation, and proprioception. Postural control and primitive reflexes also influence required movements, including the ability to place hands at midline and in line with the eyes.

Attaining control of grasp and release allows the infant to hold toys for sensory exploration, to grasp food for finger feeding, and later to hold a spoon. When infants can bring both hands together, they can then learn to transfer objects from hand to hand, hold more than one object at a time, and bang objects together. Changes in object properties elicit different motor manipulations, changes in the shape of objects leads to more rotation and transferring activities, and changes in texture stimulate more fingering play and longer play duration (Pehoski, 2006).

Development of grasp and release is essential for infants to allow the opportunity for tactile experiences and to gain self-care skills. When a child has weak or no grasp, compensation in intervention is important. Placing items in their hands that are large enough for them to grasp or strapping objects to the hand(s) to promote use and maintain contact with preferred play items provides utility. Care should be taken so the infant does not bang her head with the toys by mistake. Splints or orthotics can also assist with impaired development of holding and grasping. Continued work on

active abilities for better grasp and release is necessary because these are essential skills.

Preschoolers learn to maintain a variety of grasps on toys, depending on the size and shape of the toy, and to use tools to color, paint, snip and cut; to squeeze Play-Doh; and to begin to establish hand dominance. They also learn to hold and grasp items while walking and often experiment with how many toys they can carry at a time. Substantial increases in grip and pinch strength have been shown to occur in children during the preschool years (Lee-Valkow, 2003; Yim, 2003). The ability to sustain objects in the hand is primarily related to intact somatosensory functioning (Gordon, 1997).

School-aged children learn to use the ulnar and radial side of their hand separately and establish the ability to tuck the ring and little finger against the palm and still use the thumb with the index and/or middle finger to grasp objects, such as a cracker or a pencil. The ability to use the ulnar and radial sides of the hand is developed separately, including radial or thumb side for **precision grasp** and ulnar or little finger side for **power grasp**. **Prehensile movement**, or **prehension**, involves the grasp of an object and includes both precision and power grasps. School-aged children also continue to develop strength of grip and pincher grasp. Development of these grasps allows for experimentation with in-hand manipulation skill and writing.

**In-hand manipulation** is the unilateral hand action to manipulate materials; in other words, one hand can hold and move objects within the hand in various patterns. It includes five types of grasp patterns: palm-to-finger translation, finger-to-palm translation, shift, simple rotation, and complex rotation (Exner, 2005). Control of the hand (the arches and muscles) is necessary to allow one part of the hand to hold while the other part or side manipulates. These skills can occur with only one object in the hand or with two or more objects in the hand. The term **in-hand stabilization** indicates that an object within the palm is

| TABLE 33-4 | **Stages of Functional Hand Skills** | | | |
|---|---|---|---|---|
| | **LEARNING APPROACH** | **SENSORY FOCUS** | **ARM AND WRIST MOVEMENTS** | **HAND AND GRASP ACTIONS** |
| Stage 1 | General exploration activities; vision and feedback provided by toys sustain interest | Sensory exploration of objects; focus on perceptual learning | Limited purpose of movement: wrist rotation of visible object, arm movement of toy toward and away from body (translation), rapid movement of object by bending and extending arm (vibration) | A variety of grasp patterns; objects fixed in the hands in a power grip |
| Stage 2 | Learning is best when the activity provides interest and the skills required match the infant's abilities | Focus is on perceptual learning and feedback acquired | Continued use of previous motor patterns; newer patterns develop; bilateral holding skills; holding one toy with both hands; holding one toy with each hand | Begin use of one hand to finger and explore the textures of a toy while other hand holds it; learns to transfer toys hand to hand |
| Stage 3 | Learning is focused on discovery of the "optimal" approach as the child learns which motor actions produce the best (desired) response; infants use a wide variety of grasp patterns and explore the effects of these on the properties of toys | Continued sensory exploration with integration into more mature motor organization of actions | Normal synergy movements develop into more mature movements, organization, efficiency, and ability to generalize a movement pattern into newer tasks | Development of greater isolation of index finger and thumb movements for greater variety of grasp patterns; move from a raking grasp to a more refined lateral pincher and then tip-to-tip pincher grasp; can hold a toy without pressing it against the palm; can control release into a container; manipulation skills improve |

stabilized or kept from moving. For example, if you have several coins in your hand while at a vending machine, you may stabilize some coins while using palm-to-finger translation to move one coin from the palm of the hand to the fingers to then be placed in the coin slot and released. This would then be termed *palm-to-finger translation with stabilization.*

Exner (2005) identified several prerequisite skills for in-hand manipulation that can be incorporated into functional UE intervention, including "movement into and stability in various degrees of supination, wrist stability, opposed grasp with thumb opposition and object contact with the finger surface, isolated thumb and radial finger movement, control of the transverse metacarpal arch, disassociation of the radial and ulnar sides of the hand ..." (p. 300). These skills develop between the ages of 12 months and 12 years. Two compensatory patterns, used when an individual does not have in-hand manipulation skills, include changing of hands (putting the object in the other hand for use) and transferring from hand to hand (such as turning and placing the pencil in the other hand to erase and then switching back to the original hand to write).

**Handedness,** or the consistent and more proficient use of a preferred hand (right or left) in functional and skilled tasks, is often considered an indicator of hemispheric specialization and callosal myelination (Annett, 1998). Taking advantage of this established hand dominance is essential for successful occupational performance and development of high-level manual skills (Hurlock, 1975; Mandell, 1984; Vasconcelos, 1993). A person

is identified as either right- or left-handed when she presents with an unambiguous, obvious hand preference with superior performance. In the general population, there is a higher incidence of right-handedness. Hand preference is considered a multicausal behavior affected by genetics, the environment, intrauterine and birth-related stresses, and trauma (Kraus, 2006).

Most children demonstrate a preference for one hand by the age of 4 years (McManus, 1988). The preference may begin earlier and is often initially observed with the preferred hand used most commonly for self-feeding. Preschoolers discover one hand works better for manipulating, and they use the other hand as the helper or holding hand as they engage in a growing number of bilateral hand skills. When a child does not reach across the midline of the body to the other side to get toys, then she will always use the right hand for toys on the right and use the left hand for toys on the left. Placing items at the midline of the body allows equal opportunity for either hand use. Preschoolers demonstrate hand preference for painting, coloring, and cutting as these skills are learned and practiced. By age 6 years, children cross their midline with their preferred hand consistently (Stilwell, 1987), and handedness is established, although it continues to be refined. Hand preference continues to develop until it is fully established by age 6 to 9 years. This coincides with the time the child is expected to develop manuscript writing and later cursive writing proficiency.

Bilateral hand use, the use of two hands together, has onset at 5 to 6 months; it is necessary for many daily tasks, such as fastening a button, tying shoes, and manipulating tools (e.g., styling the hair). Functional hand use is learned with a variety of tools and evolves and changes with age, culture, context, and occupations. Utensils are utilized to eat, to interact with computers, to maintain and fix vehicles and wheelchairs, and to engage in leisure and sport activities. Frequently, very specific tools or complex tools are used in tasks at work. A high degree of cognition is required to learn to use some complex tools. A person must be motivated to achieve accuracy and efficiency in complex tool manipulation.

Knowledge of normal motor development is important for facilitating recovery in children who are born with or have early onset of a neurological injury or condition in which the recovery patterns need to mirror the normal developmental sequence. When developing long- and short-term goals based on progression of skills, it is helpful to review the normal developmental sequence presented in Chapter 13. Often, children with a disability have never acquired the skills before morbidity, so they are learning skills for the first time. In contrast, adults face the challenge of relearning UE tasks they were previously skilled in. Box 33-2 summarizes key points to remember in designing interventions for UE in the pediatric patient.

### Age-Related Changes Relevant to Upper Extremity Tasks

Aging is the process of growing old, an inevitable occurrence for everyone! By definition, to become old is to show the effects or characteristics of increasing age (Merriam-Webster, 1991). The characteristics of aging that emerge are due to a wide range of physiological and anatomical changes in body systems, many of which affect UE use. To organize this information and present it consistently with other sections of this chapter, the discussion incorporates the *Occupational Therapy Practice Framework* (AOTA, 2008) areas describing the effects of changes in vision, sensation, and the vestibular and neuromusculoskeletal systems on UE and hand use.

Vision changes from aging include decrease in pupil size, thickening of the lens, decreased corneal translucence, decreased light sensitivity, contraction of the vitreous fluid, and relaxation of the eyelids (Ferrer-Blasco, 2008; Lewis, 2003; Zoltan, 2007). These changes result in **presbyopia** (also called *farsightedness*, with decreased ability to focus on near objects) as well as increased astigmatism, decreased color discrimination, decreased figure-ground and depth perception, slower response to spatial tasks, and a decrease in "low vision" (perception of frowns, smiles, gestures) (Lewis, 2003; Zoltan, 2007). Although the consequences of these changes are more far-reaching than these sensory effects alone, the effects on UE use are primarily attributable to the loss of visual feedback for movement correction, resulting in decreased accuracy of reach, decreased coordination, and decreased motor skill performance.

The number of sensory receptors decreases with age; of those remaining, a loss of integrity results in inaccurate neural transmission (Lewis, 2003; Nusbaum, 1999). These neurological changes result in decreased discriminative touch, decreased proprioception, and decreased deep pain recognition, which affect the hand's ability to interact with the environment

---

### BOX 33-2  Key Points to Remember in Pediatric Upper Extremity Intervention

- Gaining postural control and the ability to sit upright and unsupported allows for the use of both hands. When sitting balance is impaired and the patient is not supported, she will need to use one or both hands to prop up and maintain her balance, thus eliminating the possibility of bilateral hand use.
- Hand dominance is most often established in the preschool years. When a neurological injury requires a change in hand dominance, younger children are more able to make the switch than older patients because of greater plasticity of the brain.
- The failure to establish a dominant hand usually results in performance of fine motor skills below age level.
- Very small numbers of individuals are **ambidextrous**, or equally good with each hand.
- The dominant hand becomes the precision hand, and the nondominant hand becomes the helper or stabilizer for most bilateral tasks.
- Vision is essential for the performance of reach and more refined motor prehension grips, especially the use of a pincher grasp. Impaired or absent vision often results in a raking grasp, which increases the likelihood of picking up the desired item in the palm of the hand rather than with the fingers.
- Visual impairment is often compensated for by very refined tactile discrimination through the hands, which informs the individual about her world.
- Sometimes it is very difficult for the patient to obtain both speed and precision. Often, these need to be addressed separately in interventions.
- The thumb used in opposition with other fingers is the key contributor to fine motor precision dexterity (see Fig. 33-4AB for a 3-jaw chuck grasp intervention activity).
- The thumb side of the hand is the precision side. The little finger side of the hand is the power side. Often, the little finger and ring finger are tucked into the palm, out of the way, while the precision fingers work.

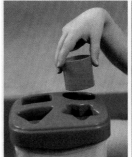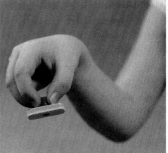

**FIGURE 33-4** "3-Jaw chuck" grasp. A therapeutic activity involving a child grasping a small object with the 3-jaw chuck grasp.

through sensation. For example, the inability to recognize the contents of one's pockets by feel or difficulty manipulating caps, pills, and other small items is due to inaccurate or absent sensory information or impaired perception of these sensations. However, the neurological changes may also increase sensitivity or decrease the threshold for pain so pain is more readily felt. Neurological changes also alter the perception of temperature. These changes often affect willingness to risk pain or the ability to handle hot items, resulting in decreased use of or injury to the UE or hand (refer to the section on safety concerns). The threshold also drops for the perception of movement; thus, reach accuracy is reduced.

The neuromusculoskeletal system exhibits characteristic aging patterns as well. In the muscular system, there is a reduction in the number and diameter of muscle fibers, an increase in fat content, a decrease in the stability of neuromuscular innervation, and an increase in time to peak tension and relaxation (Edström, 2007; Lewis, 2003). These changes cause a decline in strength, decrease in muscle mass, deconditioning, and slowed motor behavior and reaction time. Increased aging is associated with increased time to complete fine motor tasks as well as decreased hand and finger dexterity (Sebastjan, 2017). The increased time to complete fine motor tasks in older adults may be related to the resistance to reduce accuracy for speed, as commonly seen

in younger adults (Lamb, 2016). Deficits in hand function may occur as a result of deconditioning after illness or decreased physical activity rather than simply aging. It has been shown that muscles of older adults can increase in size and strength with resistance training (Forbes, 2012; Geirsdottir, 2012). UE use in skilled, coordinated actions, endurance, and power usage is directly affected by these varied neuromusculoskeletal changes.

Enlarged joints in the UE, resulting from degenerative arthritis or injury, affect physical skills such as fine motor tasks as well as self-esteem and body image. Increased risk and incidence of fractures from age-related osteoporosis have their own set of multiple effects, but just the possibility of increased risk can cause anxiety, overcautiousness, and decreased physical activity. The therapist must integrate these issues into a holistic care plan for each patient.

## Pertinent Examination/Evaluation

Examining hand and UE function in an individual is an information gathering process that helps determine areas of functional deficits and provides a foundation for developing customized treatment. Tests/measures are selected on the basis of population, purpose, and specific areas to be addressed. Table 33-5 provides information on a select group

| TABLE 33-5 | Examination Tools for Hand and Upper Extremity Function | | |
|---|---|---|---|
| EXAMINATION TOOL | POPULATION | PURPOSE | DESCRIPTION |
| Box and Block Test | Age: 6–75+ years | Evaluates gross manual dexterity | Patient is given 1 minute to move blocks from one side of the box to the other, starting with the dominant hand followed by the nondominant hand. A 15-second trial is allowed. The total number of blocks placed correctly is counted (Desrosiers, 1994). |
| Bruinicks-Oseretsky Test of Motor Proficiency (BOT-2) | Age: 4–21 years Short form for screening, long form for evaluation | To evaluate motor proficiency for gross and fine motor skills | Test contains eight subtests: fine motor precision, fine motor integration, manual dexterity, bilateral coordination, balance, running speed and agility, upper limb coordination, and strength. Scores are interpreted as age equivalents, scaled scores, percentiles, Z scores, and descriptive categories. |
| Crawford Small Parts Dexterity Test | Adolescents and adults | Evaluates eye-hand coordination and manual dexterity | The test contains two parts: (1) use tweezers to insert pins into holes and put collars over them and (2) screw small screws into a metal plate with a screwdriver (Asher, 2007). |
| Disabilities of the Arm, Shoulder and Hand (DASH) Questionnaire | Adults | Assesses musculoskeletal disorders of the upper limbs | The DASH is a 30-item self-report questionnaire that can be used to assess any joint in the upper limbs. There are optional modules to assess workers and people involved in athletics or the performing arts (Institute for Work and Health, 2011). |
| Fugl-Meyer | Adults after a cerebrovascular accident (CVA) | Designed to measure progress and recovery after a CVA | This is a 226-item sensorimotor assessment using three-point scoring in the areas of motor function, sensory function, balance, joint range of motion, and joint pain (Asher, 2007). |

| TABLE 33-5 | Examination Tools for Hand and Upper Extremity Function—cont'd | | |
|---|---|---|---|
| **EXAMINATION TOOL** | **POPULATION** | **PURPOSE** | **DESCRIPTION** |
| Jebsen-Taylor Hand Function Test | Age: 5–94 years | Evaluates hand use in everyday activities | Standardized instructions are given. The test contains seven timed manual tasks that simulate hand function, beginning with the nondominant hand (Asher, 2007). |
| Miller Fun | Age: 2 years 6 months to 7 years; children with mild to severe motor delays | Determines how motor competency effects performance, engagement, and participation | Test involves performance tasks and observation-based checklists for home and classroom and uses games to assess gross and fine motor skills. Scores are interpreted as scaled scores, percentiles, and age equivalents for visual motor, fine motor, and gross motor skills. Neurological foundation profile can be obtained. |
| Minnesota Rate of Manipulation Test (also known as the Minnesota Manual Dexterity Test) | Age: 13+ years | Evaluates gross motor dexterity | The test contains five subtests: placing, turning, displacing, one-handed turning and pacing, and two-handed turning and placing. |
| National Institutes of Health Stroke Scale | Adults after a CVA | Measures the severity of symptoms associated with cerebral infarcts; used as a quantitative measure of neurological deficit after a stroke | This 15-item impairment scale assesses level of consciousness, extraocular movements, visual fields, facial muscle function, extremity strength, sensory function, coordination (ataxia), language (aphasia), speech (dysarthria), and hemi-inattention (neglect). The scale was designed for use in clinical trials; however, it is increasingly used in clinical settings as both an initial assessment tool and for discharge planning (Kasner, 2006). |
| Nine-Hole Peg Test | Age: 4–94 years | Evaluates unilateral finger dexterity | Standardized instructions (Mathiowetz, 1985) are read. Test is timed to see how fast the patient can put the pegs into the board and remove them. |
| Peabody Development Motor Scales-2 | Birth to age 6 years; includes children with motor, speech, and hearing disorders | Evaluates gross and fine motor skills; can measure progress over time | This is a criterion-referenced task performance–based rating scale. Scores can be converted to percentiles, age-equivalent, and Z scores. Many familiar tasks such as ball play, coloring, cutting, and buttoning are included. Subtests assess reflexes, sustained control, locomotion, object manipulation, grasping, and visual-motor integration. |
| Purdue Peg Board Test | Adults | Evaluates fingertip dexterity and gross motor function of the finger, hand, and arm | Patient places pins, pins with collars, and washers onto a pegboard. A 30-second or 60-second time frame is given (Asher, 2007). |
| Stroke Impact Scale (SIS) | Adults after mild to moderate stroke | Measures changes in emotion, communication, memory, and thinking, as well as social role | Scale was developed from the perspectives of patients and caregivers rather than investigators. The SIS is a work in progress, and the number of items varies by version. A short composite physical domain score has also been developed from version 3.0 (Kasner, 2006). |
| Wolf Upper Extremity Motor Function Test | Adults after a CVA | A research tool to assess upper extremity motor function | Test is a 17-item, 6-point, function- and strength-based assessment of performance time (speed) and functional ability (movement quality) (Lin, 2009). |

of assessment tools that specifically address UE reach, grasp, pinch, sensation, overall UE function, and occupational performance. See Chapter 10 for more detailed explanations of some tests/measures for UE functional abilities.

In addition, the therapist should test underlying body system functions for impairments (including range of motion, joint mobility, muscle performance, motor control, tactile and proprioceptive sensations, postural control, and reflexes) that may limit UE functional activity.

## PATIENT APPLICATION

*Dana is the 58 year-old white female saxophone player/instructor and singer presented at the beginning of this chapter. She experienced a right hemisphere thrombolytic CVA while in surgery for a cardiac arterial shunt placement. Her medical history includes high blood pressure, coronary artery disease, and mild osteoarthritis affecting primarily her hands, knees, and hips. On initial evaluation at the outpatient rehabilitation center, she exhibited flexion synergy of the left UE. She had isolated forearm pronation and supination with the left elbow in 90 degrees of flexion and the upper arm positioned at the side of her trunk. She had extension synergy of the left lower extremity with isolated left knee flexion to 10 degrees while sitting on a plinth. She walked with a small-based quad cane, exhibiting decreased left stance time, decreased right step length and time with left circumduction, and stereotypical UE synergy as described previously. She had good static and dynamic sitting balance but exhibited poor posture and complained of decreased breath control, especially during singing exercises.*

*Collaborative goal setting for the UE included the therapist, patient, and spouse. Therapist readiness goals included an increase in coordinated movement and release from synergistic patterns of movement, adherence to a home exercise program, and increased independence in activities of daily living. Patient goals included walking from the stage wings to a chair stage-right without a cane, improved dynamic sitting balance and posture during singing, improved breath control during singing, and independent movement and coordination of the left hand digits to play the saxophone. Caregiver goals included increased independence in dressing, transfers, and walking and motivation for self-improvement.*

### Contemplate Clinical Decisions

1. *To better understand the effects of the CVA on Dana, review the hemisphere damage and describe the expected deficits.*
2. *On the basis of information obtained from the review of question #1, develop an upper extremity problem list of functional limitations in activities of daily living, instrumental activities of daily living, and work performance.*
3. *List the underlying impairments contributing to the functional limitations you identified.*
4. *Prioritize the functional problems in the order in which you would focus on them.*
5. *Write at least two appropriate goals expressing patient-centered, occupation based, realistic UE functional outcomes for this patient. Include all components of a goal.*

## ■ Functional Interventions for Upper Extremity Tasks

### General Approaches

Intervention approaches for patients with neurological impairments have changed significantly with the explosion of technology and greater understanding of how the brain works. Treatment approaches include biomechanical, motor learning and motor control, neurodevelopmental treatment, and constraint-induced (CI) movement therapy. An in-depth discussion of the theories and general treatment approaches can be found in Chapters 14 and 15. Intervention should focus on improvement in functional tasks, minimization of functional and activity limitations, optimization of health status, and prevention of disability in daily life. Compensatory techniques may be necessary in the case of permanent deficits, for either a short-term or a long-term problem, to allow active participation in desired tasks; however, it may interfere with practicing more normal aspects of the task.

Hand skills are essential to functional performance and are needed daily. The examples described in the following section are a sampling of therapeutic activities within different intervention approaches. Techniques for *positioning and postural control, transport, reaching, hand treatment, grasp, release, splinting/orthotics, constraint-induced therapy CIT), and occupational engagement* are discussed.

### Address Underlying Impairments

To optimally improve UE function and skills, it is essential that therapy focus initially on treatment of the underlying impairments detected on the neurological examination, with a quick transition toward gradually increasing the focus to functional activity with repetitions of task-specific practice, including appropriate feedback. The therapist should focus on UE impairments hypothesized to contribute to the UE functional problem specific for the patient.

For example, muscle tone can influence completion of UE functional tasks. Although flaccid muscle tone, sometimes seen in acute stroke, may not directly affect movement, it is often associated with complete paralysis of an affected limb that results in inability to move the arm. Chapter 18 discusses interventions and management strategies to address decreased and absent muscle tone as a foundation for improving function. Spastic muscle tone may interfere with voluntary movement. Although they make no long-term correction in spasticity, some of the therapeutic techniques discussed in Chapter 19 may provide a window of opportunity during which the patient can practice arm and hand movements with decreased influence of spasticity on the movements. In the context of more permanent spasticity with little chance of resolution from plasticity, the related medical and surgical interventions discussed in Chapter 19 can have a longer-term effect on minimizing spasticity and improving function, as discussed in that chapter.

When a lack of isolated or selective motor control occurs after a stroke, for example, the arm may be able to move but without precision, and the patient just cannot make the arm do exactly what she wants it to do. An intervention plan to increase selective motor control (see Chapter 25) during rehabilitation from stroke, brain injury, cerebral palsy, and multiple sclerosis, to name a few, can serve as the basis for increased precision and intentional placement during functional tasks of the arm and hand. Although weakness can prevent functional movement through the full range or against gravity in the context of disorders such as stroke, Guillain Barré syndrome, and polio, a plan of care designed to strengthen weakened muscles (Chapter 22) can improve the ability to carry out functional skills and prepare the patient for more repetitions of functional practice and endurance in functional tasks. Intervention for range-of-motion deficits (see Chapter 23), often a secondary complication after impairment of movement from neurological disorders, can dramatically improve the ability to move in functional tasks. To restate the general principle of this section another way, once an underlying impairment shows improvement, the focus must shift toward using that improved body system function in the meaningful practice of everyday tasks.

## Positioning and Postural Control

Positioning and postural control can create opportunities for and facilitation of reach and grasp in a variety of planes. Planes of movement are natural components that can be manipulated for intentional progression of the therapeutic activity from easy to more difficult (Fell, 2004). In addition, positioning is a daily consideration for those with limited mobility, with the effects of positioning considered from neuromuscular, biomechanical, cognitive, environmental interaction, and social participation standpoints. For example, a 6 year-old child with spastic quadriplegic cerebral palsy needs positioning that facilitates or supports postural control and allows the child to sit upright as much as possible during the school day to observe and participate in school tasks. However, the child may utilize a switch, controlled with the head, the elbow, the knee, the toe, the eyes, or the tongue, to complete some academic work.

Individuals with cerebral palsy, traumatic brain injuries, stroke, or near-drowning accidents, who have poor postural control because of the abnormal influence of primitive reflex patterns such as symmetrical and asymmetrical tonic neck reflexes and tonic labyrinthine reflex, may benefit from therapeutic techniques to address posture/position. Postural control and movement patterns of the head can greatly influence the tone and motor patterns of the arms, especially when primitive reflexes persist or recur after neurological injury. Primitive reflexes and delayed postural reflexes interfere with UE use during occupational activities. In addition, many individuals with central nervous system damage exhibit abnormal muscle tone and in some cases musculoskeletal abnormalities that further contribute to deficits in postural control. Poor stability and/or muscle weakness often contributes to fixing or biomechanically locking body segments, resulting in limited patterns of movement. Box 33-3 provides examples of therapeutic techniques you can implement for positioning and postural control.

---

### BOX 33-3  Examples of Interventions for Positioning and Postural Control to Enhance Upper Extremity Function

1. Adapt the immediate environment to increase stimulation and use of the affected upper extremity (UE) in the following ways:
   - Communicate with the patient while she is standing or sitting on the affected side, offering items to reach for or grasp with the affected extremity.
   - Position the television so the patient has to turn onto the affected side, increasing proprioceptive input to the affected joints (in addition, turning the head toward the affected side may enhance attention to the affected side).
   - Encourage family members or friends to hold and stroke the patient's affected hand while communicating to increase sensory input.
   - Can you think of other adaptations to the environment that would increase awareness and use of the affected side?
2. Alter the plane of movement through positioning to increase independent use of the UE in the following ways:
   - Forward reach (shoulder flexion) in sitting occurs against gravity. When only gravity-eliminated movement is possible, facilitate independent range of motion by having the patient in sidelying on the unaffected side and positioning a bedside table or other support at the level of the shoulder to facilitate gravity-eliminated movement. Powder on the support surface or arm skates may reduce friction and enhance movement to allow early practice of motor control.
   - A patient with spastic quadriplegic cerebral palsy may have the ability to perform some arm motions in a gravity-decreased plane. Evaluate active motor control and its relation to strength and look at the possibilities for positioning in supine, prone, sidelying, and supported sitting and supported standing. Each position changes the demands of the head, arms, and hands for active control. Supporting the patient in sitting and placing a lap tray on the wheelchair allows horizontal abduction and adduction movements (e.g., to pet a puppy or finger paint; slippery paint reduces friction, which also facilitates freedom of movement).
   - What other gravity-reduced positions can you imagine for this individual to facilitate functional independent UE use?

*Continued*

---

**BOX 33-3 Examples of Interventions for Positioning and Postural Control to Enhance Upper Extremity Function—cont'd**

3. Examples using Robin (see Patient Application at the end of the chapter)

3a. To reduce fixing into neck hyperextension and facilitate postural control and positioning for UE use

- To work on head control sit in long-sitting with your legs additionally flexed at the hip and knees and the child reclining on your legs. Robin is seated in your lap, facing you, and is propped on the your thighs with his head toward your knees. This allows you to control the degree of patient recline by changing the angle of knee flexion.
- Continue to work on head control, this time on neck flexors, by encouraging Robin to hold his head in a slightly chin-tucked position while you hold his hands and gently lower his back toward your legs. This could be an activity later shown to the parents as part of a home program and play ideas.
- Once Robin is upright, encourage him to hold his head there while using his eyes to visually track a slowly moving toy or soap bubbles. Placing your hand on the child's head and providing some joint compression through the spine may assist with tone enhancement and head alignment.

3b. Moving on to upright sitting and grasping and reaching techniques

- Play a game with some intermittent compression and traction to the UE by holding the child's hands and doing some gentle pulling and releasing, encouraging him to hold with his fingers and pull with his arms.
- Place the child in the familiar ring sitting posture, placing your hand on his lower back to facilitate the lumbar spine from the rounded and flexed alignment to the more upright position. Keep moving your hand so he will not "sink" into it and depend on it, but instead, will need to continue to respond to the changing sensory input of your moving hand. Also, assist him in pulling his shoulders back and spreading his chest. Encourage reach within his range of control, offering toys to grasp and reach. Allow success, but continually increase the challenge.
- Once upright sitting is acquired with your supports, provide intermittent joint compression from the shoulders and head down through the spine. Encourage increased upper extremity range of motion through task-specific training during reach and play activities.

---

## Therapeutic Functional Activities

In addition to addressing known underlying impairments and applying general principles as an initial foundation for improving UE functional skills, designing opportunities for multiple repetitions of functional practice for the skill that needs to be improved is a key aspect of intervention. Functional practice should be task specific but should incorporate variety in the task and environment and allow rich feedback (see Chapter 14). Also, many general approaches to therapeutic intervention are applicable to UE functional intervention (see Chapter 15). A variety of specific functional intervention activities, including functional reaching, functional hand skills such as grasp, and electromechanical, robotic and orthotic applications to enhance these functional skills, are described in this section.

### Functional Reaching Skills

In populations with neuromuscular disorders, UE reaching skills are most commonly affected by a deficit in range of motion, strength, and/or motor control. Limitations in strength may indicate a need for functional movement in altered planes (as discussed in the previous section) while beginning strengthening activities. Limitations in range and motor control should be evaluated to determine the nature of the problem. Determination of the severity of the limitation as well as its acute-versus-chronic nature will assist with treatment decisions related to ameliorating the underlying deficit, working on alternative methods, using task-specific training, or incorporating compensatory modifications in the environment.

Box 33-4 provides examples of functional UE intervention activities to improve reaching ability, with a focus on task-specific activities.

### Functional Hand Skills

During normal motor development, infants weight-bear and weight shift on their hands during multiple transitional movements, including pushing up on extended arms and crawling. These actions develop the hand arches and prepare the muscles for elongation and movement (Boehme, 1988). Individuals who do not experience this normal motor development do not receive the needed stimulation and muscle preparation.

To improve hand skills of patients across the lifespan, you must first determine the impairments limiting the ability to grasp. Proper positioning of trunk and proximal girdles, as discussed previously, is the first step in facilitating optimal use of the UEs. The hands should then be positioned in line with the eyes to allow visual feedback and to facilitate eye-hand coordination. When underlying abnormal tone is interfering with hand function, it should be addressed as a preparatory intervention, before functional activities; specific techniques may be used to either promote opening of the tight hand or grasping and holding of the low-tone hand (see Chapter 18 for preparatory interventions for hypotonicity and Chapter 19 for preparatory interventions for spasticity). Grasp develops and becomes more refined, from a large whole hand grasp to smaller and smaller items to more thumb/finger grasps, such as the three-jaw chuck and lateral pinch.

**BOX 33-4  Examples of Interventions for Reaching Activities**

Examples of reaching activities:

1. **Increase the functional reach of patients with decreased strength (or endurance).**
   - Patients who have decreased reach due to reduced strength from conditions such as polio, Charcot-Marie-Tooth disease, or deconditioning may benefit from functional upper extremity (UE) practice with assistance or guidance initially. The patient's nondominant arm can help generate an active-assisted reach movement. When reaching into a cabinet to retrieve a can of food, the patient can provide support and additional lift by using the nondominant hand to grasp the dominant arm proximal to the elbow and adding either stability or "push" for the movement.

2. **Increase the functional reach of patients with nonreducible limitations.**
   - Patients who have decreased reach due to permanent impairments such as joint limitations, chronic vertigo, or hip precautions may require compensatory equipment, including reachers, sock aids, or long-handled equipment such as hairbrushes, or they may employ alternative strategies.

3. **Increase the functional reach of patients with motor control deficits.**
   - Patients may have motor control issues related to a variety of conditions, each of which must be evaluated to understand their unique presentation and needs. The effect of Parkinsonian tremors may be reduced by use of wrist weights during functional reach activities, such as bringing food from the plate to one's mouth for eating. Reaching tasks that are imprecise because of lack of isolated control (abnormal synergies) may be improved through successive shaping tasks discussed with constraint-induced movement therapy (see Chapters 15 and 25) or through manual guidance of the movement in which assistance is gradually withdrawn as the patient recovers control from plasticity.

4. **Increase the functional use of UE movement in dynamic patterns.**
   - Dynamic movement patterns with varied reach, speed, balance, and coordination demands are often difficult to simulate in a treatment environment. The use of virtual reality, such as a Wii system, provides a viable option for more dynamic movement patterns and has been shown to promote motor recovery after a stroke (Saposnik, 2010).

5. **Functional intervention examples using Robin (see Patient Application at the end of the chapter)**

5a. **Add reaching to a therapeutic activity to facilitate positioning and postural control.**
   - Placement of a toy (or reach object for the adult) is a key element in providing a "just right" challenging and dynamic reaching activity and for intentionally progressing the activity. Begin by having Robin reach for a toy just in front of his body because it is less challenging. Progress to having him reach out away from the body (more demanding) and then reaching across the body/across midline. Crossing the midline is much more demanding than reaching on the same side. Reaching up is also more demanding as it requires more spine extension and strength from the arm for antigravity reaching.

5b. **Choose a toy the child really wants to play with to increase motivation for reaching.**
   Robin can be positioned in sitting with one arm on the floor for support/weight-bearing while reaching with the other arm. You can help by continually monitoring postural control and providing intermittent assistance to facilitate stability while enhancing mobility and the skill. As Robin reaches forward for the toy, keep your hands close to his lumbar spine and the elbow of his support arm to provide sensory cues or guarding as needed. His parents may be instructed in placement of a Boppy® pillow behind him as support and in providing hands-on assist (e.g., holding one arm in a support position while providing assist at the shoulder of the reaching arm).

When loss of motor innervation occurs, an evaluation must be conducted to determine the potential for development and use of an extension-facilitated grasp. Box 33-5 presents examples of functional activities that can be used to improve functional hand use.

### Additional Techniques and Supports to Promote Function

The frequent poor outcomes and ongoing challenge of facilitating functional use of the neurologically impaired UE has led to the development of a variety of intervention techniques and supports. Electromechanical or robot-assisted devices can be used in the training of the UE and may involve passive range of motion of the upper limb as well as active assistive range during an activity. A Cochrane Database review of 19 studies found inconsistencies, suggesting caution in the interpretation that patients who received electromechanical or robot-assisted intervention were more likely to improve generic activities of daily living than patients who received traditional treatment (Mehrholz, 2012).

Mirror therapy is a technique the reader may be more familiar with as therapy for patients with an amputation; however, it has also been successful in patients after a neurological insult. Mirror therapy involves placement of a mirror midsagittally, between the patient's arms or legs so movement of the nonaffected limb provides the illusion of movement in the affected limb. A Cochrane Database review of 14 studies found that mirror therapy effectively improved UE motor function, increased performance of activities of daily living, and reduced pain in those with complex regional pain syndrome (Thieme, 2012). A Cochrane Database review on the effect of transcranial direct current stimulation (tDCS) on stroke patients'

### BOX 33-5 Examples of Activities for Interventions for Functional Use of the Hand

1. **Spinal cord injury at the C5–C7 level resulting in loss of gross grasp**
   - With a C5–C7 lesion, a patient may be evaluated for development of an extension-facilitated grasp (i.e., tenodesis). Discuss the patient's preference, and evaluate strength and muscle availability for a natural wrist extension–facilitated grasp or the need for a splint, biofeedback, or electric stimulation to facilitate the wrist extension (Thorsen, 2006).
   - Facilitate enhancement of grasp through wrist extension by having patients work on a surface that is more vertical than horizontal. For example, writing, drawing, or coloring on a chalkboard or angled tabletop promotes wrist extension more than the same activities done on a flat/horizontal surface.
   - Patients who have sustained a spinal cord injury with resulting loss of voluntary finger flexion and inability to perform grasp and release may benefit from intentional shortening of the finger flexors to take advantage of the passive finger flexion that results from active wrist extension (i.e., tenodesis).
   - Numerous adaptive cuffs are available for compensatory adaptations, such as allowing an item to be inserted into the pocket of a cuff wrapped around the hand at the metacarpal level. For example, a toothbrush may be inserted into the cuff, allowing the user to brush the teeth without the need to grasp the handle of the toothbrush.

2. **Hypotonic hands that are overexpanded and flattened, not shaped with a thenar and hypothenar eminence**
   - With the wrist in neutral, apply pressure to the patient's mid-palm with the fingers to facilitate palmar arches, and then add slight traction on the palmar skin to activate a gross grasp pattern. Provide stimulation of arches and muscles by molding the patient's hand to shape itself around a variety of objects as the first step toward developing a firm grip.
   - Roll objects from distal to proximal along the palm of the hypotonic hand to facilitate grasp. Shape the patient's fingers around a ball of yarn in a gross grasp pattern, and then play a game of tug-of-war, with gentle tugging on the yarn to increase palmar arches and holding.
   - Help the patient compensate for decreased grasp of soft objects while developing grasp by attaching a Velcro® strap to an object (or toy) and wrapping it around the hand.

3. **Treatment for the hand with spastic hypertonia**
   - In preparation for functional activities, use of a natural extension–facilitated grasp may be required to promote opening of the hand. Move the wrist into flexion to allow your fingers into the patient's palm, and then slowly work on moving the digits into extension. Do not pull forcefully on the tight thumb; rather, open the hand by expanding the thumb outward from the palm (abduction and extension), and the thumb will usually come along to a more open position. Weight-bearing may help reduce tone. (Additional techniques for addressing spastic tone can be found in Chapter 19.) A patient with one-side involvement can be taught this technique by using the unaffected hand to open her involved hand for tasks such as cleaning the hand and placing objects into the hand.
   - Have patients look at their own fingers while actively closing/opening them with control as you provide feedback on the performance.
   - Carefully monitor the position of the patient's arm during object placement and consider the demands placed on both reaching and the releasing tasks.
   - Incorporate task-specific training into activities.
   - For children, use a variety of knobbed puzzles, larger checkers, firm plastic cups, character toys, animals, and other items.
   - Developing release in the hypertonic hand is done initially with stabilization. For the patient with difficulty releasing, begin by stabilizing the object before attempting release. Later, release may be accomplished without stabilization. Thus, to improve release in the context of hypertonicity and finger flexion, the therapist needs to consider positioning, tone inhibition techniques, and placement of the object with stabilization.
   - For a child, stabilization may occur by placing a toy in the mouth, transferring it to the other hand, or placing it on a firm surface.

4. **Examples using Robin (see Patient Application at the end of the chapter). Adding grasp to the treatment activity**
   - In later stages, consider working more distally and utilize the techniques described previously to specifically improve hand grasp on the toys. Consider having Robin roll a toy from the distal finger tips to the palm. Then tap into the hand to promote the child's ability to hold an item in the fingers while you gently try to pull it away (as when playing a gentle game of tug-of-war) to build tone in the hand and shape the palmer arches to maintain grasp on the desired toy.

---

ADLs and their physical and cognitive function found low to moderate quality evidence on the effectiveness as compared to sham treatment (Elsner, 2016). The same review found 55 studies on the use of tDCS with stroke patients in progress, suggesting the quality of evidence may change as these are completed. While recent studies show UE and hand improvements after tDCS and intervention in patients post stroke, further research is needed (Ozkeskin, 2016; Tosun, 2017; Wang, 2017).

Although splinting with orthotics may be indicated to promote positions of rest and healing for the hand, some individuals may benefit from wrist and hand splinting to improve UE function (see Table 33-6 for examples of splinting to promote

| TABLE 33-6 | Examples of Splints/Orthoses to Increase Function | | |
|---|---|---|---|

| SPLINT/ ORTHOSIS | PHOTO | APPLICATION LEVEL | PURPOSE |
|---|---|---|---|
| Wrist support with palmar clip or pocket | | Wrist | Compensates for lack of grasp, supports the wrist in neutral or slight extension, provides a clip or pocket in the palm to insert tools |
| Pressure splints | | Elbow (mid-upper arm across elbow to mid-forearm) | To counter abnormal high tone, inhibit spasticity, reduce edema; provides sensory input and assists with reach/extension patterns and weight-bearing tasks |
| Mallet finger splint | | Distal digits | Supports distal interphalangeal joint in extension, allows movement of proximal interphalangeal joints |
| Swan-neck ring splint | | PIP of digits | Corrects Swan-neck deformity of the PIP joint and prevents hyperextension of PIP but allows flexion; can be used for joint stability on PIP or DIP joints |
| Thumb spica splint positioning CMC for digit opposition | | Carpal metacarpal thumb joint (may include wrist) | To provide support and positioning of the thumb in a resting or functional position including digit opposition; when in functional position, allows pincher and 3-jaw chuck finger grasp against stabilized thumb |
| Thumb spica splint for abduction | | Thumb abduction including IP joint | Facilitates thumb abduction, including the IP joint in preparation for grasp |
| Neoprene strap splint | | Thumb, wrist, and/or forearm may be included | Intended to improve thumb abduction and extension for grasp in patients with a neurological impairment through facilitation of opposition; neoprene provides compression and sensory input while allowing movement |
| SaeboFlex® | (See Fig. 23-4) | Hand and wrist (elbow) | For patients with high flexor tone; dynamic traction brings digits and wrist into extension, but allows flexion, facilitating grasp; can be used with SaeboReach® for dynamic elbow extension to increase reach |

*Continued*

| TABLE 33-6 | Examples of Splints/Orthoses to Increase Function—cont'd | | |
|---|---|---|---|
| SPLINT/ ORTHOSIS | PHOTO | APPLICATION LEVEL | PURPOSE |
| Bioness H200 | (See Fig. 24-6) | Hand, wrist, and forearm | For patients with low tone or poor wrist and digit strength; provides electrical stimulation to wrist and finger muscles to facilitate reaching, grasping, and opening and closing the hand as well as wrist extension and flexion |
| Antispasticity ball splint | | Hand, wrist, and forearm | For patients with high tone; provides inhibitory positioning of the thumb and digits to reduce tone in preparation for functional use; splint displayed has adjustable wrist angle and forearm-to-hand piece distance to accommodate patients with significant postural deformities |

CMC = carpometacarpal joint; IP = interphalangeal joint (of the thumb); PIP = proximal interphalangeal joint; DIP = distal interphalangeal joint.

functional use of the hand). A wide variety of static and dynamic orthoses is available, as well as orthoses with mechanical or electrical components. The selection, fabrication, and use of orthoses is an important consideration in therapeutic intervention. Detailed information about fabricating and applying orthoses is available in more specialized textbooks. Consider referral to a specialized professional in the local area to assist in this process.

### Constraint-Induced Therapy in Functional Skills

Morris (2006) described **constraint-induced (CI) therapy,** also sometimes called **constraint-induced movement therapy (CIMT),** as a "therapeutic package" (Box 33-6). The current protocol for CIT, most often for UE rehabilitation, requires retention of some hand and wrist movements and consists of the following elements: constraining the affected UE; repetitive, task-oriented training (of actual, meaningful functional skills); and a transfer package including daily administration of a motor activity log, a home diary, problem-solving to utilize the affected UE, a behavioral contract, a caregiver contract, a home skill assignment, home practice, and a daily schedule (Morris, 2006). The components of the "transfer package" are listed in the following sections, with a description of each along with strategies to increase UE use. Additional training beyond the entry level is required to learn and apply the full protocol.

A Cochrane Database review of 19 studies concluded that patients treated with CI therapy improved the ability to manage activities of daily living relative to those treated without CI therapy; however, no evidence of lasting benefits is available (Sirtori, 2009). A modified child-friendly CIMT that incorporated restraint of the unaffected hand and repetitive play-based practice

(cards, board games, arts, crafts, puzzles) in children with hemiplegic cerebral palsy showed positive changes in unimanual hand performance, bimanual hand performance, and functional outcomes (Gordon, 2005). Use of CI therapy in a pediatric practice-based setting resulted in statistically significant improvement in 88 children age 18 months to 12 years (DeLuca, 2016). A randomized trial combining CI therapy and peripheral nerve stimulation on 19 adults found statistically significant improvements in UE motor function as compared to treatment using CI therapy alone, immediately after treatment and at one month follow up (Carrico, 2016).

### Functional Use of the Upper Extremity in Daily Activities

Encourage the patient to use the affected UE as much as possible while engaging in all activities of daily life, consistent with the CI therapy approach to intervention and motor learning principles in general. The affected UE can be used during functional tasks for weight-bearing (see Fig. 18-8), bilateral use of the extremities, and hand-over-hand activities (Fig. 33-5). Specifically, ask the patient which daily living tasks are important to them and what related UE skills they want to improve. Box 33-7 contains some examples of treatment ideas for UE function.

## Pediatric Considerations for Intervention

To motivate a child to work consistently with her hands, we need to carefully select toys she wants to play with. This often means using multisensory toys that provide feedback such as music, lights, vibration, or pictures that move when touched.

## BOX 33-6 Components of Transfer Package Use in Constraint-Induced Therapy

1. The **constraint mitt** is a covering for the hand that is similar to a glove but has a single compartment for all the fingers. For this therapeutic application, the mitt is placed to restrict the patient from using the nonaffected limb (i.e., it is placed on the unaffected hand as a reminder to use the more affected hand during functional skills and activities). An arm sling was originally used as the constraint device, but it created a safety hazard in that the functional arm was impaired by the sling from participating in balance reactions and protective extension. The mitt can be used in various protocols to constrain the more functional arm and increase functional use of the affected upper extremity (UE), using schedules that range from 5 hours per day to 90% of waking hours. Compliance with constraint of the less-affected extremity is extremely important—even essential—as is the inclusion of **massed practice** of a functional task (i.e., a continuous form of practice without rest between repeated performances of the skill). In children, the unaffected arm is casted to make it difficult to use (see Figs. 25-4A and 25-5).

2. The Upper Extremity **Motor Activity Log** is a 30-item, scripted, structured interview that documents by rating perception of how much and how well a patient uses the affected UE during activities of daily living (Uswatte, 1999). For example, activities such as turning on a light with a switch and opening a drawer are rated by the patient using a 0 to 5 scale on their perception of how much the involved UE is used in the activity and how well the activity is done.

3. The **behavioral contract** (Morris, 2006) is a formal, signed agreement establishing what the patient is going to do routinely with the affected UE when she is not in therapy. The contract mainly emphasizes consistent use of the affected UE with no use of the less-affected UE. This component helps optimize accountability and keeps the person focused on the goal of increasing functional use of the affected UE.

4. When not in therapy, the patient is asked to keep a **home diary** of activities completed with the affected UE during all waking hours. It also holds the individual accountable for using or incorporating the affected UE into activities of daily living and adhering to the behavioral contract.

5. The **home skill assignment** (Morris, 2006) is an important way to encourage use of the affected UE during a variety of "different" functional activities outside of therapy. You should select some activities that are challenging and some that are easy to perform.

6. Feedback, coaching, modeling, and encouragement are all essential when shaping tasks are used as an intervention. **Shaping** intentionally progresses the demands in a training activity, such that the final objective is approached through successive approximations. Tasks are selected according to the needs of the individual. Start by performing the task in a way that the patient can successfully complete the action; then gradually change the parameters (e.g., distance, force, time) to increase the challenge while still allowing success at each step. Continue until the patient matches the final goal for that activity. Each task may be performed in a set of 10 trials that usually lasts 30 to 45 seconds (Taub, 1994).

7. **Home practice** (Morris, 2006) involves performing a functional task repeatedly (i.e., massed practice) with the affected UE for 15 to 30 minutes while at home.

8. **Task practice** (Morris, 1997) includes functionally based tasks performed continuously for 15 to 30 minutes using the affected UE. Therapists should provide encouragement at least once every 5 minutes and a summary of the person's performance at the end of the task. Positive feedback is emphasized (see Fig. 25-5).

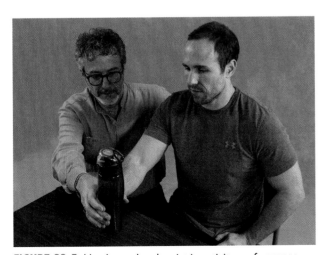

**FIGURE 33-5** Hand-over-hand assist in activity performance. An upper extremity functional treatment activity emphasizing bilateral hand use with the therapist providing assistance. The therapist's hands are placed over the patient's hands to reinforce bilateral grasp and a normal movement pattern.

Texture considerations are also motivating to children, so incorporating the exploration of items with various sizes, shapes, and textures may be educational as well as motivational. We can often incorporate playful themes into the treatment on the basis of the child's interests, such as animals, characters, vehicles, dolls, or blocks, and incorporate the themes into the need to move or place the toys. Promoting play-based interactions helps the child apply newly learned motor skills into her daily play routines.

Often children need to hold themselves up in a position that allows them to then visually explore the environment or visually track a person or toy. Weight-bearing and holding positions are often accomplished while encouraging the child to visually track items such as bubbles or balls, and then, if possible, coordinating the motor demands to weight shift and to reach out and pop a bubble or catch a ball.

Be aware of the balance of motor and cognitive demands each task places on the child. You can start with a higher cognitive demand (e.g., requiring the patient to follow

---

**BOX 33-7  Examples of Functional Intervention Activities of Daily Living for the Upper Extremities**

Note: Therapists should use task analysis skills to evaluate all upper extremity (UE) component contributions to a functional activity, including postural control, reaching, stabilizing, and hand use. A patient may have skilled UE active reach but poor control of weight-bearing through the same arm. To be maximally effective and produce coordinated motor performance, therapists should consider a patient's eccentric, concentric, and isometric control of motor actions.

1. Facilitate stability in the affected UE, with weight-bearing through the arm, by performing activities such as standing at the sink to comb the hair or brush the teeth with the unaffected UE. Also, emphasize weight-bearing during contralateral reaching tasks, including reaching for items in an upper cabinet.

2. Bilateral hand tasks increase awareness of and practice use of the affected UE while encouraging functional use and purposeful movement. For example, use both hands to perform tasks such as drinking from a cup, a real daily task. Activities such as dusting or wiping a table or scrubbing the legs with a washcloth may incorporate both UEs by interlocking the fingers so the unaffected arm (on top) can assist the affected arm (on bottom) with the movement. Can you think of other activities that can be done with bilateral hand use to incorporate the affected UE?

3. The caregiver or therapist can use hand-over-hand activities to train the patient in recovery of movement by guiding the affected UE through specific movement patterns to incorporate it in functional tasks.

---

directions with prepositions such as *in, under,* or *next to*) in an activity while the motor demand is low (e.g., reaching and releasing). Then plan the next activity to be a much higher motor control demand with less cognitive demand to balance it out (e.g., having to pick up smaller toys with a three-jaw chuck grasp and place them in cups matching by colors). Plan a sequence of activities allowing adequate rest and demands. Be aware of children who may put small objects in their mouths. Be spontaneous and incorporate actual play with the child. Make silly faces when appropriate, promote sharing and turn-taking when appropriate, and be willing to sing, laugh, and help build imaginary play when the opportunity arises. Have fun, be playful, and keep the child engaged in the activity.

## PATIENT APPLICATION

*Grayson is a 5 week-old infant. He was born at 37 weeks' gestation and weighed 10 pounds 6 ounces. His mother had gestational diabetes and experienced a long labor. Grayson was diagnosed with a brachial plexus injury called Erb palsy with C5–C6 involvement. His shoulder is held in shoulder extension, internal rotation and adduction, elbow extension, forearm pronation, and wrist and finger flexion. This is often referred to as the "waiter's tip" position. Before discharge home, therapy fitted him with a TheraTogs® immobilizer and instructed the parents in range-of-motion exercises. The physician then ordered therapy once per week.*

### Contemplate Clinical Decisions

*Pondang (2004) provided an excellent review of the natural history of obstetric brachial plexus injury (OBPI). On the basis of this chapter, the Pondang review, and other materials available to you, consider the following questions.*

1. *Consider the brachial plexus diagnosis and the specific level of involvement for Grayson. Which muscles can you expect to be impaired? What sensory impairment is likely to be detected*

*on the neurological examination? And given Grayson's young age, what functional limitations of specific activities might you anticipate?*

2. *What do you need to examine as part of your initial evaluation? Which assessment tools will you choose? What questions will you ask the parents? In what positions will you place the infant to observe his functional abilities? (Consider the Active Movement Scale for children with OBPI as a tool for measuring muscle grading [Clarke, 1995] and the Mallet classification of function in obstetrical brachial plexus palsy [Gilbert, 1993]).*

3. *Develop a problem list of functional limitations of activity in this patient.*

4. *List the underlying impairments of body systems contributing to the functional limitations.*

5. *Prioritize the problems.*

6. *Write at least two appropriate long-term goals that express realistic functional outcomes for this patient. Include all components of the goal.*

7. *What interventions are appropriate to administer this early in the diagnosis?*
   - *What developmentally appropriate positions and play should be considered?*
   - *How can you promote the use of the grasp that is just developing?*
   - *How can you provide tactile stimulation to increase awareness and increase muscle contractions?*
   - *When is the use of electrical stimulation indicated?*
   - *Might a wrist orthosis or a resting hand orthosis be indicated?*
   - *What is the expected outcome for this child?*

## ■ Considerations for Nontherapy Time and Discharge

### Aspects of Patient and Family Education

Treatment does not stop when a person leaves the clinic after a treatment session. Treatment is most effective when it is carried over into all aspects of the individual's life. It is important to educate the patient/client and family on interventions that can be implemented during nontherapy time. A home program needs to fit into the individual's and family's routine without creating more stress. Asking about the daily typical schedule and routines will help identify naturally occurring opportunities in which to insert the learned or needed skills (Rainforth, 1988). Patients should be encouraged to identify activities in which they want to engage and establish structured practice time at home to improve both performance and participation in these activities.

## Activities for Nontherapy Time

Throughout the rehabilitation process, the patient spends more time out of the therapy setting (e.g., in the car or at home, work, school, a shopping center, church, and entertainment venues) than with the therapist. Therefore, from a motor learning standpoint, it is essential to educate the patient regarding optimal positioning, weight-bearing, UE use, and UE patterns of movement both to pursue and to avoid during nontherapy times.

One of the most important aspects is to encourage neural plasticity by strongly urging the patient to use the affected UE in functional activities as frequently as possible (even when the movement is not perfect to begin with); the patient should pay attention to the outcome of each movement (feedback), reflect on what could be improved, and then attempt to incorporate these changes in subsequent attempts. This mindset helps prevent the onset of learned nonuse. In some ways, the particular tasks the patient completes may not be as important as finding ways to incorporate the affected arm(s) in functional tasks and increasing use over time.

Tasks should be specific to the occupation or activity of daily living in which the patient wants to engage. Specific tasks addressed in treatment may be carried over into the home program for continued work on either skilled use of the affected UE during the task or incorporation of the affected UE (e.g., through dynamic weight-bearing or for stabilization in bilateral UE use). Personal care tasks such as brushing the teeth, shaving, using a washcloth, and styling hair should be included. Tasks in the kitchen or around the home can include washing the dishes, stirring a pot, wiping the countertops, stabilizing a cutting board, using a remote control, dialing a phone, turning on a light switch, folding clothes, or engaging in hobbies. Home maintenance activities might include washing a window, pushing a lawn tool or cart, or weeding a garden. Work or education tasks can include keyboarding at a computer, holding a book, and using work- or school-specific tools.

To increase use of the affected UE, a child is most easily engaged in sensory rich motivational play; there are many ways for children to use their hands for play during daily tasks. A tactile exploration activity could involve placing a child in the highchair and allowing her to explore the textures of various toys and materials (e.g., finger-painting with Cool Whip), making a small suction-cup toy spin, or simply exploring various food textures.

In the bathtub, encourage the child to reach for toys on the tub wall, scribble or write with tub crayons, hold a cup and scoop up and pour out water, reach and grasp for toys as they gently float by, squeeze toys that squirt, or place characters onto a floating boat. Place small open baskets or bowls on the floor with toys in them so the child can empty, fill, explore, shake, spin, and roll the toys along the floor. Play with Play Doh® to strengthen hand muscles by squeezing, rolling, squishing, cutting, and forming various shapes and objects with the tools. Play outside with squirt guns aimed at targets. Use sidewalk chalk to scribble, draw, or write on fences and driveways.

Organize smaller toys into pouches with zippers or buttons (as appropriate), and teach the child to unzip or unbutton to get her favorite toys out to play. Create dress up corners where the child has to put on and take off hats, crowns, boots, shoes, socks, vests, shirts, and pants to learn to use her hands to pull and push on clothing and use fasteners. Create simple arts and craft projects to promote use of crayons, pencils, glue, scissors, and a puncher. Have the child string large beads or pieces of macaroni to make a bracelet or necklace. Hang a large sheet of paper on a fence and allow the child to use a paint brush and water colors to paint. Fill a small tray with sand or salt and ask the child to imitate the lines, shapes, or letters you demonstrate writing with your fingers. Play flashlight chase games by having the child hold a flashlight with one or both hands and make her light follow your light as you move it along the wall or ceiling. Suspend a beach ball and ask the child to catch it, stop it, hit it with a bat, hit it with one hand, or hit it with alternating hands.

## Illustrated Sample Home Exercise Program

Patients and caregivers enjoy handouts, pictures, and videotapes they can refer to later and review on their own time to serve as reminders. When possible, write home programs in the individual's or parent's preferred language. Pictures are considered helpful, especially for individuals who are not able to read or who do not understand written language well. The ability to take photos with cell phones and digital cameras and download them onto computers makes it easy to provide a customized home program with good quality photos.

Provide practice opportunities and feedback before the patient and/or family is expected to perform independently at home. Provide time for them to watch as you perform the activity with explanations and review the pictures and written instructions. Then allow the patient to practice with you watching and guiding. Provide positive constructive feedback, and be sure patients and/or families know what to do before the session ends. Check to see how the home program is developing, and allow another practice time if needed. When providing therapy in the home for a child, consider including siblings into selected components of the therapy session. Box 33-8 provides tips and examples of functional activities with the UE that require caregiver involvement.

## BOX 33-8  Upper Extremity Functional Interventions That Require Caregiver Involvement

Tips for upper extremity (UE) functional interventions with caregivers:

- Encourage family members to hold the person's affected hand and rub the person's arm with various textures to increase awareness.
- Encourage the family to modify the environment to stimulate and encourage awareness of the affected side.
- Educate the family on how to safely and gently perform UE passive range of motion and stretching exercises.
- Encourage the use of the affected UE by implementing a behavioral contract.
- Remind parents that they can use diaper changes to complete stretching and range of motion exercises with children.
- Have parents incorporate fingering and sensory play into the routine before meals. When the child is seated in the high chair, they can set up toys on the large tray to engage her while they finish cooking the meal.

Examples of interventions for the patient at home:

- Encourage use of the affected UE in weight-bearing as appropriate during all activities of daily living.
- Perform self-range of motion patterns.
- Open and close toothpaste tubes, drink bottles, etc., with the affected hand to develop fine motor skills.
- Use laundry time as an opportunity for sensory input, feeling the warmth of the items just out of the dryer, running hands and forearms along the different textures of the materials.
- Use cleaning activities to incorporate stretching and range-of-motion activities. Vacuuming can incorporate increased reach forward as well as light strengthening combined with balance activities. Dusting with a dust wand incorporates reach in multiple directions.
- Use family time in the park to incorporate balance and sensory input as a child is gently pushed in a swing.
- Discuss the client's daily and weekend activities to identify opportunities to incorporate therapy goals into daily life.
- Consider how you can incorporate stretching, reaching, strengthening, and fine motor movements into daily activities.

### PATIENT APPLICATION: 19 YEAR-OLD WHO SUSTAINED A TRAUMATIC BRAIN INJURY SECONDARY TO A MOTOR VEHICLE ACCIDENT

*Preston is a 19 year-old male who sustained a closed head injury/intracerebral bleed after a motorcycle wreck approximately 1 month ago. He underwent a craniotomy for evacuation of the intracranial hemorrhage. In addition to anemia, initial clinical findings included dysarthria, dysphagia, right lower extremity weakness, and extreme bilateral upper extremity weakness. Due to his upper extremity weakness, he is unable to independently perform personal care tasks or other activities of daily living. As a result of the injury, he also demonstrates cognitive deficits in orientation, initiation,*

*judgment, organization, problem-solving, sequencing memory, and decision-making. Since the injury, Preston has been taking Dilantin for a seizure disorder. He plans to return home with his mother and continue working at a local restaurant while attending college. Preston has been referred to the rehabilitation institute for further evaluation and treatment.*

*Results of the OT evaluation indicate that Preston is dependent with all eating, dressing, grooming, bathing, and toileting tasks and transfers. He is at Ranchos Los Amigos level IV. He also has no selective functional movement of his upper extremities except for approximately 10 degrees of active right elbow extension. He presents with Ashworth 1 spasticity in bilateral elbow flexors, wrist flexors, and long finger flexors and rates the pain in his left shoulder as 8 on a scale of 10.*

## HANDS-ON PRACTICE

▪▪▪ **Following is a summary of the practical skills the student should know after reading and practicing the skills described in this chapter.**

1. **Facilitation of grasp** through (1) wrist extension by having patients work on a surface that is more vertical than horizontal, (2) enhancement of the tenodesis pattern by intentional shortening of the finger flexors when there is a loss of voluntary finger flexion, and (3) dynamic orthosis or functional electrical stimulation to facilitate extension when wrist extension is not available

2. **Addressing safety issues** that occur as a result of impaired sensation (use compensatory techniques such as

visual vigilance and inspection), poor antigravity postural control (provide stability with extra trunk support as needed), poor endurance (do more difficult parts first and easier parts later), or pain (identify contributing factors and incorporate alternative strategies to minimize the pain) while involving the patient and caregiver

3. **Intervention through positioning and postural control** to enhance upper extremity (UE) use through (1) adapting the environment to increase stimulation, (2) altering the plane of movement through positioning to increase independent use of the UE, (3) reducing fixing into neck hyperextension

# HANDS-ON PRACTICE—cont'd

to facilitate postural control and positioning for UE use, and (4) facilitating grasp and reaching in upright sitting

4. **Intervention to enhance reaching** through (1) increased functional reach of patients with decreased strength (or endurance), (2) increased functional reach of patients with nonreducible limitations, and (3) increased functional reach of patients with motor control deficits

5. **Intervention for functional use of the hand** through (1) an extension-facilitated grasp, (i.e., tenodesis), (2) increasing tone in hypotonic hands that are over-expanded and flattened, not shaped with a thenar and hypothenar eminence, (3) reduction of tone for the

hand with spastic hypertonia, and (4) options for functional orthoses

6. **Intervention to enhance occupations** through (1) production of coordinated motor performance (eccentric, concentric, and isometric control of motor actions), (2) facilitation of stability in the affected UE, (3) increasing awareness of and use of the affected UE in bilateral hand tasks, (4) training the patient in recovery of movement using hand-over-hand activities

Students should refer to their training in task analysis to evaluate all of the UE component contributions to functional activities of daily life, including postural control, reaching, stabilizing, and hand use.

## Let's Review

1. Give examples of how neurological conditions can affect the upper extremity during the performance of daily tasks and life activities.

2. List typical upper extremity impairments seen in patients with neurological conditions.

3. Identify important safety considerations during management of upper extremity function in patients with neurological conditions.

4. Discuss important considerations related to age and lifespan influences for management of upper extremity function in patients with neurological conditions.

5. Compare and contrast different tests and measures used in the assessment of upper extremity impairment and function.

6. Design a plan of care inclusive of appropriate evidence-based intervention strategies at the occupational performance skill level of the upper extremity.

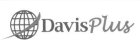 **Davis**Plus   For additional resources, including Focus on Evidence tables, case study discussions, references, and glossary, please visit http://davisplus.fadavis.com

## CHAPTER SUMMARY

Overviews of topics specific to function of the UE are presented in this chapter. For each patient, the effects of illness and injury on the functional repertoire of the hand and arm must be considered, especially as they relate to the performance of daily tasks and engagement in life activities. Lifespan factors influencing UE use must also be evaluated. Typical impairment characteristics of the hand and UE underlie abnormal function in patients with a neurological disorder, and they should be considered with each patient, including appropriate examination techniques to document these problems.

UE interventions for the basic functioning skill level as well as the more holistic occupational performance skill level are discussed in this chapter. The clinical cases, including the two

included with online resources, illustrate key concepts. The evidence basis for functional UE interventions is summarized in two online (ONL) Focus on Evidence tables: Table 33-7 (for adult patients) and Table 33-8 (for pediatric patients).

As a "bottom line," the reader must understand the therapist's obligation to take a holistic approach toward treatment of the UE; loss of the functional repertoire due to illness or injury significantly affects all aspects of performance of daily tasks and therefore the level of engagement in life. With all functional interventions to enhance motor performance, the patient must be provided feedback and encouragement to complete adequate repetitions of task-specific practice, and continually make adjustments toward motor learning.

# Functional Activity Intervention in Horizontal (Bed Mobility to Quadruped Skills)

Reva P. Rauk, PT, PhD, MMSc, NCS ▪ Randy Carson, PT, DPT, NCS, CCCE

**CHAPTER 34**

## CHAPTER OUTLINE

## CHAPTER OBJECTIVES

Upon completion of this chapter, the learner should be able to:

1. Discern which functions in horizontal are important and of most benefit to a particular patient.
2. Discuss normal movement components in horizontal functions.
3. Identify abnormal movements and function in horizontal by comparing them with normal function.
4. Identify appropriate examination strategies for function in horizontal.
5. Determine impairments contributing to abnormal function in horizontal.
6. Incorporate important safety considerations during patient management in horizontal.
7. Outline expected outcomes and prognostic indicators for function in horizontal.
8. Design appropriate interventions for an individual with abnormal function in horizontal.
9. Appropriately progress or modify a patient's treatment in horizontal.
10. Design an appropriate plan for nontherapy time motor practices or a home exercise program for a patient with abnormal function in horizontal.
11. Discuss evidence to support patient management in horizontal.

## ▪ Introduction

Although functional skills in horizontal positions are an essential component of the developmental process in children (e.g., crawling and creeping for exploration and play), mobility in horizontal postures is also important for adults (e.g., for bed mobility/scooting, crawling to play with a grandchild, or creeping to the sofa to rise from the floor). This chapter shows how the therapist can deliver therapeutic activities and interventions for underlying impairments when dysfunction is detected in activities or skills in horizontal.

## Typical Characteristics/Patterns of Movement in Horizontal

In horizontal, the head, trunk, and extremities move according to the demands of the task. Given the position or activity (e.g., supine rolling vs. bridging vs. quadruped), the therapist must consider all aspects of normal movement, as explained in Chapters 10 and 13, along with biomechanical elements such as base of support, center of gravity, number of segments involved in movement or weight-bearing, and length of the lever arm. In addition to being able to isolate and control movements of the trunk and extremities, patients must be able to do so under changing environmental contexts (e.g., the firmness or softness of the surface; type of bed sheets used; type of bedclothes worn; type of flooring, such as carpeting or linoleum).

Normal adults move using many different strategies depending on the demands or constraints of the task. As the task changes, they have the flexibility to vary their movement patterns and combinations. For example, in one analysis of rolling, 36 normal adult participants demonstrated 32 different combinations of movements (Richter, 1989). The most common combinations of trunk, upper, and lower extremity movements observed during rolling in this analysis are described in Table 34-1. Components and combinations of

| TABLE 34-1 | Patterns of Trunk and Extremity Movements in Supine, Bridging, Scooting, and Rolling |
|---|---|
| **SUPINE*†** | |
| *Trunk* | |
| Initiated from upper trunk | Upper trunk flexion with head and shoulders lifting up and away from the surface; includes cervical and upper thoracic flexion and scapular abduction (moving from supine to long sitting) |
| Upper trunk rotation (to the right) | Left arm reaches forward and across toward the right side, and the upper trunk flexes and rotates; left scapular abduction and upward rotation (reaching for an object, initiating rolling) |
| Initiated from lower trunk and body | Hip and knee flexion with feet in weight-bearing (as in moving into hooklying position) |
| Lower trunk rotation (to the right) | Left leg moves into hooklying, and the hip moves into adduction; right pelvic rotation |
| *Upper Extremity* | |
| Lifting the hand off the bed | • Shoulder and elbow flexion—reaching up toward face, pillow (adjusting pillow or reaching overhead)<br>• Shoulder flexion with elbow extension—reaching toward hip, knee (adjusting sheets) |
| Arm positioning | Alongside body, on body, over or behind head, out to side |
| Supine on elbows | • Bilateral—weight-bearing on both forearms<br>• Unilateral—weight-bearing on one forearm, usually with the opposite arm reaching across the body as in moving to get out of bed |
| *Lower Extremity* | |
| Movement in bed | Movement of the leg into abduction or adduction (sliding out to the side; moving lower leg off the edge of the bed or onto the bed) |
| Weight-bearing patterns | • Hip and knee flexion and ankle dorsiflexion with feet in weight-bearing (hooklying)<br>• Hooklying combined with lower trunk rotation—from hooklying with the knees in midline, the knees move to one side resulting in pelvic rotation to that side and lower trunk extension/rotation |
| **Bridging*†** | |
| Bilateral weight-bearing | Bridging—increased weight-bearing into the feet, hip extension, knee flexion, and lower trunk extension, resulting in lifting the buttocks off the surface |
| Unilateral weight-bearing (on right) | Half-bridging—right leg in hooklying and the left remains in extension; pushing only with the right flexed leg results in a lifting of the right side of the pelvis, right hip extension, and left pelvic rotation |
| **Scooting*†** | |
| Up in bed | • Legs positioned into hooklying with bilateral weight-bearing<br>• Arms positioned at the side; may position in weight-bearing with shoulder extension combined with elbow flexion to assist with pushing up<br>• Legs push into the surface, resulting in a partial bridge<br>• Legs (hip/knee extension) and arms (shoulder flexion with elbow extension) push upward, resulting in the body sliding up in the bed |
| Down in bed | • Legs positioned into hooklying with bilateral weight-bearing<br>• Arms positioned at the side |

*Continued*

**TABLE 34-1    Patterns of Trunk and Extremity Movements in Supine, Bridging, Scooting, and Rolling—cont'd**

### SUPINE*†

|  |  |
|---|---|
|  | • Legs push into the surface, resulting in a partial bridge<br>• Legs (hip/knee flexion, ankle dorsiflexion) and arms (shoulder extension with elbow flexion) pull body toward the feet, resulting in the body moving down in the bed |
| Sideways in bed<br>(scooting to the right) | • Legs positioned into hooklying with bilateral weight-bearing<br>• Arms positioned at the side; right arm is placed into more abduction<br>• Legs push into the surface, resulting in a partial bridge<br>• Legs push to shift the hips laterally over to the right (right hip adduction and left hip abduction)<br>• Hips settle back onto the bed<br>• Left arm pushes and right arm pulls the upper body to the right in order to align the upper body with the lower body; the head and shoulders are lifted slightly off the bed during this movement |

### Rolling (Supine to Prone)*

| Most common movement pattern<br>combinations (rolling to left) | Upper extremity (UE): right UE lifts and reaches above shoulder level across the body (rolls over left UE or shoulder)<br>Head-trunk (H-T): shoulder girdle leads (head turns to left; upper trunk flexes and rotates left; right shoulder leads right pelvis)<br>LE: unilateral lift (RLE lifts off surface before right pelvis lifts) |
|---|---|
| Second preferred pattern<br>combinations (rolling to left) | UE: RUE lifts and reaches above shoulder level across the body<br>HT: shoulder girdle leads<br>LE: unilateral push (RLE into hooklying and pushes pelvis to left—left pelvic rotation, right hip extension) |
| Third preferred pattern<br>combinations (rolling to left) | UE: RUE lifts and reaches above shoulder level across the body<br>HT: shoulder girdle leads<br>LE: bilateral lift (bilateral slight hip/knee flexion; feet may lift off the surface and follow trunk as individual rolls) |
| Fourth preferred pattern<br>combinations (rolling to left) | UE: RUE lifts and reaches above shoulder level across the body<br>HT: relationship between pelvis and shoulder girdle changes (right shoulder initially leads the rotation, then pelvis leads just before and throughout remainder of roll)<br>LE: Unilateral push |

### Crawling

| Movement pattern | Crawling—prone locomotion with abdomen on supporting surface, propelling by pulling with elbows and pushing with opposite knee; limb movement is reciprocal. Not typically used in adults unless function dictates its use (e.g., crawling under a low object). |
|---|---|

### Quadruped

| Movement pattern/position | Quadruped (pronounced KWOD-roo-ped)—prone on hands and knees with abdomen off supporting surface; individual is able to maintain static balance in order to hold position. Dynamic balance includes the ability to shift weight and rock in all directions: forward, back, to the side, diagonally; should also be able to maintain balance while lifting one arm, one leg, or one arm and one leg off supporting surface; most often used in adults as a point of transition between positions (e.g., moving from sitting on the floor to side-sitting to quadruped to kneeling, half-kneeling, and standing) |
|---|---|

### Creeping

| Movement pattern | Creeping—prone locomotion on hands and knees or hands and feet (always with abdomen off supporting surface), propelled by pulling with the hands and pushing with the opposite knee/foot; limb movement is reciprocal. In adults, used commonly as a means to move from place to place while on the floor (e.g., playing with children on the floor; walking on hands and knees to move closer to a couch or chair to use as a support to transition to standing) |
|---|---|

*Richter, 1989<br>†Ryerson, 1997

typical trunk and extremity movements for **bridging, crawling, quadruped**, and **creeping** are also included in the table (Richter, 1989; Ryerson, 1997).

## THINK ABOUT IT 34.1

Take a moment to review your day and identify the functional movements and positions you performed in horizontal over the past 24 hours.

- What activities did you do?
- How much time do you estimate you spent in horizontal?
- What movement pattern/strategy did you use to accomplish the task?
- How many times do you estimate you changed positions in horizontal or adjusted the sheets or pillow?
- If you completed an activity more than once, what different strategies did you use?
- Why did you use a different strategy? What is it about the context that required a different strategy?
- How did environmental factors help or hinder your movement?
- Note the speed at which you moved. How might different environmental factors change the efficiency of your movement?

## Clinical Picture of Activities in Horizontal

Performance of activities in horizontal is essential to daily functioning. Movement and positioning in horizontal during rest, sleep, and recreational activities are important for several functional activities: rolling, changing positions in bed, scooting, getting in/out of bed, managing sheets or pillows, reaching for the telephone on the bedside table or to set the alarm, watching television, and sexual activity, to name a few. Most commonly, we lie in horizontal when resting or sleeping. The time spent in horizontal for sleep alone varies with age (Table 34-2).

As noted previously, functional activities in horizontal use the entire body—the head, trunk, upper extremities, and lower extremities. Adult rolling movement patterns include three sequence categories: head and trunk movement, upper extremity movement, and lower extremity movement (Richter, 1989). Other movements in horizontal (e.g., scooting, crawling, creeping, quadruped) also require coordinated control of the head, trunk, and extremities.

Loss of motor control results in horizontal functional activity limitations and the inability to independently participate in daily activities. Positioning and movement in horizontal are basic prerequisites for independent functioning because we spend as much as one-third of our day in horizontal. This chapter focuses on the promotion of functional activities in horizontal, such as rolling, scooting, bridging, crawling, quadruped, and creeping.

| TABLE 34-2 | Changing Sleep Patterns With Age |
|---|---|
| **AGE** | **AVERAGE AMOUNT OF SLEEP PER DAY** |
| Newborns – 3 months | 14-17 hours; 1–3 hours awake |
| 4–11 months | 12-15 hours; 30-minute to 2-hour naps, 1–4 times per day |
| 1–2 years | 11–14 hours; 1 nap of 1–3 hours |
| 3–5 years | 10–13 hours; no naps typically after age 5 years |
| 6–13 years | 9–11 hours |
| Adolescents, 14–17 years | 8–10 hours |
| Adults, 18–25 years | 7-9 hours |
| 26–64 years | 7-9 hours |
| 65+ years | 7–8 hours |

Adapted from:
Bureau of Labor Statistics (BLS). American time use survey summary. Washington DC: United States Department of Labor; December 20, 2016.
Hirshkowitz M, Whiton K, Albert SM, et al. National Sleep Foundation's sleep time duration recommendations: methodology and results summary. *Sleep Health.* 2015; 1:40-43.
Smith M, Robinson L, Segal R. Sleep Needs: What to do if you're not getting enough sleep. June 2017. Available at: https://www.helpguide.org/articles/sleep/sleep-needs-get-the-sleep-you-need.htm. Accessed August 16, 2017.

## Possible Impairments Underlying Abnormal Function in Horizontal

Many body structure and functional impairments can contribute to abnormal function in horizontal. During the initial examination, the therapist should identify the specific impairments underlying the limitations; often, several impairments contribute to a single problem. Table 34-3 presents examples of impairments that can contribute to problems in horizontal. For example, Tanaka (1997) found that muscle performance was substantially lower in patients with hemiplegia than in controls. Kafri (2005) found that a combination of weaknesses in the external oblique, pectoralis major, and rectus femoris muscles impaired the ability to roll from supine to the uninvolved side. The study also indicated that the pectoralis major played a major role in stabilizing the paretic side when the patient rolled to the involved side.

Therapists must consider specific muscle performance when analyzing movement in horizontal, as well as which impairments are primary results of a neurological condition and which may be secondary effects.

Although normal movements in horizontal appear effortless and fluid, persons with neurological conditions and underlying impairments described previously often demonstrate abnormal postures and movements in horizontal tasks.

| TABLE 34-3 | Impairments That May Contribute to Abnormal Function in Horizontal |
|---|---|
| **CATEGORY** | **IMPAIRMENT** |
| Aerobic capacity/ endurance | Hypertension or hypotension<br>Shortness of breath<br>Oxygen saturation<br>Peak oxygen consumption ($VO_2$) values<br>Perceived exertion |
| Arousal, attention, and cognition | Ability to maintain attention<br>Level of consciousness<br>Cooperation, motivation<br>Ability to process commands<br>Orientation (person, place, time, situation)<br>Judgment, insight<br>Aphasia<br>Recall, memory |
| Cranial and peripheral nerve integrity | Vision: acuity, visual field loss<br>Vestibular |
| Joint integrity and mobility | Joint mobility in the spine, rib cage, shoulders, hips, knees |
| Motor function | Motor control: rate and frequency of neural activation<br>Coordination: timing and coordination of muscle contractions<br>Presence of atypical movements<br>Dysfunctional movement/ posture<br>Apraxia (Spinazzola, 2003) |
| Muscle performance | Weakness/paralysis (Tanaka, 1997)<br>Power<br>Endurance |
| Pain | Level of pain |
| Range of motion | Functional range of motion<br>Muscle length, extensibility, and flexibility<br>Active and passive range of motion |
| Reflex integrity | Deep tendon reflexes<br>Postural reflexes, equilibrium, and righting reactions<br>Resistance to passive stretch (tone) |
| Sensory integrity | Light touch<br>Sharp/dull<br>Vibration<br>Proprioception<br>Sensory integration/weighting<br>Perception |

Table 34-4 describes typical abnormal postures and movements that occur with a few common neurological diagnoses.

# Safety Considerations

Safety is less of a concern in horizontal compared to more upright positions. However, potential for patient injury still exists. The most obvious risk is the patient rolling off the side of the bed. When working on rolling, the therapist may guard from the side of the bed toward which the patient is rolling. This allows the therapist to use his body as a block. Therapist positioning is especially important when working with an impulsive, quick-moving patient. Particular attention is also needed with individuals with flaccid extremities, especially in conjunction with hemineglect. These individuals are at high risk for injuring their shoulders. With this population, the therapist should guide the involved arm when rolling or teach the patient to support the arm when rolling.

Another consideration is minimizing the risk of secondary complications. This is crucial for individuals who lack protective sensation. For example, bony prominences such as the heels are at high risk for pressure sores. Pillows and towels should be used to evenly distribute pressure sources. Splinting devices that "float" the heels may be indicated. These devices are also useful in preventing range-of-motion impairments. A patient is at especially high risk for tightness/contractures of the heel cords.

## Lifespan Influences

### Neonatal/Childhood Developmental Considerations

During the first 6 to 9 months of life, an infant spends the most time in horizontal positions, gradually strengthening the ability to move against gravity and work toward more upright positions (Campbell, 2011; Aubert, 2014). The first 3 months (first quarter) is dominated by flexion and working on head control and alignment. Accidental rolling from supine may occur during this time and is nonsegmental in nature. The second quarter is characterized by more extension: bridging in supine, pushing up onto the elbows and hands in prone, and crawling. Increased segmental dissociation of the spine is seen in head turns combined with trunk rotation. The third quarter brings more exploration with decreased time in supine, consistent purposeful segmental rolling, and quadruped creeping (hand and knees, hands and feet). In the fourth quarter, the supine and prone positions are seen primarily during transitions because the infant spends more time in upright. Less reliance on creeping on hands and knees or in plantigrade is seen as the infant learns to walk. Table 34-5 outlines typical horizontal postures and movements seen in the first year of life.

Neurological injury may cause impairments in selective motor control. Children and adults with significant neurological involvement may display persistence of early tonic reflexes that interfere with movement in horizontal postures. These tonic reflexes are typically integrated or disappear by 6 months

| TABLE 34-4 | Abnormal Postures and Movements in Horizontal Tasks |
|---|---|
| **NEUROLOGIC CONDITION** | **ABNORMAL POSTURES AND MOVEMENTS** |

*Supine and Rolling*

| | |
|---|---|
| Hemiplegia (Ryerson, 1997; Umphred, 2012) | The body is supported by the surface and any movement away from that surface is being resisted by gravity. Ryerson (1997) described the effect of gravity on the body in supine as follows: "[G]ravity acts to pull the whole body back into bed ... severe muscle weakness or paralysis ... exaggerates the effects of gravity on body posture." As a result, the hemiplegic side may appear to be "sunken" into the bed compared with the other side. |
| | Head: Laterally flexed to the hemiplegic side and rotated toward the noninvolved or less-involved side. In rolling, the patient may have difficulty lifting the head off the surface and may stay in extension. |
| | Arm: With hypertonicity, the arm may be held in a flexion synergy pattern. The patient may have difficulty reaching in any direction involving a combination of shoulder flexion and elbow extension; difficulty weight-bearing on the elbow/forearm (requiring shoulder abduction with shoulder depression) or on extended arm; and difficulty placing the arm in a safe comfortable position during rolling. |
| | With hypotonicity or flaccidity, the arm may be "floppy" or "lifeless" at the patient's side. The patient has difficulty lifting the arm off the bed surface and the arm is often forgotten or left behind when rolling toward the opposite side. |
| | Trunk: May present laterally flexed on the hemiplegic side; shoulder and pelvic girdles may be in retraction and in posterior rotation relative to the other side. |
| | Leg: With hypertonicity, may present in an extension synergy pattern; the patient has difficulty flexing the hip and knee for movements off the bed or placing the foot in weight-bearing. The leg may lift as a whole (stiff and straight). |
| | With hypotonicity, the leg may be floppy and heavy in bed with abnormal hip abduction and external rotation. The patient also has difficulty lifting the leg off the surface, but the therapist may see initiation of hip and knee flexion (rather than a stiffly straight leg). |
| Bridging and scooting | In bridging, the patient often has difficulty with<br>• Flexion of the hip and knee to place the foot in weight-bearing<br>• The hemiplegic side lagging behind with posterior pelvic rotation because of decreased hip extension as the patient lifts the buttocks off the surface<br>In scooting, the patient has difficulty maintaining the bridge to move the pelvis to the side. Shifting the pelvis to the involved side is easier than shifting toward the uninvolved side. Because of the weakness or lack of selective control of the hip extensors, the patient may prematurely return to the hooklying position (plopping back down to the bed). Because of the lack of selective trunk control, the patient also has difficulty shifting the trunk laterally to align the shoulders with the new position of the pelvis. The patient may have trouble lifting the head and shoulders off the surface of the bed and pulling/pushing with the upper extremities in forearm weight-bearing. |
| Quadruped and creeping | Depending on the motor control of the hemiplegic limbs, the patient may need assistance moving the limbs into proper weight-bearing alignment and maintaining position in quadruped. The hemiplegic arm may be unable to maintain extension to provide weight-bearing support. The patient may lean or lose balance toward the hemiplegic side because of difficulty maintaining cocontraction around the hip and shoulder (i.e., to hold the hip and shoulder directly over the weight-bearing knee and/or hand). The patient may also have difficulty controlling weight shifting, especially toward the hemiplegic side.<br>In creeping, the patient may manifest decreased strength and/or motor control in advancing the hemiplegic limb to the new position, holding weight-bearing support while other limbs move, and pulling or pushing as needed to propel in any direction. |
| Parkinson disease (Fredericks, 1996) | ALL movements; severity of movement abnormality depends on the disease stage.<br>The most commonly seen movement abnormalities include impaired<br>• Motor planning<br>• Initiation of movement |

*Continued*

| TABLE 34-4 | Abnormal Postures and Movements in Horizontal Tasks—cont'd |
| NEUROLOGIC CONDITION | ABNORMAL POSTURES AND MOVEMENTS |
| --- | --- |
| | • Slowness of movement (bradykinesia)<br>• Amplitude of movement (hypokinesia)<br>• Trunk rotation (may see individuals log roll rather than segmentally roll)<br>Individuals seem to have the greatest difficulty with rotational movements, such as rolling and turning over in bed or sitting up. |
| Spinal cord injury (Sisto, 2009; Somers, 2009) | Typical movement patterns vary by level of injury. In complete tetraplegia or paraplegia, individuals rely on available strength and use the momentum of upper extremity arm swing to initiate and execute rolling and other bed mobility skills. See the functional intervention section of this chapter for descriptions of movement strategies. |

| TABLE 34-5 | Typical Horizontal Postures and Movement Seen in Infants |
| --- | --- |
| **0–3 Months** | |
| Supine | Posture: predominately flexed<br>• Trunk flexed, buttocks not in contact with supporting surface<br>• Head to one side or other, moving to midline after about 1 month<br>• Arms and legs symmetrically flexed with hands to trunk and feet near buttocks<br>Movement:<br>• Moving head side-side from midline<br>• Arms and legs stretching and kicking<br>• Exploring own body, playing with hands and feet<br>• Occasional accidental rolling supine to prone |
| Prone | Posture: predominately flexed<br>• Head turned to one side<br>• Arms and legs flexed<br>Movement:<br>• Active extension of head and later upper trunk against gravity<br>• Beginning to push up on elbows |
| **4–6 Months** | |
| Supine | Posture: decreasing flexion dominance with arms and legs relaxed into more extension, with arms out away from the trunk and feet on supporting surface<br>Movement:<br>• Active lifting of legs, bringing feet to mouth<br>• Lifting legs in combination with head rotation and upper trunk extension leading to falling over into sidelying<br>• Bridging with feet on supporting surface |
| Prone | Posture:<br>Movement:<br>• Prone on elbows to prone on hands<br>• Pivot prone<br>• Reaches for toys—plays on extended arms<br>• Crawling (locomotion with abdomen on supporting surface)<br>• Hands-and-knees rocking |
| **7–9 Months** | |
| Supine | Decreased time spent in supine<br>Movement: Consistent ability to roll to sidelying and prone |
| Prone | Movement: increased isolation and dissociation of arms and legs; spends a lot of time playing in prone and sidelying |

| TABLE 34-5 | Typical Horizontal Postures and Movement Seen in Infants—cont'd |
|---|---|
| Quadruped | Movement: <br> • Achieves position easily <br> • Rocking forward/backward <br> • Creeping and bear (plantigrade) walking (hands and feet) |
| *10–12 Months* | |
| Supine/Prone/Quadruped | Positions used primarily as transitional movements; creeping on hands and knees and in plantigrade seen as primary locomotion as child learns to walk |

Adapted from: Campbell SK. *Physical Therapy for Children,* 4th edition. St. Louis, MO: Saunders Elsevier; 2011. Tecklin JS. Pediatric Physical Therapy, 5th ed. Lippincott Williams & Wilkins; New York, 2014

of age, but they may never integrate in children with developmental disability, or they may recur in adults after a cerebral neurological injury. For example, an **asymmetrical tonic neck reflex (ATNR)** may interfere with rolling, and the **tonic labyrinthine reflex (TLR)** may interfere with rolling and extension in prone. The ability to weight-bear on hands in prone and to roll from supine to prone by the age of 18 months has been significantly related to age at onset of independent walking (Fedrizzi, 2000).

### Age-Related Changes

Age-related changes influencing the ability to function in horizontal vary greatly from individual to individual (Lewis, 2008). Natural aging occurs in everyone. Even individuals dedicated to the healthiest lifestyle are unable to stop the aging process. This normal aging process is illustrated best by comparing two different species. For example, a human being has a much slower aging process than a dog does. Natural aging as well as genetic and environmental factors influence an individual's ability to maintain mobility and reserve capacities when faced with disease. Similarly, genetic factors unique to each individual are out of our control. We all have a family history that may predispose us to conditions that influence our aging process, such as diabetes, arthritis, and heart disease. We have the most influence over environmental factors, such as diet, exercise, and other lifestyle choices that may contribute to the aging process.

A progressive loss of muscle strength has been noted as an individual ages, which affects all muscles in the body including the core musculature. Most movements in the horizontal plane demand core musculature to work against gravity when performing a desired functional movement. Spinal flexibility also decreases with age. This decrease in flexibility and a corresponding decrease in strength make movement in horizontal more difficult as one ages.

### PATIENT APPLICATION

**Case – Parkinson Disease:** *The patient is a 64 year-old, average-sized Caucasian male with a 7-year history of Parkinson disease (PD). He was recently seen by his neurologist and reported increased difficulty with rolling and moving around in bed.*
**Medical History:** *hypertension, congestive heart failure, renal insufficiency, osteoporosis*

**Social History:** *The patient has lived alone the last 2 years since his wife died. He has two children who do not live in the area. His hobbies include reading, walking, woodworking, and going to the movies. The patient lives in a single-story home with five stairs at the entrance, with one handrail on the right side. His laundry room and woodshop are in the basement.*
**General Health Status:** *The patient attends a wellness group for individuals with PD two times per week and takes occasional walks around his neighborhood. He is independent with all activities of daily living (ADLs) and instrumental activities of daily living (IADLs), but he is finding everything more difficult lately. He continues to drive even though his children think he should stop.*
**Medications:** *Sinemet 10/100 tid, Eldepryl 5 mg q.a.m., amantadine 100 mg bid, Lopressor HCT (metoprolol tartrate and hydrochlorothiazide) 50/25 QD, ramipril 5 mg QD*
**Prior Therapies:** *The patient has had no therapy except for the evaluation to enter the wellness program.*
**Physical Examination:**
**Systems Review:**
- *Cardiovascular/Pulmonary: Blood Pressure 95/60mmHg; Heart Rate 78bpm; Respiratory Rate 20rpm; O$_2$ Saturation 97%*
- *Integumentary: Skin is intact; peripheral edema is noted in bilateral lower extremities.*
- *Neuromuscular: Bradykinesia, akinesia, and resting pill-rolling tremor are noted.*
- *Musculoskeletal: Height is 5 feet 11 inches and weight is 165 pounds.*
- *Communication: Patient speaks softly and is sometimes difficult to understand, but no major communication barriers are identified. He asks and responds to questions appropriately.*
**Aerobic Capacity/Endurance:** *Patient can tolerate a 60-minute evaluation session without problems. The patient walked 656 feet on the 6-minute walk test.*
**Arousal, Attention, and Cognition:** *The patient is awake and cooperative. He displays good judgment/insight. He reports having trouble learning new activities.*

1052 SECTION V  Specific Functional Intervention to Improve Activity/Participation

**Safety:** *The patient is very safety conscious and expresses tremendous fear of falling.*

**Assistive and Adaptive Devices:** *Patient has a single-point cane at home. He reports that he is constantly misplacing it around his house. He arrived without it at the evaluation.*

**Range of Motion:** *Passive range of motion: Patient is lacking 10 degrees to neutral hip extension according to the Thomas Test. He demonstrates a moderate decrease in trunk rotation and extension.*

**Motor Function:**

**Tone:** *The patient has rigidity in all four extremities and in his trunk.*

**Motor Control:** *The patient has a resting tremor in his right hand that decreases with volitional movement. All movements are bradykinetic. He had a 1- to 2-second akinesia delay during manual muscle testing. When he was asked to perform alternating movements, there was a noted decrease in amplitude of movement with each repetition.*

**Muscle Performance:** *Bilateral upper extremity and lower extremity muscle strength is 5/5.*

**Reflex Integrity:** *Deep tendon reflexes are within normal limits.*

**Sensory Integrity:** *Light touch, sharp, dull, and proprioception are intact.*

**Posture:**

- *Sitting Balance/Postural Control: The patient is independent with static sitting. His sitting functional reach is 10 inches. He exhibits a forward head posture with increased thoracic kyphosis, decreased lumbar lordosis, and a posteriorly tilted pelvis.*
- *Gait, Locomotion, and Balance: The patient walks independently without an assistive device. He has a shuffling gait, decreased arm swing, and stooped forward-flexed posture. He has freezing at initiation, when turns are required, or as he approaches thresholds. When turning, he keeps his trunk rigid and turns "en bloc." No festination is noted.*

**Self-care/Functional Skills:**

- *Bed Mobility: The patient had a 10-second delay before initiating rolling from supine to sidelying. He required 15 seconds to complete the task. When rolling, he does so "en bloc" and only slightly bends his hips and knees. When asked to bridge, the patient required 2 seconds to initiate lower extremity flexion and 20 seconds to assume the bridging position. He is able to lift his buttocks off the mat, but he is not able to scoot up on the mat. When asked to assume sitting from sidelying, he required 8 seconds to initiate the activity. He achieved the activity without assistance by bringing his legs off the side of the mat and pushing up with the upper extremity that he was lying on. The other upper extremity did not assist with the activity.*
- *Transfers: Sit pivot transfer, wheelchair to/from bed/mat, requires maximum assist in both directions.*

- *Bowel/Bladder: Patient has occasional incontinence that he attributes to not being able to get to the bathroom quickly enough. He relates that he starts walking to the bathroom, but just before he can get there he loses bladder control.*

## Contemplate Clinical Decisions

1. Develop a list of activity limitations and participation restrictions for this patient.
2. What underlying body structure and functional impairments contribute to the functional activity limitations?
3. Identify patient assets. (What does he have going for him?)
4. Prioritize the problems and underlying impairments.
5. Write at least two appropriate goals that express realistic functional outcomes for this patient.
6. How can you set the patient up to make rolling easier for him initially?
7. How might you change the activity to progress his ability to roll?

# ■ Pertinent Examination and Evaluation

## Tests and Measures

The therapist should evaluate the patient's ability to achieve a position and accomplish necessary movements in horizontal. This includes functional tasks and possible underlying impairments affecting the tasks. Table 34-6 includes several tests and measures used to evaluate function in horizontal; tests that can be used to identify impairments affecting function and tests that include aspects of horizontal function within the overall test.

A patient's ability to roll unassisted from a horizontal position should be evaluated. The type of surface should be noted and should replicate the patient's home environment as closely as possible. Most mat tables in a clinical setting are firmer than a patient's bed in the hospital or at home and therefore overestimate the individual's ability to realistically complete the task. The patient's ability to perform the task with sheets and bedding should be assessed because this typically makes the task more difficult.

Tasks to be assessed include rolling, bridging, scooting to each side, scooting up and down in the bed, and when needed for the patient's typical daily function (or safety), quadruped and creeping. When analyzing a patient's ability to complete functional tasks in horizontal, the therapist should compare normal movements (see Table 34-3) with the patient's performance. Aspects to consider when analyzing a functional task in horizontal (American Physical Therapy Association, 2000) are included in Box 34-1.

## THINK ABOUT IT 34.2

For each of the tests and measures in Table 34-6, discuss how the test assesses function in horizontal or how it contributes to your understanding of function in horizontal.

| TABLE 34-6 | **Tests and Measures for Evaluating Function in Horizontal**\* |
|---|---|

**IMPAIRMENT LEVEL**

| | |
|---|---|
| Aerobic capacity/ endurance | Blood pressure<br>Heart rate<br>Baseline Dyspnea Index (Mehler, 1988)<br>Oxygen saturation—pulse oximetry<br>Perceived exertion—Borg Scale (Dunbar, 1992) |
| Arousal, attention, and cognition | Mini-Mental Status Examination (Folstein, 1975)<br>Rivermead Behavioural Memory Test (Wilson, 1989)<br>Rivermead Perceptual Assessment Battery (Whiting, 1980)<br>Behavioral Inattention Test (Wilson, 1987) |
| Cranial and peripheral nerve integrity | Vision<br>• Broken Wheel (Acuity) Test (Richman, 1984); Snellen Chart<br>Acuity test<br>• Visual field test<br>Vestibular<br>• Dix-Hallpike test (hyperfunction, benign paroxysmal positional vertigo [BPPV]) (Epley, 1980; Kollen, 2006)<br>• Head thrust test (hypofunction) (Wrisley, 2000) |
| Balance (Sisto, 2009) | Static sitting<br>1. Poor (–): Requires Max A to maintain position<br>2. Poor: Requires Mod A to maintain position<br>3. Poor (+): Requires Min A to maintain position<br>4. Fair (–): Requires contact guard to maintain<br>5. Fair: Maintains position with close supervision (<2 min)<br>6. Fair (+): Maintains position with close supervision (>2 min)<br>7. Good (–): Maintains position with Min resistance<br>8. Good: Maintains position with Mod resistance<br>9. Good (+): Maintains position with Max resistance<br>Dynamic balance<br>1. Poor (–): Requires Max A to right; unable to move voluntarily from midline<br>2. Poor: Able to move through 25%–50% range; requires Mod A to return<br>3. Poor (+): Able to move through 50% range; requires Min A to return<br>4. Fair (–): Able to move through 50%–75% range with contact guard to return<br>5. Fair: Able to move through 75% range with contact guard or 50%–75% with close supervision<br>6. Fair (+): Able to move through full range with close supervision, all directions<br>7. Good (–): Independent in basic dynamic balance activities<br>8. Good: Independent in function dynamic balance activities<br>9. Good (+): Independent in high-level dynamic balance activities |
| Joint integrity and mobility | Joint mobility in spine, rib cage, shoulders, elbows, wrists, hips, knees, ankles |
| Motor function | Motor Assessment Scale (MAS) for Stroke (Carr, 1985)<br>Fugl-Meyer Assessment (Fugl-Meyer, 1975)<br>Test of Infant Motor Performance (Campbell, 2002)<br>Alberta Infant Motor Scale (Piper, 1995)<br>Gross Motor Function Measure (Russell, 1989)<br>Gross Motor Performance Measure (Boyce, 1991, 1995) |
| Muscle performance | Manual Muscle Test (Wadsworth, 1987)<br>Motricity Index (Wade, 1987) |
| Pain | Numerical Rating Scale, Verbal Rating Scale, Visual Analog Scale (Berthier, 1998) |
| Range of motion | Goniometry: Active and passive range of motion of trunk and extremities |

*Continued*

| TABLE 34-6 | Tests and Measures for Evaluating Function in Horizontal*—cont'd |
|---|---|
| **IMPAIRMENT LEVEL** | |
| Reflex integrity | Postural reflexes, equilibrium, and righting reactions |
| | Modified Ashworth Scale (Gregson, 2000) |
| | Milani-Comparetti Motor Development Screening Test (Stuberg, 1989) |
| Sensory integrity | Light touch |
| | Sharp/dull |
| | Pressure |
| | Proprioception—appreciation of movement, direction of movement, and joint position sense |
| | Rivermead Assessment of Somatosensory Performance (RASP) (Winward, 2002) |
| | Visuospatial neglect |
| | Bells test (Gauthier, 1989) |
| | Rivermead Behavioural Inattention Test (RBIT) (Wilson, 1987) |
| | Bodily neglect (Azouvi, 1996; Bisiach, 1986) |

**ACTIVITY LIMITATIONS LEVEL**

Standardized tests and measures that include functions in horizontal, such as rolling, bridging, and scooting

Trunk Control Test (Franchignoni, 1997)
Motor Assessment Scale (MAS) for Stroke (Carr, 1985)
Barthel Index (Loewen, 1988; Mahoney, 1965)
Rivermead Mobility Index (Lennon, 2000)
Katz Index of Independence in Activities of Daily Living (Brorsson, 1984)
Functional Independence Measure (FIM) (Dodds, 1993)
Outcome and Assessment Information Set (OASIS) (Shaughnessy, 2002)
Spinal Cord Independence Measure (Catz, 1997)

**PERFORMANCE RESTRICTIONS LEVEL**

Global outcome measures that may be affected by an individual's function in horizontal

Craig Handicap Assessment and Reporting Technique (CHART) for TBI (Whiteneck, 1992)
Disability Rating Scale (Salen, 1994)
Frenchay Activities Index (Wade, 1985)
Lawton IADLs (Lawton, 1988)
Functional Independence Measure (FIM) (Dodds, 1993)
Functional Independence Measure for Children (WeeFIM) (Msall, 1994)
Functional Assessment Measure (FAM) (Donaghy, 1998)
Functional Status Questionnaire (Jette, 1986)
Multiple Sclerosis Quality of Life Index (Vickrey, 1995)
Parkinson Disease Quality of Life (de Boer, 1996)
Stroke Impact Scale (Duncan, 1999)
Pediatric Evaluation of Disability Inventory (Feldman, 1990; Iyer, 2003)

*Not an exhaustive list.
Abbreviations: IADL = instrumental activity of daily living; TBI = traumatic brain injury.

## Expected Outcomes and Prognostic Factors

For focal injuries (e.g., multiple sclerosis, stroke, brain injury, tumor, and PD), the expected outcomes and prognosis are often dependent on the severity of the lesion or trauma and other contributing factors (Smith, 1999; Wade, 1987) (Table 34-7). In looking at functional outcomes in stroke rehabilitation, Franchignoni (1997) and more recently Kafri (2005) found that rolling to the involved side was consistently easier than rolling to the uninvolved side and that trunk muscle strength in stroke patients was impaired multidirectionally, with the greatest impairment toward flexion. In children with spastic diplegia, independent walking was significantly related to their ability to bear weight on their hands in prone and to roll supine to prone by 18 months of age (Fedrizzi, 2000).

## BOX 34-1  Questions to Consider When Analyzing a Functional Task in Horizontal (American Physical Therapy Association, 2000)

What is the patient able to do?
- Can the patient do the task?
- What assistance is required?
- Is the patient able to perform a series of increasingly demanding tasks?
- Is this a mobility, stability, controlled mobility, or skill level movement?
- Is the patient safe throughout the task?

How does the patient do it?
- What are the starting alignment and position of body segments relative to each other and are they expected for the task?
- Describe how the movement is initiated.
  - Where is the movement initiated?
  - What are the speed and direction of the component movements?
- Describe the movement sequence used to execute the task, considering
  - Head and neck position
  - Trunk segment alignment
  - Alignment of pelvis, hips, knees, and feet
  - Scapular and upper extremity position and alignment
  - Symmetry and weight distribution
- Which components of the movement are
  - Normal or almost normal?
  - Abnormal?
  - Missing or delayed?
- What muscle activity was needed to terminate the movement?

Why does the patient do it this way?
- Are movements free, stabilizing, or compensatory?
- Are movements compensatory and functional or noncompensatory and nonfunctional?
- What impairments constrain the movement (e.g., muscle strength, motor control, tone, range of motion, tissue length changes)?

What happens under changing task demands?
- What happens with fatigue? Do movements change over time?
- How do different environmental contexts affect the task?
- Is the patient able to adapt to changing task or environmental demands?
- What happens with increasing challenge to stability and decreasing base of support?

Expected functional outcomes after a traumatic spinal cord injury are dependent not only on the level of injury but also on whether the injury is complete or incomplete. Typical functional outcomes for individuals with complete spinal cord injury are found in Box 34-2 (Consortium for Spinal Cord Medicine, 1999).

| TABLE 34-7 | Prognostic Factors Influencing Expected Outcomes | |
|---|---|
| **FOCAL INJURY** | **SPINAL CORD INJURY (SCI)** |
| • Severity and location: constellation of motor, sensory, and visual deficits; severity of balance loss<br>• Prior stroke<br>• Age<br>• Loss of consciousness or coma<br>• Cognitive status<br>• Aphasia<br>• Neglect<br>• Visual-perceptual deficit<br>• Persistent tone<br>• Depression<br>• Bladder and bowel functions | • Complete versus incomplete injury<br>• Extent of zone of partial preservation (complete injuries)<br>• Level of injury<br>• Strength of innervated musculature<br>• Presence of other traumatic orthopedic injuries (e.g., fractures), secondary diagnoses, or complications<br>• Intact sensation to pinprick test below level of injury<br>• Level of spasticity<br>• Pain<br>• Body type |

Adapted from: Smith MT, Baer GD. Achievement of simple mobility milestones after stroke. *Arch Phys Med Rehabil.* 1999;80:442–447.

## BOX 34-2  Typical Functional Outcomes for Individuals With Complete SCI (Consortium for Spinal Cord Medicine, 1999)

| | |
|---|---|
| C1–C4: | Total assist |
| C5: | Total to moderate assistance |
| C6: | Minimal assistance to modified independence |
| C7 and below: | Modified independent to independent |

## PATIENT APPLICATION

### Case of individual with PD (see case presented earlier)

### *Contemplate Clinical Decisions*

*Refer to the previous case involving the individual with PD:*

1. *Identify tests and measures completed in each level of the enablement model (impairment, activity limitation, performance restrictions).*
2. *What additional tests and measures might you want to complete?*
3. *What impairments contribute to this patient's problems with horizontal bed mobility?*
4. *What environmental factors might affect this patient's function with horizontal bed mobility?*

5. *What personal factors might affect this patient's function with horizontal bed mobility?*

6. *What components of the patient's horizontal bed mobility are normal? Abnormal?*

7. *At which point(s) during the task does the patient present difficulty with horizontal bed mobility (starting alignment, initiation, execution, termination)?*

8. *How might the patient modify his movement patterns for changing tasks or environmental demands?*

9. *How would you anticipate this patient's function to change throughout his medication cycle?*

# ■ Functional Interventions in Horizontal Skills

Therapeutic interventions in horizontal help our patients to move around in bed and become more comfortable. Ideally, every time a patient moves in bed, the task should be viewed as an opportunity to practice and improve the ability to complete the task as independently as possible. The therapist should practice the tasks with the patient in bed or modify the environment to simulate the functional task as it would normally be done at home.

## General Approaches

The clinician will need to consider the patient's goals, current abilities in horizontal, and prognosis to determine whether intervention strategies should focus on compensation or remediation in horizontal. Compensatory strategies may include substituting muscles with good voluntary control to serve as the prime mover of the activity. Adaptations to the environment may include the use of adaptive equipment such as grab bars and bed ladders. When remediation of function in horizontal is a realistic goal, several intervention approaches may be considered.

As described in Chapter 15, the patient's current stage of motor control can be determined and interventions initiated at an appropriate level. For example, when the patient is very rigid and lacks mobility to segmentally move the trunk, the clinician may begin with mobility, working on increasing range of motion and flexibility. The patient needs to be able to maintain a sidelying position, reflecting the stability stage. Reaching with one upper extremity to assist with rolling is an example of the static-dynamic stage. Controlled mobility may include rolling in a segmental and controlled manner without use of momentum to achieve the task. Skill has been obtained once the patient is able to roll and make adjustments to the bedding at the same time. The task-oriented model or the systems model may include altering the firmness of the support surface and practicing horizontal activities with bed sheets, blankets, and pillows.

## Therapeutic Functional Activities

### Positioning Considerations

The therapist should consider the patient's position before applying therapeutic techniques. Will the patient be on a

firm, medium, or soft surface? How will the upper extremities be positioned to accomplish the task as well as for safety? If the individual has an affected upper extremity, how will it be positioned? Box 34-3 provides a list of possible positions for a hemiplegic upper extremity. The lower extremity position depends on the functional task: rolling or scooting.

When a patient's neurological condition is so severe that he cannot move himself in bed, the individual needs to be positioned to avoid secondary complications such as contractures or pressure sores. The therapist should determine the best positioning for each patient and communicate strategies to other health-care providers so they can be carried out throughout the day/night. The health-care team should ensure that the patient changes positions every 2 hours to prevent pressure sores. If the patient displays voluntary movement, he should be able to move as much as possible around positioning devices to encourage as much active movement as possible (i.e., to avoid being constrained by the positioning). Table 34-8 describes positioning in supine and sidelying for individuals after a stroke.

### Horizontal: Bridging

Bridging is a weight-bearing position for the lower extremities in supine. It is both a developmental and a functional activity essential for independent dressing and moving in bed. When working with a patient, immediately put the bridge into a function, such as lifting to scoot sideways or up in bed. Increased control for the stance phase of gait with pelvic rotation and weight shift in a more isolated movement combination (e.g., hip extension with knee flexion) can also be facilitated using this position. Biomechanical factors to consider are a higher base of support, a smaller center of gravity, and an increased number of joints involved compared with supine.

#### Assumption of the Position

Guide and/or resist the patient's lower extremities into a stable flexed position with feet flat on the supporting surface. Assist the patient in lifting the lower extremity with the fingers on the lateral border of the foot and the lateral popliteal fossa. When some flexion is achieved, move the proximal hand to the anterior knee, below the patella (Fig. 34-1). Place the noninvolved leg over the top of the involved foot to assist the involved leg in bending up, and place the feet flat on the surface (you may provide pressure on the tibia to assist). Placing the assistance anteriorly rather than underneath

---

**BOX 34-3 Positioning Options for an Individual With Unilateral Hemiplegia When Performing a Functional Task**

1. Cradle the involved upper extremity with the uninvolved extremity. Both extremities will be in elbow flexion and shoulder internal rotation.

2. Clasp hands together with fingers intertwined. This will allow the arm with hemiparesis to participate more in the activity.

| TABLE 34-8 | Positioning Strategies for Individuals After a Stroke |
|---|---|

**Supine (see Fig. 18-6)**

| | |
|---|---|
| Head | • Midline<br>• Slight flexion<br>• May use a rolled towel under a pillow to prevent lateral neck flexion or side rotation (in the event of hemineglect) |
| Scapula | • Mobilization in supine before positioning to address abnormal tone<br>• Place folded washcloth or small towel under affected scapula to maintain protraction but not so much as to unweight it |
| Arm | (In general, position out of abnormal synergy postures)<br>• Scapula protracted<br>• Shoulder in slight abduction<br>• Shoulder in external rotation with elbow crease facing up<br>• Forearm in neutral or pronated and resting on a pillow (from elbow distally) for slight elevation<br>• Elbow in slight flexion (avoid too much elbow extension)<br>• Hand in weight-bearing resting on a pillow in neutral or only slight extension |
| Pelvis | • Keep protracted by placing a thin towel or sheet under the pelvis on the affected side about to the spine; not too thick of a sheet or towel because this may overexaggerate hip protraction, which would unweight the hip<br>• Maintain weight-bearing |
| Leg | (In general, position out of abnormal synergy postures)<br>• For supine supported hooklying, place pillows on their edge under the knees to maintain knee flexion, give support, and allow the patient to relax the legs while keeping the heels in weight-bearing<br>• When patient is staying in supine with legs extended, place a folded towel under the distal end of the femur, maintaining the affected knee in slight flexion; a smaller towel under the heel cord or sheepskin booties will relieve pressure on the heels |
| Other | • With the head of the bed up, make sure the patient is up as high as possible so the break of the bed is at the hips; in this position, the spine and trunk can stay in alignment |

**Sidelying: Involved Side Down (see Fig. 18-7A)**

| | |
|---|---|
| Head | • Height of the pillow can be a little higher to take pressure off the involved shoulder |
| Scapula/Arm | (In general, position out of abnormal synergy postures)<br>• Avoid rolling onto the shoulder directly; roll over three-quarters of the way OR protract the shoulder so the patient can roll all the way over onto that side<br>• Position as in supine with palm up; prop the arm in a little flexion from the elbow distally |
| Trunk/Spine | • Lying on the involved side increases elongation and weight-bearing on that side |
| Legs | (In general, position out of abnormal synergy postures)<br>• Place towel (if needed) between knees for comfort of bony knees; not putting a pillow between the knees allows the patient to move around more freely with the noninvolved side<br>• Encourage the patient to move the noninvolved side, increasing movement over the weight-bearing surface; promote slight flexion at the hip and more flexion at the knee<br>• Be protective of the feet and ankles when the patient is not very active |

**Sidelying: Involved Side Up (see Fig. 18-7B)**

| | |
|---|---|
| Head | • In neutral alignment |
| Arm | (In general, position out of abnormal synergy postures)<br>• Place up on a pillow(s) to avoid too much adduction and lateral rotation; keep in neutral but do not block the patient's vision |
| Trunk/Spine | • To maintain a straight spine, a folded sheet placed at the patient's unaffected side before rolling should prevent shortening on the affected side; the width of the sheet should be such that it lies between the patient's iliac crest and the inferior angle of the scapula |
| Legs | (In general, position out of abnormal synergy postures)<br>• Bottom leg is straight with hip in extension<br>• Top leg is slightly flexed and positioned on pillows in front of the other leg to avoid excessive hip adduction and internal rotation and to support the calf and foot; build up enough pillows to keep leg and foot in neutral |

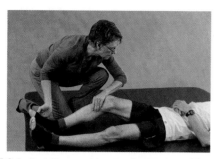

**FIGURE 34-1** Assisting a patient in placing the involved leg in a hooklying position with one hand at the lateral order of the foot to encourage dorsiflexion with eversion and the other hand at the anterior surface of the knee.

the leg encourages the patient to do as much of the work of lifting the leg as possible, rather than relying on the therapist to do most of the lifting or using the less-involved limb to lift the more-involved limb. Regarding foot placement, you may start with the feet apart for stability and progress toward a narrower base and/or start closer to the buttocks and progress to farther away.

A compensatory strategy for the patient is moving the legs into hooklying. The patient can hook the less-involved foot under the more-involved foot and use the strength of the uninvolved leg to pull the involved leg up into hooklying.

When a patient is unable to lift her buttocks off the supporting surface, you can facilitate the lift. Position yourself facing the patient's head and straddle her feet. Place your hands on the patient's distal femur, providing pressure down into the feet (cuing weight-bearing) and lightly pull the femurs forward over the feet. Then give an upward lifting cue with the fingers along the lateral aspects of the distal femur. You may lean your body back to increase weight-bearing into the patient's feet (Fig. 34-2A)

When the patient needs additional assistance, use a drawsheet around the crest of the pelvis, giving the same cues as described previously (Fig. 34-2B). Alternatively, your forearms can be placed on the patient's femurs with weight-bearing pressure given into the patient's feet. Then guiding the femurs forward over the feet, simultaneously lift the pelvis with the drawsheet.

### Stability

When the patient is able to lift into a bridge, strength is needed to hold the bridge long enough for a functional task (e.g., scooting sideways). One method for building strength and cocontraction around the hips is to apply **alternating isometrics (AIs)** and **rhythmic stabilization (RS)** with appropriate manual resistance (Fig. 34-3A). Manual contacts can begin at the pelvis; to make holding progressively more difficult, they can move to the knees and then to the ankles. To progress the level of difficulty, you can place the feet narrower and the feet farther away from the buttocks. You can add to the difficulty by placing the lower legs or feet on a Swiss ball (Fig. 34-3B).

### Controlled Mobility

The therapist can work on the patient's ability to weight shift laterally (necessary for scooting sideways in bed) and rotate the pelvis by applying **slow reversal hold (SRH)** or **slow reversal (SR)** while providing appropriate manual resistance with manual contacts at the pelvis. **Agonistic reversals** promote the strengthening of isometric, concentric, and eccentric contractions of the hip extensors.

### Static/Dynamic

The same progression of stability and controlled mobility can be done with one-legged bridging. In addition to working on hip strength and control, one-legged bridging facilitates the

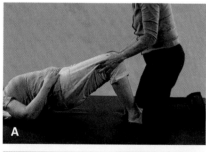

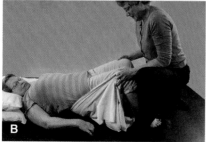

**FIGURE 34-2** (A) Facilitating bridging and (B) facilitating bridging using a drawsheet to assist.

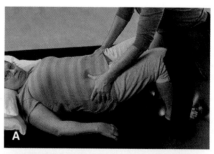

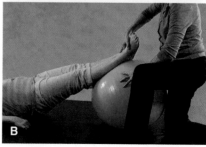

**FIGURE 34-3** Working on stability in bridging (A) applying alternating isometrics and/or rhythmic stabilization and (B) using a Swiss ball.

patient's use of one leg as the primary push for scooting sideways (Fig. 34-4).

### Horizontal: Scooting

For increased independence in bed mobility, a patient must be able to maneuver in bed. Scooting is considered a skilled movement in supine. For *scooting sideways,* begin with the patient in a bridge. With the positions and hand placements described previously in bridging (Figure 34-2A), give input with one hand toward the pelvis (as if shortening the leg) and the other toward the knee (as if lengthening the leg). Maintain the upward direction cue to keep the bridge the entire time until ready to set the hips back down. Work with the patient to control the hips descending back down to the supporting surface (rather than plopping down). Assist the patient in aligning the legs with the new position of the hips; if necessary, lean the knees together so the legs can stay propped up. The patient then aligns the upper body with the lower body by lifting the head and shoulders slightly and shifting the shoulders over. You may cue the patient at the shoulders when needing assistance with upper body alignment.

In all cases, the patient should be doing as much of the work as possible with the therapist assisting as little as possible. When the patient needs more assistance with maintaining a bridge during the sideways scooting practice, a drawsheet can be used around his pelvis as described previously in bridging, with the addition of shortening and lengthening cues.

For *scooting up in bed,* again begin with a bridge. Using the position and hand placements described previously in bridging, give input with the fingers on both hands, simultaneously giving the patient the input to move the buttocks toward the head (pushing lightly toward the patient's head). The patient can additionally assist by pushing up with both feet and hands to slide upward.

### Horizontal: Rolling

In addition to scooting, a patient needs to be able to roll in both directions for independence in bed mobility. Although typically used for bed mobility, rolling is also used for dressing in individuals who cannot dress in sitting or standing, for pressure relief in individuals who are unable to bridge, and to decrease general tone when done slowly and rhythmically.

Biomechanical factors include a large base of support that can be increased with an arm on the mat and a low center of gravity. The ATNR or TLR will interfere with normal rolling if present, whereas intact righting reflexes will assist with rolling. When moving from supine toward prone, gravity resists the supine-to-sidelying portion of the movement and assists the sidelying-to-prone movement.

Begin by asking the individual to roll. When the patient presents with hemiparesis, ask him to roll toward the less-involved side. What strategy does the patient spontaneously try to use? If possible and appropriate, help the patient to relearn his preferred rolling strategy.

Initially, it may be easier for the patient to roll from supine to sidelying "en bloc" (log roll) rather than segmentally. When considering the patient who has experienced a stroke with one side significantly more impaired than the other, rolling onto the weaker side is easier than moving onto the uninvolved side (Franchignoni, 1997; Kafri, 2005). Because the external oblique, pectoralis major, and rectus femoris muscles play significant roles in the ability to roll to either side after a stroke, any activity or isolated muscle strengthening targeting these muscles will contribute to a patient's overall functional success with rolling (Kafri, 2005).

When teaching a patient to *roll onto the involved side,* first have her place the legs in hooklying (assist as little as possible). Protract the affected scapula and slightly abduct the arm away from the body to avoid the patient lying on it when rolling. Be careful to also avoid side neck flexion toward the affected shoulder by placing the patient's head on an additional small pillow when needed to keep the head slightly tilted away from the affected shoulder; this takes pressure off the affected shoulder. With you on the patient's affected side (patient rolls toward you), one hand facilitates at the shoulder and the other hand at the legs (or pelvis) to assist/allow the body to roll onto sidelying (Fig. 34-5A). Be careful to maintain affected shoulder protraction or have the patient roll only partially onto sidelying. A caudal pressure may also be applied at the shoulder and aimed toward the pelvis to help the patient lift and turn the head toward the involved side.

For *rolling onto the less-involved side,* again begin in hooklying. The patient brings the noninvolved hand across and assists by holding the involved arm, grasping more proximally at the upper arm or scapula. The patient maintains the affected scapula in protraction. The therapist, now on the patient's uninvolved side (patient rolls toward the therapist), uses one hand at the knees (or pelvis) to bring the hips over and the other hand at the scapula to assist the upper trunk in rolling into sidelying (Fig. 34-5B).

Figure 34-5C shows an option of cradling the involved arm during the roll. The therapist may provide a caudal pressure at the shoulder and aimed toward the pelvis to help the patient lift the head and laterally flex the involved side of the trunk. The therapist can also add approximation into a weight-bearing foot (hooklying) while simultaneously providing traction of the hip to cue the patient to help push over with the involved lower extremity.

Several techniques can be used to assist a patient in maintaining sidelying once the position is attained. The therapist can use AIs, RS, and SRH by gradually decreasing the range

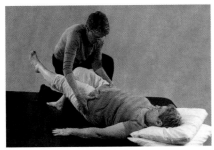

**FIGURE 34-4** Working on static-dynamic control with one-legged bridging.

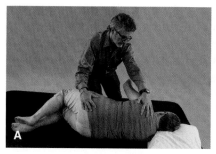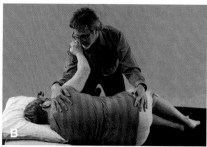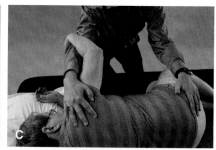

**FIGURE 34-5** Assisted rolling (A) onto the involved side, (B) onto the less-involved side, and (C) onto the less-involved side cradling the involved arm.

of movement. These techniques are especially helpful for individuals with ataxia.

A therapist can use several strategies for facilitating segmental rolling from supine to sidelying or prone. One strategy is *lower trunk rotation* (LTR). LTR works on building lower trunk–initiated segmental rolling. With the patient in the supine hook-lying position, the therapist can use any of the techniques described in Table 34-9, depending on the patient's ability to complete the LTR or her strength throughout the LTR range. When using LTR to facilitate rolling, the patient learns to lead with the legs, pelvis, and lower trunk, with the upper body following into sidelying or over into prone (Fig. 34-6A). The therapist strengthens the patient's ability to use the lower extremities to push over from supine to sidelying.

| TABLE 34-9 | Techniques to Encourage Lower Trunk Rotation (LTR) for Rolling |
|---|---|
| *Mobility* | |
| Use this technique when the patient is having difficulty initiating or sustaining movement. | |
| Rhythmic initiation | Progress from passive LTR → active assistive → active → resisted LTR; active movement is bidirectional. |
| Repeated contractions | The therapist uses repeated quick stretches to initiate, reinforce, or strengthen a muscle contraction. The quick stretch is superimposed on an existing contraction throughout the movement pattern. The technique is typically used for weak muscles that are unable to sustain a contraction throughout the range or are significantly weaker within a portion of the range. |
| Replication | The patient learns to move through progressively increasing increments of range until he gains control of the entire LTR range. The therapist passively moves the patient's knees over to the end position and asks the patient to hold in that position. The patient is then asked to slowly let go, letting the therapist move the limb back toward the beginning range a little. This elicits an eccentric contraction through a small increment of range. The patient is then asked to pull back to the starting (end) position. This process is repeated with the eccentric phase gradually lengthened until the patient has completed the entire range of LTR. Active movement is unidirectional. |
| Hold relax active movement (HRAM) | This technique is helpful when the patient is unable to initiate movement on his own. The therapist passively moves the patient over into the end (or middle) range of LTR and asks the patient to "hold" while resistance is provided in the direction of the intended movement. The patient is then asked to relax, at which time the therapist passively moves the patient into the lengthened (beginning) range. This is immediately followed by a quick stretch or series of quick stretches with active movement back toward the shortened range. Depending on the amount of muscle activation elicited, the therapist may assist, track, or resist the concentric movement. |
| *Controlled Mobility* | |
| This technique is used when the patient is having difficulty with weight shifting, strength through the range, or proximal dynamic stability. | |
| Agonistic reversal | This technique strengthens all three muscle contractions around the hip and lower trunk: isometric, concentric, and eccentric. |
| Slow reversal hold/slow reversal | This technique strengthens LTR in both directions. |

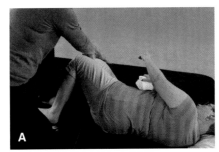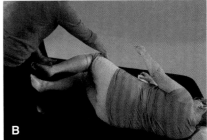

**FIGURE 34-6** Lower trunk rotation for (A) rolling and (B) use of proprioceptive neuromuscular facilitation lower extremity D1 flexion for rolling.

Another segmental rolling strategy involves using one lower extremity rather than both as in LTR. In this strategy, the patient practices reaching with the opposite leg up and over the other leg, moving into sidelying. When rolling onto the left side, the patient reaches up and over with the right leg. The therapist can use a proprioceptive neuromuscular facilitation (PNF) **D1 flexion (D1F)** pattern to practice this movement (Fig. 34-6B). Any of the techniques in Table 34-9 would also be appropriate with the D1F depending on the patient's lower extremity strength and control. The therapist may also use slow reversal, gradually increasing the range of movement. An alternative strategy is for the opposite leg to push down into the bed, using the force to push the body over into sidelying.

A third segmental strategy is to initiate the movement with bilateral or unilateral upper extremities. The therapist could use a unilateral PNF D1F pattern, maintaining the patient's elbow in extension or a bilateral pattern such as a **lift**. A momentum-based strategy works well with either a unilateral or bilateral upper extremity pattern. The movement is initiated with the patient's head turning to the side he is rolling toward. Simultaneously, the upper extremity(ies) reaches up and across the body. The lower extremity can assist by lifting and rotating over the opposite side of the body as the body moves into sidelying or prone. The patient can build momentum by rocking the upper extremities side to side before the final reach over (see Chapter 26). As noted previously, the therapist can also use SR, gradually increasing the range of movement.

Because individuals with a *complete spinal cord injury* lack the trunk motor control needed for completing the task of rolling, compensation is taught immediately. One method is to use momentum from the upper extremities to translate down through the trunk passively to create enough force to complete the task. This is accomplished by swinging the arms to one side and then to the other. When this is done with enough force, the patient's trunk will rock back and forth with increased amplitude with each repetition. The patient will then throw the upper extremities with increased effort in the desired direction of rolling one last time to accomplish the task (see Fig. 26-7ABC). When the patient is first learning this method, the therapist can facilitate by crossing the leg that is opposite the direction of rolling over the leg that is in the direction of rolling. If this is still too difficult, the therapist can provide manual assistance to the patient's legs to make the task easier.

In the patient with C5 or C6 tetraplegia, this task is more difficult because of the lack of triceps muscle control to keep the elbows straight while swinging the arms side to side to attain the momentum to roll. Keeping the arms straight can be accomplished by two methods. The first method is to have the individual externally rotate his shoulders until the elbow crease is facing upward. This allows gravity to keep the elbows straight as long as the individual does not flex the shoulders too high. The second method is to internally rotate the shoulders and lock out the hands together in shoulder flexion to allow the horizontal adductors of the shoulder to act in a closed chain manner to keep the elbow straight. After the shoulders are straight, the task can be accomplished as described previously. Another method is adapting the patient's bed to assist with rolling. Grab bars, hooks, or bed ladders can provide leverage to complete the task of rolling (see Fig. 26-9AB).

Many individuals with a spinal cord injury can perform supine to long sit with greater ease than rolling. They may choose to transition to long sitting and then cross their legs with their upper extremities and transition to sidelying from long sit. See Chapter 26 regarding the transition from supine to long sit (Fig. 26-13A–H).

## THINK ABOUT IT 34.3

- How might you alter the environment to either increase or decrease the challenge for the patient?
- How might neglect contribute to a patient's ability to relearn how to roll?
- How might bedding (sheets, comforters, etc.) or an individual's bedclothes affect the ability to roll?

### *Horizontal: Prone on Elbows*

Prone on elbows is most typically used as a key component of bed mobility in individuals with a complete cervical spinal cord injury. During prone on elbows, cocontraction of the head, neck, scapula, and shoulders is facilitated; gravity resists the head, neck, and upper trunk extensors. The position has a large base of support and a low center of gravity.

In children or adults with a head injury and abnormal tonic reflexes, prone on elbows helps them learn to vary the head position without allowing a change in posturing of the arms. Righting reactions help to maintain the head in vertical. **Caution:** This posture is not appropriate for patients with increased lordosis, respiratory dysfunction, or other conditions that make being on their stomachs stressful.

## Assumption of Position

From prone with arms in abduction and external rotation, the patient uses momentum of head side-side movement to weight shift onto one elbow and then the other while alternatively pulling each elbow into adduction until the elbows are positioned under the shoulders (walking the elbows in; see Fig. 26-10ABC). The therapist may assist with the lifting and/or the side-to-side weight shift. Another strategy is to begin from sidelying. As the patient rolls over into prone, he places the swing arm so that the elbow is under the shoulder as he completes the weight shift over. At the same time, the arm the patient was lying on pushes into abduction to complete the weight shift, followed by pulling that elbow into position.

## Stability

To help build a patient's ability to maintain prone on elbows, the therapist can apply AIs and RS with manual contacts at the shoulders, forearms, and/or hands (Fig. 34-7A). Moving more distally increases the difficulty of the task. The angle of pressure can vary from almost vertical with emphasis on approximation to almost horizontal with emphasis on resistance. When approximation is emphasized, it is important that the patient's arm be at a 90-degree angle to the shoulder joint.

## Controlled Mobility

To promote the patient's ability to control weight shifting side to side in prone on elbows, the therapist can use **SRH** or **SR**, moving through increasing increments of range (small to large) (Fig. 34-7B). Manual contacts are typically at the shoulders.

## Static/Dynamic

To move into the long sitting position, individuals with a spinal cord injury commonly begin in prone on elbows and walk on the elbows around toward the knees. This is followed by one arm hooking underneath the thigh and pulling up into sitting while the other arm provides the push from the elbow. To accomplish the skill of walking on the elbows while prone-on-elbows, the patient must build dynamic stability in the shoulder joint to allow weight-bearing on one elbow while lifting and moving the other. This static-dynamic movement can be practiced with different tasks such as reaching for objects with one arm while the other is in weight-bearing, playing one-handed catch, or providing resistance to the free arm while moving.

## Horizontal: Hands and Knees/Quadruped/All-Fours

Quadruped in adults is used most often as a position of transition between other postures or positions, such as moving from sitting on the floor to standing. This position facilitates upper and lower trunk strength and control; increased range of motion in the trunk, hips, shoulders, knees and wrists; and weight acceptance through the pelvis and shoulder girdle. It has a smaller base of support and higher center of gravity than other horizontal positions, and an increased number of joints

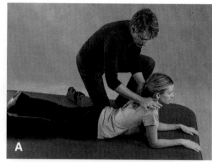
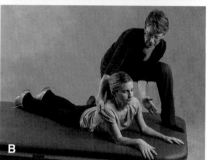

FIGURE 34-7 (A) Alternating isometrics in prone on elbows promoting stability and (B) controlled mobility in prone on elbows using slow reversal hold or slow reversal.

are needed to control the position relative to prone on elbows. To maintain and move within this position, a patient must combat the resistance of gravity. The maintained pressure on the long finger flexor and quadriceps tendon may decrease tone in these muscle groups in individuals with spasticity.

## Assumption of the Position

To assist a poststroke individual into the all-fours position, the patient should begin in the sidelying position with the involved side on top. The therapist is best positioned on the patient's involved side. The patient flexes both legs up into flexion. As the patient pushes with both the uninvolved leg and arm into abduction, the therapist helps the patient weight shift up and over onto the involved knee and helps to place the involved upper extremity in weight-bearing, supporting elbow extension as needed and trying to achieve heel of hand weight-bearing if possible (protect the functional tenodesis in individuals with tetraplegia by keeping the fingers in flexion). With weight shifted onto the involved arm and leg, the patient can finish positioning the uninvolved hand and knee into alignment under the shoulder and hip. In this transition into all-fours, the patient utilizes his stronger components.

## Stability

To help build the patient's ability to maintain quadruped, the therapist can apply AIs and RS with manual contacts at the shoulders, pelvis, or shoulders and pelvis (Fig. 34-8AB). Moving more distally increases the difficulty of the task. As with prone on elbows, the angle of pressure varies depending on the need for approximation or resistance. The therapist can utilize quick approximation and maintained approximation and also quick adjustments in this posture.

## Controlled Mobility

To promote a patient's ability to control weight shifting in all directions (side-side, forward-back, cross diagonal, around in a circle), the therapist can use SRH or SR moving through increasing increments of range (small to large). Manual contacts are typically at the shoulders. Individuals with ataxia may benefit from moving through gradually decreasing decrements of range (large to small), learning to grade forces and improve proximal stability.

## Static/Dynamic

As in prone on elbows, locomotion in quadruped (creeping) is considered a *skill* movement. To creep, the patient must be able to momentarily lift one arm and leg while weight-bearing on the others. The patient can practice lifting one arm (Fig. 34-8C),

then one leg, and then an opposite arm and leg together (Fig. 34-8D) while maintaining balance control on the remaining weight-bearing limbs. The therapist can work with the patient on reaching activities with one arm, throwing-catching, or providing resistance to the free moving arm. The patient can practice lifting the opposite leg during these activities to increase the demand and difficulty of the task.

## Skill

As stated, skill in quadruped is creeping. In adults, creeping is used as a means of locomotion while one is on the floor, usually to move toward a piece of furniture that can be used as an assist for the transition back into standing. A therapist can strengthen a patient's ability to creep by providing resistance in the form of weights or manual resistance at the ankles or pelvis.

### Contemplate Clinical Decisions

*Refer to the case of the patient with PD presented earlier:*

1. During which stage(s) of motor control (mobility, stability, controlled mobility, static-dynamic, skill) do you anticipate this patient will have the most difficulty?
2. During which functional tasks in horizontal does this patient have the most difficulty?
3. Design an initial treatment program to improve this patient's function in horizontal.
4. Design a plan for progressing your treatment.
5. How would you modify your treatment if it was too difficult for the patient?
6. How would you modify your treatment if it was too easy for the patient?
7. Given what you know about the effects of auditory and visual stimulation on movement in individuals with PD, how might you modify your program to make it more successful?
8. What aspects of your program would you include in a home program?

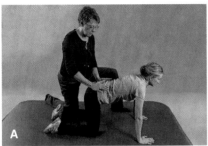
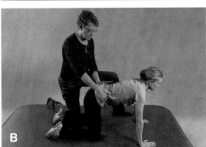
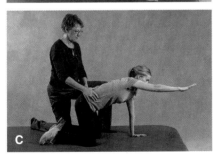
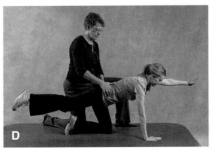

**FIGURE 34-8** Quadruped stability using (A) alternating isometrics and (B) rhythmic stabilization. Static-dynamic work in quadruped (C) lifting one arm and (D) lifting opposite arm and leg.

## Pediatric Considerations

The principles described previously also apply to the pediatric population. In general, use creativity in age-appropriate play to encourage normal developmental tasks, playing in and moving through various positions in horizontal. Progress from gravity-eliminated movements to working against gravity (e.g., it may be easier to reach for a toy in sidelying than in supine). When the child is unable to complete the movements, you can give assistance, but it should be gradually reduced to encourage the child to take on greater control (e.g., bring the child's feet to the hands to encourage body awareness/exploration).

External supports can be used to provide an opportunity for the child to practice in positions he may not be able to do by himself (e.g., prop the child on a pillow in prone on elbows, place prone on hands over a ball or wedge, or place in quadruped over a ball with rocking forward and back to encourage weight shifting). Sensory experiences may be needed for children whose motor output is affected by sensory impairment (e.g., tactile, visual, vestibular, proprioceptive, body awareness).

Initially, the newborn spends much of his time in horizontal, sleeping with intermittent bouts of wakefulness and activity. Care should be taken with positioning while sleeping or eating and during prone "tummy time." In supine, encourage the child to follow brightly colored objects with his/her head and later reaching or rolling toward those objects. Provide tummy time for the infant to practice lifting his head and upper trunk. Find interesting toys or objects to encourage the infant to lift his head and trunk, progressing to prone on elbows and prone on hands. Move objects to the side to encourage weight shifts in controlled mobility and reaching skill tasks.

For older children who need to work on these skills, interest in the activity is key for maintaining motivation. For example, playing "Superman" strengthens the extensor musculature (pivot prone), or the child can shoot Nerf basketballs while on his hands and knees over a therapy ball.

## ■ Considerations for Nontherapy Time and Discharge

### Patient and Family Education

Given the patient's limited time in therapy each day, key principles in critical horizontal skills must be practiced outside therapy time. Safety should be a primary concern whenever nontherapy-time motor practice or a home exercise program is planned.

Treatment in horizontal positions often happens early in a patient's rehabilitation process. In the poststroke patient, family members may be hesitant to handle the hemiplegic side, or they may mishandle the patient (e.g., pulling on his arm). To ensure appropriate interactions with family and friends, they should be brought in early as members of the treatment team and given instructions on the following topics:

- The nature of the movement impairments, neglect, body awareness
- Addressing the patient from the hemiplegic side (talking, placement of items the patient needs, touching, helping with feeding and other ADLs)
- Proper positioning in supine and sidelying
- Proper handling of the hemiplegic arm

- How to assist with rolling, bridging, scooting, and other bed/mat movements to encourage symmetry, control, and muscle activity
- How to judge the level of assistance needed to foster independence and motor control versus doing too much for the patient

### Activities for Home

The patient and family should be encouraged to practice sufficient repetitions of specific bed/mat/floor activities during nontherapy hours to further enhance motor learning through neural plasticity. Because of the inherent stability of the horizontal position, skills such as bridging and prone-on-elbows activities are relatively safe to practice in the home environment. Activities such as scooting and rolling require that the patient be safely positioned so the task does not move him to the edge of the bed, where he risks falling off. Moving into the quadruped position and ultimately creeping brings the center of mass away from the support surface, adding instability to the system, to which the patient must respond with increasing equilibrium reactions.

The home exercise program should be limited to three to five exercises to avoid overwhelming the patient and to improve compliance. Build exercises into everyday functional tasks and hobbies/interests. For example, place the patient's glasses, flashlight, or family pictures on the bedside table and ask him to turn his head and reach for an object during rolling. This encourages segmental upper extremity–initiated rolling. Also consider the environment, such as suggesting silk sheets to foster ease of movement in bed and decrease the chance of getting tangled in the sheets. Another suggestion is to use one top sheet along with a lightweight comforter instead of a sheet, blanket, and bedspread (i.e., decreased weight and number of items under which to maneuver).

### Contemplate Clinical Decisions

*Consider the patient with PD presented at the beginning of this chapter.*

- *What instructions would you provide to the patient?*
- *When considering a home program, what safety issues concern you?*
- *What tasks or exercises would you prescribe for him to practice at home? Why?*
- *How might you design the task practice to encourage improved initiation of horizontal movements?*
- *How many times would you want him to practice during the day?*
- *How might you alter the environment to make his movement in horizontal more efficient?*

# HANDS-ON PRACTICE

Be sure to practice the following skills from this chapter. With further practice, you should be able to:

- Position a patient who demonstrates changes in muscle tone (high or low) in supine and sidelying.
- Instruct/guide/assist a patient into bridging, prone on elbows, and quadruped.
- Use any of the following proprioceptive neuromuscular facilitation (PNF) techniques in bridging, rolling, prone on elbows, and quadruped:
  - Mobility: hold relax active movement; rhythmic initiation; repeated contractions; replication
  - Stability: alternating isometrics, rhythmic stabilization

- Controlled mobility: slow reversal hold, slow reversal, agonistic reversals
- Strengthening: appropriate resistance or assistance
- Instruct/guide/assist a patient in scooting sideways or up in bed
- Instruct/guide/assist a patient in rolling from supine to sidelying
- Use the following strategies to instruct/guide/assist a patient in rolling: lower trunk rotation; bilateral or unilateral upper or lower extremity PNF diagonal patterns (D1, D2); momentum

## Let's Review

1. Describe normal movement components of horizontal functions such as bridging, scooting, rolling, prone on elbows, and quadruped.

2. List appropriate patient examination strategies for functions in horizontal.

3. Identify impairments that may underlie movement abnormalities in horizontal.

4. Identify important safety considerations for patient function in horizontal.

5. Identify indicators for predicting prognosis of movement function in horizontal.

6. Outline appropriate treatment interventions to improve function in horizontal.

7. What evidence supports patient management in horizontal?

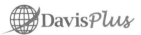 For additional resources, including Focus on Evidence tables, case study discussions, references and glossary, please visit http://davisplus.fadavis.com

## CHAPTER SUMMARY

Important functional activities during rest, sleep, and recreational activities take place in horizontal; a few examples include rolling, changing position in bed, scooting, getting in/out of bed, managing sheets or pillows, reaching for the telephone on the bedside table or setting the alarm, watching television, and sexual activity. Most commonly, we lie in horizontal when resting or sleeping.

This chapter focuses on the promotion of functional activities in horizontal to help the individual with neurological dysfunction increase independence. Typical movement patterns, impairments underlying movement problems, safety considerations, examination components, and lifespan influences are discussed. Interventions to address functional activity limitations are presented in the context of different functional activities in horizontal and stages of motor control (mobility, stability, controlled mobility and skill). Sample patient cases illustrate treating dysfunction in horizontal in individuals with different neurological diagnoses. Although evidence supporting many of the intervention techniques is lacking, the online (ONL) Focus on Evidence Tables 34-10, 34-11, and 34-12 summarize the most important recent studies addressing this topic.

# Functional Activity Intervention in Sitting

**CHAPTER 35**

Reva P. Rauk, PT, PhD, MMSc, NCS ▪ Kathy L. Mercuris, PT, DHS

## CHAPTER OUTLINE

## CHAPTER OBJECTIVES

Upon completion of this chapter, the learner should be able to:
1. Describe normal patterns of movement in sitting.
2. Describe possible impairments underlying abnormal movements in sitting.
3. Identify safety considerations for the management of individuals with altered function in sitting.
4. Identify and describe components of an evaluation of function in sitting.
5. Describe appropriate interventions for various individuals who present with altered function in sitting.
6. Design appropriate goals, expected outcomes, and plan of care for a given patient with sitting dysfunction.

## ▪ Introduction

Performing activities in sitting is essential to daily function. How much time we spend in sitting depends on our work/ play/life demands, but it can be quite significant (e.g., working at a computer, attending meetings and conferences, reading, studying, and driving). In addition, many activities of daily living (ADLs) and instrumental activities of daily living (IADLs) take place in sitting, such as eating meals, toileting, putting on socks and shoes, writing, watching movies or sporting events, and paying bills.

Take a moment to review your day and identify just how much time you spent sitting. What activities did you do in sitting? How many activities required sitting, or did you choose to do them in sitting rather than in standing or in another position?

Because we spend so much time functioning in sitting, this is an important area to remediate or restore in our patients. This chapter focuses on functional activities in sitting such as

seated scooting and transfers, as well as fostering the trunk control needed for these activities. Interventions specific to upper extremity (UE) function in sitting are addressed in Chapter 33.

## Typical Characteristics/Patterns of Movement in Sitting

The terms **sitting** and **seated position** describe a posture in which the trunk is generally upright, with the base of support consisting mostly of the ischial tuberosities and perhaps the posterior thighs and feet. During sitting activities, the trunk moves in one or a combination of three planes of movement: flexion/extension, lateral flexion, and rotation. Furthermore, the head, trunk, and extremities move together in typical patterns depending on the task demands.

In addition to being able to isolate and separate movements of the upper and lower trunk in sitting, an individual must be able to combine trunk movements with UEs or lower extremities (LEs) to perform a functional task while maintaining balance and equilibrium under changing environmental contexts (e.g., feet on the floor or dangling, sitting with or without back support, sitting on a high stool, sitting on surfaces of varying compliancy).

A variety of head movements occur normally depending on the task at hand in sitting (Campbell, 2001). Campbell identified no consistent pattern of head flexion/extension during reaching; however, subjects tended to rotate their heads opposite to the direction of the reach slightly (12 ± 10 degrees). Table 35-1 identifies components and combinations of normal trunk movements typically observed in seated activities (Ryerson, 1997).

Muscle activation patterns in the trunk and limbs during sitting depend on the base of support (whether feet or hands are in weight-bearing), how far we need to move (distance), and the speed of movement needed for a functional activity (Carr, 1998). When the feet are unsupported, the pelvis and trunk muscles control movement. Hip flexors/extensors control sagittal plane movement, and abductors/adductors control frontal plane movement. Once the feet are placed on the floor, lower leg muscles act to stabilize the body. Because of the increased base of support, patients can move much farther when their feet are in weight-bearing than when they are not (Chari, 1986). Healthy individuals are able to reach the farthest with both feet on the floor (Chari, 1986). With one foot and then both feet off the ground, reaching distance progressively decreases (Chari, 1986). Thigh support also allows for greater reach distances but only when both feet are off the ground (Chari, 1986).

| TABLE 35-1 | Patterns of Trunk Movements in Sitting* |
|---|---|
| **POSITION** | **TRUNK PATTERN OF MOVEMENT** |
| Erect sitting | "Sitting tall," the spine is in a neutral position including slight lumbar extension, with the shoulders in alignment over the hips in all planes (sagittal, coronal, and transverse) |
| Relaxed sitting | "Slumped sitting," the spine is forward flexed with the shoulders in alignment over the hips (not back, forward, or rotated) |
| Upper trunk forward (anterior) weight shift | The head and neck begin the movement with the trunk sequentially flexing forward (e.g., as in reaching straight forward to the floor with both hands to pick up a ball) |
| Upper trunk extension (posterior) weight shift | The head and neck begin the movement into extension; the shoulders may stay in line with or move posterior to the hips; weight shifts posteriorly (e.g., as in looking straight overhead at a ceiling light fixture) |
| Upper trunk lateral weight shift | The arm and shoulder on one side begin a sideways movement by dipping toward the hip; the weight shifts onto the same side hip and leg (e.g., as in reaching sideways to pick up an object off the floor) |
| Upper trunk forward flexion with rotation | The head, neck, and upper trunk begin movement with forward flexion combined with rotation to one side; the weight shifts forward onto the same side hip, leg, and foot (e.g., as in reaching down to the floor to one side) |
| Upper trunk extension with rotation | The head, neck, and upper trunk begin movement into extension with rotation; the weight shifts posteriorly onto the same side (e.g., as in reaching up and behind you) |
| Lower trunk extension (anterior) weight shift | The pelvis and lumbar spine begin movement into extension with an anterior pelvic tilt, trunk extension, and hip flexion; the weight shifts forward toward the legs and feet (e.g., as in reaching forward and up to a bookshelf) |
| Lower trunk flexion (posterior) weight shift | The pelvis and lumbar spine begin movement with a posterior pelvic tilt and trunk flexion; the weight shifts posteriorly (e.g., as in lifting a knee to the chest) |
| Lower trunk lateral weight shift | While an anterior pelvic tilt is maintained, the pelvis and lumbar spine begin movement to one side; the weight shifts to the same side hip and leg. The spine stays erect with a convexity on the weight-bearing side and a concavity on the unweighted side (e.g., as in reaching up and sideways to the right) |
| Lower trunk flexion with rotation | The pelvis and lower trunk begin movement with a posterior pelvic tilt continuing into trunk flexion and rotation to the opposite side; the weight shifts posteriorly and to one side while the trunk rotates to the opposite side (e.g., as in slumping backward to the left and turning the shoulders to the right) |
| Lower trunk extension with rotation | The pelvis and lower trunk begin movement with an anterior pelvic tilt continuing into trunk extension and rotation to the same side; the weight shifts forward and to one side while the trunk rotates to the same side (e.g., as in reaching across to the left with the right hand) |

*Adapted from Ryerson S, Levit K. *Functional Movement Reeducation.* New York, NY: Churchill Livingstone; 1997.

Depending on the speed of movement, the leg muscles also act to either assist or brake movement. The tibialis anterior muscle activates in advance of and during an arm movement (a reaching task), whereas the soleus acts to slow forward trunk movement (Crosbie, 1995). LE muscles become more involved as we move toward and outside our base of support and are also more active with faster movements (Dean, 1997). Patients can reach the farthest and the fastest when they have the most support, such as that provided by both thighs and the feet (Chari, 1986; Dean, 1997).

## Clinical Picture of Functional Activities in Sitting

Most functional activities in sitting use the UEs. Our trunk plays a critical role in providing the foundational stability we need to carry out tasks. Some activities are completed relatively close to midline and require only small adjustments in our trunk to maintain balance. Other activities, such as reaching laterally outside our base of support for an object or moving to a new position, require greater control and activity from not just our trunk but also our arms and legs. To maintain stability, we control our body segments in relation to each other, the supporting surfaces, and the environment (Perennou, 2001). The timing and degree to which our trunk and limb muscles activate depends on the distance excursion of the movement, whether we have our feet or hands in weight-bearing as part of the base of support, and the speed at which we move (Ryerson, 1997).

Loss of the ability to maintain and control movement in sitting results in functional activity limitations and the inability to independently participate in our daily roles. Sitting function is considered a key prerequisite for regaining independence in ADLs and mobility after a neurological injury (Feigin, 1996; Nichols, 1996; Smith, 1999; Tyson, 2007).

Persons with neurological conditions often demonstrate typical abnormal postures and movements in sitting. In individuals who have experienced a stroke, the major impairments in trunk muscle activity responsible for altered sitting postures and movements include decreased muscle activity in lateral trunk muscles on the paretic side, delayed muscle activity onset on the paretic side, and impaired coordination/synchronization of muscle activity (Dickstein, 2000, 2004). Typical sitting postures and movement variations seen in individuals with common neurological diagnoses are described in Box 35-1.

---

### BOX 35-1  Typical Abnormal Sitting Postures and Movements: Components That Should Be Addressed

#### Stroke—Hemiplegia

1. Spinal flexion (slump) with posterior pelvic tilt, weight-bearing shifted to unimpaired side, lateral trunk and neck flexion to the impaired side, unimpaired shoulder appears higher, and forward head; may see posterior rotation of the impaired side compared with the unimpaired side.

   After a stroke, individuals may show excessive lateral weight shift to the unimpaired side when reaching forward, decreased lateral weight shift when reaching to the unimpaired side, and decreased head movements during reaching.

2. Spinal flexion with posterior pelvic tilt, increased weight-bearing on the impaired side with lateral flexion to the unimpaired side with impaired shoulder appearing higher, forward head; may see the hemiplegic side rotated more posteriorly compared with the unimpaired side.

   With scapular abduction and downward rotation, depending on tonal abnormalities, the impaired arm may be limp at the side or held in a flexion posture.

   The hip may be abducted. Weight-bearing on the impaired foot may be decreased during forward unilateral and bilateral reaching and when reaching toward the impaired side. In one study, unilateral and bilateral reaching toward the sound side resulted in symmetrical weight-bearing on both feet (Messier, 2005).

   (Campbell, 2001; Messier, 2005; O'Sullivan, 2007; Ryerson, 1997; Tessem, 2007)

#### Stroke—Contraversive Pushing (Pusher Syndrome)

Pusher syndrome (contraversive pushing): a perceptual deficit after some strokes, with active pushing away from the unimpaired side and increasing weight shift toward the impaired side, which is unable to support the weight. Individuals sit with trunk leaning toward the impaired side and the unimpaired upper and/or lower extremity (if in weight-bearing) abducted and extended. Increased pelvic tilt with normal head orientation correlates with increased balance loss in sitting. Individuals resist passive correction of the leaning posture. (Karnath, 2003; Perennou, 2002; Roller, 2004)

#### Spinal Cord Injury (SCI)—Tetraplegia

Excessive spinal flexion with posterior pelvic tilt; flexion tends to be midline and symmetrical; shoulder protraction and forward head; and weight-bearing on bilateral upper extremities for support. Degree of forward spinal flexion depends on the level of injury. (Hobson, 1992; Sisto, 2009)

#### Parkinson Disease

Spinal flexion with posterior pelvic tilt; may see slight asymmetry of weight-bearing, forward head.

## Possible Impairments Underlying Abnormal Function in Sitting

Many body structure and functional impairments contribute to abnormal function in sitting. To design an appropriate plan of care, the therapist should identify which impairments contribute to a patient's functional limitations. Often, several impairments contribute to a single problem in sitting. Table 35-2 identifies examples of impairments that may contribute to problems in sitting. Therapists must consider which impairments are a primary result of the neurological condition and which may be secondary effects.

## Safety Considerations

A major safety consideration in sitting is a loss of balance or a potential fall. The therapist should determine the amount of assistance needed or degree of guarding required on the basis of the tasks requested and the patient's abilities. Box 35-2 includes a list of questions to consider when determining the level of assistance needed for safety.

During the initial examination and early intervention sessions, the patient should never be left alone while in an unsupported sitting position, and great care should be taken when the patient is sitting on the edge of a mat or the edge of a wheelchair. The therapist should plan ahead and have necessary equipment and support personnel available before positioning the patient in unsupported sitting. A gait belt is used to give the therapist an advantage in preventing a fall. The therapist should always have a free hand to protect against a fall or provide a manual contact for patients needing assistance to maintain unsupported sitting. The manual contacts for guarding the patient are determined by the amount of assistance needed, the task, and the location of the therapist in relation to the patient. All health-care providers and caregivers should be taught to avoid pulling on a weak impaired UE to assist with balance or transfers. For example, a patient with tetraplegia may initially require a person at both the right and left sides with manual contacts on each shoulder and on the gait belt to maintain a seated position.

The therapist may sit on either the impaired or unimpaired side of a person with hemiplegia. Patients with hemiplegia tend to lose balance toward the impaired side. When the therapist is sitting on the impaired side, manual contacts may be on the shoulder and gait belt or on the gait belt and the impaired extremity to assist or protect it during exercises. When additional support is needed, you can place the arm closest to the patient around the patient's waist to guard from posterior and lateral falls while the other arm is ready to catch any forward imbalance. You may choose to sit in front of a patient with manual contacts on the extremities or a gait belt to provide visual feedback, work on lateral weight shifts, or during anterior reaching tasks. Sitting behind the patient might be best when in **long sitting** with a posterior pelvic tilt because a posterior loss of balance is most probable. Be especially alert to potential falls when the patient is fatigued or when new tasks are attempted.

| TABLE 35-2 | Examples of Impairments That Contribute to Abnormal Function in Sitting |
|---|---|
| **CATEGORY** | **IMPAIRMENT** |
| Aerobic capacity/ endurance | Hypertension or hypotension<br>Shortness of breath<br>Impaired oxygen saturation<br>Perceived exertion<br>Note: Abnormal sitting posture and postural control may contribute to alterations in aerobic capacity and endurance |
| Arousal, attention, and cognition | Inability to maintain attention<br>Altered level of consciousness<br>Decreased cooperation, motivation<br>Inability to process commands<br>Impaired orientation (person, place, time, situation)<br>Impaired judgment/insight<br>Aphasia<br>Impaired recall, memory<br>Abnormal perception of midline/vertical |
| Cranial and peripheral nerve integrity | Impaired vision: acuity, visual field loss<br>Vestibular impairments |
| Joint integrity and mobility | Impaired joint mobility in the spine, rib cage, shoulders, and hips |
| Motor function | Impaired motor control: rate and frequency of neural activation<br>Incoordination: timing and coordination of muscle contractions<br>Presence of atypical movements<br>Dysfunctional movement/posture<br>Apraxia (Spinazzola 2003) |
| Muscle performance | Weakness/paralysis<br>Decreased power<br>Decreased muscle endurance |
| Pain | Level of pain |
| Range of motion | Limited range of motion (active and passive)<br>Impaired muscle length, extensibility, and flexibility |
| Reflex integrity | Abnormal deep tendon reflexes<br>Impaired postural reflexes, equilibrium, and righting reactions<br>Abnormal muscle tone (resistance to passive stretch) |
| Sensory integrity | Impaired light touch<br>Impaired sharp/dull<br>Impaired vibration<br>Impaired proprioception<br>Sensory integration/weighting dysfunction<br>Impaired perception |

**BOX 35-2   Questions a Therapist May Explore to Ensure Patient Safety and Identify Aspects of Intervention Needing Extra Attention**

| Patient considerations | 1. What is the patient's cognitive status? Is the patient able to follow one- or two-step commands? Does the patient have insight to his condition and abilities? Is the patient impulsive or lacking appropriate judgment? |
|---|---|
| | 2. Is the patient intrinsically motivated to remain in sitting? Is fatigue a factor in the patient's abilities? |
| | 3. Is the patient's perception altered? Does the patient recognize figure ground differences and depth perception? How is the patient's vision? Does the patient have unilateral neglect? |
| | 4. Does the patient have tactile sensory impairments affecting feedback from support surfaces? |
| Posture | 1. Does the patient need physical assistance to maintain sitting, or can the patient sit independently? |
| | 2. Given the abnormal sitting postures outlined in Table 35-3 or from your observational examination, will the resting posture predispose the patient to a loss of balance in a particular direction? |
| | 3. Does the patient exhibit any protective extension or equilibrium reactions? If yes, in what directions and how quickly are they implemented? |
| The task | 1. Can a meaningful task be safely incorporated into the treatment session? |
| | 2. Is balance difficult to maintain with volitional active movements or with unexpected perturbations (feed forward or feedback)? |
| | 3. Is the patient sitting on a stationary or moving support surface while performing tasks? |
| | 4. What speed of movement and strength are required for task completion? |
| | 5. Can the patient perform weight shifts/reaching in all planes, or do certain directions increase the risk of loss of balance? |
| Diagnosis/Prognosis | 1. Will the patient's balance improve or worsen over time? |
| | 2. What expected abnormal sitting postures might develop? |
| | 3. What assistive devices are or will be needed to maintain sitting? |
| | 4. On the basis of the patient's goals and diagnosis, what seated positions will be utilized for function? |

Other considerations for safety include protecting body parts from injury. In patients with UE paralysis/paresis, be sure to place the hand in an appropriate weight-bearing position for the functional task and avoid a dependent hanging position (see Chapter 18). In patients with tetraplegia, be sure to keep their fingers curled in flexion when their hands are in weight-bearing to preserve a functional tenodesis grip (see Chapter 26). In patients with impaired protective sensation, also work to minimize shearing forces during scooting or transfers by ensuring good clearance of the patient's buttocks and minimizing sliding across a surface, especially the edges.

## THINK ABOUT IT 35.1

1. Where would you guard the patient in the following scenarios:
   a. Patient with hemiplegia who repeatedly loses balance to the impaired side
   b. Patient with hemiplegia working on side-to-side scooting on the edge of the bed
   c. Patient with a C6 spinal cord injury who is short sitting on the edge of a therapy mat
2. How would you support the flaccid upper extremity of a person with hemiplegia during a sit-to-stand transfer?

## Lifespan Influence

### Developmental Considerations

During the first 2 weeks of life, sitting is maintained only through support offered by the caregiver or by furniture. Functional sitting is not possible for the neonate because he is unable to maintain the head in an upright position for more than a few seconds (Campbell, 2012, p. 55). Poor control is a result of the relatively large size and weight of the head, weakness in the spinal extensors resulting in a flexed "C" curve with a posterior pelvic tilt position, and lack of awareness of head and body position (Bly, 1994, p. 7). Over the first 3 months of life, the strength of the antigravity spinal extensors increases, followed by activation of the cervical flexors, so the head can be maintained in an upright position for increased periods (Bly, 1994, p. 27).

Health-care professionals often use a **pull-to-sit maneuver** as part of assessing infant development and head control. The examiner grasps the hands and forearms of the supine infant and gently pulls him to a seated position while carefully monitoring the head position. There is a gradual progression from a complete head lag to the infant attempting to assist by flexing the head, trunk, and UEs during the first 3 months of life. However, the task remains difficult and is performed inconsistently (Bly, 1994, p. 38). Once the infant is seated with handheld assist, scapular adduction increases the thoracic extension and provides stability for the head position. Even with the increasing activation of both trunk flexors and extensors, the infant remains too weak and lacks equilibrium for independent sitting. The infant maintains a slight posterior pelvic tilt with weight-bearing through the ischial tuberosities. The LEs gradually become more externally rotated and abducted, but they are still not in contact with the floor and are unable to offer stability in the seated posture (Bly, 1994, p. 39).

By the end of the fourth month of life, the infant's sternocleidomastoids, capital cervical flexors, and abdominals work together as he uses the UEs to assist with pull-to-sit. The optical and vestibular systems are maturing, and there is evidence the infant is anticipating and preparing for the pull-to-sit test. This may indicate the use of a feed-forward mechanism for motor control (Bly, 1994, pp. 66, 68). The 4 month-old is able to maintain unsupported sitting for a few seconds. The infant is positioned with the trunk slightly forward of the hips, and the spinal extensors are providing the stability for the upright posture. Therefore, any head movement results in a weight shift and a loss of balance (Bly, 1994, p. 69).

When the child is placed in a posture, the ability to maintain the position occurs before the ability to assume the posture independently. The infant is able to maintain independent ring sitting (Fig. 35-1) or static balance when placed in the posture at 5 to 6 months of age. During the fifth month, the infant is able to sit erect with only the hands held and can briefly maintain the position with UE weight-bearing in a forward propped position (Bly, 1994, p. 99).

By 6 months of age, the infant has increased trunk strength and has learned to control the degrees of freedom to allow independent sitting with UE play; however, lateral reaching with weight shift and cervical rotation may still result in a fall. The pelvis is now in a neutral position, and weight-bearing is through the ischial tuberosities. As equilibrium and righting reactions are gained over the next several months, the child learns how to transition into varied sitting postures (Figs. 35-1 to 35-6).

Postural control is gained through practice and is supported by the integration of multiple systems. Righting reactions orient the head to horizontal or move a body part into alignment with the head. Examples of **righting reactions** include optical righting, labyrinthine righting, body-on-head righting, and neck-on-body righting. The onset for these reactions is 2 to 4 months of age, and they will integrate at 5 years with the exception of the optical and labyrinthine reactions, which persist throughout life (Barnes, 1984, p. 222).

**Protective extension** reactions of the UEs, which are used to prevent a fall, develop in the anterior direction at 6 to 7 months of age and progress to lateral protection at 7 to 8 months and to posterior protection at 9 to 10 months in sitting (Barnes, 1984, p. 222). These uniplanar motions allow practice and strengthening of the trunk muscles and lead to the development of rotational and diagonal control, which is essential for equilibrium reactions. Eventually, protective responses are used only when equilibrium reactions

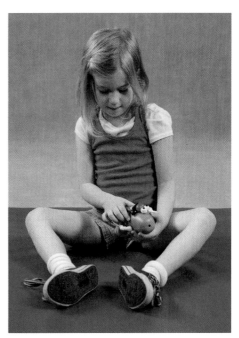

FIGURE 35-1 Ring sitting.

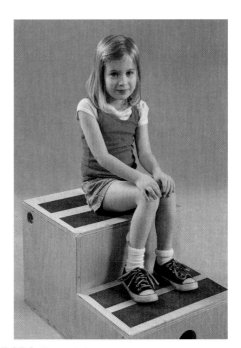

FIGURE 35-2 Short sitting.

are not sufficient to maintain postural control (Cech, 2002, p. 377). **Equilibrium reactions** result in the body moving in the opposite direction of a perturbation or weight shift and include the total body response of rotational or diagonal motions of the trunk and extremities.

The ability to dissociate trunk and LE movements, combined with the equilibrium response, is necessary for transitioning between postures. The 6 to 8 month-old becomes more proficient in independently transitioning into multiple sitting postures (described in the next paragraph) from prone,

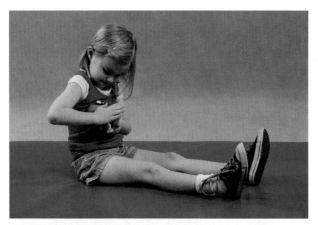

FIGURE 35-3 Long sitting.

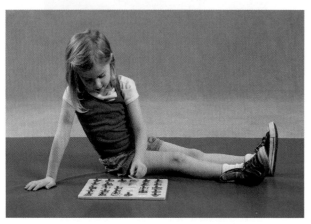

FIGURE 35-4 Long sitting with lateral weight shift and trunk rotation.

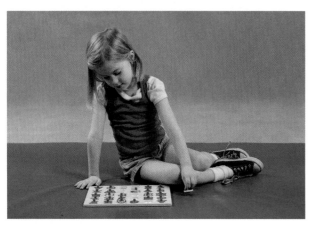

**FIGURE 35-5** Side sitting.

sidelying, or quadruped. Sitting becomes functional once the child can change positions and use the UEs for play in sitting without falling.

During the next several months, an increase in lumbar extension develops in sitting with dynamic hip-pelvic-trunk postural control (Bly, 1994, p. 148). The seated base of support narrows with a decrease in hip abduction and an increase in knee extension. Full cervical and trunk rotation

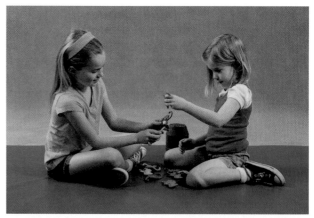

**FIGURE 35-6** The older child on the left exhibits crossed-ankle sitting while the younger child shows a W-sit position.

along with altered LE positions result in greater weight shifts and improved function. The infant explores postural control with active anterior and posterior pelvic tilts.

Development of a variety of seated positions and smooth transitions between them is expected. Seated positions include (1) **short sitting** on a chair or bench with hips and knees at 90 degrees (Fig. 35-2); (2) long sitting with slight variation of LE positions (Figs. 35-3 and 35-4); (3) symmetry in LE positions that may be seen with a **"straddle" sit**; (4) **side sitting** with both legs off to one side, which is frequently used to transition to and from sitting (Fig. 35-5); (5) **crossed-ankle sitting** (Fig. 35-6); and (5) **"W-sitting"** with the LEs positioned in a W position (bilateral hip flexion, internal rotation, and knee flexion). This LE W position provides greater stability and allows UE functional play activities (Fig. 35-6). The W position can be seen transiently as part of normal sitting variability in childhood development, but it also may be used excessively or exclusively by children with a neurological dysfunction with decreased strength and range of motion (ROM).

In summary, gravity, immaturity of the nervous system, weakness of the muscular system, and physiological flexion are a few of the variables that result in the flexed, supported, seated position of the newborn. Through practice within the environment and maturation of the various body systems, an upright posture is achieved and the spinal curves develop. Direction-specific postural adjustments, activation of dorsal muscles when the body sways forward, and activation of ventral muscles when the body sways backward are evident at birth, suggesting an innate ability to control posture through synergistic muscle activation (Hadders-Algra, 1999, 2005; Hirschfeld, 1994). A high variability of these responses exists at birth, with few adaptations to the environment (Hadders-Algra, 2005). A transition with minimal activation of postural muscles is seen at 3 months of age and lasts until a major transition occurs at 6 months. At 6 months, the infant is able to adapt postural control according to environmental demands, with gradually increasing specificity. Anticipatory postural adjustments are evident at 13 to 14 months of age.

## Age-Related Changes

Sensory, musculoskeletal, and neuromuscular changes that occur during normal aging may contribute to changes in posture and function in sitting. The musculoskeletal system experiences changes in connective, cartilage, muscle, and skeletal tissues with aging. Connective tissue becomes stiff with fiber cross-linkages and decreased elasticity. Collagenous and elastin fibers become rigid with loss of hydration, and joints become stiff. Intervertebral disks compact because of dehydration, resulting in decreased height. Muscle mass decreases with age, proximally more than distally, with a decrease in the number and size of muscle fibers. Type II muscle fibers are lost during aging, with a resultant increase in the percentage of type I muscles from 40% at age 20 years to 30% to 55% at age 60 to 65 years (Aniansson, 1981). The primary skeletal change seen is a reduction in bone mass and density, with a rate of bone loss about 1% per year in women beginning at age 30 to 35 years and in men at age 50 to 55 years. Neurological characteristics of aging include neuronal loss resulting in decreased brain mass (10% by age 90 years), decreases in nerve fiber conduction velocity (loss of the myelin sheath), and delayed synaptic transmission. Sensory changes include decreases in touch, vision, hearing, proprioception/kinesthesia, and the vestibular system.

Together, changes in normal aging influence an individual's flexibility, strength, posture, coordination, balance, and speed of movement. For example, a poor sitting posture resulting from decreased flexibility, strength, and vertebral changes combined with slower reaction times may place older individuals at a high risk for falls. Distance reached and speed of movement during reaching while in sitting decrease with age. Campbell (2001) found distance reached in sitting decreased by 4 mm and speed of movement decreased by 0.02 m/sec each year beginning at age 30 years. Lateral pelvic tilt also decreases with age, up until age 50 years (from 34 degrees at age 30 years to 16 degrees at age 80 years), after which it levels off (Campbell, 2001). Changes of normal, healthy aging are therefore compounded when a neurological disease or condition is added.

### PATIENT APPLICATION: CASE

*Medical Diagnosis: Cerebrovascular accident (CVA)*
*Reason for Referral: Inpatient rehabilitation*

#### History

Sophie is an 83 year-old, average-sized Caucasian female who experienced a right (R) middle cerebral artery CVA. Her husband (85 years old) promptly called emergency medical services upon initial symptoms, and Sophie was admitted to an acute care facility. Now at 4 days after the CVA, she is admitted to the inpatient rehabilitation unit.
**Medical/Surgical History:** Hypertension, atrial fibrillation, gallbladder removed in 1996.
**Social History (as per husband):** Husband appears healthy and physically/mentally capable of caring for her. Of her four children, three live in the local area, but they are unable to

provide much assistance because of full-time employment and young children. Both Sophie and her husband have been retired since age 65 years. Sophie's hobbies include reading, knitting, walking, and gardening. She has been active in her church community. Sophie and her husband live in a two-story home with a main floor bedroom and bath. There are four steps up into the house at both the garage and front door entrances.
**General Health Status: Before the CVA:** Sophie was a community ambulator who walked long distances and up and down stairs without assist (A) or a device. She was independent in all ADLs and IADLs.
**Medications:** Heparin, digoxin
**Prior therapies:** She received daily physical therapy (PT), occupational therapy, and speech language pathology therapy while in the acute care setting.

#### Physical Examination
**Systems Review:**
- *Cardiovascular/Pulmonary: Blood pressure, 130/80mmHg; heart rate, 80bpm; respiratory rate, 20rpm; oxygen saturation, 95%*
- *Integumentary: Skin intact; color and pliability normal for age*
- *Neuromuscular: Unable to isolate movement on left (L) side; impaired motor learning (unable to carry over task learning between sessions); dependent in bed mobility and transfers*
- *Musculoskeletal: Height 5 feet 4 inches; weight 120 pounds; ROM within functional limits (WFLs); L UE, trunk, and LE paresis*
- *Communication: Demonstrates dysarthria (slurred speech)*

**Aerobic Capacity/Endurance:** Sophie is able to tolerate 30-minute treatment sessions with adequate rest between sessions.
**Arousal, Attention, and Cognition:** Sophie is awake and cooperative. She displays L spatial neglect, decreased attention span (unable to attend to task for more than 30 seconds without verbal cues), and impaired judgment/insight (Sophie tends to reach for things and loses trunk balance). She is oriented X 2 (person, place).
**Safety:** Questionable judgment during transfers and during wheelchair (w/c) propulsion.
**ROM:** Passive WFLs bilaterally
**Motor Function:**
**Tone:** Flaccid L UE and hypotonic L trunk; L LE displays spastic tone within extensor muscle groups (1+ on Modified Ashworth Scale); no clonus present
**Motor Control:** L UE: Flaccid, unable to initiate movement, no reflex activity or associated reactions; Fugl-Meyer UE score = 0/66; L LE: able to initiate movement of hip flexion, extension, abduction, and adduction in supine; knee extension full range against gravity in supine only within extensor synergy pattern; no voluntary motion elicited in the ankle but associated reactions observed (within extension synergy movement seen with yawns, coughs, and stressful situations); Fugl-Meyer LE score = 11/34

**Trunk:** In supine, L trunk movement noted when Sophie attempts to scoot in bed. However, no active movement is noted in sitting. Ability to move in sitting is dependent on R trunk activity.
R UE and R LE: Able to isolate all movements

**Muscle Performance/Force Production:** R UE and R LE strength appears to be WFLs for her age.

**Sensory Integrity:**

- Light Touch: Intact R UE/LE; impaired L LE compared with R
- Sharp/Dull: Intact R UE/LE; L UE absent; impaired L LE compared with R
- Proprioception: R UE/LE intact; absent L UE; impaired L LE

**Posture:**

- Sitting Balance/Postural Control: Sophie is able to assume erect sitting with maximal (max) assistance of 1, but she is unable to maintain sitting without UE or back support. She is able to maintain sitting with supervision while leaning to the R with R weight shift and UE weight-bearing support. As soon as she approaches midline or attempts to weight shift to the L, she loses her balance and falls to the L (without back support). In the w/c, she is able to maintain posture once positioned: She sits with a posterior pelvic tilt and is slumped to the L.
- Gait, Locomotion, and Balance: Sophie is unable to stand or ambulate at this time.
- W/c management: Positioning in w/c requires moderate (mod) assist; however, once she is positioned, she is able to initiate propulsion only on level smooth surfaces using R UE and LE.

**Self-Care/Functional Skills:**

- Bed Positioning: Sophie is able to position herself in bed with mod to max A for use of L LE and protection of L UE. She requires verbal cues for how to use R UE/LE as an assist.
- Bed Mobility: Sophie requires minimal (min) A to roll to L sidelying from supine without bed rails; independent with bed rails. Rolling to R sidelying from supine requires max A. Sophie is dependent supine to/from prone. Sit to/from sidelying requires max A from R sidelying and mod A from L sidelying. Bridging requires mod A for L LE placement as well as lifting the buttocks. Scooting in bed requires mod A to the R with use of the bed rail and mod A to scoot up; Sophie is unable to scoot to the L. She is unable to scoot in sitting.
- Transfers: Sit pivot w/c to/from bed/mat requires max A in both directions.

## Status at 6 Weeks After stroke:

**Arousal, Attention, and Cognition:** Oriented X 4

**Motor Function:**

**Muscle Tone:** Modified Ashworth Scale: L UE: 1; L LE: 1+

**Motor Control:**

**LUE:** Sophie is able to achieve shoulder elevation with retraction. She displays one-quarter ROM antigravity into shoulder abduction, flexion, internal and external rotation. She is able to achieve three-quarter range into elbow flexion in gravity-eliminated conditions and one-quarter range into extension. She is able to initiate wrist flexion and can grasp but is unable to release. All movements are initiated at the shoulder. UE Fugl-Meyer = 13/66.

**L LE:** Sophie displays one-half range hip flexion and abduction antigravity; full-range hip adduction and extension gravity eliminated. Knee extension is full-range antigravity, and flexion is one-half range, gravity eliminated. Patient can initiate dorsiflexion and is able to plantarflex and invert one-half range without abnormal synergies.
LE Fugl-Meyer = 16/34.

**Trunk:** Sophie can assume and maintain an erect posture x 30 seconds. She is able to move in and out of anterior/posterior tilt. She is able to weight shift bilaterally, to the R better than to the L. She displays difficulty actively shortening the L trunk for weight shift onto the R and actively elongating the L for weight shift onto the L. Movements are initiated with the upper trunk.

**Posture:** In sitting, she shows a tendency to slump into flexion and L lateral bending with weight-bearing primarily on the R.

**Self-Care: Functional Skills:**

- Bed Positioning: Occasional cuing required
- Bed Mobility: Standby assist (SBA)—min A (when fatigued)
- Transfers: Sit pivot requires min A (when fatigued)—SBA
- Scooting in Sitting: Difficulty maintaining upright posture while scooting forward
- Scooting backward in sitting requires min A for equal weight-bearing while scooting forward.

**Gait, Locomotion, and Balance:**

- W/c management: SBA—occasional min A (verbal cues) secondary to L neglect
- Standing: Requires min A with tendency to weight-bear on R LE
- Gait: Wide-base quad cane used and mod A of one required for balance
- Swing on L: Hip hiking to initiate swing and attempt to clear the floor; decreased hip and knee flexion in swing; toe drag with plantar flexion and inversion
- Stance on L: Decreased terminal stance; knee hyperextension in midstance; no heel/toe off; R LE shows decreased terminal stance and excessive lateral weight shift. Sophie weight-bears primarily on the R LE and shows decreased step length of the R. Her L pelvis is rotated and retracted posteriorly throughout gait. Sophie is able to utilize a more normal pattern of swing through if she does not pick up her leg but slides it through.

## Contemplate Clinical Decisions

For the patient case described in the previous section:
Initial presentation:

1. Develop a problem list of activity limitations and participation restrictions for Sophie.
2. What are the underlying body structure and function impairments contributing to her functional activity limitations?
3. Identify environmental and personal factors that may affect Sophie's rehabilitation. Which of these factors are barriers, and which are assets?
4. Prioritize her problems and the underlying impairments.

5. *Write at least two appropriate goals expressing realistic functional outcomes for Sophie.*

*Six-week post status presentation:*

1. *Develop a new problem list of activity limitations and participation restrictions for Sophie.*
2. *What underlying body structure and function impairments are contributing to her functional activity limitations?*
3. *Prioritize her problems and the underlying impairments.*
4. *Write at least two appropriate goals expressing realistic functional outcomes for Sophie.*

## THINK ABOUT IT 35.2

1. How many ways can you position your lower extremities to vary or alter your sitting posture?
2. In a short-sitting position (feet are flat on the floor, and your hips and knees are at 90 degree angles)
   a. Describe your base of support
   b. List the joints that are weight-bearing
   c. How does your posture change when the seating surface is elevated and your feet remain on the floor?
   d. How does your posture change when the seating surface is lower than the level of your knees, and your feet remain on the floor?
   e. Complete the following table with different upper extremity positions.

| | HEAD POSITION | TRUNK POSITION | LOWER EXTREMITY POSITION |
|---|---|---|---|
| Right upper extremity reaching toward your left ear (**PNF D1 flexion**) | | | |
| Both upper extremities reaching up and out (**PNF bilateral symmetrical D2**) | | | |
| Both upper extremities reaching up and toward the right (**PNF bilateral asymmetrical pattern**) | | | |
| One hand reaching up and out and the other reaching down and out (**PNF cross diagonal**) | | | |

PNF = proprioceptive neuromuscular facilitation.

3. Imagine you are seated next to an 80 year-old person on a city bus. How would you each maintain your balance if the bus came to a sudden stop? Would your reactions be different if you were wearing a trunk orthosis that limited all trunk motions?

## ▮ Pertinent Examination/Evaluation

### Tests and Measures

The therapist should evaluate a patient's ability to (1) maintain sitting when all components are still (static); (2) control movement within a position or when the sitting surface is moving (dynamic); and (3) automatically prepare for and respond to task demands (Table 35-3). Depending on the patient's functional activity requirement and potential for active use of the legs, the therapist may want to test long sitting in addition to the short-sitting position on various surfaces. Children may be tested on an elevated surface without foot support. In analyzing a patient's ability to maintain and complete functional tasks in sitting, the therapist must compare normal movements (Table 35-1) with the patient's performance. Aspects to consider in a functional sitting task analysis (Schenkman, 2000; Tyson, 2003) are included in Table 35-4.

When a patient has difficulty performing sitting activities, the therapist should determine the underlying contributing cause(s) or impairment(s). Tables 35-5, 35-6, and 35-7 list several tests and measures for evaluating function in sitting. Table 35-5 presents tests and measures for identifying impairments related to sitting function. Few standardized tests examine only sitting. Most tests feature sitting as one aspect of a patient's overall function and therefore include other functions within the test. Table 35-6 identifies standardized tests that contain aspects of sitting. Note also that an individual's performance in sitting will most likely affect results on global outcome measures at the participation level, such as the Craig Handicap Assessment and Reporting Technique (Whiteneck, 1992), Disability Rating Scale (Salén, 1994), Frenchay Activities Index (Wade, 1985), Functional Status Questionnaire (Jette, 1986), Stroke Impact Scale (Duncan, 1999), and Parkinson's Disease Quality of Life Index (de Boer, 1996). Box 35-3 highlights standardized tests that focus primarily on sitting function.

In individuals with major loss of balance on one side in sitting, it is important to distinguish between contraversive pushing, thalamic astasia, and lateropulsion (Wallenberg syndrome). Contraversive pushing is characterized by spontaneous body positioning toward the impaired side, active pushing toward the impaired side with unimpaired extremities into abduction and extension, and resistance to passive correction of body position (Karnath, 2000, 2003; Roller, 2004). The keys in contraversive pushing are the individual's active pushing and perception of visual vertical. Individuals with this condition maintain their perception of the visual world (visual vertical), meaning they are able to see that they are tilted compared with visual cues in the environment

| TABLE 35-3 | Suggestions for Static and Dynamic Assessment of Sitting Balance* |
| --- | --- |
| **SITTING BALANCE ACTIVITY** | **ASPECTS TO CONSIDER IN ASSESSMENT** |
| Static sitting balance | • Length of time able to maintain position<br>• Amount and type of assistance required<br>• Amount of support with upper extremities<br>• Use of external support or other environmental constraints<br>• Frequency of balance loss in a given time<br>• Causes for balance loss<br>• Awareness of loss of balance<br>• Strategies used in regaining balance |
| Dynamic sitting balance | Stable surface with body moving, advancing to maintaining balance on a moving surface<br>• Excursion and direction of movement<br>• Speed of movement<br>• Frequency of balance loss in a given time<br>• Causes of balance loss<br>• Strategies for maintaining/regaining balance<br>• Environmental constraints |
| Automatic activities | Determine appropriateness of anticipatory postural adjustments (missing or delayed?) Response to unknown balance challenges<br>• Intensity of perturbation<br>• Direction of perturbation<br>• Frequency of balance loss given number of perturbations<br>• Strategies for maintaining/regaining balance<br>• Environmental constraints<br>• Presence of reactive postural control strategies<br>• Frequency or level of assist to maintain balance |

*Complete with increasing complexity: increasing challenge to stability and decreasing base of support.
Schenkman M, Gill-Body KM, Deutsch J, et al. *A Compendium for Teaching Professional Level Neurologic Content.* Alexandria, VA: Neurology Section, American Physical Therapy Association; 2000.
Tyson SF, Desouza LH. A clinical model for the assessment of posture and balance in people with stroke. *Dis Rehabil.* 2003;25(3):120–126.

| TABLE 35-4 | Considerations for Task Analysis in Sitting |
| --- | --- |
| **ASPECTS OF SITTING TASK** | **CONSIDERATIONS** |
| *Ability* to perform task | • What aspects of the task is the patient able to do?<br>• Level of assistance needed?<br>• Safety? |
| *Classification* of the task | • Mobility, stability, controlled mobility, or skill level task? |
| *How* task is performed | • Identify starting body alignments: Normal? Abnormal?<br>• Movement initiation<br>  • Movement initiates from where?<br>  • Speed and direction of movement components?<br>• Task execution—Identify the movement sequence used considering:<br>  • Presence/absence of movement components? Pieces missing?<br>  • Alignment of body segments: Normal? Abnormal?<br>  • Weight distribution: Normal? Abnormal?<br>  • Speed and timing of movement: Normal? Delayed? Abnormal sequence?<br>• Termination of movement<br>  • Alignment of body segments: Normal? Abnormal?<br>  • Weight distribution: Normal? Abnormal?<br>  • Speed and timing of movement: Normal? Delayed?<br>  • Grading of forces needed to stop movement? |
| What happens under *various conditions* or task demands? | • What happens with fatigue? Does movement change over time?<br>• How do environmental demands affect task performance? Is the patient able to adapt?<br>• What happens with increasing challenge to stability and/or decreasing base of support? |
| Evaluation of *why* patient moves this way | • Are movements isolated, compensatory, or used to stabilize self?<br>• Are movements functional? Nonfunctional?<br>• What impairments are causing the movement dysfunction (e.g., muscle strength, motor control, tone, range of motion, tissue length changes)? |

(e.g., doorway, pillars, windows). The Scale for Contraversive Pushing may help therapists identify and grade the severity of pushing (Karnath, 2003).

Individuals with Wallenberg syndrome (acute unilateral lesion in the medulla) demonstrate lateropulsion without active pushing or resistance to correction, a vertical tilt toward the unimpaired side (opposite to contraversive pushing), and perceived tilt of the world around them (impaired visual vertical)

| TABLE 35-5 | **Tests and Measures for Identifying Underlying Impairments Potentially Related to Sitting Functional Activity** |
|---|---|
| **IMPAIRMENT** | **TEST/MEASURE** |
| Aerobic capacity/endurance | Blood pressure <br> Heart rate <br> Baseline Dyspnea Index (Mehler, 1988) <br> Oxygen saturation—pulse oximetry <br> Perceived exertion—Borg Scale (Dunbar, 1992) |
| Arousal, attention, and cognition | Mini-Mental Status Examination (Folstein, 1975) <br> Rivermead Behavioural Memory Test (Wilson, 1989) <br> Rivermead Perceptual Assessment Battery (Whiting, 1980) <br> Behavioral Inattention Test (Wilson, 1987) |
| Cranial and peripheral nerve integrity | Vision <br> • Broken Wheel Acuity Test (Richman, 1984) <br> • Snellen Chart Acuity Test <br> • Visual Field Fest <br> Vestibular <br> • Dix-Hallpike Test (hyperfunction, benign paroxysmal positional vertigo [BPPV]) (Epley, 1980; Kollen, 2006c) <br> • Head Thrust Test (hypofunction) (Wrisley, 2000) |
| Balance | Static and dynamic sitting balance; refer to Chapter 9, "Balance Grading Scales" |
| Joint integrity and mobility | Joint mobility in the spine, rib cage, shoulders, hips |
| Motor function | Motor Assessment Scale (MAS) for Stroke (Carr, 1985) <br> Fugl-Meyer Assessment (Fugl-Meyer, 1975) <br> Trunk Impairment Scale (Verheyden, 2004) <br> Gross Motor Function Measure (Russell, 1989) <br> Gross Motor Performance Measure (Boyce, 1991, 1995) <br> Bruininks-Oseretsky Test of Motor Proficiency (Bruininks, 1978) |
| Muscle performance | Manual Muscle Test (Wadsworth, 1987) |
| Pain | Numerical Rating Scale, Verbal Rating Scale, Visual Analog Scale (Berthier, 1998) |
| Range of motion | Goniometry; active and passive range of motion of trunk and extremities |
| Reflex integrity | Postural reflexes, equilibrium, and righting reactions <br> Modified Ashworth Scale (Gregson, 2000) <br> Milani-Comparetti Motor Development Screening Test (Stuberg, 1989) |
| Sensory integrity | Light touch <br> Sharp/dull <br> Pressure <br> Proprioception/kinesthesia—appreciation of movement, direction of movement, and joint position sense <br> Wrist Position Sense Test (Carey, 1996) <br> Sensory integration/weighting: Clinical Test of Sensory Integration and Balance (CTSIB) (Di Fabio, 1990) <br> Rivermead Assessment of Somatosensory Performance (RASP) (Winward, 2002) <br> Visuospatial neglect <br> Bells test (Gauthier, 1989) <br> Rivermead Behavioural Inattention Test (RBIT) (Wilson, 1987) <br> Bodily neglect (Azouvi, 1996; Bisiach, 1986) |

| TABLE 35-6 | Standardized Tests That Include Aspects of Sitting Function |
|---|---|
| **SITTING FUNCTION** | **STANDARDIZED TESTS** |
| Activity limitations level | Motor Assessment Scale (MAS) for Stroke (Carr, 1985) |
| | Barthel Index (Loewen, 1988; Mahoney, 1965) |
| | Rivermead Mobility Index (Lennon, 2000) |
| | Katz Index of Activities of Daily Living (Brorsson, 1984; Vickrey, 1995) |
| | Functional Independence Measure (Dodds, 1993; Donaghy, 1998) |
| | Outcome and Assessment Information Set (OASIS) (Shaughnessy, 2002) |
| | Spinal Cord Independence Measure (Catz, 1997) |
| | Berg Balance Scale (Berg, 1989) |
| | Postural Assessment Scale for Stroke (Hsieh, 2002) |
| | Brunel Balance Assessment (Tyson, 2004a, 2004b, 2007) |
| | Ability for Basic Movement (Hashimoto, 2007) |

**BOX 35-3 Standardized Tests Specific to Sitting**

Reach Test (forward and to paretic side) (Nichols, 1996; Tyson, 2004b)

Sit-and-Reach Test (SRT) (Tsang, 2004; Tyson, 2004b)

Sitting Arm Raise Test (Tyson, 2004b)

Trunk Impairment Scale (Fujiwara, 2004; Verheyden, 2004, 2006, 2007b)

Trunk Control Test (Collin, 1990; Franchignoni, 1997; Verheyden, 2006, 2007b)

Scale for Contraversive Pushing (SCP) (Baccini, 2006; Karnath, 2003)

Lateropulsion Scale (D'Aquila, 2004)

(Dieterich, 1992). These patients fall to the side of the lesion. The Lateropulsion Scale may help therapists identify and grade lateropulsion in several functional positions or activities (supine, sitting, standing, transfers, and walking) (D'Aquila, 2004).

Patients with thalamic astasia (lesion of the posterolateral thalamus) typically have mild to no motor weakness, and when asked to sit upright, they will pull themselves up with their UEs rather than use their available trunk control (Masdeu, 1988). In contrast, when individuals with contraversive pushing are asked to sit upright, they will actively push themselves toward the impaired side, falling to the impaired side rather than coming up to vertical.

## Expected Outcomes and Prognostic Factors

With a focal injury (e.g., multiple sclerosis [MS], brain injury [BI], tumor, Parkinson's disease [PD], CVA), expected outcomes and prognosis are often cited as depending on the severity of the lesion or trauma and on other contributing factors (Table 35-7) (Smith, 1999). Several studies have cited sitting balance as predictive of overall mobility and independent ambulation after a stroke. Measures of the Trunk Control Test and Trunk Impairment Scale correlate with balance, gait, and functional ability (Kollen, 2006a; Verheyden, 2006, 2007b). Independent sitting balance 3 to 10 days after stroke onset has been correlated with independent ambulation on discharge (Hill, 1997; Kwakkel, 1996, 1999; Morgan, 1994; Nitz, 1995; Smith, 1999). Distance reached on the Sit-and-Reach Test correlates with the Functional Independence Measure mobility score on discharge and the distance achieved on the timed walk test (Tsang, 2004).

After a stroke, individuals who exhibit contraversive pushing are slower to recover but demonstrate the same ultimate functional outcomes as those without pushing behavior. Pedersen (1996) found that individuals with contraversive pushing took 63% longer (3.6 weeks) to reach the same functional outcomes as those without pusher syndrome. Prognosis is therefore good for independence in individuals with contraversive pushing (Karnath, 2002; Pedersen, 1996).

| TABLE 35-7 | Prognostic Factors Influencing Expected Outcomes |
|---|---|
| **FOCAL INJURY** | **SPINAL CORD INJURY** |
| • Severity and location: constellation of motor, sensory, and visual deficits; severity of balance loss | • Complete versus incomplete injury |
| | • Extent of zone of partial preservation (complete injuries) |
| • Prior stroke | • Level of injury |
| • Age | • Strength of innervated musculature |
| • Loss of consciousness or coma | • Presence of other traumatic orthopedic injuries (e.g., fractures), secondary diagnoses, or complications |
| • Cognitive status | |
| • Aphasia | |
| • Neglect | |
| • Visual-perceptual deficit | • Presence of intact sensation to pinprick below level of injury |
| • Persistent tone | |
| • Depression | • Level of spasticity |
| • Bladder and bowel function | • Pain |
| | • Body type |

Modified from Smith MT, Baer GD. Achievement of simple mobility milestones after stroke. *Arch Phys Med Rehabil.* 1999;80:442–447.

Expected functional outcomes after a traumatic spinal cord injury (SCI) depend on the level of injury but also on whether the injury is complete or incomplete. Typical general functional outcomes for individuals with complete SCI are shown in Box 35-4 (Consortium for Spinal Cord Medicine, 1999).

## ■ Functional Intervention for Sitting

### General Approaches

The clinician needs to consider the patient's goals, current sitting abilities, and individual prognosis to determine whether intervention strategies should focus on compensation or remediation for sitting. Compensatory strategies include the use of an abdominal binder or trunk orthosis to provide external support for the trunk musculature or instructing the patient to consistently use one UE for support. Adaptations to the environment can include use of chair backs for support or altering the seat angle or height. Furniture armrests may also provide lateral support.

When remediation of sitting is a realistic goal, several intervention approaches can be considered. As described in Chapter 15, the patient's current stage of motor control (Sullivan, 1995, p. 7) can be determined and interventions initiated at an appropriate level. Examples of applications to sitting include:

**Mobility:** Displaying passive ROM and strength to assume the seated position

---

**Stability:** Ability to maintain symmetrical static balance with erect postural alignment with or without perturbations

**Controlled Mobility** and **Static/Dynamic:** Ability to move within sitting and between different sitting postures and to lift a hand for reaching or lift a foot from the floor to complete ADLs or leisure pursuits

**Skill:** Scooting to the edge of the chair or bed and transitioning from sit-to-stand in an efficient and controlled manner.

## THINK ABOUT IT 35.3

1. Identify the mobility prerequisites for sitting.
2. Provide examples of functional tasks/activities requiring static control in sitting.
3. Provide examples of functional tasks/activities requiring dynamic postural control (during controlled mobility) in sitting.
4. Provide examples of functional tasks/activities that are classified in the static-dynamic stage of motor control.
5. Provide examples of functional tasks/activities requiring control of skilled movement in sitting.

The systems model and task-oriented interventions can be implemented by altering the task and environment. Some examples include altering the height of the support surface (e.g., from a high mat surface) with early attempts at sit-to-stand or practicing sitting activities on varied surfaces, such as the bed, dining room chair, toilet, or car seat. Sitting on dynamic surfaces such as a tilt board, therapeutic ball, moving car, subway, or boat can further challenge sitting balance. Altering the speed of motion and direction of movement adds additional challenges. Learning is enhanced with improved generalization as the UEs are used for functional and goal-directed activities in sitting. Table 35-8 shows how different sitting postures can be combined with varied surfaces and functional tasks to enhance motor learning.

---

### BOX 35-4 Typical Functional Outcomes for Individuals With a Complete Spinal Cord Injury

C1-4: Total assistance
C5: Total to moderate assistance
C6: Minimal assistance to modified independence
C7 and below: Modified independence to independent

---

**TABLE 35-8  Seated Postures, Surfaces, and Tasks That Can Be Mixed and Matched for Varied Practice**

| SEATED POSTURE | SURFACE | TASK |
|---|---|---|
| Short sitting | Sofa | Reading |
| | Dining room chair with or without armrests | Preparing, eating a meal |
| | Desk armchair | Writing or keyboarding |
| | Bar-height chair | Painting a wall |
| | Car seat | • Turning to look over your shoulder to someone calling your name or checking for oncoming traffic<br>• Moving the foot from the accelerator to the brake |
| | Rolling/swivel desk chair | Rolling a chair in the office to reach objects on a desk or nearby bookshelves |

*Continued*

**TABLE 35-8　Seated Postures, Surfaces, and Tasks That Can Be Mixed and Matched for Varied Practice—cont'd**

| SEATED POSTURE | SURFACE | TASK |
| --- | --- | --- |
| | Toilet | Reaching for toilet paper<br>Pulling slacks to the knees |
| | Tub bench | Bathing with reaching |
| | Bus seat | Reading, texting |
| | Bed | Donning socks and shoes |
| Side sitting | Floor | Playing a board game |
| Long sitting | Bed | Pulling slacks to the hips |
| | Tub | Bathing |
| | Floor | Watching TV |
| Crossed-ankle sitting | Floor | Playing a card game |
| Heel sitting | Floor | Transition between different types of sitting or surfaces or come from sit-to-stand |

## Therapeutic Activities

Guided practice allows the patient to experience the desired motion and utilize motor programs that were familiar to him before the central nervous system dysfunction. Manual cues are incorporated to enhance motor learning if the patient is unable to problem-solve the task independently. Guidance should also be combined with functional task-oriented practice in varied postures and can serve as an alternative to teaching compensatory behaviors. The current health-care environment and reimbursement plans often force focus on compensatory techniques to improve a patient's function before discharge. Although this is certainly necessary, many of the guided practice techniques demonstrated here may be incorporated to enhance movement quality. Improved quality of motions allows increased endurance/efficiency and prevents impairments caused by overuse injuries.

### Positioning Considerations

The therapist should consider the patient's sitting position before applying therapeutic techniques. Some of these considerations were suggested earlier in this chapter. Will the patient have back support? Will the patient be on a firm, soft, stable, or dynamic surface? How will the UEs be positioned? Will the patient be able to use one or both UEs for support? How will a hemiplegic UE be positioned or supported, and what positions will be avoided?

Box 35-5 lists possible positions for a hemiplegic UE. The LE position chosen depends on the functional task or therapeutic goal for the intervention session. For example, a pediatric patient may be working on the transition from side sit to quadruped, whereas a person with tetraplegia is learning how to don trousers in a long-sitting posture.

### Supine-to-Sit Transition

For normal function, a patient needs to be able to assume an upright seated posture. Individuals assume sitting with varied strategies, such as sitting directly from supine utilizing forward flexion of the trunk, pivoting into sitting with a diagonal motion over the hip, and pushing up from a sidelying posture. The therapist should be familiar with several methods of transitioning to sitting in order to provide the patient with different alternatives. These choices can be adapted on the basis of the patient's individual skills, the given task, and the environmental constraints.

Altering the environment may result in different movement strategies. For example, different patterns can be used to come to sit from supine when on the floor. The head of the bed or support surface may be elevated before asking the patient to sit. Various goal-directed tasks, such as reaching in different planes, alter the sitting strategy. The therapist may need to offer support or assistance early in the rehabilitation process with the goal of decreasing assistance as the patient gains independence.

### Hemiparesis

Figure 35-7AB illustrates an assisted diagonal pivot pattern to transition from supine to short sitting by moving toward the

**BOX 35-5　Positioning Options for a Hemiplegic or Hemiparetic Upper Extremity During Sitting**

1. Cradle the impaired upper extremity with the unimpaired extremity. Both extremities will be in elbow flexion and shoulder internal rotation.
2. Clasp the hands together with the fingers intertwined.
3. Place the hands in a weight-bearing position with the fingers extended. The hands may be placed in shoulder external rotation on a low stool lateral to the hips or placed forward in midline on a low table or chair with the unimpaired hand on top of the impaired hand. The stable surface can be progressed to an unstable surface such as a rolling table or ball.

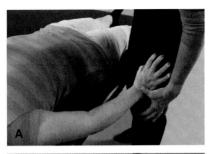
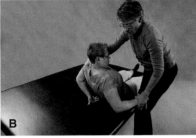

**FIGURE 35-7** Diagonal pivot supine to short-sitting transition. (A) In the starting position, the patient's hemiparetic hand placement is in weight-bearing on the therapist's thigh. (B) The therapist assists the patient during the transition.

hemiparetic side. Assist the LEs off of the bed while protecting and providing weight-bearing forces through the impaired UE. Verbally cue the patient to reach toward your shoulder with the intact UE. This motion requires the patient to activate intact musculature and assist with the transition. Make the task more goal directed with a functional focus by asking the patient to reach for an object or a phone on a bedside table. When the patient requires additional assistance to the upper trunk, place the hemiparetic lower limb off the mat table with the hip in neutral, the knee at 90 degrees, and the foot flat on the floor or a stool. The LE is now positioned so you can focus on assisting the upper trunk to come upright. A compensatory method is to have the patient assist the paretic lower limb off the mat table with the intact limb.

An alternative strategy is for the patient to come to short sitting from a sidelying position. When lying on the unimpaired side and pushing up with the intact UE, the patient must perform antigravity lateral trunk flexion with the hemiparetic side of the trunk, which can be difficult. The transition from sidelying on the impaired side to short sitting may be even more difficult. The patient may not be able to use the impaired UE to push to sitting, and the position is not biomechanically conducive to pushing with the intact UE.

When a dependent transfer is needed, place one arm beneath the patient's upper trunk and the other arm under the patient's knees by reaching over the top of the legs to place your hand near the popliteal fossa. Using good body mechanics, lift the upper trunk and swing the legs off the mat in a pivoting motion so the patient is in a short-sit position.

Common alternative strategies for the supine-to-short sit transition include rolling to sidelying first and pushing with the UEs into long sitting followed by swinging the legs over the side of the bed/mat. Some individuals lift both LEs in the air and use the momentum of dropping the legs off the side

of the bed/mat to assist the trunk coming into upright sitting. Grabbing onto the side of the bed/mat with the outside arm and pulling the trunk up while swinging the legs off the mat is yet another strategy employed by some individuals. Please refer to Chapter 14 for further discussion of these and additional strategies.

### Spinal Cord Injury

*Supine to Long Sitting.* One method for independent transition from supine to long sitting in individuals with an SCI is to come from a prone-on-elbows position (Fig. 26-13ABCDEFGH). Have the patient roll from supine to prone and then come up onto the elbows. From there, the patient "walks" on the elbows around to the side, positioning the trunk as far forward toward the legs as possible. Then the patient swings the arm closest to the legs around the thigh or knee. The patient then brings the trunk up over the legs into long sitting while pulling with the elbow flexors on the leg, pushing up with the other arm and using head momentum.

Another method is for the patient to come into long sitting from a supine-on-elbows position (Fig. 26-12ABCD). In supine, the patient can either hook the hands in the pants pockets, the thumbs in the belt loops, or the hands under the buttocks to use elbow flexors combined with shoulder extensors while alternately weight shifting side to side with momentum to pull up into supine on elbows. From supine on elbows, the patient swings one arm behind, with full shoulder external rotation to lock the elbow, into weight-bearing; the procedure is repeated with the other arm. The patient then alternately "walks" forward on the hands into a more upright long-sitting position. Please refer to Chapter 26 for a more detailed description of these strategies.

*Long Sitting to Short Sitting.* One strategy to move from long sitting to short sitting involves the patient first scooting the buttocks toward the edge of the bed/mat. While weight-bearing on one hand or elbow, the patient hooks a hand or wrist underneath the thigh closest to the edge and gradually works the foot and leg off the side of the bed using wrist extensors or elbow flexors. The patient then repeats the movement with the other leg (Fig. 35-8AB and refer to Fig. 26-15). Once both feet are off the bed, the patient can scoot around to squarely face the edge of the bed if needed.

### Sitting: Mobility

Once the patient achieves an upright, seated position, the quality of the seated position may need to be addressed. It is beneficial for the patient to learn how to sit with a neutral or slight anterior pelvic tilt with adequate lumbar extension, an erect thoracic and cervical spine, and symmetrical weight-bearing in a midline position. A sequence of cues can facilitate this erect posture and can be used for instruction to assume, maintain, and learn control for any posture (Box 35-6). Figure 35-9ABC provides suggestions for hand placement to guide the patient into this seated alignment, and Fig. 35-10ABC illustrates soft tissue mobilization methods for patients whose ROM is insufficient to assume the desired posture.

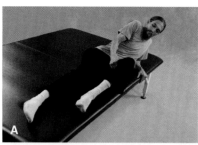

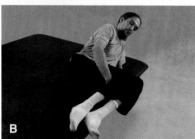

**FIGURE 35-8** Supine to short sitting in a patient with a spinal cord injury. (A) The patient hooks a hand beneath the leg closest to the edge of the mat and gradually works the foot and leg to the edge. (B) The patient then repeats the sequence with the other leg to move both legs off the mat.

---

### BOX 35-6 Cues to Facilitate Erect Sitting

**Essential Before Any Upright Functional Activity**

1. Ask the patient to sit erect in midline, or you can demonstrate the position.
2. Facilitate the posture when the patient is unable to sit erect.
   a. Demonstrate the position again.
   b. Readjust the patient's alignment to ensure that the feet are flat on the floor, the hips and knees are at 90 degrees, and the pelvis is in neutral alignment in all planes.
   c. Provide a task or visual cue that encourages the desired position.
   d. Provide manual cues to assist to the position as shown in Figs. 35-9ABC (give only the minimal amount of input necessary to gain the desired motion, and intentionally and gradually turn control over to the patient).
3. When the patient is unable to move passively into the posture (e.g., lacks sufficient lumbar extension range), perform soft tissue mobilization (see Figs. 35-10 A, B and C) and then repeat the previous steps.
4. Ask the patient to maintain the position as you remove the manual cues.
5. Once the patient can hold the position, request a controlled eccentric contraction ("slowly release") followed by a concentric contraction back into the desired erect posture.
6. To challenge the task, increase the time the position is maintained, move in and out of the position, request increased speed of movement, or alter the functional task being completed in the position.

---

Unilateral pelvic elevation is necessary for scooting in a seated position and contributes to the small lateral excursion of the pelvis during ambulation. As shown later in this chapter, active lateral tilt can be used functionally as a skill level for seated scooting forward to the edge of the chair. Figure 35-11AB illustrates examples of lateral shift–guided practice.

---

### PATIENT APPLICATION: MOBILITY

*In the clinical case presented at the beginning of the chapter, Sophie was unable to move her L trunk in sitting but could do so in supine. You have considered strengthening the trunk in the horizontal position with segmental rolling, bridging, and scooting in bed activities (see Chapter 34). When incorporating the suggestions in Box 35-6, first consider the environment and Sophie's position to create an opportunity for her to be successful. With Sophie in sitting, ensure that her feet are flat on the floor and her hips and knees are flexed at ~90 degrees with hips neither adducted nor abducted.*

*It may be easier for Sophie to accomplish an anterior tilt in sitting when she is sitting closer to the edge of the mat (because less of the femur creates friction on the support surface) and when her hips are slightly higher than her knees. Place Sophie's hands in a natural weight-bearing position, one that is appropriate for the task. Provide a task or visual cue, such as reaching overhead or looking up at a target, to encourage her movement into an anterior pelvic tilt and more erect sitting. As needed, provide manual cues to assist in the position. It is important to give only the minimal amount of cuing necessary to gain the desired motion. As Sophie can maintain erect sitting, remove your manual cues. Once she can hold the position, request a controlled posterior pelvic tilt, followed by an active return to the erect posture. Vary the task to encourage lateral pelvic tilt—controlled lateral shift to one side, eccentric return to midline, controlled weight shift in the opposite direction, and eccentric control to midline. If Sophie is unable to move passively into the posture, consider performing soft tissue mobilization and then repeat the previous steps.*

---

### Contemplate Clinical Decisions: Mobility

*When planning mobility interventions in sitting for Sophie, consider the following questions:*

1. *Where should you position yourself to guard Sophie for safety and to facilitate the movement sequence for erect short sitting?*
2. *What cues would you provide Sophie to achieve the desired movements?*
3. *What functional tasks could you incorporate?*
4. *How would you sequence your intervention session? What would you work on first?*

*For Sophie's status at 6 weeks:*

1. *How have your position and manual cues changed from those in the initial interventions?*
2. *What functional tasks can be incorporated?*

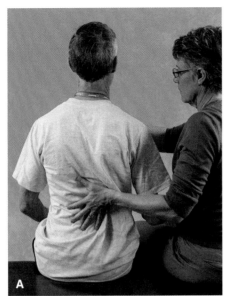
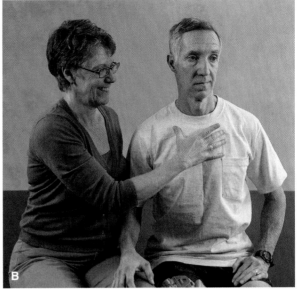
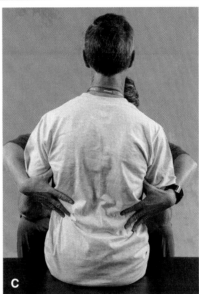

**FIGURE 35-9** In the first two photos, the therapist is sitting at the patient's side to facilitate the upright trunk. (A) A light cue is given by the therapist's posterior hand in an upward/forward direction over the patient's low back to guide the lumbar spine into extension and the pelvis out of posterior tilt. (B) At the same time, the anterior hand is placed just below the patient's clavicles and gives a light pressure laterally and upward to cue thoracic extension and facilitate an upright posture. (C) Alternatively, while seated in front of the patient, the therapist places the hands over the lateral trunk, to guide the pelvis to neutral alignment and an upright trunk.

## Sitting: Stable Postural Control

Maintaining stable postural control of the trunk and all weight-bearing components in sitting is a critical foundation for functional activities. As stated previously, activities completed relatively close to midline require only small adjustments in the trunk to maintain balance/equilibrium. Therapists should focus on functional ability to maintain erect sitting for a sufficient period to complete a task. The patient's initial position should maximize the base of support and stability. In short sitting, this entails having feet flat on the floor in weight-bearing, with the hips and knees at 90-degree flexion, the knees and ankles aligned with the hips (neutral abduction/adduction/rotation),

and the thighs fully supported by the bed or mat. The UEs may be placed in a natural weight-bearing position for the patient who needs additional support or to encourage spontaneous UE use.

Many individuals with a SCI also need stability in long sitting because this position is used for several functional activities, including scooting, dressing, repositioning the LEs, and getting in and out of bed. Long sitting is valuable because of the inherent stability from the extended base of support. Trunk posture and positioning depend on the level of injury and residual muscle control. For all patients, you can begin training by eliciting an isometric contraction on one side of

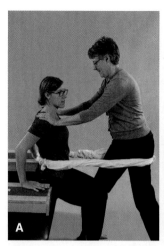
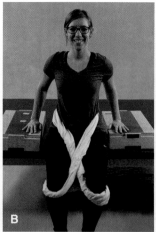
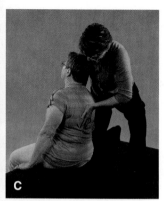

**FIGURE 35-10**  (A) A method for providing passive guidance and soft tissue mobilization into an anterior pelvic tilt is illustrated. (B) When the patient has difficulty maintaining the position and the session needs to advance to higher skills, a sheet or stadium chair can be used as an assistive device to hold the posture. (C) A method for general soft tissue mobilization of the thoracic spine into extension is illustrated. The pelvis needs to be in neutral alignment. The therapist, in a half-kneeling position at the patient's side, locates the apex of the thoracic flexion and positions the hand with the thenar/hypothenar eminences on the paraspinal muscles (i.e., the hand directed inferiorly). With the contralateral hand providing a stabilizing counterpressure to the upper anterior trunk, the therapist provides an anterior force over the spine. The hand is moved cranially, one spinal segment at a time. The thoracic spine extends between T1 and T4 (Boyle, 2002); this mobilization technique should not be performed above T4.

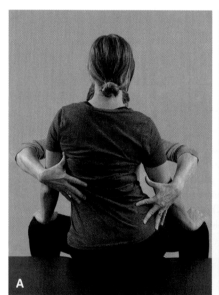
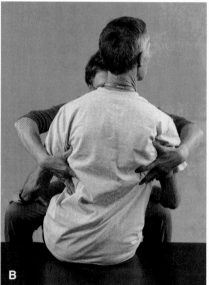

**FIGURE 35-11**  (A) Manual guidance for a passive "lift" of the pelvis into a left lateral tilt is shown. (B) Lateral shift to the patient's right with the facilitation of the left quadratus lumborum for active unilateral pelvic elevation is shown. The therapist's right hand (patient's left trunk) is giving an up-and-in cue at the quadratus lumborum (deep to the erector spinae muscles) and toward the opposite shoulder to encourage active shortening of the patient's left trunk while the therapist's left hand is providing an up-and-out cue to encourage elongation on the patient's right side. Timing of each cue (shortening then elongation) is important to encourage the right lateral weight shift rather than a left lateral side bend without weight shift. In both techniques, the lateral shift needs to be maintained for 20 to 30 seconds, followed by a request for the patient to hold the position without assistance.

the trunk and progress to the ability to hold contractions on all sides and the ability to balance the cocontractions needed to maintain sitting against challenges. A number of techniques to enhance segment stability (especially at the trunk) are discussed in the following text (Sullivan, 1995, pp. 72–77).

### Shortened Held Resisted Contraction

With the patient in upright erect sitting, place your hands on the extensor side of the patient's trunk at the shoulders, gradually increasing resistance while asking the patient to "hold" (Fig. 35-12). Gradually increase resistance to approximately 40% of the patient's maximal isometric contraction to facilitate recruitment of type I slow-twitch muscle fibers, building muscle endurance.

### Alternating Isometrics

While the patient is sitting erect, apply resistance on alternating sides of the trunk (e.g., both hands on either the front or back), with hand placements at the shoulder or pelvis depending on the need to foster controlled sitting. Maintain the contraction through the transition from side to side or front to back while asking the patient to "hold" (Fig. 35-13AB). A smooth, gradual transition to the opposite side is key, not allowing any relaxation between isometric contractions (no "letup" of the resistance). As in shortened held resisted contraction (SHRC), contractions are gradually built on each side and are kept at a moderate intensity level.

### Rhythmic Stabilization

**Rhythmic stabilization** (RS) adds a level of difficulty to alternating isometrics (AIs). Apply resistance on alternating

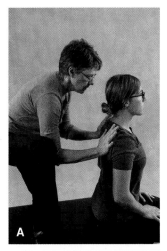

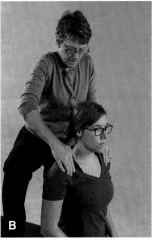

**FIGURE 35-13** Alternating isometrics in sitting with (A) resistance to the trunk extensors and transitioning to (B) resistance to the trunk flexors are performed while isometric contractions are maintained in the alternating muscle groups to encourage trunk stability in sitting.

sides of the patient's trunk with hand placements simultaneously on opposite sides of the trunk (e.g., one front and one back) (Fig. 35-14). Like AIs, the resistance is of moderate intensity, is built gradually, and is maintained through the transitions. The verbal cue to the patient is "Don't let me twist you." Transition smoothly and gradually as each hand simultaneously switches from front to back, not allowing any relaxation between contractions. It is as if you are trying to twist the patient while the patient is trying to hold still. RS begins to build cocontraction around the trunk. Hand placements may be at the pelvis or at the shoulders.

### Slow Reversal Hold or Slow Reversal Through Decrements of Range

In **slow reversal hold (SRH) or slow reversal (SR) through decrements of range**, you resist the patient's forward/backward or side/side movement, gradually decreasing the range of movement from larger to smaller, ending in a static

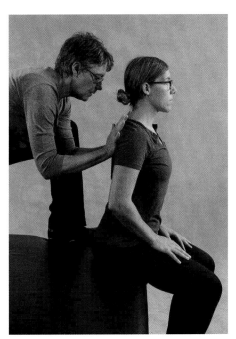

**FIGURE 35-12** Shortened held resisted contraction in sitting.

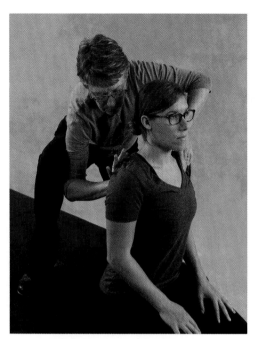

**FIGURE 35-14** Rhythmic stabilization in sitting, with manual resistance applied at two locations in the same rotary direction, encourages trunk stability in sitting. The location of the resistance is then shifted, one hand at a time, to two new locations to increase cocontraction.

---

**BOX 35-7  Intervention Plan for Individuals With Contraversive Pushing (Karnath, 2003)**

According to Karnath (2003), therapists should design interventions that proceed in the following sequence:

1. Assist the patient in realizing his misperception of upright vertical posture.
2. Provide the patient with multiple opportunities to see if current posture is oriented to upright by working in and exploring environments with many vertical structures (windows, doorways, pillars).
3. Assist the patient in learning how to move to the correct posture and achieve vertical upright status.
4. Provide the patient with multiple opportunities to practice maintaining upright while performing other functional tasks or activities.

---

hold in midline. This is often used with patients who have difficulty maintaining sitting because of poorly controlled excessive movements (e.g., ataxia, athetosis). AIs or RS may follow this technique to further build proximal stability.

### Techniques for a Midline Vertical Posture

Achieving stability in sitting can be especially challenging for patients who have impaired midline perception and body orientation. Patients with an impaired perception of vertical may push themselves with their intact extremities toward the hemiplegic side, leading to a lateral loss of balance (known as pusher syndrome, ipsilateral pushing, or contraversive pushing). Patients may strongly resist passive repositioning to midline but may be responsive to conscious strategies and visual cues (using intact visual and vestibular inputs). Repeated exposures to visually vertical surroundings and practicing maintaining vertical during functional tasks can be beneficial (Karnath, 2003). Be sure to involve the patient in active repositioning to vertical and problem-solving (see Box 35-7).

Visual cues such as mirrors are helpful for the patient to view personal posture with respect to the environment. Environmental cues are also helpful, such as sitting next to a wall or positioning the therapist on the patient's unimpaired side. The patient can be asked to reposition himself toward the wall or the therapist.

To decrease UE pushing, place the patient's intact arm on a higher surface (pillow or bed table), putting the arm at a biomechanical disadvantage for pushing. You may also choose to engage the patient in a reaching activity with the intact arm to inhibit pushing. For LE pushing, block the intact leg from migrating into abduction and extension. The intact foot can also be placed on a stool, or the stronger leg can be crossed over the hemiplegic leg to decrease pushing and add a weight-bearing component to the hemiplegic side.

### Progressing Therapeutic Activities in Sitting Stability

Gradually increase the difficulty of the task by changing the patient's base of support through altering UE and LE weight-bearing. Begin with both of the patient's hands in weight-bearing and gradually narrow the base of support to midline. Progressively decrease the base of support to one hand, to both hands non–weight-bearing, and ultimately to the hands manipulating an object in the context of a functional task. You can also progress the UE weight-bearing surface from a stable surface to a dynamic surface, such as a ball or rolling table. Similarly, begin with both of the patient's feet in weight-bearing on the floor and progress to lifting one leg off the floor, marching, and raising the height of the seated surface until the feet are dangling. After beginning balance training with the patient's eyes open, you can alter sensory input by asking the patient to perform the task with the eyes closed.

You can also increase the difficulty level by manipulating the environment. Progressively increase difficulty by changing the characteristics of the seating surface, including height or compliance (soft chair), stable or moving surface (ball, bus), and the presence or absence of a backrest or armrests. You can also challenge the patient's ability to maintain sitting stability by abruptly letting go of an isometric hold, applying unexpected perturbations from different directions, or lifting the patient's legs in different directions. Throughout these interventions, you should make the activity meaningful by incorporating everyday tasks completed in sitting on stable and unstable surfaces (Fig. 35-15).

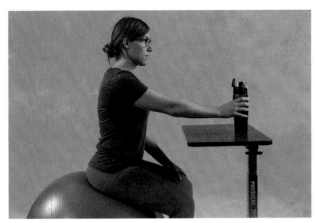

**FIGURE 35-15** Sitting on an unstable surface while completing a functional reaching task.

## PATIENT APPLICATION: MAINTAINING SITTING STABILITY

In the clinical case presented at the beginning of the chapter, Sophie was unable to maintain erect sitting once placed and required maximal assistance. Set up the environment for patient success as discussed in the first case application. Select the surface height so Sophie can have both feet in weight-bearing with her hips at 80 to 90 degrees of flexion and neutral with respect to abduction, adduction, and rotation. Identify tasks that are meaningful to Sophie and that require maintaining a sitting posture as well as providing opportunities for her to succeed when given assistance.

Manually guide Sophie into erect sitting, using as little cuing as possible. Place her hands in a natural weight-bearing position. Decrease the amount of assistance given to maintain the position, and ask her to try to keep her position. If she drifts off midline or begins to slump, ask her to correct the displacement and assist in returning to the erect sitting posture. Attempt several trials. Build isometric strength by applying slight resistance in the form of an SHRC.

A second person can help Sophie maintain sitting as she tries to counter the resistance given in the SHRC. First, give the resistance at the pelvis. With a shorter lever arm, it may be easier for Sophie to be successful than with resistance given at the shoulders. Also try alternating isometrics and RS. SR through decrements of range may help Sophie gain a feel for proprioception regarding where midline is located. Can Sophie move away from midline and then return to midline (even with assistance)? How far away from midline can she move and still return to midline?

You may also use a mirror in front of Sophie to provide visual feedback during attempts to maintain position. Can she identify midline without the mirror? Incorporate functional tasks throughout the practice session, and involve Sophie in active problem-solving. Because her attention span has decreased, have several task-related ideas ready and switch between them in order to maintain her attention and interest. Sophie also displays impaired insight and judgment into her abilities, so you will need to guard against a potential fall. What is the best position for you in order to guard Sophie safely?

### Contemplate Clinical Decisions: Maintaining Sitting Stability

*Other considerations are important in planning stability interventions:*

1. *How can you increase the challenge of maintaining sitting?*
2. *What meaningful functional tasks can you incorporate to encourage sitting stability?*
3. *How would you sequence your activities and techniques? What would you do first?*
4. *How do interventions for mobility compare with those for stability?*

*For Sophie's functional status at 6 weeks:*

1. *How should your position and manual cues change from those of the initial interventions?*
2. *What functional tasks can be incorporated now?*
3. *What are your new short-term goals for Sophie at this point?*

### Sitting: Controlled Mobility

A patient in sitting should also be able to maintain control while moving and shifting weight. Reaching and scooting in all directions, seated transfers, completing UE tasks, and responding to environmental challenges all require a patient to control a moving center of gravity over a base of support. An activity completed close to midline (e.g., reaching for something within arm's reach) requires only small adjustments in the trunk to maintain balance, whereas activities farther away from midline require greater trunk control. The timing and degree to which trunk and limb muscles activate depends on several factors, including the excursion of the movement, whether the feet or hands are in weight-bearing, and the speed of the movement (Carr, 1998; Chari, 1986; Crosbie, 1995; Dean, 1997). This section focuses on the patient's ability to maintain control during functional weight shifts in sitting.

A patient should be able to weight shift in all directions, incorporating isolated movements and normal combinations of trunk flexion, extension, and rotation as described in Table 35-1. For these activities, it is very important that a patient dissociate the upper trunk from the lower trunk so each can work independently of the other.

#### Therapeutic Activities for Controlled Mobility

Training can begin with practicing trunk movements in all directions. Provide the patient with verbal and manual cues only as needed (see the previous mobility section) to practice the movements outlined in Table 35-1. Limiting the use of manual cues as much as possible while structuring the practice environment can help the patient to personally problem-solve movement strategies. In addition, have the patient practice the movements within the context of a specific task or functional activity (e.g., turning to look over the shoulder, leaning forward as if to stand). As the patient develops psychomotor skills for moving the upper and lower trunk in the sagittal and coronal planes, increase the complexity by including rotation (extension or flexion with rotation).

Proprioceptive neuromuscular facilitation (PNF) upper trunk patterns, such as **PNF chop** (trunk flexion and rotation), **PNF reverse chop** (extension with rotation), **PNF lift** (extension and rotation), and **PNF reverse lift** (flexion and rotation), are good ways to indirectly promote trunk component movement while accentuating rotation (Sullivan, 1995, pp. 15–18). In poststroke individuals, these patterns also promote bilateral UE use and crossing midline. The lift is especially helpful for individuals with Parkinson disease to encourage extension with rotation.

In addition to isolating upper and lower trunk movements and performing movement combinations with the trunk, a patient must be able to control these movements while using the UEs and LEs. Good trunk control allows successful achievement of functional tasks using the extremities. Work with the patient to practice combined trunk and extremity movements within the context of a specific functional task. Examples include lifting a leg to take off a shoe, lifting one leg up on a stool, crossing one leg over the other, moving the feet back in preparation for standing, reaching overhead, and pouring a glass of water. The trunk also extends the reach of the arms in all directions as far as possible without losing balance. Tasks that can be used as part of treating trunk control in sitting are limitless. Work on tasks the patient would do in the course of a typical day considering his life roles, responsibilities, and hobbies or recreational activities.

The patient must also be able to withstand expected challenges (reaching for tissues in a purse while sitting on the bus) and unexpected challenges (the bus swerves to avoid a dog in the road). Work with the patient on maintaining control while sitting on a compliant (foam) or moving (tilt board, ball) surface. The patient should also be able to handle unexpected perturbations from all directions while weight shifting.

### Progressing Therapeutic Activities in Controlled Mobility

The level of challenge and task difficulty can be increased by decreasing the dimensions of the base of support, removing or disadvantaging UE or LE support (from partial support to no support), or placing the hands or feet on a dynamic surface (ball). Have the patient practice sitting weight shifting with the feet off the floor to increase workload on the trunk. Consider altering the surface upon which the patient is sitting to increase the level of difficulty, including progressing from a stable, level surface (mat) to a stable, inclined surface such as a wedge, to an unstable surface (rolling stool) or a compliant surface (bed, foam). Intervention can also be progressed by manipulating the magnitude of movement excursion (reaching farther and farther from midline), by manipulating the speed of the movement, and by implementing tasks involving both UEs and LEs (e.g., lifting the foot to put on a sock or leaning to catch a falling object). Increasing the complexity of the UE task also provides further challenge (e.g., pouring a cup of water versus dusting).

### PATIENT APPLICATION: CONTROLLED MOBILITY

To promote Sophie's ability to control balance while moving in sitting, practice trunk movements in sitting and gradually decrease the amount of assistance given. You may begin with movements such as lower trunk–initiated (Table 35-1) anterior pelvic tilt (Fig. 35-9ABC) or posterior pelvic tilt and lateral weight shift (Fig. 35-11AB) in both directions. Encourage Sophie to isolate and control movement speed and accuracy. With lateral weight shifts, have Sophie control movement to one side, return to midline, and then control movement to the other side. Movements to the R will be easier for Sophie to control than movements to the L. Upper trunk–initiated movements may also be practiced (see Table 35-1).

Incorporate practice within functional or simulated functional tasks. Most functional tasks incorporate combinations of movements, such as extension or flexion with rotation (see Table 35-1). You can also promote sitting trunk control by forcing trunk activity in a more stressful position, such as kneeling, half-kneeling, or standing. Initially, Sophie will most likely need assistance through a body weight–support overhead harness system for standing or walking.

### Contemplate Clinical Decisions: Controlled Mobility

Planning controlled mobility interventions includes the following considerations:

1. How can you increase the challenge of controlling sitting balance while moving?
2. What meaningful tasks can you choose to encourage controlled mobility?
3. How will you sequence your activities and techniques? What will you do first?
4. Why is laterally shifting to the right easier for Sophie than shifting to the left?
5. How do interventions for mobility and stability compare with those for controlled mobility?

For Sophie's functional status at 6 weeks:

1. How will your position and manual cues change from those used in the initial interventions?
2. What functional tasks can be incorporated now?
3. What are your new short-term goals for Sophie?

### Sitting: Skill

A patient needs to advance to the skill level of sitting to complete functional tasks within the environment. Skill in sitting includes the ability to scoot forward and back as well as side to side in a controlled manner while in the seated posture. The patient will need to scoot forward on a chair (or other support surface) to achieve an optimal position for transfers and transitioning from sitting to standing. The individual returning to a seated position will need to scoot backward in the chair for comfort and stability. The skill level also includes the ability to move from a seated position to stance to complete transfers and from place to place. These higher-level activities require available ROM in the trunk and extremities, strength and endurance, and equilibrium and righting reactions. The movements require the ability to rotate and dissociate the upper and lower trunk and the lower trunk/pelvis and LEs. These motions are critical for transitional movements, as discussed earlier in the chapter.

Transitions into and out of other sitting positions, such as side sitting or crossed-ankle sitting, can also be addressed at this phase of the intervention. The sequencing for scooting and 1-inch partial stands in a progression typically used in the clinic is outlined in the following section. Certainly, the sequence can be altered depending on the patient's needs; in addition, overlapping techniques before one is perfected enhances patient learning.

### Scooting

*Scooting Forward.* As a prerequisite for scooting in sitting, the patient should be instructed in how to perform a weight shift and lateral pelvic tilt (Fig. 35-11AB). The patient completes scooting through a series of steps. First, the patient laterally shifts weight while maintaining an erect sitting posture, requiring trunk lengthening on the side that is weighted and lateral trunk flexion on the unweighted side. Next, the unweighted side shifts forward. When needed, offer facilitation through manual contacts at the posterior pelvis with a forward cue on one side (Fig. 35-16) or by applying forward and midline forces on the knee. Verify that erect sitting posture

has been maintained, and repeat the shift and forward scoot with the opposite side. The patient then alternately scoots each hip forward until reaching the edge of the chair. At this point, the patient is positioned for transfer or come to standing.

*One-Inch Partial Stands in Preparation for Scooting Backward and for Transfers.* The ability to perform a **1-inch partial stand** (or 1-inch liftoff) allows the patient to begin transferring weight to the LEs in a safe semistance posture (Fig. 35-17AB). Performance of the task in midline symmetry with equal weight-bearing is very difficult and may require multiple trials over several treatment sessions. The patient must be confident that a fall will not occur in order to achieve the necessary trunk flexion, and in hemiparesis, be willing to take weight

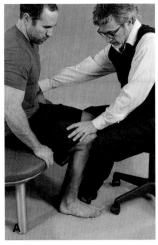

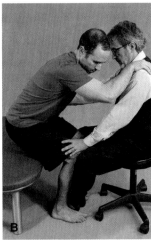

**FIGURE 35-17** One-inch partial stand. (A) In the starting position, the feet are placed posteriorly under the seating surface. (B) As the patient leans forward (hip flexion with the pelvis and lumbar spine in neutral alignment), a biomechanical balance point is reached, and the patient can lift the buttocks from the support surface with minimal effort. Ask the patient to maintain the "liftoff" posture briefly and then eccentrically slowly lower to the seated position. When the lift is too difficult for the patient to perform, consider raising the height of the support surface, changing the upper extremity position, and/or verifying the correct foot position.

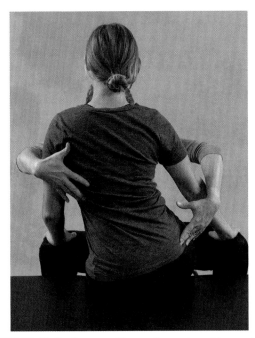

**FIGURE 35-16** Facilitation of forward scooting with anterior manual guidance of the patient's right pelvis is shown. The pattern of movement is then repeated to scoot the left side forward.

on the impaired LE. You will need to monitor the patient's trunk/pelvic alignment, symmetry, and foot position while adapting manual cues to the body area requiring the most assistance. If the patient is having difficulty, you will need to problem-solve which component is missing through careful motion analysis.

Prepare the patient by facilitating an upright sitting posture to midline with appropriate UE placement. Place the patient's feet under the chair/mat as a starting base of support for better alignment and enhance the weight shift forward and rise-to-stand (Fig. 35-17A). Encourage the patient to lean forward at the hips while maintaining pelvis, trunk, and head alignment (Fig. 35-17B). This may need to be practiced numerous times to maintain symmetry!

In patients presenting with hemiplegia, facilitation may be required to promote weight-bearing on the involved limb. For a patient with right hemiplegia, sit on a chair in front of the patient and place your left foot between the patient's feet with your leg abducted and crossing the patient's right tibia. With this positioning, you will not stop the tibia from forward translation because this is a critical biomechanical component in moving from sit-to-stand. Your right foot is placed on top of your left foot to assist in utilizing your left tibia to provide a traction force downward and encourage weight-bearing on the impaired lower limb (Fig. 35-17AB). Provide manual cues at the trunk and the LEs to enhance weight-bearing in the impaired leg and to assist the patient with knee extension as the lift is completed. As the patient gains confidence and skill, you may choose to cue the patient from the side rather than from the front (Fig. 35-18AB). This allows the patient greater freedom of movement.

Patients who are fearful of falling forward during a partial stand can first work on the leaning forward component to gain confidence. One strategy is to ask the patient to practice leaning forward and bearing weight with both hands on to a stable surface such as a chair or stacked blocks (Fig. 35-19). You can control the height of the blocks to encourage more or less forward leaning and weight shift.

*Scooting Backward.* When returning to a seated position, the patient will most likely need to scoot back into the chair for safety, comfort, and neutral positioning. This task can be accomplished by reversing the alternate hip movements used to scoot forward. However, when the patient with hemiparesis has a retracted pelvis, the task of moving the hip back may reinforce that abnormal retraction. In this case, it may be beneficial to help the patient scoot back using a symmetrical position.

Sit in front of the patient with both feet positioned between the patient's feet and with the hips abducted, resulting in your tibias crossing the patient's tibias to provide a backward/downward force and to facilitate weight-bearing. Initially, manual contacts may be at the pelvis to facilitate a liftoff. Have the patient lean forward into a 1-inch partial stand; then ask the patient to sit back into the chair. As the patient is asked to sit, you plantarflex both feet (causing your tibia to provide a posterior force on the patient's tibia), cuing the patient to sit back from the edge of the chair.

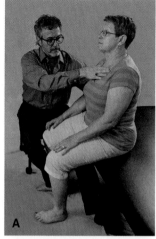

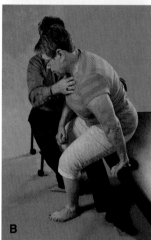

**FIGURE 35-18** Alternative partial rise or liftoff method to guide a patient into a 1-inch partial stand is shown. This technique aids symmetry by focusing on weight-bearing through the impaired lower extremity. (A) For the starting position, sit in a chair at the patient's impaired side (the patient's right side in the figures). Extend your leg closest to the mat (left lower extremity) beneath the patient's thighs to enhance your stability. Place your right foot behind the patient's heel on the affected side with your tibia crossing in front of the patient's tibia, allowing you to give input to tibia position. Use manual contacts on the trunk as needed (upper trunk, abdominals, etc.), as shown in Fig. 35-9, to maintain alignment and possibly over the knee for approximation to encourage weight-bearing through the impaired leg. (B) Completion of a partial stand is shown. Completion of this task without the patient using the upper extremity is eventually encouraged.

*Scooting to the Side.* Scooting laterally may be a necessary skill for scooting on a sofa, allowing someone to sit beside you, or moving sideways on a church bench. To perform lateral scooting, the patient once again starts from a symmetrical midline sitting position. The patient's arms may be placed in any of the positions described earlier. However, when the hands are placed lateral to the hips, the hand toward which the patient is scooting will need to be positioned in more abduction to allow room for lateral translation of the pelvis. The patient will assume a 1-inch liftoff, shift the lower trunk/hips toward

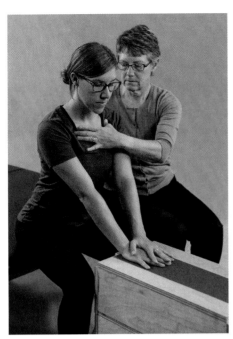

**FIGURE 35-19** The alternative upper extremity position for a partial stand shown here may be easier for the patient. This illustrates how a component part of the task may be practiced. The patient's typical environment will not facilitate this hand placement, so this position is used for training purposes and will need to be progressed.

one side, and lower the pelvis to sit again. This task requires trunk rotation. During practice, the feet may be kept in the same position as the patient repeats the sequence in reverse direction to return to the original position. The activity can be repeated to both sides with eventually wider excursions completed by moving to the right and left without stopping at midline.

These lateral movements challenge the patient to increase weight-bearing on a weakened LE and require increased balance and equilibrium reactions. Scooting in one direction for several trials can be used for transfers as described in the following section.

### Seated Transfers Requiring Skill

Ultimately, a patient should be able to transfer to both sides and to handle transfers to different heights and surfaces (e.g., a wheelchair, hospital bed, therapy mat, car seat, tub seat, kitchen chair, and soft couch). For example, a patient with left hemiplegia will transfer from the chair to the bed in very early rehabilitation by pivoting to the right on the unimpaired limb. The wheelchair will need to be repositioned to the opposite side of the bed for the same patient to transfer back from the bed to the chair with the same pivot on the right limb. Functionally, this one-sided approach to transfers is not realistic because the patient is unable to reposition the chair while in bed, and the caretaker is unlikely to move the wheelchair to the other side after transfer to the bed to allow for a same-side transfer. In addition, most bathrooms do not have ample space to place a wheelchair on both sides of the

toilet for transfers. Similar restrictions exist when transferring in/out of a car.

In addition to the functional task of moving from one seated surface to another, transfers can be used to encourage a patient's symmetrical LE weight-bearing and weight shifting to enhance sit-to-stand transition and gait. Initially after an injury, a patient may require major assistance to successfully complete a transfer. Several strategies are reviewed here for teaching transfers depending on a patient's motor control and the level of assistance needed.

In preparation for transfers:

1. Work with the patient to maintain midline symmetry in sitting.
2. Have the patient lean forward a few times to activate the LEs for weight-bearing.
3. Have the patient perform a partial stand and weight shift laterally as described previously for lateral scooting.
4. Ask the patient to remain in a partial stand and "dust" the surface by moving his lower trunk right and left for increasing weight shifts while maintaining the partial stand for longer periods.
5. Determine UE placement.
6. Determine the type of transfer to be completed:
   a. Partial stand transfer
   b. Full stand transfer (see Chapter 36)

*Squat-Pivot Partial Stand Transfer: Wheelchair to Mat Transfer.* In this transfer, the patient raises the buttocks off the surface in a "1-inch partial squat," enough to unweight the buttocks and pivot on the feet to the new surface. The transfer occurs from one edge (the wheelchair) to another edge (the mat).

Sequence:

1. Have the patient scoot forward toward the edge of the chair or mat, as previously taught.
2. Foot placement: Figure 35-20 shows how the lead foot (i.e., the foot closest to the surface the patient is transferring to) should be placed forward and turned in toward midline (i.e., aligned with the ending sitting position). The other foot is placed back and pointed outward.
3. Hand placement: The patient's hands are placed in natural weight-bearing positions.
4. The therapist may be seated in front of the patient as shown in Fig. 35-17AB, facing in the same direction as the patient's feet are pointing.
5. The patient is guided to perform a partial stand, turn, sit, and repeat in increments until the transfer is complete. Repositioning will be necessary as the patient progresses through the transfer.

Alternatives:

1. Use a transfer board for patients who are unable to complete the 1-inch partial stand but can unweight enough to move across the transfer board. Box 35-8 provides important considerations when using a transfer board.

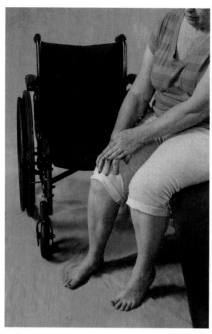

**FIGURE 35-20** Foot placement and body alignment during squat-pivot partial stand transfer is shown. The trailing foot is placed in alignment with the body's start position, and the leading foot is aligned with the end position, where the transfer will be completed.

---

**BOX 35-8    Preparation for Using a Transfer Board**

A transfer board may be helpful for patients who are unable to complete a transfer in one movement because of strength or balance impairments. Often, patients initially learn transfers using a transfer board and progress to independence. Key points for using a transfer board include the following:

- Select the appropriate transfer board on the basis of the patient's strength and control (length, width, hand cutouts, or options to decrease shearing forces).
- Place the board under the patient's buttock on the side closest to the transfer destination.
- Position the board at an angle to the mat so that it passes in front of the rear wheel of the wheelchair.
- Take care to avoid any pinching of the patient's skin. If needed, assist the patient in a lateral weight shift toward the side opposite where the board is being placed in order to allow safe and appropriate placement of the board.
- Avoid shearing forces created by "sliding" across the board; be sure the patient lifts the buttocks during the transfer.
- Warn the patient not to insert his fingers/hand into the sliding board cutouts during the transfer.

---

2. Use a second person, positioned behind and to the side of the patient toward the direction of the transfer, to provide additional assist. The second person places her hands at the patient's hips and upper thighs. During the transfer, the second person helps the patient shift body weight forward onto the feet and helps guide the lateral weight shift in the direction of the transfer. A transfer board may also be used.

3. Changing the patient's UE positioning can be useful in transferring patients who demonstrate contraversive pushing as described previously (Box 35-1) or to encourage patients to utilize the LEs more than the UEs. Stand in front of the patient in a stride position. Position the patient's UEs forward with the hands resting on your arms or waist (Fig. 35-21). Manual contacts are moved to more distal locations on the patient as a progression.

4. To encourage increased weight-bearing on the impaired LE during the squat-pivot transfer in a patient with hemiplegia:

   a. Place the impaired LE farther back under the support surface (in more knee flexion), with the unimpaired leg placed farther forward.

   b. Place the unimpaired foot up on a footstool while the impaired leg remains on the floor to receive increased weight shift.

*Transfers in Sitting for the Patient With an SCI.* Several strategies exist for individuals with an SCI to transfer between two surfaces in an upright sitting position, either independently or with assistance. In individuals with an SCI, the level of injury typically defines the level of independence a patient may achieve with transfers. Typically, the higher the level of injury, the greater the dependence on others for transfers. The therapist must consider muscle strength, motor control, sitting balance, selective muscle imbalances, ROM, body weight/mass, spasticity, the presence of orthostatic hypotension, cognition, age, fear, motivation, the presence of bracing/orthoses, the

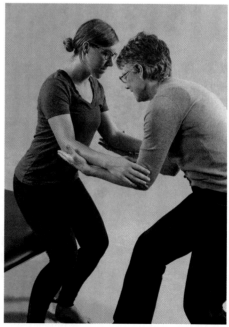

**FIGURE 35-21** Partial-squat transfer is shown with the therapist in stride stance and the patient's forearms resting on the therapist's forearms, grasping the therapist's lower arms bilaterally.

height of the surfaces, and the presence of other secondary complications in selecting the appropriate transfer strategy.

Use of the **head-hips relationship principle** is critical in a successful transfer. According to the head-hips principle, when the head is moved in one direction, the hips move in the opposite direction. For example, when the patient leans forward at the hips (head moving down), the hips will unweight (rise). When the patient wants to move his hips to the left, he can swing his head and upper torso to the right. Figure 35-22 shows a patient moving his head and upper torso down and to the right in order to move his hips forward and to the left. The head-hips principle takes advantage of momentum to control movement. The higher the level of injury, the more the patient needs to exaggerate the head-hips principle to take advantage of momentum.

The patient with weak or absent triceps will need to use the **elbow-locking mechanism** to bear weight through the UE with an extended elbow. This principle requires innervated anterior deltoid and upper pectoral muscles. With a closed kinetic chain (hand in weight-bearing), activation of the anterior deltoid and upper pectoral muscles combined with shoulder external rotation results in biomechanical locking of the elbow in extension (see Fig. 26-6AB).

You should also pay close attention to appropriate patient hand placement. In patients without selective finger control who have active wrist extension, preserve the functional **tenodesis grip** by never weight-bearing with extended fingers (see Fig. 26-8B). Also avoid extreme wrist extension to prevent increased pressure on the median nerve and carpal tunnel. To limit wrist extension, have the patient weight-bear on a closed fist with the wrist in neutral, place the fingers over the edge of the transferring surface, and combine finger flexion with limited wrist extension. Additional tips for transfer preparation are given in Box 35-9.

In each of the transfers described, you should guard the patient by sitting or standing in front. From the front, you can prevent the patient from falling in any direction. You may

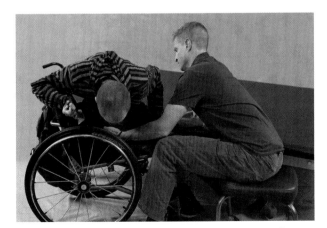

**FIGURE 35-22** Short-sit lateral transfer for a patient with a spinal cord injury is shown. Using the head-hips principle, the patient moves his head and upper torso down and to his right in order to move his hips forward and to the left.

---

**BOX 35-9  Tips for Transfer Preparation in Individuals With a Spinal Cord Injury**

- Place the patient's wheelchair as close as possible to the transferring surface with the front of the chair angled slightly toward the surface (at an approximately 30-degree angle).
- Be sure the brakes on the chair are locked.
- Rotate out of the way, lift, or remove the armrest on the transfer side.
- To assist with stability in weight-bearing, place the patient's feet on the wheelchair footrests, floor, combination of floor and footrest, or mat (see long-sit transfer).
  - If the patient's feet remain on the chair footrests, complete the transfer in increments to stop and reposition the feet during the transfer.
  - If the patient's feet are positioned on the floor and the front rigging is movable, remove the leg/foot rests or fold/swing the footrests up out of the way to avoid the rigging, which may cause patient injury or interfere with the transfer.
- Use the head-hips relationship to preposition the hips slightly forward or rotated toward the transferring surface.

---

also support in front of the patient's knees to prevent him from sliding forward, prevent the legs from extending because of a spasm, or assist with repositioning the feet during the transfer. Several alternative strategies exist for transfer with patients with an SCI. Refer to Chapter 26 for a more in-depth discussion of transfer strategies.

### Short-Sit Lateral Transfer

In this transfer, the patient with a strong upper body utilizes a push-up with full shoulder depression to clear the buttocks and head-hips momentum and move the hips toward the transferring surface (see Fig. 26-20AB). The patient may need to use the elbow-locking mechanism depending on triceps strength. When the patient does not have the strength to transfer over in one movement, transferring in smaller increments is an option.

### Long-Sit Lateral Transfer

In the long-sitting transfer, the patient places the feet and lower legs up onto the transferring surface while remaining seated in the wheelchair. With the legs already on the mat, the patient then uses the shoulder depression push-up and head-hips relationship to move the buttocks over onto the mat and vice versa when returning to the wheelchair (Fig. 35-23AB). This works well when the transferring surfaces are even and plenty of room is available for placement of the LEs. It also allows the patient to remain in a supported sitting position that assists with trunk balance while managing the LEs.

### Roll-Out Transfer

The **roll-out transfer** begins as in the long-sitting lateral transfer with the LEs up on the mat. The patient then places an

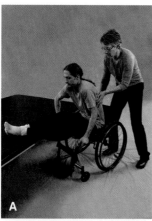

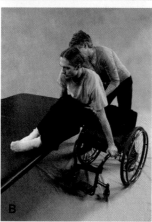

**FIGURE 35-23** Long-sit lateral transfer for a patient with a spinal cord injury is shown. (A) Starting with legs on the mat, the patient (B) uses a push-up and head-hips principle, moving the head to the left, to move the buttocks to the right over onto the mat.

outstretched arm or elbow on the mat (the arm closest to the transferring surface) and swings the other arm across the body (momentum) in order to "roll out" of the wheelchair onto the mat into a prone position. Again, this transfer is best performed when moving from the wheelchair to a bed or mat and when the surface heights are relatively even.

### Advanced Skills: Ground-to-Wheelchair Transfer

The ground-to-wheelchair transfer is essential for those with an SCI who use manual wheelchairs in the community, especially for those who are active in recreational activities. Figure 35-24ABC depicts a commonly used strategy. The individual is positioned perpendicular to the front of the wheelchair with knees to the chest and feet on the floor (Fig. 35-24A). Using the head-hips relationship and momentum, the patient transfers his weight mechanically onto the feet by ducking the head and pushing through the arms, resulting in a high lift of the buttocks (Fig. 35-24B). Using the arms and momentum of the upper torso, the patient simultaneously lifts and twists the buttocks onto the seat of the chair (Fig. 35-24C).

### Sitting: Dependent Transfers

Patients with substantial paresis and motor control deficits may not be able to assist with transfers or may be able to assist

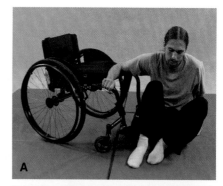

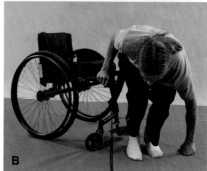

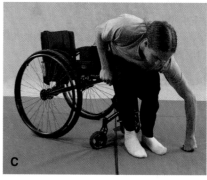

**FIGURE 35-24** Ground-to-wheelchair transfer for a patient with a spinal cord injury is shown. (A) The patient positions himself perpendicular to the front of his wheelchair with his knees to his chest and his feet on the floor. (B) Using the head-hips relationship and momentum, he transfers his weight mechanically onto his feet by ducking his head while pushing with his arms, resulting in a high lift of the buttocks. (C) Using his arms and the momentum of his upper torso, the patient simultaneously lifts and twists his buttocks onto the seat of his chair.

only minimally. Mechanical lifts can be used when manual transfer of the patient is difficult. Use of a lift is practical for the patient's family, caregivers, and health-care professionals and for long-term patient and caregiver safety. Many types of lifts are available (e.g., the Hoyer Lift) through medical equipment vendors. The suppliers are good resources for selecting the appropriate lift for a patient's particular needs.

Many hospitals are incorporating "no-lift" policies as part of an overall approach to prevent musculoskeletal injuries in staff and promote safe patient care. The no-lift policy calls for staff members to avoid manual lift techniques in virtually all patient care situations. The advent of these policies increases the number of mechanical lifts available to staff and decreases the use of dependent transfers by therapists in these settings.

A few different strategies are described here for manual one- and two-person dependent transfers. These transfers work well for many individuals with an SCI and for patients with severe impairments. Prepare for the transfer with appropriate wheelchair placement, management of the footrests and armrests, and positioning of the patient in the chair (see Boxes 35-8 and 35-9). Maintain safety at all times! This includes patient and therapist safety by utilizing proper body mechanics and transfer techniques. Use appropriate judgment in your decision to use manual versus mechanical lifts.

### One-Person Lifts

One option for a one-person lift is to position yourself in a half-kneeling position in front of the patient. Lean the patient forward and the upper torso away from the mat/chair with the patient's chest over your shoulder. The patient's arms can be in the lap or over your shoulders. Place your hands under the patient's buttocks and your forearms under the patient's thighs as much as possible. Lean back and rock the patient forward while pivoting the patient to the mat/chair (Fig. 35-25ABCDEF). In all transfers, shifting your weight back and pivoting your body as a whole avoids twisting the patient's body and maintains good body mechanics.

As an alternative to the half-kneeling transfer, position yourself on a rolling stool in front of the patient. Place the patient's knees in between your legs. Lean the patient forward and the upper torso away from the mat/chair with patient's chest over your shoulder. The patient's arms can be in the lap or over your shoulders. Place your hands under the patient's ischial tuberosities and your forearms under the patient's thighs as much as possible. Lean back and rock the patient forward while pivoting the patient to the mat/chair (Fig. 35-26ABCDEF).

As another one-person lift option, position yourself in front of the patient in a semisquat. Place the patient's legs in between your legs with your knees positioned so that the patient's knees are blocked from sliding forward. Lean the patient forward and the upper torso away from the mat/chair with the patient's chest over your shoulder or under your arm against your hip (Fig. 35-27AB). Place your hands under the patient's buttocks as much as possible. Lean back and rock the patient forward while pivoting him to the mat/chair. Plantarflex your foot to provide a posterior force along the femur to help guide the pelvis laterally and prevent the patient from sliding forward.

With all these transfers, you may use a gait belt around the patient's hips to assist with the lift, rather than reaching with your hands under the buttocks. Also, with each of the one-person lift alternatives described, a second person positioned behind the patient, half-way between both surfaces, can help with lifting the patient's hips as needed (Fig. 35-28).

### Two-Person Lifts

In some cases, the therapist cannot safely transfer a patient alone, even with a second person assisting during a one-person

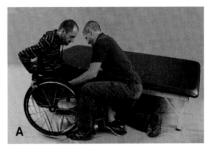
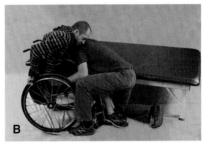
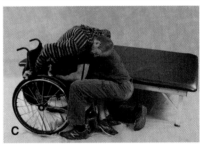
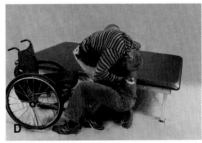
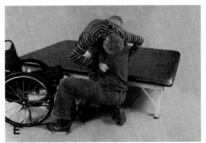
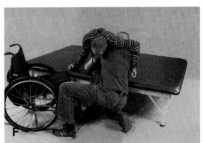

**FIGURE 35-25** The photos in A–F illustrate the steps in a one-person transfer for a patient with a spinal cord injury, with the therapist in a stable half-kneeling position.

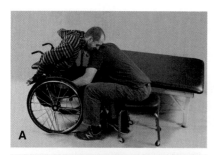
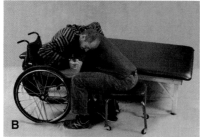
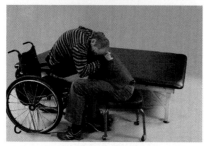
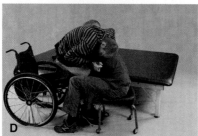
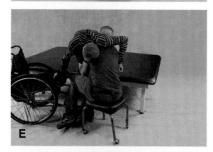
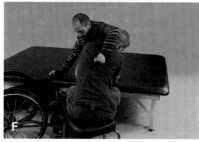

**FIGURE 35-26** The photos in A–F illustrate the steps in a one-person transfer for a patient with a spinal cord injury, with the therapist seated on a stool.

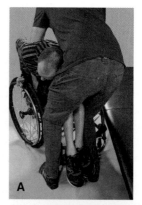
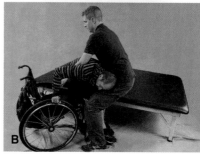

**FIGURE 35-27** The photos in A–B illustrate a one-person transfer for a patient with a spinal cord injury, with the therapist standing.

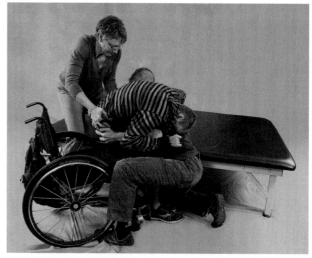

**FIGURE 35-28** Half-kneeling one-person lift for a patient with a spinal cord injury, with a second person assisting.

lift. During multiperson dependent transfers, it is important for one person to take the lead in directing the transfer. This person should communicate clearly the stepwise process and the directions to be used before starting the transfer and should call out the timing, such as "on the count of three." This enhances coordination of all persons involved. Typically, the lead person is positioned at the patient's head or torso.

In one option for a two-person dependent transfer, position yourself behind the patient and toward the transferring surface. Cross the patient's arms across the chest, bring your hands under the patient's upper arms and over the forearms, holding onto the forearms. To safely perform this body hold and prevent injury to the patient's shoulders, the patient must have enough shoulder strength to actively depress and stabilize both shoulders during the transfer. You should also squeeze the patient's ribs to avoid sliding into the axilla (which could hurt the patient's shoulders). The second person is positioned in front of the patient, supporting the patient's LEs as high under the thighs as possible. With the patient actively depressing the shoulders, the team simultaneously lifts the patient to a short-sitting position on the transferring surface (Fig. 35-29).

When moving to a long-sitting position, the person at the patient's legs should be positioned on the side of the patient farthest way from the transferring surface, with one arm cradled under the patient's thighs as high as possible and the other arm cradling the lower legs. This way, the second person can place both of the patient's legs entirely on the transferring surface without catching on the edge of the mat or bed.

When the patient does not have the shoulder strength to depress the shoulders during the transfer, the therapist in front can lean the patient forward enough so the therapist behind can get ahold of the patient underneath the buttocks, hold onto the patient's pants at the sides of the hips, or grasp a gait belt placed around the patient's hips. When holding onto pants, be sure to take up any extra material so the pants serve as a sling. Do not lift from behind the patient and pull up on his pants, or you will cause the pants to ride up, placing pressure on the buttocks and groin area. Once the therapist behind is holding the patient, the person in front can lean the patient back so he rests back on the therapist's arms. The person in front then repositions to support the LEs during the transfer.

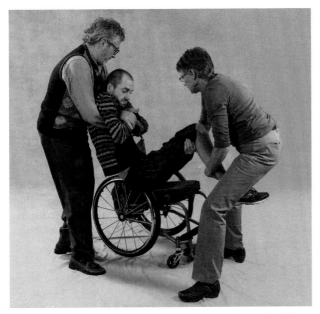

**FIGURE 35-29** Two-person transfer from ground to wheelchair.

### Contemplate Clinical Decisions: Skill

*Consider the following questions:*

1. *To which side will it be easier for Sophie to transfer?*
2. *Why do you want to incorporate transfers to both sides early on in rehabilitation?*
3. *Given Sophie's initial function, what modifications would you consider?*
4. *How would you instruct the husband in helping his wife transfer?*
5. *How could you increase the challenge of the transfer task?*
6. *How would you sequence your activities and techniques? What would you do first?*
7. *How do interventions for skill compare with previous tasks/ activities?*

*For Sophie's functional status at 6 weeks:*

1. *How will therapist position and manual cues change from the initial interventions?*
2. *How can you vary transfers to increase Sophie's function at home?*
3. *What are your new short-term goals for Sophie?*

## Pediatric Considerations

The principles described previously for the adult population also apply to the pediatric population. In children, additional varied sitting positions (straddle sit, long sit, side sit) may be incorporated. Children spend time in floor play and will need to transition between many different positions. For example, the child may move from crossed-ankle sitting to side sitting and then to quadruped to reach a toy and then rock back into a W-sit to play. Stable midline sitting symmetry is necessary for the development of UE functional tasks. Activities need to be progressed for weight shifts in controlled mobility and skill tasks.

The patient requires less assistance for transfers when sitting balance is good. Parents of young children often lift their child for transfers and do not consider how transfers will be completed as the child grows and becomes heavier. Independent transfers will allow the child to have greater independence in the school environment, including bus transfers, toileting, and play.

The therapist needs to be creative and offer play activities that encourage the child to move into varied sitting postures because the child will not follow verbal cues or stay motivated for repetitive practice. The play activities selected will depend on the child's age and interests. For example, a 5 year-old child may be willing to play "statue" and freeze while the therapist offers resistance for RS or alternating isometrics. Playing "Superman" encourages a prolonged hold of extensor musculature for strengthening. Sitting on a therapeutic ball develops trunk control and equilibrium reactions. The feet can be placed on or off the floor depending on the goals of the session. The child can look at a book, play catch, or engage in other play activities while on the ball. Varied surfaces such as swings, slides, tilt boards, and scooter boards will keep the child engaged while offering varied conditions to improve sitting postures. Children as well as adults may enjoy working on sitting while horseback riding. Ideas for exercising in sitting are limited only by one's imagination.

## Progressing Functional Interventions in Sitting

Previous sections offered several suggestions for increasing the level of challenge for the patient. In addition to altering variables relating to the patient (e.g., base of support, head movement, and eyes open or closed), the environment (e.g., stable or moving, consistent, or changing), and the task (e.g., simplicity or complexity, speed of movement), you may consider motor learning and exercise variables. Consider the frequency, timing, and scheduling of feedback. High levels of assistance throughout a task may impede learning, whereas providing the patient an opportunity to problem-solve movement enhances learning. Allowing the patient time to think about the movement rather than immediately providing your feedback may also facilitate learning. Altering practice schedules, such as planning a highly specific task and randomizing practice trials, also enhances motor learning. Figure 35-30 illustrates how intervention variables can be changed to progress treatment with increasing demand placed on the patient.

## ■ Intervention: Considerations for Nontherapy Time and Discharge

While the patient remains in an inpatient setting, he should be encouraged to practice outside the therapy environment. The patient must be able to safely and correctly perform the suggested exercises independently. The health-care team should also consider the patient's endurance level for ongoing activities throughout the day. Carryover and practice of learned tasks in therapy may be incorporated without undue fatigue on the nursing floor. Possible exercises include sitting with an erect posture at the dining room table, scooting to the edge of the chair before a transfer, and asking the health-care provider for permission to perform a couple of partial stands before completing the transfer. With supervision, the patient may don socks and shoes while seated or prepare his wheelchair for a transfer by leaning forward to lock the brakes and removing the foot pedals. As the patient nears discharge, the caregiver(s) should learn and begin to supervise and/or assist with these tasks.

## Patient and Family Education

It is beneficial for the caregiver to attend a few treatment sessions to observe the patient performing the exercise program. This allows the therapist to explain the purpose of the activities and point out when the task is performed correctly or when adjustments need to be made. The therapist can model how to best cue the patient and provide manual contacts for facilitation of a task or for safety. Caregivers will most likely need several opportunities to observe and learn how to best assist their "patient." Caregivers also need to perform the tasks in order to demonstrate their understanding and competence for the therapist. This process may be overwhelming to the caregivers, who are often undergoing numerous changes in their lives after the neurological insult to their loved one. The therapist should be understanding and patient when teaching the caregiver the skills needed.

The patient and family must also consider any needed adaptations to the home environment before discharge. For example, transfers are easier and safer when the two surfaces are equal in height. Therefore, the toilet height at home may need to be raised with a toilet raiser, or the patient's bed may have to be raised to more closely match the height of the wheelchair.

Safety continues to be a factor, and when a desk chair or table chair is on wheels, an alternative stable chair will be needed. A tub seat may be necessary for bathing. The therapist needs to consider the patient's ability to safely short sit with or without back support in order to determine the best seat. Consideration to the needs of others living in the home is necessary to ensure that everyone can function with any permanent adaptations. Universal design resources may be helpful to the patient and family.

## Activities for Home

The patient needs to practice interventions outside the therapy environment. Safety should be the first consideration when activities are being determined. The patient should not be asked to perform more than three to five exercises in the home program, and compliance is improved when activities are linked to the functional tasks built into the person's daily routine. For example, the patient may be asked to perform five 1-inch stands at the end of each meal before leaving the table. The patient may lay the newspaper on the kitchen table and then maintain a symmetrical posture while leaning forward to turn the pages. The patient may sit by the clothes dryer and remove the clothes and place them on the counter (which will be rather high when the patient is seated). This task allows for weight shifting, trunk rotation, and extension.

When the therapist understands the components needed for sitting and transfers as well as the movement patterns used during daily tasks, numerous exercises for a home program can be realized. Box 35-10 gives examples of the types of questions a therapist should consider when designing components of a home program. Box 35-11 provides a sample home exercise program.

**Changing Intervention Variables* to Progress Treatment**
(e.g., Position = Sitting)

| Motor Control Variables:<br>Task = Define the task | ↑Stability ↓Challenge ⟷ ↓Stability ↑Challenge | | | | | | | |
|---|---|---|---|---|---|---|---|---|
| **Person** — Transport (moving) | No | | | | | | | Yes |
| Base of support | Wide | | | | | | | Narrow |
| Center of mass | Low | | | | | | | High |
| # Joints involved | 1-few | | | | | | | Many |
| UE | B-WB (Wide → Narrow) | 1-WB | NWB | Manipulation: simple | Manipulation: complex | | | ↑Speed |
| LE | B-WB (Wide → Narrow) | Staggered | 1-WB | Alternative WB | NWB quiet | NWB mvmt simple | NWB mvmt complex | ↑Speed |
| Trunk | Passively placed | | | Active | Active/resistance | | | |
| Head | Stable | | | Moving | Complex visual field | | | |
| Eyes | Open | | | Closed | Complex visual field | | | |
| Cognitive challenge | Low | | | | | | | High |
| **Environment** — Seated surface | Stable (firm) | Unstable (soft/tilt) | | Moving: Consistent (e.g., car–straight road) | Moving: Variable (e.g., boat, roller coaster) | | | |
| Seat height | Low (hips > 90°) | | | Even (hips = 90°) | High (hips < 90°) | | | |
| Seat angle | Tilt posterior | | | | Tilt anterior | | | |
| Armrests | Yes | | | | None | | | |
| Back support | Yes: High | | | Yes: Low | None | | | |
| **Motor Learning** — Feedback | | | | | | | | |
| • Frequency | High<br>High levels of guidance | | | | Low<br>Discovery | | | |
| • Timing | Instantaneous KR | | | | Delayed KR | | | |
| • Scheduling | Reverse-faded | | | Constant | Faded | | | |
| Practice | | | | | | | | |
| • Specificity | Low | | | | High | | | |
| • Variability | Blocked and non-variable | | | | Random and unpredictable | | | |
| • Part/whole | Part | | | | Whole | | | |
| **Exercise Variables** — Frequency | Low (↓practice amount) | | | | High (↑practice amount) | | | |
| Duration | Short (↓practice amount) | | | | Long (↑practice amount) | | | |
| Intensity | Low | | | | High | | | |

*Note: Ideally do not alter more than one variable at a time.

**FIGURE 35-30** Treatment progression through changing intervention variables.

---

**BOX 35-10  Examples of Questions to Consider When Designing a Home Program**

Consider the patient's functional goal. For example, for a goal of returning to driving, consider the task of backing out of the driveway in your car and checking for traffic by placing your arm on the seat back and rotating your head and trunk.

- Describe the motions of your head, trunk, pelvis, and scapular girdle.
- How does your weight shift?
- How do your lower extremities move?
- How could you integrate these movements into a treatment session to improve sitting?
- What activities can the patient safely perform while at home (without excessive burden to the caregiver)?

---

**BOX 35-11  Sample Home Exercise Program for a Child**

1. Ring sitting on the floor without back support: Reach upward for a block and place it on the floor to the child's right to build a tower. When the tower falls, ask the child to reach from a seated position to retrieve the blocks. (The child may move into side sitting to reach farther.)
2. Sitting on a low stool in front of a mirror, chalkboard, or refrigerator: Ask the child to color, draw with whipped topping, or play with magnets. Incorporate reaching in all directions.
3. Sitting sideways in a rocking chair: The child will need to maintain lateral trunk control with the rocking motions. The parent may alter the speed and degree of rocking to increase the challenge. The child can turn the pages of a book during the task to limit protective extension reactions and improve equilibrium reactions.
4. Sitting on a flat scooter and holding on to the end of a rope: The parent pulls the child on the scooter. The parent may alter the speed, sudden stops/starts, and direction. The task can be made easier by using a broomstick instead of rope or made more difficult with a piece of TheraBand. This can be done in the home on level surfaces or outside on rougher sidewalks.

---

# HANDS-ON PRACTICE

Be sure to practice the following skills addressed in this chapter. With further practice, you should be able to:

- Use various positioning options for a hemiparetic upper extremity during sitting.
- Instruct/guide/assist a patient into sitting (either short sitting or long sitting) from supine.
- Use any of the following proprioception neuromuscular facilitation techniques in sitting to promote:
    - Stability: shortened held resisted contraction, alternating isometrics, rhythmic stabilization
    - Controlled mobility: slow reversal hold, slow reversal, agonistic reversals
    - Strengthening: appropriate resistance or assistance
- Apply various activities to help a patient with contraversive pushing maintain sitting.

- Instruct/guide/assist a patient to achieve the following skill activities in sitting:
    - Scooting forward
    - 1-Inch partial stands
    - Scooting backward
    - Side-to-side scooting
    - Squat-pivot transfer
    - Use of a transfer board
    - Long-sit lateral transfer for a patient with a spinal cord injury (SCI)
    - Roll-out transfer for a patient with an SCI
    - One-person dependent transfer for a patient with an SCI
    - Two-person dependent transfers for a patient with an SCI

---

## Let's Review

1. Describe normal patterns of trunk movements in sitting.

2. Describe the importance of functions in sitting as a part of normal daily life. Why is this an important position in which to function?

3. Identify impairments that may contribute to abnormal function in sitting.

4. Identify important considerations for analyzing patient function in sitting:
    a. Ability to perform task
    b. How the task is performed
    c. What happened under various conditions or task demands
    d. Evaluation of why the patient moves a particular way

5. Identify important standardized tests for measuring sitting performance.

6. Identify indicators to predict prognosis of movement function in sitting.

7. Outline appropriate treatment interventions to improve and progress function in sitting.

8. Identify activities for patients during nontherapy time and to incorporate in a home exercise program.

9. What evidence supports patient management in sitting?

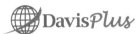 **DavisPlus**    For additional resources, including Focus on Evidence tables, case study discussions, references and glossary, please visit http://davisplus.fadavis.com

## CHAPTER SUMMARY

As noted in the scenarios described previously, key daily functional activities take place in sitting, such as playing, eating, driving, toileting, writing, and typing at the computer keyboard. This chapter focuses on the promotion of trunk control and functional activities in sitting to improve activity and general participation in individuals with dysfunction. Typical movement patterns, impairments underlying movement problems, safety considerations, examination components, and lifespan influences are discussed. Interventions to address functional activity limitations are presented within the context of stages of motor control (mobility, stability, controlled mobility, and skill). Sample patient cases (in text and in online (ONL) resources) provide illustrations for treating sitting dysfunction in individuals with different neurological diagnoses. Although evidence to support many specific intervention techniques is lacking, the online Focus on Evidence Table 35-9 (ONL) summarizes the most important recent studies addressing this topic.

## CHAPTER 36

# Functional Intervention in Sit-to-Stand, Stand-to-Sit, and Standing

Mary T. Blackinton PT, EdD, GCS, CEEAA

## CHAPTER OBJECTIVES

Upon completion of this chapter, the learner should be able to:

1. Describe the biomechanical and motor control characteristics for sit-to-stand, standing, and stand-to-sit.
2. Identify at least three control parameters for sit-to-stand, standing, and stand-to-sit.
3. Hypothesize impairments of body structure/function that will interfere with the functional skills/ activity of sit-to-stand, stand-to-sit, and standing.
4. Identify tests and measures that can be used during an examination of sit-to-stand, stand-to-sit, and standing; include both quantitative and qualitative tests.
5. Alter the biomechanics of sit-to-stand or stand-to-sit to make the task easier or harder for a patient.
6. Demonstrate a progression of standing interventions in which the patient exhibits (1) quiet standing, (2) standing with head, arms, or trunk movement, and (3) weight shift within the base of support.
7. Apply the concept of practice intensity to the skills of sit-to-stand and stand-to-sit by demonstrating a task-intensive practice session.
8. Teach a patient to move sit-to-stand or stand-to-sit with minimally explicit directions to emphasize implicit learning.
9. Design a functional therapeutic exercise program using sit-to-stand and stand-to-sit, including a progression of the activities using added weight, tubing, or changes in the biomechanics of the tasks.
10. Given a case study of a patient with hemiparesis who has difficulty standing symmetrically and moving sit-to-stand, design a plan of care that includes functional training strategies, electrotherapeutic modalities, and an orthosis or heel wedge to improve symmetry.
11. Given a case study of a patient with a progressive neurological disease, suggest two types of home modification equipment to assist with sit-to-stand and standing.
12. Develop a home exercise program to enhance the functional skills of (1) sit-to-stand, (2) stand-to-sit, and (3) standing and weight shifting.

# Introduction

When asked about their personal rehab goals, most people with neurological impairments immediately reply "I want to walk again!" Patients rarely acknowledge standing up as an important goal, despite the fact they must stand in order to walk. Clinically, it is possible to see a patient who can walk with supervision but who needs physical assistance to stand up from a chair.

Sit-to-stand (STS) and stand-to-sit (SIT) are critical functional skills and the ultimate *transitional movements* because they are the gateway between seated activities and standing/gait functions. Standing facilitates many important functions/activities: (1) the ability to access home/work/play tools or equipment that is above wheelchair height, such as a standard refrigerator and closet shelves; (2) the ability to transfer to the toilet, car, bathtub, or exercise equipment; and (3) the ability to move to a position that assists in the prevention of lower extremity (LE) contractures and ischial tuberosity/sacral pressure sores. Likewise, the ability to stand independently, even when the patient is unable to walk, allows functional independence for self-care, home/work/school management, and participation in the community with or without environmental adaptation.

This chapter focuses on the transitions from STS, SIT, and standing as key tasks crucial to functional independence and mobility for patients with neuromuscular deficits.

# Biomechanical and Motor Control Characteristics of Sit-to-Stand, Stand-to-Sit, and Standing

Movement analysis and functional training utilize principles of biomechanics and motor control. The next sections describe the biomechanical and motor control variables related to STS, standing, and SIT. Before reading on, take a moment to perform the following activities so you can appreciate these variables:

## THINK ABOUT IT 36.1

### "Take a Stand"

Ask someone to videotape you while moving from sit-to-stand:

- Stand up first without thinking. How did you stand up? How long did it take you? What were the relative positions of your feet, knees, and trunk? Did you use your arms or did you use momentum?
- Stand again: This time place your feet out in front of your knees and then stand. Was that easier or harder than when your feet were behind you? How did your speed and effort change? How did you compensate for the change in foot position?
- Sit down, but do not allow your trunk to bend forward while sitting down. How did that change the time, effort, and quality of your movement for stand-to-sit?

- Stand up again with the majority of weight on only one leg. What happened to your symmetry and posture? How balanced did you feel in standing?
- Remain standing without moving; how much muscular effort are you using? How does your effort change when you turn and look behind you or raise your hands over your head?

## Biomechanical Analysis of Sit-to-Stand

### Four Mechanical Phases of Sit-to-Stand

Unlike the clearly defined and agreed-upon phases of gait, the biomechanics of STS have been described using different classification systems (Etnyre, 2007; Fotoohabadi, 2010; Janssen, 2002b; Schenkman, 1990). Schenkman described four mechanical phases of STS: (1) flexion momentum, (2) momentum transfer, (3) extension, and (4) stabilization (Table 36-1). *Flexion momentum* is the forward motion of the trunk over the feet as the pelvis rotates forward and increases hip flexion. The center of mass (COM) in this phase moves primarily *forward*; hence, this is also referred to as the *horizontal* phase of STS. A kinematic analysis of the spine and LEs during an STS task in healthy older adults revealed that during this phase the hips moved 19.4 degrees from the starting position to their maximally flexed position, whereas the lumbar spine contributed only 4.1 degrees of flexion during this phase (Fotoohabadi, 2010).

The second phase, *momentum transfer*, is the shift of weight from the buttocks to the feet using both momentum force and hip/knee muscle forces. This phase is also called the *liftoff* phase because it refers to the point when the buttocks leave the chair surface. At this time, the thoracic spine moves into more extension while the lumbar spine is slightly more flexed (Fotoohabadi, 2010). The *momentum transfer* phase involves two strategies: (1) The momentum generated during phase I is immediately transferred to the total body to allow continued motion vertically into standing, and (2) the trunk rotates forward over the hips to the maximum hip flexion position *before* liftoff (Schenkman, 1990). The latter strategy reduces the use of momentum and thus requires greater muscle force in the legs; however, it is more stable.

The *extension* phase describes concomitant knee and hip extension that moves the COM upward, and because of this upward direction, this phase has also been referred to as the *vertical* phase of STS. During the extension phase, the lumbar spine also moves from approximately 5.9 degrees of flexion to 13.3 degrees of extension (Fotoohabadi, 2010.) The *stabilization* phase is the reestablishment of balance over a smaller base of support (BOS) once standing, with the hips, knees, and lumbar spine in relative extension.

These four phases of STS are used throughout this chapter. It is important to note that scooting forward in a chair is not a component of STS. The "ready" position for moving STS in both examination and training assumes both feet are flat on the floor. Some sitting surfaces, such as hospital beds and wheelchairs, require the patient to scoot forward so the feet

| TABLE 36-1 | Phases of Sit-to-Stand* | |
|---|---|---|
| PHASE | NAME | BIOMECHANICAL EVENTS IN PHASE |
| 1 | Flexion momentum | Trunk and pelvis rotate forward over the hips approximately 16 degrees. Upper body momentum is created when the person leans forward, reflecting upper body mass and the velocity in which it moves. The erector spinae muscles act eccentrically to control the forward momentum. It is a relatively stable phase because the COM is within the BOS. This phase can also be called the *horizontal phase* because the COM is translating horizontally. |
| 2 | Momentum transfer | This begins when the buttocks lift off the chair. Maximal motion occurs in ankle dorsiflexion, trunk flexion, and head extension. In this phase, the COM is moved vertically upward, and the BOS transfers from the buttocks to the feet. This point is described as "dynamic stability" because the COM is moving from one BOS to another. Muscle contributions include hip and knee extensor muscles such as the rectus femoris, vastus medialis, biceps femoris, and gluteus maximus. The highest ground reaction forces occur when the buttocks lift off the seat. |
| 3 | Extension | This phase begins with attainment of maximal dorsiflexion during phase 2 and ends when the hips stop moving in upright. The focus of this phase is to translate the body upward while the COM is over the feet. The muscle forces needed include continued coactivation of the knee and hip extensors as well as contraction of the abdominals. |
| 4 | Stabilization | In this phase, movement is terminated, and the body returns to normal postural sway. The key muscle groups involved in the control of quiet standing vary with the sway in the COM and include the erector spinae, iliopsoas, abdominals, gluteus medius and tensor fasciae latae, gastrocnemius/soleus, and tibialis anterior. |

BOS = base of support; COM = center of mass.

*As described by Schenkman M, Berger RA, Riley PO, Mann RW, Hodge WA. Whole-body movements during rising to standing from sitting. *Phys Ther.* 1990;70(10):638–651.

can be in this ready position and must be addressed by the therapist. However, scooting forward is NOT considered a normal biomechanical aspect of STS.

### Two-Phase System: Preextension and Extension

STS has also been described using a two-phase system that focuses on the position of the COM over the BOS (Carr, 1994, 2003; Shepherd, 1994). The two phases are called the *preextension* and *extension* phases. The purpose of the preextension phase is to move the COM over the BOS so less muscle force is needed to stand. This occurs by moving the feet posteriorly while the upper body rotates forward. The axis of rotation occurs in two places: around the hips when the trunk moves forward and around the ankle as the tibia moves forward over the foot. The anterior movement of both the trunk and tibia help to translate the COM from the chair to the feet. Muscle activity during the first phase begins with concentric activation of the iliopsoas for hip flexion and the tibialis anterior (TA) for ankle dorsiflexion (Khemlani, 1998). The abdominal and spinal muscles most likely cocontract to keep the trunk stable (Carr, 2003). Toward the end of phase 1, the biceps femoris may provide a braking action to hip/trunk flexion while assisting in hip extension (Khemlani, 1998).

The *extension phase* begins when the thighs lift off the chair and vertical motion results from concentric extensor muscle forces at the knees, hips, and ankles (Carr, 2003; Khemlani, 1998). These forces must be strong enough to move body weight vertically against gravity and are generated by combined action of the vastus lateralis and medialis, rectus femoris,

biceps femoris, gluteus maximus, and occasional gastrocnemius/soleus muscles (Carr, 2003). Knee extensor forces occur earlier than hip and ankle forces and have been predictive of independence in STS (Eriksrud, 2003).

Overall, the degree of motion and force generation required in the legs during STS is greater than that needed during ambulation (Jevsevar, 1993; Carr, 2003). This explains why some patients need assistance to stand up even though they are able to walk independently. The delineation of STS into phases is mainly for biomechanical analysis, as the movement itself does not occur in phases but is usually one continuous motion. However, identifying *where* in the STS continuum the patient is having difficulty will help therapists plan appropriate treatment strategies. For example, one patient may have difficulty standing because he does not bring the COM anteriorly during the flexion momentum phase, whereas another may need assistance because he lacks knee and hip extensor muscle strength. The phases can be used while documenting STS in a way that emphasizes your clinical reasoning about why the patient is experiencing a problem.

## THINK ABOUT IT 36.2

### Can You Picture This Patient's Sit-to-Stand Transition?

The patient needed minimal assistance (hand on back to bring trunk forward) from the therapist to move sit-to-stand (STS) from a wheelchair. During STS, the patient lacked forward flexion of the trunk and did not place the feet behind the knees. The patient's movement strategy interfered with flexion momentum and his ability to bring his center of mass over his new standing base of support. This increased the muscle force needed to rise off the seat during the momentum transfer phase, noted by pushing with his arms to assist in transferring the weight to his feet. He made three attempts before standing successfully. The overall time to stand up was 32 seconds. When given the external visual cue to move his "nose over toes," the patient could stand in 22 seconds.

## Motor Control Analysis of Sit-to-Stand

Motor control analysis adds to information from biomechanical analysis by considering how movement is organized on the basis of the specific individual, the task, and the environment in which the movement occurs (Shumway-Cook, 2012). Using motor control terminology, STS is a **discreet task** because it has a distinct beginning and end. It is also a **mobility task** because the COM moves from a relatively large and stable BOS that is close to the ground (e.g., a chair surface) to a less stable and higher position on a smaller BOS (i.e., the support area under both feet). STS can include upper extremity (UE) manipulation depending on whether the hands are used to push up from the chair or to carry an object such as a bottle of water. It is also a **closed task** because it requires relatively low attention and has little trial-to-trial variability.

**Control parameters** are defined as variables internal or external to the individual that influence the way the system organizes a particular movement (Shumway-Cook, 2012). Internal control parameters reflect the motor, sensory, and perceptual strategies of the individual, such as available motion or strength at a particular joint. External control parameters reflect the regulatory aspects of the environment, such as the size, shape, height, and firmness of objects.

In the introduction to the chapter, you were asked to stand up and sit down using slightly different positions of your feet and hands. On the basis of your experience, can you hypothesize the control parameters related to the STS task?

Janssen (2002b) reviewed the literature on the determinants of STS. The literature search indicated that chair height, foot position, and use of armrests influenced performance of STS (Table 36-2).

Chair height is an important and easy control parameter that therapists can address in retraining STS. Observe the amount of LE motion of the patient in Fig. 36-1ABC as she stands up from different seating surfaces. Which surface requires more muscle force? Other possible *external* control parameters include the firmness of the chair and the angle of the seat relative to the horizontal plane. In addition, Anan (2008) investigated the effect of cushion thickness on STS motion in older adults and found a significant increase in the amount of hip flexion needed between no cushion and a 90-mm cushion, even after controlling for overall seat height.

Foot position in patients after a stroke was analyzed by Brunt (2002) and Camargos (2009) with different results. Brunt (2002) reported greater activation of the TA and quadriceps (QD) when they were positioned behind the nonparetic limb, whereas Camargos (2009) found no significant differences in electromyography (EMG) values between symmetric and asymmetric foot positions in TA and QD muscles. Camargos (2009) reported that spontaneous strategies for foot position and symmetrical foot positions improved speed of standing and provided greater stability than asymmetrical

| **TABLE 36-2** | **Evidence-Based Control Parameters for Sit-to-Stand** |
|---|---|
| **CONTROL PARAMETER** | **EFFECT ON SIT-TO-STAND** |
| Chair height | • Lowering the height of the chair increases the difficulty and force requirements in STS. In community-dwelling and nursing home residents aged 64–105 years, a seat height of 120% of lower leg length promoted successful standing (Janssen, 2002b). |
| Foot position | • Foot and knee positions alter how far the COM must move forward. Altering the position of the feet affects the timing and amount of force generated in both healthy and impaired adults (Brunt, 2002). Placing the dominant or noninvolved leg at a biomechanical disadvantage results in greater force generation in the nondominant or involved leg in healthy adults and in people after a stroke (Brunt, 2002). |
| Armrests | • The use of armrests lowers the muscle forces required at the knee and hip (Janssen, 2002b), reduces the vertical peak ground reaction forces, increases the overall time to stand, and decreases the time needed for the flexion momentum phase (Schenkman, 1990).<br>• Keeping arms free significantly reduced leg forces needed during the events of momentum transfer, extension, and stability phases (Schenkman, 1990). |
| Chair cushion | • Greater cushion thickness (90 mm) significantly increased the amount of hip flexion required compared with thin cushion or no cushion (Anan, 2008). |
| Cane use | • In patients with hemiparesis, moving STS with a cane was faster and more symmetrical and yielded a greater extensor moment in the paretic limb than not using a cane (Hu, 2013). |

COM = center of mass; STS = sit-to-stand.

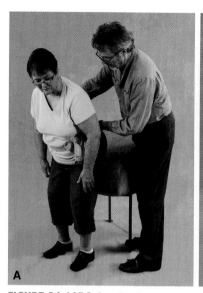
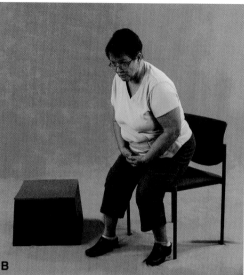
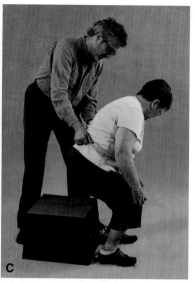

**FIGURE 36-1ABC** Seat height as a control parameter for sit-to-stand. (A) High surface, (B) standard chair height, and (C) low surface. Note the differences in the amount of knee flexion required during the momentum transfer phase of sit-to-stand.

strategies. Therefore, understanding factors that affect STS for a given patient helps direct your interventions.

Because the use of armrests changes the forces and timing of forces required at various segments of STS, the decision to retrain STS using armrests or with arms free should be made carefully and should depend on each patient's abilities. For example, a patient with LE weakness might be encouraged to use momentum-based strategies without using armrests, whereas a patient with postural instability might be encouraged to use armrests to increase stability in standing. Kinoshita (2012) investigated the kinematics of STS with and without handrails and with handrails in different locations and found a combination of high and low handrail positions increased the speed of STS and decreased LE torque compared with no handrails. Therapists should experiment with the use and position of armrests and handrails for each patient and incorporate changes as part of the progression of the plan of care.

Another caveat in STS training is that scooting forward is often trained as part of the task, even though it is only necessary in chairs that are deep. Therapists who want to encourage STS and ambulation should recommend seating that does not require the patient to scoot forward. In preparing your patients to stand, ask that they position the feet flat on the floor. This will ensure that the patient is forward in the chair when necessary and separates standing up from moving forward.

## Biomechanical and Motor Control Analysis of Standing

Standing is considered the stabilization phase of STS. In normal postural alignment using a lateral view, a standard plumb line starting slightly posterior to the apex of the coronal suture ideally falls through the external auditory meatus, midway through the shoulder, through the bodies of the lumbar vertebrae and sacral promontory, slightly posterior to the center of hip joint, slightly anterior to the axis of the knees joint, and

slightly anterior to the lateral malleolus (Kendall, 2005). Quiet standing is influenced by body alignment, muscle tone, postural tone, and muscle strength (Shumway-Cook, 2012). Muscles that are tonically active during standing include the gastrocnemius/soleus, TA, gluteus medius/tensor fasciae latae, iliopsoas, and erector spinae (Shumway-Cook, 2012).

However, altered postural alignment associated with aging, neurological deficits, or obesity can increase stability demands during quiet standing (Kendall, 2005). For example, when a patient with Parkinson disease (PD) stands with slight hip and knee flexion, the plumb line now falls posterior to the axis of the knee and requires activation of the QD muscles to maintain that position. Similarly, a unilateral deficit such as equinovarus position of the foot substantially alters the base of support and the forces needed to maintain balance in standing.

Let us proceed with motor control analysis in standing. In contrast to STS, standing is a **continuous** task because it has no beginning, middle, or end (Rose, 2006). It is also a **stability task** because the BOS is not moving. The COM moves slightly within the BOS during quiet standing in what is termed *normal postural sway*. Standing can be considered a **closed task** with little trial-to-trial variability within the same environment. Standing on a moving train or bus is considered perturbed standing or an **open task** because there is a lot of variability depending on the speed, direction, and acceleration or deceleration of the train.

What are the control parameters for standing? **External control parameters** include the firmness of the floor surface, the angle of the floor surface, the angle and firmness of the shoes, and any external forces such as wind, perturbations, or acceleration/deceleration. Figure 36-2AB demonstrates two external control parameters for standing. **Internal control parameters** include the strength of key postural control muscles such as the erector spinae or gastrocnemius/soleus muscles, the position of the COM in relation to the BOS, the reaction

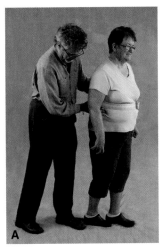

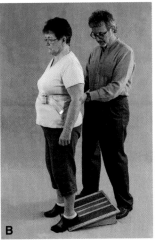

**FIGURE 36-2AB** Two external control parameters for standing. (A) Narrow base of support and (B) angle of the floor surface both affect the motor control involved in quiet standing.

time, and the sensation of the foot for detecting the center of pressure (Shumway-Cook, 2012).

The goal of standing is to keep the COM within the BOS. Standing can occur under several conditions: quiet standing with no movement other than postural strategies; standing while moving body segments such as the head, trunk, or extremities; and standing when outside forces are acting on the body, such as perturbations or catching a ball. The demands for stability *increase* in standing when the COM moves within the BOS, such as during reaching, when the BOS becomes smaller, or when the mass is increased.

What other activities might change the COM in standing? Understanding which factors increase stability demands in standing can help you plan the progression of your plan of care. Ideas to challenge your patient in standing are presented in Box 36-1.

## Biomechanical and Motor Control Analysis of Stand-to-Sit

What are some of the important biomechanics of SIT? How do they differ from the biomechanics of STS? First, the pelvis rotates forward, moving the trunk closer to the thighs than

---

### BOX 36-1 Ideas to Challenge Patients in Standing

**Moving Body Segments of Head, Arms, and Trunk**
- Looking over one shoulder, rotating trunk, side bending
- Raising the arms high in the air or reaching forward
- Bending the knees, squatting

**Change in Weight Distribution**
- Holding a weighted object

**Withstanding External Forces**
- Catching a weighted ball
- External push/nudge (perturbation)

**Changing the Base of Support**
- Gradual decrease in distance between feet
- Standing on one leg or in tandem

**CHALLENGE:** How else could you challenge a patient during standing?

---

occurs during STS; however, in SIT the COM moves *posteriorly and downward*. The knees and hip joints flex simultaneously in SIT to help move the COM in this direction. Once the buttocks touch the seat surface (initial contact), the hips extend and the pelvis rotates posteriorly over the hips. Maximal ankle dorsiflexion occurs just before this initial contact with the seat surface, whereas maximal trunk flexion occurs at initial contact with the seat (Dubost, 2005).

Second, in contrast to the momentum forces used in STS to raise the body off the chair against gravity, SIT uses controlled *eccentric* muscle forces of the hip, knee, and ankle extensors to control descent assisted by gravity (Dubost, 2005). The movement time is thus slower during SIT than during STS (Kralj, 1990) because of this controlled motion. Patients with weak knee and hip extensors tend to sit down quickly or use their arms to control descent.

The required joint motions at the hip, knee, and ankle are similar to those of STS, although maximal joint motion occurs at different points in the movement. For example, maximal trunk flexion in STS occurs when the thighs leave the chair, whereas during SIT it occurs when the thighs touch the chair (Dubost, 2005). In a study comparing the kinematics of STS and SIT in 10 healthy older adults and nine young adults, Dubost (2005) found that older adults utilized approximately 10 degrees less trunk flexion during SIT than younger counterparts. The authors suggested this change in kinematics may be a marker of reduced postural stability with aging.

Using motor control terminology, SIT is a **discreet mobility** task, as is STS. Unlike STS, however, the body moves from a relatively small BOS in standing to a larger BOS in sitting, meaning the end position is more stable than the beginning position. Sometimes, patients "plop" down to sitting very quickly, almost as if they cannot wait to be in this more secure position. SIT is also a **closed** task with relatively little variability between trials. The hands might not be used at all, or they may be used to control the descent and/or for a manipulation task.

Now that you have experience analyzing the control parameters for STS and standing, what are the most likely control parameters for SIT?

- Potential internal control parameters are eccentric strength of the hip extensors and knee extensors, range of motion of hip flexion and ankle dorsiflexion, and fear or confidence in bending forward. A good example of an internal control parameter limitation is a prohibition against bending the hip more than 70 degrees after hip arthroplasty. In this case, the strategy to move SIT would have to be altered to protect the joint from dislocation.
- Potential external control parameters are the height of the chair, height of the armrests (if applicable), firmness of the chair, and stability of the chair as a nonmoving surface (legs versus wheels).

## Impairments Influencing Sit-to-Stand, Standing, and Stand-to-Sit

According to the motor control and biomechanical descriptions of STS, standing, and SIT, which impairments could affect functional ability, postures, and quality of movement? A patient with LE weakness will certainly have difficulty during STS, standing, and SIT. Imagine trying to stand up or sit down with little assistance of the knee extensors. To stand up, you would need to increase the degree of trunk and LE flexion and momentum in the flexion momentum phase and use the arm extensors to push up out of the chair. To sit down, the UEs would have to eccentrically control descent; most likely you would see a distinct plop or letting go of the patient's eccentric control. Table 36-3 lists underlying impairments that can affect STS, standing, and SIT.

The inability of older adults to stand independently is often associated with dependence, institutionalization, and greater risk of joint contractures and pressure ulcers that can lead to additional impairments of all body systems (Dubost, 2005). For this reason, STS and standing are excellent choices in designing a home exercise program (HEP) because they are functionally relevant and can maintain strength in the LEs (Chandler, 1998; de Vreede, 2005).

## Safety Considerations

Because STS and SIT are mobility tasks, a degree of instability occurs during these transitional movements. Using the phases of STS previously described by Schenkman

| TABLE 36-3 | Impairments Affecting Sit-to-Stand, Standing, and Stand-to-Sit |
| --- | --- |
| **IMPAIRMENT** | **POTENTIAL EFFECT ON STS/SIT OR STANDING** |
| Impaired movement initiation | • Slow: more time needed to move STS<br>• Decreased ability to use momentum strategies, thus greater extension forces needed at the knee and hip or upper extremities |
| Loss of LE motor recruitment | • Increased time to rise<br>• Inability to generate enough force to move out of a chair<br>• Need to use upper extremities to assist in the movement<br>• Decreased weight-bearing on involved extremity, resulting in asymmetrical posture (Brunt, 2002; Dean, 2000) |
| Reduced muscle strength/ power of LE | • Increased time to stand or multiple attempts to stand (Bean, 2002; Chandler, 1998)<br>• Instability during momentum transfer or stabilization phase in STS<br>• Inability to control eccentric forces that break forward motion during SIT, leading to a faster or uncontrolled descent (i.e., plop)<br>• Increased sway during standing with eyes open |
| Restricted range of motion | • Altered movement pattern depending on which joints are restricted<br>• Increased time to move as efficiency decreases<br>• Use of additional forces in upper extremity or LE to overcome mechanical restrictions |
| Hypertonicity (spasticity, rigidity) | • Decreased knee and ankle flexion needed to bring COM over BOS related to increased extension force; decreased trunk mobility and control related to spasticity or rigidity<br>• Asymmetrical movement pattern during rising to stand and standing<br>• Decreased stability in standing |
| Impaired movement coordination | • Abnormal timing of movement phases (i.e., trying to lift buttocks off the chair without a flexion momentum phase)<br>• Loss of balance during extension and stabilization phases<br>• Overshooting distances during momentum phase |
| Abnormal postural alignment | • Asymmetry during STS and standing<br>• Increased muscle forces needed for stability in quiet standing<br>• Recruitment of nonpostural muscles to maintain standing, such as the gluteus maximus or quadriceps muscle |

BOS = base of support; COM = center of mass; LE = lower extremity; SIT = stand-to-sit; STS = sit-to-stand.

(1990), phases 2 (momentum transfer) and 3 (extension) are less stable than phase 1 because the COM is moving and the BOS is significantly smaller than in sitting. During the less stable phases, you can use several strategies to ensure safety:

- For patients in wheelchairs, ensure that the brakes are locked. Placing the chair-back against the wall prevents tipping backward.
- Ensure that the patient has a large BOS to increase stability during all phases of STS, standing, and SIT (see Fig. 36-3). Less effort and movement are required when the feet are under or behind the knees.
- Select a guarding strategy appropriate for the patient's abilities. One option is to position yourself on one side of the patient with one hand guarding anteriorly and the other guarding posteriorly (see Fig. 36-4A). Another option is to position yourself in front of the patient with your legs stabilizing the LEs and your arms encouraging flexion and forward momentum of the trunk on the pelvis (Fig. 36-4B). In the latter position, make sure you do not block the forward movement of the patient by keeping your own trunk lateral to midline to encourage trunk flexion. When assistance is needed to help move during momentum transfer and extension phases, remember to support close to the COM (anterior to S2) and not under the arms.

During SIT, both the therapist and the patient should ensure that the seat surface is nonmoving and at least one posterior thigh can feel the seat surface. Add stability to the task by keeping the patient's feet apart from both medial/lateral and anterior/posterior perspectives. Encourage the patient to bend the trunk and hips "like a hinge" (a great external visual cue) to bring the COM posterior and closer to the seat surface. When more stability is needed, have the patient place both hands on the armrests to help with eccentric control and increase the BOS. Remember that healthy adults do not normally use their arms to push up from a chair; however, this may be needed when patients are weak or have motor control deficits.

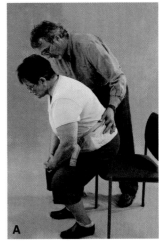

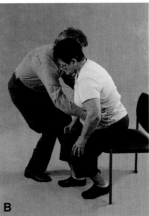

FIGURE 36-4AB Two positions to guard and guide during sit-to-stand. (A) Stand lateral and slightly anterior to the patient, making sure your hands do not block forward motion. (B) Stand anterior and slightly to one side of the patient, ensuring that your trunk does not block forward motion.

## Lifespan Influences on Sit-to-Stand

STS from a chair is not usually described in normal development from birth to 24 months; however, floor-to-standing is a component of many developmental motor scales. This chapter addresses only the age-related changes relevant to STS, standing, and SIT.

### Age-Related Changes in Standing and Sitting

Although LE strength and power decrease with age, the ability to move STS should not be impaired in healthy aging. Persons with musculoskeletal disorders such as arthritis are more likely to have difficulty moving STS and in SIT. Motion analysis of older adults with symptomatic knee osteoarthritis reveals differences in STS motion between high- and low-functioning seniors. Specifically, high-functioning men had more hip flexion and greater knee power than lower-functioning men, whereas higher-functioning females used less knee flexion than their lower-functioning counterparts (Segal, 2013).

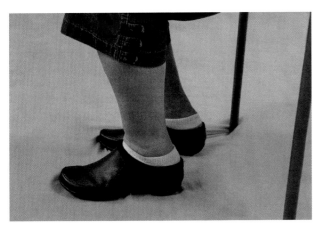

FIGURE 36-3 Feet staggered in two directions: anteroposterior and mediolateral to enlarge the BOS.

Several researchers found differences with normal aging in the STS movement pattern, including the duration of each phase of standing as well as overall body kinematics and kinetics (Ikeda, 1991). Using the Schenkman (1990) phases of STS, Ikeda (1991) noted that older adults had significantly less head extension during momentum transfer. Others found that older adults used less muscular effort in moving to standing and brought the COM farther over the BOS before moving vertically (Papa, 2000; Schultz, 1992). Some evidence indicates that older adults use less trunk flexion during SIT than younger adults do (Dubost, 2005).

The reasons underlying age-related changes in STS have not been fully investigated. The decline in muscle mass (sarcopenia) and muscle strength that occur with age have been well documented and may contribute to the change in movement strategies (Janssen, 2002a; Skelton, 1994). When STS was compared in high- and low-functioning older women, Segal (2013) noted a significant difference (decrease) in hip abductor strength in the low-functioning females but did not find a difference in knee extensor strength between these two groups. Furthermore, peak power is predictive of walking speed, distance, and number of steps in older adults with functional limitations (Puthoff, 2008); thus, it is also possible that power affects STS. Older adults who have difficulty moving STS and SIT usually have LE weakness, joint changes, or visual deficits (Schultz, 1992).

## ■ Examination of Sit-to-Stand, Stand-to-Sit, and Standing

Examination of a patient's ability to come to standing, to stand, or to sit down can be done *quantitatively*, using time-based measurements and/or rating scales describing the degree of assistance required, and *qualitatively*, using detailed descriptions or scales describing the patient's biomechanics and motor control strategies. A simple, quantitative method of documenting STS or SIT is to calculate the time it takes to perform the task in seconds and to monitor this performance over time. It is important to document the height of the chair and to start the patient with the back against the chair to improve interrater and intrarater consistency in timing the patient. Similarly, the STS Test, or Timed Chair Stands, measures how long it takes to rise from a chair five times and has been used as a test for LE strength (Bohannon, 1995; Csuka, 1985) and balance (Cheng, 1998; Lord, 2002; Whitney, 2005). The patient is instructed to stand up from a chair five times with the arms folded across the chest to eliminate UE assistance in the task (see Table 36-4). The time

| TABLE 36-4 | Standardized Tests for Sit-to-Stand, Stand-to-Sit, and Standing | |
|---|---|---|
| **TEST** | **TASK** | **ITEM** |
| Berg Balance Scale (BBS)* | Sitting to standing (Item #1) | 4: Able to stand without using hands; stabilize independently<br>3: Able to stand independently using hands<br>2: Able to stand using hands after several tries<br>1: Needs minimal aid to stand or to stabilize<br>0: Needs moderate or maximal assist to stand |
| BBS | Standing (Item #2) | 4: Able to stand safely for 2 minutes<br>3: Able to stand for 2 minutes with supervision<br>2: Able to stand 30 seconds unsupported<br>1: Needs several tries to stand 30 seconds unsupported<br>0: Unable to stand for 30 seconds unassisted |
| BBS | Stand-to-sit (Item #3) | 4: Sits safely with minimal use of hands<br>3: Controls descent by using hands<br>2: Uses back of legs against chair to control descent<br>1: Sits independently but has uncontrolled descent<br>0: Needs assistance to sit |
| BBS | Looking over shoulder in standing (Item #10) | 4: Looks behind from both sides and weight shifts well<br>3: Looks behind one side only; other side shows less weight shift<br>2: Turns sideways only but maintains balance<br>1: Needs supervision when turning<br>0: Needs assist to keep from losing balance or falling |
| Motor Assessment Scale | Sitting to standing | 1: Gets to standing with help from therapist<br>2: Gets to standing with standby help (weight unevenly distributed, uses hands for support)<br>3: Gets to standing (no uneven weight distribution/help from hands)<br>4: Gets to standing and stands for 5 seconds with hips and knees extended (do not allow uneven weight distribution) |

| TABLE 36-4 | Standardized Tests for Sit-to-Stand, Stand-to-Sit, and Standing—cont'd | |
|---|---|---|
| **TEST** | **TASK** | **ITEM** |
| | | 5: Sitting to standing to sitting with no standby help (do not allow uneven weight distribution, full extension of hips/knees)<br>6: Sitting to standing to sitting with no stand-by help three times in 10 seconds (do not allow uneven weight distribution) |
| Mobility Scale for Acute Stroke | Sit to vertical stand from a standardized stool chair with no armrests (best of three) | 1: Unable to do activity; patient makes no contribution or unable to complete<br>2: Maximum assistance of one to two people; patient makes minimal contribution to activity<br>3: Moderate assistance of one individual, hands-on for most of activity; patient able to perform some part of activity independently<br>4: Minimum assistance, hands-on for part of the activity<br>5: Supervised (verbal input, no hands-on)<br>6: Unassisted and safe; no verbal input |
| Timed Chair Stands (Whitney, 2005) | Time to stand five times | ≥60 years: ≥14.2 seconds indicates balance dysfunction<br><60 years: ≥10 seconds indicates balance dysfunction |
| Tinetti Balance | Arises | 0: Unable without help<br>1: Able; uses arms<br>2: Able without use of arms |
| | Attempts to rise | 0: Unable without help<br>1: Able; more than one attempt<br>2: Able; one attempt |
| | Immediate standing balance | 0: Unsteady, swaggers; moves feet or sways<br>1: Steady using walker or other support<br>2: Steady without support |
| | Standing balance | 0: Unsteady<br>1: Steady but wide base of support (heels >4 inches apart) or using device for support)<br>2: Narrow stance without support |
| Functional Independence Measure (FIM) | • Bed/chair or wheelchair transfers<br>• Toilet transfers<br>• Shower/tub transfers<br>• Car transfers (FIM/Functional Assessment Measure) | 7: Complete independence; timely and safely<br>6: Modified independence; extra time or device<br>5: Supervision: cuing, coaxing, prompting<br>4: Minimal assist: patient performs 75% or more of task<br>3: Moderate assist: patient performs between 50% and 74% of task<br>2: Maximal assist: patient performs 25%–49% of task<br>1: Total dependence: patient performs <25% of task |
| Parkinson Activity Scale | Chair transfers—getting up | Have patient perform two trials, first trial without hands, second trial with hands<br>4: Normal; without apparent difficulties<br>3: Without arms; mild difficulties (toes dorsiflex to maintain balance)<br>2: Without arms; impossible or several attempts needed; with arms normal<br>1: With arms; difficult (several attempts, hesitation)<br>0: Dependent on physical assistance |
| | Chair transfers—sitting down | 4: Normal; without apparent difficulties<br>3: Without arms; mild difficulties (uncontrolled landing)<br>2: Without arms; abrupt landing or ending uncomfortable; with arms normal<br>1: With arms; abrupt landing or ending uncomfortable<br>0: Dependent on physical assistance |

is stopped on the fifth stand, although some authors report stopping the time when the patient returns to sitting after the fifth stand (Whitney, 2005). Whitney reported optimal sensitivity and specificity cutoff scores to predict balance dysfunction as 10 seconds for subjects younger than 60 years and 14.2 seconds in those 60 years and older. Others have indicated scores of 12.3 in persons 70 to 79 years old (Lord, 2002) and 15 to 16 in those 80 years and older (Guralnik, 1994).

STS, standing, and SIT are also components of several standardized functional scales and outcome measures (see Table 36-4). Although some clinicians avoid using standardized measures because they perceive them as time-consuming, remember that one measure can provide insight into a variety of functional skills. For example, the Berg Balance Scale (BBS) consists of 14 items and takes between 10 and 15 minutes to complete. Within this scale, however, you can document STS, SIT, transfers, and standing in 11 different conditions such as turning, reaching, or picking an object up off the floor. The BBS is also a valid and reliable measure for assessing standing balance and fall risk in older adults as well as in people with a stroke, spinal cord injury (SCI), PD, and brain injury (Finch, 2002).

At the time of this writing, the Academy of Neurology Physical Therapy (ANPT) of the American Physical Therapy Association had developed recommended outcome measure through its EDGE imitative for six patient populations: patients with stroke, multiple sclerosis (MS), traumatic brain injury (TBI) SCI, Parkinson Disease, and Vestibular Disorders (ANPT, 2015). Four of the six workgroups highly recommended the BBS as a measure of standing activity (stroke, MS, SCI in American Spinal Injury Association [ASIA] ASIA Impairment Scale C/D categories), whereas the workgroup for TBI recommended avoiding the BBS for individuals who are severely dependent or highly functioning because of the ceiling effects of the scale (ANPT, 2015). Readers are encouraged to use this excellent evidence-based resource from ANPT.

Another strategy to assess STS, standing, and SIT is applying control parameters to the examination (see Table 36-5). In this approach, internal and external control parameters can be varied to see how they affect the patient's motor function in moving STS, standing, or SIT. Varying the control parameters of STS helps you determine the patient's functional

| TABLE 36-5 | Using Control Parameters as Variables During Examination | | |
|---|---|---|---|
| CONTROL PARAMETER | SIT-TO-STAND | STANDING | STAND-TO-SIT |
| Vary the height of the chair | X | | X |
| Vary the use of armrests for support | X | X | X |
| Change the position of the knees/ankles | X | | X |
| Modify shoe type and floor surface | | X | |
| Change the size of the base of support | X | X | X |
| Vary the speed of movement | X | | X |
| Hold a weighted object | | X | |
| Catch a weighted object | | X | |
| Move the head, trunk, or extremities | | X | |

ability in variable conditions and should influence your plan of care. For example, a patient may stand independently *only* when the chair height is 45 centimeters or higher and when using the arms to assist. The plan of care might include STS training beginning at heights of 47 centimeters, without the use of the arms, and gradually lowering the chair height to increase intensity without using the arms. At home, however, the patient would be encouraged to select chairs at least 45 centimeters high with armrests to maximize safety and independence.

## PATIENT APPLICATION

The following information documents the history, examination, evaluation, and prognosis for Mr. P, focusing primarily on his ability to move STS, SIT, and standing.

### History, Patient Goals, and Systems Screen

Mr. P is a 77 year- old male with PD who had a right total knee arthroplasty (TKA) 6 months ago. Mr. P was diagnosed with PD 2 years ago and has a history of osteoarthritis, spinal stenosis, and venous stasis. He uses a front-wheeled walker with tennis balls on the back legs to ease sliding. Although he has not fallen, his wife or daughter usually walks next to him, so much so that

he jokes, "I can't do anything without having one of these two secret service agents by my side."

Mr. P lives in a one-story house with his wife, daughter, and two grandchildren, with only one step into the house. He wears glasses for both distance and reading and compression stockings for his venous stasis condition. His wife noted that sometimes it takes him four or five attempts to stand up and that he seems to take "baby steps" when walking. Since his surgery, he has not been able to do the grocery shopping, participate in church activities, or visit friends. His day consists mostly *of sitting and watching television, interacting with family, and going out to dinner. Despite his difficulty walking and standing up, he recently resumed driving his grandchildren to school.*

*Before his TKA, Mr. P walked independently without an assistive device on level surfaces and was very active in his church and community. Mr. P's goals are as follows:*

- *"I would like to be able to go back to being a lector and Eucharistic Minister at my church."*
- *"I love my family, but they hover around too much! I need to do for myself!*
- *"I used to love to go for walks every morning and visit friends in the neighborhood. I was a free spirit until all this baloney happened. Now I'm a couch potato because there's nothing else to do!"*

- *Systems screen: Integumentary-venous stasis; cardiopulmonary-hypertension controlled with medication*
- *Musculoskeletal: Spinal stenosis and radiculopathy L1–L3*
- *Neuromuscular: History of PD*

## Pertinent Examination Findings

*Systems review:*

- *Integumentary system impaired in both legs as evidenced by redness and edema typical of venous stasis; well-healed scar anterior aspect right knee 3.8 inches long*
- *Urogenital: Occasional incontinence; reports wearing protective incontinent pads when he cannot get to bathroom fast enough*

## Examination: Tests and Measures

| CATEGORY | TEST/MEASURE AND OBSERVATIONS |
|---|---|
| Assistive devices | Front-wheeled rolling walker; glasses; wears thick, rubber-soled shoes |
| Cranial/Peripheral N | • Cranial nerves II–XII intact; peripheral nerves: decreased sensation L3–S1 on left |
| Gait, locomotion, balance | • Timed up and go (TUG) test: 34.6 seconds; TUG-c (secondary cognitive task): 48.2 seconds<br>• Tinetti balance: 6/16; difficulty arising and attempts to arise, turning; wide base 12 inches, and response to nudge<br>• Static balance: modified Clinical Test of Sensory Interaction in Balance (CTSIB): 30 seconds eyes open on firm surface (feet not totally together because of varus knees); 30 seconds eyes closed; 20 seconds eyes open on foam<br>• Perturbations: minimal ankle and hip strategies; used stepping strategy automatically |
| Joint integrity and Range of Motion | • Right (R) knee ROM deficit: –8 degrees extension to 100 degrees knee flexion, Left (L): –5 to 108 degrees<br>• Bilateral (B) ankle dorsiflexion: 4 degrees (beyond neutral)<br>• B hip flexion: 115 degrees (limited by back pain) |
| Motor function | • Unified Parkinson's Disease Rating Scale (UPDRS):<br>Mentation/Mood: 3/12; motor subscale: 25/108; ADL subscale: 9/51<br>• STS: sitting on the edge of a 40-inch-high mat, sit-to-stand took 13.7 seconds with manual contact to bring COM forward; at 42 inches took 8 seconds, and at 44 inches took 4.5 seconds; at 40 inches made three attempts before successful; COM stayed posterior even with verbal cue to "Bring nose over toes," leading to difficulty in flexion momentum and momentum transfer phases<br>• Car: needs stand-by assistance to get in/out of van primarily because of slow speed |
| Muscle performance (Manual Muscle Test grades) | Dorsiflexion R: 2+/5, L: 2/5; plantar flexion R: 2+/5, L: 2/5;<br>Knee extension B: 5-/5; knee flexion B: 3+/5; hip flexion R: 4-/5, L: 3+/5 |
| Standing posture | Forward trunk flexion and R side flexion, knee varus (L > R), wide BOS |
| Work, community, leisure integration | Drives grandchildren to school in minivan, assistance getting into the van; bed low (18 inches); not able to hand out communion or stand/sit quickly during church service |

## Evaluation, Diagnosis, Prognosis, and Expected Outcomes

### Evaluation

Mr. P has difficulty initiating movement and is hesitant to move his COM over his BOS, interfering with both flexion momentum and momentum transfer phases of STS. I believe his limitation in moving forward relates to his limited motion in the left knee and both ankles, as well as a delay in movement initiation and

bradykinesia consistent with PD. Mr. P has postural instability that is evident by his large BOS in quiet standing and instability when his BOS is narrowed (stool tapping, steps, and tandem). His thick-soled shoes may be an external factor that interferes with his ability to feel the floor and thus balance in standing. He relies on a rolling walker for balance and has difficulty reaching/turning or moving his body over his BOS. His difficulty during STS and standing has caused a significant reduction in *activity over the past 2 years and losses in aerobic endurance and independent community function. He is at risk for further aerobic deconditioning, muscle weakness, and falls secondary to inactivity and motor planning dysfunction.*

### Physical Therapy Diagnosis

*Mr. P's postural instability and difficulty standing are consistent with the movement dysfunction associated with PD and are further complicated by restricted right knee function after TKA and LE weakness related to spinal stenosis.*

### Prognosis and Expected Outcomes

*Mr. P has good potential to meet the expected functional outcomes within 20 to 30 visits. His rehabilitation time is longer because of his comorbidities of PD, TKA, spinal stenosis, and resultant muscle weakness. His prognosis is favorably affected by his strong family support, a single-story home environment, and limited disability related to PD (Hoehn and Yahr stage 2.5). He is very motivated to return to his previous social tasks, including his role in his church.*

### Expected Outcomes in 3 Months (20 to 30 Visits) and Prerequisite Goals

*Outcomes: In 3 Months*

*1. Independent STS from firm surfaces of 38 to 42 inches within 3 to 4 seconds*

*2. Improved static standing balance so he will be able to stand independently without a cane or device for periods of 3 minutes, turn, and shift weight without losing balance in order to perform self-care tasks at the sink, toilet, and kitchen*

*3. Improved dynamic balance such that the patient will be able to reach items above his head independently and without losing balance and will be able to turn and walk over an object independently without a loss of cadence*

*4. Return to his role of Eucharistic Minister at his church, which requires him to walk independently without a device and to stand for 5 to 10 minutes performing a manipulation task*

*Short-term Goals: In 1 Month Patient Will:*

*1. Increase muscle strength of hip flexors to 4/5 bilaterally and dorsiflexors to 3/5*

*2. Increase standing tolerance to 10 minutes with a BOS of 6 inches*

*3. Improve postural reaction so he can consistently use ankle and hip strategy with minimal perturbation*

*4. Improve functional mobility as evidenced by TUG time of 22 seconds and TUG-c time of 28 seconds*

### Contemplate Clinical Decisions

- *Develop an initial problem list that includes Mr. P's reported activity and participation restrictions as well as your anticipated problems related to sit to stand (STS).*
- *Write a list of STS tests and measures for incorporation into your initial examination.*
- *Hypothesize the relationships between impairments and activity restrictions in STS.*
- *Consider the pathophysiology of his medical diagnoses and hypothesize how it affects STS.*

## ■ Functional Interventions for Standing and Sitting

### General Approaches and Early Decisions

Retraining STS, standing, and SIT involves several types of rehabilitation interventions, including functional training, therapeutic exercises, and/or the prescription of devices and equipment. These interventions are discussed separately in the following paragraphs.

Several important questions should be asked before training. First, will you approach training using remediation, compensation, or perhaps a combination of the two? Remediation of STS involves retraining the task using normal biomechanics and/or reduction of impairments that interfere with the task in patients who have capacity for improvement. For example, you would practice STS using normal biomechanics and strengthen the QD both concentrically and eccentrically for a patient with LE weakness. In comparison, a compensatory approach would involve

equipment to perform the STS task in patients whose motor function will not improve over time or when safety prohibits the use of normal strategies. A combination approach employs both strategies to maximize function, safety, and independence. A patient with amyotrophic lateral sclerosis (ALS), for example, may need a chair at home with an electric STS assist mechanism. In the case of Mr. P, remediation techniques, including task-intensive training and strengthening exercises to retrain STS, would be appropriate. In addition, compensatory approaches using risers to raise the height of his bed might promote functional independence and safety at home.

The second question to consider is whether you will perform the STS and SIT training with or without the use of the UEs. As previously described, the use of armrests changes the timing and amount of forces needed at the various phases of STS (Etnyre, 2007). A patient who has instability during SIT and is fearful of falling might benefit from using the arms initially to increase the BOS and gain stability. This could be changed over time as the patient progresses.

Lastly, for patients who need moderate to maximum assistance to stand, an important question is whether to use equipment to assist. Devices that assist in STS, standing, and SIT are recommended by specialists to reduce the incidence of patient- and therapist-related injuries.

### Functional Training in Self-Care and Home Management

Functional training is influenced by a variety of factors, including the patient's biomechanics, motor control strategies, and use of adaptive devices or equipment. The following paragraphs organize the interventions according to these principles.

## Biomechanical Approach to Functional Training

As discussed previously, the biomechanics of STS are influenced by many factors including foot position, seat height, use of armrests, and muscle forces (Janssen, 2002b). Retraining STS and SIT using a **remediation approach** should promote normal biomechanics during the movement. An example is to facilitate horizontal motion of the COM forward over the feet during the momentum phase by using tactile, visual, or verbal cues. Depending on the patient's response, use your understanding of normal STS biomechanics to make the task easier or harder as needed. Raising or lowering the height of the seat surface is one example. Table 36-6 provides examples of biomechanically based strategies to retrain STS, standing, and SIT.

The biomechanical principles for SIT should also be incorporated into training. Specifically, emphasize controlled descent via eccentric contraction; use verbal cues such as "Sit down slowly" or "Let yourself down slowly." Maximal hip flexion during SIT occurs when the buttocks first touch the seat surface (Khemlani, 1998), so it also might be valuable to work on hip flexion range of motion during this functional activity. A verbal cue such as "Take a bow" or manual guidance to bend at the waist can promote greater trunk flexion, which in turn decreases the eccentric muscle force requirements of the quadriceps. You can also encourage more stability using a "foot apart" strategy (Fig. 36-1).

## Motor Learning Principles Applied to Standing

A traditional physical therapy interaction for STS training might sound something like this:

> "OK, Mr. Smith, today we're going to work on standing up from your chair. I'm going to use this gait belt around you for safety. First, you must make sure your wheelchair is locked. This is important so the chair won't roll away as you're standing up. Next, I need you to scoot to the edge of the chair. GREAT! Now put your hands on the arms of the chair. You never want to pull up on this walker because it's not stable. Now try to stand up. Well done! OK, let's do it again, but you tell me the steps you should take..."

Wow! This therapist is definitely safe, but has this interaction encouraged motor learning? For many years, physical therapists taught skills to patients from a "safety first" perspective and in a step-by-step manner, assuming that correct information given verbally is the best way to facilitate learning. In reality, most of what occurred during the encounter may have hindered learning.

Notice how the conversation was one-sided: The therapist was the teacher, and the patient was the listening student. Is this how you would learn a new dance—hearing about it instead of seeing it? The therapist relied on explicit verbal directions to promote motor learning. In subsequent paragraphs, you will read that explicit directions can sometimes impair learning, especially after a stroke or brain injury. The unspoken message in the previous example was "Don't fall" rather than "Let's stand." Also, what type of feedback did the therapist give? She used generic encouraging words such as "Great"

| TABLE 36-6 | Biomechanical Approaches for Sit-to-Stand, Stand-to-Sit, and Standing |
|---|---|
| **GOAL** | **TECHNIQUE** |
| Improve LE biomechanics to lower energy costs | • To stand, position the feet posterior to the knees so there is at least 100 degrees of knee flexion and 10–15 degrees of dorsiflexion<br>• To sit, place one leg touching the chair, keeping the second forward to increase BOS |
| Decrease force required to move sit-to-stand | • Promote forward trunk flexion of at least 15 degrees from upright sitting using momentum (rocking forward) that continues into the next phase of extension<br>• Select seat heights of at least 120% of the lower leg length and lower as tolerated (Janssen, 2002b); for example, when the distance between the heel and the popliteal fossa is 42 cm, select a seat height of at least 50 cm to begin training |
| Improve symmetry of sit-to-stand to enhance immediate standing balance | • Position the weaker leg in a position of support (100 degrees of knee flexion) while moving the stronger leg forward or elevating it (Brunt, 2002)<br>• Eccentric strengthening of weak knee extensors (Engardt, 1995)<br>• Use cane in sit-to-stand transition |
| Decrease dependence on armrests or UEs | • Practice sit-to-stand and stand-to-sit with and without armrests or gradually decrease dependence on armrests<br>• Gradually reduce the amount of UE support in quiet and perturbed standing |
| Increase use and contribution of LEs | • Enhance LE muscle force production through the affected leg through circuit training that emphasizes functional strength LE, such as sit-to-stand from various heights, step-ups in multiple directions, treadmill walking, and walking in variant conditions. When the patient cannot use momentum, increase the degree of forward bending at the hip. This increases the knee extensor forces needed during sit-to-stand. |

BOS = base of support; LE = left extremity; UE, upper extremity.

and "Well done" rather than specific feedback such as "Try to lean your nose even farther over your toes." Lastly, the discreet task of STS was broken down into four steps and was trained as "parts" rather than as a single, continuous movement. Does that really make STS easier to learn? How can a patient use the body's momentum strategies when he is stopping between steps?

Research with *healthy* young adults has revealed that motor learning is enhanced by intense practice, random and variable practice schedules, and augmented feedback that is decreased over time (Rose, 2006; Schmidt, 2005). We also know that in the early stages of learning, the role of the therapist is to encourage experimentation and practice as well as to give specific feedback about the quality of the movement (Shumway-Cook, 2012).

Motor control strategies for this chapter are based on a review by Kleim (2008) of 10 principles of experience-dependent neural plasticity as applied to patients with brain damage. These principles are based largely on the idea that training matters, such that training should be task specific, intense, meaningful to the patient, and repetitive (Kleim, 2008).

## Practice Intensity: The Most Important Treatment Parameter

Ask any coach, athlete, or physical therapy instructor, and she will tell you the most important variable in learning a new skill or relearning a skill is the intensity of practice. Imagine being taught how to perform a spinal manipulation for the first time in class and practicing it only three times before being tested. How would you perform? Would you remember it a year later if you had not practiced?

Research regarding the importance of practice intensity in patients with neurological dysfunction clearly has demonstrated that more practice results in higher function (Barreca, 2004; Boyd, 2006; Boyne, 2011; Britton, 2008; Canning, 2003). Unfortunately, the concept of intensive practice is not always applied in clinical practice. A study of STS at a stroke rehabilitation center revealed that in a standard therapy day, patients stood on average *only* 18 times (Britton, 2008). These researchers designed a quasi-experimental study in which the treatment group of nine patients were given 30 additional minutes of STS training per day, increasing the average number of STSs by 50 times per day compared with the control group. The experimental group demonstrated greater symmetry as measured by more weight on the involved LE after only 1 week of more intense practice (Britton, 2008).

Similar research revealed that three additional 45-minute sessions of STS training beyond the average inpatient therapy increased the level of independence and satisfaction with quality of life (Canning, 2003). Intensive practice should not be limited to inpatient settings, however. It has been shown that intensive STS training along with step-up exercises and calf stretches in a 3-week home health setting improved STS speed and ability and walking speed (Lang, 2007).

The benefits of task-intensive practice for STS have also been reported in patients with acquired brain injury and those with PD. Subjects with ABI residing in an inpatient rehabilitation facility were assigned to a standard therapy group or to an experimental group (Barreca, 2004). The experimental group performed up to 100 repetitions of STS per day and 60 step-ups in addition to the standardized therapy. After 4 weeks of therapy, there was a significant improvement in the number of STS repetitions performed in 3 minutes in the experimental group compared with the control group, reflecting a 62% improvement from baseline. In patients with PD, 4 weeks of task-specific STS training significantly increased the vertical and horizontal velocities generated during STS and increased the speed of standing compared with an LE strengthening program (Mak, 2008).

So how much practice is enough? Although we would all agree that 15 repetitions per day is not enough, what about 30 repetitions? Are 50 or 100 repetitions too much? Boyne (2011) used speed-dependent and body weight–supported STS training 3 days per week for 45 to 60 minutes in two persons after a stroke. These patients completed more than 750 STS repetitions and achieved independence within 8 to 11 sessions. In addition to gaining independence, the patients improved in gait velocity and quality of life measures on the Stroke Impact Scale. The aforementioned researched studies support the idea that "more is better."

The concept of task-intensive training has been well-researched with the UEs through constraint-induced movement therapy (CIMT) trials (Morris, 2006; Taub, 2002). Step training with body weight support on a treadmill is an example of task-intensive training, such that the movement of the treadmill encourages continued stepping. Some researchers have begun to apply the concept of intensive task training or CIMT to the LE (Marklund, 2006).

In reality, intensive practice means you should maximize the number of repetitions on the basis of each patient's *available* strength and cardiopulmonary endurance as well as the time allotted in therapy and the need to spend time treating other activity restrictions or impairments. Intensive practice may be contraindicated in patients with certain forms of neuropathy or demyelination disorders such as Guillain-Barré syndrome or MS.

There are many fun and interesting ways to increase the intensity of your STS, standing, and SIT practices (Box 36-2). One example is creating a "STS/SIT circuit." This involves gathering chairs of different heights, depth, and firmness and asking the patient to stand up and sit down multiple times on each surface (Fig. 36-5). Similarly, a standing circuit can be created in which a patient has to stand in five to 10 different positions for 2 minutes each, varying the surface, BOS, angle of the floor, and even movement in the environment.

Despite an abundance of literature supporting intensive practice, this idea is not always translated into clinical practice. An observational study performed in an outpatient setting revealed that on average, therapists performed only eight repetitions of LE functional movements and 12 repetitions of UE functional movements. Only gait training, with an average of 242 steps per day, demonstrated the application of task-intensive training (Lang, 2007). Using creative strategies to increase practice potentially improves patient functional outcomes.

## BOX 36-2 How Can You Increase the Intensity of Sit-to-Stand (STS), Stand-to-Sit, or Standing?

- Create an STS circuit, where the patient walks between different stations and must stand up 10 times at each chair, bench, stool, or mat (see Figure 36-5).
- Give the patient STS as homework in inpatient or outpatient situations. For safety, have him stand with a wheelchair or chair that is against a wall.
- Give the patient homework to perform mental practice of STS.
- Create a group STS class to supplement individual therapy sessions.
- Intersperse 10 STS repetitions whenever you change activities in your therapy program.
- Log the number of STSs daily using a simple recording form and chart the patient's progress.
- Create a STAND circuit, varying floor surface (foam, carpet, wood, tile, sand), varying the size of the base of support, and varying the angle of the floor surface.

Challenge: Create your own STS circuit and test it out. How many repetitions of STS will you do if you do 10 repetitions at each station of the circuit?

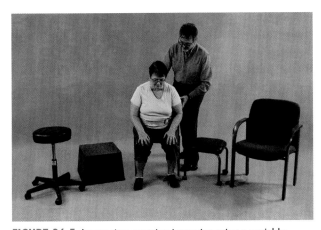

**FIGURE 36-5** Increasing practice intensity using a variable sit-to-stand circuit.

### Other Forms of Practice: Observation and Mental Practice

Observational practice and mental practice have also improved task performance in patients with neurological deficits (Celnik, 2008; Ertelt, 2007; Guttman, 2012; Malouin, 2004; Page, 2007; Sidaway, 2005). During **observational practice**, the individual learning a task observes the performance of another person performing the same task. Action observation, when provided at the same time as task practice and in the same direction of movement, significantly enhanced motor memory formation in people with mild stroke as measured by transcranial magnetic stimulation (Celnik, 2008).

To integrate the concept of observational practice into your STS or SIT training, have the model sit next to or in front of the patient while the patient is practicing. The position of the model is important because his movement should be in the same direction as the patient's movement (Page, 2007). The model can be "live" or on videotape, again ensuring that his movement is similar to that of the patient. Consider having a model of a similar age or disposition as the person learning the task.

Similarly, **mental practice** (also called *motor imagery*) combined with physical therapy has reduced impairments and increased function compared with physical therapy alone (Page, 2007). Mental practice provides a "safe" way for patients to rehearse movements when alone or when limited by fatigue. It is also an excellent method of increasing practice intensity. Two types of mental practice are described in the literature: **external imagery**, such that the patient views himself from the viewpoint of a visual observer and **internal imagery**, in which the patient imagines the sensations within his own body as a kinesthetic experience (Guttman, 2012).

Guttman (2012) investigated the effect of motor imagery on STS and reach to grasp in 13 patients with chronic stroke. They used both external and internal imagery to practice STS for 15 minutes, three times per week for 4 weeks. In addition, they changed the focus of the practice over the 4 weeks: (1) Week 1 focused on the full STS; (2) week 2 focused on the beginning portion of the movement until the buttocks left the seat; (3) week 3 focused on extension to stand and stabilization; and (4) week 4 involved practicing full STS again with varying velocities. After the mental practice intervention, the speed of both STS and transfers increased significantly. There were also significant improvements in motor function as measured by the Fugl-Meyer lower limb index and TUG scores.

Several take-home mental practice strategies can be gleaned from the aforementioned study:

- Use mental practice to increase practice intensity and make mental practice itself intense.
- Ensure that mental practice occurs in a quiet room.
- Use both internal (kinesthetic) and external (visual) imagery.
- Incorporate speed into the task by using a timer or metronome.

## THINK ABOUT IT 36.3

### Example of a Sit-to-Stand Mental Practice Session

This is a sample mental practice rehearsal. Does this use extrinsic (visual) or intrinsic (kinesthetic) cues?

As you close your eyes, imagine sitting up tall in your chair, feeling the chair beneath your bottom and against your back. Feel both feet on the floor underneath your knees. The feet are separated, and there is equal weight on both feet. Now imagine your shoulders and chest leaning forward over your knees; as you do so, there is more pressure on the soles of your feet. As you continue to move forward, you can feel your buttocks leave the seat while your legs push up against the floor equally to help stand. Imagine a string pulling you from the top of your head toward the ceiling to gracefully pull you to full standing. Once standing, notice the equal pressure on the right and left feet and how strong your legs feel.

Challenge: Using this session as a guide, write a mental practice session for sit-to-stand.

### Implicit versus Explicit Instructions

**Explicit training** refers to the use of stated directions to guide a task or skill, whereas **implicit training** refers to the use of practice and repetition to guide learning. In the previous example of a therapist directing a patient to move STS, the therapist used explicit instructions to guide the patient. Although this strategy might work with children or healthy adults, recent research has indicated that the rules of training change after a stroke. Boyd (2006) studied the effect of explicit information on learning discreet and continuous motor tasks in patients with a stroke in either the sensorimotor cortex or the basal ganglia. The UE tasks were performed on the less-involved UE in the patients with a stroke and on the dominant side of the healthy controls. The results demonstrated several important findings:

- All participants improved with practice.
- Although healthy age-matched controls improved in discreet and continuous tasks when given explicit information, performance in people with a stroke declined when given explicit information.
- With explicit instructions, negative effects occurred in both discreet and continuous tasks.
- The negative effect of explicit information was maintained during a retention test, even though the explicit information was withdrawn at the retention test.

Although the reason for these findings is unclear, there may be competition for neural resources between the implicit and explicit memory systems in the impaired brain (Boyd, 2006). Some studies suggest that explicit learning may be harmful in people after sensorimotor and basal ganglia strokes (Boyd, 2006; Orrell, 2006; Vidoni, 2007).

Although the aforementioned research on explicit versus implicit learning occurred primarily with UE tasks, we can conceptually apply similar principles to the movement of STS, standing, and SIT. How do we make our STS training more implicit than explicit? At the risk of sounding redundant, intensive practice facilitates implicit learning, so once again, focus on intensive practice. For STS and SIT, intensive practice means many repetitions. In standing, intensive practice means standing for longer periods, increasing from seconds to minutes. Another suggestion to enhance implicit learning is to encourage the patient to experiment. For example, when working on SIT, ask the patient to experiment with "hinging" the trunk forward at the hips in gradually increasing increments. Other suggestions for decreasing explicit instructions during therapy are summarized in Box 36-3.

External visual cues can decrease the need for verbal directions about movement. A great example of this for STS is to place a wooden box that is lower than the chair height in front of the patient, and ask the patient to lean on the box to stand up (Fig. 36-6). Touching the box positioned anterior and inferior to the seat causes the patient to lean forward and bring the COM over the BOS. After intensive practice using the box, eliminate the box and have the patient stand up using the same forward motion. Other externally based cues include "Nose over toes" or "Bend like a hinge" on your way to standing up. The idea in external cues is to give the patient a reference he can see or visualize.

### Practice Schedules

Practice schedules for STS training can be blocked, variable, or random. In healthy adults, variable practice enhances the ability to transfer learning to a novel movement task in the same class of movement and to generalize the ability to perform the task in different environments (Rose, 2006; Schmidt, 2005).

Motor learning theories support the use of variable practice schedules once the patient understands the basic dynamics of the task. For example, early in training, make sure the patient understands the STS movement by using a blocked practice schedule. This means repeatedly practicing STS using the same conditions, without varying the task or the environmental features. Once the patient demonstrates that the basic mechanics are present, vary the height of the sitting surface, the compliance/softness of the surface, the noise in the environment, or

---

### BOX 36-3  TALK LESS So Your Patient LEARNS MORE

- Encourage implicit learning by *speaking less* and *increasing patient practice* time. Rather than saying to the patient "You need to scoot to the edge of the chair first," say instead "Please stand up." For motor learning, less talk means more learning.
- When the patient has difficulty, modify the leg position and say "Try again." Switch positions of the feet so the back leg becomes the front leg, and say "Stand again." In this way, experimentation is encouraged without explicit instructions.
- Consider sitting next to the patient and saying, "Let's do this" while you demonstrate the full STS movement.
- If your goal is to increase hip flexion, try asking the patient to stand up quickly. You can also gently guide the trunk to move forward during the movement without using the external visual cue/demonstration, while saying "Bend forward."
- When using explicit cues, try to use an external focus of attention rather than an internal focus of attention. For example, instead of asking the patient to "Bend forward" as an internal explicit cue, use the phrase "Nose over your toes" or "Move like a hinge" to emphasize the forward rotation of the pelvis over the hips.

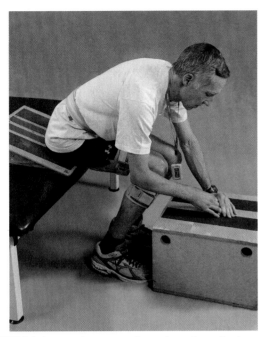

**FIGURE 36-6** Use of an external visual cue (i.e., a box) to encourage a patient to move the center of mass forward.

the speed of STS. Variable training can be organized by using an STS circuit, as previously discussed, or by varying the functional conditions of STS and SIT as follows:

- STS and SIT from a wheelchair
- STS and SIT from a bed
- STS and SIT from a commode or toilet
- STS and SIT from a car seat
- STS and SIT from a couch

The difference between a blocked practice schedule and a random practice schedule is the amount of **contextual interference**. Contextual interference refers to the interruption in learning of one skill by introducing a different skill or tasks during a given time frame (Rose, 2006; Schmidt, 2005). In a 45-minute treatment session, a blocked practice schedule can consist of practicing STS for 15 minutes, teaching a HEP for 15 minutes, followed by gait training using a cane for 15 minutes. The same 45-minute treatment using random practice might consist of 10 STS repetitions, HEP instruction, 10 STS repetitions, gait training on a level surface, 10 STS repetitions, gait training on a ramp, HEP instruction, and 10 STS repetitions. This type of practice schedule allows memory "trace decay" on a given motor skill so the learner has to dig deeper into his memory to perform the task again.

In healthy adults, random practice conditions enhance retention of motor tasks (Schmidt, 2005). Additional research is needed regarding practice conditions for adults with neurological deficits. On the contrary, people with PD retain tasks better using blocked practice. A pilot study demonstrated that people with PD were more accurate on retention tests of a motor task with blocked practice schedules than with random practice schedules, whereas the reverse was true for healthy age-matched adults (Lin, 2007).

## Feedback

What type of feedback can a therapist use when teaching STS, SIT, or a standing task? As a review, **extrinsic** (augmented) feedback refers to feedback provided from a source external to the learner, such as the therapist. The therapist who provides manual guidance or verbal cues to move the trunk farther forward during STS is using extrinsic feedback. Extrinsic feedback describing the outcome of the task is considered **knowledge of results**. The therapist might say: "Wow! You stood up in less than 5 seconds!" **Knowledge of performance** feedback describes the quality of the movement rather than the outcome, such as "Try to bend farther forward like a hinge" (the therapist demonstrates a hinge at the waist). Internal/**intrinsic** feedback is feedback generated by the learner's internal system and includes the use of sensory systems such as visual, vestibular, auditory, proprioceptive, and cutaneous receptors. The therapist can enhance a patient's use of internal feedback by asking, "Can you feel the pressure moving over your feet as you stand up?"

Most research regarding the effect of feedback on motor learning has involved healthy adults (Rose, 2006; Schmidt, 2005). A recent review of the literature synthesized research regarding external feedback variables in both healthy adults and in people with stroke (van Vliet, 2006). Table 36-7 summarizes the findings from this review.

The following bullets provide examples of appropriate feedback strategies for use with patients during STS, standing, and SIT training:

- Knowledge of performance, or specific characteristics of the patient's movement, is *more valuable* than generic phrases such as "That's great!" or "Good job!" This does not mean you should avoid encouragement; rather, be specific about what was great. For example, consider saying "I liked how you rocked your body forward to help stand up" or "Did you notice how much smoother your motion was the second time around? That's progress!"
- Do not over-rely on an internal focus of attention; try to relate the movement task to the external environment. You can say "Bend your nose over this line" as easy as "Bend farther forward." Or you can cut back on words by saying "Bend like this" while you demonstrate the hinging motion of the pelvis rotating forward.
- Avoid creating a dual task environment by giving feedback while the patient is moving. Although more research needs to be performed on the timing of feedback, let the patient complete the task first and then give feedback. This allows the patient to allocate more attention on what you are saying or showing, and attention is important for learning.
- Use videotapes to provide visual feedback or as an instructional tool (Mak, 2008).

## ■ Therapeutic Exercises to Improve Standing and Sitting

Impairments of muscle strength, power, and endurance make it difficult to move STS or SIT. As stated previously, STS uses primarily concentric muscle forces in a closed kinetic chain,

| TABLE 36-7 | Summary of Feedback Variables in Healthy Adults and People With Stroke | |
|---|---|
| **HEALTHY ADULTS (MICHAEL, 2008)** | **PEOPLE WITH NEUROLOGICAL IMPAIRMENTS (VAN VLIET, 2006)** |
| • Precise feedback describing the error and how to correct it is more effective than descriptive feedback alone<br>• Verbal feedback can override visual feedback, even when incorrect<br>• Verbal *knowledge of results* feedback can be redundant when task results are obvious<br>• Experienced learners benefit from self-review of videotapes; novice learners benefit from attention cuing during video review | • Verbal knowledge of results can be redundant in people with a stroke when a task is obvious<br>• Visual feedback about weight distribution may help balance<br>• Auditory feedback on force production may help sit-to-stand ability |
| • Too-frequent feedback impairs learning<br>• Concurrent feedback interferes with learning and transfer<br>• Summary feedback enhances learning<br>• Giving learner the ability to choose frequency of feedback enhances learning | • No significant difference between frequent and infrequent feedback, but more research is needed<br>• Some evidence that summary feedback or averaged feedback may be beneficial compared with 100% feedback after each trial |
| • External focus of attention enhances learning; internal focus of attention decreases learning<br>• Adults benefited from external focus of attention, whereas children did not show the same benefit from external focus and showed improved transfer skills with internal focus | • Some evidence exists that external focus of attention improved performance and learning |

Synthesized from Michal E, Jarus T, Bart O. Effect of focus of attention and age on motor acquisition, retention, and transfer: A randomized trial. *Phys Ther.* 2008;88(2):251–259.
van Vliet PM, Wulf G. Extrinsic feedback for motor learning after stroke: What is the evidence? *Disabil Rehabil.* 2006;28(13–14):831–840.

whereas SIT uses eccentric muscle forces in a closed kinetic chain. Therapeutic exercise serves as an important intervention to enhance STS and SIT. Although this statement should not surprise you, it raises many important questions: What types of exercises, at what intensity, in what position, and for what duration enhance STS and SIT? Should the type of exercise be different for someone with PD versus an adult with cerebral palsy (CP) if the goal is to improve STS? Although much more research is needed, most forms of strength training reported in the literature enhanced both strength and function in patients with neurological deficits and older adults with disabilities (Engardt, 1995; Krebs, 2007; Marigold, 2005; Taylor, 2004;). The following paragraphs summarize modes of therapeutic exercise to enhance STS, standing, and SIT.

## Functional Strengthening Exercise

Exercising key muscles of the LE through repetitive STS and SIT is a logical way to strengthen muscle groups needed for these tasks (Krebs, 2007; Rosie, 2007). Functional exercises have the advantage of being efficient because the patient is practicing a functional task and working on LE strength at the same time. The resistance in STS/SIT is the patient's body weight, whereas the amount of force needed to stand or sit relates to the height of the chair as well as body weight. Functional exercises have improved force production through the impaired LE during STS in people with chronic stroke, and these findings were highly correlated with improved speed in the TUG test (Leroux, 2006). Even reaching beyond arm's length in sitting has increased peak vertical force in the affected extremity during STS as

well as movement speed in people with an acute stroke (Dean, 2007).

STS, like other closed chain exercises, can be progressed by varying the percentage of body weight, narrowing the BOS, making the support surface less stable, and increasing the speed of the task (Kisner, 2007). To lower the percentage of body weight needed, provide assistance using the arms, an overhead harness, or manual assistance. Increase resistance by applying manual resistance, weighted vests, or elastic tubing. Weighted vests and a one repetition maximum (1RM) formula has been used to create a loaded STS exercise in children with spastic diplegia (Liao, 2007). Repetitive STS may also increase muscular endurance when the activity is performed with high enough number of repetitions (Kisner, 2007).

The following procedures are recommended when using STS or SIT as therapeutic exercise:

- Determine the maximum number of repetitions a patient can perform from a given chair/mat height before fatiguing. To improve muscle endurance, perform a high number of repetitions with less resistance (e.g., with a higher chair or without manual resistance). To enhance muscle strength by providing resistance, consider adding enough resistance using tubing or weights so the patient fatigues after six to 12 repetitions and performing two or three sets of this resisted exercise (Kisner, 2007).
- To emphasize power, ask the patient to do a certain number of repetitions within a specified time: "Mr. Smith, I want you to stand up five times in 10 seconds. Ready, begin." The Five Timed Chair Stands Test can be used as a baseline to compare power in the legs over time (Whitney, 2005).

## Activities to Enhance Standing Symmetry

Many patients with a neurological disorder stand asymmetrically, with uneven weight distribution between the two legs. In some cases, the cause of the asymmetry is a perceptual deficit that interferes with perceiving true vertical. Other patients may stand asymmetrically because they avoid putting weight on the weaker leg. A variety of strategies can be employed to enhance standing symmetry, ranging from very low–technical applications such as mirror feedback (Vaillant, 2004) to more technical but inexpensive options such as the Wii Fit® gaming system and expensive computerized force plate systems (Cheng, 2001; Sackley, 1997; Weinstein, 1989). Figure 36-7 demonstrates the use of a mirror to provide feedback in alignment during standing. In patients with a stroke, visual feedback using force platforms and force plates has enhanced symmetry and alignment (Cheng, 2001; Sackley, 1997; Yoo, 2006). Visual and auditory feedback using force plates has also improved balance as measured by a decreased number of falls (Cheng, 2001).

In patients with hemiparesis, use of a unilateral assistive device such as a cane is controversial because it is thought to promote asymmetry and uneven weight-bearing. However, research by Hu (2013) indicated that standing up with a cane actually improved symmetry between two limbs compared with standing without a cane in patients with hemiparesis.

What are some concrete examples of ways to improve standing symmetry? You do not need to spend a lot of money to provide feedback to the patient on how symmetrical he is when standing. You can provide visual feedback using mirrors, game systems such as the Wii Fit®, bathroom scales, and mirroring the patient's movement with your own. When the patient has perception deficits, external lines in the architecture of a room (such as a doorframe) or a vertical line of tape on the wall or mirror can be used as a visual reference. To assist the patient in seeing the relationship between the body and vertical, you can also place a piece of tape down the front of the patient's shirt and ask him to align the line on his shirt with the line on the mirror.

When a patient has a difficult time accepting weight onto a weak leg or automatically bears more weight on one side than on the other, several strategies can be tried. Use a small step under the leg that normally takes more of the weight to force weight-bearing onto the weaker or non–weight-bearing side (Fig. 36-8). When using a step to facilitate weight shift onto the weaker leg, the degree of weight-bearing on the weaker side will be influenced by the size and location of the step. Figure 36-9ABC illustrates the change in weight-bearing on the weaker side that occurs as the size of the step is progressively increased to biomechanically shift more weight onto the weaker leg. Weight acceptance can also be achieved by shifting weight forward onto the weaker LE in stride stance (Fig. 36-10). Reaching toward objects placed on the weaker side may also help achieve weight shift.

When the leg lacks the motor control to keep the knee extended, use your body or an external device such as an air splint to provide additional support to that side. Gradually reduce the amount of support you provide externally to the weaker side. When the patient is standing in the parallel bars, ask him to bring the weaker hip closer to the parallel bar on that side of the body—in essence providing an external cue to help the patient relearn the feeling of symmetry. Manual guidance and/or compression into the joint can facilitate equal weight-bearing as well. Typically, manual guidance and compression are given early in the treatment program, providing additional sensory information guided by the therapist. As the

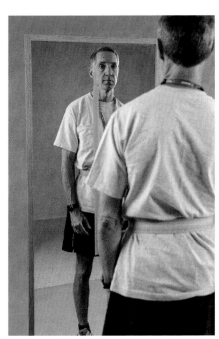

**FIGURE 36-7** Use of a mirror to work on standing symmetry and alignment.

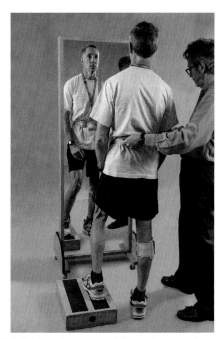

**FIGURE 36-8** Use of a step to shift weight onto the more involved extremity (left foot on the step shifts weight to right lower extremity).

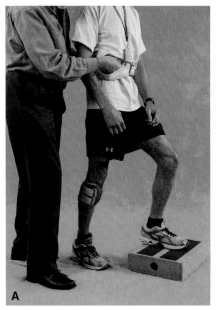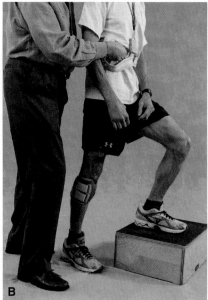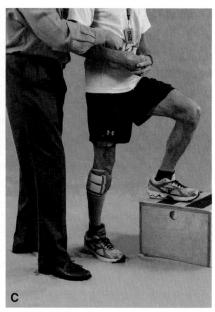

FIGURE 36-9ABC Placing the less-involved leg on boxes of various heights helps to shift weight progressively to the more-involved leg.

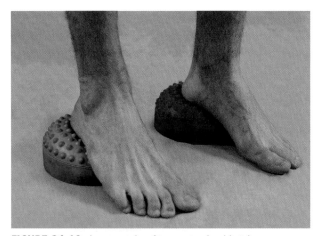

FIGURE 36-10 An example of increasing heel height to promote better weight distribution in a patient with bilateral ankle flexion contractures.

treatment progresses, offer the patient other external visual cues, even when your hands are not there to guide the movement. Pressure-sensitive door mats or even children's toys with squeaky sounds can be used to create auditory feedback regarding weight shift.

Regardless of the type of cuing used to facilitate weight shift, therapists must use intensive practice to encourage long-term changes in performance. For the task of standing, intensive practice means standing for longer periods or having more repetitions during which the patient has to stand. You can begin by asking the patient to maintain the alignment for 15 seconds, progressing to 30 seconds, 45 seconds, and so on. You can progress standing symmetry training by adding movement in the environment or by placing the patient on a more compliant surface, such as foam or a trampoline. Box 36-4 offers some examples for incorporating standing symmetry training into your plan of care.

## Standing Weight-Shift Training

Perform the following three tasks: (1) Stand in front of a sink and reach for the faucets; (2) stand in front of a door and open it; and (3) turn to shake the hand of someone standing on your left. Each of these tasks included a component of weight shifting not accompanied by walking. Weight shifting, or moving the COM within the BOS, is a normal component of standing, reaching, activities of daily living (ADLs), and gait activities. Traditionally, weight shifting was integrated into therapy as a "pregait" activity; however, we now know that weight shifting occurs during most standing activities. Weight-shift training involves encouraging patients to shift their COM within the BOS in the context of as many different tasks and directions as possible. In weight-shift training, the therapist takes on the following roles:

a) Organizing the weight-shifting practice in an intensive and progressive manner: easy to hard, small to large shifts, slow to fast shifts, and weight shifting in multiple directions

b) Providing extrinsic (augmented) feedback as needed, such as "Bring your hip closer to the wall"; manual guidance should be used judiciously to avoid the patient becoming dependent on external sensory input

c) Incorporating real-life activities into the weight-shifting practice, such as reaching for meaningful objects on a shelf overhead (salience)

d) Asking the patient to pay attention to how weight shifting changes when pressure is placed on the foot (e.g., removing the patient's socks and shoes during a forward reaching task and asking the patient "Is your weight on the ball of your foot or on the heel of your foot?")

T'ai Chi is a martial art emphasizing slow and controlled movements with weight shifting. Resources such as *T'ai Chi Fundamentals: For Health Professionals and Instructors*

---

### BOX 36-4 Standing Symmetry Training

**Preparation**

- Know your patient's sensory (visual, auditory, somatosensory) skills and impairments.
  - A patient with severe homonymous hemianopsia will have difficulty with visual feedback; a patient with hearing loss may prefer visual over auditory feedback.
- Position the equipment accurately to receive accurate feedback.
  - For left/right standing symmetry, place the mirror in front of the patient.
  - For anterior/posterior symmetry, place the mirror laterally.
  - On the Wii Fit® balance board, ensure that the patient's legs are positioned symmetrically.
  - When using bath scales, make sure the left and right feet are placed similarly on each scale.
- Safety: Use a gait belt low and snug around the patient's hips or a harness for safety; position yourself laterally and slightly posterior to the patient so your hands are free to catch either an anterior or posterior fall.

**Implementation**

- Using clear and uncomplicated language, tell the patient what will happen or what to do. Whenever possible, DEMONSTRATE rather than describe.
  - "On the screen, your body is shown as a red dot. When you move, it makes a wiggly line. The goal is to keep the dot in the center of the blue box. Let me show you."
- The mirror or screen should be the main source of feedback to the patient, but use your skills as needed to direct the patient's attention. Remember that explicit training can interfere with motor learning, so try to keep your input to a minimum.
  - "In the mirror, are you straight or leaning to one side? OK, now try to stand straight."
  - "The loud BEEP means that too much weight is on your RIGHT leg. Can you lean more to the left? Great! Now try to stay in that position."
- Use external visual cues as needed to help direct the patient's attention.
  - Tape a vertical line on the patient's shirt with blue painter's tape, and do the same on the mirror at the same height. Ask the patient to match up the line on the shirt with that on the mirror.

---

(Yu, 1999) provide text and video instruction that can be used with patients.

How do we provide augmented feedback to the patient regarding weight shifting? Mirrors, force plates, and Wii Fit® or other gaming systems can be used to track the center of pressure as it moves during an activity, just as it is used to give feedback on standing symmetry. Table 36-8 provides additional examples of weight-shifting activities in standing.

### Circuit Training

Circuit training has been effective in increasing muscle strength and STS function in both adults (Dean, 2000) and children aged 4 to 8 years (Blundell, 2003). Circuit training implies a series of activities usually performed at different stations and used for strengthening or aerobic training. Activities in the circuit should be varied, and the order should emphasize varying the primary muscle groups involved in the activity (Kisner, 2007). Circuit training for standing might include six stations with different standing tasks, as follows:

- A group exercise class for children aged 4 to 8 years utilized a circuit that included forward and lateral step-ups, STS, leg-press exercises, heel raises, crouching to pick up objects at various distances, walking on a treadmill, and walking up/down steps (Blundell, 2003).
- A circuit for adults with stroke included 10 stations: (1) sitting and reaching for objects at various distances to promote weight-bearing on the legs, (2) STS from

differing chair heights, (3) step-ups forward, backward, and sideways on a block, (4) heel lifts in standing, (5) standing while decreasing the BOS, (6) reciprocal leg flexion and extension exercise using an isokinetic computerized trainer, (7) standing from a chair and walking a short distance, then returning to the chair, (8) walking on a treadmill, (9) walking over various surfaces and obstacles, and (10) walking over slopes and stairs (Dean, 2000).

### Open Kinetic Chain Exercises

Although we intuitively think of closed chain exercises for increasing muscle strength or power for STS, research has demonstrated that open chain (OC) isokinetic exercises are also effective in improving strength and STS performance (Engardt, 1995). Patients with a stroke were trained with either eccentric OC exercises or concentric OC exercises on an isokinetic apparatus at speeds of 60, 120, and 180 degrees per second. Both groups of patients improved knee extensor strength, although the eccentrically trained group had significantly larger torque in both eccentric and concentric test positions, whereas the concentrically trained group had much lower increases in eccentric torque than in concentric torque. In addition, the eccentrically trained group showed significantly better weight-bearing on the paretic leg after training than the concentrically trained group. Although both eccentric and concentric strengthening exercises improved strength, eccentric training had more carryover into functional tasks such as STS (Engardt, 1995). However, the aforementioned

| TABLE 36-8 | Examples of Weight-Shifting Activities in Standing |
|---|---|
| **CONCEPTUAL BASIS** | **SAMPLE ACTIVITIES** |
| Sensory input and sensory attention | • In normal standing alignment, add compression into the legs by putting pressure through the iliac crests or over and downward through the greater trochanter.<br>• Use manual contacts over the anterior superior iliac crests and ask the patient to "push into your hands" while you are positioned anteriorly and slightly laterally. This facilitates a diagonal weight shift.<br>• Remove the patient's shoes and ask the patient to pay attention to where the pressure is on the foot as weight shifts anterior-posterior, medial-lateral, and diagonally. |
| External visual cue | • Patient is standing in the parallel bars with feet staggered, ask the patient to lean toward the front foot by moving that hip closer to the parallel bar; reverse to bring the other hip to the other bar.<br>• Hang a plumb line or foam "noodle" (sold in pool stores) from the ceiling just outside the patient's broadest point (usually the shoulders). Ask the patient to alternately touch one line/noodle with the left shoulder and then change directions and touch the opposite noodle with the right shoulder. Repeat in different directions. |
| Biomechanical demands | • Place the less-involved leg on a progressively large step (3-inch, 6-inch, 10-inch), forcing the COM onto the more-involved leg. Stepping up onto even small steps requires the patient to shift weight.<br>• The size of the BOS will influence how far the COM must move. Gradually increase the distance between the two feet to increase shift. |
| Games or computer | • Wii Fit®-Balance: almost all games, including Tilt Ball, Soccer, Skiing; Wii Fit®-Aerobic: Hula Hoop. |
| T'ai Chi | • All T'ai Chi movements involve a slow weight shift. |

BOS = base of support; COM = center of mass.

study trained only knee extensor muscles; it would make sense to also include knee flexion training.

Concentric and eccentric OC exercises can also improve LE strength and STS ability (Taylor, 2004). Adults with CP were given a progressive resisted strengthening program of approximately 60% to 80% of the 1RM two times per week for 10 weeks. The exercises included leg presses, knee extensions, latissimus dorsi pull-downs, a chest press, seated rows, and abdominal curls. Participants demonstrated improved leg and arm strength as well as significant improvement in speed of STS.

Lastly, patients with unilateral or bilateral LE weakness who have a difficult time standing at all may benefit from a strengthening program on a recumbent cycle. Kerr (2007) demonstrated the similarity in muscle recruitment of LE cycling with STS and step-up tasks in healthy adults. So, a recumbent bicycle could be an early impairment exercise to strengthen the ankle, knee, and hip musculature and/or as a functional training modality.

## ■ Prescription, Application, and Fabrication of Devices and Equipment

### Orthotics and Shoe Wedges

As stated previously, for a variety of reasons, asymmetrical standing is a common deficit in people with neurological conditions. Orthotics and shoe wedges have been useful in promoting standing balance symmetry in people with hemiparesis

(Chaudhuri, 2000; Rodriquez, 2002). The theoretical basis behind orthotics and shoe wedges is generally biomechanical in nature. Shoe wedges can be used to raise the shoe height on the less-involved side to shift weight onto the more-involved LE or to provide support for a patient with bilateral ankle plantar flexion contracture (Fig. 36-11).

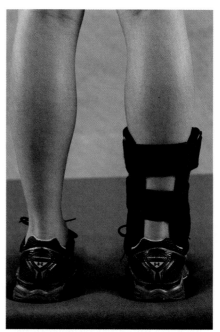

**FIGURE 36-11** Air stirrup brace used to provide medial-lateral support.

The effect of shoe wedges on symmetry during standing was investigated using 5-, 7.5-, and 12.5-degree wedges under the nonparetic leg. This research revealed that the 5- and 7.5-degree wedges improved standing symmetry, with the 5-degree wedge creating the greatest symmetry between the two limbs (Rodriquez, 2002). Even after the wedges were removed, there was improved symmetry in weight-bearing between the two limbs compared with results in the pretesting trials, suggesting a carryover effect. Similar findings have been found in shoe lifts of 0.6 centimeter, 0.9 centimeter, and 1.2 centimeters on the nonparetic side (Chaudhuri, 2000). The long-term effect of shoe wedges has not been investigated; however, the devices should be considered to address standing asymmetry.

Standing symmetry has also been enhanced with the use of an individually designed ankle-foot orthosis (AFO) in people with hemiparesis (Pohl, 2006) and children with spastic diplegia (Park, 2004). An atypical AFO that was only 8 inches high and did not cover the metatarsophalangeal joints significantly improved stance symmetry and reduced postural sway in adults with eyes open who were already able to stand and walk without assistance (Pohl, 2006). More research is needed to investigate the effect of orthotics on standing symmetry with lower-functioning patient populations.

In children with spastic diplegia, a hinged AFO significantly shortened STS time as well as increased knee flexion and ankle dorsiflexion compared with a barefoot condition (Park, 2004). Although the AFO did not reduce proximal conditions of pelvic tilt and hip flexion, the power of the hip and knee joints significantly increased with the hinged AFO. Once again, the AFO provided a biomechanical condition in the ankle and knee that promoted STS (Park, 2004).

Because orthotics provide an external mechanism of stability by altering the biomechanics of the foot/ankle complex, they are considered a compensatory strategy for enhanced standing symmetry. There are several drawbacks to the use of orthotics. They can be expensive, can be difficult to don/doff, and can cause skin irritation or breakdown. Orthotics also affect joint range of motion and muscle function. Before ordering an orthosis, create a temporary orthosis similar to that described by Pohl (2006). Another idea is to use an Ace wrap or even a prefabricated device and observe how it affects STS, standing, and SIT. After observing how the temporary orthotic affects function, weigh the benefits and drawbacks for each patient and discuss the potential effects with the patient and caregivers.

## Home and Chair Modifications and Equipment

Another compensatory approach to improving independence in STS and SIT is the modification of furniture, including chairs, beds, and wheelchairs. This approach also uses biomechanical principles to facilitate STS. As previously discussed, seat heights at 120% of the length of the lower leg have been found to decrease the work needed for STS (Janssen, 2002b). A simple and inexpensive way to raise chair height is to use furniture risers

(Fig. 36-12). Other factors affecting ease of STS include seat softness/compliance and the angle of the seat. Home or institutional furniture can also be modified to enhance the ease of STS and SIT as outlined in the following bullets.

- Purchase furniture risers (Fig. 36-13) and place them under the legs of a bed, couch, or chair. Most risers increase the height of the bed or chair by 8 inches. Ensure that the furniture is stable after the risers are in place.
- Modify wheelchair seats that are too low or not firm enough. A wooden insert can be placed on top of a sling seat, followed by a dense cushion to distribute pressure over the ischial tuberosities. When you modify the height of a wheelchair, be sure to assess how it affects the back height, armrest height, and ability of the feet to touch the floor. A wooden board can also be placed under the mattress of most beds and in some couches to increase firmness. Furniture stores that sell bunk beds often have boards designed to provide firm support under a mattress.
- Create a slight slope in a seat or chair so it is higher posteriorly than anteriorly. This places the patient in a slight anterior pelvic tilt, which facilitates forward pelvic rotation and weight transfer onto the legs during STS. This position brings the COM forward and thus is not safe for a patient with poor trunk control. Firm wedges of various degrees can be purchased from medical equipment companies. Conversely, wedge cushions in the reverse direction (the front is higher than the back) are sometimes used as a restraint-free strategy to prevent falls because it makes STS more difficult.
- Mechanical seat lifts and chairs with pneumatic lifts can also be used for patients who do not have the strength to move STS independently or who have chronic conditions in which functional improvement is not likely. Some devices

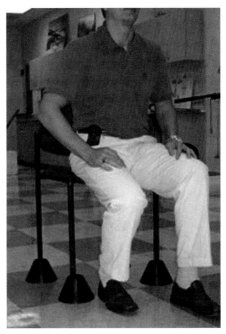

**FIGURE 36-12** Using furniture risers to raise the height of a standard chair.

are electric, providing up to 100% of the lifting force, and others are pneumatic and do not require electricity. Most seat lifts are portable and range in weight, size, and cost. Chair lifts have built-in lifts in the entire chair or in the seat of the chair. Chair lifts traditionally were built as reclining chairs that could go from reclining all the way to upright. Newer model chairs lifts include classic wing chairs in which only the seat cushion rises, as well as commode chair lifts. Chair lifts are more expensive than seat lifts, but they are more permanent and more comfortable. Chair lifts and seat lifts can also decrease the amount of assistance needed by a caregiver.

Ruszala (2005) analyzed physiotherapists' perceived rate of exertion, stability, ease of use, effectiveness, posture, and duration of the task with four STS devices for patients in an inpatient rehabilitation facility. Their findings indicated a significant difference in therapist time (duration) to complete a task among the four devices evaluated (walking harness, stand-and-walk aid, chair lifter, and stand-and-turn aid), with the walking harness and stand-and-walk aid taking longer to use than the chair lifter and stand-and-turn aid. In general, therapists in this study found that setting up the equipment was often complex and time-consuming. Focus group findings also indicated that although the devices do not promote normal biomechanics of STS, therapists believed they can complement other physical therapy interventions and promote function and weight-bearing.

When a patient cannot independently stand, adaptive devices can also assist with standing. Standing frames can be used by people with severe LE weakness or paralysis to provide daily standing for physiological benefits. Standing boxes are designed to help maintain standing once the patient is standing upright, whereas standing frames provide assistance to move to standing and then stability once standing (Fig. 36-13ABC). Standing frames are expensive; however, the high cost must be weighed against the high cost of complications from immobility, including contractures and pressure ulcers. Physiological benefits of standing include sacral/buttock pressure relief; stretching of hip flexors, knee flexors, and plantar flexors; enhanced bone density; improved cardiovascular tolerance to standing or decreased orthostatic hypotension; and improved digestive health (Eng, 2001; Kunkel, 1993).

Research on the effects of standing frames on spasticity for people with an SCI has been inconclusive. Canadians with an SCI were surveyed to determine how prolonged standing was used and its perceived effects (Kunkel, 1993). Thirty percent of the respondents reported standing almost daily and that standing was more often done by people with paraplegia than by those with quadriplegia. The perceived benefits of standing included a feeling of well-being, improved circulation such as decreased LE swelling, decreased reflex activity (muscle spasms), and better bowel/ bladder function. Respondents also reported improved self-care skills, digestion, breathing, and skin integrity. Twenty-five percent of those who stood daily also reported better sleep and decreased pain. More research on the physiological benefits of standing is needed for persons with MS, end-stage PD, ALS, and muscular dystrophy.

## ■ Electrotherapeutic Modalities

The use of functional electrical stimulation (FES) to stand people with paraplegia has been documented since 1981 (Bajd, 1981; Triolo, 1996). FES can be used as a compensatory approach to assist function much like a brace or a standing frame. When FES is used, the biomechanics of STS are different in a patient with an SCI than in healthy adults. A kinematic analysis of STS in people with paraplegia who

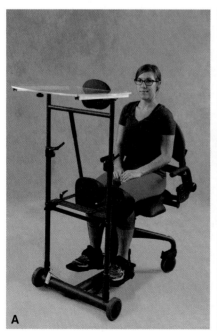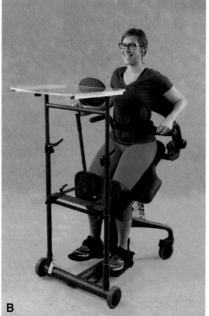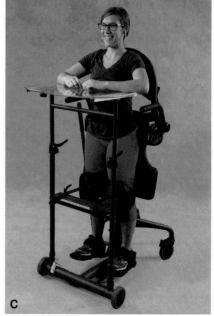

**FIGURE 36-13ABC** A standing frame provides maximal support in patients with severe lower extremity weakness or instability.

used FES demonstrated one of three strategies: (1) primary use of the arms for support despite FES; (2) arm support with better use of leg FES to unload the arms; and (3) use of the upper body/trunk to gain linear momentum along with FES of the legs (Kamnik, 1999). The latter strategy is most similar to that used in healthy adults.

There are several potential advantages to using FES for standing compared with use of standing devices and lifts: less cumbersome equipment, added versatility such as the ability to maneuver in small spaces, better appearance, and less muscle atrophy (Triolo, 1996). The outcomes of four patients with a cervical SCI who were given implanted neuromuscular electric stimulation to assist with STS and transfers have been documented. All patients progressed from percutaneous stimulation to an implanted system and from exercises to a tilt table to standing in parallel bars/a walker. The implanted FES system activated knee, hip, and trunk extensor musculature. Functional outcomes for the patients included sitting and standing independently and transferring or stepping over obstacles with significantly less effort (Triolo, 1996).

The use of an implanted FES systems is still being investigated, however, and is not ready for common clinical application.

## ■ Progression of Sit-to-Stand, Stand-to-Sit, or Standing

Therapeutic activities to enhance STS, standing, and SIT should incorporate the principles of motor learning, the unique biomechanics of each activity, and other performance-based variables such as assistance from equipment or a therapist. These criteria not only form the theoretical basis for organizing a given functional training session, but they also provide a framework for progression of an activity such as STS, standing, SIT, or weight shifting. Although the plan of care varies greatly depending on the impairments of each patient, progression principles that can be employed with any patient are described by Fell (2004). Table 36-9 provides an overview, with progression categorized on the basis of motor learning principles such as variation of feedback or environment; progression of movement characteristics such as the velocity and amplitude of the movement; and progression based on other variables such as use of assistive devices or developmental position variations. Therapists can apply principles of progression in a systematic way in order to gradually increase the difficulty of STS, standing, and SIT.

Let us apply the principle of progression using the environment as a variable in a patient who is having difficulty standing. Initially, have the patient stand with a wide BOS in a closed (nonchanging) environment (Fig. 36-14A). Progress the patient by gradually decreasing the BOS by moving the feet closer together, then next to one another, then in tandem, and even onto one leg if possible (Fig. 36-14B). To further progress this patient, add an environmental perturbation (Fig. 36-14C). Throwing a weighted ball provides an external perturbation that is unpredictable; when combined with a narrow BOS, it provides a major postural control challenge to standing (Fig. 36-14D). The ball could even be thrown against a trampoline for additional variability.

| TABLE 36-9 | Progression of Therapeutic Activities as Applied to Sit-to-Stand, Standing, and Stand-to-Sit |
|---|---|
| *Motor Learning Progression* | |
| Variability of practice | • Vary the task by standing up from many different chairs/surfaces<br>• Begin with using armrests; progress to standing without<br>• Alter feet position: right foot behind, left foot behind, symmetrical<br>• Vary the size of the base of support<br>• Alter movements of the head, trunk, and arms during standing |
| Feedback | • Decrease reliance on verbal feedback; use visual feedback when possible<br>• Gradually decrease the amount/frequency of feedback over time<br>• Utilize video recorders and ask the patient to self-assess |
| Environment progression | • Decrease the height of the seat to increase difficulty<br>• Angle the seat higher anteriorly than posteriorly<br>• Create a softer seat surface or a soft/uneven floor surface<br>• Progress to a less stable seat surface, such as a chair with wheels (if safe)<br>• Start with a quiet environment and add distractions<br>• Reach farther and in multiple directions<br>• Add a dual motor task, such as standing up with a purse or wallet<br>• Add a dual cognitive task, such as a mental calculation |
| *Movement Characteristics* | |
| Amplitude of movement | • Begin with a large amplitude of movement (nose over toes) and progress to smaller amplitudes, requiring more strength and power of the legs |

*Continued*

| TABLE 36-9 | Progression of Therapeutic Activities as Applied to Sit-to-Stand, Standing, and Stand-to-Sit—cont'd |
|---|---|
| Velocity of movement | • Begin using momentum to make STS easier; progress by slowing the speed<br>• Slow the speed of motion on returning to sit, which also increases the difficulty<br>• Move the head or arms quickly or shift weight quicker to make movement harder |
| Amount of work | • Lower the height of the seat and increase the number of repetitions to add work<br>• Add a weighted vest or resistive tubing to increase work in STS or standing |
| Endurance | • Increase the total amount of time (minutes) practicing STS, SIT, and standing<br>• Perform more repetitions in a given period |
| Regional | • Increase use of the involved LE by positioning the less-involved LE anteriorly<br>• Increase weight-bearing on the involved leg by elevating the stronger leg on a step or with a shoe wedge |
| | **Other Variables** |
| Development positions | • Begin with a larger base of support via a modified plantigrade position, allowing the patient to push up from a weight-bearing surface placed anteriorly<br>• Progress by removing the box and unweighting the arms; this increases the degrees of freedom the patient must control and makes the task harder |
| Assistive devices | • Early in training, add support by blocking the knees or assisting in the forward flexion or flexion momentum phase<br>• Decrease the amount of assistance or support over time, including verbal cues |

LE = lower extremity; SIT, stand-to-sit; STS, sit-to-stand.
Modified from Fell D. Progressing therapeutic interventions in patients with neuromuscular disorders: A framework to assist clinical decision making. *J Neurol Phys Ther.* 2004;28(1):35.

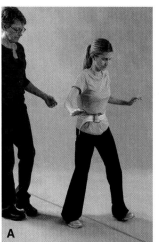 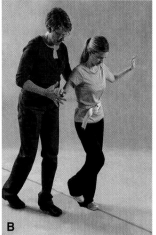 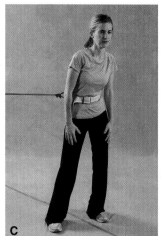 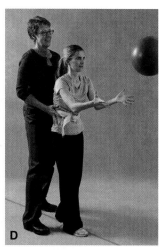

**FIGURE 36-14ABCD** Progression of standing (A) from wide base of support and closed environment, (B) to narrow base of support standing on one leg, and (C) to external perturbation (see the cord attached at trunk), (D) to throwing a weighted ball.

## PATIENT APPLICATION: INTERVENTIONS

*Let us return to our patient, Mr. P, and select interventions to enhance his ability to move STS, SIT, and standing.*

### Therapeutic Exercise
- *Warm-up activity: 10 to 20 minutes of gentle LE warm-up on an LE cycle or elliptical machine*
- *Passive stretching and range of motion*
  - *Bilateral dorsiflexion, standing stretches immediately after warm-up*

- *Strengthening LE musculature for motion: total gym squats; progress to wall squats with resistance plus body weight (60%–80% 1RM)*
  - *Muscles for STS-concentric, closed chain*
    - *TA, gluteus maximus, QD*
  - *Muscles for SIT: eccentric, closed chain*
    - *QD, gluteus maximus, gastrocnemius/soleus*
- *Strengthening trunk/LE for stability (60%–80% 1RM)*
  - *Gluteus medius, tensor fasciae latae, abdominals, back extensors; postural control: TA, gastrocnemius/soleus, iliopsoas*
    - *Rhythmic stabilization in standing*

- - Slow reversals and slow reversal hold of trunk/UE rotation
    - Variation in standing surface
  - Increase environmental variability or task conditions
    - Vary BOS, surface, amount of resistance
    - Sudden letting go of TheraBand/resistance, standing on incline board
- T'ai Chi pull and press

## Functional Training in Self-Care and Home Management, Including ADLs and Instrumental ADLs

- STS training and SIT training
  - Begin with wedge elevating to 46-inch height seat, no UEs
  - Decrease incline and height of matt gradually; vary speed (fast/slow)
  - Change surface of seat and floor; use visual cues
- Standing home tasks: shaving in standing, setting the table, trimming plants
  - Standing in front of a mirror, shaving, or brushing the teeth
  - Vary the BOS, surface conditions, environmental conditions
  - Reaching while standing (setting the table), multiple directions
  - Outside on uneven terrain; trimming or shaping plants

## Functional Training in Work (Job/School/Play), Community, and Leisure Integration

- Church-related activities
  - Standing, handing out communion wafers, moving the head, arms, trunk over the feet
  - Perturbations with varying BOS from variety of directions

## Prescription, Application, and Fabrication of Devices and Equipment (Assistive, Adaptive, Orthotic, Protective, Supportive)

- Gradually reduce use of armrests during STS; reduce UE support in standing
- Raise the bed height using risers

## Electrotherapeutic Modalities

- Electrical stimulation to the TA during STS

### Contemplate Clinical Decisions

This plan of care is by no means the only approach to Mr. P and his ability to move sit-to-stand (STS) and stand-to-sit and to stand. Test your understanding by answering the following questions:

#### Review the Selection of Therapeutic Exercises:

1. What other exercise techniques would you use to strengthen Mr. P's lower extremities? Trunk?
2. How would you emphasize power versus endurance?
3. How would you calculate a one-repetition maximum on the Total Gym ®?
4. What exercises would you prescribe for his home exercise program?

#### Consider the Functional Training Strategies:

5. When is it most appropriate to select a momentum strategy over a nonmomentum strategy in retraining STS?
6. What strategies would MAXIMIZE implicit learning for Mr. P in his ability to move STS? Would any techniques interfere with implicit learning?
7. Use the principles of progression to develop three different ways to modify the patient's progression of STS and standing.
8. What type of external auditory cues or external visual cues could you use to increase the ease of initiation to stand for Mr. P?
9. What tests and measures would you use to document changes in his functional ability to move STS or to stand over time?

## ■ Patient-/Client-Related Instruction

The *Guide to Physical Therapist Practice* (APTA, 2015) outlines important considerations for patient-related instruction, including the need for:

- Instruction designed to decrease impairments, functional limitations, or disabilities
- Instruction designed to reduce risk factors
- Instruction appropriate for impaired arousal, attention, cognition, and senses
- Instructional or assistive technology needed to enhance learning, such as large-print text
- Identification of potential learning barriers (beliefs, cultural expectations, language)
- Identification of assistance from caregivers, family, equipment
- Identification of patient's/client's personal goals

Patient-related instruction *specific to standing* includes three key goals: (1) making the patient aware of the critical importance or *value* of standing as both a functional task and as a preventive measure; (2) instruction in a standing HEP that enhances function, strength, and fitness; and (3) safety considerations, including the use of equipment or personnel to prevent injury. Placing an armchair in front of a wall, for example, improves the stability of the chair for home practice of STS and SIT exercises.

How can we apply these principles to our patient, Mr. P? The Patient Application highlights patient-related instructions based on the benefits of standing, a HEP related to standing, and overall safety guidelines for standing.

### PATIENT APPLICATION

#### Benefits of Standing
#### Relate STS to the Patient's Key Functional Goals

- Independent mobility at home
- Role of lector and Eucharistic Minister at his church

#### Relate STS to Terms of Prevention

- Prevention of muscle stiffness, joint contractures, and spine stiffness seen in people with PD

- Prevention of pressure sores
- Maintenance of circulation, prevention of deep vein thrombosis
- Prevention of deconditioning related to sitting
  - Keep STS log

### Home Exercise Program
### STS and SIT

- Before each meal in the kitchen, perform three sets of 12 standing up and sitting down
- During TV watching, stand up and sit down five times during commercials

### Standing Activities

- Quiet standing: in front of the counter not holding on
  - Play solitaire or other games with grandchildren
  - Wash dishes
- Dynamic standing: in front of sink, counter, or table
  - Lift light objects from left to right side of sink

- Set three places at the table when standing in one position
- Sand wood projects while standing at a counter
  - Three sets of 20 heel raises

### Safety
### Equipment for Home

- Bed risers to increase height of the bed
- Selection of chair(s) with armrests and at ample height for independence; may modify this over time as patient progresses
- Use of external visual cues (14-inch step stool) that encourage patient to bring weight forward during standing

### Assistance From Wife/Daughter

- Allow patient to perform independently or with supervision
- Helpful verbal cues standing up: Stagger Feet, Nose Over Toes
- Helpful hints: use momentum, stand to the side of the patient
- Avoid talking to the patient during a task; wait until finished

# HANDS-ON PRACTICE

### Practical Skills for Sit-to-Stand (STS), Stand-to-Sit (SIT), and Standing Symmetry

- Practice different guarding positions with a patient who needs minimal to moderate assistance with STS
- Perform the following tests and outcome measures for STS, SIT, and standing:
  - Berg Balance Scale
  - Timed Chair Stands
  - Tinetti Balance
  - Mobility Scale for Acute Stroke
- Demonstrate three ways to decrease the level of difficulty for STS and three ways to progress the

level of difficulty for STS using the control parameters described in this chapter.
- Create an STS circuit to increase practice intensity and variability.
- Conduct a 15-minute mental practice session to practice STS/SIT or standing symmetry.
- Demonstrate two exercises that improve STS through:
  - Functional strengthening
  - Standing symmetry using visual feedback
  - An open kinetic chain
- Use a wedge to improve symmetry in a patient standing asymmetrically.

## Let's Review

1. Explain the four phases of sit-to-stand (STS) as described by Schenkman (1990), noting which phase is the most stable and which phases are less stable and why.

2. Compare and contrast the biomechanics of STS and stand-to-sit (SIT). What are the implications for functional training and therapeutic exercises?

3. According to the principles of motor control and motor learning, how would you teach a patient with Parkinson disease to move STS? Consider the following questions:
   a. What type of instructions will you give?
   b. What type of cues (internal, visual, external) will you use?
   c. What type of practice schedule and feedback will you provide?
   d. How will you increase practice intensity when the patient is in an inpatient setting? An outpatient setting? A home-health setting?

4. Describe three ways to approach a patient who stands asymmetrically with more of her weight on the nonparetic side of her body.

5. Compare and contrast compensatory approaches for STS, SIT, and standing symmetry, including assistive equipment, braces or wedges, and environmental changes.

6. A patient needs minimal assistance to move STS and SIT after an exacerbation of multiple sclerosis with left-sided weakness. Describe a plan of care that includes **two** of the following elements: functional training, therapeutic exercises, prescription of assistive/adaptive devices, patient-related instruction, and electrotherapeutic interventions.

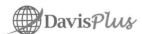

For additional resources, including Focus on Evidence tables, case study discussions, references, and glossary, please visit http://davisplus.fadavis.com

## CHAPTER SUMMARY

Moving SIT, standing, and moving STS are three distinct functional tasks that are essential for independent function and the prevention of complications related to immobility. Biomechanical and motor control analyses of these activities provide an important framework for examination and intervention. STS and SIT are discreet mobility tasks; STS uses primarily concentric muscle forces to move from a large to a small BOS, whereas SIT uses eccentric muscle forces to move from a small to a large BOS. In contrast, standing is a continuous stability task that requires ongoing postural control and cocontraction of muscles in the trunk and LEs. Using the arms during STS and SIT changes the force requirements; it increases stability, slows movement time, and decreases the use of momentum. External control parameters, such as chair height and floor compliance, and internal control parameters, such as knee extensor force, can be used to develop and progress a patient's skills over time.

Examination strategies for standing include quantitative and qualitative descriptions of function and portions of standardized tools such as the Berg Balance Scale as well as measurement of underlying impairments such as strength and range of motion. The most important intervention for STS, standing, and SIT is functional training with an emphasis on normal biomechanics, motor control strategies, and motor

learning principles, such as intensive practice and the avoidance of concurrent feedback.

Online (ONL) Table 36-10 in the online supplemental material is the Focus on Evidence (FOE) table that summarizes evidence for some of the most important interventions to improve STS function. Ample evidence demonstrates the value of task-intensive practice for STS regardless of the patient's neurological diagnosis or age. Motor control strategies can also be used to progress the plan of care, such as decreasing the chair height, changing the speed of movement, and decreasing the amount of verbal cues or feedback. The Focus on Evidence Table 36-11 ONL summarizes evidence on interventions to improve symmetry in the standing position. Therapeutic exercises using the principles of specificity and overload through various equipment, body weight, or circuit-training also enhance standing skills regardless of age or diagnosis. Other evidence-based interventions include the use of motor imagery, shoe wedges, and orthotics; electrical stimulation; and assistive devices such as mechanical lifts, chair lifts, and standing frames. Patient-/client-related instruction includes educating patients about the value of these functional tasks for daily activities and prevention, instruction in home exercises that enhance strength or function, and guidance on safety precautions, including caregiver assistance and home equipment.

# Functional Activity Intervention in Upright Mobility

**CHAPTER 37**

Susan Diane Simpkins, PT, EdD ▪ Genevieve Pinto Zipp, PT, EdD ▪ Dennis W. Fell, PT, MD

## CHAPTER OBJECTIVES

Upon completion of this chapter, the learner should be able to:

1. Describe the biomechanical and motor control characteristics of gait.
2. List the primary impairments that affect upright mobility in patients with neurological disorders.
3. Select tests and measures to examine upright mobility across the International Classification of Functioning Disability and Health (ICF) domains of impairments in body structure and function, activity limitations, and participation restrictions.
4. Discuss the clinical management of patients with disorders of upright mobility.
5. Explain the evidence that supports the use of body weight–supported treadmill training for patients with upright mobility disorders.
6. Design an intervention using functional mobility activities to address a specific patient's mobility disorder.
7. Explain how to modify upright mobility activities to vary task complexity.
8. Describe factors that contribute to dual task control and explain how to use Gentile's Taxonomy of Tasks to train dual task performance.

## ▮ Introduction

*Mrs. Z is an 81 year-old female who sustained an infarct to the right middle cerebral artery 3 days ago, resulting in left hemiplegia. She is in a local hospital and has been receiving physical therapy and occupational therapy daily for 30 to 45 minutes each. Her medical history includes hypertension, which has been pharmacologically managed since its onset at age 40 years. Her vision and hearing are within functional limits. Before the injury, Mrs. Z lived at home with her husband and was independent in all activities of daily living. She enjoys cooking, cleaning, and shopping. She resides in a ranch-style home; however, five steps must be climbed to enter the home. There is one bathroom with a tub-shower stall combination.*

**Upright mobility** includes all forms of moving the body from one place to another while in an upright position. Upright mobility tasks include walking on level surfaces, walking on a ramp, stepping over obstacles, and climbing stairs. Walking, the most common form of upright mobility, is a complex task typically affected in patients with progressive and nonprogressive nervous system disorders. Gait disturbances may signal the onset of a progressive neurological disease, such as multiple sclerosis or Parkinson disease (PD). Gait disturbances can also be a hallmark of nonprogressive neurological disorders such as stroke, traumatic brain injury, and cerebral palsy. Because the ability to walk contributes substantially to one's quality of life and is highly valued by patients, families, and caregivers, therapists typically devote considerable treatment time to developing, improving, or preserving a patient's upright mobility skills.

Mobility tasks such as walking, stair climbing, and obstacle negotiation share common basic features: forward propulsion, postural control and balance, and adaptation to environmental conditions (Patla, 1997; Shumway-Cook, 2007). These basic features are essential for successful locomotion and can be viewed as goals for movement organization (Higgins, 1995). Effective achievement of these goals is determined by the individual's unique abilities and resources, the requirements of the task, and the characteristics of the environment. When these goals are not met, the therapist must identify factors contributing to the problem. The therapist then develops an evidence-based plan of care to promote the best possible match between the abilities and resources of the individual and the requirements of the task and environment. This includes progressively challenging the patient to meet varying task and environment demands (Fig. 37-1).

This chapter focuses on functional activities in upright mobility. As used here, the term *functional* means any action or skill that supports an individual's ability to carry out meaningful activities and participate in life roles. An activity limitation due to a mobility deficit not only compromises how individuals maneuver within and outside their home, but it may also limit performance of other functional activities, such as personal care and household tasks, not to mention participation in vocational, recreational, and leisure activities.

The effect of a mobility disorder on an individual's level of function not only affects activity and participation, but also can lead to **secondary impairments,** such as obesity, osteoporosis, hypertension, and depression. According to the Centers for Disease Control and Prevention (CDC, 1998), individuals with activity limitations experience pain, depression, anxiety, and sleeplessness on more days per month than people without activity limitations. Consequently, mobility problems affect not only the patient's immediate needs but also the risk for secondary health conditions.

## ■ General Characteristics of Normal Gait

Gait is perhaps the most extensively studied pattern of functional human movement. Research into human gait has resulted in the development of models and frameworks describing the biomechanical characteristics and motor control processes underlying this functional movement pattern. The gait model presented here was developed by Jacqueline Perry (2010), a physician and researcher who devoted much of her career to the study of normal and pathological gait. Perry's model, developed at the Rancho Los Amigos National Rehabilitation Center in California, led to a systematic approach to observational gait analysis (OGA) referred to as the Rancho Los Amigos OGA system (Perry, 2010).

### Gait Terminology

**Gait** is a rhythmical, repetitive movement pattern distinguished by a characteristic sequence of limb and trunk movements. The term **gait cycle** describes the events of one complete sequence of movements in ambulation and is defined as the time from the **initial contact (IC)** of one foot to the next IC of the same foot. The gait cycle, which is also termed a **stride,** is divided into two periods: stance and swing. The **stance phase** is defined as the period when the foot is in contact with the ground, whereas the **swing phase** is the period when the foot is not in contact with the ground.

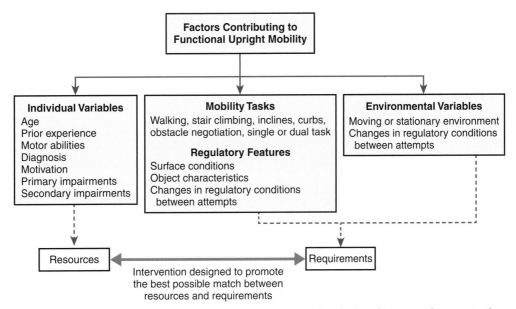

**FIGURE 37-1**  Variables that constrain movement must be considered when designing a therapeutic plan of care to improve walking. The goal of intervention is to match the abilities and resources of the individual with the characteristics of the task and environment.

A consecutive sequence of one stance and one swing phase of the same limb is called a *step*.

The gait cycle is divided into stance phase and swing phase, with four stance key events, and four swing key events (Table 37-1), as illustrated in Fig. 10-8. The eight phases of the gait cycle can be categorized as two stance period tasks, **weight acceptance (WA)** and **single-limb support (SLS)**, and one swing period task, **swing limb advancement (SLA)** (Perry, 2010). **WA** occurs when the swing limb touches down at IC and body weight is quickly transferred to the stance leg. This is also known as the **loading response (LR)**. **SLS** occurs when full body weight is supported in stance by a single stance limb while the other limb is in the swing phase. When the stance limb is in SLS, the contralateral lower extremity (LE) completes **SLA** as it moves under and then ahead of the body (Perry, 2010).

So, how do the tasks of WA, SLS, and SLA contribute to designing successful upright mobility intervention? First, each of these tasks (WA, SLS, and SLA) makes a unique contribution to progression. During the stance period, progression—which is the movement of the body in the desired direction—occurs as the weight-bearing limb is loaded (WA) and then continues as body weight is transferred along the foot and a propulsive force is generated (SLS) to move the body in the planned direction (Perry, 2010). During SLA, forward progression occurs as the reference limb is unloaded, the foot is elevated and moves forward under the body, and then the foot is lowered and contacts the ground to initiate the next stance period (Perry, 2010).

The tasks of WA and SLS contribute to postural control and balance by ensuring that the LE is in a stable position at **IC**, or the moment when the foot first contacts the surface. As weight is transferred onto the stance limb, known as the **LR**, a flexion moment at the knee quickly shifts to an extension moment as the limb is loaded at midstance. It is important to note which part of the foot makes IC (heel, flat foot, lateral foot,

forefoot, or toe) because this can influence the success of the LR and can provide clues about the abnormal motor control that is causing limitations in ambulation. During SLS, postural control is maintained by an extension moment at the hip and knee and a plantar flexion moment at the ankle (Perry, 2010). This muscle activity is designed to prevent collapse of the LE as the limb is loaded and the body continues to move forward and ahead of the foot.

Control of the head, arms, and trunk (HAT) as a unit is another postural control and balance requirement for successful upright mobility. Control of the HAT occurs primarily by hip muscle activity, with compensatory changes in knee muscle activity ensuring that an adequate net extensor moment is maintained in the LE (Winter, 1984).

Finally, control of the swing limb (SLA) contributes to the goal of adaptability. **Adaptability** in gait refers to global modifications of the basic locomotor pattern that are designed to specifically match the regulatory features of the task and the environment (Patla, 1997). Adaptability in ambulation includes changes in speed, direction, step length and step width, limb elevation, and foot placement at IC. With the exception of changing direction, these adaptations can be carried out in one step cycle. Directional changes must be planned one step before they occur because they usually require a change in speed and orientation of the body (Patla, 1997).

Although many of the described adaptations result in modifications to the swing limb, changes in muscle activation also occur in the stance limb (Patla, 1997). Think for a minute about a situation that requires you to increase your step length to avoid an obstacle. Provided your gait speed remains constant, taking a longer or higher step to clear the obstacle increases the time spent in SLS. This requires changes in muscle activity in the opposite, stance limb to ensure that your stability is preserved while the swing limb advances (Patla, 1997).

| TABLE 37-1 | Eight Phases of the Gait Cycle (compare to Figure 10-8) |
|---|---|
| **PHASE: KEY EVENTS** | **DEFINITION** |
| ***Stance Phase (60% of Gait Cycle)*** | |
| • Initial Contact (IC) | The moment when the foot contacts the ground |
| • Loading Response (LR) | When weight is rapidly transferred onto the stance limb. This is the first period of double support. |
| • Mid Stance (MSt) | The body progresses over a single, stable limb. |
| • Terminal Stance (TSt) | Progression over the stance limb continues. The body moves ahead of the limb, and weight is transferred onto the forefoot. |
| ***Swing Phase (40% of Gait Cycle)*** | |
| • Pre-Swing (PSw) | A rapid unloading of the stance limb occurs as weight is transferred onto the contralateral limb. This is the second period of double support. |
| • Initial Swing (ISw) | The thigh begins to advance as the foot comes up off the floor. |
| • Mid Swing (MSw) | The thigh continues to advance as the knee begins to extend and the foot clears the ground in forward progression. |
| • Terminal Swing (TSw) | The knee extends; the limb prepares to contact the ground for initial contact. |

(*Observational Gait Analysis Handbook.* Downey, CA: Los Amigos Research and Education Institute; 2001. p. 7).

## Biomechanics of Normal Gait

Gait can also be described using distance (spatial) and time (temporal) measures, which are referred to as **spatiotemporal parameters**. Spatial parameters include stride length, step length, and step width/base of support. Temporal parameters include step and stride times and double and single support times. Parameters derived as a composite of spatial and temporal measures include gait velocity and cadence.

Parameters such as velocity and cadence are easy to measure and are good indicators of an individual's level of functional upright mobility; however, they are too often neglected in clinical settings. Gait velocity is typically measured by having patients walk a known distance at a (1) comfortable or usual pace, (2) slow pace, and (3) fast but safe pace. Normative data for spatiotemporal gait parameters, including gait velocity, are shown in Table 10-3 with terms defined in Tables 10-8 (temporal parameters) and 10-9 (spatial parameters). These reference values should be compared with an individual's actual gait parameters to determine the extent of mobility disorder, to provide direction in planning intervention, to indicate potential for rehabilitation (in some patients), and to determine functional outcomes after treatment (Schmid, 2007).

Walking velocity in patients after stroke is a meaningful outcome measure because it predicts rehabilitation potential and correlates well with muscle strength and balance (Richards, 1995). Adults with cerebral palsy showed significant improvements in walking velocity after participating in a 10-week strength training program (Andersson, 2003). Similar findings have been reported for older adults (Richards, 1995), for adolescents with cerebral palsy (Eagleton, 2004), and for patients with stoke (Scianni, 2010), PD (Dibble, 2006), and multiple sclerosis (White, 2004).

## THINK ABOUT IT 37.1

Walking velocity is easy to measure, but interpreting a patient's walking velocity requires knowledge of age-matched normative values from healthy individuals. These data are available for persons from 1 to 90 years of age.

Where can you obtain age-matched normative values for your patient? Once you obtain the normative data, you can determine your patient's level of impairment. You can also determine how fast your patient walks "relative" to a healthy individual by dividing your patient's gait velocity by the normative value. For example, if your patient walked at 0.9 m/s and the normative value for her age is 1.4 m/s, your patient is walking at 65% of the expected velocity for her age.

The understanding of gait biomechanics has been greatly enhanced by use of computerized motion analysis equipment, which enables therapists to look beyond the spatiotemporal parameters of gait. Specifically, information on the kinematics, kinetics, and muscle activation patterns used during gait has improved understanding of the gait deviations associated with neurological disorders and the efficacy of interventions aimed at improving functional mobility.

**Kinematic** variables describe segmental and joint linear and angular displacements, velocity, and acceleration without considering the forces that cause the movement. Figure 37-2AB shows average joint angle data for the hip, knee, and ankle during nine walking trials recorded over several days for a single subject. Note the low values for the coefficient of variation (CV) over repeated trials, indicating that hip, knee, and ankle kinematics during gait are fairly consistent cycle to cycle in a healthy individual. Figure 37-3 shows the consistent relationship between hip and knee movement over several gait cycles in healthy adults.

In contrast, **kinetic** analyses, which describe the forces acting to produce the kinematics or observed movement patterns, have showed much higher variability cycle to cycle within and between individuals (Winter, 1991). Kinetic variables of gait include joint moments, power, and work, as well as **center of pressure (COP)** and ground reaction forces. A **joint moment** is force application that results in a rotational force around an axis. The COP is the center of the distribution of the total force applied to the supporting surface. The **ground reaction force** is the force exerted by the ground when the foot contacts it; it is equal in amount and opposite in direction to the force applied by the foot onto the ground. Figure 37-2B shows joint moments of force for the hip, knee, and ankle and the net support moment for the same trials as shown in Fig. 37-2A.

Stated another way, the variability of joint forces and moments (kinetic data) at the hip, knee, and ankle is much greater than the variability of joint movements (kinematic data) from the corresponding joints. It is interesting to note that walking pace has a strong bearing on the variability of LE joint moments. Variability of the joint moments increases substantially at the hip and knee when subjects walk slower than their comfortable pace (Fig. 37-4), and it decreases significantly when subjects walk faster than their comfortable pace. The CVs for the joint moments at the ankle remain essentially the same across walking speeds.

Activation patterns for individual muscles of the LE are studied using electromyography (EMG), which enhances understanding and guides intervention for gait improvement. **EMG** is an instrument that measures muscle activity by reading the electrical signals via a needle that is inserted into the muscle or a sensor that is placed on the skin. EMG can be used to assess the health of the muscle itself as well as the innervation. EMG variables include the timing (onset and offset) and amplitude (intensity) of muscle activity during movement. Figure 37-5 shows the timing pattern of muscles that are active during the stance and swing phases of gait. The black bars represent the time a muscle is active.

These data are used for comparison with EMG data from individuals with pathological gait. Timing errors in EMG activity may reflect a premature or delayed onset of muscle activity, prolonged activity, or absent activity (Perry, 2010). Amplitude (intensity) errors may include muscle activity that is greater than normal, less than normal, or insufficient. Timing and amplitude comparisons can aid decision-making on the value and

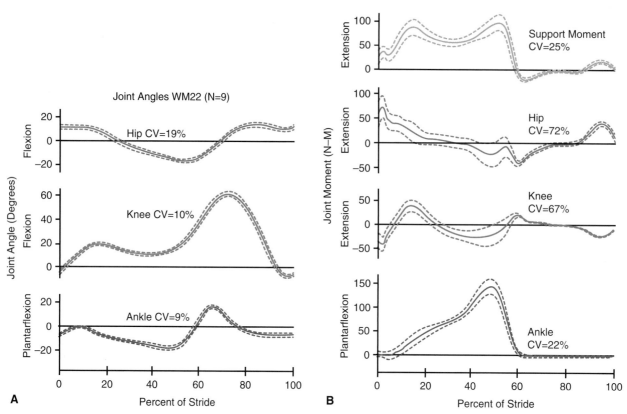

**FIGURE 37-2** (A) Average joint angles of the hip, knee, and ankle from nine trials in the same subject. (B) Joint moments for nine trials with the same subject walking at a comfortable pace. Note the low coefficient of variation for joint angles of the hip, knee, and ankle and high coefficient of variation for average joint moments. *(adapted from Winter, 1984.)*

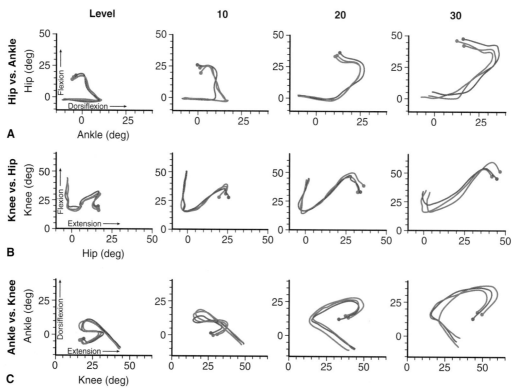

**FIGURE 37-3** Angle-angle diagrams showing consistent patterns of interlimb coordination for subjects walking on a level surface and on progressively steeper inclines of 10, 20, and 30 degrees. Note the overlap of the profiles, indicating a consistent pattern of intralimb coordination from trial to trial.

effectiveness of physical rehabilitation and medical and surgical interventions in the management of pathological gait.

## Motor Control Analysis of Gait

An understanding of the motor control aspects of human ambulation is essential in designing an intervention program to improve gait and independence in walking. As described in the following sections, many factors positively influence the understanding of gait components and how best to provide intervention and warrant consideration.

### Central Pattern Generator

Gait is a **continuous task**, or a motor task with an arbitrary beginning and end point, that requires the coordination and control of essentially all limbs and body segments. In nonhuman mammals, the rhythmical, cyclical flexion and extension patterns that characterize gait are organized by neural networks in the central nervous system called central pattern generators (CPGs). More than a hundred years ago, Graham Brown demonstrated that cats with spinal cord transection could produce rhythmical, alternating flexion and extension

movements of their hind limbs when supported on a moving treadmill (Stuart, 2008). Since then, an extensive body of research on CPGs in cats and monkeys has confirmed and extended Brown's findings (Stuart, 2008).

Although it is generally accepted that CPGs exist in some form in humans, research support is equivocal. Human bipedal gait has higher strength and balance requirements than quadruped gait and is thus more complex. The human CPG model favored today is McCrea and Rybak's two-stage model (McCrea, 2008). According to this model, each CPG has both a rhythm generator, which controls the pace of gait, and a pattern formation, which generates the sequence or pattern of limb movement. These two stages require input centrally, which modulates either or both the pattern or the rhythm (McCrea, 2008).

The best support for CPG networks in humans comes from research on patients with spinal cord injuries (SCIs). Patients with incomplete injuries of the spinal cord can relearn the ability to walk with extensive task-specific training. For example, Behrman (2008) reported that a 4.5 year-old boy with an incomplete SCI at the cervical level learned to walk with a reverse rolling walker after an intensive 16-week intervention program. Treatment began with body weight–supported

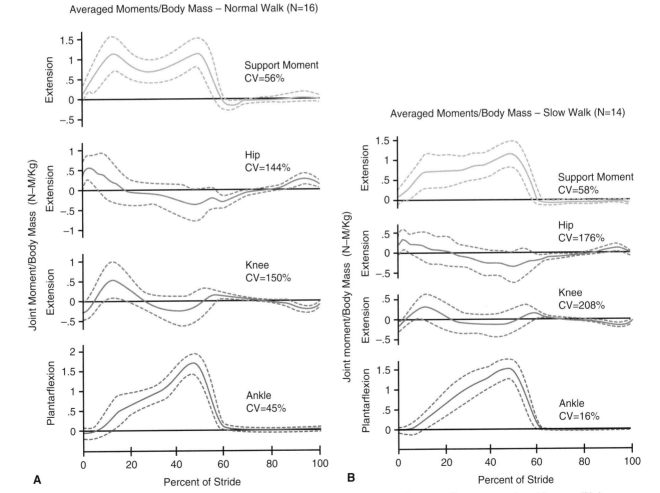

**FIGURE 37-4** (A) Average joint moments for the hip, knee, and ankle from 16 subjects walking at a comfortable pace. (B) Average joint moments from 14 subjects walking at a slow pace.

*Continued*

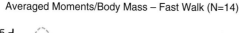

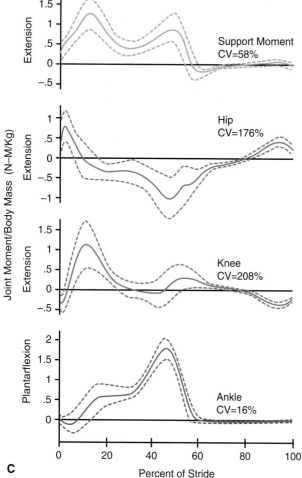

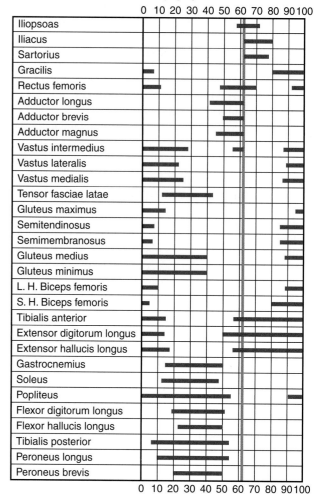

**FIGURE 37-4—cont'd** (C) Average joint moments from 14 subjects walking at a fast pace. Note the much higher coefficient of variation for joint moments when subjects walked at a slow pace compared with a fast pace. *(Winter, 1984.)*

**FIGURE 37-5** Phasic electromyography activity of lower extremity muscles showing when each muscle is active throughout the gait cycle. Red bars indicate the extent of time a muscle is active during the gait cycle (percent of stride).

treadmill training (BWSTT) and progressed to overground walking with a walker. Treadmill training is thought to activate CPG networks through the sensory input produced by walking (Behrman, 2008). Research findings such as these support the notion that CPGs underlie the rhythmical, repetitive LE movements that contribute to forward progression in upright mobility and characterize human locomotion; as such, they should be considered when designing interventions to improve walking ability.

## Gait Initiation and Termination

Locomotor control also includes the ability to initiate and terminate a step. During both the initiation and termination of a step, a time of postural instability presents a balance challenge. Initiating a step requires a smooth transition from a position of a bilateral stance (a relatively large base of support) to a unilateral stance (a relatively small base of support). This transition is associated with a predictable pattern of muscle relaxation and activation that results in unloading of the limb

that is preparing to swing and loading of the stance limb. Initial unloading involves a posterior-lateral weight shift toward the limb that is preparing to swing followed by a medial weight shift toward the new stance limb. Immediately before toe-off of the swing limb, there is an anterior weight shift over the stance limb and generation of a propulsive force that initiates leg movement in the intended direction. Steady-state velocity is typically achieved within two steps: 90% of steady-state velocity in the first step and the remaining 10% in the second step (Jian, 1993).

The termination of gait is a transition between steady-state walking and a complete stop. This transition requires a breaking force to slow down the body's momentum and attain a stable final position with the center of mass (COM) over the base of support. The process can be characterized by three periods: preparatory braking, fast braking, and final braking (Jian, 1993). **Preparatory braking** is associated with a small reduction in velocity (<10%) and a postural adjustment in preparation for fast breaking. In the **fast break** period, velocity is markedly reduced by about 90%, with the final 10% reduction occurring in the final break period. Coming to a stop requires the coordinated action of both limbs. There is an increase in vertical and anterior-posterior braking forces by the lead foot and a reduction in propulsive forces by the trailing foot. Forward progression can usually be stopped within two steps.

## Complexity and Organization

Upright mobility tasks are complex and organized skills. Upright mobility is complex because of the number of contributing components or parts and the information processing demands of the task as a whole. Essentially all upright mobility tasks require whole body control and ongoing information processing. As a person moves through space by walking, running, or stair climbing, for example, the environment expands around her. The faster the person moves, the faster the environment changes. The ability to respond to changes in the environment as quickly as needed means the individual must pay close attention to surface conditions and the movement of other people and objects.

**Organization** describes the relationship among the component parts of a skill. The stronger the relationship between the components, the higher the degree of organization (Magill, 2011).

Walking is a perfect example of an organized task because a high degree of spatial and temporal coordination is seen both within and between the LEs (Haddad, 2006). In walking and running, the joints of the LE are tightly coupled, which means they function together as a unit. A tight coupling also exists between the LEs of the two sides. This is demonstrated during gait by a consistent, relative phase relationship between the two LEs.

A **relative phase relationship** describes the position or action of one leg *relative* to the other leg. In walking and running, the LEs demonstrate a consistent out-of-phase relationship cycle after cycle because the swing phase in one leg is always associated with the stance phase in the opposite leg. This means one leg is halfway through its cycle (180 degrees) as the other leg begins its cycle (0 degrees).

Relative phase is a good index of coordination between two limb segments or two limbs. The tight coupling within and between the LEs may be due to the CPG networks that apparently underlie rhythmic leg movement in humans.

## Arm Swing

Arm swing is a characteristic feature of human gait. Under normal conditions, the arms and legs move in an *out-of-phase* (i.e., opposite and alternating) pattern during which the right arm swings forward in synchrony with the forward swing of the left leg, then the left arm moves forward in synchrony with the right leg. Although this pattern of interlimb coordination is a characteristic feature of normal gait, it is not essential for successful locomotion. Humans are quite skilled at walking while carrying objects with one or both arms without any *apparent* disruption to the gait pattern.

Interestingly, when arm swing is limited, changes in LE gait parameters are noted, including a tendency to shorten stride length and decrease stride frequency and gait velocity (Wagenaar, 2000). Furthermore, when arm swing is constrained, there is less trunk rotation than with typical walking (Eke-Okoro, 1997). Changes in stride frequency and stride length as a result of changes in arm swing suggest the existence of a coupling between the arms and legs.

The amplitude and coordination of arm swing varies with walking velocity. At velocities of less than 0.8 m/sec (slow pace), arm swing is minimal and arms generally move in phase with the LEs, synchronized with step frequency. At velocities of greater than 0.8 m/sec (comfortable pace), the arms move out of phase and are synchronized with stride frequency (Ford, 2007a). Thus, in a person with a neurological disorder who has a very slow gait, normal arm swing should not be expected until gait speed has been restored to more normal levels.

Although arm swing is not essential for successful locomotion, research indicates that it plays a role in metabolic efficiency by contributing to stability (Ortega, 2008). Arm swing reduces both momentum in the transverse plane and vertical movement of the body's COM (Ortega, 2008). When arm swing is limited, metabolic cost increases by 5% to 6%. Changes in arm swing are commonly observed in persons with neurological disorders such as PD, stroke, and cerebral palsy, related to motor control impairment as well as slow gait velocity. Indeed, it has been suggested that asymmetry in arm swing may be an early sign of PD and can be useful in differential diagnosis (Lewek, 2010).

Arm swing is disrupted after a stroke. The amplitude of arm movement is reduced on the hemiplegic side, which results in decreased thoracic and pelvic transverse rotation. This condition leads to a shorter stride length and reduced walking velocity (Ford, 2007b). After a stroke, arm swing of the hemiplegic upper extremity (UE) lacks the typical out-of-phase coordination pattern seen in adults, and arm movement is no longer synchronized with stride frequency. Ford (2007b) reported that patients with a stroke can produce a more normal arm swing during treadmill walking when instructed to move their arms in a typical out-of-phase pattern. However, more research is needed to determine whether this type of intervention improves limb coordination and gait velocity in overground walking.

In a pilot study of children with hemiplegia, Zipp (2012) reported significant improvements in cadence and gait velocity after the children completed a 3-week program of constraint-induced movement therapy (CIMT). CIMT is an intervention designed to improve functional use of the involved UE in a child or adult with hemiplegia. The authors speculated that improvement in UE control and a "more normal arm swing" may have contributed to better rhythmical interlimb coordination and, as a result, changes in gait efficiency.

## Upright Mobility in a Holistic Context

The ability to walk contributes substantially to an individual's capacity to carry out a wide range of tasks for participation in life roles. Although individuals can participate in daily work, social, and leisure activities using power mobility devices, the ability to walk for even short distances may increase a patient's efficiency and independence and reduce caregiver assistance.

In addition, walking is a convenient and effective form of exercise that should be encouraged when feasible (Myers, 2003). A walking program can prevent deconditioning and the development of secondary impairments, such as obesity and cardiovascular disease, in persons with neurological disorders (Gordon, 2004). The sedentary lifestyle adopted by many patients after stroke is associated with an increase in fall risk and recurrence of stroke, which contributes to the high mortality rates among stroke survivors (Gordon, 2004). Remember, a stroke is a cardiovascular event. The American Heart Association has recommended physical activity, including walking, as a means of reducing the risk for cardiac problems and recurrent strokes (Stroke, 2014). Thus, walking can prevent both the occurrence and recurrence of chronic health conditions.

## Primary Impairments Underlying Abnormal Upright Mobility

Neurological disorders result in a wide range of primary impairments that directly limit upright mobility. These impairments frequently include perceptual and cognitive deficits, sensory loss, weakness of affected muscles, abnormal muscle tone, balance problems, poor selective control of body segments for stability or movement, and difficulty with multijoint coordination (Scheets, 2007). Secondary impairments such as limited range of motion and deconditioning can also limit upright mobility skills. The effects of these impairments on upright mobility depend on the nature and extent of the patient's condition. Furthermore, patients with neurological disorders usually have more than one of the aforementioned impairments, which complicates determining how one particular impairment affects functional mobility.

It is also important to remember that the relationship between impairments, activity limitations, and participation restrictions is not completely understood or defined. As a result, the therapist must be cautious about attributing a patient's mobility problems to only one impairment or to a cluster of impairments. For this reason, we suggest that intervention should focus primarily on task-specific functional training when possible.

## Safety Considerations

Walking is an inherently unstable task because of the small, ever-changing base of support and the antigravity control needed to maintain the body's vertical orientation against gravity. Fall risk is the primary safety concern when evaluating a patient's potential for functional ambulation. Clinicians should utilize proper guarding techniques at all times and use a harness system when necessary to prevent a fall and patient injury.

However, determining risk is complicated by the multifactorial nature of falls. A patient's likelihood of falling varies depending on the nature and extent of the disability, the characteristics of the upright mobility task, and the complexity of the performance environment. The physical abilities needed to walk short distances on a level surface within a familiar indoor environment, such as one's home, are much different from the abilities needed to walk in a grocery store or on a busy, uneven city sidewalk. Other forms of upright mobility, such as stair climbing, walking on a ramp (incline), and walking under **dual task** conditions (i.e., walking while performing another task), present greater safety hazards than walking on level indoor surfaces. This is due to greater balance and attentional requirements.

The factors contributing to fall risk are divided into two broad categories: intrinsic and extrinsic factors (detailed in Table 37-2). Intrinsic factors are characteristics of the individual that contribute to fall risk, including increased age, decreased functional level, and chronic conditions such as PD or multiple sclerosis. So older adults with a neurological condition are at particularly increased risk for falling. Extrinsic factors include features of the environment that create hazardous conditions, such as slippery ground or uneven surfaces. Because patients are invariably concerned about regaining the ability to walk, safety in upright mobility should be assessed and discussed at the first patient encounter and should continue until the time of discharge.

The first step in reducing a patient's likelihood of falling is to quantify the risk as part of the examination process.

| TABLE 37-2 | Intrinsic and Extrinsic Risk Factors for Falls |
|---|---|
| **INTRINSIC FACTORS** | **EXTRINSIC FACTORS** |
| Older age | Environmental conditions |
| Sex (female) | Unlevel surfaces |
| Health conditions affecting gait and balance | Slippery surfaces |
| | Cluttered walkways |
| Cognitive impairment | Poor lighting |
| Dementia | Loose rugs/carpet |
| Slow walking speed | Exposed cords/wires on the floor |
| Inadequate/poorly fitting shoes | |
| Sensory loss | Use of an assistive device (increases cognitive load) |
| Acute and chronic illness | |
| Number of medications (polypharmacy) | Open environments |
| Depression | |
| Previous falls | |
| Fear of falling | |

Information adapted from Curtin A. Prevention of falls in older adults. *Med Health R I.* 2005;88(1):22–25.
Rose D. *Fall Proof a Comprehensive Balance and Mobility Training Program.* Champaign, IL: Human Kinetics; 2003.
Stolze H, Klebe S, Zechlin C, Baecker C, Friege L, Deuschl G. Falls in frequent neurological diseases: Prevalence, risk factors and aetiology. *J Neurol.* 2004;251:79–84.

Standardized tools with good sensitivity and specificity are available to assess fall risk (see Chapter 9 for details). Because impairments in gait, balance, and strength are also related to the occurrence of falls, tests and measures to assess these components of movement should be included as well (see Box 37-1).

Patient education is an important aspect of any intervention to reduce fall risk. Educating the patient on the extrinsic factors associated with falls, especially those found in the home, can increase awareness of hazardous environmental conditions. A safety assessment can be completed to identify and correct potentially unsafe conditions in and around the patient's home (see Table 30-7 in the Balance Intervention chapter). Once unsafe conditions have been identified, they can typically be remedied with simple modifications.

## Lifespan Influences on Upright Mobility

### Early Development of Gait

Bipedal locomotion is a uniquely human form of mobility. On average, the Peabody Developmental Motor Scale–2 indicates that children take their first independent steps between the ages of 9 and 15 months (Folio, 2000). Leading up to the acquisition of this important developmental milestone, the systems that contribute to independent ambulation undergo major changes; these include (1) increased formation of connections between neurons throughout the nervous system, (2) antigravity control due to improvements in strength and balance, (3) changes in sensory-perceptual processing, (4) skeletal growth and development, (5) the ability to organize a movement to achieve a goal, and (6) the ability to use feedback to adapt gait to task and environmental demands (Herzia, 1991). A child must also be motivated to explore the environment and understand the value of mobility as a means to an end (Higgins, 1995), pointing to the role of cognitive function in mobility development. Varied movement experiences offer opportunities for the infant to explore, discover, and select effective and efficient movement patterns.

Shortly after birth, infants demonstrate reflexive stepping movements when held in an upright position with the feet contacting a solid horizontal surface. Kinematic analysis has revealed a similarity between the spatiotemporal pattern of flexion and extension movements of infant stepping and mature walking (Thelen, 1995). A similar relationship has been found between supine kicking movements in infants and walking. The similarity between the spatiotemporal coordination of infant stepping, supine kicking, and mature walking further supports the existence of CPG networks in humans (Thelen, 1995).

The gait pattern of a child who is first learning to walk is very different from that of an older child or adult. A toddler's first independent steps are characterized by a high step frequency, lack of reciprocal arm swing, ankle plantar flexion at initial contact, knee flexion throughout stance, limited dorsiflexion during swing, increased hip and knee flexion during swing, and hip external rotation and abduction in stance and swing, which creates a wide base of support for stability (Sutherland, 1980). In addition, within the first year of walking, toddlers spend less time in SLS because of the strength and balance needed to successfully achieve this stance period task (Sutherland, 1980).

As the toddler gains walking experience and strength and balance improves, stance width decreases and step length increases (Breniere, 1986). These changes contribute to sagittal plane progression, an increase in SLS time, and faster walking velocity. At around 24 months, most young walkers demonstrate IC with the heel and the beginning of a reciprocal arm swing (Sutherland, 1980). By the time a child is 3.5 years old, gait appears adultlike; however, a child's gait does not resemble the kinematic, kinetic, and muscle activation patterns of adults until approximately age 7 years. Table 37-3 lists the five determinants of mature gait as defined by Sutherland (1980).

## Age-Related Changes in Gait

During early and middle adulthood, gait and other forms of upright mobility are relatively stable. Between the ages of 20 years and approximately 60 years, self-selected gait velocity remains relatively constant, ranging from 82 to 86 meters per minute (1.37–1.43 m/sec) (Bohannon, 1997). After age 60 years, walking velocity decreases, especially in women, with less decline in men. In addition to walking more slowly, older adults show reduced toe clearance and arm swing and less pelvic rotation. These changes are associated with a shorter stride length and a compensatory increase in cadence in order to maintain velocity. Gait velocity is described as the "sixth vital sign" because it correlates with functional ability and can predict health status, potential for rehabilitation, and fall risk (Fritz, 2009).

Research into changes in upright mobility in later adulthood must include a thorough screening process to distinguish healthy older adults from those with early clinical pathology and to account for the influence of disease on gait

### BOX 37-1 Commonly Used Tests That Assess Fall Risk

- Activities-Specific Balance Confidence Scale (Powell, 1995)
- Berg Balance Scale (Berg, 1992)
- Balance Evaluation Systems Test (Horak, 2009)
- Dynamic Gait Index (Shumway-Cook, 1997)
- Functional Gait Assessment (Wrisley, 2004)
- Falls Efficacy Scale (Tinetti, 1990)
- Multidirectional Functional Reach Test (Newton, 2001)
- Modified Clinical Test of Sensory Interaction in Balance (Shumway-Cook, 1986)
- Performance-Oriented Mobility Assessment (Tinetti, 1986)
- Timed Up-and-Go (Podsiadlo, 1991)
- Timed Up-and-Go Cognitive (TUG$_{cognitive}$) and Manual (TUG$_{manual}$) (Shumway-Cook, 2000a)

| TABLE 37-3 | **Five Determinants of Mature Gait** |
| --- | --- |
| **DETERMINANT** | **CHANGES IN DETERMINANTS** |
| Duration of single-limb stance (as a percentage of gait cycle) | Increases from 32% at age 1 year to 38% at age 7 years |
| Walking velocity | Increases steadily, especially before 3.5 years: from 60 cm/sec at age 1 year, to about 100 cm/sec at age 3.5 years, to 120 cm/sec by age 7 years |
| Cadence (steps per minute) | Decreases with age from about 180 steps/min at age 1 year to about 140 steps/min at age 7 years |
| Step length | Increases rapidly until age 2.5 years, then increases more slowly: from 20 cm at age 1 year, to 33 cm at age 2.5 years, to 47 cm at age 7 years |
| Ratio of pelvic span to ankle spread | Increases rapidly until age 2.5 years, then more slowly until age 3.5 years, with little increase to age 7 years: from 1.2% at age 1 year, to 2.3% at age 2.5 years, to 2.4% at age 7 years (reflects decrease in base of support) |

Adapted from Sutherland D, Olshen R, Cooper L, Woo S. The development of mature gait. *J Bone Joint Surg.* 1980;62:336–353.

parameters. In a recent investigation of gait in older adults, participants were carefully screened for dementia and disability to ensure that they were free of any conditions that affected gait parameters when baseline data were collected (i.e., conventional normal group). A subset of participants was then followed up for 1 year to ensure that they remained free of any clinically diagnosed gait disorders. Gait parameters collected at baseline from all subjects were compared with parameters for the subset of subjects (i.e., robust normal group) that remained disease-free at the 1-year follow-up. The robust normal group demonstrated better performance on all measured gait parameters including velocity, cadence, and stride length (Oh-Park, 2010). This supports the view that normative data from cross-sectional studies may have included findings from older adults with undiagnosed pathological conditions that affected gait and therefore may underestimate the mobility level of healthy, community-dwelling older adults.

Age-related changes in upright mobility can be attributed to a combination of primary and secondary aging. **Primary aging**, which is largely unavoidable, is due to an individual's genetic predisposition to bodily deterioration over a lifetime. In contrast, **secondary aging** describes changes in body systems due to avoidable factors such as inactivity, poor nutrition, stress, and exposure to environmental toxins.

The relative contribution of each of these factors to age-related changes in gait varies across individuals. For example, muscle weakness due to selective loss of type II muscle fibers (fast twitch fibers) is a common cause of age-related changes in mobility (Williams, 2002). Sarcopenia, the loss of muscle mass, also results in muscle weakness and is a normal part of primary aging. However, in older adults, the effects of sarcopenia can be accelerated by physical inactivity (secondary aging). Thus, the effects of primary aging can be compounded by the effects of secondary aging.

Two main causes of age-related changes in mobility that must be addressed in the treatment plan are muscle weakness and impaired balance. In addition to sarcopenia and physical

inactivity, muscle strength is affected by the age-related loss of alpha motor neurons, poor nutrition, and decreased cardiovascular endurance (Williams, 2002). Muscle weakness and changes in motor unit size interfere with the ability to generate enough force to maintain a functional walking velocity and dynamic balance control. The ability to react to a postural perturbation and avert a fall depends in part on rapidly generating adequate LE joint moments. Falls may occur when the rate of force is too slow or the level of force is too low to overcome and compensate for the postural disturbance. Interventions to increase muscle strength are presented in Chapter 22.

Impairments in dynamic balance are also due to deterioration in the acuity of the sensory systems that are important for postural control and safe mobility. The visual, vestibular, and somatosensory systems give the brain information about where the body is located in space and thus detect postural disturbances during movement activities. A loss of receptors in the eye diminishes visual acuity, making it difficult to detect changes in surface conditions to proactively avoid unsafe environments. A narrowing of the peripheral visual field can interfere with the ability to detect movement of self in the environment, which may diminish responsiveness to a postural disturbance. A loss of hair cells (sensory receptors) in the semicircular canals and saccule and utricle of the otoliths reduces the vestibular system's sensitivity to head movement and head position relative to gravity and the response of the vestibulo-ocular reflex. As a result, the individual has difficulty knowing the speed and direction of head movement or the exact position of the head relative to gravity and decreased ability to keep objects stable in the field of vision.

Finally, skin, muscle, and joint receptors decline with age and limit information about joint position and movement (Shaffer, 2007). A decrement in function of one or more of these sensory systems reduces the availability of information needed for safe and efficient upright mobility (Patla, 1995). Interventions to address underlying balance impairments are described in Chapter 30.

# ▉ Pertinent Examination

The *Guide to Physical Therapist Practice* states that examination must take place before the initial intervention and should be performed for all patients/clients (APTA, 2015). This section addresses factors to consider when selecting, administering, and interpreting tests and measures to quantify the impairments, activity limitations, and participation restrictions that are interfering with a patient's functional upright mobility.

Selection of the most appropriate tests and measures for a specific examination depends on the information gathered during the initial interview and a systems review, including the patient's age, medical diagnosis or condition, cognitive level, extent of impairments, and goals. See Table 37-4 for questions to guide the examination and other components of patient management.

Factors such as duration of the disorder, stage of recovery, and comorbidities are also important to consider when developing an examination strategy. For example, a patient with a neurological disorder in addition to a condition such as arthritis may not be able to walk the distance needed to complete a mobility test such as the 6-minute walk. Although this is a reliable test of endurance for individuals with stroke (Kosak, 2005), it is not appropriate for this particular patient at this time.

In addition to reviewing the aforementioned patient-specific information when selecting appropriate tests and measures, the physical or occupational therapist should also understand the intended purpose of the assessment tool and its psychometric properties.

## THINK ABOUT IT 37.2

- A child's gait pattern undergoes major changes over the first few years of life. When doing an observational gait analysis on a young child with a neurological condition, you must determine which gait determinants indicate an immature gait pattern and which indicate a pathological gait pattern. In contrast to Table 37-3, can you discuss which gait observations might indicate a pathological gait pattern?
- What are some specific ways you would adapt the questions in Table 37-4 to issues related to ambulation and development of a treatment plan to improve gait after a neurological disorder?

The tests and measures section of an examination provides detailed information about the consequences of the patient's disorder on body structure and function, daily activity, and participation in life roles. Specific tests and measures for examining an individual with a mobility disorder can be selected according to the International Classification of Functioning, Disability and Health (ICF) component that the tool assesses. For example, the Dynamic Gait Index (DGI) can be used to gather valid and reliable information about the activity of walking under varied conditions for persons with chronic stroke (Jonsdottir, 2007). Although information from the DGI may be useful in planning interventions, the index does not inform the therapist about how deficits in the patient's upright mobility skills affect participation or which neuromuscular and/or

| **TABLE 37-4** | **Guiding Questions in Patient Management** |
|---|---|

*Determining what questions to ask a patient depends on factors such as age, diagnosis, time since onset of condition, extent of primary and secondary impairments, cognitive status, comorbidities, and family involvement. Following is a representative (not exhaustive) list of questions a therapist may ask the patient in order to gather information important in clinical reasoning.*

*Note: If the patient is a child or an adult who cannot reliably respond, questions may be directed to the family or other involved individuals. For example, parents may be asked to describe their child's typical day in terms of activities and participation and the amount of assistance the child needs.*

| PATIENT MANAGEMENT | THERAPIST DETERMINES | QUESTIONS FOR PATIENT |
|---|---|---|
| Initial interview | 1. Why is the patient seeking services, or why was he/she referred for services?<br>2. How do the patient's mobility problems affect his/her daily life?<br>3. What are the patient's goals for therapy? | 1. What brings you to physical therapy? Therapist may ask follow-up question:<br>a. How is your condition affecting your daily life?<br>2. Can you describe the difficulties you have moving inside your home, outside your home, in your workplace or school, and in the community? Therapist may ask follow-up questions about:<br>a. Use of assistive devices, orthotics, adaptive equipment, need for assistance from others<br>b. Patient's ability to use public transportation<br>c. Patient's ability to care for himself/herself<br>3. What specific activities would you like to do more easily? Follow-up question:<br>a. In what contexts? |

*Continued*

| TABLE 37-4 | Guiding Questions in Patient Management—cont'd | |
| --- | --- | --- |
| **PATIENT MANAGEMENT** | **THERAPIST DETERMINES** | **QUESTIONS FOR PATIENT** |
| Systems review | Are there comorbidities, or cautionary signs and symptoms that require closer examination or referral to another health-care provider? | 1. Tell me about any other health/medical problems you are having.<br>2. What medications are you taking? |
| Tests and measures | 1. Is participation affected?<br>2. Are there tasks the patient can and cannot perform?<br>3. What is the patient's ability to adapt his/her upright mobility skills to task and environmental conditions?<br>4. What is the extent of the patient's impairments, and how do they constrain upright mobility? | 1. Patient/family can be asked to complete participation measures:<br>  a. The Activities-specific Balance Confidence (ABC) Scale,<br>  b. 36-Item Short Form Survey (SF-36), or<br>  c. Pediatric Quality of Life Inventory. |
| Evaluation | 1. What are the patient's specific mobility problems?<br>2. What movement systems diagnosis or practice pattern best fits the patient's impairments and level of function?<br>3. Does the patient have the potential to make functional improvements in upright mobility skills?<br>4. Is remediation possible?<br>  a. Are impairments likely to improve with intervention?<br>  b. Does the patient have the support needed to regularly attend therapy and implement a home exercise program?<br>5. Is compensation indicated?<br>6. How much time will it take for outcomes and goals to be achieved?<br>7. Is referral or consultation needed? | 1. Do you understand the findings of the examination?<br>2. Have we set goals that reflect your needs?<br>3. Are you able to regularly attend treatment sessions with help from your family if necessary?<br>4. Will you be able to practice specific activities at home with help from your family or caregiver? |
| Plan of care | 1. What specific functional tasks and activities will the patient practice in treatment and at home?<br>2. How should practice be organized to promote motor learning/drive neural plasticity to optimize the patient's time in treatment? | 1. How often are you carrying out your home exercise program (HEP)?<br>2. Are you having difficulty with any of your HEP activities?<br>3. Can you tell me what tasks are getting easier for you to carry out at home? Are you moving more easily at home? |
| Outcomes assessment | 1. According to outcome measures, did the patient achieve his/her desired goals?<br>  a. Did the patient make clinically significant improvements in upright mobility skills? | 1. Are you satisfied with the outcome of your treatment program?<br>2. Where have you noticed the greatest improvement in your mobility skills?<br>3. What can you do now that you had difficulty with before you began treatment? |

musculoskeletal system impairments may be contributing to the patient's mobility disorder. The Balance Evaluation Systems Test (BESTest) is better suited for planning interventions because it can help identify what neuromuscular and/or musculoskeletal system impairments are contributing to your patient's mobility disorder (See Chapter 9 for more details).

Selecting tests and measures from each ICF component ensures that the examination is complete and patient centered. When patients are asked what outcomes they expect to achieve in physical therapy, most want to improve their ability to perform a specific activity, particularly walking, for a specific purpose such as returning to work or leisure interests (participation). Rarely does a patient frame a goal

## BOX 37-2 Examples of Tests and Measures Used to Examine Functional Mobility Problems in Individuals With Neurological Impairments

### Body Structure and Function

Flexibility
Range of motion
Manual muscle testing
Sensory testing
Reflex testing
Fatigue Impact Scale (Fisk, 1994)
Perceptual testing
Single-limb stance
Modified Ashworth Scale (Bohannon, 1987)
Mini-Mental State Examination (Folstein, 1975)
Rancho Levels of Cognitive Function
Spatiotemporal gait parameters
Observational Gait Analysis

### Activity

Berg Balance Scale (Berg, 1992)
Multidirectional Functional Reach Test (Newton 2001)
Timed Up-and-Go (Podsiadlo, 1991)
Dynamic Gait Index (Shumway-Cook, 1997)
Functional Gait Assessment
Walk tests (2-, 3-, 6-, 12-minute)
10 Meter walk test; 4 Meter walk test
High Level Mobility Assessment Tool (Williams, 2006)
Functional Independence Measure (Uniform Data Set, 1996)
Modified Emory Functional Ambulation Profile (Baer, 2001)
Gross Motor Function Measure (Russell, 2002)
Peabody Developmental Motor Scale-2 (Folio, 2000)
Pediatric Evaluation of Disability Inventory (Haley, 1992)

### Participation

Stroke Impact Scale (Duncan, 2003)
SF-36® (Ware, 1992)
Activities-Specific Balance Confidence Scale (Powell, 1995)
Falls Efficacy Scale (Tinetti, 1990)
School Function Assessment (Coster, 1998)
Impact of Participation and Autonomy (Cardol, 1999)
Pediatric Quality of Life Inventory (Varni, 1998)

Summarized from Academy of Neurologic Physical Therapy. Outcome Measures Recommendations. Available at: http://www.neuropt.org/professional-resources/neurology-section-outcome-measures-recommendations. Accessed August 28, 2017.

A patient examination should include tests and measures from each of these ICF components. Many of the tests and measures used in the initial examination can be readministered at reevaluation and later at discharge as objective outcome assessments to determine how the patient has changed over time.

A therapist can increase the likelihood of accurately documenting change in the patient's mobility status by selecting a test with a scale of measure precise enough to detect the expected degree of change. For example, a timed walking test (ratio scale) is more sensitive to change than a walking test that uses an ordinal scale. An ordinal scale ranks behavior according to categories with predefined performance criteria. A patient may make gains in therapy but not meet the criterion needed to change rank, which means the change in performance is not reflected by the test score. In contrast, tests that measure time or distance (ratio scale) can identify smaller changes and are more precise than an ordinal scale, which improves the likelihood that changes will be detected. A ratio scale also eliminates the floor and ceiling effects seen in ordinal scale tests.

In a clinical setting, gait is assessed most often by OGA, the most widely used clinical tool to examine pathological gait. OGA involves the systematic visual inspection of the posture and displacement of limb and trunk segments and joints during the eight phases of the gait cycle. Figure 10-9 shows the OGA form developed at Rancho Los Amigos on the basis of Perry's model of gait (Perry, 2010), with sample data from a patient with cerebrovascular accident (CVA) or stroke. A form such as this directs a therapist's observation of a patient's posture and movement through each of the eight phases of the gait cycle.

Research on OGA used in patients with neurological and orthopedic conditions has reported only moderate levels of inter- and intrarater reliability (Brunnekreef, 2005; Krebs, 1985; McGinley, 2003). The moderate reliability of OGA is explained, as least in part, by the difficulty associated with assessing a complex, whole body task such as walking using visual inspection.

The reliability of OGA may be improved when therapists adopt a structured, systematic approach to gait examination. One approach includes using a form to guide and record your observations, starting the visual observation distally at the foot and systematically scanning proximally to the head, observing one segment at a time. Observe each segment over several complete gait cycles before proceeding to the next segment. Also, consider the use of video to record gait and allow playback to enhance intrarater reliability. OGA may be conducted under conditions that require gait adaptations by varying walking speed from internally (self) paced to externally paced or by incorporating directional changes and varied surfaces. The standard walking obstacle course includes many of these conditions and offers a systematic approach to assessing gait adaptations in children and adults (Held, 2006; Taylor, 1997).

Knowledge of pathological gait and the deviations commonly associated with specific impairments and neurological diagnoses (see Table 10-9) can direct the therapist's attention to specific limb and body segments at specific points in the gait cycle and promote greater efficiency and accuracy in OGA.

in impairment-level terms, such as increasing range of motion. Selecting tests and measures across ICF (World Health Organization, 2001) components ensures that information about activity and participation is gathered in addition to relevant impairment-level information.

The ICF (WHO, 2001) classifies the effect of a health condition across three components: impairments in body structure and function, activity limitations, and participation restrictions.

# ■ Evaluation

Examination findings can be clustered by the ICF components of impairment, activity limitation, and participation restriction. The therapist can then carefully analyze the findings across ICF components to develop a working hypothesis for why the patient is experiencing functional mobility problems (see Hypothesis-Oriented Algorithm for Clinicians in Chapter 2: Figs. 2-6, 2-7, 2-8, and 2-9). The results of a specific examination can then be evaluated and used for diagnosis, prognosis, and treatment planning.

It must be noted, however, that working only on underlying impairments without shifting focus to task-specific functional training may not optimize improvements in activity and participation. Consequently, the therapist must use sound clinical reasoning skills when evaluating the findings of an examination. Ultimately, the therapist must incorporate the gains achieved in the impairment domain into the practice of task-specific functional activities.

## THINK ABOUT IT 37.3

Many of the standardized tests we use to assess a patient's mobility, such as the Dynamic Gait Index, are composed of multiple test items. Each test item is scored on the basis of the patient's performance and then summed for a total score. Although the total score of a test provides important information about a patient's mobility, such as fall risk, remember to look at how the patient performed on *each individual item*.

- On the basis of the gait/mobility tools you know, give an example of when looking at individual item scores will help you identify the types of tasks that are most challenging for the patient in order to inform your plan of care.

Scheets (1999, 2007) proposed a diagnostic system for describing motor system problems in patients with neuromuscular disorders. This scheme describes the primary movement system problems (impairments) associated with neurological disorders (see Table 37-5). The findings of the examination are compared with the inclusion criteria for a specific diagnostic category. Each diagnosis is coupled with a specific cluster of impairment-level signs. For example, key signs for the category *movement pattern coordination deficit* include altered sequence of movement components during tasks such as sit-to-stand, slow or awkward reach-to-grasp movements, and increased postural sway. Expected outcomes for patients within this movement system diagnosis include ambulation without an assistive device and improvements in gait speed and standing balance. The medical diagnoses associated with this movement system diagnosis include mild stroke, mild PD, and remitting multiple sclerosis (Scheets, 2007).

These movement system diagnoses are used to characterize clusters of impairments commonly observed in persons with neurological disorders across the lifespan (Scheets, 2007). For example, *hypermetria* describes an inability to grade forces appropriately for the distance and speed aspects of a task (Scheets, 2007). Patients with this diagnosis may walk with variable step length and step width and overshoot or undershoot when reaching for an object. This movement system problem may be seen in patients with lesions to the cerebellar system, which can occur with disorders such as multiple sclerosis, traumatic brain injury, stroke, cerebral palsy, or cerebellar degeneration.

Although not exhaustive, descriptions of the diagnosis, key signs, and associated signs do offer a framework to guide the examination and intervention. For example, patients with hypermetria have associated problems with balance and gait; therefore, a test such as the Performance-Oriented

| TABLE 37-5 | Movement System Diagnoses | |
|---|---|
| **MOVEMENT SYSTEM DIAGNOSIS** | **POSSIBLE EFFECTS ON GAIT** |
| Movement pattern coordination deficit | Variable foot placement; slow, small steps; may need assistance |
| Force production deficit | May need assistive device or assistance; may have severe gait deviations such as crouched gait, or knee buckling in mid-stance; may not be able to ambulate |
| Sensory detection deficit | Variable foot placement; may require assistance; gait may improve with vision |
| Sensory selection and weighting deficit | Deviation from straight path; difficulty with changes in sensory environment |
| Perceptual deficit | Variable gait impairment; asymmetrical posture |
| Fractioned movement deficit | Slow, stiff movement; marked gait deviations; may need ankle foot orthosis or assistive device |
| Hypermetria | Variable foot placement; may need assistance |
| Hypokinesia | Difficulty initiating gait; variable step length; may need assistance |
| Cognitive deficit | Unable to modify movement based on instructions; poor memory for movement-related instruction |

Adapted from Scheets P, Sahrmann S, Norton B. Diagnosis for physical therapy for patients with neuromuscular conditions. *Neurol Rep.* 1999;23:158–169. Scheets P, Sahrmann S, Norton B. Use of movement system diagnoses in the management of patient with neuromuscular conditions. *Phys Ther.* 2007;87:654–699.

Mobility Assessment (POMA) (Tinetti, 1986) is appropriate to include in the examination. The balance subscale of the POMA measures steadiness in sitting and standing and reactive balance control, whereas the gait subscale measures step length, step continuity, path, and step width (Tinetti, 1986). The POMA provides valid and reliable information about balance and gait that can be used to develop task-specific interventions targeting the movement problems associated with hypermetria.

Predicting the amount of time or the number of sessions a patient needs in order to achieve the expected level of function is challenging, particularly for students and novice therapists. The challenge is due to the numerous factors influencing the patient's response to intervention and ultimate prognosis. These factors include the nature and course of the patient's condition; age at onset; extent of sensory, motor, and cognitive impairment; stage of recovery (nonprogressive disorders); and disease stage (progressive disorders). However, factors external to the individual may also affect the response to intervention.

A unique aspect of the ICF model is that context (personal and environmental factors) plays an important role in how a health condition affects an individual's functioning and disability. The level of functional change a patient makes during physical therapy is influenced by personal factors such as coping style, education, and social background in addition to environmental factors, such as the physical environment, social attitudes, social network, and availability of medical and rehabilitation services. Consequently, the prognosis must also consider contextual factors within the patient's life.

## PATIENT APPLICATION

### History, Patient Goals, and Systems Screen

*Mrs. Z has been admitted to your inpatient rehabilitation facility, and you are completing her initial evaluation. Currently, Mrs. Z presents with slurred speech. She understands one- and two-step verbal and nonverbal commands. At times, she gets frustrated by the lack of clarity of her speech, and so she prefers not to speak. She is oriented to person, place, and time and appears cooperative during therapy. She does a stand pivot transfer to a wheelchair, with moderate assistance of one. She is able to stand for 10 seconds with minimum assistance and sit with minimum assistance on a chair without arms for 5 minutes. Her posture during standing and in the chair is characterized by asymmetry, with trunk leaning to the L (left).*

*She is unable to ambulate or step up onto a step without maximum assistance from the therapist for L LE advancement and stabilization during the stance phase. She uses a wide cane in her right (R) hand for additional external support. Upon voluntary effort, she exhibits flexion synergy of the L UE with no isolated movements. She is unable to reach across midline or past her base of support in either sitting or standing with her L UE; however, she can do it with the R UE. She presents with L LE flexion synergy with the initial signs of isolated movements at the knee.*

*Systems Screen: Integumentary—venous stasis; cardiopulmonary—hypertension controlled with medication; musculoskeletal—spinal stenosis C1–C3; neuromuscular: history of infarct to the right middle cerebral artery. Mrs. Z's personal goals include the following:*

- *"I would like to be able to go back to caring for my husband and our home."*
- *"I want to do as much as I can without help from anyone!"*
- *"I want to be able to walk again—by myself!"*

### Systems Review:

- *Integumentary system impaired in both legs as evidenced by edema typical of venous stasis*
- *Urogenital: Mrs. Z is continent.*

### Examination: Tests and Measures

| CATEGORY | TEST/MEASURE AND OBSERVATIONS |
|---|---|
| Cranial/peripheral nerves | • Cranial nerves intact II–XII bilaterally; sensation: intact |
| Muscle performance | • R LE and R UE: grossly 5/5 all joints/planes<br>• L LE: able to complete three-quarters of range antigravity in hip and knee, one-half of antigravity range in ankle<br>• L UE: shoulder and elbow able to complete one-half of antigravity range, only trace movements noted at wrist, hand, thumb, and fingers<br>• L UE and LE flexor synergy present throughout with the initial observation of knee isolated movements |
| Motor function | • Full isolated movements throughout each joint in the R UE and LE present<br>• Absence of full-range isolated movements at each joint in the L UE and LE<br>• Poor bilateral motor coordination in both UE and LE, resulting from L-side motor control issues |
| Standing posture | Forward trunk flexion and L-side lateral flexion, L knee hyperextension in standing with moderate assistance at the pelvis to maintain upright posture, wide base of support (BOS) with R LE leading, L-sided pelvic retraction |

*Continued*

| CATEGORY | TEST/MEASURE AND OBSERVATIONS |
|---|---|
| Gait, locomotion, balance | • Timed up-and-go (TUG) test: 34.6 seconds; TUG$_{cognitive}$: 48.2 seconds; gait speed is 0.16 m/s<br>• Ambulates with maximal assistance of one for L LE advancement during swing and stability during stance at the knee and hip with the use of cane in R UE for a distance of 10 feet on level surfaces<br>• Patient required maximal assistance at the knee and hip for L LE advancement and stability during ascending and descending one step with the R UE on the R handrail<br>• Sit-to-stand: sitting on the edge of a 25-inch-high mat, sit-stand took 13.7 seconds with moderate assistance to bring COM forward<br>• Car transfer: needs moderate assistance to get in/out of car primarily b/c limited motor control on the L side and postural control<br>Wheelchair propulsion: patient propels wheelchair with R LE and R UE with minimal assistance for turns, 50 feet |

## Evaluation, Diagnosis, Prognosis, and Expected Outcomes

### Evaluation

*Mrs. Z has difficulty initiating and maintaining control of movements on her left side. She is hesitant to move her COM over her BOS and to cross midline, thus interfering with transferring from sit-to-stand, standing, and walking. Mrs. Z presents with postural control limitations evident in her large BOS in quiet standing and L-leaning trunk. She relies on a wheelchair for mobility at this time. In standing, she has difficulty reaching across midline and forward over her BOS because of decreases in strength and motor control on the L side. Her inability to stand independently or advance her L LE to take a step has resulted in a significant reduction in her activity level and ability to independently function. Her endurance is compromised, and she requires frequent rest periods. Although she is motivated to participate in motor tasks to the best of her ability, she does not always recognize her level of fatigue. On the basis of the impairments noted, she is at risk for further aerobic deconditioning, muscle weakness, range of motion limitations, and decreased overall flexibility secondary to her level of inactivity.*

### Diagnosis

*Mrs. Z's motor control impairments, postural instability, and limitations of functional abilities (difficulty in transferring, sitting, standing, and ambulating) are consistent with the movement dysfunction associated with a R CVA. The primary practice patterns based on her movement dysfunction include:*

- *Neuromuscular 5D: impaired motor function and sensory integrity associated with nonprogressive disorders of the nervous system—acquired in adolescence or adulthood*
- *Neuromuscular 5A: primary prevention/risk reduction for loss of balance and falling*

### Prognosis and Expected Outcomes

*Mrs. Z has the potential to meet the expected functional outcomes within 2 weeks with daily visits of intensive inpatient physical rehabilitation followed by outpatient rehabilitation services twice weekly for 6 to 8 weeks to ensure participation*

*within her community. Her prognosis is favorable because she has family support, lives in a ranch-style home with limited stairs, understands one- and two-step commands, and is very motivated to regain her functional independence.*

### (a) Expected Outcomes/Goals in 6 Weeks and Prerequisite Objectives

#### Outcomes/Goals Long Term Goal (LTG): in 6 weeks

1. *Transition from sitting to standing independently from a firm seat of 21 to 25 inches from the floor in <4 seconds*
2. *Stand independently with a cane in R hand with sufficient static balance for periods of 3 minutes without falling (improve static balance)*
3. *Stand independently with a cane in R hand, turn L or R, and shift weight without losing balance in order to perform self-care tasks at the sink, on the toilet, and in the kitchen (improve dynamic standing balance)*
4. *Reach items overhead independently with L UE and without losing balance (improve dynamic standing balance)in order to perform household tasks*
5. *Reach across midline to touch items placed at waist height independently with L UE and without losing balance (improved dynamic standing balance)*
6. *Ambulate independently a distance of 20 feet on level surfaces with the use of a cane in the R UE (improve L LE motor control and walking function) with gait velocity of at least 0.8 m/s*
7. *Ambulate independently on level surfaces a distance of 20 feet with the use of a cane in the R UE, and turn and walk over a 6-inch-high, 6-inch-wide object independently without a loss of cadence, on command*
8. *Rise from a chair, ambulate independently a distance of 10 feet, turn, and then return to the chair in less than 20 seconds with the use of a quad cane in R UE*
9. *Stand independently for 5 to 10 minutes while performing a manipulation task*
10. *Ascend five steps independently and nonreciprocally (step-to pattern) with the use of R handrail*

11. *Descend five steps independently and nonreciprocally (step-to pattern) with the use of R handrail*

**Prerequisite Objectives Short Term Goal (STG): in 1 week, patient will:**

1. *Increase static standing to 10 minutes with a BOS of 6 inches*
2. *Ambulate a distance of 10 feet or 12 steps with the use of a cane and minimal support for L LE advancement and verbal cues with gait velocity of at least 0.3 m/s*
3. *Improve postural reaction to consistently use ankle and hip strategy with minimal perturbation*

4. *Ascend two steps nonreciprocally with the use of R handrail and minimal assistance for L LE advancement*
5. *Descend two steps nonreciprocally with the use of R handrail and minimal assistance for L LE stability at the knee*
6. *Improve functional mobility as evidenced by TUG time of 22 seconds and TUG-cognitive time of 28 seconds with the use of a cane in R UE and minimal assistance for L LE advancement*
7. *Score 42 on the Berg Balance Scale 45 by 6-weeks*
8. *Score 18 on the DGI 21 by 6-weeks*

## *Contemplate Clinical Decisions*

1. *Consider Mrs. Z and the previously described goals and objectives and select a guide practice pattern to address them. Visit the online supplement for additional feedback.*
2. *Mrs. Z has met the expected functional outcomes in the 6 weeks with daily intensive inpatient physical rehabilitation. She was discharged to home with a referral for outpatient rehabilitation twice a week for 8 weeks. You are asked to develop her outpatient rehabilitation program to promote her participation within the community. Develop/design the following:*
   - *Two long-term goals*
   - *Four objectives*
   - *A progressive treatment intervention plan*
   - *A home program*
3. *According to findings from Mrs. Z's examination, which movement system diagnosis from Table 37-5 best fits her movement dysfunction?*

## ■ Functional Interventions for Upright Mobility

### General Approaches

Over recent decades, neuroscience research has revealed important information on the role of experience in **neural plasticity**. Table 14-2 lists 10 principles to encourage experience-dependent plasticity, all of which have strong implications for clinical practice in physical and occupational therapy (Kleim, 2008) and obvious application to gait rehabilitation. These principles emphasize that patients must be engaged in the intense, repetitive, task-specific practice of meaningful activities in order to drive neural plasticity and functional change. Neural plasticity research using both animal and human models indicates that it takes hundreds, if not thousands, of repetitions of a task to promote neural adaptation (Lang, 2007). Given the extensive practice needed to promote neuroplastic changes, how can therapists ensure that their patients benefit from the time spent in rehabilitation? Also, how can therapists ensure enough repetitions of stepping in patients who have weakness, impaired endurance, and perhaps pain? Currently, the translational and clinical research needed

to answer these questions is limited; however, evidence does support the use of task-specific interventions that adhere to the principles of experience-dependent neural plasticity described by Kleim (2008) and summarized in Table 14-2.

The retraining of upright mobility involves several types of rehabilitation interventions, including three broad areas: (1) therapeutic exercises to address identified underlying impairments, (2) functional training that is task specific and personally meaningful, and/or (3) the use of devices and equipment to augment or support functional ability.

When designing a training session, consider whether you are approaching training from a remediation or compensation perspective. As discussed in Chapter 36, remediation involves retraining the task using normal biomechanics and/or reduction of impairments that interfere with the task in patients who have the capacity for improvement. When a training session for upright mobility in a patient with weakness secondary to a stroke is organized, the remediation model recommends practicing upright standing using normal biomechanics and strengthening the muscles of the UE, LE, and trunk. Alternatively, the compensatory approach used as a framework for a training session focuses on movement substitution, alternative strategies, and the utilization of devices or equipment that enable the patient to perform the upright mobility tasks, particularly when there is poor prognosis for any recovery of underlying impairments.

Given the emergence of evidence supporting the role of neural plasticity (see Chapter 1) and the promotion of motor control via principles of motor learning (see Chapter 15), therapists frequently use an eclectic approach. When using a combination of strategies associated with the remediation and compensation models to help patients attain functional mobility, therapists have the unique problem of balancing the two models to maximize functional independence in upright mobility activities with optimal efficiency. For example, a patient with a progressive condition such as PD may need a wheelchair for long-distance activities in the community to ensure safety and monitor fatigue; however, she may ambulate at home with a walker.

For Mrs. Z, it is appropriate to use remediation strategies, including intensive task-specific training and strengthening exercises to retrain motor control for upright mobility activities.

Nevertheless, compensatory strategies that incorporate a wheelchair for long-distance mobility and tools for UE reaching may also be indicated to ensure functional independence and safety in all environments.

As stated in Chapter 36, the second question to consider is whether you will incorporate the UEs, one side or bilateral, into the training session. A patient who is unstable during upright mobility activities because of limited LE motor control may benefit from using the arms, at least intermittently, either unilaterally or bilaterally to promote upright stability, with the support gradually withdrawn over time. However, when a patient has limited or unequal motor control in both UEs, as is the case with Mrs. Z, requiring the use of bilateral UEs during upright mobility may stress the motor control system beyond her ability. This task may limit her ability to decrease the degrees of freedom in the UE in order to focus on the motor control required in the LEs.

Therapists can use motor learning principles, such as practice organization and feedback, as an underlying framework for designing and reassessing training sessions as the patient progresses in her motor control to maximize ability and flexibility in upright mobility tasks. Figure 37-6 shows Mrs. Z engaging in a bilateral upright task that requires differing degrees of freedom in the UE and LE depending on the size and shape of the object being pushed.

## Therapeutic Activities to Improve Upright Mobility

Upright mobility involves the coordinated motor control of the LEs, trunk, and UEs in order to interact safely and effectively while addressing the demands of the task, including the learner characteristics and environmental conditions. The foundational elements associated with the execution of upright mobility tasks include (1) LE and trunk muscle strength and range of motion needed to support one's body over the body mass, (2) coordinated LE motor control/force to generate and sustain a rhythmical locomotor pattern, (3) dynamic and static standing balance, and (4) the ability to adapt to environmental demands that may alter the task requirements,

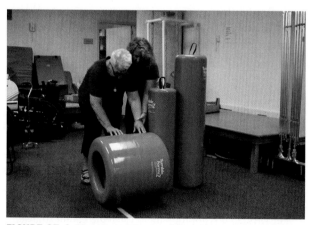

**FIGURE 37-6** Mrs. Z engaging in a bilateral upper extremity task in an upright position.

including unlevel surfaces, path alterations, and dual task performance.

The underlying foundational questions one must ask when designing a training session to address upright mobility are "What type of exercises—with what degree of intensity, for how long, and in what specific position—is best?" and "How should I intentionally progress these exercises and activities to place optimal demand on the system for optimal improvement?" To effectively address these questions, we must use the available evidence and research from practice-based studies. Preceding chapters of this text have focused on functional interventions for the UE, horizontal skill (prone and supine), sitting skill, sit-to-stand, stand-to-sit, and standing activities. The following section includes information on specific interventions for improving upright mobility skills.

### Body Weight–Supported Treadmill Training

Recent evidence reinforces the use of **body weight–supported treadmill training (BWSTT)** as an intervention to develop (Dodd, 2007), improve (McCain, 2008), and preserve ambulation (Herman, 2007) in patients with acute or chronic neurological disorders across the lifespan. This intervention requires a body weight–supported (BWS) system and a treadmill. Another form of this intervention involves ambulation training using a body weight–supported system that allows the patient to ambulate overground rather than on a treadmill. Sometimes, the more generic term **body weight–supported ambulation training** is used.

The rational for this intervention is based on research conducted with deafferented spinal cats who recovered locomotor control after body weight–supported treadmill (BWST) walking (Barbeau, 1987). Findings such as this, along with a growing emphasis on the importance of task-specific training, contributed to the development of BWSTT in patients with incomplete SCIs (Dobkin, 1999) and stroke (Richards, 1993). This intervention is now used with children and adults with a wide range of conditions.

The improvements in locomotion seen with BWSTT are believed to result at least in part from activation of CPGs in the spinal cord, perhaps through sensory information associated with locomotion (Van de Crommert, 1998). When the limb is loaded during gait, proprioceptors from the LE extensors and hip and mechanoreceptors from the foot signal limb position and may contribute to phase transitions between the flexor and extensor movements of gait (Van de Crommert, 1998).

A body weight system consists of a harness that attaches around the patient's low trunk and pelvis. The harness is suspended from an overhead support and mounted on a mobile frame (Figs. 25-10 and 37-7) or in some cases a ceiling mount from which a variety of challenging functional activities can be performed (Fig. 37-8ABCD). The amount of BWS can range from full weight support to no weight support depending on the needs of the patient. Providing support in this way decreases the initial demands for postural control, balance, strength, and endurance from the patient for successful ambulation (Sullivan, 2002). In other words, the patient can practice the ambulation task without fear of falling or collapse

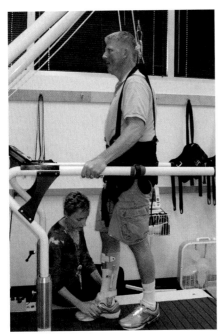

FIGURE 37-7 Patient with traumatic brain injury walking on a treadmill in a body weight–supported system with therapist assistance for foot placement on the affected side.

of the leg, allowing her to practice specific motor patterns that she otherwise would not be able to practice safely so early in the rehabilitation. In fact, in the early stages of BWSTT, components of gait may improve; however, because there is no opportunity to practice balance skills with the optimal BWS, dynamic standing balance may not improve without the progressive intentional withdrawal of BWS.

The adjustability of the system provides a safe environment that allows the therapist to easily vary the demands of a mobility task to match the patient's initial resources and increase demands as the patient improves. This variability enables a patient to begin task-specific rehabilitation within weeks of incurring a neurological impairment.

For patients with stroke, the amount of treatment time spent in gait activities during inpatient rehabilitation is associated with outcome at discharge. Horn (2005b) found that in patients with moderate and severe stokes, the sooner they started rehabilitation, specifically gait activities, the better the outcome regardless of initial Functional Independence Measure score. The authors also reported that earlier participation in challenging activities resulted in better outcomes and a greater likelihood of discharge to home, even in patients with more severe impairments. Thus, early and aggressive treatment focused on "high-order" gait activities resulted in better recovery of function (Horn S, 2005b). These encouraging findings suggest that well-timed and intense gait intervention using meaningful upright mobility activities can drive experience-dependent neural plasticity in persons with stroke.

Duncan (2011) investigated the effects of BWSTT on functional level of walking after 1 year in 408 persons who began training 2 and 6 months after a stroke. The Locomotor Experience Applied Post-Stroke (LEAPS) trial compared a standardized clinic-based BWS gait training protocol with a program of strength and balance exercises that were carried out in the participant's homes. Both groups of participants were seen three times per week for 12 to 16 weeks and were required to complete between 30 and 36 exercise sessions within that time. After completion of the program, half of all participants demonstrated a higher level of functional walking as measured by gait velocity, independent of intervention and time after stroke. The authors noted that the participants who began BWST or home intervention at 2 months showed functional gains earlier that were retained at 1-year follow-up than participants who began training at 6 months. It may be that onset of intervention was too late, even at 2 months, for participants to gain the optimal benefit of the BWS protocol. Indeed, after onset of stroke "time matters" is one of the 10 key principles of experience-dependent neuroplasticity (Kleim, 2008).

The use of BWSTT in the acute stage of rehabilitation enables the therapist to engage a patient in meaningful,

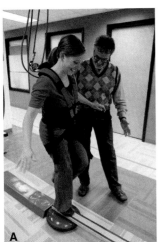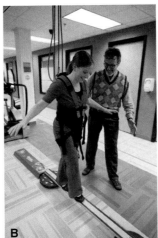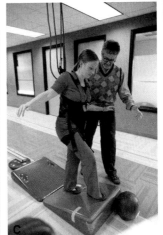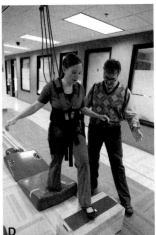

FIGURE 37-8ABCD This patient is performing challenging upright mobility tasks with the security of partial body weight support through a ceiling-mounted overhead track and harness system and close supervision by the therapist.

challenging, task-specific gait training shortly after neurological injury and before the patient develops ineffective movement strategies that cannot be easily changed (i.e., neuroplastic interference). BWS typically starts at up to 40% of body weight; you can observe the patient at 10%, 20%, 30%, and 40% and then select the percentage that facilitates proper trunk and limb alignment (Visintin, 1998); over time, you can gradually withdraw the support while increasing treadmill speed in increments of 10%.

McCain (2008) implemented early task-specific gait training on a treadmill starting with 30% BWS for 30 minutes daily with overground ambulation, initiated only after patients can walk on the treadmill for 3 minutes at a speed of 1.3 km/h with no more than 10% BWS. The authors reported that after an average of 13 sessions, patients who began receiving treadmill training 12 days after a stroke developed significantly better gait kinematics, symmetry, velocity, and endurance than patients in the comparison group (McCain, 2008).

BWSTT has been used in patients with PD (Miyai, 2002), traumatic brain injury (Scherer, 2007), SCI (Behrman, 2008), cerebral palsy (Dodd, 2007), and Down syndrome (Ulrich, 2001). Ulrich (2001) showed that infants with Down syndrome who walked on a treadmill with support by a parent for 8 minutes a day started walking 101 days earlier than infants who did not have this experience. Although results of some BWSTT studies have been inconclusive, in general the therapy shows promise as a task-specific intervention that allows patients to safely practice gait as a continuous task. Specific evidence supporting use of BWSTT is summarized in the online (ONL) Focus on Evidence –Upright Mobility Table available in the online supplemental material. However, more research is needed to establish guidelines for optimal initial percentage of BWS, when and how much to reduce BWS, and when to transition to overground walking.

When applying BWS ambulation training, it is important to consider the specific roles and tasks of the therapist, with attention to your own body mechanics as you provide support and manual guidance. Because the harness is providing the support and preventing loss of balance and falls, you can focus on providing manual guidance for appropriate lower limb progression, including optimal hip, knee, and ankle kinematics, with attention to step length and optimal foot placement at initial contact. One therapist therefore has to be down at ground level to control the distal LE and foot position.

To position yourself effectively to assist the patient and maintain proper body mechanics, it is helpful to sit on a stool or on the edge of the harness system. In optimal situations, the treadmill is surrounded by a sunken floor or "moat," allowing you to sit with your hands comfortably at the level of the patient's foot while maintaining a healthy position and body mechanics for your own spine. Without such a "moat," extreme hip and trunk flexion is required for the therapist. In many cases, a second therapist is required to help control pelvic position, weight shift, and COM oscillations.

BWS systems can also be used to promote LE weight-bearing and standing balance. A patient can safely practice balance tasks such as weight shifting, reaching for objects within and beyond

arm's length, and reacting to external perturbations. The Zero-G™ (Zero-G, 2017) BWS system is suspended from an overhead track with a trolley that follows the patient at a preprogrammed speed. This type of system allows patients to safely practice activities such as sit-to-stand and stair climbing much earlier in therapy than would otherwise be possible.

### Exoskeleton-Assisted Gait Training

The Lokomat® (www.hocoma.com/solutions/lokomat) is a robotic gait training system used with a treadmill to train or retrain locomotor control in children and adults with neurological injuries. The Lokomat® includes a BWS system designed to simulate LE loading and unloading and computerized robotic legs that attach to and guide the patient's legs through the gait cycle (Fig. 37-9). Unlike a manual BWS system, for which one or two therapists are needed to guide a patient's movement, the Lokomat® moves the patient's legs in a consistent preprogrammed pattern at a consistent pace. Because the device both supports the patient and moves the patient's legs, the physical demands on the therapist are markedly reduced. This means that the patient can spend more treatment time engaged in the task-specific practice of walking.

Evidence from studies comparing BSWTT and robotic-assisted training is equivocal. Hornby (2008) demonstrated superior gait outcomes with BWSTT versus robotic-assisted training in patients with chronic stroke while Tong (2006) demonstrated no difference between conventional gait training and robotic gait training (both with and without functional electrical stimulation) in patients with subacute stroke.

Portable and adjustable LE robotic exoskeletons are now available (see Fig. 26-27A and 26-27B) with powered hip and knee motions to help patients walk (Geigle, 2017; Jayaraman,

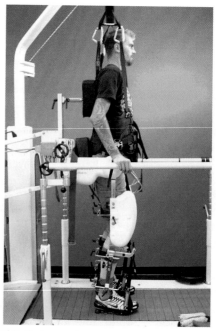

**FIGURE 37-9** Patient with an incomplete spinal cord injury ambulating in the Lokomat® with body weight support.

2017), even those with LE paralysis or weakness from a SCI, motor complete and incomplete (Kozlowski, 2015); stroke; and multiple sclerosis (Chang, 2017). The bionic systems fit over clothes and can assist the patient in rise-to-stand and ambulation. In addition to supporting greater independence in ambulation, these systems may improve spasticity and bowel function (Miller, 2016). The usefulness of these exoskeletons for general community ambulation still needs to be investigated (Lajeunesse, 2016).

The Ekso™ system (http://eksobionics.com/eksohealth/products/) includes LE exoskeleton components that strap on over the clothes, with the computer mechanism carried as a backpack and operated with a remote control to make real-time adjustments. The Ekso™ system also purports to transfer its 50-pound load directly to the ground, so the individual does not have to bear the weight. Patients with a motor complete or incomplete cervical SCI can learn to walk with the assistance of the Ekso™ exoskeleton, perhaps with no assistance and with light to moderate self-reported effort (Kozlowski, 2015). It is highly accepted and embraced by patients and helps reduce pain and spasticity in SCI (Stampacchia, 2016) and improves gait, including gait velocity and step lengths (Sale, 2016).

The ReWalk™ System (www.rewalk.com), a robotic exoskeleton that fits over the clothes, has had a positive effect on quality of life (Raab, 2016) and has even restored ambulation in persons with thoracic-level motor complete SCI (Esquenazi, 2012, 2013).

### Virtual Reality and Gaming Platforms

The use of virtual reality and gaming activities has gained popularity in the rehabilitation arena; however, more clinical evidence of its efficacy is needed. In one study, robots interfaced with virtual reality activities, which resulted in robust clinical improvements in the UEs of stroke survivors after intensive training bouts (Merians, 2011). Observable clinical changes such as these have been associated with changes in brain activity, resulting in what has been termed "neural reorganization," thus making virtual reality and gaming platforms a promising rehabilitation technique to address impairments and promote functional mobility.

The elaborate, costly gaming platforms used in most research are not frequently available to the treating therapist. Thus, therapists working with patients have begun modifying commercially available gaming systems. Regardless of the platform used, experiences are being designed to target specific impairments and/or promote specific movements. In the absence of evidence, principles of motor learning can effectively guide one's thought processes when using these platforms. In addition, when designing virtual gaming platforms and activities, one must keep in mind the need to motivate the patient to engage in active learning; thus, tasks should be creative and functionally relevant and meaningful to the patient. Although the roles of virtual reality and gaming in rehabilitation are not fully understood, emerging evidence suggests they can complement other rehabilitation techniques.

### Complex Walking Activities

Complex walking activities, often referred to as "dynamic gait" activities, require the patient to adapt the movement strategies used in less-demanding walking situations to more challenging unpredictable conditions. Patla (1999b) described locomotor adaptation under eight environmental dimensions associated with community mobility. Patla's framework (Table 37-6) has been expanded to include specific activities for promoting locomotor adaptation within these dimensions (Patla, 1999b; Shumway-Cook, 2005). The framework includes distance, temporal characteristics, ambient features, terrain, physical load, postural transitions, attentional demands, and avoidance awareness. These environmental dimensions can be used to systematically vary the complexity of a walking activity. For example, you can increase the postural demands of a walking task by changing the terrain (support surface) from level to uneven or by placing obstacles on the travel path (steps, ramps). Changing a walking task in this way increases the attentional demands of the task and requires both anticipatory and reactive postural control. In Figs. 37-10 and 37-11, we see Mrs. Z ambulating over grass and descending a curb, two activities that require increased postural control.

Progressively challenging a patient's adaptive locomotor control by modifying the distance and timing of a walking activity advances task complexity. Gait asymmetry in patients with stroke depends on walking speed, with faster walking speeds resulting in less asymmetry (Andriacchi, 1977). You can intentionally adjust movement speed or movement pacing to train a patient to adopt an external speed. When you ask a patient to walk and "keep up," you are asking her to match an externally driven pace. Another simple method to increase gait speed with an externally driven pace is to use manual cues. By increasing the speed of reciprocal arm swing or by guiding the patient at the arm, you can make her walk at a speed that is faster than what she would self-select. To match the therapist's pace, the patient must alter her force-control strategy, probably several times, to meet the new task demands. Because you can easily speed up and slow down the

| TABLE 37-6 | Locomotor Adaptation Under Eight Environmental Dimensions Associated With Community Mobility |
|---|---|
| **DIMENSIONS** | |
| Distance | *Systematically vary the complexity of a walking activity by modifying these 8 dimensions individually and concurrently* |
| Temporal characteristics | |
| Ambient features | |
| Terrain | |
| Physical load | |
| Postural transitions | |
| Attentional demands | |
| Avoidance awareness | |

Adapted from Patla A, Shumway-Cook A. Dimensions of mobility: Defining the complexity and difficulty associated with community mobility. *J Aging Phys Act.* 1999b;7:7–19.

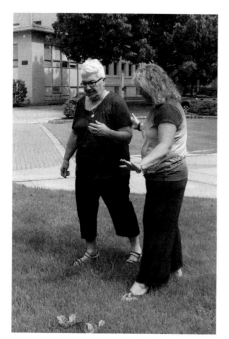

**FIGURE 37-10** Mrs. Z ambulating over grass.

ambulation pace, the patient must constantly monitor the pace to ensure a match.

When using a treadmill for walking practice, you are setting the speed that the patient must match with her pace. The treadmill speed remains constant until either you or the patient adjusts it. Thus, the patient does not need to anticipate changes in speed, which reduces her need to modulate force and the attentional demands of the task. Although both overground and treadmill walking requires the patient to adjust her walking pace to an external cue, overground walking gives

the therapist greater flexibility to vary the task demands, thereby ensuring that the patient is appropriately challenged.

Although an overground pacing task provides practice in modulating walking speed, a treadmill provides practice in the initiation and termination of gait. In daily life, the initiation of gait can be either internally (self) or externally (mechanically) driven, depending on the task. For example, when asked to keep pace during overground walking, the patient chooses when to initiate the first step (self-initiated). However, there are no real consequences if the patient does not initiate the movement when requested. In contrast, when the patient is standing on a treadmill and the treadmill begins to move, the patient must begin to move or incur a postural perturbation. In this example, the treadmill is used as an externally paced operating system that promotes a type of "**forced use**," or a situation in which the patient is required to use her involved extremity rather than her noninvolved limb. Although not consistent with traditional strategies, this required movement can be used with the current approach of **CIMT**, in that the patient must generate a strategy with her impaired limb to meet the demands of the task while her uninvolved limb is constrained. Although the strategy might not be "normal" initially, it is the patient's best attempt to organize a movement to meet the demands of the task and environment given the current state of her motor system.

Although CIMT studies have focused specifically on the UE effects of this approach, one question has recently been asked: "Does increasing the functional mobility of one's UE further enhance one's overall balance capabilities, quality of gait, and functional gross motor skill level?" Preliminary data support the premise that because the motor system is a dynamic system, improvements in UE functioning resulting from CIMT positively influence interlimb coordination and

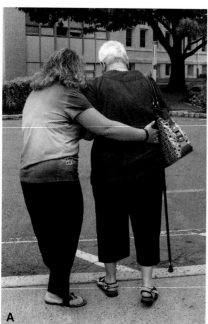
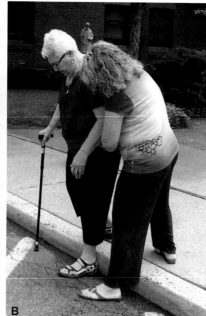
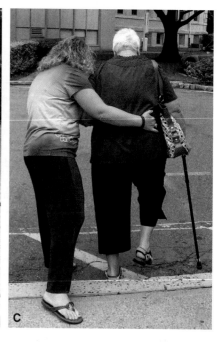

**FIGURE 37-11ABC** Mrs. Z descending a curb.

can enhance gait efficiency. However, given that speed influenced interlimb coordination in the treadmill training experiments without a speed requirement, interlimb coordination may not be retained in patients who have learned to avoid using an extremity. Therefore, combining CIMT and treadmill training may provide the environmental requirements needed to promote a positive interlimb response.

Another strategy that may indirectly force interlimb coordination is to place a rocker bottom shoe (sneaker) or boot on the patient's noninvolved LE, thereby requiring her to spend less time in single-leg stance on the noninvolved extremity and encouraging more time on the involved LE. Figure 37-12 shows Mrs. Z wearing a rocker bottom sneaker on her uninvolved foot while engaging in upright mobility activities.

Patients must also be able to safely terminate gait under both self-initiated and externally driven conditions. Pacing and speed are important variables to monitor. When self-initiating a reduction in speed before terminating gait, the patient must modulate force output to gradually slow the forward progression of the body's COM while maintaining postural control. When termination of gait is externally paced (e.g., when a treadmill is stopped without warning or without ramping down the speed), the patient must be able to react

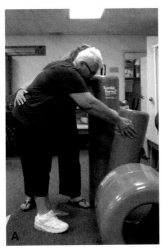
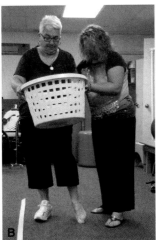

**FIGURE 37-12AB** Mrs. Z wearing a rocker bottom sneaker on her uninvolved foot during upright mobility activities.

quickly to stop on command. The patient must generate a postural strategy in real time to offset the reactive forces associated with the sudden stop of the treadmill. For carryover of these strategies into real life, the patient should practice both the gradual slowing of the COM and quick reactions in the clinic. You can use these activities to challenge the patient's attention and the ability to react quickly to a potential postural threat.

A patient's ability to change direction while walking should also be addressed. Think about how many times you change direction while walking—completing simple daily activities, such as dressing, bathing, and cooking, and more complex mobility activities, such as walking around school. Using video analysis, Glaister (2007) examined the frequency of turns in common community mobility settings such as a cafeteria and convenience store and when walking from one office to another or from an office to a parking lot. The authors found that turning steps constituted the following percentages of total steps in these situations: cafeteria (50%), office (45%), convenience store (35%), and office to car (8%). Because turning steps constitute a large percentage of movement in common activities, it is important that patients practice directional changes during ambulation.

Incorporating changes in direction during walking also promotes a patient's visual attention to the environment and ability to use environmental information to make visually guided real-time adjustments to the gait pattern. Changing direction while walking requires that patients control medial-lateral movement of their COM. This is accomplished through a complex sequence of movements involving changes in foot placement, turning of the head toward the new travel direction, and reorientation of the trunk (Patla, 1999b). Using an obstacle course is an excellent way to practice both directional and timing changes. You can grade the level of task complexity by varying the number and type of obstacles and by using verbal cues to pace the patient's walking speed.

Introducing task-relevant changes, including changes in environmental lighting, can also require alterations in locomotor control. When walking in reduced lighting conditions, the patient must slow down and attend more closely to the travel path. You can incorporate walking on a variety of terrains, including ambulating on ramps, curbs, stairs, and uneven surfaces, such as sand, grass, and rugs, to modify the parameters of the patient's walking strategy without requiring generation of a totally new strategy. You can further modify walking tasks by (1) incorporating pushing, pulling, or carrying of objects of different weights, shapes, and configurations; (2) concurrent performance of cognitive and/or motor tasks such as talking on the phone (Fig. 37-13A); and (3) maneuvering over or around obstacles. Modifying walking tasks in this way enables progression of the intervention to ensure the patient is performing at an optimal level. Of course, you must always consider patient safety in such activities and guard appropriately. In Fig. 37-13B, Mrs. Z is walking while carrying a clothes basket, which not only requires the use of bilateral UEs but also visually obstructs her walking path.

Stair ambulation is one of many complex functional walking activities a patient must achieve to maneuver effectively

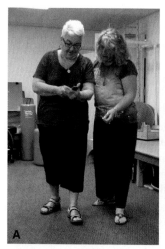 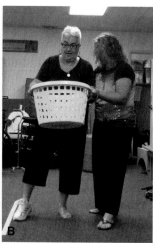 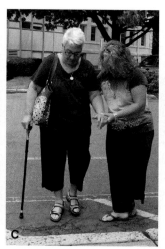 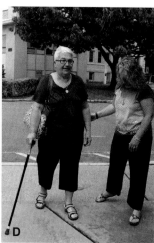

**FIGURE 37-13** Mrs. Z performing dual task activities during walking: (A) talking on the cellphone, (B) carrying a clothes basket, and (C and D) stepping up on a curb.

in the home and community. Although stair climbing, like walking, requires forward progression, stability, and adaptation, the control strategy used for stair climbing is quite different from that used for walking (Patla, 1999b). Stair ascent is accomplished through concentric LE control during antigravity movements to lift the body up to the next step. Stair ascent requires twice as much muscle force as level walking, with most of the force generated by the quadriceps (Craik, 1982). Conversely, during stair descent, eccentric LE contractions of the same muscle groups control the body as it is lowered or descends against gravity (Simoneau, 1991). Effective and efficient integration of available sensory information also influences successful stair ambulation (Craik, 1982; Simoneau, 1991).

The stair ambulation retraining strategies presented in the literature have focused primarily on stroke rehabilitation. Manual assistance is often given by the therapist to promote LE flexion control for effective swing and LE extensor control for effective single-limb stance (Davies, 1985). Traditional strategies recommend advancing the nonhemiplegic leg first when ascending stairs and the hemiplegic leg first when descending (Bobath, 1978; Davies, 1985; Voss, 1985). Using this notion of *"up with the good, down with the bad"* for stair ambulation, O'Sullivan (2007) provided detailed guarding techniques for working on progressive stair climbing with canes and crutches. Ultimately, however, the patient should be able to step up with either leg in real-life situations.

When safe and clinically appropriate, you should train ascending and descending stairs leading with both LEs. Progressing from manual assistance to partial guidance to active movements during "retraining" is advocated (Shumway-Cook, 2007). The specific pattern used during stair ambulation varies with the strength and balance capabilities of the patient. Regardless of the foot with which the patient first steps up, the second foot should step to the same step, a nonreciprocal **"step-to pattern"**; when patients have the strength, balance, and control, they may step up past the first step to the next higher step, a reciprocal **"step-through pattern."**

Individuals without impairment typically use a step-through pattern, with a particular foot making contact only with every other stair step.

A possible progression for stair ambulation includes (1) nonreciprocal LE advancement ("step-to pattern") with bilateral UE support, (2) nonreciprocal LE advancement with unilateral UE support, (3) nonreciprocal LE advancement without UE support, (4) reciprocal LE advancement ("step-through pattern") with bilateral UE support, (5) reciprocal LE advancement with unilateral UE support, and finally (6) reciprocal LE advancement without UE support. Depending on the patient's motor control needs, you can assist by varying your hand placement. However, it is imperative that you recognize when your hands, feet, etc., come in contact with the patient to either provide support or guide advancement of the patient's extremities; your hands are now part of the environment that the patient's movement must respond to or match, thus altering the task requirements. When patients are subsequently asked to generate a movement without therapist support or assistance, the task demands are different and the patients must reorganize their strategy to be successful. Ongoing monitoring of the patient's ability to execute the movement, as well as the contribution of the therapist to that movement, is needed to continually modify the task and challenge the patient's system to promote independent execution that is also safe and efficient.

Figure 37-14 shows an intervention progression on a stairwell as Mrs. Z ascends a flight of stairs while carrying a bag in her involved UE, with contact guard and minimal assistance as needed from the therapist to maintain upright stability and advance her left LE.

Task-oriented treatment activities that focus on improving motor skill learning of the patient are the foundation of an effective rehabilitation plan (Carr, 1992). Capitalizing on the patient's potential and encouraging active patient participation promote an optimal environment for motor learning to occur (Carr, 1992). When your patient is unsuccessful with a movement or activity, encourage her to utilize self-assessment

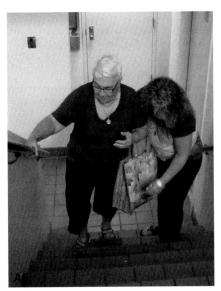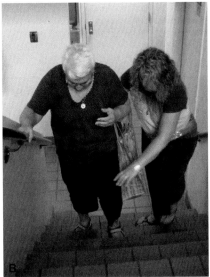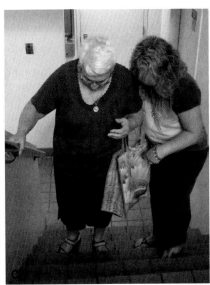

**FIGURE 37-14ABC** Mrs. Z ascending a flight of stairs while carrying a bag.

of critical elements and mistakes during the activity to maximize learning. When the patient is unable to accurately self-assess mistakes, you can highlight the critical elements for successful motor skill attainment. By using these two strategies, you can enhance the patient's ability to develop effective strategies for task completion.

During stair ambulation, the patient must match her movements with many relevant environmental features. These include the height, depth, and width of the stairs, overall width of the stair well, texture of the step surface, number of steps, availability of handrails (on one or both sides), availability of a landing, and presence or absence of stationary or moving objects on the stairs. Intentionally design your stair intervention activities to bring these factors to the patient's awareness and incorporate a variety of these conditions for practice.

Practicing upright mobility skills such as stair climbing as a whole task provides an opportunity for the patient to relearn the whole movement sequence while incorporating the balance and strengthening needed for the task (Magill, 2011). Initially, structure the environment in such a way that the task as a whole can be accomplished and practiced by the patient. For example, simplify the task by changing its regulatory features, such as decreasing the step height or using stairs with a flat, smooth surface texture to start. As the patient performs the movement with greater ease, change the environmental structure to make the task more challenging, including taller step height, textured surfaces, and working toward reciprocal stair climbing, with the patient holding the railing with one hand while repeatedly stepping up and down one step. As the patient progresses and gains control, increase the number of stair steps and reduce support until the patient is able to ascend several steps without support.

Although designing treatment plans that focus on whole-task practice is preferred, some patients may not be able to perform the whole task initially. For these patients, you can use a partial approach initially, practicing individual components of

the task that the patient can complete, with progression to whole-task practice as soon as the patient is ready, even when assistance is required. Naylor (1963) suggested that part-task training may be more effective for **serial tasks,** saving whole-task training for continuous tasks such as ambulation; however, no data support this notion. Therefore, you must continually test hypotheses in each patient and, when indicated, update the patient's plan of care. Select and modify tasks on the basis of the patient's functional level, the requirements of the task, and the environmental demands likely to be encountered in the real world.

Table 37-7 lists a variety of upright mobility tasks and potential modifications to progress intervention in patients with neurological disorders. For each task, one variable is highlighted to demonstrate how a therapist might modify the task according to the level of complexity. The tasks in the table are arranged in order of increasing difficulty, but the difficulty level in any given situation depends on the performer's motor control, distribution and severity of impairments, and cognitive status.

As therapists, we understand that the functional tasks utilized during upright mobility training support the patient's therapeutic goals; however, many times our patients or students fail to see their relatedness. In our role as educators, we must help to make the connection for patients and students so they ultimately see the therapeutic benefits and carryover of the tasks into functional activities. For example, in the following table, the functional task of lifting an object is listed as addressing upright mobility. A patient or student may question how lifting tasks can support a mobility goal. Generally, one can address this question by pointing out the interrelated, dynamic nature of our system. One can also be very specific by explaining that when we lift an object from the floor, we bend at our knees and our trunk; in doing so, our muscles grade our strength so we have enough control to bend down and enough force generated to lift the object and still return to standing without losing our balance.

**TABLE 37-7  Functional Task-Oriented Activities for Training Upright Mobility**

| TASK | MODIFICATION/PROGRESSION TO VARY TASK COMPLEXITY | EXAMPLE OF LOW COMPLEXITY → HIGH COMPLEXITY |
|---|---|---|
| *Pointing with foot:* • Position foot (dorsiflexion [DF] or plantar flexion [PF]), specified hip, and knee to make contact with **an object** | • Incorporate variability in object size, shape, and distance from individual, stationary, or moving object, with or without upper extremity (UE) support unilaterally or bilaterally<br>• Incorporate modifications to speed, vision, and attentional demands; degree of intertrial variability; externally or internally paced, continuous, or noncontinuous performance | A stationary object → a moving object |
| *Sliding the foot:* • Position of the foot (DF or PF), specified hip, and knee for **directional sliding** | • Incorporate variability in direction, required distance traveled of the sliding foot from the stationary foot, with or without UE support unilaterally or bilaterally<br>• Incorporate modifications to speed, vision, and attentional demands; degree of intertrial variability; externally or internally paced, continuous, or noncontinuous performance | One-directional sliding → bidirectional sliding |
| *Standing reach with point/grasp:* Pointing to or grasping **an object** | • Incorporate variability in object size, shape, and distance from individual; stationary or moving object; position of feet (tandem, narrow, or wide base of support); specified hip and knee position; unidirectional, bidirectional, unilateral, or bilateral reaching; required distance traveled of the reaching arm, with or without UE support unilaterally or bilaterally<br>• Incorporate modifications to speed, surface firmness, vision, and attentional demands; degree of intertrial variability; externally or internally paced, continuous, or noncontinuous performance | Stationary object → moving object |
| *Lifting:* Lifting **an object** | • Incorporate variability in object size, shape, weight, and distance from individual; stationary or moving object; position of feet (tandem, narrow or wide base of support); specified hip and knee position; unidirectional, bidirectional, unilateral or bilateral lifting; required distance traveled of the reaching arm, with or without UE support unilaterally or bilaterally<br>• Incorporate modifications to speed, vision, and attentional demands; degree of intertrial variability; externally or internally paced, continuous, or noncontinuous performance | Stationary object → moving object |
| *Pushing:* Pushing **an object** | • Incorporate variability in object size, weight, shape and distance from individual; stationary or moving object; position of feet (tandem, narrow, or wide base of support); specified hip and knee position; unidirectional or bidirectional stepping; unilateral or bilateral lifting; required distance traveled pushing, with or without UE support unilaterally or bilaterally<br>• Incorporate modifications to speed, vision, and attentional demands; degree of intertrial variability; externally or internally paced, continuous, or noncontinuous performance | Stationary object → moving object |
| *Pulling:* Pulling **an object** | • Incorporate variability in object size, weight, shape and distance from individual; stationary or moving object; position of feet (tandem, narrow or wide base of support); specified hip and knee position; unidirectional or bidirectional stepping; unilateral or bilateral lifting; required distance traveled pulling, with or without UE support, unilaterally or bilaterally<br>• Incorporate modifications to speed, vision, and attentional demands; degree of intertrial variability; externally or internally paced, continuous, or noncontinuous performance | Stationary object → moving object |

| TABLE 37-7 | Functional Task-Oriented Activities for Training Upright Mobility—cont'd | |
|---|---|---|
| **TASK** | **MODIFICATION/PROGRESSION TO VARY TASK COMPLEXITY** | **EXAMPLE OF LOW COMPLEXITY → HIGH COMPLEXITY** |
| *Marching:* Marching with specified ankle, hip, and knee position in specified directions | • Incorporate variability in direction, with or without UE support unilaterally or bilaterally; carrying objects unilaterally or bilaterally; weighted lower extremities (LEs)<br>• Incorporate modifications to speed, surface firmness, vision, and attentional demands; degree of intertrial variability; externally or internally paced, continuous, or noncontinuous performance | Forward → backward or sideways, one-directional or bidirectional |
| *Bending down:* Bending with specified position of foot, hip, and knee and varying UE support | • Incorporate variability with unilateral or bilateral UE support<br>• Incorporate modifications to speed, vision, and attentional demands; degree of intertrial variability; externally or internally paced, continuous, or noncontinuous performance | With UE support → without UE support |
| *Stepping:* Stepping (1 step) while varying UE support | • Incorporate variability in step height, depth, length; direction of ascent and descent (forward, backward, sideways); UE support unilaterally or bilaterally; carrying objects unilaterally or bilaterally<br>• Incorporate modifications to speed, surface firmness, vision, and attentional demands; degree of intertrial variability; externally or internally paced, continuous, or noncontinuous performance | With UE support → without UE support |
| *Kicking:* Kicking an object | • Incorporate variability in object weight, height, and shape; required distance traveled and direction<br>• Incorporate modifications to speed, surface firmness, vision, and attentional demands; degree of intertrial variability; externally or internally paced, continuous, or noncontinuous performance | Light object weight → heavier object weight |
| *Sit-to-stand:* Sit-to-stand from chairs with differing stability | • Incorporate variability in chair type, chair height, depth, number, with or without UE support unilaterally or bilaterally; carrying objects unilaterally or bilaterally<br>• Incorporate modifications to speed, surface firmness, vision, and attentional demands; degree of intertrial variability; externally or internally paced, continuous, or noncontinuous performance | Standard chair → rolling chair |
| *Side stepping:* Side stepping while varying UE support | • Incorporate variability with unidirectional or bidirectional stepping; specified ankle, hip, and knee position; UE support unilaterally or bilaterally; carrying objects unilaterally or bilaterally; weighted LEs<br>• Incorporate modifications to speed, surface firmness, vision, and attentional demands; degree of intertrial variability; externally or internally paced, continuous, or noncontinuous performance | With UE support → without UE support |
| *Walking:* Walking on different surfaces | • Incorporate variability including obstacles (over, around, under, through); dual tasking with cognitive or motor tasks; pace (internal and external), with or without UE support unilaterally or bilaterally; carrying objects unilaterally or bilaterally; weighted LEs<br>• Incorporate modifications to speed, surface firmness, vision, and attentional demands; degree of intertrial variability; externally or internally paced, continuous, or noncontinuous performance | Level surfaces → unlevel surfaces |
| *Treadmill:* Treadmill ambulation in various directions | • Incorporate variability including direction of ambulation, treadmill width, length, speed, incline, with or without UE support unilaterally or bilaterally; carrying objects unilaterally or bilaterally<br>• Incorporate modifications to speed, vision, and attentional demands; degree of intertrial variability; externally or internally paced, continuous, or noncontinuous performance | Forward → sideways and backward |

*Continued*

| TABLE 37-7 | Functional Task-Oriented Activities for Training Upright Mobility—cont'd | |
| --- | --- | --- |
| **TASK** | **MODIFICATION/PROGRESSION TO VARY TASK COMPLEXITY** | **EXAMPLE OF LOW COMPLEXITY → HIGH COMPLEXITY** |
| *Ramps:* Ambulation on ramps or inclines **in various directions** | • Incorporate variability including direction of step (up, down, sideways, diagonal), ramp height, width, depth, length, with or without UE support unilaterally or bilaterally; carrying objects unilaterally or bilaterally<br>• Incorporate modifications to speed, vision, and attentional demands; degree of intertrial variability; externally or internally paced, continuous, or noncontinuous performance | Forward → sideways and backward |
| *Stair:* Ambulate on stairs **in various directions and in dual task** | • Incorporate variability including pace: internal and external, step height, depth, length, number, direction of ascent, and descent (forward, backward, sideways); dual task incorporation, with or without UE support unilaterally or bilaterally; carrying objects unilaterally or bilaterally; weighted LEs<br>• Incorporate modifications to speed, surface firmness, vision, and attentional demands; degree of intertrial variability; externally or internally paced, continuous, or noncontinuous performance | Ascend, descend, side step, backward → dual tasking (cognitive and motor) |
| *Curbs:* Stepping up on a curb while **varying UE support** | • Incorporate variability including stepping direction (forward, sideways, backward), distance, speed, UE support unilaterally or bilaterally; carrying objects unilaterally or bilaterally<br>• Incorporate modifications to speed, vision, and attentional demands; degree of intertrial variability; externally or internally paced, continuous, or noncontinuous performance | With UE support → without UE support |
| *Braiding:* Ambulation with a weaving pattern of the LEs (see Fig. 30-20) while **varying UE support** | • Incorporate variability in direction (forward, backward, or sideways, one-directional, or bidirectional); UE support unilaterally or bilaterally; carrying objects unilaterally or bilaterally; weighted LEs<br>• Incorporate modifications to speed, vision, and attentional demands; degree of intertrial variability; externally or internally paced, continuous, or noncontinuous performance | With UE support → without UE support |
| *Obstacle course:* Ambulation through an obstacle course **in various directions** | • Incorporate variability in direction (forward, sideways, backward, figure-of-eight), distance, speed, with or without UE support unilaterally or bilaterally; obstacle height, length, width, depth, and number of; carrying objects unilaterally or bilaterally<br>• Incorporate modifications to speed, vision, and attentional demands; degree of intertrial variability; externally or internally paced, continuous, or noncontinuous performance | Forward, sideways → backward, figure-of-eight |
| *Hopping:* Hopping **in various directions** | • Incorporate variability in intended location (stationary or to a new location), direction of hop, distance (height of the hop), speed; with or without UE support unilaterally or bilaterally; carrying objects unilaterally or bilaterally; bilateral or one-legged<br>• Incorporate modifications to speed, vision, and attentional demands; degree of intertrial variability; externally or internally paced, continuous, or noncontinuous performance | Forward → backward |
| *Skipping:* Skipping **in various directions** | • Incorporate variability in direction (forward, backward), distance, speed; with or without UE support unilaterally or bilaterally; carrying objects unilaterally or bilaterally<br>• Incorporate modifications to speed, vision, and attentional demands; degree of intertrial variability; externally or internally paced, continuous, or noncontinuous performance | Forward → backward |

| | | EXAMPLE OF LOW COMPLEXITY → HIGH COMPLEXITY |
|---|---|---|
| **TASK** | **MODIFICATION/PROGRESSION TO VARY TASK COMPLEXITY** | |
| *Jogging:* Jogging in various directions | • Incorporate variability in direction (forward, backward), distance, speed; with or without UE support unilaterally or bilaterally; carrying objects unilaterally or bilaterally<br>• Incorporate modifications to speed, vision, and attentional demands; degree of intertrial variability; externally or internally paced, continuous, or noncontinuous performance | Forward → backward |
| *Running:* Running in various directions | • Incorporate variability in direction (forward, sideways, backward), distance, speed; with or without UE support unilaterally or bilaterally; carrying objects unilaterally or bilaterally<br>• Incorporate modifications to speed, vision, and attentional demands; degree of intertrial variability; externally or internally paced, continuous, or noncontinuous performance | Forward → sideways, backward |

**TABLE 37-7   Functional Task-Oriented Activities for Training Upright Mobility—cont'd**

In Fig. 37-15, Mrs. Z is approaching a curb with the use of a straight cane for support and contact guard provided by the therapist. Figure 37-16 displays Mrs. Z's progression in side-stepping up and down a curb. During both tasks, we see Mrs. Z using her visual system to effectively survey the stationary environment. Once Mrs. Z is able to deal with the high attentional demands required in these stationary environments, these tasks can be practiced in a more open environment.

### Attention and Dual Task Control

Although upright mobility tasks such as walking can be performed as a single task, the realities of everyday life require we perform under dual and multitask conditions. Incorporating

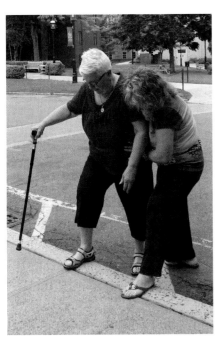

**FIGURE 37-15** Mrs. Z approaching a curb with the use of a straight cane.

practice of specific functional skills in a dual task paradigm is important for most patients because this ability is typically compromised in those with neurological disorders, including stroke (Bowen, 2001; Hyndman, 2006; McDowd, 2003; Plummer-D'Amato, 2008; Yang, 2007), Alzheimer disease (Sheridan, 2003), PD (Bloem, 2001; Camicioli, 1998; Morris, 1996; 2000; O'Shea, 2002), and in the neurological changes of general aging (Brown, 1999; Lundin-Olsson, 1998; Shumway-Cook, 2000b; Toulotte, 2006).

Walking and balance were once thought of as automatic tasks; however, we now know that some attention is allocated to those tasks. Therefore, when another task is added to walking, there is potential for a decrement in walking and/or task performance. When more than one task is performed at a time, attention capacity emerges as a key interfering factor. When the successful performance of one or both tasks is limited, the decrement in performance is referred to as **dual task interference** (Schmidt, 1999). The degree of dual task interference may be influenced by the attentional requirements of the two tasks being performed concurrently (Pellecchia, 2005). This phenomenon has been investigated using a specific paradigm in which the primary task (postural or walking) is the task of interest and the secondary task (cognitive) is the task used to cause inference with attentional resources. Depending on the instructions given to the performer, the attentional focus shifts from emphasis on the primary task to equal emphasis on both tasks (primary and secondary), thus altering the way the performer allocates attentional resources. These concepts should be kept in mind as you design a dual task intervention.

The negative effects of the primary task (motor/postural task) on the secondary (cognitive) task has been well documented in young healthy adults (Kerr, 1985; Lajoie, 1993). Conversely, the effects of a secondary task on the primary task also have been reported in the literature. Specifically, postural sway increased when performance was concurrent with a cognitive task (Andersson, 2002, 2003; Maylor, 2001; Pellecchia, 2005; Swan, 2004).

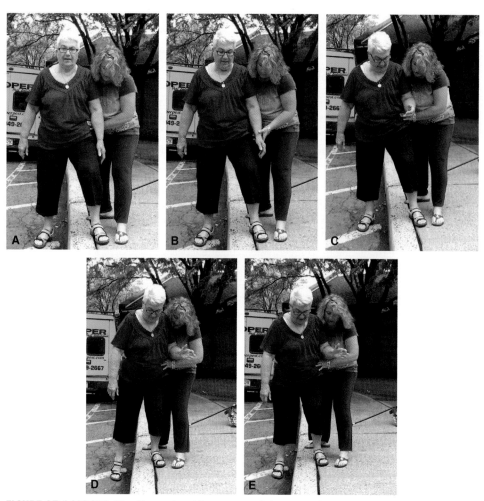

**FIGURE 37-16ABCDE** Mrs. Z stepping sideways up and down a curb, including use of visual input.

As we age, the attention needed to perform relatively automatic tasks during quiet standing, such as the control of posture, increases to compensate for deterioration in the visual, auditory, and sensory/motor systems. Research into the effects of dual task training on postural control revealed that after training, both young and older adults decreased their postural sway under dual task conditions (Pellecchia, 2005). This research supports the need to provide dual task practice as part of a customized therapeutic intervention plan. Dual task practice should work toward the patient's goals and include varying levels of combined cognitive and motor demands. Table 37-8 presents ideas for dual task interventions using Gentile's Taxonomy of Tasks as a framework for organizing and intentionally progressing the activities of patients with neurological conditions.

By categorizing tasks according to "action function" and "environmental context," you can organize teaching and learning environments to appropriately challenge your patient's performance throughout an episode of care. Addressing dual task performance using Gentile's Taxonomy of Tasks provides insights into the cumulative task demands placed on a learner when performing dual tasks and assists with progressing the intervention. Table 37-9 lists other secondary tasks that can be incorporated into a dual task

paradigm to improve ambulation or other complex upright mobility skills during therapeutic intervention.

## Contemplate Clinical Decisions

*Look at Mrs. Z in Fig. 37-17 and classify the task she is performing according to Gentile's Taxonomy of Tasks. Once you determine which box this tasks falls into, modify the task so that it falls into two other boxes. Once you have done that, think about why it is important for Mrs. Z to successfully complete the tasks that fell into the three boxes you have identified.*

Context-specific tasks should be used to assess and promote motor skill development in patients with neurological disorders. Research on obstacle courses as a context-specific modality demonstrated that they are a valid and reliable way to address the interaction between the individual and the environment during task performance (Means, 2000; Rubenstein, 1997). Obstacle courses require the patient to follow and/or remember multiple steps for successful completion of individual tasks; as a result, the attentional and cognitive demands associated with the concurrent performance of motor tasks are more naturally stimulated. In addition, an obstacle course can incorporate the

| TABLE 37-8 | Dual Task Motor Skill Categorization Using Gentile's Taxonomy of Motor Skills (With Upright-Mobility Examples) | | | |
|---|---|---|---|---|
| | **BODY STABILITY** | | **BODY TRANSPORT** | |
| **ACTION FUNCTION** | *No Object Manipulation* | *Object Manipulation* | *No Object Manipulation* | *Object Manipulation* |
| ***Environmental Context*** | | | | |
| Stationary regulatory conditions No intertrial variability | Standing and reading a sign | Standing in front of a TV pressing the "Enter" button on a TV remote | Walking and reading a sign | Walking and pressing the "Enter" button on a TV remote |
| Stationary regulatory conditions / Intertrial variability | Standing on a variety of surfaces reading a sign | Sitting in front of a TV on a stool playing an interactive video game with a handheld remote control | Walking on a variety of surfaces and reading a sign | Walking on a variety of surfaces and texting on a cell phone |
| In-motion regulatory conditions No intertrial variability | Walking on an inclined treadmill with consistent speed while talking on a hands-free cell phone | Walking on an inclined treadmill with constant speed while talking on a handheld cell phone | Walking in a shopping mall with a friend while carrying on a conversation | Walking in a shopping mall with a friend while carrying on a conversation and carrying shopping bags |
| In-motion regulatory conditions Intertrial variability | Walking on an inclined treadmill with speed varied by a trainer while talking on a hands-free cell phone | Walking on an inclined treadmill with speed varied by a trainer while talking on a handheld cell phone | Walking in a crowded shopping mall with a group of friends while carrying on a conversation | Walking in a crowded shopping mall with a group of friends while carrying on a conversation and carrying shopping bags |

| TABLE 37-9 | Secondary Tasks That Can Be Part of a Dual Task Intervention |
|---|---|

| SECONDARY COGNITIVE TASKS | SECONDARY PHYSICAL/MOTOR TASKS |
|---|---|
| • Continuously repeat a simple phrase: "Where is the child?" (Morris, 1996)<br>• Repeat the word "Apple apple, apple…" with one syllable per step while walking (which the patient can match to the cadence)<br>• Repeat the word "Banana banana banana…" with one syllable per step while walking (which does not match a right-left cadence as easily)<br>• Identify shapes or common objects (dog, comb, cat…) from photo cue cards (Huang, 2003)<br>• Identify environmental sounds (cow, whistle, bird, doorbell) from a sound effects CD (Huang 2003) | • Coin transference: use the hand to transfer coins from one pocket across the midline to the opposite pocket (O'Shea, 2002) |
| • Ask the patient to talk (answer questions or carry on a conversation) while walking<br>• Progress to asking more complex questions<br>• Listing tasks (80s movies, fruits, etc.) | • Read a sign on the wall while walking |
| • Counting forward 1–10<br>• Progress to counting backward from 100<br>• Progress to counting backward from 100 by sevens (100, 93, 86, 79…) or counting backward by threes starting at a random number between 20 and 100 (e.g., 46, 43, 40, 37, 34, 31…) (Shumway-Cook, 2000a) | • Carry a glass in the hand (start with an empty glass)<br>• Progress to carrying the glass half-full of water<br>• Progress ultimately to carrying the glass full of water (Lundin-Olsson, 1998, Shumway-Cook, 2000a) |

*Continued*

| TABLE 37-9 | Secondary Tasks That Can Be Part of a Dual Task Intervention—cont'd | |
|---|---|---|
| **SECONDARY COGNITIVE TASKS** | | **SECONDARY PHYSICAL/MOTOR TASKS** |
| • Digit recall/digit span: repeat a sequence of random single-digit numbers forward<br>• Start with two digits and progress up to eight<br>• Progress to backward digit recall, asking the patient to repeat the digits but in reverse order<br>• Repeat the days of the week in reverse order beginning with Sunday (Morris, 1996) | | • Carry a tray<br>• Progress to carrying a tray with items on it, including ultimately unstable items that roll around or a glass full of water<br>• Carry an empty backpack and then increase the weight while carrying the backpack over bilateral shoulders or one shoulder (Bond, 2000; Canning 2005) |
| • Traffic light color verbal response (when shown a color, verbally state what you are expected to do at that color when crossing the street while maintaining your posture) (Pinto Zipp, 2006) | | • Use a cell phone while walking (combines the motor task of holding the phone to the ear and the cognitive task of problem-solving about the call and conversation) |
| • Modified Stroop test: present subjects with printed color names (the words), but printed in a variety of colors of ink (i.e., ink color is always inconsistent with the color name; for example, the word "blue" may be printed in red ink). The patient is asked to verbally state the color of the ink, ignoring the word (i.e., the color name) (Jensen, 1966; Stroop, 1935). | | • Video game manipulation (Pinto Zipp, 2011) |

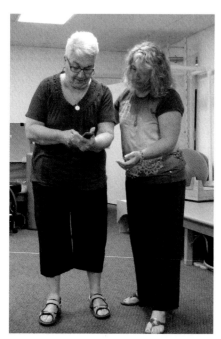

**FIGURE 37-17** Mrs. Z dual tasking.

physical features of the environment described by Shumway-Cook (2002) and presented earlier in this chapter. When you incorporate an obstacle course into an intervention, you can modify distance traveled, temporal characteristics, ambient features, terrain, physical load, postural transitions, attentional demands, and avoidance awareness. When you incorporate any activity that challenges the patient's balance, remember it is always imperative to guard the patient carefully, including use of a gait belt, to ensure safety.

A standardized obstacle course can also provide an objective measure of how well a patient manages varied environmental conditions and components. The standardized walking obstacle course (SWOC), which has high inter- and intrarater reliability and moderate concurrent validity with the TUG test in children (Held, 2006), requires that the patient ambulate along a carpeted path from a chair with armrests to a chair without armrests while encountering a 30-degree turn to the right, a 90-degree turn to the left, a visually stimulating mat, a 70-degree turn to the right around a tall object, and a shag rug. The patient is then instructed to sit down on the armless chair to rest. Once the patient feels capable of moving through the obstacle course, she travels in the reverse order along the carpeted path to the armchair. The patient can also traverse the obstacle course under three different conditions: arms at the side, holding a tray (which blocks vision of the feet), and walking with shaded glasses with arms at the side.

Obstacle courses such as the SWOC efficiently incorporate multiple tasks into an intervention session. Furthermore, when a valid and reliable standardized obstacle course is used as an outcome measure, changes in the patient's score or time to completion can be more confidently attributed to changes in the patient's performance abilities than to the tool or the tester.

### Addressing Underlying Impairments

Nonspecific task training or training at the impairment level—including stretching, strengthening, motor control training, and pregait activities, which have been covered in earlier chapters—further equips the therapist to develop an effective plan of care to meet the patient's individualized needs. However, therapy that addresses underlying impairments should be transitioned as early as possible to functional task-specific gait activities. For example, although LE strengthening is very important as a preparatory activity, a systematic review with meta-analysis demonstrated that even properly dosed strength training was not as effective as task-specific gait training that focused on velocity and electromyographic biofeedback training at improving functional gait speed in children with cerebral palsy (Moreau, 2016).

When a patient's plan of care is developed, all body system impairments must be considered and addressed to effectively and efficiently support functional upright mobility. Therefore, it is imperative to carefully consider and integrate the material covered in prior chapters as you move forward in addressing upright control and mobility issues. Using the various process-oriented approaches covered in Chapter 2 will provide a framework as you critically reflect upon and process the patient's data and make sound informed clinical decisions.

### Management Strategies to Facilitate Upright Mobility

Because many of the tasks previously described in this chapter to address upright mobility are highly coordinated and may be difficult for patients to learn, therapists frequently use motor learning principles in conjunction with manual contacts to guide and facilitate missing elements in a functional movement. Table 37-10 outlines several types of assistance that you may provide to a patient. When using adjunctive strategies such as manual contacts, remind yourself that the patient's environment for performing the task now includes the manual contact you provide. Subsequently, when you withdraw these manual contacts or conjunctive strategies, the patient may not be able to perform the task. Therefore, you must continually reassess the benefits of such conjunctive strategies in promoting patient motor skill learning and have a clear, intentional plan for gradual, systematic withdrawal of these external inputs (Fell,

2004). Your ultimate goal should be to maximize the patient's functional independence and promote flexibility and adaptability to perform motor skills.

Clearly, the role of the therapist has evolved to that of a coach who has the knowledge required to (1) critically evaluate the patient's abilities, (2) design intervention training sessions that are structured and based upon available evidence, and (3) provide adequate feedback when needed to promote function-induced recovery.

## ■ Intervention: Considerations for Nontherapy Time and Discharge

Although the time in therapy is very important, it is also critical to consider what forms of upright mobility the patient is practicing when she is not in a treatment session. If you teach patients a more efficient strategy for ambulation in a treatment session, but then they leave the clinic and immediately revert back to their dysfunctional, inefficient gait pattern, they will spend much more time per day ambulating with the dysfunctional, inefficient gait pattern than they spend practicing an efficient pattern in the clinic. Because the principle of task-specificity tells us the patient will learn whatever they practice with repetitions and feedback this patient will get "better" at walking with the dysfunctional, inefficient pattern. Therefore, we must teach patients the importance of meaningful practice of functional tasks throughout the day, using optimal patterns of movement. This is such an important concept. We must convince our patients of the importance of optimal practice throughout the day!

### PATIENT APPLICATION: INTERVENTIONS

*Regarding Mrs. Z, our patient presented earlier in the chapter, let us design a training session to enhance her ability to perform upright mobility tasks. Use the information presented in this chapter as well as the other chapters in this text as a frame of reference for your training session design. Use the following questions to stimulate your thinking.*

| TABLE 37-10 | Adjunctive Strategies to Guide Movements and Facilitate Missing Elements in Upright Mobility Tasks |
|---|---|
| **STRATEGY** | **PURPOSE** |
| Manual contacts (manual assistance, manual guidance) | • Provides an initial understanding of the task requirements<br>• Provides assisted experience with the tactile and kinesthetic inputs inherent in the movement<br>• May allay patient fears associated with moving |
| Verbal cues | • Provides focus on the critical task elements<br>• Assists the patient in understanding what she needs to do and when she needs to do it<br>• Provides feedback to the patient on how she did and what she may need to do differently |
| Modeling | • Demonstrates the critical task elements<br>• Assists the patient in understanding what she needs to do and when she needs to do it<br>• Provides feedback to the patient on how she did and what she may need to do differently |

## Contemplate Clinical Decisions

- Will you use therapeutic exercise in preparation for gait activities? If so, which ones, why, and for how long?
- How will you progress the patient?
- How will you ensure transfer of learning to the functional tasks important to the patient?
- Will you use a functional training approach?
- What will be the focus of your home exercise program?
- What feedback techniques will you use initially? How will this change as the patient progresses?
- Will you use modeling, mental practice, and manual guidance? When and for what?
- Will you design a random or blocked practice session?
- Will you practice part- or whole-task training?
- Will you work through the developmental sequence?
- Will you recommend an assistive device and/or equipment (assistive, adaptive, orthotic, protective, or supportive)?

Although this list is by no means exhaustive, the questions will help you develop a treatment framework to meet the needs of the patient.

Now that you have designed a training session to enhance Mrs. Z's ability to perform upright mobility tasks, reflect on the plan of care and ask yourself if other pieces of information from the patient's history or examination would have been helpful when you developed the plan. Here are some additional questions for your consideration.

1. Can complementary therapies be used to address underlying impairments of body structure/body function, such as strength, balance, and coordination?
2. Are issues surrounding Mrs. Z's endurance and cardiovascular status addressed in the current plan of care?
3. When is it appropriate to introduce walking over unlevel surfaces, and how would you do this?
4. What strategies would promote Mrs. Z's ability to ambulate while carrying an object?
5. How can you use the principles of task complexity to advance through different levels of ascending four steps?
6. Will you use external auditory cues or external visual cues in the training session so that Mrs. Z can ascend and descend stairs more automatically?
7. What tests and measures will you use to document change in her upright mobility?

# HANDS-ON PRACTICE

### Practical Skills

- Select tests and measures for an examination across the International Classification of Functioning, Disability and Health domains of body structure and function, activity, and participation.
- Utilize a systematic approach to improve the reliability of observational gait analysis.
- Develop a plan of care for a patient with a neurological disorder using knowledge of motor control and the principles of neuroplasticity.

- Progress a patient's plan of care by varying task and environmental conditions and by incorporating dual task practice.
- Maintain safe body mechanics when manually guiding a patient's lower extremity movement during body weight–supported treadmill training.
- Ensure patient safety during intervention by employing appropriate guarding techniques, using a gait belt, and requesting the assistance of other trained professionals when needed.

## Let's Review

1. What are the eight phases of the gait cycle, and how is each defined?

2. How do the gait tasks of weight acceptance, single-limb support, and swing limb advancement contribute to progression, postural control and balance, and adaptation in a therapeutic plan of care?

3. How do gait parameters differ between children and adults, and why is it important to know these differences?

4. What are some intrinsic factors that contribute to fall risk? Which tests and measures can you incorporate into an examination to assess these factors? How will you assess the extrinsic factors of fall risk?

5. Identify the primary impairments associated with a neurological condition. How do these primary impairments interfere with upright mobility skills? Over time, what secondary impairments may develop that will further interfere with functional upright mobility? And what would you do to provide intervention for these impairments?

6. You have a new patient who is 18 years old and presents 1 year after a traumatic brain injury. His primary goal is to walk faster and fall less. Use Box 37-2 to select two tests/measures from each of

the International Classification of Functioning, Disability and Health components that are appropriate to include in the examination. What is the rationale for your choices? How would the results help to guide your intervention plan?

7.  You found that your new patient has specific difficulty with dual tasks, particularly when negotiating obstacles. You plan to use a standard walking obstacle course and gradually add cognitive and manual dual tasks. Use the suggested cognitive and manual dual tasks in Table 37-11 to show how you would progress the intervention as your patient's dual task performance improves.

8.  How can you use Gentile's Taxonomy of Tasks to guide the progression of a stair-climbing task? Be specific about how you would adapt the task to progress your patient from the easiest to the most difficulty form of the task.

9.  What must you keep in mind when using manual contacts and assistance to guide your patient's movements?

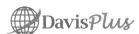 For additional resources, including Focus on Evidence tables, case study discussions, references, and glossary, please visit http://davisplus.fadavis.com

## CHAPTER SUMMARY

In this chapter, key concepts regarding upright mobility were presented and discussed to provide practicing clinicians, clinical researchers, and especially students a comprehensive understanding of its importance in the patient's ability to participate in her community. As discussed, safe and independent negotiation of the environment contributes substantially to an individual's quality of life. In both adults and children, limitations in upright mobility due to progressive or nonprogressive neurological disorders typically restrict activity and participation. As with all interventions discussed in this book, a rehabilitation program to develop, improve, or preserve a patient's functional mobility skill begins with a thorough examination and evaluation. Once the patient's problems are identified and outcomes and goals are established, the therapist develops an individualized intervention plan to address underlying impairments that are hypothesized to contribute to the functional limitation and provide meaningful practice of functional skills with appropriate repetitions and feedback to maximize outcomes. Throughout this process, therapists must use both evidence-based and practice-based, patient-centered approaches to inform and direct clinical decision-making. The information provided in this chapter supports one overriding tenet: Therapists can maximize recovery and learning by engaging patients in meaningful functional activities using practice strategies that drive neural plasticity.

Tables 37-9 and 37-10 offer a wide range of functional upright mobility tasks with suggested modifications to ensure that the patient is practicing at an optimal level of intensity throughout the episode of care (Fell, 2004). The Focus on Evidence (FOE) Table for Upright Mobility, available in the online supplemental material, summarizes important scientific articles related to the techniques or treatment methods discussed in this chapter. It is the role of the health-care community, including academicians, clinical researchers, clinical specialists, senior-level therapists, entry-level therapists, and students, to continually search for and use both evidenced- and practice-based approaches when designing a plan of care. Therefore, therapists must continually modify and challenge their clinical decision-making on the basis of an emerging and expanding body of knowledge.

Finally, therapists must seek effective ways to promote and develop clinical decision-making skills. Figure 37-18 presents a mind map that graphically represents the clinical reasoning related to intervention planning for upright mobility and ambulation for Mrs. Z. By reflecting on this mind map, we see how this technique, presented in Chapter 2, can be a tool to assist a therapist in organizing and integrating patient information in order to develop a plan of care based upon sound evidenced. For health-care professionals, the key to continued growth, development, and effectiveness is being open to life-long learning.

To provide optimal therapeutic care to our patients, we must listen to and understand the individual as a whole, identify and measure components of the movement system that are limiting the person's functional activity, use objective and standardized measures—along with observation—to document current functional and participation status, and then use that data to design a patient-centered, individualized plan of care. Implementation of the therapeutic intervention must be driven by sound clinical decision-making based on the best evidence and intentionally progressed as the patient improves, always requiring work and practice at an optimal level to enhance neuroplasticity and functional recovery, with the ultimate goal being greater independence and enjoyment of all the things we do in life!

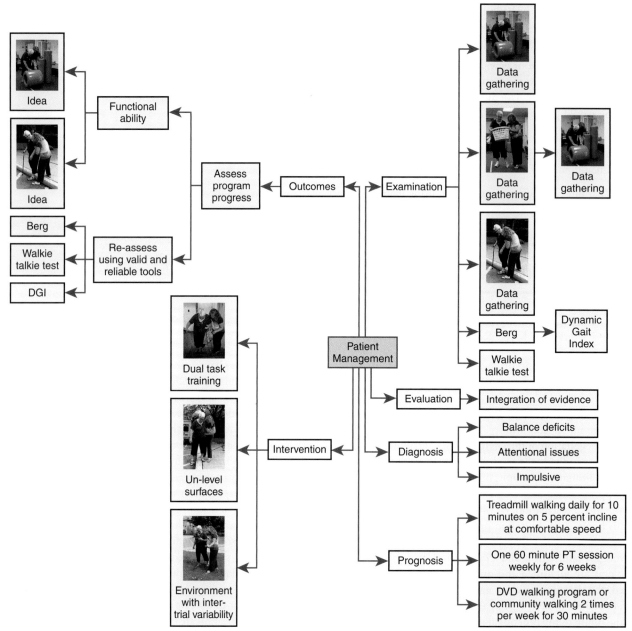

**FIGURE 37-18** Mind map showing how one therapist might view patient management elements for Mrs. Z.

# Subject Index

Page numbers followed by f indicate figures; t, tables; b, boxes

## A